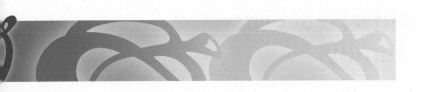

Vascular Medicine

A Companion to Braunwald's Heart Disease

Look for These Other Titles in the Braunwald's Heart Disease Family

Braunwald's Heart Disease Companions

Pierre Théroux
Acute Coronary Syndromes

Elliott M. Antman and Marc S. Sabatine
Cardiovascular Therapeutics

Christie M. Ballantyne
Clinical Lipidology

Ziad Issa, John M. Miller, and Douglas Zipes
Clinical Arrhythmology and Electrophysiology

Douglas L. Mann
Heart Failure

Henry R. Black and William J. Elliott
Hypertension

Robert L. Kormos and Leslie W. Miller
Mechanical Circulatory Support

Catherine M. Otto and Robert O. Bonow
Valvular Heart Disease

Braunwald's Heart Disease Imaging Companions

Allen J. Taylor
Atlas of Cardiac Computed Tomography

Christopher M. Kramer and W. Gregory Hundley
Atlas of Cardiovascular Magnetic Resonance

Ami E. Iskandrian and Ernest V. Garcia
Atlas of Nuclear Cardiology

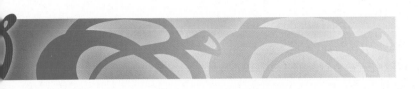

Vascular Medicine
A Companion to Braunwald's Heart Disease
SECOND EDITION

Mark A. Creager, MD
Professor of Medicine
Harvard Medical School
Director, Vascular Center
Simon C. Fireman Scholar in Cardiovascular Medicine
Brigham and Women's Hospital
Boston, Massachusetts

Joshua A. Beckman, MD, MS
Associate Professor
Harvard Medical School
Director, Cardiovascular Fellowship Program
Cardiovascular Division
Department of Medicine
Brigham and Women's Hospital
Boston, Massachusetts

Joseph Loscalzo, MD, PhD
Hersey Professor of the Theory and Practice of Medicine
Harvard Medical School
Chairman, Department of Medicine
Physician-in-Chief
Brigham and Women's Hospital
Boston, Massachusetts

ELSEVIER
SAUNDERS

1600 John F. Kennedy Blvd.
Ste 1800
Philadelphia, PA 19103-2899

VASCULAR MEDICINE: A COMPANION TO BRAUNWALD'S HEART DISEASE   ISBN:978-1-4377-2930-6

Copyright © 2013, 2006 by Saunders, an imprint of Elsevier Inc.

All rights reserved. No part of this publication may be reproduced or transmitted in any form or
by any means, electronic or mechanical, including photocopying, recording, or any information
storage and retrieval system, without permission in writing from the publisher. Details on how
to seek permission, further information about the Publisher's permissions policies and our
arrangements with organizations such as the Copyright Clearance Center and the Copyright
Licensing Agency, can be found at our website: www.elsevier.com/permissions.

This book and the individual contributions contained in it are protected under copyright by the
Publisher (other than as may be noted herein).

Notices

Knowledge and best practice in this field are constantly changing. As new research and
experience broaden our understanding, changes in research methods, professional
practices, or medical treatment may become necessary.

Practitioners and researchers must always rely on their own experience and knowledge
in evaluating and using any information, methods, compounds, or experiments described
herein. In using such information or methods they should be mindful of their own safety
and the safety of others, including parties for whom they have a professional responsibility.

With respect to any drug or pharmaceutical products identified, readers are advised
to check the most current information provided (i) on procedures featured or (ii) by
the manufacturer of each product to be administered, to verify the recommended dose
or formula, the method and duration of administration, and contraindications. It is the
responsibility of practitioners, relying on their own experience and knowledge of their
patients, to make diagnoses, to determine dosages and the best treatment for each individual
patient, and to take all appropriate safety precautions.

To the fullest extent of the law, neither the Publisher nor the authors, contributors, or
editors assume any liability for any injury and/or damage to persons or property as a matter
of products liability, negligence or otherwise, or from any use or operation of any methods,
products, instructions, or ideas contained in the material herein.

Library of Congress Cataloging-in-Publication Data
Vascular medicine : a companion to Braunwald's heart disease / [edited
by] Mark A. Creager, Joshua A. Beckman, Joseph Loscalzo. – 2nd ed.
    p. ; cm.
  Companion v. to: Braunwald's heart disease.
  Includes bibliographical references and index.
  ISBN 978-1-4377-2930-6 (hardback : alk. paper)
  I. Creager, Mark A. II. Beckman, Joshua A. III. Loscalzo, Joseph. IV.
Braunwald's heart disease.
  [DNLM: 1. Vascular Diseases–diagnosis. 2. Vascular
Diseases–therapy. WG 500]
  LC classification not assigned
  616.1'3–dc23
                                                        2012018965

Executive Content Strategist: Dolores Meloni
Content Development Specialist: Julia Bartz
Content Coordinator: Brad McIlwain
Publishing Services Manager: Anne Altepeter
Production Manager: Hemamalini Rajendrababu
Team Leader: Srikumar Narayanan
Project Manager: Cindy Thoms
Designer: Steve Stave

Printed in China

Last digit is the print number: 9 8 7 6 5 4 3 2 1

Working together to grow
libraries in developing countries

www.elsevier.com | www.bookaid.org | www.sabre.org

ELSEVIER   BOOK AID
            International   Sabre Foundation

To our wives, Shelly, Lauren, and Anita, and to our children, Michael and Alyssa Creager, Benjamin and Hannah Beckman, and Julia Giordano and Alex Loscalzo

CONTRIBUTORS

Mark J. Alberts, MD
Professor of Neurology
Northwestern University Feinberg School of Medicine
Director, Stroke Program
Northwestern Memorial Hospital
Chicago, Illinois

Elisabeth M. Battinelli, MD, PhD
Associate Physician
Division of Hematology
Brigham and Women's Hospital
Instructor
Harvard Medical School
Boston, Massachusetts

Joshua A. Beckman, MD, MS
Associate Professor
Harvard Medical School
Director, Cardiovascular Fellowship Program
Cardiovascular Division
Department of Medicine
Brigham and Women's Hospital
Boston, Massachusetts

Michael Belkin, MD
Division Chief
Professor of Surgery
Harvard Medical School
Vascular and Endovascular Surgery
Brigham and Women's Hospital
Boston, Massachusetts

Francine Blei, MD, MBA
Medical Director
Vascular Birthmark Institute of New York
Roosevelt Hospital
New York, New York

Peter Blume, DPM
Assistant Clinical Professor of Surgery
Orthopedics and Rehabilitation
Yale University School of Medicine
Director of Limb Preservation
Department of Orthopedics and Rehabilitation
Yale-New Haven Hospital
New Haven, Connecticut

Eric P. Brass, MD, PhD
Professor of Medicine
David Geffen School of Medicine at UCLA
Torrance, California

Christina Brennan, MD
Department of Cardiovascular Medicine
North Shore LIJ/Lenox Hill Hospital
New York, New York

Naima Carter-Monroe, MD
Staff Pathologist
CVPath Institute, Inc.
Gaithersburg, Maryland

Billy G. Chacko, MD, RVT, MRCP(UK)
Vascular Medicine Fellow
Vascular and Endovascular Surgery, Section on Vascular Medicine
Wake Forest University School of Medicine
Winston-Salem, North Carolina

Veerendra Chadachan, MD
Vascular Medicine Program
Boston University Medical Center
Boston, Massachusetts

Stephen Y. Chan, MD, PhD
Assistant Professor of Medicine
Harvard Medical School
Associate Physician
Division of Cardiovascular Medicine
Brigham and Women's Hospital
Boston, Massachusetts

Maria C. Cid, MD
Associate Professor
Department of Medicine
University of Barcelona
Senior Consultant
Department of Autoimmune Diseases
Hospital Clinic
Barcelona, Spain

Joseph S. Coselli, MD
Chief, Adult Cardiac Surgery
St. Luke's Episcopal Hospital
Professor and Chief, Division of Cardiothoracic Surgery
Director, Thoracic Surgery Residency Program
Baylor College of Medicine
Houston, Texas

Mark A. Creager, MD
Professor of Medicine
Harvard Medical School
Director, Vascular Center
Simon C. Fireman Scholar in Cardiovascular Medicine
Brigham and Women's Hospital
Boston, Massachusetts

Michael H. Criqui, MD, MPH
Distinguished Professor and Chief
Division of Preventive Medicine
Family and Preventive Medicine
University of California, San Diego
School of Medicine
La Jolla, California

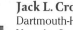

Jack L. Cronenwett, MD
Dartmouth-Hitchcock Medical Center
Vascular Surgery
Lebanon, New Hampshire

Michael D. Dake, MD
Professor, Cardiothoracic Surgery
Adult Cardiac Surgery
Stanford University Medical School
Stanford, California

Rachel C. Danczyk, MD
Resident
Department of Surgery
Oregon Health and Science University
Portland, Oregon

Mark D.P. Davis, MD
Professor
Chair
Division of Clinical Dermatology
Department of Dermatology
Mayo Clinic
Rochester, Minnesota

Cihan Duran, MD
Associate Professor
Department of Radiology
Istanbul Bilim University
Istanbul, Turkey
Associate Professor
Applied Imaging Science Laboratory
Department of Radiology
Harvard Medical School
Boston, Massachusetts

Matthew J. Eagleton, MD
Staff, Department of Vascular Surgery
Cleveland Clinic Foundation
Assistant Professor
Cleveland Clinic Lerner College of Medicine
Case Western Reserve University
Cleveland, Ohio

Robert T. Eberhardt, MD
Associate Professor of Medicine
Department of Medicine
Boston University School of Medicine
Boston, Massachusetts

John W. Eikelboom, MD
Associate Professor of Medicine
Hematology and Thromboembolism Department
McMaster University
Hamilton, Ontario, Canada

Marc Fisher, MD
Professor
Department of Neurology
University of Massachusetts School of Medicine
Worcester, Massachusetts

Jane E. Freedman, MD
Professor of Medicine
Director
Translational Research
UMass Memorial Heart and Vascular Center
Department of Medicine
University of Massachusetts Medical School
Worcester, Massachusetts

Julie Ann Freischlag, MD
Department Director and Surgeon-in-Chief
Surgery
Johns Hopkins Medical Institutions
Baltimore, Maryland

David R. Fulton, MD
Associate Chief, Administration
Chief, Outpatient Cardiology Services
Department of Cardiology
Children's Hospital
Boston, Massachusetts

Nitin Garg, MBBS, MPH
Assistant Professor
Surgery and Radiology
Medical University of South Carolina
Attending
Ralph H. Johnson VA Medical Center
Charleston, South Carolina

Marie Gerhard-Herman, MD, MMSc
Associate Professor
Department of Medicine
Harvard Medical School
Medical Director, Vascular Diagnostic Laboratory
Cardiovascular Division
Brigham and Women's Hospital
Boston, Massachusetts

Peter Gloviczki, MD
Vascular Surgery
Mayo Clinic
Rochester, Minnesota

Samuel Z. Goldhaber, MD
Professor of Medicine
Harvard Medical School
Director
Venous Thromboembolism Research Group
Medical Co-Director
Anticoagulation Management Service
Brigham and Women's Hospital
Boston, Massachusetts

Larry B. Goldstein, MD, FAAN, FAHA
Professor of Medicine
Department of Medicine
Duke University
Attending Neurologist, Medicine
Durham VA Medical Center
Durham, North Carolina

Heather L. Gornik, MD, MHS
Assistant Professor of Medicine
Cleveland Clinic Lerner College of Medicine of Case Western Reserve
    University
Medical Director
Non-Invasive Vascular Laboratory and Staff Physician
Heart and Vascular Institute and Department of Cardiovascular
    Medicine
Cleveland Clinic
Cleveland, Ohio

Daniel M. Greif, MD
Assistant Professor
Cardiovascular Section, Department of Internal Medicine
Yale University School of Medicine
New Haven, Connecticut

Kathy K. Griendling, PhD
Professor of Medicine
Division of Cardiology
Department of Medicine
Emory University
Atlanta, Georgia

Jonathon Habersberger, MBBS, BSc
Department of Cardiovascular Medicine
North Shore LIJ/Lenox Hill Hospital
New York, New York

Jonathan L. Halperin, MD
Robert and Harriet Heilbrunn Professor of Medicine
Director, Clinical Cardiology Services
Mount Sinai Medical Center
New York, New York

Kimberley J. Hansen, MD
Department of Vascular Surgery
Bowman Gray Medical Center
Wake Forest University
Winston-Salem, North Carolina

Omar P. Haqqani, MD
Tufts Medical Center
Division of Vascular Surgery
Boston, Massachusetts

David G. Harrison, MD
Betty and Jack Bailey Professor of Medicine
Clinical Pharmacology
Department of Medicine
Vanderbilt University
Nashville, Tennessee

Nancy Harthun, MD
Associate Professor
Department of Vascular Surgery and Endovascular Therapies
Johns Hopkins Medical Institutions
Baltimore, Maryland

William R. Hiatt, MD
Professor of Medicine
Division of Cardiology
University of Colorado School of Medicine
Aurora, Colorado

Lula L. Hilenski, PhD
Assistant Professor of Medicine
Director, Internal Medicine Imaging Core
Medicine
Emory University
Atlanta, Georgia

Gary S. Hoffman, MD, MS
Professor of Medicine
Medicine, Rheumatic, and Immunologic Diseases
Cleveland Clinic
Lerner College of Medicine
Cleveland, Ohio

Joseph Huh, MD
Chief, Cardiothoracic Surgery
The Permanente Medical Group, Inc.
Sacramento, California

Mark D. Iafrati, MD
Tufts Medical Center
Division of Vascular Surgery
Boston, Massachusetts

Sriram S. Iyer, MD, FACC
Department of Cardiovascular Medicine
North Shore LIJ/Lenox Hill Hospital
New York, New York

Kirk A. Keegan, MD
Clinical Instructor
Urologic Surgery
Vanderbilt University School of Medicine
Nashville, Tennessee

Christopher J. Kwolek, MD
Assistant Professor of Surgery
Harvard Medical School
Program Director, Vascular Fellowship
Division of Vascular and Endovascular Surgery
Massachusetts General Hospital
Boston, Massachusetts
Chief of Vascular Surgery
Department of Surgery
Newton-Wellesley Hospital
Newton, Massachusetts

Gregory J. Landry, MD
Associate Professor of Surgery
Division of Vascular Surgery
Oregon Health and Science University
School of Medicine
Portland, Oregon

Joe F. Lau, MD, PhD, FACC
Assistant Professor of Cardiology and Vascular Medicine
Department of Cardiology
Hofstra North Shore-Long Island Jewish School of Medicine
New Hyde Park, New York

Scott A. LeMaire, MD
Professor of Surgery, Molecular Physiology and Biophysics
Division of Cardiothoracic Surgery
Michael E. DeBakey Department of Surgery
Baylor College of Medicine
Attending Surgeon
Cardiovascular Surgery Service
Texas Heart Institute at St. Luke's Episcopal Hospital
Houston, Texas

Jane A. Leopold, MD
Associate Professor of Medicine
Harvard Medical School
Associate Physician
Cardiovascular Division
Brigham and Women's Hospital
Boston, Massachusetts

Peter Libby, MD
Mallinckrodt Professor of Medicine
Harvard Medical School
Chief, Cardiovascular Division
Brigham and Women's Hospital
Boston, Massachusetts

Judith H. Lichtman, PhD, MPH
Associate Professor
Department of Epidemiology and Public Health
Yale University School of Medicine
New Haven, Connecticut

Chandler A. Long, MD
Vascular Surgery Research Fellow
Department of Surgery
University of Tennessee Health Science Center
Knoxville, Tennessee
Visiting Research Fellow
Department of Vascular Surgery
Massachusetts General Hospital
Boston, Massachusetts

Joseph Loscalzo, MD, PhD
Hersey Professor of the Theory and Practice of Medicine
Harvard Medical School
Chairman, Department of Medicine
Physician-in-Chief
Brigham and Women's Hospital
Boston, Massachusetts

James M. Luther, MD
Assistant Professor of Medicine and Pharmacology
Division of Clinical Pharmacology
Vanderbilt University Medical Center
Nashville, Tennessee

Herbert I. Machleder, MD
Emeritus Professor
Department of Surgery
University of California
Los Angeles, California

Ryan D. Madder, MD
Interventional Cardiology Fellow
Department of Cardiovascular Medicine
Beaumont Health System
Royal Oak, Michigan

Amjad Al Mahameed, MD
Associate Staff
Cardiovascular Medicine
Cleveland Clinic Foundation
Cleveland, Ohio

Kathleen Maksimowicz-McKinnon, DO
Assistant Professor of Medicine
Medicine – Rheumatology and Clinical Immunology
University of Pittsburgh
Pittsburgh, Pennsylvania

Bradley A. Maron, MD
Instructor in Medicine
Harvard Medical School
Cardiovascular Division
Brigham and Women's Hospital
Boston, Massachusetts

James T. McPhee, MD
Vascular Surgery Fellow
Division of Vascular Surgery
Brigham and Women's Hospital
Boston, Massachusetts

Matthew T. Menard, MD
Instructor in Surgery
Harvard Medical School
Associate Surgeon and Co-Director
Division of Vascular and Endovascular Surgery
Brigham and Women's Hospital
Boston, Massachusetts

Peter A. Merkel, MD, MPH
Chief of Rheumatology, Professor of Medicine and Epidemiology
University of Pennsylvania
Philadelphia, Pennsylvania

Gregory L. Moneta, MD
Professor and Chief
Division of Vascular Surgery
Staff Surgeon
Department of Surgery
Oregon Health and Science University
Staff Surgeon
Operative Care Division
Portland Department of Veterans Affairs Hospital
Portland, Oregon

Wesley S. Moore, MD
Professor and Chief Emeritus
Division of Vascular Surgery
Department of Surgery
David Geffen School of Medicine at UCLA
Los Angeles, California

Jane W. Newburger, MD, MPH
Commonwealth Professor of Pediatrics
Harvard Medical School
Associate Cardiologist-in-Chief for Academic Affairs
Department of Cardiology
Boston Children's Hospital
Boston, Massachusetts

William B. Newton III, MD
Internal Medicine
Wake Forest University Baptist Medical Center
Winston-Salem, North Carolina

Patrick T. O'Gara, MD
Professor of Medicine
Harvard Medical School
Executive Medical Director of the Carl J. and Ruth Shapiro
    Cardiovascular Center
Brigham and Women's Hospital
Boston, Massachusetts

Jeffrey W. Olin, DO
Professor of Medicine
Zena and Michael A. Wiener Cardiovascular Institute
Mount Sinai School of Medicine
New York, New York

Mehmet Zülküf Önal, MD
Medical Faculty
Department of Neurology
TOBB ETÜ University of Economics and Technology
Ankara, Turkey

Reena L. Pande, MD
Instructor in Medicine
Harvard Medical School
Cardiovascular Division
Brigham and Women's Hospital
Boston, Massachusetts

David F. Penson, MD, MPH
Professor of Urologic Surgery
Vanderbilt University
Director, Center for Surgical Quality
    and Outcomes Research
Vanderbilt Institute
Staff Physician
Geriatric Research Education and Clinical Center
VA Tennessee Valley Healthcare System
Nashville, Tennessee

Todd S. Perlstein, MD
Instructor in Medicine
Harvard Medical School
Cardiovascular Division
Brigham and Women's Hospital
Boston, Massachusetts

Gregory Piazza, MD, MS
Instructor in Medicine
Harvard Medical School
Cardiovascular Division
Brigham and Women's Hospital
Boston, Massachusetts

Mitchell M. Plummer, MD
Associate Professor
Division of Vascular Surgery
University of Texas Southwestern Medical Center
Dallas, Texas

Rajendra Raghow, PhD
Professor
Department of Pharmacology
University of Tennessee Health Science Center
Senior Research Career Scientist
Department of Veterans Affairs Medical Center
Memphis, Tennessee

Sanjay Rajagopalan, MD, FACC, FAHA
John W. Wolfe Professor of Cardiovascular Medicine
Director, Vascular Medicine and Co-Director, MR/CT
    Imaging Program
Internal Medicine, Cardiology
Wexner Medical Center at Ohio State University School of Medicine
Columbus, Ohio

Suman Rathbun, MD, MS
Professor of Medicine
University of Oklahoma Health Sciences Center
Oklahoma City, Oklahoma

Stanley G. Rockson, MD
Allan and Tina Neill Professor of Lymphatic Research and Medicine
Division of Cardiovascular Medicine
Stanford University School of Medicine
Stanford, California

Thom W. Rooke, MD
Krehbiel Professor of Vascular Medicine
Vascular Center
Mayo Clinic
Rochester, Minnesota

Gary Roubin, MD, PhD
Department of Cardiovascular Medicine
North Shore LIJ/Lenox Hill Hospital
New York, New York

Frank J. Rybicki, MD, PhD
Associate Professor
Harvard Medical School
Director, Applied Imaging Science Laboratory
Director, Cardiac CT and Vascular CT/MRI
Brigham and Women's Hospital
Boston, Massachusetts

Robert D. Safian, MD
Professor of Medicine
Oakland University William Beaumont
School of Medicine
Director, Center for Innovation and Research
Department of Cardiovascular Medicine
William Beaumont Hospital
Royal Oak, Michigan

Roger F.J. Shepherd, MBBCh
Assistant Professor of Medicine
Division of Cardiovascular Medicine
Mayo Clinic College of Medicine
Rochester, Minnesota

Piotr S. Sobieszczyk, MD
Instructor in Medicine
Harvard Medical School
Attending Physician
Cardiovascular Division
Brigham and Women's Hospital
Boston, Massachusetts

David H. Stone, MD
Assistant Professor of Surgery
Section of Vascular Surgery
Dartmouth-Hitchcock Medical Center
Lebanon, New Hampshire

Bauer E. Sumpio, MD, PhD
Professor, Surgery and Radiology
Yale University School of Medicine
Chief, Vascular Surgery
Director, Vascular Center
Program Director, Vascular Surgery Integrated and Independent
    Training Programs
Yale New Haven Medical Center
New Haven, Connecticut

Alfonso J. Tafur, MD, RPVI
Assistant Professor of Medicine
Department of Medicine, Cardiology, Vascular Medicine
Oklahoma University Health and Science Center
Oklahoma City, Oklahoma

Allen J. Taylor, MD
Director, Cardiology Service
Walter Reed Army Medical Center
Washington, DC

Stephen C. Textor, MD
Professor of Medicine
Division of Nephrology and Hypertension
Mayo Clinic College of Medicine
Rochester, Minnesota

Gilbert R. Upchurch, Jr., MD
William H. Muller Professor of Surgery
Chief of Vascular and Endovascular Surgery
Department of Surgery
University of Virginia
Charlottesville, Virginia

R. James Valentine, MD
Professor and Chair
Division of Vascular Surgery
Department of Surgery
University of Texas Southwestern Medical Center
Attending Staff
Surgery
University Hospital – St. Paul
Parkland Memorial Hospital
Dallas VA Medical Center
Dallas, Texas

Renu Virmani, MD
Clinical Research Professor
Department of Pathology
Vanderbilt University
Nashville, Tennessee
President and Medical Director
CVPath Institute, Inc.
Gaithersburg, Maryland

Jiri Vitek, MD
Department of Cardiovascular Medicine
North Shore LIJ/Lenox Hill Hospital
New York, New York

Michael C. Walls, MD
Cardiologist
Cardiology
Saint Vincent Medical Group
Lafayette, Indiana

Michael T. Watkins, MD
Associate Professor of Surgery
Harvard Medical School
Director
Vascular Surgery Research Laboratory
Massachusetts General Hospital
Boston, Massachusetts

Jeffrey I. Weitz, MD, FCRP, FACP
Professor
Medicine and Biochemistry
McMaster University
Executive Director
Thrombosis and Atherosclerosis Research Institute
Hamilton, Ontario, Canada

Christopher J. White, MD
Chairman and Professor of Medicine
Department of Cardiovascular Diseases
Ochsner Medical Institutions
New Orleans, Louisiana

Timothy K. Williams, MD
Fellow
Department of Vascular Surgery and Endovascular Therapies
Johns Hopkins Medical Institutions
Baltimore, Maryland

FOREWORD

With the aging of the population and the greatly increasing prevalence of diabetes mellitus, extracoronary vascular disease is a serious and rapidly growing health problem. Clinical manifestations of compromised blood flow in all arterial beds, including those of the extremities, kidneys, central nervous system, viscera, and lungs, as well as in the venous bed, occur frequently and often present immense challenges to clinicians. Diseases of vessels of all sizes are responsible for clinical manifestations ranging from annoyances and discomfort to life-threatening emergencies.

Fortunately, our understanding of the underlying pathobiology of these conditions and their diagnoses – using both clinical and modern imaging techniques – is advancing rapidly and on many fronts. Simultaneously, treatment of vascular diseases is becoming much more effective. Catheter-based surgical and pharmacologic interventions are each making important strides. Because vascular diseases affect a large number of organ systems and are managed by a variety of therapeutic approaches, it is not within the domain of a single specialty. Medical vascular specialists, vascular surgeons, radiologists, interventionalists, urologists, neurologists, neurosurgeons, and experts in coagulation are just some of those who contribute to the care of these patients. There are few fields in medicine in which the knowledge and skills of so many experts are needed for the provision of effective care.

Because the totality of important knowledge about vascular diseases has increased enormously in the past decade, there is a pressing need for a treatise that is at once scholarly and thorough and at the same time up to date and practical. Drs. Creager, Beckman, and Loscalzo have combined their formidable talents and experiences in vascular diseases to provide a book that fills this important void. Working with a group of talented authors, they have provided a volume that is both broad and deep, and that will be immensely useful to clinicians, investigators, and trainees who focus on these important conditions.

The second edition of *Vascular Medicine* has incorporated the many advances that have occurred in this important field in the past six years, since publication of the first edition. In addition to Dr. Joshua Beckman joining the editorial team, 19 authors are also new to this edition. *Vascular Medicine* is becoming the "bible" in this important field, and I am especially proud of its role as a companion book to *Braunwald's Heart Disease: A Textbook of Cardiovascular Medicine*.

Eugene Braunwald, MD
Boston, Massachusetts

PREFACE

The vessels communicate with one another and the blood flows from one to another...they are the sources of human nature and are like rivers that purl through the body and supply the human body with life.

Hippocrates

Life's tragedies are often arterial.

William Osler

Vascular diseases constitute some of the most common causes of disability and death in Western society. More than 25 million people in the United States are affected by clinically significant sequelae of atherosclerosis and thrombosis. Many others suffer discomfort and disabling consequences of vasospasm, vasculitis, chronic venous insufficiency, and lymphedema. Important discoveries in the field of vascular biology have enhanced our understanding of vascular diseases. Technological achievements in vascular imaging, novel medical therapies, and advances in endovascular interventions provide an impetus for an integrative view of the vascular system and vascular diseases. Vascular medicine is an important and dynamic medical discipline, well poised to facilitate the transfer of information acquired at the bench to the bedside of patients with vascular diseases.

The second edition of *Vascular Medicine: A Companion to Braunwald's Heart Disease* integrates a contemporary understanding of vascular biology with a thorough review of clinical vascular diseases. Nineteen new authors have contributed chapters to this edition. Novel discoveries in vascular biology are highlighted, and all of the clinical chapters include recent developments in diagnosis and treatment. The second edition also includes access to the Expert Consult website, which provides images, videos, and other features to inform the reader.

As in the previous edition, the book is organized into major parts that include important precepts in vascular biology, principles of the evaluation of the vascular system, and detailed discussions of both common and unusual vascular diseases. The authors of each of the chapters are recognized experts in their fields. The tenets of vascular biology are provided in Part I, which includes chapters on vascular embryology and angiogenesis (a new chapter), endothelium, smooth muscle, connective tissue of the subendothelium, hemostasis, vascular pharmacology, and pharmacology of antithrombotic drugs (another new chapter). Part II, Pathobiology of Blood Vessels, includes updated chapters on atherosclerosis, vasculitis, and thrombosis. Part III, Principles of Vascular Evaluation, provides tools for the approach to the patient with vascular disease, beginning with the history and physical examination, and comprises illustrated chapters on noninvasive vascular tests,

magnetic resonance imaging, computed tomographic angiography, and catheter-based angiography. The parts that follow cover major vascular diseases, including peripheral artery disease, renal artery disease, mesenteric vascular disease, cerebrovascular disease, aortic dissection, and aortic aneurysms and include updated chapters that elaborate on the epidemiology, pathophysiology, clinical evaluation, and medical, endovascular, and surgical management of these specific vascular disorders. A unique and newly authored chapter reviews vasculogenic erectile dysfunction.

Part XI, Vasculitis, features an overview of all vasculitides and chapters that elaborate on the presentation, evaluation, and management of Takayasu arteritis, giant cell arteritis, thromboangiitis obliterans, and Kawasaki disease. Newly authored chapters in Part XII, Acute Limb Ischemia, provide contemporary discussions of acute arterial occlusion and atheroembolism. An entire part is devoted to vasospastic disease, such as Raynaud's phenomenon, and other temperature-related vascular diseases, such as acrocyanosis, erythromelalgia, and pernio.

Venous and pulmonary vascular diseases are featured prominently in this book. Part XIV, which discusses venous thromboembolism, includes chapters on venous thrombosis and pulmonary embolism by experts in the field who integrate pathophysiologic precepts with a contemporary approach to diagnosis and management. Contemporary management of chronic venous disorders including varicose veins and chronic venous insufficiency is reviewed in Part XV. Part XVI, Pulmonary Hypertension, comprises comprehensive chapters on both pulmonary arterial hypertension and secondary pulmonary hypertension. The management of lymphedema is broadly covered in Part XVII, Lymphatic Disorders. The final part of the book includes chapters on other important vascular diseases, including ulcers, infection, trauma, compression syndromes, congenital vascular malformations, and neoplasms.

This textbook will be useful for vascular medicine physicians as well as clinicians, including internists, cardiologists, vascular surgeons, and interventional radiologists, who care for patients with vascular disease. We anticipate that it will serve as an important resource and reference for medical students and trainees. The information is presented in a manner that will enable readers to understand the relevant concepts of vascular biology and to use these concepts in a rational approach to the broad range of vascular diseases that confront them frequently in their daily practice. The vasculature is an organ system in its own right, and we believe that the approach presented in this textbook will place physicians in a better position to evaluate patients with a broad and complex range of vascular diseases, and to implement important diagnostic and therapeutic strategies in the care of these patients.

Mark A. Creager, MD

Joshua A. Beckman, MD, MS

Joseph Loscalzo, MD, PhD

ACKNOWLEDGMENTS

We are extremely grateful for the editorial assistance provided by Joanne Normandin and Stephanie Tribuna.

CONTENTS

CONTENTS

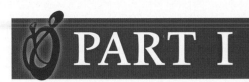

PART I

BIOLOGY OF BLOOD VESSELS

CHAPTER **1**

Vascular Embryology and Angiogenesis

Daniel M. Greif

In simple terms, the cardiovascular system consists of a sophisticated pump (i.e., the heart) and a remarkable array of tubes (i.e., blood and lymphatic vessels). Arteries and arterioles (*efferent* blood vessels in relation to the heart) deliver oxygen, nutrients, paracrine hormones, blood and immune cells, and many other products to capillaries (small-caliber, thin-walled vascular tubes). These substances are then transported through the capillary wall into extravascular tissues where they participate in critical physiological processes. In turn, waste products are transported from the extravascular space back into blood capillaries and returned by venules and veins (*afferent* vessels) to the heart. Alternatively, about 10% of the fluid returned to the heart courses via the lymphatic system to the large veins.[1] To develop normally, the embryo requires delivery of nutrients and removal of waste products beginning early in development; indeed, the cardiovascular system is the first organ to function during morphogenesis.

The fields of vascular embryology and angiogenesis have been revolutionized through experimentation with model organisms. In particular, this chapter focuses on key studies using common vascular developmental models that include the mouse, zebrafish, chick, and quail-chick transplants, each of which has its advantages. Among mammals, the most powerful genetic engineering tools and the greatest breadth of mutants are readily available in the mouse. Furthermore, the mouse is a good model of many aspects of human vascular development; in particular, the vasculature of the mouse retina is a powerful model because it develops postnatally and is visible externally. The zebrafish is a transparent organism that develops rapidly with a well-described pattern of cardiovascular morphogenesis, and sophisticated genetic manipulations are readily available. The chick egg is large, with a yolk sac vasculature that is easily visualized and develops rapidly. And finally, the coupling of quail-chick transplants with species-specific antibodies allows for cell tracing experiments. The combination of studies with these powerful model systems as well as others has yielded key insights into human vascular embryology and angiogenesis.

Although blood vessels are composed of three tissue layers, the vast majority of vascular developmental literature has focused on morphogenesis of the *intima*, or inner layer. This intima consists of a single layer of flat endothelial cells (ECs) that line the vessel lumen and are elongated in the direction of flow. Moving radially outward, the next layer is the *media*, consisting of layers of circumferentially oriented vascular smooth muscle cells (VSMCs) and extracellular matrix (ECM) components, including elastin and collagen. In smaller vessels such as capillaries, the mural cells consist of pericytes instead of VSMCs. Finally the outermost layer of the vessel wall is the *adventitia*, a collection of loose connective tissue, fibroblasts, nerves, and small vessels known as the *vaso vasorum*.

This chapter summarizes many key molecular and cellular processes and underlying signals in the morphogenesis of the different layers of the blood vessel wall and of the circulatory system

in general. Specifically, for intimal development, it concentrates on early EC patterning, specification and differentiation, lumen formation, co-patterning of vessels and nonvascular tissues, and briefly discusses lymphatic vessel development. In the second section, development of the tunica media is divided into subsections examining components of the media, VSMC origins, smooth muscle cell (SMC) differentiation, and patterning of the developing VSMC layers and ECM. Finally, the chapter concludes with a succinct summary of the limited studies of morphogenesis of the blood vessel adventitia. Understanding these fundamental vascular developmental processes are important from a pathophysiological and therapeutic standpoint because many diseases almost certainly involve recapitulation of developmental programs. For instance, in many vascular disorders, mature VSMCs dedifferentiate and exhibit increased rates of proliferation, migration, and ECM synthesis through a process termed *phenotypic modulation*.[2]

Tunica Intima: Endothelium

Early Development

Development begins with fertilization of the ovum by the sperm. Chromosomes of the ovum and sperm fuse, and then a mitotic period ensues. The early 16- to 32-cell embryo, or *morula*, consists of a sphere of cells with an inner core termed the *inner cell mass*. The first segregation of the inner cell mass generates the *hypoblast* and *epiblast*. The hypoblast gives rise to the *extraembryonic yolk sac* and the epiblast to the *amnion* and the three germ layers of the embryo known as the *endoderm*, *mesoderm*, and *ectoderm*. The epiblast is divided into these layers in the process of gastrulation, when many of the embryonic epiblast cells invaginate through the cranial-caudal primitive streak and become the mesoderm and endoderm, while the cells that remain in the embryonic epiblast become the ectoderm. Most of the cardiovascular system derives from the mesoderm, including the initial ECs, which are first observed during gastrulation. A notable exception to mesodermal origin is SMCs of the aortic arch and cranial vessels, which instead derive from the neural crest cells of the ectoderm.[3]

Although ECs are thought to derive exclusively from mesodermal origins, the other germ layers may play an important role in regulating differentiation of the mesodermal cells to an EC fate. In a classic study of quail-chick intracoelomic grafts, host ECs invaded limb bud grafts, whereas in internal organ grafts, EC precursors derived from the graft itself.[4] The authors hypothesized that the endoderm (i.e., from internal organ grafts) stimulates emergence of ECs from associated mesoderm, whereas the ectoderm (i.e., from limb bud grafts) may have an inhibitory influence.[4] Yet the endoderm does not appear to be absolutely required for initial formation of EC precursors.[5,6]

The initial primitive vascular system is formed prior to the first cardiac contraction. This early vasculature develops through vasculogenesis, a two-step process in which mesodermal cells differentiate into angioblasts in situ, and these angioblasts subsequently coalesce into blood vessels.[7] Early in this process, many EC progenitors apparently pass through a bipotential hemangioblast stage in which they can give rise to endothelial or hematopoietic cells. Furthermore, early EC precursors may in fact be multipotent; there is controversy whether ECs and mural cells share a common lineage.[8,9]

Following formation of the initial vascular plexus, more capillaries are generated through sprouting and nonsprouting angiogenesis, and the vascular system is refined through pruning and regression (reviewed in[10]). In the most well studied form of angiogenesis, existing blood vessels sprout new vessels, usually into areas of low perfusion, through a process involving proteolytic degradation of surrounding ECM, EC proliferation and migration, lumen formation, and EC maturation. Nonsprouting angiogenesis is often initiated by EC proliferation, which results in lumen widening.[10] The lumen then splits through transcapillary ECM pillars or fusion and splitting of capillaries to generate more vessels.[10] In addition, the developing vascular tree is fine-tuned by the pruning of small vessels. Although not involved in construction of the initial vascular plan, flow is an important factor in shaping vascular system maturation, determining which vessels mature and which regress. For instance, unperfused vessels will regress.

Arterial and Venous Endothelial Cell Differentiation

Classically it was thought that arterial and venous blood vessel identity was established as a result of oxygenation and hemodynamic factors such as blood pressure, shear stress, and the direction of flow. However, over the last decade, it has become increasingly evident that arterial-specific and venous-specific markers are segregated to the proper vessels quite early in the program of vascular morphogenesis. For instance, ephrinB2, a transmembrane ligand, and one of its receptors, the EphB4 tyrosine kinase, are expressed in the mouse embryo in an arterial-specific and relatively venous-specific manner, respectively, prior to the onset of angiogenesis.[11-13] EphrinB2 and EphB4 are each required for normal angiogenesis of both arteries and veins.[12,13] However, in mice homozygous for a *tau-lacZ* knock-in into the *ephrinB2* or *EphB4* locus (which renders the mouse null for the gene of interest), lacZ staining is restricted to arteries or veins, respectively.[12,13] This result indicates that neither of these signaling partners is required for arterial and venous specification of ECs.

Furthermore, even before initial ephrinB2 and EphB4 expression and prior to the first heart beat, Notch pathway members delta C and gridlock mark presumptive ECs in the zebrafish.[14-16] In this model, *deltaC* is a homolog of the Notch ligand gene *Delta*, and *gridlock* (*grl*) encodes a basic helix-loop-helix protein that is a member of the Hairy-related transcription factor family and is downstream of Notch. The lateral plate mesoderm (LPM) contains artery and vein precursors,[17] and prior to vessel formation, the *grl* gene is expressed as two bilateral stripes in the LPM.[16] Subsequently, gridlock expression is limited to the trunk artery (dorsal aorta) and excluded from the trunk vein (cardinal vein).[16]

In a lineage tracking experiment of the zebrafish LPM, Zhong et al. loaded one- to two-cell embryos with 4,5-dimethoxy-2-nitrobenzyl-caged fluorescent dextran.[15] Between the 7- and 12-somite stage of development, a laser was used to activate a patch of 5 to 10 LPM cells with pulsations and thereby "uncage" the dye.[15] The contribution of the uncaged cells and their progeny to the dorsal aorta and cardinal vein was assayed the next day.[15] Among all the uncaging experiments, marked cells were found in the artery in 20% of experiments and in the vein in 32% of experiments.[15] Interestingly, within a single uncaging experiment, the group of marked cells never included both arterial and venous cells, suggesting to the authors that by the 7- to 12-somite stage, an individual angioblast is destined to contribute in a mutually exclusive fashion to the arterial or venous system.[15]

In addition to being an early marker of arterial ECs, the Notch pathway is a key component of a signaling cascade that regulates arterial EC fate. In zebrafish, down-regulating the Notch pathway through genetic means or injection of messenger ribonucleic acid (mRNA) encoding a dominant-negative Suppressor of Hairless, a known intermediary in the Notch pathway, results in reduced ephrinB2 expression with loss of regions of the dorsal aorta.[15,18] Reciprocally, contiguous regions of the cardinal vein expand and EphB4 expression increases.[15] By contrast, activation of the Notch pathway results in reduced expression of flt4, a marker of venous cell identity, without an effect on arterial marker expression or dorsal aorta size.[15,18] Furthermore, Lawson et al. followed up on these findings to describe a signaling cascade in which vascular endothelial growth factor (VEGF) functions upstream of Notch, and Sonic hedgehog (Shh) is upstream of VEGF.[19] Taken together, these results suggest that the Shh-VEGF-Notch axis is necessary for arterial EC differentiation; however, Notch is not sufficient to induce arterial EC fate.

These studies of EC fate raise the issues of when the arterial-venous identities of ECs are specified and whether and/or when these identities become fixed. To examine these issues, Moyon et al. dissected the dorsal aorta, carotid artery, cardinal vein, or jugular vein from the embryonic day 2 to 15 (E2-15) quail and grafted the vessel into the E2 chick coelom.[20] On E4, the host embryos were immunostained with arterial-specific antibodies and the quail-specific anti-EC antibody QH1 to determine whether the grafted vessels yielded ECs that colonized host arteries, veins, or neither.[20] Quail vessels that were harvested until around E7 and then grafted into the chick colonized ECs in both host arteries and veins, but if harvesting was delayed after E7, plasticity of the grafted vessels decreased.[20] Indeed, quail arteries or veins that were isolated after E10 and subsequently grafted almost exclusively contributed to host arteries (>95% of QH1+ ECs) or veins (~90% of QH1+ ECs), respectively.[20] Interestingly, when ECs were isolated by collagenase treatment from the quail E11 dorsal aorta wall and then grafted, plasticity of the ECs was restored to that of an E5 aorta (~60% of QH1+ EC contribution to arteries and ~40% contribution to veins).[20] The authors reasoned that an unknown signal from the vessel wall regulates EC identity.[20] A recent investigation of the origins of the coronary vascular endothelium also highlights the plasticity of ECs during early mouse development.[21] This study suggests that EC sprouts from the sinus venous, the structure that returns blood to the embryonic heart, dedifferentiate as they migrate over and through the myocardium.[21] Endothelial cells that invade the myocardium differentiate into the coronary arterial and capillary ECs, while those that remain on surface of the heart will redifferentiate into the coronary veins.[21]

Endothelial Tip and Stalk Cell Specification in Sprouting Angiogenesis

Tubular structures are essential for diverse physiological processes, and proper construction of these tubes is critical. Tube morphogenesis requires coordinated migration and growth of cells that compose the tubes; the intricate modulation of the biology of these cells invariably uses sensors that detect external stimuli.[22] This information is then integrated and translated into a biological response. Important examples of such biological sensors include the growth cones of neurons and the terminal cells of the *Drosophila* tracheal system. Both of these sensors have long dynamic filopodia that sense and respond to external guidance cues and are critical in determining the ultimate pattern of their respective tubular structures.

Similarly, endothelial tip cells are located at the ends of angiogenic sprouts and are polarized with long filopodia that play both a sensory and motor role[22] (Fig. 1-1). In a classic study published over 30 years ago, Ausprunk and Folkman reported that on the day after V2 carcinoma implantation into the rabbit cornea, ECs of the host limbal vessels displayed surface projections that resembled "regenerating ECs,"[23] consistent with what is now classified as *tip cell*

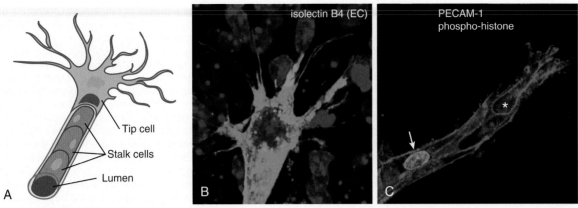

FIGURE 1-1 **Endothelial tip and stalk cells. A,** Graphic illustration of tip and stalk cells of an endothelial sprout. **B,** Endothelial tip cell with filopodia from a mouse retina stained to mark endothelial cells (ECs) (isolectin B4, *green*) and nuclei *(blue)*. **C,** Vascular sprout labeled with markers for ECs (PECAM-1, *red*), mitosis (phospho-histone, *green*), and nuclei *(blue)*. Arrow indicates a mitotic stalk cell nucleus;* indicates tip cell nucleus. *(Redrawn with permission from Gerhardt H, Golding M, Fruttiger M, et al: VEGF guides angiogenic sprouting utilizing endothelial tip cell filopodia. J Cell Biol 161:1163–1177, 2003.)*

filopodia. Tip cells are post-mitotic and express high levels of actin, platelet derived growth factor-β (PDGF-β), and vascular endothelial growth factor receptor-2 (VEGFR-2).[22] Proximal to the tip cells are stalk cells that also express VEGFR-2 but, unlike tip cells, are proliferative[22] (see Fig. 1-1). During initiation of sprouting angiogenesis, endothelial tip cells develop initial projections prior to stalk cell proliferation.[23]

The mouse retina model has been widely utilized in studies of angiogenesis and is an excellent model for studying different aspects of blood vessel development: retinal vasculature is visible externally and develops postnatally through a stereotyped sequence of well-described steps. In addition, at most time points, the retina simultaneously includes sprouting at the vascular front and remodeling at the core. The VEGF pathway is critical for guiding angiogenic sprouts, and in the retina, expression of the ligand VEGF-A is limited to astrocytes, with the highest levels at the leading edge of the front of the extending EC plexus,[22] suggesting that the astrocytes lay down a road map for the ECs to follow.[24] Vascular endothelial growth factor-A signals through VEGFR-2 on tip and stalk cells. Interestingly, proper distribution of VEGF-A is required for tip cell filopodia extension and tip cell migration, while the absolute concentration, but not the gradient, of VEGF-A appears to be critical for stalk cell proliferation.[22]

Similar to sprouting angiogenesis, budding *Drosophila* trachea airways encompass tip cells that lead branch outgrowth and lagging cells that form the branch tube. Ghabrial and Krasnow used this system to address a fundamental question that commonly

arises in a variety of disciplines ranging from politics to sports, and in this case to biology: "What does it take to become a leader?"[25] An elegant genetic mosaic analysis showed that tracheal epithelial cells are assigned to the role of tip (i.e., leader) or stalk (i.e., follower) cell in the dorsal branch as a result of a competition for FGF activity.[25] Those cells with the highest FGF activity become tip cells, and those with lower activity are relegated to the stalk position.[25] Furthermore, Notch pathway–mediated lateral inhibition plays an important role in limiting the number of leading cells.[25]

Similarly, the Notch pathway is also critical in assigning ECs in sprouting angiogenesis to tip and stalk positions (Fig. 1-2; reviewed in[26]). The Notch ligand Dll4 is specifically expressed in arterial and capillary ECs, and in the developing mouse retina, Dll4 is enriched in tip cells, while Notch activity is greatest in stalk cells.[26–28] Attenuation of Notch activity through genetic (i.e., *dll4*[+/−]) or pharmacological (i.e., γ-secretase inhibitors) approaches results in increased capillary sprouting and branching, filopodia formation, and tip cell marker expression.[26,29] Importantly, VEGF appears to induce *dll4* expression in vivo; injection of soluble VEGFR1, which functions as a VEGF sink, into the eyes of mice reduces Dll4 transcript levels.[29]

Furthermore, as with the investigations of tip and stalk cells in the *Drosophila* dorsal airway branches,[25] mosaic analyses indicate that competition between cells (in this case for Notch activity) is critical in determining the division of labor in sprouting angiogenesis. Genetic mosaic analysis involves mixing at least two populations of genetically distinct cells in the early embryo, and

FIGURE 1-2 **Notch-mediated lateral inhibition of neighboring endothelial cells (ECs). A,** Lateral inhibition gives rise to a nonuniform population of ECs. **B,** Schematic illustration of vascular endothelial growth factor-A (VEGF-A)-Notch feedback loop controlling tip-stalk specification: purple stalk cells receive high Notch signal, which represses transcription of VEGF receptors Kdr (VEGFR2), Nrp1, and Flt4, while stimulating expression of the decoy receptor (s)Flt1 (soluble VEGFR1). Green tip cells receive low Notch signal, allowing for high Kdr, Nrp1, and Flt4 expression but low (s)Flt1 expression. *(Redrawn with permission from Phng LK, Gerhardt H: Angiogenesis: a team effort coordinated by notch. Dev Cell 16:196–208, 2009.)*

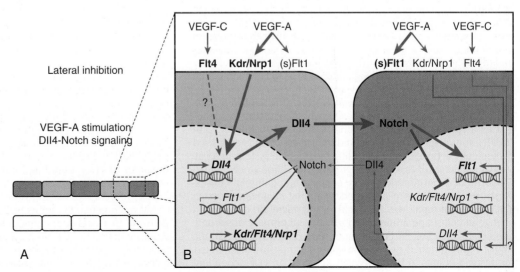

subsequently comparing the contribution of each cell population to a specific structure or process. Notably, mosaic analysis is usually complementary to experiments with total knockouts and in fact can often be more informative because complete removal of a gene may impair interpretation by grossly distorting the tissue architecture or eliminating competition between cells that harbor differing levels of a gene product.

Experiments using mosaic analysis of Notch pathway mutants in a *wildtype* background indicate that the Notch pathway acts in a cell autonomous fashion to limit the number of tip cells. In comparison to *wildtype* ECs in the mouse retina, ECs that are genetically engineered to have reduced or no *notch1* receptor expression are enriched in the tip cell population.[27]

Mosaic studies of Notch signaling components in the developing zebrafish intersegmental vessels (ISVs) are also informative. ISVs traverse between the somites from the dorsal aorta to the dorsal longitudinal anastomotic vessel (DLAV) and are widely used in investigation of blood vessel development. The ISV has been classified as consisting of three (or four) cells in distinct positions: a base cell that contributes to the dorsal aortic cell, a connector cell that courses through the somites, and the most dorsal cell that contributes to the DLAV.[30,31] Lateral plate mesoderm angioblasts contribute to the ECs of all the trunk vasculature, including the dorsal aorta, posterior cardinal vein, ISVs, DLAV, and the subintestinal venous vessels. Precursors destined for the ISVs and DLAV initially migrate to the midline dorsal aorta and then between somites to their ultimate positions.[30,31] Siekmann and Lawson generated mosaic zebrafish by transplanting into early *wildtype* embryos marked cells from embryos either lacking the key Notch signaling component recombining protein suppressor of hairless (Rbpsuh) or expressing an activated form of Notch.[31] Interestingly, *rbpsuh*-deficient cells were excluded from the dorsal aorta and enriched in the DLAV position.[31] In turn, transplanted cells harboring activated Notch mutations were excluded from the DLAV in mosaics and instead preferentially localized to the base cell and dorsal aorta positions.[31]

Taken together, the findings indicate that in sprouting angiogenesis, ECs compete for the tip position through Notch-mediated lateral inhibition of neighboring cells[26] (see Fig. 1-2). Tip cells express high levels of Dll4, which engages Notch receptors on neighboring cells and thereby inhibits these neighboring cells from developing tip cell characteristics. Furthermore, in the developing retina, the expression of Dll4 is regulated by VEGF-A, which is secreted by astrocytes in response to hypoxia.

Molecular Determinants of Branching

The pattern of many branched structures, such as the vasculature, is critical for function; diverse branched structures use similar signaling pathways to generate their specific patterns. A number of well-studied systems such as the *Drosophila* trachea, mammalian lung, ureteric bud (UB), and the vasculature consist of hierarchical tubes, progressing from larger to smaller diameter, that transport important gas and/or fluid constituents. The molecular strategies underlying morphogenesis of these patterns often include receptor tyrosine kinase–mediated signaling as well as fine-tuning with inhibitors of these signaling pathways.[32,33]

In the *Drosophila* embryo, *trachealess* selects the trachea primordia and induces conversion of planar epithelium into tracheal sacs that express *breathless* (*btl*), the fibroblast growth factor receptor (FGFR) homolog.[33,34] The FGF ligand *branchless* (*bnl*) is expressed dynamically at positions surrounding the tracheal system, in a pattern which determines where and in which direction a new branch will form.[35] Furthermore, loss of *bnl* prevents branching, and misexpression of *bnl* induces mislocalized branching.[35] Signaling through this FGF receptor pathway is critical for the migration of cells and change in cell shape inherent in formation of primary or secondary airway branches.[33,34] Furthermore, tertiary airways consist of a single highly ramified cell whose pattern is not inherently fixed, but instead adapts to tissue oxygen needs in an FGF-dependent

manner.[36] Finally, as a means of fine-tuning *Drosophila* airway patterning, branchless induces *sprouty*, an inhibitor of FGFR signaling, which blocks branching.[37,38]

Evolutionary conservation of these signaling pathways is striking because the FGF pathway is also essential for determining branch patterning in the mammalian airway system (e.g., the lung). In the mouse, trachea and lung bronchi bud from gut wall epithelium at about E9.5.[39] Subsequently, three distinct branching subroutines are repeated in various combinations to generate a highly stereotyped, complex, tree-like structure[40] that facilitates gas exchange. In early embryogenesis, the visceral mesenchyme adjacent to the heart expresses FGF10, and FGF10 binds endodermal FGFR2b, the mouse ortholog of *Drosophila* breathless.[32] *FGF10* null mice lack lungs and have a blind trachea.[41] Similarly, *FGFR2b*[(−/−)] mice form underdeveloped lungs that undergo apoptosis.[42] Akin to the *Drosophila* tracheal system, sprouty is a key component of an FGF-induced negative-feedback loop in the lung.[38] In response to FGF10, FGFR2b induces Sprouty2 tyrosine phosphorylation and activation, and active Sprouty2 inhibits signaling downstream of FGFR2b.[32] In addition, carefully regulated levels of the morphogens sonic hedgehog and bone morphogenic protein (BMP) 4 modulate the branching of lung airways.[32]

As with the *Drosophila* and mammalian airway systems, generation of the metanephric kidney requires signals conveyed through epithelial receptor tyrosine kinase. The metanephric mesenchyme secretes glial-derived neurotrophic factor (GDNF), which activates the receptor tyrosine kinase Ret and its membrane-anchored co-receptor Gdnf family receptor alpha 1 (Gfra1), thereby inducing the UB to evaginate from the nephric duct.[43,44] These components are required for UB branching because UB outgrowth fails in mice null for *Gdnf*, *Gfra1*, or *Ret*.[43] Furthermore, *RET* is frequently mutated in humans with renal agenesis.[45] In addition, FGFR2b is also highly expressed on UB epithelium, and FGFR2b-mediated signaling regulates UB branching.[32] FGF7 and FGF10 are expressed in mesenchymal tissue surrounding the UB, and FGFR2b binds with comparable affinity to these ligands.[32] As with lung development, BMP4-mediated signaling modulates the branching of the renal system.[32]

The most well-studied molecular determinants of vascular branching are the VEGF family of ligands (VEGF-A, -B, -C, and -D) and endothelial receptor tyrosine kinases (VEGFR1, 2, and 3).[46] VEGF has been shown to be a potent EC mitogen and motogen and vascular permeability factor, and the level of VEGF is strictly regulated in development; VEGF heterozygous mice die around E11.5 with impaired angiogenesis and blood island formation.[47,48] During embryogenesis, VEGFRs are expressed in proliferating ECs and the ligands in adjacent tissues. For instance, secretion of VEGF by the ventricular neuroectoderm is thought to induce capillary ingrowth from the perineural vascular plexus.[49] Mice null for *VEGFR2* or *VEGFR1* die around E9.0, with *VEGFR2*[(−/−)] mice lacking yolk-sac blood islands and vasculogenesis[50] and *VEGFR1*[(−/−)] mice displaying disorganized vascular channels and blood islands.[51] Although VEGFR3 expression eventually restricts to lymphatic ECs, its broad vascular endothelial expression early in development is critical for embryonic morphogenesis. Indeed, *VEGF3* null mice undergo vasculogenesis and angiogenesis; however, the lumens of large vessels are defective, resulting in pericardial effusion and cardiovascular failure by E9.5.[52] As with hypoxia-induced FGF-dependent tertiary branching in the *Drosophila* airway,[36] low oxygen levels induce vascular EC branching through hypoxia-inducible factor-1 alpha (HIF-1α)-mediated expression of VEGFR2.[53] VEGFR1 is thought to largely function as a negative regulator of VEGF signaling by sequestering VEGF-A. The affinity of VEGFR1 for VEGF-A is higher than that of VEGFR2, and VEGFR1 kinase domain mutants are viable.[46]

Although generally not as well studied as the role of the VEGF pathway in vessel branching, other signaling pathways, such as those mediated by FGF, Notch, and other guidance factors, are also likely to play important roles. For instance, transgenic FGF expression in myocardium augmented coronary artery branching and blood flow, whereas expression of a dominant-negative FGFR1 in retinal pigmented epithelium reduced the density and branching of retinal vessels.[32] Furthermore, a murine homolog of *sprouty* was shown to inhibit small blood vessel branching and sprouting in mouse embryo cultures.[54] The role of the Notch pathway was discussed earlier in the section on endothelial tip and stalk cells. The role of guidance cues initially described in the nervous system is discussed later in the section on neurons and vessels. Finally, the maturation of branches to a more stable state that is resistant to pruning is thought to largely be regulated by signaling pathways that modulate EC branch coverage by mural cells. Interestingly, two of the most important such pathways involve receptor tyrosine kinases such as the angiopoietin-Tie and PDGF ligand receptor pathways.

Vascular Lumenization

Endothelial cells at the tips of newly formed branches lack lumens, but as the vasculature matures, formation of a lumen is an essential step in generating tubes that can transport products. Angioblasts initially migrate and coalesce to form a solid cord that is subsequently hollowed out to generate a lumen through a mechanism that has recently become controversial. Around 100 years ago, researchers first suggested that vascular lumenization in the embryo occurs through an intracellular process involving vacuole formation.[55] Seventy years later, Folkman and Haudenschild developed the first method for long-term culture of ECs, and bovine or human ECs cultured in the presence of tumor-conditioned medium were shown to form lumenized tubes ([56]and references therein). In this and similar in vitro approaches, an individual cell forms Cdc42[+] pinocytic vacuoles that coalesce, extend longitudinally, and then join the vacuole of neighboring ECs to progressively generate an extended lumen.[56-58] Subsequently, a study using two-photon high-resolution time-lapse microscopy suggested that the lumens of zebrafish ISVs are generated through a similar mechanism of endothelial intracellular vacuole coalescence, followed by intercellular vacuole fusion.[59]

Recently, however, a number of studies have called this intracellular vacuole coalescence model into question, and instead support an alternate model in which the lumen is generated extracellularly (reviewed in[60]). One such investigation[61] suggests that in contrast to what had been thought previously,[30,31] ECs are not arranged serially along the longitudinal axis of the zebrafish ISV, but instead overlap with one another substantially; the circumference of an ISV at a given longitudinal position usually traverses multiple cells. If the lumen of a vessel were derived intracellularly in a unicellular tube, the tube would be "seamless" (as in the terminal cells of *Drosophila* airways[62]) and only have intercellular junctions at the proximal and distal ends of the cells. However, in the 30 hours post fertilization zebrafish, junctional proteins zona occludens 1 (ZO-1) and VE-cadherin are co-expressed, often in two medial "stripes" along the longitudinal axis of the ISV, suggesting that ECs align and overlap along extended regions of the ISV.[61] Thus, the lumen is extracellular—that is, in between adjacent cells, not within the cytoplasm of a single cell.

In addition, recent investigations show that EC polarization is a prerequisite for lumen formation, and both the Par3 complex and VE-cadherin play a critical role in establishing polarity.[63] Endothelial-specific knockdown of β_1-integrin reduces levels of Par3 and leads to a multilayered endothelium with cuboidal-shaped ECs and frequent occlusion of midsized vascular lumens.[63] VE-cadherin is a transmembrane EC-specific cell adhesion molecule that fosters homotypic interactions between neighboring ECs, and in vascular cords, VE-cadherin is distributed broadly in the apical membrane (reviewed in[60]). VE-cadherin deletion is embryonic lethal in the mouse; development of *VE-cadherin*[(-/-)] embryonic vessels arrests at the cord stage and does not proceed to lumenization.[60,64,65] Under normal conditions, during polarization, junctions form at the lateral regions of the apical membrane as VE-cadherin translocates to these regions, which also

harbor ZO-1.[60] VE-cadherin is required for the apical accumulation of de-adhesive molecules, such as the highly glycosylated podocalyxin/gp135, which likely contributes to lumen formation through cell-cell repulsion. In addition to anchoring neighboring ECs, VE-cadherin also is linked through β-catenin, plakoglobin, and α-catenin to the F-actin cytoskeleton.[60]

Although establishing polarity of the ECs is a critical step, it is insufficient to induce lumen formation. Indeed, in *VEGF-A*[(+/-)] mice, ECs of the dorsal aorta polarize, but this vessel does not lumenize.[65] VEGF-A activates Rho-associated protein kinases (ROCKs) that induce nonmuscle myosin II light chain phosphorylation, thereby enhancing recruitment of nonmuscle myosin to the apical membrane.[65] Actomyosin complexes at the apical surface are thought to play an important role in pulling the apical membranes of neighboring cells apart, thus generating an extracellular lumen.[63]

Another important component of the process of EC cord lumenization is the dynamic dissolution and formation of inter-EC junctions. Egfl7 is an EC-derived secreted protein that promotes EC motility and is required for tube formation.[66] The knockdown of *Egfl7* in zebrafish impairs angioblasts from dissolving their junctions, preventing them from separating, which is required for tube formation.[66] Interestingly, a recent study suggests that excessive cell-cell junctions in migratory angioblasts may explain the delayed migration of these cells in endodermless zebrafish.[5]

Neurons and Vessels

The similarities between the vasculature and neurons extend well beyond the cell biology of their respective sensors (i.e., tip cells, growth cones). Interestingly, in many organs, vascular and neural networks are closely aligned[67] (Fig. 1-3). In a landmark paper, Mukouyama et al. investigated vascular and neural development of the mouse limb, in which skin arteries but not veins are specifically aligned with peripheral nerves.[68] As in many developing vascular beds, the vasculature of the mouse limb initially consists of an EC plexus that, in the case of the limb bud, is present prior to peripheral nerve invasion. Subsequently, nerve invasion and vascular plexus remodeling ensue, resulting in formation of larger vessels, and most nerve-associated vessels express arterial markers such as ephrinB2, Neuropilin1 (Nrp1), and/or Connexin40 (CX40).[68] The semaphorins are a family of important axon guidance factors, and mice null for *Semaphorin3A* (*Sema3A*) display disorganized peripheral nerve growth. Interestingly, in *Sema3A*[(-/-)] mice, small-diameter blood vessels align with this disorganized array of peripheral nerves and express Nrp1 and CX40.[68] In contrast, *Neurogenin1/Neurogenin2* compound homozygous nulls have essentially no peripheral nerves or associated Schwann cells in the limb skin and have markedly reduced arterial marker expression in small-diameter vessels.[68] Finally, to specifically examine the role of Schwann cells, the authors investigated mice with homozygous null mutations in *erbB3*, a co-receptor for the axon-derived signal Neuregulin-1.[68] These *erbB3*[(-/-)] mice lack peripheral Schwann cells and, similar to *Sema3A* null mice, have a disordered pattern of axon growth. However, in contrast to *Sema3A* null mice, there is a marked reduction in both arterial marker expression and association of blood vessels with the disordered peripheral nerves in *erbB3*[(-/-)] limb skin. Furthermore, Schwann cells isolated from *wildtype* limb skin express VEGF, and in co-culture, Schwann cells induce undifferentiated ECs to express ephrinB2 in a VEGFR2-dependent manner.[68] Taken together, the mouse limb skin provides an example of how neurons and/or neural-associated tissues such as Schwann cells can modulate the patterning and differentiation of arterial networks.

An alternative compelling potential mechanism underlying the alignment of vascular and neural networks is *mutual guidance*, in which the patterning of these tissues is regulated by a third structure. For instance, in the developing lung, some airways are

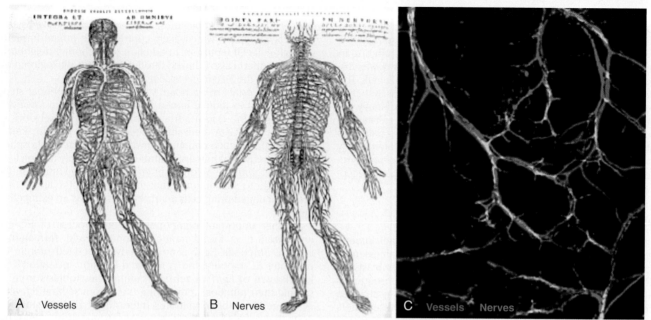

A Vessels

B Nerves

C Vessels Nerves

FIGURE 1-3   Parallels in vessel and nerve patterning. A-B, Drawings highlight similar arborization of vascular and nervous networks. **C,** Vessels *(red)* and nerves *(green)* in skin of mouse limb track together. *(Redrawn with permission from Carmeliet P, Tessier-Lavigne M: Common mechanisms of nerve and blood vessel wiring. Nature 436:193–200, 2005; and Mukouyama YS, Shin D, Britsch S, et al: Sensory nerves determine the pattern of arterial differentiation and blood vessel branching in the skin. Cell 109:693–705, 2002.)*

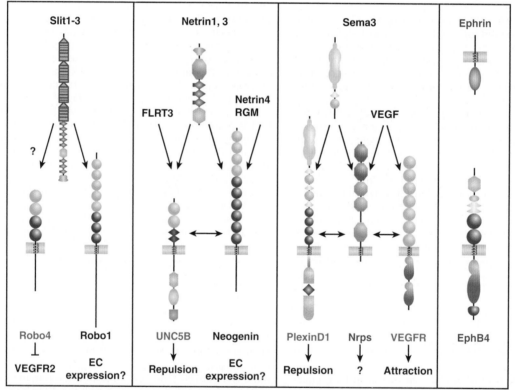

FIGURE 1-4   Endothelial cell (EC) expression of axon guidance receptors. Schematic representation of the four families of axon guidance cues and their receptors. Receptors predominantly expressed in ECs are labeled in red, receptors with shared expression in nervous and vascular systems in blue, and molecules without known expression in vascular system in black. Note that at least one member of each axon guidance receptor family is expressed in vasculature. VEGF, vascular endothelial growth factor; VEGFR, vascular endothelial growth factor receptor. *(Redrawn with permission from Adams RH, Eichmann A: Axon guidance molecules in vascular patterning. Cold Spring Harb Perspect Biol 2:a001875, 2010.)*

accompanied by a closely juxtaposed artery and neuron (unpublished results). Guidance cues are integral in regulating neural patterning through their actions as attractants or repellants in short (cell- or matrix-bound) or long (diffusible) range,[67] and a wealth of recent investigations have demonstrated that members of the four families of axon guidance cues (i.e., netrins, semaphorins, ephrins,

slits) and their receptors play critical roles in vascular patterning.[67,69] Both the nervous and vascular systems express Nrps and Eph receptors, whereas Robo4, UNC5B, and PlexinD1 expression is mostly confined to the vasculature[69] (Fig. 1-4). Thus, in some locations, neurons and vessels may be co-patterned by similar guidance cues emitted by adjacent non-neuronal, nonvascular structures.

Vascular Induction of Nonvascular Tissue Development

In addition to neural patterning of the vasculature and mutual guidance of neurons and vessels, signals emitted from cells of the developing vasculature may modulate development of neurons and other nonvascular tissues. Studies with artemin (ARTN), a member of the GDNF family of ligands, and GDNF family receptor (GFR) α3/ret receptor complexes implicate vessels as playing a critical role in patterning sympathetic neurons.[70,71] In mice with the *tau-lacZ* gene "knocked in" to the *ARTN* or *GFRα3* locus, X-gal and anti-lacZ immunohistochemical stains indicate that ARTN is expressed in VSMCs, and GFRα3 is expressed throughout the sympathetic nervous system.[71] *ARTN* null mice have disrupted sympathetic neuroblast migration and impaired target tissue innervation, resulting in ptosis.[71] Because blood vessels may indirectly influence development of adjacent nonvascular tissues through delivery of growth factors or inhibitors, it is imperative to evaluate the role of vascular tissues and/or vessel-derived signals in the absence of blood flow. Cultured rat VSMCs and sympathetic ganglia express ARTN and GFRα3, respectively, and co-culturing femoral arteries with sympathetic ganglia promotes neurite growth in a largely ARTN-dependent manner.[70] Furthermore, ARTN-coated beads placed adjacent to sympathetic chains in whole embryo mouse cultures induce robust neurite outgrowth towards the ectopic source of ARTN.[71]

In addition to induction of neural networks, the vasculature plays an important role in shaping morphogenesis of other tissues, including endodermal-derived organs. For instance, shortly after the initial specification and proliferation of hepatic cells in the endodermal epithelium, the early nascent liver bud invades the adjacent septum transversum mesenchyme. Prior to invasion, discontinuous angioblasts that have not yet formed tubes comprise a loose network located between the early epithelial and mesenchymal layers.[72] Matsumoto et al. argue that this primitive vasculature interacts with nascent liver cells "prior to blood vessel formation and function."[72] *VEGFR-2*$^{(-/-)}$ embryos lack ECs,[50] and their early hepatic endodermal cells fail to both proliferate adequately and invade the septum transversum mesenchyme.[72] Furthermore, experiments with liver bud explants isolated from *VEGFR-2* null mice or cultured in the presence of EC inhibitors show that ECs specifically induce hepatic cell proliferation.[72] Similarly, the dorsal aorta has been implicated as playing an important role in development of the dorsal pancreatic bud, which gives rise to the body and tail of the pancreas.[73] In co-culture experiments, dorsal aortic tissue induces dorsal endodermal expression of pancreatic transcription factors as well as hormones such as insulin.[73-75] Removal of aortic precursors in *Xenopus* embryos or deletion of *VEGFR-2* in mice results in failure to form the dorsal pancreatic bud or to express insulin, respectively.[74,75] In addition to directly influencing pancreatic morphogenesis, aortic ECs have an indirect effect by promoting survival of nearby mesenchymal cells, which in turn signal to the dorsal pancreatic bud.[76] Furthermore, a case study of a patient with coarctation of the aorta and dorsal pancreas agenesis demonstrates the clinical relevance of these developmental studies.[77]

Lymphatic Vessel Development

Complementing the veins, the lymphatic system plays a critical role in transporting lymph (i.e., fluid, macromolecules, cells) from the interstitial space to the subclavian veins and thereby back to the heart. Lymphatic capillaries are highly permeable by virtue of their structure: a single layer of discontinuous lymphatic endothelial cells (LECs) without mural cells or basement membrane. Lymph drains from lymphatic capillaries into precollector vessels and then into collecting lymphatic vessels that have valves, continuous inter-EC junctions, basement membrane, and SMC layer. These collecting vessels drain into the right lymphatic trunk or thoracic duct and then into the right or left subclavian vein, respectively.

Based on her experiments over 100 years ago, Florence Sabin proposed the "centrifugal model" in which lymphatic sacs derive from veins, and vessels sprouting from these sacs give rise to the lymphatic vasculature.[78,79] Recently, histological, marker, and lineage studies have yielded findings supportive of Sabin's model (reviewed in[1]). The homeobox transcription factor Sox18 (sex-determining region Y box 18) is a molecular switch that turns on the differentiation of venous ECs to a lymphatic EC fate,[80] and mutations in *SOX18* underlie lymphatic abnormalities in the human disorder hypotrichosis-lymphedema-telangectasia.[81] Sox18 induces expression of a number of lymphatic markers, including the homeobox gene *Prox1*,[80] which is absolutely required to initiate lymphatic vessel morphogenesis.[1] Lymphatic development begins in the lateral parts of the cardinal veins with EC expression of *Sox18*, followed by *Prox1* expression, and subsequently these Sox18$^+$/Prox1$^+$ ECs sprout laterally and form lymph sacs.[1,80] The peripheral lymphatic vasculature then results from centrifugal sprouting from the lymph sacs and remodeling of the LEC capillary plexus. The *Tie2-GFP* transgene is expressed specifically in blood ECs and not in LECs or undifferentiated mesenchyme, whereas lineage tracing with the transgenic *Tie2-Cre* strain and the *R26R lacZ* cre reporter marks LECs, further supporting a venous origin for lymphatics.[82] Interestingly, the venous identity of lymphatic precursors is critical; deletion of *COUP-TFII* in ECs results in arterialization of veins and inhibition of LEC specification of cardinal vein ECs.[82,83]

Tunica Media: Smooth Muscle and Extracellular Matrix

Cellular and Extracellular Matrix Components

In large and medium-sized vessels, radially outward from the EC layer is the tunica media, consisting of VSMCs and ECM components including elastin and collagen. The dynamic contraction and relaxation of VSMCs allows for the tone of the blood vessel to be adjusted to the physiological demands of the relevant tissue and to maintain blood pressure and perfusion. Collagen provides strength to the vessel wall, and elastin is largely responsible for its elasticity, such that upon receiving cardiac output in systole, the arterial wall stretches to increase the lumen volume, and subsequently, in diastole, it recoils to help maintain blood pressure. The capillary wall is substantially thinner than that of larger vessels, facilitating the transfer of substances to and from the vascular compartment. Capillary mural cells consist of pericytes rather than VSMCs. Pericytes, VSMCs, and the ECM play critical roles in many vascular diseases, but there are strikingly few studies of the development of these components in comparison to the vast number of investigations of the morphogenesis of EC networks and tubes.

Although differences exist between VSMCs and pericytes (Table 1-1), in general these mural cell types are considered to exist along a continuum and lack rigid distinctions (reviewed in[84]). Pericytes are imbedded in the basement membrane of capillary ECs, and thus may be characterized as having an intimal location, whereas VSMCs are separated from the basement membrane in the media. Vascular smooth muscle cells are oriented circumferentially around the vessel, whereas pericytes have an irregular orientation. Pericytes contact multiple ECs and are thought to play important roles in intercellular communication, microvessel structure, and phagocytosis; VSMCs are important in regulating vascular tone. Molecular markers of these cell types are overlapping, but the commonly used markers of pericytes include platelet-derived growth factor receptor beta (PDGFR-β), neuron glial 2 (NG2), and regulator of G-protein signaling 5 (RGS5). The markers of VSMCs include alpha–smooth muscle actin (αSMA) and smooth muscle myosin heavy chain (SMMHC).

TABLE 1-1	Vascular Mural Cells: Pericytes and Vascular Smooth Muscle Cells*	
CHARACTERISTIC	**PERICYTE**	**VSMC**
Vessel size	Smaller	Larger
Vascular wall location	Within endothelial BM	Media
Orientation in vessel wall	Irregular	Circumferential
"Function"	Intercellular communication Microvessel structure Phagocytosis (in CNS)	Vascular tone
"Canonical" markers	PDGFR-β, NG2, RGS5	αSMA, SMMHC

*Differences between pericytes and VSMCs are noted, but in general, these mural cell types lack rigid distinctions and are considered to exist along a continuum.[62] See text for details. BM, basement membrane; CNS, central nervous system; NG2, neuron glial 2; PDGFR-β, platelet derived growth factor receptor beta; RGS5, regulator of G-protein signaling; αSMA, alpha-smooth muscle actin; SMMHC, smooth muscle myosin heavy chain; VSMC, vascular smooth muscle cell.

Vascular Smooth Muscle Cell Origins

The origins of VSMCs are diverse and differ among blood vessels and even within specific regions of individual blood vessels (Fig. 1-5; reviewed in[3]). Interestingly, the borders between SMCs of different lineages are sharp, with little mixing among cells of different origins. Smooth muscle cells of the aorticopulmonary septum, aortic arch, and cranial vessels derive from neural crest cells of the ectoderm, and descending aorta SMCs originate from the mesoderm.[3] Using hoxB6-cre to mark cells derived from the LPM, Wasteson et al. suggest that these cells are the source of descending aortic ECs and that the ventral wall of the descending aorta is temporarily inhabited at around E9.5 for about 1 day with early SMCs that derive from the LPM.[85] Subsequently, Meox1-cre, which

labels cells derived from both the presomitic paraxial mesoderm and the somites, marks SMCs that replace the LPM-derived aortic wall cells.[85] Thus, in the adult descending aorta, ECs and SMCs derive from distinct mesodermal populations, the LPM and the presomitic/somitic mesoderm, respectively. Importantly, another investigation using a powerful and distinct approach, clonal analysis, previously showed that aortic SMCs share a lineage with paraxial mesoderm-derived skeletal muscle cells.[86] Here, a nlaacZ reporter containing a duplication of the lacZ coding sequence that yields a truncated inactive β-galactosidase enzyme was targeted to the α-cardiac actin locus.[86] The nlaacZ reporter requires a very rare intragenic recombination event that is heritable and random in order to generate a functional lacZ gene.[86] X-gal staining showed that only 2% of *nlaacZ* embryos analyzed had labeled cells in the dorsal aorta; of these, two thirds had concomitant labeling in the somitic-derived myotome.[86] Finally, Topouzis and Majesky suggest that the lineage of SMC populations has important functional implications.[87] In response to transforming growth factor (TGF)-β stimulation, ectodermally-derived E14 chick embryo aortic arch SMCs increase deoxyribonucleic acid (DNA) synthesis, while the growth of mesodermally derived abdominal aortic SMCs was inhibited.[87]

Coronary artery SMCs are critical players in atherosclerotic heart disease, and there has been significant investigation into their origin from the proepicardium (reviewed in[88]). The *proepicardium* is a transient tissue that forms on the pericardial surface of the septum transversum in the E9.5 mouse and, through a fascinating process, gives rise to epicardial cells that migrate as a mesothelial sheet over the myocardium. Signals emanating from the myocardial cells induce an epithelial-to-mesenchymal transition (EMT) in which some epicardial cells lose their cell-cell adhesion and invade the myocardium. Furthermore, lineage labeling with dyes and viral vectors and more recently with genetic approaches

Neural Crest

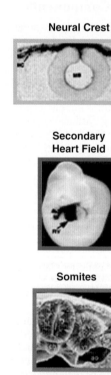

Secondary Heart Field

Somites

Various Stem Cells

Mesoangioblasts

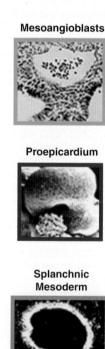

Proepicardium

Splanchnic Mesoderm

Mesothelium

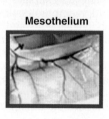

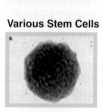

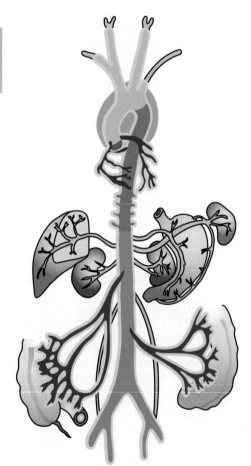

FIGURE 1-5 Developmental origins of vascular smooth muscles. Colors represent specific origins for vascular smooth muscle cells (VSMCs) as indicated in boxed images. Yellow outline indicates additional contributions from various sources of vascular stem cells. Boundaries between different lineages of VSMCs are approximated in the figure because, in general, they are not precisely known and may shift with growth and aging. *(Redrawn with permission from Majesky MW: Developmental basis of vascular smooth muscle diversity. Arterioscler Thromb Vasc Biol 27:1248–1258, 2007.)*

using the Wilms tumor1 (Wt1)-cre has illustrated that the proepicardium and epicardium contribute to the coronary artery SMC lineage.[88,89]

Similar to these studies of the coronary artery, investigations of other organs suggest the mesothelium could more generally be an important source of VSMCs. For instance, Wilm et al. showed that expression of the Wt1 protein in the developing gut is limited to the serosal mesothelium, and a Wt1-cre yeast artificial chromosome (YAC) transgene marked a lineage of cells that includes the SMCs of gut and mesenteric major blood vessels.[90] Using the Wt1-cre YAC transgene and a panel of cre reporters, lung mesothelium was implicated as the source of about a third of all pulmonary vascular cells expressing αSMA.[91]

More recently, the etiology of pulmonary artery SMCs has become controversial. Morimoto et al. reported that embryos with the same Wt1-cre YAC transgene and a R26R-YFP cre reporter have only rare YFP+ lung VSMCs.[92] Furthermore, using the Tie1-cre, these authors suggest that most SMCs of the proximal pulmonary arteries arise from ECs.[92] Transdifferentiation of ECs into VSMCs has been raised previously in developmental and disease contexts.[8,9,93] For instance, embryonic stem cell–derived Flk1+ cells have the potential to differentiate into ECs or mural cells.[9] However, our recent results with the VE-cadherin-cre[94] and mTomato/mGFP cre reporter[95] indicate that ECs are not a significant source of the E18.5 pulmonary arterial SMCs. Additional experiments indicate that instead, these cells largely derive from local mesenchyme.[96]

Smooth Muscle Cell Differentiation

A critical component of characterizing the morphogenesis of any tissue (e.g., vascular smooth muscle) is defining morphological and molecular criteria that constitute the differentiated phenotype of specific cell types (e.g., VSMCs) that make up the tissue. Early undifferentiated cells that are presumed to be destined to the VSMC fate have prominent endoplasmic reticulum and Golgi, a euchromatic nucleus, and lack a distinctly filamentous cytoplasm.[97] In contrast, mature VMSCs have a heterochromatic nucleus, myofilaments, and decreased synthetic organelles.[97] In addition to these morphological changes, differentiation of SMCs is marked by expression of a number of contractile and cytoskeletal proteins. αSMA is the most abundant protein of SMCs, comprising 40% of the total protein in a differentiated SMC.[2] αSMA is an early marker of SMCs but is nonspecific; it is expressed in skeletal muscle and a variety of other cell types, and is temporarily expressed in cardiac muscle during development.[2,98] The actin and tropomyosin binding protein transgelin (also known as SM22α) is another early marker of SMCs and a more specific marker of adult SMCs; however, it also is expressed in the other muscle types during development.[98] The two isoforms of SMMHC are expressed slightly later during development than αSMA and SM22α, and in contrast to these other markers, SMMHC expression is limited to the SMC lineage.[99] Smoothelin is another cytoskeletal protein that is also specific for SMCs but is not expressed until very late in the differentiation process when the cells are part of a contractile tissue.[100]

Studies of VSMC development or even SMCs in the mature blood vessel are challenging because these cells can assume a variety of phenotypes, depending on their environment.[2] During the early stages of blood vessel development, many VSMCs rapidly proliferate, migrate substantial distances, and synthesize large amounts of ECM components. In contrast, more mature VSMCs are predominantly sedentary and nonproliferative and express contractile proteins but do not generate significant ECM. However, the distinctions between these synthetic and contractile states are not always firm. Even adult VSMCs are not terminally differentiated, so in many vascular diseases, extracellular cues are implicated in inducing VSMCs to assume a dedifferentiated state through a process termed *phenotypic modulation*.[2]

Underlying these phenotypes, the gene expression program of SMCs toggles between a differentiated contractile set of genes and a distinct, undifferentiated, synthetic and proliferative set of genes.[101] Expression of almost all smooth muscle contractile and cytoskeletal genes is modulated by the ubiquitous transcription factor serum response factor (SRF). Serum response factor binds the 10-base-pair DNA consensus sequence CC(A/T)$_6$GG known as the *CArG box* (i.e., C, AT rich, G box), which is found in the regulatory regions of virtually all smooth muscle genes. In fact, for most SMC genes, there are at least two CArG boxes. However, the CArG box sequence is also found within the 23-base-pair serum response enhancer element of early growth response genes such as the c-fos proto-oncogene.[101] Because SRF is ubiquitous and the *cis*-regulatory CArG element is present in both growth and differentiation genes, a higher order of control is required to determine which of these disparate gene sets are expressed in a specific cell at a given time period.

Control of expression of contractile and cytoskeletal SMC genes is regulated through a competition for SRF between the transcriptional coactivator myocardin and ternary complex factors.[102] Myocardin is a master regulator of SMC differentiation in that ectopic expression of this factor in nonmuscle cells is sufficient to induce activation of the SMC differentiation gene program.[103] In addition, murine embryos null for myocardin lack VSMC differentiation and die at mid-gestation.[104] Counterbalancing this effect of myocardin is the ternary complex factor Elk-1, which acts as a myogenic repressor by competing with myocardin for a common docking site on SRF, thereby preventing induction of SMC differentiation gene expression.[102]

Patterning of Developing Vascular Smooth Muscle Cell Layers

Although a number of recent investigations describe the molecular mechanisms regulating SMC differentiation, there are relatively few studies of the patterning of morphogenesis of SMC layers of a developing blood vessel (reviewed in[97]). Consequently, little is known about recruitment of SMCs and/or their precursors to the vascular wall, investment of these cells around the nascent EC tube, and the pattern of differentiation of VSMC precursors within or in proximity to the vascular wall. Limited relevant studies have mostly focused on histology and αSMA expression in the developing aortic wall. Early in development, the dorsal aortae exist as parallel tubes that subsequently fuse to generate the single descending aorta. The early EC tube is surrounded by loose undifferentiated mesenchymal cells, and as the aorta matures, expression of αSMA proceeds in a cranial-to-caudal direction.[105,106] Within a cross-section of the descending aorta, the location of initial mesenchymal cell consolidation and αSMA expression depends on the cranial-caudal position: proximally these processes initially occur on the dorsal aspect of the aorta, whereas more distally they are first noted on the ventral side.[105,106] Studies published 40 years ago indicate that within the chick aortic media, outer layers mature initially with condensation and elongation of early presumptive SMCs and accumulation of elastic tissue.[107,108] In contrast, in rodent or quail aortae, cells immediately adjacent to the EC layer are the first to consolidate and express SMC markers; subsequently, additional layers of SMCs are added.[105,106,109,110]

Recently we have undertaken a meticulous investigation of murine pulmonary artery morphogenesis and found that the medial and adventitial wall of this vessel is constructed radially from inside out by sequential induction and recruitment of successive layers.[96] The inner layer undergoes a series of morphological and molecular transitions that lasts about 3 days in order to build a relatively mature SMC layer. After this process commences in the first layer, the next layer initiates and completes a similar process. Finally, this developmental program arrests midway through construction of the outer layer to generate a relatively "undifferentiated" adventitial cell layer.

This inside-outside radial patterning is likely to involve an EC-derived signal and result from one or more potential mechanisms. For instance, in the morphogen gradient model,[111] an

EC-derived signal diffuses through the media and adventitia and, depending on discrete concentration thresholds, induces responses in the cells of these compartments, such as changes in morphology, gene expression, and/or proliferation. Alternatively, in the relay mechanism,[112] a short-range or plasma membrane-bound EC signal induces adjacent cells, which in turn propagate the signal through either secreting a morphogen or inducing their neighbors, and so on (i.e., "the bucket brigade model"). Such a bucket brigade mediated by the Notch ligand Jagged1 on SMCs is implicated in regulating ductus arteriosus closure in a recently published report.[113] Finally, our recent results suggest a third mechanism in which some of the progeny of inner-layer SMCs migrate radially outward to contribute to the next layer(s) of SMCs.[96]

A number of signaling pathways involving an EC-derived signal and mesenchymal receptors have been implicated in vascular wall morphogenesis (reviewed in[114]). The PDGF pathway is perhaps the most well-studied pathway in vascular mural cell development, with a ligand expressed in ECs (PDGF-β) and receptors expressed in undifferentiated mesenchyme (PDGFR-α and -β) and pericytes (PDGFR-β). Mice null for *PDGF-β* or *PDGFR-β* have reduced SMC coverage of medium-sized arteries and lack pericytes, which results in microvascular hemorrhages and perinatal lethality.[115–118] In addition, when co-cultured with ECs, undifferentiated embryonic mesenchymal 10T1/2 cells are induced to express SMC markers and elongate in a TGF-β-dependent manner.[119] Similar changes are also induced by directly treating 10T1/2 cells with TGF-β₁.[119] Furthermore, the Notch pathway has been shown to play important roles in arterial SMC differentiation in vivo (reviewed in[120]), and EC-derived Jagged1 is required for normal aortic and yolk sac vessel SMC differentiation.[121] In human adults, the receptor Notch3 is specifically expressed in arterial SMCs, and at birth, blood vessels of *Notch3* null mice and *wildtype* mice are indistinguishable.[122,123] However, Notch3 is required for postnatal maturation of the tunica media of small vessels in mice.[122] Furthermore, *NOTCH3* mutations in humans cause the CADASIL (cerebral autosomal dominant arteriopathy with stroke and dementia) syndrome, characterized clinically by adult-onset recurrent subcortical ischemic strokes and vascular dementia, and pathologically by degeneration and eventual loss of VSMCs.[123,124] Finally, it is important to note that other signaling pathways, such as those mediated by angiopoietin-Tie and S1P ligand-receptor pairs, do not involve an EC-derived ligand and/or mesenchymal receptors but play important roles in SMC development.[114]

Extracellular Matrix: Collagen and Elastic Fibers

In addition to maturation of cellular constituents of the blood vessel wall, proper formation of the ECM is also critical for vascular function. Gene expression profiling of the developing mouse aorta revealed dynamic expression of most structural matrix proteins: an initial major increase of expression at E14 is often followed by a brief decrease at postnatal day 0 (P0), and then a steady rise for about 2 weeks, and finally a decline to low levels at 2 to 3 months that persist into adulthood.[125,126] Within the tunica media, circumferential collagen fibers have high tensile strength and bear most of the stressing forces at or above physiological blood pressures.[126] Seventeen collagens are expressed in the developing murine aortic wall, and deletions in a number of them result in vascular phenotypes.[126] Furthermore, *COLLAGEN3A1* mutations in humans are responsible for Ehlers-Danlos syndrome type IV, with vascular manifestations that include vessel fragility and large-vessel aneurysm and rupture.[126]

In contrast to collagen, elastin has low tensile strength, is distensible, and distributes stress throughout the wall, including onto collagen fibers.[126] Elastin is the major protein of the arterial wall, comprising up to 50% of the dry weight of the aorta.[127] Vascular smooth muscle cells secrete tropoelastin monomers that undergo posttranslational modifications, cross-linking, and are organized into circumferential elastic lamellae in the tunica media. These elastic lamellae alternate with rings of VSMCs to form lamellar units. *Eln*$^{(+/-)}$ mice have a normal lifespan despite being hypertensive and having a 50% reduction in elastin mRNA.[128,129] In comparison to *wildtype*, the *Eln*$^{(+/-)}$ aorta has thinner elastic lamellae but a 35% increase in the number of lamellar units, which results in a similar tension per lamellar unit.[129,130] More dramatically, humans hemizygous for the ELN-null mutant have a 2.5-fold increase in lamellar units and suffer an obstructive arterial disease, supravalvular aortic stenosis.[129] Similarly, at the end of gestation in the mouse, subendothelial cells of *Eln*$^{(-/-)}$ arteries are hyperproliferative, resulting in increased numbers of αSMA⁺ cells and reduced luminal diameter, with lethality by P4.5.[131] Furthermore, it is conceivable that localized disruption of elastin in the mature artery results in focal SMC phenotypic modulation and consequent neointima formation[132] (Fig. 1-6).

Finally, *microfibrils* are fibrous structures intimately associated with elastic fibers surrounding the elastin core. Fibrillin1 is the major structural component of microfibrils, and its temporal pattern of expression during aortic development is similar to that of most structural proteins (e.g., elastin), except the peak expression of fibrillin1 occurs at P0.[125] Mutations in the human *FBN1* gene result in Marfan syndrome, with vascular manifestations that include aortic root aneurysm and dissection.[133]

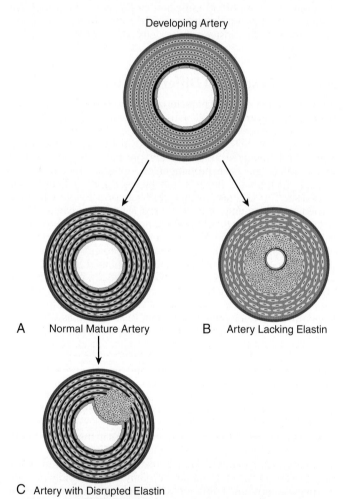

FIGURE 1-6   Elastin–vascular smooth muscle cell (VSMC) interactions in development and disease. A, During normal development, concentric rings of elastic lamellae form around arterial lumen. Elastin signals VSMCs to localize around elastic lamellae and remain in a quiescent, contractile state. **B,** In the absence of elastin, this morphogenic signal is lost, resulting in pervasive subendothelial migration and proliferation of VSMCs that occlude vascular lumen. **C,** Karnik et al. propose that vascular injury of the mature artery may focally disrupt elastin, releasing smooth muscle cells (SMCs) to dedifferentiate, migrate, and proliferate and thereby contribute to neointimal formation.[132] *(Redrawn with permission from Karnik SK, Brooke BS, Bayes-Genis A, et al: a critical role for elastin signaling in vascular morphogenesis and disease. Development 130:411–423, 2003.)*

Tunica Adventitia: Fibroblasts and Loose Connective Tissue

Owing to a striking paucity of studies, very little is known about development of the outer layer of blood vessels, which is referred to as the *tunica adventitia* or *tunica externa*. The tunica externa is composed of loose connective tissue (mostly collagen), and the predominant cell type is the fibroblast. Diffusion of nutrients from the lumen to the adventitia and outer media is inadequate in larger vessels, so the adventitia of these vessels also includes small arteries known as the *vaso vasorum* that supply a capillary network extending through the adventitia and into the media. The adventitia of coronary vessels is thought to arise from the epicardium, based on experiments with quail-chick transplants.[134] Quail epicardial cells grafted into the pericardial space of the E2 chick undergo EMT and contribute to both coronary vascular SMCs (consistent with findings discussed earlier regarding VSMC origins in the tunica media) and coronary perivascular fibroblasts.[134]

Recently a number of studies have investigated a population of adventitial cells expressing stem cell markers. These investigations are largely a result of a paradigm shift: classically, the adventitia was considered a passive supportive tissue, but more recently, adventitial fibroblast and progenitor cells have been implicated as playing an important role in neointimal formation during vascular disease.[135,136] A niche for cells expressing the stem cell marker CD34 (but not the EC marker CD31) has been identified in the interface between the media and adventitia of human internal thoracic arteries.[137] The intensively studied growth factor Shh is expressed in this vascular "stem cell" niche of medium and large-sized arteries of the perinatal mouse.[138] *Patched-1* (*Ptc1*) and *patched-2* (*Ptc2*) are Shh target genes, and their gene products are Shh receptors. β-Galactosidase staining in Shh reporter mice, *Ptc1lacZ* or *Ptc2lacZ*, suggests that Shh signaling is active in the adventitia during the late embryonic period and early postnatal period.[138] Cells expressing the stem cell marker Sca1 are located in the adventitia of the mouse between the aortic and pulmonary trunks, initially in the late embryonic stages and persisting into adulthood, and Shh signaling appears to be critical for this population of cells because the number of adventitial Sca1+ cells is greatly diminished in *Shh* null mice.[138] In sum, the adventitia is likely to be an important tissue in vascular development and disease; however, its role in these processes is critically understudied.

REFERENCES

1. Tammela T, Alitalo K: Lymphangiogenesis: molecular mechanisms and future promise, *Cell* 140(4):460–476, 2010.
2. Owens GK, Kumar MS, Wamhoff BR: Molecular regulation of vascular differentiation in development and disease, *Physiol Rev* 84(3):767–801, 2004.
3. Majesky MW: Developmental basis of vascular smooth muscle diversity, *Arterioscler Thromb Vasc Biol* 27(6):1248–1258, 2007.
4. Pardanaud L, Yassine F, Dieterlen-Lievre F: Relationship between vasculogenesis, angiogenesis and haemopoiesis during avian ontogeny, *Development* 105(3):473–485, 1989.
5. Jin SW, Beis D, Mitchell T, et al: Cellular and molecular analyses of vascular tube and lumen formation in zebrafish, *Development* 132(23):5199–5209, 2005.
6. Vokes SA, Krieg PA: Endoderm is required for vascular endothelial tube formation, but not for angioblast specification, *Development* 129(3):775–785, 2002.
7. Risau W, Flamme I: Vasculogenesis, *Annu Rev Cell Dev Biol* 11:73–91, 1995.
8. DeRuiter MC, Poelmann RE, VanMunsteren JC, et al: Embryonic endothelial cells transdifferentiate into mesenchymal cells expressing smooth muscle actins in vivo and in vitro, *Circ Res* 80(4):444–451, 1997.
9. Yamashita J, Itoh H, Hirashima M, et al: Flk1-positive cells derived from embryonic stem cells serve as vascular progenitors, *Nature* 408(6808):92–96, 2000.
10. Risau W: Mechanisms of angiogenesis, *Nature* 386(6626):671–674, 1997.
11. Adams RH, Wilkinson GA, Weiss C, et al: Roles of ephrinB ligands and EphB receptors in cardiovascular development: demarcation of arterial/venous domains, vascular morphogenesis, and sprouting angiogenesis, *Genes Dev* 13(3):295–306, 1999.
12. Gerety SS, Wang HU, Chen ZF, et al: Symmetrical mutant phenotypes of the receptor EphB4 and its specific transmembrane ligand ephrin-B2 in cardiovascular development, *Mol Cell* 4(3):403–414, 1999.
13. Wang HU, Chen ZF, Anderson DJ: Molecular distinction and angiogenic interaction between embryonic arteries and veins revealed by ephrin-B2 and its receptor Eph-B4, *Cell* 93(5):741–753, 1998.
14. Smithers L, Haddon C, Jiang YJ, et al: Sequence and embryonic expression of deltaC in the zebrafish, *Mech Dev* 90(1):119–123, 2000.
15. Zhong TP, Childs S, Leu JP, et al: Gridlock signalling pathway fashions the first embryonic artery, *Nature* 414(6860):216–220, 2001.
16. Zhong TP, Rosenberg M, Mohideen MA, et al: Gridlock, an HLH gene required for assembly of the aorta in zebrafish, *Science* 287(5459):1820–1824, 2000.
17. Noden DM: Embryonic origins and assembly of blood vessels, *Am Rev Respir Dis* 140(4):1097–1103, 1989.
18. Lawson ND, Scheer N, Pham VN, et al: Notch signaling is required for arterial-venous differentiation during embryonic vascular development, *Development* 128(19):3675–3683, 2001.
19. Lawson ND, Vogel AM, Weinstein BM: Sonic hedgehog and vascular endothelial growth factor act upstream of the Notch pathway during arterial endothelial differentiation, *Dev Cell* 3(1):127–136, 2002.
20. Moyon D, Pardanaud L, Yuan L, et al: Plasticity of endothelial cells during arterial-venous differentiation in the avian embryo, *Development* 128(17):3359–3370, 2001.
21. Red-Horse K, Ueno H, Weissman IL, et al: Coronary arteries form by developmental reprogramming of venous cells, *Nature* 464(7288):549–553, 2010.
22. Gerhardt H, Golding M, Fruttiger M, et al: VEGF guides angiogenic sprouting utilizing endothelial tip cell filopodia, *J Cell Biol* 161(6):1163–1177, 2003.
23. Ausprunk DH, Folkman J: Migration and proliferation of endothelial cells in preformed and newly formed blood vessels during tumor angiogenesis, *Microvasc Res* 14(1):53–65, 1977.
24. Stone J, Itin A, Alon T, et al: Development of retinal vasculature is mediated by hypoxia-induced vascular endothelial growth factor (VEGF) expression by neuroglia, *J Neurosci* 15(7 Pt 1):4738–4747, 1995.
25. Ghabrial AS, Krasnow MA: Social interactions among epithelial cells during tracheal branching morphogenesis, *Nature* 441(7094):746–749, 2006.
26. Phng LK, Gerhardt H: Angiogenesis: a team effort coordinated by notch, *Dev Cell* 16(2):196–208, 2009.
27. Hellstrom M, Phng LK, Hofmann JJ, et al: Dll4 signalling through Notch1 regulates formation of tip cells during angiogenesis, *Nature* 445(7129):776–780, 2007.
28. Shutter JR, Scully S, Fan W, et al: Dll4, a novel Notch ligand expressed in arterial endothelium, *Genes Dev* 14(11):1313–1318, 2000.
29. Suchting S, Freitas C, le Noble F, et al: The Notch ligand delta-like 4 negatively regulates endothelial tip cell formation and vessel branching, *Proc Natl Acad Sci U S A* 104(9):3225–3230, 2007.
30. Childs S, Chen JN, Garrity DM, et al: Patterning of angiogenesis in the zebrafish embryo, *Development* 129(4):973–982, 2002.
31. Siekmann AF, Lawson ND: Notch signalling limits angiogenic cell behaviour in developing zebrafish arteries, *Nature* 445(7129):781–784, 2007.
32. Horowitz A, Simons M: Branching morphogenesis, *Circ Res* 103(8):784–795, 2008.
33. Affolter M, Caussinus E: Tracheal branching morphogenesis in *Drosophila*: new insights into cell behaviour and organ architecture, *Development* 135(12):2055–2064, 2008.
34. Metzger RJ, Krasnow MA: Genetic control of branching morphogenesis, *Science* 284(5420):1635–1639, 1999.
35. Sutherland D, Samakovlis C, Krasnow MA: Branchless encodes a *Drosophila* FGF homolog that controls tracheal cell migration and the pattern of branching, *Cell* 87(6):1091–1101, 1996.
36. Jarecki J, Johnson E, Krasnow MA: Oxygen regulation of airway branching in *Drosophila* is mediated by branchless FGF, *Cell* 99(2):211–220, 1999.
37. Hacohen N, Kramer S, Sutherland D, et al: Sprouty encodes a novel antagonist of FGF signaling that patterns apical branching of the *Drosophila* airways, *Cell* 92(2):253–263, 1998.
38. Mason JM, Morrison DJ, Basson MA, et al: Sprouty proteins: multifaceted negative-feedback regulators of receptor tyrosine kinase signaling, *Trends Cell Biol* 16(1):45–54, 2006.
39. Cardoso WV, Lu J: Regulation of early lung morphogenesis: questions, facts and controversies, *Development* 133(9):1611–1624, 2006.
40. Metzger RJ, Klein OD, Martin GR, et al: The branching programme of mouse lung development, *Nature* 453(7196):745–750, 2008.
41. Min H, Danilenko DM, Scully SA, et al: Fgf-10 is required for both limb and lung development and exhibits striking functional similarity to *Drosophila* branchless, *Genes Dev* 12(20):3156–3161, 1998.
42. De Moerlooze L, Spencer-Dene B, Revest JM, et al: An important role for the IIIb isoform of fibroblast growth factor receptor 2 (FGFR2) in mesenchymal-epithelial signalling during mouse organogenesis, *Development* 127(3):483–492, 2000.
43. Costantini F, Kopan R: Patterning a complex organ: branching morphogenesis and nephron segmentation in kidney development, *Dev Cell* 18(5):698–712, 2010.
44. Dressler GR: Advances in early kidney specification, development and patterning, *Development* 136(23):3863–3874, 2009.
45. Skinner MA, Safford SD, Reeves JG, et al: Renal aplasia in humans is associated with RET mutations, *Am J Hum Genet* 82(2):344–351, 2008.
46. Olsson AK, Dimberg A, Kreuger J, et al: VEGF receptor signalling in control of vascular function, *Nat Rev Mol Cell Biol* 7(5):359–371, 2006.
47. Carmeliet P, Ferreira V, Breier G, et al: Abnormal blood vessel development and lethality in embryos lacking a single VEGF allele, *Nature* 380(6573):435–439, 1996.
48. Ferrara N, Carver-Moore K, Chen H, et al: Heterozygous embryonic lethality induced by targeted inactivation of the VEGF gene, *Nature* 380(6573):439–442, 1996.
49. Breier G, Albrecht U, Sterrer S, et al: Expression of vascular endothelial growth factor during embryonic angiogenesis and endothelial cell differentiation, *Development* 114(2):521–532, 1992.
50. Shalaby F, Rossant J, Yamaguchi TP, et al: Failure of blood-island formation and vasculogenesis in Flk-1-deficient mice, *Nature* 376(6535):62–66, 1995.
51. Fong GH, Rossant J, Gertsenstein M, et al: Role of the Flt-1 receptor tyrosine kinase in regulating the assembly of vascular endothelium, *Nature* 376(6535):66–70, 1995.
52. Dumont DJ, Jussila L, Taipale J, et al: Cardiovascular failure in mouse embryos deficient in VEGF receptor-3, *Science* 282(5390):946–949, 1998.
53. Coulon C, Georgiadou M, Roncal C, et al: From vessel sprouting to normalization: role of the prolyl hydroxylase domain protein/hypoxia-inducible factor oxygen-sensing machinery, *Arterioscler Thromb Vasc Biol* 30(12):2331–2336, 2010.

54. Lee SH, Schloss DJ, Jarvis L, et al: Inhibition of angiogenesis by a mouse sprouty protein, *J Biol Chem* 276(6):4128–4133, 2001.

55. Downs KM: Florence Sabin and the mechanism of blood vessel lumenization during vasculogenesis, *Microcirculation* 10(1):5–25, 2003.

56. Folkman J, Haudenschild C: Angiogenesis by capillary endothelial cells in culture, *Trans Ophthalmol Soc U K* 100(3):346–353, 1980.

57. Davis GE, Bayless KJ: An integrin and Rho GTPase-dependent pinocytic vacuole mechanism controls capillary lumen formation in collagen and fibrin matrices, *Microcirculation* 10(1):27–44, 2003.

58. Bayless KJ, Davis GE: The Cdc42 and Rac1 GTPases are required for capillary lumen formation in three-dimensional extracellular matrices, *J Cell Sci* 115(Pt 6):1123–1136, 2002.

59. Kamei M, Saunders WB, Bayless KJ, et al: Endothelial tubes assemble from intracellular vacuoles in vivo, *Nature* 442(7101):453–456, 2006.

60. Zeeb M, Strilic B, Lammert E: Resolving cell-cell junctions: lumen formation in blood vessels, *Curr Opin Cell Biol* 22(5):626–632, 2010.

61. Blum Y, Belting HG, Ellertsdottir E, et al: Complex cell rearrangements during intersegmental vessel sprouting and vessel fusion in the zebrafish embryo, *Dev Biol* 316(2):312–322, 2008.

62. Lubarsky B, Krasnow MA: Tube morphogenesis: making and shaping biological tubes, *Cell* 112(1):19–28, 2003.

63. Zovein AC, Luque A, Turlo KA, et al: Beta1 integrin establishes endothelial cell polarity and arteriolar lumen formation via a Par3-dependent mechanism, *Dev Cell* 18(1):39–51, 2010.

64. Carmeliet P, Lampugnani MG, Moons L, et al: Targeted deficiency or cytosolic truncation of the VE-cadherin gene in mice impairs VEGF-mediated endothelial survival and angiogenesis, *Cell* 98(2):147–157, 1999.

65. Strilic B, Kucera T, Eglinger J, et al: The molecular basis of vascular lumen formation in the developing mouse aorta, *Dev Cell* 17(4):505–515, 2009.

66. Parker LH, Schmidt M, Jin SW, et al: The endothelial-cell-derived secreted factor Egfl7 regulates vascular tube formation, *Nature* 428(6984):754–758, 2004.

67. Carmeliet P, Tessier-Lavigne M: Common mechanisms of nerve and blood vessel wiring, *Nature* 436(7048):193–200, 2005.

68. Mukouyama YS, Shin D, Britsch S, et al: Sensory nerves determine the pattern of arterial differentiation and blood vessel branching in the skin, *Cell* 109(6):693–705, 2002.

69. Adams RH, Eichmann A: Axon guidance molecules in vascular patterning, *Cold Spring Harb Perspect Biol* 2(5):a001875, 2010.

70. Damon DH, Teriele JA, Marko SB: Vascular-derived artemin: a determinant of vascular sympathetic innervation? *Am J Physiol Heart Circ Physiol* 293(1):H266–H273, 2007.

71. Honma Y, Araki T, Gianino S, et al: Artemin is a vascular-derived neurotropic factor for developing sympathetic neurons, *Neuron* 35(2):267–282, 2002.

72. Matsumoto K, Yoshitomi H, Rossant J, et al: Liver organogenesis promoted by endothelial cells prior to vascular function, *Science* 294(5542):559–563, 2001.

73. Eberhard D, Kragl M, Lammert E: "Giving and taking": endothelial and beta-cells in the islets of Langerhans, *Trends Endocrinol Metab* 21(8):457–463, 2010.

74. Lammert E, Cleaver O, Melton D: Induction of pancreatic differentiation by signals from blood vessels, *Science* 294(5542):564–567, 2001.

75. Yoshitomi H, Zaret KS: Endothelial cell interactions initiate dorsal pancreas development by selectively inducing the transcription factor Ptf1a, *Development* 131(4):807–817, 2004.

76. Jacquemin P, Yoshitomi H, Kashima Y, et al: An endothelial-mesenchymal relay pathway regulates early phases of pancreas development, *Dev Biol* 290(1):189–199, 2006.

77. Kapa S, Gleeson FC, Vege SS: Dorsal pancreas agenesis and polysplenia/heterotaxy syndrome: a novel association with aortic coarctation and a review of the literature, *JOP* 8(4):433–437, 2007.

78. Sabin FR: On the origin of the lymphatic system from the veins and the development of the lymph hearts and thoracic duct in the pig, *Am J Anat* 1:367–391, 1902.

79. Sabin FR: The lymphatic system in human embryos, with a consideration of the morphology of the system as a whole, *Am J Anat* 9:43–91, 1909.

80. Francois M, Caprini A, Hosking B, et al: Sox18 induces development of the lymphatic vasculature in mice, *Nature* 456(7222):643–647, 2008.

81. Irrthum A, Devriendt K, Chitayat D, et al: Mutations in the transcription factor gene SOX18 underlie recessive and dominant forms of hypotrichosis-lymphedema-telangiectasia, *Am J Hum Genet* 72(6):1470–1478, 2003.

82. Srinivasan RS, Dillard ME, Lagutin OV, et al: Lineage tracing demonstrates the venous origin of the mammalian lymphatic vasculature, *Genes Dev* 21(19):2422–2432, 2007.

83. You LR, Lin FJ, Lee CT, et al: Suppression of Notch signalling by the COUP-TFII transcription factor regulates vein identity, *Nature* 435(7038):98–104, 2005.

84. Armulik A, Abramsson A, Betsholtz C: Endothelial/pericyte interactions, *Circ Res* 97(6):512–523, 2005.

85. Wasteson P, Johansson BR, Jukkola T, et al: Developmental origin of smooth muscle cells in the descending aorta in mice, *Development* 135(10):1823–1832, 2008.

86. Esner M, Meilhac SM, Relaix F, et al: Smooth muscle of the dorsal aorta shares a common clonal origin with skeletal muscle of the myotome, *Development* 133(4):737–749, 2006.

87. Topouzis S, Majesky MW: Smooth muscle lineage diversity in the chick embryo. Two types of aortic smooth muscle cell differ in growth and receptor-mediated transcriptional responses to transforming growth factor-beta, *Dev Biol* 178(2):430–445, 1996.

88. Majesky MW: Development of coronary vessels, *Curr Top Dev Biol* 62:225–259, 2004.

89. Zhou B, Ma Q, Rajagopal S, et al: Epicardial progenitors contribute to the cardiomyocyte lineage in the developing heart, *Nature* 454(7200):109–113, 2008.

90. Wilm B, Ipenberg A, Hastie ND, et al: The serosal mesothelium is a major source of smooth muscle cells of the gut vasculature, *Development* 132(23):5317–5328, 2005.

91. Que J, Wilm B, Hasegawa H, et al: Mesothelium contributes to vascular smooth muscle and mesenchyme during lung development, *Proc Natl Acad Sci U S A* 105(43):16626–16630, 2008.

92. Morimoto M, Liu Z, Cheng HT, et al: Canonical Notch signaling in the developing lung is required for determination of arterial smooth muscle cells and selection of Clara versus ciliated cell fate, *J Cell Sci* 123(Pt 2):213–224, 2010.

93. Arciniegas E, Frid MG, Douglas IS, et al: Perspectives on endothelial-to-mesenchymal transition: potential contribution to vascular remodeling in chronic pulmonary hypertension, *Am J Physiol Lung Cell Mol Physiol* 293(1):L1–L8, 2007.

94. Alva JA, Zovein AC, Monvoisin A, et al: VE-cadherin-Cre-recombinase transgenic mouse: a tool for lineage analysis and gene deletion in endothelial cells, *Dev Dyn* 235(3):759–767, 2006.

95. Muzumdar MD, Tasic B, Miyamichi K, et al: A global double-fluorescent Cre reporter mouse, *Genesis* 45(9):593–605, 2007.

96. Greif DM, Hum JN, An AC, et al: Radial construction of the arterial wall. Manuscript in preparation.

97. Hungerford JE, Little CD: Developmental biology of the vascular smooth muscle cell: building a multilayered vessel wall, *J Vasc Res* 36(1):2–27, 1999.

98. Li L, Miano JM, Cserjesi P, et al: SM22 alpha, a marker of adult smooth muscle, is expressed in multiple myogenic lineages during embryogenesis, *Circ Res* 78(2):188–195, 1996.

99. Miano JM, Cserjesi P, Ligon KL, et al: Smooth muscle myosin heavy chain exclusively marks the smooth muscle lineage during mouse embryogenesis, *Circ Res* 75(5):803–812, 1994.

100. van der Loop FT, Schaart G, Timmer ED, et al: Smoothelin, a novel cytoskeletal protein specific for smooth muscle cells, *J Cell Biol* 134(2):401–411, 1996.

101. Miano JM: Serum response factor: toggling between disparate programs of gene expression, *J Mol Cell Cardiol* 35(6):577–593, 2003.

102. Wang Z, Wang DZ, Hockemeyer D, et al: Myocardin and ternary complex factors compete for SRF to control smooth muscle gene expression, *Nature* 428(6979):185–189, 2004.

103. Wang Z, Wang DZ, Pipes GC, et al: Myocardin is a master regulator of smooth muscle gene expression, *Proc Natl Acad Sci U S A* 100(12):7129–7134, 2003.

104. Li S, Wang DZ, Wang Z, et al: The serum response factor coactivator myocardin is required for vascular smooth muscle development, *Proc Natl Acad Sci U S A* 100(16):9366–9370, 2003.

105. de Ruiter MC, Poelmann RE, van Iperen L, et al: The early development of the tunica media in the vascular system of rat embryos, *Anat Embryol (Berl)* 181(4):341–349, 1990.

106. Hungerford JE, Owens GK, Argraves WS, et al: Development of the aortic vessel wall as defined by vascular smooth muscle and extracellular matrix markers, *Dev Biol* 178(2):375–392, 1996.

107. el-Maghraby AA, Gardner DL: Development of connective-tissue components of small arteries in the chick embryo, *J Pathol* 108(4):281–291, 1972.

108. Kadar A, Gardner DL, Bush V: The relation between the fine structure of smooth-muscle cells and elastogenesis in the chick-embryo aorta, *J Pathol* 104(4):253–260, 1971.

109. Nakamura H: Electron microscopic study of the prenatal development of the thoracic aorta in the rat, *Am J Anat* 181(4):406–418, 1988.

110. Takahashi Y, Imanaka T, Takano T: Spatial and temporal pattern of smooth muscle cell differentiation during development of the vascular system in the mouse embryo, *Anat Embryol (Berl)* 194(5):515–526, 1996.

111. Turing AM: The chemical basis of morphogenesis, *Philos Trans R Soc Lond B Biol Sci* 237(641):37–72, 1952.

112. Reilly KM, Melton DA: Short-range signaling by candidate morphogens of the TGF beta family and evidence for a relay mechanism of induction, *Cell* 86(5):743–754, 1996.

113. Feng X, Krebs LT, Gridley T: Patent ductus arteriosus in mice with smooth muscle-specific Jag1 deletion, *Development* 137:4191–4199, 2010.

114. Gaengel K, Genove G, Armulik A, et al: Endothelial-mural cell signaling in vascular development and angiogenesis, *Arterioscler Thromb Vasc Biol* 29(5):630–638, 2009.

115. Hellstrom M, Kalen M, Lindahl P, et al: Role of PDGF-β and PDGFR-beta in recruitment of vascular smooth muscle cells and pericytes during embryonic blood vessel formation in the mouse, *Development* 126(14):3047–3055, 1999.

116. Leveen P, Pekny M, Gebre-Medhin S, et al: Mice deficient for PDGF B show renal, cardiovascular, and hematological abnormalities, *Genes Dev* 8(16):1875–1887, 1994.

117. Lindahl P, Johansson BR, Leveen P, et al: Pericyte loss and microaneurysm formation in PDGF-B-deficient mice, *Science* 277(5323):242–245, 1997.

118. Soriano P: Abnormal kidney development and hematological disorders in PDGF beta-receptor mutant mice, *Genes Dev* 8(16):1888–1896, 1994.

119. Hirschi KK, Rohovsky SA, D'Amore PA: PDGF, TGF-beta, and heterotypic cell-cell interactions mediate endothelial cell-induced recruitment of 10T1/2 cells and their differentiation to a smooth muscle fate, *J Cell Biol* 141(3):805–814, 1998.

120. Gridley T: Notch signaling in vascular development and physiology, *Development* 134(15):2709–2718, 2007.

121. High FA, Lu MM, Pear WS, et al: Endothelial expression of the Notch ligand Jagged1 is required for vascular smooth muscle development, *Proc Natl Acad Sci U S A* 105(6):1955–1959, 2008.

122. Domenga V, Fardoux P, Lacombe P, et al: Notch3 is required for arterial identity and maturation of vascular smooth muscle cells, *Genes Dev* 18(22):2730–2735, 2004.

123. Wang T, Baron M, Trump D: An overview of Notch3 function in vascular smooth muscle cells, *Prog Biophys Mol Biol* 96(1–3):499–509, 2008.

124. Joutel A, Corpechot C, Ducros A, et al: Notch3 mutations in CADASIL, a hereditary adult-onset condition causing stroke and dementia, *Nature* 383(6602):707–710, 1996.

125. McLean SE, Mecham BH, Kelleher CM, et al: Extracellular matrix gene expression in the developing mouse aorta, *Adv Dev Biol* 15:81–128, 2005.

126. Kelleher CM, McLean SE, Mecham RP: Vascular extracellular matrix and aortic development, *Curr Top Dev Biol* 62:153–188, 2004.

127. Parks WC, Pierce RA, Lee KA, et al: Elastin, *Adv Mol Cell Biol* 6:133–181, 1993.

128. Faury G, Pezet M, Knutsen RH, et al: Developmental adaptation of the mouse cardiovascular system to elastin haploinsufficiency, *J Clin Invest* 112(9):1419–1428, 2003.

129. Li DY, Faury G, Taylor DG, et al: Novel arterial pathology in mice and humans hemizygous for elastin, *J Clin Invest* 102(10):1783–1787, 1998.

130. Wagenseil JE, Nerurkar NL, Knutsen RH, et al: Effects of elastin haploinsufficiency on the mechanical behavior of mouse arteries, *Am J Physiol Heart Circ Physiol* 289(3):H1209–H1217, 2005.

131. Li DY, Brooke B, Davis EC, et al: Elastin is an essential determinant of arterial morphogenesis, *Nature* 393(6682):276–280, 1998.

132. Karnik SK, Brooke BS, Bayes-Genis A, et al: A critical role for elastin signaling in vascular morphogenesis and disease, *Development* 130(2):411–423, 2003.

133. Ramirez F, Dietz HC: Marfan syndrome: from molecular pathogenesis to clinical treatment, *Curr Opin Genet Dev* 17(3):252–258, 2007.

134. Dettman RW, Denetclaw W, Ordahl CP, et al: Common epicardial origin of coronary vascular smooth muscle, perivascular fibroblasts, and intermyocardial fibroblasts in the avian heart, *Dev Biol* 193(2):169–181, 1998.

135. Hu Y, Zhang Z, Torsney E, et al: Abundant progenitor cells in the adventitia contribute to atherosclerosis of vein grafts in ApoE-deficient mice, *J Clin Invest* 113(9):1258–1265, 2004.

136. Sartore S, Chiavegato A, Faggin E, et al: Contribution of adventitial fibroblasts to neointima formation and vascular remodeling: from innocent bystander to active participant, *Circ Res* 89(12):1111–1121, 2001.

137. Zengin E, Chalajour F, Gehling UM, et al: Vascular wall resident progenitor cells: a source for postnatal vasculogenesis, *Development* 133(8):1543–1551, 2006.

138. Passman JN, Dong XR, Wu SP, et al: A sonic hedgehog signaling domain in the arterial adventitia supports resident Sca1+ smooth muscle progenitor cells, *Proc Natl Acad Sci U S A* 105(27):9349–9354, 2008.

VASCULAR EMBRYOLOGY AND ANGIOGENESIS

CHAPTER **2** # The Endothelium

Jane A. Leopold

In 1839, the German physiologist Theodor Schwann became the first to describe a "thin, but distinctly perceptible membrane" that he observed as part of the capillary vessel wall that separated circulating blood from tissue.[1,2] The cellular monolayer that formed this membrane would later be named the *endothelium*; however, the term *endothelium* did not appear until 1865 when it was introduced by the Swiss anatomist Wilhelm His in his essay, "Die Häute und Höhlen des Körpers (The Membranes and Cavities of the Body)."[2,3] Owing to its anatomical location, the endothelium was believed initially to be a passive receptacle for circulating blood, cells, and macromolecules. It is now known that the endothelium is a dynamic cellular structure, and its biological and functional properties extend beyond that of a physical anatomical boundary. In its totality, the endothelium comprises approximately 10 trillion (10^{13}) cells with a surface area of 7 m^2, weighs 1.0 to 1.8 kilograms, and contributes 1.4% to total body mass.[4,5] Endothelium exists as a monolayer of cells that is present in all arteries, veins, capillaries, and the lymphatic system, and lies at the interface of the bloodstream or lymph and the vessel wall.

The paradigm shift in our understanding of the role of the endothelium in vascular function has occurred over the past half century and continues to evolve. As a cellular structure with its luminal surface in continuous contact with flowing blood, the endothelium serves as a thromboresistant, semipermeable barrier, and governs interactions with circulating inflammatory and immune cells. In response to pulsatile flow and pressure, the endothelium mechanotransduces these hemodynamic forces to synthesize and release vasoactive substances that regulate vascular tone as well as signals for compensatory vessel wall remodeling. This chapter will focus on the biology of the endothelium to provide insight into how perturbations of these homeostatic functions result in (mal)adaptive responses that determine vascular health or disease.

Homeostatic Functions of the Endothelium

The endothelium exhibits considerable regional heterogeneity that reflects its arterial or venous location in the vascular tree, as well as the specialized metabolic and functional demands of the underlying tissues.[5-7] Despite this heterogeneity, there are basal homeostatic properties that are common to all endothelial cell (EC) populations, although some of these functions may achieve greater importance in selected vascular beds[7] (Box 2-1).

Maintenance of a Thromboresistant Surface and Regulation of Hemostasis

The endothelium was first recognized as a cellular structure that compartmentalizes circulating blood.[4] As such, the endothelial luminal surface is exposed to cells and proteins in the bloodstream that possess prothrombotic and procoagulant activity and, when necessary, support hemostasis. Normal endothelium preserves blood fluidity by synthesizing and secreting factors that limit activation of the clotting cascade, inhibit platelet aggregation, and promote fibrinolysis.[8] These include the cell surface–associated anticoagulant factors thrombomodulin, protein C, tissue factor pathway inhibitor (TFPI), and heparan sulfate proteoglycans (HSPG) that act in concert to limit coagulation at the luminal surface of the endothelium.[8-10] For instance, thrombin-mediated activation of protein C is accelerated 10^4-fold by binding to thrombomodulin, Ca^{2+}, and the endothelial protein C receptor. Activated protein C (APC) engages circulating protein S, which is also synthesized and released by the endothelium, to inactivate factors Va and VIIIa proteolytically.[8,11] Tissue factor pathway inhibitor is a Kunitz-type protease inhibitor

that binds to and inhibits factor VIIa; about 80% of TFPI is bound to the endothelium via a glycosylphosphatidylinositol anchor and forms a quaternary complex with tissue factor – factor VIIa to diminish its procoagulant activity.[12,13] Proteoglycan heparan sulfates that are present in the EC glycocalyx attain anticoagulant properties by catalyzing the association of the circulating serine protease inhibitor antithrombin III to factors Xa, IXa, and thrombin.[8] Thus, these anticoagulant factors serve to limit activation and propagation of the clotting cascade at the endothelial luminal surface and thereby maintain vascular patency.

The endothelium also synthesizes and secretes tissue plasminogen activator (tPA) and the ecto-adenosine diphosphatase (ecto-ADPase) CD39 to promote fibrinolysis and inhibit platelet activation, respectively. Tissue plasminogen activator is produced and released into the bloodstream continuously, but unless tPA binds fibrin, it is cleared from the plasma within 15 minutes by the liver.[8] Fibrin binding accelerates tPA amidolytic activity by increasing the catalytic efficiency for plasminogen activation and plasmin generation. Platelet activation at the endothelial luminal surface is inhibited by the actions of the ectonucleotidase CD39/NTPDase1 that hydrolyzes adenosine diphosphate (ADP), prostacyclin (PGI_2), and nitric oxide (NO).[8,14,15] Together these agents maintain an environment on the endothelial surface that is profibrinolytic and antithrombotic.

By contrast, in the setting of an acute vascular injury or trauma, the endothelium initiates a rapid and measured hemostatic response through regulated synthesis and release of tissue factor and von Willebrand factor (vWF). Tissue factor is a multidomain transmembrane glycoprotein (GP) that forms a complex with circulating factor VIIa to activate the coagulation cascade and generate thrombin.[16] Tissue factor is expressed by vascular smooth muscle cells (VSMCs) and fibroblasts and by ECs only after activation. Tissue factor acquires its biological activity by phosphatidylserine exposure, dedimerization, decreased exposure to TFPI, or posttranslational modification(s) including disulfide bond formation between Cys186 and Cys209.[17-19] This disulfide bond is important for tissue factor coagulation activity and may be reduced by protein disulfide isomerase, which is located on the EC surface.

The endothelium also synthesizes and stores vWF, a large polymeric GP that is expressed rapidly in response to injury. Propeptides and multimers of vWF are packaged in Weibel-Palade bodies that are unique to the endothelium. Once released, vWF multimers form elongated strings that retain platelets at sites of endothelial injury. Weibel-Palade bodies also contain P-selectin, angiopoietin-2, osteoprotegerin, the tetraspanin CD63/Lamp3, as well as cytokines, which are believed to be present as a result of incidental packaging.[20] The stored pool of vWF may be mobilized quickly to the endothelial surface, where it binds to exposed collagen and participates in formation of a primary platelet hemostatic plug. The endothelium modulates this response further by regulating vWF size, and thereby its activity, through the action of the EC product ADAMTS13 (a disintegrin and metalloproteinase with thrombospondin type I motif, number 13).[21] This protease cleaves released vWF at Tyr1605-Met1606 to generate smaller-sized polymers and decrease the propensity for platelet thrombus formation.[21] Thus, the endothelium uses geographical separation of factors that regulate its anti- and prothrombotic functions to maintain blood fluidity yet allow for a hemostatic response to vascular injury.

Semipermeable Barrier and Transendothelial Transport Pathways

The endothelial monolayer serves as a size-selective semipermeable barrier that restricts the free bidirectional transit of water, macromolecules, and circulating or resident cells

Box 2-1 Homeostatic Functions of the Endothelium

Maintenance of a thromboresistant surface
Regulate hemostasis
Function as a semipermeable barrier
Modulate transendothelial transport of fluids, proteins, and cells
Regulate vascular tone
Regulate inflammation and leukocyte trafficking
Participate in vascular repair and remodeling
Sense and mechanotransduce hemodynamic forces

between the bloodstream and underlying vessel wall or tissues. Permeability function is determined in part by the architectural arrangement of the endothelial monolayer, as well as the activation of pathways that facilitate the transendothelial transport of fluids, molecules, and cells. This transport occurs via either transcellular pathways that involve vesicle formation, trafficking, and transcytosis, or by the loosening of interendothelial junctions and paracellular pathways[22] (Fig. 2-1). Molecules that traverse the endothelium by paracellular pathways are size restricted to a radius of 3 nm or less, whereas those of larger diameter may be actively transported across the cell in vesicles.[23] Although the diffusive flux of water occurs in ECs through aquaporin transmembrane water channels, the

contribution of these channels to hydraulic conductivity and cellular permeability is limited.[24]

There is significant macrostructural heterogeneity of the endothelial monolayer that reflects the functional and metabolic requirements of the underlying tissue and has consequences for its permeability function. Endothelium may be arranged in either a continuous or discontinuous manner: continuous endothelium is either nonfenestrated or fenestrated.[4–6]

Continuous nonfenestrated endothelium forms a highly exclusive barrier and is found in the arterial and venous blood vessels of the heart, lung, skin, connective tissue, muscle, retina, spinal cord, brain, and mesentery.[4–6] By contrast, continuous fenestrated endothelium is located in vessels that supply organs involved in filtration or with a high demand for transendothelial transport, including renal glomeruli, the ascending vasa recta and peritubular capillaries of the kidney, endocrine, and exocrine glands, intestinal villi, and the choroid plexus of the brain.[4–6] These ECs are characterized by fenestrae, or transcellular pores, with a diameter of 50 to 80 nm that, in the majority of cells, has a 5- to 6-mm nonmembranous diaphragm across the pore opening.[4–6,22] The distribution of these fenestrae may be polarized within the EC and allow for enhanced barrier size selectivity owing to the diaphragm.[4–6]

Discontinuous endothelium is found in the bone marrow, spleen, and liver sinusoids. This type of endothelial monolayer is

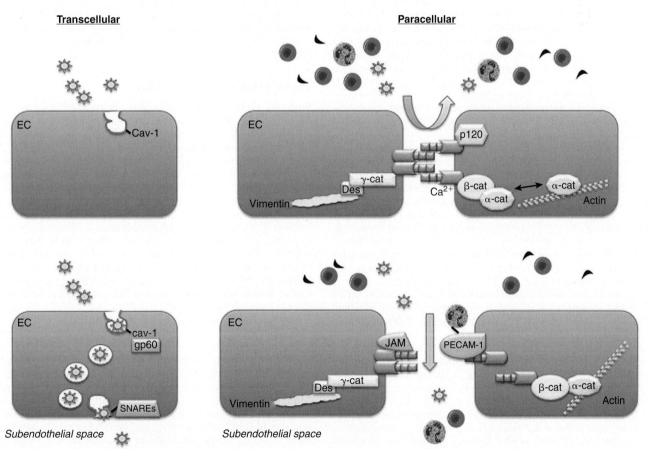

FIGURE 2-1 Transendothelial transport mechanisms. The endothelium is a semipermeable membrane that facilitates transendothelial transport of solutes, macromolecules, and cells via a transcellular pathway (left) or a paracellular pathway (right). The transcellular pathway allows for transit of albumin and other large molecules across the endothelium using caveolae as the transport mechanism. Once caveolin-1 (cav-1) interacts with gp60, caveolae separate from cell surface to form vesicles that undergo vectorial transit to the endoluminal surface. Here, the vesicles fuse with soluble N-ethylmaleimide-sensitive factor attachment receptors (SNAREs) and release their cargo to the subendothelial space. By contrast, the paracellular pathway relies on the integrity of adherens junctions between endothelial cells (EC). Vascular endothelial (VE)-cadherin molecules from adjacent ECs form a barrier that is maintained by β-catenin (β-cat), α-catenin (α-cat), and γ-catenin (γ-cat). Some mediators that increase permeability do so by promoting actin cytoskeletal rearrangement, leading to physical separation of the VE-cadherin molecules and passage of solutes and proteins. Platelet–endothelial cell adhesion molecule-1 (PECAM-1) and junctional adhesion molecules (JAM) present in the adherens junction also allow leukocytes to traffic through the adherens junction. (Adapted from Komarova Y, Malik AB: Regulation of endothelial permeability via paracellular and transcellular transport pathways. Annu Rev Physiol 72:463–493, 2010.)

notable for its large-diameter fenestrae (100-200 nm) with absent diaphragms and gaps, and a poorly organized underlying basement membrane that is permissive for transcellular flow of water and solutes as well as cellular trafficking.[4-6]

Transcellular and paracellular pathways are two distinct routes by which plasma proteins, solutes, and fluids traverse the endothelial monolayer. The transcellular pathway provides a receptor-mediated mechanism to transport albumin, lipids, and hormones across the endothelium.[22,25,26] The paracellular pathway is dependent upon the structural integrity of adherens, tight, and gap junctions and allows fluids and solutes to permeate between ECs but restricts passage of large molecules.[22,25,26] Although these pathways were believed to function independently, it is now recognized that they are interrelated and together modulate permeability under basal conditions.

The transcellular transport of albumin and albumin-bound macromolecules is initiated by albumin binding to gp60, or albondin, a 60-kDa albumin-binding protein located in flask-shaped caveolae that reside at the cell surface.[27,28] These caveolae are cholesterol- and sphingolipid-rich structures that contain caveolin-1. Once activated, gp60 interacts with caveolin-1, followed by constriction of the caveolae neck and fission from the cell surface.[29,30] These actions lead to formation of vesicles with a diameter of about 70 nm and vesicle transcytosis. Caveolae may contain as much as 15% to 20% of the cell volume, so they are capable of moving significant amounts of fluid across the cell through this mechanism.[29,30] Once vesicles have detached from the membrane, they undergo vectorial transit to the abluminal membrane, where they dock and fuse with the plasma membrane by interacting with vesicle-associated and membrane-associated target soluble *N*-ethylmaleimide-sensitive factor attachment receptors (SNAREs).[31] Once docked, the vesicles release their cargo to the interstitial space. Vesicles may traverse the cell as individual structures or cluster to form channel-like structures with a diameter of 80 to 200 nm that span the cell.[5,6] Although transcellular vesicle trafficking is the predominant mechanism by which cells transport albumin, it is now appreciated that this pathway is not absolutely necessary for permeability function, owing to the compensatory capabilities of the paracellular pathway.

The junctions between ECs include the adherens, tight, and gap junctions; only the former two modulate permeability and comprise the paracellular pathway.[32] Adherens junctions are normally impermeant to albumin and other large molecules and are the major determinant of endothelial barrier function and permeability. The expression of tight junctions, by contrast, is limited to the blood-brain or blood-retinal barriers where they restrict or prevent passage of small molecules (<1 kDa) and some inorganic ions.[22] Gap junctions are composed of connexins that form a channel between adjacent cells to enhance cell-cell communication and facilitate the transit of water, small molecules, and ions.[22]

Adherens junctions are critical for maintaining endothelial barrier functional integrity and are composed of complexes of vascular endothelial (VE)-cadherin and catenins. Vascular endothelial cadherin is a transmembrane GP with five extracellular repeats, a transmembrane segment, and a cytoplasmic tail. The external domains mediate the calcium-dependent hemophilic adhesion between VE-cadherin molecules expressed in adjacent cells.[25,26,33] The cytoplasmic tail interacts with β-catenin, plakoglobin (γ-catenin), and p120 catenin to control the organization of VE-cadherin and the actin cytoskeleton at adherens junctions. The actin binding proteins α-actinin, annexin 2, formin-1, and eplin may further stabilize this interaction. Other proteins located in adherens junctions thought to provide stability include junctional adhesion molecules (JAMs) and platelet–EC adhesion molecule 1 (PECAM-1).[22]

Endothelial permeability may be increased or decreased through mechanisms that involve adherens junction remodeling or through interactions with the actin cytoskeleton.[25,26,34] These events may occur rapidly, be transient or sustained, and are reversible. Most commonly, mediators that increase endothelial permeability either destabilize adherens junctions through phosphorylation, and thereby internalization, of VE-cadherin or by RhoA activation and actin cytoskeletal rearrangement to physically pull apart VE-cadherin molecules and adherens junctions, resulting in intercellular gaps.[22] To counteract these effects, other mediators that attenuate permeability are present in the plasma or interstitial space. Fibroblast growth factor (FGF) stabilizes VE-cadherin by stabilizing VE-cadherin-gp120-catenin interaction. Sphingosine-1-phosphate, generated by breakdown of the membrane phospholipid sphingomyelin or released from activated platelets, also stabilizes adherens junctions. This effect occurs through activation of Rac1/Rap1/Cdc42 signaling and reorganization of the actin cytoskeleton, recycling of VE-cadherin to the cell surface, and (re)assembly of adherens junctions. The cytokine angiopoietin-1 stabilizes adherens junctions by inhibiting endocytosis of VE-cadherin.[22,25,26,35,36]

Endothelial tight junctions predominate in specialized vascular beds that require an impermeable barrier. These tight junctions are composed of the specific tight junction proteins occludin, claudins (3/5), and JAM-A.[22,33,36,37] Occludin and claudins are membrane proteins that contain four transmembrane and two extracellular loop domains. The extracellular loop domains of these proteins bind similar domains on neighboring cells to seal the intercellular cleft and prevent permeability. Occludin, claudins, and JAM-A are also tethered to the actin cytoskeleton by α-catenin and zona occludens proteins (ZO-1, ZO-2).[22] The ZO proteins also function as guanylyl kinases or scaffolding proteins and use PDZ and Sc homology 3 (SH3)-binding domains to recruit other signaling molecules. Connections between tight junctions and the actin cytoskeleton are stabilized further via the actin cross-linking proteins spectrin or filamen or by the accessory proteins cingulin and AF-6.[22,36] In this manner, the junctions remain stabilized and sealed to limit or prevent transendothelial transport of fluids and molecules.

Regulation of Vascular Tone

Since the early seminal studies of Furchgott and Zawadski, it has been increasingly recognized that the endothelium regulates vascular tone via endothelium-derived factors that maintain a balance between vasoconstriction and vasodilation[38,39] (Fig. 2-2). The endothelium produces both gaseous and peptide vasodilators, including NO, hydrogen sulfide, PGI_2, and endothelium-derived hyperpolarizing factor (EDHF). The effects of these substances on vascular tone are counterbalanced by vasoconstrictors that are either synthesized or processed by the endothelium, such as thromboxane A_2 TxA_2, a product of arachidonic acid metabolism, and the peptides endothelin-1 (ET-1) and angiotensin II (Ang-II). The relative importance of these vasodilator or vasoconstrictor substances for maintaining vascular tone differs between vascular beds, with NO serving as the primary vasodilator in large conduit elastic vessels and non-NO mechanisms playing a greater role in the microcirculation.

Nitric oxide is synthesized by three structurally similar NO synthase (NOS) isoenzymes: the constitutive enzyme identified in the endothelium (eNOS or NOS3) and neuronal cells (nNOS or NOS1) or the inducible enzyme (iNOS or NOS2) found in smooth muscle cells (SMCs), neutrophils, and macrophages following exposure to endotoxin or inflammatory cytokines.[40-42] Nitric oxide is generated via a five-electron oxidation reaction of L-arginine to form L-citrulline and stoichiometric amounts of NO, and requires molecular oxygen and NADPH as co-substrates and flavin adenine dinucleotide, flavin mononucleotide, heme, and tetrahydrobiopterin as cofactors.[43-45] In the endothelium, eNOS expression is up-regulated by a diverse array of stimuli including transforming growth factor (TGF)-β1, lysophosphatidylcholine, hydrogen peroxide, tumor necrosis factor (TNF)-α, oxidized low-density lipoprotein (LDL) cholesterol, laminar shear stress, and hypoxia, and is subject to both posttranscriptional and posttranslational modifications that influence activity, including phosphorylation, acetylation, palmitoylation and myristolation, as well as

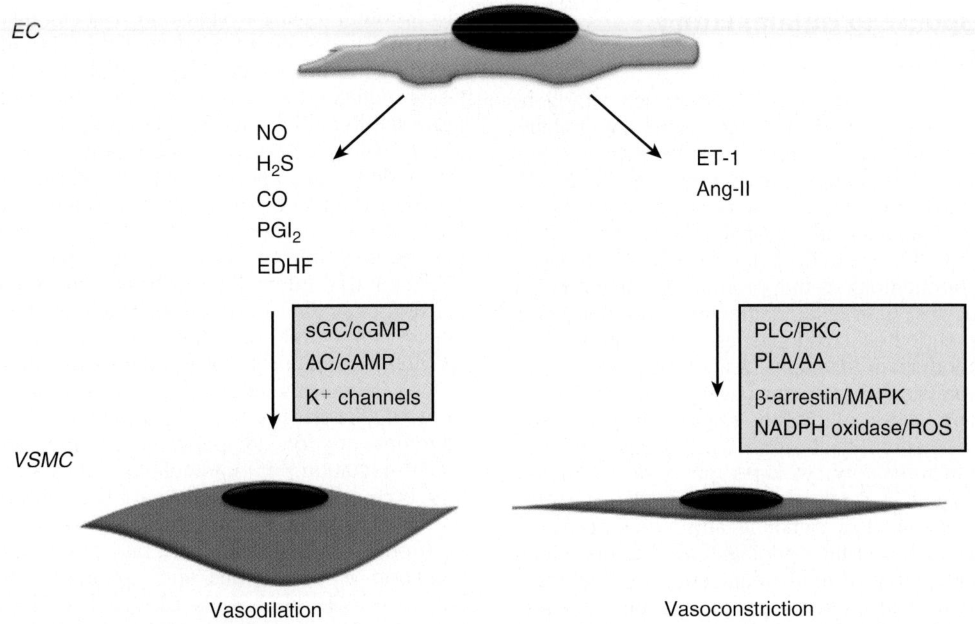

FIGURE 2-2 Endothelium-derived vasoactive factors. Endothelium modulates vascular tone by synthesizing or participating in activation of vasoactive peptides that promote vascular smooth muscle cell (VSMC) vasodilation or relaxation. The vasodilator gases nitric oxide (NO) and carbon monoxide (CO) activate soluble guanylyl cyclase (sGC) to increase cyclic guanosine monophosphate (cGMP) levels, although NO has a far greater affinity for sGC than CO. Hydrogen sulfide (H_2S), similar to endothelium-derived hyperpolarizing factor (EDHF) activates potassium channels. Prostacyclin (PGI_2) promotes vasodilation by activating adenylyl cyclase (AC) to increase cyclic adenosine monophosphate (cAMP) levels that influence calcium handling by sarcoplasmic reticulum calcium ATPase. Endothelium also synthesizes the vasoconstrictor peptide endothelin-1 (ET-1) and metabolizes angiotensin I (Ang-I) to angiotensin II (Ang-II). These vasoconstrictor peptides activate phospholipase C (PLC) and protein kinase C (PKC) signaling, phospholipase A (PLA) and arachidonic acid (AA) metabolism, activate mitogen-activated protein kinase (MAPK) signaling through β-arrestin-cSrc signaling, or increase NADPH oxidase activity and reactive oxygen species (ROS) levels.

localization to caveolae.[45] Once generated, NO diffuses into SMCs and reacts with the heme iron of guanylyl cyclase to increase cyclic guanosine monophosphate (cGMP) levels and promote vasodilation.[42] Nitric oxide can also react with SH-containing molecules and proteins (e.g., peroxynitrite, N_2O_2) to generate S-nitrosothiols, a stable reservoir of bioavailable NO with recognized antiplatelet and vasodilator effects.[46-48] In the presence of oxygen, NO can be oxidized to nitrite and nitrate, which are stable end-products of NO metabolism; nitrite serves as a vasodilator, predominantly in the pulmonary and cerebral circulations.[48,49] In addition to vasodilator and antiplatelet effects, NO has other paracrine effects that include regulation of VSMC proliferation and migration, and leukocyte adhesion and activation.[15]

Hydrogen sulfide gas generated by the endothelium also possesses vasodilator properties. Hydrogen sulfide is membrane permeable and released as a byproduct of cysteine or homocysteine metabolism via the transulfuration/cystathionine-β-synthase and cystathionine-γ-lyase pathway or by the catabolism of cysteine via cysteine aminotransferase and 3-mercaptopyruvate sulfur transferase. Hydrogen sulfide–mediated vasodilation results from activation of K_{ATP} and transient receptor membrane channel currents.[50-52]

Prostacyclin is an eicosanoid generated by cyclooxygenase (COX) and arachidonic acid metabolism in the endothelium. It promotes vasodilation via adenylyl cyclase/cyclic adenosine monophosphate (cAMP) signal transduction pathways. Prostacyclin also induces smooth muscle relaxation by reducing cytoplasmic Ca^{2+} availability; decreases VSMC proliferation through a cAMP–peroxisome proliferator-activated receptor (PPAR)-γ-mediated mechanism, and limits inflammation by decreasing interleukin (IL)-1 and IL-6.[53] Importantly, PGI_2 has significant antiplatelet effects and by decreasing TxA_2 levels, limits platelet aggregation. Because both COX-1 (constitutively expressed) and COX-2 (induced) contribute to basal PGI_2 production, selective pharmacological inhibition of either isoform may result in diminished PGI_2 levels, increased platelet aggregation, and impaired vasodilation.[54]

No single molecule has been identified as the vasodilator referred to as *endothelium-derived hyperpolarizing factor*, and the effects attributed to Endothelium-derived hyperpolarizing factor likely represent the composite actions of several agents that share a common mechanism. Endothelium-derived hyperpolarizing factor is an important vasodilator in the microcirculation and acts by opening K^+ channels to allow for K^+ efflux, hyperpolarization, and vascular smooth muscle relaxation. Candidate EDHFs include the 11, 12-epoxyeicosatrienoic acids and hydrogen peroxide.[39,55-58]

To counterbalance the effects of endothelium-derived vasodilators, the endothelium also synthesizes the vasoconstrictor ET-1 and metabolizes Ang I to Ang II. Endothelin-1, a 21-amino-acid peptide, is synthesized initially as inactive pre-proET-1 that is processed by endothelin-converting enzymes to its active form.[59,60] Endothelin-1 binds to the G protein–coupled receptors (GPCRs) ET_A and ET_B: ECs express ET_B, whereas SMCs express both receptors. Although activation of endothelial ET_B increases NO production, concomitant activation of SMC ET_A and ET_B results in prolonged and long-lasting vasoconstriction that predominates.[61]

There is no evidence that ET-1 is stored for immediate early release in the endothelium, indicating that acute stimuli such as hypoxia, TGF-β, and shear stress that increase ET-1 production do so via a transcriptional mechanism; however, ET-1 and endothelin-converting enzyme are packaged in Weibel-Palade bodies.[62] Endothelium also expresses angiotensin-converting enzyme (ACE) and, as such, modulates processing of Ang-I to the vasoconstrictor peptide Ang-II.[63] Ang-II–stimulated activation of the Ang-I receptor results in vasoconstriction and SMC hypertrophy and proliferation, in part, by activating NADPH oxidase to increase reactive oxygen species (ROS) production.[64-66] Vascular tone, therefore, is determined by the balance of vasodilator and vasoconstrictor substances synthesized or processed by the endothelium in response to stimuli: each vasoactive mediator may attain individual importance in a different vascular bed.

Regulating Response to Inflammatory and Immune Stimuli

The endothelium monitors circulating blood for foreign pathogens and participates in immunosurveillance by expressing Toll-like receptors (TLRs) 2, 3, and 4.[67-69] These TLRs identify pathogen-associated molecular patterns that are common to bacterial cell wall proteins or viral deoxyribonucleic acid (DNA) and ribonucleic acid (RNA) in the bloodstream. Once activated, TLRs elicit an inflammatory response through activation of nuclear factor (NF)-κB and generation of chemokines that promote transendothelial migration of leukocytes, have chemoattractant and mitogenic effects, and increase endothelial oxidant stress and apoptosis.[67,68]

The quiescent endothelium maintains its antiinflammatory phenotype through expression of cytokines with antiinflammatory properties and cytoprotective antioxidant enzymes that limit oxidant stress. The endothelium synthesizes TGF-β1, which inhibits synthesis of the proinflammatory cytokines monocyte chemotactic protein-1 (MCP-1) and IL-8; expression of the TNF-α receptor; NF-κB-mediated proinflammatory signaling; and leukocyte adherence to the luminal surface of the endothelium.[70,71] Endothelium also expresses a wide array of antioxidant enzymes, including catalase, the superoxide dismutases, glutathione peroxidase-1, peroxiredoxins, and glucose-6-phosphate dehydrogenase.[48] Through the actions of these antioxidant enzymes, ROS are reduced, and the redox environment remains stable. This homeostatic redox modulation also limits activation of ROS-stimulated transcription factors such as NF-κB, activator protein-1, specificity protein-1, and PPARs.[48] The inflammatory phenotype of the endothelium is also influenced by other circulating or paracrine factors that have antioxidant or antiinflammatory properties, such as high-density lipoprotein (HDL) cholesterol, IL-4, IL-10, IL-13, and IL-1 receptor antagonist.[5,6,72,73]

The endothelium is capable of mounting a rapid inflammatory response that involves the actions of chemoattractant cytokines, or chemokines, and their associated receptors to facilitate interactions between leukocytes and the endothelium. Endothelial cells express the chemokine receptors CXCR4, CCR2, and CCR8 on the luminal or abluminal surface of cells.[74] These receptors bind and transport chemokines to the opposite side of the cell to generate a chemoattractant gradient for inflammatory cell homing. Heparan sulfate (HS), which is present in the endothelial glycocalyx, may serve as a chemokine presenter and is necessary for the action of some chemokines such as CXCL8, CCL2, CCL4, and CCL5.[75,76]

Endothelial cells also express the Duffy antigen receptor for chemokines (DARC) that participates in chemokine transcytosis across cells. Duffy antigen receptor for chemokines is a member of the silent chemokine receptor family that has high homology to GPCRs and can bind a broad spectrum of inflammatory CC and CXC chemokines, including MCP-1, IL-8, and CCL5 or Regulated upon Activation, Normal T-cell Expressed, and Secreted (RANTES), but does not activate G-protein signaling.[77-79] Exposure to chemokines, in turn, activates cellular signaling pathways that promote EC–leukocyte interactions; however, homing of leukocytes to tissues is mediated directly by cell surface adhesion molecules.

Endothelium expresses selectins and immunoglobulin (Ig)-like cell surface adhesion molecules that regulate endothelial-leukocyte interactions. P-selectin and E-selectin are lectin-like transmembrane GPs. These selectins mediate leukocyte adhesion through Ca^{2+}-dependent binding of their N-terminal C-type lectin-like domain with a sialyl-Lewis X capping structure ligand present on leukocytes.[80-82] P-selectin is stored in Weibel-Palade bodies where it can be mobilized rapidly to the cell surface in response to thrombin, histamine, complement activation, ROS, and inflammatory cytokines. Cell surface expression of P-selectin is limited to minutes.[80,82] By contrast, E-selectin requires de novo protein synthesis for its expression. E-selectin is expressed on the cell surface, but it may also be found in its biologically active form in serum as a result of proteolytic cleavage from the cell surface.[5,81,82] These selectins bind the leukocyte ligands P-selectin glycoprotein ligand-1 (PSGL-1), E-selectin-ligand-1, and CD44, each of which appears to have a distinct function: PSGL1 is implicated in the initial tethering of leukocytes to the endothelium, E-selectin-ligand-1 converts transient initial tethers to slower and more stable rolling, and CD44 controls the speed of rolling.[81,82]

The Ig-like cell surface adhesion molecules expressed by the endothelium are intercellular adhesion molecule (ICAM)-1, ICAM-2, vascular cell adhesion molecule (VCAM)-1, and PECAM-1. Intercellular adhesion molecule-1 is expressed at low levels in the endothelium, but its expression is up-regulated several-fold by TNF-α or IL-1. Intercelluar adhesion molecule-1 is active when it exists as a dimer and is able to bind macrophage adhesion ligand-1 or lymphocyte function–associated antigen-1 on leukocytes to facilitate transendothelial migration.[82,83] Clustering of ICAM-1 stimulates endothelial cytoskeletal rearrangements to form cuplike structures on the endothelial surface and remodel adherens junction complexes to enhance leukocyte transendothelial migration.[82,84,85] Intercellular adhesion molecule-2, by contrast, is constitutively expressed at high levels by the endothelium, but its expression is down-regulated by inflammatory cytokines; however, ICAM-2 is believed to play a role in cytokine-stimulated migration of eosinophils and dendritic cells.[86,87] Vascular cell adhesion molecule-1 is also up-regulated by inflammatory cytokines, binds to very late antigen-4 on leukocytes, and activates Rac-1 to increase NADPH oxidase activity and ROS production.[82] PECAM-1 is expressed abundantly in adherens junctions and is involved in homophilic interaction between endothelial and leukocyte PECAM-1. This interaction stimulates targeted trafficking of segments of EC membrane to surround a leukocyte in preparation for transendothelial migration and typically occurs within 1 or 2 μm of an intact endothelial junction.[82] The determination as to whether a leukocyte migrates paracellularly or transcellularly, therefore, appears to be dependent upon the relative tightness of endothelial junctions.

Vascular Repair and Remodeling

The vessel wall undergoes little proliferation or remodeling under ambient conditions, with the exception of repair or remodeling associated with physiological processes such as wound healing or menses. When the endothelial monolayer sustains a biochemical or biomechanical injury resulting in EC death and denudation, loss of contact inhibition stimulates the normally quiescent adjacent ECs to proliferate. If the injury is limited, locally proliferating ECs will cover the injured site. However, if the area of injury is larger, circulating blood cells are recruited to aide proliferating resident ECs and reestablish vascular integrity.[88]

A subset of circulating blood cells that participate in vascular repair expresses cell surface proteins that were thought to be endothelial-specific and subsequently referred to as endothelial progenitor cells (EPCs). These cells could be expanded in vitro to phenotypically resemble mature ECs, and when given in vivo could promote vascular repair and regeneration at sites of ischemia. It is now recognized that these putative EPCs are likely not true progenitor cells for the endothelium, but represent a mixed population of cells that include proangiogenic hematopoietic cells (myeloid or monocyte lineage), circulating ECs that that are viable but nonproliferative, and endothelial colony-forming cells that are viable, proliferative, and emerge at day 14 when cultured in vitro.[88-90] These cells reside in the bone marrow as well as in specific niches in postnatal organs and vessel wall. Within blood vessels, it is believed that they are located in niches in the subendothelial matrix or in the vasculogenic zone in the adventitia.[91]

Putative EPCs were initially thought to promote vascular repair by incorporating into and contributing structurally to the vessel wall, but more recent evidence supports a paracrine role. Once these cells are recruited to sites of injury, they secrete growth and angiogenic factors that promote and support endothelial proliferation. In fact, these cells are known to secrete high levels of vascular endothelial growth factor (VEGF), hepatocyte growth factor

(HGF), granulocyte colony-stimulating factor, and granulocyte-macrophage colony-stimulating factor.[88,89] These cells also provide transient residence as immediate placeholders at the site of endothelial injury and may reside there until proliferation of the endothelial monolayer is complete.[89]

Mechanotransduction of Hemodynamic Forces

The endothelium is subjected to the effects of hemodynamic forces such as hydrostatic pressure, cyclic stretch, and fluid shear stress, which occur as a consequence of blood pressure and pulsatile blood flow in the vasculature (Fig. 2-3). In the vascular tree, there is a gradient of pulsatile pressure that is proportional to vessel diameter, ranges from around 120 to 100 mmHg in the aorta to about 0 to 30 mmHg in the microcirculation, and modulates other hemodynamic forces.[92] Endothelial cells mechanotransduce these forces into cellular responses via ion channels, integrins, and GPCRs, as well as cytoskeletal deformations or displacements.[92,93]

The endothelial monolayer is exposed to variable levels of shear stress in the vascular tree that are inversely proportional to the radius of the vessel and range from 1 to $6 \, \text{dyn/cm}^2$ in veins and from 10 to $70 \, \text{dyn/cm}^2$ in arteries.[93] Physiological shear stress promotes a quiescent endothelial phenotype with cells that are aligned morphologically in the direction of flow, owing to the influence of laminar flow and shear on NO release. Increases in shear stress stimulate compensatory EC and SMC hypertrophy to expand the vessel and thereby return shear forces to basal levels. Conversely, a decrease in shear can narrow the lumen of the vessel in an endothelium-dependent manner.[93] Flow in tortuous vessels or at bifurcations is characterized by flow reversals, low flow velocities, and flow separation that cause shear stress gradients. Here, ECs acquire a polygonal shape with diminished cell and cytoskeletal alignment with flow.[5–7] This disturbed flow profile contributes to development of endothelial dysfunction at these susceptible locations.[6,7,93]

Cyclic strain is circumferential deformation of the blood vessel wall associated with distension and relaxation with each cardiac cycle.[92] Under ambient conditions, cyclic strain averages roughly 2% at 1 Hz in the aorta, but may increase to over 30% when hypertension is present.[94,95] In the endothelial monolayer, individual cells are typically arranged so they are oriented perpendicular to the stretch axis. However, when strain levels are increased to pathophysiological levels, this orientation is lost, and stress fibers parallel the direction of stretch.[96,97] Elevated levels of cyclic strain increase endothelial matrix metalloproteinases (MMPs) and induce remodeling of the extracellular matrix (ECM) as well as VE-cadherin and adherens junctions.[98]

In addition to physical forces imposed upon them, ECs are capable of generating traction stress and exerting force against the extracellular environment. These traction forces are mediated by stress fibers, actin-myosin interactions, and other proteins that anchor cells to focal adhesions. These self-generated forces are important for cell shape stability, regulate endothelial permeability and connectivity by applying force to cell junctions, and promote endothelial network formation by creating tension-based guidance pathways by which ECs sense each other at a distance.[92,99–102]

Endothelial Heterogeneity

Within the vascular tree, there is significant regional heterogeneity of the endothelium that occurs as a result of differences in developmental assignment, cellular structure, and surrounding environmental factors.[5,6,103] This heterogeneity exists to support the specialized functions of the underlying vascular beds and tissues. As a result of these differences, the normal adult endothelium also exhibits functional heterogeneity in the homeostatic properties common to all ECs (Fig. 2-4). For instance, the endothelium functions as a semipermeable membrane that regulates transport of fluid, proteins, and macromolecules. Under basal conditions, this takes place primarily across capillaries, albeit at differing rates throughout the vascular beds. However, when stimulated with histamine, serotonin, bradykinin, or VEGF, the endothelium in postcapillary venules responds by increasing permeability either through retraction of adherens junctions and formation of interendothelial gaps, or via increased transendothelial transcytosis. This phenomenon is supported by increased expression of receptors for these agonists in the postcapillary venules.[5–7,104,105]

Transendothelial migration of leukocytes occurs as postcapillary venules in the skin, mesentery, and muscle, whereas in the lung and liver, this function takes place mostly at the level of the capillaries. In lymph nodes, this function occurs at the high endothelial venules.[106] Activated ECs that are largely restricted to

Atheroprotective

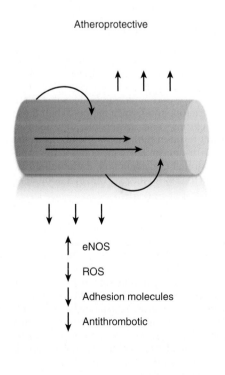

↑ eNOS

↓ ROS

↓ Adhesion molecules

↓ Antithrombotic

Atheroprone

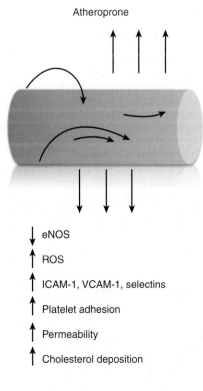

↓ eNOS

↑ ROS

↑ ICAM-1, VCAM-1, selectins

↑ Platelet adhesion

↑ Permeability

↑ Cholesterol deposition

FIGURE 2-3 Effects of hemodynamic forces on endothelial functions. Endothelium is subjected to the effects of hemodynamic forces such as shear stress, cyclic strain, and pulsatile pressure. Under ambient conditions, these forces are generally atheroprotective and increase expression of nitric oxide synthase (eNOS) to generate nitric oxide (NO), decrease reactive oxygen species (ROS) and oxidant stress, decrease expression of proinflammatory adhesion molecules, and maintain an antithrombotic surface. When these forces are increased or perturbed, loss of laminar shear stress, increased cyclic strain, or increased pulse pressure leads to a decrease in eNOS expression, an increase in ROS levels, and up-regulation of proinflammatory and prothrombotic mediators that can lead to cholesterol oxidation and deposition to initiate atherosclerosis. ICAM-1, intercellular adhesion molecule-1; VCAM-1, vascular cell adhesion molecule-1.

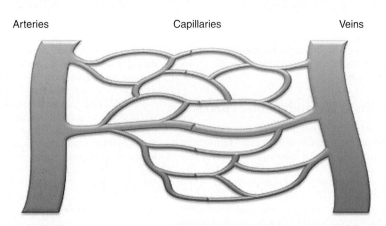

	Arteries	Capillaries	Veins
Hemostasis	TM t-PA EPCR	TM TFPI	TM EPCR vWF
Inflammation	ICAM-1 VCAM-1	ICAM-1 VCAM-1	E-selectin P-selectin ICAM-1 VCAM-1
Permeability	+	+	++
Vascular tone	++	−	−

FIGURE 2-4 Functional heterogeneity of the endothelium. The endothelium is adapted both structurally and functionally to serve the needs of underlying vascular bed. Between the arterial, capillary, and venous systems, there are regional differences in expression of anticoagulant and antithrombotic factors and inflammatory adhesion molecules. Permeability tends to be increased preferentially at postcapillary venules, whereas vascular tone is regulated by arterioles. EPCR, endothelial protein C receptor; ICAM-1, intercellular adhesion molecule-1; TFPI, tissue factor plasminogen inactivator; TM, thrombomodulin; tPA, tissue plasminogen activator; VCAM-1, vascular cell adhesion molecule-1; vWF, von Willebrand factor.

postcapillary venules and express E-selectin mediate this function.[107] P-selectin, which is stored in Weibel-Palade bodies, is also preferentially expressed by endothelium in postcapillary venules, with levels of highest expression in the lung and mesentery.[108] By contrast, ICAM-1 and VCAM-1 may be expressed throughout the vasculature and respond rapidly to induction by lipopolysaccharide or cytokines. Although interactions between leukocytes and the endothelium occur typically in postcapillary venules, they can also occur in arterioles, capillaries, and large veins.[5-7]

The endothelium regulates hemostatic functions largely through expression of both anticoagulant and antiplatelet factors that are unevenly distributed throughout the vasculature. For instance, endothelium in the arterial system expresses thrombomodulin, tPA, and the endothelial protein C receptor; capillaries express thrombomodulin and TFPI; and thrombomodulin, the endothelial protein C receptor, and vWF are typically expressed in veins.[5-7,109] Endothelium also regulates vascular tone and does so at the level of the resistance arterioles through release of site-specific vasodilator and vasoconstrictor molecules. The endothelium is the predominant source of NO generated by eNOS, and expression of eNOS is greater in the arterial than the venous system.[7] Thus, many of these functional heterogeneities allow the endothelium to respond to (patho)physiological stimuli and adapt to a changing environment.

Endothelial Dysfunction and Vascular Disease

Although the endothelium that resides at different locations within the vascular tree may be uniquely adapted to suit the local environment, there are circumstances where a prolonged or aberrant stimulus may lead to phenotype transition, endothelial dysfunction, and progress to frank vascular disease. When challenged with these (patho)physiological stimuli, the endothelium undergoes phenotype transition to an activated state. Activated ECs modulate their basal homeostatic functions to adapt to the aberrant stimuli and may display a broad spectrum of responses.

The endothelial monolayer can demonstrate increased permeability to plasma proteins and transendothelial migration of leukocytes, increased adhesion of inflammatory cells, and fluctuating imbalances in pro- and antithrombotic substances, vasodilators and vasoconstrictors, and growth factors. When these phenotypic changes are chronic and irreversible, they lead to maladaptive responses that result in permanent alterations in the structure and function of the endothelial monolayer; this phenomenon is known as endothelial dysfunction. Endothelial dysfunction is now understood to play an integral role in a number of vascular disease processes.

Thrombosis

Thrombus formation at sites of vascular injury is a physiological process localized to the endothelial surface. In contrast, intravascular thrombosis is a pathophysiological event that occurs at sites of vascular injury, and the response is augmented by concomitant endothelial dysfunction. These events may be associated with a chronic vascular injury process such as atherosclerosis and plaque erosion, or with a more acute injury pattern that occurs with infection/autoimmune reactions, vascular compromise resulting from atherosclerotic encroachment on the vessel lumen, or percutaneous coronary intervention (PCI)–associated mechanical trauma to the endothelial monolayer.

In conjunction with exposure to these pathophysiological stimuli, the activated endothelium is faced with loss of its anticoagulant cell surface–associated molecules, lower levels of antithrombotic NO, and expression of the prothrombotic factors tissue factor and vWF, as well as platelets that are recruited to the site of injury.[40,42,110-113] Thrombosis is augmented further by increases in endothelial ROS and oxidant stress, inhibition of tPA activity by plasminogen activator inhibitor-1 (PAI-1) generated by activated ECs, and alterations in shear and other mechanical forces as blood fluidity is diminished.[8,81,93]

Vasculitis

The primary systemic vasculitides differentially affect vessels based on size and, as such, are grouped accordingly. Takayasu's arteritis is a large-vessel type that affects the aorta and its major branches, whereas granulomatosis with polyangiitis (formerly known as Wegener's granulomatosis) affects mostly small vessels and occurs as a vasculitis that primarily affects the kidneys and lungs.[114,115] Although these vasculitides represent heterogeneous disease processes, they share the endothelium as the common target and propagator of an immuno-inflammatory reaction that occurs in the vessel wall. This immuno-inflammatory reaction may be so profound, as is seen in systemic lupus erythematosus (SLE), that antiendothelial antibodies are generated. These processes result in vascular immune-complex deposition, complement activation, and neutrophil-induced injury to the endothelial monolayer that results in EC activation, apoptosis, and in some areas, denudation.[116,117] Other resident activated ECs synthesize and secrete cytokines, growth factors, and chemokines that include IL-1, IL-6, IL-8, and MCP-1.[110] Repeated injury to the endothelium from prolonged attack by immune and inflammatory cells can stimulate a prothrombotic and profibrotic response that ultimately leads to vessel occlusion and abnormal vascular remodeling.

Atherosclerosis

Atherosclerosis is a progressive disease of blood vessels that is initiated by endothelial dysfunction and is now recognized as a chronic inflammatory and immune process. Atherosclerosis is characterized by the accumulation of lipid, thrombus, and inflammatory cells within the vessel wall.[48,118-120] This process may acutely occlude the vessel lumen, as occurs with plaque rupture and thrombosis, or result in a more chronic but stable process that eventually encroaches on the vessel lumen. In either event, atherosclerosis can lead to end-organ ischemia and ensuing infarction of the heart, brain, vital organs, or extremities. Early endothelial dysfunction associated with atherosclerosis is evidenced by the presence of a subendothelial accumulation of lipids and infiltration of monocyte-derived macrophages and other immune cells to form the fatty streak. Among the risk factors associated with development of atherosclerosis, diabetes mellitus, tobacco use, hyperlipidemia, and hypertension are all known to induce endothelial dysfunction.[121] Within the vasculature, however, the branch points and bifurcations tend to be the most atherosclerosis-prone segments, indicating that hemodynamic profiles and complex non-uniform flow is also of importance for endothelial dysfunction.[93,122] Once atherosclerosis is established, the endothelium continues to modify the progression of disease by recruiting inflammatory and immune cells and platelets; diminished NO production, enhanced permeability, and the production of prothrombotic species are believed to contribute to plaque progression.[48,118-120,123]

Functional Assessment of the Endothelium

Nitric Oxide—Mediated Vasodilation

Owing to the importance of endothelial function for vascular health, assessments of endothelial-dependent vasodilator responses, which reflect endothelial NO generation and NO bioavailability, have been advanced as predictors of adverse cardiovascular events. These studies are based on the principle that a healthy endothelium, when challenged with a physiological stress such as shear stress or an endothelium-dependent vasodilator such as acetylcholine, will release NO, leading to a measurable vasodilatory response. In contrast, when the endothelium is dysfunctional or diseased, these stimuli will elicit a vasoconstrictor or significantly diminished vasodilator response. In humans, this phenomenon, which recapitulates the preclinical studies of Furchgott and Zawadski, was first demonstrated following the intracoronary administration of acetylcholine to patients with angiographically diseased or normal epicardial coronary arteries. Here, the patients with prevalent atherosclerosis demonstrated paradoxical vasoconstriction when infused with acetylcholine, but normal vasodilator responses when challenged with the NO donor nitroglycerin. Patients with normal vessels dilated appropriately to both agents.[124]

Subsequently, a close correlation between coronary artery vasodilation in response to acetylcholine and noninvasive measurements of flow-mediated dilation of the brachial artery was demonstrated. Imaging of the brachial artery with high-resolution vascular ultrasound to detect flow-mediated dilation or the use of strain-gauge forearm plethysmography to assess forearm blood flow in response to pharmacological stimuli that release NO are both accepted methodologies for evaluating endothelial function.[125-127] To date, these methods have been used to demonstrate impaired endothelium-dependent vascular reactivity in adults with risk factors for atherosclerosis in the absence of overt atherothrombotic cardiovascular disease; in children with diabetes mellitus, hypercholesterolemia, and congenital heart disease; and to demonstrate improved function in patients treated with 3-hydroxy-3-methylglutaryl-coenzyme A reductase inhibitors (statins) or ACE inhibitors.[128-133]

Measurement of peripheral arterial tonometry is emerging as a newer methodology to examine endothelial function. This device utilizes finger-mounted probes with an inflatable membrane that record a pulse wave in the presence and absence of flow-mediated dilation. This method has been shown to correlate well with endothelial dysfunction assessed by brachial artery flow-mediated dilation.[134]

ADMA as a Biochemical Marker of Nitric Oxide Bioavailability

The endogenous competitive NOS inhibitor asymmetrical dimethylarginine (ADMA) has been suggested as a biomarker for decreased NO bioavailability and endothelial function. Asymmetrical dimethylarginine generated by the hydrolysis of methylated arginine residues is subject to intracellular degradation by dimethylarginine dimethylaminohydrolase (DDAH), but the activity of this enzyme is decreased significantly by oxidant stress.[135-138] This in turn leads to increases in plasma ADMA levels, a finding that has been demonstrated in patients with risk factors for atherosclerosis or established coronary artery disease (CAD).[139-142]

With respect to endothelial function, a cross-sectional study of individuals enrolled in the Cardiovascular Risk in Young Finns Study confirmed a significant, albeit modest, inverse relationship between ADMA levels and endothelial function assessed by flow-mediated vasodilation.[143] Despite these findings, in a community-based sample, ADMA levels were not associated with cardiovascular disease incidence or all-cause mortality in diabetic patients.[144] Based on these observations, in certain populations, ADMA levels alone may not provide a full assessment of endothelial function; direct measurements of endothelial vasodilator capacity may be required.

Endothelial Microparticles

Endothelial microparticles are emerging as a surrogate biomarker for endothelial dysfunction.[145] Endothelial cells can release membrane vesicles with a diameter of approximately 0.1 to 1.0 μm that include microparticles, exosomes, and apoptotic bodies.

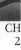

These microparticles are formed from plasma membrane blebbing and package endothelial proteins that include VE-cadherin, PECAM-1, ICAM-1, E-selectin, endoglin, VEGF receptor-2, S-endo, α_v integrin, and eNOS.[145,146] Although many of these proteins are expressed by microparticles derived from other cell types, the presence of VE-cadherin and E-selectin indicates EC origin. Endothelial microparticle formation is stimulated by TNF-α, ROS, inflammatory cytokines, lipopolysaccharides, thrombin, and low shear stress.[146] They have procoagulant properties as a result of exposed phosphatidylserines and tissue factor that is present in the microparticle, as well as proinflammatory properties.

Techniques to measure circulating endothelial microparticles rely on differential centrifugation in platelet-free plasma and on the identification of cell-surface CD antigens.[145,146] Thus, they may not be as convenient a measure of endothelial function as currently available noninvasive imaging techniques. Nonetheless, circulating endothelial microparticles have been measured and found to be elevated in a number of patient populations with risk factors or diseases associated with endothelial dysfunction.[146] Increased levels of endothelial microparticles have been demonstrated and shown to correlate with flow-mediated dilation in individuals with end-stage renal disease, acute coronary syndromes (ACS), metabolic syndrome, diabetes, and systemic and pulmonary hypertension.[147-152]

Conclusions

The endothelium is a structurally and metabolically dynamic interface that resides between circulating blood elements, the vascular wall, and the underlying tissues served by these blood vessels. Owing to its unique anatomical location, the endothelium regulates thrombosis and hemostasis, immuno-inflammatory responses, vascular permeability, and vascular tone. These homeostatic functions are responsive to alterations in the local and systemic environments. Failure to adapt to (patho)physiological stimuli may activate aberrant compensatory mechanisms that alter the endothelial phenotype and promote endothelial dysfunction. As techniques to assess endothelial function advance, the clinical utility of this measure, coupled with biochemical and molecular assessments to define an endothelial phenotype profile, will provide a unique understanding of an individual's vascular endothelial function and guide both prognosis and therapeutic interventions.

REFERENCES

1. Schwann T: *Microscopical researches into the accordance in the structure and growth of animals and plants*, London, 1847, Syndenham Society.
2. Hwa C, Aird WC: The history of the capillary wall: doctors, discoveries, and debates, *Am J Physiol Heart Circ Physiol* 293:H2667–H2679, 2007.
3. His W: *Die häute und höhlen des körpers*, Basel, 1865, Schwighauser.
4. Gimbrone M: *Vascular endothelium: Nature's blood container. Vascular endothelium in hemostasis and thrombosis*, New York, 1986, Churchill Livingstone, pp 1–13.
5. Aird WC: Phenotypic heterogeneity of the endothelium: I. Structure, function, and mechanisms, *Circ Res* 100:158–173, 2007.
6. Aird WC: Phenotypic heterogeneity of the endothelium: II. Representative vascular beds, *Circ Res* 100:174–190, 2007.
7. dela Paz NG, D'Amore PA: Arterial versus venous endothelial cells, *Cell Tissue Res* 335:5–16, 2009.
8. van Hinsbergh VW: Endothelium-role in regulation of coagulation and inflammation, *Semin Immunopathol* 2011.
9. Navarro S, Bonet E, Estelles A, et al: The endothelial cell protein C receptor: Its role in thrombosis, *Thromb Res* 128:410–416, 2011.
10. Rezaie AR: Regulation of the protein C anticoagulant and antiinflammatory pathways, *Curr Med Chem* 17:2059–2069, 2010.
11. Conway EM: Thrombomodulin and its role in inflammation, *Semin Immunopathol* 2011.
12. Kasthuri RS, Glover SL, Boles J, et al: Tissue factor and tissue factor pathway inhibitor as key regulators of global hemostasis: Measurement of their levels in coagulation assays, *Semin Thromb Hemost* 36:764–771, 2010.
13. Zhang J, Piro O, Lu L, et al: Glycosyl phosphatidylinositol anchorage of tissue factor pathway inhibitor, *Circulation* 108:623–627, 2003.
14. Atkinson B, Dwyer K, Enjyoji K, et al: Ecto-nucleotidases of the cd39/ntpdase family modulate platelet activation and thrombus formation: potential as therapeutic targets, *Blood Cells Mol Dis* 36:217–222, 2006.
15. Welch G, Loscalzo J: Nitric oxide and the cardiovascular system, *J Card Surg* 9:361–371, 1994.
16. Bazan JF: Structural design and molecular evolution of a cytokine receptor superfamily, *Proc Natl Acad Sci U S A* 87:6934–6938, 1990.
17. Jasuja R, Furie B, Furie BC: Endothelium-derived but not platelet-derived protein disulfide isomerase is required for thrombus formation *in vivo*, *Blood* 116:4665–4674, 2010.
18. Breitenstein A, Tanner FC, Luscher TF: Tissue factor and cardiovascular disease: quo vadis? *Circ J* 74:3–12, 2010.
19. Bach RR: Tissue factor encryption, *Arterioscler Thromb Vasc Biol* 26:456–461, 2006.
20. Valentijn KM, Sadler JE, Valentijn JA, et al: Functional architecture of Weibel-Palade bodies, *Blood* 117:5033–5043, 2011.
21. Lowenberg EC, Meijers JC, Levi M: Platelet-vessel wall interaction in health and disease, *Neth J Med* 68:242–251, 2010.
22. Komarova Y, Malik AB: Regulation of endothelial permeability via paracellular and transcellular transport pathways, *Annu Rev Physiol* 72:463–493, 2010.
23. Pappenheimer JR, Renkin EM, Borrero LM: Filtration, diffusion and molecular sieving through peripheral capillary membranes; a contribution to the pore theory of capillary permeability, *Am J Physiol* 167:13–46, 1951.
24. Fischbarg J: Fluid transport across leaky epithelia: central role of the tight junction and supporting role of aquaporins, *Physiol Rev* 90:1271–1290, 2010.
25. Dejana E, Orsenigo F, Molendini C, et al: Organization and signaling of endothelial cell-to-cell junctions in various regions of the blood and lymphatic vascular trees, *Cell Tissue Res* 335:17–25, 2009.
26. Dejana E, Tournier-Lasserve E, Weinstein BM: The control of vascular integrity by endothelial cell junctions: molecular basis and pathological implications, *Dev Cell* 16:209–221, 2009.
27. Tiruppathi C, Finnegan A, Malik AB: Isolation and characterization of a cell surface albumin-binding protein from vascular endothelial cells, *Proc Natl Acad Sci U S A* 93:250–254, 1996.
28. Tiruppathi C, Song W, Bergenfeldt M, et al: Gp60 activation mediates albumin transcytosis in endothelial cells by tyrosine kinase-dependent pathway, *J Biol Chem* 272:25968–25975, 1997.
29. Predescu D, Palade GE: Plasmalemmal vesicles represent the large pore system of continuous microvascular endothelium, *Am J Physiol* 265:H725–H733, 1993.
30. Predescu SA, Predescu DN, Palade GE: Endothelial transcytotic machinery involves supramolecular protein-lipid complexes, *Mol Biol Cell* 12:1019–1033, 2001.
31. Hu C, Ahmed M, Melia TJ, et al: Fusion of cells by flipped SNAREs, *Science* 300:1745–1749, 2003.
32. Mehta D, Malik AB: Signaling mechanisms regulating endothelial permeability, *Physiol Rev* 86:279–367, 2006.
33. Weber C, Fraemohs L, Dejana E: The role of junctional adhesion molecules in vascular inflammation, *Nat Rev Immunol* 7:467–477, 2007.
34. Spindler V, Schlegel N, Waschke J: Role of GTPases in control of microvascular permeability, *Cardiovasc Res* 87:243–253, 2010.
35. Mochizuki N: Vascular integrity mediated by vascular endothelial cadherin and regulated by sphingosine 1-phosphate and angiopoietin-1, *Circ J* 73:2183–2191, 2009.
36. Curry FR, Adamson RH: Vascular permeability modulation at the cell, microvessel, or whole organ level: towards closing gaps in our knowledge, *Cardiovasc Res* 87:218–229, 2010.
37. Taddei A, Giampietro C, Conti A, et al: Endothelial adherens junctions control tight junctions by VE-cadherin-mediated upregulation of claudin-5, *Nat Cell Biol* 10:923–934, 2008.
38. Furchgott RF, Zawadzki JV: The obligatory role of endothelial cells in the relaxation of arterial smooth muscle by acetylcholine, *Nature* 288:373–376, 1980.
39. Triggle CR, Ding H: The endothelium in compliance and resistance vessels, *Front Biosci (Schol Ed)* 3:730–744, 2011.
40. Michel T, Vanhoutte PM: Cellular signaling and no production, *Pflugers Arch* 459:807–816, 2010.
41. Searles CD, Miwa Y, Harrison DG, et al: Posttranscriptional regulation of endothelial nitric oxide synthase during cell growth, *Circ Res* 85:588–595, 1999.
42. Walford G, Loscalzo J: Nitric oxide in vascular biology, *J Thromb Haemost* 1:2112–2118, 2003.
43. Bredt DS, Hwang PM, Glatt CE, et al: Cloned and expressed nitric oxide synthase structurally resembles cytochrome p-450 reductase, *Nature* 351:714–718, 1991.
44. Bredt DS, Hwang PM, Snyder SH: Localization of nitric oxide synthase indicating a neural role for nitric oxide, *Nature* 347:768–770, 1990.
45. Dudzinski DM, Michel T: Life history of eNOS: Partners and pathways, *Cardiovasc Res* 75:247–260, 2007.
46. Handy DE, Loscalzo J: Nitric oxide and posttranslational modification of the vascular proteome: S-nitrosylation of reactive thiols, *Arterioscler Thromb Vasc Biol* 26:1207–1214, 2006.
47. Upchurch GR, Welch GN, Loscalzo J: The vascular biology of S-nitrosothiols, nitrosated derivatives of thiols, *Vasc Med* 1:25–33, 1996.
48. Leopold JA, Loscalzo J: Oxidative risk for atherothrombotic cardiovascular disease, *Free Radic Biol Med* 47:1673–1706, 2009.
49. Stamler JS, Singel DJ, Loscalzo J: Biochemistry of nitric oxide and its redox-activated forms, *Science* 258:1898–1902, 1992.
50. Bhatia M: Hydrogen sulfide as a vasodilator, *IUBMB Life* 57:603–606, 2005.
51. Wang R: Hydrogen sulfide: A new EDRF, *Kidney Int* 76:700–704, 2009.
52. Li L, Rose P, Moore PK: Hydrogen sulfide and cell signaling, *Annu Rev Pharmacol Toxicol* 51:169–187, 2011.
53. Parkington HC, Coleman HA, Tare M: Prostacyclin and endothelium-dependent hyperpolarization, *Pharmacol Res* 49:509–514, 2004.
54. Feletou M, Huang Y, Vanhoutte PM: Endothelium-mediated control of vascular tone: COX-1 and COX-2 products, *Br J Pharmacol* 164:894–912, 2011.
55. Matoba T, Shimokawa H, Nakashima M, et al: Hydrogen peroxide is an endothelium-derived hyperpolarizing factor in mice, *J Clin Invest* 106:1521–1530, 2000.
56. Edwards G, Dora KA, Gardener MJ, et al: K+ is an endothelium-derived hyperpolarizing factor in rat arteries, *Nature* 396:269–272, 1998.
57. Campbell WB, Fleming I: Epoxyeicosatrienoic acids and endothelium-dependent responses, *Pflugers Arch* 459:881–895, 2010.
58. Shimokawa H: Hydrogen peroxide as an endothelium-derived hyperpolarizing factor, *Pflugers Arch* 459:915–922, 2010.
59. Kohan DE, Rossi NF, Inscho EW, et al: Regulation of blood pressure and salt homeostasis by endothelin, *Physiol Rev* 91:1–77, 2011.
60. Yanagisawa M, Kurihara H, Kimura S, et al: A novel potent vasoconstrictor peptide produced by vascular endothelial cells, *Nature* 332:411–415, 1988.

61. Watts SW: Endothelin receptors: what's new and what do we need to know? *Am J Physiol Regul Integr Comp Physiol* 298:R254–R260, 2010.
62. Rondaij MG, Bierings R, Kragt A, et al: Dynamics and plasticity of Weibel-Palade bodies in endothelial cells, *Arterioscler Thromb Vasc Biol* 26:1002–1007, 2006.
63. Danser AH, Saris JJ, Schuijt MP, et al: Is there a local renin-angiotensin system in the heart? *Cardiovasc Res* 44:252–265, 1999.
64. Griendling KK, Minieri CA, Ollerenshaw JD, et al: Angiotensin II stimulates NADH and NADPH oxidase activity in cultured vascular smooth muscle cells, *Circ Res* 74:1141–1148, 1994.
65. Zafari AM, Ushio-Fukai M, Akers M, et al: Role of NADH/NADPH oxidase-derived h2o2 in angiotensin II-induced vascular hypertrophy, *Hypertension* 32:488–495, 1998.
66. Garrido AM, Griendling KK: NADPH oxidases and angiotensin II receptor signaling, *Mol Cell Endocrinol* 302:148–158, 2009.
67. Tobias PS: TLRS in disease, *Semin Immunopathol* 30:1–2, 2008.
68. Tobias PS, Curtiss LK: Toll-like receptors in atherosclerosis, *Biochem Soc Trans* 35: 1453–1455, 2007.
69. Zimmer S, Steinmetz M, Asdonk T, et al: Activation of endothelial Toll-like receptor 3 impairs endothelial function, *Circ Res* 108:1358–1366, 2011.
70. Feinberg MW, Jain MK: Role of transforming growth factor-beta1/smads in regulating vascular inflammation and atherogenesis, *Panminerva Med* 47:169–186, 2005.
71. Kofler S, Nickel T, Weis M: Role of cytokines in cardiovascular diseases: a focus on endothelial responses to inflammation, *Clin Sci (Lond)* 108:205–213, 2005.
72. Haas MJ, Mooradian AD: Inflammation, high-density lipoprotein and cardiovascular dysfunction, *Curr Opin Infect Dis* 24:265–272, 2011.
73. de Vries JE: The role of IL-13 and its receptor in allergy and inflammatory responses, *J Allergy Clin Immunol* 102:165–169, 1998.
74. Speyer CL, Ward PA: Role of endothelial chemokines and their receptors during inflammation, *J Invest Surg* 24:18–27, 2011.
75. Lortat-Jacob H: The molecular basis and functional implications of chemokine interactions with heparan sulphate, *Curr Opin Struct Biol* 19:543–548, 2009.
76. Celie JW, Beelen RH, van den Born J: Heparan sulfate proteoglycans in extravasation: assisting leukocyte guidance, *Front Biosci* 14:4932–4949, 2009.
77. Peiper SC, Wang ZX, Neote K, et al: The Duffy antigen/receptor for chemokines (DARC) is expressed in endothelial cells of Duffy-negative individuals who lack the erythrocyte receptor, *J Exp Med* 181:1311–1317, 1995.
78. Schnabel RB, Baumert J, Barbalic M, et al: Duffy antigen receptor for chemokines (DARC) polymorphism regulates circulating concentrations of monocyte chemoattractant protein-1 and other inflammatory mediators, *Blood* 115:5289–5299, 2010.
79. Horne K, Woolley IJ: Shedding light on DARC: the role of the Duffy antigen/receptor for chemokines in inflammation, infection and malignancy, *Inflamm Res* 58:431–435, 2009.
80. Huo Y, Xia L: P-selectin glycoprotein ligand-1 plays a crucial role in the selective recruitment of leukocytes into the atherosclerotic arterial wall, *Trends Cardiovasc Med* 19:140–145, 2009.
81. Langer HF, Chavakis T: Leukocyte-endothelial interactions in inflammation, *J Cell Mol Med* 13:1211–1220, 2009.
82. Muller WA: Mechanisms of leukocyte transendothelial migration, *Annu Rev Pathol* 6: 323–344, 2010.
83. Miller J, Knorr R, Ferrone M, et al: Intercellular adhesion molecule-1 dimerization and its consequences for adhesion mediated by lymphocyte function associated-1, *J Exp Med* 182:1231–1241, 1995.
84. Shaw SK, Ma S, Kim MB, et al: Coordinated redistribution of leukocyte LFA-1 and endothelial cell ICAM-1 accompany neutrophil transmigration, *J Exp Med* 200:1571–1580, 2004.
85. Yang L, Froio RM, Sciuto TE, et al: ICAM-1 regulates neutrophil adhesion and transcellular migration of TNF-alpha-activated vascular endothelium under flow, *Blood* 106:584–592, 2005.
86. Woodfin A, Voisin MB, Imhof BA, et al: Endothelial cell activation leads to neutrophil transmigration as supported by the sequential roles of ICAM-2, JAM-A, and PECAM-1, *Blood* 113:6246–6257, 2009.
87. Huang MT, Larbi KY, Scheiermann C, et al: ICAM-2 mediates neutrophil transmigration *in vivo*: evidence for stimulus specificity and a role in PECAM-1-independent transmigration, *Blood* 107:4721–4727, 2006.
88. Becher MU, Nickenig G, Werner N: Regeneration of the vascular compartment, *Herz* 35:342–351, 2010.
89. Richardson MR, Yoder MC: Endothelial progenitor cells: quo vadis? *J Mol Cell Cardiol* 50:266–272, 2011.
90. Torsney E, Xu Q: Resident vascular progenitor cells, *J Mol Cell Cardiol* 50:304–311, 2011.
91. Watt SM, Athanassopoulos A, Harris AL, et al: Human endothelial stem/progenitor cells, angiogenic factors and vascular repair, *J R Soc Interface* 7(Suppl 6):S731–S751, 2010.
92. Califano JP, Reinhart-King CA: Exogenous and endogenous force regulation of endothelial cell behavior, *J Biomech* 43:79–86, 2010.
93. Chiu JJ, Chien S: Effects of disturbed flow on vascular endothelium: pathophysiological basis and clinical perspectives, *Physiol Rev* 91:327–387, 2011.
94. Lee T, Sumpio BE: Cell signalling in vascular cells exposed to cyclic strain: the emerging role of protein phosphatases, *Biotechnol Appl Biochem* 39:129–139, 2004.
95. Wedding KL, Draney MT, Herfkens RJ, et al: Measurement of vessel wall strain using cine phase contrast MRI, *J Magn Reson Imaging* 15:418–428, 2002.
96. Iba T, Sumpio BE: Morphological response of human endothelial cells subjected to cyclic strain *in vitro*, *Microvasc Res* 42:245–254, 1991.
97. Kaunas R, Nguyen P, Usami S, et al: Cooperative effects of Rho and mechanical stretch on stress fiber organization, *Proc Natl Acad Sci U S A* 102:15895–15900, 2005.
98. Cummins PM, von Offenberg Sweeney N, Killeen MT, et al: Cyclic strain-mediated matrix metalloproteinase regulation within the vascular endothelium: a force to be reckoned with, *Am J Physiol Heart Circ Physiol* 292:H28–H42, 2007.
99. Lu L, Feng Y, Hucker WJ, et al: Actin stress fiber pre-extension in human aortic endothelial cells, *Cell Motil Cytoskeleton* 65:281–294, 2008.
100. Lu L, Oswald SJ, Ngu H, et al: Mechanical properties of actin stress fibers in living cells, *Biophys J* 95:6060–6071, 2008.
101. Costa KD, Sim AJ, Yin FC: Non-hertzian approach to analyzing mechanical properties of endothelial cells probed by atomic force microscopy, *J Biomech Eng* 128:176–184, 2006.
102. Kniazeva E, Putnam AJ: Endothelial cell traction and ECM density influence both capillary morphogenesis and maintenance in 3-D, *Am J Physiol Cell Physiol* 297:C179–C187, 2009.
103. Atkins GB, Jain MK, Hamik A: Endothelial differentiation: molecular mechanisms of specification and heterogeneity, *Arterioscler Thromb Vasc Biol* 31:1476–1484, 2011.
104. McDonald DM, Thurston G, Baluk P: Endothelial gaps as sites for plasma leakage in inflammation, *Microcirculation* 6:7–22, 1999.
105. Feng D, Nagy JA, Hipp J, et al: Reinterpretation of endothelial cell gaps induced by vasoactive mediators in guinea-pig, mouse and rat: many are transcellular pores, *J Physiol* 504(Pt 3):747–761, 1997.
106. Miyasaka M, Tanaka T: Lymphocyte trafficking across high endothelial venules: dogmas and enigmas, *Nat Rev Immunol* 4:360–370, 2004.
107. Petzelbauer P, Bender JR, Wilson J, et al: Heterogeneity of dermal microvascular endothelial cell antigen expression and cytokine responsiveness *in situ* and in cell culture, *J Immunol* 151:5062–5072, 1993.
108. McEver RP, Beckstead JH, Moore KL, et al: Gmp-140, a platelet alpha-granule membrane protein, is also synthesized by vascular endothelial cells and is localized in Weibel-Palade bodies, *J Clin Invest* 84:92–99, 1989.
109. Laszik Z, Mitro A, Taylor FB Jr, et al: Human protein C receptor is present primarily on endothelium of large blood vessels: implications for the control of the protein C pathway, *Circulation* 96:3633–3640, 1997.
110. Levi M: The coagulant response in sepsis and inflammation, *Hamostaseologie* 30: 10–12,14–16, 2010.
111. Granger DN, Rodrigues SF, Yildirim A, et al: Microvascular responses to cardiovascular risk factors, *Microcirculation* 17:192–205, 2010.
112. Antoniades C, Bakogiannis C, Tousoulis D, et al: Platelet activation in atherogenesis associated with low-grade inflammation, *Inflamm Allergy Drug Targets* 9:334–345, 2010.
113. Freedman JE, Loscalzo J, Barnard MR, et al: Nitric oxide released from activated platelets inhibits platelet recruitment, *J Clin Invest* 100:350–356, 1997.
114. Arnaud L, Haroche J, Mathian A, et al: Pathogenesis of Takayasu's arteritis: a 2011 update, *Autoimmun Rev* 11:61–67, 2011.
115. Jennette JC: Nomenclature and classification of vasculitis: lessons learned from granulomatosis with polyangiitis (Wegener's granulomatosis), *Clin Exp Immunol* 164(Suppl 1):7–10, 2011.
116. Duval A, Helley D, Capron L, et al: Endothelial dysfunction in systemic lupus patients with low disease activity: evaluation by quantification and characterization of circulating endothelial microparticles, role of anti-endothelial cell antibodies, *Rheumatology (Oxford)* 49:1049–1055, 2010.
117. Savage CO: Vascular biology and vasculitis, *APMIS Suppl* 37–40, 2009
118. Libby P: Molecular and cellular mechanisms of the thrombotic complications of atherosclerosis, *J Lipid Res* 50(Suppl):S352–S357, 2009.
119. Libby P, Ridker PM, Hansson GK: Inflammation in atherosclerosis: from pathophysiology to practice, *J Am Coll Cardiol* 54:2129–2138, 2009.
120. Libby P, Ridker PM, Hansson GK: Progress and challenges in translating the biology of atherosclerosis, *Nature* 473:317–325, 2011.
121. Reriani MK, Lerman LO, Lerman A: Endothelial function as a functional expression of cardiovascular risk factors, *Biomark Med* 4:351–360, 2010.
122. Kwon GP, Schroeder JL, Amar MJ, et al: Contribution of macromolecular structure to the retention of low-density lipoprotein at arterial branch points, *Circulation* 117:2919–2927, 2008.
123. Borissoff JI, Spronk HM, ten Cate H: The hemostatic system as a modulator of atherosclerosis, *N Engl J Med* 364:1746–1760, 2011.
124. Ludmer PL, Selwyn AP, Shook TL, et al: Paradoxical vasoconstriction induced by acetylcholine in atherosclerotic coronary arteries, *N Engl J Med* 315:1046–1051, 1986.
125. Charakida M, Masi S, Luscher TF, et al: Assessment of atherosclerosis: the role of flow-mediated dilatation, *Eur Heart J* 31:2854–2861, 2010.
126. Corretti MC, Anderson TJ, Benjamin EJ, et al: Guidelines for the ultrasound assessment of endothelial-dependent flow-mediated vasodilation of the brachial artery: a report of the international brachial artery reactivity task force, *J Am Coll Cardiol* 39:257–265, 2002.
127. Joyner MJ, Dietz NM, Shepherd JT: From Belfast to Mayo and beyond: the use and future of plethysmography to study blood flow in human limbs, *J Appl Physiol* 91:2431–2441, 2001.
128. Jarvisalo MJ, Lehtimaki T, Raitakari OT: Determinants of arterial nitrate-mediated dilatation in children: role of oxidized low-density lipoprotein, endothelial function, and carotid intima-media thickness, *Circulation* 109:2885–2889, 2004.
129. Jarvisalo MJ, Raitakari M, Toikka JO, et al: Endothelial dysfunction and increased arterial intima-media thickness in children with type 1 diabetes, *Circulation* 109:1750–1755, 2004.
130. Pasquali SK, Marino BS, Powell DJ, et al: Following the arterial switch operation, obese children have risk factors for early cardiovascular disease, *Congenit Heart Dis* 5:16–24, 2010.
131. Wallace SM, Maki-Petaja KM, Cheriyan J, et al: Simvastatin prevents inflammation-induced aortic stiffening and endothelial dysfunction, *Br J Clin Pharmacol* 70:799–806, 2010.
132. Ostad MA, Eggeling S, Tschentscher P, et al: Flow-mediated dilation in patients with coronary artery disease is enhanced by high dose atorvastatin compared to combined low dose atorvastatin and ezetimibe: results of the CEZAR study, *Atherosclerosis* 205:227–232, 2009.
133. Shahin Y, Khan JA, Samuel N, et al: Angiotensin converting enzyme inhibitors effect on endothelial dysfunction: a meta-analysis of randomised controlled trials, *Atherosclerosis* 216:7–16, 2011.
134. Lekakis J, Abraham P, Balbarini A, et al: Methods for evaluating endothelial function: a position statement from the European Society of Cardiology Working Group on Peripheral Circulation, *Eur J Cardiovasc Prev Rehabil* 2011.
135. Cooke JP: Asymmetrical dimethylarginine: the uber marker? *Circulation* 109:1813–1818, 2004.

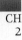

136. Cooke JP, Ghebremariam YT: DDAH says NO to ADMA, *Arterioscler Thromb Vasc Biol* 31:1462–1464, 2011.

137. Teerlink T: ADMA metabolism and clearance, *Vasc Med* 10(Suppl 1):S73–S81, 2005.

138. Ito A, Tsao PS, Adimoolam S, et al: Novel mechanism for endothelial dysfunction: dysregulation of dimethylarginine dimethylaminohydrolase, *Circulation* 99:3092–3095, 1999.

139. Sibal L, Agarwal SC, Home PD, et al: The role of asymmetric dimethylarginine (ADMA) in endothelial dysfunction and cardiovascular disease, *Curr Cardiol Rev* 6:82–90, 2011.

140. Abbasi F, Asagmi T, Cooke JP, et al: Plasma concentrations of asymmetric dimethylarginine are increased in patients with type 2 diabetes mellitus, *Am J Cardiol* 88:1201–1203, 2001.

141. Kielstein JT, Donnerstag F, Gasper S, et al: ADMA increases arterial stiffness and decreases cerebral blood flow in humans, *Stroke* 37:2024–2029, 2006.

142. Kielstein JT, Impraim B, Simmel S, et al: Cardiovascular effects of systemic nitric oxide synthase inhibition with asymmetrical dimethylarginine in humans, *Circulation* 109:172–177, 2004.

143. Juonala M, Viikari JS, Alfthan G, et al: Brachial artery flow-mediated dilation and asymmetrical dimethylarginine in the cardiovascular risk in Young Finns study, *Circulation* 116:1367–1373, 2007.

144. Boger RH, Sullivan LM, Schwedhelm E, et al: Plasma asymmetric dimethylarginine and incidence of cardiovascular disease and death in the community, *Circulation* 119:1592–1600, 2009.

145. Dignat-George F, Boulanger CM: The many faces of endothelial microparticles, *Arterioscler Thromb Vasc Biol* 31:27–33, 2010.

146. Chironi GN, Boulanger CM, Simon A, et al: Endothelial microparticles in diseases, *Cell Tissue Res* 335:143–151, 2009.

147. Amabile N, Guerin AP, Leroyer A, et al: Circulating endothelial microparticles are associated with vascular dysfunction in patients with end-stage renal failure, *J Am Soc Nephrol* 16:3381–3388, 2005.

148. Mallat Z, Benamer H, Hugel B, et al: Elevated levels of shed membrane microparticles with procoagulant potential in the peripheral circulating blood of patients with acute coronary syndromes, *Circulation* 101:841–843, 2000.

149. Arteaga RB, Chirinos JA, Soriano AO, et al: Endothelial microparticles and platelet and leukocyte activation in patients with the metabolic syndrome, *Am J Cardiol* 98:70–74, 2006.

150. Sabatier F, Darmon P, Hugel B, et al: Type 1 and type 2 diabetic patients display different patterns of cellular microparticles, *Diabetes* 51:2840–2845, 2002.

151. Preston RA, Jy W, Jimenez JJ, et al: Effects of severe hypertension on endothelial and platelet microparticles, *Hypertension* 41:211–217, 2003.

152. Bakouboula B, Morel O, Faure A, et al: Procoagulant membrane microparticles correlate with the severity of pulmonary arterial hypertension, *Am J Respir Crit Care Med* 177:536–543, 2008.

CHAPTER 3

Vascular Smooth Muscle

Lula L. Hilenski, Kathy K. Griendling

With the evolution of an enclosed circulatory system to transport oxygenated blood, hormones, immune cells, metabolites, and waste products to and from cells in distal sites within the vertebrate body, blood vessels evolved adaptations necessary for repeated cycles of contraction and extension resulting from cardiac-driven pulsatile blood flow. These adaptations for blood vessel distensibility allow elastic conductance arteries in the macrocirculation, under the influence of the pulsatile cardiac cycle, to provide blood flow to end organs by altering the luminal diameter of the vessel. They also allow resistance arteries in the microcirculation, which experience steady flow, to regulate vasomotion at the organ level to maintain blood pressure homeostasis.[1] The cells that primarily establish and orchestrate these contraction and distensible properties are vascular smooth muscle cells (VSMCs), the majority cell type within the normal vessel wall. VSMCs maintain contractile tone by a highly organized architecture of contractile/cytoskeletal proteins and associated regulatory components within the cell cytoplasm and establish distensibility by synthesis, secretion, and organization of extracellular matrix (ECM) components with elastic recoil and resilience properties.[1] VSMCs within the vascular continuum have the ability to adapt expression of proteins involved in contraction and ECM synthesis according to extrinsic and intrinsic cues during different developmental stages and in disease or response to injury. This ability is due to a phenomenon known as *VSMC phenotypic modulation* and is a major feature that distinguishes VSMCs from terminally differentiated cells.[2]

Vascular smooth muscle cell phenotypic modulation is the ability to switch phenotypic characteristics from a migratory synthetic phenotype in embryonic tissue patterning to a quiescent, contractile phenotype in maintenance of vascular tone in mature vessels. Importantly, during vascular remodeling in response to injury, VSMCs can switch back to a synthetic phenotype characterized by increased VSMC proliferation and ECM synthesis. Although the ability to switch phenotypes may have evolved as an adaptive survival mechanism for VSMCs to adjust physiological responses due to changing hemodynamic demands or to repair damage after vascular injury, phenotypic modulation has important implications both during development and during vascular disease.[2]

This chapter will highlight how these diverse functions of VSMCs arise from both innate genetic programs and a range of diverse environmental cues that include soluble signaling factors, insoluble ECM components, physical mechanical forces, and interactions with other cell types.[3] Discussion will center on the complex webs of signaling networks generated by these diverse external factors, and how these networks are regulated and integrated at multiple transcriptional and posttranslational levels to mediate the diverse functions of VSMCs in normal physiology and disease/injury pathology.

Origins of Vascular Smooth Muscle Cells During Embryonic Development

Initially in embryonic vasculature development, endothelial precursor cells form a common progenitor vessel which then gives rise to the first artery (dorsal aorta) and vein (cardinal vein) by selective sprouting and subsequent arterial-venous cell segregation[4] (see also Chapter 1). The distinct molecular identities of arteries and veins are regulated by complex interactions of several signaling pathways, including sonic hedgehog (Shh), a member of the hedgehog (Hh) family of secreted morphogens; secreted growth factors in the vascular endothelial growth factor family (VEGFs)[5]; Notch receptors (Notch 1-4) and Notch ligands (Jagged1,2); and transmembrane proteins that can transduce cell-cell interactions into signals determining cell fates.[6] Interactions of these signals

induce differential expression of VEGF receptors, Ephrin ligands, and tyrosine kinase Eph receptors on the segregating arterial/venous cells, with ephrin B2 and EphB4 as markers expressed in arteries and veins, respectively.[4,5] In response to VEGF signaling, endothelial cells (ECs) within these primordial vascular networks recruit mural cells, including nascent VSMCs.[7]

Nascent VSMCs derive from multiple and nonoverlapping embryonic origins that are reflected in different anatomical locations within the adult. Ectodermal cardiac neural crest cells give rise to the large elastic arteries (e.g., ascending and arch portions of the aorta), ductus arteriosus, and carotid arteries; proepicardium mesothelial cells produce the coronary arteries; mesodermal cells are origins for the abdominal aorta and small muscular arteries; the mesothelium forms the mesenteric vasculature; secondary heart field cells form the base of the aorta and pulmonary trunk; somite-derived cells produce the descending thoracic aorta; and satellite-like mesoangioblasts give rise to the medial layers of arteries.[8] The heterogeneous mosaic of VSMCs in the vessel wall may be due in part to these diverse embryological origins of VSMCs and could be reflected in the presence of phenotypically distinct subpopulations within the media that account for VSMC plasticity.[9] There is some evidence that VSMCs derived from different lineages exhibit morphologically and functionally distinct properties and respond differently to soluble factors *in vitro* and to morphogenetic cues *in vivo*,[8] suggesting that the major determinants of VSMC responses to signals in vascular development are principally lineage-dependent rather than environment-dependent.[8]

Vascular Smooth Muscle Cell Phenotypic Modulation

Characterization of Vascular Smooth Muscle Cell Phenotypes

Given the multiple origins and distinct subpopulations of VSMCs, a compelling central question for understanding VSMC biology is how cells from these diverse embryonic origins, initially expressing lineage-specific pathways, differentiate to express the same marker genes specifically characteristic of VSMCs.[8,10] Another question is how these same VSMCs, responding to both extrinsic and intrinsic cues, can alter expression of these genes (and thus molecular pathways), leading to diverse phenotypes with distinct and diverse functions. VSMC phenotypes can be loosely divided into three types: contractile/differentiated, synthetic/dedifferentiated, and inflammatory.

CONTRACTILE, DIFFERENTIATED VASCULAR SMOOTH MUSCLE CELLS

Contractile or differentiated VSMCs are characterized by a repertoire of contractile proteins, contractile-regulating proteins, contractile agonist receptors, and signaling proteins responsible for contraction and maintenance of vascular tone.[3,11,12] Of the VSMC "marker" proteins expressed in the contractile phenotype repertoire (Fig. 3-1), the most discriminating markers are smooth muscle myosin heavy chain (SMMHC) in conjunction with alpha-smooth muscle actin (αSMA), smoothelin, SM-22α, h1-calponin, and h-caldesmon.[2] In addition to expressing these proteins associated with contractile function, contractile VSMCs exhibit differential levels of ECM components (increased collagen types 1 and IV) and matrix-modifying enzymes (decreased matrix metalloproteinases [MMPs] and increased tissue inhibitors of matrix metalloproteinases [TIMPs]). Contractile VSMCs are further characterized by an elongated spindle-shaped morphology in culture, a low

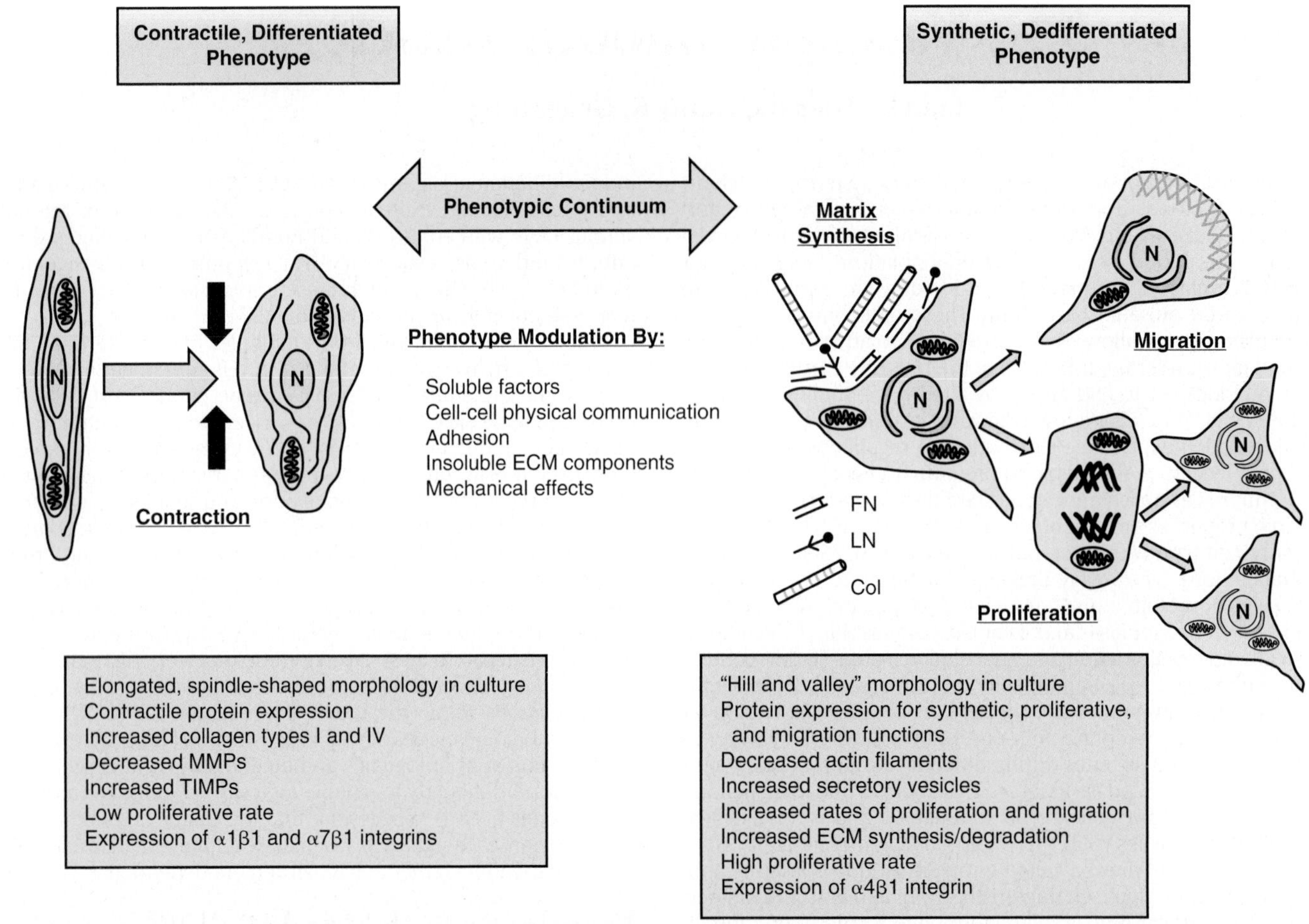

| Contractile, Differentiated Phenotype | | Synthetic, Dedifferentiated Phenotype |

Phenotypic Continuum

Phenotype Modulation By:

Soluble factors
Cell-cell physical communication
Adhesion
Insoluble ECM components
Mechanical effects

Contraction

Matrix Synthesis

Migration

FN
LN
Col

Proliferation

Elongated, spindle-shaped morphology in culture
Contractile protein expression
Increased collagen types I and IV
Decreased MMPs
Increased TIMPs
Low proliferative rate
Expression of α1β1 and α7β1 integrins

"Hill and valley" morphology in culture
Protein expression for synthetic, proliferative, and migration functions
Decreased actin filaments
Increased secretory vesicles
Increased rates of proliferation and migration
Increased ECM synthesis/degradation
High proliferative rate
Expression of α4β1 integrin

FIGURE 3-1 Summary of VSMC phenotype characteristics along the phenotypic continuum between contractile, differentiated phenotype on left and synthetic, dedifferentiated phenotype on right, with some of the environmental cues that modulate this continuum. Col, collagen; ECM, extracellular matrix; FN, fibronectin; LN, laminin; MMPs, matrix metalloproteinases; TIMPs, tissue inhibitors of MMPs. (Adapted from Beamish JA, He P, Kottke-Marchant K, et al: Molecular regulation of contractile smooth muscle cell phenotype: implications for vascular tissue engineering. Tissue Eng Part B Rev 16:467–491, 2010; Moiseeva EP: Adhesion receptors of vascular smooth muscle cells and their functions. Cardiovasc Res 52:372–386, 2001; Rensen SS, Doevendans PA, van Eys GJ: Regulation and characteristics of vascular smooth muscle cell phenotypic diversity. Neth Heart J 15:100–108, 2007; and Raines EW, Bornfeldt KE: Integrin α7β1 COMPels smooth muscle cells to maintain their quiescence. Circ Res 106:427–429, 2010.)

proliferative rate, and expression of α1β1, α7β1 integrins and the dystrophin-glycoprotein complex (DGPC).[3,13]

SYNTHETIC, DEDIFFERENTIATED VASCULAR SMOOTH MUSCLE CELLS

Synthetic or dedifferentiated VSMCs have decreased expression of SMC-related genes for contractile proteins (e.g., SMMHC), with concomitant increased osteopontin, l-caldesmon, nonmuscle myosin heavy chain B, vimentin, tropomyosin 4, and cellular-retinal binding-protein-1 (CRBP-1) (see Fig. 3-1). "Positive" marker genes, such as nonmuscle myosin heavy chain (NM-B MHC) or SMMHC embryonic (SMemb) expressed specifically in embryonic or phenotypically modified VSMCs, are characteristic of dedifferentiated VSMCs in association with vascular injury.[2] Other characteristics of synthetic VSMCs include decreased number of actin filaments, an increase in secretory vesicles, increased rates of proliferation and migration, extensive ECM synthesis/degradation capabilities, increased cell size and "hill-and-valley" morphology in culture, high proliferative rate, and increased expression of α4β1 integrin.

INFLAMMATORY VASCULAR SMOOTH MUSCLE CELLS

In addition to the phenotypic continuum between contractile and synthetic phenotypes, VSMCs can also express markers of an inflammatory phenotype in response to EC-induced recruitment of monocytes and macrophages during the progression of atherosclerosis.[14] Various stimuli, including secretion of cytokines

by these inflammatory cells, changes in ECM composition, oxidized low density lipoprotein (oxLDL), and VSMC interactions with monocytes/macrophages, induce expression of inflammatory cytokines, vascular cell adhesion molecule (VCAM-1) and transcription factors (NFκB) in VSMCs, leading to recruitment of inflammatory cells into the vessel wall.

Each of these types of VSMCs has a distinct response to microenvironmental chemical, structural, and mechanical cues. Not only do these cues initiate phenotypic modulation, but they also initiate specific intracellular signaling events that control the functional response of VSMCs in specific environments.

Upstream Mediators of Phenotypic Modulation

GROWTH-INDUCING FACTORS

Soluble factors that include growth factors, hormones, and reactive oxygen species (ROS) serve as upstream mediators of the phenotypic switch from contractile to synthetic VSMCs, which results in large part from coordinate activation/repression of VSMC marker genes important in the contractile response[2,3,15,16] (Fig. 3-2). Some of the most important growth-inducing factors include platelet-derived growth factor (PDGF), epidermal growth factor (EGF), insulin-like growth factor (IGF), and basic fibroblast growth factor (bFGF). Growth factors bind to surface membrane receptor tyrosine kinases (RTKs), triggering sequential downstream signaling pathways mediated through complex formation of activated RTKs with adaptor and signaling proteins Grb2/Shc/Sos, and activation

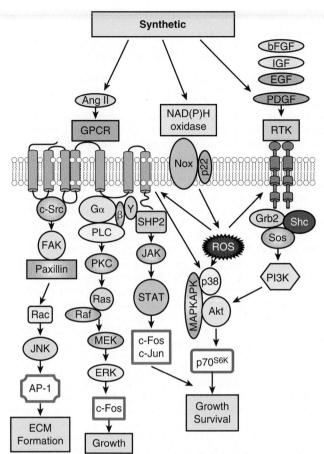

FIGURE 3-2 Summary of multiple soluble extracellular factors, their receptors, their interacting signaling pathways, and various transcription factors responsible for expression of the synthetic/dedifferentiated VSMC phenotype, characterized by growth/survival pathways and ECM formation. Details are outlined in text. (*Adapted from Owens GK, Kumar MS, Wamhoff BR: Molecular regulation of vascular smooth muscle cell differentiation in development and disease. Physiol Rev 84:767–801, 2004; Berk BC: Vascular smooth muscle growth: autocrine growth mechanisms. Physiol Rev 81:999–1030, 2001; Griendling K, Harrison D, Alexander R: Biology of the vessel wall. In Fuster V, Walsh R, O'Rourke R, Poole-Wilson P, editors: Hurst's the heart. 12th ed. New York, 2008, McGraw-Hill, pp 135–154; Mehta PK, Griendling KK: Angiotensin II cell signaling: physiological and pathological effects in the cardiovascular system. Am J Physiol Cell Physiol 292:C82–C97, 2007; and Hilenski L, Griendling K, Alexander R: Angiotensin AT1 receptors. In Re R, DiPette D, Schiffrin E, Sowers J, editors. Molecular mechanisms in hypertension. London, 2006, Taylor and Francis, pp 25–40.)*

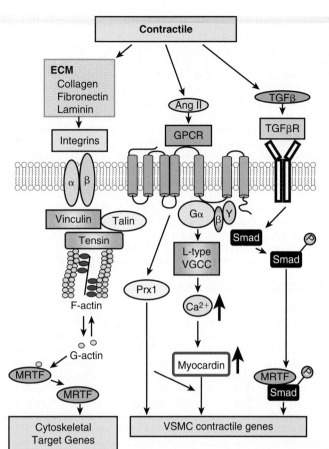

FIGURE 3-3 Summary of soluble and insoluble extracellular factors, their receptors, their interacting signaling pathways, and transcription factors responsible for expression of the contractile/differentiated VSMC phenotype. Details are outlined in text. (*Adapted from Owens GK, Kumar MS, Wamhoff BR: Molecular regulation of vascular smooth muscle cell differentiation in development and disease. Physiol Rev 84:767–801, 2004; Berk BC: Vascular smooth muscle growth: autocrine growth mechanisms. Physiol Rev 81:999–1030, 2001; Griendling K, Harrison D, Alexander R: Biology of the vessel wall. In Fuster V, Walsh R, O'Rourke R, Poole-Wilson P, editors. Hurst's the heart. 12th ed. New York, 2008, McGraw-Hill, pp 135–154; Mehta PK, Griendling KK: Angiotensin II cell signaling: physiological and pathological effects in the cardiovascular system. Am J Physiol Cell Physiol 292:C82–C97, 2007; and Hilenski L, Griendling K, Alexander R: Angiotensin AT1 receptors. In Re R, DiPette D, Schiffrin E, Sowers J, editors. Molecular mechanisms in hypertension. London, 2006, Taylor and Francis, pp 25–40.)*

of intracellular kinases, including phosphatidylinositol 3-kinase (PI3K), mitogen-activated protein kinases (MAPKs: extracellular signal regulated kinase, ERK1/2, p38MAPK, and c-jun NH2-terminal kinase, JNK), Akt, MAPKAPK2, and p70S6 kinase (p70S6K). These signals not only transcriptionally mediate the switch to the synthetic phenotype, but also serve to promote growth and survival. In addition, ROS such as hydrogen peroxide (H_2O_2) produced by activation of NADPH oxidases, multimeric enzymes containing p22phox and other subunits depending upon the specific isoform, can act as second messengers for canonical G protein–coupled receptor (GPCR) and RTK pathways.[17]

DIFFERENTIATION-INDUCING FACTORS

In contrast to growth factor–stimulated proliferation, the cytokine transforming growth factor β (TGF-β) and members of the bone morphogenetic protein (BMP) subgroup of this family promote the differentiated, contractile phenotype in VSMCs by inducing expression of the VSMC contractile genes αSMA and calponin (Fig. 3-3). Transforming growth factor β binds to a tetrameric complex consisting of two type I and two type II receptors, resulting in phosphorylation of Smads, transcription factors named for

Caenorhabditis elegans Sma and *Drosophila* Mad (mothers against decapentaplegic).[18] Within the TGF-β signaling pathway itself, different Smads control expression of different markers. For example, Smad3 transactivates the SM22α promoter, while Smad2 activates the αSMA gene. Other soluble factors that inhibit proliferation and increase differentiation include heparin and retinoic acid.[9] Most smooth muscle differentiation markers share additional common transcriptional pathways, discussed in more detail later. For example, both TGF-β-induced phosphorylated Smads and ECM-induced activation of integrins, mediated through focal adhesion components vinculin, talin, and tensin, in concert with changes in cytoskeletal F/G actin dynamics, result in myocardin-related transcription factor (MRTF) induction of cytoskeletal/contractile genes (see Fig. 3-3).

DUAL FACTORS

One factor with a potential dual role, depending upon initial phenotype/developmental stage, is the octapeptide hormone angiotensin II (Ang II), the effector molecule of the renin–angiotensin II system.[19] Angiotensin II can induce either contractile or synthetic phenotypes, with differential responses depending upon cell context and locations within the artery (see Figs. 3-2 and 3-3). Angiotensin II, binding to its GPCR AT1R, activates VSMC marker gene expression indicative of the contractile phenotype through L-type voltage-gated Ca²⁺ channel–induced elevations in intracellular Ca²⁺ concentrations, and subsequent increased myocardin transcription coactivator expression dependent upon Prx1, a homeodomain protein that promotes serum response factor (SRF) binding to conserved elements in VSMC marker gene promoters.[20] In addition, Ang II binding to AT₁R can induce signatures of the synthetic phenotype by activation of multiple kinase and enzyme pathways that are interconnected in signaling networks (see Fig. 3-2). These include the MAPKs; RTKs, including ROS-sensitive transactivation of epidermal growth factor receptor (EGFR); nonreceptor tyrosine kinases (c-Src/focal adhesion kinase [FAK]/paxillin/Rac/JNK/AP-1) and tyrosine phosphatases; SHP2/Janus kinase and signal transducers and activators of transcription (JAK/STAT); and GPCR classic signaling cascades (phospholipase C [PLC]/protein kinase C [PKC]/Ras/Raf/ mitogen extracellular signal regulated kinase [MEK]/ERK) leading to stimulation of early growth-response genes (c-fos, c-jun), survival pathways (e.g., Akt), and ECM formation (JNK/AP-1).

NOTCH COMMUNICATION

In addition to its critical function in development, Notch signaling is also important in defining VSMC differentiation.[21,22] Downstream Notch effector gene activation results in activation of "master regulators" of VSMC differentiation (myocardin, MRTFs, or SRF) or direct induction of contractile proteins SMMHC and αSMA, as well as the VSMC specific differentiation marker SM22α (also known as *transgelin*).[6] Data regarding Notch signaling on VSMC differentiation, however, are conflicting, with some studies supporting a repressive effect, while others indicate a promoting effect on expression of VSMC marker genes SMMHC and αSMA.[22] These discrepancies may be due to the antagonistic roles of Notch and the Notch effector Hairy-related transcription factor 1 (HRT1) on markers of VSMC differentiation, specifically αSMA and SMMHC.[23] Hairy-related transcription factor 1 inhibits Notch/RBP-Jκ binding to the αSMA promoter in a histone deacetylase-independent manner. The context-dependent roles of Notch and HRT1 on markers of VSMC differentiation may serve to fine-tune VSMC phenotypic modulation during vascular development, injury, and disease.

There is considerable cross-talk between Notch and other signaling pathways. Notch and TGF-β cooperatively induce a functional contractile, differentiated phenotype through parallel signaling axes,[24] while HRT factors block VSMC differentiation in both pathways. Other examples of cross-talk among key signaling pathways for morphogenesis (Hh, Notch) and mitogenesis (VEGF-A, PDGF) include a Shh/VEGF-A/Notch signaling axis in VSMCs in the neointima to increase growth and survival,[25] and Notch-induced up-regulation of PDGFR-β to mediate growth and migration.[26]

Homotypic VSMC-VSMC Notch-mediated signaling pathways are also apparent in adult vascular pathologies and response to injury.[22] After injury, Notch receptors are increased, along with elevated levels of HRT. Negative feedback between HRT and Notch may account for the adaptive response to injury in which initial Notch/HRT-induced suppression of the contractile phenotype is followed by arterial remodeling. As Notch/HRT signaling decreases, the contractile phenotype is reestablished.[24]

Transcriptional Regulation of Vascular Smooth Muscle Cell Diversity

The complex web of signaling pathways induced by these external signals—whether they are soluble, insoluble, structural, or mechanical—converge on a network of transcription factors (TFs) that coordinately regulate gene expression and act as "master switches" for growth and differentiation[27] (Fig. 3-4). Transcription of VSMC-specific differentiation or proliferative genes is regulated by cooperative interaction of TFs and their coregulators, including SRF,[28] myocardin and myocardin-related TFs (MRTF-A and -B),[29] Ets domain transcription factors known as *ternary complex factors*

(TCFs),[30] zinc finger factors GATA6[30] and PRISM/PRDM6,[31] and Krüppel-like factors (KLFs).[32,33]

SERUM RESPONSE FACTOR/MYOCARDIN AXIS

Serum response factor, a widely expressed member of the MADS (MCM1, agamous, deficien, SRF) box of TFs, is a nodal point linking signaling pathways to differential gene expression related either to growth or differentiation, depending upon which transcriptional partner is bound to SRF.[28] Serum response factor self-dimerizes and binds with high affinity and specificity to a consensus deoxyribonucleic acid (DNA) sequence CArG box found in the promoters of cyto-contractile genes.[34] More than half of the VSMC "marker" genes that define VSMC molecular signature contain CArG boxes.[34] Included in these genes are three categories modulating actin filament dynamics: (1) structural (e.g., αSMA-actin, SM22α, caldesmon, SMMHC); (2) effectors of actin turnover (e.g., cofilin, gelsolin); and (3) regulators of actin dynamics (four-and-a-half LIM domains proteins [FHL1 and 2], MMP9, and myosin light chain kinase).[35]

Serum response factor itself is a weak activator of CArG-dependent genes.[30] Potent SRF-dependent transcriptional activation is therefore dependent upon regulation at several levels: by interaction with different signal-regulated or tissue-specific regulatory SRF transcription cofactors/corepressors; by posttranslational phosphorylation, acetylation, and sumoylation, modifications that affect these interactions; and by epigenetic alterations in chromatin structure in which myocardin serves as a scaffold for recruitment of chromatin-remodeling enzymes[36] that enable SRF and its cofactors to gain access to SRF target genes.[8] Myocardin association with histone acetyltransferases (HATs), including p300, enhances transcription of VSMC-restricted genes, whereas association with class II histone deacetylases (HDACs) suppresses myocardin-induced transcription of VSMC marker genes[36] (see Fig. 3-4).

Serum response factor interacts with cofactors in two principal families: the TCF family of Ets-domain proteins (Elk, SAP-1, and Net)[37] activated by the MAPK pathway, leading to SRF binding to immediate early growth factor-inducible genes such as c-fos[28]; and the myocardin/MRTF-A/MRTF-B family[35] to promote activation of VSMC-specific marker genes, most of which code for filamentous proteins that function in contractile activities or proteins that function in cell-matrix adhesions.[10] These alternative pathways provide the "plasticity" associated with VSMC phenotypic modulation ranging from contractile functions to maintain vascular tone to synthetic or proliferative functions in response to vascular injury.[29]

Discovery of the cell-restricted SRF transcriptional coactivator myocardin, expressed specifically in cardiac and VSMCs, resolved the paradoxical observations that SRF can regulate mutually exclusive gene expression programs for growth or differentiation.[30,34] In VSMCs, myocardin is a master regulator of SMC marker gene expression and sufficient for the smooth muscle–like contractile phenotype. Myocardin competes with Elk-1 for direct binding to SRF in VSMCs; thus, myocardin and Elk-1 can act as binary transcriptional switches that may regulate contractile vs. synthetic VSMC phenotypes[30] (see Fig. 3-4). In addition, myocardin transduction leads to lower levels of the cell cycle–associated gene cyclin D1, resulting in repression of growth. Therefore, myocardin is a nodal point for two features indicative of SMC differentiation: expression of the contractile apparatus and suppression of growth.[30]

While myocardin functions exclusively as a transcriptional coactivator,[38] additional proteins function to regulate transcriptional activity of myocardin. Hairy-related transcription factor 2 and GATA factors repress or enhance myocardin-induced transcriptional activity, depending upon cell context.[30] In addition, activation of Notch receptors by Jagged1 endogenous ligand induces translocation of Notch intracellular domain (ICD) to the nucleus where it inhibits myocardin-induced SMC gene expression.[29] Angiotensin II stimulation, as well as activation of L-type voltage-gated Ca²⁺ channels, activates SMC marker genes by inducing myocardin expression and, in the case of Ang II, increasing SRF binding to CArG elements in the promoter regions of VSMC marker genes such as αSMA.[20]

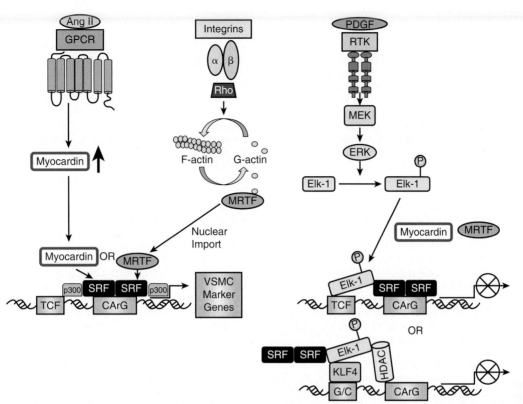

FIGURE 3-4   Model for opposing roles of transcription factors, their coregulators, and chromatin remodeling enzymes in control of vascular smooth muscle cell (VSMC) growth or differentiation. Differentiation-inducing extracellular cues such as G protein–coupled receptor (GPCR) or integrin activation, which increase myocardin or modulate Rho-mediated actin dynamics, respectively, stimulate signaling pathways leading to the transcription factor serum response factor (SRF). SRF binds to a CArG deoxyribonucleic acid (DNA) sequence found in promoters of many cytocontractile genes and interacts with myocardin/MRTF/p300 histone acetylase to promote VSMC marker gene expression. Growth factor signaling through the mitogen extracellular signal regulated kinase (MEK)/extracellular signal regulated kinase (ERK) pathway represses VSMC marker genes by phosphorylation of the ternary complex factor (TCF) Elk-1 and by increasing KLF4 expression. Phospho-Elk-1 inhibits SRF interaction with myocardin and KLF4, which binds to G/C-rich elements located in regulatory elements controlling expression of VSMC contractile genes, recruits histone deacetylase (HDAC), and reduces SRF binding to CArG elements. Ang II, angiotensin II; MRTF, myocardin-related transcription factor; PDGF, platelet-derived growth factor; RTK, receptor tyrosine kinase. *(Adapted from Wang D-Z, Olson EN: Control of smooth muscle development by the myocardin family of transcriptional coactivators. Curr Opin Genet Dev 14:558–566, 2004; and Pipes GC, Creemers EE, Olson EN: The myocardin family of transcriptional coactivators: versatile regulators of cell growth, migration, and myogenesis. Genes Dev 20:1545–1556, 2006.)*

Serum response factor transcriptional activity is also controlled by Rho-induced actin dynamics that facilitate movement of MRTFs into or out of the nucleus[29] (see Fig. 3-4). In most cell types, MRTFs form a stable complex with monomeric G-actin and remain sequestered in the cytoplasm. Myocardin-related transcription factors in VSMCs, however, are localized in the nucleus where binding to SRF in the basal state promotes contractile gene expression, and the differentiated phenotype. In response to growth factors or vascular injury, extracellular signals transduced through the Rho-actin pathway result in nuclear export of MRTF, down-regulation of SRF/MRTF-induced VSMC contractile gene expression, and promotion of mitogen-induced ERK1/2 phosphorylation of TCFs, resulting in TCF displacement of MRTFs and SRF/TCF-mediated activation of growth-responsive genes.[29] These differential pathways provide a switch in which SRF target genes are differentially regulated through growth factor–induced signaling for growth (active TCF, MRTF blocked) or Rho-actin signaling for differentiation (inactive TCF, MRTF active)[30] (see Fig. 3-4).

ZINC FINGER PROTEINS

GATA6, a zinc finger transcription factor expressed in VSMCs, induces growth arrest by increasing expression of the general cyclin-dependent kinase inhibitor (CDKI) p21[CIP1] and inhibiting S-phase entry.[30] PRISM is a smooth muscle–restricted member of zinc finger proteins belonging to the PRDM (PR domain in smooth muscle) family and acts as a transcriptional repressor by interacting with class I histone deacetylases and G9a histone methyltransferases. PRISM induces the proliferative phenotype while repressing differentiation regulators myocardin and GATA6.[31]

One of the most intensely studied zinc finger transcriptional regulators in VSMCs is the KLF subfamily that binds to the TGF-β control element (TCE) in the regulatory sequences of target genes (reviewed in[32,33,39]). Vascular smooth muscle cells express four KLFs (KLF4, KLF5, KLF13, and KLF15), each with individual biological functions implicated in regulating a range of processes in both growth and differentiation.[32] Individual KLFs may have opposing functions, depending upon temporal and developmental expression patterns and interactions with other factors. For example, KLF4 inhibits, whereas KLF5 and KLF13 induce, VSMC marker gene expression. Mechanisms that may account for these opposing functions of KLF factors include posttranslational modifications, interaction with specific cofactors, differential expression by growth factors, cytokines and differentiation state, or regulation by another KLF.[32]

KLF4 functions as both a VSMC growth repressor and a repressor for VSMC differentiation, although data on the effect of KLF4 on VSMC differentiation are conflicting[33] (see Fig. 3-4). As a growth repressor, KLF4 inhibits PDGF-BB-induced mitogenic signaling and induces expression of the negative cell cycle regulator p53 and its target gene p21[CIP1]. As a differentiation repressor, KLF4 prevents SRF from binding to the TCE in promoters of VSMC marker genes, suppresses expression of myocardin, inhibits myocardin-induced activation of SMC marker genes, reduces SRF binding to CArG elements in SMC contractile gene promoters,[33] and induces histone hypoacetylation at SMC CArG regions associated with gene silencing.[40] On the other hand, there is evidence that KLF4 promotes VSMC differentiation by directly activating VSMC marker gene transcription of SM22α and αSMA.[33] KLF4 thus functions as a bifunctional TF or "molecular switch" that can both activate and repress VSMC marker genes, depending upon regulation of KLF4.[33]

Even though the closely homologous KLF4 and KLF5 TFs share similar developmental and tissue pattern expression, they exert different, often opposing, effects on gene regulation and proliferation/differentiation.[33] Whereas KLF4 is associated with growth arrest, KLF5 exerts pro-proliferative effects, particularly in vascular remodeling in response to injury. KLF5 expression, abundant in fetal VSMCs but down-regulated in the adult (reviewed in[39]), is induced after vascular injury by activation of immediate early response genes by Ang II and ROS.[41] KLF5 in turn mediates re-expression of SMemb/NMHC-B, a marker for the dedifferentiated phenotype, and activates other critical injury response genes involved in remodeling, such as PDGF-A/B, Egr-1, plasminogen activator inhibitor 1 (PAI-1), inducible nitric oxide synthase (iNOS), and VEGFR, implicating KLF5 as a key regulator for VSMC response to injury.[39] In additional injury responses, KLF5 increases cyclin D1 expression and inhibits the cyclin kinase inhibitor p21, thus leading to vascular remodeling by increased cell proliferation.[42] Similar to KLF4 regulation, KLF5 expression and activity are regulated at multiple levels, including upstream Ras/MAPK, PKC, and TGF-β signaling pathways; downstream interactions with TFs, including retinoic acid receptor α (RARα), NF-κB, and peroxisome proliferator–activated receptor gamma (PPARγ); as well as posttranslational modifications that can positively or negatively regulate KLF activity.[39] In addition, KLF5 activity is regulated in the nucleus by chromatin remodeling factors such as SET, a histone chaperone that inhibits the DNA binding activity of KLF5,[43] p300 (a coactivator/acetylase that coactivates KLF5 transcription), and HDAC1, which inhibits KLF5 binding to DNA.[32]

Two additional KLFs have been identified in VSMCs: KLF13 and KLF15.[32] After vascular injury, KLF13 is induced and activates the promoter for the VSMC differentiation marker SM22α, while KLF15 expression is down-regulated, implicating KLF15 as a negative regulator of VSMC proliferation and a counterbalance to the growth-promoting effects of KLF5 in vascular injury response.

Posttranscriptional Regulation of Vascular Smooth Muscle Cell Diversity: Noncoding microRNAs

Upstream signaling and downstream transcriptional pathways in VSMCs are intertwined with a multitude of micro ribonucleic acid (miRNAs) that act as "rheostats" and "switches" in regulating protein activity in development, function, and disease.[44] miRNAs are small, noncoding RNAs (20-25 nucleotides in length) that associate with a miRNA-induced silencing complex (miRISC) of regulatory proteins, including Argonaute family proteins, Argonaute interacting proteins of the GW182 family, eukaryotic initiation factors (eIFs), polyA-binding complexes, decapping enzymes/activators, and deadenylases, to induce posttranscriptional silencing of their target genes.[45] These multiple components are assembled and interact in a multistep process with components of the translational machinery to inhibit translation initiation, mark mRNAs for degradation through deadenylation, and sequester targets into cytoplasmic P bodies.[44] Multiple mechanistic models for miRNA-induced gene silencing have been proposed that provide insights into the molecular mechanisms of translational inhibition, deadenylation, and mRNA decay, but questions remain concerning the kinetics and ordering of these translational events and whether they are coupled or independent.[45] A recent unifying model for miRNA-regulated gene repression is an attempt to reconcile the often conflicting existing data. It proposes that recruitment of Argonaute and associated GW182 proteins to miRNA induces binding to the mRNA 5′m[7] Gcap, thus blocking translation initiation, potentially by mRNA deadenylation. Subsequent to miRNA-mediated deadenylation, mRNA is degraded through recruitment of decapping proteins.[46] In this model, inhibition of translation initiation is linked to subsequent rapid mRNA decay in a coupled process. Because miRNAs—which in general are negative regulators of gene expression—may be almost as important as transcription factors in controlling gene expression in the pathogenesis of human diseases,[47] insights into the functions of this class of noncoding RNAs are important in evaluating their potential use as therapeutic targets.[45]

Cardiovascular-specific, highly conserved miRNAs miR-143 and miR-145, the most abundant miRNA in the vascular wall,[48] are key players in programming VSMC fate from multipotent progenitors in embryonic development and in reprogramming VSMCs during phenotypic modulation in the adult[44,49] (Fig. 3-5). miR-143 and miR-145 have distinct sequences but are clustered together and transcribed as a bicistronic unit. Upstream in the genomic sequence of miR-143/145 is a conserved SRF-binding CArG box site, indicating control by SRF and myocardin.[49,50] These miRNAs cooperatively feed back to modulate the actions of SRF by

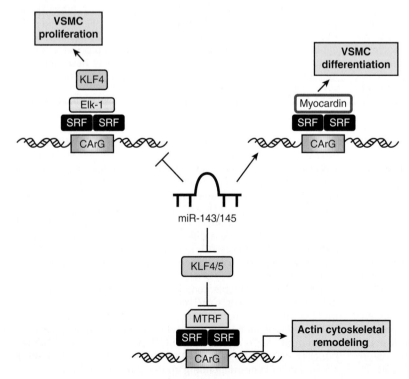

FIGURE 3-5 Model for regulation of vascular smooth muscle cell (VSMC) phenotypes by cardiovascular-specific micro ribonucleic acids (microRNAs) miR-143 and miR-145. These miRNAs act as signaling nodes to modulate serum response factor (SRF)-dependent transcription by regulating coactivators and co-repressors to control VSMC proliferation or differentiation. miR-145 represses proliferation by repressing KLF4 and promotes differentiation by stimulating myocardin; miR-143 represses proliferation by repressing Elk-1. miR-143/145 also controls actin/cytoskeletal remodeling by repressing KLF4/5 and regulators of actin dynamics, including MTRF/SRF activity. *(Adapted from Liu N, Olson EN: MicroRNA regulatory networks in cardiovascular development. Dev Cell 18:510–525, 2010; Cordes KR, Sheehy NT, White MP, et al: MiR-145 and miR-143 regulate smooth muscle cell fate and plasticity. Nature 460:705–710, 2009; and Xin M, Small EM, Sutherland LB, et al. MicroRNAs miR-143 and miR-145 modulate cytoskeletal dynamics and responsiveness of smooth muscle cells to injury. Genes Dev 23:2166–2178, 2009.)*

targeting a network of transcription factors/coactivators/core-pressors. This network includes miR-145-induced repression of KLF4, a positive regulator of proliferation and myocardin repressor; miR-143-induced repression of Elk-1, a myocardin competitor and positive regulator of proliferation; and, contrary to the usual inhibitory role of miRNA, miR-145-induced stimulation of myocardin, a positive regulator of differentiation. Thus, miR-145 is necessary and sufficient for VSMC differentiation, and the miR-143/miR-145 cluster acts as an integrated signaling node to promote differentiation while concurrently repressing proliferation.[49] Although mice with genetic deletions for miR-143/145 show no obvious abnormalities in early development, VSMCs in the adult exhibit both structural and phenotypic differences in injury- or stress-induced vascular remodeling. Ultrastructural analysis of arteries from miR-143/145 knockout mice shows reduced numbers of medial VSMCs with a contractile appearance, and an increase in synthetic VSMCs.[51] These results suggest that miR-143 and miR-145 modulate cytoskeletal structure, actin dynamics, and modulation to a dedifferentiated phenotype[50] (see Fig. 3-5). Importantly, miR-143/145 knockout mice with increased synthetic VSMCs develop spontaneous neointimal lesions in the femoral artery in the absence of hyperlipidemia and inflammation, supporting a key role for phenotypically altered VSMCs in the pathogenesis of lesion formation.[51]

While miR-143 and miR-145 play keys roles in the contractile phenotype of VSMCs and the response to injury,[52] miR-221 and miR-222 are modulators of VSMC proliferation, although largely by affecting growth-related signaling pathways rather than by controlling VSMC phenotype. miR-221 and miR-222, encoded by a gene cluster on the X chromosome, are up-regulated in VSMCs in neointimal lesions and in proliferating cultured VSMCs stimulated by PDGF-BB.[53] Studies show that two CDKIs, p27[KIP1] and p57[KIP2], have miR-221 and miR-222 binding sites and are gene targets for miR-221 and miR-222 in the rat carotid artery *in vivo*.[53] Thus, miR-221 and miR-222 are pro-proliferative because they repress two CDKIs, p27[KIP1] and p57[KIP2]. Furthermore, PDGF, via miR-221 induction, inhibits VSMC differentiation via c-kit-induced inhibition of myocardin.[54]

Posttranslational Regulation of Vascular Smooth Muscle Cell Diversity: Epigenetics

The "epigenetic landscape" controls gene expression by chemical modifications that mark regions of chromosomes either by methylation of promoter CpG sequences in the DNA itself, or by covalent modification of histone proteins that package DNA by posttranslational addition of methyl, acetyl, phosphoryl, ubiquityl, or sumoyl groups, leading to expression/repression of transcription (reviewed in[55]). In VSMCs, multiple levels of epigenetic controls exist for gene expression leading to differentiation or dedifferentiation programs in healthy cells and for dysregulated gene expression in vascular disease. These epigenetic changes in VSMCs involve both DNA and histone methylation as well as histone acetylation/deacetylation. Methylation of histones, catalyzed by histone methyltransferases (HMTs), results in a tight, stable epigenetic mark between methylated histones and chromatin that can be passed to daughter cells, thus providing "epigenetic memory" that defines cell lineage and identity by controlling SRF access to VSMC-specific marker genes.[55] Acetylation is controlled by HATs, which promote gene transcription by destabilizing chromatin structure to an "open," transcriptionally active conformation, and HDACs, which promote chromatin condensation to a "closed," transcriptionally silent conformation with restricted access to DNA. Histone acetylation/deacetylation thus serves to regulate transcription in a rapid and "on/off" manner in response to dynamic environmental changes and links the cell's genome with new extrinsic signals.[55]

In VSMCs, SRF binding to CArG boxes in the promoters of SMC marker genes to promote the VSMC differentiated phenotype depends upon alterations of chromatin structure, including histone methylation and acetylation. In a model for epigenetic regulation of VSMC phenotype,[56] SRF binding to CArG boxes in VSMC marker gene promoters is blocked by conditions such as PDGF-BB exposure or vascular injury. Such conditions promote KLF4-induced myocardin suppression as well as KLF4-induced recruitment of HDACs, resulting in "closed" deacetylated chromatin and transcriptional repression of VSMC marker genes. Histone methylation, in contrast, is not affected by PDGF-BB and may serve as a permanent "memory" for VSMC identity during repression of SRF-dependent transcription and can, once repressive signals are terminated, reactivate the differentiation program by recruiting myocardin/SRF complexes or HATs to VSMC marker genes for reexpression. In the absence of KLF4 activation, SRF/myocardin can bind to HAT-induced acetylated "open" chromatin at CArG boxes for transcriptional activation of VSMC marker genes, thus promoting VSMC differentiation. In addition, myocardin induces acetylation of histones in the vicinity of SRF-binding promoters in VSMC marker genes by association with p300, a ubiquitous transcriptional coactivator with its own intrinsic HAT activity, leading to synergistic activation of VSMC marker gene expression. This pro-myogenic program is antagonized and repressed by myocardin binding to class II HDACs, which strongly inhibits expression of marker genes αSMA, SM22α, SMMLCK and SMMHC. These opposing actions of HATs and HDACs on SRF/myocardin function to activate or repress, respectively, VSMC differentiation and serve to regulate transcription in a rapid and reversible manner in response to dynamic changes in the environment.[55]

Often, transcription mediators play roles in both classic signal transduction pathways and epigenetic programming.[57] Smad proteins, for example, transmit TGF-β signals from the membrane to the nucleus to mediate gene transcription and VSMC differentiation. The balance between Smad-induced recruitment of corepressors or coactivators to TGF-β-responsive genes is associated with activation of HDAC or HAT (p300), which then alters histone acetylation. Transforming growth factor β induces histone hyperacetylation at the VSMC marker gene SM22 promoter through recruitment of HATs, Smad3, SRF, and myocardin, demonstrating a role for HATs and HDACs in TGF-β activation of VSMC differentiation.[58]

A proposed example of metabolic memory stored in the histone code of VSMCs is found in the dysregulation of histone H3 methylation, an epigenetic mark usually associated with transcriptional repression in type 2 diabetes.[59] In VSMCs derived from type 2 diabetic db/db mice, levels of H3K9me3 (H3 lysine-9 trimethylation), as well as its HMT, are both reduced at the promoters of inflammatory genes. This loss of repressive histone marks, leading to increased inflammatory gene expression, is sustained in VSMCs from db/db mice cultured *in vitro*, suggesting persistence of metabolic memory. These results suggest that dysregulation in the histone code in VSMCs is a potential mechanism for increased and sustained inflammatory response in diabetic patients who continue to exhibit "metabolic memory" and vascular complications after glucose normalization.[60]

Influence of Cell-Cell and Cell-Matrix Interactions

Many differential VSMC functions are influenced by cell-cell and cell-matrix adhesion receptors that are altered during phenotypic modulation and during response to injury or disease. Cell-cell adhesion receptors include cadherins and gap junction connexins; cell-matrix interactions are dependent upon combinations of integrins, syndecans, and α-dystroglycan.[11]

Cell-Cell Adhesion Molecules: Cadherins and Gap Junction Connexins

After investment of VSMCs to the EC layer of nascent vessels, *vascular stabilization*, also known as *maturation*,[61] is regulated by the sphingosine 1-phosphate (S1P) receptor S1P1, a GPCR on ECs. S1P1 activates the cell-cell adhesion molecule N-cadherin in ECs and induces formation of direct N-cadherin-based junctions between ECs and VSMCs required for vessel stabilization.[61] To maintain VSMC quiescence within the vascular wall, cadherin-mediated cell-cell adherens-type junctions between VSMCs inhibit VSMC proliferation, possibly by inhibiting the transcriptional activity of β-catenin, a component of the Wnt signaling pathway, which interacts with the intracellular domain of cadherins.[62] Inhibition of β-catenin or stabilization of cadherin junctions in VSMCs may be useful in treating vascular disease or injury.

Another type of direct intercellular junction between cells in the vasculature is the gap junction.[63] Gap junctions, formed by connexin proteins between ECs and VSMCs and between VSMCs, are intercellular channels that allow movement of metabolites, small signaling molecules, and ions between cells.[63–65] Of the four connexin proteins expressed in VSMCs (Cx37, Cx40, Cx43, and Cx45), Cx45 is exclusively found in VSMCs, while Cx43 is the most prominent and is essential for coordination of proliferation and migration.[63] Homotypic gap junctions between VSMCs coordinate changes in membrane potential and intracellular Ca^{2+}, and heterotypic contacts between ECs and VSMCs at the myoendothelial junction control vascular tone by EC-mediated VSMC hyperpolarization. Notably, expression and/or activity of vascular connexins are altered in vascular diseases such as hypertension, atherosclerosis, or restenosis[64] and in diabetes.[63]

Cell-Matrix Adhesion Molecules: Integrins and Syndecans

INTEGRINS

Transmembrane integrin receptors are composed of combinations of α and β subunits, each combination with its own ligand-binding specificity and signaling properties. Integrins link the ECM with the actin cytoskeleton within VSMCs. The β1 subunit is the main β subunit in VSMCs *in vivo* and *in vitro*; the major α integrin subunits expressed in VSMCs *in vivo* are α1, α3, and α5.[11] Integrin α1β1 is involved in collagen remodeling after injury, and integrin α5β1 binds to fibronectin (FN) and effects FN polymerization.

Activation of different VSMC integrins results in expression of differential phenotypic programs. Beta-1 expression contributes to maintenance of the VSMC contractile phenotype, whereas integrins α2β1, α5β1, α7β1, and αvβ3 participate in SMC migration indicative of the synthetic phenotype.[11] Neointimal formation after vessel injury is reduced by blocking αvβ3, but apoptosis in the injured vessel is increased, potentially promoting plaque rupture. In addition, neointimal formation is prevented and the VSMC contractile phenotype is maintained by binding of α7β1 integrins to COMP (cartilage oligomeric matrix protein), a macromolecular ECM protein.[66]

SYNDECAN CORECEPTOR

Syndecans are members of a family of four transmembrane heparan sulfate proteoglycans (HSPGs) consisting of a core protein covalently coupled with (GAGs).[67,68] Syndecans function as coreceptors with growth factor or adhesion receptors and function to "tune" extracellular signal transfer across the cell surface to the cytoskeleton and cytoplasmic mediators to effect activation of a variety of intracellular signaling cascades. All four syndecans are expressed in the artery, and VSMC syndecans bind to ECM proteins, cell adhesion molecules, heparin-binding growth factors such as fibroblast growth factor (FGF) and EGF, lipoproteins, lipoprotein lipases, and components of the blood coagulation cascade.[11] Syndecan-1 inhibits VSMC growth in response to PDGF-BB and FGF2 after vascular injury.[69] Syndecan-4 has been implicated in thrombin-induced VSMC migration and proliferation by acting both as a mediator for bFGF signaling and as a cofactor for fibroblast growth factor receptor 1 (FGFR-1), suggesting that syndecan-4 is an early response gene after injury, whereas syndecan-1 is active during the proliferative and migratory phase.[68]

INSOLUBLE EXTRACELLULAR MATRIX COMPONENTS

One of the most important functions of VSMCs is to secrete, organize, and maintain an elaborate ECM architecture, an "extended cytoskeleton" that varies according to the biomechanical stresses of the differing vascular beds. Large elastic arteries (e.g., thoracic aorta, carotid, renal arteries) are characterized by multiple concentric elastic lamellae that distribute cardiac-driven pulsatile stress evenly throughout the vessel wall. Smaller muscular arteries that experience less force (e.g., coronary, cerebral, mesenteric) contain only two elastic laminae. Elaboration of the ECM synthesized and organized by VSMCs is considered to be a major part of their "differentiated" phenotype[70] because ECM components influence the same pathways regulated by growth/differentiation factors (see Fig. 3-3). Changes acquired by VSMCs during acquisition of contractile properties are in turn maintained by the ECM in "dynamic reciprocity" between the matrix and gene expression. In addition to providing a structural elastic scaffold for the extensible vessels, the ECM regulates gene expression through binding of matrix receptors on the cell surface and through acting as a reservoir for growth factors such as PDGF and FGF that regulate cell function (reviewed in[71]).

Extracellular matrix components are classified as fiber-forming molecules (certain collagens and elastin), non-fiber-forming or interfibrillar molecules (proteoglycans and glycoproteins), and matricellular proteins (thrombospondin-1 and -2, secreted protein acidic and rich in cysteine [SPARC/osteonectin], tenascin-C, and osteopontin) that modulate cell-matrix interactions and tissue repair.[72] A list of ECM molecules and diseases resulting from ECM alterations can be found in a recent review[72] (also see Chapter 4).

BASEMENT MEMBRANE

Vascular smooth muscle cells in the intact vessel are surrounded by a basement membrane composed primarily of type IV collagen and laminin.[11] *Laminins* are basement membrane modular glycoproteins that interact with both cells and ECM to affect proliferation, migration, and differentiation.[70] Evidence from cultured VSMCs suggests that laminin induces expression of contractile proteins and moderates the proliferative response to mitogens such as PDGF through a mechanism involving the laminin receptor α7β1, which links the basement membrane to the VSMC contractile apparatus.[3]

FIBRONECTIN

Fibronectin is present in developing tissues prior to collagen, and there is evidence that FN has an organizing role in ECM assembly as a "master orchestrator" for matrix assembly, organization, and stability.[73,74] Fibronectin binding to α5β1 induces integrin-bound FN clustering, resulting in activation of actin polymerization, actin-myosin interactions, and signaling through kinase cascades. Thus, FN modulates VSMCs toward the synthetic phenotype.[12]

COLLAGENS

Differential phenotypic modulation of VSMCs in response to different forms of collagen or to different isotypes of collagen illustrates the importance of cues from the physical and chemical ECM environment that regulate VSMC physiology in normal and disease states.[75] Cells cultured on fibrillar vs. monomeric collagen type 1 exhibit very different gene expression profiles, responses to growth factors such as PDGF-BB, and migration properties.[12] Fibrillar collagen type 1 promotes the contractile phenotype, whereas monomeric collagen type 1, found in the degraded matrix of vascular lesions ("atherosclerotic matrix"), activates proliferation,[76] reduces contractile gene expression, and promotes a VSMC inflammatory phenotype with increased VCAM-1 expression.[75] Vascular smooth muscle cells also exhibit different phenotypic profiles depending upon contact with different collagen isotypes: collagen type IV, a component of the basement membrane surrounding VSMCs ("protective" matrix), promotes expression of contractile proteins by regulating the SRF coactivator myocardin expression and mediating recruitment of SRF to CArG boxes in αSMA and SMMHC promoters.[75]

ELASTINS AND ELASTIN-ASSOCIATED PROTEINS

Elastic fibers are composed of tropoelastin, fibrillin-1, and fibrillin-2 and are assembled and deposited in a tightly regulated, hierarchical manner.[77,78] They provide not only unique elastomeric properties to the vessel wall but also influence phenotypes of VSMCs, directly through adhesion and indirectly through TGF-β signaling,[77] to regulate migration, survival, and differentiation.[78] Elastin maintains the quiescent, contractile phenotype of VSMCs by specifically regulating actin polymerization and organization via a signal transduction pathway involving Rho GTPases and their effector proteins.[79] Mechanical injury or inflammation that results in focal destruction of insoluble elastin into soluble elastin-derived peptides induces VSMC dedifferentiation and migration. Elastin-derived peptides can activate cyclins/cyclin-dependent kinases, leading to cell cycle progression and proliferation found in neointimal formation.

FIBRILLINS

Fibrillins are large cysteine-rich glycoproteins that serve dual roles: (1) providing stability and elasticity to tissues and (2) sequestering TGF-β and BMP complexes in the ECM to limit their bioavailability, providing for spatial and temporal growth factor signaling during remodeling or repair.[80,81] Mutations in the fibrillin-1 gene are found in Marfan syndrome, a heritable disease associated with disorganized elastic fibers in defective aorta and excess TGF-β signaling.[78]

FIBULINS

Fibulins are elastic fiber–associated proteins.[78] Vascular smooth muscle cells from fibulin-5 null mice exhibit enhanced proliferation and migration, indicating an inhibitory role for fibulin-5 in VSMC response to mitogenic stimuli.[82] Vascular smooth muscle cell-specific deletion of the fibulin-4 gene results in large aneurysm formation exclusively in the ascending aorta and down-regulation of SMC-specific contractile proteins and transcription factors for SMC differentiation. Thus fibulin-4 may serve a dual role in both elastic fiber formation and SMC differentiation, and therefore may protect the aortic wall against aneurysm formation *in vivo* and may also maintain an ECM environment for VSMC differentiation. Fibulin-2 and fibulin-5 double knockout mice have vessels that exhibit disorganized internal elastic lamina and an inability to remodel after carotid artery ligation-induced injury,[83] which was not observed in single knockout mice for fibulin-2 or fibulin-5. These data suggest that fibulins 2 and 5 function cooperatively to form the internal elastic laminae and protect vessel integrity.

EMILINS

EMILINs (elastin microfibril interface-located proteins) act as an extracellular negative regulator of TGF signaling.[84] EMILIN null mice (*Emilin1[−/−/−]*) exhibit inhibition of cell proliferation, smaller blood vessels, altered elastic fibers,[85] and increased peripheral resistance, causing hypertension.[84] These data indicate a role for EMILIN in elastogenesis, maintenance of VSMC morphology, and—importantly—in blood pressure control.

GLYCOSAMINOGLYCANS, PROTEOGLYCANS, AND MATRICELLULAR PROTEINS

Glycosaminoglycans in the vascular ECM, including heparin and the related heparan sulfate, inhibit VSMC migration and proliferation. Heparin also induces expression of contractile markers for maintenance of the differentiated phenotype.[3] Proteins bearing GAG chains, the proteoglycans,[86] which include syndecan transmembrane HSPG and perlecan basement membrane HSPG,

interact with FN in matrix assembly.[74] Different proteoglycans can have opposing effects on VSMCs: the HSPG perlecan inhibits VSMC proliferation and intimal thickening by sequestering FGF-2,[12,69] while versican, a chondroitin sulphate proteoglycan, promotes VSMC proliferation.[87] Vasoactive agents acting through GPCRs such as endothelin-1 and Ang II stimulate elongation of GAG chains on the proteoglycan core proteins.[88] These elongated GAG chains exhibit enhanced binding to low-density lipoprotein (LDL), providing a mechanism for atherogenic lipid retention in the vessel wall. Finally, matricellular proteins (e.g., thrombospondins, tenascins, SPARC), are thought to be "antiadhesive proteins" with effects on VSMC migration and adhesion.[70] CCN (cysteine-rich protein, Cyr 61/CCN1) is a family of secreted matricellular proteins that mediate cellular responses to environmental stimuli through interaction with a variety of cell surface proteins and adhesion receptors including Notch receptors and integrins.[89] CCN1, which is up-regulated in the VSMCs of injured arteries, stimulates VSMC proliferation through CCN1/α6β1 integrin interactions.[90] Knockdown of CCN1 in injury models suppresses neointimal hyperplasia. In contrast, CCN3 protein inhibits VSMC proliferation in a TGF-β-independent manner by increasing the CDKI p21, partly through Notch signaling, thus suppressing neointimal thickening.[91] These contrasting roles for pro-proliferative CCN1/α6β1 integrin signaling and antiproliferative CCN3/Notch signaling in VSMCs offer therapeutic strategies for reducing neointimal hyperplasia.[91]

MATRIX METALLOPROTEINASES AND TISSUE INHIBITORS OF MATRIX METALLOPROTEINASES

Matrix metalloproteinases are zinc-containing enzymes that, along with extracellular proteases in the plasminogen activation system, induce remodeling of VSMC cell-matrix and cell-cell interactions (reviewed in[92–94]) and release ECM-bound growth factors, cytokines, and proteolyzed ECM fragments, or "matrikines," with cytokine-like properties into the ECM. Members of the MMP family found in vascular tissues (listed in Ref. 95) include interstitial collagenases, basement membrane gelatinases, stromelysins, matrilysins, and membrane type (MT)-MMPs and metalloelastase (see Chapter 4). In the vascular wall, production of pro-MMP-2, MMP-14, and TIMP-1 and -2 is constitutive,[96] while other MMPs can be induced by inflammatory cytokines (interleukin [IL]-1 and -4 and tumor necrosis factor α [TNF-α]), hemodynamics, vessel injury, and ROS.[93] In addition, MMPs can act synergistically with growth factors such as PDGF and FGF-2.

Matrix metalloproteinase induced remodeling of basement membrane components laminin, polymerized type IV collagen, and HSPGs promotes a VSMC migratory phenotype. In addition, MMP cleavage and shedding of non-matrix substrates—in particular, adherens junction cadherins—act to remove physical constraints on cell movement.[93] Furthermore, ECM remodeling enables integrin signaling from the cell surface to focal adhesions, modulating cell cycle components cyclin D1 and p21/p27 CDKIs.[96]

In vascular remodeling, MMP activities are tightly regulated at several levels: transcriptional level, activation of pro-forms, interaction with specific ECM components, and inhibition by TIMPs. Modulation of MMP activity is evident in VSMC migration and neointima formation after injury, plaque destabilization in atherosclerosis, aneurysm formation, hypertension, and coronary restenosis.[95] In atherosclerosis, MMPs have potential either to promote plaque instability, as in advanced plaques of hypercholesterolemia models, or to stabilize plaques by increasing VSMC migration/proliferation. Up-regulation of MMPs in VSMCs may contribute to aneurysm formation.[3]

MECHANICAL EFFECTS

Data on VSMC phenotypic modulation by the mechanical environment indicate that continuous cyclic mechanical strain acting directly on VSMCs increases collagen and fibronectin synthesis, possibly by paracrine release of TGF-β1, resulting in increased ECM remodeling indicative of a VSMC synthetic phenotype.[12] In contrast, some studies have shown that mechanical strain can also stimulate expression of contractile genes.[3] Although MAPK signaling pathways are induced following initiation of cyclic strain, mechanisms for this induction are unclear. Activation of ion channels and tyrosine kinases, and paracrine release of soluble mediators such as Ang II, PDGF, and IGF, are postulated to play a role.[3]

Mechanical signals play a role in stimulating cell cycle progression. Actin filament polymerization and organization induced by integrin ligation generate intracellular mechanical tensional forces that promote cell cycle progression.[97] In addition, "stiffness," or compliance of the ECM, can direct cellular functions through integrin-dependent signaling pathways involving FAK, the canonical mediator of integrin signaling, Rho family GTPase Rac and cyclin D1.[98]

Phenotype-Specific Vascular Smooth Muscle Cell Functions

Contraction

The primary function of differentiated VSMCs is to maintain vascular tone. This is an active process requiring significant energy expenditure, especially in resistance arterioles. A number of hormones and peptides regulate VSMC contraction, including catecholamines, Ang II, and endothelin-1. Contractions can be phasic, lasting only minutes, or tonic, depending on the stimulus.

In nearly all cases, stimulation of VSMC with contractile agents results in activation of a specific GPCR (Fig. 3-6). The immediate response is activation of PLC, which cleaves the membrane phospholipid phosphatidylinositol 4,5-bisphosphate (PIP_2) to release

inositol 1,4,5-trisphosphate (IP_3) and diacylglycerol (DAG). IP_3, in turn, binds to its receptor (a channel) on the sarcoplasmic reticulum (SR), creating an open conformation and translocating Ca^{2+} to the cytoplasm. Simultaneously, receptor activation depolarizes the plasma membrane by altering the activity of pumps such as the sodium/potassium–adenosine triphosphate (Na^+/K^+-ATPase), and channels that include Ca^{2+}-sensitive K^+ channels and TRP channels.[99] Membrane depolarization leads to activation of voltage-dependent L-type Ca^{2+} channels, calcium influx, and a more sustained but less robust elevation of cytosolic calcium. Moreover, Ca^{2+} entry through these channels activates ryanodine receptors on the SR, further increasing Ca^{2+} release into the cytosol.

The increased cytoplasmic calcium binds to calmodulin (CaM) at a ratio of four calcium ions to one CaM molecule. Calmodulin then undergoes a conformational change, and binds to and activates myosin light chain kinase (MLCK), the enzyme responsible for phosphorylation of the 20-kD regulatory myosin light chain (LC20) on serine 19. Activated LC20 facilitates actin-mediated myosin adenosine triphosphate (ATPase) activity and cyclic interaction of myosin and actin,[100] leading to contraction. Contraction is maintained even when calcium drops, suggesting that LC20 becomes sensitized to calcium, likely by inhibition of myosin phosphatase (see later discussion).[101]

Because the increase in intracellular calcium caused by vasoconstrictors is largely responsible for activation of the contractile apparatus, essential mechanisms exist to limit Ca^{2+} entry and clear Ca^{2+} from the cytosol. Ryanodine receptors cluster to release calcium sparks, which in turn stimulate Ca^{2+}-activated large conductance K channels (BK channels) to cause hyperpolarization and limit L-type calcium channel activity.[102]

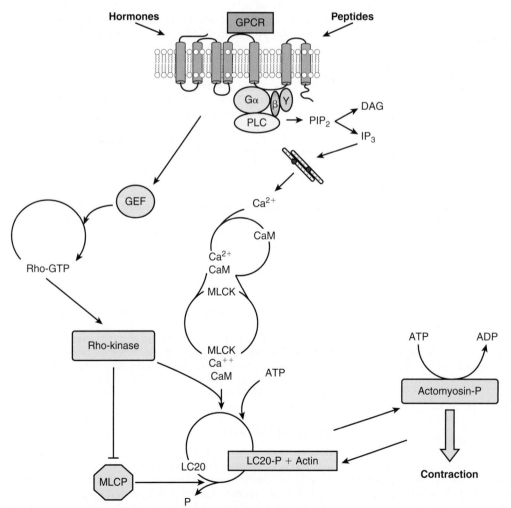

FIGURE 3-6 Model for contraction cascade in vascular smooth muscle cell (VSMC). Binding of contractile agonists to G protein-coupled receptors (GPCRs) activates phospholipase C (PLC) and subsequent PLC-mediated hydrolysis of phosphatidylinositol 4,5-bisphosphate (PIP_2) to release inositol 1,4,5-trisphosphate (IP_3) and diacylglycerol (DAG), leading to increased mobilization of Ca^{2+}. Ca^{2+} combines with calmodulin (CaM) and activates myosin light chain kinase (MLCK)-induced phosphorylation of myosin light chain (MLC), which, together with actin, initiates contraction. In addition, guanine nucleotide exchange factor (GEF) activation of Rho leads to Rho kinase stimulation and inhibition of myosin light chain phosphatase (MLCP), resulting in enhancement of contraction. ADP, adenosine diphosphate; ATP, adenosine triphosphate; GTP, guanosine triphosphate. (Adapted from Griendling K, Harrison D, Alexander R: Biology of the vessel wall. In Fuster V, Walsh R, O'Rourke R, Poole-Wilson P, editors. Hurst's the heart. 12th ed. New York, 2008, McGraw-Hill, pp 135–154.)

Additionally, the sarcoplasmic reticulum Ca^{2+}-ATPase (SERCA) mediates Ca^{2+} reuptake into the SR and serves to maximize Ca^{2+} extrusion from the cell because the newly taken-up SR Ca^{2+} is released in a directed manner towards the plasma membrane, where a plasma membrane Ca^{2+}-ATPase extrudes Ca^{2+} from the cell. Importantly, SERCA is inhibited by CaM kinase II–mediated phosphorylation.[103]

Recently, ROS and reactive nitrogen species (RNS) have emerged as effective modulators of contractile signaling.[104] Specifically, high levels of ROS oxidize SERCA, thereby inhibiting its activity. Hydrogen peroxide applied externally increases IP_3 receptor-mediated release of Ca^{2+} into the cytosol, and activation of NADPH oxidases by contractile agonists sensitizes the IP_3 receptor to IP_3. Ryanodine receptors are also redox-sensitive. S-nitrosylation activates them, and exposure to endogenous levels of ROS and RNS can protect these receptors from inhibition by CaM at high concentrations of calcium. Both hydrogen peroxide and superoxide can stimulate Ca^{2+} entry via L-type or T-type calcium channels (including TRP channels), but S-nitrosylation by nitric oxide (NO) is inhibitory. Thus, in general, ROS and RNS inhibit Ca^{2+} pumps and activate Ca^{2+} entry and release, resulting in an increase in intracellular Ca^{2+} concentration.

Myosin light chain phosphatase (MLCP) is also a vital regulator of vascular contraction. It is a multimeric enzyme composed of a regulatory myosin-binding subunit (MYPT1), a catalytic subunit (PP1c), and a 20-kD protein (M20). The activity of MLCP is largely regulated by Rho kinase-mediated phosphorylation of MYPT1 on Thr695, either directly or via Rho-kinase activation of ZIP kinase.[101] Myosin light chain phosphatase activity can also be inhibited by CPI-17 (PKC-potentiated PP1 inhibitory protein of 17 kD), which when phosphorylated by PKC, acts as a pseudosubstrate, binds to PP1c, and competes with LC20 for phosphorylation. Inhibition of MLCP activity enhances contraction, as mentioned, by inducing Ca^{2+} sensitization of the contractile apparatus.[105]

Rho kinase has thus emerged as an important part of the contraction cascade.[106] In addition to its role in enhancing contraction, such as in response to Ang II, it is a major regulator of relaxation. Its activator, the small-molecular-weight GTPase RhoA, is a target of NO, which by activating protein kinase G (PKG), inactivates Rho, thus indirectly inhibiting Rho kinase, increasing MLCP activity, and inhibiting contraction.

It is noteworthy that paracrine factors such as NO secreted by neighboring ECs represent the major mechanism of vasorelaxation. Shear stress forces and hormones such as acetylcholine or bradykinin stimulate ECs to secrete NO, which in turn initiates VSMC relaxation.[3,107,108] Nitric oxide induces relaxation of smooth muscle potentially via a number of pathways, the most important of which depend on its ability to release cyclic guanosine monophosphate (cGMP). It can directly (via S-nitrosylation of cysteine residues) or indirectly (through PKG) activate BK channels,[109] thus causing membrane hyperpolarization and reducing influx through L-type Ca^{2+} channels. In addition, PKG phosphorylates IP_3 receptor-associated PKG-I substrate (IRAG), which inhibits Ca^{2+} release from IP_3 receptors. Nitric oxide also increases Ca^{2+} uptake via S-glutathionylation of SERCA and decreases the Ca^{2+} sensitivity of contractile proteins. This pathway is perturbed in diabetic animal models, in which high levels of ROS derived from NADPH oxidase 4 irreversibly oxidize SERCA, rendering it insensitive to NO.[110] In addition to regulating Ca^{2+} levels, NO-mediated activation of PKG can phosphorylate PP1c and/or MYPT1 to block vasoconstrictor-mediated inhibition of MLCP.

Other relaxing factors secreted by endothelial cells include hydrogen peroxide, prostaglandins, and epoxyeicosatrienoic acids (EETs). In addition, perivascular adventitial adipocytes (PVAs) have also been shown to secrete factors that influence contractility (reviewed in[111]). These cytokines, collectively known as *adipokines*, are both vasoactive and pro- and antiinflammatory, and include cytokines TNF-α, IL-6, chemokines (IL-8 and monocyte chemoattractant protein [MCP-1]) and hormones (leptin, resistin, and adiponectin).[111,112]

Proliferation

Vascular smooth muscle cell proliferation is important in early vascular development and in repair mechanisms in response to injury. However, excessive VSMC proliferation contributes to pathology, not only in vascular proliferative diseases such as atherosclerosis but also, ironically, as a consequence of the intervention procedures used to treat these occlusive atherosclerotic diseases and their complications, including postangioplasty restenosis, vein bypass graft failure, and transplant failure.[113]

Vascular smooth muscle cell proliferation can be regulated by myriad soluble and insoluble factors that activate a variety of intracellular signaling pathways such as MAPK or Janus kinase/signal transducers, tyrosine phosphorylation, and mitogen-activated proteins.[114,115] Regardless of the initial proliferative stimulus, these signaling pathways ultimately converge onto the cell cycle[116] (Fig. 3-7). The four distinct phases of the cell cycle are: (1) Gap 1 (G1) in which factors necessary for DNA replication are assembled; (2) DNA replication or S phase; (3) Gap 2 (G2) in preparation for mitosis; and (4) mitosis or M phase. Restriction points in the cell cycle exist at transitions between G1/S and G2/M. Progression through the cell cycle phases is regulated by cyclin-dependent kinases (CDKs) and their regulatory cyclin subunits. Cyclins D/E and CDK2, 4, and 5 control G1, cyclin A and CDK2 control the S phase along with the DNA polymerase cofactor PCNA, and cyclins A/B and CDK1 control the M phase. Cyclin-dependent kinases such as $p27^{KIP1}$ and $p21^{CIP1}$ bind to and inhibit the activation of cyclin-CDK complexes (see Fig. 3-7). Activities of these enzymes depend upon phosphorylation status of CDKs, levels of expression of cyclins, and nuclear translocation of cyclin-CDK complexes. One regulatory protein is survivin, which competitively interacts with the CDK4/$p16^{INK4a}$ complex to form a CDK4/survivin complex, thus inducing CDK2/cyclin E activation and S-phase entry and cell cycle progression.[117] Transcription factors that transactivate CDKs and CDKIs also mediate cell cycle progression. It is known that p53, GAX, and GATA-6 induce $p21^{CIP1}$ expression, leading to G1 phase arrest, and E2F transcription factors control the G1/S transition regulated by the retinoblastoma protein Rb, the product of the rb tumor suppressor gene. Rb exerts its negative regulation on the cell cycle by binding to E2F transcription factors, rendering them ineffective as transcription factors. When the Rb/E2F complex is phosphorylated by CDKs in early G1, the complex is dissociated, leaving E2F available to activate genes required for S-phase DNA synthesis.[116] It is worth noting that the HDAC inhibitor trichostatin A blocks proliferation by induction of the cell cycle inhibitor $p21^{CIP1}$ and suppression of Rb protein phosphorylation, leading to subsequent cell cycle arrest at the G1/S phase.[117]

In addition to cell cycle regulatory proteins, telomerase activity is required for VSMC proliferation. Telomeres are noncoding DNA TTAGGG repeat sequences at the ends of chromosomes that cap and stabilize chromosomes against degradation, recombination, or fusion.[118] Associated with telomeric DNA are protein complexes, including telomerase, that synthesize new telomeric DNA in cells with high proliferative potential. Telomerase consists of an RNA component and two protein components, one of which is telomerase reverse transcriptase (TERT), the catalytic component and limiting factor for telomerase activation. When telomerase expression is low, telomere attrition with each mitotic cycle results in chromosome shortening and instability, replicative senescence, and growth arrest. In VSMCs, posttranslational phosphorylation of TERT is linked to telomerase activation, and levels of telomerase expression and activity correlate with proliferation.[118] Importantly, telomerase activation and telomere maintenance have been associated with excessive VSMC proliferation in both animal and human vascular injury and disease;[118] disruption of telomerase activity reduces this proliferative response.

Growth of VSMC is initiated by exposure of the cells to proproliferative signals. Classical growth factors activate RTKs, either directly or via GPCR-mediated transactivation.[116,117] Growth factors in VSMCs binding to RTKs include PDGF, bFGF, IGF-1, TGF-β, EGF,

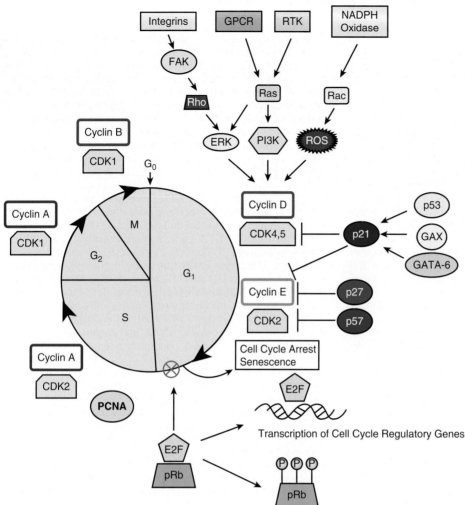

FIGURE 3-7 Model for cell cycle regulation in Vascular smooth muscle cells (VSMCs). Mitogens activate growth factor receptor tyrosine kinase (RTKs), G protein-coupled receptors (GPCRs), NADPH oxidase, and integrins to stimulate extracellular signal regulated kinase (ERK), phosphatidylinositol 3-kinase (PI3K) and Rho/Rac pathways, which converge onto cell cycle components, especially cyclin D, to regulate proliferation. Cyclin regulatory subunits and cyclin-dependent kinases (CDKs) catalytic subunits form holoenzymes that are phase-specific for the four phases of the cell cycle: G1, deoxyribonucleic acid (DNA) replication or S phase, G2, and mitosis or M phase. Endogenous cyclin-dependent kinase inhibitors (CDKIs), including p21, p27, and p57, inactivate cyclin/CDKs and therefore block cell cycle progression and proliferation. Other cell cycle regulators include the tumor suppressor p53 and the transcription factors GAX and GATA-6 that stimulate CDKI p21[CIP1] and induce cell cycle arrest. Cooperating with cyclin/CDKs is proliferating cell nuclear antigen (PCNA) for transition through G1 and S phases. Hyperphosphorylation of the retinoblastoma protein (pRb) releases elongation factor 2F (E2F), allowing cell cycle progression through the G1 phase restriction point and expression of genes required for DNA synthesis. Activation of p53 or Rb pathways results in cell cycle arrest and senescence. (*Adapted from Fuster JJ, Fernandez P, Gonzalez-Navarro H, et al: Control of cell proliferation in atherosclerosis: insights from animal models and human studies. Cardiovasc Res 86:254–264, 2010; and Dzau VJ, Braun-Dullaeus RC, Sedding DG: Vascular proliferation and atherosclerosis: new perspectives and therapeutic strategies. Nat Med 8:1249–1256, 2002.*)

and hypoxia-inducible factor (HIF), and mitogens that activate GPCRs include hormones such as Ang II,[15] endothelin, or oxidized LDL. Activation of these receptors stimulates sequential signaling cascades mediated by Ras, p70[S6K], Rac/NADPH/ROS, PI3K/Akt, MEK/ERK, or MAPKK/p38MAPK, which induce cyclin D1 expression.[115] Src homology 2–containing protein tyrosine phosphatase 2 (SHP2), a member of the non-receptor protein tyrosine phosphatase family, dephosphorylates tyrosine residues on target proteins in response to growth factors, hormones, and cytokines.[119] In VSMCs, SHP2 is a positive mediator of IGF-1- and LPA-induced MAPK signaling pathways; SHP2 has negative effects on EGF- and Ang II-induced Akt signaling, implicating SHP2 in modulating cell cycle progression, growth, and migration.

An important integration point in growth factor signaling is mTOR (mammalian target of rapamycin), which regulates protein synthesis, cell cycle progression, and proliferation.[117] Mammalian target of rapamycin is a protein kinase that regulates translation initiation through effectors p70[S6K] and eIF4E, leading to protein synthesis necessary for cell division. Rapamycin, an immunosuppressive macrolide antibiotic, inhibits mTOR downstream signaling cascades, with reductions in protein synthesis leading to cell cycle arrest.[116] In VSMCs, rapamycin inhibits the mTOR/p70[S6K] signaling axis, promotes a VSMC differentiated, contractile phenotype by regulating transcription of contractile proteins, and induces expression of the antiproliferative CDKIs p21[CIP] and p27[KIP] to inhibit cell cycle progression.[117] Use of rapamycin (sirolimus)-coated coronary stents is highly effective in reducing the postangioplasty restenosis rate in interventional cardiology.[120]

Ion channels for Ca[2+], Mg[2+], and K[+] are also activated by growth factors and mediate proliferation. Transient increases in Ca[2+]

concentration, together with subsequent Ca[2+] binding to its intracellular receptor CaM, are universally required for proliferation.[121] The mechanism for the Ca[2+] sensitivity of this G1-to-S transition involves the Ca[2+]-dependent binding of CaM to cyclin E and activation of CDK2 to promote G1/S transition and VSMC proliferation (reviewed in[122,123]). Elevated levels of Mg[2+] increase expression of cyclin D1 and CDK4 and decrease activation of p21[CIP1] and p27[KIP1] through an ERK1/2-dependent, p38 MAPK-independent pathway.[124] Changes in VSMC K[+] channel expression profiles and activity are linked to cell cycle progression, implicating these ion channels as "internal timers" of VSMC cell division.[125] Growth factor–induced release of Ca[2+] from intracellular Ca[2+] storage organelle activates and up-regulates intermediate-conductance Ca[2+]-activated K[+] (IK$_{Ca}$)-type K[+] channels, the predominant Ca[2+]-sensitive K[+] channel in proliferating VSMCs.[126] In addition, voltage-gated K[+] channels K$_V$1.3[127] and K$_V$3.4[128] are up-regulated in proliferating VSMCs. Blockade of these Ca[2+]-activated and voltage-gated K[+] channels inhibits proliferation and attenuates vascular disease/injury–induced remodeling in rodents.[129]

Signals from insoluble ECM-activated integrins and from soluble growth factor mitogens converge and jointly regulate upstream cytoplasmic signaling networks to mediate expression of cyclin D1 and cyclin E and associated CDK4/6 and CDK2 in the G1 phase, the part of the cell cycle most affected by extracellular stimuli.[130] In addition, joint RTK/integrin complex signaling networks impact G1 phase regulation by inhibiting p21[CIP1] and p27[KIP1], resulting in Rb phosphorylation and induction of E2F-dependent genes, with progression to autonomous stages of the cell cycle (S, G2, and M) that are independent of external stimuli.

As noted previously, Notch proteins are also important regulators of VSMC proliferation (reviewed in[22]). Notch4/HRT-induced repression of p27[KIP1] and Notch3/HRT1-induced repression of p21[CIP1], as well as up-regulation of Akt signaling, an anti-apoptosis pathway, result in promotion of VSMC proliferation. Furthermore, Notch1 is critical in mediating neointimal formation and remodeling after vascular injury.

Peroxisome proliferator-activated receptors (PPARs), nuclear hormone receptors with regulatory roles in lipid and glucose metabolism, are beneficial in VSMCs by targeting genes for cell cycle progression, cellular senescence, and apoptosis to inhibit proliferation and neointimal formation in atherosclerosis and postangioplasty restenosis (reviewed in[131]). Activation of PPARα suppresses G1-to-S progression by inducing expression of p16[INK4a] (a CDKI), thereby inhibiting phosphorylation of Rb.[132] This antiproliferative effect is mediated by repression of telomerase activity by inhibiting E2F binding sites in the TERT promoter.[133] Another PPAR isotype, PPARγ, also blocks G1-to-S cell cycle transition by preventing degradation of p27[KIP1], resulting in inhibition of pRb phosphorylation and suppression of E2F-regulated genes responsible for DNA replication.[131] Similar to PPARα, PPARγ also inhibits telomerase activity in VSMCs by inhibition of early response gene Ets-1-dependent transactivation of the TERT promoter.[131] Thiazolidinediones (TZD), PPARγ agonists used clinically in the treatment of type 2 diabetes mellitus, decrease VSMC proliferation and prevent atherosclerosis in murine models of the disease.[131]

Cyclic adenosine 3′,5′-monophosphate (cAMP) and cGMP are second messengers in myriad signal transduction pathways.[134] In VSMCs, cAMP serves as an antagonist both to mitogenic signaling pathways (by inhibiting MAPK, PI3 kinase, and mTOR signaling axes) and to cell cycle progression (by down-regulating cyclins or up-regulating CDKI p27[KIP1]). An additional antiproliferative effect is due to down-regulation of S-phase kinase-associated protein-2 (Skp2) mediated by inhibition of FAK phosphorylation and adhesion-dependent signaling. Skp2 is a ubiquitin ligase subunit that targets p27[KIP1] for proteasomal degradation, thus promoting VSMC proliferation.[135]

A more recently appreciated pathway that controls VSMC growth involves miRNAs. The potential involvement of these molecules was first noted in balloon-injured rat carotid arteries, where several miRNAs, including miR-21, are up-regulated compared with control arteries (reviewed in[136]). Cell culture models show that miR-21 is a pro-proliferative and anti-apoptotic regulator of VSMCs, with target genes phosphatase and tensin homology deleted from chromosome 10 (PTEN), programmed cell death 4 (PDCD4), and Bcl-2. miR-21 has opposite effects on PTEN and Bcl-2: overexpression down-regulates PTEN and up-regulates Bcl-2. PTEN modulates VSMCs through PI3K and Akt signaling pathways, while Bcl-2 mediates its downstream signaling through AP-1.

Finally, cell-cell junctions, as described above for cadherins and gap junction connexins, and cell-matrix contacts can greatly influence VSMC proliferation (reviewed in[115]). Normally, resident VSMCs, surrounded by and binding to polymerized collagen type 1 fibrils through α2β1 integrins, exhibit low proliferation indices, are arrested in the G1 phase of the cell cycle, and are refractory to mitogenic stimuli. In this quiescent state, levels of cell cycle regulatory proteins are modulated to inhibit the G1/S transition: cyclin E and CDK2 phosphorylation is inhibited, while CDKIs are up-regulated and suppress cyclin E/CDK2 activity. Additionally, p70[S6K], a potent stimulator of mitogenesis and a regulator of p27[KIP1], is suppressed. In contrast, VSMCs on monomeric collagen matrices are responsive to growth factor signals which result in increased cyclin E-associated kinase activity and cell proliferation. These differential responses of VSMCs to structurally distinct forms of collagen type 1 are reflected in the differential regulation of cell cycle proteins and the differential response to mitogenic stimuli. Therefore, perturbations or degradation of the collagen matrix, as found in sites of monomeric collagen in vascular lesions, result in altered VSMC proliferation, response to mitogens, and neointimal formation.[76]

Migration

Smooth muscle migration is an essential element of wound repair, but unchecked migration and proliferation can contribute to neointimal thickening and development of atherosclerotic plaques. A number of promigratory and antimigratory molecules regulate VSMC migration, including peptide growth factors, ECM components, and cytokines.[137] The extent of migration is also influenced by physical factors such as shear stress, stretch, and matrix stiffness. PDGF-BB, bFGF, and S1P are among the most potent promigratory stimuli in the vascular system. Intracellular signaling cascades initiated by these growth factors act in concert with those activated by integrin receptor interaction with matrix to mediate the migratory response. Matrix surrounding the migrating cell must be degraded by MMPs to allow a pathway into which the cell can protrude. Important promigratory matrix components include collagen I and IV, osteopontin, and laminin. Matrix interactions can also be antimigratory, as with the formation of stable focal adhesions, activation of TIMPs, and heparin.

When a cell begins to migrate, a number of coordinated events must take place in a cyclic fashion[138] (Fig. 3-8). Signaling mechanisms that regulate migration have mostly been studied in fibroblasts, but recently many have been confirmed in VSMCs. Migration requires specialized signaling domains at the front and rear of the cell. When confronted with a migratory stimulus, the cell senses the gradient and establishes polarity. Plasma membrane in the form of lamellipodia is then extended in the direction of movement. This process is controlled by reorganization of the actin cytoskeleton just under the protruding membrane. New focal complexes are formed in the lamellipodia via cytoskeletal remodeling and integrin interaction with the matrix. The cell body begins to contract, powered by engagement and phosphorylation of myosin II, and focal adhesions in the rear of the cell become detached, leading to retraction of the "tail" of the cell. Finally, adhesion receptors are recycled by endocytosis and vesicular transport. Successful migration is thus dependent on proper temporal and spatial activation of many molecules, most of which are related to cytoskeletal elements.

Much is known or inferred about the signaling mechanisms activated by PDGF in migrating cells.[137] When PDGF-BB binds to PDGFRs, receptor autophosphorylation creates binding sites for phospholipase Cγ, which mobilizes calcium; PI3K, which forms the membrane-targeting lipid PIP$_2$; and Ras, which activates MAPKs. Nucleation of new actin filaments at the leading edge is initiated by binding of nucleation promoting factors verprolin-homologous protein (WAVE) and Wiskott-Aldrich's syndrome protein (WASP) to actin-related protein ARP2/3; phosphorylation of the actin binding coronin; and dissociation of actin capping proteins, many of which are regulated by PIP$_2$. Extension of new actin filaments is promoted by formins (mDia1 and mDia2), which act on the plus end of actin filaments in coordination with profilin. Regulation of mDia proteins is largely via conformational changes induced by the small G-proteins RhoA and cdc42. Profilin increases nucleotide exchange on G-actin monomers, thus enhancing actin polymerization. Severing of existing actin filaments is a consequence of activation of gelsolin and cofilin, which limit filament length and initiate turnover of existing filaments. Rac also regulates actin reorganization in the lamellipodium, perhaps by activation of p21-activated kinase (PAK)-mediated phosphorylation of actin binding proteins. The result of these complicated, coordinated events is protrusion of lamellipodia in the direction of the detected migratory stimulus (see Fig. 3-8).

Once lamellipodial protrusion has occurred, it is necessary for the cell to create new contacts with the matrix and dissolve ones no longer needed. These nascent focal contacts provide traction for eventual contraction of the cell body and propulsion of the cell forward.[137] Very little is known about focal adhesion composition in VSMCs, but signaling at focal adhesions is coordinated by integrin interaction with the matrix, integrin clustering, activation of a series of protein tyrosine kinases including integrin-linked

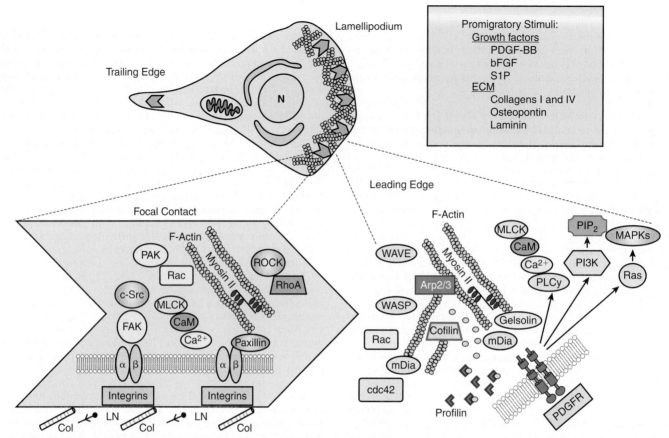

FIGURE 3-8 **Summary of signaling and effectors molecules leading to remodeling of actin cytoskeleton at the leading edge and in focal contacts in migrating vascular smooth muscle cells (VSMCs).** In response to promigratory stimuli and activation of multiple intracellular signaling pathways (details given in text), cells extend lamellipodia and form new focal contacts, areas of dynamic actin turnover. Coordination of actin dynamics depends upon multiple actin binding and associated proteins for actin filament nucleation and extension (actin-related protein [Arp2/3], WAVE, Wiskott-Aldrich's syndrome [WASP], mDia, profilin) and actin filament depolymerization (cofilin) and filament capping and severing (gelsolin), remodeling events regulated by small G-proteins Rho, Rac, and cdc42 and Rho-activated protein kinase (ROCK). Myosin II activation by Ca²⁺/calmodulin (CaM)/myosin light chain kinase (MLCK) and p21-activated kinase (PAK) generates traction forces on the matrix to move the cell forward. In turn, matrix components exert tractile forces by matrix/integrin binding-induced phosphorylation of focal contact components such as paxillin, focal adhesion kinase (FAK) and c-Src, which induce actomyosin motor protein interaction to move the cell forward. *(Adapted from Gerthoffer WT: Mechanisms of vascular smooth muscle cell migration. Circ Res 100:607–621, 2007.)*

kinase (ILK), FAK and Src, and interaction with the cortical F-actin cytoskeleton. Phosphorylation of focal adhesion components including FAK and paxillin occurs during VSMC migration, as does turnover of focal adhesion proteins by membrane-type metalloproteinases. Regulation of focal adhesion turnover is also intimately related to the microtubular network.

The final major event in cell migration is contraction of the cell body. Similar to contraction in differentiated cells, cell body contraction is initiated through calcium-mediated activation of MLCK and MLC phosphorylation following matrix interaction. RhoA and Rho kinase may also play a role because pharmacological inhibition of Rho kinase blocks migration of VSMCs.[139] Current theory suggests that myosin II generates traction forces on the matrix, and the matrix in turn regulates myosin II activation.[137]

Much research remains to fully understand the mechanisms underlying VSMC migration, but the potential for identifying new targets for prevention of restenosis and plaque formation is obvious.

Inflammation

As noted earlier, VSMCs can assume an inflammatory phenotype that is found primarily in atherosclerotic lesions. These cells are found in the media of the vessel wall and express both markers of differentiation and inflammatory genes such as VCAM-1 and exhibit activated NF-κB signaling.[140] One of the primary stimuli for development of this inflammatory phenotype is oxidized LDL, but ECs activated by disturbed flow also contribute to inflammatory changes in VSMC by secreting proinflammatory cytokines.[14]

Oxidized LDL and other cytokines like IL-1β and TNF-α stimulate VSMC expression of chemokines such as MCP-1, TNF-α, and chemokine (C-X-C motif) ligand 1 (CXCL1), as well as adhesion molecules such as VCAM-1, ICAM-1, and CCR-2, the receptor for MCP-1. Because many of these molecules activate NF-κB, exposure to one of them often induces the expression of others, resulting in propagation of a positive feedback signaling mechanism to enhance the local inflammatory response. The end result is recruitment and adhesion of T cells and monocytes to smooth muscle cells (SMCs) in the vessel wall.

Proinflammatory gene expression in VSMC, as in other cell types, is largely a consequence of posttranscriptional regulation of inflammatory gene expression by the stress-activated protein kinase p38MAPK and transcriptional regulation by proinflammatory transcription factors such as NF-κB and STAT1/3. Both of these pathways are activated by ROS, which have been shown to be increased in inflammatory regions of plaques as a result of macrophage infiltration as well as direct stimulation of VSMCs by cytokines. Stimulation of cytokine receptors activates p38MAPK, which controls proinflammatory protein levels by MAPKAPK-2 mediated phosphorylation of adenylate uridylate–rich elements (AREs) binding proteins such as tristetraprolin (TTP), thus promoting mRNA stability of TNF-α.[141] Many other inflammatory gene mRNAs, including MCP-1, IL-1β, IL-8, intercellular adhesion molecule 1 (ICAM-1), and VCAM-1, also contain AREs. It should be noted that ARE binding proteins can both stabilize and destabilize mRNA: HuR protects ARE-containing transcripts from degradation, but AUF1 destabilizes its targets. p38MAPK can also regulate inflammatory protein expression by translational regulation via activation of MAPK signal-integrating kinase-1 (Mnk-1), which phosphorylates the translation initiation factor eIF-4E and enhances its affinity for the mRNA cap.[142] Transcriptional regulation of proinflammatory gene expression is largely a consequence of activation of the NF-κB pathway. Commonly, the p65-p50 heterodimer is the transactivating factor that binds to NF-κB-containing elements to increase proinflammatory gene transcription. Regulation of gene expression by STATs is a consequence of the canonical tyrosine kinase receptor activation of JAK, and subsequent phosphorylation of STAT followed by translocation to the nucleus.

Another major environmental factor that contributes to maintenance of the VSMC proinflammatory phenotype is the matrix milieu in which cells exist. In atherosclerotic plaques, VSMCs begin to secrete collagen I and collagen III, but also, as a result of NF-κB activation, express MMP-1, MMP-3, and MMP-9, which degrade collagen fibrils to the monomeric form, thus promoting an inflammatory phenotype, as evidenced by an increase in VCAM-1 expression.[75] A similar response is seen to osteopontin, which is also increased in atherosclerosis.[143] The effects of these matrix proteins on VSMCs are mediated by binding to specific integrins, most likely α5β1 or αvβ3.[14] The nonintegrin matrix receptor CD44, which binds to hyaluronic acid in the matrix, has also been implicated in the transition to the proinflammatory phenotype, as shown by its ability to stimulate VCAM-1 expression.[144]

Senescence, Apoptosis, and Autophagy

In response to aging and oxidative stress, cells that have accumulated damaged organelles/proteins/DNA due to limitations in DNA repair or antioxidant mechanisms rely on two processes to avoid replication and passing the damage to daughter cells: permanently arresting the cell cycle (senescence), or programmed cell death, including apoptosis (self-killing) or autophagy (self-eating).[145]

Senescent cells are permanently arrested in the G1 phase of the cell cycle and exhibit specific senescence-associated markers such as β-galactosidase, heterochromatin foci, and accumulation of lipofuscin granules. Unlike quiescent cells, senescent cells are not responsive to growth factors.[146] Multiple stresses, including DNA-damaging radiation or chemicals, mitochondrial dysfunction, and oxidant stress, can invoke two types of senescence programs: stress-induced premature senescence (SIPS) and replicative senescence associated with accelerated telomere uncapping or shortening.[147] These diverse stimulatory pathways converge onto two effector pathways: the tumor suppressor protein p53 and the Rb pathways; p53 is normally targeted to proteasome-mediated degradation by mouse double minute 2 MDM2. Mitogenic stress or DNA damage suppresses MDM2 activity, resulting in p53-mediated activation of the CDKI p21 and cell cycle arrest.[145] In the second pathway, stress or damage activates Rb, which then binds to and inhibits E2F, a transcription factor required for the G1 phase/S phase transition to cell cycle progression (see Fig. 3-7). These two senescence pathways exhibit cross-talk at the level of p53 and can overlap death pathways. Senescent cells release degradative proteases, growth factors, and inflammatory cytokines, which impact on neighboring cells.

In VSMCs, DNA damage caused by ROS (e.g., superoxide, hydrogen peroxide, hydroxyl radicals) incites rapid (within days) SIPS. There are increased levels of ROS in all diseased layers of an atherosclerotic lesion, particularly in the plaque itself,[147] and senescent VSMCs have been identified in injured arteries and in the intima of atherosclerotic plaques.[148]

Many of the changes in senescent VSMCs are reminiscent of changes indicative in age-related vascular disease, implicating cellular senescence in vascular pathologies.[148] Therefore, a model for how senescence contributes to vascular disease emerges. Atherogenic stimuli such as Ang II initially stimulate proliferation, followed by mitogen-induced SIPS or replicative senescence via telomere uncapping. Inflammatory cytokine/chemokine release by senescent VSMCs results in ECM degradation. The decreased cellularity and increased inflammation contribute to plaque instability.[148]

Senescent VSMCs are also implicated in vascular calcification. They exhibit enhanced expression of osteoblastic genes such as alkaline phosphatase (ALP), type 1 collagen, and RUNX-2, while expression of matrix Gla protein (MGP), an anticalcification factor, is down-regulated.[149]

Apoptosis, the controlled activation of proteases and hydrolases within an intact cell's plasma membrane boundary so that neighboring cells are not affected and an immune response is not triggered,[150] is an important mechanism for blood vessel remodeling during proliferative vascular disease and after therapeutic interventions (e.g., angioplasty/stenting of arteries, vein bypass graft surgery).[151] Mitogens such as thrombin or PDGF can induce proliferative episodes in VSMCs within atherosclerotic lesions (reviewed in[152]). Proliferation is counterbalanced by death-inducing VSMC apoptosis triggered by a variety of proinflammatory mediators, cytokines, oxidized lipids, and free radicals produced by immune cells within the plaque. These proinflammatory mediators activate caspases, components of the extrinsic death receptor pathway (e.g., Fas/CD95 TRAIL [TNF-related apoptosis-inducing ligand]), and/or cause intrinsic mitochondrial dysfunction in VSMCs under the control of Bcl family members (reviewed in[153]).

Interactions among mitogenic, apoptotic, and survival signals produce a variety of lesion characteristics and determine whether there is a fragile fibrous cap poised for rupture, a lipid-rich necrotic core, or a fibrotic and calcified core (reviewed in[152]). High percentages of apoptotic VSMCs within atherosclerotic plaques are one of the major causes of plaque rupture due to decreased cellularity in the media and thinning of the fibrous cap. In addition, reduced phagocytotic clearance of apoptotic VSMCs, resulting in necrotic VSMCs, and low levels of VSMC apoptosis over extended periods of hyperlipidemia induce viable VSMC release of IL-6 and MCP-1 to produce chronic inflammation.[154] Apoptotic VSMCs also generate thrombin, promoting coagulation.[152]

Vascular smooth muscle cell apoptosis has also been associated with other lesion characteristics including inflammation, calcification, thrombosis, and aneurysms (reviewed in[156]). In vivo, VSMC apoptosis causes release of cytokines and MCP-1, recruiting macrophages. Vascular calcification has been associated with inorganic phosphate–induced VSMC apoptosis and subsequent generation of VSMC-derived matrix vesicles that serve as the nidus for calcification (reviewed in[156]). Statins restore the Gas6-mediated survival pathway and inhibit VSMC calcification by preventing apoptosis.

In addition to apoptosis, autophagy, a survival process by which the cell degrades its own components, such as damaged organelles or long-lived aberrant or aggregated proteins,[145] contributes to pathology in atherosclerotic plaques. Ultrastructural analysis of VSMCs in the fibrous cap of advanced plaques reveals characteristics of cells undergoing autophagic degradation.[157] Because autophagy is a survival mechanism and not a death pathway, VSMC autophagy in the fibrous cap may function in plaque stability and protection from oxidative stress.[157] If oxidative stress damages lysosomal membranes, lysosome/autophagic vacuole fusion is impaired and apoptosis ensues.

Stem/Progenitor Cells

The ability of stem cells to differentiate into a variety of cell types has led to research on the potential efficacy of using pluripotent embryonic stem cells as a source of VSMCs for regenerative cell-based therapies and tissue engineering in injury/disease repair. Research on the role of putative resident adult stem cells in bone marrow and/or unipotent lineage committed VSMC progenitor cells within the circulating blood, vascular wall, or other peripheral tissues in the development of the neointima in atherosclerotic lesions is also ongoing.[158-161]

Pluripotent embryonic stem cells (ESCs) form embryoid bodies *in vitro* that contain isolated areas of contractile SMCs induced by endogenous TGF-β.[162] Because undifferentiated ESCs have the potential to form teratocarcinomas, the ability to isolate pure populations of differentiated cells is essential for use of ESCs in tissue-engineering applications. An alternative method for tissue regeneration is to reprogram somatic cells to resemble ESCs. Somatic cells can be induced to form pluripotent stem cells (iPS) by addition of defined factors such as Sox2, Oct4, KLF4, and c-myc (reviewed in[163]).

Multipotent adipose-derived mesenchymal stem cells (MSCs) are candidates for a VSMC source for tissue-engineered blood vessels because these MSCs can be easily obtained from human lipoaspirate, readily expanded in culture, and differentiated into contractile VSMC-like cells in culture media containing both TGF-β and BMP-4.[164]

Initial hypotheses for the origin of neointimal VSMCs proposed that injury-induced growth factors and ECM proteolysis caused a VSMC phenotypic switch from a quiescent, contractile phenotype to a synthetic type, resulting in proliferation and migration of a small number of clonal or oligoclonal VSMCs from the underlying media into the intima where remodeling led to plaque formation and lumen occlusion. Subsequent evidence suggested that circulating bone marrow–derived SMC progenitor cells may contribute to normal vascular injury repair and formation of the neointima in vascular lesions.[2,158] However, the origin of intimal VSMCs from bone marrow–derived progenitor cells in the blood in response to injury or disease has been disputed.[165,166] In long-term studies of transplanted bone marrow cells into lethally irradiated mice with wire injury, the bone marrow–derived cells, initially found in high numbers in the neointima, were not stable residents, and the few remaining after 16 weeks did not exhibit definitive VSMC marker proteins calponin and SM MHC. Additionally, the adventitial layer of the wall serves as a niche for wall-derived MSCs and VSMC progenitor cells,[161] including resident stem cell antigen-1 (Sca-1)-positive cells, maintained in the adventitia by Shh signaling and myocardin transcriptional corepressors, which are capable of differentiating into VSMCs.[167] This population of Sca1+ progenitor cells in the arterial adventitia could contribute to vessel wall remodeling in injury/disease. The prevailing hypothesis is that neointimal VSMCs originate from the injured media and also from local resident progenitors in the adventitia.[166]

The nature of VSMC phenotype plasticity, exemplified in distinct genetic expression patterns of marker genes and thus in differential functions, complicates the definition and identification of VSMCs derived from bone marrow resident and circulating stem/progenitor cells.[168] The safe and effective use of regenerative VSMCs in translational clinical therapy for cardiovascular disease awaits further methodologies for identifying, producing, and isolating cells that will differentiate into VSMCs.

Conclusions

The protean nature of VSMCs is fundamental not only to their contractile and synthetic functions within the normal vessel wall during development and maturation, but also to vascular remodeling in response to injury and disease. As evidenced in this chapter, recent advances in studies from animal models, the clinic, and basic cell biology laboratories have enhanced our understanding of the factors, both intrinsic in the genetic code and extrinsic in environmental cues, that regulate and control VSMC plasticity. Future challenges include how to translate this understanding into developing clinically effective pharmacological interventions for treatment of cardiovascular disease and into producing functional tissue-engineered vascular constructs for diseased/injured vessel replacement.

REFERENCES

1. Wagenseil JE, Mecham RP: Vascular extracellular matrix and arterial mechanics, *Physiol Rev* 89(3):957–989, 2009.
2. Owens GK, Kumar MS, Wamhoff BR: Molecular regulation of vascular smooth muscle cell differentiation in development and disease, *Physiol Rev* 84(3):767–801, 2004.
3. Beamish JA, He P, Kottke-Marchant K, et al: Molecular regulation of contractile smooth muscle cell phenotype: implications for vascular tissue engineering, *Tissue Eng Part B Rev* 16(5):467–491, 2010.
4. Herbert SP, Huisken J, Kim TN, et al: Arterial-venous segregation by selective cell sprouting: an alternative mode of blood vessel formation, *Science* 326(5950):294–298, 2009.
5. Swift MR, Weinstein BM: Arterial-venous specification during development, *Circ Res* 104(5):576–588, 2009.
6. Anderson LM, Gibbons GH: Notch: a mastermind of vascular morphogenesis, *J Clin Invest* 117(2):299–302, 2007.
7. Jain RK: Molecular regulation of vessel maturation, *Nat Med* 9(6):685–693, 2003.
8. Majesky MW: Developmental basis of vascular smooth muscle diversity, *Arterioscler Thromb Vasc Biol* 27(6):1248–1258, 2007.
9. Hao H, Gabbiani G, Bochaton-Piallat M-L: Arterial smooth muscle cell heterogeneity: implications for atherosclerosis and restenosis development, *Arterioscler Thromb Vasc Biol* 23(9):1510–1520, 2003.
10. Larsson E, McLean SE, Mecham RP, et al: Do two mutually exclusive gene modules define the phenotypic diversity of mammalian smooth muscle? *Mol Genet Genomics* 280(2):127–137, 2008.
11. Moiseeva EP: Adhesion receptors of vascular smooth muscle cells and their functions, *Cardiovasc Res* 52(3):372–386, 2001.
12. Rensen SS, Doevendans PA, van Eys GJ: Regulation and characteristics of vascular smooth muscle cell phenotypic diversity, *Neth Heart J* 15(3):100–108, 2007.
13. Rzucidlo EM: Signaling pathways regulating vascular smooth muscle cell differentiation, *Vascular* 17(Suppl 1):S15–S20, 2009.
14. Orr AW, Hastings NE, Blackman BR, et al: Complex regulation and function of the inflammatory smooth muscle cell phenotype in atherosclerosis, *J Vasc Res* 47(2):168–180, 2010.
15. Berk BC: Vascular smooth muscle growth: autocrine growth mechanisms, *Physiol Rev* 81(3):999–1030, 2001.
16. Griendling K, Harrison D, Alexander R: Biology of the vessel wall. In Fuster V, Walsh R, O'Rourke R and Poole-Wilson P, editors: *Hurst's the heart*, ed 12, New York, 2008, McGraw Hill, pp 135–154.
17. Garrido AM, Griendling KK: NADPH oxidases and angiotensin II receptor signaling, *Mol Cell Endocrinol* 302(2):148–158, 2009.
18. Pardali E, Goumans M-J, ten Dijke P: Signaling by members of the TGF-β family in vascular morphogenesis and disease, *Trends Cell Biol* 20(9):556–567, 2010.
19. Mehta PK, Griendling KK: Angiotensin II cell signaling: physiological and pathological effects in the cardiovascular system, *Am J Physiol Cell Physiol* 292(1):C82–C97, 2007.
20. Yoshida T, Owens GK: Molecular determinants of vascular smooth muscle cell diversity, *Circ Res* 96(3):280–291, 2005.
21. High FA, Zhang M, Proweller A, et al: An essential role for Notch in neural crest during cardiovascular development and smooth muscle differentiation, *J Clin Invest* 117(2):353–363, 2007.
22. Gridley T: Notch signaling in the vasculature, *Curr Top Dev Biol* 92:277–309, 2010.
23. Tang Y, Urs S, Liaw L: Hairy-related transcription factors inhibit Notch-induced smooth muscle α-actin expression by interfering with Notch intracellular domain/CBF-1 complex interaction with the CBF-1-binding site, *Circ Res* 102(6):661–668, 2008.
24. Tang Y, Urs S, Boucher J, et al: Notch and transforming growth factor-beta (TGFβ) signaling pathways cooperatively regulate vascular smooth muscle cell differentiation, *J Biol Chem* 285(23):17556–17563, 2010.
25. Morrow D, Cullen JP, Liu W, et al: Sonic hedgehog induces Notch target gene expression in vascular smooth muscle cells via VEGF-A, *Arterioscler Thromb Vasc Biol* 29(7):1112–1118, 2009.
26. Jin S, Hansson EM, Tikka S, et al: Notch signaling regulates platelet-derived growth factor receptor-β expression in vascular smooth muscle cells, *Circ Res* 102(12):1483–1491, 2008.
27. Wang D-Z, Olson EN: Control of smooth muscle development by the myocardin family of transcriptional coactivators, *Curr Opin Genet Dev* 14(5):558–566, 2004.
28. Miano JM, Long X, Fujiwara K: Serum response factor: master regulator of the actin cytoskeleton and contractile apparatus, *Am J Physiol Cell Physiol* 292(1):C70–C81, 2007.
29. Parmacek MS: Myocardin-related transcription factors: critical coactivators regulating cardiovascular development and adaptation, *Circ Res* 100(5):633–644, 2007.
30. Pipes GC, Creemers EE, Olson EN: The myocardin family of transcriptional coactivators: versatile regulators of cell growth, migration, and myogenesis, *Genes Dev* 20(12):1545–1556, 2006.
31. Davis CA, Haberland M, Arnold MA, et al: PRISM/PRDM6, a transcriptional repressor that promotes the proliferative gene program in smooth muscle cells, *Mol Cell Biol* 26(7):2626–2636, 2006.
32. Haldar SM, Ibrahim OA, Jain MK: Kruppel-like factors (KLFs) in muscle biology, *J Mol Cell Cardiol* 43(1):1–10, 2007.
33. Zheng B, Han M, Wen JK: Role of Krüppel-like factor 4 in phenotypic switching and proliferation of vascular smooth muscle cells, *IUBMB Life* 62(2):132–139, 2010.
34. Miano JM: Deck of CArGs, *Circ Res* 103(1):13–15, 2008.
35. Olson EN, Nordheim A: Linking actin dynamics and gene transcription to drive cellular motile functions, *Nat Rev Mol Cell Biol* 11(5):353–365, 2010.
36. Liu N, Olson EN: Coactivator control of cardiovascular growth and remodeling, *Curr Opin Cell Biol* 18(6):715–722, 2006.
37. Posern G, Treisman R: Actin' together: serum response factor, its cofactors and the link to signal transduction, *Trends Cell Biol* 16(11):588–596, 2006.
38. Parmacek MS: Myocardin: dominant driver of the smooth muscle cell contractile phenotype, *Arterioscler Thromb Vasc Biol* 28(8):1416–1417, 2008.

39. Dong J-T, Chen C: Essential role of KLF5 transcription factor in cell proliferation and differentiation and its implications for human diseases, *Cell Mol Life Sci* 66(16):2691–2706, 2009.
40. Kawai-Kowase K, Owens GK: Multiple repressor pathways contribute to phenotypic switching of vascular smooth muscle cells, *Am J Physiol Cell Physiol* 292(1):C59–C69, 2007.
41. Liu Y: Wen J-K, Dong L-H, et al: Kruppel-like factor (KLF) 5 mediates cyclin D1 expression and cell proliferation via interaction with c-Jun in Ang II-induced VSMCs, *Acta Pharmacol Sin* 31(1):10–18, 2009.
42. Suzuki T, Sawaki D, Aizawa K, et al: Kruppel-like factor 5 shows proliferation-specific roles in vascular remodeling, direct stimulation of cell growth, and inhibition of apoptosis, *J Biol Chem* 284(14):9549–9557, 2009.
43. Nagai R, Suzuki T, Aizawa K, et al: Significance of the transcription factor KLF5 in cardiovascular remodeling, *J Thromb Haemost* 3(8):1569–1576, 2005.
44. Liu N, Olson EN: MicroRNA regulatory networks in cardiovascular development, *Dev Cell* 18(4):510–525, 2010.
45. Eulalio A, Huntzinger E, Izaurralde E: Getting to the root of miRNA-mediated gene silencing, *Cell* 132(1):9–14, 2008.
46. Djuranovic S, Nahvi A, Green R: A parsimonious model for gene regulation by miRNAs, *Science* 331(6017):550–553, 2011.
47. Bartel DP: MicroRNAs: target recognition and regulatory functions, *Cell* 136(2):215–233, 2009.
48. Cheng Y, Liu X, Yang J, et al: MicroRNA-145, a novel smooth muscle cell phenotypic marker and modulator, controls vascular neointimal lesion formation, *Circ Res* 105(2):158–166, 2009.
49. Cordes KR, Sheehy NT, White MP, et al: miR-145 and miR-143 regulate smooth muscle cell fate and plasticity, *Nature* 460(7256):705–710, 2009.
50. Xin M, Small EM, Sutherland LB, et al: MicroRNAs miR-143 and miR-145 modulate cytoskeletal dynamics and responsiveness of smooth muscle cells to injury, *Genes Dev* 23(18):2166–2178, 2009.
51. Boettger T, Beetz N, Kostin S, et al: Acquisition of the contractile phenotype by murine arterial smooth muscle cells depends on the Mir143/145 gene cluster, *J Clin Invest* 119(9):2634–2647, 2009.
52. Song Z, Li G: Role of specific microRNAs in regulation of vascular smooth muscle cell differentiation and the response to injury, *J Cardiovasc Transl Res* 3(3):246–250, 2010.
53. Liu X, Cheng Y, Zhang S, et al: A necessary role of miR-221 and miR-222 in vascular smooth muscle cell proliferation and neointimal hyperplasia, *Circ Res* 104(4):476–487, 2009.
54. Davis BN, Hilyard AC, Nguyen PH, et al: Induction of microRNA-221 by platelet-derived growth factor signaling is critical for modulation of vascular smooth muscle phenotype, *J Biol Chem* 284(6):3728–3738, 2009.
55. McDonald OG, Owens GK: Programming smooth muscle plasticity with chromatin dynamics, *Circ Res* 100(10):1428–1441, 2007.
56. McDonald OG, Wamhoff BR, Hoofnagle MH, et al: Control of SRF binding to CArG box chromatin regulates smooth muscle gene expression *in vivo*, *J Clin Invest* 116(1):36–48, 2006.
57. Mohammad HP, Baylin SB: Linking cell signaling and the epigenetic machinery, *Nat Biotech* 28(10):1033–1038, 2010.
58. Qiu P, Ritchie RP, Gong XQ, et al: Dynamic changes in chromatin acetylation and the expression of histone acetyltransferases and histone deacetylases regulate the SM22α transcription in response to Smad3-mediated TGFβ_1 signaling, *Biochem Biophys Res Commun* 348(2):351–358, 2006.
59. Villeneuve LM, Reddy MA, Lanting LL, et al: Epigenetic histone H3 lysine 9 methylation in metabolic memory and inflammatory phenotype of vascular smooth muscle cells in diabetes, *Proc Natl Acad Sci U S A* 105(26):9047–9052, 2008.
60. Ceriello A, Ihnat MA, Thorpe JE: The "metabolic memory": is more than just tight glucose control necessary to prevent diabetic complications? *J Clin Endocrinol Metab* 94(2): 410–415, 2009.
61. Paik JH, Skoura A, Chae SS, et al: Sphingosine 1-phosphate receptor regulation of N-cadherin mediates vascular stabilization, *Genes Dev* 18(19):2392–2403, 2004.
62. George SJ, Dwivedi A: MMPs, cadherins, and cell proliferation, *Trends Cardiovasc Med* 14(3):100–105, 2004.
63. Figueroa XF, Duling BR: Gap junctions in the control of vascular function, *Antioxid Redox Signal* 11(2):251–266, 2009.
64. Brisset AC, Isakson BE, Kwak BR: Connexins in vascular physiology and pathology, *Antioxid Redox Signal* 11(2):267–282, 2009.
65. Johnstone S, Isakson B, Locke D: Biological and biophysical properties of vascular connexin channels, *Int Rev Cell Mol Biol* 278:69–118, 2009.
66. Wang L, Zheng J, Du Y, et al: Cartilage oligomeric matrix protein maintains the contractile phenotype of vascular smooth muscle cells by interacting with $\alpha7\beta1$ integrin, *Circ Res* 106(3):514–525, 2010.
67. Tkachenko E, Rhodes JM, Simons M: Syndecans: new kids on the signaling block, *Circ Res* 96(5):488–500, 2005.
68. Alexopoulou AN, Multhaupt HAB, Couchman JR: Syndecans in wound healing, inflammation and vascular biology, *Int J Biochem Cell Biol* 39(3):505–528, 2007.
69. Fukai N, Kenagy RD, Chen L, et al: Syndecan-1: an inhibitor of arterial smooth muscle cell growth and intimal hyperplasia, *Arterioscler Thromb Vasc Biol* 29(9):1356–1362, 2009.
70. Kelleher CM, McLean SE, Mecham RP: Vascular extracellular matrix and aortic development, *Curr Top Dev Biol* 62:153–188, 2004.
71. Hynes RO: The extracellular matrix: not just pretty fibrils, *Science* 326(5957):1216–1219, 2009.
72. Järveläinen H, Sainio A, Koulu M, et al: Extracellular matrix molecules: potential targets in pharmacotherapy, *Pharmacol Rev* 61(2):198–223, 2009.
73. Mao Y, Schwarzbauer JE: Fibronectin fibrillogenesis, a cell-mediated matrix assembly process, *Matrix Biol* 24(6):389–399, 2005.
74. Singh P, Carraher C, Schwarzbauer JE: Assembly of fibronectin extracellular matrix, *Annu Rev Cell Dev Biol* 26:397–419, 2010.
75. Orr AW, Lee MY, Lemmon JA, et al: Molecular mechanisms of collagen isotype-specific modulation of smooth muscle cell phenotype, *Arterioscler Thromb Vasc Biol* 29(2):225–231, 2009.
76. Koyama H, Raines EW, Bornfeldt KE, et al: Fibrillar collagen inhibits arterial smooth muscle proliferation through regulation of Cdk2 inhibitors, *Cell* 87(6):1069–1078, 1996.
77. Kielty CM, Sherratt MJ, Shuttleworth CA: Elastic fibres, *J Cell Sci* 115(14):2817–2828, 2002.
78. Kielty CM: Elastic fibres in health and disease, *Expert Rev Mol Med* 8(19):1–23, 2006.
79. Karnik SK, Brooke BS, Bayes-Genis A, et al: A critical role for elastin signaling in vascular morphogenesis and disease, *Development* 130(2):411–423, 2003.
80. Ramirez F, Rifkin DB: Extracellular microfibrils: contextual platforms for TGFβ and BMP signaling, *Curr Opin Cell Biol* 21(5):616–622, 2009.
81. Ramirez F, Sakai L: Biogenesis and function of fibrillin assemblies, *Cell Tissue Res* 339(1): 71–82, 2010.
82. Yanagisawa H, Davis EC: Unraveling the mechanism of elastic fiber assembly: the roles of short fibulins, *Int J Biochem Cell Biol* 42(7):1084–1093, 2010.
83. Chapman SL, Sicot F-X, Davis EC, et al: Fibulin-2 and fibulin-5 cooperatively function to form the internal elastic lamina and protect from vascular injury, *Arterioscler Thromb Vasc Biol* 30(1):68–74, 2010.
84. Zacchigna L, Vecchione C, Notte A, et al: Emilin1 links TGF-β maturation to blood pressure homeostasis, *Cell* 124(5):929–942, 2006.
85. Zanetti M, Braghetta P, Sabatelli P, et al: EMILIN-1 deficiency induces elastogenesis and vascular cell defects, *Mol Cell Biol* 24(2):638–650, 2004.
86. Couchman JR: Transmembrane signaling proteoglycans, *Annu Rev Cell Dev Biol* 26:89–114, 2010.
87. Wight TN: Arterial remodeling in vascular disease: a key role for hyaluronan and versican, *Front Biosci* 13:4933–4937, 2008.
88. Ballinger ML, Ivey ME, Osman N, et al: Endothelin-1 activates ETA receptors on human vascular smooth muscle cells to yield proteoglycans with increased binding to LDL, *Atherosclerosis* 205(2):451–457, 2009.
89. Chen C-C, Lau LF: Functions and mechanisms of action of CCN matricellular proteins, *Int J Biochem Cell Biol* 41(4):771–783, 2009.
90. Matsumae H, Yoshida Y, Ono K, et al: CCN1 knockdown suppresses neointimal hyperplasia in a rat artery balloon injury model, *Arterioscler Thromb Vasc Biol* 28(6):1077–1083, 2008.
91. Shimoyama T, Hiraoka S, Takemoto M, et al: CCN3 inhibits neointimal hyperplasia through modulation of smooth muscle cell growth and migration, *Arterioscler Thromb Vasc Biol* 30(4):675–682, 2010.
92. Newby AC: Dual role of matrix metalloproteinases (matrixins) in intimal thickening and atherosclerotic plaque rupture, *Physiol Rev* 85(1):1–31, 2005.
93. Newby AC: Matrix metalloproteinases regulate migration, proliferation, and death of vascular smooth muscle cells by degrading matrix and non-matrix substrates, *Cardiovasc Res* 69(3):614–624, 2006.
94. Nagase H, Visse R, Murphy G: Structure and function of matrix metalloproteinases and TIMPs, *Cardiovasc Res* 69(3):562–573, 2006.
95. Raffetto JD, Khalil RA: Matrix metalloproteinases and their inhibitors in vascular remodeling and vascular disease, *Biochem Pharmacol* 75(2):346–359, 2008.
96. Newby AC: Metalloproteinases and vulnerable atherosclerotic plaques, *Trends Cardiovasc Med* 17(8):253–258, 2007.
97. Assoian RK, Klein EA: Growth control by intracellular tension and extracellular stiffness, *Trends Cell Biol* 18(7):347–352, 2008.
98. Klein EA, Yin L, Kothapalli D, et al: Cell-cycle control by physiological matrix elasticity and *in vivo* tissue stiffening, *Curr Biol* 19(18):1511–1518, 2009.
99. Watanabe H, Murakami M, Ohba T, et al: TRP channel and cardiovascular disease, *Pharmacol Ther* 118(3):337–351, 2008.
100. Akata T: Cellular and molecular mechanisms regulating vascular tone. Part 1: basic mechanisms controlling cytosolic Ca^{2+} concentration and the Ca^{2+}-dependent regulation of vascular tone, *J Anesth* 21(2):220–231, 2007.
101. Kim HR, Appel S, Vetterkind S, et al: Smooth muscle signalling pathways in health and disease, *J Cell Mol Med* 12(6A):2165–2180, 2008.
102. Essin K, Gollasch M: Role of ryanodine receptor subtypes in initiation and formation of calcium sparks in arterial smooth muscle: comparison with striated muscle, *J Biomed Biotechnol* 2009.
103. Sathish V, Thompson MA, Bailey JP, et al: Effect of proinflammatory cytokines on regulation of sarcoplasmic reticulum Ca^{2+} reuptake in human airway smooth muscle, *Am J Physiol Lung Cell Mol Physiol* 297(1):L26–L34, 2009.
104. Trebak M, Ginnan R, Singer HA, et al: Interplay between calcium and reactive oxygen/nitrogen species: an essential paradigm for vascular smooth muscle signaling, *Antioxid Redox Signal* 12(5):657–674, 2010.
105. Berk B: Vascular smooth muscle. In Creager M, Dzau V, Loscalzo J, editors: *Vascular medicine: a companion to Braunwald's heart disease*, ed 1, Philadelphia, 2006, Saunders-Elsevier, pp 17–30.
106. Hilgers RHP, Webb RC: Molecular aspects of arterial smooth muscle contraction: focus on Rho, *Exp Biol Med* 230(11):829–835, 2005.
107. Masaki T: Historical review: endothelin, *Trends Pharmacol Sci* 25(4):219–224, 2004.
108. Tsutsui M, Shimokawa H, Otsuji Y, et al: Pathophysiological relevance of NO signaling in the cardiovascular system: novel insight from mice lacking all NO synthases, *Pharmacol Ther* 128(3):499–508, 2010.
109. Gao Y, Yang Y, Guan Q, et al: IL-1beta modulate the Ca(2+)-activated big-conductance K channels (BK) via reactive oxygen species in cultured rat aorta smooth muscle cells, *Mol Cell Biochem* 338(1–2):59–68, 2010.
110. Tong X, Hou X, Jourd'heuil D, et al: Upregulation of Nox4 by TGFβ1 oxidizes SERCA and inhibits NO in arterial smooth muscle of the prediabetic Zucker rat, *Circ Res* 107(8):975–983, 2010.
111. Rajsheker S, Manka D, Blomkalns AL, et al: Crosstalk between perivascular adipose tissue and blood vessels, *Curr Opin Pharmacol* 10(2):191–196, 2010.
112. Zhang H, Cui J, Zhang C: Emerging role of adipokines as mediators in atherosclerosis, *World J Cardiol* 2(11):370–376, 2010.
113. Fuster JJ, Fernandez P, Gonzalez-Navarro H, et al: Control of cell proliferation in atherosclerosis: insights from animal models and human studies, *Cardiovasc Res* 86(2):254–264, 2010.
114. Griendling KK, Ushio-Fukai M, Lassegue B, et al: Angiotensin II signaling in vascular smooth muscle: new concepts, *Hypertension* 29(1):366–370, 1997.

115. Schwartz MA, Assoian RK: Integrins and cell proliferation: regulation of cyclin-dependent kinases via cytoplasmic signaling pathways, *J Cell Sci* 114(14):2553–2560, 2001.

116. Dzau VJ, Braun-Dullaeus RC, Sedding DG: Vascular proliferation and atherosclerosis: new perspectives and therapeutic strategies, *Nat Med* 8(11):1249–1256, 2002.

117. Marsboom G, Archer SL: Pathways of proliferation: new targets to inhibit the growth of vascular smooth muscle cells, *Circ Res* 103(10):1047–1049, 2008.

118. Fuster JJ, Andres V: Telomere biology and cardiovascular disease, *Circ Res* 99(11):1167–1180, 2006.

119. Kandadi MR, Stratton MS, Ren J: The role of Src homology 2 containing protein tyrosine phosphatase 2 in vascular smooth muscle cell migration and proliferation, *Acta Pharmacol Sin* 31(10):1277–1283, 2010.

120. Abizaid A: Sirolimus-eluting coronary stents: a review, *Vasc Health Risk Manag* 3(2):191–201, 2007.

121. Kahl CR, Means AR: Regulation of cell cycle progression by calcium/calmodulin-dependent pathways, *Endocr Rev* 24(6):719–736, 2003.

122. Koledova VV, Khalil RA: Ca²⁺, calmodulin, and cyclins in vascular smooth muscle cell cycle, *Circ Res* 98(10):1240–1243, 2006.

123. Choi J, Husain M: Calmodulin-mediated cell cycle regulation: new mechanisms for old observations, *Cell Cycle* 5(19):2183–2186, 2006.

124. Touyz RM, Yao G: Modulation of vascular smooth muscle cell growth by magnesium—role of mitogen—activated protein kinases, *J Cell Physiol* 197(3):326–335, 2003.

125. Burg ED, Remillard CV, Yuan JXJ: Potassium channels in the regulation of pulmonary artery smooth muscle cell proliferation and apoptosis: pharmacotherapeutic implications, *Br J Pharmacol* 153(S1):S99–S111, 2008.

126. Neylon CB: Potassium channels and vascular proliferation, *Vasc Pharmacol* 38(1):35–41, 2002.

127. Cidad P, Moreno-Dominguez A, Novensa L, et al: Characterization of ion channels involved in the proliferative response of femoral artery smooth muscle cells, *Arterioscler Thromb Vasc Biol* 30(6):1203–1211, 2010.

128. Miguel-Velado E, Perez-Carretero FD, Colinas O, et al: Cell cycle-dependent expression of Kv3.4 channels modulates proliferation of human uterine artery smooth muscle cells, *Cardiovasc Res* 86(3):383–391, 2010.

129. Jackson WF: KV1.3: a new therapeutic target to control vascular smooth muscle cell proliferation, *Arterioscler Thromb Vasc Biol* 30(6):1073–1074, 2010.

130. Assoian RK, Schwartz MA: Coordinate signaling by integrins and receptor tyrosine kinases in the regulation of G1 phase cell-cycle progression, *Curr Opin Genet Dev* 11(1):48–53, 2001.

131. Gizard F, Bruemmer D: Transcriptional control of vascular smooth muscle cell proliferation by peroxisome proliferator-activated receptor-gamma: therapeutic implications for cardiovascular diseases, *PPAR Res* 2008.

132. Gizard F, Amant C, Barbier O, et al: PPARα inhibits vascular smooth muscle cell proliferation underlying intimal hyperplasia by inducing the tumor suppressor p16INK4a, *J Clin Invest* 115(11):3228–3238, 2005.

133. Gizard F, Nomiyama T, Zhao Y, et al: The PPARα/p16INK4a pathway inhibits vascular smooth muscle cell proliferation by repressing cell cycle-dependent telomerase activation, *Circ Res* 103(10):1155–1163, 2008.

134. Koyama H, Bornfeldt KE, Fukumoto S, et al: Molecular pathways of cyclic nucleotide-induced inhibition of arterial smooth muscle cell proliferation, *J Cell Physiol* 186(1):1–10, 2001.

135. Wu Y-J, Sala-Newby GB, Shu K-T, et al: S-phase kinase-associated protein-2 (Skp2) promotes vascular smooth muscle cell proliferation and neointima formation in vivo, *J Vasc Surg* 50(5):1135–1142, 2009.

136. Cheng Y, Zhang C: MicroRNA-21 in cardiovascular disease, *J Cardiovasc Trans l Res* 3(3):251–255, 2010.

137. Gerthoffer WT: Mechanisms of vascular smooth muscle cell migration, *Circ Res* 100(5):607–621, 2007.

138. San Martín A, Griendling KK: Redox control of vascular smooth muscle migration, *Antioxid Redox Signal* 12(5):625–640, 2010.

139. Seasholtz TM, Majumdar M, Kaplan DD, et al: Rho and Rho kinase mediate thrombin-stimulated vascular smooth muscle cell DNA synthesis and migration, *Circ Res* 84(10):1186–1193, 1999.

140. Landry DB, Couper LL, Bryant SR, et al: Activation of the NF-kappa B and I kappa B system in smooth muscle cells after rat arterial injury. Induction of vascular cell adhesion molecule-1 and monocyte chemoattractant protein-1, *Am J Pathol* 151(4):1085–1095, 1997.

141. Sun L, Stoecklin G, Van Way S, et al: Tristetraprolin (TTP)-14–3–3 complex formation protects TTP from dephosphorylation by protein phosphatase 2a and stabilizes tumor necrosis factor-alpha mRNA, *J Biol Chem* 282(6):3766–3777, 2007.

142. Pyronnet S: Phosphorylation of the cap-binding protein eIF4E by the MAPK-activated protein kinase Mnk1, *Biochem Pharmacol* 60(8):1237–1243, 2000.

143. Yin BL, Hao H, Wang YY, et al: Downregulating osteopontin reduces angiotensin II-induced inflammatory activation in vascular smooth muscle cells, *Inflamm Res* 58(2):67–73, 2009.

144. Cuff CA, Kothapalli D, Azonobi I, et al: The adhesion receptor CD44 promotes atherosclerosis by mediating inflammatory cell recruitment and vascular cell activation, *J Clin Invest* 108(7):1031–1040, 2001.

145. Vicencio JM, Galluzzi L, Tajeddine N, et al: Senescence, apoptosis or autophagy? When a damaged cell must decide its path–a mini-review, *Gerontology* 54(2):92–99, 2008.

146. Campisi J, d'Adda di Fagagna F: Cellular senescence: when bad things happen to good cells, *Nat Rev Mol Cell Biol* 8(9):729–740, 2007.

147. Gorenne I, Kavurma M, Scott S, et al: Vascular smooth muscle cell senescence in atherosclerosis, *Cardiovasc Res* 72(1):9–17, 2006.

148. Minamino T, Miyauchi H, Yoshida T, et al: Vascular cell senescence and vascular aging, *J Mol Cell Cardiol* 36(2):175–183, 2004.

149. Burton DG, Matsubara H, Ikeda K: Pathophysiology of vascular calcification: pivotal role of cellular senescence in vascular smooth muscle cells, *Exp Gerontol* 45(11):819–824, 2010.

150. Taylor RC, Cullen SP, Martin SJ: Apoptosis: controlled demolition at the cellular level, *Nat Rev Mol Cell Biol* 9(3):231–241, 2008.

151. Muto A, Fitzgerald TN, Pimiento JM, et al: Smooth muscle cell signal transduction: implications of vascular biology for vascular surgeons, *J Vasc Surg* 45(6 Suppl 1):A15–A24, 2007.

152. Geng Y-J, Libby P: Progression of atheroma: a struggle between death and procreation, *Arterioscler Thromb Vasc Biol* 22(9):1370–1380, 2002.

153. Gupta S, Kass GE, Szegezdi E, et al: The mitochondrial death pathway: a promising therapeutic target in diseases, *J Cell Mol Med* 13(6):1004–1033, 2009.

154. Clarke MCH, Talib S, Figg NL, et al: Vascular smooth muscle cell apoptosis induces interleukin-1-directed inflammation: effects of hyperlipidemia-mediated inhibition of phagocytosis, *Circ Res* 106(2):363–372, 2010.

155. Clarke M, Bennett M: Defining the role of vascular smooth muscle cell apoptosis in atherosclerosis, *Cell Cycle* 5(20):2329–2331, 2006.

156. Son BK, Akishita M, Iijima K, et al: Mechanism of pi-induced vascular calcification, *J Atheroscler Thromb* 15(2):63–68, 2008.

157. Martinet W, De Meyer GR: Autophagy in atherosclerosis, *Curr Atheroscler Rep* 10(3):216–223, 2008.

158. Hirschi KK, Majesky MW: Smooth muscle stem cells, *Anat Rec Part A: Disc Mol Cell Evo Biol* 276A(1):22–33, 2004.

159. Margariti A, Zeng L, Xu Q: Stem cells, vascular smooth muscle cells and atherosclerosis, *Histol Histopathol* 21(9):979–985, 2006.

160. Orlandi A, Bennett M: Progenitor cell-derived smooth muscle cells in vascular disease, *Biochem Pharmacol* 79(12):1706–1713, 2010.

161. Ergün S, Tilki D, Klein D: Vascular wall as a reservoir for different types of stem and progenitor cells, *Antioxid Redox Signal* 2011 Jan 7.

162. Sinha S, Wamhoff BR, Hoofnagle MH, et al: Assessment of contractility of purified smooth muscle cells derived from embryonic stem cells, *Stem Cells* 24(7):1678–1688, 2006.

163. Nandan MO, Yang VW: The role of Kruppel-like factors in the reprogramming of somatic cells to induced pluripotent stem cells, *Histol Histopathol* 24(10):1343–1355, 2009.

164. Wang C, Yin S, Cen L, et al: Differentiation of adipose-derived stem cells into contractile smooth muscle cells induced by transforming growth factor-beta1 and bone morphogenetic protein-4, *Tissue Eng Part A* 16(4):1201–1213, 2010.

165. Daniel J-M, Bielenberg W, Stieger P, et al: Time-course analysis on the differentiation of bone marrow-derived progenitor cells into smooth muscle cells during neointima formation, *Arterioscler Thromb Vasc Biol* 30(10):1890–1896, 2010.

166. Hoglund VJ, Dong XR, Majesky MW: Neointima formation: a local affair, *Arterioscler Thromb Vasc Biol* 30(10):1877–1879, 2010.

167. Passman JN, Dong XR, Wu SP, et al: A sonic hedgehog signaling domain in the arterial adventitia supports resident Sca1+ smooth muscle progenitor cells, *Proc Natl Acad Sci U S A* 105(27):9349–9354, 2008.

168. Dotsenko O: Stem/Progenitor cells, atherosclerosis and cardiovascular regeneration, *Open Cardiovasc Med J* 4:97–104, 2010.

169. Raines EW, Bornfeldt KE: Integrin α7β1 COMPels smooth muscle cells to maintain their quiescence, *Circ Res* 106(3):427–429, 2010.

170. Hilenski L, Griendling K, Alexander R: Angiotensin AT1 receptors. In Re R, DiPette D, Schiffrin E, Sowers J, editors: *Molecular mechanisms in hypertension*, London, 2006, Taylor and Francis, pp 25–40.

CHAPTER 4

Connective Tissues of the Subendothelium

Rajendra Raghow

Varieties of Blood Vessels and Their Connective Tissue

The vascular system consists of a massive network of tubular channels that circulate blood to transport nutrients and oxygen to the tissues; blood vessels also serve as conduits for leukocytes that carry on immunological surveillance and need to move rapidly to sites of injury and inflammation. The vascular endothelium and its specialized extracellular matrix (ECM), owing to their location between circulating blood and underlying tissues, have evolved with unique structural and functional properties that ensure optimal tissue homeostasis. The elastic fibers and tensile forces–bearing networks of ECM that reside in the vessel wall maintain their histological integrity in the face of enormous mechanical load. Yet, the organization of the vessel walls allows leukocytes to move through them without any obvious leakage. The mechanical function of the vascular ECM has been recognized for a long time. In recent years, compelling data have accumulated to indicate that molecular components of ECM provide informational cues to the endothelial cells (ECs) and vascular smooth muscle cells (VSMCs) to regulate their proliferation, differentiation, and death. Additionally, ECM can sequester a number of growth factors and cytokines, thereby modulating their spatial and temporal actions to regulate disparate physiological and pathological responses of the vascular tissues.

The evolutionary transition from an open to a closed circulatory system is clearly reflected in the architecture of the blood vessels.[1,2] The size and anatomical organization of individual vessels vary with their specific locations and functions in the body. The major vessels that carry blood directly from the heart are capable of storing and releasing large amounts of energy during the cardiac cycle. As a result, the walls of large arteries are relatively thick and more elastic to allow their expansion and contraction in response to the systolic and diastolic cycles of the heart. Without such elasticity, the intense surge in pressure as blood is ejected from the heart would inhibit its emptying, and the pressure in the vessels would fall too low for the heart to refill. The elasticity of large arteries enables them to store a portion of the stroke volume with each systole and discharge that volume with diastole. Thus, the unique structure of large arteries allows the flow of blood from the heart to be continuous, smooth, and efficient.

The smaller arteries are more rigid. Regulation of blood flow in small arteries is facilitated by the contractile activity of their smooth muscle cells (SMCs), which control the size of the vessel lumen, depending on the rate of blood flow in a given location. Capillaries contain only one layer of endothelial cells (ECs) with an underlying basement membrane. This thin-walled structure of capillaries permits rapid exchange of water, nutrients, and metabolic products between blood and interstitial fluids. Capillaries deliver blood to the venous system at a much lower pressure. Consequently, veins and venules have thinner walls, less ECM, and a larger lumen than their arterial counterparts. They also have far fewer SMCs and are equipped with valves to prevent reversal of blood flow due to hydrostatic forces.

The walls of the large arteries contain three identifiable layers. The luminal surface of arteries contains a single layer of polygonal ECs connected by gap junctions. This cell layer rests on a basement membrane, which in turn is supported by a network of elastic fibers in a fenestrated plate called the *internal elastic lamina*. This region of the wall is called the *tunica intima*. The middle layer, called the *tunica media*, represents the bulk of the vessel wall, contains few elastic fibers

but has a large number of VSMCs, with their long axes perpendicular to the lumen axis.[3] Smooth muscle cells residing in the tunica media synthesize the major components of ECM that ultimately define the mechanical properties of the vessel. The extracellular space contains a variable mixture of collagen fibers in a continuous sheath adjacent to the elastic fibers. The external elastic lamina separates the medial and adventitial layers of the vessel wall. The outermost layer of the vessel wall, the *tunica adventitia*, consists primarily of collagen-rich ECM and the *vasa vasorum*, a network of vessels that supplies nutrients and O_2 to the outer portion of arterial walls. Although the unique anatomy and high collagen content of the tunica adventitia help prevent arterial rupture at extremely high pressures, the adventitia is highly susceptible to vascular inflammation.

The walls of smaller arteries are intermediate in size. The tunica intima is relatively thin, as is the medial layer. The tunica adventitia of small arteries usually contains more densely packed collagen fibers arranged longitudinally along the vessel axis. Arterioles have simpler walls; their EC layer is surrounded by VSMCs, and the adventitia is smaller and more pliable compared with those of larger arteries.[1,3] Capillaries adjoining the arterioles are surrounded by a few SMCs that control the amount of blood passing through them. The walls of arterial and venous capillaries are lined with flat ECs surrounded by a basement membrane; a discontinuous sheath of pericytes and a fibrous reticulum, made primarily of type III collagen, are attached to the basement membrane. The walls of venules also contain a reticular network of collagen fibers derived from type III collagen, along with smaller quantities of type I collagen fibers.

Vascular Morphogenesis and Extracellular Matrix

Two distinct processes, vasculogenesis and angiogenesis, are involved in the formation of blood vessels in vertebrates. Vasculogenesis is de novo vessel formation that primarily occurs in the developing embryo. Conversely, angiogenesis is the process by which new vessels are sprouted from preexisting blood vessels throughout life. During early embryogenesis, ECs begin the process of vasculogenesis by forming a network of capillaries in the absence of blood flow. Following the onset of blood circulation, primitive capillary networks are transformed into arteries and veins to form the fully functional closed circulatory system in the developing fetus. For obvious reasons, the mechanisms of vasculogenesis and angiogenesis have received intense scrutiny in recent years. Although both vasculogenesis and angiogenesis are orchestrated by interactions among the ECs, hematopoietic cells, and VSMCs, the detailed molecular mechanisms involved in these processes are distinct.

The preceding overview underscores the striking structural and phenotypic diversity of different branches of the vascular tree. Therefore it is not surprising that the vascular ECM displays similar complexity depending on its location in the vasculature.[2-5] This caveat notwithstanding, all vascular ECM is composed of fibrillar and nonfibrillar components. The fibrillar component of the vascular connective tissue is mainly collagen, and a diversity of proteins and proteoglycans (PGs) make up the rest. What follows is an overview of the structural and functional properties of the major macromolecules that characterize the vascular ECM. For a more detailed discussion of the individual classes of ECM macromolecules, astute readers will need to consult specialized reviews and critical commentaries, a number of which are cited in the chapter.

Collagens

Twenty-eight genetically distinct types of collagen comprising 43 unique α chains have been identified in vertebrates (Table 4-1). The vast majority of these collagens exist in humans.[6-9] Based on their domain organization and other structural features (Fig. 4-1), collagens may be categorized as (1) fibril-forming collagens represented by types I, II, III, V, XI, XXIV, and XXVII; (2) fibril-associated collagens with interrupted triple helices (FACIT; e.g., IX, XII, XIV, XVI, XIX, XX, XXI, XXII, and XXVI collagens); (3) collagens capable of forming hexagonal network (e.g., VIII, X); (4) basement membrane collagens represented by IV collagen; (5) collagens that assemble into beaded filaments (e.g., type VI); (6) anchoring fiber-forming collagens (e.g., VII); (7) plasma membrane-spanning types XIII, XVII, XXIII, and XXV collagens; and (8) collagens with unique domain organization, represented by types XV and XVIII.

We should note that the nomenclature of proteins as collagens and their classification into different types is somewhat arbitrary, since collagen fibrils invariably consist of more than one type of collagen. For instance, type I collagen fibrils contain small amounts of type III, V, and XII; similarly, type II collagen fibrils contain significant amounts of collagen types IX and XI. Even more strikingly, types V and IX collagen are known to form hybrid fibrils. The discovery of collagens that have extensive non-triple-helical domains and several proteins that contain triple-helical domains, such as C1q, adiponectin, acetyl cholinesterase, and ectodysplasin (see Fig. 4-1), further challenge the notion of what constitutes a "true collagen" and how it should be classified. Although several collagen types are found in the vasculature, collagen types I and III are the dominant constituents of the blood vessel wall.[6,7,9] Collagen types II and X are excluded from our discussion because they are not relevant to the ECM of the vascular endothelium.

Fibrillar Collagens

The collagen molecule, the basic unit of collagen fibers, has an asymmetrical, rodlike structure composed of three polypeptide chains called α *chains*. Because of the Gly-X-Y repeating units and their stereochemistry, each α chain forms a minor helix (Fig. 4-2). Three α chains wind around a common axis to form a right-handed triple helix. In some collagens, all three α chains are identical, while in others two or three unique α chains form the triple-helical molecule. Type I and type III collagens are the most abundant collagens in the blood vessel and together form the striated fibrils. With the exception of types XXV and XXVII, fibrillar collagens form an uninterrupted triple-helical domain of approximately 300 nm. The type I collagen α chains contain 338 Gly-X-Y repeats, and there are 341 such triplets in type III α chains. At both the NH_2 and COOH ends of each α chain are short segments of nonhelical sequences of approximately 15 to 20 amino acid residues, referred to as *telopeptides*.

Because of their similarities, type I and type III collagens are discussed together here. The type I collagen molecule is a heterotrimer of two identical α chains, α1(I), and a different α chain, α2(I), and has the chain structure $[\alpha1(I)]_2\alpha2(I)$. The type III collagen molecule is formed by three identical α chains and has the chain structure $[\alpha I(III)]_3$. The helical domain of the α chain contains a repeating triplet sequence of $[Gly-X-Y]_n$, where X and Y may be any amino acid but are most frequently proline or hydroxyproline. The amino acid residues in the Y position are nearly always hydroxylated (4-hydroxyproline). The configuration of the amino acids forces the α chain to assume a left-handed helix, thus allowing α chains to form a right-handed supercoil with a one-amino-acid stagger between adjacent chains. The presence of glycine (without a bulky side chain) as every third amino acid is critical because it will occupy the center position within the triple helix. Substitution of any other amino acid for glycine in the Gly-X-Y leads to disruption of the triple helix.

The collagen triple helix is further stabilized by interchain hydrogen bonds contributed by hydroxyproline residues. Thus, the collagen molecule is a long cylindrical rod with dimensions of 1.5 nm × 300 nm. Under physiological conditions of ionic strength, pH, and temperature, collagen molecules spontaneously aggregate into striated fibrils. Fibril formation occurs by lateral aggregation of collagen molecules, in which each neighboring row of molecules is displaced along its long axis by a distance of 68 nm. In addition, within the same row, there is a gap of approximately 40 nm between the end of one molecule and the beginning of the next (see Figs. 4-1 and 4-2). The short nonhelical telopeptides at the NH_2 and COOH ends of each α chain are located in the gap or hole zone of the fibril and are therefore accessible to enzymes that regulate collagen cross-linking.

Network-Forming Collagens

As shown in Figure 4-1, collagen types IV (α1-α6 chains), VI (α1-α5 chains), VIII (α1-α2 chains) and X are known to form networks in the ECM of basement membranes. The supramolecular organization and function of type IV collagen has been extensively characterized. Six different α polypeptide chains of collagen IV are each encoded by an evolutionary conserved gene. The amino and carboxyl propeptides of type IV collagen remain as integral parts of the molecules when they are deposited in the basement membrane. As a result, rather than forming a quarter-stagger, side-by-side alignment of individual molecules, as seen in types I, II, and III collagens, type IV collagen α chains form chicken-wire structures by end-to-end associations stabilized by lysine-derived cross-linking and interchain disulfide bonds (Fig. 4-3). The α1(IV) and α2(IV) collagen chains are more closely related to each other than to α3(IV)1, α4(IV), α5(IV), and α6(VI); the latter share a high degree of sequence homology with each other. The amino terminal domains of α1(IV) and α2(IV) collagen chains are 143 and 167 amino acids, respectively; the NH_2-termini of the other four α chains are much smaller (ranging in size from 13 to 19 amino acids). Theoretically, all six α chains of type IV collagen may combine randomly to generate 56 unique triple-helical permutations. However, as shown in Figure 4-4, in vascular basement membranes the most common composition of triple-helical fibrils is $[\alpha1(IV)]_2\alpha2(IV)$. The $[\alpha3(IV)1]_2\alpha4(IV)$ and $[\alpha5(IV)1]_2\alpha6(IV)$ are also present in basement membrane.[9,10]

Organization of the type IV collagen genes is unusual. The COLA4A1 and COLA4A2 genes are paired head-to-head on the same chromosome and are transcribed in opposite directions. The pairs of COLA3A4 and COLA4A4 and COLA4A5 and COLA4A6 genes are similarly arranged, except each pair is located on a different chromosome. Type IV collagen genes are very large, as exemplified by COLA4A1 and COLA4A5 genes that exceed 100 kb in size.

Type VI collagen, another network-forming molecule, is represented by six distinct α chains in the mouse and five α chains in humans; the gene encoding the putative α4(VI) collagen chain is not functional in humans. Heterotrimers of different α chains, encoded by unique genes, form the basic unit of type VI collagen. Alternate splicing of messenger ribonucleic acids (mRNAs) generates additional variants of α2 (VI) and α3 (VI) chains.[7,9] The Gly-X-Y domains of α chains of type VI collagen microfibrils are rather short (about 330 amino acid residues) and are flanked by a number of von Willebrand factor (vWF) A domains.

Type VI collagen forms relatively unusual aggregates by a stepwise assembly into the triple-helical monomeric units that form dimers in an antiparallel fashion. The dimers in turn form tetramers, held together by disulfide bonds, to create scissors-like structures. The supramolecular assemblies of type VI collagen, formed by end-to-end associations of tetramers, appear as beads on a string, as revealed by electron microscopy.[9] These characteristic structures have been observed in vascular subendothelium and skeletal muscle basement membranes. Type VI collagen microfibrils exhibit unique adhesive properties to other ECM components,

TABLE 4-1   Collagen Types, Constituent α-Chains, and Their Genes*

TYPE	α-CHAINS	GENE	# AMINO ACIDS	TISSUE DISTRIBUTION
I	α1(I) α2(I)	COL1A1 COL1A2	1464 1366	Most connective tissues, especially in bone, tendon, ligament
II	α1(II)	COL2A1	1487	Cartilage, vitreous humor, cornea
III	α1(III)	COL3A1	1466	Tissues containing collagen I, except bone and tendon
IV	α1(IV) α2(IV) α3(IV) α4(IV) α5(IV) α6(IV)	COL4A1 COL4A2 COL4A3 COL4A4 COL4A5 COL4A6	1669 1712 1670 1690 1685 1691	Basement membranes (BM)
V	α1(V) α2(V) α3(V)	COL5A1 COL5A2 COL5A3	1838 1499 1745	Tissues containing collagen I
VI	α1(VI) α2(VI) α3(VI) α4(VI)	COL6A1 COL6A2 COL6A3 COL6A4	1028 1019 3177 2611	Most connective tissues
VII	α1(VII)	COL7A1	2944	Anchoring fibrils
VIII	α1(VIII) α2(VIII)	COL8A1 COL8A2	744 703	Many tissues
IX	α1(IX) α2(IX) α3(IX)	COL9A1 COL9A2 COL9A3	921 869	Tissues containing collagen II
X	α1(X)	COL10A1	680	Hypertrophic cartilage
XI	α1(XI) α2(XI) α3(XI)	COL11A1 COL11A2 COL11A3	1806 1736 1806	Tissues containing collagen II
XII	α1(XII)	COL12A1	3063	Tissues containing collagen I
XIII	α1(XIII)	COL13A1	717	Many tissues
XIV	α1(XIV)	COL14A1	1796	Tissues containing collagen I
XV	α1(XV)	COL15A1	1388	Many tissues in the BM zone
XVI	α1(XVI)	COL16A1	1604	Many tissues
XVII	α1(XVII)	COL17A1	1497	Skin hemidesmosomes
XVIII	α1(XVIII)	COL18A1	1516	Many tissues in the BM zone
XIX	α1(XIX)	COL19A1	1142	Many tissues in the BM zone
XX				
XXI	α1(XXI)	COL21A1	957	Fetal tissues and blood vessels
XXII	α1(XXII)	COL22A1	1626	BM of myotendinous junctions
XXIII	α1(XXIII)	COL23A1	540	Lung, kidney, brain, tumor cells
XXIV	α1(XXIV)	COL24A1	1714	
XXV	α1(XXV)	COL25A1	654	Amyloid plaques
XXVI	α1(XXVI)	COL26A1	439	Testis and ovaries
XXVII	α1(XXVII)	COL27A1	1630	Early development of many tissues
XXVIII	α1(XXVIII)	COL28A1	1125	Dorsal root ganglia

*Adapted from Myllyharju J, Kivirikko KI: Collagens, modifying enzymes and their mutations from humans, flies and worms. Trends Genet 20:33–43, 2004; and Gordon MK, Hahn RK: Collagens. Cell Tissue Res 339:247–257, 2010.

such as other collagens, heparin, and vWF, and may be involved in the adhesion of platelets and SMCs. In the medial layer, type VI collagen facilitates interaction between SMCs and elastin by bridging the elastin fibers and cells.[11]

As illustrated in Figure 4-5 (see discussion in "Metalloproteinases"), types VIII and X collagens comprise a unique subfamily of collagens that form hexagonal networks. These relatively short collagens, containing noncollagenous domains on their NH$_2$ and COOH termini, are collectively known as the *multiplexin family* of collagens. Type VIII collagen is expressed in many tissues, especially in the endothelium, while type X is exclusively associated with hypertrophic chondrocytes during cartilage and bone development. The preponderance of evidence to date indicates that the two α chains of collagen VIII, encoded by COL8A1 and COL8A2,

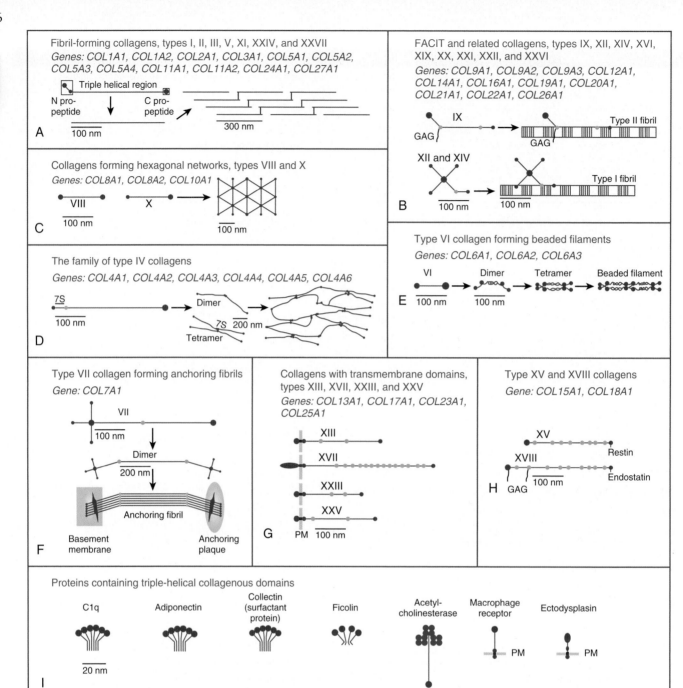

FIGURE 4-1   Classification of superfamily of vertebrate collagens. Based on their primary structure, domain organization, and ability to form supramolecular assemblies, all currently known collagens may be divided into nine families. These include **(A)** fibril-forming collagens, **(B)** fibril-associated collagens with interrupted triple helices (FACIT collagens), located on the surface of collagen fibrils, and structurally related collagens, **(C)** collagens capable of forming hexagonal networks, **(D)** the family of type IV collagens located in the basement membranes, **(E)** type VI collagen that forms beaded filaments, **(F)** collagen that forms anchoring filaments of basement membranes, **(G)** collagens with transmembrane domains, and **(H)** the family of XV and XVIII collagens. The supramolecular organization of collagens in **(G)** and **(H)** are not known. Polypeptide chains found in the 27 collagen types, each consisting of three chains, are encoded by 42 unique genes *(written in blue)*. A number of proteins possess collagenous domains **(I)** but are not considered to be bona fide collagens. The N- and C-terminal noncollagenous domains of these proteins are shown in dark pink, and noncollagenous domains interrupting the collagen triple helix in light blue. For acetylcholinesterase, the catalytic domain *(shown in green)* and the tail domain are encoded by separate exons. GAG, glycosaminoglycan. *(From Myllyharju J, Kivirikko KI: Collagens, modifying enzymes and their mutations in humans, flies and worms. Trends Genet 20:33–43, 2004.)*

assemble into homotrimers of α1(VIII) and α2(VIII) (Fig. 4-6). Hexagonal aggregates of type VIII collagen have been observed both *in vivo* (e.g., Descemet's membrane of the cornea) and *in vitro* with purified protein. It is believed that type VIII collagen is capable of assuming other forms of macromolecular aggregates, since hexagonal lattices have yet to be observed in the subendothelial ECM.[9]

Fibril-Associated Collagens with Interrupted Triple Helices

As the name suggests, the FACIT collagens (types IX, XII, XIV, XVI, XIX, XX, XXI, XXII, and XXVI) do not form fibrils themselves but associate with other fibril-forming collagens.[9] Type IX collagen, the prototype of this group, is cross-linked to the surface of type II

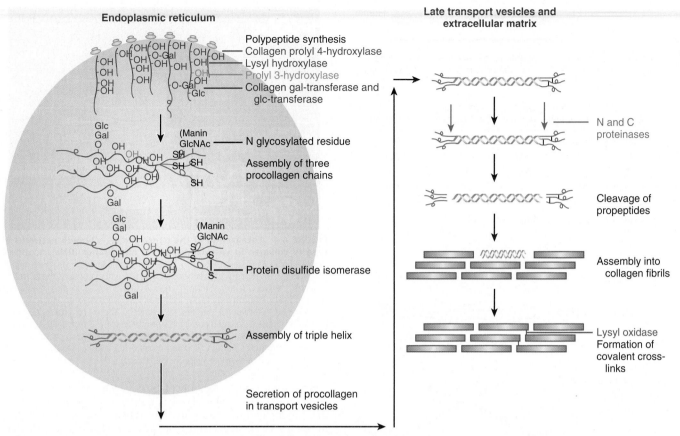

FIGURE 4-2 **An overview of the main steps involved in the synthesis of fibril-forming collagens.** The α-polypeptide chains are synthesized on membrane-bound ribosomes and secreted into the lumen of the endoplasmic reticulum (ER). The main steps in collagen biosynthesis are (i) cleavage of the signal peptide (not shown), (ii) hydroxylation of specific proline and lysine residues, (iii) glycosylation of certain asparagine residues in the C-peptide, and (iv) formation of intramolecular and intermolecular disulfide bonds. A nucleus for the assembly of the triple helix is formed in the C-terminal region after the C propeptides of three α-chains become registered with each other and ~100 proline residues in each α-chain have been hydroxylated to 4-hydroxyproline. The triple helix formation proceeds toward the N-terminus in a zipper-like fashion. Procollagen molecules are transported from the ER to Golgi, where they begin to associate laterally and exit the cell via secretory vesicles. This is followed by cleavage of N and C propeptides, spontaneous self-assembly of the collagen molecules into fibrils, and formation of cross-links. *(From Myllyharju J, Kivirikko KI: Collagens, modifying enzymes and their mutations in humans, flies and worms. Trends Genet 20:33–43, 2004.)*

collagen fibrils in cartilage (see Fig. 4-1); type XII and type XIV collagens are found in both cartilage and noncartilaginous tissues, where they are involved in controlling the diameter of collagen fibrils (see Fig. 4-1). The other FACIT-like collagens (e.g., types XVI, XIX, and XXII) are localized in specialized basement membranes. For instance, XVI collagen is associated with fibrillin 1 near the epidermal basement membrane. Collagen types XXI and XXII are closely related to each other in structure and are involved in formation of supramolecular aggregates in the basement membranes of myotendinous junctions.[12,13] As a key constituent of cutaneous basement membranes, anchoring fibrils of type VII collagen form a structural continuum between the dermis and epidermis of normal human skin. The vWF A–like domain in collagen VII binds to fibrils of type I collagen *in vitro*.[14]

Minor Collagen Types with Unique Structures

As illustrated in Figure 4-1, the transmembrane collagens (types XIII, XVII, XXIII, and XXV) contain a cytoplasmic domain, a membrane-spanning hydrophobic domain, and extracellular triple-helical domains interspersed with noncollagenous domains; these collagens may also exist in a soluble form. Type XVII collagen is a unique member of this group that is expressed on the basal surface of keratinocytes that bind to laminin found in the basement membrane; compared with the other three members of this group, type XVII has a rather large intracellular domain whose function remains unknown. Collagen types XIII, XXIII, and XXV are similar

to each other in their primary structure, but the patterns of their expression appear to be unique. Type XXV collagen is enriched in the senile plaques of Alzheimer's disease brains.[9,12,13,15] High expression of full-length collagen XXIII is found in the lungs, whereas its shed form is enriched in brain, suggesting that shedding of XXIII collagen occurs in a tissue-specific manner.

Collagen types XV and XVIII are highly pertinent to the EC biology in several ways.[16,17] The full-length types XV and XVIII collagen are basement membrane components; their triple-helical domains share a high degree of homology. Collagen types XV and XVIII were initially identified as PG core proteins containing chondroitin sulfate and heparan sulfate (HS) side chains, respectively. The COOH-terminal domains of XV and XVIII collagens can be cleaved to generate biologically active peptides, endostatin and restin, respectively; these peptides inhibit migration of ECs and thus potently block angiogenesis. *In vitro*, recombinant collagen XV binds to fibronectin (FN), laminin, and vitronectin (VN) but not to fibrillar collagens, fibril-associated collagens, or decorin.[18]

Finally, collagens XXVI and XXVIII are newly discovered collagens that are unique both with regard to their structures and tissue-specific distributions. The triple-helical domain of type XXVI is rather small, with only 146 Gly-X-Y repeats. Expression of type XXVI collagen occurs predominantly in testis and ovary. The von Willebrand factor–A domains flank the triple-helical structure of type XXVIII collagen that is almost exclusively expressed in the peripheral nerves.[19,20]

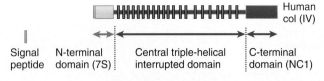

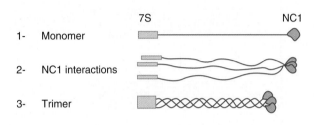

A

Chain	N-terminal 7S domain	Central domain	C-terminal NC1 domain	Interruptions
α1	143 aa	1271 aa	228 aa	21
α2	157	1303	227	26
α3	13	1398	231	26
α4	26	1396	230	25
α5	15	1416	228	23
α6	29	1407	227	25

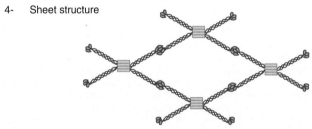

B

FIGURE 4-3 **A,** Linear structures of human collagen IV α-chains. Six different genes encode collagen IV α-chains. Each polypeptide is composed of three distinct domains: a cysteine-rich N-terminal 7S domain, a central triple-helical domain with multiple small interruptions (boxes), and a globular C-terminal noncollagenous NC1 domain. The NC1 and central triple-helical domains are of an equivalent size, whereas 7S domains are shorter in the cases of α3, α4, α5, and α6 compared with α1 and α2. On the basis of sequence homology, type IV collagen α-chains can be divided in two groups: the α1-like (α1, α2, α5) and the α2-like (α2, α4, α6). **B,** Assembly of collagen IV α chains. Assembly of trimers is dependent on the association of NC1 domains, followed by formation of triple-helical structure and 7S domains in a spider-shaped structure; the two trimers interact head-to-head through their NC1 domains, forming a sheet structure. Several trimers can also lace together along their triple-helical domains, thickening the structure. (Adapted from Company of Biologists Ltd., Ortega N, Werb Z: New functional roles for noncollagenous domains of basement membrane collagens. J Cell Sci 115:4201, 2002.)

Regulation of Collagen Biosynthesis

Collagen chains are synthesized as prepro-α chains from which the hydrophobic leader sequence is removed prior to secretion, and the pro-α chains are secreted into the extracellular space (see Fig. 4-2). The pro-α1(I) chain contains an NH$_2$ propeptide (N-peptide) and a COOH propeptide (C-peptide). The N-peptide consists of a 139-residue sequence that precedes a 17-residue sequence of nonhelical telopeptide. This is followed by a 1014 amino acids-long Gly-X-Y helical sequence attached sequentially to a 26 residues-long COOH telopeptide and a 262-residues-long nonhelical C-peptide. The domain organization of pro-α2(I) and pro-α1(III) chains are similar except for minor variations in the number of amino acid residues.[6,7,21]

The genomic organization and chromosomal locations for genes that encode collagens have been studied. In humans, the genes encoding 43 distinct α chains are dispersed on at least 15

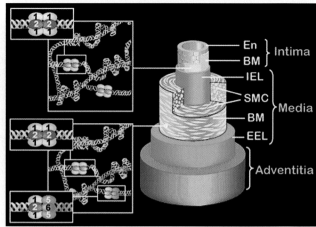

FIGURE 4-4 **Localization of the α1·α2 and α1·α2·α5·α6 networks of type IV collagen in vascular basement membranes (BMs).** Schematic diagram of a large artery (aorta) depicts its multilayered structure (right). Endothelial cells (En) rest on a subendothelial BM, which contains the α1·α2(IV) collagen network (right). Smooth muscle cells (SMCs) in the media are surrounded by smooth muscle BM and are sandwiched between an internal and external elastic lamina (IEL and EEL, respectively). The α1·α2 and α1·α2·α5·α6 networks of type IV collagen coexist in smooth muscle BM (right). (Adapted from Borza DB, Bondar O, Ninomya Y, et al: The NC1 domain of collagen IV encodes a novel network composed of the alpha-1, alpha-2, alpha-5, and alpha-6 chains in smooth muscle basement membranes. J Biol Chem 276:28532, 2001.)

chromosomes. Unlike majority of the collagen-encoding genes, the six homologous α-chains of type IV collagen are encoded by genes that are located in pairs with head-to-head orientation on chromosomes 13 (COL4A1 and COL4A2), 2 (COL4A3 and COL4A4), and the X chromosome (COL4A5 and COL4A6). Interestingly, the promoters of these pairs of type IV collagens overlap, suggesting a coordinate regulation of the gene pairs. The precise molecular mechanisms of this regulation, however, remain incompletely known.[6,7,9,21,22]

The molecular events involved in procollagen biosynthesis, from transcription and splicing of mRNA to its transport and translation in the cytoplasm, are nearly identical to most other proteins synthesized by eukaryotic cells. Regulation at the level of transcription and mRNA turnover appears to be involved in the coordinated synthesis of two pro-α1(I) chains for every one of pro-α2(I) chain. Most cells that produce type I collagen also produce type III collagen in variable amounts, depending on the specific type of tissue, its age, and the physiological and pathological situations.

The molecular mechanisms of regulation of biosynthesis of a number of collagens have been studied to varying degrees, both in physiological and pathological settings. Regulation of genes that encode α chains of type I collagen has been studied extensively and is briefly summarized. Transcriptional regulation of genes that generate fibrillar (COL1A1, COL1A2, COL3A1) and basement membrane (e.g., COL4A1-6) collagens evidently involves both genomic and epigenomic (deoxyribonucleic acid [DNA] methylation and posttranslational modification of histones) mechanisms. Although collagen genes are predominantly regulated at the level of transcription, a number of reports indicate that posttranscriptional regulation is also exerted under some conditions.

The cis-acting elements of COLA1 and COLA2 genes are modularly organized on either side of the transcription start point (TSP). The regulatory elements are distributed over a distance of 100 to 150 kb of genomic DNA, depending on the specific gene and the assays used to study their transcriptional and posttranscriptional regulation. The tissue-specific and inducible activation of collagen genes involves complex interactions among the cis-acting modules of their promoters and enhancers. Promoters of COLA1 and COLA2 genes contain TATA boxes located 25 to 35 bp upstream of the TSP. Existence of a number of enhancer and repressor cis-elements around the TSP and in the first intron of COLA1 gene has been demonstrated.

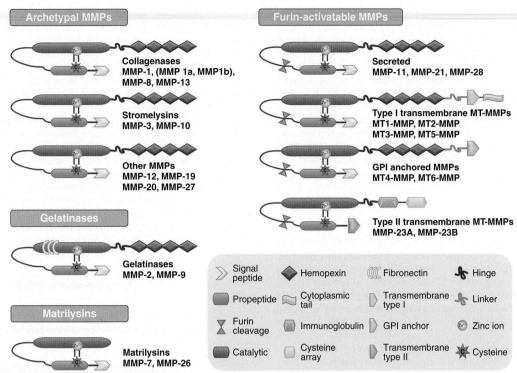

FIGURE 4-5   Domain structure of matrix metalloproteinases (MMPs). The MMPs are multidomain enzymes that have a pro-domain, an enzymatic domain, a zinc-binding domain, and a hemopexin/vitronectin (VN)-like domain (except in MMP-7 and MMP-26). Additionally, membrane-type MMPs contain membrane anchor, with some membrane type (MT)-MMPs also possessing a cytoplasmic domain and a carboxyl terminus. Gelatinases contain a gelatin-binding domain with three fibronectin (FN)-like repeats. In particular, MMP-9 also contains a serine- threonine- and O-glycosylated domain. N-glycosylated sites, one of which is conserved in most MMPs, are denoted with a Y symbol. Part of the propeptide, which contains the chelating cysteine, and part of the zinc-binding domain with three histidines are indicated with one letter code for amino acids. *(Adapted from Hu J, et al: Matrix metalloproteinase inhibitors as therapy for inflammatory and vascular disease. Nat Rev Drug Discov 6:480–498, 2007.)*

A key role for CAAT-binding factor, Sp1, Sp3, Ap1, nuclear factor (NF)-κB, and SMADs has been reported for several collagen genes; a number of orientation-dependent enhancer-like elements have also been documented.[23,24]

Fibrillar and nonfibrillar collagens found in subendothelial ECM are regulated by many cytokines and growth factors; collagen gene expression in response to cytokines (e.g., transforming growth factor [TGF]-β, tumor necrosis factor [TNF]-α, interleukins [ILs]), glucocorticoids, estrogen, androgen, and retinoids has been reported. The signaling cascades initiated by intrinsic and exogenous regulators impinge on a distinct set of *cis*-acting elements that bind to constitutive and inducible transcription factors. The emerging theme from these studies is that various *cis*- and *trans*-acting factors interact to recruit selective transcriptional coactivators and co-repressors in response to specific stimuli.[23,24] However, the precise mechanisms that determine combinatorial interactions under physiological and inflammatory conditions remain to be elucidated.

Following translation, pre-procollagen α chains are chaperoned from the endoplasmic reticulum (ER) to the Golgi. It has been reported that the heat shock protein-47 (Hsp47) functions as a collagen-specific chaperone; thus, hsp47 is presumed to provide a quality control mechanism needed for proper maturation of newly synthesized procollagen chains. To demonstrate a role of hsp47 *in vivo* Nagai and coworkers[25] inactivated Hsp47 gene by homologous recombination. The mutant embryos died in utero before 11.5 days of postcoitus development as a result of severely reduced levels of mature type I collagen in their tissues.

As shown in Figure 4-2, fibrillar and nonfibrillar collagens also undergo a number of posttranslational modifications for proper maturation; these include proteolysis of signal peptides, hydroxylation of key proline and lysine residues, glycosylation, and formation of interchain and intrachain disulfide bridges.[6,7,21] Thus, optimal biosynthesis and assembly of collagens depends on a

number of key enzymes. These include three hydroxylases, two collagen-specific glycosyl transferases, two unique proteinases that cleave the NH_2- and COOH-termini, and a collagen-specific oxidase that is needed for cross-link formation. The posttranslational processing of the procollagen molecules also needs a peptidyl proline *cis-trans* isomerase and a protein disulfide isomerase (PDI).

Vitamin C–dependent 4-prolyl hydroxylase, an $\alpha_2\beta_2$-tetramer located in the ER, plays a central role in collagen synthesis because 4-proline hydroxylation is obligatory for cross-link formation. In humans, there are three known isozymes of 4-prolyl hydroxylases, each with a distinct α subunit, but all contain PDI as their β subunit. Hydroxylation of lysine is carried out by lysyl hydroxylase, which also uses the same cofactors as prolyl hydroxylase and reacts only with a lysine residue in the Y position of the Gly-X-Y triplets. There are three known isozymes of lysyl hydroxylase in humans. The under-hydroxylation of procollagen leads to reduced secretion and rapid degradation. Deficiency of lysine hydroxylase is associated with skeletal deformities, tissue fragility, and vascular malformations.[6,7,21]

Several collagens undergo glycosylation; both galactose and glucose residues are attached to some hydroxylysine residues during pre-procollagen biosynthesis. The enzyme UDP galactose:hydroxylysine galactosyltransferase adds a galactose residue to the hydroxyl group of hydroxylysine. The UDP glucose galactosyl:hydroxylysine glucosyltransferase then transfers a glucose residue to the hydroxylysine-linked galactose. The two enzymes act in sequence so that galactose is added first, with glucose added only to galactose. Glycosylation occurs during nascent chain synthesis and before the formation of triple helices. Only two of seven hydroxylysine residues of α1(I), α2(I), and α1(III) contain the disaccharide; most of the hydroxylysine residues are glycosylated in other collagens. Glycosylation of some hydroxylysine residues imparts stability to the cross-link.

Assembly of procollagen chains into triple-helical molecules is directed by the COOH-terminal propeptide, with formation of interchain disulfide bonds (see Fig. 4-2). There is a high degree of structural conservation within the propeptide of fibrillar collagens across species. Following its triple-helical assembly, the procollagen molecule is secreted into the extracellular space. Once secreted, however, the NH$_2$ and COOH propeptides are removed by the actions of N- and C-specific peptidases to yield the collagen molecule. The two proteinases that remove the NH$_2$ and COOH propeptides from the newly synthesized collagen are represented by three isozymes each. The C-specific peptidases, members of the tolloid family, also cleave a number of other ECM proteins, and fragments of the propeptides can inhibit procollagen synthesis by a feedback mechanism.[26,27]

Extracellular Maturation of Collagens

During collagen fibril formation, lysyl oxidase catalyzes the oxidative deamination of specific lysine or hydroxylysine residues in the NH$_2$- or COOH-terminal telopeptides to yield allysine and hydroxyallysine, respectively.[28] These reactive aldehydes, being located in the hole zone of the fibril, are free to react with the ε-amino group of lysine or hydroxylysine residues on adjacent chains to form a Schiff base, which undergoes Amadori rearrangement to form ketoimine. With time, two ketoimine structures condense to form a trivalent cross-link, 4-hydroxy-pyridinium. All three types of cross-link may coexist in different fibrils.

A second type of cross-link seen in collagen originates from the condensation of two aldehydes in allysine or hydroxyallysine on adjacent chains. The resulting aldol condensate has a free aldehyde that reacts with other ε-amino groups of lysine or histidine, thus potentially linking three or four collagen chains.[29] Once the aldehydes of allysine and hydroxyallysine are formed, subsequent aldamine and aldol condensation reactions proceed spontaneously. Thus, inter- and intramolecular cross-linking of fibrillar collagens results in formation of insoluble macromolecular aggregates that possess high tensile strength.

Turnover of Collagen

Metabolic turnover of collagens in intact tissues during adulthood is extremely low. In contrast, a very rapid breakdown and synthesis of collagen takes place during tissue remodeling. In their native fibrillar state, collagens are quite resistant to the action of proteases, yet once their helical structure is disrupted, they are readily degraded by a number of proteases. The FACITs such as types IX, XII, and XIV and other collagens containing noncollagenous domains (e.g., type VI collagen) are relatively more susceptible to proteases. After cleavage of the nonhelical segments, the triple-helical domains of collagens denature at 37°C and become susceptible to nonspecific proteases. Additionally, a specific class of proteinases, the matrix metalloproteinases (MMPs), degrades collagens in vivo and in vitro (see later discussion). For example, MMPs cleave the native type I collagen molecule at a single position within its triple helix, between amino acid residues 775 and 776, and the resulting collagen fragments denature spontaneously at body temperature and pH and become highly susceptible to the actions of many other proteases.

Metalloproteinases

The structural and functional diversity of MMPs rivals that of the superfamily of collagens. The MMPs belong to a large family of zinc-dependent endopeptidases, the first of which was described nearly a half century ago. To date, the presence of 23 distinct MMPs has been reported in human tissues. Based on their cellular localization, these enzymes can be broadly subdivided into secreted and membrane-bound MMPs. However, a more detailed analysis of their structural organization and substrate specificities indicates that MMPs may be better classified as collagenases, gelatinases, stromelysins, metrilysins, and membrane-type MMPs.[30–33]

The architectural blueprint of a prototype MMP consists of three subdomains: the Pro-domain, the catalytic domain, and the hemopexin-like C-domain, connected to the catalytic domain via a short linker region (see Fig. 4-5). The catalytic domain of MMPs contains a Zn^{++} ion-binding amino acid sequence motif and a substrate-specific site. The prototypic MMP is synthesized as a pre-proenzyme and is maintained in latent conformation by the Pro-domain via interaction between a cysteine (located in the cysteine switch region of the Pro-domain) and Zn^{++} ion in the catalytic domain. Only when this interaction is disrupted, either by proteolysis of the Pro-domain or by a chemical modification of the cysteine, MMP becomes activated.[32] A number of intracellular and extracellular proteinases, including other MMPs, are known to specifically degrade the Pro-domain to activate MMPs in vivo.

Although in vitro studies have identified numerous substrates for various MMPs (Table 4-2), the precise identities of their in vivo targets remain largely elusive. A number of macromolecules associated with ECM of the endothelium are potential

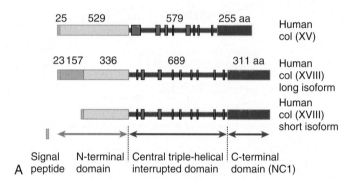

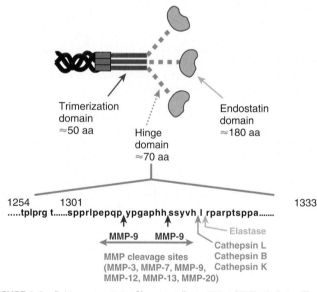

FIGURE 4-6 **A,** Linear structure of human collagen XV and XVIII α1 chains. The α1 chains of collagen XV and XVIII are structurally homologous; they comprise the multiplexin family on the basis of their central triple-helical domain with multiple long interruptions. They are also characterized by a long noncollagenous N-terminal domain–containing thrombospondin sequence motif, with two splicing variants in human collagen XVIII and long, noncollagenous, globular C-terminal domain or NCl domain. **B,** Functional subdomains of human NCl (XVIII) and protease cleavage sites. The NCl domain contains three functionally different subdomains: these domains consist of an N-terminal noncovalent domain involved in trimerization, a hinge domain containing multiple sites that are sensitive to different proteases, and an endostatin globular domain covering a fragment of 20 kD with antiangiogenic and antivessel sprouting activities. Numerous enzymes can generate fragments containing endostatin. Cathepsin L and elastase are the most efficient, but in contrast to matrix metalloproteinase (MMP) cleavage, which leads to accumulation of endostatin, cathepsins L and B degrade the molecule. *(Adapted from Company of Biologists Ltd., Ortega N, Werb Z: New functional roles for non-collagenous domains of basement collagens. J Cell Sci 115:4201, 2002.)*

CONNECTIVE TISSUES OF THE SUBENDOTHELIUM

TABLE 4-2 Members of the Matrix Metalloproteinase Family in Representative Vascular and Nonvascular Tissues*

MMPS	OTHER NAMES	MOL. WT. KDa		TISSUE DISTRIBUTION/DISEASE CONDITION	COLLAGEN SUBSTRATE	OTHER SUBSTRATES
		PROFORM	ACTIVE			
Vascular						
Collagenases MMP-1	Collagenase-1	55	45	Fibroblast, interstitial, tissue collagenase	I, II, III, VII, X	Aggrecan, gelatin, MMP-2, MMP-9
MMP-8	Collagenase-2	75	58	Neutrophil or PMNL collagenase	I, II, III, V, VII, VIII, X	Aggrecan, elastin, FN, gelatin, laminin
MMP-13	Collagenase-3	60	48	SMC, varicose veins, preeclampsia, breast cancer	I, II, III, IV	Aggrecan, gelatin
Gelatinases						
MMP-2	Gelatinase-A	72	66	Aortic aneurysm, varicose veins	I, II, III, IV, V, VII, XI	Aggrecan, elastin, FN, gelatin, laminin, PG, MMP-9, MMP-13
MMP-9	Gelatinase-B	92	86	Aortic aneurysm, varicose veins	IV, V, VII, XIV	Aggrecan, elastin, FN, gelatin
Stromelysins						
MMP-3	Stromelysin-1	57	45	SMC, synovial fibroblasts, CAD, HTN, tumor invasion	II, III, IV, IX, X, XI	Aggrecan, elastin, FN, gelatin, laminin, PG, MMP-7, MMP-8, MMP-13
MMP-10	Stromelysin-2	57	44	Uterine, preeclampsia, arthritis, atherosclerosis, carcinoma cells	III, IV, V	Aggrecan, elastin, FN, gelatin, laminin, MMP-1, MMP-8
Matrilysins						
MMP-7	Matrilysin-1	28	19	Uterine	IV, X	Aggrecan, elastin, FN, gelatin, laminin, PG, MMP-1, MMP-2, MMP-9
Membrane-Type MMPs						
MMP-14	MT1-MMP	66	56	Human fibroblasts, SMC, VSMC, uterine, angiogenesis	I, II, III	Aggrecan, elastin, FN, gelatin, laminin, MMP-2, MMP-13
MMP-15	MT2-MMP	72	50	Fibroblasts, leukocytes, preeclampsia, cancer (breast, prostate, colon)	I	FN, gelatin, laminin, MMP-2
MMP-16	MT3-MMP	64	52	Leukocytes, angiogenesis, human cancer	I	MMP-2
MMP-24	MT5-MMP	57	53	Leukocytes, brain tumor, astrocytoma/glioblastoma	None identified	Fibrin, gelatin
Other MMPs						
MMP-11	Stromelysin-3	51	44	Uterine, angiogenesis, hepatocellular carcinoma	Does not cleave	Aggrecan, FN, laminin
MMP-12	Metalloelastase	54	45 and 22	Macrophage	IV	Elastin, FN, gelatin, laminin
MMP-21	XMMP	62	49	Human placenta		α_1-Antitrypsin
Non-Vascular						
MMP-18	Xenopus collagenase-4	70	53	Xenopus (amphibian)	I	Gelatin
MMP-26	Matrilysin-2, endometase	28	19	Human endometrial tumor	IV	Gelatin, FN
MMP-17	MT4-MMP	57	53	Brain-specific cerebellum, breast cancer	None identified	Fibrin, gelatin
MMP-25	MT6-MMP, leukolysin	34	28	Leukocytes, anaplastic astrocytomas, glioblastomas	IV	Gelatin, FN, laminin, fibrin
MMP-19	RASI-1	54	45	Liver	IV	FN, aggrecan, COMP, laminin, gelatin
MMP-20	Enamelysin	54	22	Tooth enamel	V	Aggrecan, amelogenin, COMP
MMP-22	CMMP	51		Chicken fibroblasts	Unknown	Gelatin
MMP-23	Cysteine array MMP	28	19	Reproductive tissues	Unknown	Unknown
MMP-28	Epilysin	56	45	Skin keratinocytes	Unknown	Unknown

CAD, coronary artery disease; CMMP, Chicken metalloproteinase; COMP, cartilage oligomeric matrix protein; FN, fibronectin; HTN, Hypertension; MMP, matrix metalloproteinase; MT, membrane-type; PG, proteoglycan; PMNL, Polymorphonuclear leukocyte; RASI-1, Rheumatoid arthritis inflamed-1; SMC, smooth muscle cell; VSMC, vascular smooth muscle cell.
*From Raffetto JD, Khalil RA: Matrix metalloproteinases and their inhibitors in muscular remodeling and vascular disease. Biochem Pharmacol 75:346–359, 2008.

in vivo targets of MMPs. For example, MMP-1 (collagenase 1) readily degrades collagen types I, II, and III, whereas MMP-8 (collagenase 2) digests types I, III, IV, V, VII, X, and XI collagen. Similarly MMP-2 (gelatinase A) degrades types I, III, IV, V, VII, X, and XI collagens, whereas gelatinase B (MMP-9) can degrade collagen types IV, V, XI, and XIV preferentially. MMP-13 (collagenase 3) is also capable of degrading collagens that are prevalent in subendothelial ECM (types I, III, VI, IX, and XIV). Many collagenous and noncollagenous ECM components are readily degraded by stromelysin-1 (MMP-3) and stromelysin-2 (MMP-10), whereas stromelysin-3 (MMP-11) does not degrade known collagens but readily breaks down laminin. Matrix metalloproteinases are also capable of digesting a number of other constituents of ECM, such as FN and elastin, and a variety of other cell- and ECM-associated molecules (see Table 4-2). The actions of some MMPs are likely to mediate highly regulated processing of ECM-bound pro-TGF-β and pro-IL-1.

Numerous studies have been undertaken to elucidate the molecular mechanisms by which the actions of MMPs are regulated in the tissues under physiological and pathological conditions.[32] Two major mechanistic themes have emerged from these studies to explain the exquisite specificity of various MMPs. First, synthesis and localization of various pro-MMPs and their highly tissue-specific inhibitors (TIMPs) are regulated by autocrine and paracrine factors. Thus, cytokines such as IL-1 and TNF-α and a number of other circulating factors regulate expression of various MMPs at the transcriptional and posttranscriptional levels.

The second type of regulation of MMPs is exerted via the unique organization of their functional domains. As outlined earlier, the Pro-domain plays a critical role in maintaining the MMPs in a latent state that is altered by a number of physiological and pathological stimuli. Similarly, the presence of three cysteine-rich repeats, akin to those found in FN (see later discussion) in gelatinase A and gelatinase B, determines their affinities for elastin and collagen. The domain organization of MMPs allows them to be regulated by TIMPs; these inhibitors reversibly bind to MMPs in a 1:1 stoichiometry and inhibit enzymatic activity.[34] Tissue inhibitors of MMPs, represented by four homologous proteins (TIMP1 to 4), preferentially inhibit various MMPs.[35,36] For example, whereas TIMP3 potently inhibits MMP-9, both TIMP2 and TIMP3 inhibit membrane-type 1 (MT1)-MMP. In contrast, TIMP1 is a very poor inhibitor of MT-3-MMP but a potent inhibitor of MMP-3.[34]

Concerted actions of various MMPs and their TIMPs regulate key events in the formation of blood vessels in the developing embryo, and the processes of neovasculogenesis and angiogenesis in the adult in response to injury and regeneration (Table 4-3). Formation of new blood vessels from existing vessels is dependent on extensive turnover of subendothelial ECM. This process enables migration of blood vessel–associated cells, liberation of angiogenic factors sequestered in the ECM, and exposure of cryptic cell-regulatory domains found in the intact fibrillar and nonfibrillar components of connective tissue. Therefore, a crucial balance between MMPs and TIMPs is essential for maturation of newly formed blood vessels and ongoing maintenance of their structural integrity. These processes are known to play a critical role during embryogenesis; the formation of solid tumors and their acquisition of invasive, metastatic phenotype is also vitally dependent on the emergence of new blood vessels.[37] MMP-2 binds to the $\alpha_v\beta_3$ integrin and promotes angiogenesis and tumor growth.[38] In contrast, the transmembrane MMP, MT1-MMP, cleaves $\alpha_v\beta_3$ integrin and enhances its affinity for its ligands containing arginine-glycine-aspartic acid (RGD) sequences.

Elastin

Blood vessels are endowed with a high degree of elasticity, and subendothelial elastic fibers are responsible for the resilience of the vasculature to cycles of deformity and passive recoil during diastole and systole, respectively. The elastic fiber consists of an insoluble core of polymerized tropoelastin surrounded by a

TABLE 4-3	The Effect of Matrix Turnover on Vascular Pathologies*	
	MODEL	**EFFECTS**
Aneurysm	MMP-3$^{-/-}$ / ApoE$^{-/-}$	↓ Aneurysm
	MMP-9$^{-/-}$	↓ Aneurysm
	MMP-12$^{-/-}$	↔ Aneurysm
	Broad-range MMP inhibitor LDLR$^{-/-}$	↓ Aneurysm
	TIMP-1$^{-/-}$ / ApoE$^{-/-}$	↑Aneurysm
	TIMP-1 ↑ rat	↓ Aneurysm
Neointima formation	MMP-9 ↑rat	↑SMC migration ↓ matrix content ↑Luminal diameter
	Broad-range MMP inhibitor	↓ Early and ↔ late neo-intima formation
	LDLR$^{-/-}$ Doxycycline, MMP inhibition rat	↓ Neointima formation
	TIMP-1 ↑human vein	↓ Neointima formation
	TIMP-2 ↑human vein	↓ Neointima formation
	TIMP-3 ↑human and pig veins	↓ Neointima formation
	MMP-9$^{-/-}$, mouse carotid ligation	↓ Intimal hyperplasia, ↑ collagen content
Remodeling	MMP-12 ↑	↓ Luminal diameter
	MMP inhibitor pig	↓ Constrictive remodeling
Atherosclerosis	MMP-1 ↑/ ApoE$^{-/-}$	↓ Plaque size ↓ collagen content
	MMP-3$^{-/-}$ / ApoE$^{-/-}$	↑ Plaque size ↑ collagen content
	MMP-3 ↓ human, promoter polymorphism	↑Plaque progression
	MMP-9 ↑ human, promoter polymorphism	↑Triple-vessel disease
	MMP-9 ↑ human promoter polymorphism	↔ Coronary artery stenosis
	Broad-range MMP inhibitor LDL$^{-/-}$	↔ Plaque size
	TIMP-1$^{-/-}$ / ApoE$^{-/-}$	↓ Plaque size ↑ lipid core content
	TIMP-1$^{-/-}$ / ApoE$^{-/-}$	↔ Plaque size, medial rupture, micro aneurysms
	TIMP-1 ↑/ ApoE$^{-/-}$	↓ Plaque size ↑ collagen content
	TGF-β inhibition ApoE$^{-/-}$	↑ Plaque vulnerability, intra-plaque hemorrhage

MMP, matrix metalloproteinase; Apo, apolipoprotein; LDLR, LDL receptor; TIMP, tissue inhibitor of matrix metalloproteinase; SMC, smooth muscle cell; TGF, transforming growth factor; +/+, transgenic overexpressing mice; –/–, knock-out or homozygous deficient mice; ↑, upregulation or increased; ↓, downregulated or decreased.
*Adapted from Heeneman S, Cleutjens JP, Faber BC, et al: The dynamic extracellular matrix: intervention strategies during heart failure and atherosclerosis. J Pathol 2003:516, 2003.

mantle of microfibrils. A schematic representation of the modular organization of human tropoelastin is shown in Figure 4-7. The primary structure of tropoelastin consists of hydrophilic and hydrophobic domains; these may be further divided into subdomains based on the composition of their amino acid sequences (see Fig. 4-7). The mechanical properties of the elastic fiber are similar to rubber (i.e., the degree of elongation without irreversible changes per unit force applied to unit cross-sectional areas is high).

Organization of the elastic fibers has been studied by electron microscopic, biochemical, and genetic approaches, and a number of key insights have been gathered in recent years.[3] Elastin is a major constituent of the elastic fiber and may contribute as much as 50% of the dry mass of large arteries.[39] The elastic fibers begin to form at mid-gestation by deposition of tropoelastin, the soluble precursor of the cross-linked mature elastin, on a template of fibrillin-rich microfibers. The cross-linked elastin contained in the elastic fibers produced during late fetal and postnatal development generally lasts a lifetime.

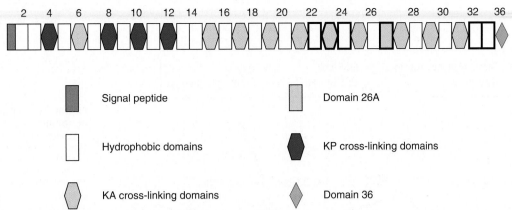

FIGURE 4-7   Domain organization of human tropoelastin, containing all possible exons. The NH$_2$-terminus of tropoelastin contains the signal peptide, whereas exon 36 encoded sequences with highly conserved two-cysteine residues and RKRK form the COOH-terminus. Hydrophilic cross-linking domains are further divided into KP- and KA-rich regions. Alternative splicing is a hallmark of tropoelastin biosynthesis; at least 11 human tropoelastin splice variants have been characterized, resulting from developmentally regulated alternative splicing of domains 22, 23, 24, 26A, 32, and 33 *(highlighted in bold)*.

Elastin has an amorphous appearance in the electron microscope; microfibrils appear as 10- to 15-nm diameter filaments. The assembly of elastic fibers occurs via a stepwise process that includes formation of a scaffold of microfibrils that facilitate deposition of tropoelastin monomers (Fig. 4-8), followed by extensive cross-linking to form the functional polymer.[3,40,41] Tropoelastin is the soluble monomer of elastin that is one of the most apolar and insoluble proteins in nature. Although the glycine and proline content of elastin is similar to fibrillar collagens, elastin contains no hydroxyproline or hydroxylysine, and very small amounts of polar amino acids. Elucidation of the molecular organization of elastin has been difficult because of the technical problems in obtaining large quantities of tropoelastin. Therefore, scientists have relied mainly on the structure of fragments of hydrolyzed soluble elastin and recombinant tropoelastin produced in bacteria.

As illustrated in Figure 4-7, human tropoelastin is encoded as a 72-kD polypeptide that is characterized by a series of tandem repeats. The tropoelastin amino acid sequence is divided into hydrophobic domains that are rich in nonpolar amino acids (glycine, valine, and proline) that typically occur as repeating units; these sequences alternate with hydrophilic domains that are enriched in lysine and alanine. *In vitro*, elastin undergoes a process of ordered self-aggregation called *coacervation* (aligning and concentrating the protein in unit spheres) prior to cross-linking. Tropoelastin binds to cell surface glycosaminoglycans as well as to αvβ3 integrins.[42] Although the sequential interactions of tropoelastin with fibrillins and its associated molecules are poorly defined, it is thought that the process of elastic fiber assembly is initiated on the cell surface.[43,44] This is caused by specific interactions of the individual hydrophobic domains of tropoelastin, since it has an intrinsic ability to organize into polymeric structures.[39]

In vivo, tropoelastin probably interacts with microfibrils prior to aggregation and becomes cross-linked by lysyl oxidase.[40,41,45] Soluble precursors of elastin are not found in extracts of normal tissues. This provides a clue as to the rapid formation of mature, highly cross-linked elastin fibers and the low rate of tropoelastin synthesis. In experimental conditions such as copper deficiency or lathyrism induced by β-aminopropionitrile, which inhibits lysyl oxidase activity and thus cross-link formation, a soluble 72 kD tropoelastin can be extracted from the aorta. Like collagens, newly synthesized tropoelastin undergoes posttranslational modifications before its assembly into elastic fibers; in fact, the same lysyl oxidase reacts with both collagens and elastin.[46] In contrast to collagen, however, reduction of double bonds in the elastin cross-link occurs spontaneously, and the quantity of lysine involved in cross-linking is much larger in elastin than in collagen (see Fig. 4-8). Oxidative deamination of lysine residues, followed by subsequent condensation reactions, creates

$$>—CH_2—CH_2—CH_2—CH=N—CH—CH_2—CH_2—CH_2—<$$

Dehydrolysinonorleucine

$$>—CH_2—CH_2—\underset{\underset{CHO}{|}}{C}=CH—CH_2—CH_2—CH_2—<$$

Allysinealdol

$$>—CH_2—CH_2—\underset{\underset{\underset{N—CH_2—CH_2—CH_2—CH_2—<}{|}}{\underset{CH}{|}}}{C}=CH—CH_2—CH_2—CH_2—<$$

Dehydromerodesmosine

Desmosine

Isodesmosine

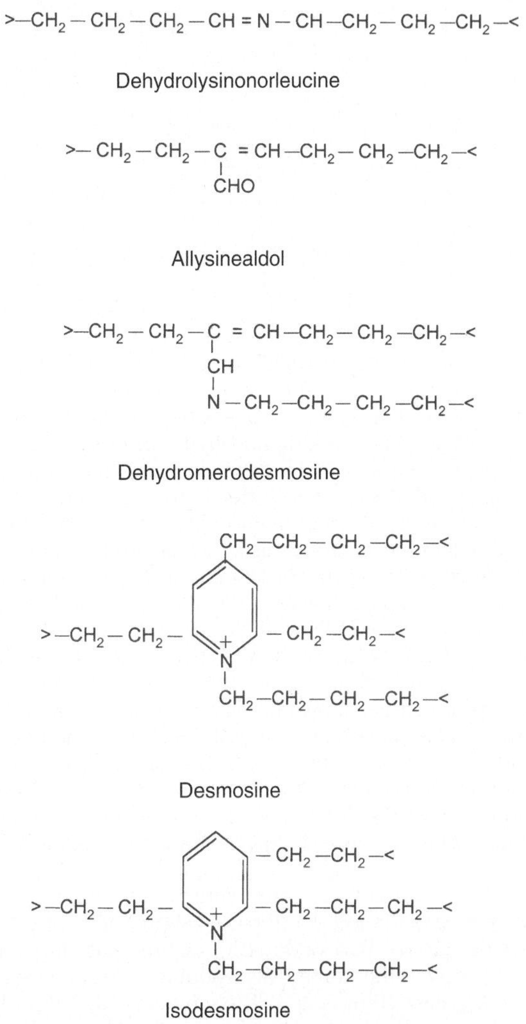

FIGURE 4-8   The structures of cross-links found in elastin. Desmosine and isodesmosine represent final products of lysine-derived cross-links.

the unusual cross-links found in elastin. All of the cross-links in elastin are derived from lysyl residues through allysine (Fig. 4-9). However, the precise molecular reactions needed to form desmosine remain to be elucidated. Cross-linking in elastin occurs frequently, not only between peptide chains but also within the same polypeptide chain, producing intrapolypeptide links.

Fibrillin

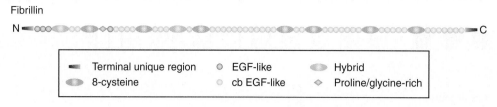

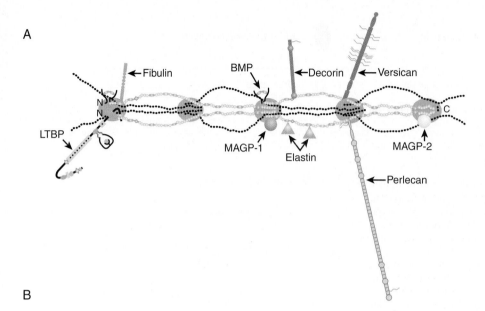

B

FIGURE 4-9 **A, Domain organization of fibrillin.** All three fibrillins have a similar modular organization, with strong homologies with each other. Fibrillin-1 has a proline-rich region, whereas fibrillin-2 has a glycine-rich sequence; in contrast, fibrillin-3 has a region that is both proline- and glycine-rich. This region lies between the first 8-cysteine module and the fourth epidermal growth factor (EGF)-like domain. **B,** Schematic of various ligands that bind to fibrillin to assemble microfibrils. Putative binding sites for various ligands are based on *in vitro* observations; association of various molecules with fibrillins is most likely regulated dynamically by physiological and pathological stimuli. BMP, bone morphogenetic protein; LTBP, latent transforming growth factor β-binding protein; MAGP, microfibril-associated glycoprotein. *(Adapted from Ramirez F, Sakai LY: Biogenesis and function of fibrillin assemblies. Cell Tissue Res 339:71–82, 2010.)*

The cross-linking process is highly efficient, and it is unclear how the cross-linking sites in the monomer get aligned.

Genomic organization of the tropoelastin gene indicates that functionally distinct cross-linking and hydrophobic domains of tropoelastin may be encoded by distinct exons. Short segments rich in alanine and lysine are clustered to apparently delimit the cross-linked region. These amino acids are clustered in the α-helical configuration of tropoelastin, where each begins with tyrosine followed by Ala-Ala-Lys or Ala-Ala-Ala-Lys. In humans, several distinct tropoelastin polypeptides may be generated by alternative splicing (see Fig. 4-7). Space-filling atomic models indicate that lysines separated by two or three alanyl residues in α-helical conformation protrude on the same side of the helix. Hence, the sequence Lys-Ala-Ala-Lys allows formation of dehydrolysinonorleucine, whereas the sequence Lys-Ala-Ala-Ala-Lys accommodates either aldol condensation or dehydrolysinonorleucine formation. Condensation of the two intrachain cross-links could result in the formation of the interchain desmosine cross-links. The alanine- and lysine-rich cross-linking segments are separated by large hydrophobic segments of 6 to 8 kD, which are in a β-spiral structure with elastomeric properties. Within the hydrophobic segments, a repeating pentapeptide (Pro-Gly-Val-Gly-Val) is present. A collagen-like sequence (Gly-Val-Pro-Gly) occurs quite frequently, which would explain the limited susceptibility of tropoelastin to bacterial collagenase (Pro-Gly-X-Y). The sequence Gly-X-Pro-Gly is recognized by the prolyl hydroxylase involved in the cross-linking of collagens (see earlier discussion).

Elastin Metabolism and Vascular Homeostasis

After deposition, tropoelastin production is strikingly reduced; the half-life of elastin in normal humans has been estimated in years. In the event of injury, production of elastin can be quickly initiated. A number of growth factors and cytokines induce biosynthesis of tropoelastin. Under these conditions, a very specific set of proteinases named *elastases* are responsible for elastin remodeling.

Elastin fibers may be degraded by a number of MMPs, particularly MMP-2,-3,-9 and -12, that are present as latent enzymes under physiological conditions but are activated following vessel wall injury.[47] The MMPs from neutrophils or macrophages are believed to degrade the elastin-rich ECM found in inflamed tissues. A hereditary defect in circulating elastase inhibitors is associated with a progressive destruction of the elastin-rich alveolar wall, resulting in premature emphysema. Furthermore, experimental instillation of elastase into the lungs of animals causes destruction of the lung similar to that seen in patients with α1-proteinase inhibitor deficiency.

Mice with a disrupted elastin gene have provided important insights into the function of elastin protein. Heterozygous (elastin[+/-] mice) had decreased arterial compliance and were hypertensive. The homozygous elastin-null mice died young due to arterial obstruction caused by uncontrolled proliferation of smooth muscle cells (SMCs).[39,48] A direct link between occlusive vascular diseases and perturbation in the organization of the elastic fibers in the vessels has also been established.[49] Mutations in the elastin gene are associated with supravalvular aortic stenosis (SVAS) and Williams-Beuren's syndrome (WBS), pediatric disorders characterized by hemodynamic stress and loss of elasticity.[49] Furthermore, haploinsufficiency of elastin resulting from aberrant degradation of mutated protein in humans or ablation of the elastin gene in transgenic mice caused intimal hyperplasia and thickened arteries.[40,45,50-52] Apparently, VSMCs, the primary producers of elastin, organized more cell layers to compensate for lost elasticity and biomechanical support in developing blood vessels of elastin haploinsufficient patients and transgenic mice.

Vascular smooth muscle cells from SVAS patients, WBS patients, and elastin[-/-] mice show increased rates of proliferation and chemotactic migration, and reduced rates of elastin synthesis *in vitro*.[50-52] Exogenous supplementation of recombinant tropoelastin and α-elastin to these cultures reversed their phenotype. The elastin-rich ECM serves as an autocrine regulator of VSMC; Karnik et al.[53] inserted elastin-coated stents in a porcine coronary injury model of restenosis and found that intimal thickness and arterial stenosis were significantly reduced. Although the identities of the specific receptors mediating elastin VSMC interactions and the signaling mechanisms underlying vascular remodeling remain obscure,[54] restoring elastin to an injured arterial wall is known to reduce obstructive vascular pathology.[55,56] Inhibitors of MMPs have been shown to prevent degradation of elastic fibers after vascular injury and ameliorate neointimal thickening.[47]

Fibrillins and Other Microfibril-Associated Proteins

Fibrillins, the major constituent of microfibers, are large glycoproteins that form loosely packed bundles in the tissues. The fibrillin superfamily also includes the structurally related latent TGF-β-binding proteins (LTBP1, 2, 3, and 4) and fibulins.[40,45,57] Fibrillins are represented by three homologous proteins: fibrillin-1, fibrillin-2, and fibrillin-3. All three fibrillins are approximately 350-kD glycoproteins that display similar modular organization (see Fig. 4-9) that consists of 46/47 epidermal growth factor (EGF)-like domains (42/43 of these are calcium-binding type; cbEGF) interspersed with seven 8-cysteine-containing TGF-β-binding (TB) modules found in LTBPs. Additionally, fibrillins contain two hybrid domains composed of TB/8Cys and cbEGF-like sequences and NH_2- and COOH-termini with sequence homologies with respective segments of LTBPs and fibulins. The structural versatility of elastic fibers (e.g., concentric rings in arterial walls vs. parallel bundles in the ocular ligament that anchors the lens to the ciliary body) most probably reflects a selective use of different fibrillins in different locations. Importantly, the function of fibrillin-3 remains to be established, and thus the following narrative is restricted to fibrillin-1 and fibrillin-2.

Fibrillins are thought to organize into microfibrils in which individual molecules are organized in a head-to-tail arrangement as well as sideways. The precise molecular architecture of fibrillins within the microfiber and how its elasticity is regulated are incompletely understood. The developmental role of fibrillins has become evident from studies in transgenic mice. Thus, fibrillin-1-deficient mice display frequent dissecting aneurysm and die soon after birth.[58,59] This is in contrast to the vessels of fibrillin-2−/− mice that appear to be structurally and functionally normal. However, mice with haploinsufficiency of both fibrillin-1 and fibrillin-2 elicit variable phenotypes, although many die in utero. These studies indicate that fibrillin-1 and -2 play somewhat unique context-dependent instructive and mechanical roles in the developing vasculature. The four known LTBPs with multiple EGF-repeats of fibrillin-1 and fibrillin-2 and their associated ligands (e.g., perlecan, elastin, fibulin) are mechanistically involved in the developmental actions of these versatile ECM proteins.[40,45,57]

Fibrillin-rich microfibrils play a vital role in extracellular regulation of TGF-βs and bone morphogenetic proteins (BMPs) by modulating their storage, release, and activation in response to various stimuli.[3,40,41,45,49,57] Apparently, LTBP1, 3, and 4 elicit functional redundancy and target the latent TGF-β to elastin-rich microfibrils; LTBP2 does not bind TGF-β but is highly expressed in response to arterial injury. Fibrillins appear to play a direct role in TGF-β signaling, as revealed by fibrillin-1 knockout mice that were born with impaired lungs and emphysema, without measurable signs of inflammation. A detailed analysis of these animals revealed that aberrant TGF-β (Smad2/3) signaling in the developing lungs was responsible for the observed pulmonary phenotype.[58,59] More recently, a role of fibrillin-1 mutations in the development of mitral valve prolapse and aortic aneurysm was also reported.

The microfibril-associated glycoproteins MAGP-1 and MAGP-2 are also believed to impart structural integrity to microfibrils.[60,61] The expression profile of MAGP-1 in the aorta resembles that of fibrillin-2; both are thought to be critical for embryonic and fetal development of the aorta. Additionally, PGs (e.g., biglycan, decorin, versican) are also associated with microfibrils and are believed to facilitate their incorporation into surrounding ECM.[3,40,41,45,49,57]

Fibulins represent a family of ECM proteins with cbEGF-like domains and a distinctive COOH-terminal module.[57] Seven fibulins have been identified since the discovery of the prototype, fibulin-1. The unique distribution of various fibulins suggests that their contribution to the organization of various types of the elastic fibers may be tissue specific. Based on their length and domain organization, fibulins are classified into two groups. The short fibulins (fibulin-3, -4, -5, and -7) are elastogenic and contain tandem repeats of cbEGF. How various fibulins modify endothelial ECM has been investigated *in vitro* and in transgenic mice. Whereas fibulin-1 is located in the elastin core, fibulin-2 and -4 are found at the interface between the central elastic core and the mantle of microfibrils. Fibulin-1 knockout mice have dysfunctional vasculature and die of spontaneous bleeding. Mice that lack a functional fibulin-4 gene are also born with severe vascular defects.

The preceding description of microfibrils underscores the notion that the elastic fiber and its associated ECM are molecular integrators of extrinsic and intrinsic mechanical signals that impinge on TGF-β and BMP as focal points of tissue homeostasis. Therefore, it is mechanistically probable that diverse assemblies of fibrillin-associated molecules are involved in translating environmental inputs into physiological and pathological responses of the endothelium. Suffice to say, however, that the molecular interactions that regulate the putative extracellular inputs, as well as their corresponding responses both in time and space that mediate remodeling the vasculature during embryogenesis and in the adult, remain to be elucidated.[62]

Fibronectin

Fibronectin is one of the best characterized molecules of the vascular ECM.[63,64] Evolutionary emergence of FN correlates with the appearance of EC lined vasculature in vertebrates.[65] There is high degree of interspecies homology and conservation of domain organization of the FN gene across species.[65,66] Fibronectin dynamically partners with multiple macromolecules to promote adhesion and spreading of cells, trigger chemotaxis of leukocytes towards injured tissue, and facilitate nonimmune opsonization and phagocytosis of bacteria. Some biologically active modules of FN are normally cryptic and are only exposed under special circumstances. Crosstalk between FN and growth factor/cytokine-mediated signals modulates tissue repair and regeneration and is involved in anchorage-independent growth of cancer cells. Fibronectin is especially abundant in the ECM of the embryo, where it plays a crucial role in phenotypic differentiation of vascular and nonvascular tissues. A functional FN gene is obligatory for development of the cardiovascular system.

Fibronectin Structure

In blood plasma, FN exists in a soluble state, synthesized and secreted by the liver, and is converted into an insoluble supramolecular complex in the ECM. The soluble FN is made of two disulfide-linked monomers of similar or identical mass (220-255 kD). As shown in Figure 4-10, each FN monomer is a mosaic of repeating modules termed *type I, II,* and *III* repeats that are 40, 60, and 90 amino acids long, respectively.[67,68] A cluster of 15 to 17 type III repeats (depending on alternative splicing) located in the middle of the molecule represents 90% of the FN monomer. In addition, there are 12 type I and 2 type II repeats in each monomer of FN. The type III repeats fold into nearly identical shapes despite having only 20 to 40 amino acid sequence identity (see Fig. 4-10). The striking modular organization of the repeated peptide sequences in FN is reflected in the organization of its gene. The FN gene consists of 47 exons spanning nearly 100 kb in the human genome and generates multiple alternatively spliced mRNAs.[69–72] A single gene thus generates about 20 variants of FN protein that may be preferentially synthesized under various physiological and pathological situations.[68] Fibronectin monomers containing or lacking the extra domain A (EDA) or B (EDB) are particularly significant

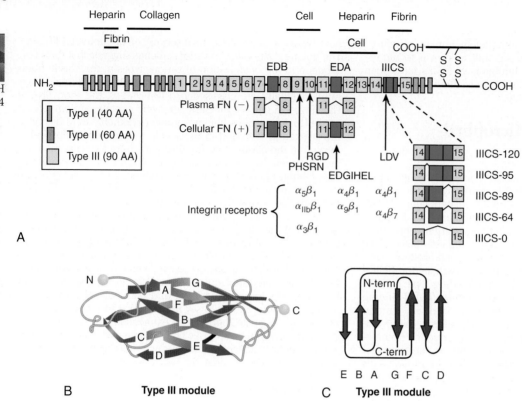

FIGURE 4-10 **Primary structure of fibronectin (FN) and its modular organization.** Hypothetical scheme represents an FN dimer with various sequence modules. **A,** Different types of homologous domains (12 type I, 2 type II, and 15 type III) are shown. Numbering of type III homologies excludes extra domain (ED)A and EDB domains. Types I, II, and III domains are made of 40, 60, and 90 amino acids, respectively. Constitutively expressed (RGD), alternatively spliced (LDV), synergy (PHSRN) and EDA (EDGIHEL) cell-binding sites are indicated, together with integrin receptors to which they bind. EDA and EDB splicing is similar in all species, whereas the IIICS region is spliced in a species-specific (five variants in humans, three in rodents, and two in chickens) manner. Type III homologies are organized in seven antiparallel β strands. Spatial and planar representations of type III module are shown in **B** and **C**, respectively. (Adapted from White ES, Baralle FE, Muro AF: New insights into form and function of fibronectin splice variants. J Pathol 216:1–14, 2008.)

with regard to their biological functions. Plasma FN (soluble) lacks both EDA and EDB domains; in contrast, FN assembled into ECM contains variable mixtures of cellular FN with or without EDA and EDB domains (see Fig. 4-10).

Functional Domains of Fibronectin

Fibronectin is a multifunctional molecule with a series of specialized modules.[67,68] Proteolysis of FN generates a number of fragments that bind to specific ligands. The NH₂-terminal 70-kD fragment of FN binds to a surprisingly large number of ECM ligands that include collagen, gelatin, fibrin, and heparin. The 70-kD FN also binds to some gram-positive bacteria (e.g., *Staphylococcus aureus, Streptococcus pyogenes, Streptococcus pneumoniae*) via the so-called microbial surface components recognizing adhesive matrix molecules (MSCRAMM). Thus lipoteichoic acid, M proteins, and several other bacterial adhesins anchored in the cell wall bind to FN and enhance opsonization and phagocytosis of bacteria.[73] Gram-negative bacteria do not bind to FN.

THE COLLAGEN-BINDING DOMAIN

The collagen-binding domain of FN includes type I repeats 6 to 9 and type II repeats 1 and 2.[74,75] The first component of complement C1q, which contains a collagen-like structure, also binds FN.[76] Denatured collagen (gelatin) has a much greater affinity for FN. Several FN binding sites exist along the collagen α chain, including a high-affinity site in type I collagen in the amino acid sequence targeted for cleavage by MMP-1 and MMP-2. It has been posited that the gelatin-binding domain of FN facilitates clearance of denatured collagen from circulating plasma. However, since triple-helical domains of fibrillar collagens may be partially unwound at body temperature, such local unraveling of the triple helix facilitates FN binding to native collagen and modulates its interactions with other molecules.[31,33]

THE CELL-BINDING DOMAIN

Fibronectin binds to cell surfaces via specific heterodimeric receptors called *integrins* that initiate intracellular signal transduction.[68,77,78] Although FN binds to a number of integrins (e.g., $\alpha_4\beta_1, \alpha_5\beta_1, \alpha_v\beta_3, \alpha_v\beta_1$), most FN functions in vascular development may be mediated via $\alpha_5\beta_1$ integrin.[67] Studies in transgenic mice have demonstrated that specific ablation of α_5 integrin causes the most severe defects in vessel formation. The mechanistic relationship between α_5 integrin and FN is further highlighted by the observation that the vascular phenotypes of $\alpha_5\beta_1$ integrin knockout and FN-ablated mice are extremely similar.[79–81] The RGD site, located in the tenth type III repeat of FN, binds to $\alpha_5\beta_1$ integrin, and this interaction is obligatory for intracellular signaling. The alternatively spliced variants of FN bind to other integrins. For example, a segment of EDA binds to $\alpha_4\beta_1$ integrin, whereas a peptide located in the IIICS segment can bind to both $\alpha_5\beta_1$ and $\alpha_4\beta_7$ integrins.

Based on a number of *in vitro* assays, subdomains of FN, particularly EDA and EDB, have been ascribed many functions that include cellular adhesion, mitogenic signal transduction, dimer formation, matrix assembly, and regulation of cytokine-dependent secretion of MMPs.[68,77,78] However, these studies must be interpreted with caution and need *in vivo* corroboration. This caveat is highlighted by the observation that mice engineered to express FN without either EDA- or EDB-encoding exons develop normally. Conversely, deletion of both EDA and EDB exons leads to severe cardiovascular anomalies and premature death.[82,83]

Incorporation of FN into insoluble ECM is a cell-mediated process that is obligatory for vasculogenesis. The NH₂-terminal domain of soluble FN binds to the cell surface and is converted into disulfide-linked polymers. Polymerization of FN occurs at specialized surfaces of many cells, including SMCs and fibroblasts, and is coordinated by integrins.[84] Since integrins $\alpha_5\beta_1, a_{IIb}\beta_3$, or $\alpha_v\beta_3$ can polymerize FN and incorporate it into larger ECM aggregates, different integrins appear to be functionally redundant.[64]

THE HEPARIN-BINDING DOMAIN

The heparin-binding domain of FN is located at the NH$_2$ terminus and overlaps the fibrin-binding site (see later discussion). Several polyanionic molecules (e.g., heparin, heparan sulfate, dextran sulfate, DNA) bind to FN; this binding is specific, since other polyanionic molecules (e.g., chondroitin sulfates, dermatan sulfate [DS]) do not. Some of these macromolecules bind to FN in a cooperative fashion. For example, the presence of heparan sulfate or hyaluronic acid enhances the association between FN and gelatin. Similarly, FN causes precipitation of type I or type III collagens, but only in the presence of heparin. Such cooperative binding of diverse ligands to various modules of FN is likely to facilitate its incorporation into a tissue-selective ECM *in vivo*.[68]

THE FIBRIN-BINDING DOMAINS AND CLOTTING

The highly organized architecture of blood vessels and their cellular elements are perturbed by persistent hypertension, atherosclerosis, and other vascular pathologies. At these putative sites of injury, thrombus formation is invariably initiated by platelets. Fibronectin participates in blood coagulation and thrombosis.[85-87] The human FN monomer contains a fibrin-binding domain at its carboxyl end, and the complex of FN and fibrin is cross-linked by factor XIIIa. The integrin $\alpha_{IIb}\beta_3$ found on platelets is recognized by fibrin and FN. Under static conditions, FN binds to $\alpha_{IIb}\beta_3$, $\alpha_v\beta_3$, and $\alpha_5\beta_1$ integrins on platelets; glycoprotein Ib on platelets also binds FN *in vitro*. The known interactions of various types of FN (e.g., plasma, cellular, basement membrane, α granule stored FN in platelets) with platelets and ECM macromolecules suggest that FN might engage in thrombus formation by both direct and indirect mechanisms.[85-87]

Clot formation serves a dual function of restoration of vascular integrity and assembly of provisional ECM needed in the initial phase of remodeling and regeneration of injured tissues.[88] The provisional ECM assembled in a clot that is also enriched in growth promoting factors facilitates phenotypic transformation of fibroblasts into myofibroblasts. This is followed by deposition of a more permanent ECM that is primarily laid down by myofibroblasts. Thus, an optimal wound healing and repair is dependent on sequential maturation of the ECM. Somewhat similar cell-ECM interactions are believed to occur in atherosclerotic lesions, where VSMCs acquire a proliferative and highly synthetic phenotype not unlike that of myofibroblasts. Increased expression of EDA and EDB domain–containing FN is often associated with a phenotypic transformation of VSMC and transdifferentiation of fibroblasts into myofibroblasts. It is interesting to note that $\alpha_9\beta_1$ and $\alpha_4\beta_3$ integrins that specifically recognize the EDA domain are present on ECs but absent on the surface of platelets.

Laminin

Laminins belong to an ancient family of glycoproteins that polymerize into cruciform structures that form the structural scaffold of all vascular basement membranes. Each laminin molecule is a trimer that consists of one α, one β, and one γ laminin chain. Individual polypeptide chains are joined via a long coiled coil to produce a molecule with one long arm and up to three short arms.[89-91] The basement membranes of *Hydra* contain primordial laminin-like proteins, and there are at least four genes that encode laminins in *Caenorhabditis elegans* and *Drosophila melanogaster*. As shown in Figure 4-11, in mammals, there are five distinct α, three β, and three γ chains of laminin that are encoded by LAMA1-5, LAMB1-3, and LAMC1-3 genes, respectively.[92,93] Thus, it is theoretically possible to generate more than 45 different laminin trimers; at least 18 distinct isoforms of mammalian laminins have been described to date.[90] It is likely that additional isoforms of laminins remain to be discovered.

The process of trimer formation is not random and is likely to be tissue- and cell-specific. According to a recently adopted system of nomenclature,[89] laminin isoforms are named according to their

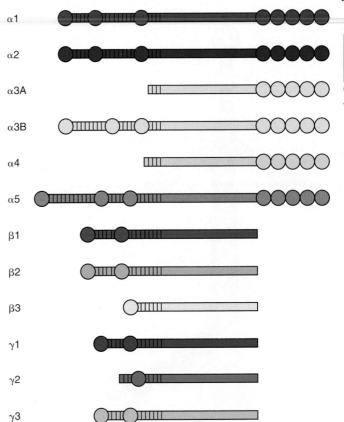

FIGURE 4-11   Structural motifs found in various laminin subunits. The α, β, and γ chains of laminins consist of tandem arrays of globular and rodlike motifs. N-terminal and internal short-arm globular modules are indicated by ovals. The rodlike epidermal growth factor (EGF) repeats are shown as vertical rectangles. *(Adapted from Durbeej M: Laminins. Cell Tissue Res 339:259–268, 2010.)*

chain composition; for instance, LM-111 consists of α1, β1, and γ1 chains, whereas laminin-511 is made of α5, β1, and γ1 chains. A single type of chain may be incorporated into more than one laminin isoform; for example, laminin-411, laminin-421, and laminin-423 laminins all contain α4 chain.

Various laminin α-chains show tissue-specific expression and are involved in formation of unique basement membranes at different locations in the body.[94-96] Laminin-111 ($\alpha_1\beta_1\gamma_1$), the most abundant and best studied laminin, is highly expressed during embryogenesis; laminin-332 ($\alpha_3\beta_3\gamma_2$) and laminin-311 ($\alpha_3\beta_1\gamma_1$) are found preferentially in the basement membranes underlying stratified epithelia of the skin. Basement membranes of the vascular endothelium are enriched in laminins containing α_4 or α_5 chains.[97] The basement membranes of most vessels contain laminin-411 ($\alpha_4\beta_1\gamma_1$) and laminin-421 ($\alpha_4\beta_2\gamma_1$). The laminin α_5 chain is expressed by endothelium of the capillaries and venules that contain laminin-511 and laminin-521 in their basement membranes.

All laminin chains share a common structure, with a tandem array of globular and rodlike domains that invariably fold into a cruciform shape, as seen in the prototype, laminin-111 (Fig. 4-12). The NH$_2$-termini of all laminin chains contain globular domains (LG) separated by laminin EGF-like (LEa, LEb, LEc) motifs. The α chain also contains two additional globular domains named *L4a* and *L4b*. Similarly, the β and γ chains contain unique LF and L4 domains, respectively. The shaft of the cross is a helical coiled coil formed by one α, one β, and one γ chain of laminin (see Fig. 4-12). The five LG domains of the laminin α chain are attached at the base of the cross. The polymerization of laminin and its incorporation into the supramolecular scaffolds of basement membranes is a cell surface receptor–mediated process, a situation reminiscent of the supramolecular assembly of FN.

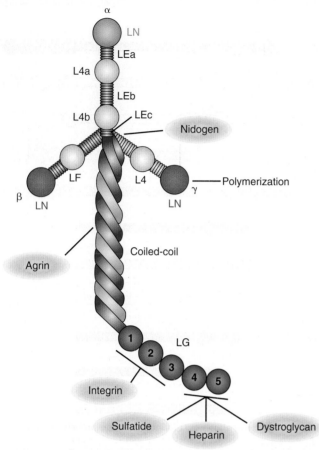

FIGURE 4-12 Representative cruciform shape of laminin proteins; α, β, and γ chains of laminin are shown in red, blue, and cyan colors, respectively. Rod-shaped and Y-shaped laminins are formed as a result of incorporation of truncated α3 and α4 and γ2 chains, respectively. Globular domains at the N-terminal end of chains are separated by laminin epidermal growth factor (EGF)-like repeats (LEa, LEb, and LEc). Laminin N-terminal domains (LN), which are important for laminin self-assembly and network formation, are present in all chains. The α-chains contain L4a and L4b globular domains. The β and γ chains contain LF and L4 domains, respectively. The C-terminal end of the α-chain forms five globular LG domains, numbered 1-5. Binding sites for various molecules involved in the supramolecular assemblies of laminin-111 and its integrin-binding modules are denoted. (*Adapted from Agtmael TV, Bruckner-Tuderman L: Basement membranes and human disease. Cell Tissue Res 339:167–188, 2010.*)

As illustrated in Figure 4-12, various domains of laminin possess unique functional properties that include promotion of architectural scaffolding, binding to cell surfaces via sulfated carbohydrates, or interacting with specific integrins and α-dystroglycan.[90,91] Thus, the LN domain, which is present in the α1, α2, α3B, α5, β1, β2, β3, γ1, and γ3 chains, is needed for self-assembly of laminins into trimers that further aggregate into a large network to which additional ECM molecules bind. At least eight unique integrins (α1β1, α2β2, α3β1, α6β1, α6β4, α7β1, α9β1, and αvβ3) and four different types of syndecans bind to laminin.[90,91] Similarly, the Lutheran blood group glycoprotein binds to laminins containing the α5 chain, whereas nidogen-1 and -2 bind to a specific region in the laminin γ1 and γ3 chains. Finally, the HS PG agrin binds the central region of the coiled coil domain of laminin (see Fig. 4-12).

Intact laminin is specifically cleaved by a number of proteases (e.g., furin, MT1-MMP, MMP-2, BMP1, plasmin). Controlled proteolysis may uniquely fragment laminin to release its functional domains as well as uncover additional biologically active domains that remain cryptic in the intact molecule. Intact laminin or its proteolytic fragments can modulate adhesion, migration, and phenotypic differentiation of many cell types, hence affecting disparate physiological and pathological

events.[98,99] These actions of laminins are mediated via their ability to ligate cell surface receptors that trigger intracellular signaling pathways (see later discussion).

The biological functions of laminin isoforms have been deduced from *in vitro* studies as well as from transgenic mice in which one or both alleles of a particular laminin chain are mutated or deleted.[96,100] Congenital ablation of laminin-111 and laminin-511 leads to embryonal death in mice.[90] Mice containing dysfunctional α4 or γ1 genes have defective kidneys, placenta, brain, lungs, and limbs. A number of mutations in the human LAMB2 gene are associated with Pierson's syndrome, an autosomal recessive disorder characterized by ocular and renal defects.[101] A deletion of the Lamb2 gene in mice resulted in renal and ocular defects reminiscent of the Pierson's syndrome.[102] Even more significantly, the mutant phenotype in the transgenic mice could be rescued by exogenous expression of the laminin β2 chain.

Laminins are a key determinant of the structure and function of basement membranes and are therefore essential for optimal performance of the vascular tree.[91,101] In addition to contributing to the formation of the blood vessels, laminins (1) impart structural and mechanical stability to mature blood vessels, (2) modulate the barrier function of vessel walls, and (3) act as mechanosensors of shear stress relayed by ECs. In the developing embryo, the cell-attached scaffold of polymerized laminin nucleates the formation of basement membranes that acquire structural maturity, ligand diversity, and functional complexity as other ECM molecules (e.g., IV collagen, PGs) are incorporated into the laminin scaffold.[96]

The barrier function of blood vessel walls is facilitated by laminins that directly and indirectly regulate movement of charged macromolecules, leukocytes, and tumor cells through subendothelial basement membranes.[90,91,101,103] LM-411 was shown to facilitate extravasation of T cells, whereas their transmigration through the vessel wall was restricted by LM-511. Similarly, the growth of primary tumors and metastasis were accelerated in α4−/− mice that elicited defective angiogenesis (e.g., irregular growth of vessel sprouts, dilated vessels). Signaling mechanisms induced by the α4 chain that binds to EC-specific integrins (α6β1 and α3β1) play a vital role in angiogenesis. It is therefore significant that not only intact laminin but also its subfragments may be functionally relevant for angiogenesis under physiological and pathological conditions. The COOH-terminal LG4-LG5 domains of α4 laminin inhibit EC migration and blood vessel sprouting *in vitro*. Mice lacking α4 are born with widespread defects in their vasculature.[104] Expression of endothelial laminins is induced by proinflammatory cytokines that may promote transmigration of circulating leukocytes and tumor cells.

Endothelial cells lining the luminal surfaces of blood cells are ideally located to act as mechanosensors of shear stress and relay this information to other compartments of the vessel wall. A laminin network, in addition to providing a structural scaffold, links the basement membrane to the cell surface via integrins. Sensing and relaying of shear stress is mediated via focal adhesions formed by ECs on the subluminal side. Focal adhesions are formed by ECM-linked aggregated integrins whose cytoplasmic tails are connected to the cytoskeleton. Enhanced shear stress promotes formation of focal adhesions that activate specific signaling kinases such as focal adhesion kinase (FAK) that relay intracellular signals to induce gene expression needed for cellular response to exogenous stressors (see later discussion).

Proteoglycans

The amorphous ground substance in the interfibrillar milieu of subendothelial ECM is composed mainly of PGs. With the exception of hyaluronan (HA), PGs consist of a protein core substituted with covalently linked glycosaminoglycan (GAG) chains of disaccharide units in which one of the sugars is always an amino sugar (e.g., N-acetylglucosamine, N-acetylgalactosamine) the second sugar is usually a uronic acid (e.g., glucuronic acid, iduronic acid). Hyaluronan consists of an extremely long polysaccharide chain (containing up to 25,000 nonsulfated disaccharide units); it exists in most connective tissues but is critical for optimal functioning of articular cartilage.

Glycosaminoglycan are linear chains of negatively charged polysaccharides that may be divided into (1) sulfated GAGs such as chondroitin-4 and -6 sulfates (CS), DS, HS, heparin, keratan sulfate (KS), and (2) nonsulfated GAGs represented by hyaluranan.[105–107] The repeating disaccharide unit of a GAG contains one sugar that is invariably a glucosamine or a galactosamine, and the other is either a glucuronic or an L-iduronic acid; KS contains a galactose in the place of the hexuronic acid. Hexosamine is, as a rule, N-acetylated except in HS, where it may be N-sulfated. The structures of the repeating units of GAGs are presented in Figure 4-13.

The uronic acid linkage in CS and HA is β1,3, and the analogous linkage in DS is α1,3 because of the presence of L-iduronic acid; the hexosaminidic linkage in all three GAGs is β1,4. The disaccharide unit of KS is β-galactosyl (1,4)-N-acetylglucosamine that is polymerized by a β1,3 glucosaminidic bond. The structure of HS contains some disaccharide units composed of D-glucosamine and D-glucuronic acid and others of D-glucosamine and L-iduronic acid. The uronyl linkage in HS is α1,4 rather than β1,3, and the hexosaminidic linkage is α1,4 rather than β1,4. The glucosamine residues are partly N-sulfated as well as O-sulfated. Heparan sulfate is structurally related to the anticoagulant heparin, which actually has a higher sulfate content than HS. The GAG chains range in molecular weights from several thousand to several million daltons. All hexosamine residues are N-substituted with either acetyl or sulfate groups. In addition, most GAGs have ester O-sulfate on one or both sugars of the disaccharide unit.[105–108]

The superfamily of PGs consists of about 30 members that are subdivided into three classes: modular PGs, small leucine-rich PGs (SLRPs) and cell surface PGs. Modular PGs are further subdivided into hyalectans and non-HA-binding PGs (Table 4-4 and Fig. 4-14). A number of recent reviews[105–109] may be consulted for more comprehensive structural and functional descriptions of various classes of PGs. Following is a brief outline of the major PGs, with an emphasis on their function in subendothelial ECM.

Modular Proteoglycans

Modular PGs consist of a heterogeneous group of highly glycosylated PGs characterized by a tripartite structure of their core proteins. This group is further divided into two subfamilies represented by HA- and lectin-binding PGs, hyalectans and non-HA-binding PGs.

Hyaluronan- and Lectin-Binding Proteoglycans

Four distinct PGs—versican, aggrecan, neurocan, and brevican—constitute the hyalectan family of PGs.[105–109] The tripartite organization of their core proteins consists of the NH$_2$- and COOH-terminal domains separated by a distinct central domain where GAGs are attached. The amino terminal domain of these PGs binds to HA and their carboxyl termini contain lectin-like domains, thus the name hyalectans (see Table 4-4). The central domain of hyalectans contains variable numbers of GAG chains, ranging from 3 seen in brevican to around 100 found in aggrecan. Versican, the largest member of the hyalectan family, may be considered a prototype[109,110] (see Fig. 4-14 and Table 4-4). Versican and other hyalectans are believed to connect lectin-containing proteins on the cell surface with HA in the intercellular space. Versican has an immunoglobulin (Ig)-like motif and two tandem HA-binding domains near the NH$_2$-terminus; an EGF-like domain and a lectin-like motif are located near the COOH-terminus of versican. Four alternatively spliced versican isoforms (V0, V1, V2, and V3) are preferentially expressed in different tissues. Versican binds to numerous cell-associated and ECM molecules that include type I collagen, tenascin, fibulins, fibrillin-1, FN, selectins, chemokines, CD-44, integrin β1, EGF, and Toll-like receptors.[109–113]

Aggrecan typically contains around 100 CS-enriched and 30 KS-enriched GAGs that are covalently linked to about a 220-kD core protein (see Table 4-4). As the most abundant constituent of cartilage ECM, aggrecan is found in giant aggregates with link proteins and HA, and occupies a large hydrodynamic volume (2×10^{-12} cm^3) that may be equivalent to a bacterium.[108] The lectin modules of both versican and aggrecan can interact with simple sugars found in glycoproteins; this binding is calcium dependent.[114] Defective cartilage and shortened limb development have been demonstrated in mice, chickens, and humans that contain mutated aggrecan genes.[115,116]

Neurocan and brevican, with tripartite organization of core proteins characteristic of hyalectans, are the most abundant PGs of this class in the central nervous system.[117] Brevican is synthesized in the brain as a secreted full-length molecule, as well as a truncated form that lacks the COOH-terminal domain. The short form of brevican is attached to the plasma membrane via a GPI anchor. Neurocan and brevican promote neuronal attachment and outgrowth of neurites in developing neurons. Brevican activates EGF receptor (EGFR) signaling that results in enhanced expression of cell adhesion molecules such as FN. Highly aggressive central nervous system tumors elicit accelerated synthesis and proteolysis of brevican and thus may promote tumor metastasis.

Non-Hyaluronan-Binding (Basement Membrane) Proteoglycans

Perlecan, agrin, and bamacan are usually present in the vascular and epithelial basement membranes of mammalian tissues.[97,109] Whereas the three GAG chains of perlecan and agrin consist primarily of HS and CS, the three bamacan GAG chains contain only CS. The core protein of the human perlecan is about 470 kD in size and contains five well-defined domains (I through V) that

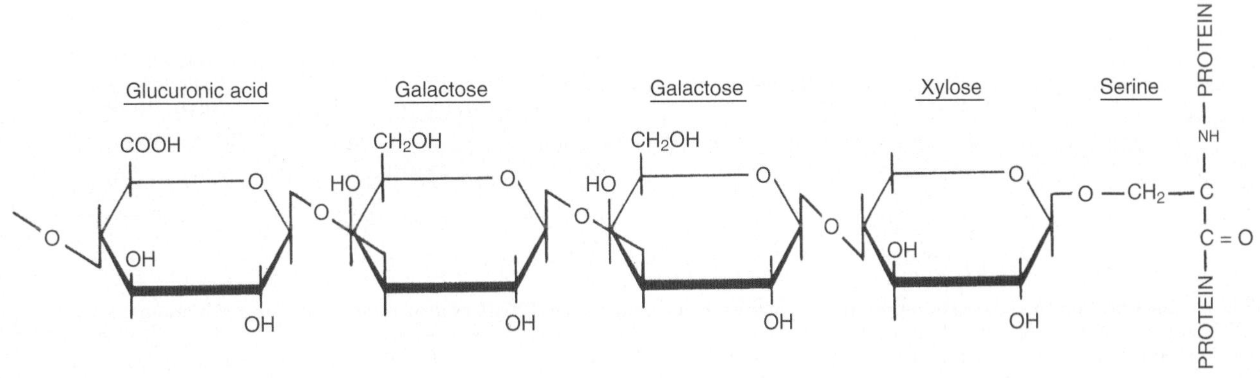

FIGURE 4-13 Oligosaccharide linkage between glycosaminoglycans (GAGs) and protein core. *(Adapted from Silber JE: Structure and metabolism of proteoglycans and glycosaminoglycans. J Invest Dermatol 79:31, 1982. Copyright by Williams & Wilkins.)*

TABLE 4-4 General Characteristics of Major Proteoglycans*

PROTEOGLYCAN	GENE	CHROMOSOME	PROTEIN CORE (KD)	GAG TYPE (NO. OF CHAINS)
BM Type				
Perlecan	HSPG2	1p36	400-467	HS/CS (3)
Agrin	AGRN	1p32-pter	250	HS (3)
Bamacan			138	CS (3)
Hyalectans				
Versican	CSPG2	5q13.2	265-370	CS/DS (10-30)
Aggrecan	AGC1	15q26	~220	CS (~100)
Neurocan	NCAN		~136	CS (3-7)
Brevican	BCAN	1q25-q31	~100	CS (1-3)
SLRPs				
Decorin	DCN	12q23	40	DS/CS (1)
Biglycan	BGN	X128	40	DS/CS (2)
Fibromodulin	FMOD	1q32	42	KS (2-3)
Lumican	LIM	12q21.3-22	38	KS (3-4)
Keratocan			38	KS (3-5)
PRELP	PRELP	1q32	44	KS (2-3)
Osteoadherin			42	KS
Epiphycan	ESPG3	12q21	35	Dermatan/chondroitin
Osteoglycin	OG		35	KS

*BM, basement membrane; GAG, glycosaminoglycan; SLRP, small leucine-rich proteoglycan; PRELP, prokine/arginine-rich end leucin-rich protein.
Adapted from Iozzo RV: Matrix proteoglycans: from molecular design to cellular function. Annu Rev Biochem 67:609, 1998.

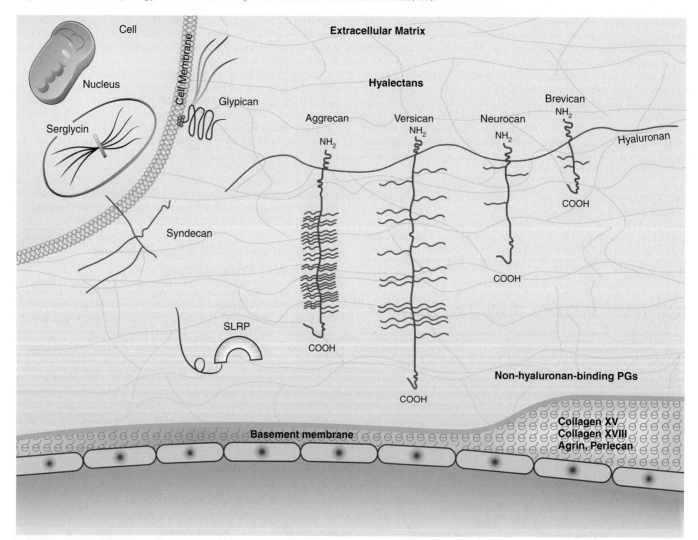

FIGURE 4-14   Classification and schematic representation of the major proteoglycans (PGs) based on cellular location and binding. The heterogeneous group of PGs includes those of the extracellular matrix (ECM) such as small leucine-rich PGs (SLRPs) (decorin) and modular PGs. Modular PGs are divided into hyaluronan-binding, hyalectans (e.g., aggrecan, versican), and non-hyalectans (e.g., perlecan, agrin) of the basement membranes. The third group of cell surface PGs encompasses mainly the membrane-spanning syndecans (e.g., syndecan-4) and GPI-anchored glypican. Serglycin is an intracellular PG found in hematopoietic and endothelial cells (ECs). *(From Schaefer L, Schaefer RM: Proteoglycans: from structural compounds to signaling molecules. Cell Tissue Res 339:237–246, 2010.)*

are mosaics of sequences found in other proteins. Thus, domain I of perlecan consists of three serine-glycine-asparagine triplets to which HS side chains are covalently attached, and an SEA module (containing sperm protein, enterokinase, and agrin homology sequence). Domain II contains four low-density lipoprotein (LDL) receptor class-A repeats located next to IgG-like motifs. Three laminin IV globular domains interspersed with nine laminin EGF-like motifs comprise the domain III of perlecan. Domain IV contains 21 IgG-like motifs that share homology with neural cell adhesion molecules (N-CAM). Finally, domain V is made of three laminin G motifs separated by two sets of EGF-like repeats; the 85-kD COOH-terminal fragment of perlecan called *endorepellin* is a potent anti-angiogenic molecule.[97,109,118]

Agrin is a major PG of basement membranes of the renal glomerulus and nerve-muscle junctional synapses. Although the four-domain structure of agrin, with three HS–rich GAG chains, resembles perlecan, there are critical structural differences between perlecan and agrin. The amino terminus of agrin is required for binding to laminin-111 as well as for secretion of the newly synthesized agrin. Agrin is essential to aggregate acetylcholine receptors at the neuromuscular synapse and facilitates synaptogenesis during neuromuscular junction development. Although originally isolated from the Reichert membrane, CS-rich bamacan is found in variable amounts in most basement membranes.

In addition to imparting structural integrity to the basement membranes, PGs modulate cellular behavior because of their ability to interact with a large number of molecules, as exemplified by perlecan.[97,109,110,118] Although perlecan is embedded within the subendothelial basement membranes, it binds to fibroblast growth factor 2 (FGF-2), vascular endothelial growth factor (VEGF), platelet-derived growth factor (PDGF), several cell surface molecules, and ECM proteins. Heparan sulfate GAGs of perlecan associate with FGF-2 and serve as its reservoir in blood vessel walls. During aortic morphogenesis, there is an inverse correlation between perlecan expression and smooth muscle proliferation in the rat. Perlecan interacts with $\alpha_1\beta_2$ integrin, an integrin that also binds to fibrillar collagens. Dynamic interactions of perlecan and fibrillar collagens with integrins potentiate atherosclerosis, angiogenesis, and carcinogenesis. Perlecan regulates the motility of ECs and transformed cells and promotes metastasis.[119] Perlecan-null mice die in utero or shortly after birth.

Small Leucine-Rich Proteoglycans

Nine known members of this family of PGs, characterized by central leucine-rich domains and DS/KS GAG chains, are currently known.[120] Based on their primary structures and evolutionary relationships, SLRPs may be further divided into three subclasses (see Table 4-4). Members of the SLRP family have been[121] implicated in diverse functions that include regulation of growth factor accessibility (e.g., TGF-β) and control of collagen fibrillogenesis.[119] Presence of decorin, fibromodulin, or lumican retards collagen fibrillogenesis in vitro.[122-125] A reciprocal relationship between the amount of decorin and rate of collagen fibril growth in the developing tendon of the chicken was also demonstrated.[126] The abnormal collagen fibril formation and reduced tensile strength of the skin seen in decorin knockout mice support a functional role for decorin in proper collagen fibrillogenesis.[122]

Decorin, a prototype of the SLRP, is organized into four discernible domains.[109] Core protein of decorin binds TGF-β1, -2, and -3 with high affinity. Because the TGF-β/decorin complex is incapable of intracellular signaling, decorin is believed to facilitate deposition of inactive TGF-βs at specific tissue locations. Perturbation of this interaction and activation of TGF-βs may occur in response to inflammatory reactions. Decorin itself has been shown to regulate cell proliferation, and ectopic expression of decorin could

suppress the growth of cancer cells. Decorin directly interacts with EGFR with a 1:1 stoichiometry; this interaction inactivates EGFR and its downstream signaling.[127] Vascular ECs undergoing cord formation that precedes angiogenesis *in vitro* synthesize decorin, whereas proliferating ECs showed enhanced synthesis of biglycan; these two structurally similar SLRPs appear to regulate EC phenotype in an opposite manner.

Cell Surface Proteoglycans

Two main classes of cell surface PGs are membrane-spanning syndecans and GPI-linked PGs represented by glypicans.[109,128,129] There are four members of the syndecan subfamily. Syndecan-4 is distributed ubiquitously, but syndecan-1, -2, and -3 have more restricted tissue- or development-specific expression.[128-130] For example, syndecan-1 is highly expressed in the developing embryo, and syndecan-3 is primarily enriched the neural tissue. Syndecans are involved in multiple signaling pathways to regulate cell proliferation, adhesion, motility, and differentiation. The cell surface HS-enriched syndecans serve as co-receptors for FGF and EGF to facilitate their binding and signal transduction. Syndecan-1 is cleaved by MMPs, and the soluble ectodomain of syndecan promotes tumor growth and invasiveness *in vitro*.[121,131,132] Exogenous treatment of microvascular ECs with EGF and FGF leads to shedding of syndecan-2 that in turn affects EC behavior.[133]

The subfamily of GPI-linked cell surface PGs includes six member glypicans and a splicing variant of brevican that lacks the COOH-terminal lectin binding and EGF motifs. While most tissues express glypican-1, expression of glypican-3, -4, and -5 is restricted to the central nervous system. In contrast, glipican-2 is expressed abundantly in the embryo, whereas glypican-6 is found mainly in the heart, kidney, and intestine. Glypican-3, which inhibits hedgehog (Hh) signaling by competing for its receptor Patched, is upregulated in neuroblastoma and Wilms tumor. Glypican regulates binding and signaling of a number of other morphogens and growth factors that include Wnts, slit, FGFs, insulin-like growth factors (IGFs), and BMPs. The regulatory actions of glypicans on proliferation and differentiation of cells appear to be context dependent.[129,134,135]

Biosynthesis of Proteoglycans

Biosynthesis of all PGs involves similar steps, the rate-limiting step being translation of the core protein.[119,136,137] Following its synthesis, core protein undergoes covalent modification with GAG chains that begins with the linkage of xylose to a specific serine(s). Proteoglycan synthesis occurs in late ER and the Golgi with attachment of a xylose residue to the OH group of serine in the protein core.[138] Linking of galactose to xylose is carried out by galactosyl transferase. A second galactose is then transferred by a distinct galactosyl transferase that is followed by addition of the first glucuronic acid by UDP–glucuronic acid transferase. Growth of the GAG chain then occurs by alternating transfer of hexosamine and uronic acid residues. Thus, the UDP derivatives of *N*-acetylglucosamine and glucuronic acid are precursors for HA, heparin, and HS; whereas *N*-acetylgalactosamine and glucuronic acid are precursors for CS and DS. After addition of the first sugar, elongation occurs by the same *N*-acetyl-hexosaminyltransferase and glucuronosyltransferase, regardless of which chain is being synthesized. The respective chains are variably modified by pathway-specific epimerization and sulfation reactions to yield iduronic acid and sulfation.[107,127]

Nonspecific sulfotransferases transfer a sulfate group from 3-phosphoribosyl phosphoadenosine 5-phosphoribosyl phosphosulfate to the appropriate site on the GAG. Because no partial sulfation occurs, it is believed the GAG may become attached to the particulate-bound sulfotransferases and glycosyl transferases and are completely sulfated before release. This N-sulfation is unique to heparin and HS; all other PGs contain an O-linked sulfate group. The synthesis of this N-sulfate linkage proceeds through the N-acetylglucosamine addition to the GAG chain, deacetylation, and replacement of the acetyl group by sulfate. Iduronic acid formation in heparin, HS, and DS takes place after polysaccharide synthesis by epimerization of glucuronic acid. Proteoglycan size is extremely heterogenous and mainly reflects Gag chain length.

Degradation of Proteoglycans

Compared to collagen and elastin, PGs have more rapid rates of turnover, with turnover of 2 to 10 days in younger animals.[97,109,110,119] Degradation of the PGs involves proteolysis of the core protein by MMPs, breakdown of the sugar chain, and desulfation of sugars. The dramatic loss of cartilage matrix that results from experimental intravenous injection of papain illustrates the importance of the protein core to the structural integrity of PGs. Fibroblasts, macrophages, and neutrophils produce a variety of enzymes that can degrade PGs at neutral pH. Degradation of sugar chains occurs mainly in lysosomes. Perhaps the best characterized GAG-degrading enzyme is testicular hyaluronidase, which degrades HA, CS, and DS to oligosaccharides. Other glycosidases are required to complete the breakdown of oligosaccharides to monosaccharides. Lysosomes contain glucuronidase and N-acetylhexosaminidases that remove the terminal glucuronic acid and hexosamine residues, respectively. Lysosomes also contain β-xylosidase, β-galactosidase, and α-iduronidase, which complete the breakdown. Lysosomal sulfatases are responsible for removal of sulfate groups from oligosaccharides. Inherited defects in the activity of various GAG-degrading enzymes cause mucopolysaccharidoses, characterized by faulty catabolism of one or another type of GAGs.[97,109,110,119]

Subendothelial Extracellular Matrix as a Regulator of Cell Signaling

The central role of ECM, to endow blood vessels with the mechanical ability to undergo repeated cycles of extension and passive recoil throughout the life of the organism, has been appreciated for nearly a century. However, in recent years we have also discovered that ECM, beyond providing scaffolding for the vascular walls, has many effects on their cellular inhabitants. Thus ECs, pericytes, and VSMCs dynamically sense their physical (e.g., shear stress) and biochemical microenvironment and adjust cellular behavior accordingly.[139–141] Numerous experimental observations indicate that ECM is a key component of this bidirectional communication between cells and their microenvironment.[142]

Vascular cells actively synthesize and mold their ECM into unique configurations to ensure it optimal stiffness and deformability; molecular constituents of the subendothelial ECM in turn profoundly modulate the adhesion, polarity, motility, survival, proliferation, and differentiation of vascular cells. The fibrillar and nonfibrillar ECM interact with dozens of cell-associated and extracellular molecules that alter the signaling repertoire of ECs, VSMCs, and platelets.[139,143,144]

The functional diversity of ECM emanates from the architectural complexity of its molecular constituents, which have myriad specifically folded domains, some uniquely juxtaposed in the basement membranes of the vascular tree. Subendothelial ECM, in addition to forming an adhesive scaffold via integrins that are capable of bi-directional intracellular signal transduction, serves as a reservoir of growth factors.[78,145] The anchorage-dependent survival and growth of normal epithelial cells, ECs, and VSMCs depends on their adhesive interactions with ECM. When this adhesive normalcy is lost, cells acquire anchorage-independent growth potential, a hallmark of cancerous transformation and metastasis.[146] Thus, as highly organized solid-phase signal inducers, ECM molecules can integrate numerous signals in the microenvironment of the blood vessels to regulate their development, maturation, and homeostasis. The following is a brief summary of the mechanisms that underlie the dynamic two-way signaling between cells and their ECM.

Extracellular Matrix—Integrin Bi-Directional Signaling

Each of the many molecules found in the vascular ECM recognizes a variety of cell surface proteins predominated by integrins, a superfamily of heterodimeric transmembrane receptors (Fig. 4-15). Integrins are assembled by selective pairings of 18 individual α and 8 unique β chains. Twenty-four integrin receptors with distinct ligand selectivity, cell-specific expression, and signaling properties have been described in mammals.[147,148] The extracellular segment of the α subunit of integrin consists of a β-propeller domain, an I-domain, and three Ig-like domains. The ectodomain of the integrin β subunit also has a modular organization, with two tandem I-domains, an Ig hybrid motif, a plexin-semaphorin-integrin (PSI) domain, and four EGF-like domains. Integrins specifically bind to several ECM molecules, their subfragments, and divalent cations. With respect to vasculature, ECs express integrins that specifically bind to collagen ($\alpha_1\beta_1$, $\alpha_2\beta_1$, $\alpha_{10}\beta_1$, and $\alpha_{11}\beta_1$), FN ($\alpha_4\beta_1$ and $\alpha_4\beta_1$), and laminin ($\alpha_3\beta_1$, $\alpha_6\beta_1$, and $\alpha_6\beta_4$). Based on a number of $in vitro$ and $in vivo$ observations, at least eight integrins (α_{1_7}, $\alpha_2\beta_1$, $\alpha_3\beta_1$, $\alpha_4\beta_1$, $\alpha_5\beta_1$, $\alpha_6\beta_1$, $\alpha_v\beta_3$, and $\alpha_v\beta_5$) have been implicated in the process of angiogenesis.[149,150] In contrast, leukocytes express a number of unique integrins on their surface that include $\alpha_4\beta_7$, $\alpha_L\beta_2$, and $\alpha_M\beta_2$ integrins. We should note that the ligand selectivity of integrins is far from absolute, as exemplified by $\alpha_v\beta_3$, which binds to several RGD sequence–containing proteins and peptides.[147,148] The following discussion summarizes numerous observations that underscore the fact that integrins lie at a unique crossroads of extracellular microenvironment, cytoskeleton mechanics, and intracellular signaling networks to alter the behavior of vascular walls in health and disease (see Fig. 4-15).

Integrins are unusual proteins among the transmembrane receptors, with an ability to relay signals in both directions.[147,148,151] The intracellular changes induced by ECM-liganded integrins are referred to as *outside-in signaling*. Conversely, *inside-out signaling* occurs when intracellular biochemical changes trigger reorganization of the cytoskeleton, which alters the shape of the ectodomain of integrin and its affinity for the ligand. The ECM-liganded integrins are clustered as dot-like foci that sequentially evolve into focal adhesions, fibrillar adhesions, and finally into supramolecular three-dimensional adhesions. Such mass clustering of integrins into focal adhesions results in summation of numerous weak-affinity interactions of individual integrins into an adhesive unit with high affinity and high avidity.

Clustering and activation of integrins induce a number of characteristic biochemical and physical changes in the cells that are collectively referred to as *outside-in signal transduction*.[143,144,152] Since integrins themselves lack catalytic activity, they signal indirectly via a host of accessory proteins that assemble multi-protein platforms to recruit bona fide signaling catalysts into the focal adhesions. The assembly of bi-directional signaling complexes depends on interactions among a large number of integrin-binding proteins (e.g., talin), adapter molecules (e.g., vinculin, paxillin), and signaling enzymes (e.g., FAK, RhoA-kinase [ROCK], myosin phosphatase). It has been estimated that the "integrin adhesome" consists of more than 150 unique proteins; therefore it is conceivable that recruitment of unique sets of adapter and signaling molecules to focal adhesions might be different under differing physiological and pathological conditions.[153,154]

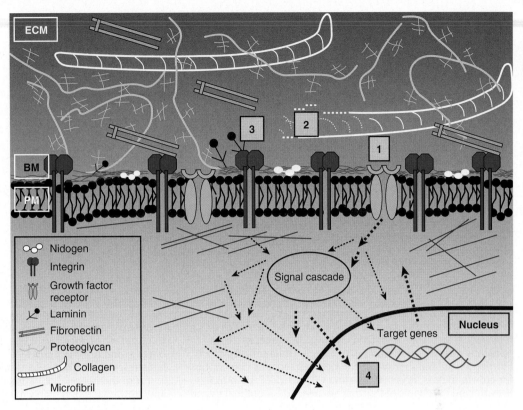

FIGURE 4-15 Illustration of various components of extracellular matrix (ECM), their cell surface receptors, and major intracellular signaling molecules. Potential steps that may be exploited for pharmacotherapy include: (1) Blocking synthesis of ECM by blocking specific growth factors such as transforming growth factor beta (TGF-β), their receptor molecules, or intracellular signal transduction. (2) Blocking degradation of ECM by interfering with enzymes involved in its remodeling (e.g., matrix metalloproteinases (MMPs), ADAMTS, cathepsins) and/or their inhibitors (tissue inhibitor of MMP [TIMPs]). (3) Interfering with ECM signaling pathways (e.g., via integrins) either by blocking ECM and integrin interactions or subsequent signal transduction cascades. (4) Influencing transcription of specific ECM molecules (e.g., by siRNA). Please note that that purple rods in cytoplasm, marked as microfibrils, are in fact actin cytoskeleton intimately involved in intracellular signing by ECM. BM, basement membrane; PM, plasma membrane. *(From Jarvelainnen H, Sainio A, Koulu M, et al: Extracellular matrix molecules: potential targets in pharmacotherapy. Pharmacol Rev 61:198–223, 2009.)*

The inside-out signaling of integrins is best exemplified by their own activation, particularly on the surface of leukocytes, where integrins are normally present as inactive receptors.[143,144,152] This mechanism enables the immune cells and platelets to circulate through the bloodstream without undesirable adherence to the vessels or causing premature thrombosis, respectively. The activation of T cells, neutrophils, and platelets can occur by integrin-independent pathways (i.e., occupancy of the T-cell receptor by MHC-loaded antigenic peptides, ligation of selectins on the surface of neutrophils, and interaction between platelet glycoprotein IV and collagen. Such activation initiates a series of intracellular reactions that lead to binding of kindlin and talin to intracellular tails of β-integrin and its conformation-dependent activation. As a consequence, the affinity of integrin for its ligands is greatly enhanced, as is its signaling strength.

Integrin signaling is mainly propagated by kinases and phosphatases that, by dynamic phosphorylation and dephosphorylation, alter protein-protein interactions of their substrates and catalytic activities of signaling enzymes in focal adhesions.[143,144,152,155] The major enzymes involved in this process include tyrosine kinase, FAK, protein kinase C (PKC; a serine/threonine kinase), a lipid kinase (PI3-kinase), and the receptor protein tyrosine phosphatase α (PTPα). Activation of integrin immediately initiates tyrosine phosphorylation of specific substrates that include the integrin β tails. Concomitantly, there is a surge in intracellular concentration of lipid second messengers, phosphatidylinositol-4,5-bisphosphates and phosphatidylinositol-3,4,5-trisphosphates, and a reorganization of the cytoskeleton.

As shown in Figure 4-16, the characteristic physical link between integrins and cytoskeleton is initiated and maintained by integrin-bound proteins that also bind to actin (e.g., talin, filamin) in collaboration with other proteins that regulate the structure of cytoskeleton indirectly (e.g., paxillin, FAK, kindlin). Additionally, the integrin-cytoskeleton linkage and signal propagation is critically dependent on actin-binding proteins (e.g., vinculin) and several signaling adapters (e.g., RhoA, Rac1,

cdc42). Numerous biochemical and biophysical analyses have revealed that talin, vinculin, α-actinin, and integrin-linked kinase (ILK) are indispensable for bidirectional signaling of focal adhesions.[143,144,152,155]

Integrin activation leads to a sequence of biochemical and biophysical reactions that may be divided into three temporal phases. First, high-affinity ligand-integrin association leads to immediate activation of phosphatidylinositol 3-kinase (PI3K) and concomitant phosphorylation of several proteins. The second stage of signaling, observable within half an hour, proceeds to activation of the Rho family of GTPases that are crucial for the architectural reshaping of the cytoskeleton. The final phase of signaling—executed over many hours—culminates in the nucleus, with reprogramming of gene expression carried out by transcription factors and their coactivators.

The unique molecular composition of focal adhesions at different locations in the vasculature is likely to affect signal strength and quality.[77,78,154] The striking diversity of signal transduction cascades documented in various cell types also involves crosstalk among the canonical and alternative signaling pathways (see Fig. 4-16). Finally, the growth factor microenvironment (see later discussion) greatly influences the mechanisms that control attachment, polarity, and directional motility of vascular cells. Aberration of these signals leads to dramatic changes in the ability of cells to attach, polarize, and migrate, as well as their growth factor– and anchorage-independent proliferation.

Signaling Triad of Extracellular Matrix, Integrin, and Growth Factors

Although the ECM-integrin signaling axis has been the focus of most investigations, it has become evident in recent years that subendothelial connective tissues make additional contributions to the bidirectional signaling of vascular and nonvascular cells. A number of growth factors and developmental morphogens are sequestered in the fibrillar and nonfibrillar constituents of ECM.

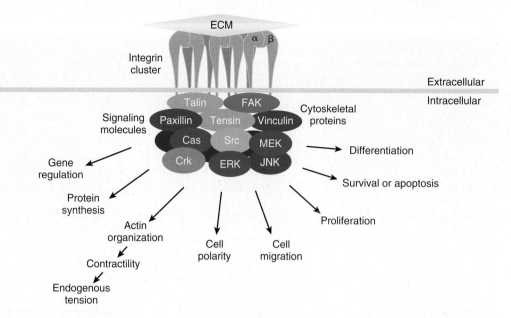

FIGURE 4-16 General model of cell–extracellular matrix (ECM) adhesions and downstream signaling pathways. Cell-ECM adhesions containing clusters of integrins recruit cytoplasmic proteins (e.g., talin, paxillin, vinculin) and kinases (focal adhesion kinase [FAK], Src, and c-jun NH 2-terminal kinase [JNK]), which in cooperation with other cell surface receptors (growth factor receptors; see Fig. 4-17) control diverse cellular processes, functions, and phenotypes. Details of these interactions are described in text. ERK, extracellular signal regulated kinase; MEK, mitogen extracellular signal regulated kinase. *(Adapted from Berrier AL, Yamada KM: Cell-matrix adhesion. J Cell Physiol 213:565–573, 2007.)*

Presumably, such ECM-bound factors have the potential to be released in a highly regulated manner in response to developmental cues or tissue injury and inflammation.[78,145,146] Furthermore, a number of ECM molecules serve as coreceptors for growth factors, as is the case for FGF and VEGF; both bind to heparin and HS chains of PGs that are needed for optimal ligand presentation and signal transduction. Proteoglycans modulate TGF-β signaling in a number of ways. Transforming growth factor beta binds to decorin in the ECM and in this state cannot bind to its cell surface receptors. Additionally, the binding of TGF-β to its signaling receptors is dependent on a plasma membrane-bound PG (β-glycan) and the cell surface glycoprotein endoglin, both of which serve as co-receptors. Finally, some growth factors can independently activate a number of downstream effectors of integrin signaling (FAK, Src, PI3-K, MAPK); this is exemplified by synergistic modulation of ECM-integrin signaling by IGF-1 and PDGF (Fig. 4-17).

Comodulation of integrin and growth factor signaling has been documented for EGF, hepatocyte growth factor (HGF), IGF-1, and PDGF, both during early development of model organisms and in cell lines.[156–162] Evidently, a trimolecular interaction among the BMP homolog DPP, its cell surface receptor, and type IV collagen is crucial for optimal relay of signals involved in morphogenesis of the dorso-ventral axis in *Drosophila*. A similar mechanistic interaction of HGF with two other proteins has been reported. Apparently, fibronectin- or VN-bound HGF forms a trimolecular complex that contains (FN or VN)-HGF, c-Met (HGF receptor), and $\alpha_3\beta_4$ integrin. A functional role of these interactions was corroborated by showing that ligand-independent activation of c-Met by cellular adhesion plays a crucial role in the growth and invasive potential of epithelial cells in response to HGF. Finally, it has been reported that the downstream signaling evoked by the tyrosine kinase transmembrane glycoprotein EGFR was complemented by integrins; thus, EGFR was shown to laterally coaggregate with $\alpha_v\beta_3$, $\alpha_2\beta_1$, and $\alpha_6\beta_4$ integrins.

As reviewed in a number of excellent publications,[78,144] the crosstalk between growth factors and integrins involves a number of mechanisms (see Fig. 4-17). First, it involves integrin's ability to concentrate signaling adapters in close proximity of growth factor receptors to enhance their intracellular signaling ability. An additional mechanism of crosstalk may be dependent on lateral mass aggregation of integrins, a process posited to alter the location and/or concentration of growth factor receptors on the cell surface. The observation that $\alpha_1\beta_2$ integrin and EGFRs were coaggregated at the foci of cell-cell contact bolsters such a mechanism. Furthermore, integrin-mediated adhesive interactions may alter the rate of internalization and degradation of some receptors (e.g., PDGFR).

Conversely, integrin activation may lead to enhanced expression of some growth factors; thus, it was shown that increased biosynthesis of VEGF and IGF-2 occurred via the actions of $\alpha_6\beta_4$ and $\alpha_1\beta_{1A}$ integrins, respectively. These observations and many others are consistent with the notion that bidirectional crosstalk between integrins and growth factors is highly relevant to cellular behavior and phenotype. However, the relative contribution of these two processes to bidirectional signaling remains controversial. Similarly, the hierarchical relationship between integrin and growth factor signaling pathways remains to be sorted out.[78,143,145]

Vascular Extracellular Matrix and Platelet Interaction

Circulating platelets act as sentinels of vascular integrity and do not attach to vessel walls under normal conditions. However, upon injury of blood vessel walls, platelets rapidly adhere to ECM of the subendothelium and neointima (formed after repeated damage to vessel wall) and aggregate with each other at the site of injury. The adhesive interactions between subendothelial ECM and platelets and thrombus formation have been extensively studied.[86,163–165] Binding and activation of platelets by the subendothelial ECM is modulated by hemodynamic stress, composition of the vascular tissue, and extent and depth of the lesion.

The fibrillar collagens, of which types I, III, IV, V, and VI are widely distributed in the vascular ECM, are key initiators of thrombosis in injured vessels.[7,9,166] The hemostatic cascade begins when platelets adhere to the exposed subendothelial collagens via vWF, a large glycoprotein that is constitutively synthesized by ECs.[86,87] The vWF both circulates in plasma as a soluble molecule and is stored in the α granules of platelets. Endothelial or plasma vWF, which forms multimeric aggregates, binds to collagen. It is believed that high hemodynamic stress causes local uncoiling of multimeric vWF, further facilitating its binding to platelet GPIbα and collagen.[167,168] Additional interactions of collagen with $\alpha_2\beta_1$ integrin and glycoprotein VI (GPVI) synergize the binding of platelets to vascular ECM. Although a pivotal role of collagens in thrombosis is borne out by numerous observations, the relative contributions of individual fibrillar collagens to this process appears to be highly context dependent.[86,87,169] This view is supported by the observation that platelets adhere to and are activated by types I-V collagens under relatively high and moderate hemodynamic stress. In contrast, binding and activation of platelets by type V-VIII collagens occurs at much lower shear stress, and type V collagen binds to platelets only under static conditions.

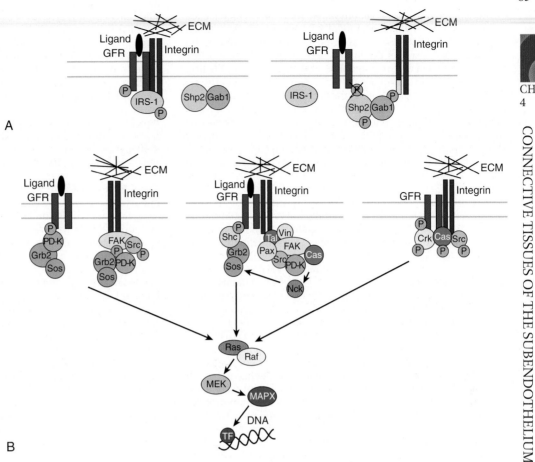

FIGURE 4-17 Regulation of growth factor receptor (GFR) signaling by integrins. Several mechanisms by which integrins might control GFR activity have been proposed. **A,** The first potential mechanism by which integrins control GFR activity involves recruitment of specific adapters (Shp2 and Gab1) to plasma membrane (left). Integrins are thought to recruit adapters to plasma membrane and concentrate them in close proximity to GFRs (right), thus enhancing their signaling. **B,** The second proposed mechanism is that integrins, upon close association with GFRs, change their subcellular localization of these receptors. Thus, coaggregation of integrins and GFRs in focal adhesions may alter the quality and/or strength of downstream signaling cascades that culminate in altered gene expression. There are compelling data to suggest that an association between GFRs and integrins may also facilitate crosstalk between extracellular matrix (ECM) liganded integrin and GFRs. DNA, deoxyribonucleic acid; FAK, focal adhesion kinase; MAPK, mitogen-activated protein kinase; MEK, mitogen extracellular signal regulated kinase; TF, transcription factor. *(Adapted from Alam N, Goel HL, Zarif MJ, et al: The integrin–growth factor receptor duet. J Cell Physiol 213:649–653, 2007.)*

Over the years, many platelet-associated proteins have been claimed as candidate collagen receptors.[170–178] However, a careful review of the literature would suggest that some of these claims reflect vagaries of different experimental models (*in vivo* vs. *ex vivo*), while others may have emanated from a lack of technical or interpretational rigor.[87,166,169] Historically, the search for collagen receptors on platelets began with studies using purified type I and III collagens or their cyanogen bromide (CB) subfragments that were tested for their ability to bind and activate platelets. These studies led to the discovery that purified native type I/III collagens and some of their CB fragments interacted with platelet integrin $\alpha_2\beta_1$. More recently, a series of overlapping triple-helical peptides spanning human collagen types I and III have been systematically tested for their ability to bind and activate platelets.[179–181] These elegant studies have unraveled discrete sequence motifs on types I and III collagen that interact with receptors on the surface of platelets and vWF. Based on these analyses, it has been surmised that type I collagen contains four $\alpha_2\beta_1$ integrin-binding sites of varying affinities; apparently, similar sequence motifs are also conserved in type III collagen. The molecular interactions between high-affinity type I collagen triple-helical peptide and $\alpha_2\beta_1$ integrin have been elucidated with precision. These and related studies have shown that fibrillar collagens also interact with $\alpha_{IIb}\beta_3$, albeit indirectly. Finally, the use of well-defined triple-helical collagen peptides has led to the discovery of amino acid sequence motifs in types I and III collagen that specifically bind to the platelet surface GPVI, as well as to vWF.[86,87,180]

How collagen-platelet interactions culminate in the formation of a thrombus has been investigated in considerable detail.[86,87,180] Under high shear stress, the obligatory first step is co-engagement of $\alpha_2\beta_1$ integrin and vWF by collagens. Platelet proteins GPVI and GPIV (CD36) strengthen the initial encounter with collagen. Glycoprotein VI has a modular organization that is composed of 2 Ig domains,

an O-linked glycosylated stalk, an intramembrane domain, and an intracellular tail. In platelets, GPVI exists in association with the FcR γ-chain, a transmembrane protein containing an immunoreceptor tyrosine activation motif (ITAM) motif. Interaction of platelets with collagen triggers phosphorylation of the FcR γ-chain and signaling that mimics signaling cascades associated with T-cell activation. The intracellular signaling is mainly driven by Ca++ mobilization that also occurs in response to other platelet-activating stimuli (e.g., thrombin, adenosine diphosphate [ADP]). The role of CD36 in thrombosis is somewhat debatable in light of the observation that nearly 5% of Japanese lack functional CD36 protein in their platelets without overt complications of hemostasis.

Platelets also adhere to other components of ECM, particularly to FN and laminin, both of which are essential ECM components of the subendothelial connective tissues.[86,87,182,183] Since the original 1978 report of Hynes et al. supporting a role of FN in platelet adhesion, a number of apparently conflicting data have muddled this issue.[86,87,182,183] There is little doubt that platelets adhere to FN; platelets possess two integrin receptors that bind FN (i.e., $\alpha_5\beta_1$, $\alpha_{IIb}\beta_3$). Depletion of FN from plasma reduced the ability of platelets for thrombus formation on fibrillar substratum or subendothelium, and if FN was restored, interplatelet aggregation and activation was restored. The NH_2-terminal 70-kD fragment of FN could be incorporated in the clot and was cross-linked to fibrin. Further bolstering a positive role of FN in thrombosis is the phenotype of mice with various gene knockouts. Thus, $FN^{-/-}$ mice were shown to elicit defective thrombus formation. Similarly, mice lacking both fibrinogen and vWF elicited thrombosis primarily driven by FN and other proteins at the sites of blood vessel injury. However, it was noted that FN-platelet interactions were apparently too weak to withstand the normal shear stress. Based on these observations, it has been posited that FN plays a complementary role in thrombus formation in the presence of fibrinogen and vWF.[184,185]

These paradoxical observations on the role of FN in platelet activation may be reconciled in a model that suggests that the ultimate response of platelets may be determined by their initial encounter with different sets of ECM molecules in the endothelium. It is known that platelets can assemble a fibrillar network of FN from soluble FN. However, when platelets attach to vWF, it suppresses their ability to deposit FN. Under these conditions, aggregation and activation of platelets may be driven mainly by fibrinogen-$\alpha_{IIb}\beta_3$ integrin interaction. In contrast, if fibrin or collagen initiates adhesion of platelets, they acquire a greater ability to convert plasma FN into supramolecular FN that gets incorporated it into thrombi. It follows then that aggregation and clustering of platelets via fibrinogen or assembled FN may be regulated in a mutually exclusive manner.[86,87]

In the injured vessel wall, platelets are exposed to various forms of laminin; thus, laminin-411 and laminin-511 are present not only in the vascular ECM but also in platelets that contain laminin-522. Laminins bind to platelets and thus may play a role in their adhesion and activation. Despite the presence of laminin-binding integrin receptors on the platelet surface, the relative role of laminin-mediated adhesion in thrombus formation remains to be more precisely delineated. Analogous to more nuanced regulation of FN-platelet interaction, where interplay among fibrinogen, vWF, and VN negatively regulate FN assembly, interactions among laminin, fibrin, and collagen elicit an opposite effect on FN. Thus, it is not unreasonable to conclude that the precise outcome of platelets' encounter with the endothelium is highly context dependent.[186,187]

Finally, we should note that nonfibrillar constituents of the subendothelium might also impinge on the function of platelets in a number of ways. For instance, heparin binds to serine protease inhibitors (SERPINS), antithrombin III, and heparin cofactor II and thus accelerates formation of the thrombin-antithrombin complex. Thrombin is a pivotal serine protease of the coagulation pathway, and it also exerts a positive feedback effect on its own biogenesis by activating factors V and VIII. Inhibition of thrombin by GAGs is a key mechanism in the regulation of blood clotting.[188–191] Platelets contain platelet factor 4 (PF4) in α granules, where it is stored in a complex with chondroitin-4-sulfate PG. When released, PF4 has the ability to neutralize the anticoagulant effects of heparin and heparan. The PG-PF4 complex is dissociated by conditions of high ionic strength and by GAGs. Based on these interactions, it is conceivable that any HS– and DS–containing PGs present in blood vessel walls could serve to control deposition of PF4 locally by competitively dissociating the PG-PF4 complex.

Perspectives

This brief discussion of the subendothelial connective tissues is intended to underscore their pivotal role in developmental patterning of the vascular system, and maturation and maintenance of its functional integrity. Extracellular matrix molecules are involved in the regulation of adhesion, motility, growth, differentiation, and death of ECs, pericytes, and VSMCs. Such functional versatility of ECM is derived from the modular organization of its constituent molecules that contain assorted, independently folded, and evolutionarily conserved sequence motifs. While some domains of the fibrillar and nonfibrillar proteins facilitate supramolecular assemblies that characterize ECM, others bind to cell adhesion receptors and growth factors and modulate intracellular signal transduction pathways. Thus, by acting as a solid-phase multivalent ligand and as a reservoir of growth factors, ECM can integrate numerous complex signaling pathways elicited by physiological and pathological stimuli. Unsurprisingly, many genetic and acquired vascular diseases can be directly or indirectly linked to dysfunctional ECM molecules.

Consistent with their role in imparting mechanical integrity and tensile strength to blood vessels, a spectrum of recessive mutations in genes that encode fibrillar collagens and elastic fiber-associated proteins has been reported. Thus, haploinsufficiency of types I and III collagen have been associated with arterial aneurysms

and Ehlers Danlos syndrome (EDS) type IV in patients. Ablation of type I collagen expression in mice led to death due to rupture of large vessels between day 12 and 14 of gestation. Although mutations in type I collagen gene were mainly associated with osteogenesis imperfecta (OI), a number of OI patients were predisposed to dissection and rupturing of their aorta. Finally, Biswas et al. reported that a point mutation in the COL8A2 gene (encodes transmembrane collagen type VIII) was associated with two different types of endothelial dystrophy in the cornea.[192] It is noteworthy that aberrant turnover of ECM as a result of mutations in MMPs or TIMPs also yielded vascular phenotypes in transgenic mice. Mice deficient in either MMP-2 or MMP-9 are resistant to $CaCl_2$-induced formation of aneurysm; conversely, disruption of TIMP-1, an inhibitor of MMP-9, leads to enhanced propensity of mice to develop aneurysms.

A direct role of FN and its receptor integrins in the development of blood vessels has been most clearly demonstrated by gene knockout studies in mice. Ablation of either FN or the α5 subunit of $\alpha_5\beta_1$ integrin (major FN receptor) led to defective vasculogenesis that resulted in embryonic and prenatal death. Similarly, the angiogenesis response in adult mice was greatly blunted if these animals had haploinsufficiency of expression of either FN, $\alpha_4\beta_1$, or $\alpha_5\beta_1$ integrin. The angiogenesis response was particularly compromised in mice expressing truncated FN lacking EDA and EDB modules, thus corroborating a vital role of the alternatively spliced form of FN (see earlier discussion).

Experimental ablation of various laminin α chains has been accomplished in mice. Consistent with their integral role in basement membrane formation in many tissues and an apparent overlap in their functions, haploinsufficiency of a particular laminin results in diverse phenotypes. Thus, depending on laminin type, knockout may result in embryonic lethality (e.g., α3, β3, and γ2 chains of laminin) in mice; alternatively, these animals develop renal, skin, or neuromuscular complications as they grow. Skin blistering seen in mice that lack the α3 or β3 laminin chain resembles junctional epidermolysis bullosa seen in humans with analogous mutations in laminin genes. Finally, mice that fail to express laminin-411, laminin-421, or laminin-511 do not die in utero but show aberrant development of blood vessels in various organs.

The complex structural and signaling defects caused by mutations in an ECM molecule are most vividly illustrated by the clinical manifestations in Marfan's syndrome patients. In such patients, mutations in fibrillin-1 and -2 genes have been associated with progressive aortic dissection, vascular aneurysms, and abnormally thick and elongated cardiac valve leaflets. It was noted that there was apparent breakdown and disarray of elastic fibers in various tissues of Marfan's syndrome patients. Accumulation of inflammatory cells and elaboration of MMP-2 and MMP-9 in the elastic tissues were also a common occurrence. Similar pathological findings were also corroborated in Marfan's syndrome mouse models, where aortic walls showed aberrant elastic fibers coexisting with excessive ECM and enhanced expression of MMPs. For many years, these common pathological findings in patients and mouse models were interpreted as telltale signs of a structural deficit in the ECM caused by reduced levels of fibrillin. However, an astute set of observations made while studying the pulmonary pathology in a Marfan's syndrome mouse model led to the discovery that rather than playing a structural role, fibrillin-1 was needed for an obligatory signaling step in lung morphogenesis. These investigations elucidated an important connection between the fibrillin-1 gene and TGF-β signaling. Evidently, insufficient sequestration of TGF-β in the lungs of fibrillin-1 deficient mice led to excessive action of this cytokine that was responsible for the pulmonary pathology. These elegant experiments followed by many others led to the conclusion that TGF-β signaling was a key player in the multiorgan manifestations of Marfan's syndrome.

Maintenance of the functional integrity of blood vessels by ECM is fundamental for both human health and disease. Therefore, a comprehensive understanding of the vast array of biological mechanisms impacted by the subendothelial ECM is indispensable if we seek novel diagnoses and therapies for diseases caused by aberrant vascular ECM. This is a daunting goal in the face of the complexity and redundancy of signal transduction pathways elicited by the subendothelial ECM. To achieve this objective, we will need to further refine the reductionist methods of the "one gene/ one disease" phenotype that have been extremely successful in the past. Such experimental and analytical maneuvers would enable us to rigorously evaluate the redundancies in genetic networks, and the consequential compensatory responses mounted by the organism in response to haploinsufficiency of a particular gene. Finally, a combined approach from bedside to bench and back would be highly desirable to attain these objectives.

REFERENCES

1. Burton AC: Relation of structure to function of the tissues of the wall of blood vessels, *Physiol Rev* 34(4):619–642, 1954.
2. Eble JA, Niland S: The extracellular matrix of blood vessels, *Curr Pharm Des* 15(12):1385–1400, 2009.
3. Wagenseil JE, Mecham RP: Vascular extracellular matrix and arterial mechanics, *Physiol Rev* 89(3):957–989, 2009.
4. Davis GE: The development of the vasculature and its extracellular matrix: a gradual process defined by sequential cellular and matrix remodeling events, *Am J Physiol Heart Circ Physiol* 299(2):H245–H247, 2010.
5. Davis GE, Senger DR: Endothelial extracellular matrix: biosynthesis, remodeling, and functions during vascular morphogenesis and neovessel stabilization, *Circ Res* 97(11):1093–1107, 2005.
6. Myllyharju J, Kivirikko KI: Collagens and collagen-related diseases, *Ann Med* 33(1):7–21, 2001.
7. Myllyharju J, Kivirikko KI: Collagens, modifying enzymes and their mutations in humans, flies and worms, *Trends Genet* 20(1):33–43, 2004.
8. Kadler KE, Baldock C, Bella J, et al: Collagens at a glance, *J Cell Sci* 120(Pt 12):1955–1958, 2007.
9. Gordon MK, Hahn RA: Collagens, *Cell Tissue Res* 339(1):247–257, 2010.
10. Khoshnoodi J, Pedchenko V, Hudson BG: Mammalian collagen IV, *Microsc Res Tech* 71(5):357–370, 2008.
11. Murakami M, Simons M: Regulation of vascular integrity, *J Mol Med* 87(6):571–582, 2009.
12. Koch M, Schulze J, Hansen U, et al: A novel marker of tissue junctions, collagen XXII, *J Biol Chem* 279(21):22514–22521, 2004.
13. Koch M, Veit G, Stricker S, et al: Expression of type XXIII collagen mRNA and protein, *J Biol Chem* 281(30):21546–21557, 2006.
14. Villone D, Fritsch A, Koch M, et al: Supramolecular interactions in the dermo-epidermal junction zone: anchoring fibril-collagen VII tightly binds to banded collagen fibrils, *J Biol Chem* 283(36):24506–24513, 2008.
15. Hashimoto T, Wakabayashi T, Watanabe A, et al: CLAC: a novel Alzheimer amyloid plaque component derived from a transmembrane precursor, CLAC-P/collagen type XXV, *EMBO J* 21(7):1524–1534, 2002.
16. Sasaki T, Larsson H, Tisi D, et al: Endostatins derived from collagens XV and XVIII differ in structural and binding properties, tissue distribution and anti-angiogenic activity, *J Mol Biol* 301(5):1179–1190, 2000.
17. Li D, Clark CC, Myers JC: Basement membrane zone type XV collagen is a disulfide-bonded chondroitin sulfate proteoglycan in human tissues and cultured cells, *J Biol Chem* 275(29):22339–22347, 2000.
18 Hurskainen M, Ruggiero F, Hagg P, et al: Recombinant human collagen XV regulates cell adhesion and migration, *J Biol Chem* 285(8):5258–5265.
19. Sato K, Yomogida K, Wada T, et al: Type XXVI collagen, a new member of the collagen family, is specifically expressed in the testis and ovary, *J Biol Chem* 277(40):37678–37684, 2002.
20 Grimal S, Puech S, Wagener R, et al: Collagen XXVIII is a distinctive component of the peripheral nervous system nodes of Ranvier and surrounds nonmyelinating glial cells, *Glia* 58(16):1977–1987.
21. Prockop DJ, Kivirikko KI: Collagens: molecular biology, diseases, and potentials for therapy, *Annu Rev Biochem* 64:403–434, 1995.
22. Plenz GA, Deng MC, Robenek H, et al: Vascular collagens: spotlight on the role of type VIII collagen in atherogenesis, *Atherosclerosis* 166(1):1–11, 2003.
23. Ghosh AK: Factors involved in the regulation of type I collagen gene expression: implication in fibrosis, *Exp Biol Med (Maywood)* 227(5):301–314, 2002.
24. Ghosh AK, Varga J: The transcriptional coactivator and acetyltransferase p300 in fibroblast biology and fibrosis, *J Cell Physiol* 213(3):663–671, 2007.
25. Nagai N, Hosokawa M, Itohara S, et al: Embryonic lethality of molecular chaperone hsp47 knockout mice is associated with defects in collagen biosynthesis, *J Cell Biol* 150(6):1499–1506, 2000.
26. Aycock RS, Raghow R, Stricklin GP, et al: Post-transcriptional inhibition of collagen and fibronectin synthesis by a synthetic homolog of a portion of the carboxyl-terminal propeptide of human type I collagen, *J Biol Chem* 261(30):14355–14360, 1986.
27. Bornstein P: Regulation of expression of the alpha 1 (I) collagen gene: a critical appraisal of the role of the first intron, *Matrix Biol* 15(1):3–10, 1996.
28. Fujii K, Tanzer ML, Cooke PH: Collagen fibrogenesis and the formation of complex cross-links, *J Mol Biol* 106(1):223–227, 1976.
29. Bernstein PH, Mechanic GL: A natural histidine-based imminium cross-link in collagen and its location, *J Biol Chem* 255(21):10414–10422, 1980.
30 Bourboulia D, Stetler-Stevenson WG: Matrix metalloproteinases (MMPs) and tissue inhibitors of metalloproteinases (TIMPs): positive and negative regulators in tumor cell adhesion, *Semin Cancer Biol* 20(3):161–168.
31 Kessenbrock K, Plaks V, Werb Z: Matrix metalloproteinases: regulators of the tumor microenvironment, *Cell* 141(1):52–67.
32. Fanjul-Fernandez M, Folgueras AR, Cabrera S, et al: Matrix metalloproteinases: evolution, gene regulation and functional analysis in mouse models, *Biochim Biophys Acta* 1803(1):3–19.
33. Raffetto JD, Khalil RA: Matrix metalloproteinases and their inhibitors in vascular remodeling and vascular disease, *Biochem Pharmacol* 75(2):346–359, 2008.
34. Brew K, Nagase H: The tissue inhibitors of metalloproteinases (TIMPs): an ancient family with structural and functional diversity, *Biochim Biophys Acta* 1803(1):55–71.
35. Sternlicht MD, Werb Z: How matrix metalloproteinases regulate cell behavior, *Annu Rev Cell Dev Biol* 17:463–516, 2001.
36. Woessner J, Nagase H: *matrix metalloproteinases and TIMPs*, New York, 2002, Oxford University Press.
37. Ruoslahti E: Specialization of tumour vasculature, *Nat Rev Cancer* 2(2):83–90, 2002.
38. Silletti S, Kessler T, Goldberg J, et al: Disruption of matrix metalloproteinase 2 binding to integrin alpha vbeta 3 by an organic molecule inhibits angiogenesis and tumor growth in vivo, *Proc Natl Acad Sci U S A* 98(1):119–124, 2001.
39. Wise SG, Weiss AS: Tropoelastin, *Int J Biochem Cell Biol* 41(3):494–497, 2009.
40. Ramirez F, Dietz HC: Fibrillin-rich microfibrils: structural determinants of morphogenetic and homeostatic events, *J Cell Physiol* 213(2):326–330, 2007.
41. Royce PM, Steinmann B, Kielty CM, et al: The collagen family: structure, assembly, and organization in the extracellular matrix, In Royce PM, Steinmann B, editors: *Connective tissue and its heritable disorders: molecular, genetic, and medical aspects*, ed 2, New York, 2002, Wiley & Sons, p 159.
42. Broekelmann TJ, Kozel BA, Ishibashi H, et al: Tropoelastin interacts with cell-surface glycosaminoglycans via its COOH-terminal domain, *J Biol Chem* 280(49):40939–40947, 2005.
43. Czirok A, Zach J, Kozel BA, et al: Elastic fiber macro-assembly is a hierarchical, cell motion-mediated process, *J Cell Physiol* 207(1):97–106, 2006.
44. Kozel BA, Rongish BJ, Czirok A, et al: Elastic fiber formation: a dynamic view of extracellular matrix assembly using timer reporters, *J Cell Physiol* 207(1):87–96, 2006.
45. Ramirez F, Sakai LY: Biogenesis and function of fibrillin assemblies, *Cell Tissue Res* 339(1):71–82, 2010.
46. Sato F, Wachi H, Ishida M, et al: Distinct steps of cross-linking, self-association, and maturation of tropoelastin are necessary for elastic fiber formation, *J Mol Biol* 369(3):841–851, 2007.
47. Galis ZS, Khatri JJ: Matrix metalloproteinases in vascular remodeling and atherogenesis: the good, the bad, and the ugly, *Circ Res* 90(3):251–262, 2002.
48. Pezet M, Jacob MP, Escoubet B, et al: Elastin haploinsufficiency induces alternative aging processes in the aorta, *Rejuvenation Res* 11(1):97–112, 2008.
49. Brooke BS, Bayes-Genis A, Li DY: New insights into elastin and vascular disease, *Trends Cardiovasc Med* 13(5):176–181, 2003.
50. Li DY, Brooke B, Davis EC, et al: Elastin is an essential determinant of arterial morphogenesis, *Nature* 393(6682):276–280, 1998.
51. Li DY, Faury G, Taylor DG, et al: Novel arterial pathology in mice and humans hemizygous for elastin, *J Clin Invest* 102(10):1783–1787, 1998.
52. Urban Z, Riazi S, Seidl TL, et al: Connection between elastin haploinsufficiency and increased cell proliferation in patients with supravalvular aortic stenosis and Williams-Beuren syndrome, *Am J Hum Genet* 71(1):30–44, 2002.
53. Karnik SK, Brooke BS, Bayes-Genis A, et al: A critical role for elastin signaling in vascular morphogenesis and disease, *Development* 130(2):411–423, 2003.
54. Raines EW: The extracellular matrix can regulate vascular cell migration, proliferation, and survival: relationships to vascular disease, *Int J Exp Pathol* 81(3):173–182, 2000.
55. Waugh JM, Li-Hawkins J, Yuksel E, et al: Therapeutic elastase inhibition by alpha-1-antitrypsin gene transfer limits neointima formation in normal rabbits, *J Vasc Interv Radiol* 12(10):1203–1209, 2001.
56. Zaidi SH, You XM, Ciura S, et al: Overexpression of the serine elastase inhibitor elafin protects transgenic mice from hypoxic pulmonary hypertension, *Circulation* 105(4):516–521, 2002.
57 Yanagisawa H, Davis EC: Unraveling the mechanism of elastic fiber assembly: the roles of short fibulins, *Int J Biochem Cell Biol* 42(7):1084–1093.
58. Arteaga-Solis E, Gayraud B, Lee SY, et al: Regulation of limb patterning by extracellular microfibrils, *J Cell Biol* 154(2):275–281, 2001.
59. Carta L, Smaldone S, Zilberberg L, et al: p38 MAPK is an early determinant of promiscuous Smad2/3 signaling in the aortas of fibrillin-1 (Fbn1)-null mice, *J Biol Chem* 284(9):5630–5636, 2009.
60. Trask BC, Trask TM, Broekelmann T, et al: The microfibrillar proteins MAGP-1 and fibrillin-1 form a ternary complex with the chondroitin sulfate proteoglycan decorin, *Mol Biol Cell* 11(5):1499–1507, 2000.
61. Trask TM, Trask BC, Ritty TM, et al: Interaction of tropoelastin with the amino-terminal domains of fibrillin-1 and fibrillin-2 suggests a role for the fibrillins in elastic fiber assembly, *J Biol Chem* 275(32):24400–24406, 2000.
62. Ramirez F, Dietz HC: Extracellular microfibrils in vertebrate development and disease processes, *J Biol Chem* 284(22):14677–14681, 2009.
63. Hynes RO: *Fibronectins*, New York, 1990, Springer.
64. Magnusson MK, Mosher DF: Fibronectin: structure, assembly, and cardiovascular implications, *Arterioscler Thromb Vasc Biol* 18(9):1363–1370, 1998.
65. Hynes RO, Zhao Q: The evolution of cell adhesion, *J Cell Biol* 150(2):F89–F96, 2000.
66. Whittaker CA, Bergeron KF, Whittle J, et al: The echinoderm adhesome, *Dev Biol* 300(1):252–266, 2006.
67. Pankov R, Yamada KM: Fibronectin at a glance, *J Cell Sci* 115(Pt 20):3861–3863, 2002.
68. White ES, Baralle FE, Muro AF: New insights into form and function of fibronectin splice variants, *J Pathol* 216(1):1–14, 2008.
69. Gutman A, Kornblihtt AR: Identification of a third region of cell-specific alternative splicing in human fibronectin mRNA, *Proc Natl Acad Sci U S A* 84(20):7179–7182, 1987.
70. Kornblihtt AR, Vibe-Pedersen K, Baralle FE: Human fibronectin: molecular cloning evidence for two mRNA species differing by an internal segment coding for a structural domain, *EMBO J* 3(1):221–226, 1984.
71. Schwarzbauer JE, Patel RS, Fonda D, et al: Multiple sites of alternative splicing of the rat fibronectin gene transcript, *EMBO J* 6(9):2573–2580, 1987.

CH 4

72. Schwarzbauer JE, Tamkun JW, Lemischka IR, et al: Three different fibronectin mRNAs arise by alternative splicing within the coding region, *Cell* 35(2 Pt 1):421–431, 1983.
73. Bisno AL, Brito MO, Collins CM: Molecular basis of group A streptococcal virulence, *Lancet Infect Dis* 3(4):191–200, 2003.
74. Klebe RJ: Isolation of a collagen-dependent cell attachment factor, *Nature* 250(463):248–251, 1974.
75. Kleinman HK, Klebe RJ, Martin GR: Role of collagenous matrices in the adhesion and growth of cells, *J Cell Biol* 88(3):473–485, 1981.
76. Engvall E, Ruoslahti E, Miller EJ: Affinity of fibronectin to collagens of different genetic types and to fibrinogen, *J Exp Med* 147(6):1584–1595, 1978.
77. Hynes RO: Cell-matrix adhesion in vascular development, *J Thromb Haemost* 5(Suppl 1): 32–40, 2007.
78. Hynes RO: The extracellular matrix: not just pretty fibrils, *Science* 326(5957):1216–1219, 2009.
79. George EL, Georges-Labouesse EN, Patel-King RS, et al: Defects in mesoderm, neural tube and vascular development in mouse embryos lacking fibronectin, *Development* 119(4):1079–1091, 1993.
80. Astrof S, Kirby A, Lindblad-Toh K, et al: Heart development in fibronectin-null mice is governed by a genetic modifier on chromosome four, *Mech Dev* 124(7–8):551–558, 2007.
81. Francis SE, Goh KL, Hodivala-Dilke K, et al: Central roles of alpha5beta1 integrin and fibronectin in vascular development in mouse embryos and embryoid bodies, *Arterioscler Thromb Vasc Biol* 22(6):927–933, 2002.
82. Astrof S, Crowley D, Hynes RO: Multiple cardiovascular defects caused by the absence of alternatively spliced segments of fibronectin, *Dev Biol* 311(1):11–24, 2007.
83. Astrof S, Crowley D, George EL, et al: Direct test of potential roles of EIIIA and EIIIB alternatively spliced segments of fibronectin in physiological and tumor angiogenesis, *Mol Cell Biol* 24(19):8662–8670, 2004.
84. Wierzbicka-Patynowski I, Schwarzbauer JE: The ins and outs of fibronectin matrix assembly, *J Cell Sci* 116(Pt 16):3269–3276, 2003.
85. Cho J, Mosher DF: Role of fibronectin assembly in platelet thrombus formation, *J Thromb Haemost* 4(7):1461–1469, 2006.
86. Lowenberg EC, Meijers JC, Levi M: Platelet-vessel wall interaction in health and disease, *Neth J Med* 68(6):242–251, 2010.
87. Ruggeri ZM, Mendolicchio GL: Adhesion mechanisms in platelet function, *Circ Res* 100(12):1673–1685, 2007.
88. Raghow R: The role of extracellular matrix in postinflammatory wound healing and fibrosis, *FASEB J* 8(11):823–831, 1994.
89. Aumailley M, Bruckner-Tuderman L, Carter WG, et al: A simplified laminin nomenclature, *Matrix Biol* 24(5):326–332, 2005.
90. Durbeej M: Laminins, *Cell Tissue Res* 339(1):259–268, 2010.
91. Miner JH, Yurchenco PD: Laminin functions in tissue morphogenesis, *Annu Rev Cell Dev Biol* 20:255–284, 2004.
92. Aumailley M, Pesch M, Tunggal L, et al: Altered synthesis of laminin 1 and absence of basement membrane component deposition in (beta)1 integrin-deficient embryoid bodies, *J Cell Sci* 113(Pt 2):259–268, 2000.
93. Colognato H, Yurchenco PD: Form and function: the laminin family of heterotrimers, *Dev Dyn* 218(2):213–234, 2000.
94. Scheele S, Falk M, Franzen A, et al: Laminin alpha1 globular domains 4–5 induce fetal development but are not vital for embryonic basement membrane assembly, *Proc Natl Acad Sci U S A* 102(5):1502–1506, 2005.
95. Scheele S, Nystrom A, Durbeej M, et al: Laminin isoforms in development and disease, *J Mol Med* 85(8):825–836, 2007.
96. Tzu J, Marinkovich MP: Bridging structure with function: structural, regulatory, and developmental role of laminins, *Int J Biochem Cell Biol* 40(2):199–214, 2008.
97. Van Agtmael T, Bruckner-Tuderman L: Basement membranes and human disease, *Cell Tissue Res* 339(1):167–188, 2010.
98. Engbring JA, Kleinman HK: The basement membrane matrix in malignancy, *J Pathol* 200(4):465–470, 2003.
99. Kleinman HK, Koblinski J, Lee S, et al: Role of basement membrane in tumor growth and metastasis, *Surg Oncol Clin N Am* 10(2):329–338, ix, 2001.
100. Miner JH: Laminins and their roles in mammals, *Microsc Res Tech* 71(5):349–356, 2008.
101. Gubler MC: Inherited diseases of the glomerular basement membrane, *Nat Clin Pract Nephrol* 4(1):24–37, 2008.
102. Patton BL, Wang B, Tarumi YS, et al: A single point mutation in the LN domain of LAMA2 causes muscular dystrophy and peripheral amyelination, *J Cell Sci* 121(Pt 10):1593–1604, 2008.
103. Timpl R, Tisi D, Talts JF, et al: Structure and function of laminin LG modules, *Matrix Biol* 19(4):309–317, 2000.
104. Thyboll J, Kortesmaa J, Cao R, et al: Deletion of the laminin alpha4 chain leads to impaired microvessel maturation, *Mol Cell Biol* 22(4):1194–1202, 2002.
105. Esko JD, Lindahl U: Molecular diversity of heparan sulfate, *J Clin Invest* 108(2):169–173, 2001.
106. Gandhi NS, Mancera RL: The structure of glycosaminoglycans and their interactions with proteins, *Chem Biol Drug Des* 72(6):455–482, 2008.
107. Bulow HE, Hobert O: The molecular diversity of glycosaminoglycans shapes animal development, *Annu Rev Cell Dev Biol* 22:375–407, 2006.
108. Roughley PJ: The structure and function of cartilage proteoglycans, *Eur Cell Mater* 12: 92–101, 2006.
109. Schaefer L, Schaefer RM: Proteoglycans: from structural compounds to signaling molecules, *Cell Tissue Res* 339(1):237–246, 2010.
110. Theocharis AD, Skandalis SS, Tzanakakis GN, et al: Proteoglycans in health and disease: novel roles for proteoglycans in malignancy and their pharmacological targeting, *FEBS J* 277(19):3904–3923, 2010.
111. Wu YJ, La Pierre DP, Wu J, et al: The interaction of versican with its binding partners, *Cell Res* 15(7):483–494, 2005.
112. Kim S, Takahashi H, Lin WW, et al: Carcinoma-produced factors activate myeloid cells through TLR2 to stimulate metastasis, *Nature* 457(7225):102–106, 2009.
113. Iozzo RV, Zoeller JJ, Nystrom A: Basement membrane proteoglycans: modulators par excellence of cancer growth and angiogenesis, *Mol Cells* 27(5):503–513, 2009.
114. Drickamer K: A conserved disulphide bond in sialyltransferases, *Glycobiology* 3(1):2–3, 1993.
115. Li H, Schwartz NB, Vertel BM: cDNA cloning of chick cartilage chondroitin sulfate (aggrecan) core protein and identification of a stop codon in the aggrecan gene associated with the chondrodystrophy, nanomelia, *J Biol Chem* 268(31):23504–23511, 1993.
116. Watanabe H, Kimata K, Line S, et al: Mouse cartilage matrix deficiency (cmd) caused by a 7 bp deletion in the aggrecan gene, *Nat Genet* 7(2):154–157, 1994.
117. Kwok JC, Afshari F, Garcia-Alias G, et al: Proteoglycans in the central nervous system: plasticity, regeneration and their stimulation with chondroitinase ABC, *Restor Neurol Neurosci* 26(2–3):131–145, 2008.
118. Iozzo RV: Basement membrane proteoglycans: from cellar to ceiling, *Nat Rev Mol Cell Biol* 6(8):646–656, 2005.
119. Iozzo RV: Matrix proteoglycans: from molecular design to cellular function, *Annu Rev Biochem* 67:609–652, 1998.
120. Iozzo RV, Schaefer L: Proteoglycans in health and disease: novel regulatory signaling mechanisms evoked by the small leucine-rich proteoglycans, *FEBS J* 277(19):3864–3875, 2010.
121. Brule S, Charnaux N, Sutton A, et al: The shedding of syndecan-4 and syndecan-1 from HeLa cells and human primary macrophages is accelerated by SDF-1/CXCL12 and mediated by the matrix metalloproteinase-9, *Glycobiology* 16(6):488–501, 2006.
122. Danielson KG, Baribault H, Holmes DF, et al: Targeted disruption of decorin leads to abnormal collagen fibril morphology and skin fragility, *J Cell Biol* 136(3):729–743, 1997.
123. Hedbom E, Heinegard D: Binding of fibromodulin and decorin to separate sites on fibrillar collagens, *J Biol Chem* 268(36):27307–27312, 1993.
124. Nurminskaya MV, Birk DE: Differential expression of fibromodulin mRNA associated with tendon fibril growth: isolation and characterization of a chicken fibromodulin cDNA, *Biochem J* 317(Pt 3):785–789, 1996.
125. Vogel KG, Paulsson M, Heinegard D: Specific inhibition of type I and type II collagen fibrillogenesis by the small proteoglycan of tendon, *Biochem J* 223(3):587–597, 1984.
126. Birk DE, Nurminskaya MV, Zycband EI: Collagen fibrillogenesis *in situ*: fibril segments undergo post-depositional modifications resulting in linear and lateral growth during matrix development, *Dev Dyn* 202(3):229–243, 1995.
127. Goldoni S, Iozzo RV: Tumor microenvironment: modulation by decorin and related molecules harboring leucine-rich tandem motifs, *Int J Cancer* 123(11):2473–2479, 2008.
128. Heinegard D: Proteoglycans and more–from molecules to biology, *Int J Exp Pathol* 90(6):575–586, 2009.
129. Filmus J, Capurro M, Rast J: Glypicans, *Genome Biol* 9(5):224, 2008.
130. Alexopoulou AN, Multhaupt HA, Couchman JR: Syndecans in wound healing, inflammation and vascular biology, *Int J Biochem Cell Biol* 39(3):505–528, 2007.
131. Li Q, Park PW, Wilson CL, et al: Matrilysin shedding of syndecan-1 regulates chemokine mobilization and transepithelial efflux of neutrophils in acute lung injury, *Cell* 111(5):635–646, 2002.
132. Endo K, Takino T, Miyamori H, et al: Cleavage of syndecan-1 by membrane type matrix metalloproteinase-1 stimulates cell migration, *J Biol Chem* 278(42):40764–40770, 2003.
133 Manon-Jensen T, Itoh Y, Couchman JR: Proteoglycans in health and disease: the multiple roles of syndecan shedding, *FEBS J* 277(19):3876–3889.
134. Rodgers KD, San Antonio JD, Jacenko O: Heparan sulfate proteoglycans: a GAGgle of skeletal-hematopoietic regulators, *Dev Dyn* 237(10):2622–2642, 2008.
135. Beckett K, Franch-Marro X, Vincent JP: Glypican-mediated endocytosis of hedgehog has opposite effects in flies and mice, *Trends Cell Biol* 18(8):360–363, 2008.
136. Kjellen L, Lindahl U: Proteoglycans: structures and interactions, *Annu Rev Biochem* 60:443–475, 1991.
137. Lindahl U, Kusche-Gullberg M, Kjellen L: Regulated diversity of heparan sulfate, *J Biol Chem* 273(39):24979–24982, 1998.
138. Ruoslahti E: Structure and biology of proteoglycans, *Annu Rev Cell Biol* 4:229–255, 1988.
139. Geiger B, Spatz JP, Bershadsky AD: Environmental sensing through focal adhesions, *Nat Rev Mol Cell Biol* 10(1):21–33, 2009.
140. Lock JG, Wehrle-Haller B, Stromblad S: Cell-matrix adhesion complexes: master control machinery of cell migration, *Semin Cancer Biol* 18(1):65–76, 2008.
141. Delon I, Brown NH: Integrins and the actin cytoskeleton, *Curr Opin Cell Biol* 19(1):43–50, 2007.
142. Tilghman RW, Parsons JT: Focal adhesion kinase as a regulator of cell tension in the progression of cancer, *Semin Cancer Biol* 18(1):45–52, 2008.
143. Berrier AL, Yamada KM: Cell-matrix adhesion, *J Cell Physiol* 213(3):565–573, 2007.
144. Legate KR, Wickstrom SA, Fassler R: Genetic and cell biological analysis of integrin outside-in signaling, *Genes Dev* 23(4):397–418, 2009.
145. Alam N, Goel HL, Zarif MJ, et al: The integrin-growth factor receptor duet, *J Cell Physiol* 213(3):649–653, 2007.
146. Xu R, Boudreau A, Bissell MJ: Tissue architecture and function: dynamic reciprocity via extra- and intra-cellular matrices, *Cancer Metastasis Rev* 28(1–2):167–176, 2009.
147. Hynes RO: Integrins: bidirectional, allosteric signaling machines, *Cell* 110(6):673–687, 2002.
148. Humphries JD, Byron A, Humphries MJ: Integrin ligands at a glance, *J Cell Sci* 119(Pt 19): 3901–3903, 2006.
149. Astrof S, Hynes RO: Fibronectins in vascular morphogenesis, *Angiogenesis* 12(2):165–175, 2009.
150. Gui P, Chao JT, Wu X, et al: Coordinated regulation of vascular Ca^{2+} and K^{+} channels by integrin signaling, *Adv Exp Med Biol* 674:69–79, 2010.
151. Luo BH, Carman CV, Springer TA: Structural basis of integrin regulation and signaling, *Annu Rev Immunol* 25:619–647, 2007.
152. Jarvelainen H, Sainio A, Koulu M, et al: Extracellular matrix molecules: potential targets in pharmacotherapy, *Pharmacol Rev* 61(2):198–223, 2009.
153. Zaidel-Bar R, Itzkovitz S, Ma'ayan A, et al: Functional atlas of the integrin adhesome, *Nat Cell Biol* 9(8):858–867, 2007.
154. Lo SH: Focal adhesions: what's new inside, *Dev Biol* 294(2):280–291, 2006.
155. Li S, Guan JL, Chien S: Biochemistry and biomechanics of cell motility, *Annu Rev Biomed Eng* 7:105–150, 2005.
156. Goel HL, Breen M, Zhang J, et al: Beta1A integrin expression is required for type 1 insulin-like growth factor receptor mitogenic and transforming activities and localization to focal contacts, *Cancer Res* 65(15):6692–6700, 2005.
157. Goel HL, Moro L, King M, et al: Beta1 integrins modulate cell adhesion by regulating insulin-like growth factor-II levels in the microenvironment, *Cancer Res* 66(1):331–342, 2006.

158. Sridhar SC, Miranti CK: Tetraspanin KAI1/CD82 suppresses invasion by inhibiting integrin-dependent crosstalk with c-Met receptor and Src kinases, *Oncogene* 25(16):2367–2378, 2006.

159. Baron V, Schwartz M: Cell adhesion regulates ubiquitin-mediated degradation of the platelet-derived growth factor receptor beta, *J Biol Chem* 275(50):39318–39323, 2000.

160. Cabodi S, Moro L, Bergatto E, et al: Integrin regulation of epidermal growth factor (EGF) receptor and of EGF-dependent responses, *Biochem Soc Trans* 32(Pt3):438–442, 2004.

161. Bill HM, Knudsen B, Moores SL, et al: Epidermal growth factor receptor-dependent regulation of integrin-mediated signaling and cell cycle entry in epithelial cells, *Mol Cell Biol* 24(19):8586–8599, 2004.

162. Chen X, Abair TD, Ibanez MR, et al: Integrin alpha1beta1 controls reactive oxygen species synthesis by negatively regulating epidermal growth factor receptor-mediated Rac activation, *Mol Cell Biol* 27(9):3313–3326, 2007.

163. Hawiger: Adhesive interactions of blood cells and vascular wall in hemostasis and thrombosis, In Coleman R, Hirsch J, Marder V, et al, editors: *Hemostasis and thrombosis: basic principles and clinical practices*, ed 3, Philadelphia, 1994, JB Lippincott, pp 639–653.

164. Ruggeri ZM: Platelets in atherothrombosis, *Nat Med* 8(11):1227–1234, 2002.

165. Gawaz M, Langer H, May AE: Platelets in inflammation and atherogenesis, *J Clin Invest* 115(12):3378–3384, 2005.

166. Nieswandt B, Watson SP: Platelet-collagen interaction: is GPVI the central receptor? *Blood* 102(2):449–461, 2003.

167. Wagner DD: Cell biology of von Willebrand factor, *Annu Rev Cell Biol* 6:217–246, 1990.

168 McGrath RT, McRae E, Smith OP, et al: Platelet von Willebrand factor--structure, function and biological importance, *Br J Haematol* 148(6):834–843.

169. Farndale RW, Sixma JJ, Barnes MJ, et al: The role of collagen in thrombosis and hemostasis, *J Thromb Haemost* 2(4):561–573, 2004.

170. Asch AS, Liu I, Briccetti FM, et al: Analysis of CD36 binding domains: ligand specificity controlled by dephosphorylation of an ectodomain, *Science* 262(5138):1436–1440, 1993.

171. Chiang TM, Rinaldy A, Kang AH: Cloning, characterization, and functional studies of a nonintegrin platelet receptor for type I collagen, *J Clin Invest* 100(3):514–521, 1997.

172. Kato K, Kanaji T, Russell S, et al: The contribution of glycoprotein VI to stable platelet adhesion and thrombus formation illustrated by targeted gene deletion, *Blood* 102(5):1701–1707, 2003.

173. Kunicki TJ, Nugent DJ, Staats SJ, et al: The human fibroblast class II extracellular matrix receptor mediates platelet adhesion to collagen and is identical to the platelet glycoprotein Ia-IIa complex, *J Biol Chem* 263(10):4516–4519, 1988.

174. Moroi M, Jung SM, Okuma M, et al: A patient with platelets deficient in glycoprotein VI that lack both collagen-induced aggregation and adhesion, *J Clin Invest* 84(5):1440–1445, 1989.

175. Moroi M, Jung SM, Shinmyozu K, et al: Analysis of platelet adhesion to a collagen-coated surface under flow conditions: the involvement of glycoprotein VI in the platelet adhesion, *Blood* 88(6):2081–2092, 1996.

176. Nieswandt B, Brakebusch C, Bergmeier W, et al: Glycoprotein VI but not alpha2beta1 integrin is essential for platelet interaction with collagen, *EMBO J* 20(9):2120–2130, 2001.

177. Nieuwenhuis HK, Akkerman JW, Houdijk WP, et al: Human blood platelets showing no response to collagen fail to express surface glycoprotein Ia, *Nature* 318(6045):470–472, 1985.

178. Santoro SA: Identification of a 160,000 dalton platelet membrane protein that mediates the initial divalent cation-dependent adhesion of platelets to collagen, *Cell* 46(6): 913–920, 1986.

179. Smethurst PA, Onley DJ, Jarvis GE, et al: Structural basis for the platelet-collagen interaction: the smallest motif within collagen that recognizes and activates platelet glycoprotein VI contains two glycine-proline-hydroxyproline triplets, *J Biol Chem* 282(2):1296–1304, 2007.

180. Farndale RW, Lisman T, Bihan D, et al: Cell-collagen interactions: the use of peptide toolkits to investigate collagen-receptor interactions, *Biochem Soc Trans* 36(Pt 2):241–250, 2008.

181. Herr AB, Farndale RW: Structural insights into the interactions between platelet receptors and fibrillar collagen, *J Biol Chem* 284(30):19781–19785, 2009.

182. Gardner JM, Hynes RO: Interaction of fibronectin with its receptor on platelets, *Cell* 42(2):439–448, 1985.

183. Ni H, Yuen PS, Papalia JM, et al: Plasma fibronectin promotes thrombus growth and stability in injured arterioles, *Proc Natl Acad Sci U S A* 100(5):2415–2419, 2003.

184. Hynes RO: A reevaluation of integrins as regulators of angiogenesis, *Nat Med* 8(9): 918–921, 2002.

185. Ginsberg MH, Partridge A, Shattil SJ: Integrin regulation, *Curr Opin Cell Biol* 17(5): 509–516, 2005.

186 White-Adams TC, Berny MA, Patel IA, et al: Laminin promotes coagulation and thrombus formation in a factor XII-dependent manner, *J Thromb Haemost* 8(6):1295–1301.

187. Bennett JS, Berger BW, Billings PC: The structure and function of platelet integrins, *J Thromb Haemost* 7(Suppl 1):200–205, 2009.

188. Carrell RW, Huntington JA, Mushunje A, et al: The conformational basis of thrombosis, *Thromb Haemost* 86(1):14–22, 2001.

189. Casu B: Structural features and binding properties of chondroitin sulfates, dermatan sulfate, and heparan sulfate, *Semin Thromb Hemost* 17(Suppl 1):9–14, 1991.

190. Furie B, Furie BC: Molecular and cellular biology of blood coagulation, *N Engl J Med* 326(12):800–806, 1992.

191. Warkentin TE, Greinacher A: Heparin-induced thrombocytopenia and cardiac surgery, *Ann Thorac Surg* 76(2):638–648, 2003.

192. Biswas S, Munier FL, Yardley J, et al: Missense mutations in COL8A2, the gene encoding the alpha2 chain of type VIII collagen, cause two forms of corneal endothelial dystrophy, *Hum Mol Genet* 10(21):2415–2423, 2001.

CONNECTIVE TISSUES OF THE SUBENDOTHELIUM

CHAPTER 5

Normal Mechanisms of Vascular Hemostasis

Elisabeth M. Battinelli, Joseph Loscalzo

Hemostasis occurs in response to vessel injury. The clot is essential for both prevention of blood loss and initiation of the wound repair process. When there is a lesion present in the blood vessel, the response is rapid, highly regulated, and localized. If the process is not balanced, abnormal bleeding or nonphysiological thrombosis can result. In cardiovascular disease, formation of abnormal thrombus at the area of an atherosclerotic plaque results in significant morbidity and mortality. This chapter will focus on normal mechanisms of hemostasis, with specific attention to the role of the platelet in the process, the coagulation cascade, and fibrinolytic mechanisms as a basis for understanding how abnormalities in these processes can lead to thrombotic and hemorrhagic disorders.

Endothelial Function and Platelet Activation

Platelets are anucleate cells produced by megakaryocytes in the bone marrow. Once they have traversed from the bone marrow to the general circulation, their lifespan is approximately 10 days. They function mainly to limit hemorrhage after trauma resulting in vascular injury. Normally in the vasculature, platelets are in a resting state and only become activated after exposure to a stimulus leads to a shape change and release reaction that causes the platelet to export many of its biologically important proteins. Some of the agonists that can initiate this response include thromboxane A_2, adenosine diphosphate (ADP), thrombin, and serotonin. In areas of vascular injury, platelets are attracted to the impaired site by collagen through binding with von Willebrand factor (vWF) via the glycoprotein (GP) Ib/V/IX complex. This initial binding results in platelet activation, with a subsequent feedback mechanism in which ADP, thrombin, and thromboxane A_2 further activate the platelets and recruit additional platelets to the area. The complex firmly binds the platelet to the area of injury so there is no disruption by the high shear forces of turbulent blood flow that occur with vessel disruption. This amplification of the response is essential to form a hemostatic plug and represents the first stage in the hemostatic process. When vWF is not present, hemostatic abnormalities result, with deficiencies leading to von Willebrand's disease, which can be associated with severe bleeding. Hemostasis issues also arise when the platelet receptor complex GPIb/V/IX is mutated, resulting in inability of vWF to bind, a disorder termed *Bernard-Soulier's syndrome*.[1,2]

Additional platelet aggregation occurs through activation of G protein–coupled receptors (GPCRs), with the final pathway relying on the GP IIb/IIIa complex, the main receptor for platelet aggregation and adhesion.[3,4] Fibrinogen tethers GP IIb/IIIa complexes on different platelets, stabilizing the clot. The integral role of this receptor is manifest in *Glanzmann thrombasthenia*, a disorder in which fibrinogen binding is impaired, leading to spontaneously occurring mucocutaneous bleeding episodes.[5]

Vascular endothelium is essential to this hemostatic process; this is the cellular site where regulation and initiation of coagulation begins. Endothelial cells (ECs) modulate vascular tone, generate mediators of inflammation, and provide a resistant surface that allows for platelets to experience laminar flow with minimal shear. Endothelial cells regulate hemostasis by releasing a number of inhibitors of platelets and inflammation. Vascular endothelium is essential for regulating uncontrolled platelet activity through mechanisms of inhibition including the arachidonic acid–prostacyclin pathway, L-arginine–nitric oxide pathway, and endothelial ectoadenosine diphosphatase (ecto-ADPase) pathway[6] (Table 5-1).

Nitric oxide (NO) is produced constitutively by (ECs) via an endothelial isoform of nitric oxide synthase (eNOS) in a process dependent on conversion of L-arginine to L-citrulline. Vascular tone is regulated by NO as it controls smooth muscle cell (SMC) contraction. It also inhibits platelets directly, blocking platelet aggregation through stimulation of guanylyl cyclase and cyclic guanosine monophosphate (cGMP) and inhibition of platelet phosphoinositol-3-kinase (PI-3 kinase). Nitric oxide functions by decreasing the intracellular Ca^{2+} level through cGMP, which inhibits the conformational change in GP IIb/IIIa suppressing fibrinogen's ability to bind to the receptor, thereby attenuating platelet aggregation.[7]

Prostacyclin, which is synthesized in the ECs from arachidonic acid through cyclooxygenase-1 or -2 (COX-1, COX-2)-dependent pathways, inhibits platelet function by increasing cyclic adenosine monophosphate (cAMP). This is essential for aspirin's ability to diminish platelet function through acetylation of platelet COX1 at serine 529.

The last pathway important in modulating vascular endothelium's interaction with platelets is the endothelial ecto-ADPase pathway, which impairs ADP-mediated platelet activation. By hydrolyzing ADP, this enzyme inhibits the critical state of platelet recruitment to a growing aggregate, thereby limiting thrombus formation. Once the platelet aggregate has been stabilized by fibrin with red cells to the vessel wall, the next stage of hemostasis involves activation of the highly regulated coagulation cascade (Fig. 5-1).

Coagulation Cascade Leading to Fibrin Formation

Disruption in the endothelium not only recruits platelets for plug formation, it also stimulates activation of the coagulation cascade, which is essential for secondary clot formation through fibrin generation. The coagulation cascade is a dynamic integrated process in which each step is dependent on another step for activation of proenzymes or zymogens to their active forms through proteolytic cleavage. This process is dependent upon calcium and the phospholipid bilayer allowing inactive clotting factors to be converted to active enzymes through serine protease activity. These coagulation proteins function in a step-by-step fashion to activate downstream members of the cascade, leading to production of the penultimate clotting factor, thrombin. Thrombin is versatile, playing a role in many of the essential stages of hemostasis. Not only is it important for platelet activation, it is also necessary for the cross-linking of fibrin. Recently there have been attempts to limit thrombus formation by directly inhibiting thrombin activity through anticoagulants such as ximelagatran and the oral medication, dabigatran, which is now available for clinical use.[8]

The *clotting cascade* is divided into two main pathways, the *intrinsic* and *extrinsic pathways*. The extrinsic pathway begins with establishment of a complex between tissue factor, found on the cell surface or on microparticles, and factor VIIa. This complex leads to activation of factor X to Xa, which can then further the response by looping back and converting factor VII to VIIa in a feedback mechanism. When factor Xa is present, it binds to factor Va on the membrane surface and again generates prothrombinase, which converts prothrombin to thrombin and then generates fibrin as detailed earlier. The activity of factor Xa is accelerated by the presence of factor Va through calcium and formation of a noncovalent association γ-carboxyglutamate residues of factor Xa and the phospholipid surface of activated platelets.[9]

TABLE 5-1 Factors Involved in Fibrinolysis

PROHEMOSTATIC	ANTIHEMOSTATIC
Circulating	
α₂-Antiplasmin	Antithrombin III
Thrombin	Protein C
Thrombin-activatable fibrinolysis inhibitor (TAFI)	Protein S
	Tissue factor pathway inhibitor (TFPI)
Endothelium-Derived	
Plasminogen activator inhibitor-1 (PAI-1)	Ectoadenosine diphosphatase (Ecto-ADPase)/CD39
Tissue factor (TF)	Heparan sulfate (HS)
von Willebrand factor (vWF)	Nitric oxide (NO)
	Thrombomodulin
	Tissue plasminogen activator (tPA)
	Urokinase plasminogen activator (uPA)

may have a role in these allosteric changes; however, recent studies have questioned the importance of "de-encryption" in this process.[11–14] Tissue factor functions through activation of factors X and IX after interactions with factor VII as a complex. Factor VII, although at low levels in an active state (factor VIIa) in the circulation, only becomes biologically important after it is bound to tissue factor in complex with factors X and IX. This complex formation is essential for activation of thrombin.[9]

The role of tissue factor has recently been expanded. It circulates in the blood in association with microvesicles that are derived from cellular membranes produced from lipid rafts on monocytes and macrophages.[15] These tissue factor–bearing microvesicles can directly initiate the coagulation cascade on activated platelets in a process that may be important for understanding the hypercoagulable state.[16,17]

Once thrombin is activated in the tissue factor X/IX/VIIa complex, it initiates further activation within the coagulation cascade. In addition to activating platelets and factor V, it also activates factor VIII, which exists in the circulation in association with vWF. Activated factor VIII (factor VIIIa) works in a feedback loop with factor IXa to activate further factor X to Xa and thereby yield more thrombin to accelerate its own activation. Factors VIII and IX are essential in coagulation, as is evident in patients who suffer deficiencies of these factors leading to hemophilia A and B, respectively. These disorders lead to severe bleeding due to loss of activation of factor X, leading to decreased thrombin formation. Another deficiency that is seen occurs when factor XI is mutated, resulting in a disorder associated with delayed bleeding in the postoperative setting. The importance of this coagulation cascade is highlighted by the severity of this disorder, suggesting that the feedback mechanism by which thrombin activates factor XI, with subsequent activation of IX and then further generation of thrombin, is an essential stage of amplification necessary for hemostasis.

The extrinsic pathway is measured by prothrombin time (PT), which is determined by adding an extrinsic substance such as tissue factor or thromboplastin.[10]

The extrinsic pathway, which is dependent on tissue factor, appears to be the main pathway responsible for hemostasis, with the intrinsic pathway playing a supporting role. Tissue factor is a membrane-bound GP that is constitutively expressed by SMCs and fibroblasts but selectively expressed by ECs when there is vessel wall injury. The "encrypted" activated form of factor VIIa is made functional through a conformational change that occurs at cysteines 186 and 209, leading to disulfide bond formation upon vessel wall injury. Protein disulfide isomerase, glutathione, and NO all

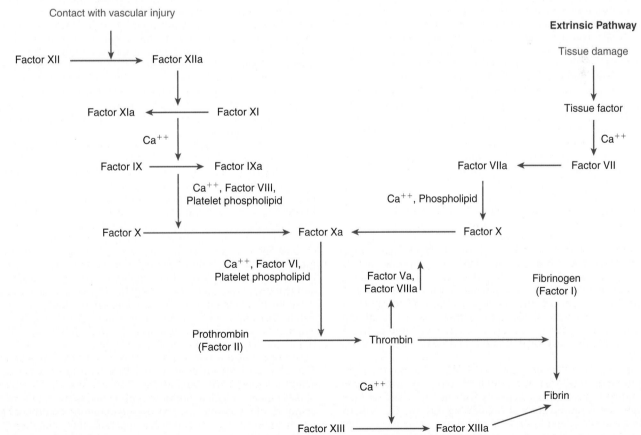

FIGURE 5-1 Coagulation cascade.

The extrinsic pathway, described earlier, joins up with the intrinsic pathway through factor X to form the *common pathway*. The intrinsic pathway is initiated by contact and results in activation of factor IXa, which then goes on to activate factor X as described. It is generally accepted that the intrinsic pathway is of less importance in coagulation than the tissue factor–mediated extrinsic pathway, although it plays an essential role in inflammation and fibrinolysis. The intrinsic pathway is based on exposure of blood to a negatively charged surface, and is classically initiated by activation of factor XIIa by kallikrein, which is facilitated by kininogen. Kallikrein is generated from prekallikrein through proteolytic cleavage by activated factor XII in a reaction dependent on the presence of high-molecular-weight kininogen (HMWK). When kallikrein has been generated, it also functions to cleave HMWK to bradykinin, which functions as an inflammatory mediator to potentiate vasodilation and vascular permeability, thereby expanding the role of factor XIIa to inflammation, regulation of vascular tone, and fibrinolysis.[18] Activated factor XII catalyzes conversion of factor XI to the active enzyme form, factor XIa. When calcium is present, factor XIa next functions to convert IX to IXa, which then binds to VIIIa on membrane surfaces, converting X to its active form, factor Xa. Factor Xa then binds to Va on the membrane surface to generate prothrombinase, which converts prothrombin to thrombin. As thrombin is formed, two small prothrombin fragments, termed *molecules F1 and F2*, are released and can be used as markers of serum thrombin formation.[19] The intrinsic pathway is monitored through the activated partial thromboplastin time (APTT), which relies on foreign substances such as glass or silicates to activate factor XII to initiate the pathway. Deficiencies in the earliest states of the intrinsic pathway, when prekallikrein, HMWK, and factor XII are involved, are not associated with bleeding tendencies and therefore do not lead to a bleeding diathesis, even though there is an elevation in partial thromboplastin time. Mutations in factor XII have been reported in a group of patients with hereditary angioedema, although there does not appear to be a bleeding diathesis with this disorder. Some initial studies have suggested that factor XII polymorphisms may be associated with an increased propensity for thrombosis, but this has not been validated.[20,21]

When factor Xa generates thrombin, the intrinsic and extrinsic pathways have merged into the common pathway. Thrombin is essential for fibrinogen to generate fibrin, which is released through proteolytic cleavage.[22] The fibrin molecules that are generated have polymerization sites exposed, making it easier for fibrin to cross-link noncovalently. This cross-linking enables platelets to be entrapped in a meshwork of fibrin strands to form the secondary clot through the action of factor XIII, activated by thrombin.[23] In the process of cross-linking, there is also an inherent mechanism of autoregulation, with the binding sites necessary to initiate fibrinolysis being blocked so the clot does not self-destruct.

This process of platelet activation and up-regulation of the coagulation cascade occurs in a swift and efficient manner to prevent excessive bleeding. It can, however, lead to thrombosis if left unchecked, so there are other mechanisms in place whose main role is to modulate coagulation activities to avoid such complications. These mechanisms involve mechanical means such as dilution of coagulation factors in blood and removal of factors after activation through the reticuloendothelial system, as well as antithrombotic pathways that are separate from the coagulation cascade. Patients with deficiencies in these natural antithrombotic mechanisms often present with thrombosis. These pathways include antithrombin, protein C and S, and tissue factor pathway inhibitor (TFPI).

Antithrombin is a serine protease inhibitor that binds specifically to factors IXa, Xa, and thrombin, thereby inactivating them. Antithrombin has two main binding sites that maintain its functionality: the reactive center at Arg 393/Ser 394 and the heparin binding site at the amino-terminal end of the molecule. Binding of both endogenous and exogenous heparins at this site causes a conformational change in antithrombin that enables it to inactivate its targets at an accelerated rate. The glycosaminoglycan heparan sulfate (HS), present on the surface of ECs, mediates antithrombin's ability to increase its activity and functions as the physiological equivalent to heparin.[24] Deficiency of antithrombin is associated with a genetic propensity to form venous thrombosis, discussed in Chapter 10.[25]

Activated protein C (APC) and protein S are also important mechanisms for preventing excessive clotting. During the clotting process, thrombin binds to thrombomodulin, which is also present on the EC surface. It then undergoes a conformational change leading to activation of protein C.[26] Activated protein C complexes with protein S and proteolytically cleaves factors Va and VIIIa, resulting in their inactivation and a decrease in generation of factors Xa and thrombin. Cleavage of factor Va occurs at Arg 506, Arg 306, and Arg 679 by APC in a sequential manner such that the cleavage at Arg 506 exposes cleavage sites at the other sites through a conformational change. Mutation of the arginine located at position 506 to glutamine leads to factor V Leiden, which is associated with a hypercoagulable state.

Another important natural anticoagulant is TFPI, which acts as a multivalent protease inhibitor to inactivate both factor Xa and IXa. Tissue factor pathway inhibitor is also present within ECs, with the majority remaining localized to the endothelial surface and very little circulating in plasma. The concentration in plasma, however, is increased in the presence of heparin, which modulates its release from the endothelial surface.

Fibrinolysis

The importance of fibrinolysis lies in its removing blood clots and maintaining hemostasis without excessive clotting. The mechanism of serine protease activity is preserved in the fibrinolytic system and accounts for the mechanism of action of many of its components (Fig. 5-2). The main factor responsible for fibrinolysis is plasmin. The process begins when plasminogen in its inactive form is converted to the active enzyme, plasmin, which functions to covert fibrin to soluble fibrin degradation products. Two molecules that mimic this function include tissue-type plasminogen activator (tPA) and urokinase-type plasminogen activator (uPA). The motif responsible for its action is the *kringle domain*, which resides in the amino-terminal end. Kringles are 80 amino acids in length and have a unique folded sheet structure that results from disulfide linkages, which yields a homotypic binding site specific for plasminogen, fibrinogen, and fibrin. There is homology between the kringles contained in all three of these molecules.

These kringle domains are essential for providing a mechanism for binding many components of the developing thrombus, including fibrinogen and fibrin. The kringle domains shared by tPA and plasminogen allow fibrinogen and fibrin to bind and therefore be incorporated into the developing clot. Plasminogen is converted to plasmin through the proteolytic cleavage achieved by tPA and uPA at the Arg 560 and Val 561 sites.[27] The plasmin generated can then bind to a number of proteins involved in the process of fibrinolysis. Relevant properties include its high affinity for fibrin, ability to cleave Glu-plasminogen to Lys-plasminogen, ability to activate factor XII, and ability to inactivate factors V and VIII in the coagulation cascade. Plasmin cleaves the fibrin molecule into differentially sized degradation or split products (FDP), the smallest of which is D-dimer, which is used as a marker of venous thromboembolism and disseminated intravascular coagulopathy (DIC).

The plasminogen pathway is complex and tightly regulated.[28] The main proteins involved in its modulation are plasminogen activator inhibitors (PAI)-1 and PAI-2. The activators and inhibitors of plasminogen regulate fibrinolysis upon release from ECs. These activators of the fibrinolytic process are under the control of PAIs, which complex with tPA and uPA to inactivate them and therefore block plasmin generation.

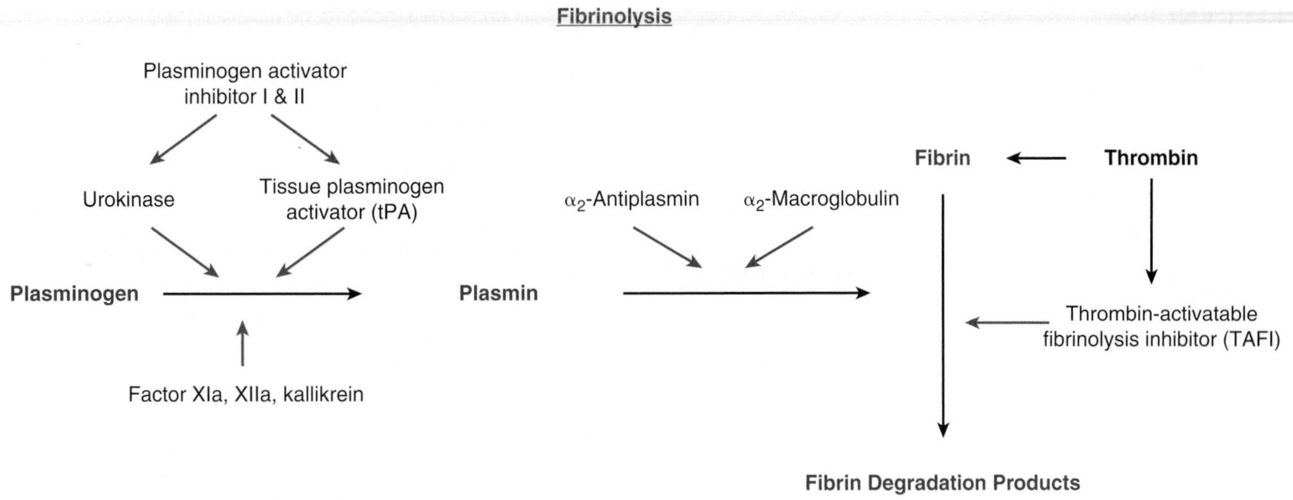

Fibrinolysis

FIGURE 5-2 Pathway of fibrinolysis. Inhibition is signified by red arrows and stimulation is signified by green arrows.

Evidence for why tPA is more important than uPA for normal hemostasis is how ECs up-regulate production of this protein when injured. It is stimulated by a variety of substances, including thrombin, serotonin, bradykinin, cytokines, and epinephrine. This binding affords tPA some protection from degradation and enables it to survive for longer than its expected half-life of only 4 minutes. Its role in hemostasis is of such significance that recombinant tPA (alteplase) and its derivatives that incorporate the kringle domains (e.g., reteplase, tenecteplase) are used as thrombolytic agents in patients with acute thrombotic events, including myocardial infarction.[29]

The other essential plasminogen activator in this process is uPA, which exists in a high-molecular-weight and a low-molecular-weight form, both of which have the ability to activate plasminogen through cleavage at Arg 560/Val 561. Urokinase is present in high concentration in urine. Whereas tPA is mainly important for intravascular fibrinolysis, urokinase has more of a role in the extravascular compartment. Unlike tPA, however, uPA does not bind to fibrin and therefore is not involved in activation of plasminogen incorporated into clots through fibrin binding.[30] As its name implies, uPA is derived from urokinase, which consists of a single-chain precursor molecule termed *scuPA* that is hydrolyzed by plasmin or kallikrein to the two-chain active uPA, which is biologically active.[31] In plasma, scuPA does not activate plasminogen, but in the presence of fibrin, it is actually scuPA that induces clot lysis. Interestingly, the role of urokinase has been expanded to include support of invasion and metastasis in malignancy[32,33]; uPA has been shown to play a role in extracellular matrix degradation, allowing for migration and invasion of metastatic cells. There is now a growing interest in developing targeted therapy that blocks this pathway as a means of controlling metastasis.

Streptokinase does not participate in normal hemostasis but is used as a therapeutic agent for acute thrombosis. It is isolated from β-hemolytic streptococci, and since it is not an enzyme, must complex with plasminogen to form an active molecule which then has the ability to cleave plasminogen to plasmin.[34] Its use as a therapeutic agent, however, is limited; as a foreign substance, it is often recognized by the immune system, and antistreptokinase antibodies are generated.

There are multiple endogenous proteins that can rapidly inhibit the fibrinolytic response. These include PAI-1, α_2-antiplasmin, α_2-antitrypsin, and C1 inhibitor. Most of these inhibitors act through serine protease inhibition (serpin) and therefore affect many aspects of coagulation. The most important of these inhibitors is PAI-1, which is expressed by ECs or platelets after exposure to thrombin; inflammatory mediators such as tumor necrosis factor alpha (TNF-α); and growth factors, lipids, insulin, angiotensin II (ANGII), and endotoxin.[35] Recently the role of PAI-1 as an inhibitor of tissue factor has been postulated to regulate hemostasis in inflammatory conditions such as sepsis or acute lung injury.[36] It has been shown that platelets release PAI-1 as a mechanism of preventing premature clot dissolution. Patients who are deficient in PAI-1 have a bleeding diathesis when confronted with trauma or surgery.

Another important mechanism for regulation of fibrinolysis is thrombin-activatable fibrinolysis inhibitor (TAFI), which is not a member of the serpin family. It is known for its ability to cleave the carboxy-terminal lysine in fibrin, impairing plasminogen binding.[37] Activation of TAFI is dependent upon the thrombin-thrombomodulin complex, which can expedite the inhibitory process in a similar manner to thrombin.[38] This process has recently been shown to be inhibited by platelet factor 4, which is secreted by activated platelets.[39] If the feedback mechanisms of thrombin generation through factors V, VIII, and XI is impaired—leading to diminution of the thrombin-thrombomodulin complex and therefore decreased activation of TAFI—clinical consequences can occur. It has been suggested that in chronic liver disease where coagulation factors are decreased, low amounts of TAFI may account for the low-grade fibrinolysis typically observed.[40] The opposite can also occur, as is seen in patients with the G20210A prothrombin gene mutation in which thrombin generation is increased leading to increased activation of TAFI and an increased thrombotic propensity through a inhibition of fibrinolysis.[41]

Recently it has been shown that there is yet another important mechanism by which to regulate the fibrinolytic process via matrix metalloproteinases (MMPs). Matrix metalloproteinases (including MMP-3, -7, -9, and -12) are found in ECs and have the ability to cleave uPA and plasminogen. The importance of MMPs in down-regulating cellular fibrinolysis remains to be elucidated, but it is clear they function by reducing availability of plasminogen. MMP-3 and -7 also have the ability to degrade fibrinogen and cross-linked fibrin; MMP-11 can degrade fibrinogen but not fibrin. Matrix metalloproteinases also can modulate the activity of many inhibitors of fibrinolysis, including α_2-antiplasmin and PAI-1.[42,43]

Summary

In this chapter, we have described the intricate pathways involved in coagulation and fibrinolysis, with specific emphasis on regulation of hemostasis. Future endeavors focused on understanding the complex nature of these processes and how they relate to human disease processes, including inflammation, malignancy, and arterial and venous thrombotic events, will provide targeted therapies to modulate hemostasis and thrombosis.

74

CH
5

REFERENCES

1. Kunishima S, Kamiya T, Saito H: Genetic abnormalities of Bernard-Soulier syndrome, *Int J Hematol* 76(4):319–327, 2002.
2. Sadler JE: Von Willebrand disease type 1: a diagnosis in search of a disease, *Blood* 101(6):2089–2093, 2003.
3. Offermanns S: Activation of platelet function through G protein-coupled receptors, *Circ Res* 99(12):1293–1304, 2006.
4. Kulkarni S, Dopheide SM, Yap CL, et al: A revised model of platelet aggregation, *J Clin Invest* 105(6):783–791, 2000.
5. Bellucci S, Caen J: Molecular basis of Glanzmann's thrombasthenia and current strategies in treatment, *Blood Rev* 16(3):193–202, 2002.
6. Davi G, Patrono C: Platelet activation and atherothrombosis, *N Engl J Med* 357(24): 2482–2494, 2007.
7. Moncada S: Adventures in vascular biology: a tale of two mediators, *Philos Trans R Soc Lond B Biol Sci* 361(1469):735–759, 2006.
8. Mehta RS: Novel oral anticoagulants. Part II: direct thrombin inhibitors, *Expert Rev Hematol* 3(3):351–361, 2010.
9. Mann KG, Butenas S, Brummel K: The dynamics of thrombin formation, *Arterioscler Thromb Vasc Biol* 23(1):17–25, 2003.
10. Bajaj SP, Joist JH: New insights into how blood clots: implications for the use of APTT and PT as coagulation screening tests and in monitoring of anticoagulant therapy, *Semin Thromb Hemost* 25(4):407–418, 1999.
11. Mandal SK, Pendurthi UR, Rao LV: Cellular localization and trafficking of tissue factor, *Blood* 107(12):4746–4753, 2006.
12. Chen VM, Ahamed J, Versteeg HH, et al: Evidence for activation of tissue factor by an allosteric disulfide bond, *Biochemistry* 45(39):12020–12028, 2006.
13. Kothari H, Nayak RC, Rao LV: Cystine 186-cystine 209 disulfide bond is not essential for the procoagulant activity of tissue factor or for its de-encryption, *Blood* 115(21):4273–4283, 2010.
14. Bach RR, Monroe D: What is wrong with the allosteric disulfide bond hypothesis? *Arterioscler Thromb Vasc Biol* 29(12):1997–1998, 2009.
15. Bogdanov VY, Balasubramanian V, Hathcock J, et al: Alternatively spliced human tissue factor: a circulating, soluble, thrombogenic protein, *Nat Med* 9(4):458–462, 2003.
16. Del Conde I, Shrimpton CN, Thiagarajan P, et al: Tissue-factor-bearing microvesicles arise from lipid rafts and fuse with activated platelets to initiate coagulation, *Blood* 106(5):1604–1611, 2005.
17. Panes O, Matus V, Saez CG, et al: Human platelets synthesize and express functional tissue factor, *Blood* 109(12):5242–5250, 2007.
18. Skidgel RA, Alhenc-Gelas F, Campbell WB: Prologue: kinins and related systems. New life for old discoveries, *Am J Physiol Heart Circ Physiol* 284(6):H1886–H1891, 2003.
19. Horan JT, Francis CW: Fibrin degradation products, fibrin monomer and soluble fibrin in disseminated intravascular coagulation, *Semin Thromb Hemost* 27(6):657–666, 2001.
20. Cochery-Nouvellon E, Mercier E, Lissalde-Lavigne G, et al: Homozygosity for the C46T polymorphism of the F12 gene is a risk factor for venous thrombosis during the first pregnancy, *J Thromb Haemost* 5(4):700–707, 2007.
21. Reuner KH, Jenetzky E, Aleu A, et al: Factor XII C46T gene polymorphism and the risk of cerebral venous thrombosis, *Neurology* 70(2):129–132, 2008.
22. Mosesson MW, Siebenlist KR, Meh DA: The structure and biological features of fibrinogen and fibrin, *Ann N Y Acad Sci* 936:11–30, 2001.
23. Ariens RA, Lai TS, Weisel JW, et al: Role of factor XIII in fibrin clot formation and effects of genetic polymorphisms, *Blood* 100(3):743–754, 2002.
24. Weitz JI: Heparan sulfate: antithrombotic or not? *J Clin Invest* 111(7):952–954, 2003.
25. Patnaik MM, Moll S: Inherited antithrombin deficiency: a review, *Haemophilia* 14(6):1229–1239, 2008.
26. Esmon CT: The protein C pathway, *Chest* 124(3 Suppl):26S–32S, 2003.
27. Miles LA, Castellino FJ, Gong Y: Critical role for conversion of glu-plasminogen to Lys-plasminogen for optimal stimulation of plasminogen activation on cell surfaces, *Trends Cardiovasc Med* 13(1):21–30, 2003.
28. Kolev K, Machovich R: Molecular and cellular modulation of fibrinolysis, *Thromb Haemost* 89(4):610–621, 2003.
29. Kunadian V, Gibson CM: Thrombolytics and myocardial infarction, *Cardiovasc Ther* doi: 10.1111/j.1755-5922.20a0.00239.x. [Epub ahead of print].
30. Rijken DC, Sakharov DV: Basic principles in thrombolysis: regulatory role of plasminogen, *Thromb Res* 103(Suppl 1):S41–S49, 2001.
31. Colman RW: Role of the light chain of high molecular weight kininogen in adhesion, cell-associated proteolysis and angiogenesis, *Biol Chem* 382(1):65–70, 2001.
32. Mekkawy AH, Morris DL, Pourgholami MH: Urokinase plasminogen activator system as a potential target for cancer therapy, *Future Oncol* 5(9):1487–1499, 2009.
33. Hildenbrand R, Allgayer H, Marx A, et al: Modulators of the urokinase-type plasminogen activation system for cancer, *Expert Opin Investig Drugs* 19(5):641–652, 2010.
34. Bell WR: Present-day thrombolytic therapy: therapeutic agents–pharmacokinetics and pharmacodynamics, *Rev Cardiovasc Med* 3(Suppl 2):S34–S44, 2002.
35. Kohler HP, Grant PJ: Plasminogen-activator inhibitor type 1 and coronary artery disease, *N Engl J Med* 342(24):1792–1801, 2000.
36. Sen P, Komissarov AA, Florova G, et al: Plasminogen activator inhibitor-1 inhibits factor VIIa bound to tissue factor, *J Thromb Haemost* 9:531–539, 2010.
37. Zhao L, Buckman B, Seto M, et al: Mutations in the substrate binding site of thrombin-activatable fibrinolysis inhibitor (TAFI) alter its substrate specificity, *J Biol Chem* 278(34):32359–32366, 2003.
38. Mosnier LO, Meijers JC, Bouma BN: Regulation of fibrinolysis in plasma by TAFI and protein C is dependent on the concentration of thrombomodulin, *Thromb Haemost* 85(1):5–11, 2001.
39. Mosnier LO: Platelet factor 4 inhibits thrombomodulin-dependent activation of thrombin-activatable fibrinolysis inhibitor (TAFI) by thrombin, *J Biol Chem* 286:502–510, 2010.
40. Van Thiel DH, George M, Fareed J: Low levels of thrombin activatable fibrinolysis inhibitor (TAFI) in patients with chronic liver disease, *Thromb Haemost* 85(4):667–670, 2001.
41. Colucci M, Binetti BM, Tripodi A, et al: Hyperprothrombinemia associated with prothrombin G20210A mutation inhibits plasma fibrinolysis through a TAFI-mediated mechanism, *Blood* 103(6):2157–2161, 2004.
42. Lijnen HR, Van Hoef B, Collen D: Inactivation of the serpin alpha(2)-antiplasmin by stromelysin-1, *Biochim Biophys Acta* 1547(2):206–213, 2001.
43. Lijnen HR, Arza B, Van Hoef B, et al: Inactivation of plasminogen activator inhibitor-1 by specific proteolysis with stromelysin-1 (MMP-3), *J Biol Chem* 275(48):37645–37650, 2000.

CHAPTER 6

Vascular Pharmacology

David G. Harrison, James M. Luther

Vascular pharmacology has traditionally focused on drugs that modulate vasomotion, and such agents continue to be commonly used for treatment of disorders such as hypertension, myocardial ischemia, vasospasm, cardiovascular shock, and orthostatic hypotension. In the past 2 decades, new drug targets have been recognized, including inflammation, angiogenesis, and thrombosis. In some cases, drugs affect these targets by unexpected off-target effects that are nevertheless pharmacologically important.

Vascular Smooth Muscle Activation

The actions of many drugs discussed in this chapter affect vascular smooth muscle cell (VSMC) contraction, and a basic understanding of contractile regulation is essential to understanding their mechanism of action. Contraction of vascular smooth muscle involves a sliding filament mechanism similar to that observed in other smooth muscle or in skeletal muscle. This topic has been reviewed in depth previously,[1] is covered in detail in Chapter 3, and is therefore only briefly discussed here. The classical paradigm, depicted in Figure 6-1, is that increases in intracellular calcium lead to formation of a calcium-calmodulin complex. Calcium–CaM then binds and activates myosin light chain kinase (MLCK), which then phosphorylates myosin light chain (LC-20). Phosphorylation of LC-20 increases myosin adenosine triphosphatase (ATPase) activity, which leads to cross-bridge cycling and contraction. Myosin light chain phosphatase negatively regulates this process by dephosphorylating LC-20. Myosin light chain phosphatase is in turn inhibited by the small G-protein Rho and Rho kinase, which phosphorylates a subunit of myosin light chain phosphatase known as the *myosin-binding subunit* (MBS), leading to inhibition of phosphatase activity and favoring contraction. Myosin phosphatase is also inhibited by a 17-kDa protein known as *CPI-17* (protein kinase C [PKC]–potentiated inhibitory protein of 17 kDa) that in turn is activated by PKC. Thus, activation of PKC can indirectly reduce myosin phosphatase activity, increase myosin phosphorylation, and promote vasoconstriction.

An important counterregulatory pathway in this scheme is the nitric oxide (NO) pathway. Nitric oxide acts on soluble guanylyl cyclase (sGC), which catalyzes the conversion of guanosine triphosphate (GTP) to cyclic guanosine monophosphate (cGMP). In turn, cGMP acts as the only substrate for type 1 protein kinase G (PKG), which phosphorylates MBS, increasing its phosphatase activity and promoting vasodilation. Protein kinase G also phosphorylates and inhibits Rho, further reducing the propensity for vasoconstriction and promoting vasodilation. These pathways are targets of myriad vasoactive drugs that will be considered in greater depth in this chapter and are depicted in Figure 6-1.

Traditionally, precapillary arterioles with diameters of approximately 25 μm were thought to regulate blood flow. While this is true in some organs such as the kidney, in many organs, vascular resistances are distributed over a wider range of vessel sizes. In the coronary circulation, fully half of this resistance lies in vessels between 100 and 300 μm in diameter, and the remainder exists in vessels smaller than 100 μm and in venules. Interestingly, many vasoactive agents variably affect these different-sized vessels. As an example, organic nitrates act predominantly on the larger arteries and veins and have minimal effect on arterioles. In contrast, adenosine potently dilates resistance vessels and has less effect on larger vessels. Vasopressin is a potent constrictor of resistance arterioles and causes endothelium-dependent vasodilation of conductance arteries. These differential effects cause various drugs and hormones to selectively affect factors such as venous capacitance, large (conductance) vessel diameter, and blood flow in the intact circulation.

It is now apparent that many pharmacological agents not only modulate vascular tone but also vascular growth, remodeling, inflammation, thrombosis, and vascular repair. As examples, many components of the contractile pathway discussed earlier exist in endothelial cells (ECs), including actin, myosin light chain, MLCK, Rho, and Rho kinase. These regulate endothelial shape, migration, cell-cell contact, and permeability. Myosin light chain kinase activation controls EC calcium entry, NO production, and release of endothelium-derived hyperpolarizing factor (EDHF).[2] The Rho/Rho kinase pathway works in concert with other GTPases to modulate endothelial production of NO and reactive oxygen species (ROS) and gene expression.[3] These aspects of vascular control have been the subject of substantial recent research, and new drugs have been developed to affect these targets. In addition, these pathways seem to be affected in an off-target fashion by several existing pharmacological agents.

Pharmacokinetics and Pharmacodynamics

Before discussing specific pharmacological agents, the basic concepts of pharmacology should be reviewed. Drug absorption, distribution, metabolism, and clearance are the principal concepts of *pharmacokinetics*, and these concepts are detailed elsewhere in pharmacology texts. Certain disease states, such as renal insufficiency, liver insufficiency, or heart failure, may have important effects on drug pharmacokinetics within individuals, and relevant situations will be discussed with specific drugs. *Pharmacodynamics* is the study of drug mechanism of action and physiological effects. Because some agents produce persistent effects beyond their clearance from the circulation, a drug with a short half-life can have a longer dosing interval than that predicted by its clearance. For example, aspirin irreversibly inactivates the cyclooxygenase (COX) enzyme and achieves long-lasting platelet inhibition despite rapid clearance from the circulation. Diuretic agents may have a persistent antihypertensive effect after drug cessation, at least until a new level of sodium balance is achieved. Other effects may become evident only after drug withdrawal. For example, β-blockers increase receptor sensitivity as well as circulating catecholamines, and sudden drug withdrawal of their β-blockade can result in rebound hypertension. Therefore, consideration of both pharmacokinetic properties and pharmacodynamic effects is essential for understanding drug action.

The nature of a drug response helps classify the drug as a full or partial agonist, antagonist, or an inverse agonist (Fig. 6-2A) and may provide insight into the mechanism of drug action. For receptor conformation–specific drugs, pure antagonists stabilize the active and inactive conformations equally and have no net effect on basal activity. Inverse agonists preferentially stabilize the receptor's inactive form, and agonists stabilize the active conformation.

The *potency* of a drug refers to the molar concentration necessary to achieve a desired response (e.g., 50% maximal stimulation or inhibition; Fig. 6-2B), whereas *efficacy* reflects the drug's maximal response relative to other agents (Fig. 6-2C). Clinical differences in drug potency may be overcome by increasing the dosage, whereas differences in drug efficacy cannot.

Receptor antagonists can be assessed by the response to a known stimulus in the presence of increasing antagonist concentration (Fig. 6-3). Antagonists that reversibly bind to the receptor can be overcome with increasing concentration of agonist (Fig. 6-3A). Antagonists that irreversibly bind their target impair the maximal response with increasing concentration (Fig. 6-3B). A number of drugs act in an allosteric manner by binding to a site

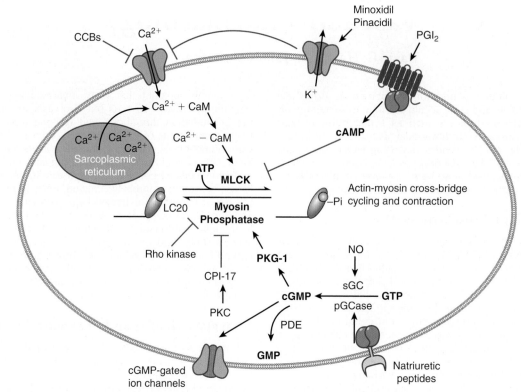

FIGURE 6-1   Vascular smooth muscle contractile regulation. ATP, adenosine triphosphatase; CaM, calmodulin; cAMP, cyclic adenosine monophosphate; CCB, calcium channel blocker; cGMP, cyclic guanosine monophosphate; CPI-17, protein kinase C-potentiated inhibitory protein of 17 kDa; GMP, Guanosine monophosphate; GTP, guanosine triphosphate; MLCK, myosin light chain kinase; NO, nitric oxide; PDE, phosphodiesterase; pGCase, particulate guanylyl cyclase; PGI₂, prostacyclin; PKC, protein kinase C; PKG-1, type 1 protein kinase G; sGC, soluble guanylyl cyclase.

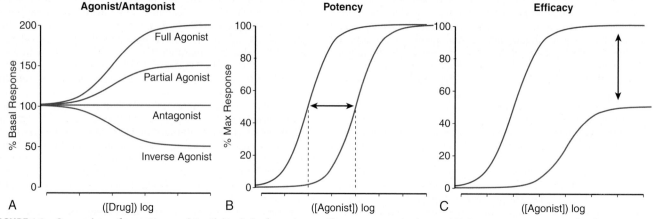

FIGURE 6-2   Comparison of receptor agonist activity. A, Conformation-specific receptor agonists (see text). **B,** Drug potency is compared by the concentration necessary to achieve 50% maximal drug response (EC₅₀). **C,** Drug efficacy is compared by the observed maximal response achieved.

on the receptor that is distinct from the native ligand, inducing a conformational change. Allosteric modulators can either increase or decrease agonist response by binding to a site distinct from the agonist binding site. An allosteric antagonist dose-response curve appears similar to that of a noncompetitive antagonist. Allosteric potentiators shift the agonist curve to the left (see Fig. 6-3A), while competitive antagonists shift the curve to the right.

Drugs That Affect Nitric Oxide/Guanylyl Cyclase/cGMP–Dependent Protein Kinase Pathway

The NO pathway plays a major role in modulating vascular reactivity; however, NO represents only one step in a complex pathway that can be affected by a variety of signaling molecules.

This pathway is illustrated in the right portion of Figure 6-1, and involves the guanylyl cyclase enzymes, cGMP, and the binding targets of cGMP, which include the cGMP-dependent PKGs, ion channels regulated by cGMP, and phosphodiesterases (PDEs). The guanylyl cyclase/cGMP pathway is affected by a variety of agents, including NO and NO donors (the nitrovasodilators); other agents that activate guanylyl cyclase; agents that modulate degradation of cGMP; and agents that directly activate PKG.

Endogenously, NO is produced by the nitric oxide synthase (NOS) enzymes, and serves myriad signaling roles depending on the cell and tissue in which it is produced.[4] Experimental studies have shown that NO produced by the endothelium not only mediates vasodilation, but also inhibits expression of adhesion molecules, reduces platelet adhesion, inhibits vascular smooth muscle growth and hypertrophy, and prevents vascular remodeling.

Competitive Antagonist

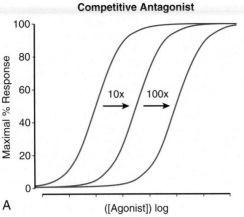

Non-Competitive Antagonist

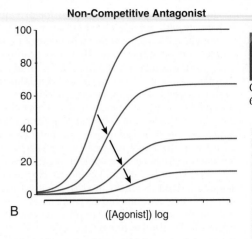

FIGURE 6-3 Receptor antagonism. A, With increasing concentration of a competitive antagonist, the agonist dose response curve is shifted to the right. Allosteric potentiators produce a left shift of this curve. **B,** Noncompetitive antagonists and allosteric antagonists shift the agonist response curve to the right and impair maximal response in a nonlinear manner.

Guanylyl cyclases convert GTP to cGMP. When first discovered, this enzymatic activity was found in both the particulate or membrane fractions and in the soluble or cytoplasmic fractions of cell homogenates. Shortly after this first discovery, it was recognized that the soluble enzyme was activated by sodium azide, sodium nitroprusside, and nitroglycerin in a heme-dependent fashion. It has subsequently been confirmed that NO allosterically binds a prosthetic heme group in sGC, which in turn alters enzyme conformation and activates the enzyme. Removal of the heme group eliminates the ability of NO to stimulate enzyme activity. Ten years later, the particulate form was found to be activated not by NO-like compounds but by atrial natriuretic peptide (ANP), and that the particulate forms are in fact receptors for the natriuretic peptides. Thus, NO donors and the natriuretic peptides share common downstream signaling pathways, albeit via activation of different upstream enzymes.

Nitrovasodilators

The nitrovasodilators produce their biological effects either by releasing NO or closely related molecules that are converted to NO in cells. The most commonly employed nitrovasodilators are the organic nitrates and sodium nitroprusside. It is useful to begin a discussion of these agents by comparing sodium nitroprusside and nitroglycerin, which are illustrated in Figure 6-4. As apparent, the oxidation state of the nitrogen that is ultimately released as NO differs in these molecules, and this basic structural property provides insight into their pharmacological profiles. Sodium nitroprusside requires a one-electron reduction to release NO, and this is readily accomplished nonenzymatically by a variety of reductants in the circulation, the interstitial space, and the cell. Thus, when infused intravenously, nitroprusside begins to release NO throughout the circulation and potently dilates all vessels. Moreover, given

the short half-life of NO, the vasodilation caused by nitroprusside is short-lived once its infusion is discontinued.

As is apparent from its structure, nitroprusside possesses five cyanide groups in each molecule (highlighted in red in Fig. 6-4), and prior studies have shown that each of these is reduced prior to the release of NO. The cyanide radicals react with hemoglobin (Hb) to form methemoglobin and are converted to thiocyanate in the liver. When these metabolic pathways are depleted, cyanide toxicity occurs, characterized by central nervous system (CNS) dysfunction, metabolic acidosis with a base deficit, and elevated plasma lactic acid concentrations.[5] Fortunately, cyanide toxicity is infrequent during brief administration of sodium nitroprusside but occurs more commonly when infusion rates exceed 2 µg/kg/min and when the drug is infused for prolonged periods. In addition, the risk of cyanide toxicity is increased in patients with renal or hepatic failure, so sodium nitroprusside should be avoided in patients with these conditions. Owing to its capacity to rapidly release NO, sodium nitroprusside produces potent systemic vasodilation and is effective as an antihypertensive. It is still used for treatment of severe hypertension and, in some cases, for afterload reduction in patients with severe heart failure; however, newer agents with less potential toxicity are now more commonly used.

In contrast to sodium nitroprusside, nitroglycerin and other organic nitrates require a 3-electron reduction to yield NO. In the last several years, it has become clear that this is in large part accomplished by the action of the mitochondrial enzyme aldehyde reductase-2 (ADH2).[6] Mice lacking this enzyme are resistant to the actions of nitroglycerin. Notably, about 40% of East Asians have a dominant negative mutation of ADH2 that causes intolerance to ethanol and markedly impaired vasodilator responses to nitroglycerin.[7]

As mentioned earlier, organic nitrates preferentially dilate larger arteries and veins while having less effect on arterioles, particularly at lower doses.[8] This response profile is likely beneficial in alleviating angina because potent arteriolar dilators are prone to cause coronary steal and paradoxically worsen myocardial ischemia. Moreover, venous dilatation reduces left ventricular (LV) filling, alleviates pulmonary congestion, and can improve subendocardial perfusion in ischemic regions of the myocardium.

Traditionally, organic nitrates have been employed to either alleviate or prevent the chest pain associated with myocardial ischemia. For acute angina, nitroglycerin is administered either as a sublingual tablet or an oral spray. For prevention of angina, long-acting nitroglycerin preparations or related organic nitrates (e.g., isosorbide mononitrate, isosorbide dinitrate, pentaerythritol tetranitrate, transdermal nitrates) are commonly employed. Nitroglycerin is often administered intravenously for treatment of acute coronary syndromes (ACS).

Experimental studies have shown that NO inhibits platelet adhesion, expression of adhesion molecules, and vascular smooth muscle proliferation and migration. Thus, one might expect that NO donors such as nitroglycerin would reduce atherosclerosis

FIGURE 6-4 Nitrovasodilator agents. Structure of nitric oxide (NO) donor agents. The nitroprusside cyanide ligands (C≡N) are highlighted in red.

Nitroglycerin   Nitroprusside   Molsidomine

progression and potentially reduce major cardiovascular events in patients with coronary artery disease (CAD). Despite extensive use for alleviation of myocardial ischemia for almost a century and a half, no clinical trials have shown that these drugs reduce ischemic cardiovascular events. The GISSI-3 and ISIS-4 trials examined the effect of nitrates following myocardial infarction (MI) but failed to show a significant improvement in outcome.[9,10] These trials only observed patients for 5 weeks to 6 months following MI, and therefore did not determine whether long-term nitrates might have a beneficial effect on outcome in patients with ischemic heart disease. Given the many putative beneficial effects of NO on vascular function, longer-term treatment might impart a beneficial effect on atherosclerosis, inflammation, vascular remodeling, or plaque stability. Indeed, a recent analysis of the GRACE registry, which includes patients admitted for ACS, showed that chronic nitrate users were much more likely to present with non–ST-segment elevation MI NSTEMI) than non-nitrate users.[11] These data must be interpreted with caution because the use of nitrates was not randomized, and conclusions were derived from a retrospective analysis.

In addition to their use as antianginal agents, the long-acting nitrates are now often employed for treatment of congestive heart failure (CHF), commonly in combination with hydralazine. Unlike the case for treatment of CAD, prospective randomized trials have shown that long-acting nitrates improve survival, reduce hospitalizations, and enhance quality of life in patients with CHF, particularly among African Americans.[12] Precise mechanisms underlying the beneficial effects are unclear; however, long-acting nitrates appear to synergize with hydralazine as afterload- and preload-reducing agents. These agents might also improve renal hemodynamics and promote diuresis and, via release of NO, have beneficial effects on vascular and cardiac remodeling.

A major limitation to prolonged use of organic nitrates is development of tolerance. Within about 12 hours of administration, the hemodynamic effects of organic nitrates begin to abate, in part due to extravascular adaptations such as volume redistribution and neurohormonal activation. After several days of continuous nitrate therapy, the direct vascular actions of nitrates are lost, even when vessels are removed from the animal or human. The mechanisms of nitrate tolerance, and in particular this latter form of true vascular tolerance, remain uncertain but have been attributed to formation of ROS, nitrosation and oxidation of guanylyl cyclase, and changes in activity of ADH2.[13] A number of strategies have been proposed to prevent nitrate tolerance, but the only approach accepted clinically is to allow a drug "holiday"; that is, to withdraw the nitrate for about 12 hours daily. The commonly employed isosorbide mononitrate preparations accomplish this by increasing blood levels of the drug for about 12 hours during waking hours, after which blood levels fall to near-undetectable levels. Experimental studies have shown that hydralazine prevents nitrate tolerance by reducing oxidative stress,[13] which might explain the benefit of hydralazine when added to long-acting nitrates in the treatment of heart failure. The long-acting nitrate pentaerythritol tetranitrate seems not to cause tolerance in experimental animals, but this has not been proven in clinical studies.

Intravenous nitroglycerin has occasionally been used for treatment of hypertensive emergencies. This condition is often associated with a contracted blood volume. Owing to nitroglycerin's propensity to produce venular dilation rather than arteriolar dilation, it has the potential to reduce cardiac output in this setting and may produce untoward effects in patients with compromised coronary, renal, or cerebral perfusion.[14] Low-dose nitroglycerin might be useful in combination with other agents in treating a hypertensive emergency, particularly in patients with acute pulmonary edema, but other agents are available and likely more effective.

In addition to its reaction with sGC, NO can react with other heme proteins and radicals. Higher oxides of NO can also react with thiols, leading to formation of nitrosothiols.[15] An important example of these reactions is the reversible NO reaction with cytochrome C, which modulates mitochondrial respiration and superoxide production.[16] It is uncertain as to how important these reactions are in the overall response to nitrovasodilators.

Related to the chemistry mentioned earlier are reactions of inorganic nitrate (NO_3^-) and nitrite (NO_2^-). Although these are oxidation products of endogenously produced NO, they are also derived from dietary sources such as green leafy vegetables. Nitrate is rapidly converted to nitrite by bacteria in the oral cavity and gastrointestinal tract. Nitrite, in turn, can be reduced by various heme proteins, including deoxyhemoglobin, to NO. Studies have shown that the reaction of nitrite with deoxyhemoglobin promotes NO formation and vasodilation in regions of the circulation where oxygen tension is low, thereby improving oxygenation of hypoxic tissues.[17] Thus, once considered an inactive metabolite of NO, nitrite likely has physiological significance and might have therapeutic utility.[18]

Molsidomine (see Fig. 6-4) has also been used as an NO donor for treatment of angina, but it is not commonly employed clinically. The liver metabolizes molsidomine to release SIN-1, which in turn decomposes to NO and superoxide in equimolar amounts. These species can react rapidly with one another to yield the strong oxidant peroxynitrite. Because of this chemistry, SIN-1 oxidizes lipoproteins, damages DNA, and depletes antioxidants. This capacity to generate peroxynitrite has dampened enthusiasm for clinical use of molsidomine and related drugs, but SIN-1 is commonly used to produce peroxynitrite in experimental settings.

There are other agents used experimentally as NO donors. Two classes that deserve mention are the S-nitrosothiols (SNOs) and the NONOates. S-nitrosothiols can be formed either by reactions of thiols with higher oxides of NO or by the reaction of NO with thiyl radicals. There is substantial evidence that SNOs are found in vivo, where they serve as reservoirs for NO, and that the attachment of NO to thiols in proteins affects protein function. As an example, S-nitrosylation of Hb has been implicated in oxygen affinity and delivery. S-nitrosothiols are simple to synthesize and, depending on the thiol backbone, have different stabilities such that they can release NO in times ranging from seconds to minutes. S-nitrosothiols can also undergo heterolytic scission, yielding the nitrosonium cation (NO^+), which acts as a nitrosating agent to form various nitroso compounds. The NONOates are commercially available nucleophilic/NO complexes often used experimentally as NO donors. These release only NO and are very useful because their varying structures permit controlled NO delivery over widely varying times, ranging from seconds to hours. Neither SNOs nor NONOates are clinically used at present.

Unique Modulators of Soluble Guanylyl Cyclase

Soluble guanylyl cyclase contains a heme group that is responsible for binding and activation by NO. Agents such as 1H-[1,2,4] oxadiazolo[4,3-a]quinoxalin-1 (ODQ), ferricyanide, or methylene blue can inactivate sGC by oxidizing the heme group. Owing to this enzymology, ODQ and methylene blue have been used as pharmacological probes to prove that a biological response is dependent on guanylyl cyclase. In a similar vein, oxidation of the heme group by superoxide or hydrogen peroxide might alter NO-dependent enzyme activity and therefore impair endothelium-dependent vasodilation under conditions where endogenous production of ROS is increased. Thus, in addition to oxidative inactivation of NO, superoxide and related oxidants can impair NO function by inactivating sGC.

Compounds have been developed that activate sGC in an NO-independent fashion.[19] Some of these, such as the pyrazolopyridine BAY 41-2272 and YC-1, interact with the heme group independent of NO, or can markedly enhance NO-stimulated enzyme activity. Others, such as BAY 58-2667 and HMR-1766, activate sGC in a heme-independent fashion and can stimulate cGMP formation even when the heme group is oxidized. Because these agents do not depend on endogenous production of NO, they have potential advantages over PDE inhibitors (see later discussion) in diseases where NO production is impaired. They also potentially bypass the problem of tolerance observed with various NO donors. These agents produce vasodilation, lower blood pressure, inhibit platelet aggregation, and have been shown to have therapeutic benefit in experimental models of systemic hypertension, pulmonary hypertension (PH), and heart failure.[19] Like NO, they inhibit neointima formation following balloon injury in rats and therefore might be effective in treatment or prevention of restenosis and atherosclerosis. They also hold promise for treatment of erectile dysfunction (ED), liver fibrosis, and renal disease. Currently, clinical trials are underway to examine the efficacy of some of these agents in the treatment of heart failure and PH.

Natriuretic Peptides

Natriuretic peptides, including atrial (ANP), brain (BNP), and C-type (CNP) natriuretic peptides, are 17-amino-acid ring structures with an internal disulfide bond and are secreted as prohormones. Atrial natriuretic peptide and BNP are predominantly produced by atrial and ventricular myocytes; CNP is produced by vascular endothelial cells, the brain, and other peripheral tissues.[20] Urodilatin, a related peptide processed from the ANP prohormone, is released from distal tubular cells of the kidney.[21] The A and B natriuretic peptide receptors are homodimers that are widely distributed, particularly in the cardiovascular system and kidney.[21] The cytoplasmic tails of these contain a guanylyl cyclase domain that is activated by binding with natriuretic peptides.[20] There also exists a C-type natriuretic receptor that has a short cytoplasmic tail without a guanylyl cyclase domain and seems predominantly involved in clearing natriuretic peptides from the circulation.

As mentioned, ANP and BNP are produced predominantly in atrial myocytes. In the setting of a variety of conditions (e.g., heart failure, cardiac inflammation, fibrosis, hypoxia), BNP is expressed in large amounts by ventricular myocytes, leading to an elevation of circulating BNP. Thus, BNP and pro-BNP are commonly used as biomarkers for detection of various cardiac pathologies, and in particular for diagnosis and management of volume overload states.[22]

Activation of the A- and B-type natriuretic receptors leads to vasodilation and a variable diuretic and natriuretic response, depending on volume status. For this reason, a synthetic form of BNP known as *nesiritide* has been marketed and employed for treatment of decompensated heart failure. Like the nitrovasodilators, nesiritide infusion lowers pulmonary capillary wedge pressure (PCWP), right atrial pressure, and systemic vascular resistance, and improves symptoms of dyspnea.[23] This agent also lowers circulating catecholamines, aldosterone, and angiotensin-(Ang) II levels, and aids diuresis. One study suggested that nesiritide was more effective than intravenous nitroglycerin treatment of patients with severe heart failure.[23] An early meta-analyses suggested that nesiritide therapy was associated with an increase in mortality within 30 days of treatment, for uncertain reasons[24]; however, more recent meta-analysis of six randomized clinical trials showed no change in outcome at 10, 30, or 180 days following administration of this agent.[25] A randomized trial of more than 7000 subjects has shown that treatment with nesiritide acutely improves patients with class IV heart failure, without worsening long-term outcome.[26] This positive study is tempered by a very recent large study of 7143 patients with acute heart failure that showed no benefit of nesiritide in reducing symptoms or improving outcome at 30 days.[27]

Phosphodiesterase Inhibitors

As reflected in Figure 6-1, cGMP is rapidly inactivated to GMP by cellular PDEs. There are 11 PDE isoenzymes with varying specificities for the different cyclic nucleotides. Phosphodiesterases 5, 6, and 9 are highly selective for cGMP, while PDEs 3 and 10 are preferentially activated by cyclic adenosine monophosphate (cAMP). Phosphodiesterases 1, 2, and 11 have dual substrate specificity.[28] In the cardiovascular system, the predominant PDEs are PDE1, 2, and 5. The PDEs are subject to substantial posttranslational regulation. As examples, PDE1 is calcium/CaM-dependent, cGMP stimulates PDE2 inactivation of cAMP, and binding of cAMP to PDE3 is inhibited by cGMP.

Several naturally occurring PDE inhibitors, such as caffeine, theophylline, and theobromines, are present in coffee, chocolates, and tea, and have been used since antiquity as stimulants.[29] These are among the most widely distributed drugs in the world. Like cAMP and cGMP, the PDE inhibitors commonly contain a purine structure with linked pyrimidine and imidazole rings. These agents occupy the cAMP or cGMP PDE binding sites and inhibit respective PDE isoenzymes with varying degrees of selectivity.[29] The immediate cardiovascular effects of nonselective PDE inhibition include vasodilation due to accumulation of cGMP and cAMP, increases in cardiac contractility due to accumulation of cAMP, and improvement in diastolic relaxation (lusitrophy) mediated by cAMP and cGMP.

In the past 30 years, a variety of PDE5 inhibitors, including sildenafil, tadalafil, and vardenafil, have been developed and are now used clinically (Table 6-1). Experimental studies have shown that the vasodilator effect of PDE5 inhibitors is almost exclusively dependent on endogenous NO release, and is prevented by inhibition of NOS and in conditions in which endogenous NO production is impaired.[28] These agents also affect cardiac function. The PDE5 inhibitors acutely reduce cardiac contractility and precondition cardiac myocytes to reduce necrosis and apoptosis caused by experimental ischemia.[30,31] Chronic PDE5 inhibition with sildenafil prevents experimental cardiac hypertrophy caused by transaortic constriction.[32]

The PDE5 inhibitors were developed as antihypertensive agents, but because of their potent effect on the corpus cavernosa, they were initially approved and have become widely employed for treatment of erectile dysfunction. These agents are also potent dilators of the pulmonary circulation. Sildenafil and tadalafil been approved by the U.S. Food and Drug Administration (FDA) for treatment of pulmonary arterial hypertension (PAH). This disorder, defined by the hemodynamic parameters of a mean pulmonary artery pressure (PAP) above 25 mmHg and a PCWP 15 mmHg or lower, occurs as a primary condition and in the setting of a variety of diseases that affect the pulmonary circulation.[33] (Also see Chapters 56 and 57.) A single dose of sildenafil was found to reduce PAP in patients with both primary and secondary PH and to augment the effect of inhaled NO in these subjects.[34] Clinical studies have shown that chronic administration of PDE5 inhibitors reduces PAP and right ventricular (RV) mass, and improves exercise tolerance and functional status in patients with PAH.[35] The recent SUPER-2 clinical trial showed that sildenafil improved 3-year survival in patients with PAH compared to historical controls.[36] For these reasons, PDE5 inhibitors are now considered a mainstay of therapy for PAH. They have also been

	DRUG	$T_{1/2}$	DOSE	DOSE RANGE	DOSING INTERVAL
CLASS	(TRADE NAME)	(HOURS)	ADJUSTMENT	(TOTAL mg/DAY)	(HOURS)
PDE5 inhibitor	Sildenafil (Viagra)	4	L, R	25-100	24
	Tadalafil (Cialis)	17.5	L, R	2.5-20	24
	Vardenafil (Levitra)	4-5	L	10-20	24

TABLE 6-1 Phosphodiesterase-5 Inhibitors

L, liver failure; PDE5, phosphodiesterase type 5; R, renal failure; $T_{1/2}$, half-life.

used with some success in neonates with persistent pulmonary hypertension of the newborn (PPHN).[37]

Phosphodiesterase type 5 inhibition has beneficial effects on hemodynamics and cardiac function in heart failure. In various experimental models of heart failure, PDE inhibitors prevent and reverse cardiac hypertrophy, reduce remodeling, and decrease myocardial fibrosis.[38,39] In a recent placebo-controlled clinical trial of patients with severe heart failure, sildenafil treatment for 1 year improved ejection fraction, improved parameters of diastolic function, and reduced left atrial size while improving functional capacity and clinical status.[40] This study was not designed to determine whether sildenafil improves survival; larger studies are needed with longer-term follow-up to discern whether PDE5 inhibition provides survival benefit. Nevertheless, these orally available agents, which avoid the problem of tolerance encountered with the nitrovasodilators, have substantial promise in treating ventricular dysfunction.

Prostaglandins and Thromboxane Agonists and Antagonists

Release of lipids from the cell membrane upon receptor binding or mechanical stimulation is a major signaling event in mammalian cells. One major class of lipid metabolites is the prostanoids, which include the prostaglandins (PGs) and thromboxane. The pathway leading to formation of these lipids is illustrated in Figure 6-5. They are formed from arachidonic acid, released from membrane phospholipids via the action of phospholipase A_2. The initial step in prostanoid synthesis is conversion of arachidonic acid to the endoperoxide prostaglandin H_2 (PGH_2) by COX

enzymes. Prostaglandin H_2 is in turn a substrate for several enzymes including various PG synthases and thromboxane synthases (see Fig. 6-5), which leads to formation of multiple PG metabolites including PGE_2, prostacyclin (PGI_2), $PGF_{2\alpha}$, PGD_2, and thromboxane A_2 TxA_2. Each of these has several G protein–linked receptors that are widely distributed and modulate myriad physiological and pathophysiological responses that include inflammation, vasomotor tone, hemostasis, renal function, and blood pressure.[41,42] Vascular response to the various prostanoids depends on the category of the heterotrimeric G-protein receptor to which it binds. Vasodilator prostanoids, including PGI_2 and PGD_2, activate G_s, which leads to an increase in intracellular cAMP. The contractile prostanoids, including TxA_2 and $PGF_{2\alpha}$, activate G_q, which leads to increased intracellular calcium. There are both G_s and G_q receptors for PGE_2, which can therefore both vasodilate and vasoconstrict.

There are two isoforms of the COX enzymes: COX-1 and COX-2. Cyclooxygenase-1 is constitutively expressed and exerts housekeeping functions in many cells, including vascular cells. Cyclooxygenase-2 is generally considered an inducible enzyme, and its levels increase in the settings of inflammation, in particular when inflammatory cells enter the affected tissue.[42] Cyclooxygenase-2 is also constitutively expressed in some cells, including ECs. The preferred substrate of COX-1 is arachidonic acid, but COX-2 can also produce unique antiinflammatory products from the endogenous cannabinoid 2-arachidonyl glycerol.[43] Both COX-1 and COX-2 are activated by shear stress in the endothelium.[44] The downstream products of COX are highly dependent on the cell type. In healthy blood vessels, the predominant arachidonic acid metabolite is PGI_2, whereas platelets predominantly produce TxA_2. In a variety

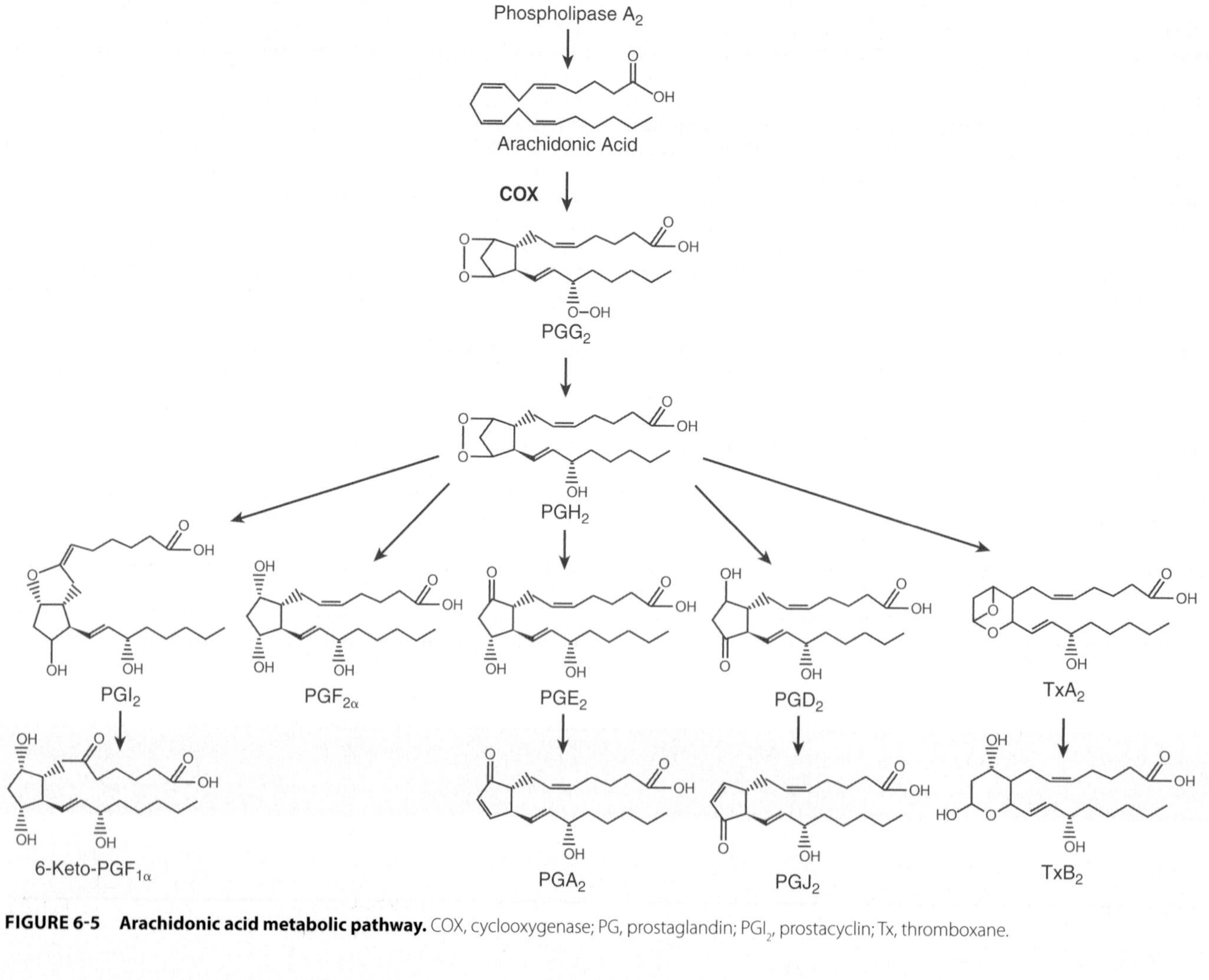

FIGURE 6-5 **Arachidonic acid metabolic pathway.** COX, cyclooxygenase; PG, prostaglandin; PGI_2, prostacyclin; Tx, thromboxane.

of common cardiovascular diseases, however, vascular production of prostanoids can be shifted toward proinflammatory, procoagulant, and vasoconstrictor prostanoids.[44] As an example, Ang-II stimulates COX-2 expression and production of PGE_2 in VSMCs, and this response contributes to VSMC proliferation and migration in response to this hormone.[45] In several experimental models of hypertension, obesity, and aging, the endothelium begins to produce prostanoid-contracting factors including PGH_2, TxA_2, and ROS generated as byproducts of COX activity.[46]

Cyclooxygenase Inhibitors

Cyclooxygenase inhibitors have been used since antiquity to alleviate pain and fever. Salicylic acid was purified from willow bark in the 18th and 19th centuries and was further modified to acetylsalicylic acid (ASA) in 1897. A large number of nonsteroidal antiinflammatory drugs (NSAIDs) have been developed to specifically inhibit COX enzymes, and together with ASA are the most commonly used drugs in the world. Drugs that specifically inhibit COX-2 were subsequently developed. These were intended to reduce gastrointestinal side effects and block inflammation caused by COX-2, although as mentioned later, they have unexpected and untoward effects that have reduced their popularity.

Aspirin has been studied extensively since the 1950s as a means of reducing cardiovascular events.[47] Numerous large clinical trials performed in the 1980s supported the concept that aspirin decreases the occurrence of MI and stroke. A recent large metaanalysis showed that aspirin was effective in both primary and secondary prevention of total coronary events, ischemic stroke, and serious vascular events, with the greatest benefit observed in the case of secondary prevention.[48] Another recent meta-analysis of nine trials that included 90,000 patients showed that aspirin is effective for primary prevention of nonfatal MI and total cardiovascular events, but not for stroke, cardiovascular mortality, or all-cause mortality.[49] Of interest, several recent meta-analyses have suggested that aspirin might not be useful for primary prevention of events in the diabetic population.[50,51]

The beneficial effects of aspirin are generally considered a consequence of its antiplatelet effects and reduction of thrombosis. However, aspirin reduces levels of C-reactive protein (CRP) in patients with recent unstable coronary syndromes,[52] and in experimental models of atherosclerosis, reduces atheroma burden, decreases inflammation, and improves endothelial function,[53,54] suggesting that it might also have direct vascular effects.

Although aspirin has proven effective in reducing cardiovascular events, there are no clinical trials showing that other COX inhibitors convey similar cardiovascular benefit, and paradoxically, there is substantial evidence that these agents are harmful. The most striking example is that of the COX-2 inhibitor rofecoxib, which was withdrawn from the market because of increased thrombotic events[55]; however, other COX inhibitors might also increase cardiovascular risk, depending upon the relative COX-2–to–COX-1 selectivity.[56,57] The precise mechanisms underlying this increased risk remain undefined, and it is unclear why aspirin, which inhibits the same enzyme, albeit via different mechanisms, is beneficial. These differences might relate to inhibition of vascular PGI_2 and perhaps renal COX, which in turn could promote sodium retention and blood pressure elevation and worsen cardiovascular outcome. As previously mentioned, the downstream products and their receptors are myriad, so the in vivo actions of these agents are complex and difficult to predict. Nevertheless, NSAIDs other than aspirin should be used sparingly in patients with known cardiovascular diseases and currently have no role in preventing cardiovascular events.

Prostacyclin Analogs as Therapeutic Agents

Given its potent vasodilator effects, there is enormous interest in therapeutic use of PGI_2 and its analogs. Several preparations have been developed. The most commonly employed are epoprostenol,

a freeze-dried synthetic preparation of PGI_2, and the PGI_2 analogs iloprost, treprostinil, and beraprost. These agents have become a mainstay of treatment for PAH. Epoprostenol was initially approved for treatment of PAH following a 12-week trial in 81 patients prospectively randomized to either epoprostenol or conventional therapy.[58] Among those treated with epoprostenol, there was improvement in exercise capacity and a decline in PAP. This was in contrast to those receiving conventional therapy, in whom walk time decreased and PAP increased. Patients treated with epoprostenol had greater symptomatic improvement, and most strikingly in this small study, eight patients died, all in the conventional therapy group. A second study showed that epoprostenol improved exercise duration and lowered PAP in patients with PH associated with scleroderma.[59] Interestingly, these subjects showed a trend toward improvement of digital ulcers, suggesting that systemic vasodilation caused by this drug might also be beneficial. Subsequent long-term follow-up in large registries have confirmed a beneficial effect of continuous intravenous epoprostenol in PAH.

A downside of epoprostenol therapy is that it requires chronic central line placement, which is accompanied by risk of infection that might be related in part to prostanoid-mediated immunosuppression. The drug also often requires up-titration to overcome tachyphylaxis and is expensive.[60] Owing to its short half-life, there is rebound PH that develops shortly after discontinuing the drug, which can have serious consequences. Common side effects include headaches, occasional cases of thyrotoxicosis, nausea, jaw pain, thrombocytopenia (in up to 34% of patients), flushing, skin rash, anorexia, arthralgias, and myalgias.

For the reasons mentioned, PGI_2 analogs (i.e., iloprost, treprostinil, beraprost) have been developed. These have longer half-lives and can be given intravenously, subcutaneously, via nebulizer, and in some cases orally. Numerous studies have shown that these improve exercise tolerance and quality of life, either alone or in combination with endothelin blockade and PDE5 inhibitors in patients with PAH. The subcutaneous and, intravenous forms of administration are frequently complicated by local pain, induration, and inflammation at injection sites. Inhaled forms avoid these complications but require frequent administration. Despite their limitations, these agents improve hemodynamics, increase exercise tolerance, and enhance quality of life.

Although these agents are potent vasodilators and have the potential to reduce pulmonary vascular resistance (PVR), it is actually unclear as to how they impart therapeutic benefit. Hemodynamic studies have shown that the decrease in pulmonary pressure following inhalation therapy is brief and unlikely to account for sustained benefit. Moreover, the pulmonary vasculature in these patients is often extensively occluded, questioning the potential benefit of vasodilation. These agents enhance RV performance, and they might decrease fibrosis and thrombosis within the pulmonary vasculature.

There is also lack of consensus on how to use these agents, which agents to use, and what dosing regimen is optimal.[48] As discussed elsewhere in this chapter, these agents are often used in conjunction with PDE5 inhibitors and endothelin-1 (ET-1) receptor antagonists, again without uniformity across various centers.

Sympathetic and Parasympathetic Nervous Systems

Abrupt changes in blood pressure are buffered by the sympathetic and parasympathetic nervous system (Fig. 6-6). The baroreflex response helps integrate blood pressure detection and CNS response, and impairment of this response produces profound orthostatic intolerance and inability to maintain upright posture.[61] Increased blood pressure stimulates baroreceptors located in the carotid sinus and aortic arch, which transmit their signals to the nucleus tractus solitarius in the CNS. The transmitted signal inhibits sympathetic outflow from the rostral ventrolateral medulla (RVLM). Sympathetic efferent preganglionic axons extend to the

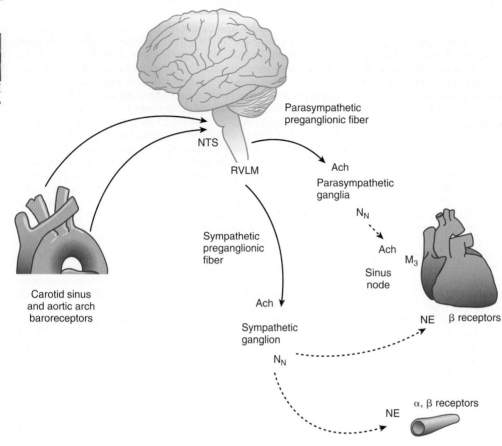

FIGURE 6-6 Baroreceptors and the autonomic nervous system. Ach, acetylcholine; M₃, muscarinic acetylcholine receptor; NE, norepinephrine; N_N neuronal nicotinic acetylcholine receptor; NTS, nucleus tractus solitarius; RVLM, rostral ventrolateral medulla.

sympathetic ganglion, where acetylcholine serves as the principal neurotransmitter to postganglionic nicotinic receptors. Postganglionic sympathetic fibers extend to effector organs such as the heart and vasculature and release norepinephrine (NE) to produce vasoconstriction and increased contractility. The adrenal medulla is innervated directly by preganglionic sympathetic neurons and releases both NE and epinephrine into the circulation. At the same time, the reflex activates parasympathetic system and reduces heart rate via innervation of the cardiac conduction system. Therefore, the net effect of an abrupt increase in blood pressure is inhibition of the sympathetic system and activation of the parasympathetic nervous system.

Vascular Parasympathetic System

Postganglionic parasympathetic fibers release acetylcholine, which stimulates muscarinic and nicotinic receptors. Most blood vessels lack parasympathetic innervation, although some notable exceptions exist (e.g., coronary arteries), and the physiological role of endogenous acetylcholine in vasodilation is uncertain.[62] The vasculature does contain muscarinic receptors and responds to exogenously administered acetylcholine or mimetics (e.g., methacholine). Exogenous acetylcholine dilates blood vessels by its actions on the vascular endothelium, but it produces vasoconstriction if the endothelial layer is injured or removed. This discovery demonstrated the importance of the endothelium as an active participant in vascular reactivity and eventually led to the discovery of endothelium-derived relaxing factors (e.g., NO, PGI₂[63]). Patients with cardiovascular disease exhibit an impaired vasodilatory response to acetylcholine (endothelial dysfunction) but often have a normal response to direct vasodilators such as nitroprusside. Impaired vascular reactivity in both the coronary and forearm vasculature predicts future cardiovascular events,[64,65] and the endothelium-dependent response may be improved with drug therapy, exercise, or risk factor modification (e.g., smoking cessation).[66–68]

Acetylcholine receptors (AchRs) are classified by their ability to respond to either muscarine (M₁-M₅) or nicotine (nAchR). Muscarinic receptors are classic G protein–coupled receptors (GPCRs), coupled to G_i, which inhibits cAMP production. Nicotinic AchRs are ligand-gated voltage channels. Vascular M₁, M₂, and M₃ receptors have been described and produce vasodilation via endothelial, or vasoconstriction via VSMC, receptors[69] (Table 6-2). Acetylcholine is a nonselective agonist; there are no clinically available subtype-selective agents, although a number of investigational drugs exist. Methacholine is frequently used in clinical research because of its longer half-life and stability. Atropine is a nonselective muscarinic antagonist used mainly to increase heart rate by its effects on cardiac M₂ and M₃ receptors. Muscarinic receptors are also located on postsynaptic sympathetic nerve terminals and inhibit NE release. Peripheral neuronal nicotinic AchRs (N_N) transmit sympathetic impulses in autonomic ganglia and adrenal medulla to stimulate NE and epinephrine release. Trimethaphan inhibits N_N and was one of the earliest antihypertensive agents available, although it is no longer used, owing to resulting severe autonomic impairment and intolerable side effects.

Adrenergic Receptors and Agonist Selectivity

Sympathetic postganglionic neurons richly innervate the vasculature and release NE, whereas the adrenal medulla secretes epinephrine in addition to NE. These catecholamines activate adrenergic receptors, which are classic seven-transmembrane receptors coupled to G proteins. They are further classified as either α (α₁ and α₂) or β receptors (β₁, β₂, and β₃). α-Receptor subtypes have also been identified (α_{1A}, α_{1B}, α_{1D}, α_{2A}, α_{2B}, and α_{2C}), although no subtype-specific antagonists are available. Their physiological effects have been determined in part by the study of receptor knockout models.[70,71] In general, α₁ is coupled to G_q (stimulation of phospholipase C/D/A₂), α₂ to G_i (inhibition of adenylate cyclase), and β-receptors to G_s (stimulation of adenylate cyclase).

TABLE 6-2 Vascular Adrenergic and Muscarinic Receptor Actions

RECEPTOR	TISSUE	ACTION	AGONIST	ANTAGONIST
α_1	VSMC	Vasoconstriction	Phenylephrine Methoxamine Midodrine Amphetamine	Phenoxybenzamine Phentolamine Tolazoline α-Blockers Vasodilator β- blockers
α_{2A}	Sympathetic nerve terminal	Inhibition of NE release	Clonidine α-Methyldopa Dexmedetomidine Guanabenz Guanfacine Tizanidine	Phentolamine Tolazoline Phenoxybenzamine Yohimbine Rauwolfia alkaloids Piperazine
α_{2B}	VSMC Placental vasculature	Vasoconstriction Placental angiogenesis	Oxymetazoline Etomidate	
α_{2C}	VSMC Adrenal medulla	Vasoconstriction Inhibition of NE/E release	Oxymetazoline	
β_1	Cardiac conduction system Cardiac myocytes Coronary arteries Kidney: afferent arteriole	Increased heart rate Increased contractility Vasodilation Stimulation of renin release	Isoproterenol Dobutamine	β-Blockers
β_2	VSMC	Vasodilation	Isoproterenol Terbutaline Ritodrine	β-Blockers
β_3	Cardiac myocytes Vascular ECs	Decreased contractility Vasodilation		
M_1	Vascular endothelium VSMC Sympathetic neurons	Vasodilation Vasoconstriction Stimulate NE release	Acetylcholine Muscarine Methacholine Carbachol Arecoline Mc-N-A-343	Atropine Pirenzepine Telenzepine
M_2	VSMC Sympathetic neurons Cardiac conduction system	Vasoconstriction Inhibit NE release Slow conduction	Acetylcholine Muscarine Methacholine Carbachol Arecoline L-660,863	Atropine AF-DX-116 AQ-RA 741 Methoctramine BIBN 99
M_3	Vascular endothelium VSMC Cardiac conduction system	Vasodilation Vasoconstriction Slow conduction	Acetylcholine Muscarine Methacholine Carbachol Arecoline	Atropine 4-DAMP p-F-HHSiD HHSiD
M_4	Sympathetic neurons	Inhibit NE release	Acetylcholine Muscarine Methacholine Carbachol Arecoline	Atropine

EC, endothelial cell; NE, norepinephrine; VSMC, vascular smooth muscle cell.

Distribution of tissue adrenergic receptors is a major determinant of the agonist response because they are relatively nonselective for epinephrine and NE (see Table 6-2). Vascular smooth muscle cells (venous, arterial, and arteriolar) are richly innervated by sympathetic nerve terminals and possess adrenergic receptors (α_1, α_2, and β_2). These receptors can have opposing actions within the vasculature, as demonstrated by α-mediated vasoconstriction and β_2-mediated vasodilation, and the vascular response is determined by the relative activation of α_1, α_2, and β_2 receptors. Vascular α_1 receptors produce vasoconstriction, whereas presynaptic α_2 receptors suppress NE release. Cardiovascular β_1 receptors are expressed primarily within the cardiac conduction system and cardiomyocytes, rather than in the vascular bed. However, vascular β_1 receptors mediate vasodilation within coronary arteries and stimulate renin secretion in the renal juxtaglomerular apparatus.[72] The β_3 receptor is primarily expressed on adipocytes, where it stimulates lipolysis; β_3 receptors may counteract adrenergic stimulation via β_1 receptors in cardiac myocytes and contribute to control of vasodilation by vascular ECs.

Pharmacological Interruption of Catecholamine Metabolism

Catecholamine metabolism is an important target of therapeutic drugs and other chemical agents. Catecholamines are produced locally within the sympathetic neurons by metabolism of tyrosine (Fig. 6-7) to dopamine. Dopamine is concentrated into vesicles via vesicular monoamine transporters. Once in the vesicles, dopamine is converted into NE. Norepinephrine is then secreted and activates adrenergic receptors, provides positive or negative feedback, or is taken back up into the cell via NE transporter (NET). Norepinephrine transporters and similar transporters also

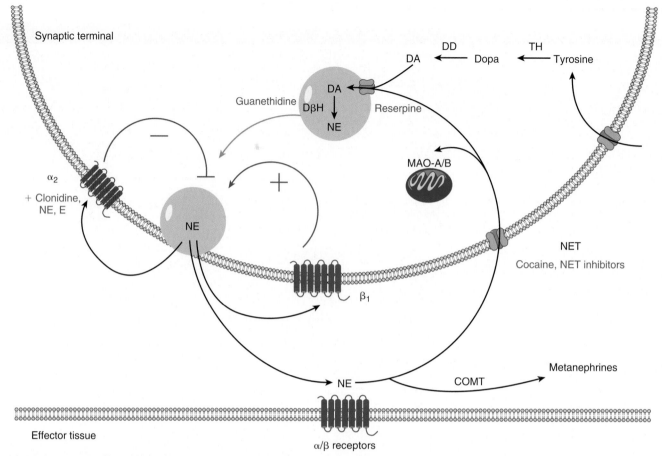

FIGURE 6-7   Norepinephrine (NE) release and reuptake. NE is released from the sympathetic nerve terminal and can signal via vascular α or β receptors. NE also provides positive and/or negative feedback. NE is rapidly taken back up into the nerve terminal via NE transporters (NETs) and can be recycled into granules or metabolized via monoamine oxidase (MAO). Metabolism and/or receptor signaling can be interrupted at multiple steps in the pathway. COMT, catechol-*O*-methyl transferase; DA, dopamine; DβH, dopamine β-hydroxylase; DD, dopamine decarboxylase; E, epinephrine; TH, tyrosine hydroxylase.

transport other neurotransmitters such as epinephrine, dopamine, and serotonin. Norepinephrine is metabolized via monoamine oxidases (MAO-A and MAO-B) after reuptake into the cell, or by catechol-*O*-methyltransferase (COMT) after diffusion into the circulation.

Pharmacological agents that affect this pathway are used clinically for treatment of hypertension, depression, and movement disorders. Reserpine blocks vesicular dopamine/NE transport and depletes NE from the nerve terminals: Guanethidine is an antihypertensive agent that is taken up into vesicles, displaces NE, and reduces NE release during long-term therapy. Many herbal, over-the-counter, or illicit medications act by stimulating NE release (e.g., amphetamine, pseudoephedrine), activating adrenergic receptors (phenylephrine), or acting via mixed mechanisms (ephedrine). Cocaine and tricyclic antidepressants block NE reuptake into the cell and may transiently increase NE and produce hypertension. Antidepressant medications such as selective serotonin reuptake inhibitors (SSRIs) act similarly, and may also nonselectively block NET. Sibutramine is a nonselective serotonin reuptake/NET inhibitor previously used for appetite suppressant effects, but it has been withdrawn from the market because of increased risk of cardiovascular events. Monoamine oxidase inhibitors (MAOIs) are occasionally used to treat depression and can cause marked hypertension during ingestion of tyramine-containing foods, which stimulates NE release. COMT inhibitors and dopa are used to treat movement disorders and can cause orthostatic hypotension and blood pressure dysregulation.

Many weight-loss supplements, decongestant preparations, and herbal supplements act as α₁-agonists (direct sympathomimetics)

or stimulate release of catecholamines (indirect sympathomimetics).[73–75] Whereas epinephrine and NE are rapidly metabolized via COMT, many synthetic sympathomimetic drugs are resistant to this effect, and are therefore effective when ingested by mouth. Ephedra (or ma huang) is a sympathomimetic herbal extract used for asthma treatment, weight loss, and enhanced athletic performance. It can cause severe hypertension, cardiovascular events, and even death in young, apparently healthy individuals. Caffeine coadministration likely exacerbates ephedra-related complications.[76] Performance athletes or enthusiastic weight lifters may also take sympathomimetic supplements, which comprise many of the medications banned by the World Anti-Doping Agency.[74]

Adrenergic Agonists and Antagonists

Vascular α- and β-receptor agonists and antagonists are listed in Table 6-2, and their vascular actions can generally be inferred from the respective receptor actions. Physiological effects of endogenous and synthetic catecholamines are complex because they activate multiple receptors, exhibit dose-dependent responses, and activate compensatory reflexes.

Epinephrine is primarily secreted by the adrenal medulla, where it constitutes roughly 80% of total catecholamine content. Depending on the dose and route of administration, epinephrine may produce divergent vascular responses (Table 6-3). Acute intravenous administration produces marked vasoconstriction, tachycardia, and elevated blood pressure. Continuous infusion or subcutaneous administration of epinephrine increases heart rate and cardiac contractility, systolic blood pressure, and mean

TABLE 6-3 Receptor Activity and Hemodynamic Effects of Commonly Used Adrenergic Agonists

RECEPTOR	EPI	NE	DA*	ISOPROTERENOL	DOBUTAMINE	PHENYLEPHRINE
α_1	+++	++	+++	+	↔	+++
α_2	+++	++	↔	+	↔	↔
β_1	++	++	+++	+++	+++	↔
β_2	++	+/↔	+	+++	+/↔	↔
Physiological Effects						
HR	↑↑	↓	↑↑	↑	↑↑	↔/↓
SBP	↑	↑↑	↑	↔/↑	↔/↓	↑↑
MAP	↔/↑	↑↑	↑	↓	↔/↓	↑↑
DBP	↑/↔/↓	↑	↑	↓	↔/↓	↑↑
CO	↑↑	↔/↓		↑↑	↑↑	↔/↓
PVR	↔/↓	↑↑	↔/↑	↓↓	↓	↑↑

*Dopamine effects are dose-dependent. Effects at maximal dose are presented.
+ Indicates degree of receptor activation, and ↔ indicates minimal effect.
CO, cardiac output; DA, dopamine; DBP, diastolic blood pressure; EPI, epinephrine; HR, heart rate; MAP, mean arterial pressure; NE, norepinephrine; PVR, peripheral vascular resistance; SBP, systolic blood pressure.

arterial blood pressure. Diastolic blood pressure is affected to a lesser extent, resulting in a marked increase in pulse pressure. At lower doses, epinephrine reduces vascular resistance secondary to β_2-receptor stimulation and vasodilation, which may reduce blood pressure. Epinephrine is commonly used to treat anaphylactic reactions, bronchoconstriction, and refractory bradycardia and hypotension. Epinephrine is less often used than NE for treatment of septic shock because of tachycardia and concerns for worsened splanchnic ischemia compared to other agents.

Norepinephrine produces vasoconstriction with lesser direct cardiac effects and β_2 activity than epinephrine, which increases both blood pressure and peripheral vascular resistance. Heart rate decreases due to the baroreflex response. Norepinephrine is useful for treating hypotension refractory to fluid resuscitation (e.g., septic shock). Although there is debate regarding the optimal vasopressor in septic shock, NE has proven as effective as comparable agents, possibly with fewer complications.[77-81] Norepinephrine appears to produce less splanchnic vasoconstriction and intestinal ischemia than epinephrine or phenylephrine.

Isoproterenol is a nonselective β_1/β_2 agonist that is commonly used to increase heart rate for treatment of sinus bradycardia or torsades de pointes. Although its predominant effect is to increase heart rate, vasodilation is also produced by vascular β_2 receptors. Dobutamine is more β_1 selective and is used for its relative selective effects on cardiac contractility.

α_1-Antagonists

Most clinically available α-antagonists are α_1-selective and produce vascular relaxation, vasodilation, and reduction in blood pressure (Table 6-4). These agents are most commonly used for treatment of urinary retention in prostatic hypertrophy because of their inhibitory actions on the prostatic urethra smooth muscle. They are therefore useful for hypertension treatment in patients with concomitant chronic urinary retention. Side effects are nasal congestion, fatigue, and those in common with other vasodilators (peripheral edema, reflex tachycardia, and postural hypotension). The major dose-limiting side effects are postural hypotension and fluid retention. α-Blockers have also been linked to the rare occurrence of "intraoperative floppy iris syndrome," which may result in permanent vision loss after eye surgery. α-Blockers are not generally recommended as hypertension monotherapy, owing to side effects and increased occurrence of cardiovascular events, compared to the thiazide diuretic chlorthalidone in the Antihypertensive and Lipid-Lowering Treatement to Prevent Heart Attack Trial (ALLHAT) trial.[82]

Nonselective α-antagonists (phenoxybenzamine and phentolamine) are used primarily for preoperative treatment of pheochromocytoma. Phenoxybenzamine is administered orally, produces irreversible inhibition, and has a long half-life, whereas phentolamine is given intravenously, acts competitively, and is

TABLE 6-4 α-Agonists and Antagonists

CLASS	DRUG (TRADE NAME)	$T_{1/2}$ (HOURS)	DOSE ADJUSTMENT	DOSE RANGE (TOTAL mg/DAY)	DOSING INTERVAL (HOURS)
Selective α_1-antagonist	Alfuzosin (Uroxatral)	10	L, R	10	24
	Doxazosin (Cardura)	22	L	1-8	24
	Tamsulosin (Flomax)	15	—	0.4-0.8	24
	Prazosin (Minipress)	2-4	L	3-15	8-12
	Silodosin (Rapaflow)	24	L, R	4-8	24
	Terazosin	12	—	1-20	24
Nonselective α_1-antagonist	Phenoxybenzamine (Dibenzyline)	24	—	10-40	12-24
	Phentolamine (Regitine, OraVerse)	15-30 minutes	—	5-20	2-4
α_2-Agonist	Clonidine (Catapres)	4	—	0.3-0.9	6-8
	Guanfacine (Tenex)	16	—	0.5-2	24
	Guanabenz	10	L	4-32	12
	Methyldopa (Aldomet)	*	R	250-3000	8-12

L, liver failure; R, renal failure; $T_{1/2}$, half-life (includes active metabolites as appropriate).

rapidly cleared. When used for treatment of pheochromocytoma, α-blockade should be achieved *before* starting β-blockers because of the risk of unopposed α-receptor activation during β-blocker monotherapy. Some β-blockers also have α-blocking effects (e.g., carvedilol, labetalol), but they should not be used for sole therapy of pheochromocytoma or cocaine overdose because of the relatively low-potency α effects.

α₁-Agonists

Activation of the α_1 receptor stimulates vascular smooth muscle contraction and vasoconstriction. These agents are most commonly used in over-the-counter sinus preparations to treat nasal congestion. Phenylephrine is commonly used for treatment of hypotension in intensive care settings because of its relatively selective vascular effect without increasing heart rate.

α₂-Agonists

Activation of the α_2 receptor within the CNS provides negative feedback inhibition of sympathetic activity and NE release. Clonidine and other α_2-agonists (see Table 6-4) suppress sympathetic and increase parasympathetic activity by actions within the CNS. Evidence for the central effect is obtained from *in vivo* studies demonstrating no effect of clonidine after spinal cord transection. Clonidine can also produce vasoconstriction via activation of peripheral α_{2B} receptors, although this usually only occurs after intravenous administration or accidental overdose.[83] However, this effect may be evident after oral clonidine administration in some patients with autonomic dysfunction.[84] Methyldopa is metabolized similarly to NE and acts as a false transmitter and α_2-agonist. Methyldopa is commonly used in pregnancy for its history of safety, and also remains an effective alternative in resistant hypertension. Other α_2-agonists, such as tizanidine and dexmedetomidine, are used for their sedative effects but may affect blood pressure regulation as a side effect. Etomidate is a sedative with pressor effects that appear to be mediated via α_{2B}.

All α_2-agonists can produce sedation, fatigue, dry mouth, bradycardia, and orthostatic hypotension. Transdermal clonidine frequently produces localized skin irritation due to the adhesive, rather than a drug reaction. Methyldopa carries additional risks of hepatic dysfunction, hemolytic anemia, lupus-like syndrome, and thrombocytopenia. Long-term use of clonidine results in receptor hypersensitivity and rebound hypertension due to exaggerated sympathetic discharge after abrupt drug withdrawal. This syndrome is accompanied by sympathetic hyperactivity and can be minimized by gradual taper or treated with combined α- and

β-blockade. Methyldopa is less likely to produce rebound, owing to the longer half-life of active metabolites, but caution should still be used when stopping this drug.

α₂-Antagonists

Antagonists of α_2-receptors are infrequently used in clinical practice but have a few specific clinical applications. Yohimbine is an α_2-antagonist that increases sympathetic activity in patients with orthostatic hypotension and may also be useful for treatment of ED. Subtype-specific antagonists are not available. Although these drugs are not available commercially, herbal supplements with α_2-antagonist activity are commonly available.

β-Adrenergic Antagonists

Historically, β-adrenergic antagonists (β-blockers) have been classified by receptor subtype specificity and intrinsic sympathomimetic activity (ISA). In addition, some β-blockers also inhibit α_1 receptors, producing a vasodilatory effect. Intrinsic sympathomimetic activity reflects the drug's ability to activate receptors when administered in the absence of any endogenous sympathetic activity (e.g., sympathetic denervation). This effect likely reflects the relative stabilization of the inactive/active receptor conformations as discussed in the pharmacodynamics section. Drugs with ISA tend to produce less bradycardia and may directly reduce vascular resistance, although evidence that this translates into hard clinical outcomes remains debatable. Analyses suggest that β-blockers with ISA do not reduce cardiovascular mortality and may actually worsen outcomes.[85]

Drugs with β-blocking ability are summarized in Table 6-5. Propranolol was the first clinically available β-blocker, and is nonselective. Second-generation agents offer increased β_1 selectivity. Recently, vasodilatory β-blockers entered the market and produce additional blood pressure lowering effects via α_1 blockade and possibly via β_3 activation.[86] β-Blockers are commonly used to treat hypertension, acute MI, heart failure, angina, and supraventricular arrhythmias. In acute MI, atenolol reduces in-hospital mortality by 15%, although benefit with prolonged therapy is less well established. Perioperative β-adrenergic blockade also reduces in-hospital mortality in patients with high cardiovascular risk.[85]

In the past, β-blockers were withheld in patients with systolic heart failure, owing to concerns of worsening contractile function and intolerance. However, the observation that the sympathetic nervous system is activated in severe heart failure and predicted mortality supported the concept of sympathetic blockade in CHF.[87] Randomized clinical trials have definitively

TABLE 6-5 β-Blockers

CLASS	DRUG (TRADE NAME)	ISA	T₁/₂ (HOURS)	DOSE ADJUSTMENT	DOSE RANGE (TOTAL mg/DAY)	DOSING INTERVAL (HOURS)
Nonselective β₁/β₂-antagonists	Propranolol (Inderal)	—	3-6	L	20-240	8-12
	Nadolol (Corgard)	—	10-24	L, R	40-320	24
	Pindolol (Visken)	++	3-4	L, R	10-60	12
	Penbutolol (Levatol)	+	5	—	10-40	24
	Sotalol* (Betapace)	—	12	R	80-240	24
Selective β₁-antagonists	Acebutolol (Sectral)	+	8-13	R	200-800	12
	Atenolol (Tenormin)	—	7	R	25-100	12-24
	Betaxolol (Kerlone)	—	14-22	L, R	5-20	24
	Bisoprolol (Zebeta)	—	9-12	R	2.5-20	24
	Esmolol (Brevibloc)	—	9 min	—	150-300 μg/kg/min	Continuous infusion
	Metoprolol (Toprol, Lopressor)	—	3-8	L	25-400	12
	Nebivolol (Bystolic)	—	10-36	L, R	5-40	24
Nonselective β₁/β₂/α₁-antagonists	Carvedilol (Coreg)	—	7-10	L	6.25-80	12
	Labetalol (Normodyne, Trandate)	+	6-8	—	200-800	12

"+"just refers to the presence and strength of intrinsic sympathomimetic activity.
*Sotalol has additional potassium channel blocking effects.
ISA, intrinsic sympathomimetic activity; L, liver failure; R, renal failure; T₁/₂, half-life (includes active metabolites as appropriate).

demonstrated that metoprolol, bisoprolol, and carvedilol improve systolic function and reduce mortality in CHF. These agents should be introduced gradually and titrated upwards as tolerated in patients with severe CHF.

All β-blockers can produce side effects related to their mechanism of action (bradycardia, heart block, hypotension). β-Blockers can also worsen hyperglycemia (especially when combined with thiazide diuretics) or blunt the compensatory response to hypoglycemia. They should not be used as primary treatment for pheochromocytoma, cocaine intoxication, clonidine-withdrawal hypertension, or other hyperadrenergic crises, owing to the possibility of unopposed α-receptor activation. Sotalol is a unique β-blocker with antiarrhythmic effects due to potassium channel blocking activity, which requires close monitoring for QT prolongation and proarrhythmia.

Dopamine and Dopaminergic Agonists

Dopamine is endogenously produced in both peripheral and central neuronal cells and in the adrenal gland via the action of dopa decarboxylase on dopa (see Fig. 6-7). Dopamine acts on one of 5 G protein–linked receptors, termed *D1* through *D5*, which are further classified into two major groups termed *D1* and *D2*. The D1 class of dopamine receptors, D1 and D5, are $G_{\alpha s}$-linked receptors that activate adenylyl cyclase; the D2 class receptors are linked to $G_{\alpha i/o}$ and inhibit adenylyl cyclase. Perturbations of dopamine signaling in the CNS have been linked with a variety of disorders, including Parkinson's disease, Huntington's disease, Tourette's syndrome, schizophrenia, and major depression. In addition to CNS receptors, dopamine receptors are widely present in peripheral tissues including the kidney, gastrointestinal tract, heart, adrenal glands, and vasculature. Dopamine receptor signaling has recently been reviewed in depth.[88]

The predominant clinical use of dopamine has been for circulatory support in critically ill patients in settings such as shock or the postoperative period. The clinical response to dopamine is complex and depends on the dose. At low doses (1-4 µg/kg/min), often referred to as "renal doses," dopamine acts on D1-like receptors and β-adrenergic receptors to promote renal arterial vasodilation and improve renal blood flow. As the dose is increased, dopamine begins to exert greater effects at β- and α-adrenergic receptors, and the α-adrenergic effects begin to predominate at doses exceeding 10 µg/kg/min. There is also substantial variability in these responses, such that the precise effect of dopamine in an individual patient is difficult to predict. The potential increase renal blood flow, due to D1-like receptor activation, has not proven to have significant clinical benefit. Recent clinical trials have shown no benefit of dopamine over NE infusion in patients with septic shock, with substantially more cardiac arrhythmias and sinus tachycardia caused by dopamine.[89,90]

Owing to the mixed effects of dopamine on multiple receptors, agonists have been developed that have greater specificity for D1-like receptors, and therefore would serve as potent vasodilators with limited off-target effects. Fenoldopam is such an agent that has been approved by the FDA for treatment of severe hypertension. This agent is a potent vasodilator with rapid onset of action that produces dose-dependent reductions in blood pressure when administered intravenously to patients with hypertension. It is devoid of the α- and β-adrenergic effects of dopamine, so less prone to cause off-target effects. Early studies showed that it preferentially increased renal plasma flow, in keeping with preferential dilation of the renal vasculature, and dramatically enhanced renal sodium excretion.

Despite these potentially beneficial effects of fenoldopam, its clinical use in severe hypertension remains limited, largely because several other drugs are quite effective. In prior clinical trials, fenoldopam showed no benefit over sodium nitroprusside in lowering blood pressure,[91] and it is considerably more expensive.

Based on its ability to enhance renal perfusion and sodium excretion, fenoldopam has been used as a renal protectant in critically ill patients. A recent meta-analysis of 16 randomized trials involving 1290 patients indicated that fenoldopam reduced the need for renal replacement therapy, in-hospital mortality, and length of stay in the intensive care unit in postoperative or critically ill patients.[92] Similar results were obtained from a meta-analysis of patients undergoing cardiovascular surgery.[93] Such analyses can be flawed by publication bias, and prospective trials are needed to establish a benefit of fenoldopam in this setting.

There was initial enthusiasm for use of fenoldopam to prevent contrast-induced nephropathy. However, a rigorous randomized prospective trial showed no benefit of this agent in preventing changes in renal function in patients undergoing angiography procedures,[94] and its use in this setting is no longer recommended. Dopexamine, which is a combined D1-like and β2-adrenergic agonist, has been studied in a variety of settings involving critically ill patients, but it has not proven beneficial in randomized prospective trials.[95,96]

Vascular Potassium and Calcium Channels

Direct vasodilators reduce blood pressure by acting on vascular smooth muscle and ultimately impair myosin light chain phosphorylation and contraction (see Fig. 6-1). Minoxidil, for example, activates K_{ATP} channels, which hyperpolarizes the cell and prevents calcium entry and contraction.[97,98] Channel blocking agents are presented in Table 6-6.

Calcium channel blockers (CCBs) decrease intracellular calcium entry via the L-type calcium channels on the vasculature and cardiac conduction system. L-type calcium channels are located on cardiac myocytes, vascular smooth muscle, and the cardiac conduction system. Blockade of these channels reduces cardiac and vascular smooth muscle contraction and slows conduction. Calcium channel blockers can be classified broadly as dihydropyridines (DHP; e.g., amlodipine, nifedipine) and non-dihydropyridines (verapamil and diltiazem). Dihydropyridines are more potent vasodilators than non-DHP, whereas verapamil and diltiazem also slow cardiac conduction.

Dihydropyridines produce relatively selective vascular effects *in vivo* and do not significantly slow cardiac conduction. In some patients, vasodilation may produce reflex tachycardia and vasodilatory edema. This may cause tachycardia and rarely precipitate angina, especially if given acutely. The rapid hypotensive effect of immediate-release nifedipine, particularly when given sublingually, can actually increase cardiovascular events and should be avoided by using only slow-release formulations.[99] In contrast, long-acting DHPs have a good safety profile and reduce hypertensive complications.[97] Because multiple other agents have proven effectiveness in CHF, and CCBs may worsen cardiac function, they should not be used in this class of patients. Vasodilatory edema during treatment with CCBs is typically refractory to diuretic treatment, but the incidence is reduced by concomitant treatment with an angiotensin-converting enzyme inhibitor (ACEI) or angiotensin receptor blocker (ARB).

Verapamil and diltiazem slow cardiac conduction in addition to their vasodilatory effect, and are frequently used for control or prevention of supraventricular arrhythmias. These agents also impair cardiac contractility and should be avoided in patients with impaired systolic function. Both drugs also inhibit CYP3A4, and attention to avoid significant drug interactions is needed. In particular, caution should be given to patients receiving statins, owing to increased risk of rhabdomyolysis. Vasodilatory edema occurs less often than with DHPs. All CCBs may produce constipation.

Because of their frequent side effects, minoxidil and hydralazine are direct vasodilators typically reserved for refractory hypertension.[100] Minoxidil acts on the sulfonylurea receptor-2 (SUR2) component of the K_{ATP} channel in VSMCs, and in turn increases K^+ flux, hyperpolarizes the cell, and produces vasodilation. Although sulfonylurea drugs (e.g., glibenclamide, glyburide, glipizide) stimulate insulin secretion via opposite effects on SUR1, evidence

TABLE 6-6 Channel Blocking Agents

CLASS	DRUG (TRADE NAME)	$T_{1/2}$(HOURS)	DOSE ADJUSTMENT	DOSE RANGE (TOTAL mg/DAY)	DOSING INTERVAL (HOURS)
Ca²⁺ CCB: DHPs	Amlodipine (Norvasc)	40-50	L	2.5-10	24
	Felodipine (Plendil)	11-16	L	30-120	12-24
	Isradipine (DynaCirc)	8	R	2.5-10	12
	Nicardipine (Cardene)	11.5	—	60-120	8
	Nifedipine (Adalat, Procardia)	2-5	L	30-120	12-24
	Nimodipine (Nimotop)	2.8	L	180-360	4
	Nisoldipine (Sular)	15	L	20-60	24
Ca²⁺ CCB: non-DHPs	Diltiazem (Cardizem, Dilacor, Tiazac)	3-5	L	120-480	24
	Verapamil (Calan, Isoptin)	8-12	L, R	80-480	8-24
K_{ATP} openers	Hydralazine (Apresoline)	2-8	R	10-300	8-12
	Minoxidil (Loniten)	4	R	2.5-80	
	Pinacidil*			12.5-150	12

*Not available in the United States.

Ca²⁺ CCB, calcium channel blocker; DHP, dihydropyridine; K_{ATP}, ATP-sensitive potassium channel; L, liver failure; R, renal failure; $T_{1/2}$, half-life.

that they cause vasoconstriction via SUR2 *in vivo* is lacking. Hydralazine is a direct vasodilator, although the exact mechanism of action is poorly understood. Minoxidil is more effective than hydralazine and can be effective in patients who have not responded to hydralazine. They must be administered with a rate-controlling agent and diuretic to prevent reflex tachycardia and fluid retention, which limit their antihypertensive effectiveness. Minoxidil may worsen LV hypertrophy despite adequate hypertension control, in part because of these compensatory responses. During long-term use, excessive hair growth also occurs and is particularly worrisome to female patients. Hydralazine may also produce a lupus-like syndrome. Both drugs may also produce pericardial or pleural effusions. Reflex sympathetic activation may precipitate cardiac ischemia in some patients. Use of these agents in the setting of acute aortic dissection should be avoided because of reflex sympathetic activation. Hydralazine has been approved for treatment of heart failure in African Americans in combination with a nitrate, as discussed earlier.[12]

Renin-Angiotensin-Aldosterone System

Regulation of the Renin-Angiotensin-Aldosterone System

The renin-angiotensin-aldosterone system (RAAS) is highly coordinated to maintain blood volume and blood pressure, and is of major importance during sodium and/or fluid depletion (Fig. 6-8). The RAAS is stimulated under pathological conditions that cause reduced renal perfusion, such as heart failure, aortic coarctation, or renal artery stenosis. In addition, this system is inappropriately activated in obesity and diabetes.

Renin secretion by renal juxtaglomerular cells, the rate-limiting step in the RAAS cascade, is stimulated by reduced sodium chloride delivery to the macula densa, reduced renal perfusion pressure, and sympathetic stimulation.[101] Upon release into the circulation, renin cleaves circulating angiotensinogen to angiotensin (Ang-I). Although Ang-I is inactive, it is rapidly converted into Ang-II by angiotensin-converting enzyme (ACE), which is abundantly expressed within the pulmonary vasculature and to a lesser extent in the peripheral circulation. In addition to the endothelial membrane-bound form, ACE also circulates in a soluble form. Angiotensin-II is a potent vasoconstrictor, acting directly on the Ang-II type 1 receptors (AT₁) on VSMCs. Within the kidney, Ang-II acts upon the renal afferent and efferent arteriole, to a greater extent on the efferent arteriole. During periods of volume depletion, this efferent selectivity serves to preserve glomerular filtration by increasing intraglomerular pressure. Angiotensin-II also stimulates aldosterone secretion from the

adrenal gland. Aldosterone reinforces the vasoconstrictor effect of Angiotensin-II by increasing renal sodium reabsorption and expanding intravascular volume via the mineralocorticoid receptor (MR) in principal cells of the kidney and activation of the epithelial sodium channel (ENaC). Angiotensin-converting enzyme is the principal metabolizing enzyme for a number of

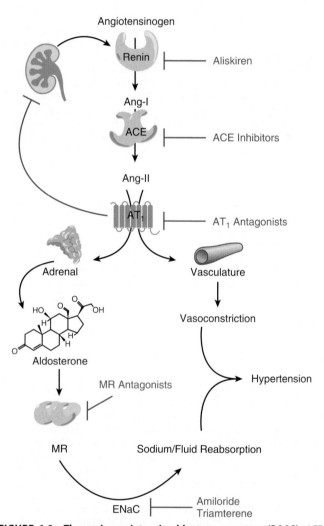

FIGURE 6-8 The renin-angiotensin-aldosterone system (RAAS). ACE, angiotensin-I converting enzyme; Ang, angiotensin; AT₁, angiotensin-II type 1 receptor; ENaC, epithelial sodium channel; MR, mineralocorticoid receptor.

other vasoactive peptides, notably bradykinin, which may confer some of the beneficial antihypertensive and antithrombotic effects observed during ACE inhibition.

Receptors and Novel Mediators in RAAS Signaling

The AT_1 and AT_2 receptors are the principal Ang-II receptors in humans and are widely expressed, including in areas important for blood pressure regulation (vascular smooth muscle, kidney, adrenal cortex, brain). AT_1 is a classic seven-transmembrane domain GPCR that signals via $G_{\alpha q}$ and phospholipase C, as well as other G protein–independent pathways.[102,103] Upon Ang-II binding, angiotensin receptor–associated protein (ATRAP) facilitates AT_1 internalization and desensitization.[104] AT_1 mediates the classic Ang-II effects including vasoconstriction, adrenal aldosterone secretion, and renal proximal tubule sodium reabsorption. In addition, Ang-II participates in a negative feedback loop in the kidney to inhibit renin secretion via AT_1. In mice, two AT_1 receptors have been identified, AT_{1a} and AT_{1b}, with AT_{1a} responsible for most of the pressor and mitogenic effects, although a single AT_1 receptor is present in humans.

In general, the actions of the AT_2 receptor tend to oppose those of the AT_1 receptor, although some effects are inconsistent with this generalization.[105,106] AT_2 stimulation produces vasodilation, in part via an increase in bradykinin and receptor heterodimerization with the bradykinin receptor. AT_2 has an antinatriuretic effect within renal tubules. However, AT_2 and AT_1 similarly suppress renin secretion. Although investigational agonists and antagonists for the AT_2 receptor are available, these agents are not available clinically. Therefore, the clinical implication of the AT_2 receptor remains unproven. Angiotensin-II decreases during ACE inhibition but increases during AT_1 antagonism. However, the AT_2 receptor remains available for Ang-II activation during chronic AT_1 antagonism and may promote beneficial effects. This rationale has led some to argue the benefit of AT_1 antagonism over ACE inhibition.

Aldosterone and other corticosteroids activate the MR within principal cells in the cortical collecting duct. Angiotensin-II, aldosterone, and MR activation induce multiple proteins that coordinate to increase renal sodium and water reabsorption.[107–109] The MR is a classic nuclear receptor localized to the cytosol in its inactive form, which dimerizes and translocates to the nucleus and activates nuclear transcription when activated. Although aldosterone appears to be the critical physiological stimulus, cortisol, corticosterone, and other steroids have a similar affinity for the MR. However, within epithelial target tissues, 11-β-hydroxysteroid dehydrogenase type 2 (11βHSD2) inactivates these hormones and prevents inappropriate MR activation. Either inhibition of this enzyme by licorice or genetic deficiency produces unregulated MR activation and hypertension with metabolic alkalosis and hypokalemia. The MR is also expressed within vascular smooth muscle and ECs, where it may contribute to vascular injury via activation of NADPH oxidase, generation of ROS, and inflammation.

Greater complexity of the RAAS has emerged with the discovery of novel angiotensin peptides and receptors. Angiotensin-(1-7) is formed by cleavage of Ang-I by neprilysin or prolyl-endopeptidase or from cleavage of Ang-II by ACE2.[110] Angiotensin-(1-7) acts via the Mas receptor, a G protein–coupled cell-surface receptor generally opposing AT_1 effects.[111] Angiotensin-(1-7) and ACE2 confer protection against Ang-II–mediated cardiovascular injury, and ACE2-deficient mice have accentuated Ang-II–induced injury.[112] Angiotensin-II is also metabolized in vivo by aminopeptidase A to Ang-III and Ang-IV, which may have important physiological effects within the CNS.[103]

Additional interest has focused on the (pro)-renin receptor (PRR), which binds either renin or prorenin.[113] The PRR can exist as a full-length transmembrane protein, a soluble circulating form, or a truncated protein (transmembrane/ cytoplasmic portion). The full-length transmembrane PRR can bind and activate prorenin by inducing a conformational change that exposes the catalytic site. In addition, (pro)-renin activates PRR and cellular signaling events (e.g., mitogen-activated protein kinase [MAPK] pathways) independent of renin activity.[114] Prorenin circulates in marked excess of active renin, and the prorenin/renin ratio is further increased in diabetes, raising the possibility that (pro)renin-PRR signaling or PRR-induced activation of prorenin and local angiotensin production could contribute to cardiovascular injury.

Drugs That Inhibit the Renin-Angiotensin-Aldosterone System

The first ACE inhibitor was serendipitously discovered as a bradykinin-potentiating factor isolated from venom of the pit viper *Bothrops jararaca*. Subsequent studies demonstrated its activity against ACE, suggesting that this enzyme played a key role in regulating both the RAAS and the kallikrein-kinin systems. Isolation of the responsible peptide sequences led to development of captopril, one of the earliest examples of structure-based drug design.[115] Captopril's success in treatment of cardiovascular disease was critical to the development of other drugs that block the RAAS (Table 6-7). Drugs are now clinically available to block the RAAS cascade at nearly every level (see Fig. 6-8).

Direct renin inhibitors are the most recent class of RAAS blocking agents. Although renin is the rate-limiting enzyme in the RAAS pathway and a logical drug target, development of clinical renin inhibitors was hindered by poor potency, stability, and oral bioavailability.[116] Development of aliskiren overcame these issues, and other agents are in clinical studies. Aliskiren selectively inhibits renin activity and dose-dependently reduces Ang-I and Ang-II production and blood pressure. Renin secretion markedly increases during aliskiren therapy, and attention to the assay method is needed if plasma renin concentration is measured.[117] Plasma renin activity (assessed by in vitro Ang-I generation) remains inhibited, and thus compensatory renin secretion does not appear to overcome the effect of aliskiren or increase blood pressure.[118] Aliskiren is well tolerated and has a low rate of side effects, which are principally gastrointestinal. Aliskiren effectively reduces blood pressure when used in alone or in combination with diuretic therapy, ACE inhibitors, or ARBs.[116,119–121] Addition of aliskiren to maximal-dose losartan reduced proteinuria compared to placebo in a population with diabetic proteinuira.[122] Aliskiren provided similar LV mass reduction compared to losartan in a group of overweight subjects with hypertension but provided no additional benefit in combination.[123] Further studies are needed to investigate hard cardiovascular endpoints.

Angiotensin-converting enzyme inhibitors are used to treat hypertension, diabetic nephropathy, CHF, and prior MI or stroke. Their antihypertensive effect is generally less effective in African Americans because of a higher prevalence of low-renin hypertension, but concurrent thiazide diuretic administration improves responsiveness. Many orally administered ACE inhibitors are given as a prodrug, which are rapidly metabolized into active metabolite via enteric metabolism (e.g., enalapril to enalaprilat). Enalaprilat is the active metabolite of enalapril and is available for intravenous administration. Most ACE inhibitors are renally excreted and require careful monitoring in patients with renal insufficiency.

Angiotensin-II can also be generated by enzymes other than ACE (e.g., chymase, cathepsin G), providing a rationale for combination therapy with ARBs and ACE inhibitors. Angiotensin-II type 1 receptor antagonists (ARBs) also provide an alternative treatment option for patients who are intolerant of ACE inhibitors. Early studies were done with saralasin, an intravenous peptide Ang-II analog, which demonstrated effectiveness of ARBs and led to the development of orally available agents.[124] Since then, multiple agents have been developed and approved for hypertension treatment and prevention of cardiovascular complications (see Table 6-7). Angiotensin receptor blockers are remarkably well tolerated and may even

TABLE 6-7 Drugs That Interrupt the Renin-Angiotensin-Aldosterone System

DRUG CLASS	DRUG (TRADE NAME)	$T_{1/2}$ (HOURS)	DOSE ADJUSTMENT	DOSE RANGE (mg/DAY)	DOSING INTERVAL (HOURS)
Direct renin inhibitors	Aliskiren (Tekturna)	24-48	—	150-300	Once daily
ACE inhibitors	Benazepril (Lotensin)	10-11	R	20-40	24
	Captopril (Capoten)	2	R	12.5-100	8-12
	Enalapril (Vasotec)	2	—	5-40	12-24
	Enalaprilat[†]	35*	—	0.625-5	6
	Fosinopril (Monopril)	12	—	10-40	24
	Lisinopril (Prinivil, Zestril)	12	R	2.5-40	24
	Moexipril (Univasc)	2-9*	R	7.5-30	24
	Perindopril (Aceon)	3-10	R	2-16	24
	Quinapril (Accupril)	3*	R	5-80	24
	Ramipril (Altace)	13-17	R	2.5-20	24
	Trandolapril (Mavik)	22.5*	L, R	1-8	24
AT$_1$ antagonists	Azilsartan (Edarbi)	11	—	40-80	24
	Candesartan (Atacand)	5-9	L	4-16	12-24
	Eprosartan (Teveten)	5-9	—	400-800	12-24
	Irbesartan (Avapro)	11-15	—	150-300	24
	Losartan (Cozaar)	6-9*	L	50-100	12-24
	Olmesartan (Benicar)	12-15	—	5-40	24
	Telmisartan (Micardis)	24	L	20-80	24
	Valsartan (Diovan)	6	L	80-320	24
MR antagonists	Spironolactone (Aldactone)	10-23*	R	12.5-100	24
	Eplerenone (Inspra)	4-6	R	25-200	12-24

*Elimination half-life includes active metabolites.
[†]Intravenous formulation.
ACE, angiotensin-converting enzyme; AT$_1$, angiotensin-II type 1; L, liver failure; MR, mineralocorticoid receptor; R, renal failure; $T_{1/2}$, half-life.

reduce the incidence of some complaints such as headache. All of the ARBs are reliably absorbed, highly protein bound, and selective for the AT$_1$ receptor. Telmisartan and the losartan metabolite EXP3174 can also activate peroxime proliferator-activated receptor gamma (PPARγ), which may explain improvement in insulin sensitivity.[125,126] Losartan has a short half-life, but has an active metabolite (EXP3174) with a long half-life. Elimination is primarily hepatic for most ARBs, but dose adjustment is usually needed only in severe liver impairment.

RAAS blockade with any of these drugs (ACE inhibitors, ARBs, or renin inhibitors) is contraindicated during pregnancy because of the risk of congenital renal and other malformations and should be used with extreme caution in women of childbearing potential.[127] These agents also carry a risk of hyperkalemia and worsening renal insufficiency.[128] RAAS blockade should not be used in the setting of bilateral renal artery stenosis because of the risk of worsening renal failure. Angiotensin-converting enzyme inhibitors rarely cause potentially fatal angioedema, which is more frequent in African Americans. Angiotensin-converting enzyme inhibitors commonly cause a cough, which may be bothersome enough to require cessation, but is a separate pathogenesis than angioedema.[129]

Spironolactone and eplerenone are MR antagonists whose main effect is mediated by antagonizing MR activity in the distal kidney. These agents also produce systemic vascular effects such as reducing inflammation, improving vascular endothelial function, and promoting fibrinolysis. Mineralocorticoid receptor antagonists reduce mortality in patients with chronic heart failure and after acute MI, and are very effective in the treatment of drug-resistant hypertension.[130-133] Spironolactone possesses progesterone-like activity and can cause gynecomastia and/or breast tenderness in 5% to 10% of patients, which resolves upon cessation. Eplerenone does not cause gynecomastia because it is MR specific and therefore provides an alternative for those who are spironolactone intolerant. As opposed to other diuretics, MR antagonists do not require filtration into the urinary space to achieve their effect, but renal insufficiency carries an increased risk of hyperkalemia, and they should be used with caution if at all in this setting. Eplerenone

carries additional risk of drug interactions due to moderate CYP3A4 inhibition.

Endothelin Receptor Antagonists

Endothelin-1 is a vasoactive peptide initially described in 1988, and among the most potent vasoconstrictor substances known.[134,135] Endothelin-1 is converted by endothelin-converting enzyme from a precursor protein, big ET-1, and is secreted from the cell. Although multiple isoforms exist, ET-1 produces most of the important cardiovascular effects. Endothelin-1 is secreted abluminally (e.g., by ECs toward VSMC) and produces responses that are highly tissue dependent. Although ET-1 is found in the circulation, local paracrine and autocrine actions are more important than endocrine effects. Endothelin-1 acts via ET-1 type A (ET$_A$) and B (ET$_B$) receptors that are widely distributed throughout the body. In vascular smooth muscle, ET$_A$ and ET$_B$ produce vasoconstriction, whereas endothelial ET$_B$ mediates NO-dependent vasodilation. ET$_B$ also contributes to clearance of ET-1 by internalization and cellular degradation.

Vascular bed–specific differences exist, with the renal vasculature being exquisitely sensitive to the effects of ET-1. However, the predominant effect of ET-1 within the kidney is to increase natriuresis and free water excretion. Renal ET-1 is produced predominantly in the medulla, which contributes to long-term blood pressure control via ET$_B$ in the distal nephron.[134] Knockout of ET-1 within the cortical collecting duct results in hypertension and inability to excrete a sodium load, which is improved by ENaC blockade with amiloride.

In the pulmonary vasculature, ET$_A$ acts as a potent vasoconstrictor and also promotes vascular smooth muscle hypertrophy and proliferation, making the endothelin system a logical pharmacological target. Endothelin receptor antagonists (ETRAs) achieved initial clinical success in patients with PAH. Bosentan was the first ETRA and blocks both ET$_A$ and ET$_B$. Ambrisentan is ET$_A$ selective. Bosentan and ambrisentan are effective in PH and have demonstrated improved exercise capacity and hemodynamics.[136,137] Improved long-term survival has been suggested by observational studies but not in randomized clinical trials.

TABLE 6-8 Endothelin Receptor Antagonists

DRUG (TRADE NAME)	RECEPTOR SELECTIVITY	$T_{1/2}$(HOURS)	DOSE ADJUSTMENT	DOSE RANGE (TOTAL mg/DAY)	DOSING INTERVAL (HOURS)
Ambrisentan (Letairis)	ET_A	9	L	5-10	24
Atrasentan*	ET_A	20-24	L	*	*
Avosentan*	ET_A	7-10	L	*	*
Bosentan (Tracleer)	$ET_A > ET_B$	5	L	62.6-250	12
Darusentan*	ET_A	16-18	L	*	*
Sitaxsentan (Thelin) *	ET_A	6-7	L	*	*

*Not U.S. Food and Drug Administration (FDA) approved in the United States.
ET, endothelin; L, liver failure; $T_{1/2}$, half-life.

The role of ETRAs in hypertension, diabetic nephropathy, and heart failure is still developing and has mainly been tested using experimental agents (Table 6-8). Clinical trials in hypertension have demonstrated that the ET_A-selective antagonist darusentan is effective in patients with resistant hypertension.[138] The ET_A-selective antagonist avosentan reduced albuminuria by 40% to 50% in patients with diabetic nephropathy, but also significantly increased the occurrence of fluid overload and clinical heart failure. In heart failure, ETRAs appear to improve hemodynamic endpoints, but in longer-term trials do not improve clinical symptoms or mortality.[139,140] Endothelin receptor antagonists commonly produce edema, headache, and a decrease in Hb. Hepatic toxicity (increase in serum transaminase) is the most serious adverse effect and requires close monitoring.

REFERENCES

1. Kim HR, Appel S, Vetterkind S, et al: Smooth muscle signalling pathways in health and disease, *J Cell Mol Med* 12(6A):2165–2180, 2008.
2. Watanabe H, Tran QK, Takeuchi K, et al: Myosin light-chain kinase regulates endothelial calcium entry and endothelium-dependent vasodilation, *FASEB J* 15(2):282–284, 2001.
3. Budzyn K, Sobey CG: Vascular Rho kinases and their potential therapeutic applications, *Curr Opin Drug Discov Devel* 10(5):590–596, 2007.
4. Bryan NS, Bian K, Murad F: Discovery of the nitric oxide signaling pathway and targets for drug development, *Front Biosci* 14:1–18, 2009.
5. Friederich JA, Butterworth JF: Sodium nitroprusside: twenty years and counting, *Anesth Analg* 81(1):152–162, 1995.
6. Chen Z, Zhang J, Stamler JS: Identification of the enzymatic mechanism of nitroglycerin bioactivation, *Proc Natl Acad Sci U S A* 99(12):8306–8311, 2002.
7. Li Y, Zhang D, Jin W, et al: Mitochondrial aldehyde dehydrogenase-2 (ALDH2) Glu504Lys polymorphism contributes to the variation in efficacy of sublingual nitroglycerin, *J Clin Invest* 116(2):506–511, 2006.
8. Chihara E, Manyari DE, Isaac DL, et al: Comparative effects of nitroglycerin on intestinal vascular capacitance and conductance, *Can J Cardiol* 18(2):165–174, 2002.
9. ISIS-4: a randomised factorial trial assessing early oral captopril, oral mononitrate, and intravenous magnesium sulphate in 58,050 patients with suspected acute myocardial infarction. ISIS-4 (Fourth International Study of Infarct Survival) Collaborative Group, *Lancet* 345(8951):669–685, 1995.
10. Six-month effects of early treatment with lisinopril and transdermal glyceryl trinitrate singly and together withdrawn six weeks after acute myocardial infarction: the GISSI-3 trial. Gruppo Italiano per lo Studio della Sopravvivenza nell'Infarto Miocardico, *J Am Coll Cardiol* 27(2):337–344, 1996.
11. Ambrosio G, Del PM, Tritto I, et al: Chronic nitrate therapy is associated with different presentation and evolution of acute coronary syndromes: insights from 52,693 patients in the Global Registry of Acute Coronary Events, *Eur Heart J* 31(4):430–438, 2010.
12. Taylor AL, Ziesche S, Yancy C, et al: Combination of isosorbide dinitrate and hydralazine in blacks with heart failure, *N Engl J Med* 351(20):2049–2057, 2004.
13. Daiber A, Munzel T, Gori T: Organic nitrates and nitrate tolerance--state of the art and future developments, *Adv Pharmacol* 60:177–227, 2010.
14. Rhoney D, Peacock WF: Intravenous therapy for hypertensive emergencies, part 2, *Am J Health Syst Pharm* 66(16):1448–1457, 2009.
15. Thomas DD, Miranda KM, Colton CA, et al: Heme proteins and nitric oxide (NO): the neglected, eloquent chemistry in NO redox signaling and regulation, *Antioxid Redox Signal* 5(3):307–317, 2003.
16. Erusalimsky JD, Moncada S: Nitric oxide and mitochondrial signaling: from physiology to pathophysiology, *Arterioscler Thromb Vasc Biol* 27(12):2524–2531, 2007.
17. Lundberg JO, Weitzberg E, Gladwin MT: The nitrate-nitrite-nitric oxide pathway in physiology and therapeutics, *Nat Rev Drug Discov* 7(2):156–167, 2008.
18. Dejam A, Hunter CJ, Tremonti C, et al: Nitrite infusion in humans and nonhuman primates: endocrine effects, pharmacokinetics, and tolerance formation, *Circulation* 116(16):1821–1831, 2007.
19. Evgenov OV, Pacher P, Schmidt PM, et al: NO-independent stimulators and activators of soluble guanylate cyclase: discovery and therapeutic potential, *Nat Rev Drug Discov* 5(9):755–768, 2006.
20. Misono KS, Philo JS, Arakawa T, et al: Structure, signaling mechanism and regulation of the natriuretic peptide receptor guanylate cyclase, *FEBS J* 278(11):1818–1829, 2011.
21. Clerico A, Giannoni A, Vittorini S, et al: Thirty years of the heart as an endocrine organ: Physiological role and clinical utility of cardiac natriuretic hormones, *Am J Physiol Heart Circ Physiol* 2011.
22. Palazzuoli A, Gallotta M, Quatrini I, et al: Natriuretic peptides (BNP and NT-proBNP): measurement and relevance in heart failure, *Vasc Health Risk Manag* 6:411–418, 2010.
23. Colucci WS, Elkayam U, Horton DP, et al: Intravenous nesiritide, a natriuretic peptide, in the treatment of decompensated congestive heart failure. Nesiritide Study Group, *N Engl J Med* 343(4):246–253, 2000.
24. Sackner-Bernstein JD, Kowalski M, Fox M, et al: Short-term risk of death after treatment with nesiritide for decompensated heart failure: a pooled analysis of randomized controlled trials, *JAMA* 293(15):1900–1905, 2005.
25. Abraham WT, Trupp RJ, Jarjoura D: Nesiritide in acute decompensated heart failure: a pooled analysis of randomized controlled trials, *Clin Cardiol* 33(8):484–489, 2010.
26. Hernandez AF, O'Connor CM, Starling RC, et al: Acute Study of Clinical Effectiveness of Nesiritide in Decompensated Heart Failure Trial (ASCEND-HF), *Circulation* 122(21):2217, 2010.
27. O'Connor CM, Starling RC, Hernandez AF, et al: Effect of nesiritide in patients with acute decompensated heart failure, *N Engl J Med* 365(1):32–43, 2011.
28. Kass DA, Takimoto E, Nagayama T, et al: Phosphodiesterase regulation of nitric oxide signaling, *Cardiovasc Res* 75(2):303–314, 2007.
29. Francis SH, Sekhar KR, Ke H, et al: Inhibition of cyclic nucleotide phosphodiesterases by methylxanthines and related compounds, *Handb Exp Pharmacol* (200):93–133, 2011.
30. Das A, Xi L, Kukreja RC: Phosphodiesterase-5 inhibitor sildenafil preconditions adult cardiac myocytes against necrosis and apoptosis. Essential role of nitric oxide signaling, *J Biol Chem* 280(13):12944–12955, 2005.
31. Borlaug BA, Melenovsky V, Marhin T, et al: Sildenafil inhibits beta-adrenergic-stimulated cardiac contractility in humans, *Circulation* 112(17):2642–2649, 2005.
32. Takimoto E, Champion HC, Li M, et al: Chronic inhibition of cyclic GMP phosphodiesterase 5A prevents and reverses cardiac hypertrophy, *Nat Med* 11(2):214–222, 2005.
33. Badesch DB, Abman SH, Simonneau G, et al: Medical therapy for pulmonary arterial hypertension: updated ACCP evidence-based clinical practice guidelines, *Chest* 131(6):1917–1928, 2007.
34. Michelakis E, Tymchak W, Lien D, et al: Oral sildenafil is an effective and specific pulmonary vasodilator in patients with pulmonary arterial hypertension: comparison with inhaled nitric oxide, *Circulation* 105(20):2398–2403, 2002.
35. Benedict N, Seybert A, Mathier MA: Evidence-based pharmacologic management of pulmonary arterial hypertension, *Clin Ther* 29(10):2134–2153, 2007.
36. Rubin LJ, Badesch DB, Fleming TR, et al: Long-term treatment with sildenafil citrate in pulmonary arterial hypertension: SUPER-2, *Chest* 2011.
37. Cruz-Blanquel A, Espinosa-Oropeza A, Romo-Hernandez G, et al: Persistent pulmonary hypertension in the newborn: therapeutic effect of sildenafil, *Proc West Pharmacol Soc* 51:73–77, 2008.
38. Fisher PW, Salloum F, Das A, et al: Phosphodiesterase-5 inhibition with sildenafil attenuates cardiomyocyte apoptosis and left ventricular dysfunction in a chronic model of doxorubicin cardiotoxicity, *Circulation* 111(13):1601–1610, 2005.
39. Nagayama T, Hsu S, Zhang M, et al: Sildenafil stops progressive chamber, cellular, and molecular remodeling and improves calcium handling and function in hearts with pre-existing advanced hypertrophy caused by pressure overload, *J Am Coll Cardiol* 53(2):207–215, 2009.
40. Guazzi M, Vicenzi M, Arena R, et al: PDE5 inhibition with sildenafil improves left ventricular diastolic function, cardiac geometry, and clinical status in patients with stable systolic heart failure: results of a 1-year, prospective, randomized, placebo-controlled study, *Circ Heart Fail* 4(1):8–17, 2011.
41. Hao CM, Breyer MD: Physiological regulation of prostaglandins in the kidney, *Annu Rev Physiol* 70:357–377, 2008.
42. Tilley SL, Coffman TM, Koller BH: Mixed messages: modulation of inflammation and immune responses by prostaglandins and thromboxanes, *J Clin Invest* 108(1):15–23, 2001.
43. Rockwell CE, Raman P, Kaplan BL, et al: A COX-2 metabolite of the endogenous cannabinoid, 2-arachidonyl glycerol, mediates suppression of IL-2 secretion in activated Jurkat T cells, *Biochem Pharmacol* 76(3):353–361, 2008.
44. Feletou M, Huang Y, Vanhoutte PM: Endothelium-mediated control of vascular tone: COX-1 and COX-2 products, *Br J Pharmacol* 2011.
45. Hu ZW, Kerb R, Shi XY, et al: Angiotensin II increases expression of cyclooxygenase-2: implications for the function of vascular smooth muscle cells, *J Pharmacol Exp Ther* 303(2):563–573, 2002.

46. Tang EH, Leung FP, Huang Y, et al: Calcium and reactive oxygen species increase in endothelial cells in response to releasers of endothelium-derived contracting factor, Br J Pharmacol 151(1):15–23, 2007.

47. Bunimov N, Laneuville O: Cyclooxygenase inhibitors: instrumental drugs to understand cardiovascular homeostasis and arterial thrombosis, Cardiovasc Hematol Disord Drug Targets 8(4):268–277, 2008.

48. Baigent C, Blackwell L, Collins R, et al: Aspirin in the primary and secondary prevention of vascular disease: collaborative meta-analysis of individual participant data from randomised trials, Lancet 373(9678):1849–1860, 2009.

49. Bartolucci AA, Tendera M, Howard G: Meta-analysis of multiple primary prevention trials of cardiovascular events using aspirin, Am J Cardiol 107(12):1796–1801, 2011.

50. Stavrakis S, Stoner JA, Azar M, et al: Low-dose aspirin for primary prevention of cardiovascular events in patients with diabetes: a meta-analysis, Am J Med Sci 341(1):1–9, 2011.

51. Simpson SH, Gamble JM, Mereu L, et al: Effect of aspirin dose on mortality and cardiovascular events in people with diabetes: A meta-analysis, J Gen Intern Med 2011.

52. Kronish IM, Rieckmann N, Shimbo D, et al: Aspirin adherence, aspirin dosage, and C-reactive protein in the first 3 months after acute coronary syndrome, Am J Cardiol 106(8):1090–1094, 2010.

53. Yamamoto Y, Yamashita T, Kitagawa F, et al: The effect of the long term aspirin administration on the progress of atherosclerosis in apoE-/- LDLR-/- double knockout mouse, Thromb Res 125(3):246–252, 2010.

54. Cyrus T, Sung S, Zhao L, et al: Effect of low-dose aspirin on vascular inflammation, plaque stability, and atherogenesis in low-density lipoprotein receptor-deficient mice, Circulation 106(10):1282–1287, 2002.

55. Bresalier RS, Sandler RS, Quan H, et al: Cardiovascular events associated with rofecoxib in a colorectal adenoma chemoprevention trial, N Engl J Med 352(11):1092–1102, 2005.

56. Mitchell JA, Warner TD: COX isoforms in the cardiovascular system: understanding the activities of nonsteroidal antiinflammatory drugs, Nat Rev Drug Discov 5(1):75–86, 2006.

57. Antman EM, DeMets D, Loscalzo J: Cyclooxygenase inhibition and cardiovascular risk, Circulation 112(5):759–770, 2005.

58. Barst RJ, Rubin LJ, Long WA, et al: A comparison of continuous intravenous epoprostenol (prostacyclin) with conventional therapy for primary pulmonary hypertension. The Primary Pulmonary Hypertension Study Group, N Engl J Med 334(5):296–302, 1996.

59. Badesch DB, Tapson VF, McGoon MD, et al: Continuous intravenous epoprostenol for pulmonary hypertension due to the scleroderma spectrum of disease. A randomized, controlled trial, Ann Intern Med 132(6):425–434, 2000.

60. Chen YF, Jowett S, Barton P, et al: Clinical and cost-effectiveness of epoprostenol, iloprost, bosentan, sitaxentan and sildenafil for pulmonary arterial hypertension within their licensed indications: a systematic review and economic evaluation, Health Technol Assess 13(49):1–320, 2009.

61. Freeman R: Clinical practice. Neurogenic orthostatic hypotension, N Engl J Med 358(6):615–624, 2008.

62. Sequeira IM, Haberberger RV, Kummer W: Atrial and ventricular rat coronary arteries are differently supplied by noradrenergic, cholinergic and nitrergic, but not sensory nerve fibres, Ann Anat 187(4):345–355, 2005.

63. Murad F: Shattuck Lecture. Nitric oxide and cyclic GMP in cell signaling and drug development, N Engl J Med 355(19):2003–2011, 2006.

64. Schachinger V, Britten MB, Zeiher AM: Prognostic impact of coronary vasodilator dysfunction on adverse long-term outcome of coronary heart disease, Circulation 101(16):1899–1906, 2000.

65. Perticone F, Ceravolo R, Pujia A, et al: Prognostic significance of endothelial dysfunction in hypertensive patients, Circulation 104(2):191–196, 2001.

66. Pretorius M, Rosenbaum DA, Lefebvre J, et al: Smoking impairs bradykinin-stimulated t-PA release, Hypertension 39(3):767–771, 2002.

67. Pretorius M, Rosenbaum D, Vaughan DE, et al: Angiotensin-converting enzyme inhibition increases human vascular tissue-type plasminogen activator release through endogenous bradykinin, Circulation 107(4):579–585, 2003.

68. DeSouza CA, Shapiro LF, Clevenger CM, et al: Regular aerobic exercise prevents and restores age-related declines in endothelium-dependent vasodilation in healthy men, Circulation 102(12):1351–1357, 2000.

69. van Zwieten PA, Doods HN: Muscarinic receptors and drugs in cardiovascular medicine, Cardiovasc Drugs Ther 9(1):159–167, 1995.

70. Brede M, Philipp M, Knaus A, et al: Alpha2-adrenergic receptor subtypes--novel functions uncovered in gene-targeted mouse models, Biol Cell 96(5):343–348, 2004.

71. Civantos CB, Aleixandre de AA: Alpha-adrenoceptor subtypes, Pharmacol Res 44(3):195–208, 2001.

72. Gao F, de Beer VJ, Hoekstra M, et al: Both beta1- and beta2-adrenoceptors contribute to feedforward coronary resistance vessel dilation during exercise, Am J Physiol Heart Circ Physiol 298(3):H921–H929, 2010.

73. Davis E, Loiacono R, Summers RJ: The rush to adrenaline: drugs in sport acting on the beta-adrenergic system, Br J Pharmacol 154(3):584–597, 2008.

74. Docherty JR: Pharmacology of stimulants prohibited by the World Anti-Doping Agency (WADA), Br J Pharmacol 154(3):606–622, 2008.

75. Grossman E, Messerli FH: Secondary hypertension: interfering substances, J Clin Hypertens (Greenwich) 10(7):556–566, 2008.

76. Haller CA, Benowitz NL: Adverse cardiovascular and central nervous system events associated with dietary supplements containing ephedra alkaloids, N Engl J Med 343(25):1833–1838, 2000.

77. Morelli A, Ertmer C, Rehberg S, et al: Phenylephrine versus norepinephrine for initial hemodynamic support of patients with septic shock: a randomized, controlled trial, Crit Care 12(6):R143, 2008.

78. De BD, Creteur J, Silva E, et al: Effects of dopamine, norepinephrine, and epinephrine on the splanchnic circulation in septic shock: which is best? Crit Care Med 31(6):1659–1667, 2003.

79. Nygren A, Thoren A, Ricksten SE: Vasopressors and intestinal mucosal perfusion after cardiac surgery: norepinephrine vs. phenylephrine, Crit Care Med 34(3):722–729, 2006.

80. Levy B, Perez P, Perny J, et al: Comparison of norepinephrine-dobutamine to epinephrine for hemodynamics, lactate metabolism, and organ function variables in cardiogenic shock. A prospective, randomized pilot study, Crit Care Med 39(3):450–455, 2011.

81. Russell JA, Walley KR, Singer J, et al: Vasopressin versus norepinephrine infusion in patients with septic shock, N Engl J Med 358(9):877–887, 2008.

82. Furberg CD, Wright JT, Davis BR,et al: Major cardiovascular events in hypertensive patients randomized to doxazosin vs. chlorthalidone: the antihypertensive and lipid-lowering treatment to prevent heart attack trial (ALLHAT). ALLHAT Collaborative Research Group, JAMA 283(15):1967–1975, 2000.

83. Frye CB, Vance MA: Hypertensive crisis and myocardial infarction following massive clonidine overdose, Ann Pharmacother 34(5):611–615, 2000.

84. Robertson D, Goldberg MR, Hollister AS, et al: Clonidine raises blood pressure in severe idiopathic orthostatic hypotension, Am J Med 74(2):193–200, 1983.

85. Cruickshank JM: Are we misunderstanding beta-blockers, Int J Cardiol 120(1):10–27, 2007.

86. Dessy C, Balligand JL: Beta3-adrenergic receptors in cardiac and vascular tissues emerging concepts and therapeutic perspectives, Adv Pharmacol 59:135–163, 2010.

87. Schrier RW, Abraham WT: Hormones and hemodynamics in heart failure, N Engl J Med 341(8):577–585, 1999.

88. Beaulieu JM, Gainetdinov RR: The physiology, signaling, and pharmacology of dopamine receptors, Pharmacol Rev 63(1):182–217, 2011.

89. De BD, Biston P, Devriendt J, et al: Comparison of dopamine and norepinephrine in the treatment of shock, N Engl J Med 362(9):779–789, 2010.

90. Patel GP, Grahe JS, Sperry M, et al: Efficacy and safety of dopamine versus norepinephrine in the management of septic shock, Shock 33(4):375–380, 2010.

91. Devlin JW, Seta ML, Kanji S, et al: Fenoldopam versus nitroprusside for the treatment of hypertensive emergency, Ann Pharmacother 38(5):755–759, 2004.

92. Landoni G, Biondi-Zoccai GG, Tumlin JA, et al: Beneficial impact of fenoldopam in critically ill patients with or at risk for acute renal failure: a meta-analysis of randomized clinical trials, Am J Kidney Dis 49(1):56–68, 2007.

93. Landoni G, Biondi-Zoccai GG, Marino G, et al: Fenoldopam reduces the need for renal replacement therapy and in-hospital death in cardiovascular surgery: a meta-analysis, J Cardiothorac Vasc Anesth 22(1):27–33, 2008.

94. Stone GW, McCullough PA, Tumlin JA, et al: Fenoldopam mesylate for the prevention of contrast-induced nephropathy: a randomized controlled trial, JAMA 290(17):2284–2291, 2003.

95. Gopal S, Jayakumar D, Nelson PN: Meta-analysis on the effect of dopexamine on in-hospital mortality, Anaesthesia 64(6):589–594, 2009.

96. Davies SJ, Yates D, Wilson RJ: Dopexamine has no additional benefit in high-risk patients receiving goal-directed fluid therapy undergoing major abdominal surgery, Anesth Analg 112(1):130–138, 2011.

97. Basile J: The role of existing and newer calcium channel blockers in the treatment of hypertension, J Clin Hypertens (Greenwich) 6(11):621–629, 2004.

98. Abernethy DR, Schwartz JB: Calcium-antagonist drugs, N Engl J Med 341(19):1447–1457, 1999.

99. Grossman E, Messerli FH, Grodzicki T, et al: Should a moratorium be placed on sublingual nifedipine capsules given for hypertensive emergencies and pseudoemergencies? JAMA 276(16):1328–1331, 1996.

100. Sica DA: Minoxidil: an underused vasodilator for resistant or severe hypertension, J Clin Hypertens (Greenwich) 6(5):283–287, 2004.

101. Peti-Peterdi J, Harris RC: Macula densa sensing and signaling mechanisms of renin release, J Am Soc Nephrol 21(7):1093–1096, 2010.

102. Crackower MA, Sarao R, Oudit GY, et al: Angiotensin-converting enzyme 2 is an essential regulator of heart function, Nature 417(6891):822–828, 2002.

103. Oliveira L, Costa-Neto CM, Nakaie CR, et al: The angiotensin II AT1 receptor structure-activity correlations in the light of rhodopsin structure, Physiol Rev 87(2):565–592, 2007.

104. Oppermann M, Gess B, Schweda F, et al: Atrap deficiency increases arterial blood pressure and plasma volume, J Am Soc Nephrol 21(3):468–477, 2010.

105. Carey RM, Padia SH: Angiotensin AT2 receptors: control of renal sodium excretion and blood pressure, Trends Endocrinol Metab 19(3):84–87, 2008.

106. Porrello ER, Delbridge LM, Thomas WG: The angiotensin II type 2 (AT2) receptor: an enigmatic seven transmembrane receptor, Front Biosci 14:958–972, 2009.

107. Butterworth MB, Edinger RS, Frizzell RA, et al: Regulation of the epithelial sodium channel by membrane trafficking, Am J Physiol Renal Physiol 296(1):F10–F24, 2009.

108. Hoorn EJ, Nelson JH, McCormick JA, et al: The WNK Kinase Network Regulating Sodium, Potassium, and Blood Pressure, J Am Soc Nephrol 22(4):605–614, 2011.

109. Vallon V, Schroth J, Lang F, et al: Expression and phosphorylation of the Na+-Cl-cotransporter NCC in vivo is regulated by dietary salt, potassium, and SGK1, Am J Physiol Renal Physiol 297(3):F704–F712, 2009.

110. Ferrario CM, Varagic J: The ANG-(1-7)/ACE2/mas axis in the regulation of nephron function, Am J Physiol Renal Physiol 298(6):F1297–F1305, 2010.

111. Alenina N, Xu P, Rentzsch B, et al: Genetically altered animal models for Mas and angiotensin-(1-7), Exp Physiol 93(5):528–537, 2008.

112. Zhong J, Basu R, Guo D, et al: Angiotensin-converting enzyme 2 suppresses pathological hypertrophy, myocardial fibrosis, and cardiac dysfunction, Circulation 122(7):717–728, 18, 2010.

113. Nguyen G: Renin, (pro)renin and receptor: an update, Clin Sci (Lond) 120(5):169–178, 2011.

114. Feldt S, Batenburg WW, Mazak I, et al: Prorenin and renin-induced extracellular signal-regulated kinase 1/2 activation in monocytes is not blocked by aliskiren or the handle-region peptide, Hypertension 51(3):682–688, 2008.

115. Cushman DW, Ondetti MA: History of the design of captopril and related inhibitors of angiotensin converting enzyme, Hypertension 17(4):589–592, 1991.

116. Jensen C, Herold P, Brunner HR: Aliskiren: the first renin inhibitor for clinical treatment, Nat Rev Drug Discov 7(5):399–410, 2008.

117. Campbell DJ: Interpretation of plasma renin concentration in patients receiving aliskiren therapy, Hypertension 51(1):15–18, 2008.

118. Stanton AV, Gradman AH, Schmieder RE, et al: Aliskiren monotherapy does not cause paradoxical blood pressure rises: meta-analysis of data from 8 clinical trials, Hypertension 55(1):54–60, 2010.

119. Oparil S, Yarows SA, Patel S, et al: Efficacy and safety of combined use of aliskiren and valsartan in patients with hypertension: a randomised, double-blind trial, Lancet 370(9583):221–229, 2007.

120. Nussberger J, Wuerzner G, Jensen C, et al: Angiotensin II suppression in humans by the orally active renin inhibitor aliskiren (SPP100): comparison with enalapril, *Hypertension* 39(1):E1–E8, 2002.

121. Stanton A, Jensen C, Nussberger J, et al: Blood pressure lowering in essential hypertension with an oral renin inhibitor, aliskiren, *Hypertension* 42(6):1137–1143, 2003.

122. Parving HH, Persson F, Lewis JB, et al: Aliskiren combined with losartan in type 2 diabetes and nephropathy, *N Engl J Med* 358(23):2433–2446, 2008.

123. Solomon SD, Appelbaum E, Manning WJ, et al: Effect of the direct renin inhibitor aliskiren, the angiotensin receptor blocker losartan, or both on left ventricular mass in patients with hypertension and left ventricular hypertrophy, *Circulation* 119(4):530–537, 2009.

124. Burnier M: Angiotensin II type 1 receptor blockers, *Circulation* 103(6):904–912, 2001.

125. Benson SC, Pershadsingh HA, Ho CI, et al: Identification of telmisartan as a unique angiotensin II receptor antagonist with selective PPARgamma-modulating activity, *Hypertension* 43(5):993–1002, 2004.

126. Kappert K, Tsuprykov O, Kaufmann J, et al: Chronic treatment with losartan results in sufficient serum levels of the metabolite EXP3179 for PPARgamma activation, *Hypertension* 54(4):738–743, 2009.

127. Cooper WO, Hernandez-Diaz S, Arbogast PG, et al: Major congenital malformations after first-trimester exposure to ACE inhibitors, *N Engl J Med* 354(23):2443–2451, 2006.

128. Palmer BF: Managing hyperkalemia caused by inhibitors of the renin-angiotensin-aldosterone system, *N Engl J Med* 351(6):585–592, 2004.

129. Sica DA: Angiotensin-converting enzyme inhibitors side effects--physiologic and non-physiologic considerations, *J Clin Hypertens (Greenwich)* 6(7):410–416, 2004.

130. Zannad F, McMurray JJ, Krum H, et al: Eplerenone in patients with systolic heart failure and mild symptoms, *N Engl J Med* 364(1):11–21, 2011.

131. Pitt B, Remme W, Zannad F, et al: Eplerenone, a selective aldosterone blocker, in patients with left ventricular dysfunction after myocardial infarction, *N Engl J Med* 348(14):1309–1321, 2003.

132. Pitt B, Zannad F, Remme WJ, et al: The effect of spironolactone on morbidity and mortality in patients with severe heart failure. Randomized Aldactone Evaluation Study Investigators, *N Engl J Med* 341(10):709–717, 1999.

133. Vaclavik J, Sedlak R, Plachy M, et al: Addition of Spironolactone in Patients With Resistant Arterial Hypertension (ASPIRANT): a randomized, double-blind, placebo-controlled trial, *Hypertension* 57(6):1069–1075, 2011.

134. Kohan DE, Rossi NF, Inscho EW, et al: Regulation of blood pressure and salt homeostasis by endothelin, *Physiol Rev* 91(1):1–77, 2011.

135. Dhaun N, Goddard J, Kohan DE, et al: Role of endothelin-1 in clinical hypertension: 20 years on, *Hypertension* 52(3):452–459, 2008.

136. Channick RN, Simonneau G, Sitbon O, et al: Effects of the dual endothelin-receptor antagonist bosentan in patients with pulmonary hypertension: a randomised placebo-controlled study, *Lancet* 358(9288):1119–1123, 2001.

137. Anderson JR, Nawarskas JJ: Pharmacotherapeutic management of pulmonary arterial hypertension, *Cardiol Rev* 18(3):148–162, 2010.

138. Weber MA, Black H, Bakris G, et al: A selective endothelin-receptor antagonist to reduce blood pressure in patients with treatment-resistant hypertension: a randomised, double-blind, placebo-controlled trial, *Lancet* 374(9699):1423–1431, 2009.

139. Anand I, McMurray J, Cohn JN, et al: Long-term effects of darusentan on left-ventricular remodelling and clinical outcomes in the EndothelinA Receptor Antagonist Trial in Heart Failure (EARTH): randomised, double-blind, placebo-controlled trial, *Lancet* 364(9431):347–354, 2004.

140. McMurray JJ, Teerlink JR, Cotter G, et al: Effects of tezosentan on symptoms and clinical outcomes in patients with acute heart failure: the VERITAS randomized controlled trials, *JAMA* 298(17):2009–2019, 2007.

VASCULAR PHARMACOLOGY

CHAPTER 7 | # Pharmacology of Antithrombotic Drugs

Omar P. Haqqani, Mark D. Iafrati, Jane E. Freedman

Atherothrombotic disease and atherosclerotic plaque rupture is the leading cause of death worldwide. Its prevalence among adults in the United States is estimated at over 81 million, with costs exceeding $503 billion annually.[1] Thrombus and clot formation involved in atherothrombotic disease develop as a complex and dynamic interaction between platelets, blood vessel wall, and coagulation cascades. Increased understanding of the mechanism of these interactions has provided for the development of novel drugs. Antiplatelet drugs have come to the forefront in managing atherothrombotic disease, owing in large part to platelets' involvement in the initiation and propagation of thrombus. Our understanding of platelet function has expanded from a rudimentary knowledge of aspirin as a cyclooxygenase (COX) inhibitor within the arachidonic acid pathways, to a more complex picture of multiple receptor-modulating agents including thienopyridines, glycoprotein (GP)IIb/IIIa receptor antagonists, von Willebrand factor (vWF)-GPIb/IX, and collagen-GPVI inhibitors. Despite advances with newer inhibitors and combinations, treatment failures persist, necessitating development of new antiplatelet agents.

Also contributing to thrombus formation, the coagulation cascade is intimately linked with platelet activation and continues to be an area of therapeutic interest. Our deeper understanding of coagulation pathway targets has channeled numerous novel agents that regulate coagulation, limiting thrombus propagation and atherosclerotic plaque rupture. Synergistic effects of novel antiplatelet and anticoagulation therapies have provided new options for evaluating clinical outcomes in the management of cardiovascular disease.

Platelets, Thrombosis, Coagulation, and Atherothrombotic Vascular Disease

Atherosclerotic plaque rupture and endothelial cell (EC) disruption lead to platelet activation and formation of occlusive thrombi, triggering acute ischemic events in patients with atherothrombotic disease. Platelet activation and aggregation involve multiple signaling molecules and their receptors. Initially, platelets adhere to the subendothelial proteins vWF and collagen), which are exposed at sites of vascular injury. Adenosine diphosphate (ADP), thromboxane A_2 (TxA_2), serotonin, collagen, and thrombin activate platelets through unique intracellular signaling pathways, resulting in further platelet activation and secretion of mediators, thus further amplifying and sustaining the initial platelet response.[2] Adenosine diphosphate, serotonin, and calcium are released by activated platelets via degranulation; thromboxane from arachidonic acid; and thrombin from activated coagulation cascade pathways.[3] Activation of platelets occurs through binding of their primary blood-soluble agonists to their respective platelet receptors: ADP binds P2Y1 and P2Y12, thrombin binds to protease-activated receptor 1 (PAR1) and PAR4, and thromboxane binds to the thromboxane/prostanoid (TP) receptor.[4] The final common pathway for all autocrine and paracrine activation signals is GPIIb/IIIa activation, which mediates fibrinogen and vWF binding to platelets and contributes to platelet aggregation. Thus, in both physiological hemostasis and pathological states, platelets are recruited to form a platelet-fibrin thrombus.[3,4] Various classes of antiplatelet drugs act synergistically through complementary yet independent mechanisms, preventing platelet aggregation and thus acute thrombus formation. Currently available drugs and those under investigation target the thromboxane-induced (aspirin, sulfinpyrazone, indobufen, and triflusal) and ADP-induced (ticlopidine,

clopidogrel, prasugrel, ticagrelor, cangrelor and elinogrel) pathways of platelet activation and their final common pathway of GPIIb/IIIa-induced (abciximab, eptifibatide, and tirofiban) platelet aggregation.[4,5] The processes of platelet adhesion, activation, and aggregation, along with the targets of platelet-inhibiting drugs, are shown in Figure 7-1. Antiplatelet drugs, in addition to inhibiting acute arterial thrombosis, interfere with the physiological role of platelets in hemostasis. Thus the range of adverse effects, particularly bleeding, is a major factor in evaluating the utility of available and upcoming antiplatelet drugs and their combination regimens. Coagulation cascades are intimately activated through atherosclerotic plaque rupture and platelet activation. Targets of drug therapy to regulate the effects of thrombus formation and propagation are accomplished through oral anticoagulation (warfarin); thrombin inhibitors, both direct and indirect (heparin, low-molecular-weight heparin [LMWH], fondaparinux, hirudins, bivalirudin, argatroban, ximelagatran, dabigatran, etexilate, rivaroxaban, apixaban, DU-176b, LY517717, betrixaban, and YM150); factor IX inhibitors; and factor Xa inhibitors.

Pharmacology of Platelet Inhibitors

Platelets circulate in blood with their activation inhibited by both nitric oxide (NO) and prostaglandin I_2 released from ECs.[6,7] Activated platelets prevent bleeding by catalyzing the formation of stable blood clot in conjunction with activated coagulation pathways. In the initiation phase of primary hemostasis, platelets roll, adhere, and spread along the exposed collagen matrix of injured blood vessels to form an activated platelet monolayer.[8] During the rolling phase, platelet adhesion and tethering is mediated by the platelet GPIb/V/IX receptor complex and vWF, which itself is bound to collagen (see Fig. 7-1). Additional tethering is accomplished between the GPVI and GPIa proteins directly with collagen at sites of vascular injury.[6–8] The binding of GPIb/V/IX to vWF has a fast off rate insufficient to mediate stable adhesion, but instead, able to maintain platelets in close contact with the endothelial surface. Platelet activation stimulates high-affinity integrins to form stable adhesion complexes.

Blood flows with greater velocity in the center of the vessel than near the wall, thereby generating shear forces between adjacent layers of fluid. In conditions of high shear, such as those of small arteries, arterioles, and stenosed arteries, the tethering process is integral in the mechanisms of platelet adhesion. von Willebrand factor binds to collagen within the extracellular matrix (ECM) and to platelet receptors (GPIb/V/IX and GPIIb/IIIa [$\alpha IIb\beta 3$ integrin]).[8] Binding of ECM collagen triggers intracellular signals that shift platelet integrins to a higher-affinity state and induce release of the secondary mediators ADP and TxA_2. Both ADP and TxA_2, along with thrombin produced from the coagulation cascade, synergistically induce full platelet activation. Upon platelet activation, arachidonic acid is liberated from membrane phospholipids by phospholipase A_2 and C, thereby producing TxA_2. Aspirin and other agents, such as sulfinpyrazone, indobufen, and triflusal, act to inhibit enzymes within the arachidonic acid cascade, thereby limiting production of TxA_2. Adenosine diphosphate binds to $P2Y_1$ and $P2Y_{12}$ surface platelet receptors, which are targets of clopidogrel, prasugrel, and ticagrelor.

Thrombin is produced at the surface of activated platelets by tissue factor and is responsible for generating fibrin from fibrinogen, which contributes to formation of the hemostatic plug and platelet thrombus growth. Thrombin also directly activates platelets through stimulation of the PAR1.[7] Both direct and indirect

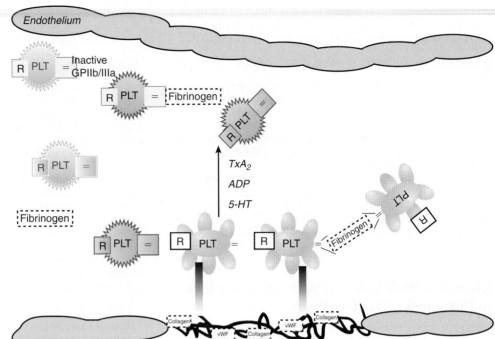

FIGURE 7-1 Platelet activation and thrombosis. Platelets circulate in an inactive form in vasculature. Damage to endothelium and/or external stimuli activate platelets that adhere to exposed subendothelial von Willebrand factor (vWF) and collagen. This adhesion leads to platelet activation, shape change, and synthesis and release of thromboxane A₂ (TxA₂, serotonin (5-HT), and adenosine diphosphate (ADP). Platelet stimuli cause conformational change in platelet integrin glycoprotein (GP) IIb/IIIa receptor, leading to high-affinity binding of fibrinogen and formation of a stable platelet thrombus.

inhibitors of thrombin inhibit thrombin and affect thrombin activation, respectively. Release of ADP and TxA₂ from adherent platelets contributes to recruitment of circulating platelets, thereby inducing a change in platelet shape, increased expression of proinflammatory molecules (P-selectin, CD40 ligand), expression of platelet procoagulant activity, and conversion of the GPIIb/IIIa receptor into an active form, leading to pathological thrombosis.[6–8] Activation of GPIIb/IIIa (αIIβ3 integrin) mediates platelet aggregation and spreading on the exposed ECM of the injured vessel wall by means of fibrinogen bridges.[8]

Fibrinogen bridges activated platelets and contributes to thrombus stabilization.[8] Activation of platelets results in a conformational change in the αIIβ3 integrin (IIb/IIIa) receptor, enabling it to bind fibrinogen-enhancing cross-links to adjacent platelets, resulting in aggregation and formation of a platelet plug. Simultaneous activation of the coagulation system results in thrombin generation and fibrin clot formation, which further stabilizes the platelet plug. Abciximab, eptifibatide, and tirofiban inhibit GPIIb/IIIa, thereby inhibiting platelet aggregation.

Cyclooxygenase Inhibitors and the Arachidonic Acid Cascade

Arachidonic acid is liberated from membrane phospholipids by phospholipase A₂ and C upon platelet stimulation[9] (Fig. 7-2). Prostaglandin (PG) H-synthase catalyzes the conversion of arachidonic acid to PGG₂ and PGH₂.[10] Prostaglandin-synthase possesses two catalytic sites, a COX site, responsible for the formation of PGG₂ and a hydroperoxidase site, which reduces the 15-hydroperoxyl group of PGG₂ to produce PGH₂.[11] Subsequent enzymatic catalyzation of PGH₂ generates PGs, D₂, E₂, F₂α, I₂, and TxA₂.[11] Aspirin irreversibly binds and inhibits the COX site by acetylating the hydroxyl group of a serine residue at position 529 (Ser 529) without affecting the hydroperoxidase activity of the enzyme, thus inhibiting production of PGG₂ and therefore PGH₂ circumventing TxA₂ production.[12]

ASPIRIN

Aspirin produces dose-dependent inhibition of platelet COX activity after a single oral dose. A single dose of 100 mg effectively suppresses biosynthesis of TxA₂ within several minutes of administration via acetylation of platelet COX in the presystemic

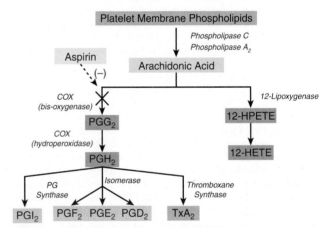

FIGURE 7-2 Metabolism of arachidonic acid in platelets. Arachidonic acid is metabolized through two catalytic pathways mediated by cyclooxygenase (COX) and lipoxygenase generating thromboxane A₂ (TxA₂) and 12-hydroxyeicosatetraenoic (12-HETE), respectively. PG, prostaglandin.

circulation.[13] Owing to aspirin's irreversible inhibition of COX and the inability of platelets to synthesize new proteins, aspirin's effect is maintained for the lifespan of the platelet (7-10 days). Cyclooxygenase activity returns only as new platelets are generated.

Aspirin reduces acute coronary and cerebrovascular events such as unstable angina, myocardial infarction (MI), sudden cardiac death, and stroke.[13] Its utility is enhanced by its modest cost and nominal side effects. Although aspirin effectively reduces platelet secretion and aggregation, it is a relatively weak platelet inhibitor. The inhibitory effects of aspirin are pronounced when using relatively weak platelet agonists, but less so against stronger agonists like thrombin that can induce platelet activation in the absence of TxA₂. Importantly, the majority of platelet responses remain unaffected by aspirin treatment. Aspirin does not inhibit shear stress–induced platelet activation and platelet adhesion. In addition to its antiplatelet properties, aspirin also exerts antiinflammatory effects.[14] In a meta-analysis of antiplatelet therapy studies in patients with acute coronary syndrome (ACS), administration of several doses of aspirin (from 75 mg/day up to 150 mg/day) significantly decreased the overall risk of nonfatal MI, nonfatal stroke, and death rates.[15] Several studies, however, have demonstrated that aspirin monotherapy is inadequate because of high intraindividual variability to aspirin response, as well as increased aspirin resistance, especially observed in patients with diabetes mellitus.[16]

NONSTEROIDAL ANTIINFLAMMATORY DRUGS

There are several nonsteroidal antiinflammatory drugs (NSAIDs) that act as competitive reversible inhibitors of PGH-synthase. Sulfinpyrazone, indobufen, and triflusal are several of the drugs in this class evaluated for their antithrombotic activity in randomized clinical trials. The active sulfide metabolite of sulfinpyrazone administered in the highest dose allowable (200 mg four times a day) inhibits only 60% of platelet COX activity, with results suggesting no significant clinical efficacy.[17] The clinical, biochemical, and functional effects of the more effective inhibitor, indobufen, are similar to those of aspirin. An oral dose of indobufen 200 mg twice daily inhibits 95% of platelet TxA_2 synthesis.[18] Triflusal, a derivative of salicylic acid, is also able to inhibit platelet COX, but only after conversion to a longer-lasting metabolite.[19] None of the three are currently approved for use as antiplatelet drugs in the United States.

Adenosine Diphosphate, Purinergic Receptors, and Thienopyridine Inhibitors

Adenosine diphosphate is a key mediator in activating platelet aggregation and thrombus formation. Inhibiting the effects of ADP activity has lead to development of numerous $P2Y_{12}$ receptor–targeting antiplatelet drugs. Adenosine diphosphate is released from dense granules of activated platelets, providing a soluble positive feedback mediator binding to the receptors $P2Y_1$ and $P2Y_{12}$. Both $P2Y_1$ and $P2Y_{12}$ are platelet surface-bound purinoreceptors belonging to the G protein–coupled receptor (GPCR) class, with $P2Y_1$ being coupled to G_q and $P2Y_{12}$ to G_i. Adenosine diphosphate binding to both $P2Y_1$ and $P2Y_{12}$ receptors activates distinct intracellular signaling pathways.[20] Binding of ADP to the $P2Y_1$ receptor and its G_q protein mobilizes intracellular calcium, triggering a change in the platelet shape and rapid, reversible aggregation.[21] Adeosine diphosphate binding through the $P2Y_{12}$ receptor and its G_i protein results in reduced levels of cyclic adenosine monophosphate (cAMP), resulting in amplification of the platelet response, stabilization of resulting aggregates, and secretion of further mediators from platelet granules.[22] Binding of ADP to both $P2Y_1$ and $P2Y_{12}$ purinoreceptors is necessary for normal ADP-induced aggregation. $P2Y_{12}$ is considered the major platelet ADP receptor and, since it is more restricted in its expression throughout cell lines, has become an attractive therapeutic target for antithrombotic agents.[20]

THIENOPYRIDINE PLATELET P2Y12 RECEPTOR ANTAGONISTS

The thienopyridine class of antiplatelets (ticlopidine, clopidogrel, and prasugrel) selectively and irreversibly inhibit the $P2Y_{12}$ purinoreceptor throughout the life of the platelet. Clopidogrel is the dominant member within the class and provides for modest platelet inhibition, delayed onset of action, and significant interpatient variability, including nonresponsiveness to the drug, which necessitated the search for more potent and stable alternatives.[23] Ticlopidine has been eclipsed because of its adverse hematological side effects, including neutropenia and thrombotic thrombocytopenic purpura.[24] The opposite, however, is true of third-generation thienopyridines, namely prasugrel.

Oral thienopyridines are prodrugs that require conversion into their active metabolites by hepatic cytochrome P450 (CYP) enzymes (CYP3A4 isozyme). Whereas clopidogrel requires esterase inactivation and a two-step CYP-dependent activation, prasugrel requires only one reaction to yield its active metabolite.[25] This difference in metabolism translates into different patient responses and drug interactions. Genetic variations of P450 (CYP) enzymes affect clopidogrel's active metabolite formation, resulting in lower platelet inhibition and, most importantly, a higher rate of major adverse cardiovascular events. Prasugrel's pharmacology, however,

is not affected by CYP polymorphisms and provides a stable platform for antiplatelet therapy. Prasugrel has a faster onset of action and a tenfold higher potency than clopidogrel.[26]

CLOPIDOGREL

Clopidogrel is metabolized by CYP P450. Its active metabolite irreversibly binds to the platelet $P2Y_{12}$ receptor, thus inhibiting the effect of ADP on platelets. As a result, GPIIb/IIIa receptors have decreased activation, thereby resulting in reduced platelet function. The Clopidogrel versus Aspirin in Patients at Risk of Ischemic Events (CAPRIE) study, a randomized trial that included patients with ischemic stroke, MI, or symptomatic atherosclerotic peripheral artery disease, showed that clopidogrel-treated patients had an 8.7% relative risk reduction for acute MI, stroke, or vascular death, compared to those patients treated with aspirin.[27] The Clopidogrel in Unstable Angina to Prevent Recurrent Events (CURE) trial was the first study establishing the significance of dual antiplatelet therapy (acetylsalicylic acid [ASA] plus clopidogrel) in patients with ACS[28] and involved a population of 12,562 patients presenting with non-ST-elevation ACS who were randomized to receive either a combination of ASA (75-325 mg/day) and clopidogrel (300 mg loading dose, followed by 75 mg/day) or ASA and placebo for 3 to 12 months. At 12 months, a lower incidence of MI, stroke, or cardiovascular death was observed in the clopidogrel plus ASA group compared to the placebo group; however, the risk of major bleeding was increased among patients treated with clopidogrel plus ASA.

Similar results were reported by the COMMIT study.[29] Patients received either a combination of clopidogrel (75 mg/day) and ASA (162 mg/day) or placebo and ASA for 28 days or until hospital discharge. There was a 9% relative risk reduction in the composite endpoint of stroke, vascular reinfarction, or death and a 7% relative risk reduction for death in the group receiving dual antiplatelet therapy. In the CREDO study, which was the first to evaluate the significance of dual antiplatelet therapy pre- and post-percutaneous coronary intervention (PCI), patients undergoing PCI received either a 300-mg loading dose of clopidogrel 3 to 24 hours before the procedure and then 75 mg/day for 12 months, or 75 mg/day for 30 days after the procedure without a loading dose.[30] All patients also received a 325 mg/day dose of ASA during the 12-month follow-up period. A 27% relative risk reduction for death, MI, or stroke was observed in the group receiving long-term dual antiplatelet therapy. Given the established antiplatelet effect of clopidogrel, the Clopidogrel for High Atherothrombotic Risk and Ischemic Stabilization Management and Avoidance (CHARISMA) study investigated the potential benefit from 28-month dual antiplatelet therapy (75 mg/day clopidogrel and 75-162 mg/day ASA) in patients 45 years of age or older who experienced one of the following conditions: multiple atherothrombotic risk factors, documented coronary disease, documented cerebrovascular disease, or documented symptomatic peripheral artery disease.[31] The control group received ASA and placebo. No benefit was observed in the primary endpoint of MI, stroke, or cardiovascular death in the dual antiplatelet therapy group. By contrast, asymptomatic patients of the group with risk factors but without clinical evidence of CAD had a higher risk of bleeding.[32] A further analysis in the subgroup of patients with documented atherothrombotic cardiovascular disease showed a significant risk reduction for new MI, stroke, or cardiovascular death in those patients compared with controls.[33]

PRASUGREL

Prasugrel is a $P2Y_{12}$ inhibitor acting similarly to clopidogrel. Prasugrel is rapidly converted to its active metabolite by the P450 cytochrome and has higher bioavailability than clopidogrel.[26] Recently, a 60-mg loading dose of prasugrel achieved high platelet inhibition both in healthy subjects and in patients scheduled for PCI, whereas healthy clopidogrel poor-responders achieved satisfactory platelet inhibition of up to 80% after prasugrel administration.[26] The beneficial effect of prasugrel was also established in the TRITON-TIMI 38 study.[34] Patients scheduled for PCI were randomized to receive either clopidogrel (300-mg loading dose and 75 mg/day afterwards) or prasugrel (60-mg loading dose and 10 mg/day afterwards). All patients also received ASA, and about half the patients from each group were treated with a GPIIb/IIIa inhibitor as well. The prasugrel group demonstrated a significant risk reduction for the composite primary endpoint of death, nonfatal MI, and nonfatal stroke. In addition, risk was significantly lower in the diabetes mellitus patient subgroup[34]; however, incidence of major hemorrhagic events was more frequent in the prasugrel group, but even when this parameter was added to the study's primary endpoints, the net clinical benefit findings still favored prasugrel compared to clopidogrel. Subgroup analysis demonstrated a higher rate of major bleeding in those with body weight of less than 60 kg, history of stroke or transient ischemic attack, and age older than 75 years.[34]

NON-THIENOPYRIDINE PLATELET P2Y12 RECEPTOR ANTAGONISTS

Novel non-thienopyridine platelet $P2Y_{12}$ receptor antagonists include ticagrelor, cangrelor, and elinogrel, which are direct and reversible $P2Y_{12}$ antagonists with rapid onsets and short durations of action. Ticagrelor is highly selective and very specific for the $P2Y_{12}$ receptor, and it exhibits a greater, more consistent inhibition of platelet aggregation than clopidogrel.[35] Ticagrelor is administered orally and does not require metabolic activation, providing a rapid onset peaking within 2 to 4 hours of dosing. The metabolism of ticagrelor yields an active molecule (AR-C124910XX) that has similar $P2Y_{12}$-blocking activity as its parent molecule. Ticagrelor's plasma half-life is approximately 12 hours, which corresponds to twice-daily dosing and a 1- to 2-day restoration of normal platelet-mediated hemostasis upon discontinuation. These pharmacokinetics are in contrast to clopidogrel and prasugrel, which require discontinuation approximately 5 days before restoration of normal platelet-mediated hemostasis is achieved. Ticagrelor's potential advantage in plasma half-life also carries the risk of increased thrombotic events if patients miss a dose.[36]

Multiple trials have demonstrated the benefits of ticagrelor in clinical practice. The Dose Confirmation Study Assessing Antiplatelet Effects of AZD6140 vs. Clopidogrel in Non-ST-Segment Elevation Myocardial Infarction (DISPERSE-2) trial showed no difference in major bleeding or MI, with an increase in minor bleeding at higher doses of ticagrelor in 990 patients with non-ST-segment elevation ACS.[37] In the PLATO (the Study of Platelet Inhibition and Patient Outcomes) trial comparing ticagrelor and clopidogrel with respect to their efficacy in preventing cardiovascular events and safety showed ticagrelor significantly reduced the rate of death from vascular causes, MI, or stroke, without an increase in the rate of overall major bleeding compared to clopidogrel in 18,624 patients with ACS.[38] Ticagrelor is the first investigational antiplatelet drug to demonstrate a reduction in cardiovascular death when compared to clopidogrel in patients with ACS.

Finally, research has shown ticagrelor to produce platelet inhibition regardless of genotypic variations in the three genes that had been associated with variability to clopidogrel in platelet inhibition.[39] All these trials underline the potential for ticagrelor to achieve a rapid and sustained antiplatelet effect that could be reversed and could overcome nonresponsiveness and interpatient variability to clopidogrel, thus addressing the main limitations of clopidogrel therapy.[24] Nonetheless, its adverse effects (e.g., dyspnea, bradycardia) and weight-based dosing require further investigation before ticagrelor may advance toward routine use in antiplatelet therapy.[38]

Role of Integrin Receptors in Platelet Function

Platelet activation leads to the final activation of GPIIb/IIIa receptors that bind adhesion molecules such as fibrinogen and vWF, thereby enhancing platelet aggregation. By competing with fibrinogen and vWF for GPIIb/IIIa binding, GPIIb/IIIa antagonists interfere

with platelet cross-linking and clot formation. Inhibition of approximately 80% of GPIIb/IIIa receptors results in clinically relevant inhibition of platelet-dependent thrombus formation. Investigation of oral GPIIb/IIIa inhibitors has been halted because of negative outcomes from several large trials in patients with ACS or undergoing PCI. Parenteral GPIIb/IIIa inhibitors are associated with an increased risk of bleeding and are only administered within the hospital setting; they are not used in the long-term care of patients with atherothrombotic disease. There are currently three parenteral GPIIb/IIIa antagonists in clinical use, indicated only in patients with ACS: abciximab, eptifibatide, and tirofiban.

ABCIXIMAB

Abciximab is a large chimeric monoclonal antibody Fab fragment with high affinity for the GPIIb/IIIa receptor.[40] Abciximab is the largest agent with binding sites located on the β-chain of the GPIIb/IIIa receptor which, because of its large size, causes a steric hindrance to ligand access.

Abciximab has the strongest affinity for the GPIIb/IIIa receptor and dissociates at a slower rate than other GPIIb/IIIa antagonists. Unbound abciximab is rapidly cleared from plasma by proteolytic degradation, resulting in a very short plasma half-life (several minutes), whereas the biological half-life ranges from 8 to 24 hours. As such, some GPIIb/IIIa receptors may still be occupied by drug up to 2 weeks after discontinuation of drug infusion. In the event of bleeding, the antithrombotic effects of abciximab cannot be rapidly reversed by discontinuing therapy, but rather are diminished by exogenous platelet transfusion.

The efficacy and safety of abciximab in patients undergoing PCI has been evaluated in several trials, including EPIC, EPILOG, and EPISTENT.[41–43] The Intracoronary Stenting and Antithrombotic Regimen–Rapid Early Action for Coronary Treatment (ISAR-REACT) trial demonstrated that the rate of death, MI, and urgent revascularization at 30 days was low and comparable between patients undergoing elective PCI after pretreatment with clopidogrel 600 mg and allocated to abciximab vs. placebo.[44] Rates of major bleeding were similar between groups, although abciximab was associated with a significantly higher rate of thrombocytopenia. ISAR-REACT-2 evaluated the same abciximab and clopidogrel treatment regimens in high-risk patients with non-ST-segment elevation ACS undergoing PCI.[45] Death, MI, and urgent revascularization at 30 days occurred significantly less frequently with abciximab compared to placebo; however, the treatment benefit of abciximab was confined to patients with elevated troponin levels. Rates of major bleeding were similar between groups. Overall, the findings suggest that in the modern era of interventional cardiology using high clopidogrel dosing regimens, GPIIb/IIIa inhibition should be reserved only for high-risk ACS patients with positive cardiac markers.

EPTIFIBATIDE

Eptifibatide is a competitive antagonist of the GPIIb/IIIa receptor. It is a synthetic small-molecule inhibitor that fits directly into the Arg-Gly-Asp binding pocket of the GPIIb/IIIa receptor, directly competing with the binding of ligands such as fibrinogen and vWF.[46] Eptifibatide rapidly dissociates from its receptor, is cleared by the kidney largely as active drug, and has a plasma half-life of approximately 1.5 to 2.5 hours. The return of hemostatic platelet function is largely dependent on clearance of the drug from plasma. Cessation of drug infusion restores platelet function and, in patients with normal renal function, normal hemostasis returns within 15 to 30 minutes after drug discontinuation. Unlike abciximab, however, the platelet inhibitory effect of eptifibatide is not significantly influenced by platelet transfusion.[46]

Eptifibatide has demonstrated efficacy and safety in patients with non-ST-segment elevation ACS or undergoing PCI in a number of randomized clinical trials. Most recently, the Early Glycoprotein IIb/IIIa Inhibition in Non-ST-Segment Elevation

Acute Coronary Syndrome (EARLY ACS) trial demonstrated that early administration of eptifibatide vs. provisional eptifibatide after angiography (delayed eptifibatide) resulted in similar 30-day rates of death, MI, urgent revascularization, or thrombotic complications during PCI in patients with non-ST-segment elevation ACS undergoing invasive management.[47] Major and minor bleeding rates were significantly higher with early eptifibatide vs. delayed eptifibatide. Overall, these findings do not support the use of upstream compared with ad hoc GPIIb/IIIa inhibition in ACS patients undergoing PCI.

TIROFIBAN

Tirofiban is a tyrosine-derived nonpeptide inhibitor associated with rapid onset and short duration of action, with a plasma half-life of approximately 2 hours. Tirofiban, like eptifibatide, is a competitive inhibitor of the GPIIb/IIIa receptor that has high specificity but relatively low affinity.[46] Tirofiban is excreted by the kidney, predominantly as unchanged drug; it rapidly dissociates from the receptor and has a biological half-life of 1.5 to 2.5 hours. Restoration of hemostasis is best achieved by discontinuing the drug infusion. Efficacy and safety of tirofiban in PCI patients has been investigated in several trials.

Platelet Adhesion

Over the past few years, interest has been directed toward other platelet adhesion mechanisms that might permit platelet inhibition while mitigating the untoward effects of bleeding. Two such adhesion pathways are the vWF/GPIba and GPVI pathways.

von Willebrand factor is present in plasma, platelets, and vascular subendothelium, and is synthesized and stored by megakaryocytes and ECs.[48] von Willebrand factor can be released into the circulation by ECs upon activation by vasopressin (desmopressin/DDAVP [1-deamino-8-D-arginine-vasopressin]) or thrombin, for example.[48] von Willebrand factor serves two important functions in the hemostatic response of platelets: initially through platelet/platelet binding (GPIba/vWF A1 domain), and subsequently through collagen/platelet binding (GPIba/vWF A3 domain). The vWF A1 domain specifically serves to assist with platelet aggregation by binding to platelet GPIba in the GPIb/V/IX complex for platelet/platelet adhesion, especially under conditions of high shear stress. von Willebrand factor additionally promotes platelet adhesion by binding to collagen in exposed vascular subendothelium via the vWF A3 domain. The adhesion function of the GPIb/V/IX complex that interacts with vWF resides in the GPIba chain; mutations within this segment may alter its affinity for the vWF A1 domain.[49]

von Willebrand factor is integrally involved in the pathogenesis of atherosclerosis and arterial thrombosis. Disruption of the ECs lining the artery wall, such as with plaque rupture, exposes subendothelial collagen to arterial blood flow. Exposed collagen captures circulating vWF, causing accumulation of vWF at subendothelial sites. von Willebrand factor becomes a receptor for platelet GPIba, which supports platelet rolling along the damaged artery and eventually promotes platelet adhesion. This process, along with conversion of circulating fibrinogen to fibrin and up-regulation of GPIIb/IIIa receptor on platelets, promotes local thrombus formation. The vWF/GPIba interaction is an adhesive event under high shear conditions, such as at sites of atherosclerosis. Under low shear conditions, such as in flowing venous blood, the vWF/GPIba adhesion mechanism is less important, and other adhesion receptors, such as GPIIb/IIIa and platelet collagen receptors, can independently mediate platelet adhesion. Therefore, agents that inhibit the vWF/GPIba interaction will have selectivity for blocking high-shear arterial platelet adhesion and minimal impact in low-shear blood flow states. Clinical studies have routinely demonstrated that inhibition of GPIba/platelet interactions has profound antithrombotic effects, with low to moderate effects on bleeding time, and can have positive therapeutic benefit for patients with ACS.

VON WILLEBRAND FACTOR – GPIP/IX INHIBITORS

A number of vWF-GPIb/IX inhibitors, including aurin tricarboxylic acid, peptide fragments from vWF A1 domain, and a soluble GPIb-immunoglobulin (Ig)G, have been examined for inhibiting vWF and platelet interactions.[50] Glycoprotein-290 is a recombinant protein consisting of a 290 amino acids sequence of the N-terminal of human GPIba, with two gain-of-function mutations that increase the affinity for the vWF A1 domain. The in vivo antithrombotic and antihemostatic effects have been evaluated with good GPIba/vWF inhibition, which could be reversed with a currently approved (DDAVP) treatment regimen. A lower clopidogrel dose combined with GPIba/vWF inhibition could theoretically have improved efficacy with less bleeding risk.

AJvW-2 is a murine monoclonal antibody to human vWF A1 domain that blocks the GPIba/vWF interaction and has demonstrated antithrombotic activity in animal models.[51] In order to reduce immunological response, AJvW-2 was humanized and converted from an IgG1 to an IgG4.[52] This humanized antibody (AJW200) exhibited similar inhibition of in vitro vWF-mediated platelet activation to AJvW-2. In human volunteer studies, AJW200 demonstrated no clinically significant adverse events or immunogenicity. Ristocetin cofactor (Ri:CoF) assays showed a significant reduction at 1 hour post infusion compared with baseline that lasted for up to 12 hours. The template bleeding time was not significantly prolonged at any time or dose of AJW200. Platelet function as measured by the PFA-100 was reduced by up to 3 to 6 hours at the lower dose and 12 hours at the highest dose administered.

ARC1779 is an aptamer that blocks the GPIba/vWF A1 domain interaction. Aptamers are nucleic acid molecules with high affinity and specificity for a selected target molecule, discovered through in vitro selection on the basis of their ability to fold into unique three-dimensional structures that promote binding to that target.[53] ARC1779 is a modified deoxyribonucleic acid/ribonucleic acid (DNA/RNA) oligonucleotide composed of hybrid terminal ends to minimize endonuclease and exonuclease digestion, with nucleotide segments designed to enhance affinity for vWF. ARC1779 has demonstrated efficacy comparable or superior to that of previously published dosing regimens of abciximab with respect to protection from thrombus formation and average time to occlusion. ARC1779 was evaluated in a randomized double-blind placebo-controlled study that demonstrated it was well tolerated, and no bleeding was observed.[54] An S-nitroso derivative of a mutated fragment of the A1 domain (S-nitroso-AR545C) was shown to inhibit effectively arterial thrombosis in the carotid artery.[55] In unpublished observations, it has also been reported that targeting the vWF A1 domain with the recombinant nanobody ALX-0081, a novel class of antibody therapeutics, resulted in inhibition of vWF-mediated platelet activation, providing novel options for future therapies.

COLLAGEN-GPVI INHIBITORS

Glycoprotein VI is also expressed on the surface of platelets. Signaling by GPVI is via an immunoreceptor tyrosine activation motif (ITAM) promoting phosphorylation and initiating the syk signaling cascade. Syk activation results in activation of integrin-induced platelet aggregation, release of ADP and thromboxane, and procoagulant activity.[56] Rat monoclonal antibody (JAQ1) to mouse GPVI results in inhibition of collagen-induced aggregation.[57] In animal models, JAQ1 caused mild thrombocytopenia and resulted in a 34% decrease in platelet counts within 24 hours of treatment, which returned to normal levels within 3 days of treatment. Platelets showed no indication of activation or change in surface protein expression. A single dose of JAQ1 resulted in 14 days of inhibition of ex vivo collagen-induced aggregation. Further evaluation of in vivo response determined that binding of antibody to the platelet GPVI resulted in depletion of platelet GPVI. Collagen-induced adhesion was significantly reduced in these GPVI-depleted platelets. Bleeding times of JAQ1-treated mice were significantly elevated over control mice (330 seconds vs. 158 seconds), but less than that seen following inhibition of GPIIb/IIIa (330 seconds vs. > 600 seconds).

Pharmacology of Antithrombotics and Thrombin Inhibitors

Overview of Coagulation

Hemostasis is accomplished by a complex sequence of interactions among platelets, endothelium, and multiple circulating and membrane-bound coagulation factors. As shown in Figure 7-3, the coagulation cascade typically has two intersecting pathways. The intrinsic pathway is initiated with factor XII and involves a cascade of enzymatic reactions that activate factors XI, IX, and VII. In the intrinsic pathway, all factors leading to fibrin clot formation are intrinsic to the circulating plasma, and no surface is required to initiate the process. The extrinsic pathway, however, requires exposure of tissue factor on the surface of the injured vessel wall to initiate the cascade, beginning with factor VII. The two arms of the coagulation cascade merge to a common pathway at factor X, which activates factors II (prothrombin) and I (fibrinogen). The formation of clot is dependent upon the proteolytic conversion of fibrinogen to fibrin.

An elevated activated partial thromboplastin time (APTT) is associated with abnormal function of the intrinsic arm of the cascade, whereas an elevated prothrombin time (PT) is associated with abnormal function of the extrinsic arm. Vitamin K deficiency and warfarin use affect factors II, VII, IX, and X. Fibrinogen levels below 50 mg/dL cause prolongation of the PT and APTT.

The physiological pathway for coagulation is initiated by exposure of subendothelial tissue factor when the luminal surface of a vessel is injured. Propagation of the clotting reaction occurs with a sequence of four enzymatic reactions. Each reaction involves a proteolytic enzyme that generates a subsequent enzyme in the cascade by cleavage of a proenzyme and a phospholipid surface, such as the platelet membrane. Many reactions are dependent upon an additional protein. Initially, factor VIIa binds to tissue factor when the luminal surface of a vascular wall is injured. The tissue factor/VIIa complex catalyzes the activation of factor X to factor Xa, which may occur on the phospholipid surface of activated platelets. The tissue factor/VIIa complex also activates factor IX to factor IXa, demonstrating crosstalk between the intrinsic and extrinsic pathways.

Factor Xa, together with factor Va, Ca²⁺, and phospholipid, comprise the prothrombinase complex that converts prothrombin to thrombin. Thrombin has multiple functions in the clotting process, including conversion of fibrinogen to fibrin and activation of factors V, VII, VIII, XI, and XIII, as well as activation of platelets. Factor VIIIa combines with factor IXa to form the intrinsic factor complex, which catalyzes conversion of factor X to Xa. This intrinsic complex (VIIIa/IXa) is approximately 50 times more effective at catalyzing factor X activation as compared to the extrinsic (tissue factor VIIa) complex.

Factor Xa combines with factor Va to form the prothrombinase complex, which converts prothrombin to thrombin. Thrombin, once formed, dissociates from the membrane surface and converts fibrinogen by two cleavage steps into fibrin and two small peptides (fibrinopeptides A and B). Removal of fibrinopeptide A permits end-to-end polymerization of the fibrin molecules, whereas cleavage of fibrinopeptide B allows side-to-side polymerization of the fibrin clot. This latter step is facilitated by thrombin-activatable fibrinolysis inhibitor (TAFI), which acts to stabilize the resulting clot.

The coagulation system is exquisitely regulated. Clot formation must occur to prevent bleeding at the time of vascular injury; however, two related processes must exist to prevent propagation of the clot beyond the site of injury. First, there is a feedback inhibition on the coagulation cascade, which deactivates the enzyme complexes for thrombin formation. Second, fibrinolysis allows for breakdown of the fibrin clot and subsequent repair of the injured vessel with deposition of connective tissue.

Tissue factor pathway inhibitor (TFPI) blocks the extrinsic tissue factor/VIIa complex formation, eliminating production of factors Xa and IXa. Antithrombin III neutralizes the procoagulant serine proteases and only weakly inhibits the tissue factor/VIIa complex. The primary effect of antithrombin III is to halt the production of thrombin. A third major mechanism of inhibition of thrombin formation is the protein C system. Once formed, thrombin binds to thrombomodulin and activates protein C to an activated protein C (APC) complex. Activated protein C forms a complex with protein S on phospholipid surfaces to cleave factors Va and VIIIa, preventing further formation of tissue factor/VIIa or prothrombinase complexes. Through these systems, feedback inhibition of thrombin formation exists to "turn off" thrombin procoagulant activation.

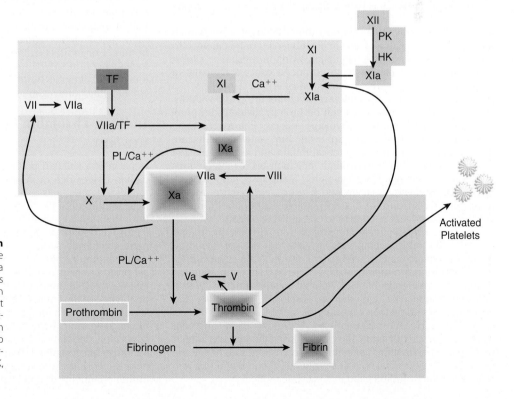

FIGURE 7-3 **Summary of the coagulation pathways.** Specific coagulation factors are responsible for conversion of soluble plasma fibrinogen into insoluble fibrin. This process occurs via a series of linked reactions in which the enzymatically active product subsequently converts downstream inactive protein into active serine protease. In addition, activation of thrombin leads to stimulation of platelets. HK, high-molecular-weight kininogen ("a" is activated form); PK, prekallikrein; TF, tissue factor.

The thrombin-thrombomodulin complex also activates TAFI. TAFI removes terminal lysine on the fibrin molecules, rendering the clot more susceptible to lysis by plasmin. Degradation of the fibrin clot is accomplished by plasmin, a serine protease derived from the proenzyme plasminogen. Plasmin formation occurs as a result of one of several plasminogen activators. Tissue plasminogen activator (tPA) is synthesized by the endothelium and other cells of the vascular wall and is the main circulating form of this family of enzymes. Tissue plasminogen activator is relatively selective for fibrin-bound plasminogen, so that endogenous fibrinolytic activity occurs predominately at the site of clot formation. The other major plasminogen activator, urokinase-type plasminogen activator (uPA), is also produced by ECs, as well as by urothelium; uPA is less selective than tPA for fibrin-bound plasminogen.

Pharmacology of Oral Anticoagulants

Warfarin currently is the most commonly used oral anticoagulant and blocks γ-carboxylation of several glutamate residues in prothrombin and factors VII, IX, and X as well as proteins C and S. Blocking γ-carboxylation results in biologically inactive coagulation factors, and the carboxylation reaction is coupled to the oxidation of vitamin K. Warfarin prevents reductive metabolism of the inactive vitamin K epoxide back to its active hydroquinone form. The specific anticoagulant effect of warfarin results from inhibited synthesis and degradation of the four vitamin K–dependent clotting factors. The resulting inhibition of coagulation is dependent on the half-lives, which are 6, 24, 40, and 60 hours for factors VII, IX, X, and II, respectively. Warfarin has several well-characterized side effects. It is known to cross the placenta and cause a hemorrhagic disorder in the fetus. Fetal proteins with γ-carboxylation residues found in bone and blood may be affected by warfarin, causing birth defects characterized by abnormal bone formation. Cutaneous necrosis with reduced activity of protein C can occur during the first weeks of therapy, as can venous thrombosis.

The therapeutic range for oral anticoagulant therapy is defined in terms of an international normalized ratio (INR). The INR is the PT ratio (patient PT/mean of normal PT for lab)[ISI], where the ISI exponent refers to the International Sensitivity Index and is dependent on the specific reagents and instruments used for the determination.

Occasionally, patients exhibit *warfarin resistance*, defined as progression or recurrence of a thrombotic event while in the therapeutic range. These individuals may have their INR target raised (which is accompanied by an increase in bleeding risk) or be changed to an alternative form of anticoagulation. Warfarin resistance is most commonly seen in patients with advanced cancers, typically of gastrointestinal origin (Trousseau's syndrome).

Oral anticoagulants often interact with other drugs and with disease states. These interactions can be broadly divided into pharmacokinetic and pharmacodynamic effects. Pharmacokinetic mechanisms for drug interaction with oral anticoagulants are mainly enzyme induction, enzyme inhibition, and reduced plasma protein binding. Pharmacodynamic mechanisms for interactions with warfarin are synergism (impaired hemostasis, reduced clotting factor synthesis, as in hepatic disease), competitive antagonism (vitamin K), and an altered physiological control loop for vitamin K (hereditary resistance to oral anticoagulants).

The most serious interactions with warfarin are those that increase the anticoagulant effect and the risk of bleeding. Serious pharmacokinetic interactions are with the pyrazolones phenylbutazone and sulfinpyrazone. These drugs not only augment hypoprothrombinemia but also inhibit platelet function. Metronidazole, fluconazole, amiodarone, disulfiram, cimetidine, and trimethoprim-sulfamethoxazole inhibit metabolic transformation of warfarin. Hepatic disease and hyperthyroidism augment warfarin pharmacodynamically by increasing the turnover rate of clotting factors. The third-generation cephalosporins eliminate the bacteria in the intestinal tract that produce vitamin K and, like warfarin, also directly inhibit vitamin K epoxide reductase.

Barbiturates and rifampin cause a marked decrease of the anticoagulant effect by induction of hepatic enzymes that transform warfarin. Cholestyramine binds warfarin in the intestine and reduces its absorption and bioavailability.

Pharmacodynamic reductions of anticoagulant effect occur with vitamin K (increased synthesis of clotting factors), the diuretics chlorthalidone and spironolactone (clotting factor concentration), hereditary resistance (due to genetic variation related to vitamin K reactivation), and hypothyroidism (decreased turnover rate of clotting factors).

Excessive anticoagulant effect and bleeding from warfarin can be reversed by stopping the drug and administering oral or parenteral vitamin K_1 (phytonadione), fresh frozen plasma, prothrombin complex concentrates such as Bebulin and Proplex T, and recombinant factor VIIa (rFVIIa). A modest excess of anticoagulant effect without bleeding may require no more than cessation of the drug. The effect of warfarin can be rapidly reversed in the setting of severe bleeding by administering prothrombin complex or rFVIIa coupled with intravenous vitamin K. It is important to note that owing to the long half-life of warfarin, a single dose of vitamin K or rFVIIa may not be sufficient.

Warfarin has several important limitations: (1) delayed onset of anticoagulation because it takes several days to lower the levels of the vitamin K–dependent clotting factors into the therapeutic range; (2) multiple drug and food interactions, rendering the anticoagulant response unpredictable and coagulation monitoring essential; (3) slow reversal of the anticoagulant effect of vitamin K antagonists upon cessation of their use, unless supplemental vitamin K and/or fresh frozen plasma is given; and (4) decreases in the levels of protein C or protein S upon initiation of oral anticoagulant therapy can cause skin necrosis in individuals whose baseline levels of proteins C or S are reduced.

Pharmacology of Thrombin Inhibitors: Indirect and Direct

Thrombin is essential to hemostasis. It is responsible for fibrin formation; activation of factor XIII and feedback activation of other coagulation factors such as factors V, VIII, and IX; platelet activation and subsequent aggregation; and it can also act as an anticoagulant by binding to thrombomodulin. Thrombin's ubiquitous role in maintaining hemostasis makes it a prime target for newer, more specific anticoagulant drugs. Thrombin inhibitors can either be direct or indirect in their action. Indirect thrombin inhibitors include heparin, LMWH, and fondaparinux. Direct thrombin inhibitors (DTIs) include hirudins, bivalirudin, argatroban, dabigatran etexilate, and ximelagatran.

Indirect Thrombin Inhibitors

HEPARIN

Heparin is a sulfated polysaccharide and is isolated from mammalian tissues rich in mast cells, most notably porcine intestinal mucosa. Heparin acts as an anticoagulant by activating antithrombin (antithrombin III), thereby accelerating the rate at which antithrombin inhibits clotting enzymes, particularly thrombin and factor Xa. Heparin activates antithrombin by binding to a unique pentasaccharide sequence to induce a conformational change within antithrombin, rendering it more readily accessible to its target proteases (Fig. 7-4). This conformational change enhances the rate at which antithrombin inhibits factor Xa but has little effect on the rate of thrombin inhibition. To catalyze thrombin inhibition, heparin serves as a template that simultaneously binds antithrombin and thrombin. Formation of this ternary structure allows close apposition, promoting formation of a stable covalent thrombin-antithrombin complex. Heparin additionally causes release of TFPI from the endothelium, a tissue factor–bound factor VIIa inhibitor, further enhancing its anticoagulant effects.

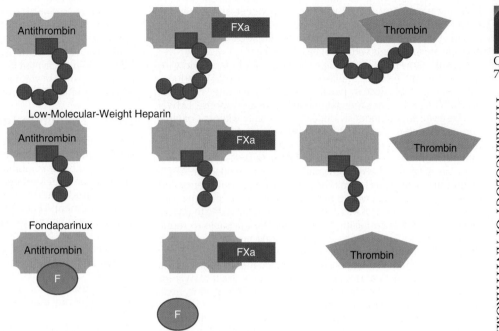

Unfractionated Heparin

FIGURE 7-4   Comparative mechanisms of action of selected anticoagulants.

PHARMACOLOGY OF ANTITHROMBOTIC DRUGS

Heparin binds to the endothelium and to plasma proteins, explaining its dose-dependent clearance. At low doses, the half-life of heparin is short because it binds rapidly to the endothelium. Clearance is mainly extrarenal, as heparin binds to macrophages, which internalize and depolymerize the long heparin chains and secrete shorter chains back into the circulation. Because of its dose-dependent clearance mechanism, the plasma half-life of heparin ranges from 30 to 60 minutes.

Heparins binding to plasma proteins, especially acute-phase reactants whose levels are elevated in ill patients, may make the anticoagulant response unpredictable to fixed or weight-adjusted doses. Consequently, coagulation monitoring is essential to ensure that a therapeutic response is obtained. This is particularly important when heparin is administered for treatment of established thrombosis because a subtherapeutic anticoagulant response may render patients at risk for recurrent thrombosis, whereas excessive anticoagulation increases bleeding risk. Heparin therapy can be monitored using the APTT or anti–factor Xa level. Anti–factor Xa levels also can be used to monitor heparin therapy. Although gaining in popularity, anti–factor Xa assays have yet to be standardized, and results can vary widely between laboratories.

The most common side effect of heparin is bleeding. Other complications include thrombocytopenia, osteoporosis, and elevated levels of transaminases. The risk of heparin-induced bleeding increases with higher heparin doses. Concomitant administration of drugs that affect hemostasis, such as antiplatelet or fibrinolytic agents, increases bleeding risk, as does recent surgery or trauma. Heparin-treated patients with serious bleeding can be given protamine sulfate to neutralize the heparin. Protamine sulfate binds heparin with high affinity, and the resultant protamine-heparin complexes are then cleared. Typically, 1 mg of protamine sulfate neutralizes 100 units of heparin. Anaphylactoid reactions to protamine sulfate can occur, and drug administration by slow IV infusion is recommended to reduce the risk.

Heparin can cause a drop in platelet count in the form of heparin-induced thrombocytopenia (HIT). Heparin-induced thrombocytopenia is an antibody-mediated process triggered by antibodies directed against neoantigens on platelet factor 4 (PF4). These antibodies (IgG isotype) bind simultaneously to the heparin-PF4 complex and to platelet Fc receptors. Such binding activates the platelets and generates platelet microparticles. Circulating microparticles are prothrombotic and can bind clotting factors and promote thrombin generation. Typically, HIT occurs 5 to 14 days after initiation of heparin therapy, but it can manifest earlier. It is rare for the platelet count to fall below 100,000/mL in patients with HIT, and even a 50% decrease in platelet count from the pretreatment value should raise the suspicion of HIT in those receiving heparin. The diagnosis of HIT is established using enzyme-linked assays to detect antibodies against heparin-PF4 complexes or with platelet activation assays. Enzyme-linked assays are sensitive but can be positive in the absence of any clinical evidence of HIT. Another diagnostic test is the serotonin release assay. This test is performed by quantifying serotonin release when washed platelets loaded with labeled serotonin are exposed to patient serum in the absence or presence of varying concentrations of heparin. If the patient serum contains the HIT antibody, heparin addition induces platelet activation and serotonin release.

Heparin is stopped in patients with suspected or documented HIT, and an alternative anticoagulant should be administered to prevent or treat thrombosis. The agents most often used for this indication are parenteral DTIs (e.g., lepirudin, argatroban, bivalirudin) or factor Xa inhibitors (e.g., fondaparinux, danaparoid). Patients with HIT, particularly those with associated thrombosis, often have evidence of increased thrombin generation that can lead to consumption of protein C; if given warfarin without a concomitant parenteral anticoagulant, this can trigger skin necrosis.

LOW-MOLECULAR-WEIGHT HEPARIN

Low-molecular-weight heparin consists of smaller fragments of heparin and is prepared from unfractionated heparin (UFH) by controlled enzymatic depolymerization. Low-molecular-weight heparin provides advantages over heparin in that it has better bioavailability and longer half-life, simplified dosing, predictable anticoagulant response, lower risk of HIT, and lower risk of osteoporosis.

Like heparin, LMWH exerts its anticoagulant activity by activating antithrombin. Even though LMWH consists of shorter pentasaccharide-containing chains, they retain greater capacity to accelerate factor Xa inhibition by antithrombin (see Fig. 7-4). Consequently, many forms of LMWH catalyze factor Xa inhibition by antithrombin more than thrombin inhibition.

Since LMWH contains shorter chains, they bind less avidly to ECs, macrophages, and heparin-binding plasma proteins. Reduced binding to ECs and macrophages eliminates the rapid dose-dependent and saturable mechanism of clearance that is a characteristic of UFH. Instead, clearance of LMWH is dose independent, and its plasma half-life is longer at approximately 4 hours. Low-molecular-weight heparin is cleared almost exclusively by the kidney, and the drug can accumulate in patients with renal insufficiency.

Because Low-molecular-weight heparin binds less avidly to heparin-binding proteins in plasma than heparin, LMWH produces a more predictable dose response, and resistance is rare. With a longer half-life and more predictable anticoagulant response, LMWH can be given subcutaneously once or twice daily without coagulation monitoring, even when the drug is given in treatment doses. In the majority of patients, LMWH does not require coagulation monitoring. If monitoring is necessary, anti–factor Xa levels must be measured because most LMWH preparations have little effect on APTT.

Indications for LMWH monitoring include renal insufficiency and obesity. Low-molecular-weight heparin monitoring in patients with a creatinine clearance of less than 50 mL/min is advisable to ensure there is no drug accumulation. It may also be advisable to monitor the anticoagulant activity of LMWH during pregnancy, because dose requirements can change, particularly in the third trimester. Monitoring should also be considered in high-risk settings, such as in patients with mechanical heart valves who are given LMWH for prevention of valve thrombosis, and when LMWH is used in treatment doses in infants or children.

The major complication of LMWH is bleeding. Meta-analyses suggest that the risk of major bleeding is lower with LMWH than with UFH. Heparin-induced thrombocytopenia and osteoporosis are less common with LMWH than with UFH. As with heparin, bleeding with LMWH is more common in patients receiving concomitant therapy with antiplatelet or fibrinolytic drugs. Recent surgery, trauma, or underlying hemostatic defects also increase the risk of bleeding with LMWH. Although protamine sulfate can be used as an antidote for LMWH, it incompletely neutralizes the anticoagulant activity of LMWH because it only binds the longer chains of LMWH and is only partially reversed.

The risk of HIT is about fivefold lower with LMWH than with heparin. Low-molecular-weight heparin binds less avidly to platelets and causes less PF4 release. Furthermore, with lower affinity for PF4 than heparin, LMWH is less likely to induce the conformational changes in PF4 that trigger the formation of HIT antibodies. Low-molecular-weight heparin should not be used to treat HIT patients because most HIT antibodies exhibit cross-reactivity with LMWH. This *in vitro* cross-reactivity is not simply a laboratory phenomenon; there are case reports of thrombosis when HIT patients are treated with LMWH.

FONDAPARINUX

Fondaparinux is a synthetic analog of the antithrombin-binding pentasaccharide sequence that differs from LMWH in several ways. As a synthetic analog of the antithrombin-binding pentasaccharide sequence found in heparin and LMWH, fondaparinux binds only to antithrombin and is too short to bridge thrombin to antithrombin (see Fig. 7-4). Consequently, fondaparinux catalyzes factor Xa inhibition by antithrombin and does not enhance the rate of thrombin inhibition. Fondaparinux is licensed for thromboprophylaxis in general surgical and high-risk orthopedic patients and as an alternative to heparin or LMWH for initial treatment of patients with established venous thromboembolism (VTE).

Fondaparinux does not bind to ECs or plasma proteins. Clearance of fondaparinux is dose independent, and its plasma half-life is 17 hours. Because fondaparinux is cleared unchanged via the kidney, it is contraindicated in patients with a creatinine clearance below 30 mL/min and should be used with caution in those with a creatinine clearance below 50 mL/min. Fondaparinux produces a predictable anticoagulant response after administration in fixed doses because it does not bind to plasma proteins.

Fondaparinux does not cause HIT because it does not bind to PF4. In contrast to LMWH, there is no cross-reactivity of fondaparinux with HIT antibodies. Consequently, fondaparinux appears to be effective for treatment of HIT patients, although large clinical trials supporting its use are lacking.

The major side effect of fondaparinux is bleeding. There is no antidote for this drug. Protamine sulfate has no effect on the anticoagulant activity of fondaparinux because it fails to bind to the drug. Recombinant activated factor VII reverses the anticoagulant effects of fondaparinux in volunteers, but it is unknown whether this agent will control fondaparinux-induced bleeding.

Direct Thrombin Inhibitors

Direct thrombin inhibitors bind thrombin with high affinity, preventing the interaction of thrombin with its substrates. Direct thrombin inhibitors inhibit platelet PAR receptors, without interfering with the platelet hemostatic role. Licensed DTIs include hirudin, bivalirudin, and argatroban; a number of novel products are in development. Theoretical advantages of DTIs include activity against fibrin-bound thrombin, less nonspecific binding to proteins and platelets, lack of a requirement for a cofactor, an absence of natural inhibitors, and a wider therapeutic window. As a result of their predictable pharmacokinetic profile and reduced specific and nonspecific protein binding, the oral DTIs also have the potential to be used without laboratory monitoring—a major advantage over current oral anticoagulants.

Parenteral Direct Thrombin Inhibitors

HIRUDINS

Hirudin consists of a single polypeptide chain of 65 amino acids with increased affinity for thrombin. Various recombinant hirudins have since been developed (lepirudin and desirudin). They are bivalent DTIs and bind thrombin with high affinity, forming noncovalent irreversible complexes. Their plasma half-life is approximately 1 to 2 hours, and they distribute widely in the extravascular space. Clearance is primarily through the kidney, so dose adjustment is required in the setting of impaired renal function.[58] Monitoring hirudin is challenging, since plasma levels must be determined using enzyme-linked immunosorbent assays (ELISA), which are costly and limited in availability. Hirudins are associated with bleeding, thus requiring monitoring to avoid excessive anticoagulation. Since hirudin prolongs APTT, it is widely used to monitor therapy. Lepirudin is licensed for use in patients with HIT with thrombosis. Major bleeding occurs in 18% to 20% of patients receiving lepirudin for treatment of HIT. Clinical use of commercially available hirudins is complicated by the development of antibodies. Studies have shown that over 40% of lepirudin-treated patients develop IgG antibodies against lepirudin.[59] Antilepirudin antibodies typically form 1 to 4 weeks after initiation of treatment and in most cases are not associated with any adverse clinical outcomes. In 10% of lepirudin-treated patients, however, formation of antibodies delay clearance of lepirudin, enhancing its anticoagulant effect.[59] Anaphylaxis, which can be fatal, has also been reported in patients receiving intravenous bolus lepirudin for treatment of HIT.[60] Lepirudin use in patients with HIT is based on the findings of three prospective, historically controlled cohort studies, HAT-1, HAT-2, and HAT-3. These studies found that compared with historical controls, lepirudin reduced the frequency of the composite endpoint of all-cause mortality, new thrombosis, or limb amputation in patients with HIT.[61] Lepirudin was also associated with significantly reduced new thrombosis. Lepirudin additionally has been studied in the setting of non-ST-segment ACS. When compared with heparin, 10,141 patients with ACS lepirudin significantly reduced the incidence of cardiovascular death, refractory angina, or new MI at 7 days from 6.7% to 5.6%, but also significantly increased the rate of major bleeding from 0.7% to 1.2%.[62] Lepirudin has not been approved for use in ACS, but such results support the hypothesis that hirudins are superior to heparin in preventing recurrent ischemia; however, they do so within a narrow therapeutic window.

Desirudin is a hirudin used for thromboprophylaxis in patients undergoing elective hip or knee surgery. Desirudin is used for 9 to 12 days, or until the patient is fully ambulatory. Unlike lepirudin, desirudin monitoring is unnecessary. Like lepirudin, bleeding is the most common side effect. When receiving desirudin for thromboprophylaxis, approximately 10% of patients also develop antibodies of the IgG class against hirudin. These antibodies have not been associated with altered plasma concentrations of desirudin, deep vein thrombosis (DVT), pulmonary embolism (PE), allergic reactions, or hemorrhage.[63] Desirudin is currently approved in Europe for thromboprophylaxis in patients undergoing elective hip or knee surgery. Approval is based on findings of two multicenter randomized double-blind trials. In the first study, desirudin 15 mg subcutaneously twice daily was compared to UHF, 5000 international units, three times daily in patients undergoing primary elective total hip replacement (THR). Desirudin was associated with a significantly lower rate of all DVT and proximal DVT.[64] In the second study, desirudin 15 mg subcutaneously twice daily was compared to enoxaparin 40 mg subcutaneously once daily in patients undergoing elective THR. Duration of treatment was 8 to 12 days, and DVT during the treatment period was verified by mandatory bilateral venography. Desirudin was associated with a significantly lower rate of proximal DVT and overall DVT. There was no significant difference in bleeding, transfusion requirements, or thrombocytopenia between the groups.[65]

BIVALIRUDIN

Bivalirudin is a hirudin analog with high-affinity binding to thrombin. Once bound, however, thrombin cleaves the Arg-Pro in the N-terminus of bivalirudin, allowing for recovery of thrombin activity and subsequent competing of fibrinogen with the bivalirudin remnant for thrombin.[66] Unlike hirudin, only 20% of bivalirudin is excreted via the kidney; the remainder is eliminated by proteolytic enzymatic degradation. Both APTT and activated clotting time (ACT) have been used to monitor bivalirudin. Bivalirudin has been licensed as an alternative to heparin in patients undergoing PCI and for patients with HIT who require PCI. A prospective trial comparing bivalirudin with high-dose heparin in 1261 patients demonstrated a lower rate of death, MI, or repeat revascularization.[67] The REPLACE-1 trial compared bivalirudin to heparin in 1056 patients undergoing coronary stenting with GPIIb/IIIa inhibitors. There was a trend toward a reduction in the combined endpoint of death, MI, or revascularization with bivalirudin at 48 hours; there was no difference in major bleeding.[68] In REPLACE-2, bivalirudin was as effective as heparin plus GPIIb/IIIa inhibition in reducing death, MI, and revascularization. Bivalirudin was also associated with significant reduction in the incidence of bleeding and thrombocytopenia.[69] In the Acute Catheterization and Urgent Intervention Triage Strategy (ACUITY) trial, patients with moderate- to high-risk unstable angina or non-ST-segment elevation myocardial infarction (NSTEMI) undergoing early invasive management[70] demonstrated that bivalirudin alone was noninferior to heparin (either UFH or enoxaparin) plus GPIIb/IIIa inhibitors in terms of mortality and the primary endpoint. It was also associated with significantly less bleeding. At 1 year, bivalirudin was still noninferior to heparin in terms of the primary endpoint and mortality rates; however, bivalirudin, either alone or with GPIIb/IIIa inhibitors, continued to be associated with significantly less bleeding. Results were similar in patients triaged to medical management, PCI, or coronary artery bypass surgery. The ACUITY trial showed a strong association between major bleeding in the first 30 days and risk of death over 1 year.[70]

ARGATROBAN

Argatroban is a potent agent that differs from parenteral DTIs in that it binds reversibly to the active site of both free and clot-bound thrombin.[71] Argatroban is metabolized by the liver, and its clearance is reduced in patients with moderate hepatic impairment (Child-Pugh > 6). Thus, significant reductions in argatroban dose are required for individuals with moderate hepatic impairment, and the drug is contraindicated in patients with severe hepatic dysfunction.

No dose adjustment is needed in the setting of renal impairment.[72] Argatroban increases APTT, PT/INR, thrombin time, ecarin clotting time, and ACT in a dose-dependent fashion.

The major side effect of argatroban is bleeding. Because there is no specific antidote, excessive bleeding can only be managed by stopping the argatroban infusion and providing supportive therapy. In patients with normal hepatic function, the anticoagulant effect of argatroban disappears 2 to 4 hours after stopping the infusion. However, the anticoagulant effects of argatroban may persist for up to 24 hours in patients with hepatic impairment. A major challenge of argatroban is its effect on PT/INR. When overlapped with warfarin, PT/INR is prolonged beyond what would be expected with warfarin alone, making dose adjustment of either drug difficult.[73]

Two multicenter phase III prospective trials of argatroban in HIT have been completed. When compared with historical controls, patients on argatroban had reduced rates of thrombosis and death due to thrombosis, without an increase in bleeding.[74] On the basis of these findings, argatroban has been approved for treatment of thrombosis and for thromboprophylaxis in patients with HIT, including those undergoing PCI with HIT.[75] Increasing data supporting the use of argatroban in patients without HIT undergoing PCI has been emerging. A 2007 multicenter prospective pilot study evaluated efficacy and safety of argatroban in combination with the GPIIb/IIIa inhibitors abciximab or eptifibatide in 152 patients. The primary efficacy endpoint (a composite of death, MI, or urgent revascularization at 30 days) occurred in 2.6% of patients, and major bleeding occurred in 1.3% of patients.[76] This study also showed that argatroban in combination with GPIIb/IIIa inhibition was an adequate anticoagulant with an acceptable bleeding risk.

Oral Direct Thrombin Inhibitors

XIMELAGATRAN

Because of the significant limitations of warfarin, alternative oral DTIs have undergone significant development and clinical study. Ximelagatran, the orally available prodrug of the univalent DTI melagatran, was the first drug in this class to generate widespread interest.[77] Although ximelagatran was shown to be as effective as warfarin in preventing stroke or systemic embolism in the setting of atrial fibrillation,[78] there were questions about its safety profile. The open-label SPORTIF III trial compared ximelagatran with warfarin for prevention of stroke and systemic embolism, and although ximelagatran was shown to be noninferior to warfarin in preventing stroke and systemic embolism, serum alanine aminotransferase levels rose to greater than three times the upper limit of normal in 6% of individuals in the ximelagatran group and greater than five times the upper limit of normal in 3.4% of individuals in the ximelagatran group.[79] Significant safety concerns regarding increased liver toxicity without a significant offsetting advantage in major bleeding led the U.S. Food and Drug Administration (FDA) to reject the sponsor's application for ximelagatran in 2004.

DABIGATRAN ETEXILATE

Like ximelagatran, dabigatran etexilate is a prodrug. Once absorbed, the drug is rapidly converted by esterases to dabigatran, whose levels peak in approximately 1 to 2 hours. Dabigatran is a small-molecule reversible inhibitor that binds to the active site of thrombin. The half-life of dabigatran is approximately 12 hours, and it is primarily eliminated via the kidney.[80] The half-life is prolonged in the elderly, reflecting their impaired renal function.[81] The pharmacokinetics and pharmacodynamics of dabigatran are not influenced by CYP P450 enzymes and other hepatic oxidoreductases and thus do not interfere with drugs that are metabolized by the P450 enzyme system.[80] Dabigatran produces a predictable anticoagulant response. Therefore, routine coagulation monitoring is not necessary. Dabigatran prolongs ecarin clotting time, APTT, and PT/INR in a dose-dependent fashion.[81] Because these widely available tests have not been used in the clinical setting for monitoring, target levels are unknown.

The major side effect of dabigatran is hemorrhage. No specific antidote is available. Consequently, bleeding complications must be managed symptomatically. Although not well studied, dialysis or hemoperfusion likely removes this compound from the circulation, and administration of activated coagulation factor complexes such as FEIBA, Autoplex, or rFVIIa may overcome its anticoagulant effect.[82] Several clinical trials have demonstrated dabigatran's antithrombotic effect. The phase II Boehringer Ingelheim Study in Thrombosis II (BISTRO II) trial compared oral dabigatran with enoxaparin as thromboprophylaxis after total hip or total knee replacement.[83] Dabigatran was administered at doses of 50 mg, 150 mg, or 225 mg twice daily, or 300 mg once daily for 6 to 10 days. A significant dose-dependent decrease in VTE occurred with increasing doses of dabigatran etexilate. Overall VTE rates were 28.5% in patients receiving 50 mg of dabigatran twice daily, 17.4% in patients receiving 150 mg of dabigatran twice daily, 13.1% in patients receiving 225 mg of dabigatran twice daily, 16.6% in patients receiving 300 mg of dabigatran once daily, and 24% in patients receiving enoxaparin. The risk of serious bleeding with dabigatran increased in a dose-dependent manner as well, but did not reach statistical significance at any dose. Serious bleeding occurred in 0.3% of patients receiving 50 mg of dabigatran twice daily, 4.1% of patients receiving 150 mg of dabigatran twice daily, 4.8% of patients receiving 225 mg of dabigatran twice daily, and 4.7% of patients receiving 300 mg of dabigatran once daily. Serious bleeding occurred in 2.0% of patients receiving enoxaparin.

The RE-NOVATE study demonstrated that dabigatran etexilate was as effective as enoxaparin for preventing VTE after THR, with a similar safety profile.[84] This double-blind, noninferiority trial randomized 3494 patients to treatment for 28 to 35 days with dabigatran etexilate 220 mg or 150 mg once daily, or subcutaneous enoxaparin 40 mg once daily. The primary efficacy outcome was the composite of total VTE and all-cause mortality. Both doses of dabigatran etexilate were noninferior to enoxaparin, with the primary efficacy outcome occurring in 6.7% of patients in the enoxaparin group vs. 6.0% of patients in the dabigatran etexilate 220-mg group, and 8.6% of patients in the 150-mg group. There was no significant difference in major bleeding rates with either dose of dabigatran etexilate compared to enoxaparin. There was no difference in the frequency of liver enzyme elevation.

The subsequent REMODEL trial reproduced these results in 2076 patients undergoing total knee replacement (TKR).[85] The primary efficacy outcome occurred in 37.7% of the enoxaparin group vs. 36.4% of the dabigatran etexilate 220-mg group and 40.5% of the 150-mg group. Both doses of dabigatran etexilate were thus noninferior to enoxaparin. Incidence of major bleeding did not differ significantly between the three groups (1.3% vs. 1.5% and 1.3%, respectively), and there were no significant differences in liver enzyme elevation.

The RE-MOBILIZE trial was similar in design to the RE-MODEL and, in contrast to REMODEL, failed to show equivalence for a composite endpoint of proximal DVT, distal DVT, PE, and all-cause mortality.[84] Warfarin is often used for thromboprophylaxis after knee arthroplasty in centers in North America, but it has not been directly compared to dabigatran in a clinical trial. Dabigatran has undergone study for initial and long-term treatment of patients with established VTE. The Randomised Evaluation of Long-Term Anticoagulant Therapy (RE-LY) trial demonstrated that in 18,133 patients with atrial fibrillation, primary outcome of stroke or embolism was lower in patients on dabigatran as compared to warfarin, as was bleeding.[86] Dabigatran has been approved for use in the United States and is in use in Europe.

Oral Factor Xa Inhibitors

RIVAROXABAN

Rivaroxaban is in development for prevention and treatment of thromboembolic disorders, including VTE prevention following orthopedic surgery, treatment of DVT and PE, ACS, and stroke prevention in patients with atrial fibrillation. Rivaroxaban is a potent inhibitor of factor Xa and does not inhibit thrombin-induced platelet aggregation, but it attenuates tissue factor–induced platelet aggregation indirectly through inhibition of thrombin generation.[87] The antithrombotic efficacy of rivaroxaban has been demonstrated in various animal models of arterial or venous thrombosis across doses that do not prolong bleeding times.[87] When combined with ASA or clopidogrel, the antithrombotic potency of rivaroxaban is enhanced.[88]

In healthy subjects and patients undergoing orthopedic surgery, rivaroxaban displays predictable pharmacokinetics and pharmacodynamics.[89] The half-life is between 7.6 and 9.1 hours. Plasma levels of rivaroxaban correlate well with both inhibition of factor Xa activity and prolongation of PT, as assessed in healthy subjects who received multiple doses of rivaroxaban across a wide dose range.[90] The pharmacodynamic effects of rivaroxaban (as measured by endogenous thrombin potential) are sustained for 24 hours after single oral doses, thus supporting once-daily dosing.[91] Age, gender, and body weight have not been shown to exert clinically significant effects on the pharmacokinetic or pharmacodynamic profiles of rivaroxaban. Rivaroxaban has a dual mode of elimination: one third is excreted unchanged via the kidneys and the remaining two thirds of the drug is metabolized by the liver; there are no major or active circulating metabolites.[92] It does not interact with or mobilize PF4 on platelets, and is therefore unlikely to induce the conformational changes in PF4 necessary for cross-reaction with HIT antibodies.

Four dose-finding clinical studies (one phase IIa and three phase IIb) have assessed the potential efficacy and safety of rivaroxaban for thromboprophylaxis in patients undergoing major orthopedic surgery.[84,93–95] All four studies assessed rivaroxaban relative to conventional anticoagulants and measured the composite of the incidence of any DVT or objectively confirmed nonfatal PE or all-cause mortality as the primary endpoint and major bleeding as the primary safety endpoint. Results from these studies support the feasibility of daily dosing. The 10 mg daily dose provided the optimal balance between efficacy and safety in the phase II trials and was therefore selected for further study in phase III trials. There has been no evidence of liver toxicity. The RECORD program (Regulation of Coagulation in Major Orthopedic Surgery Reducing the Risk of DVT and PE) was initiated in December 2005 and enrolled more than 12,500 patients worldwide to participate in four multicenter randomized, active-controlled, double-blind studies of rivaroxaban prophylaxis in patients undergoing THR (RECORD1 and RECORD2) and TKR (RECORD3 and RECORD4).[96–99] Rivaroxaban was significantly more effective in prevention of VTE after TKR and THR. These three phase III studies demonstrate that a fixed daily unmonitored dose of rivaroxaban provides a safe and effective option for short-term and extended thromboprophylaxis after major orthopedic surgery.

Rivaroxaban was also assessed for treatment of VTE in two randomized phase IIb double-blind, dose-ranging studies of rivaroxaban administered for 12 weeks in patients with acute symptomatic proximal DVT (without PE) vs. parenteral UFH or LMWH and a vitamin K antagonist.[100] These two studies of more than 1150 patients suggested that efficacy of rivaroxaban for treatment of proximal DVT was similar to that achieved with standard anticoagulation therapy, with no significant dose-response relationship for the primary efficacy endpoints and low rates of VTE recurrence and bleeding events. Following on from the promising findings in the VTE treatment studies, phase III studies of long-term rivaroxaban for stroke prevention in patients with atrial fibrillation are underway. ROCKET-AF is a randomized double-blind study designed to assess efficacy and safety of rivaroxaban (20 mg daily) relative to dose-adjusted warfarin for stroke prevention in approximately 14,000 patients with atrial fibrillation. A large dose-finding randomized, double-blind, placebo-controlled phase II study is also underway to investigate the efficacy and safety of rivaroxaban alone or in combination with ASA or ASA and thienopyridine, for secondary prevention of fatal and nonfatal cardiovascular events in patients with recent ACS.

APIXABAN

Apixaban is in clinical development for prevention of VTE in patients undergoing THR and TKR, in patients with advanced metastatic cancer and in medically ill patients, secondary prevention in patients with ACS, prevention of stroke in nonvalvular atrial fibrillation, and treatment of VTE. Apixaban is a follow-up to razaxaban. Clinical development of razaxaban was stopped following a phase II trial in patients undergoing TKR, in which the three higher dosages of razaxaban caused major bleeding. Apixaban has an improved pharmacological profile relative to razaxaban.

Apixaban is a highly potent and selective direct inhibitor of factor Xa. Apixaban is eliminated via multiple pathways; 70% of the compound is eliminated in feces, and 25% is eliminated via the renal pathway. In two double-blind randomized, placebo-controlled, dose-escalation studies in healthy males, oral apixaban demonstrated predictable pharmacokinetics with single doses, with maximum plasma concentrations achieved 1.5 to 3.5 hours after oral administration of the drug.

Efficacy and safety of apixaban for prevention of VTE in patients undergoing TKR was evaluated in a phase IIb trial (APROPOS). [101] In this study, 1217 patients were randomized to receive one of six doses of apixaban (5 mg, 10 mg, or 20 mg, administered once or twice daily), open-label enoxaparin 30 mg twice daily, or warfarin for 10 to 14 days. Apixaban and enoxaparin were initiated 12 to 24 hours after surgery, whereas warfarin was started in the evening of the day of surgery. Rates of VTE and all-cause mortality, the primary efficacy endpoint, were significantly lower in the combined apixaban groups (8.6%) than in either the enoxaparin or warfarin groups (15.6% [$P < 0.02$] and 26.6% [$P < 0.001$], respectively). The primary safety endpoint of major bleeding was similar between treatment groups.

A recent double-blind randomized dose-finding trial investigated the efficacy and safety of apixaban in patients with confirmed DVT (proximal DVT or extensive calf DVT). Frequency of the primary efficacy endpoint (composite of symptomatic recurrent VTE and deterioration of the thrombotic burden, as assessed by repeat bilateral compression ultrasound and perfusion lung scan) was similar in the apixaban 5 mg twice daily and 10 mg twice daily groups (6.0% and 5.6%, respectively) and lower in the apixaban 20 mg daily group (2.6%). Early evaluation of results from phase III study of apixaban for prevention of VTE in patients undergoing TKR, however, indicate that the primary endpoint was not met. [102]

A placebo-controlled phase II pilot study is in progress to investigate apixaban for prevention of thromboembolic events in patients undergoing treatment for advanced cancer (ADVOCATE). Efficacy and safety of a 30-day regimen of apixaban compared with enoxaparin for prevention of VTE in acutely medically ill patients has been initiated in a phase III study. Two phase III studies of apixaban for stroke prevention in atrial fibrillation are in progress. One is designed to evaluate efficacy and safety of apixaban vs. warfarin in preventing stroke and systemic embolism in 15,000 patients with nonvalvular atrial fibrillation and at least one additional risk factor for stroke (ARISTOTLE). The second trial is assessing whether apixaban is superior to ASA in preventing stroke or systemic embolism in 5600 patients with atrial fibrillation and at least one additional risk factor for stroke who refuse or are unsuitable for treatment with a vitamin K antagonist (AVERROES). A large phase II placebo-controlled study is examining the efficacy and safety of apixaban in patients with recent ACS (APPRAISE-2).

DU-176b

DU-176b is an oral direct factor Xa inhibitor in early clinical development for prophylaxis and treatment of thrombotic disorders. It is a potent inhibitor of factor Xa, with a 10,000-fold higher selectivity for factor Xa than for thrombin. DU-176b dose-dependently prolongs clotting times and decreases thrombin generation and platelet aggregation. A phase I study in 12 healthy adults demonstrated that DU-176b was able to reduce thrombus formation ex vivo in a Badimon chamber. The antithrombotic effects of DU-176b were sustained for up to 5 hours, with maximum inhibition of factor Xa activity occurring 1.5 hours after administration. [103] A recent phase II study evaluating the efficacy and safety of DU-176b for prevention of VTE in patients undergoing total knee arthroplasty demonstrated significant dose-dependent reductions in VTE in patients undergoing total knee arthroplasty, with a bleeding incidence similar to placebo. [104] In a phase II study of prevention of stroke in atrial fibrillation, patients will receive DU-176b or warfarin for 3 months.

LY517717

LY517717 is an indol-6-yl-carbonyl derivative in development for treatment and prophylaxis of thromboembolic disorders. It is a factor Xa inhibitor with 1000-fold higher selectivity for factor Xa than other serine proteases, and high oral availability. [105] In humans, anticoagulant activity of LY517717 peaked within 0.5 to 4 hours of administration, and a terminal half-life of approximately 27 hours was observed, with the gastrointestinal tract as the main elimination route. A phase II double-blind parallel-group, dose-ranging study of LY517717 was undertaken in 511 patients undergoing THR or TKR. LY517717 was investigated relative to enoxaparin. [106] The primary efficacy endpoint was a composite of DVT, and for the higher doses of LY517717, incidences of VTE were 19% (100 mg), 19% (125 mg), and 16% (150 mg), compared to 21% for enoxaparin, indicating that LY517717 at these doses was noninferior to enoxaparin according to prespecified criteria. Further development of LY517717 is planned, with phase III trials for prevention of VTE.

BETRIXABAN

Betrixaban is a potent inhibitor of factor Xa, with a half-life of 19 hours. The antithrombotic activity of betrixaban, demonstrated in different animal models of arterial and venous thrombosis, has been shown to occur at doses that inhibit thrombin generation in human blood. A phase I dose-escalation study in 64 subjects revealed that betrixaban had minimal interactions with food and predictable pharmacokinetics and pharmacodynamics. [107] Furthermore, betrixaban undergoes minimal renal excretion because it is predominantly eliminated unchanged in bile. In a phase IIa proof-of-concept study (EXPERT), betrixaban was investigated relative to enoxaparin administered for 10 to 14 days. [108] The primary efficacy endpoint was the incidence of VTE (symptomatic DVT or PE or asymptomatic DVT on a mandatory venogram) on days 10 to 14. Rates of VTE were 20% and 15%, respectively, in patients receiving betrixaban, and 10% in patients receiving enoxaparin. Further clinical studies for prevention and treatment of VTE, stroke prevention in atrial fibrillation, and secondary prevention of stroke and MI are planned.

YM150

YM150 is in development for prevention of VTE. YM150 has a major active metabolite, YM-222741, against factor Xa. A randomized open-label, phase IIa dose-escalation trial in 178 patients undergoing THR assessed YM150 for 7 to 10 days after surgery, relative to enoxaparin. [109] The primary endpoint was major and/or clinically relevant nonmajor bleeding, and the main efficacy endpoint was the composite of DVT detected by mandatory bilateral venography, confirmed symptomatic DVT, PE, and all-cause mortality. There were no major bleeding events during the study and three clinically relevant nonmajor bleeding events. Venous thromboembolism incidence was dose dependent, ranging from 52% for 3-mg dosing to 19% at 60 mg; incidence of VTE in the enoxaparin group was 39%. [110] A phase IIb study of YM150 (5-120 mg daily) for prevention of VTE after THR has been completed recently. [110] Incidence of the primary efficacy endpoint (composite of DVT, symptomatic VTE, PE, and death up to day 7 to 10 of treatment) ranged from 31.7% to 13.3% and decreased significantly with increasing doses of YM150 ($P < 0.0002$). A further phase II study will assess the pharmacokinetics, pharmacodynamics, safety, and tolerability of YM150 in an atrial fibrillation patient population.

Factor IX Inhibitors

Coagulation is a complex process in which circulating soluble proteins, cellular elements, and tissue-based proteins interface to form an insoluble clot at sites of vascular injury. Thrombin generation is maximized on the platelet surface during the propagation phase of clot formation. Activated platelets bind the factor IXa/VIIIa complex. Additional IXa is generated by factor XIa on the platelet surface.[111] The factor IXa/VIIIa complex, in physical proximity to factor Va, recruits factor X for activation. The Xa/Va complex on the platelet surface is protected from inhibition by TFPI and AT. Activation of factor X by the factor IXa/VIIIa complex is nearly 50 times more efficient than its activation by the TF/VIIa complex.[112] The platelet factor Xa/Va complex then catalyzes thrombin formation, resulting in a stable fibrin-platelet clot.[113] A severe bleeding tendency is typically associated with less than 1% factor IX activity. A moderate bleeding risk is incurred among individuals with 1% to 5% FIX activity, and a 5% to 40% factor IX activity causes a relatively modest hemostatic defect. Factor IXa plays a role in angiogenesis, wound healing, vascular repair, and platelet-mediated hemostasis. Factor IXa/VIIIa complex may play a pivotal role in amplifying thrombin generation initiated by the TF-VIIa complexes after vascular injury. Binding of factors IX and IXa to thrombin-activated human platelets is well described. In the presence of factors VIII and X, the affinity of receptors for factor IXa increases fivefold.

ACTIVE-SITE COMPETITIVE ANTAGONISTS

The earliest investigation of FIXa inhibitors was based on an active-site competitive antagonist, IXai, a protein without functional anticoagulant activity.[114] Intravenous infusion of IXai inhibited thrombosis in animal models of coronary thrombosis and stroke in a dose-dependent fashion and produced less bleeding than UFH.[114-118] To date, clinical trials of factor IXai have not been conducted.

MONOCLONAL ANTIBODIES AS ANTICOAGULANTS

Monoclonal antibodies are currently used to treat cancer, autoimmune disease, and allergy. Several antibodies directed against the Gla domain of factor IX have been developed. The 10C12 clone was an effective anticoagulant, prolonging APTT as well as inhibiting platelet-mediated clotting *in vitro*.[119] It effectively inhibited arterial thrombosis in a rabbit model of carotid artery injury, without increasing blood loss from a standardized cutaneous incision.[120] A humanized monoclonal antibody, SB 249417, is a chimeric molecule directed against the human FIX Gla domain. In a rat arterial thrombosis model, the antibody produced significant reductions in thrombus formation, with modest APTT prolongation. In a murine stroke model, SB 249417 reduced infarct volume and was associated with reduced neurological deficits compared to tPA.[121] Suppression of FIX activity and APTT prolongation were rapid and dose dependent. A phase I clinical trial with SB 249417 has been completed. Designed as a single-blind randomized placebo-controlled, single intravenous infusion dose-escalating trial, the study was undertaken to establish pharmacokinetic and pharmacodynamic properties. The antibody displayed a dose-dependent effect on clotting times, with a maximal effect at completion of a 50-minute continuous infusion.[122] There were no major safety concerns.

RIBONUCLEIC ACID APTAMERS AS ANTICOAGULANTS

Aptamers are short oligonucleotides (<100 bases) selected for their ability to bind a chosen target, typically a protein or small molecule.[123] A complex between RNA and the selected target protein (or small molecule) involves a three-dimensional folding of the RNA such that it is complementary with the surface of the target protein. Molecular recognition of a target protein by an aptamer can involve several types of RNA protein interactions, including hydrogen bonding, salt bridges, van der Waals forces, and stacking with aromatic amino acids.[124]

Aptamer 9.3t, specific for factor IXa, showed that the aptamer bound factors IX and IXa with high affinity but exhibited minimal affinity for the structurally related proteins, factors VII, X, or XI, or protein C.[125] Since factor VIIa binds FIX via the Gla and EGF domains, the aptamer may interact with the EGF domain.[126] An RNA antidote (5.2) to the FIXa aptamer has been made and can reverse 9.3t-induced anticoagulation in human plasma.[127] Other advantages of the aptamer/antidote pair include reduced generation of thrombin and inflammatory mediators (interleukin [IL]-1b, IL-6), reduced postoperative hemorrhage, and improved cardiac output.[128] The anti-IX aptamer/antidote pair 9.3t and its antidote 5-2 were subsequently optimized for *in vivo* stability and manufacturability to generate the REG-1 anticoagulation system. Regado-1A was a subject-blinded dose-escalation placebo-controlled study that randomized 85 healthy volunteers to receive a bolus of drug (FIX aptamer RB006) or placebo, followed 3 hours later by a bolus of antidote (RB007) or placebo.[129] Among subjects treated with RB006, APTT and ACT increased rapidly in a dose-dependent fashion, and the observed pharmacodynamic effect was stable over a 3-hour time period. The Regado-1C study randomized 39 healthy human subjects in a double-blind fashion to either three consecutive weight-adjusted drug/antidote treatment cycles or double placebo. Each treatment cycle consisted of an intravenous bolus of RB006, followed an hour later by an ascending dose of RB007. There was a graded response to varying doses of antidote, showing an ability to titrate anticoagulant response and reversibility. There were no major bleeding or other serious adverse events.[130] Potential clinical applications for this injectable factor IXa–specific drug antidote system include percutaneous and surgical coronary revascularization procedures, bridging therapy for elective noncardiac surgery in patients on Coumadin therapy, prophylaxis and treatment of venous and arterial thromboembolic disorders, and maintenance of hemodialysis circuit patency. A subcutaneous formulation that is currently being studied may extend the pharmacodynamic half-life of the drug, minimizing the number of daily injections and enabling home use. A key concern will be the potential for equipment-related thrombosis, a phenomenon that has hindered clinical development of other specific coagulation protease inhibitors.[131]

TTP889

TTP889 is an orally available small-molecule selective partial antagonist of factor IX/IXa. The FIXIT study group conducted a phase II clinical trial to determine the safety and antithrombotic efficacy of TTP889 in patients at risk for VTE. This multicenter placebo-controlled trial enrolled 261 hip fracture surgery patients,[132] and there was no significant difference between treatment groups in the composite primary outcome of venographic or symptomatic DVT or PE at the end of the study period. However, TTP889 had no effect on markers of thrombin generation and fibrin degradation (D-dimer) compared with placebo, despite the use of TTP889 dose levels considered sevenfold higher than that required to prevent venous thrombosis in animal models. This apparent lack of pharmacodynamic effect raises concerns about the appropriateness of the dose of TTP889 selected.

FACTOR IX-BINDING PROTEINS

It is known that natural anticoagulants occur from snake venom, including a family of homologous proteins that complex with factor IX (IX-binding proteins [bp]), factor X (X-bp), or both (IX/X-bp). The family includes habu IX-bp and habu IX/X-bp of *Trimeresurus flavoviridis*, echis IX/X-bp of *Echis carinatus leucogaster*, and acutus X-bp of *Deinagkistrodon acutus*.[133] The venom of *Agkistrodon acutus* contains agkisacutacin, a homologous protein that binds both platelet GPIb and coagulation factors IX and X.[134] These proteins have structures similar to disulfide-linked heterodimers of C-type lectin-like subunits. *In vitro* studies with IX-bp from *T. flavoviridis* showed anticoagulant activity, with prolongation of APTT and interference of FIXa binding to phosphatidyl serine on the plasma membrane.

Summary

Over the past several years, a variety of new antiplatelet and antithrombotic agents have been developed and investigated. Each agent presents clinical benefits that must be weighed against notable side effects, highlighting the complex nature of platelet activation and control of thrombosis. Many of these new therapies appear promising, but continuing studies are required to evaluate the role of existing antiplatelet and antithrombotic strategies, as well as determine the additive side effects, most notably increased bleeding. Evolution of antiplatelet and antithrombotic therapies plus our growing understanding of the delicate balance between vascular occlusive disease and the side effect of bleeding have great potential for improving future treatment of thrombosis.

REFERENCES

1. Writing Group Members, Lloyd-Jones D, Adams RJ, et al: Heart disease and stroke statistics--2010 update: a report from the American Heart Association, *Circulation* 121:e46–e215, 2010.
2. Kamath S, Blann AD, Lip GY: Platelet activation: assessment and quantification, *Eur Heart J* 22:1561–1571, 2001.
3. Quinton TM, Murugappan S, Kim S, et al: Different G protein-coupled signaling pathways are involved in α granule release from human platelets, *J Thromb Haemost* 2:978–984, 2004.
4. Hamilton JR: Protease-activated receptors as targets for antiplatelet therapy, *Blood Rev* 23:61–65, 2009.
5. Sabatine MS: Novel antiplatelet strategies in acute coronary syndromes, *Cleve Clin J Med* 76:S8–S15, 2009.
6. Davì G, Patrono C: Platelet activation and atherothrombosis, *N Engl J Med* 357:2482–2494, 2007.
7. LF B: Thrombin and platelet activation, *Chest* 124:18S–25S, 2003.
8. Varga-Szabo DP, Irina, Nieswandt B: Cell adhesion mechanisms in platelets, *Arterioscler Thromb Vasc Biol* 28(3):403–412, 2008.
9. Smith JB, Dangelmaier C, Mauco G: Measurement of arachidonic acid liberation in thrombin-stimulated human platelets. Use of agents that inhibit both the cyclooxygenase and lipoxygenase enzymes, *Biochim Biophys Acta* 835:344–351, 1985.
10. Smith WL: Prostanoid biosynthesis and mechanisms of action, *Am J Physiol* 263:F181–F191, 1992.
11. Smith WL, Marnett LJ: Prostaglandin endoperoxide synthase: structure and catalysis, *Biochim Biophys Acta* 1083:1–17, 1991.
12. Funk CD, Funk LB, Kennedy ME, et al: Human platelet/erythroleukemia cell prostaglandin G/H synthase: cDNA cloning, expression, and gene chromosomal assignment, *FASEB J* 5:2304–2312, 1991.
13. Pedersen AK, FitzGerald GA: Dose-related kinetics of aspirin. Presystemic acetylation of platelet cyclooxygenase, *N Engl J Med* 311:1206–1211, 1984.
14. Awtry EH, Loscalzo J: Aspirin, *Circulation* 101:1206–1218, 2000.
15. Berge E, Sandercock P: Anticoagulants versus antiplatelet agents for acute ischaemic stroke, *Cochrane Database Syst Rev* 2002:CD003242.
16. DiChiara J, Bliden KP, Tantry US, et al: The effect of aspirin dosing on platelet function in diabetic and nondiabetic patients: an analysis from the aspirin-induced platelet effect (ASPECT) study, *Diabetes* 56:3014–3019, 2007.
17. Pedersen AK, FitzGerald GA: Cyclooxygenase inhibition, platelet function, and metabolite formation during chronic sulfinpyrazone dosing, *Clin Pharmacol Ther* 37:36–42, 1985.
18. Rebuzzi AG, Natale A, Bianchi C, et al: Effects of indobufen on platelet thromboxane B2 production in patients with myocardial infarction, *Eur J Clin Pharmacol* 39:99–100, 1990.
19. Ramis J, Torrent J, Mis R, et al: Pharmacokinetics of triflusal after single and repeated doses in man, *Int J Clin Pharmacol Ther Toxicol* 28:344–349, 1990.
20. Marczewski MM, Postula M, Kosior D: Novel antiplatelet agents in the prevention of cardiovascular complications–focus on ticagrelor, *Vasc Health Risk Manag* 6:419–429, 2010.
21. Mangin P, Ohlmann P, Eckly A, et al: The P2Y1 receptor plays an essential role in the platelet shape change induced by collagen when TxA2 formation is prevented, *J Thromb Haemost* 2:969–977, 2004.
22. Storey RF: Biology and pharmacology of the platelet P2Y12 receptor, *Curr Pharm Des* 12:1255–1259, 2006.
23. Schomig A: Ticagrelor–is there need for a new player in the antiplatelet-therapy field? *N Engl J Med* 361:1108–1111, 2009.
24. Patrono C, Coller B, FitzGerald GA, et al: Platelet-active drugs: the relationships among dose, effectiveness, and side effects: the Seventh ACCP Conference on Antithrombotic and Thrombolytic Therapy, *Chest* 126:234S–264S, 2004.
25. Wallentin L, Varenhorst C, James S, et al: Prasugrel achieves greater and faster P2Y12 receptor-mediated platelet inhibition than clopidogrel due to more efficient generation of its active metabolite in aspirin-treated patients with coronary artery disease, *Eur Heart J* 29:21–30, 2008.
26. Brandt JT, Payne CD, Wiviott SD, et al: A comparison of prasugrel and clopidogrel loading doses on platelet function: magnitude of platelet inhibition is related to active metabolite formation, *Am Heart J* 153(66):e9–e16, 2007.
27. CAPRIE Steering Committee: A randomised, blinded, trial of clopidogrel versus aspirin in patients at risk of ischaemic events (CAPRIE), *Lancet* 348:1329–1339, 1996.
28. Yusuf S, Zhao F, Mehta SR, et al: Effects of clopidogrel in addition to aspirin in patients with acute coronary syndromes without ST-segment elevation, *N Engl J Med* 345:494–502, 2001.
29. Chen ZM, Jiang LX, Chen YP, et al: Addition of clopidogrel to aspirin in 45,852 patients with acute myocardial infarction: randomised placebo-controlled trial, *Lancet* 366:1607–1621, 2005.
30. Steinhubl SR, Berger PB, Mann JT, et al: Early and sustained dual oral antiplatelet therapy following percutaneous coronary intervention: a randomized controlled trial, *JAMA* 288:2411–2420, 2002.
31. Bhatt DL, Topol EJ: Current role of platelet glycoprotein IIb/IIIa inhibitors in acute coronary syndromes, *JAMA* 284:1549–1558, 2000.
32. Wang TH, Bhatt DL, Fox KA, et al: An analysis of mortality rates with dual-antiplatelet therapy in the primary prevention population of the CHARISMA trial, *Eur Heart J* 28:2200–2207, 2007.
33. Bhatt DL, Flather MD, Hacke W, et al: Patients with prior myocardial infarction, stroke, or symptomatic peripheral arterial disease in the CHARISMA trial, *J Am Coll Cardiol* 49:1982–1988, 2007.
34. Wiviott SD, Trenk D, Frelinger AL, et al: Prasugrel compared with high loading- and maintenance-dose clopidogrel in patients with planned percutaneous coronary intervention: the Prasugrel in Comparison to Clopidogrel for Inhibition of Platelet Activation and Aggregation-Thrombolysis in Myocardial Infarction 44 Trial, *Circulation* 116:2923–2932, 2007.
35. Tantry US, Bliden KP, Gurbel PA: Azd6140, *Expert Opin Investig Drugs* 16:225–229, 2007.
36. Sabatine MS: Novel antiplatelet strategies in acute coronary syndromes, *Cleve Clin J Med* 76(Suppl 1):S8–S15, 2009.
37. Cannon CP, Husted S, Harrington RA, et al: Safety, tolerability, and initial efficacy of AZD6140, the first reversible oral adenosine diphosphate receptor antagonist, compared with clopidogrel, in patients with non-ST-segment elevation acute coronary syndrome: primary results of the DISPERSE-2 trial, *J Am Coll Cardiol* 50:1844–1851, 2007.
38. Wallentin L, Becker RC, Budaj A, et al: Ticagrelor versus clopidogrel in patients with acute coronary syndromes, *N Engl J Med* 361:1045–1057, 2009.
39. Gurbel PA, Bliden KP, Butler K, et al: Randomized double-blind assessment of the ONSET and OFFSET of the antiplatelet effects of ticagrelor versus clopidogrel in patients with stable coronary artery disease: the ONSET/OFFSET study, *Circulation* 120:2577–2585, 2009.
40. Schror K, Weber AA: Comparative pharmacology of GP IIb/IIIa antagonists, *J Thromb Thrombolysis* 15:71–80, 2003.
41. Moliterno DJ, Califf RM, Aguirre FV, et al: Effect of platelet glycoprotein IIb/IIIa integrin blockade on activated clotting time during percutaneous transluminal coronary angioplasty or directional atherectomy (the EPIC trial). Evaluation of c7E3 Fab in the Prevention of Ischemic Complications trial, *Am J Cardiol* 75:559–562, 1995.
42. Roe MT, Moliterno DJ: The EPILOG trial. Abciximab prevents ischemic complications during angioplasty. Evaluation in PTCA to improve long-term outcome with abciximab GP IIb/IIIa blockade, *Cleve Clin J Med* 65:267–272, 1998.
43. Lincoff AM, Califf RM, Moliterno DJ, et al: Complementary clinical benefits of coronary-artery stenting and blockade of platelet glycoprotein IIb/IIIa receptors. Evaluation of Platelet IIb/IIIa Inhibition in Stenting Investigators, *N Engl J Med* 341:319–327, 1999.
44. Kastrati A, Mehilli J, Schuhlen H, et al: A clinical trial of abciximab in elective percutaneous coronary intervention after pretreatment with clopidogrel, *N Engl J Med* 350:232–238, 2004.
45. Kastrati A, Mehilli J, Neumann FJ, et al: Abciximab in patients with acute coronary syndromes undergoing percutaneous coronary intervention after clopidogrel pretreatment: the ISAR-REACT 2 randomized trial, *JAMA* 295:1531–1538, 2006.
46. Tcheng JE: Differences among the parenteral platelet glycoprotein IIb/IIIa inhibitors and implications for treatment, *Am J Cardiol* 83:7E–11E, 1999.
47. Giugliano RP, White JA, Bode C, et al: Early versus delayed, provisional eptifibatide in acute coronary syndromes, *N Engl J Med* 360:2176–2190, 2009.
48. Ruggeri ZM, Ware J: von Willebrand factor, *FASEB J* 7:308–316, 1993.
49. Weiss HJ, Sussman II, Hoyer LW: Stabilization of factor VIII in plasma by the von Willebrand factor. Studies on posttransfusion and dissociated factor VIII and in patients with von Willebrand's disease, *J Clin Invest* 60:390–404, 1977.
50. Hennan JK, Swillo RE, Morgan GA, et al: Pharmacologic inhibition of platelet vWF-GPIb alpha interaction prevents coronary artery thrombosis, *Thromb Haemost* 95:469–475, 2006.
51. Montalescot G, Philippe F, Ankri A, et al: Early increase of von Willebrand factor predicts adverse outcome in unstable coronary artery disease: beneficial effects of enoxaparin. French Investigators of the ESSENCE Trial, *Circulation* 98:294–299, 1998.
52. Kageyama S, Yamamoto H, Nakazawa H, et al: Pharmacokinetics and pharmacodynamics of AJW200, a humanized monoclonal antibody to von Willebrand factor, in monkeys, *Arterioscler Thromb Vasc Biol* 22:187–192, 2002.
53. Brody EN, Gold L: Aptamers as therapeutic and diagnostic agents, *J Biotechnol* 74:5–13, 2000.
54. Gilbert JC, DeFeo-Fraulini T, Hutabarat RM, et al: First-in-human evaluation of anti von Willebrand factor therapeutic aptamer ARC1779 in healthy volunteers, *Circulation* 116:2678–2686, 2007.
55. Gurevitz O, Eldar M, Skutelsky E, et al: S-nitrosoderivative of a recombinant fragment of von Willebrand factor (S-nitroso-AR545C) inhibits thrombus formation in guinea pig carotid artery thrombosis model, *Thromb Haemost* 84:912–917, 2000.
56. Samaha FF, Kahn ML: Novel platelet and vascular roles for immunoreceptor signaling, *Arterioscler Thromb Vasc Biol* 26:2588–2593, 2006.
57. Nieswandt B, Schulte V, Bergmeier W, et al: Long-term antithrombotic protection by in vivo depletion of platelet glycoprotein VI in mice, *J Exp Med* 193:459–469, 2001.
58. Markwardt F, Nowak G, Sturzebecher J: Clinical pharmacology of recombinant hirudin, *Haemostasis* 21(Suppl 1):133–136, 1991.
59. Eichler P, Friesen HJ, Lubenow N, et al: Antihirudin antibodies in patients with heparin-induced thrombocytopenia treated with lepirudin: incidence, effects on aPTT, and clinical relevance, *Blood* 96:2373–2378, 2000.
60. Greinacher A, Lubenow N, Eichler P: Anaphylactic and anaphylactoid reactions associated with lepirudin in patients with heparin-induced thrombocytopenia, *Circulation* 108:2062–2065, 2003.

61. Lubenow N, Eichler P, Lietz T, et al: Lepirudin in patients with heparin-induced thrombocytopenia - results of the third prospective study (HAT-3) and a combined analysis of HAT-1, HAT-2, and HAT-3, *J Thromb Haemost* 3:2428–2436, 2005.
62. Organisation to Assess Strategies for Ischemic Syndromes (OASIS-2) Investigators: Effects of recombinant hirudin (lepirudin) compared with heparin on death, myocardial infarction, refractory angina, and revascularisation procedures in patients with acute myocardial ischaemia without ST elevation: a randomised trial, *Lancet* 353:429–438, 1999.
63. Greinacher A, Eichler P, Albrecht D, et al: Antihirudin antibodies following low-dose subcutaneous treatment with desirudin for thrombosis prophylaxis after hip-replacement surgery: incidence and clinical relevance, *Blood* 101:2617–2619, 2003.
64. Eriksson BI, Ekman S, Lindbratt S, et al: Prevention of thromboembolism with use of recombinant hirudin. Results of a double-blind, multicenter trial comparing the efficacy of desirudin (Revasc) with that of unfractionated heparin in patients having a total hip replacement, *J Bone Joint Surg Am* 79:326–333, 1997.
65. Eriksson BI, Wille-Jorgensen P, Kalebo P, et al: A comparison of recombinant hirudin with a low-molecular-weight heparin to prevent thromboembolic complications after total hip replacement, *N Engl J Med* 337:1329–1335, 1997.
66. Bates SM, Weitz JI: Direct thrombin inhibitors for treatment of arterial thrombosis: potential differences between bivalirudin and hirudin, *Am J Cardiol* 82:12P–18P, 1998.
67. Bittl JA, Chaitman BR, Feit F, et al: Bivalirudin versus heparin during coronary angioplasty for unstable or postinfarction angina: final report reanalysis of the Bivalirudin Angioplasty Study, *Am Heart J* 142:952–959, 2001.
68. Lincoff AM, Bittl JA, Kleiman NS, et al: Comparison of bivalirudin versus heparin during percutaneous coronary intervention (the Randomized Evaluation of PCI Linking Angiomax to Reduced Clinical Events [REPLACE]-1 trial), *Am J Cardiol* 93:1092–1096, 2004.
69. Lincoff AM, Kleiman NS, Kereiakes DJ, et al: Long-term efficacy of bivalirudin and provisional glycoprotein IIb/IIIa blockade vs heparin and planned glycoprotein IIb/IIIa blockade during percutaneous coronary revascularization: REPLACE-2 randomized trial, *JAMA* 292:696–703, 2004.
70. Stone GW, Ware JH, Bertrand ME, et al: Antithrombotic strategies in patients with acute coronary syndromes undergoing early invasive management: one-year results from the ACUITY trial, *JAMA* 298:2497–2506, 2007.
71. Berry CN, Girardot C, Lecoffre C, et al: Effects of the synthetic thrombin inhibitor argatroban on fibrin- or clot-incorporated thrombin: comparison with heparin and recombinant Hirudin, *Thromb Haemost* 72:381–386, 1994.
72. Swan SK, St Peter JV, Lambrecht LJ, et al: Comparison of anticoagulant effects and safety of argatroban and heparin in healthy subjects, *Pharmacotherapy* 20:756–770, 2000.
73. Sheth SB, DiCicco RA, Hursting MJ, et al: Interpreting the International Normalized Ratio (INR) in individuals receiving argatroban and warfarin, *Thromb Haemost* 85:435–440, 2001.
74. Lewis BE, Wallis DE, Leya F, et al: Argatroban anticoagulation in patients with heparin-induced thrombocytopenia, *Arch Intern Med* 163:1849–1856, 2003.
75. Lewis BE, Matthai WH Jr, Cohen M, et al: Argatroban anticoagulation during percutaneous coronary intervention in patients with heparin-induced thrombocytopenia, *Catheter Cardiovasc Interv* 57:177–184, 2002.
76. Cruz-Gonzalez I, Sanchez-Ledesma M, Baron SJ, et al: Efficacy and safety of argatroban with or without glycoprotein IIb/IIIa inhibitor in patients with heparin-induced thrombocytopenia undergoing percutaneous coronary intervention for acute coronary syndrome, *J Thromb Thrombolysis* 25:214–218, 2008.
77. Francis CW, Davidson BL, Berkowitz SD, et al: Ximelagatran versus warfarin for the prevention of venous thromboembolism after total knee arthroplasty. A randomized, double-blind trial, *Ann Intern Med* 137:648–655, 2002.
78. Albers GW, Diener HC, Frison L, et al: Ximelagatran vs warfarin for stroke prevention in patients with nonvalvular atrial fibrillation: a randomized trial, *JAMA* 293:690–698, 2005.
79. Olsson SB: Stroke prevention with the oral direct thrombin inhibitor ximelagatran compared with warfarin in patients with non-valvular atrial fibrillation (SPORTIF III): randomised controlled trial, *Lancet* 362:1691–1698, 2003.
80. Blech S, Ebner T, Ludwig-Schwellinger E, et al: The metabolism and disposition of the oral direct thrombin inhibitor, dabigatran, in humans, *Drug Metab Dispos* 36:386–399, 2008.
81. Stangier J, Stahle H, Rathgen K, et al: Pharmacokinetics and pharmacodynamics of the direct oral thrombin inhibitor dabigatran in healthy elderly subjects, *Clin Pharmacokinet* 47:47–59, 2008.
82. Wienen W, Stassen JM, Priepke H, et al: Effects of the direct thrombin inhibitor dabigatran and its orally active prodrug, dabigatran etexilate, on thrombus formation and bleeding time in rats, *Thromb Haemost* 98:333–338, 2007.
83. Eriksson BI, Dahl OE, Buller HR, et al: A new oral direct thrombin inhibitor, dabigatran etexilate, compared with enoxaparin for prevention of thromboembolic events following total hip or knee replacement: the BISTRO II randomized trial, *J Thromb Haemost* 3:103–111, 2005.
84. Eriksson BI, Dahl OE, Rosencher N, et al: Dabigatran etexilate versus enoxaparin for prevention of venous thromboembolism after total hip replacement: a randomised, double-blind, non-inferiority trial, *Lancet* 370:949–956, 2007.
85. Eriksson BI, Dahl OE, Rosencher N, et al: Oral dabigatran etexilate vs. subcutaneous enoxaparin for the prevention of venous thromboembolism after total knee replacement: the RE-MODEL randomized trial, *J Thromb Haemost* 5:2178–2185, 2007.
86. Connolly SJ, Ezekowitz MD, Yusuf S, et al: Dabigatran versus warfarin in patients with atrial fibrillation, *N Engl J Med* 361:1139–1151, 2009.
87. Perzborn E, Strassburger J, Wilmen A, et al: *In vitro* and *in vivo* studies of the novel antithrombotic agent BAY 59–7939–an oral, direct factor Xa inhibitor, *J Thromb Haemost* 3:514–521, 2005.
88. Gerotziafas GT, Elalamy I, Depasse F, et al: *In vitro* inhibition of thrombin generation, after tissue factor pathway activation, by the oral, direct factor Xa inhibitor rivaroxaban, *J Thromb Haemost* 5:886–888, 2007.
89. Kubitza D, Becka M, Mueck W, et al: Rivaroxaban (BAY 59–7939)–an oral, direct factor Xa inhibitor–has no clinically relevant interaction with naproxen, *Br J Clin Pharmacol* 63:469–476, 2007.
90. Kubitza D, Becka M, Wensing G, et al: Safety, pharmacodynamics, and pharmacokinetics of BAY 59–7939–an oral, direct factor Xa inhibitor–after multiple dosing in healthy male subjects, *Eur J Clin Pharmacol* 61:873–880, 2005.
91. Graff J, von Hentig N, Misselwitz F, et al: Effects of the oral, direct factor xa inhibitor rivaroxaban on platelet-induced thrombin generation and prothrombinase activity, *J Clin Pharmacol* 47:1398–1407, 2007.
92. Weinz C, Schwarz T, Kubitza D, et al: Metabolism and excretion of rivaroxaban, an oral, direct factor Xa inhibitor, in rats, dogs, and humans, *Drug Metab Dispos* 37:1056–1064, 2009.
93. Eriksson BI, Dahl OE, Buller HR, et al: A new oral direct thrombin inhibitor, dabigatran etexilate, compared with enoxaparin for prevention of thromboembolic events following total hip or knee replacement: the BISTRO II randomized trial, *J Thromb Haemost* 3:103–111, 2005.
94. Eriksson BI, Dahl OE, Rosencher N, et al: Oral dabigatran etexilate vs. subcutaneous enoxaparin for the prevention of venous thromboembolism after total knee replacement: the RE-MODEL randomized trial, *J Thromb Haemost* 5:2178–2185, 2007.
95. Ginsberg JS, Davidson BL, Comp PC, et al: Oral thrombin inhibitor dabigatran etexilate vs. North American enoxaparin regimen for prevention of venous thromboembolism after knee arthroplasty surgery, *J Arthroplasty* 24:1–9, 2009.
96. Eriksson BI, Borris LC, Friedman RJ, et al: Rivaroxaban versus enoxaparin for thromboprophylaxis after hip arthroplasty, *N Engl J Med* 358:2765–2775, 2008.
97. Lassen MR, Ageno W, Borris LC, et al: Rivaroxaban versus enoxaparin for thromboprophylaxis after total knee arthroplasty, *N Engl J Med* 358:2776–2786, 2008.
98. Kakkar AK, Brenner B, Dahl OE, et al: Extended duration rivaroxaban versus short-term enoxaparin for the prevention of venous thromboembolism after total hip arthroplasty: a double-blind, randomised controlled trial, *Lancet* 372:31–39, 2008.
99. Turpie AG, Lassen MR, Davidson BL, et al: Rivaroxaban versus enoxaparin for thromboprophylaxis after total knee arthroplasty (RECORD4): a randomised trial, *Lancet* 373:1673–1680, 2009.
100. Agnelli G, Gallus A, Goldhaber SZ, et al: Treatment of proximal deep-vein thrombosis with the oral direct factor Xa inhibitor rivaroxaban (BAY 59–7939): the ODIXa-DVT (Oral Direct Factor Xa Inhibitor BAY 59–7939 in Patients With Acute Symptomatic Deep-Vein Thrombosis) study, *Circulation* 116:180–187, 2007.
101. Lassen MR, Davidson BL, Gallus A, et al: The efficacy and safety of apixaban, an oral, direct factor Xa inhibitor, as thromboprophylaxis in patients following total knee replacement, *J Thromb Haemost* 5:2368–2375, 2007.
102. Pfizer B-MSa: *Bristol-Myers Squibb and Pfizer provide update on apixaban clinical development program* [press release], 2008, August 26, 2008.
103. Zafar MU, Vorchheimer DA, Gaztanaga J, et al: Antithrombotic effects of factor Xa inhibition with DU-176b: phase-I study of an oral, direct factor Xa inhibitor using an ex-vivo flow chamber, *Thromb Haemost* 98:883–888, 2007.
104. Fuji T, Fujita S, Tachibana S, et al: A dose-ranging study evaluating the oral factor Xa inhibitor edoxaban for the prevention of venous thromboembolism in patients undergoing total knee arthroplasty, *J Thromb Haemost* 8:2458–2468, 2010.
105. Spyropoulos AC: Investigational treatments of venous thromboembolism, *Expert Opin Investig Drugs* 16:431–440, 2007.
106. Agnelli G, Haas S, Ginsberg JS, et al: A phase II study of the oral factor Xa inhibitor LY517717 for the prevention of venous thromboembolism after hip or knee replacement, *J Thromb Haemost* 5:746–753, 2007.
107. Turpie AG: Oral, direct factor Xa inhibitors in development for the prevention and treatment of thromboembolic diseases, *Arterioscler Thromb Vasc Biol* 27:1238–1247, 2007.
108. Turpie AG, Bauer KA, Davidson BL, et al: A randomized evaluation of betrixaban, an oral factor Xa inhibitor, for prevention of thromboembolic events after total knee replacement (EXPERT), *Thromb Haemost* 101:68–76, 2009.
109. Eriksson BI, Turpie AG, Lassen MR, et al: Prevention of venous thromboembolism with an oral factor Xa inhibitor, YM150, after total hip arthroplasty. A dose finding study (ONYX-2), *J Thromb Haemost* 8:714–721, 2010.
110. Eriksson BI, Turpie AG, Lassen MR, et al: A dose escalation study of YM150, an oral direct factor Xa inhibitor, in the prevention of venous thromboembolism in elective primary hip replacement surgery, *J Thromb Haemost* 5:1660–1665, 2007.
111. Oliver JA, Monroe DM, Roberts HR, et al: Thrombin activates factor XI on activated platelets in the absence of factor XII, *Arterioscler Thromb Vasc Biol* 19:170–177, 1999.
112. Lawson JH, Kalafatis M, Stram S, et al: A model for the tissue factor pathway to thrombin. I. An empirical study, *J Biol Chem* 269:23357–23366, 1994.
113. Bowen DJ: Haemophilia A and haemophilia B: molecular insights, *Mol Pathol* 55:1–18, 2002.
114. Benedict CR, Ryan J, Wolitzky B, et al: Active site-blocked factor IXa prevents intravascular thrombus formation in the coronary vasculature without inhibiting extravascular coagulation in a canine thrombosis model, *J Clin Invest* 88:1760–1765, 1991.
115. Spanier TB, Oz MC, Madigan JD, et al: Selective anticoagulation with active site blocked factor IXa in synthetic patch vascular repair results in decreased blood loss and operative time, *ASAIO J* 43:M526–M530, 1997.
116. Wong AG, Gunn AC, Ku P, et al: Relative efficacy of active site-blocked factors IXa Xa in models of rabbit venous and arterio-venous thrombosis, *Thromb Haemost* 77:1143–1147, 1997.
117. Spanier TB, Oz MC, Minanov OP, et al: Heparinless cardiopulmonary bypass with active-site blocked factor IXa: a preliminary study on the dog, *J Thorac Cardiovasc Surg* 115:1179–1188, 1998.
118. Choudhri TF, Hoh BL, Prestigiacomo CJ, et al: Targeted inhibition of intrinsic coagulation limits cerebral injury in stroke without increasing intracerebral hemorrhage, *J Exp Med* 190:91–99, 1999.
119. Suggett S, Kirchhofer D, Hass P, et al: Use of phage display for the generation of human antibodies that neutralize factor IXa function, *Blood Coagul Fibrinolysis* 11:27–42, 2000.
120. Refino CJ, Jeet S, DeGuzman L, et al: A human antibody that inhibits factor IX/IXa function potently inhibits arterial thrombosis without increasing bleeding, *Arterioscler Thromb Vasc Biol* 22:517–522, 2002.

121. Toomey JR, Valocik RE, Koster PF, et al: Inhibition of factor IX(a) is protective in a rat model of thromboembolic stroke, *Stroke* 33:578–585, 2002.
122. Benincosa LJ, Chow FS, Tobia LP, et al: Pharmacokinetics and pharmacodynamics of a humanized monoclonal antibody to factor IX in cynomolgus monkeys, *J Pharmacol Exp Ther* 292:810–816, 2000.
123. Ellington AD, Szostak JW: *In vitro* selection of RNA molecules that bind specific ligands, *Nature* 346:818–822, 1990.
124. Hermann T, Patel DJ: Adaptive recognition by nucleic acid aptamers, *Science* 287:820–825, 2000.
125. Rusconi CP, Scardino E, Layzer J, et al: RNA aptamers as reversible antagonists of coagulation factor IXa, *Nature* 419:90–94, 2002.
126. Gopinath SC, Shikamoto Y, Mizuno H, et al: A potent anti-coagulant RNA aptamer inhibits blood coagulation by specifically blocking the extrinsic clotting pathway, *Thromb Haemost* 95:767–771, 2006.
127. Nimjee SM, Keys JR, Pitoc GA, et al: A novel antidote-controlled anticoagulant reduces thrombin generation and inflammation and improves cardiac function in cardiopulmonary bypass surgery, *Mol Ther* 14:408–415, 2006.
128. Rusconi CP, Roberts JD, Pitoc GA, et al: Antidote-mediated control of an anticoagulant aptamer *in vivo*, *Nat Biotechnol* 22:1423–1428, 2004.
129. Dyke CK, Steinhubl SR, Kleiman NS, et al: First-in-human experience of an antidote-controlled anticoagulant using RNA aptamer technology: a phase 1a pharmacodynamic evaluation of a drug-antidote pair for the controlled regulation of factor IXa activity, *Circulation* 114:2490–2497, 2006.
130. Chan MY, Rusconi CP, Alexander JH, et al: A randomized, repeat-dose, pharmacodynamic and safety study of an antidote-controlled factor IXa inhibitor, *J Thromb Haemost* 6:789–796, 2008.
131. Califf RM: Fondaparinux in ST-segment elevation myocardial infarction: the drug, the strategy, the environment, or all of the above? *JAMA* 295:1579–1580, 2006.
132. Eriksson BI, Dahl OE, Lassen MR, et al: Partial factor IXa inhibition with TTP889 for prevention of venous thromboembolism: an exploratory study, *J Thromb Haemost* 6:457–463, 2008.
133. Atoda H, Kaneko H, Mizuno H, et al: Calcium-binding analysis and molecular modeling reveal echis coagulation factor IX/factor X-binding protein has the Ca-binding properties and Ca ion-independent folding of other C-type lectin-like proteins, *FEBS Lett* 531:229–234, 2002.
134. Li WF, Chen L, Li XM, et al: A C-type lectin-like protein from Agkistrodon acutus venom binds to both platelet glycoprotein Ib and coagulation factor IX/factor X, *Biochem Biophys Res Commun* 332:904–912, 2005.

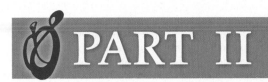

PART II

PATHOBIOLOGY OF BLOOD VESSELS

CHAPTER **8**   # Atherosclerosis

Peter Libby

Knowledge of the pathobiology of atherosclerosis has continued to evolve at a rapid pace. Previously regarded as a mainly segmental disease, we now increasingly appreciate its diffuse nature. The traditional clinical focus on atherosclerosis has emphasized coronary artery disease (CAD). The attention of physicians in general, and of cardiovascular specialists in particular, now embraces other arterial beds, including the peripheral and cerebrovascular arterial beds.

Formerly considered an inevitable and relentlessly progressive degenerative process, we now recognize that quite to the contrary, atherogenesis progresses at varied paces. Increasing clinical and experimental evidence indicates that atheromatous plaques can evolve in vastly different fashions. Atheromata behave much more dynamically than traditionally conceived, from both structural and biological points of view. Plaques not only progress, but also may regress, and/or alter their qualitative characteristics in ways that decisively influence their clinical behavior.

Concepts of the pathobiology of atherosclerosis have likewise undergone perpetual revision. During much of the 20th century, most considered atherosclerosis a cholesterol storage disease. Recognition of the key role of interactions of vascular cells, blood cells (including leukocytes and platelets), and lipoproteins challenged this model later in the 20th century.[1] Current thinking further broadens this schema, incorporating an appreciation of the global metabolic status of individuals, extending far beyond traditional risk factors as triggers to the atherogenic process.

This chapter will delineate the concepts of the widespread and diffuse distributions of atherosclerosis and its clinical manifestations, and also will describe progress in understanding its fundamental biology.

Risk Factors for Atherosclerosis: Traditional, Emerging, and Those on the Rise

Traditional Risk Factors for Atherosclerosis

CHOLESTEROL

Experimental data have repeatedly shown a link between plasma cholesterol levels and the formation of atheromata. Pioneering work performed in Russia in the early 20th century showed that consumption by rabbits of a cholesterol-rich diet caused formation of arterial lesions that shared features with human atheromata.[2] By mid-century, application of the ultracentrifuge to analysis of plasma proteins led to the recognition that various classes of lipoproteins transported cholesterol and other lipids through the aqueous medium of blood. Multiple epidemiological studies verified a link between one cholesterol-rich lipoprotein particle in particular— low-density lipoprotein (LDL)—and the risk for coronary heart disease.[3] The characterization of familial hypercholesterolemia as a genetic disease provided further evidence linking LDL cholesterol levels with coronary heart disease. Heterozygotes for this condition

had markedly elevated risk for atherosclerotic disease. Individuals homozygous for familial hypercholesterolemia commonly develop coronary heart disease within the first decade of life.

Elucidation of the LDL-receptor pathway and that mutations in the LDL receptor cause familial hypercholesterolemia provided proof positive of LDL's role in atherogenesis.[4] Yet the cholesterol hypothesis of atherogenesis still encountered skepticism. Many critics—some laypersons and some respected professionals— questioned aspects of the theory, pointing out that dietary cholesterol levels did not always correlate with cholesterolemia. Lack of proof that either dietary or drug intervention could modify outcomes dogged proponents of the cholesterol hypothesis of atherogenesis.[5]

Ultimately, controlled clinical trials that lowered LDL by interventions including partial intestinal bypass, bile acid–binding resins, and statin drugs showed reductions in coronary events and vindicated the cholesterol hypothesis. In appropriately powered trials conducted with sufficiently potent agents, lipid lowering also reduced overall mortality. Yet the very success of these interventions suggested there must be more to atherogenesis than cholesterol because a majority of events still occurred despite increasingly aggressive control of LDL cholesterol levels. Identification of proprotein convertase subtilisin/kexin type 9 (PCSK9) as the gene involved in autosomal dominant hypercholesterolemia has furnished new insight in this regard. Reduced function of this enzyme raises cellular LDL receptor numbers, and hence augments LDL clearance, leading to lower plasma LDL levels. Individuals with reduced function variants of PCSK9 who experience lifelong lower exposure to LDL show protection from atherosclerotic events even in the presence of other cardiovascular risk factors. These observations strengthen the case for involvement of LDL in atherogenesis, and for aggressive management of LDL in practice.[6]

Of course, aspects of the lipoprotein profile other than LDL can influence atherogenesis (see later discussion).[3] Yet, because atherosclerotic events commonly occur in individuals with average levels of the major lipoprotein classes, a full understanding of atherogenesis requires consideration of factors other than blood lipids.

SYSTEMIC ARTERIAL HYPERTENSION

The relationship between arterial blood pressure and mortality emerged early from actuarial studies. Insurance underwriters had a major financial stake in mortality prediction. A simple measurement of blood pressure with a cuff sphygmomanometer powerfully predicted longevity. Data emerging from the Framingham Study and other observational cohorts verified a relationship between systemic arterial pressure and coronary heart disease events.[7] Concordant observations from experimental animals and epidemiological studies bolstered the link between hypertension and atherosclerosis.

As in the case of high cholesterol, clinical evidence that pharmacological reduction in blood pressure could reduce coronary heart disease events proved fairly elusive. Early-intervention studies readily showed decreases in stroke and congestive heart failure endpoints following administration of antihypertensive drugs. Studies indicating clear-cut reductions in coronary heart disease events with antihypertensive treatment have accumulated much more recently.[8]

Mechanistically, antihypertensive drug therapy likely benefits atherosclerosis and its complications principally by lowering blood pressure, although some have posited other beneficial actions of various antihypertensive agents. A large randomized clinical trial, the Antihypertensive and Lipid-Lowering Treatment to Prevent Heart Attack Trial (ALLHAT), showed no advantage over a 5-year period of a thiazide diuretic over an angiotensin receptor blocker, a calcium channel antagonist, or a β-adrenergic blocking agent.[9,10]

Clinical observations provide strong additional support for the concept that hypertension itself can promote atherogenesis. Atherosclerosis of the pulmonary arteries seldom occurs in individuals with normal pulmonary artery pressures, but even in relatively young patients with pulmonary hypertension, pulmonary arterial atheromata occur quite commonly. This "experiment of nature" supports the direct proatherogenic effect of hypertension in humans.

CIGARETTE SMOKING

Tobacco abuse, and cigarette smoking in particular, accentuates the risk of cardiovascular events.[11] In the context of noncoronary arterial disease, cigarette smoking appears particularly important. The rapid return toward baseline rates of cardiovascular events after smoking cessation suggests that tobacco use alters the risk of thrombosis as much or more than it may accentuate atherogenesis per se. Classic studies in nonhuman primates have shown little effect of 2 to 3 years of cigarette smoke inhalation on experimental atherosclerosis in the presence of moderate hyperlipidemia.

Both first-hand and second-hand tobacco smoke impairs endothelial vasodilator functions—an index of arterial health.[12] Smoking has many other adverse systemic effects, including eliciting a chronic inflammatory response implicated in atherothrombosis.[13] Cigarette smoking seems to contribute particularly to abdominal aortic aneurysm formation. The mechanistic link between cigarette smoking and arterial aneurysm formation may resemble that invoked in the pathogenesis of smoking-related emphysema. Studies in genetically altered mice that inhale tobacco smoke have delineated a role for elastolytic enzymes such as matrix metalloproteinase (MMP)-12 in the destruction of lung extracellular matrix (ECM). Smoke-induced inflammation appears to release tumor necrosis factor (TNF)-α from macrophages that can elevate activity of elastolytic enzymes and promote pulmonary emphysema.[14] A similar mechanism might well promote destruction of elastic laminae in the tunica media of the abdominal aorta, which characterizes aneurysm formation.

AGE

Multiple observational studies have identified age as a potent risk factor for atherosclerotic events.[15] Indeed, in the current cardiovascular risk algorithm based on the Framingham Study, age contributes substantially to risk calculation. Demographic trends portend a marked expansion in the elderly population, particularly women, in coming years. Although age-adjusted rates of cardiovascular disease may appear stable or even declining in men, the actual burden of disease in the elderly will increase because of their sheer number. In view of the expanding elderly population, evidence that supports the mutability of atherosclerosis assumes even greater importance (see later discussion).

SEX

Male sex contributes to heightened cardiovascular risk in numerous observational studies. Mechanisms for this increased burden of disease may reflect male-related proatherogenic factors and/or lack of protection conferred by female sex. Cardiovascular risk increases after menopause in women; many previously attributed the vascular protection enjoyed by premenopausal women to estrogen. But estrogen therapy in women (in more recent large-scale clinical trials) and in men (in the older Coronary Drug Project study) seems to confer hazard rather than benefit in the circumstances studied.[16] Thus estrogen, certainly in combination with progesterone, does not provide a panacea for protection against cardiovascular events. Decreased in high-density lipoprotein (HDL) levels in blood after menopause might explain part of the apparent premenopausal protection from cardiovascular risk.

HIGH-DENSITY LIPOPROTEIN

The Framingham risk algorithm recognizes lower strata of HDL—below 40 mg/dL in both women and men—as a risk factor. Numerous concordant population studies have pointed to the importance of HDL as an atheroprotective lipoprotein fraction. Indeed, in patients who undergo cardiac catheterization and display angiographically significant (CAD), low HDL is more common than high LDL.

Numerous animal studies have established the antiatherogenic effects of HDL or its major apolipoprotein (apo) AI, as have small biomarker studies in humans. Mechanisms by which HDL may protect against atherosclerosis include promotion of reverse lipid transport.[17,18] Furthermore, nascent HDL particles can take up cholesterol from macrophages and other cells in a process that depends on the adenosine triphosphate (ATP) binding cassette transporter 1 (ABCA1). Mature HDL particles can also take up cholesterol through the related transporter ABCG1.[19] In addition, HDL can have antiinflammatory effects.[20] Mechanisms of HDL's arterial protective effect may relate to its ability to bind and carry numerous proteins that may regulate lipid metabolism, oxidative stress, inflammation, and proteolysis.[21]

High-density lipoprotein's metabolism is quite complex—more so in many respects than LDL.[22] The steady-state level of HDL cholesterol, therefore, does not accurately predict cardiovascular protection. Although baseline levels of HDL cholesterol quite consistently track inversely with cardiovascular events, interventions that raise HDL cholesterol levels do not necessarily reduce event rates. Moreover, recent data challenge the extent to which HDL levels influence outcomes on individuals taking potent LDL-lowering treatment.[23,24] The ability of HDL particles to effect cholesterol efflux from macrophages in vitro correlates with CAD status and the biomarker of risk, carotid intima media thickness.[18] Yet the ability of pharmacologically induced increases in HDL to confer clinical benefit remains unproven. Several large-scale trials currently in progress should clarify whether drugs of several classes that elevate HDL can reduce clinical events.[25,26]

Emerging Risk Factors for Atherosclerosis

HOMOCYSTEINE

Homocysteine, a product of amino acid metabolism, may contribute to atherothrombosis.[27] Individuals with genetic defects that lead to elevated homocysteine levels (e.g., homocystinuria, commonly due to deficiency in cystathionine β-synthase) have a thrombotic diathesis. In vitro, treatment with homocysteine and related compounds can alter aspects of vascular cell function related to atherogenesis. Reliable clinical tests for hyperhomocysteinemia exist. Although clearly associated with elevated thrombotic risk in patients with homocystinuria, elevated levels of homocysteine in unselected populations only weakly predict cardiovascular risk (Fig. 8-1). Moreover, randomized trials that have used vitamin treatments to lower homocysteine levels have not documented improvements in cardiovascular outcomes.[28-30] Enrichment of cereals and flour with folate in the United States has shifted dietary intake and should lower blood homocysteine levels in the American population.

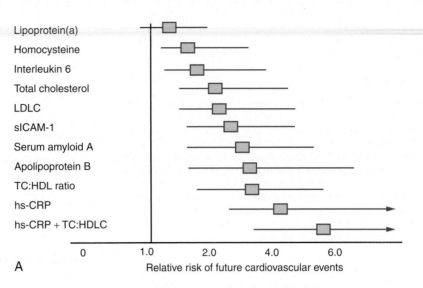

A
Relative risk of future cardiovascular events

Novel risk factors as predictors of peripheral arterial disease

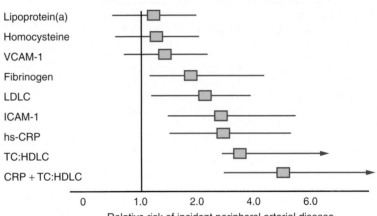

B
Relative risk of incident peripheral arterial disease
(Adjusted for age, smoking, DM, HTN, family history, exercise level, and BMI)

C-reactive protein concentration and risk of cardiovascular events: 2010
Direct comparison of hsCRP, SBP, total cholesterol, and non-HDLC

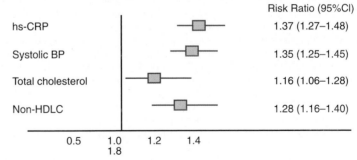

	Risk Ratio (95%CI)
hs-CRP	1.37 (1.27–1.48)
Systolic BP	1.35 (1.25–1.45)
Total cholesterol	1.16 (1.06–1.28)
Non-HDLC	1.28 (1.16–1.40)

Risk ratio (95%CI) per 1-SD higher usual values

Adjusted for age, sex, smoking, diabetes, BMI, BP, triglycerides, alcohol, lipid levels, and hsCRP
Emerging Risk Factor Collaborators, Lancet Jan 2010

C

FIGURE 8-1 Predictive power of some established and emerging risk markers for coronary and peripheral atherosclerosis. Relative risk for overall cardiovascular events **(A)** and incidence of peripheral artery disease **(B)** from the Women's Health Study and the Physicians' Health Study, respectively. Whisker plots show point estimates and confidence intervals (CIs) for various emerging and established risk factors for atherosclerotic complications. Rank, order, and magnitude of risk of peripheral artery disease in the Women's Health Study and of cardiovascular events in the Physicians' Health Study due to these established and emerging risk factors resembles that reported earlier (not shown). **C,** Direct comparison of hsCRP, systolic blood pressure, BP, total cholesterol, and non-HDLC adjusted for age, sex, smoking, diabetes, BMI, BP, triglycerides, alcohol, lipid levels, and hsCRP. Comparisons use data from 91,990 participants (5373 CHD events) from 31 studies. hs-CRP, C-reactive protein measured by the high-sensitivity assay; HTN, hypertension; LDLC, low-density lipoprotein cholesterol; sICAM-1, soluble intercellular adhesion molecule-1; TC:HDL ratio, total cholesterol/high-density lipoprotein ratio; TC:HDLC, total cholesterol/high-density lipoprotein cholesterol; VCAM-1, soluble vascular cell adhesion molecule. *(Reproduced with permission from Ridker PM: Clinical application of C-reactive protein for cardiovascular disease detection and prevention. Circulation 107:363, 2003; Ridker PM, Stampfer MJ, Rifai N: Novel risk factors for systemic atherosclerosis: a comparison of C-reactive protein, fibrinogen, homocysteine, lipoprotein(a), and standard cholesterol screening as predictors of peripheral artery disease. JAMA 285:2481, 2001; and The Emerging Risk Factors Collaboration: C-reactive protein concentration and risk of coronary heart disease, stroke, and mortality: an individual participant meta-analysis. Lancet 375:132, 2010.)*

LIPOPROTEIN(a)

Lipoprotein(a) (Lp[a]—commonly pronounced "L P little A") consists of a low-density lipoprotein particle with apolipoprotein a (apo a) covalently attached to apo B, the major apolipoprotein of LDL particles. Apo a should not be confused with apo A, the family that includes apolipoprotein A-I, the principal apolipoprotein of HDL. Lipoprotein(a) has considerable heterogeneity, determined genetically and related to the number of repeats of a structural motif known as a *kringle* in the apo a moiety of the special lipoprotein particle. The structural resemblance of apo a to plasminogen suggests that Lp(a) may inhibit fibrinolysis. Lipoprotein(a) levels in the general population have high skew. Most individuals lie in the lower range of distribution, with a few "outliers" in the higher levels of Lp(a). Black Americans have a higher frequency of elevated Lp(a). Those with Lp(a) levels substantially above normal appear to have increased cardiovascular risk. As in the case of homocysteine,

Lp(a) in large populations only weakly predicts future cardiovascular disease,[31] but genetic studies suggest a causal role of Lp(a) in provoking cardiovascular events[32] (see Fig. 8-1).

FIBRINOGEN

Fibrinogen, the substrate of thrombin, provides the major meshwork of arterial thrombi. Levels of fibrinogen increase in inflammatory states as part of the acute-phase response. A consistent body of observational evidence links elevated levels of fibrinogen with cardiovascular risk.[33,34] Standardization of assays for fibrinogen has proved difficult. Moreover, diurnal variation in plasma fibrinogen levels weakens its potential as a biomarker of cardiovascular risk, despite its obvious biological plausibility as a major participant in thrombosis. Fibrin deposition in plaques, first hypothesized by von Rokitansky in the mid-19th century, provides evidence of fibrinogen's involvement in atherogenesis.[35]

INFECTION

The possibility that infectious agents or responses to infection may contribute to atherogenesis or precipitate atherosclerotic events has periodically captured the fancy of students of atherosclerosis. Many infectious agents could contribute to aspects of atherogenesis by direct cytopathic effect or through mediators they release or elicit as part of a host defense.[36–41] The hemodynamic stresses of acute infection, and accentuated thrombotic risk or impaired fibrinolysis due to acute-phase reactants such as fibrinogen or plasminogen activator inhibitor (PAI)-1, might transiently heighten the risk for thrombotic complications of atherosclerosis.[42] Some seroepidemiological studies have suggested links between exposure to viral and bacterial pathogens and various measures of atherosclerosis or risk of atherosclerotic events. Prospective studies properly controlled for confounding factors have shown weak, if any, correlation of antibody titers against various microbial or viral pathogens and cardiovascular events. Trials of various antibiotic regimens in patients with CAD have not shown reductions in recurrent events.[43]

INFLAMMATION AND ATHEROSCLEROSIS

Recognition that inflammation provides a unifying theme for many of the pathophysiological alterations that occur during atherogenesis has provoked both interest and controversy.[44–46] A subsequent section of this chapter will discuss in detail the links between inflammatory processes and risk factors, and atherogenesis and complications of atherosclerosis. Emergence of C-reactive protein (CRP) as a validated marker of prospective cardiovascular risk has spawned countless studies proposing other inflammatory markers as potential predictors of atherosclerotic risk.[47–49] Although some markers of inflammation (e.g., fibrinogen, PAI-1) have defined roles as mediators and markers, evidence regarding CRP as an effector rather than a marker remains unsettled. Despite some laboratory evidence that CRP can produce some effects that may promote atherothrombosis, genetic data do not support a causal role for CRP in cardiovascular events.[50–52] Of course, biomarkers need not participate directly in pathogenic pathways to have utility as gauges of risk, as illustrated by the case of CRP.[53–55]

GENETIC PREDISPOSITION

The example of familial hypercholesterolemia recounted earlier irrefutably illustrates the link between gene mutation and atherosclerosis. The accelerated development of molecular genetic technology and the increasing ease of identifying and cataloging genetic polymorphisms have facilitated the search for genetic variants that predispose toward atherosclerosis or its complications.[56] Monogenic conditions such as familial hypercholesterolemia do not appear to explain the majority of the burden or risk of atherosclerotic disease. The quest for genetic polymorphisms that predispose toward atherosclerosis has yielded many potential

candidates. Genome-wide association studies have identified reproducible regions of the genome associated with increased cardiovascular risk.[57–61] Some of the genes at locations so identified have well-established functions in pathogenic pathways for atherosclerosis.[62,63] Other sites emerging from genome-wide association studies have unknown functions and have not been previously associated with cardiovascular disease. Notably, the chromosome 9p21 region concordantly associates with cardiovascular events in several independent large population studies. Yet even combinations of well-validated genetic markers may fail to improve estimation of cardiovascular risk beyond a simple query regarding family history of premature CAD (at <60 years of age).[64,65] Genetic markers of atherosclerotic risk should nonetheless prove useful in providing new understanding of disease mechanisms and may identify new avenues for intervention, even if they do not add substantially to risk stratification.

Risk Factors on the Rise

We are witnessing a transition in the pattern of atherosclerotic risk factors in the United States, and indeed worldwide.[66] Certain traditional atherosclerotic risk factors are on the wane. For example, rates of smoking in the United States are declining, particularly in men. Dissemination of effective antihypertensive therapies has provided a means to reduce the degree or prevalence of this traditional atherosclerotic risk factor. Although many patients do not achieve the currently established targets for blood pressure, effective therapies have become much more widely implemented in recent decades.

We have made striking progress in combating high levels of LDL, a major traditional risk factor for atherosclerosis, as discussed earlier. In particular, the introduction of statins and accumulating evidence of their effectiveness as preventive therapies, combined with their relative ease of use and tolerability, should foster a secular trend toward lower LDL levels in the higher-risk segments of our population.

Although we justly derive considerable satisfaction from these pharmacological inroads into the traditional profile of cardiovascular risk, we are rapidly losing ground in other respects.[66,67] The astounding increase in obesity in the U.S. population in the last decade alone represents a change in body habitus of substantial proportion in an instant on an evolutionary timescale. Short of major disasters or famines, this kind of rapid shift in body habitus may have no precedent in the history of our species. From the perspective of cardiovascular risk, the metabolic alterations that accompany this increased girth of our population should sound an alarm. Current data point to a significant increase in the prevalence of the components of the clustered risk factors often referred to as the *metabolic syndrome*.

The National Cholesterol Education Project Adult Treatment Panel III (ATP III) arbitrarily defined five components of the metabolic syndrome[68] (Table 8-1); individuals with any three components have the syndrome, according to the ATP III criteria. There is disparity in the definitions of the metabolic syndrome among varied constituencies.[69] Some have voiced cogent objections to the concept; for example, it is not clear that the sum of the risk of the metabolic syndrome components exceeds that of the individual factors combined, or that the components comprise a true syndrome, being linked mechanistically.[70,71] But many clinicians find the construct practically useful insofar as it reflects the type of individuals seen more and more in practice.

Note that LDL, the traditional focus of guidelines and therapies, does not figure among the metabolic syndrome criteria; instead, lower ranges of HDL and higher levels of triglycerides characterize the syndrome. Thus, we may witness a shift in lipid risk factor burden from primarily LDL to the dyslipidemia associated with obesity and/or insulin resistance, characterized by lower HDL and higher triglycerides. The success of statins in reducing LDL cholesterol will likely contribute to the increased importance of such dyslipidemia in the future. Although individuals with the metabolic syndrome

TABLE 8-1	Criteria for the "Metabolic Syndrome"*
RISK FACTOR	**DEFINING LEVEL**
Abdominal Obesity† (Waist Circumference‡)	
Men	>102 cm (>40 in)
Women	>88 cm (>35 in)
Triglycerides	≥150 mg/dL
HDLC	
Men	<40 mg/dL
Women	<50 mg/dL
Blood pressure	≥130/≥85 mm Hg
Fasting glucose	≥110 mg/dL

*Diagnosis is established when ≥3 of these risk factors are present.
†Abdominal obesity is more highly correlated with metabolic risk factors than is increased body mass index (BMI).
‡Some men develop metabolic risk factors when circumference is only marginally increased.
HDLC, high-density lipoprotein cholesterol.
From the Expert Panel on Detection, Evaluation, and Treatment of High Blood Cholesterol in Adults. JAMA 285:2486, 2001.

cluster commonly have dyslipidemia, their levels of LDL cholesterol may be average or even below average. This finding may provide false reassurance to physicians and patients alike. Although LDL cholesterol levels in such patients may not be especially elevated, the quality of the lipoprotein particles may prove particularly atherogenic.[72] Low-density lipoprotein particles in those with high levels of triglycerides and low levels of HDL tend to be small and dense. Such small, dense LDL particles appear to bind to proteoglycans in the arterial intima with more avidity. Their retention in the intima may facilitate their oxidative modification, so small, dense LDL particles may have particularly atherogenic properties.[73] Prolonged retention and increased entry may promote lipoprotein accumulation in the artery wall.[74]

HYPERGLYCEMIA

Hyperglycemia may contribute independently to the pathogenesis of atherosclerosis.[75] In the presence of higher levels of glucose, nonenzymatic glycation and other types of oxidative posttranslational modification of various macromolecules increases. Hemoglobin A_{1c}, a glycated form of this oxygen-carrying pigment, reflects this biochemical process. Accumulation of glycated macromolecules ultimately leads to the formation of complex condensates known as *advanced glycation end products* (AGEs) that may trigger inflammatory and oxidative responses implicated in atherogenesis.[76] A cell surface receptor for AGEs known as *RAGE* may transduce proinflammatory signals when occupied by AGE-modified ligands[77] (Fig. 8-2). This and other mechanisms link hyperglycemia and insulin resistance to aspects of host defenses considered essential for the atherogenic process, but strict glycemic control does not necessarily improve cardiovascular outcomes, as shown in several recent large clinical trials.[78–81]

INTERACTIONS OF RISK FACTORS WITH CELLS IN THE ARTERIAL WALL AND LEUKOCYTES DURING ATHEROGENESIS

We increasingly understand atherosclerosis as a process that involves cellular interactions with risk factors such as high levels of LDL. This contemporary view contrasts with previous notions that the arterial wall passively accumulated cholesterol. This crosstalk among cells of varying types during atherogenesis involves more than just the intrinsic cells of the arterial wall, endothelium, and vascular smooth muscle cells (VSMCs) (see Chapters 2 and 3).[44,82] Indeed, the mononuclear phagocyte also contributes importantly to atherogenesis. Normal endothelium resists prolonged contact with leukocytes, including blood monocytes, precursors of the tissue macrophages that accumulate in atheromata. A mechanism involving expression of particular leukocyte adhesion molecules on the endothelial surface likely mediates recruitment of blood monocytes to sites of formation of the earliest atherosclerotic lesions.[83]

The heterogeneity of monocytes and the macrophages to which they give rise has generated considerable recent interest.[84–87] A particularly proinflammatory subset of monocytes accumulate in the blood of hypercholesterolemic mice. Macrophages exhibiting atherogenic functions also appear to accumulate in atherosclerotic lesions, and therapeutic interventions may modulate these functions.[88]

Adhesion molecules considered important in this process include members of the selectin superfamily, such as P-selectin. Leukocytes passing through the arterial circulation can bind to patches of endothelial cells (ECs) expressing P-selectin, which mediates a rolling or saltatory slowing of leukocytes. The more permanent adhesion of the tethered white cell depends on expression of another category of leukocyte adhesion molecule expressed on the endothelial surface at sites prone to lesion

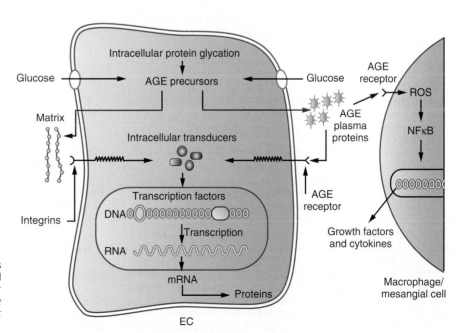

FIGURE 8-2 Cellular and molecular mechanisms of transmembrane signaling due to advanced glycation end products (AGEs). NFκB, nuclear factor κB. *(Reproduced with permission from Brownlee M: Biochemistry and molecular cell biology of diabetic complications. Nature 414:813, 2001.)*

formation: members of the immunoglobulin (Ig)G superfamily, including vascular cell adhesion molecule-1 (VCAM-1). Both P-selectin and VCAM-1, among other adhesion molecules, show increased expression in regions of human atherosclerotic plaques and on the macrovascular endothelium overlying nascent atherosclerotic plaques in experimental animals. Other leukocyte adhesion molecules certainly participate in this capture of blood leukocytes, but considerable evidence from genetically altered mice supports the essential involvement of P-selectin and VCAM-1 in lesion formation.

Once firmly bound to the endothelial surface, white blood cells must receive chemoattractant stimuli to penetrate into the intima. Among such signals, monocyte chemoattractant protein-1 (MCP-1) may be particularly important. Again, experiments in genetically altered mice support the involvement of MCP-1 in the formation of experimental atherosclerotic lesions. Other chemokines, such as the cell surface–associated molecule fractalkine, also may contribute to this process. In addition to mononuclear phagocytes, T lymphocytes accumulate in human atherosclerotic plaques, where they may play important regulatory roles. Adhesion molecules such as intracellular adhesion molecule-1 (ICAM-1), overexpressed by ECs overlying atheromata, may participate with VCAM-1 in the adhesion of T lymphocytes. Moreover a trio of chemokines induced by the T-cell activator interferon (IFN)-γ may promote chemoattraction of adherent T cells into the arterial intima.[89] Mast cells, long recognized in the leukocyte population of the arterial adventitia, also localize within the intimal lesions of atherosclerosis. Although vastly outnumbered by macrophages, mast cells may also contribute to lesion formation or complication.[82,90–92] The chemokine exotaxin may participate in recruiting mast cells to the arterial intima.

Once present in the arterial intima, these various classes of leukocytes undergo diverse activation reactions that may potentiate atherogenesis. For example, monocytes mature into macrophages in the atherosclerotic plaque, where they overexpress a series of scavenger receptors that can capture modified lipoproteins that accumulate in the atherosclerotic intima. Because their levels do not decrease as cells accumulate cholesterol, these scavenger receptors permit formation of foam cells, a hallmark of the atheromatous plaque. Macrophages within the atherosclerotic intima proliferate and become a rich source of mediators, including reactive oxygen species and proinflammatory cytokines, that may contribute to progression of atherosclerosis.[93]

One of the key signals for macrophage activation, macrophage colony-stimulating factor (M-CSF), can enhance scavenger receptor expression and promote replication of macrophages and their production of proinflammatory cytokines. Experiments in mutant mice have shown an important role for M-CSF in the formation of atheromata.

The T cells in the atherosclerotic plaque also appear to modulate aspects of atherogenesis.[45,94] Interferon-γ, a strong activating stimulus for macrophages produced by activated type 1 helper T (T$_H$1) cells, localizes in plaques. Indicators of the action of IFN-γ, such as induction of the class II major histocompatibility antigen molecules, provide evidence for the biological activity of IFN-γ in atherosclerotic plaques.

Once recruited to the intima, white blood cells can perpetuate, amplify, or mollify the ongoing inflammatory response that led to their recruitment. The function of the "professional phagocytes" adds to the proinflammatory mediators elaborated by the intrinsic vascular wall cells, and perpetuates and amplifies the local inflammatory response. T lymphocyte subsets may also quell inflammation. T helper 2 cells that produce interleukin (IL)-10, a putative antiatherosclerotic cytokine, also localize in plaques. Regulatory T cells (T$_{reg}$) produce transforming growth factor (TGF)-β, another antiinflammatory and fibrogenic mediator that may modulate plaque biology.[95] The role in atherogenesis of another T-cell subset, T$_H$17, remains unsettled.[96–98] Dendritic cells specialized in surveying the environment and presenting antigens to T cells arrive early in the arterial intima of mice subjected to hyperlipidemia.[99–101]

The nature of the antigenic stimulus to T-cell activation remains speculative, although animal experiments have suggested some candidates.[102]

ATHEROSCLEROSIS PROGRESSION

Recruitment of blood leukocytes and their activation in the arterial intima sets the stage for progression of atherosclerosis. Proinflammatory mediators produced by these various cell types lead to elaboration of factors that can stimulate migration of smooth muscle cells (SMCs) from the tunica media into the intima.[103] The normal human tunica intima contains resident SMCs. Growth factors produced locally by activated leukocytes provide a paracrine stimulus to SMC proliferation. Activated SMCs also appear capable of producing growth factors that can stimulate their own proliferation or that of their neighbors, an autocrine pathway of proliferation.[104] Smooth muscle cells also die in atheromata.[105,106] Depletion of SMCs may influence the biology of plaques by disturbing repair and maintenance of the fibrous cap.[107,108]

Other mediators present in atheromatous plaques, such as TGF-β, can augment production of macromolecules of the ECM, including interstitial collagen.[109,110] Thus, "maturing" atherosclerotic lesions assume fibrous as well as fatty characteristics. Ultimately, the established atherosclerotic plaque develops a central lipid core encapsulated in fibrous ECM. In particular, the fibrous cap— the layer of connective tissue overlying the lipid core and separating it from the arterial lumen—forms during this phase of lesion progression.

Calcification, another characteristic of the advancing atherosclerotic plaque, also involves tightly regulated biological functions. The expression of certain calcium-binding proteins within the plaque may sequester calcium hydroxyapatite. Such deposits, far from fixed, can undergo resorption as well as deposition. Inflammatory pathways participate in regulating mineralization of atheromata.[111] Reminiscent of bone metabolism, activated macrophages within the plaque appear to function as osteoclasts. Indeed, mice deficient in M-CSF, the macrophage activator, show increased accumulation of calcified deposits.[112] This observation supports the dynamic nature of calcium accretion in the plaque.

The atheroma eventually develops a central region filled with lipid, inflammatory cells, and cellular debris. Macrophage death, including apoptotic (programmed) death, contributes to formation of this lipid-rich core.[105,113] Indeed, classical pathologists often referred to this region of the plaque as the *necrotic core* of atheroma. Defective clearance of apoptotic cells, a process denoted *efferocytosis*, may contribute to the formation of the plaque's lipid core.[114]

During the progression of atherosclerotic plaques, migration and proliferation of SMCs, accumulation of ECM, and calcification lead to the transition from the fatty streak, dominated by the lipid-laden macrophages known as *foam cells*, to the fibrocalcific plaque that can produce arterial stenoses and other complications. Although this phase of lesion progression in humans may begin in youth, it often continues for many decades. Notably, atherosclerotic plaques often produce no symptoms during this generally prolonged phase of lesion evolution. Although traditionally viewed as a disease of middle and later life, the seeds of atherosclerosis are sown much earlier. This recognition highlights the importance of early and aggressive reduction of risk factors, best accomplished by lifestyle modification rather than pharmacological intervention during the formative phase of the disease process.

The Diversity of Atherosclerosis

Heterogeneity of Atherosclerosis Lesions

Although in the past we have focused on atherosclerosis of the coronary arteries, we now recognize increasingly that atherosclerosis reaches beyond the coronary bed. For example, atherosclerosis underlies many ischemic strokes. Although peripheral artery disease jeopardizes limb more than life, the limitation of exercise capacity and the considerable burden of nonhealing ulcers and other complications render this manifestation of atherosclerosis important from both medical and economical points of view (see Chapter 17). In addition, atherosclerotic involvement of the renal arteries contributes to end-stage renal disease and refractory hypertension in many instances (see Chapter 22).

From a pathophysiological perspective, atherosclerosis in different distributions of the arterial tree overlap considerably. Although the fundamental cellular and molecular events that underlie atherosclerosis in various arterial trees seem similar, certain complications appear distinct. For example, ectasia and eventual aneurysm formation affect the atherosclerotic abdominal aorta more commonly than do stenosis and thrombosis leading to total aortic occlusion. In addition, the aorta, and particularly the proximal portions of its trunk, appears especially important as a source for atheroemboli that may cause cerebral or renal infarctions.[115] Atherosclerosis of the extracranial vessels that perfuse the brain often develop stenosis, but ulceration of carotid plaques with embolization of atheromatous material commonly causes transient ischemic attacks or monocular blindness.[116]

Some of the regional variations in the expressions of atherosclerosis may depend on embryological factors. Endothelial cells in different regions of the arterial tree can display considerable heterogeneity, as determined by a variety of markers.[117] Developmental biologists have long recognized that SMCs found in various segments of the arterial tree may have distinct embryological origins. For example, SMCs in the ascending aorta and other arteries of the upper body derive from neural crest cells rather than mesenchyme.[118] Thus, SMCs can arise even from different germ layers in the lower body and neurectoderm in certain upper body arteries. The developmental biology of arteriogenesis and the determination of smooth muscle and EC lineages constitute a frontier of contemporary vascular biology research. For example, some but not all recent work suggests that both endothelial cells and smooth muscle cells, for example, may derive from bone marrow postnatally in injured, diseased, or transplanted arteries.[119–123] This recognition not only has intrinsic scientific interest but also may have therapeutic implications for regenerative medicine.

Atherosclerosis: a Focal or Diffuse Disease?

We classically understand atherosclerosis as a segmental process. Much of our traditional diagnostic armamentarium and treatment modalities aim to identify stenoses and restore flow by revascularization. Nonetheless, we recognize increasingly the diffuse nature of atherosclerosis. Classic comparison of histopathological examination with angiograms showed that the arteriogram vastly underestimates involvement of coronary arteries by atherosclerosis. More recently, the application of intravascular ultrasound has renewed our appreciation of the diffuse nature of coronary atherosclerosis. Arterial stenoses often cause ischemia and bring the patient to the attention of clinicians. Various noninvasive modalities can disclose ischemia. Contrast angiography readily localizes the focal stenoses that most often cause demand ischemia. Yet cross-sectional images obtained by intravascular ultrasound reveal that segments of arteries that appear absolutely normal by angiogram may nonetheless harbor a substantial burden of atherosclerotic disease.[124]

The process of arterial remodeling during atherogenesis explains this apparent paradox. During much of its life history, an atherosclerotic plaque grows in an outward, or abluminal, direction. Thus the plaque can grow silently without producing stenosis. Morphometric studies in nonhuman primates by Clarkson et al. first called attention to this compensatory enlargement of arteries that preserves the lumen during atherogenesis.[125] Oft-cited studies by Glagov et al. established the relevance of this process to human coronary atherosclerosis.[126] Remodeling also occurs in atherosclerotic peripheral arteries.[127] Expansive arterial remodeling can

influence the clinical manifestations of atheromata, with those with increased compensatory enlargement more prone to cause clinical events.[128] Luminal encroachment usually occurs relatively late in the life history of an atheromatous plaque.

Well-performed and systematic histopathological studies have shown that atherosclerotic disease begins early in life. In the Pathobiological Determinants of Atherosclerosis in Youth (PDAY) study, the aortas and coronary arteries of Americans 34 years of age or younger who died of noncardiac causes revealed consistent involvement of the dorsal surface of the abdominal aorta by both fatty and raised arterial plaques.[129] The coronary arteries, including the proximal portion of the left anterior descending (LAD) coronary artery, also disclosed involvement, even in this young population. The Bogalusa Heart Study also showed a correlation between risk factors during life and the degree of atherosclerotic involvement at autopsy.[130] These systematic observations agree with reports of a substantial burden of coronary arterial atherosclerosis in young American male casualties during the Korean and Vietnam wars.[131] Indeed, maternal hypercholesterolemia associates with fatty streak formation in fetuses.[132]

These various data indicate that atherosclerosis affects arteries far more diffusely than we believed only a few years ago. The process begins much earlier in life than generally acknowledged. Indeed, intravascular ultrasound studies have shown that 1 in 6 American teenagers has significant atherosclerotic involvement of the coronary arteries.[133] These findings have considerable importance for understanding the pathophysiology of the clinical manifestations of atherosclerosis. They also have important implications for the management of this disease (see later discussion).

Shear Stress and Atheroprotection: Why Atherosclerosis Begins Where It Does

The foregoing section emphasizes the diffuse nature of atherosclerosis in adults. Yet in both humans and experimental animals, atherosclerosis begins in certain stereotyped locales. The predilection of atherosclerosis for branch points and flow dividers appears quite consistent across species.

Why do these sites have a predisposition to early atherogenesis? Decades of sophisticated biomechanical analysis have established that atheromata tend to form at sites of disturbed blood flow, particularly areas of low shear stress.[134,135] Endothelial cells somehow can sense shear stress; in areas of laminar shear stress *in vivo* and in monolayers of cultured cells *in vitro*, for example, ECs align their long axes parallel to the direction of flow. At branch points and dividers in the arterial tree, the well-ordered cobblestone array of the endothelial monolayer changes—cells appear more polygonally and irregularly shaped. Areas of low shear stress show heightened EC turnover, increased permeability, and prolonged retention of lipoprotein particles in the subendothelial regions of the intima. Such data, accumulated over many decades, provide answers to the question of what goes awry at sites of lesion predilection.

More recent data have inspired a different and complementary hypothesis to explain the focality of atherosclerosis initiation. Transcriptional profiling provides a "snapshot" of the expression of a large number of genes in a single experiment. The pattern of genes expressed by ECs subjected to controlled physiological levels of laminar shear stress *in vitro* differs strikingly from that of resting ECs *in vitro*. Several of genes differentially expressed by ECs experiencing laminar shear stress appear to have "atheroprotective" functions. A number of putative atheroprotective genes rise selectively under conditions of physiological laminar shear stress. These findings suggest that regions of undisturbed laminar shear stress enjoy tonic endogenous antioxidant, vasodilatory, and antiinflammatory properties conferred by the function of these putative "atheroprotective" genes.[136]

For example, superoxide dismutase can catabolize the highly reactive superoxide anion (O_2^-). Cyclooxygenase (COX)-2 can give rise to the vasodilatory and antiaggregatory arachidonic acid

CH
8

metabolite prostacyclin. The endothelial isoform of nitric oxide synthase (eNOS) produces the endogenous vasodilator, antithrombotic, and antiinflammatory mediator nitric oxide (NO), which exerts antiinflammatory actions by combating leukocyte adhesion to the activated EC. The transcription factor Krüppel-like factor 2 (KLF-2) has emerged as an integrator of shear stress and altered endothelial functions implicated in "atheroprotection."[137] Flow-mediated stimulation of adenosine monophosphate (AMP)-dependent protein kinase may in turn signal activation of KLF-2.[138]

At regions of disturbed flow—for example, near branch points and flow dividers—expression of these endogenous atheroprotective genes should decline. Indeed, regions predisposed to early lesion formation show activation of nuclear factor (NF)κB, the master regulator of inflammatory gene expression.[139] Because NO can antagonize activation of NFκB, absence of laminar flow in these regions may explain, at least in part, the tendency of nascent atheromata to form at such sites.[140]

Thus, atherosclerosis is both a focal and diffuse disease. It begins focally for reasons we understand in increasing detail. The stenoses that cause flow-limiting lesions tend to localize in similar regions. Much of our diagnostic and therapeutic activity in contemporary cardiology and vascular medicine has traditionally focused on these stenoses. Advances in both arterial biology and clinical science heighten our appreciation of the diffuse distribution of atherosclerosis and the systemic nature of the risk factors that promote its development. These considerations help us understand how optimum medical management with systemic therapies can confer benefits on par with those derived from revascularization procedures in many patients.[141]

Pathophysiology of Thrombotic Complications of Atherosclerosis

As noted, flow-limiting stenoses have driven much of the diagnostic and therapeutic activity in clinical atherosclerosis for many decades. Patients with flow-limiting lesions often experience symptoms due to ischemia (e.g., angina pectoris in the coronary circulation, intermittent claudication in peripheral artery disease). We can readily diagnose ischemia by various noninvasive modalities. We can localize stenoses through invasive and noninvasive angiographic techniques. Percutaneous and surgical approaches can effectively relieve ischemia due to focal stenoses, but do not address lesions that do not limit flow.

We recognize increasingly that in many cases, acute thrombosis does not occur in the most tightly narrowed segments of an artery. The best illustration of this counterintuitive observation arises from analyses of fatal coronary thromboses. Clinical evidence suggests that a minority of fatal coronary thrombi occur where stenoses exceed 60%.[142,143] Thus, many occlusive thrombi complicate lesions that neither limit flow nor meet traditional angiographic criteria for "significance." Fewer data exist regarding the substrates for thrombosis in noncoronary arteries. But in peripheral and carotid arteries, inflammation—tightly linked to mechanisms of thrombosis—characterizes atherosclerotic lesions. Intraplaque hemorrhage appears quite common in carotid plaques that cause cerebral ischemic disease as well.

Although most fatal myocardial infarctions (MIs) occur at sites of noncritical stenosis, it does not follow that high-grade stenoses cause fewer heart attacks than less obstructive lesions. Indeed, on a "per-lesion basis," tighter stenoses are more likely to give rise to acute MIs.[144] Because the noncritically stenotic lesions outnumber "tight" stenoses, the total risk attributable to less stenotic lesions exceeds the risk due to the less numerous lesions that cause higher-grade stenoses.

A common confusion surrounds the distinction between lesion size and degree of stenosis. Based on our traditional angiographically centered view of atherosclerosis, many assume that lesions that cause high-grade stenoses are larger than those that cause less obstruction. This fallacy fails to consider the importance of outward remodeling or compensatory enlargement. The outward growth of most atherosclerotic plaques before they begin to encroach on the lumen protects the lumen from obstruction and conceals the growing lesion from visualization by angiography until the latter stages of its evolution. Thus, low-grade stenoses do not equate with smaller plaques. Indeed, larger and eccentrically remodeled plaques may cause acute coronary syndromes (ACSs) more frequently than smaller plaques that do not exhibit compensatory enlargement and/or produce greater degrees of stenosis.[145]

Concordant evidence from several avenues of investigation suggests that a physical disruption of the atherosclerotic plaque, rather than a critical degree of stenosis, commonly precipitates arterial thromboses. Four mechanisms of plaque disruption may cause thrombosis or rapid plaque expansion[146,147] (Fig. 8-3). A through-and-through fracture of the plaque's fibrous cap causes most fatal coronary thromboses (see Fig. 8-3). Our group hypothesized a model of the pathophysiology of this common

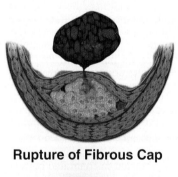

Rupture of Fibrous Cap

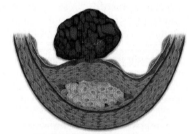

Superficial Erosion

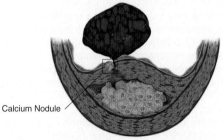

Calcium Nodule

Erosion of Calcium Nodule

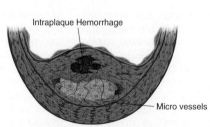

Intraplaque Hemorrhage

Micro vessels

Intraplaque Hemorrhage

FIGURE 8-3 Mechanisms of plaque disruption. Rupture of fibrous cap *(upper left)* causes two thirds to three quarters of fatal coronary thrombosis. Superficial erosion *(upper right)* occurs in one fifth to a one quarter of all cases of fatal coronary thrombosis. Certain populations, such as diabetic individuals and women, appear more susceptible to superficial erosion as a mechanism of plaque disruption and thrombosis. Erosion of a calcium nodule may also cause plaque disruption and thrombosis *(lower left)*. In addition, friable microvessels in the base of an atherosclerotic plaque may rupture and cause intraplaque hemorrhage *(lower right)*. Consequent local generation of thrombin may stimulate smooth muscle proliferation, migration, and collagen synthesis, promoting fibrosis and plaque expansion on a subacute basis. Severe intraplaque hemorrhage also can cause sudden lesion expansion by a mass effect acutely. *(Reproduced with permission from Libby P, Theroux P: Pathophysiology of coronary artery disease. Circulation 111:3481, 2005).*

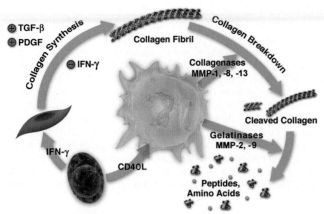

FIGURE 8-4 Relationship between inflammation and collagen metabolism in the atherosclerotic plaque. T lymphocytes can elaborate interferon (IFN)-γ, which reduces ability of smooth muscle cell (SMC) to synthesize new collagen. T cell also can stimulate the macrophage through CD40 ligand to elaborate interstitial collagenases, matrix metalloproteinase MMP-1, -8, -13—enzymes that affect initial cleavage in the collagen fibril. Elaboration of gelatinases such as MMP-2, -9 can contribute to further cleavage of collagen fragments to peptides and amino acids. Transforming growth factor (TGF)-β and platelet-derived growth factor (PDGF) from autocrine or paracrine sources, including degranulating platelets, can promote collagen synthesis by SMCs.

mechanism of atherosclerotic plaque disruption that focused on the metabolism of interstitial collagen. This ECM macromolecule accounts for much of the biomechanical strength of the plaque's fibrous cap. Further hypothesizing that inflammation regulates the metabolism of interstitial forms of collagen and might regulate the stability of an atherosclerotic plaque (Fig. 8-4), we found that certain proinflammatory cytokines expressed in the atherosclerotic plaque can inhibit the ability of the SMC to synthesize new collagen required to repair and maintain the integrity of the plaque's fibrous cap. Notably, the signature T_H1 cytokine IFN-γ can inhibit interstitial collagen gene expression in human VSMCs.[109]

The interstitial collagen triple helix resists breakdown by most proteinases. We described the overexpression of proteolytic enzymes specialized in the catabolism of collagen in the atherosclerotic plaque, and further demonstrated that inflammatory mediators found in the atheroma can enhance the expression of these collagenolytic enzymes, members of the MMP family. Cells in human atheromata overexpress all three members of the human interstitial collagenase family (MMP-1, MMP-13, and MMP-8). We have furnished evidence that collagen breakdown occurs *in situ* in human atherosclerotic plaques.[148,149] These findings indicate that the interstitial collagenase MMPs exist in their active forms rather than their precursor zymogen forms. Furthermore, demonstration of collagenolysis *in situ* indicates that these collagenases overwhelm their endogenous inhibitors, including tissue inhibitors of MMPs (TIMPs).[150] We also ascribed a hitherto unknown function to tissue factor pathway inhibitor (TFPI)-2 as a potent collagenase inhibitor.[151] Although we find little regulation of TIMPs in atherosclerotic lesions, TFPI-2, abundant in normal arteries, shows decreased levels in atherosclerotic lesions. Thus, a preponderance of proteinases over their inhibitors prevails in the atherosclerotic plaque.

Colocalization of proteinases with inflammatory cells, and regulation of their expression by products of inflammatory cells, strongly implicate disordered collagen metabolism as a key mechanism for atherosclerotic plaque destabilization. Experiments using genetically altered mice have demonstrated the importance of collagen catabolism due to MMP collagenases in the regulation of the steady-state level of this ECM macromolecule in experimental atheromata using both loss-of-function and gain-of-function strategies.[152–154] The finding that inflammatory mediators elicit overexpression of MMP collagenases from macrophages supports the view that inflammation promotes the thrombotic complications of atherosclerosis. This mechanistic insight aids the understanding of how biomarkers of inflammation can help predict such events.

Superficial erosion of the endothelial monolayer constitutes an important cause of a minority of coronary thromboses[155,156] (see Fig. 8-3). Women, the elderly, patients with diabetes, and patients with hypertriglyceridemia appear to have a higher frequency of superficial erosion as a cause of fatal thrombosis than do younger, male hypercholesterolemic individuals. Various molecular and cellular mechanisms may underlie superficial erosion. Excessive proteolysis of ECM macromolecules that make up the subendothelial basement membrane may predispose toward endothelial desquamation and superficial erosion. Apoptosis of ECs may also promote superficial erosion. Various proinflammatory stimuli can sensitize ECs to apoptosis. In addition, hypochlorous acid, a product of myeloperoxidase—an enzyme found in leukocytes in atherosclerotic plaques—can provoke EC apoptosis.[157] Local generation of tissue factor from dying ECs may also contribute to thrombosis at sites of superficial erosion.

Atherosclerotic plaques often harbor rich plexi of microvessels. Neovascularization of plaques provides an additional portal for trafficking of leukocytes that may promote the inflammatory process.[158] Neovessels in the plaque, like those in the diabetic retina, may be friable and fragile. Intraplaque hemorrhage due to disruption of microvessels may cause sudden plaque expansion (see Fig. 8-3). Local generation of thrombin and other mediators associated with coagulation *in situ* may promote lesion growth. For example, platelet-derived growth factor (PDGF), TGF-β, and platelet factor 4 (PF4), released by platelets at sites of microvascular hemorrhage and intramural thrombosis, may hasten local fibrosis. Thrombin can stimulate SMC migration, division, and collagen synthesis. Thus, microvascular disruption, while not provoking an occlusive thrombus, may promote lesion evolution nonetheless.

Erosion through the intima of a calcified nodule represents another less common form of atherosclerotic plaque disruption associated with thrombosis (see Fig. 8-3). The active metabolism of calcium hydroxyapatite, with its accretion and removal as described earlier, can contribute to calcium accumulation in regions of atherosclerotic plaques. The tendency of atheromata to accumulate calcium has given rise to clinical testing. Increasing evidence supports the contention that the amount of coronary artery calcification correlates with the burden of atherosclerotic disease. Moreover, emerging data suggest a correlation between calcium score and risk of future cardiovascular events.

The degree to which calcium scoring or any other imaging modality (such as computed tomographic coronary angiography) can provide prognostic information beyond that available from risk algorithms based on traditional risk factors and selected emerging biomarkers, such as CRP measured with the high-sensitivity assay (hsCRP), remains uncertain. The notion that arterial calcification bears a relationship to atherosclerosis complication holds considerable sway. Yet, current biological understanding and preliminary clinical evidence suggest that coronary lesions most likely to cause thrombosis contain less calcium than lesions that cause flow-limiting stenoses and ischemia.[159,160] Thus, the calcified lesions may have *less* propensity to disrupt and provoke coronary thrombosis than those with little calcium.

Mutability of the Atherosclerotic Plaque

The classic concept of atherosclerosis assumed a steady, relentless, and continuous progression of the disease. But serial angiographic studies suggest that stenoses evolve in a discontinuous fashion, with periods of relative quiescence punctuated by spurts in growth. Our current understanding of plaque pathobiology suggests a plausible mechanism to explain this angiographically discontinuous evolution of arterial stenoses. Careful study of the coronary arteries of individuals who succumb to noncardiac death, and of coronary arteries perfusion-fixed in the operating room from hearts of transplantation recipients with ischemic cardiomyopathy, as well as observations of cholesterol-fed non-human primates, all indicate that areas of plaque disruption or superficial erosion with nonocclusive mural thrombus formation occur frequently. The picture that arises from an amalgamation of these human and experimental observations indicates that most plaque disruptions with thrombosis *in situ* do not proceed to a total occlusion and, indeed, usually pass unnoticed by the patient or physician (Fig. 8-5). For various reasons, plaque disruptions with mural thrombosis may not proceed to a disastrous total thrombosis in all events. In many patients, the endogenous fibrinolytic mechanisms or antithrombotic effects of dietary or pharmacological intervention may prevent thrombi from propagating. Larger

arteries such as the aorta have sufficient flow to prevent mural thrombi from progressing to total occlusion in most instances. Indeed, although inspection of the aortas of many patients with atherosclerosis discloses many ulcerated lesions with mural thrombi, aortic occlusion due to thrombosis fortunately occurs relatively rarely (Fig. 8-6).

The failure of most mural thrombi to progress to total occlusion does not imply that such events have a benign course. Although subclinical at the time that they occur, the mural thrombi elicit a local "wound-healing" response that tends to promote plaque progression. Indeed, one of the types of "crisis" in the history of a plaque that can lead to its sudden evolution, as disclosed by serial angiographic studies, likely reflects such a scenario (see Fig. 8-5). A localized plaque disruption with mural thrombus can engender

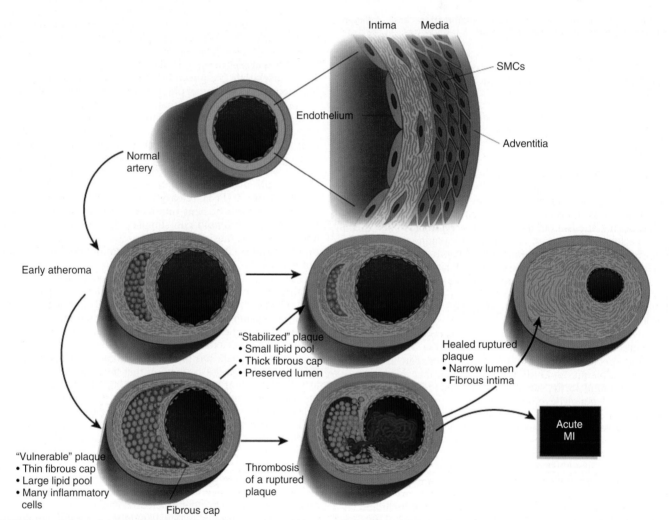

FIGURE 8-5 Schematic of the life history of an atheroma. A normal human coronary artery has a typical trilaminar structure. Endothelial cells (ECs) in contact with blood in arterial lumen rest on a basement membrane. Intimal layer in adult humans generally contains a small amount of smooth muscle cells (SMCs) scattered within intimal extracellular matrix (ECM). Internal elastic lamina forms a barrier between the tunica intima and underlying tunica media. Tunica media consists of multiple layers of SMCs much more tightly packed than in diffusely thickened intima, and embedded in a matrix rich in elastin and collagen. In early atherogenesis, recruitment of inflammatory cells and accumulation of lipids leads to formation of a lipid-rich core, as artery enlarges in an outward (abluminal) direction to accommodate intimal expansion. If inflammatory conditions prevail and risk factors such as dyslipidemia persist, lipid core can grow, and proteinases secreted by activated leukocytes can degrade extracellular matrix; whereas proinflammatory cytokines such as interferon (IFN)-γ can limit synthesis of new collagen. These changes can thin the fibrous cap and render it friable and susceptible to rupture. When a plaque ruptures, blood coming in contact with tissue factor in plaque coagulates; platelets activated by thrombin generated from coagulation cascade, and by contact with collagen in intimal compartment, instigate thrombus formation. If thrombus occludes the vessel persistently, acute myocardial infarction (MI) can result (dusky blue area in anterior wall of left ventricle *[lower right]*). Thrombus may eventually resorb secondary to endogenous or therapeutic thrombolysis, but a wound-healing response triggered by thrombin generated during blood coagulation can stimulate smooth muscle proliferation. Platelet-derived growth factor (PDGF) released from activated platelets stimulates SMC migration. Transforming growth factor (TGF)-β, also released from activated platelets, stimulates interstitial collagen production. This increased migration, proliferation, and ECM synthesis by SMCs thickens fibrous cap and causes further intimal expansion, often in an inward direction, constricting lumen. Such stenotic lesions produced by luminal encroachment of fibrosed plaque may restrict flow—particularly under situations of increased cardiac demand—leading to ischemia, commonly provoking symptoms such as angina pectoris. Such advanced stenotic plaques, being more fibrous, may prove less susceptible to rupture and renewed thrombosis. Lipid lowering can reduce lipid content and calm intimal inflammatory response, yielding a more stable plaque with a thick fibrous cap and preserved lumen *(center)*. *(Reproduced with permission from Libby P: Inflammation in atherosclerosis. Nature 420:868, 2002.)*

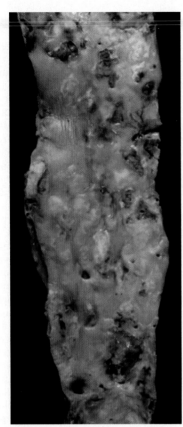

FIGURE 8-6 Widespread atheromatous involvement of abdominal aorta in patient with atherosclerosis. Note the variety of atheromata in different stages of evolution within a few centimeters of one another. There are ulcerated plaques, raised lesions, and fatty streaks among other types of lesions demonstrated in this example.

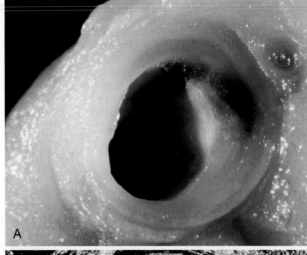

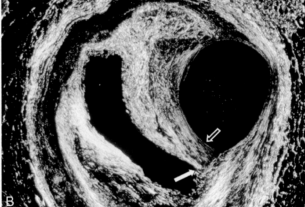

FIGURE 8-7 Hemorrhage, thrombosis, and plaque healing as a mechanism of atheroma progression. A, Photograph of coronary artery with plaque rupture that has led to an intraplaque hematoma without an occlusive thrombus. As explained in text, thrombin and platelet products such as platelet-derived growth factor (PDGF) and transforming growth factor (TGF)-β, elaborated locally at the site of microthrombosis and hematoma formation, can stimulate fibrosis. **B,** This Sirius red–stained preparation of cross-section of coronary artery shows an area of plaque rupture *(solid arrow)* that healed to cause further accretion of a layer of collagen *(open arrow)* and luminal encroachment. This example illustrates the "archaeology" of the atherosclerotic plaque: distant plaque rupture, followed by healing and fibrosis, with progression of the lesion to stenosis. Note that the arterial lumen at the time of the original plaque rupture would not have shown a critical narrowing. *(These figures were kindly provided by the late Prof. Michael J. Davies.)*

a healing response induced by platelet products released at short range, such as TGF-β, a potent stimulus to collagen gene expression by SMCs. Platelet-derived growth factor, also released during platelet aggregation, stimulates SMC migration. Thrombin locally generated at sites of thrombosis can stimulate SMC proliferation, migration, and collagen gene expression.

All these molecular and cellular mechanisms conspire to promote a cycle of SMC migration, proliferation, and local collagen synthesis. Quite plausibly, this scenario leads to evolution from a lipid-rich plaque with abundant inflammatory cells to a more fibrous lesion, rich in connective tissue, often with a paucity of inflammatory cells due to their death or departure, accretion of calcium deposits, and a relative lack of lipid accumulation. Careful study of atheromata obtained at autopsy shows signs of healed plaque disruption in some fibrous lesions[161,162] (Fig. 8-7).

The biological scenario just described depicts a more dynamic life history of the atherosclerotic plaque than that heretofore recognized (see Fig. 8-5). The heterogeneity of human atherosclerotic plaques, a concept now gaining considerable currency, highlights the importance of the qualitative characteristics of a lesion, not just its size. Whereas previous concepts emphasized the structure of atherosclerotic plaques, contemporary thinking accords a greater contribution to the biological characteristics of the plaque.

"Stable" vs. "Vulnerable" Plaques

Recognition of the heterogeneity of atherosclerotic plaques has fostered adoption of a dichotomous view of atheromata: "stable" versus "vulnerable" plaques. The notion of the vulnerable plaque has engendered considerable interest from pathologists and practitioners alike. Current cardiologic parlance uses the term

"vulnerable plaque" to designate a lesion characterized by a thin fibrous cap, a large lipid core, and a surfeit of inflammatory cells. Use of this term and its opposite, the "stable plaque," extends findings largely obtained at postmortem examination of humans who succumbed to acute MI. Although the dichotomization of plaques into vulnerable and stable provides a useful shorthand, we should exercise care in uncritically extrapolating morphological findings to foretell clinical complications.[147]

This pigeon-holing of plaques has engendered considerable effort to develop methods for identifying vulnerable or high-risk lesions, but such a view of atherosclerosis oversimplifies a disease of staggering complexity. For example, considerable evidence suggests that a given arterial tree has not one but many vulnerable plaques. Angioscopic and intravascular ultrasonographic study of coronary arteries, as well as interpretation of angiographic observations, support the multiplicity of disrupted plaques in patients with ACSs.[163]

Inflammation may provide a mechanistic link between "instability" of coronary and carotid plaques in the same individuals.

As previously mentioned, the aorta in an atherosclerotic individual often shows multiple ulcerated lesions, often within millimeters of fatty streaks, raised fibrous lesions, and resorbing healing thrombi (see Fig. 8-5). Thus, the quest to identify a single vulnerable plaque underestimates the complexity of the clinical challenge. Our broader view of the risk of atherosclerotic complications seeks the "vulnerable patient" and targets intervention more widely than to a single vulnerable plaque.

How could one approach such a vulnerable patient? Experimental and clinical consideration provide grounds for considerable optimism in this regard. Atherosclerosis exhibits considerable mutability; lipid lowering and other manipulations can alter features of plaques paramount to the clinical expression of the disease. Preclinical studies have shown that lipid lowering by diet or by treatment with statins can alter features of plaques associated with vulnerability in humans, such as proteinase activity or collagen content.[164-166] Likewise, treatment with angiotensin-converting enzyme (ACE) inhibitors can confer characteristics of stability on experimentally produced plaques in rabbits.[167] Studies in atherosclerosis-prone mice have demonstrated that interruption of inflammatory signaling pathways or manipulation of TGF-β can alter features of plaques associated with their propensity to rupture and provoke thrombosis. In addition to structural changes relating to the collagen content of plaques that may determine their biomechanical integrity, interventions such as lipid lowering can reduce expression of tissue factor, hence lowering the thrombogenic potential of the atherosclerotic plaque.

Clinical studies also support the mutability of atherosclerosis, abundantly demonstrated in animals by the experiments described earlier. Infusion of forms of apo A-I can cause modest reductions in the volume of atherosclerotic plaques, as monitored by intravascular ultrasound.[168,169] Aggressive lipid-lowering therapy with a statin can arrest or even reverse accumulation of atherosclerotic plaque, as determined by serial ultrasonographic study.[170] Careful histological correlations with magnetic resonance imaging (MRI) disclose evidence of the mutability of atherosclerotic plaques in intact humans.[171] These preclinical and clinical observations inspire considerable optimism regarding our ability to manipulate atherosclerotic plaques to benefit patient outcomes. The disease appears much more mutable than generally appreciated in the past.

Atherosclerosis: a Systemic Disease

Our traditional medical focus on atherosclerosis as a segmental disease caused by cholesterol accumulation has undergone an accelerated revision. We increasingly understand the global nature of factors that encompass the entire metabolic state of the patient, not just the serum cholesterol level. As the spectrum of risk factors in our population shifts, our attention must likewise broaden to encompass not just hypercholesterolemia but also the dyslipidemia associated with the metabolic syndrome and diabetes. As elevated LDL cholesterol and smoking recede as risk factors in our society, we must acknowledge the increasing contribution of obesity and insulin resistance.

We also recognize increasingly the importance of atherosclerosis beyond the coronary arteries. Our purview should now embrace the entire arterial tree with all its beds. We must strive to fill knowledge gaps about regional differences in human atherosclerosis, as well as differences in the biology and clinical manifestations of atherosclerosis associated with the shifting pattern of risk factors.

Our comprehension of the pathophysiology of atherosclerosis has undergone a revolution in recent decades. Emerging data and deeper understanding of this process will continue to change our concepts of this disease in the future. We should take immense satisfaction in the therapeutic inroads furnished by contemporary pharmacological tools. Reduction in coronary heart disease and cerebrovascular events accruing from treatments like statins and ACE inhibitors has changed medicine irrevocably, and provides striking benefits to patients. Therapeutic advances that have emerged from the application of progress in basic science, and have proved effective in randomized clinical trials, furnish cardiovascular medicine with an enviable and unparalleled database for the practice of evidence-based medicine.

Yet despite the victory of clinical science, much remains undone. The majority of cardiovascular events still occur despite optimal therapy that addresses multiple facets of our current understanding of the pathophysiology of this disease. Our challenge for the future is clear. We must strive to turn the tide on the alarming trends toward increased cardiovascular risk due to obesity and physical inactivity. We must not relent in our quest to advance the scientific understanding of atherogenesis and the translation to innovative therapies that address the residual and ever-growing burden of disease.

Many of the current landmark studies in the cardiovascular arena have focused on death and ACSs as "major adverse coronary events." These endpoints offer relative ease of study, adjudication, and quantification. But we must not lose sight of the enormous impediment to quality of life due to intermittent claudication caused by peripheral artery disease, and the loss of ability to communicate and live independently due to cerebrovascular disease. In addition to the human costs of these manifestations of noncoronary atherosclerosis, our society shoulders a substantial economic burden owing to the ravages of peripheral artery and cerebrovascular disease. We must pursue these issues with the same fervor we have accorded to CAD. This goal will become even more important as elder segments of our population continue to increase in numbers. The powerful tools available to investigators today provide grounds for optimism. Further inroads against the residual morbidity and mortality from atherosclerosis will emerge from future application of basic science to alter the biology of this disease, regarded not so long ago as an inevitable companion of the aging process.

REFERENCES

1. Libby P, Ridker PM, Hansson GK: Progress and challenges in translating the biology of atherosclerosis, Nature 473:317–325, 2011.
2. Anitschkow N, Chalatow S: On experimental cholesterin steatosis and its significance in the origin of some pathological processes (1913), Reprinted in Arteriosclerosis 3:178–182, 1983.
3. Di Angelantonio E, Sarwar N, Perry P, et al: Major lipids, apolipoproteins, and risk of vascular disease, JAMA 302(18):1993–2000, 2009.
4. Goldstein JL, Brown MS: The LDL receptor, Arterioscler Thromb Vasc Biol 29(4):431–438, 2009.
5. Steinberg D: The cholesterol wars: the skeptics vs. the preponderance of evidence, ed 1, San Diego, CA, 2007, Elsevier Academic Press.
6. Horton JD, Cohen JC, Hobbs HH: PCSK9: a convertase that coordinates LDL catabolism, J Lipid Res (50 Suppl):S172–S177, 2009.
7. Lloyd-Jones DM, Evans JC, Levy D: Hypertension in adults across the age spectrum: current outcomes and control in the community, JAMA 294(4):466–472, 2005.
8. Wang JG, Staessen JA, Franklin SS, et al: Systolic and diastolic blood pressure lowering as determinants of cardiovascular outcome, Hypertension 45(5):907–913, 2005.
9. Major outcomes in high-risk hypertensive patients randomized to angiotensin-converting enzyme inhibitor or calcium channel blocker vs. diuretic: The Antihypertensive and Lipid-Lowering Treatment to Prevent Heart Attack Trial (ALLHAT), JAMA 288(23):2981–2997, 2002.
10. Onuigbo MA: ALLHAT findings revisited in the context of subsequent analyses, other trials, and meta-analyses, Arch Intern Med 169(19):1810, 2009; author reply 1810–1811.
11. Smoking-attributable mortality, years of potential life lost, and productivity losses—United States, 2000–2004, MMWR Morb Mortal Wkly Rep 57(45):1226–1228, 2008.
12. Thomas GN, Chook P, Yip TW, et al: Smoking without exception adversely affects vascular structure and function in apparently healthy Chinese: implications in global atherosclerosis prevention, Int J Cardiol 128(2):172–177, 2008.
13. Yanbaeva DG, Dentener MA, Creutzberg EC, et al: Systemic effects of smoking, Chest 131(5):1557–1566, 2007.
14. Churg A, Wang RD, Tai H, et al: Macrophage metalloelastase mediates acute cigarette smoke-induced inflammation via tumor necrosis factor-alpha release, Am J Respir Crit Care Med 167(8):1083–1089, 2003.
15. Marma AK, Berry JD, Ning H, et al: Distribution of 10-year and lifetime predicted risks for cardiovascular disease in US adults: findings from the National Health and Nutrition Examination Survey 2003 to 2006, Circ Cardiovasc Qual Outcomes 3(1):8–14, 2010.
16. Magliano DJ, Rogers SL, Abramson MJ, et al: Hormone therapy and cardiovascular disease: a systematic review and meta-analysis, BJOG 113(1):5–14, 2006.
17. Rye KA, Bursill CA, Lambert G, et al: The metabolism and anti-atherogenic properties of HDL, J Lipid Res (50 Suppl):S195–S200, 2009.
18. Khera AV, Cuchel M, de la Llera-Moya M, et al: Cholesterol efflux capacity, high-density lipoprotein function, and atherosclerosis, N Engl J Med 364(2):127–135, 2011.

19. Tall AR, Yvan-Charvet L, Terasaka N, et al: ABC transporters, and cholesterol efflux: implications for the treatment of atherosclerosis, *Cell Metab* 7(5):365–375, 2008.

20. Rye KA, Barter PJ: Antiinflammatory actions of HDL: a new insight, *Arterioscler Thromb Vasc Biol* 28(11):1890–1891, 2008.

21. Vaisar T, Pennathur S, Green PS, et al: Shotgun proteomics implicates protease inhibition and complement activation in the antiinflammatory properties of HDL, *J Clin Invest* 117(3):746–756, 2007.

22. Brewer HB Jr: HDL metabolism and the role of HDL in the treatment of high-risk patients with cardiovascular disease, *Curr Cardiol Rep* 9(6):486–492, 2007.

23. Barter P, Gotto AM, LaRosa JC, et al: HDL cholesterol, very low levels of LDL cholesterol, and cardiovascular events, *N Engl J Med* 357(13):1301–1310, 2007.

24. Ridker PM, Genest J, Boekholdt M, et al: HDL cholesterol and residual risk of first cardiovascular events after treatment with potent statin therapy: an analysis from the JUPITER trial, *Lancet* 376(9738):333–339, 2010.

25. Duffy D, Rader DJ: Update on strategies to increase HDL quantity and function, *Nat Rev Cardiol* 6(7):455–463, 2009.

26. Cannon CP, Shah S, Dansky HM, et al: Safety of anacetrapib in patients with or at high risk for coronary heart disease, *N Engl J Med* 363(25):2406–2415, 2010.

27. Handy DE, Loscalzo J: Homocysteine and atherothrombosis: diagnosis and treatment, *Curr Atheroscler Rep* 5(4):276–283, 2003.

28. Lonn E, Yusuf S, Arnold MJ, et al: Homocysteine lowering with folic acid and B vitamins in vascular disease, *N Engl J Med* 354(15):1567–1577, 2006.

29. Bonaa KH, Njolstad I, Ueland PM, et al: Homocysteine lowering and cardiovascular events after acute myocardial infarction, *N Engl J Med* 354(15):1578–1588, 2006.

30. Armitage JM, Bowman L, Clarke RJ, et al: Effects of homocysteine-lowering with folic acid plus vitamin B12 vs placebo on mortality and major morbidity in myocardial infarction survivors: a randomized trial, *JAMA* 303(24):2486–2494, 2010.

31. Erqou S, Kaptoge S, Perry PL, et al: Lipoprotein(a) concentration and the risk of coronary heart disease, stroke, and nonvascular mortality, *JAMA* 302(4):412–423, 2009.

32. Clarke R, Peden JF, Hopewell JC, et al: Genetic variants associated with Lp(a) lipoprotein level and coronary disease, *N Engl J Med* 361(26):2518–2528, 2009.

33. Danesh J, Lewington S, Thompson SG, et al: Plasma fibrinogen level and the risk of major cardiovascular diseases and nonvascular mortality: an individual participant meta-analysis, *JAMA* 294(14):1799–1809, 2005.

34. Mora S, Rifai N, Buring JE, et al: Additive value of immunoassay-measured fibrinogen and high-sensitivity C-reactive protein levels for predicting incident cardiovascular events, *Circulation* 114(5):381–387, 2006.

35. Bini A, Kudryk BJ: Fibrinogen in human atherosclerosis, *Ann N Y Acad Sci* 748:461–471, 1995, discussion 471–463.

36. Libby P, Egan D, Skarlatos S: Roles of infectious agents in atherosclerosis and restenosis: an assessment of the evidence and need for future research. [Review] [91 refs], *Circulation* 96(11):4095–4103, 1997.

37. Muhlestein JB: Bacterial infections and atherosclerosis. [Review] [31 refs], *J Invest Med* 46(8):396–402, 1998.

38. Ridker PM: Are associations between infection and coronary disease causal or due to confounding?, *Am J Med* 106(3):376–377, 1999 (editorial, comment).

39. Zhu J, Nieto FJ, Horne BD, et al: Prospective study of pathogen burden and risk of myocardial infarction or death, *Circulation* 103(1):45–51, 2001.

40. Danesh J, Whincup P, Lewington S, et al: *Chlamydia pneumoniae* IgA titres and coronary heart disease; prospective study and meta-analysis, *Eur Heart J* 23(5):371–375, 2002.

41. Kalayoglu MV, Libby P, Byrne GI: *Chlamydia pneumoniae* as an emerging risk factor in cardiovascular disease, *JAMA* 288(21):2724–2731, 2002.

42. Corrales-Medina VF, Madjid M, Musher DM: Role of acute infection in triggering acute coronary syndromes, *Lancet Infect Dis* 10(2):83–92, 2010.

43. Andraws R, Berger JS, Brown DL: Effects of antibiotic therapy on outcomes of patients with coronary artery disease: a meta-analysis of randomized controlled trials, *JAMA* 293(21):2641–2647, 2005.

44. Libby P, Ridker PM, Hansson GK: Inflammation in atherosclerosis: from pathophysiology to practice, *J Am Coll Cardiol* 54(23):2129–2138, 2009.

45. Andersson J, Libby P, Hansson GK: Adaptive immunity and atherosclerosis, *Clin Immunol* 134(1):33–46, 2010.

46. Libby P, Crea F: Clinical implications of inflammation for cardiovascular primary prevention, *Eur Heart J* 31(7):777–783, 2010.

47. Ridker PM: C-reactive protein: eighty years from discovery to emergence as a major risk marker for cardiovascular disease, *Clin Chem* 55(2):209–215, 2009.

48. Ridker PM, MacFadyen JG, Libby P, et al: Relation of baseline high-sensitivity C-reactive protein level to cardiovascular outcomes with rosuvastatin in the Justification for Use of statins in Prevention: an Intervention Trial Evaluating Rosuvastatin (JUPITER), *Am J Cardiol* 106(2):204–209, 2010.

49. Kaptoge S, Di Angelantonio E, Lowe G, et al: Emerging risk factors collaboration. C-reactive protein concentration and risk of coronary heart disease, stroke, and mortality: an individual participant meta-analysis, *Lancet* 375(9709):132–140, 2010.

50. Zacho J, Tybjaerg-Hansen A, Jensen JS, et al: Genetically elevated C-reactive protein and ischemic vascular disease, *N Engl J Med* 359(18):1897–1908, 2008.

51. Elliott P, Chambers JC, Zhang W, et al: Genetic loci associated with C-reactive protein levels and risk of coronary heart disease, *JAMA* 302(1):37–48, 2009.

52. Nordestgaard BG: Does elevated C-reactive protein cause human atherothrombosis? Novel insights from genetics, intervention trials, and elsewhere, *Curr Opin Lipidol* 2009.

53. Ridker PM, Buring JE, Rifai N, et al: Development and validation of improved algorithms for the assessment of global cardiovascular risk in women: the Reynolds Risk Score, *JAMA* 297(6):611–619, 2007.

54. Ridker PM, Paynter NP, Rifai N, et al: C-reactive protein and parental history improve global cardiovascular risk prediction: the Reynolds Risk Score for men, *Circulation* 118(22):2243–2251, 2008.

55. Wilson PW, Pencina M, Jacques P, et al: C-reactive protein and reclassification of cardiovascular risk in the Framingham heart study, *Circ Cardiovasc Qual Outcomes* 1(2):92–97, 2008.

56. Hamsten A, Eriksson P: Identifying the susceptibility genes for coronary artery disease: from hyperbole through doubt to cautious optimism, *J Intern Med* 263(5):538–552, 2008.

57. Samani NJ, Erdmann J, Hall AS, et al: Genomewide association analysis of coronary artery disease, *N Engl J Med* 357(5):443–453, 2007.

58. Schunkert H, Gotz A, Braund P, et al: Repeated replication and a prospective meta-analysis of the association between chromosome 9p21.3 and coronary artery disease, *Circulation* 117(13):1675–1684, 2008.

59. Kathiresan S, Melander O, Guiducci C, et al: Six new loci associated with blood low-density lipoprotein cholesterol, high-density lipoprotein cholesterol or triglycerides in humans, *Nat Genet* 40(2):189–197, 2008.

60. Palomaki GE, Melillo S, Bradley LA: Association between 9p21 genomic markers and heart disease: a meta-analysis, *JAMA* 303(7):648–656, 2010.

61. Teslovich TM, Musunuru K, Smith AV, et al: Biological, clinical and population relevance of 95 loci for blood lipids, *Nature* 466(7307):707–713, 2010.

62. Burkhardt R, Toh SA, Lagor WR, et al: Trib1 is a lipid- and myocardial infarction-associated gene that regulates hepatic lipogenesis and VLDL production in mice, *J Clin Invest* 120(12):4410–4414, 2010.

63. Musunuru K, Pirruccello JP, Do R, et al: Exome sequencing, ANGPTL3 mutations, and familial combined hypolipidemia, *N Engl J Med* 363(23):2220–2227, 2010.

64. Ripatti S, Tikkanen E, Orho-Melander M, et al: A multilocus genetic risk score for coronary heart disease: case-control and prospective cohort analyses, *Lancet* 376(9750):1393–1400, 2010.

65. Paynter NP, Chasman DI, Pare G, et al: Association between a literature-based genetic risk score and cardiovascular events in women, *JAMA* 303(7):631–637, 2010.

66. Gaziano JM: Fifth phase of the epidemiologic transition: the age of obesity and inactivity, *JAMA* 303(3):275–276, 2010.

67. Lloyd-Jones D, Adams RJ, Brown TM, et al: Heart disease and stroke statistics–2010 update: a report from the American Heart Association, *Circulation* 121(7):e46–e215, 2010.

68. Grundy SM, Cleeman JI, Daniels SR, et al: Diagnosis and management of the metabolic syndrome: an American Heart Association/National Heart, Lung, and Blood Institute Scientific Statement, *Circulation* 112(17):2735–2752, 2005.

69. Alberti KG, Eckel RH, Grundy SM, et al: Harmonizing the metabolic syndrome: a joint interim statement of the International Diabetes Federation Task Force on Epidemiology and Prevention; National Heart, Lung, and Blood Institute; American Heart Association; World Heart Federation; International Atherosclerosis Society; and International Association for the Study of Obesity, *Circulation* 120(16):1640–1645, 2009.

70. Kahn R, Buse J, Ferrannini E, et al: The metabolic syndrome: time for a critical appraisal: joint statement from the American Diabetes Association and the European Association for the Study of Diabetes, *Diabetes Care* 28(9):2289–2304, 2005.

71. Mente A, Yusuf S, Islam S, et al: Metabolic syndrome and risk of acute myocardial infarction a case-control study of 26,903 subjects from 52 countries, *J Am Coll Cardiol* 55(21):2390–2398, 2010.

72. Berneis KK, Krauss RM: Metabolic origins and clinical significance of LDL heterogeneity, *J Lipid Res* 43(9):1363–1379, 2002.

73. Ai M, Otokozawa S, Asztalos BF, et al: Small dense LDL cholesterol and coronary heart disease: results from the Framingham Offspring Study, *Clin Chem* 56(6):967–976, 2010.

74. Tabas I, Williams KJ, Boren J: Subendothelial lipoprotein retention as the initiating process in atherosclerosis: update and therapeutic implications, *Circulation* 116(16):1832–1844, 2007.

75. Selvin E, Steffes MW, Zhu H, et al: Glycated hemoglobin, diabetes, and cardiovascular risk in nondiabetic adults, *N Engl J Med* 362(9):800–811, 2010.

76. Giacco F, Brownlee M: Oxidative stress and diabetic complications, *Circ Res* 107(9):1058–1070, 2010.

77. Yan SF, Ramasamy R, Schmidt AM: The RAGE axis: a fundamental mechanism signaling danger to the vulnerable vasculature, *Circ Res* 106(5):842–853, 2010.

78. Gerstein HC, Miller ME, Byington RP, et al: Effects of intensive glucose lowering in type 2 diabetes, *N Engl J Med* 358(24):2545–2559, 2008.

79. Patel A, MacMahon S, Chalmers J, et al: Intensive blood glucose control and vascular outcomes in patients with type 2 diabetes, *N Engl J Med* 358(24):2560–2572, 2008.

80. Duckworth W, Abraira C, Moritz T, et al: Glucose control and vascular complications in veterans with type 2 diabetes, *N Engl J Med* 360(2):129–139, 2009.

81. Holman RR, Paul SK, Bethel MA, et al: 10-year follow-up of intensive glucose control in type 2 diabetes, *N Engl J Med* 359(15):1577–1589, 2008.

82. Libby P, Shi GP: Mast cells as mediators and modulators of atherogenesis, *Circulation* 115(19):2471–2473, 2007.

83. Mestas J, Ley K: Monocyte-endothelial cell interactions in the development of atherosclerosis, *Trends Cardiovasc Med* 18(6):228–232, 2008.

84. Swirski FK, Libby P, Aikawa E, et al: Ly-6Chi monocytes dominate hypercholesterolemia-associated monocytosis and give rise to macrophages in atheromata, *J Clin Invest* 117(1):195–205, 2007.

85. Tacke F, Alvarez D, Kaplan TJ, et al: Monocyte subsets differentially employ CCR2, CCR5, and CX3CR1 to accumulate within atherosclerotic plaques, *J Clin Invest* 117(1):185–194, 2007.

86. Libby P, Nahrendorf M, Pittet MJ, et al: Diversity of denizens of the atherosclerotic plaque: not all monocytes are created equal, *Circulation* 117:3168–3170, 2008.

87. Woollard KJ, Geissmann F: Monocytes in atherosclerosis: subsets and functions, *Nat Rev Cardiol* 7(2):77–86, 2010.

88. Bouhlel MA, Derudas B, Rigamonti E, et al: PPARgamma activation primes human monocytes into alternative M2 macrophages with anti-inflammatory properties, *Cell Metab* 6(2):137–143, 2007.

89. Bromley SK, Mempel TR, Luster AD: Orchestrating the orchestrators: chemokines in control of T cell traffic, *Nat Immunol* 9(9):970–980, 2008.

90. Kovanen PT: Mast cells: multipotent local effector cells in atherothrombosis, *Immunol Rev* 217:105–122, 2007.

91. Bot I, de Jager SC, Zernecke A, et al: Perivascular mast cells promote atherogenesis and induce plaque destabilization in apolipoprotein E-deficient mice, *Circulation* 115(19):2516–2525, 2007.

92. Sun J, Sukhova GK, Wolters PJ, et al: Mast cells promote atherosclerosis by releasing proinflammatory cytokines, *Nat Med* 13(6):719–724, 2007.

93. Libby P: Inflammation in atherosclerosis, *Nature* 420(6917):868–874, 2002.

94. Mallat Z, Taleb S, Ait-Oufella H, et al: The role of adaptive T cell immunity in atherosclerosis, *J Lipid Res* 2008.

95. Taleb S, Tedgui A, Mallat Z: Regulatory T-cell immunity and its relevance to atherosclerosis, *J Intern Med* 263(5):489–499, 2008.

96. van Es T, van Puijvelde GH, Ramos OH, et al: Attenuated atherosclerosis upon IL-17R signaling disruption in LDLr deficient mice, *Biochem Biophys Res Commun* 388(2):261–265, 2009.

97. Smith E, Prasad KM, Butcher M, et al: Blockade of interleukin-17A results in reduced atherosclerosis in apolipoprotein E-deficient mice, *Circulation* 121(15):1746–1755, 2010.

98. Taleb S, Tedgui A, Mallat Z: Interleukin-17: friend or foe in atherosclerosis? *Curr Opin Lipidol* 21(5):404–408, 2010.

99. Packard RRS, Maganto-Garcia E, Gotsman I, et al: CD11c+ dendritic cells maintain antigen processing, presentation capabilities, and CD4+ T-cell priming efficacy under hypercholesterolemic conditions associated with atherosclerosis, *Circ Res* 103:965–973, 2008.

100. Randolph GJ, Potteaux S: Vascular dendritic cells as gatekeepers of lipid accumulation within nascent atherosclerotic plaques, *Circ Res* 106(2):227–229, 2010.

101. Paulson KE, Zhu SN, Chen M, et al: Resident intimal dendritic cells accumulate lipid and contribute to the initiation of atherosclerosis, *Circ Res* 106(2):383–390, 2010.

102. Hermansson A, Ketelhuth DF, Strodthoff D, et al: Inhibition of T cell response to native low-density lipoprotein reduces atherosclerosis, *J Exp Med* 207(5):1081–1093, 2010.

103. Bentzon JF, Weile C, Sondergaard CS, et al: Smooth muscle cells in atherosclerosis originate from the local vessel wall and not circulating progenitor cells in ApoE knockout mice, *Arterioscler Thromb Vasc Biol* 26(12):2696–2702, 2006.

104. Orlandi A, Bochaton-Piallat ML, Gabbiani G, et al: Aging, smooth muscle cells and vascular pathobiology: implications for atherosclerosis, *Atherosclerosis* 188(2):221–230, 2006.

105. Geng YJ, Libby P: Progression of atheroma: a struggle between death and procreation, *Arterioscler Thromb Vasc Biol* 22(9):1370–1380, 2002.

106. Kavurma MM, Tan NY, Bennett MR: Death receptors and their ligands in atherosclerosis, *Arterioscler Thromb Vasc Biol* 28(10):1694–1702, 2008.

107. Clarke MC, Figg N, Maguire JJ, et al: Apoptosis of vascular smooth muscle cells induces features of plaque vulnerability in atherosclerosis, *Nat Med* 12(9):1075–1080, 2006.

108. Clarke MC, Littlewood TD, Figg N, et al: Chronic apoptosis of vascular smooth muscle cells accelerates atherosclerosis and promotes calcification and medial degeneration, *Circ Res* 102(12):1529–1538, 2008.

109. Amento EP, Ehsani N, Palmer H, et al: Cytokines and growth factors positively and negatively regulate interstitial collagen gene expression in human vascular smooth muscle cells, *Arterioscler Thromb Vasc Biol* 11:1223–1230, 1991.

110. Robertson AK, Rudling M, Zhou X, et al: Disruption of TGF-beta signaling in T cells accelerates atherosclerosis, *J Clin Invest* 112(9):1342–1350, 2003.

111. Hjortnaes J, Butcher J, Figueiredo JL, et al: Arterial and aortic valve calcification inversely correlates with osteoporotic bone remodelling: a role for inflammation, *Eur Heart J* 31(16):1975–1984, 2010.

112. Rajavashisth T, Qiao JH, Tripathi S, et al: Heterozygous osteopetrotic (op) mutation reduces atherosclerosis in LDL receptor- deficient mice, *J Clin Invest* 101(12):2702–2710, 1998.

113. Gautier EL, Huby T, Witztum JL, et al: Macrophage apoptosis exerts divergent effects on atherogenesis as a function of lesion stage, *Circulation* 119(13):1795–1804, 2009.

114. Tabas I: Macrophage death and defective inflammation resolution in atherosclerosis, *Nat Rev Immunol* 10(1):36–46, 2010.

115. Russo C, Jin Z, Rundek T, et al: Atherosclerotic disease of the proximal aorta and the risk of vascular events in a population-based cohort: the Aortic Plaques and Risk of Ischemic Stroke (APRIS) study, *Stroke* 40(7):2313–2318, 2009.

116. Takaya N, Yuan C, Chu B, et al: Association between carotid plaque characteristics and subsequent ischemic cerebrovascular events: a prospective assessment with MRI–initial results, *Stroke* 37(3):818–823, 2006.

117. Aird WC: Mechanisms of endothelial cell heterogeneity in health and disease, *Circ Res* 98(2):159–162, 2006.

118. Majesky MW: Developmental basis of vascular smooth muscle diversity, *Arterioscler Thromb Vasc Biol* 27(6):1248–1258, 2007.

119. Dong C, Crawford LE, Goldschmidt-Clermont PJ: Endothelial progenitor obsolescence and atherosclerotic inflammation, *J Am Coll Cardiol* 45(9):1458–1460, 2005.

120. Werner N, Kosiol S, Schiegl T, et al: Circulating endothelial progenitor cells and cardiovascular outcomes, *N Engl J Med* 353(10):999–1007, 2005.

121. Shantsila E, Watson T, Lip GY: Endothelial progenitor cells in cardiovascular disorders, *J Am Coll Cardiol* 49(7):741–752, 2007.

122. Bentzon JF, Falk E: Circulating smooth muscle progenitor cells in atherosclerosis and plaque rupture: current perspective and methods of analysis, *Vasc Pharmacol* 52(1–2):11–20, 2010.

123. Hagensen MK, Shim J, Thim T, et al: Circulating endothelial progenitor cells do not contribute to plaque endothelium in murine atherosclerosis, *Circulation* 121(7):898–905, 2010.

124. Lavoie AJ, Bayturan O, Uno K, et al: Plaque progression in coronary arteries with minimal luminal obstruction in intravascular ultrasound atherosclerosis trials, *Am J Cardiol* 105(12):1679–1683, 2010.

125. Clarkson TB, Prichard RW, Morgan TM, et al: Remodeling of coronary arteries in human and nonhuman primates, *JAMA* 271(4):289–294, 1994.

126. Glagov S, Weisenberg E, Zarins C, et al: Compensatory enlargement of human atherosclerotic coronary arteries, *N Engl J Med* 316:371–375, 1987.

127. Vink A, Schoneveld AH, Borst C, et al: The contribution of plaque and arterial remodeling to de novo atherosclerotic luminal narrowing in the femoral artery, *J Vasc Surg* 36(6):1194–1198, 2002.

128. Schoenhagen P, Sipahi I: Arterial remodelling: an independent pathophysiological component of atherosclerotic disease progression and regression. Insights from serial pharmacological intervention trials, *Eur Heart J* 28(19):2299–2300, 2007.

129. McGill HC Jr, McMahan CA, Zieske AW, et al: Associations of coronary heart disease risk factors with the intermediate lesion of atherosclerosis in youth. The Pathobiological Determinants of Atherosclerosis in Youth (PDAY) Research Group, *Arterioscler Thromb Vasc Biol* 20(8):1998–2004, 2000.

130. Li S, Chen W, Srinivasan SR, et al: Childhood cardiovascular risk factors and carotid vascular changes in adulthood: the Bogalusa Heart Study, *JAMA* 290(17):2271–2276, 2003.

131. Virmani R, Robinowitz M, Geer JC, et al: Coronary artery atherosclerosis revisited in Korean war combat casualties, *Arch Pathol Lab Med* 111(10):972–976, 1987.

132. Palinski W: Maternal-fetal cholesterol transport in the placenta: good, bad, and target for modulation, *Circ Res* 104(5):569–571, 2009.

133. Tuzcu EM, Kapadia SR, Tutar E, et al: High prevalence of coronary atherosclerosis in asymptomatic teenagers and young adults: evidence from intravascular ultrasound, *Circulation* 103(22):2705–2710, 2001.

134. Gimbrone MA Jr, Topper JN, Nagel T, et al: Endothelial dysfunction, hemodynamic forces, and atherogenesis, *Ann N Y Acad Sci*, 902:230–239, 2000 discussion 239–240.

135. Libby P, Aikawa M, Jain MK: Vascular endothelium and atherosclerosis, *Handb Exp Pharmacol* (176 Pt 2):285–306, 2006.

136. Dai G, Vaughn S, Zhang Y, et al: Biomechanical forces in atherosclerosis-resistant vascular regions regulate endothelial redox balance via phosphoinositol 3-kinase/Akt-dependent activation of Nrf2, *Circ Res* 101(7):723–733, 2007.

137. Parmar KM, Nambudiri V, Dai G, et al: Statins exert endothelial atheroprotective effects via the KLF2 transcription factor, *J Biol Chem* 289:26714–26719, 2005.

138. Young A, Wu W, Sun W, et al: Flow activation of AMP-activated protein kinase in vascular endothelium leads to Kruppel-like factor 2 expression, *Arterioscler Thromb Vasc Biol* 29(11):1902–1908, 2009.

139. Hajra L, Evans AI, Chen M, et al: The NF-kappa B signal transduction pathway in aortic endothelial cells is primed for activation in regions predisposed to atherosclerotic lesion formation, *Proc Natl Acad Sci U S A* 97(16):9052–9057, 2000.

140. Peng HB, Libby P, Liao JK: Induction and stabilization of I kappa B alpha by nitric oxide mediates inhibition of NF-kappa B, *J Biol Chem* 270(23):14214–14219, 1995.

141. Boden WE, O'Rourke RA, Teo KK, et al: Optimal medical therapy with or without PCI for stable coronary disease, *N Engl J Med* 356(15):1503–1516, 2007.

142. Corti R, Fuster V, Badimon JJ: Pathogenetic concepts of acute coronary syndromes, *J Am Coll Cardiol* 41(4 Suppl S):7S–14S, 2003.

143. Libby P: The molecular mechanisms of the thrombotic complications of atherosclerosis, *J Int Med* 263:517–527, 2008.

144. Fuster V: Mechanisms leading to myocardial infarction: insights from vascular biology, *Circulation* 90(4):2126–2146, 1994.

145. Schoenhagen P, Ziada KM, Kapadia SR, et al: Extent and direction of arterial remodeling in stable versus unstable coronary syndromes: an intravascular ultrasound study, *Circulation* 101(6):598–603, 2000.

146. Libby P, Theroux P: Pathophysiology of coronary artery disease, *Circulation* 111:3481–3488, 2005.

147. Finn AV, Nakano M, Narula J, et al: Concept of vulnerable/unstable plaque, *Arterioscler Thromb Vasc Biol* 30(7):1282–1292, 2010.

148. Galis Z, Sukhova G, Lark M, et al: Increased expression of matrix metalloproteinases and matrix degrading activity in vulnerable regions of human atherosclerotic plaques, *J Clin Invest* 94:2493–2503, 1994.

149. Sukhova GK, Schonbeck U, Rabkin E, et al: Evidence for increased collagenolysis by interstitial collagenases-1 and -3 in vulnerable human atheromatous plaques, *Circulation* 99(19):2503–2509, 1999.

150. Dollery CM, Libby P: Atherosclerosis and proteinase activation, *Cardiovasc Res* 69(3):625–635, 2006.

151. Herman MP, Sukhova GK, Kisiel W, et al: Tissue factor pathway inhibitor-2 is a novel inhibitor of matrix metalloproteinases with implications for atherosclerosis, *J Clin Invest* 107(9):1117–1126, 2001.

152. Fukumoto Y, Deguchi JO, Libby P, et al: Genetically determined resistance to collagenase action augments interstitial collagen accumulation in atherosclerotic plaques, *Circulation* 110(14):1953–1959, 2004.

153. Deguchi JO, Aikawa E, Libby P, et al: Matrix metalloproteinase-13/collagenase-3 deletion promotes collagen accumulation and organization in mouse atherosclerotic plaques, *Circulation* 112(17):2708–2715, 2005.

154. Schneider F, Sukhova GK, Aikawa M, et al: Matrix-metalloproteinase-14 deficiency in bone-marrow-derived cells promotes collagen accumulation in mouse atherosclerotic plaques, *Circulation* 117(7):931–939, 2008.

155. van der Wal AC, Becker AE, van der Loos CM, et al: Site of intimal rupture or erosion of thrombosed coronary atherosclerotic plaques is characterized by an inflammatory process irrespective of the dominant plaque morphology, *Circulation* 89:36–44, 1994.

156. Virmani R, Burke AP, Farb A, et al: Pathology of the vulnerable plaque, *J Am Coll Cardiol* 47(8 Suppl):C13–C18, 2006.

157. Sugiyama S, Kugiyama K, Aikawa M, et al: Hypochlorous acid, a macrophage product, induces endothelial apoptosis and tissue factor expression: involvement of myeloperoxidase-mediated oxidant in plaque erosion and thrombogenesis, *Arterioscler Thromb Vasc Biol* 24(7):1309–1314, 2004.

158. Moulton KS: Angiogenesis in atherosclerosis: gathering evidence beyond speculation, *Curr Opin Lipidol* 17(5):548–555, 2006.

159. Beckman JA, Ganz J, Creager MA, et al: Relationship of clinical presentation and calcification of culprit coronary artery stenoses, *Arterioscler Thromb Vasc Biol* 21(10):1618–1622, 2001.

160. Bayturan O, Tuzcu EM, Nicholls SJ, et al: Attenuated plaque at nonculprit lesions in patients enrolled in intravascular ultrasound atherosclerosis progression trials, *JACC Cardiovasc Interv* 2(7):672–678, 2009.

161. Mann J, Davies MJ: Mechanisms of progression in native coronary artery disease: role of healed plaque disruption, *Heart* 82(3):265–268, 1999.

162. Burke AP, Kolodgie FD, Farb A, et al: Healed plaque ruptures and sudden coronary death: evidence that subclinical rupture has a role in plaque progression, *Circulation* 103(7):934–940, 2001.

163. Libby P: Act local, act global: inflammation and the multiplicity of "vulnerable" coronary plaques, *J Am Coll Cardiol* 45(10):1600–1602, 2005.

164. Aikawa M, Rabkin E, Okada Y, et al: Lipid lowering by diet reduces matrix metalloproteinase activity and increases collagen content of rabbit atheroma: a potential mechanism of lesion stabilization, *Circulation* 97:2433–2444, 1998.

165. Libby P, Aikawa M: Stabilization of atherosclerotic plaques: New mechanisms and clinical targets, *Nat Med* 8(11):1257–1262, 2002.

166. Libby P, Sasiela W: Plaque stabilization: can we turn theory into evidence? *Am J Cardiol* 98:S26–S33, 2006.

167. Hernandez-Presa MA, Bustos C, Ortego M, et al: ACE inhibitor quinapril reduces the arterial expression of NF-kappaB-dependent proinflammatory factors but not of collagen I in a rabbit model of atherosclerosis, *Am J Pathol* 153(6):1825–1837, 1998.

168. Nissen SE, Tsunoda T, Tuzcu EM, et al: Effect of recombinant ApoA-I Milano on coronary atherosclerosis in patients with acute coronary syndromes: a randomized controlled trial, *JAMA* 290(17):2292–2300, 2003.

169. Tardif JC, Gregoire J, L'Allier PL, et al: Effects of reconstituted high-density lipoprotein infusions on coronary atherosclerosis: a randomized controlled trial, *JAMA* 297(15):1675–1682, 2007.

170. Nissen SE, Nicholls SJ, Sipahi I, et al: Effect of very high-intensity statin therapy on regression of coronary atherosclerosis: the ASTEROID trial, *JAMA* 295(13):1556–1565, 2006.

171. Nicholls SJ, Ballantyne CM, Barter PJ, et al: Effect of two intensive statin regimens on progression of coronary disease, *N Engl J Med* 365(22):2078–2087, 2011.

172. Zhao XQ, Yuan C, Hatsukami TS, et al: Effects of prolonged intensive lipid-lowering therapy on the characteristics of carotid atherosclerotic plaques in vivo by MRI: a case-control study, *Arterioscler Thromb Vasc Biol* 21(10):1623–1629, 2001.

ATHEROSCLEROSIS

CHAPTER 9

Pathophysiology of Vasculitis

Peter Libby

The pathophysiological mechanisms that underlie vasculitis include elements of virtually all effector limbs of host defenses, including innate and adaptive immunity. Various classification schemes separate the vasculitides into primary and secondary families, and categorize them by size of the afflicted vessel. Classification of vasculitides is currently in ferment, with the classical American College of Rheumatology classification and the Chapel Hill Consensus Conference criteria under reconsideration from several fronts and for various reasons.[1-3] Epidemiological studies and clinical trials, for example, require standardized definitions of these diseases, and these may overlap considerably. The confusion that reigns in this field reflects in part an incomplete understanding of the fundamentals of the pathogenesis of human vasculitides—an endeavor still in considerable flux. Whereas Chapter 41 provides a detailed classification of the vasculitides, this chapter focuses on the primary vasculitides and, for pedagogical purposes, considers the pathophysiological mechanisms of vasculitis in two broad categories: (1) mechanisms that underlie small-vessel vasculitis, and (2) mechanisms involved in medium- and large-sized arteritides (Fig. 9-1). Although this is an oversimplified categorization, it provides an organizational framework for discussing elements of *humoral immunity* involved chiefly in primary small-vessel vasculitides, and *cellular immunity*, likely the central mechanism underlying vasculitides of medium- and large-sized arteries (Table 9-1).

Pathophysiology of Small-Vessel Vasculitis

Small-vessel vasculitides include Wegener granulomatosis, Churg-Strauss' syndrome, microscopic polyangiitis, Henoch-Schönlein purpura, and essential cryoglobulinemic vasculitis.[2,3] Recognition that antineutrophil cytoplasmic antibodies (ANCAs) associate with many (but not all) small-vessel vasculitides has advanced understanding of their pathophysiology. In particular, Wegener granulomatosis, microscopic polyangiitis, and Churg-Strauss' syndrome associate strongly with ANCA. Many of the ANCA-positive small-vessel vasculitides involve the kidney.[4]

The principal antigens recognized by ANCA are the neutrophil enzymes myeloperoxidase (MPO) and proteinase-3 (PR3) (see Table 9-1); some ANCA may recognize human neutrophil elastase as well. Anti-PR3 antibodies also may recognize plasminogen.[5] Antigens recognized by ANCA usually localize within polymorphonuclear (PMNs) leukocytes. When primed by stimuli such as tumor necrosis factor (TNF)-α or when undergoing apoptosis or NETosis (release of chromatin fibers called *neutrophil extracellular traps* (NETs) that trap and kill microbes extracellularly), PMN leukocytes can release these antigens. These antigens in turn can bind back to the cell surface—in the case of PR3, through CD177[6]—or decorate NETs.[7] Binding of ANCAs to cell surface–associated MPO and PR3 on intact neutrophils leads to further activation of these leukocytes (i.e., generation of reactive oxygen species [ROS], release of lytic enzymes, binding of cells to the endothelium), as does engagement of the surface-bound Fc-portion of immunoglobulin (Ig)G in immune complexes with FcγRs on neighboring cells. Uptake of neutrophil-released MPO and PR3 by endothelial cells (ECs) also may impair the viability and vasomotor responses of ECs.[8] These events together aggravate the local inflammatory response. As opposed to secondary vasculitides, which characteristically have substantial immune complex deposition upon histological examination, lesions of ANCA-associated conditions show modest Ig deposits.[9] When released in soluble form, proteinases such as PR3 and neutrophil elastase readily bind to widely distributed and abundant antiproteinases that may mask their recognition by ANCA. Circulating ANCA can also complex with these antigens, but such complexes form preferentially when proteinase antigens remain associated with the neutrophil cell surface (Fig. 9-2).

Individuals who express primarily MPO-directed ANCA (vs. PR3-directed ANCA) may have distinct clinical courses.[10] Microscopic polyangiitis associates particularly with anti-MPO ANCA, while Wegener granulomatosis typically associates with anti-PR3 ANCA (see Table 9-1). The possible clinical dichotomy between these patient categories may relate to the functions of target antigens. For example, binding to ANCA may protect MPO from clearance and inactivation by ceruloplasmin, increasing the ability of this enzyme to produce the highly oxidant species, hypochlorous acid (HOCl). Hypochlorous acid has many properties that may contribute to the pathophysiology of vasculitis, including stimulation of endothelial apoptosis.[11]

Not all patients with small-vessel vasculitis have ANCA-positive serology, indicating that some small-vessel vasculitides may involve other mechanisms or have low titer antibodies. Additionally, "atypical" ANCA directed against antigens other than MPO or PR3 may participate in the pathogenesis of vasculitis. Recent studies have implicated lysosomal-associated membrane protein-2 (LAMP-2) as a novel autoantigen in vasculitis.[6,12,13] In addition to neutrophils, endothelial and other cells express LAMP-2, a recognition target for ANCA.

Antineutrophil cytoplasmic antibodies have proven unequivocally pathogenic in mice. In a landmark investigation, Xiao et al. immunized mice lacking endogenous MPO, owing to targeted gene inactivation, with exogenous mouse MPO.[14] Transfer of splenocytes from these MPO-immunized mice into immunodeficient mice caused severe necrotizing crescentic glomerulonephritis. In some cases, a systemic necrotizing and granulomatous vasculitis affected lung capillaries as well as the renal microvasculature (see Fig. 9-2). Purified anti-MPO IgG isolated from the MPO-immunized mice caused renal, pulmonary, and cutaneous small-vessel vasculitis. Experimental depletion of neutrophils abrogated formation of glomerular lesions in anti-MPO IgG-treated mice, thus implicating granulocytes in the pathogenesis of ANCA-induced angiitis.[15] Moreover, studies in bone marrow chimeric mice (transplantation of MPO wild-type or MPO-deficient bone marrow into MPO-immunized MPO-null animals) suggest that leukocytes are targets of anti-MPO ANCA.[16]

Immunization of PR3-deficient mice with PR3 yielded circulating anti-PR3 antibodies and modest renal and pulmonary vasculitis.[17] These mice with anti-PR3 antibodies developed cutaneous vasculitis at sites of TNF-α injection. While not directly comparable to the passive/adoptive transfer studies in MPO-deficient mice, these results support different pathogenic capabilities of these two major classes of ANCA in terms of severity and localization of vasculitis, at least in mice. Plasma exchange causes improvement in patients with ANCA-associated disease exacerbation, supporting the causal role of antibody in these conditions.[6]

Antineutrophil cytoplasmic antibodies may provoke vasculitis in several ways (Figs. 9-3 and 9-4). These autoantibodies may increase activation and adherence of neutrophils to ECs.[18] When neutrophils "primed" by exposure to TNF-α encounter MPO-ANCA, a respiratory burst can ensue and produce ROS such as superoxide anion and hydrogen peroxide—proinflammatory mediators that can injure ECs and activate smooth muscle cells (SMCs).[19,20] Antineutrophil cytoplasmic antibodies promote neutrophil degranulation, and can activate intracellular signaling pathways and heighten sensitivity of PMN leukocytes to classic stimulants, such as formyl peptides.[21] The mechanism of vascular damage in immune complex disease also involves complement activation (see Fig. 9-4).[6] Antigen-antibody complexes (immune

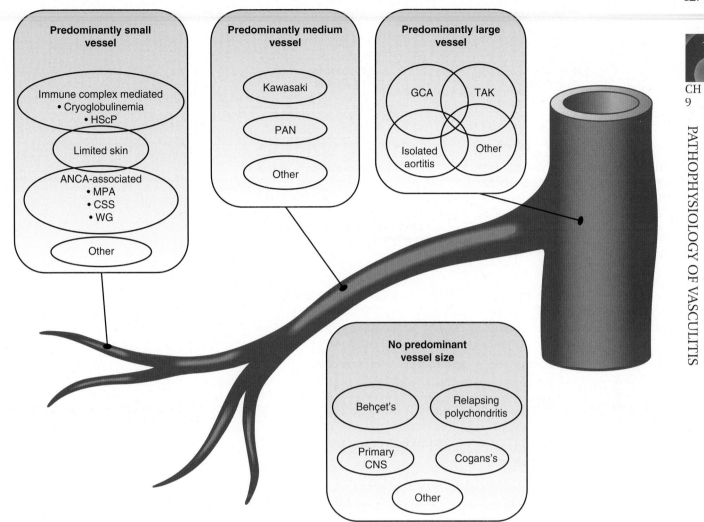

FIGURE 9-1   Classification scheme for the primary vasculitides. CNS, central nervous system; CSS, Churg-Strauss syndrome; GCA, giant-cell arteritis; HScP, Henoch-Schönlein purpura; MPA, microscopic polyangiitis; PAN, polyarterits nodosa; TAK, Takayasu arteritis; WG, Wegener granulomatosis. *(Modified from Suppiah R, Basu N, Watts RA, et al: Advances in the classification of primary systemic vasculitis. Int J Adv Rheumatol 7:10, 2009. Reproduced with permission from Watts RA, Suppiah R, Merkel PA, et al: Systemic vasculitis—Is it time to reclassify? Rheumatology 50:643, 2011.)*

complexes) containing IgM or IgG can bind to complement factor 1 (C1), lead to assembly of C3 convertase, and yield activation of C3, C4, and C5. Ultimately, assembly of the membrane attack complex (MAC, composed of oligomers of C9 and other terminal complement components) can damage ECs by forming pores in their plasma membranes. Circulating immune complexes can sequester in subendothelial basement membranes at sites where

interendothelial separation has occurred. These trapped immune complexes then activate complement, and can engage neutrophils and monocytes via their Fc and complement receptors. Anaphylatoxins (fragments of C3a, C4a, and C5a) generated during activation of the classical complement pathway can recruit granulocytes and monocytes and activate mast cells at sites of immune complex deposition in vessels. These leukocytes can amplify local inflammation and aggravate and perpetuate the vasculitic response.

Some pathogenic schemes for vasculitis invoke the participation of viruses—in some cases well substantiated, such as the association of hepatitis C and cryoglobulinemia. Given the ubiquity of viral infections and antigen-specific antibody responses, circulation of viral antigen-antibody complexes probably occurs frequently. Yet, most common viral infections do not produce clinically evident or sustained vasculitis. The relative rarity of symptomatic or sustained vasculitis in common viral infections probably relates to tight control of the complement system—which, like many protease cascades, undergoes intricate regulation by endogenous inhibitors.

The ANCA-positive vasculitides have a solid experimental and clinical evidence base that supports a pathogenic role for ANCA in the development of vasculitis. These findings illustrate the importance of humoral immunity in the pathogenesis of this category of vasculitides, but the cellular immune response may regulate aspects of the primarily humoral immune pathogenesis of the small-vessel vasculitides. For example, the balance between type 1 helper T cell (T_H1 cell, interferon [IFN]-γ predominant) responses and type 2

TABLE 9-1	Pathophysiological Mechanisms of Some Primary Vasculitides
	PUTATIVE PATHOGENIC EFFECTORS
Large-Artery Arteritides	
Takayasu arteritis	γδ T cells
Giant-cell arteritis	T_H1 and T_H17 helper T cells
Small-Artery Arteritides	
Microscopic polyangiitis	Anti-MPO ANCA > Anti-PR3 ANCA
Wegener granulomatosis	Anti-PR3 ANCA > Anti-MPO ANCA
Henoch-Schönlein purpura	Viral infections, food allergies (?)
Churg-Strauss' syndrome	Eosinophils, CD95
Cryoglobulinemia	IgM > IgG, hepatitis C virus infection

ANCA, antineutrophil cytoplasmic antibody; Ig, immunoglobulin; MPO, myeloperoxidase; PR3, proteinase-3; T_H, helper T cell.

CH
9

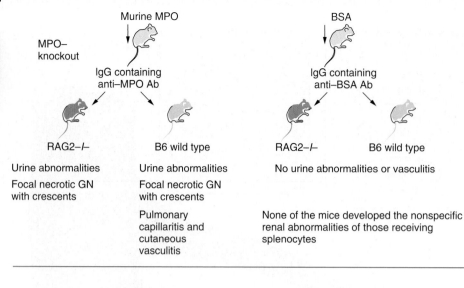

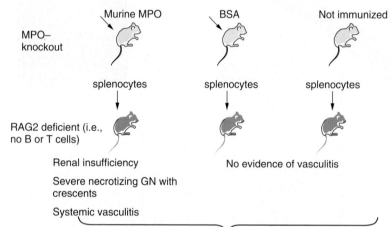

FIGURE 9-2 MPO-ANCA mice cause small-vessel arteritis. ANCA, antineutrophil cytoplasmic antibody; BSA, bovine serum albumin; GN, glomerulonephritis; IgG, immunoglobulin G; MPO, myeloperoxidase; RAG2, recombination activating gene 2. *(Data from Xiao H, Herringa P, Hu P, et al: Antineutrophil cytoplasmic autoantibodies specific for myeloperoxidase cause glomerulonephritis and vasculitis in mice. J Clin Invest 110:955, 2002. Reproduced with permission from Day CJ, Hewins P, Savage CO: New directions in the pathogenesis of ANCA-associated vasculitis. Clin Exp Rheumatol 21:S35, 2003.)*

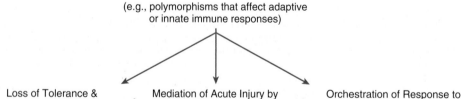

FIGURE 9-3 Pathogenic events during the evolution of ANCA disease. Production of pathogenic amounts of ANCA requires loss of tolerance. ANCAs activate neutrophils and monocytes, which results in acute inflammation and necrosis, eliciting a response orchestrated by macrophages and T cells. Multiple environmental and genetic factors modulate each pathogenic step from onset to outcome. ANCA, antineutrophil cytoplasmic antibody. *(Reproduced with permission from Jennette JC, Xiao H, Falk RJ. Pathogenesis of vascular inflammation by anti-neutrophil cytoplasmic antibodies. J Am Soc Nephrol 17:1235, 2006.)*

helper T cell (T$_H$2 cell, interleukin [IL]-4 predominant) slanted reactions may modulate expression of small-vessel vasculitides; a T$_H$1 response may associate with the localized variant of Wegener granulomatosis rather than with the generalized form.[22] Indeed, T cells appear to modulate the consequences of the antibody-induced disease.[6,23] In later stages of ANCA-induced vasculitides, T cells and

their mediators may promote granulomatous features of lesions that are more necrotizing and destructive of elastic fibers in their earlier phases. Some even speculate that such granulomatous lesions may constitute a local lymphoid tissue that can perpetuate the disease through augmented production of autoantibodies and by presenting antigens regionally via abundant dendritic cells.[23,24]

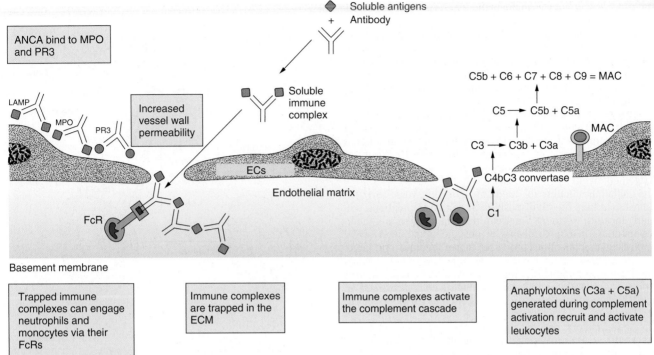

ANCA bind to MPO and PR3

Soluble antigens
+ Antibody

Soluble immune complex

Increased vessel wall permeability

$C5b + C6 + C7 + C8 + C9 = MAC$

$C5 \longrightarrow C5b + C5a$

$C3 \longrightarrow C3b + C3a$

MAC

C4bC3 convertase

C1

LAMP
MPO
PR3

ECs

Endothelial matrix

FcR

Basement membrane

Trapped immune complexes can engage neutrophils and monocytes via their FcRs

Immune complexes are trapped in the ECM

Immune complexes activate the complement cascade

Anaphylotoxins (C3a + C5a) generated during complement activation recruit and activate leukocytes

FIGURE 9-4 **Some mechanisms of small-vessel vasculitides.** In resting polymorphonuclear (PMN) leukocytes, antigens such as myeloperoxidase (MPO) or proteinase-3 (PR3) remain localized within cells in millimolar quantities and hidden from the immune system. On priming or activation, neutrophils can release or exteriorize MPO or PR3. In addition, dying PMN leukocytes can furnish externally disposed MPO, PR3, or lysosomal-associated membrane protein-2 (LAMP-2) to the immune system. Binding of antibodies known as *antineutrophil cytoplasmic antibodies* (ANCA) can activate PMN leukocytes, enhancing their adhesion to endothelial cells, (ECs) (middle EC). Activated PMN leukocytes can undergo an oxidative burst, producing high levels of reactive oxygen species (ROS) such as superoxide anion or hypochlorous acid (HOCl), which can injure ECs. Release of neutrophil elastase and other hydrolases can digest basement membrane, leading to the classic picture of a necrotizing vasculitis affecting small vessels of the glomerulus, lung, or skin. Formation of immune complexes can directly activate cells by binding to Fc receptors (FCRs), and can unleash complement which, in turn, can bind complement receptors. Activation of the complement pathway can also generate anaphylotoxins, which can recruit and activate additional leukocytes. Similar mechanisms are involved in the secondary vasculitides (e.g., those associated with endocarditis and serum sickness), systemic lupus erythematosus, and rheumatoid arthritis. ECM, extracellular matrix; MAC, membrane attack complex.

Churg-Strauss' syndrome, which characteristically occurs in individuals with asthma, comprises a special case of small-vessel vasculitis. Tissue accumulation of eosinophils and peripheral blood eosinophilia characterize this disease. This form of small-vessel vasculitis appears to result from prolonged eosinophil survival due to an excess of soluble CD95, which antagonizes apoptosis usually mediated by engagement of CD95 on the eosinophil surface—a mechanism that usually holds the eosinophil population tonically in check. Indeed, patients with Churg-Strauss' syndrome have elevated levels of soluble CD95, and CD95 ligation appears important in regulating eosinophil apoptosis.[25,26]

Observations in some secondary vasculitides further support the involvement of antibodies in vasculitis. In particular, the cryoglobulinemic vasculitis associated with hepatitis C virus infection frequently involves a polyclonal elevation of IgG and IgM antibodies, perhaps in response to polyclonal activation of B cells. In some cases, the mixed cryoglobulins in patients with chronic hepatitis C virus infection may contain ANCA, illustrating the overlap between primary and secondary vasculitides.[27]

Mechanisms that give rise to ANCA (primum movens) remain speculative. The association of *Staphylococcus aureus* nasal infections and serological evidence of exposure to Ross River virus and other viruses with Wegener granulomatosis suggests that infection may trigger ANCA formation. Antigenic mimicry with such pathogens might explain selective induction of ANCA.[12,28] A novel complex pathogenic model invokes autoantigenic complementarity rather than strict antigenic mimicry: PR3-ANCA patients have antibodies against a product of PR3 antisense ribonucleic acid (RNA) with sequence similarity to microbial and viral proteins. About half of ANCA-positive patients transcribe the complementary protein's antisense RNA. This protein product elicits antibodies that in turn provoke an antiidiotype immune response.

Antiidiotypic antibodies bind the autoantigen, raising the possibility that autoantigen complement, rather than the autoantigen itself, initiates the autoimmune response.[29] Mouse experiments have shown important influences of genetic background on expression of ANCA-related vasculitis, suggesting that modifier genes or immunogenetic mechanisms modulate individual responses to ANCA— mechanisms that might explain the daunting clinical heterogeneity of these conditions in terms of severity and organ involvement.[4]

Pathogenesis of Medium- and Large-Sized Arterial Vasculitides

The pathological hallmark of medium- and large-sized artery vasculitides—fibroproliferation with or without granuloma formation—implicates a chronic cellular immune response in their pathogenesis. In contrast to the ANCA-associated small-vessel arteritides considered previously, current evidence implicates a primary role for cellular immunity rather than humoral immunity in large-vessel arteritis (see Table 9-1).

The stimuli driving arteritis in Takayasu's disease, Kawasaki disease, and polyarteritis nodosa remain unknown. Among the many mechanisms proposed for Takayasu's disease, evidence has accumulated for T-cell involvement.[30] Recent work has implicated heat shock protein 60 (hsp60)-reactive γδ T cells in the pathogenesis of Takayasu's disease.[31] Other studies have pointed to antiendothelial cell antibodies in Takayasu arteritis.[32] In this and other arterial diseases, whether such antibodies cause or result from the disease remains unknown.

Understanding of the pathogenesis of giant-cell arteritis as T cell–mediated disease has continued to evolve. Weyand et al. have provided strong experimental evidence for the critical involvement of

CD4-positive T lymphocytes in the pathogenesis of giant-cell arteritis. Their approach involved grafting human temporal artery specimens from patients with giant-cell arteritis into immunodeficient mice. Ablation of the human T lymphocytes by administering anti–T-cell antibodies to these mice halts the inflammatory process in the xenografted human arterial specimen.[33]

Analysis of T-cell populations in human peripheral blood has shown high levels of T_H1 and T_H17 lymphocytes in untreated patients with active giant-cell arteritis.[34] These T-cell subtypes produce IFN-γ, a cytokine implicated in many aspects of arterial pathophysiology that might promote vasculitis.[35,36] Using the human-mouse chimera preparation, glucocorticoid treatment could inhibit IL-17 but not IFN-γ production. These results have clinical implications for the management of giant-cell arteritis.

The initiating stimulus for medium- and large-vessel arteritis remains uncertain. The predisposition of certain populations, particularly those of Northern European descent, suggests a genetic component. As in other diseases of obscure origin, many have hypothesized that infectious processes trigger medium- and large-artery vasculitides, but recovery of infectious agents from lesions has not proven reproducible. Some experimental results support the presence of antigens that can stimulate T cells in extracts of lesions of giant-cell or Takayasu arteritis, such as members of the hsp60 family.

The inflammatory process that initiates medium- and large-sized artery vasculitis may originate in the adventitia. Normal arterial adventitia contains resting dendritic cells. When activated, dendritic cells function importantly as antigen-presenting cells (Fig. 9-5); they patrol their environment, engulfing and presenting antigens to T helper cells that typically bear the CD4 marker. Unactivated dendritic cells usually inhibit T-cell stimulation, a process known as *tolerization*, but activated dendritic cells can trigger the cellular immune response. Normal arterial tunica media appears "immunoprivileged"—it usually does not support afferent signaling to the cellular immune system. The "break" in medial immunoprivilege may result from local expression of the characteristic T_H1 cytokine, IFN-γ.[37]

In arteries affected by giant-cell arteritis, dendritic cells become activated, as disclosed by their expression of the markers CD86 and CD83. Dendritic cells can accumulate in the media and intima of the artery. Activated dendritic cells express the chemokine receptor CCR-7, which can bind a trio of chemokine ligands, CCL-18, -19, and -21. These chemoattractant cytokines, overexpressed in the inflamed artery wall, can attract dendritic cells into the nascent vasculitic lesion. Recruited and activated dendritic cells can now effectively present antigen to T lymphocytes and stimulate the afferent limb of cellular immunity.

When activated, T cells can secrete cytokines such as IFN-γ and express CD40 ligand on their surface. These effectors of the activated T lymphocyte act as strong stimuli for macrophage activation; activated macrophages then can form granulomas. Accumulating macrophages can fuse into multinucleated giant cells, one of the histological hallmarks of granuloma formation. T cell–driven macrophage activation classically instigates the delayed-type hypersensitivity (DTH) response characteristic of granulomatous disease. For example, the cutaneous reaction to injected purified protein derivative from tubercle bacilli elicits a T cell–driven macrophage response believed to replicate the initial steps in formation of granulomas (e.g., those characteristic of infection with the tubercle bacillus).

Activated macrophages can release multiple mediators that participate in the fibroproliferative process characteristic of medium- and large-artery vasculitis. Production of mediators such as transforming growth factor (TGF)-β can stimulate collagen synthesis, as well as that of other constituents of the extracellular matrix (ECM).[38] This fibrogenic response contributes to expansion of intimal volume, characteristic of these arteritides. Mitogenic and chemoattractant factors released from activated macrophages can also stimulate SMC migration and proliferation. For example, activated macrophages can produce platelet-derived

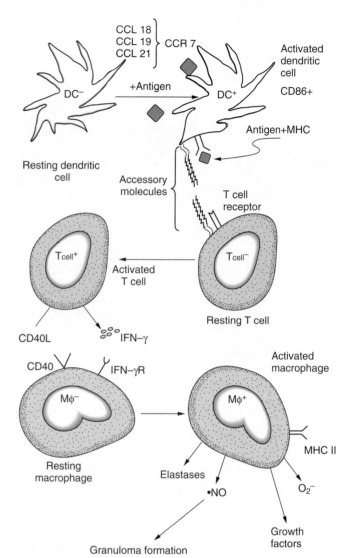

FIGURE 9-5 Some mechanisms of large-vessel vasculitides. Resting dendritic cells *(DC⁻)* can exert an inhibitory influence on T cells. DC⁻ localized in adventitia may provide a check on T-cell activation in the normal arterial wall. When appropriately stimulated, activated dendritic cells *(DC⁺)* express markers such as CD86. Expression of chemokine receptor-7 *(CCR-7)* allows recruitment of DC⁺ by the chemokine ligands CCL-18, -19, and -21. High levels of expression of class II histocompatibility antigens facilitate presentation of foreign peptides to T lymphocytes. When activated, the CD4-positive T cell *(T cell⁺)* augments production of interferon-γ *(IFN-γ)* and expresses high levels of CD40 ligand on its surface. These and other stimuli can activate the resting macrophage *(Mφ⁻)* by engaging cognate receptors on its surface. The stimulated macrophage *(Mφ⁺)* can secrete multiple mediators of the fibroproliferative response involved in intimal expansion characteristic of large- and medium-cell arteritides, including growth factors and cytokines, reactive oxygen species (ROS) such as superoxide anion *(O₂⁻)*, or reactive nitrogen species such as nitric oxide *(•NO)*. The activated macrophage also augments expression of class II major histocompatibility antigens (MHC) that enhance the cell type's antigen-presenting function. Elastolytic and other proteinases secreted by activated macrophages can contribute to arterial remodeling in inflamed vessels. Coalescence of activated macrophages creates the multinucleated giant cell characteristic of granulomata that form in these arteritides. These mechanisms participate in the pathogenesis of giant-cell arteritis and other medium- and large-vessel arteritides.

growth factor (PDGF), fibroblast growth factor (FGF) family members, and other stimulators of SMC multiplication and directed migration.[39] Activated macrophages also produce ROS and lipid hydroperoxides that can injure ECs and further amplify arterial injury.

The elastic laminae in medium- and large-sized arteries affected by giant-cell arteritis typically do not show severe dissolution, but fragmentation of the internal elastic lamina can occur. Elastolysis mediated by elastolytic enzymes of the matrix metalloproteinase (MMP) family (e.g., MMP-9, MMP-12), or by elastolytic cathepsins secreted by macrophages stimulated by CD40 ligand or other pro-inflammatory cytokines, contributes to elastic fiber fragmentation. This elastolysis can promote migration of SMCs and remodeling characteristic of intima expansion. Arterial ectasia or aneurysm formation sometimes occur in advanced giant-cell arteritis, or frequently as a chronic complication of Kawasaki disease. In this case, elastin destruction and digestion of other ECM macromolecules likely pave the way for arterial expansion. Compared with small-vessel vasculitides, medium- and large-sized arteritides do not involve extensive necrosis. A concentric fibroproliferative expansion of the intima with or without granuloma formation, rather than cell death, predominates.

Summary of Pathogenic Mechanisms in Vasculitides

This chapter has dichotomized the pathophysiological mechanisms of vasculitis—those that affect primarily small vessels, and those that characteristically involve medium- and large-sized arteries (see Table 9-1). Although exceptions and overlap clearly exist, the small-vessel vasculitides appear more driven by antibodies and activated PMN leukocytes than by cells of the adaptive immune response, such as T cells and dendritic cells involved in the initiation of medium- and large-sized arteritis. Activated PMN leukocytes appear to act as the major effector in small-vessel vasculitides. In contrast, the macrophage, recruited in response to dendritic cell–T lymphocyte control, likely accounts for much of the tissue response in medium- and large-vessel arteritides. The immunoprivilege of the arterial media provides a fertile field for dendritic cells to survey for, and to present, antigens to incite the cellular immune response. Antigens that drive small-vessel vasculitides include MPO and PR3, common stimuli for ANCA development. The antigenic drivers of medium- and large-sized arteritides remain unknown.

Necrosis, the histological hallmark of small-vessel vasculitides, occurs in all lesions, whether they affect glomerular capillaries, pulmonary microvasculature, or small vessels in the skin. In contrast, rapid formation of concentric intimal lesions, characterized by accumulation of ECM and SMCs, occurs during the formation of medium- and large-sized arteritides. The histological hallmark of these arteritides, the granuloma, usually does not involve necrosis or widespread elastolysis, but instead involves formation of giant cells derived from macrophages. Pathogenesis of both types of vasculitis appears to involve oxidative stress, as exemplified by the production of ROS including superoxide anion and MPO-derived HOCl. But elastolysis in small-vessel vasculitides probably involves neutrophil elastase, rather than the metalloelastases or cysteinyl elastases characteristically elaborated by mononuclear phagocytes stimulated by T_H1 cytokines.

Future goals of the investigation in this field include delineation of the antigens involved in instigating medium- and large-sized arteritides. We should aim to achieve a greater understanding of the differences between giant-cell arteritis, polymyalgia rheumatica (which in some ways resembles a forme fruste of giant-cell arteritis), and Takayasu arteritis. Immunogenetic components may participate in these distinct manifestations of arteritis. The current practicality of high-throughput genome sequencing may facilitate identification of susceptibility and modifier genes. Yet low numbers of patients, heterogeneity and overlap of the vasculitic syndromes, and attendant nosological controversies will likely hamper this effort.

Individuals of Northern European descent display the greatest susceptibility to giant-cell arteritis, whereas Asian and Hispanic populations seem most at risk for Takayasu arteritis. As we understand better the specific triggers for inflammatory processes involved in these various forms of vasculitis, we should strive to target therapies more precisely and develop finer diagnostic tools.

Ultimately, deeper insight into pathogenesis may guide clinical trials, inform management guidelines, and enable us to prevent and effectively treat these often serious and debilitating diseases of the vasculature.[40,41]

ACKNOWLEDGMENTS

I thank Dr. Tanya Mayadas for her critical reading of this manuscript and helpful comments and suggestions, and Ms. Sara Karwacki for her editorial expertise.

REFERENCES

1. Watts R, Lane S, Hanslik T, et al: Development and validation of a consensus methodology for the classification of the ANCA-associated vasculitides and polyarteritis nodosa for epidemiological studies, *Ann Rheum Dis* 66(2):222–227, 2007.
2. Watts RA, Suppiah R, Merkel PA, et al: Systemic vasculitis--is it time to reclassify? *Rheumatology (Oxford)* 2010.
3. Basu N, Watts R, Bajema I, et al: EULAR points to consider in the development of classification and diagnostic criteria in systemic vasculitis, *Ann Rheum Dis* 69(10):1744–1750, 2010.
4. Jennette JC, Xiao H, Falk R, et al: Experimental models of vasculitis and glomerulonephritis induced by antineutrophil cytoplasmic autoantibodies, *Contrib Nephrol* 169:211–220, 2011.
5. Bautz DJ, Preston GA, Lionaki S, et al: Antibodies with dual reactivity to plasminogen and complementary PR3 in PR3-ANCA vasculitis, *J Am Soc Nephrol* 19(12):2421–2429, 2008.
6. Chen M, Kallenberg CG: New advances in the pathogenesis of ANCA-associated vasculitides, *Clin Exp Rheumatol* 27(1 Suppl 52):S108–S114, 2009.
7. Kessenbrock K, Krumbholz M, Schonermarck U, et al: Netting neutrophils in autoimmune small-vessel vasculitis, *Nat Med* 15(6):623–625, 2009.
8. Preston GA, Yang JJ, Xiao H, et al: Understanding the pathogenesis of ANCA: where are we today? *Cleve Clin J Med* 69(Suppl 2):SII51–SII54, 2002.
9. Jennette JC, Xiao H, Falk RJ: Pathogenesis of vascular inflammation by anti-neutrophil cytoplasmic antibodies, *J Am Soc Nephrol* 17(5):1235–1242, 2006.
10. Franssen CF, Stegeman CA, Kallenberg CG, et al: Antiproteinase 3- and vasculitis, *Kidney Int* 57(6):2195–2206, 2000.
11. Sugiyama S, Kugiyama K, Aikawa M, et al: Hypochlorous acid, a macrophage product, induces endothelial apoptosis and tissue factor expression: involvement of myeloperoxidase-mediated oxidant in plaque erosion and thrombogenesis, *Arterioscler Thromb Vasc Biol* 24(7):1309–1314, 2004.
12. Kain R, Exner M, Brandes R, et al: Molecular mimicry in pauci-immune focal necrotizing glomerulonephritis, *Nat Med* 14(10):1088–1096, 2008.
13. Wilde B, Thewissen M, Damoiseaux J, et al: T cells in ANCA-associated vasculitis: what can we learn from lesional versus circulating T cells? *Arthritis Res Ther* 12(1):204, 2010.
14. Xiao H, Heeringa P, Hu P, et al: Antineutrophil cytoplasmic autoantibodies specific for myeloperoxidase cause glomerulonephritis and vasculitis in mice, *J Clin Invest* 110(7):955–963, 2002.
15. Xiao H, Heeringa P, Liu Z, et al: The role of neutrophils in the induction of glomerulonephritis by anti-myeloperoxidase antibodies, *Am J Pathol* 167(1):39–45, 2005.
16. Schreiber A, Xiao H, Falk RJ, et al: Bone marrow-derived cells are sufficient and necessary targets to mediate glomerulonephritis and vasculitis induced by anti-myeloperoxidase antibodies, *J Am Soc Nephrol* 17(12):3355–3364, 2006.
17. Pfister H, Ollert M, Frohlich LF, et al: Antineutrophil cytoplasmic autoantibodies against the murine homolog of proteinase 3 (Wegener autoantigen) are pathogenic *in vivo*, *Blood* 104(5):1411–1418, 2004.
18. Nolan SL, Kalia N, Nash GB, et al: Mechanisms of ANCA-mediated leukocyte-endothelial cell interactions *in vivo*, *J Am Soc Nephrol* 19(5):973–984, 2008.
19. Little MA, Savage CO: The role of the endothelium in systemic small vessel vasculitis, *Clin Exp Rheumatol* 26(3 Suppl 49):S135–S140, 2008.
20. Guilpain P, Servettaz A, Goulvestre C, et al: Pathogenic effects of antimyeloperoxidase antibodies in patients with microscopic polyangiitis, *Arthritis Rheum* 56(7):2455–2463, 2007.
21. Hattar K, Sibelius U, Bickenbach A, et al: Subthreshold concentrations of anti-proteinase 3 antibodies (c-ANCA) specifically prime human neutrophils for fMLP-induced leukotriene synthesis and chemotaxis, *J Leukoc Biol* 69(1):89–97, 2001.
22. Mueller A, Holl-Ulrich K, Feller AC, et al: Immune phenomena in localized and generalized Wegener's granulomatosis, *Clin Exp Rheumatol* 21(6 Suppl 32):S49–S54, 2003.
23. Tervaert JW: Translational mini-review series on immunology of vascular disease: accelerated atherosclerosis in vasculitis, *Clin Exp Immunol* 156(3):377–385, 2009.
24. Voswinkel J, Muller A, Lamprecht P: Is PR3-ANCA formation initiated in Wegener's granulomatosis lesions? Granulomas as potential lymphoid tissue maintaining autoantibody production, *Ann N Y Acad Sci* 1051:12–19, 2005.
25. Muschen M, Warskulat U, Perniok A, et al: Involvement of soluble CD95 in Churg-Strauss syndrome, *Am J Pathol* 155(3):915–925, 1999.
26. Hellmich B, Ehlers S, Csernok E, et al: Update on the pathogenesis of Churg-Strauss syndrome, *Clin Exp Rheumatol* 21(6 Suppl 32):S69–S77, 2003.
27. Lamprecht P, Gutzeit O, Csernok E, et al: Prevalence of ANCA in mixed cryoglobulinemia and chronic hepatitis C virus infection, *Clin Exp Rheumatol* 21(6 Suppl 32):S89–S94, 2003.
28. Pendergraft WF 3rd, Pressler BM, Jennette JC, et al: Autoantigen complementarity: a new theory implicating complementary proteins as initiators of autoimmune disease, *J Mol Med* 83(1):12–25, 2005.
29. Pendergraft WF, Alcorta DA, Segelmark M, et al: ANCA antigens, proteinase 3 and myeloperoxidase, are not expressed in endothelial cells, *Kidney Int* 57(5):1981–1990, 2000.
30. Seko Y: Giant cell and Takayasu arteritis, *Curr Opin Rheumatol* 19(1):39–43, 2007.
31. Chauhan SK, Singh M, Nityanand S: Reactivity of gamma/delta T cells to human 60-kd heat-shock protein and their cytotoxicity to aortic endothelial cells in Takayasu arteritis, *Arthritis Rheum* 56(8):2798–2802, 2007.

132

32. Chauhan SK, Tripathy NK, Nityanand S: Antigenic targets and pathogenicity of anti-aortic endothelial cell antibodies in Takayasu arteritis, *Arthritis Rheum* 54(7):2326–2333, 2006.

33. Brack A, Geisler A, Martinez-Taboada VM, et al: Giant cell vasculitis is a T cell-dependent disease, *Mol Med* 3(8):530–543, 1997.

34. Deng J, Younge BR, Olshen RA, et al: Th17 and Th1 T-cell responses in giant cell arteritis, *Circulation* 121(7):906–915, 2010.

35. Nagano H, Mitchell RN, Taylor MK, et al: Interferon-gamma deficiency prevents coronary arteriosclerosis but not myocardial rejection in transplanted mouse hearts, *J Clin Invest* 100(3):550–557, 1997.

36. Tellides G, Tereb DA, Kirkiles-Smith NC, et al: Interferon-gamma elicits arteriosclerosis in the absence of leukocytes, *Nature* 403(6766):207–211, 2000.

37. Dal Canto AJ, Swanson PE, O'Guin AK, et al: IFN-gamma action in the media of the great elastic arteries, a novel immunoprivileged site, *J Clin Invest* 107(2):R15–R22, 2001.

38. Amento EP, Ehsani N, Palmer H, et al: Cytokines and growth factors positively and negatively regulate intersitial collagen gene expression in human vascular smooth muscle cells, *Arterioscler Thromb Vasc Biol* 11:1223–1230, 1991.

39. Raines E, Rosenfeld M, Libby P: The role of macrophages. In Fuster V, Topol EJ, Nabel EG, editors: *Atherothrombosis and coronary artery disease*, ed 2, Philadelphia, 2004, Lippincott Williams & Wilkins, pp 505–520.

40. Jones RB, Tervaert JW, Hauser T, et al: Rituximab versus cyclophosphamide in ANCA-associated renal vasculitis, *N Engl J Med* 363(3):211–220, 2010.

41. JCS Joint Working Group: Guideline for Management of Vasculitis Syndrome (JCS 2008), *Circ J* 75(2):474–503, 2011.

CH
9

CHAPTER 10

Thrombosis

Elisabeth M. Battinelli, Jane E. Freedman, Joseph Loscalzo

Overview of Thrombosis

Abnormal hemostasis leads to thrombus formation. Thrombosis in either the arterial or venous system is a leading cause of significant morbidity and mortality. When thrombosis occurs in the arterial system, myocardial infarction (MI) and stroke may result, whereas thrombosis in the venous system leads to venous thromboembolic disease. Thrombosis and thrombotic-related events are among the most common causes of mortality in the Western World. It is estimated that 785,000 people in the United States had new thrombotic events within the coronary circulation in 2009, and that over 450,000 had recurrent events. Stroke also accounts for significant morbidity, with 795,000 people per year suffering from a thrombotic event within the cerebral circulation. There are 200,000 new cases of venous thromboembolism each year, 30% of which result in death in the first 30 days after diagnosis, the majority of deaths being sudden in the setting of a pulmonary embolism (PE).

The pathogenesis of thrombosis was elucidated as early as 1856 when Virchow first described its major determinants, including abnormalities in the vessel wall, platelets, and coagulation proteins as essential for establishing a thrombus. The composition of arterial thrombi is distinct from that of thrombi that form in the venous circulation. Arterial thrombi are composed mainly of platelets and occur in areas of vascular wall injury; venous thrombi, by contrast, are rich in fibrin and dependent on a hypercoagulable response associated with individual coagulation factor abnormalities or mechanical issues related to blood flow limitation. Under normal circumstances, the endothelial lining is not a thrombotic surface, with endothelial cells (ECs) constantly interacting with other cell types, including platelets, to directly *inhibit* thrombus formation through release of antithrombotic factors such as thrombomodulin, tissue factor pathway inhibitor (TFPI), plasmin, and antithrombin systems. At the same time, platelet aggregation is inhibited through prostacyclins and nitric oxide (NO) released directly from platelets.

When the endothelial surface becomes damaged, however, release of many procoagulant proteins (especially tissue factor) and activation of platelets result in uncontrolled hemostasis at the site of vascular injury.[1] As the thrombus begins to form, it recruits additional platelets to the area, leading to further platelet activation. Initially, tethering of platelets is dependent upon exposure of glycoprotein (Gp)Ib-V-IX in damaged collagen, which binds to von Willebrand factor (vWF), resulting in adhesion of platelets to the area of injury. Further recruitment of platelets is mediated through activation of the GPIIb-IIa platelet receptor, which

undergoes a conformational change leading to increased affinity for fibrinogen. These events culminate with further platelet activation that results in release of many essential components for thrombus formation, including adenosine diphosphate (ADP), serotonin, and thromboxane A_2 (TxA$_2$).

Exposure of vascular collagen also leads to activation of the normal mechanisms of hemostasis—including the coagulation cascade—through exposure of tissue factor, leading to "hemostasis in the wrong place." The coagulation regulatory system is outlined in Figure 10-1 and discussed in detail in Chapter 5. Briefly, both the tissue factor–mediated pathway (extrinsic) and the contact-mediated pathway (instrinsic pathway) rely on activation of inactive enzyme precursors of serine proteases, which then reflexively lead to activation of another protein within the cascade. The ultimate step results in cross-linking of fibrin to stabilize a platelet plug, leading to thrombus formation. The tissue factor–initiated pathway is essential for thrombus formation. When tissue factor is released during cellular injury, factor VII is activated and complexes. This complex next activates factors X and XI. Activation of factor X is essential for conversion of prothrombin (factor II) to thrombin through the prothrombinase complex on activated platelets. This cascade of coagulation proteins is essential for hemostasis but also can have deleterious affects when it occurs unregulated, leading to unwanted thrombotic complications.

Platelets, Thrombosis, and Vascular Disease

Venous Thrombosis

It is estimated that between 100,000 and 180,000 deaths due to a venous thromboembolic event occur annually. These events occur mainly in the vasculature at the area of the vessel sinus where stasis can lead to a hypercoagulable microenvironment. The hemostatic process is activated when tissue factor is exposed at the site of vascular injury; initiation of the coagulation cascade follows, with subsequent formation of thrombin and conversion of fibrinogen to fibrin. This process evolves at the same time platelets are actively being recruited to the area of injury through collagen exposure, leading to platelet and fibrin thrombus formation. A number of physiological anticoagulants are also present and modulate this response: antithrombin, TFPI, and activated protein C (APC) and its cofactor protein S. Defects in these hemostatic proteins can lead to disorders that elevate the risk of thrombus formation.

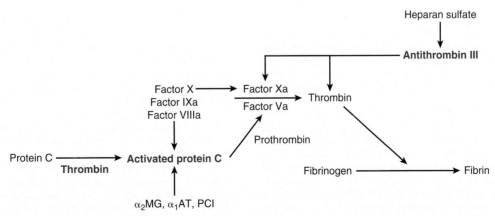

FIGURE 10-1 **Physiological regulation of blood coagulation.** α_2MG, α_2-macroglobin; α_1AT, α_1-antitrypsin; PCI, protein-C inhibitor.

Risk factors for venous thromboembolism are associated with venous stasis or acquired and congenital hypercoagulable states and include obesity, smoking, malignancy, pregnancy, hormone therapy, and recent trauma or surgery. Immobilization due to prolonged hospitalization following surgical intervention, and during long-distance air travel also contribute to the risk of VTE.

Genetic risk factors associated with increased risk of VTE include mutations in factor V (Leiden) and prothrombin 20210, as well as mutations leading to deficiencies in antithrombin, protein C, and protein S. Approximately 5% of the Caucasian population has at least one mutation for factor V Leiden, and 15% to 20% of patients who present with a VTE carry the mutation.[2–5] Approximately 2% of the population carry the prothrombin gene mutation, but it may be present in approximately 5% to 15% of persons with VTE.[6] The population frequencies of mutations in other genes responsible for other coagulation factors (e.g., protein C) are estimated to be 1 in 500 individuals. Antithrombin III deficiency is associated with a frequency of 1 in 300 in the general population, and in 3% to 5% of those with thrombotic events. Previously it was thought that genetic mutations in genes important for methylene tetrahydrofolate reductase and hyperhomocysteinemia increased the risk of VTEs; however, recently this association has been shown to be less likely.[7]

One of the acquired risk factors known to be important in both venous and arterial thrombosis is acquisition of antiphospholipid antibodies, which represent a family of antibodies against phospholipids (e.g., cardiolipins) and phospholipid binding proteins (e.g., GpI β_2). Mechanisms responsible for thrombosis are still speculative but may include inhibition of protein C, antithrombin, and annexin A_5 expression; binding and activation of platelets; enhanced EC tissue factor expression; and activation of the complement cascade.[8] Criteria for diagnosis of the associated disorder, antiphospholipid syndrome, includes the presence of both clinical events and laboratory evidence for the presence of antiphospholipid antibodies.[9]

Arterial Thrombosis

Arterial thrombosis, which accounts for MI and thrombotic cerebrovascular events, initiates from damage to the vessel wall, leading to a cascade of platelet-mediated cellular interactions. Endothelial injury resulting from plaque rupture with exposure of subendothelial collagen and vWF is the core event that leads to arterial thrombosis. Platelet activation through direct interaction with exposed collagen or thrombin generated by tissue factor leads to thrombus formation. Important in this process are platelet factors that are released with activation, including ADP, serotonin, and TxA. Recruitment of additional platelets leads to thrombus growth as platelets aggregate through bridges formed from the binding of fibrinogen to the platelet receptor GpIIb-IIIa. Recruitment and activation of platelets is modulated by a tightly regulated process that involves factors released from the platelet as well as the endothelium, including prostacyclin, NO, and ecto-AD (T)Pase. Prostacyclin, which is generated from arachidonic acid by the endothelium works through cyclic adenosine monophosphate (cAMP) to inhibit platelet function. Nitric oxide, through stimulation of the soluble guanylyl cyclase to produce cyclic guanosine monophosphate (cGMP), directly inhibits platelet activation and prevents thrombosis; cGMP signaling cascades lead to a decrease in fibrinogen binding to GpIIb-IIIa and inhibits the phospholipase A_2 and C pathways.

A primary mechanism of arterial thrombosis is rupture of atherosclerotic plaques, precipitating platelet-rich aggregates. Arterial thrombosis can have catastrophic consequences when it occurs in the coronary or carotid artery circulation. Factors that can exacerbate these types of thrombotic events include smoking, diabetes, hypertension, and hyperlipidemia. Thrombosis generally occurs when there is disruption in the hemostatic balance that results when pro- and anticoagulant molecules are at disequilibrium. Endothelial damage shifts this balance towards a more

---

Box 10-1 Genetic Polymorphisms and Arterial Thrombosis

Polymorphism
Coagulation Factors
Fibrinogen beta chain 455 G/A
Fibrinogen beta chain 854 G/A
Fibrinogen beta chain Bcl1
Fibrinogen alpha chain Thr312 Ala
FVII Arg353Gln
FVII HVR4
FVII 401 G/T
FV Leiden
Prothrombin 20210 G/A
FXIII Val34Leu

Platelet Receptors
GPIIIa Leu33Pro
GPIb alpha VNTR
GPIb alpha Thr145Met
GPIa/IIa alpha$_2$ 807 C/T
GPIa/IIa alpha$_2$ 1648A/G

Fibrinolytic System
PAI-1 675 4G/5G
PAI-1 (CA)$_n$
PAI-1 HindIII
tPA Alu insertion/deletion
tPA 7351 C/T
TAFI ala147Thr
TAFI 1542 C/G

---

procoagulant force, leading to exposure of collagen and tissue factor. Collagen that is now exposed can activate platelets in the blood flowing through the vessel, and concomitantly thrombin is generated as the coagulation cascade is initiated in the presence of tissue factor. Genetic modifications of proteins important in coagulation can alter this process, creating a propensity to form thrombi in the arterial system (Box 10-1). These mutations affect platelet function, leading to increased propensity to aggregation.

Polymorphisms in the endothelial nitric oxide synthase (eNOS) gene, which is essential for NO production by ECs, have been described. The 894-G/T polymorphism I exon 7 results in a glutamate-to-aspartate change at position 298. This polymorphism is associated with increased levels of nitrogen oxides that increase risk of hypertension, MI, and stroke in patients who are homozygous for the abnormality.[10,11] A unique polymorphism in the promoter of the glutathione peroxidase-3 gene has been associated with thrombotic strokes in children. Genome-wide associations have identified other loci associated with cardiovascular thrombotic disease.[12]

Increased levels of fibrinogen have been associated with an increased risk of MI, ischemic stroke, and peripheral artery disease.[13] Age, elevated lipids, and smoking increase the risk associated with fibrinogen. β-Chain variants, such as Arg448Lys, Bcl1, -148 C/T, -455 G/A, and -854 G/A, with the -455 G/A polymorphism, is present in 10% to 20% of the population and is associated with a significant rise in fibrinogen levels.[14] Studies, however, have not been consistent, and the association between this polymorphism and risk of arterial thrombosis is not established.[15] Another site of potential polymorphisms in the fibrinogen gene is the Thr312Ala substitution in the α chain. When this polymorphism is present, the fibrin stranding is thicker, and there is increased cross-linking that may predispose to an increased thrombotic risk.[16]

Other potential associations between arterial thrombosis and increased risk include hyperhomocysteinemia, elevated C-reactive protein (CRP), factor VII polymorphisms, increased plasminogen activator inhibitor (PAI)-1, and platelet hyperreactivity. Wald et al. performed a meta-analysis of 72 prospective cohort studies focusing on a mutation in the methylenetetrahydrofolate reductase (MTHFR) C677T gene and the occurrence of various thrombotic events, including stroke and cardiovascular disease, and found a mild association between the mutation and risk of arterial events.[17] Other factors including CRP, factor VII, and PAI-1 have shown even less promising results.[14]

DRUGS THAT MODULATE ARTERIAL THROMBOSIS

Since arterial thrombi are mainly composed of platelets, and platelet activation is key to their formation, manipulation of platelet function is central to preventing arterial thrombosis. The most commonly used drugs that effect platelet function include aspirin, thienopyridines (clopidogrel and ticlopidine), dipyridamole, and GPIIb-IIIa antagonists.

Aspirin's mechanism of action is to irreversibly inhibit acetylation at serine-529 in the active site of platelet cyclooxygenase (COX)-1. In this manner, the COX-1 enzyme is unable to interact with arachidonic acid, so generation of prostaglandin H_2 and TxA are inhibited. Thromboxane A_2 plays an essential role in regulating platelet activation and aggregation upon stimulation with platelet agonists, including collagen, thrombin, and ADP. When TxA binds to its receptor, phospholipase C is activated, and intracellular calcium increases; this leads to amplification of platelet aggregation and feedback-dependent release of more ADP and TxA. Aspirin functions by producing a dose-dependent inhibition of COX, which prevents the described feedback loop leading to platelet aggregation.

Use of aspirin to prevent arterial thrombosis was first established in the ISIS-2 trial in which aspirin was shown to reduce the mortality rate associated with MI. Other studies showed that aspirin resulted in a 25% relative risk reduction from all vascular-associated events, including MI and stroke, and the benefit occurred with treatment with low-dose aspirin.[18] Although the half-life of aspirin is only 20 minutes, and inhibitory effects of aspirin on COX occur as quickly as 5 minutes after administration, irreversible inhibition of COX ensures that its effects are preserved for the lifespan of the platelet (7-10 days) such that COX activity does not return to normal levels until a new generation of platelets is produced. Interestingly, aspirin's inhibitory properties appear to be most effective when exposed to weak platelet agonists (e.g., TxA, ADP), whereas exposure to stronger agonists (e.g., thrombin) leaves platelet function, as measured by aggregation, intact. For this reason, many of the essential functions of platelets, such as platelet adhesion to vWF or activation by thrombin, are not inhibited by aspirin. Aspirin resistance may explain some of the clinical failure seen with its use. Two recent meta-analyses regarding aspirin resistance have shown that laboratory evidence of unresponsiveness to aspirin may be associated with a high risk of recurrent thrombotic cardiovascular events.[19,20]

Another important modulator of platelet function is ADP, which acts as a weak platelet agonist through two different platelet membrane receptors, P2Y1 and P2Y12.[21] When ADP stimulates the P2Y1 receptor, the platelet undergoes a shape change and Ca^{2+} is mobilized through activation of phospholipase C to initiate platelet aggregation in a reversible manner. The P2Y12 receptor is essential for secretion and stabilization of platelet aggregation by lowering cAMP levels.

There are two available thienopyridine derivatives that act as inhibitors of ADP-induced platelet aggregation: ticlopidine and clopidogrel. Clopidogrel is metabolized by cytochrome P450 (CYP450) into an active metabolite that irreversibly blocks the P2Y12 receptor. Clopidogrel reduces recurrent thrombotic events in patients with cardiovascular disease.[22–24] The Clopidogrel vs. Aspirin in Patients at Risk of Ischemic Events (CAPRIE) trial found that clopidogrel is more effective than aspirin in reducing the risk of cardiovascular events in patients with recent MI, recent ischemic stroke, and established peripheral artery disease. Ticlopidine is also metabolized by CYP450 to an active metabolite that functions to block the PGY12 receptor. Although it functions in a similar manner to clopidogrel, it is associated with a higher degree of neutropenia and thrombotic thrombocytopenic purpura and is therefore

not used as readily as clopidogrel.[25,26] Other antiplatelet drugs in clinical development include ticagrelor, cangrelor, and elinogrel, all of which reversibly inhibit the P2Y12 receptor.[27]

Another class of drugs in the armamentarium of antithrombotic agents is that which specifically targets the GpIIb-IIIa receptor to prevent the binding of fibrinogen essential for platelet aggregation. This approach blocks platelet aggregation independently of the platelet agonist; GPIIb-IIIa activation is a final common pathway for almost all platelet agonists. The GPIIb-IIIa receptor is the most abundant receptor on platelets and is also found on the surface of megakaryocytes. Under normal circumstances, this Gp receptor is inactive, but when platelets become activated, a signal transduction cascade is initiated that leads to a conformational change and activation of the receptor, allowing it to bind to fibrinogen or, if high-shear conditions are in place, vWF. Binding is mediated by the Arg-Gly-Asp (RGD) and the Lys-Gly-Asp (KGD) sequences in both macromolecules. Drugs that inhibit GPIIb-IIIa include abciximab, eptifibatide, and tirofiban. Abciximab is derived from a murine monoclonal antibody and was one of the first GpIIb-IIIa receptor antagonists to be developed. It functions as a high-affinity antibody to inhibit platelet function through binding to the GpIIb-IIIa receptor, thereby blocking fibrinogen from interacting with its binding site. Abciximab also binds to integrins in the vitronectin receptor, as well as MAC1 and CD11b-CD18, although the clinical significance of these interactions is not understood. Eptifibatide is a cyclic heptapeptide which binds to GPIIb-IIIa through the KGD motif. Tirofiban is a tyrosine derivative that functions as an RGD mimetic.

These drugs work on the final common pathway of platelet aggregation to inhibit binding to fibrinogen in a similar manner to abciximab. They also appear to have anticoagulant activity because there is evidence of prolongation of the activated clotting time. These actions are thought to be regulated by inhibition of thrombin generation via tissue factor and a decrease in microparticle formation. Multiple clinical trials have shown that inhibition of GpIIb-IIIa is effective in preventing recurrent thrombotic events. Use of these drugs leads to a 35% decrease in acute ischemic events and a 26% decrease in recurrent events within 6 months. Long-term use of these drugs was shown to be efficacious in the EPILOG (Evaluation of PTCA to Improve Long-Term Outcome by c7E3 GpIIb-IIIa Receptor Blockade) trial, with a reduction in the incidence of death. Other trials have supported use of GpIIb-IIIa blockade in management of acute coronary syndromes (ACSs).[28,29] Their use, however, has been reserved for high-risk circumstances such as percutaneous coronary intervention (PCI) in ACSs, owing to the recent finding of long-term benefits of ADP receptor antagonists.[30]

Oral GpIIb-IIIa inhibitors have not been shown to limit cardiovascular events to date.[31] This may be due to conformational changes in the GpIIb-IIIa receptor after antagonist dissociation from it. In this case, the receptor remains active and increases binding to fibrinogen and vWF, leading to a paradoxical thrombotic effect. Novel GpIIb-IIIa antagonists that do cause such conformational changes are under development. In one study, RUC-1, which is a novel compound discovered through high-throughput screening, induced partial exposure of the binding site yet still led to decreased platelet aggregation without enhanced fibrinogen binding. RUC-1 may represent a prototype molecule for these types of derivative drugs.[32]

Other antiplatelet agents that may inhibit thrombus formation yet preserve hemostasis so bleeding complications do not result are under investigation. One potential new therapeutic target is the GPIb-V-IX complex. Initial studies of patients who have Bernard-Soulier's syndrome identified a deficiency of the GPIb complex. The GPIb complex is important for building a platelet bridge through vWF at areas of endothelial damage. Drugs under development act as antagonists for the GPIb-vWF interaction, including specific monoclonal antibodies, the GpIb complex antagonists isolated from snake venoms,[33,34] and the Fab fragment of 6B4, which is a murine monoclonal antibody that targets human GPIb and prevents binding to vWF. Early nonhuman primate studies have suggested that thrombus formation can be attenuated using these drugs.[35]

Inflammation and Thrombosis

Recent evidence has clearly established a role for inflammation in the atherothrombotic process. Patients with ACSs have increased interactions between platelets and leukocytes forming detectable aggregates. The process of inflammation involves a variety of cell types, including leukocytes, ECs, and platelets. The endothelium becomes activated, and multiple cell-adhesion molecules are released, including P-selectin, which essentially has two important roles in inflammation: recruitment of proinflammatory cells and establishing signaling cascades leading to increased expression of CD11b/CD18 (MAC-1).[36]

Platelets are instrumental in the inflammatory aspects of atherosclerosis. Thrombin activation of platelets leads to release of many procoagulant molecules and release of inflammatory molecules, including platelet factor 4 (PF4), platelet-derived growth factor (PDGF), and RANTES, which is regulated upon activation of normal T-cell expression. In addition, platelets that have been activated in the presence of thrombin secrete CD40 ligand (CD40L). This chemoattractant is key to the recruitment of ECs, smooth muscle cells (SMCs), and macrophages. CD40 ligand also recruits a variety of proinflammatory cytokines (e.g., interleukin [IL]-1, IL-6, and IL-8) and increases expression of the adhesion molecules intercellular adhesion molecule (ICAM)-1, vascular (V)CAM-1, and P-selectin.[37] CD40 ligand is also important for release of matrix metalloproteinases (MMPs), which are needed for plaque progression, neovascularization, and plaque rupture. CD40 ligand also initiates release of tissue factor, which then interacts with other cells to create a thrombogenic microenvironment. T lymphocytes orchestrate an inflammatory cascade that begins by binding to VCAM-1 through signaling regulated by interferon (IFN)-γ-inducible chemokine ligands (CXCLs), protein-10, and chemoattractant (I-TAC). Through this binding, a number of inflammatory cytokines are released, including the CD40 ligand; CD154, which leads to metalloproteinase generation; and tissue factor expression, which initiates the coagulation cascade. Mice that lack the CD40L have less atherothrombosis. Patients with ACSs have elevated levels of CD40L, and plasma levels of CD40L predict the risk of future cardiovascular events.[38-40] It has been shown that elevated soluble CD40L levels can be decreased by treatment with abciximab.[41]

Our understanding of the role of inflammation in the thrombotic response has been expanded by many clinical studies that have shown an association between bacterial infections and increased risk of MI or stroke, although more studies are needed to prove this association.[42,43] One possible mechanism is through Toll-like receptors (TLRs), which are present in platelets. Platelet activation through stimulation of TLR2 activates signaling mechanisms responsible for both thrombotic and inflammatory responses. These effects are responsible for the mechanism by which bacteria induce a proinflammatory cascade in platelets, suggesting that bacteria can directly activate platelet-dependent thrombotic responses.[44] Recently this process was further refined by demonstrating that TLR2 stimulation leads to platelet activation through PI3-kinase, which is known to be important in platelet activation–associated shape change, calcium release, and granular content secretion.[45]

In summary, as our understanding of hemostasis and thrombosis continues to evolve, so does development of novel agents directed at treating thromboembolic diseases. This development continues to be driven by scientific discovery, growing numbers of patients, and indications for antithrombotics. Targets for antiplatelet drugs continue to be defined, leading to novel therapies as well as development of additional agents in already successful classes.

REFERENCES

1. Alfirevic Z, Alfirevic I: Hypercoagulable state, pathophysiology, classification and epidemiology, *Clin Chem Lab Med* 48(Suppl 1):S15–S26, 2010.
2. Prandoni P: Acquired risk factors for venous thromboembolism in medical patients, *Hematology Am Soc Hematol Educ Program* 458–461, 2005.
3. Rosendaal FR: Venous thrombosis: the role of genes, environment, and behavior, *Hematology Am Soc Hematol Educ Program* 1–12, 2005.
4. Cushman M: Inherited risk factors for venous thrombosis, *Hematology Am Soc Hematol Educ Program* 452–457, 2005.
5. Vossen CY, Conard J, Fontcuberta J, et al: Risk of a first venous thrombotic event in carriers of a familial thrombophilic defect. The European Prospective Cohort on Thrombophilia (EPCOT), *J Thromb Haemost* 3(3):459–464, 2005.
6. Kottke-Marchant K: Genetic polymorphisms associated with venous and arterial thrombosis: an overview, *Arch Pathol Lab Med* 126(3):295–304, 2002.
7. Ray JG: Hyperhomocysteinemia: no longer a consideration in the management of venous thromboembolism, *Curr Opin Pulm Med* 14(5):369–373, 2008.
8. Lim W: Antiphospholipid antibody syndrome, *Hematology Am Soc Hematol Educ Program* 233–239, 2009.
9. Cohen D, Berger SP, Steup-Beekman GM, et al: Diagnosis and management of the antiphospholipid syndrome, *BMJ* 340:c2541, 2010.
10. Elbaz A, Poirier O, Moulin T, et al: Association between the Glu298Asp polymorphism in the endothelial constitutive nitric oxide synthase gene and brain infarction. The GENIC Investigators, *Stroke* 31(7):1634–1639, 2000.
11. Hingorani AD, Liang CF, Fatibene J, et al: A common variant of the endothelial nitric oxide synthase (Glu298->Asp) is a major risk factor for coronary artery disease in the UK, *Circulation* 100(14):1515–1520, 1999.
12. Malarstig A, Hamsten A: Genetics of atherothrombosis and thrombophilia, *Curr Atheroscler Rep* 12(3):159–166, 2010.
13. Scarabin PY, Arveiler D, Amouyel P, et al: Plasma fibrinogen explains much of the difference in risk of coronary heart disease between France and Northern Ireland. The PRIME study, *Atherosclerosis* 166(1):103–109, 2003.
14. Voetsch B, Loscalzo J: Genetic determinants of arterial thrombosis, *Arterioscler Thromb Vasc Biol* 24(2):216–229, 2004.
15. Endler G, Mannhalter C: Polymorphisms in coagulation factor genes and their impact on arterial and venous thrombosis, *Clin Chim Acta* 330(1–2):31–55, 2003.
16. Standeven KF, Grant PJ, Carter AM, et al: Functional analysis of the fibrinogen Aalpha Thr312Ala polymorphism: effects on fibrin structure and function, *Circulation* 107(18):2326–2330, 2003.
17. Wald DS, Law M, Morris JK: Homocysteine and cardiovascular disease: evidence on causality from a meta-analysis, *BMJ* 325(7374):1202, 2002.
18. Jneid H, Bhatt DL: Advances in antiplatelet therapy, *Expert Opin Emerg Drugs* 8(2):349–363, 2003.
19. Snoep JD, Hovens MM, Eikenboom JC, et al: Association of laboratory-defined aspirin resistance with a higher risk of recurrent cardiovascular events: a systematic review and meta-analysis, *Arch Intern Med* 167(15):1593–1599, 2007.
20. Krasopoulos G, Brister SJ, Beattie WS, et al: Aspirin "resistance" and risk of cardiovascular morbidity: systematic review and meta-analysis, *BMJ* 336(7637):195–198, 2008.
21. Daniel JL, Dangelmaier C, Jin J, et al: Role of intracellular signaling events in ADP-induced platelet aggregation, *Thromb Haemost* 82(4):1322–1326, 1999.
22. Yusuf S, Zhao F, Mehta SR, et al: Effects of clopidogrel in addition to aspirin in patients with acute coronary syndromes without ST-segment elevation, *N Engl J Med* 345(7):494–502, 2001.
23. Mehta SR, Yusuf S, Peters RJ, et al: Effects of pretreatment with clopidogrel and aspirin followed by long-term therapy in patients undergoing percutaneous coronary intervention: the PCI-CURE study, *Lancet* 358(9281):527–533, 2001.
24. Steinhubl SR, Berger PB, Mann JT 3rd, et al: Early and sustained dual oral antiplatelet therapy following percutaneous coronary intervention: a randomized controlled trial, *JAMA* 288(19):2411–2420, 2002.
25. Michelson AD: P2Y12 antagonism: promises and challenges, *Arterioscler Thromb Vasc Biol* 28(3):s33–s38, 2008.
26. Bertrand ME, Rupprecht HJ, Urban P, et al: Double-blind study of the safety of clopidogrel with and without a loading dose in combination with aspirin compared with ticlopidine in combination with aspirin after coronary stenting: the clopidogrel aspirin stent international cooperative study (CLASSICS), *Circulation* 102(6):624–629, 2000.
27. Michelson AD: Antiplatelet therapies for the treatment of cardiovascular disease, *Nat Rev Drug Discov* 9(2):154–169, 2010.
28. van 't Hof AW, Valgimigli M: Defining the role of platelet glycoprotein receptor inhibitors in STEMI: focus on tirofiban, *Drugs* 69(1):85–100, 2009.
29. Tamhane UU, Gurm HS: GP IIb/IIIa inhibitors during primary percutaneous coronary intervention for STEMI: new trial and registry data, *Curr Cardiol Rep* 10(5):424–430, 2008.
30. Mukherjee D, Roffi M: Glycoprotein IIb/IIIa receptor inhibitors in 2008: do they still have a role? *J Interv Cardiol* 21(2):118–121, 2008.
31. Chew DP, Bhatt DL, Sapp S, et al: Increased mortality with oral platelet glycoprotein IIb/IIIa antagonists: a meta-analysis of phase III multicenter randomized trials, *Circulation* 103(2):201–206, 2001.
32. Blue R, Murcia M, Karan C, et al: Application of high-throughput screening to identify a novel alphaIIb-specific small-molecule inhibitor of alphaIIbbeta3-mediated platelet interaction with fibrinogen, *Blood* 111(3):1248–1256, 2008.
33. Chang MC, Lin HK, Peng HC, et al: Antithrombotic effect of crotalin, a platelet membrane glycoprotein Ib antagonist from venom of Crotalus atrox, *Blood* 91(5):1582–1589, 1998.
34. Yeh CH, Chang MC, Peng HC, et al: Pharmacological characterization and antithrombotic effect of agkistin, a platelet glycoprotein Ib antagonist, *Br J Pharmacol* 132(4):843–850, 2001.
35. Fontayne A, Meiring M, Lamprecht S, et al: The humanized anti-glycoprotein Ib monoclonal antibody h6B4-Fab is a potent and safe antithrombotic in a high shear arterial thrombosis model in baboons, *Thromb Haemost* 100(4):670–677, 2008.

36. Neumann FJ, Zohlnhofer D, Fakhoury L, et al: Effect of glycoprotein IIb/IIIa receptor blockade on platelet-leukocyte interaction and surface expression of the leukocyte integrin Mac-1 in acute myocardial infarction, *J Am Coll Cardiol* 34(5):1420–1426, 1999.

37. Schonbeck U, Libby P: The CD40/CD154 receptor/ligand dyad, *Cell Mol Life Sci* 58(1):4–43, 2001.

38. Aukrust P, Muller F, Ueland T, et al: Enhanced levels of soluble and membrane-bound CD40 ligand in patients with unstable angina. Possible reflection of T lymphocyte and platelet involvement in the pathogenesis of acute coronary syndromes, *Circulation* 100(6):614–620, 1999.

39. Schonbeck U, Varo N, Libby P, et al: Soluble CD40L and cardiovascular risk in women, *Circulation* 104(19):2266–2268, 2001.

40. Varo N, de Lemos JA, Libby P, et al: Soluble CD40L: risk prediction after acute coronary syndromes, *Circulation* 108(9):1049–1052, 2003.

41. Freedman JE: CD40 ligand—assessing risk instead of damage? *N Engl J Med* 348(12):1163–1165, 2003.

42. Fagoonee S, De Angelis C, Elia C, et al: Potential link between Helicobacter pylori and ischemic heart disease: does the bacterium elicit thrombosis? *Minerva Med* 101(2):121–125, 2010.

43. Stassen FR, Vainas T, Bruggeman CA: Infection and atherosclerosis. An alternative view on an outdated hypothesis, *Pharmacol Rep* 60(1):85–92, 2008.

44. Balogh S, Kiss I, Csaszar A: Toll-like receptors: link between "danger" ligands and plaque instability, *Curr Drug Targets* 10(6):513–518, 2009.

45. Rex S, Beaulieu LM, Perlman DH, et al: Immune versus thrombotic stimulation of platelets differentially regulates signalling pathways, intracellular protein-protein interactions, and alpha-granule release, *Thromb Haemost* 102(1):97–110, 2009.

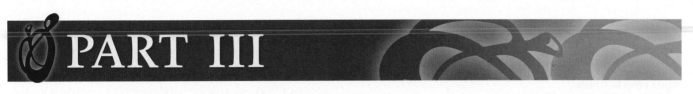

PART III

PRINCIPLES OF VASCULAR EXAMINATION

CHAPTER **11**   The History and Physical Examination

Joshua A. Beckman, Mark A. Creager

The ubiquitous nature of arteries, veins, and lymphatic vessels allows for any region of the body to develop vascular disease. This chapter describes the vascular medical history and physical examination—the core components of evaluating patients with vascular diseases. Application of these methods and tailored use of special examination maneuvers facilitate the diagnosis of vascular disease, especially when used in conjunction with vascular tests described elsewhere in this section. This chapter will review the cardinal complaints of patients with vascular disease, and then the physical findings associated with common arterial, venous, and lymphatic diseases. More specific features of the vascular history and examination are discussed in the relevant chapters of each vascular disease.

Vascular History

The medical history is the foundation of the physician-patient interaction, guiding the physical examination, testing, and treatment decisions. A comprehensive medical history can identify the diagnosis the vast majority of the time, but an inadequate one can result in excess testing and inappropriate therapy.

Arterial Disease

Symptoms of arterial disease typically arise as a result of either arterial stenoses or occlusions, though aneurysms also may cause symptoms. The important historical features of arterial disease in selected regional circulations are reviewed first.

PERIPHERAL ARTERY DISEASE

In addition to carotid and coronary artery disease (CAD), peripheral artery disease (PAD) is one of the most common clinical manifestations of atherosclerosis. Approximately 50% of patients with PAD have symptoms, described in the following discussion as typical or atypical, and the remainder are asymptomatic. The importance of making the diagnosis of PAD, even in the absence of symptoms, derives from the prognostic information implicit with its diagnosis (see Chapter 16). Notably, patients with PAD often have coexisting coronary and cerebrovascular atherosclerosis, and are two- to fourfold more likely than patients without PAD to die of cardiovascular disease.[1]

Therefore, the history of patients with PAD should seek to determine whether the patient has known risk factors for atherosclerosis, and whether or not there are concomitant clinical manifestations of atherosclerosis. The historian should elicit information regarding dyslipidemia, diabetes mellitus, hypertension, family history of premature atherosclerosis, and cigarette smoking. Historical evidence of CAD, including prior myocardial infarction (MI), symptoms of angina, or prior coronary revascularization procedures and history of stroke or symptoms of cerebrovascular ischemia, including hemiparesis, hemiparesthesia, aphasia, or amaurosis fugax, should be sought and documented.

Intermittent Claudication

A cardinal symptom of PAD is intermittent claudication (see Chapter 18). Claudication occurs when limb skeletal muscle ischemia is produced with effort because increased muscle energy requirements are not served by sufficient augmentation in blood supply. Symptoms develop *intermittently* with activity; the blood flow limitation imposed by peripheral artery stenosis typically does not compromise muscular function at rest. Claudication is variably described as aching, heaviness, burning, fatigue, cramping, and/or tightness in the affected limb. Symptoms occur with reproducible amounts of exercise: one block of walking, one flight of stairs, or 5 minutes on a bicycle, for example. Discomfort may develop in any muscular portion of the leg—buttocks, hip, thigh, calf, or foot. Areas of the limb to develop discomfort are related to the arterial segments with stenoses. Iliac artery disease typically produces hip or buttock claudication, whereas femoral artery disease causes thigh or calf claudication. Arm claudication is unusual, but may occur in patients with innominate, subclavian, axillary, or brachial artery stenosis. Cessation of activity relieves the exercising muscle's demand-supply mismatch and enables restoration of oxidative metabolism. Therefore, patients typically report that discontinuation of activity relieves the discomfort after several minutes.

Atypical symptoms also occur and may include reduction of leg discomfort despite continued effort, gait disturbance, and slower walking speed.[2] Atypical claudication may be more common than traditional symptoms because of the high frequency of other conditions present in this older age group: spinal stenosis, venous insufficiency, and degenerative join disease. Patients with intermittent claudication often slow their walking speed by a third to regulate muscle use and prolong walking distance. Thus, when a physician solicits the history of walking impairment, patients may report no change in distance walked before symptoms occur, despite a progressive decline in functional ability.[3]

Several questionnaires for PAD have been devised and validated. These provide a standard to accompany the interview when querying patients about symptoms of PAD. The Rose questionnaire was the initial PAD-related questionnaire, but limited diagnostic sensitivity minimized its utility.[4,5] The San Diego questionnaire is a modified version of the Rose Questionnaire and a more reliable instrument to assess intermittent claudication (see Chapter 16).[6] The disease-specific Walking Impairment Questionnaire has been validated and can be used to assess walking difficulty in patients with PAD. It has four subscales: severity of pain with walking, distance, speed, and stair climbing.[7]

Critical Limb Ischemia

Critical limb ischemia (CLI) occurs when limb blood flow is inadequate to meet the metabolic demands of the tissues at rest.[8] This may result in persistent pain, especially in the acral portions of the leg (toes, ball of the foot, heel). Additional foot symptoms include sensitivity to cold, joint stiffness, and hypesthesia. As a consequence of the effects of gravity on perfusion pressure, patients may report worsening of pain with leg elevation, or even when lying in bed, and reduction in pain with limb dependency (e.g., when the feet hang over the bed onto the floor). Critical limb ischemia may cause tissue breakdown (ulceration) or gangrene.

Acute Limb Ischemia

Acute limb ischemia is most often due to embolism or *in situ* thrombosis (see Chapter 46).[9] Other causes include arterial dissection or trauma. The presentation of acute arterial occlusion ranges from asymptomatic loss of a pulse, to worsened claudication, to sudden onset of severe pain at rest. Symptoms may develop suddenly over several hours, or over several days. Acute ischemic symptoms are more likely to occur when no or few collateral vessels are present, rather than when there is a well-developed collateral network. Acute arterial occlusion may cause symptoms in any portion of the leg distal to the obstruction. The five Ps—pain, pallor, poikilothermia, paresthesias, and paralysis—characterize the historical features and findings of patients with acute limb ischemia. Severity of symptoms does not discriminate among etiologies.

Atheroembolism

Atheroembolism is embolization of atherosclerotic debris that compromises distal arteries (TAO) (see Chapter 47). Atheroemboli vary in composition, from larger fibroplatelet particles that occlude small arteries to cholesterol emboli, nanometers in size, that occlude arterioles. Causes of atheroemboli include catheterization and cardiovascular surgery, but approximately half of such events occur without a known precipitant.[10]

Symptoms reflect occlusion of the small distal vessels in the limb, and patients will commonly present with calf, foot, or toe pain and areas of violaceous discoloration or cyanosis in the toes (*blue toe syndrome*). Symptoms develop hours to days after the event; ulcerations may develop and are slow to resolve. Symptoms may be unilateral or bilateral, depending upon the origin of emboli proximal to or beyond the aortic bifurcation. If atheroemboli arise proximal to the renal arteries, renal insufficiency is a potential sequela.

Other Peripheral Artery Diseases

Uncommon diseases of the peripheral arteries should be considered in patients with claudication or evidence of ischemia, but whose age falls below that typically affected by atherosclerosis or in those with atypical symptoms. These diseases include thromboangiitis obliterans (TAO) (see Chapter 44), Takayasu arteritis (see Chapter 42), and giant-cell arteritis (see Chapter 43), and vascular compression syndromes, such as those affecting the thoracic outlet, iliac artery, and popliteal artery (see Chapter 62).

Takayasu arteritis is a large-vessel vasculitis that generally occurs between the ages of 20 and 40 years. Women are more likely to develop the disease than men. Constitutional and vascular symptoms occur (e.g., fevers, weight loss, fatigue, arthralgias, myalgias) and may be present months to years without overt evidence of vascular disease. About 50% of patients complain of muscle or joint pains, and headache has been reported in up to 40%. More than 50% of patients will have a diminished pulse or claudication of an upper extremity. Approximately 30% of patients will report neck pain and have a tender carotid artery (i.e., *carotidynia*). Lightheadedness is also common and may be secondary to vertebral artery involvement.

Patients with *giant-cell arteritis* (GCA) are typically older than 50 years of age. Giant-cell arteritis predominantly affects the branches of the thoracic aorta and the intracranial arteries. Some 50% of patients have constitutional symptoms related to inflammation, and 50% have coexisting polymyalgia rheumatica. The most common complaint is headache that typically affects the occipital or temporal region; it occurs in over 60% of patients with GCA. In patients with headache, scalp tenderness may be present. Partial or complete vision loss develops in 20% of patients, and approximately 50% of these individuals report *amaurosis fugax* (i.e., transient episodes that involve one eye and last 10 minutes or less [see Chapter 43]). Patients may present with upper limb claudication, and 40% report jaw claudication. Tongue claudication and swallowing difficulties are less common.

Thromboangiitis obliterans (*Buerger's disease*) is a small- to medium-vessel vasculitis that affects the distal vessels of the arms or legs, and usually occurs before 40 years of age in cigarette smokers.[11] It affects more men than women. The classic triad of TAO is claudication, Raynaud phenomenon, and superficial thrombophlebitis. Claudication of the hands or feet may progress to ulceration of the fingers or toes.[11]

Neurovascular Compression Syndromes

Claudication in the upper extremities raises the possibility of *thoracic outlet syndrome* (see Chapter 62).[12] Compression of the axillary or subclavian artery by a cervical rib, abnormal insertion of the scalene anticus muscle, or apposition of the clavicle and first rib may result in arterial compression during head turning, arm use above or behind the head, or arm extension. Weakness, burning, aching, or fatigue in the arms can result. Examples of triggers include wall painting, hair washing, and housecleaning.

Popliteal artery entrapment should be considered in a young person with leg claudication but preserved pulses at rest.[13] Anatomical variants in the course of the popliteal artery may result in its compression by the gastrocnemius muscle during exercise and can cause symptoms of claudication.

VASOSPASTIC AND RELATED DISEASES

Raynaud phenomenon is the most common vasospastic disorder encountered in clinical practice[14] (see Chapter 48). Patients typically report that the digits become pale or cyanotic during cold exposure. Fingers are most commonly affected, but the toes develop symptoms in 40% of affected individuals. Less commonly involved areas include the tongue, nose, and ear lobes. Patients may experience paresthesias or pain in the digits if ischemia persists. With rewarming and release of vasospasm, digital rubor due to reactive hyperemia may develop. A pulsating or flushed feeling may accompany the hyperemic phase. All color phases are not required for diagnosis. Indeed, with an appropriate history, the diagnosis can be made with only one color change.

There are two categories of Raynaud phenomenon: primary and secondary. Differentiating between the two is important because of the information it provides about cause and prognosis. *Primary Raynaud's disease* is benign, typically affects fingers (and toes) symmetrically, and recovery is predictable with rewarming. Some 70% to 80% of patients with primary Raynaud's disease are women. In patients with *secondary Raynaud phenomenon*, pallor may occur in only one or several digits. In severe cases, cyanosis is unremitting and tissue loss may occur. Raynaud phenomenon that has its onset after age 45 years should prompt an investigation for an underlying cause. The history should include questions to elicit evidence of disease or conditions that cause secondary Raynaud phenomenon, including connective tissue disorders, arterial occlusive disease, trauma (vibration, hypothenar hand injury), neurovascular compression syndromes, blood dyscrasias, and drug use.

Acrocyanosis is a vascular disorder characterized by bluish discoloration of the hands and feet exacerbated by cold exposure (see Chapter 49). Unlike Raynaud phenomenon, the discoloration is not confined to the digits, and pallor does not occur. Warming, however, can ameliorate cyanosis and restore normal skin color. Acrocyanosis typically occurs in persons aged 20 to 45 years, and women are affected more often than men.

Pernio is a vascular inflammatory disorder in which skin lesions and swelling occur in fingers and toes, particularly in cold moist climates (see Chapter 51). Other exposed portions of the body may be affected. The typical lesions described by the patient are pruritic and painful blisters or superficial ulcers.

The *complex regional pain syndromes*, reflex sympathetic dystrophy (RSD), and causalgia are associated with limb symptoms, often following a relatively minor injury. Hand or foot pain is a frequent complaint. This may be associated with hyperpathia, hyperesthesias, coolness, cyanosis, hyperhidrosis, and swelling. Symptoms are typically out of proportion to severity of the initial injury. Patients may observe brittle nails that develop ridges, and report muscle, skin, and subcutaneous tissue wasting and limited joint mobility in the affected limb.

RENAL ARTERY DISEASE

No symptoms specific to renal artery stenosis are elicited by history. Unlike other end organs, symptoms of chronic renal ischemia are not localized to the kidney, but reflect systemic pathophysiological alterations that result from activation of the renin angiotensin system and disturbances of salt and water balance. Historical clues that raise suspicion of renal artery stenosis include onset of hypertension before age 30 or after age 55, malignant hypertension, hypertension refractory to three concurrently prescribed antihypertensive medications, azotemia subsequent to administration of an angiotensin-converting enzyme (ACE) inhibitor or angiotensin receptor blocker, unexplained azotemia, recurrent congestive heart failure, and episodic pulmonary edema (see Chapter 23). Renal artery stenosis should be considered in patients with these clinical clues, particularly if they have evidence of atherosclerosis in other regional circulations (e.g., CAD, PAD, aortic disease).

MESENTERIC ARTERY DISEASE

Most patients with atherosclerosis of the celiac, superior mesenteric, or inferior mesenteric arteries are asymptomatic unless two or all three of these arteries are occluded. Symptoms of chronic mesenteric ischemia include postprandial epigastric or midabdominal pain that may radiate to the back (see Chapter 27). Onset of abdominal discomfort is 15 to 30 minutes after eating, and symptoms may persist for several hours. Patients tend to avoid food to prevent these symptoms, and weight loss ensues.

CAROTID ARTERY DISEASE

The majority of patients with significant stenoses of the common or internal carotid arteries are asymptomatic (see Chapter 30). When they do occur, symptoms may be temporary (minutes to hours) or fixed, indicating a transient ischemic attack (TIA) or stroke, respectively. Symptoms of carotid artery disease reflect compromise of the neural territory subtended by its principal intracranial branch, the middle cerebral artery, and include contralateral hemiparesis, hemiparesthesia, and aphasia. Ipsilateral amaurosis fugax or blindness may also occur because the ophthalmic artery is supplied by the internal carotid artery.

The prevalence of carotid artery disease is increased in patients with CAD or PAD, both of which increase the risk of stroke by two- to fourfold.

Venous and Lymphatic Systems

A history soliciting evidence of venous and lymphatic diseases is required when patients complain of leg pain or swelling, or express concerns regarding leg ulcers, varicose veins, or localized inflammation on a limb. In patients presenting with leg edema, the history should seek to determine whether the swelling is secondary to venous or lymphatic diseases, trauma, arthritis, or whether it is associated with a systemic condition such as congestive heart failure, cirrhosis, nephrotic syndrome, renal insufficiency, or endocrinopathy (e.g., hypothyroidism, Cushing's syndrome).

DEEP VEIN THROMBOSIS

Patients with thrombosis of a deep vein of a limb may present with swelling or discomfort, or no symptoms at all (see Chapter 52). Symptoms are usually but not always unilateral. Historical queries should seek potential causes of deep vein thrombosis (DVT) when it is suspected. Information regarding recent trauma, surgery, hospitalization, prolonged period of immobility, cancer,

thrombophilic disorder, or family history of venous thrombosis should be acquired. An uncommon cause of left leg DVT is May-Thurner syndrome, in which the left iliac vein is compressed by the right iliac artery. In patients with arm symptoms, questions should seek evidence of indwelling catheters or cancer, since these are the most common causes of upper extremity DVT. In addition, a history of repetitive arm motion should be sought when considering the possibility of Paget-Schroetter syndrome, in which compression of the axillosubclavian vein by muscular, tendinous, or bony components of the thoracic outlet may cause thrombosis. Thrombosis or extrinsic compression of the superior vena cava may cause symptoms of superior vena cava syndrome, which include headache, face and neck fullness and flushing, and bilateral arm swelling.

SUPERFICIAL THROMBOPHLEBITIS

Thrombosis of a superficial vein is a local phenomenon that presents with pain and tenderness over the affected vein. Predisposing factors sought by history include intravenous catheters, varicose veins, injury, and malignancy. It is important to consider the possibility of malignancy, especially pancreatic, lung, and ovarian cancers in patients with recurrent or migratory superficial thrombophlebitis (i.e., Trousseau's syndrome). Uncommon disorders associated with superficial thrombophlebitis include TAO and Behçet's syndrome.

CHRONIC VENOUS INSUFFICIENCY

Venous insufficiency should be considered in patients who present with chronic unilateral or bilateral leg swelling. Causes of venous insufficiency include deep venous obstruction and deep venous valvular incompetence (also see Chapter 55). Approximately 30% of patients with DVT will ultimately develop chronic venous insufficiency.[15] Valvular incompetence may be a consequence of recanalized venous thrombus or a primary valvular abnormality. Queries should address the duration of leg swelling, knowledge of prior DVT, presence of focal hyperpigmentation, pain, pruritus, or ulcers. Symptoms may include a heavy, dull, or "bursting" sensation of the edematous leg. Patients may report that discomfort in the affected leg increases with dependency and improves with leg elevation. Some individuals with severe leg swelling note that calf discomfort worsens with walking, a symptom termed *venous claudication*.

VARICOSE VEINS

Most patients with varicose veins do not have specific symptoms, but present to a physician's office with cosmetic concerns. Symptoms of varicose veins include leg discomfort or aching, particularly with prolonged standing. These symptoms are most likely to occur along long segments of the greater and lesser saphenous veins and their tributaries. Burning or pruritus may develop, particularly if complicated by accompanying skin ulceration.

LYMPHEDEMA

Lymphedema should be considered in patients who present with limb swelling (see Chapter 58). This condition may affect the arms or legs and is usually unilateral, although it can be bilateral. Lymphedema should be suspected if limb swelling occurs early in life, particularly during childhood or adolescence. Congenital lymphedema typically appears at birth or shortly thereafter. Lymphedema praecox often presents around puberty but can occur anytime before age 35. Lymphedema tarda generally occurs after age 35. Lymphedema is also associated with genetic disorders such as Turner's and Noonan's syndromes. It is important to elicit history of conditions that may predispose a patient to lymphedema, including recurrent skin infection, lymphangitis, filariasis, trauma, malignancy of the lymphatic system, and radiation or surgical resection of lymph nodes and lymphatic vessels as adjunctive therapy for cancer.

LYMPHANGITIS

Patients with lymphangitis may report an erythematous patch or linear streak that affects the limb and tends to propagate proximally over time. The erythematous area may be painful and tender. These patients usually present with systemic signs of infection, including fever and shaking chills. History might determine whether lesions induced by trauma or infection may have served as a portal of entry.

Vascular Examination

As in any comprehensive physical examination, vital signs (blood pressure, heart rate, respiratory rate) should be assessed and recorded. Blood pressure should be measured in both arms and preferably in supine, seated, and upright positions. Overall appearance of the patient should be noted.

The vascular examination includes inspection, palpation, and auscultation of vascular structures in many areas of the body. A systematic approach ensures a complete evaluation, so the examination described in this chapter will cover principal anatomical regions that are particularly relevant to the peripheral vasculature. The heart, lungs, and neurological and musculoskeletal systems should be examined, but details of these examinations are beyond the scope of this chapter.

Limbs

The limbs should be inspected carefully, assessing their appearance, symmetry, color, and evidence of edema or muscle wasting.

PULSE EXAMINATION

The pulse examination of the arms and legs is a critical part of the vascular examination. Asymmetry, decreased intensity, or absence of pulses provide clinical evidence of PAD and indicate the location of stenotic lesions. Some examiners describe pulses as absent, diminished, or normal, or use a numerical scale (e.g., from 0 [absent] to 2+ [normal]). Bounding pulses may be evidence of aortic valve insufficiency, and dilated expansive pulses a sign of ectasia or aneurysm.

Pulses of the arms—brachial, radial, and ulnar pulses—should be palpated using two or three fingertips. The brachial pulse is superficial and in the medial third of the antecubital fossa. The radial pulse, also superficial, can be found over the stylus of the radius near the base of the thumb (Fig. 11-1). The ulnar pulse is palpated on the volar aspect of the wrist, over the head of the ulnar bone. Wrist support by the examiner improves pulse detection by decreasing overlying muscle tension.

Pulse examination of the leg (femoral, popliteal, posterior tibial, and dorsalis pedis pulses) should be undertaken with the patient supine. The femoral pulse is located deep, below the inguinal ligament, about midway between the symphysis pubis and iliac spine. Obesity may obscure local landmarks. Lateral rotation of the leg, pannus retraction, and two hands may be required for adequate palpation. On occasion, the increase in flow velocity caused by a stenosis may create a thrill in the common or superficial femoral artery that is appreciated by palpation of the femoral pulse, or a bruit that can be heard with auscultation.

Palpation of the popliteal pulse can be difficult. The leg should be straight yet relaxed to decrease overlying muscle stiffness. The popliteal pulse should be palpated with three fingers from each hand while the thumbs are applying moderate opposing force to the top of the knee (Fig. 11-2). The popliteal pulse typically can be found at the junction of the medial and lateral thirds of the fossa. In contrast to superficial pulses like the radial or dorsalis pedis pulse, the popliteal pulse is diffuse and deep. Widened popliteal pulses may be indicative of popliteal artery aneurysm.

The posterior tibial pulse can be found slightly below and behind the medial malleolus. Counterpressure with the thumb and passive dorsiflexion of the foot may increase the likelihood of

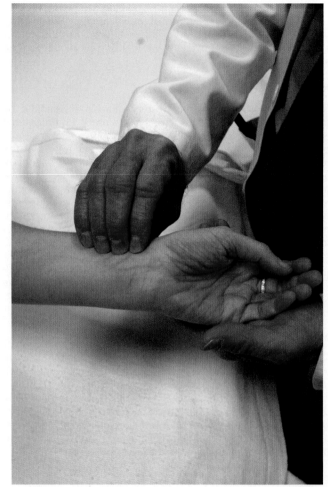

FIGURE 11-1 Palpating radial pulse. Examiner, using three or four fingers, lightly palpates the superficial radial pulse over stylus of radius near base of thumb.

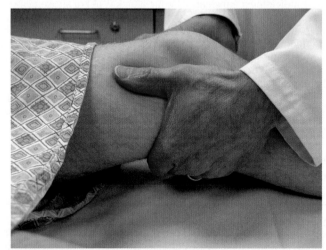

FIGURE 11-2 Palpating popliteal pulse. Popliteal pulse requires moderate pressure for its appreciation. Examiner uses both thumbs for moderate opposing force while placing digits two, three, and four in lateral third of popliteal fossa. Patient's leg should be relaxed while examiner induces mild flexion. A widened popliteal artery pulse may indicate presence of aneurysm.

palpation (Fig. 11-3). The posterior tibial pulse should be present. Its absence is diagnostic for PAD. In contrast, the dorsalis pedis pulse, which can be appreciated just lateral to the extensor tendon on the dorsum of the foot, normally may be absent in 2% to 12% of persons.

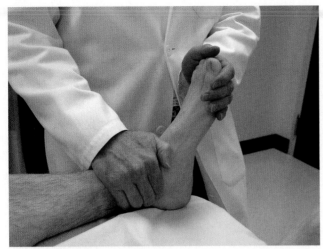

FIGURE 11-3 **Palpating posterior tibial pulse.** Posterior tibial pulse resides slightly below and behind medial malleolus. It should be approached from the lateral aspect, with digits applied to lower curvature of malleolus. Passive foot dorsiflexion may enhance appreciation of pulse.

THE ALLEN TEST

The radial and ulnar arteries supply blood flow to the hand. Within the hand, these arteries form the superficial and deep palmar arches, enabling blood supply to the digits from either vessel; 5% to 10% of the population has a congenitally incomplete arch. Disease states associated with interruption of the palmar arch include connective tissue diseases like the CREST variant (calcinosis, Raynaud phenomenon, esophageal dysmotility, sclerodactyly, telangiectasia) of scleroderma, vasculitides like TAO, and thromboemboli. The Allen test can differentiate between a complete and incomplete palmar arch. The examiner occludes both the radial and ulnar pulses (Fig. 11-4), and the patient then opens and closes the fist several times, creating palmar pallor. Upon release of one pulse, normal skin color should return within seconds. The other artery is then tested and observed similarly. Persistent pallor is indicative of an incomplete palmar arch or occluded artery distal to the remaining pulse occluded by the examiner.

Nearly three quarters of all patients with TAO, will have a positive Allen test, and 50% will report Raynaud phenomenon. Digital ischemia in these patients is more likely to progress and cause persistent cyanosis and lead to digital ulcers. Patients with TAO also may develop migratory superficial thrombophlebitis, which appears as painful, tender, red nodules.

THORACIC OUTLET MANEUVERS

Thoracic outlet syndrome results from compression of the neurovascular bundle as it leaves the thoracic cavity. Each component of the bundle may be affected, including the brachial plexus, subclavian/axillary artery, and subclavian/axillary vein.

Thoracic outlet maneuvers seek to elicit positional interruption of arterial flow. During the examination, the physician holds the radial pulse in one hand and maneuvers the arm with the other. The subclavian artery is auscultated in the supraclavicular fossa. An abnormal thoracic outlet maneuver is characterized by development of a subclavian bruit followed by loss of the radial pulse. Several thoracic outlet maneuvers have been described, and each may be relevant to compression at different sites in the thoracic outlet. Each side is examined in sequence. The *Adson maneuver* assesses the segment of the subclavian artery in the scalene triangle. The patient rotates his/her head toward the symptomatic side, extends the neck (i.e., looking up and over the shoulder), and simultaneously performs an exaggerated inspiration. The *costoclavicular maneuver* assesses the segment of the subclavian artery coursing between the clavicle and first rib. The patient thrusts the shoulders back and inferiorly. The *hyperabduction maneuver* evaluates the subclavian artery as it courses near the insertion of the pectoralis major muscle. The patient is seated and the head is looking forward. The arm is abducted 180 degrees to a position along the side of the head. Abduction of the arm to 90 degrees may be combined with external rotation in evaluating symptoms suggestive of thoracic outlet syndrome (Fig. 11-5). This maneuver is often used to assess subclavian venous or arterial compression during ultrasonography or angiography.

For patients in whom clinical suspicion for thoracic outlet syndrome is present, sensitivity and specificity for these provocative tests are 72% and 53%, respectively.[16] Routine application of these maneuvers is not warranted, however, since up to 50% of the population may have a positive finding. Indeed, in one study of 64 randomly selected subjects, application of these maneuvers in a nonspecific manner overdiagnosed the syndrome more than threefold.[17] Patients with carpal tunnel syndrome present a particularly difficult group for these maneuvers and generate a false-positive rate of nearly 50%.[18]

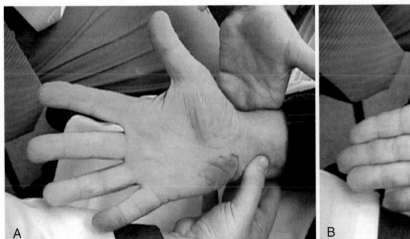
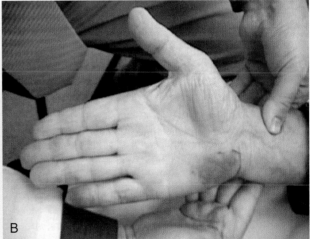

FIGURE 11-4 **Allen test.** The Allen test determines presence or absence of a complete palmar arch. Both radial and ulnar pulses are occluded while patient opens and closes hand to create palmar pallor. Once pallor is evident, examiner releases one pulse. In this example, patient presented with persistent fifth digit and hypothenar cyanosis. **A,** Release of radial artery pulse results in expected hyperemia and palmar erythema. **B,** In contrast, release of ulnar artery pulse does *not* result in palmar erythema, indicating proximal occlusion in ulnar segment of palmar arch. This test is considered a positive Allen test.

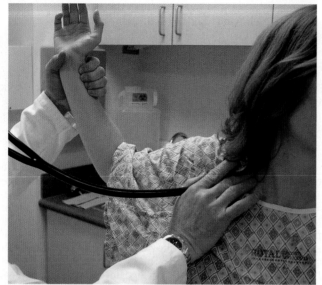

FIGURE 11-5 Elevated Arm Stress Test (EAST) may be used to evaluate subclavian artery as it courses near insertion of pectoralis major muscle. Patient initially sits looking forward while arms are abducted 90 degrees, elbows are abducted 90 degrees, and patient repeatedly makes a clenched fist. During maneuver, radial pulse should be palpated while subclavian artery is auscultated. Loss of pulse or development of subclavian artery bruit is a positive study.

LIMB ISCHEMIA

Skin color and temperature can provide information about severity of limb arterial perfusion. The feet, hands, fingers and toes should be examined for temperature and skin color, and the nails for evidence of fragility and pitting. Limb temperature can best be appreciated using the back of the examiner's hand. Temperature changes of adjacent segments on the ipsilateral limb and comparisons with the contralateral limb can be made. Presence of foot pallor while the leg is horizontal is indicative of poor perfusion and may be a sign of ischemia. Foot pallor may be precipitated in patients with PAD (who do not have CLI) by elevating the patient's leg to 60 degrees for 1 minute. Repetitive dorsiflexion and plantar flexion of the foot may also precipitate pallor on the sole of the foot when PAD is present. To qualitatively assess collateral blood flow, the leg is then lowered as the patient moves to the seated position. This is done to elicit rubor, indicative of reactive hyperemia, and determine pedal vein refill time. The time to development of dependent rubor is indicative of the severity of PAD. Severe PAD and poor collateral blood flow may prolong reactive hyperemia by more than 30 seconds. Normally, pedal venous refill occurs in less than 15 seconds. Moderate PAD subserved by collateral vessels is suspected if venous refill is 30 to 45 seconds; severe disease with poor collateral development is likely when venous filling time is longer than 1 minute.

ULCERS

Ischemia arising from arterial occlusive disease or emboli may cause formation of ischemic ulcers (see Chapter 60). They tend to be small, annular, pale, and desiccated (Fig. 11-6) and are usually located in distal areas of the limbs (e.g., toes, heels, fingertips). Ischemic ulcers vary in size but may be as small as 3 mm in diameter. Arterial ischemic ulcers are tender. Neurotrophic ulcers that develop in patients with diabetes typically occur at sites of trauma, such as areas of callus formation, bony prominence, or parts of the foot exposed to mild chronic trauma caused by ill-fitting shoes. Ischemic ulcers also develop in diabetic patients with PAD and may have features of neuropathic ulcers. Without proper treatment, ulceration may progress to tissue necrosis and gangrene. *Gangrene* can be characterized as an area of dead tissue that blackens, mummifies, and sloughs.

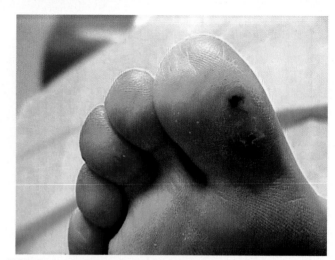

FIGURE 11-6 Digital ulceration. Pernio is associated with persistent sensation of cold, with pain in the toes. Painful blue nodules are noted in association with a discrete ulcer.

DIGITAL VASOSPASM

It is unusual for patients with Raynaud phenomenon to present to the physician's office during an attack in which the fingers are blanched. Moreover, it is difficult to precipitate digital ischemia in these patients, even with local cold exposure, such as placing the hands in ice water. Digital ischemia may be apparent in patients with fixed obstructive lesions of the digital arteries. Persistent digital ischemia may occur in patients with connective tissue disorders such as scleroderma or systemic lupus erythematosus, atheroemboli, TAO, or atherosclerosis. The fingers and toes are cool and appear cyanotic or pale. Fissures, pits, ulcerations, or necrosis or gangrene may be evident on the ischemic digits (see Fig. 11-6).

LIVEDO RETICULARIS

Livedo reticularis can be described as a lacelike or netlike pattern in the skin (Fig. 11-7). The "laces" may vary in color from red to blue and surround a central area of clearing. Cold exposure exacerbates the changes in hue. Both primary and secondary forms may occur and may be complicated by ulceration. The primary benign form is more common in women. The secondary forms are usually associated with vasculitis, atheroemboli, hyperviscosity syndromes, endocrine abnormalities, and infections. In the secondary forms of livedo reticularis, lesions may be more diffuse and ominous. Purpuric lesions and cutaneous nodules that progress to ulceration in response to cold may develop.

EDEMA

The limbs should be evaluated for edema. The most common location is in the legs, adjacent to the malleoli and over the tibia. With deep digital palpation, development of a divot or finger impression is indicative of pitting edema. Edema can be graded in each leg or arm as absent, mild, moderate, or severe or on a numerical scale of 4, with 0 being the absence of edema. Unilateral edema may be evidence of DVT, chronic venous insufficiency, or lymphedema.

The most common physical findings of DVT include unilateral leg swelling, warmth, and erythema. The affected vein may be tender. A common femoral vein cord is detected by palpating along its course just below the inguinal ligament vein, and a femoral vein cord would be appreciated along the anteromedial aspect of the thigh. In the absence of obvious edema, a subtle clue may be unilateral absence of contours of the thigh, calf, or ankle. Muscular groups subtended by the thrombosed vein may be edematous due to poor venous drainage, conferring a boggy feeling to the affected calf or thigh muscles. Inflammation associated with a thrombosis may make the leg feel warm.

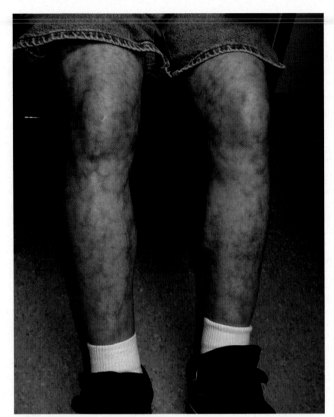

FIGURE 11-7 Livedo reticularis. Note lacelike pattern of superficial skin vessels surrounding a clear area.

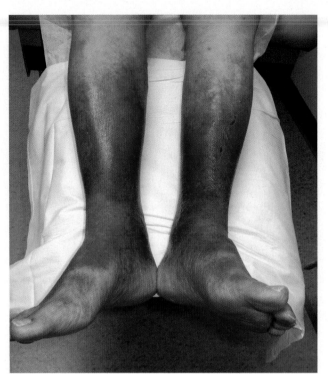

FIGURE 11-8 Skin changes of chronic venous insufficiency. Chronic venous insufficiency and edema result in deposition of hemosiderin, causing darkening and toughening of skin and giving calf a brawny appearance. Note small superficial venous ulcers mid-calf above shin.

Homans sign is nonspecific and misses the diagnosis as commonly as it makes it. In John Homans's essay on lower extremity venous thrombosis, he states, "The clinical signs of a deep thrombosis of the muscles of the calf are entirely lacking when the individual lies or even reclines in bed. It is possible there may be a little discomfort upon forced dorsiflexion of the foot (tightening of the posterior muscles) but it is not yet clear whether or not this is a sign upon which to depend."[19]

Presence of thrombus just below the skin makes the diagnosis of superficial thrombophlebitis relatively easy. The patient may present with local venous engorgement, a palpable cord, warmth, erythema, or tenderness.

CHRONIC VENOUS INSUFFICIENCY

With chronic venous insufficiency, the physical examination may demonstrate fibrosis, tenderness, excoriation, and skin induration from hyperkeratosis, cellulitis, and ulceration (Fig. 11-8). Chronic venous edema may impart hemosiderin deposition in the skin and confer a brawny appearance, typically in the pretibial calf. The severity of chronic venous disease may be classified using the CEAP (clinical signs, etiology, anatomy, pathophysiology) classification[20] (Table 11-1).

In contrast to arterial ulcers, which are circumscribed and pallid, venous ulcers are large with irregular borders, erythematous, and moist, giving the skin a shiny appearance. They are usually located near the medial or lateral malleolus. Venous ulcers may be painless, but many are associated with pain.[21,22]

VARICOSE VEINS

Varicose veins are dilated, serpentine, superficial veins. If they cluster, they may feel and appear like a bunch of grapes (Fig. 11-9). Varicose veins should be inspected and palpated. Areas of erythema, tenderness, or induration may identify superficial thrombophlebitis. Varicose veins are most prominent with leg dependence (e.g., with standing). Once filled, the veins may be balloted, and a fluid wave may be detected. Venous telangiectasias, also known as *spider veins*,

TABLE 11-1 CEAP Clinical Classification

CLASS	CLINICAL SIGNS
0	No visible or palpable signs of venous disease
1	Telangiectasis or reticular veins
2	Varicose veins
3	Edema
4	Skin changes ascribed to venous disease (e.g., pigmentation, venous eczema, lipodermatosclerosis)
5	Skin changes as defined above, with healed ulceration
6	Skin changes as defined above, with active ulceration

CEAP, clinical signs, etiology, anatomy, pathophysiology.

are commonly confused with varicose veins. Spider veins are typically small, cutaneous veins in a caput medusa pattern.

Superficial venous varicosities may be primary or result from deep venous thrombosis or insufficiency. An examiner can distinguish between superficial venous insufficiency and deep venous insufficiency at the bedside using the *Brodie-Trendelenburg test*. With the patient lying supine, the leg is elevated to 45 degrees and a tourniquet applied after the veins have drained. The patient then stands. The veins below the tourniquet should fill slowly. If venous refill distal to the site of tourniquet application occurs in less than 30 seconds, this is evidence of an incompetent deep and perforator system. Slower refills suggest a competent deep and perforator system. The varicose veins are examined upon tourniquet release. Superficial venous insufficiency will be confirmed with rapid retrograde superficial venous filling.

The *Perthes test* can differentiate between deep venous insufficiency and a deep venous obstruction as the cause of varicose veins. The patient is asked to stand, and once the superficial veins are engorged, a tourniquet is applied around the mid-thigh. The patient then walks for 5 minutes. If the varicose veins collapse below the level of the tourniquet, the perforator veins are

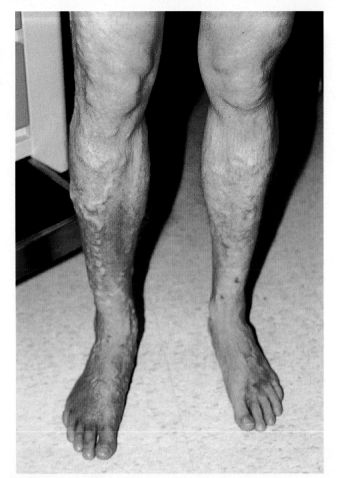

FIGURE 11-9 **Varicose veins.** Severe bilateral varicose veins with extension into both feet.

presumed competent and the deep veins patent. If the superficial veins remain engorged, either the superficial and/or communicating veins are incompetent. If the varicose veins increase in prominence, and walking causes leg pain, the deep veins are occluded.

LYMPHEDEMA

During the initial stages of lymphedema, leg swelling will be similar to venous insufficiency: soft and pitting. Extension of edema into the foot to the origin of the toes may help differentiate lymphedema from venous edema (Fig. 11-10). In addition, the inability to

pinch skin on the toes, the *Stemmer sign*, also may differentiate early lymphedema from venous edema. Subsequently, the limb becomes wooden as progressive deposition of protein-rich fluid causes induration and fibrosis of affected tissues. Lymphedema increases production of subcutaneous and adipose tissue, thickening the skin. Advanced disease may be identified when the leg feels wooden, edema is no longer pitting, and the limb is enlarged; the skin may appear verrucous at the toes. Palpation for lymphadenopathy should be performed when considering secondary causes of lymphedema.

LYMPHANGITIS

Lymphangitis can usually be visualized as a red streak that extends proximally from an inciting lesion. If left untreated, the entire limb may become edematous, erythematous, and warm, without evidence of venous congestion or impairment of arterial flow. Commonly, the regional lymph nodes are indurated.

Neck Examination

The neck is inspected for any areas of swelling or asymmetry. Jugular venous pressure is assessed to investigate the possibility of a volume overloaded state or congestive heart failure. Patients typically are placed at 45 degrees and the height of jugular venous pressure estimated. If necessary, the angle of head elevation should be adjusted to see the top of the jugular venous column.

The carotid arteries are palpated between the trachea and the sternocleidomastoid muscles. In older patients especially, the carotid body may be sensitive, and carotid pulses may induce bradycardia and hypotension. Pulses should be symmetrical with a rapid upstroke. Pulse asymmetry may indicate a proximal carotid or brachiocephalic stenosis. Parvus and tardus pulses (decreased amplitude and a delayed slow upstroke) may indicate aortic valve stenosis or proximal occlusive disease. Stenosis of the carotid bifurcation or internal carotid artery usually does not affect carotid pulse contour or amplitude. Occasionally, severe stenosis will create a thrill that can be appreciated by palpation.

The carotid pulses are auscultated to elicit evidence of bruits. Bruits are caused by blood flow turbulence as a result of arterial stenosis, extrinsic compression, aneurysmal dilation, or arteriovenous connection. The bell of the stethoscope is recommended to appreciate low-frequency bruits and eliminate any adventitious sounds heard through the diaphragm. The entire cervical portion of each carotid artery should be auscultated, including the segment near the angle of the jaw where the carotid bifurcation is often located (Fig. 11-11). Auscultation of the subclavian arteries for bruits is performed in the supraclavicular fossa and between the lateral aspect of the clavicle and pectoralis muscle. Although the proximal location of a bruit defines the area

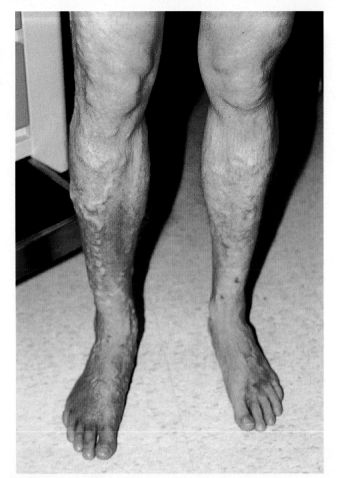

FIGURE 11-10 **Lymphedema.** Extension of edema into foot to level of toe is a useful physical sign to differentiate between venous edema and lymphedema. Foot swelling ending abruptly at toes is called *squared toe sign*.

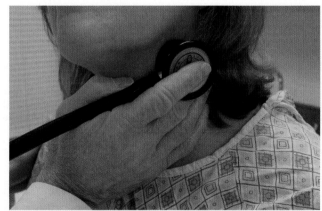

FIGURE 11-11 **Auscultation of carotid artery.** To appreciate low-tone bruits, examiner should use stethoscope bell and apply mild to moderate pressure. Entire length of artery should be examined, with particular attention paid to region just below jaw, at approximation of carotid artery bifurcation.

of turbulent flow, a bruit may be appreciated for an additional several centimeters. The sensitivity and specificity of a carotid bruit for the presence of stenosis ranges from 50% to 79% and 61% to 91%.[23] The pitch of bruits increases with worsening severity. Continuation of the bruit into diastole is another marker of severity and implies advanced stenosis. Paradoxically, severe stenosis causing subtotal arterial occlusion may not evoke an audible bruit.

Abdominal Vascular Examination

Vascular examination of the abdomen is performed as the patient lies supine on the examining table, with legs outstretched. From this position, the abdominal wall should be relaxed and not rigid. Prior to palpation, the abdomen should be inspected. Engorged superficial veins in the abdomen indicate the possibility of inferior vena cava obstruction. After inspection, all four quadrants are auscultated with the stethoscope. The presence of bruits is indicative of aortic or branch vessel occlusive disease. Bruits may arise as a result of mesenteric, renal, or aortic disease. Following auscultation, the abdomen is palpated for masses and to detect an aortic aneurysm. Deepest palpation can generally be obtained by gradually increasing pressure in the midline using both hands (Fig. 11-12). In asthenic patients, the aorta can be palpated. In subjects with a waist size greater than 40 inches, the likelihood of palpating an aneurysm is quite limited.

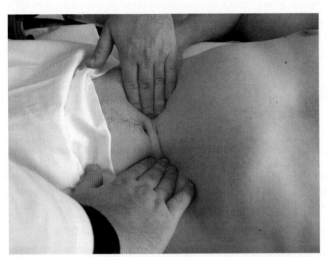

FIGURE 11-12 Abdominal palpation for aneurysm. Examiner, using progressively increasing force, palpates until aorta can be defined between both sets of fingers. Examiner should appreciate lateral pulsation with every heart beat. Aneurysm sizing is performed by estimating distance between closest fingers of each hand.

Presence of an aneurysm can be determined when there is a distinct and expansive pulsatile configuration to the aorta. An aneurysm should be sized by determining the lateral borders with both hands, and the space estimated with a measuring tape. Tenderness during the abdominal vascular examination is unusual and may suggest aneurysmal expansion, an inflammatory aneurysm, or a contained rupture. Nonaortic pathology, including appendicitis, cholecystitis, diverticulitis, and peritonitis, are more common causes of tenderness.

REFERENCES

1. Fowkes FG, Murray GD, Butcher I, et al: Ankle brachial index combined with Framingham risk score to predict cardiovascular events and mortality: a meta-analysis, *JAMA* 300: 197–208, 2008.
2. McDermott MM, Greenland P, Liu K, et al: Leg symptoms in peripheral arterial disease: associated clinical characteristics and functional impairment, *JAMA* 286:1599–1606, 2001.
3. McDermott MM, Liu K, Greenland P, et al: Functional decline in peripheral arterial disease: associations with the ankle brachial index and leg symptoms, *JAMA* 292: 453–461, 2004.
4. Rose GA: The diagnosis of ischaemic heart pain and intermittent claudication infield surveys, *Bull World Health Org* 27:645–658, 1962.
5. Coyne KS, Margolis MK, Gilchrist KA, et al: Evaluating effects of method of administration on walking impairment questionnaire, *J Vasc Surg* 38:296–304, 2003.
6. Criqui MH, Denenberg JO, Bird CE, et al: The correlation between symptoms and non-invasive test results in patients referred for peripheral arterial disease testing, *Vasc Med* 1:65–71, 1996.
7. Regensteiner JG, Gardner A, Hiatt WR: Exercise testing and exercise rehabilitation for patients with peripheral arterial disease: status in 1997, *Vasc Med* 2:147–155, 1997.
8. Rajagopalan S, Grossman PM: Management of chronic critical limb ischemia, *Cardiol Clin* 20:535–545, 2002.
9. Jaffery Z, Thornton SN, White CJ: Acute limb ischemia, *Am J Med Sci* 342:226–234, 2011.
10. Fukumoto Y, Tsutsui H, Tsuchihashi M, et al: The incidence and risk factors of cholesterol embolization syndrome, a complication of cardiac catheterization: a prospective study, *J Am Coll Cardiol* 42:211–216, 2003.
11. Olin JW: Thromboangiitis obliterans (Buerger's disease), *N Engl J Med* 343:864–869, 2000.
12. Mackinnon SE, Novak CB: Thoracic outlet syndrome, *Curr Probl Surg* 39:1070–1145, 2002.
13. Levien LJ: Popliteal artery entrapment syndrome, *Semin Vasc Surg* 16:223–231, 2003.
14. Wigley FM: Clinical practice. Raynaud's phenomenon, *N Engl J Med* 347:1001–1008, 2002.
15. Bergan JJ, Schmid-Schonbein GW, Smith PD, et al: Chronic venous disease, *N Engl J Med* 355:488–498, 2006.
16. Gillard J, Perez-Cousin M, Hachulla E, et al: Diagnosing thoracic outlet syndrome: contribution of provocative tests, ultrasonography, electrophysiology, and helical computed tomography in 48 patients, *Joint Bone Spine* 68:416–424, 2001.
17. Warrens AN, Heaton JM: Thoracic outlet compression syndrome: the lack of reliability of its clinical assessment, *Ann R Coll Surg Engl* 69:203–204, 1987.
18. Nord KM, Kapoor P, Fisher J, et al: False positive rate of thoracic outlet syndrome diagnostic maneuvers, *Electromyogr Clin Neurophysiol* 48:67–74, 2008.
19. Homans J: Venous thrombosis in the lower limbs: its relation to pulmonary embolism, *Am J Surg* 38:316–326, 1937.
20. Beebe HG, Bergan JJ, Bergqvist D, et al: Classification and grading of chronic venous disease in the lower limbs, A consensus statement, *Int Angiol* 14:197–201, 1995.
21. de Araujo T, Valencia I, Federman DG, et al: Managing the patient with venous ulcers, *Ann Intern Med* 138:326–334, 2003.
22. Nemeth KA, Harrison MB, Graham ID, et al: Pain in pure and mixed aetiology venous leg ulcers: a three-phase point prevalence study, *J Wound Care* 12:336–340, 2003.
23. Magyar MT, Nam EM, Csiba L, et al: Carotid artery auscultation–anachronism or useful screening procedure? *Neurol Res* 24:705–708, 2002.

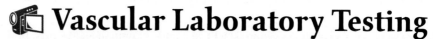 Vascular Laboratory Testing

Marie Gerhard-Herman, Joshua A. Beckman, Mark A. Creager

Vascular laboratory technology offers many cost-effective applications in the practice of vascular medicine.[1] Vascular testing includes both physiological testing and duplex ultrasonography. Physiological testing includes segmental pressure measurements, pulse volume recordings, continuous wave Doppler, and plethysmography. These tests employ sphygmomanometric cuffs, Doppler instruments, and plethysmographic recording devices. Duplex ultrasonography combines gray-scale and Doppler imaging with spectral and color Doppler and is used for the majority of vascular laboratory tests. An ultrasound machine should be equipped with vascular software and two transducers/probes, 5- to 12-MHz transducers for the neck and extremities, and 2.25- to 3.5-MHz transducers for the abdomen.

Limb Pressure Measurement and Pulse Volume Recordings

Limb segmental systolic blood pressure measurements and pulse volume recordings are used to confirm a clinical diagnosis of peripheral artery disease (PAD) and further define the level and extent of the obstruction. Segmental pressures are typically measured in conjunction with segmental limb plethysmography (pulse volume recordings). These techniques are used predominantly in the lower extremities, but are also applicable to the arms. Both procedures are performed using sphygmomanometric cuffs appropriately sized to the diameter of the limb segment under study. The patient rests in the supine position for at least 10 minutes prior to measuring limb pressures. Commercially available machines with automatic cuff inflation are able to digitally store the pressures and waveforms. A continuous-wave (CW) Doppler instrument with a 4- to 8-MHz transducer frequency is used to detect the arterial flow signal. The cuff is quickly inflated to a suprasystolic pressure and then slowly deflated until a flow signal occurs. The cuff pressure at which the flow signal is detected is the systolic pressure in the arterial segment beneath the cuff. For example, if the cuff is on the high thigh and the sensor is over the posterior tibial artery at the ankle, the measured pressure is reflective of the proximal superficial and deep femoral arteries (DFAs) beneath the cuff, as well as any collateral arteries, and not the posterior tibial artery. The Doppler flow signal from an artery at the ankle is typically used for all limb measurements. It is more accurate, although less convenient, to place the Doppler transducer probe close to the cuff being inflated.

Sphygmomanometric cuffs are positioned on each arm above the antecubital fossa, on the upper portion of each thigh (high thigh), on the lower portions of the thighs above the patella (low thigh), on the calves below the tibial tubercle, and on the ankles above the malleoli. Typically, foot pressures are measured by insonating the posterior tibial and anterior tibial arteries at the ankle level. Both arm pressures at the brachial artery are determined. A difference of greater than 20 mmHg between the arm pressures indicates the presence of stenosis on the side of the lower pressure. Pressure measurements are made at the high thigh, low thigh, calf, and ankle levels with a tibial or dorsalis pedis signal selected as the flow indicator. A second method uses one long, contoured thigh cuff rather than two separate thigh cuffs. The lower-extremity pressure evaluation should begin at the ankle level and proceed proximally. Patients who are found to have a normal pressure measurement at rest may require a treadmill exercise test to detect PAD. If disease distal to the ankle is suspected, pedal or digital artery obstruction can be evaluated with cuffs sized appropriately for the toes.

Segmental Doppler Pressure Interpretation

Segmental limb pressures are compared with the highest arm pressure. Ankle pressures are used to calculate the ankle-brachial indices (ABI) for each extremity. This is accomplished by dividing each of the ankle pressures by the higher of the brachial artery pressures.[2] A normal ABI is between 1.0 and 1.4, whereas an ABI above 0.9 to 1.0 is borderline abnormal.[3] Studies that evaluated the ABI in healthy subjects and patients with PAD confirmed by arteriography found that an ABI of 0.9 or lower was diagnostic of PAD with 79% to 95% specificity and 96% to 100% sensitivity.[4] Pressures are compared between levels. A 20-mmHg or greater reduction in pressures from one level to the next is considered significant and indicates stenosis between those two levels. In healthy subjects, the high thigh pressure determined by cuff typically exceeds the brachial artery pressure by approximately 30 mmHg. A thigh/brachial index above 1 is interpreted as normal, and an index of 1 or less indicates stenosis proximal to the thigh (Fig. 12-1). When high thigh pressures are low compared with arm pressure, the site of obstruction could be in the aorta or ipsilateral iliac artery, common femoral artery (CFA), or proximal superficial femoral artery (SFA) (see Fig. 12-1). If only one high thigh pressure is less than the brachial pressure, an ipsilateral iliofemoral artery stenosis is inferred.

In the presence of severe vascular calcification, systolic pressures cannot be determined because the vessels are noncompressible. An index of 1.4 or greater suggests vascular calcification artifact and makes interpretation of the pressure measurement unreliable. Presence or absence of a significant pressure gradient cannot be determined in the presence of vascular calcification artifact. In this setting, the toe brachial index (TBI) is a useful measurement. Toe brachial index is the ratio of the systolic pressure in the toe to the brachial artery systolic pressure. This should be performed in a warm room; cold-induced vasospasm may lower the digital pressure. To perform the procedure, a cuff is placed on a toe. Typically, the great toe is used. The pulse waveform is obtained by photoplethysmography or Doppler. The cuff is inflated to suprasystolic pressure and then deflated. Systolic pressure is determined as the pressure at which the waveform reappears. A normal value for TBI is 0.70.

Pulse Volume Recording Interpretation

The same cuffs used to measure segmental pressures may be attached to a plethysmographic instrument and used to record the change in volume of a limb segment with each pulse, designated the *pulse volume*. Pulse volume waveform evaluation allows assessment of arterial flow in regions of calcified vessels because the test does not rely on cuff occlusion of the calcified artery.[5] Each cuff is inflated in sequence to a predetermined reference pressure up to 65 mmHg. The change in volume in the limb segment causes a corresponding change in pressure in the cuff throughout the cardiac cycle. Interpretation of the pulse volume recording (PVR) requires calibration of the amount of air in the cuff.

A pulse volume waveform is recorded for each limb segment. Pulse volume recording analysis is based on evaluation of waveform shape, signal, and amplitude (Fig. 12-2). The configuration of the normal pulse volume waveform resembles the arterial pressure waveform, and is composed of a sharp systolic upstroke followed by a downstroke that contains a prominent dicrotic notch. A hemodynamically significant stenosis manifests as a change in the PVR contour toward a tardus parvus waveform. Both the slope and amplitude decrease when there is more severe disease. Severity of PAD can be defined by the slope of the upstroke and amplitude of the pulse volume (see Fig. 12-2).

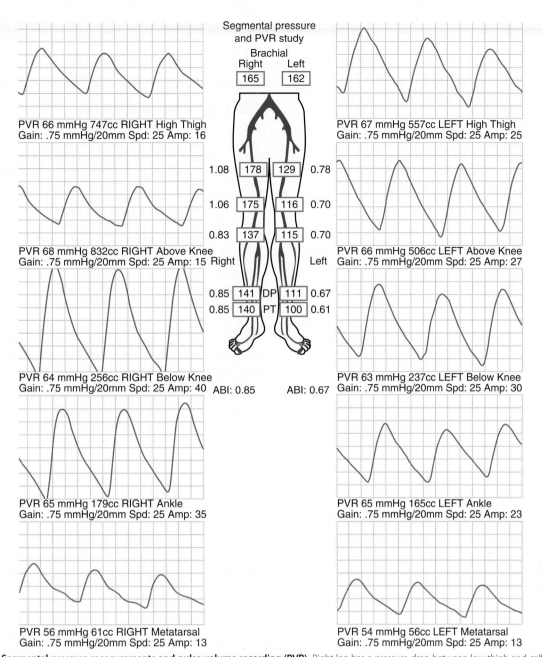

FIGURE 12-1   Segmental pressure measurements and pulse volume recording (PVR). Right leg has a pressure drop between low thigh and calf consistent with superficial femoral/popliteal artery stenosis. Left leg has a pressure drop at level of high thigh consistent with iliofemoral artery stenosis. ABI, ankle-brachial index.

Pulse waveforms can also be obtained using photoplethysmography, recording reflected infrared light. In photoplethysmography, the signal is proportional to the quantity of red blood cells in the cutaneous circulation; it does not measure volume changes. Waveform shape is assessed in a similar fashion in pulse volume and photoplethysmography recordings. Low photoplethysmographic waveforms in the toes identify increased risk of amputation, in addition to the toe pressure.[5]

Exercise Testing for Peripheral Artery Disease

Exercise testing is an adjunctive physiological test to evaluate PAD. It is useful to assess functional capacity and determine the distance patients with claudication are able to walk. Moreover, it can be used to clarify whether leg symptoms are related to PAD. This is relevant in patients with symptoms that are atypical for claudication and in those who have a history of intermittent claudication, yet normal ABIs at rest.[6] Relative contraindications to treadmill exercise testing for PAD include rest pain in the leg,

shortness of breath with minimal exertion, or unstable angina. The test cannot be performed if the patient cannot walk on a treadmill.

Patients are instructed to fast for 12 hours prior to walking on the treadmill. The constant-load treadmill test is performed at a speed of 2 mph and an incline of 12%. Graded exercise protocols increase the grade and/or speed in 2- to 3-minute stages. The Gardner protocol is the most commonly used graded protocol to evaluate walking exercise capacity.[7] It begins at a speed of 2 mph and an incline of 0%, and the grade progressively increases by 2% every 2 minutes, allowing for a wider range of responses to be measured. It is often used to determine clinical trial end points such as change in walking time in response to therapy. Other graded exercise protocols, such as the Bruce protocol, are not commonly used because the rapid rate of speed and incline limits assessment of exercise capacity in claudicants.

The treadmill exercise test is terminated when the patient cannot continue owing to leg claudication or chest pain, or is limited by other symptoms such as shortness of breath or fatigue. The patient then immediately lies down on the stretcher. Ankle pressures are

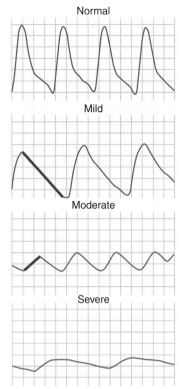

Normal

Mild

Moderate

Severe

FIGURE 12-2 **Pulse volume recording (PVR).** Normal waveform has a sharp upstroke, dicrotic notch, and a period of diastasis. Mildly abnormal waveform has a delay in upstroke and a straightened downslope *(blue line)*. Moderately abnormal waveform has a delay in upstroke *(blue line)*, flat systolic peak, and diminished amplitude. Severely abnormal waveform has a flat systolic peak and very diminished amplitude.

obtained starting with the symptomatic leg, followed by the highest brachial pressure. Pressures are repeated approximately every 1 to 2 minutes until they return to baseline. Data recorded from the exercise test should include ankle pressures, length of time the patient was able to walk, time required for pressures to return to baseline, nature and location of the patient's symptoms, and reason for discontinuing the test. A decrease in ABI of more than 20% immediately following exercise is diagnostic for PAD. The time before ankle pressure returns to normal is increased in more severe disease (e.g., from 1 minute in mild disease to 10 minutes in more severe disease).

Transcutaneous Oximetry

By exploiting variations in color absorbance of oxygenated and deoxygenated hemoglobin (Hb), transcutaneous oximetry can determine the state of blood oxygenation. Oximeters use two light frequencies, red at 600 to 750 nm and infrared at 800 to 1050 nm, to differentiate oxygenated and deoxygenated Hb. Deoxygenated blood absorbs more red light, whereas oxygenated blood absorbs more infrared light. Oximeters typically employ both an emitter and receiver. Red and infrared light is emitted and passes through a relatively translucent structure such as the finger or earlobe. A photodetector determines the ratio of red and infrared light received to derive blood oxygenation. When measured continuously, oxygenation peaks with each heartbeat as fresh oxygenated blood arrives in the zone of measurement. Normal values for oxygen tension are from 50 to 75 mmHg. One probe is placed on the chest as a control to ensure that oxygen tension is from 50 to 75 mmHg. A second probe is placed on the limb in the area of interest. Measurements are obtained from the probe, which is sequentially positioned from proximal to distal segments of the limb. Normal limb Tco_2 should approximate that of the chest. Transcutaneous oximetry is most often used to determine the

level of amputation. A value above 20 mmHg can predict healing at the site with 80% accuracy.[7] This measurement is not affected by arterial calcification.

Physical Principles of Ultrasonography

Ultrasound Image Creation

An ultrasound transducer, or probe, emits sound waves in discrete bundles or pulses into the tissue of interest. On encountering a tissue, a portion of the waves is reflected back to the transducer. The fraction of returning waves depends on density and size of the tissue examined. The depth of tissue is determined by the time required for pulse emission and return. Thus, by integrating the number of returning pulses and the time required for return, a B-mode, or gray-scale image may be created. The time for wave reflection decreases with higher ultrasound probe frequencies. Transducer probes with higher frequencies image superficial tissues better than probes with lower frequencies, but lose depth imaging because of attenuation of the returning emitted pulses.

Improvements in technology have permitted band-width widening of vascular transducers, facilitating analysis of harmonics of the fundamental frequency. A *harmonic* represents a whole-number multiple of the emitted frequency. Because the tissue compresses and expands in response to the application of ultrasound, the fundamental wave may become distorted, impairing image quality. The distortion, however, also creates harmonics of the original frequency that can be detected by the transducer. By detecting only the fundamental frequency and its harmonics, artifact such as speckle and reverberation may be reduced to create a clearer image.

Detection of Blood Flow

Normal blood flow is laminar in a straight segment of an artery. If thought of as a telescopic series of flow rings, blood moves forward most rapidly in the middle ring, and velocity decreases in the outer rings as blood comes closer to the vessel wall. The cardiac cycle, defined by its pulsatile nature of flow, causes a continual variation in blood flow velocity, highest with systole and lowest with diastole. The concentric or laminar flow of blood may be disturbed at a normal branching point or with abnormal vessel contours, such as those caused by atherosclerotic plaque. Disturbed or turbulent flow causes a much greater loss of pressure than laminar flow.

Determining flow velocity is a mainstay of vascular ultrasonography. Abnormalities in the vessel wall cause changes in flow velocity and permit detection and assessment of stenotic regions within the vessel. Flow in a normal vessel is proportional to the difference of pressure between the proximal and distal end of the vessel. The prime determinant or limitation of flow is the radius of the vessel because volume of blood flow is determined by the fourth power of the radius. For example, a 50% reduction in vessel radius causes a greater than 90% reduction in blood flow. Thus, blood flow represents an example of Poiseuille's law, which determines flow of a viscous fluid through a tube. Specifically,

$$Q = \frac{\pi \times \Delta P \times r^4}{8 \eta L}$$

where Q denotes volume of flow, ΔP is pressure at inflow minus the pressure at outflow, r is the radius, η is viscosity, and L is tube length. Because blood viscosity, blood vessel length, and pressure remain relatively stable, the most important determinant of blood flow is vessel lumen size.

Vascular ultrasonography can depict flow velocity by taking advantage of Doppler shift frequencies. Frequency will shift either positively or negatively, depending on direction of blood flow. Variables that determine the size of the shift include the speed of sound, speed of the moving object, and angle between the transmitted beam and moving object. Christoph Doppler described this relationship using the following equation:

$$F_d = (2 F_t \cdot V \cdot \cos\theta) \div c$$

where F_d is the Doppler frequency shift, F_t is the Doppler frequency transmitted from the probe, V is the velocity of flow, cos is the cosine, θ is the angle between the beam and direction of the moving object, and c is the velocity of sound.

Artifact

Although a highly reliable imaging modality, ultrasound does suffer from occasional image artifact.[8] Dense objects like vessel-wall calcium deposits permit few sound waves to penetrate, resulting in acoustic shadowing and diminishing imaging of deeper tissues. Tissue imaging enhancement may be noted on the far side of echo-free or liquid-filled zones. Tissue interfaces may generate multiple sound wave reflections, causing "additions" to the tissue termed *reverberation artifact*. Refraction of the sound pulse may cause improper placement of a structure of an image and shadowing at the edge of a large structure. Highly reflective surfaces may create mirror images because the reflecting tissue alters the timing of the returning sound wave. The mirror image should be equidistant from the reflecting surface or tissue.

Gray-Scale (B Mode) Imaging

Ultrasound images are generated using a pulse echo system. The position of the tissue interface is determined by the time between pulse generation and returning echo. Each returning echo is displayed as a gray dot on a video screen using a brightness mode (B mode) in which the brightness of the dot depends on the strength of the reflected wave. A two-dimensional (2D) image is created by sequentially transmitting waves in multiple directions within a single plane and combining the reflected echoes into a single display. The image can be refreshed rapidly, permitting real-time display of the gray-scale image. The surface of interest should be perpendicular to the ultrasound beam to obtain the brightest echo with B-mode imaging. This is readily achieved in vascular imaging because the neck, extremity, and visceral vessels generally lie parallel to the surface of the transducer. Higher-frequency probes are used to image vessels close to the surface, and lower-frequency probes are used to image deeper vessels. Details of the vessel wall can be seen more clearly with the use of harmonics. The wide band width of transducers allows analysis of returning harmonics (whole-number multiples) of the fundamental frequency.

Spectral Doppler Waveform Analysis

Velocity recordings are obtained with an angle of 60 degrees between the Doppler insonation beam and the flow. In ultrasound practice, the optimal angle of measurement between the beam and blood flow is 60 degrees. Although maximal shift is detected at 0 degrees, this angle cannot be reliably obtained in vascular imaging because the vessels are parallel to the surface of the body. Insonation angles below and above 60 degrees influence the measurement such that small reductions in the insonation angle may alter velocity by 10%, whereas small increases in insonation angle may change flow velocity by 25% (Fig. 12-3). Thus, the sample-volume cursor is placed parallel to the inner wall, and a Doppler[9,10] angle from 30 to 60 degrees between the wall and the insonation beam (or flow jet) is used. A normal peripheral artery Doppler waveform consists of a narrow, sharply defined tracing. This indicates that all blood cells are moving at an equivalent speed at any time in the cardiac cycle.[11] Waveforms are also characterized as high resistance due to limited flow during diastole (e.g., normal peripheral arterial Doppler velocity waveform), or low resistance with continuous flow during diastole, as when downstream resistance arterioles are widely dilated or there is contiguity with

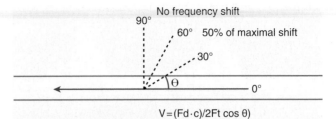

$$V = (Fd \cdot c)/2Ft \cos\theta)$$

FIGURE 12-3 **Doppler angle is the angle between insonation beam and sample cursor aligned with flow.** Dashed lines represent different insonation beams. Solid arrow represents direction of flow and position of Doppler sample cursor. Velocity is determined using the Doppler equation, with the cosine (cos) in the denominator. The cos θ degrees = 1, cos 30 degrees = 0.86, cos 60 degrees = 0.5, and cos 90 degrees = 0. c, velocity of sound; F_d, Doppler frequency shift; F_t, transmitted Doppler frequency; V, velocity.

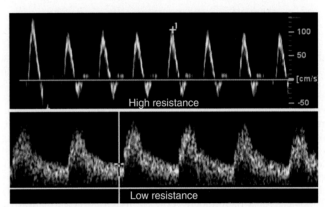

FIGURE 12-4 **High- and low-resistance waveforms.** These two waveforms are distinguished by the absence (high resistance) and presence (low resistance) of flow during diastole.

low-resistance circuits (e.g., normal internal carotid artery [ICA] velocity waveform) (Fig. 12-4). The normal high resistance waveform is typically triphasic. The first component is caused by initial high-velocity forward flow during ventricular systole. A range of normal peak systolic velocity (PSV) measurements have been defined[12] for each arterial segment, described later in this chapter.

The second phase of the waveform consists of early diastolic flow reversal as left ventricular (LV) pressure falls below aortic pressure prior to aortic valve closure.[13] The final or third component is a small amount of forward flow when there is elastic recoil of vessel walls. Flow is typically not uniform or laminar at bifurcations and sites of stenosis; at these sites flow becomes turbulent. For these locations, the spectral Doppler waveform reflects the fact that blood cells move with varying velocities. Instead of a narrow well-defined tracing (see Fig. 12-4), spectral broadening becomes evident (Fig. 12-5), with partial or complete filling-in of the area under the spectral waveform. This third, or late, diastolic component is usually absent in atherosclerotic vessels that have lost compliance or elasticity.

Color Doppler

Color Doppler is the phase or frequency shift information contained in the returning echoes and processed in real time to form a velocity map over the entire imaging field.[14] Doppler frequency-shift data are available for every point imaged. This information is then superimposed on the gray-scale image to provide a composite real-time display of both anatomy and flow. When motion is detected, it is assigned a color, typically red or blue, determined by whether the frequency shift is toward or away from the probe. Color assignment is arbitrary and can be altered by the user, but most choose to assign the color red to arteries and blue to veins. With increasing Doppler frequency shifts, the hue and intensity of the color display change, with progressive desaturation of the color and a shift toward white at the highest detectable velocities.

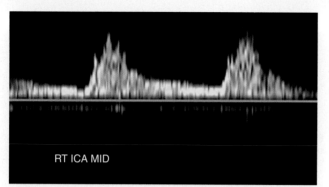

FIGURE 12-5 Post-stenotic waveform has a delay in upstroke, diminished amplitude, and marked turbulence. *RT ICA MID* denotes midportion of right internal carotid artery.

The *pulse repetition frequency* (velocity) scale determines the degree of color saturation and filling of the vessel lumen. The pulse repetition frequency (radio frequency pulses per second from the probe) is adjusted so that in a normal vessel, laminar flow appears as a homogeneous color. The color appearance changes throughout the cardiac cycle. Increasing flow velocity and turbulence in the region of a stenosis results in production of a high-velocity jet and an abrupt change in color-flow pattern (Fig. 12-6). *Color aliasing* occurs at the site of stenosis when flow velocity exceeds the Nyquist limit (i.e., when Doppler frequency shift exceeds half the pulse repetition frequency). Aliasing causes the color display to appear as if there is an abrupt reversal in direction of flow (*wraparound*). This suggests a high-velocity flow jet, requiring confirmation by pulsed-wave Doppler analysis. *Color persistence* is a continuous flow signal that is the color of the forward direction only, in contrast to the alternating color in normal arteries. There is loss of early

diastolic flow reversal. Color persistence corresponds to the monophasic spectral Doppler waveform and is indicative of severe stenosis. Post-stenotic regions display *mosaic patterns* indicating turbulent flow (see Fig. 12-6). A *color bruit* in the surrounding soft tissue also indicates flow disturbance. This color artifact is associated with turbulence and occurs with flow disturbances associated with high-velocity jets. The color bruit is particularly useful in locating postcatheterization arteriovenous fistulae (AVF).

Assessment of Arterial Stenosis

Characteristic duplex ultrasound features of a stenosis include elevated systolic velocity, elevated end-diastolic velocity (EDV), color aliasing, color bruit, spectral broadening of the Doppler waveform, post-stenotic flow, and post-stenotic turbulence. An auditory "thump" occurs in the presence of total arterial occlusion. Doppler velocity measurements are the main tools used to evaluate stenosis severity. When flow rate is constant, a decrease in vessel cross-sectional area is balanced by an increase in velocity.[13] As blood flow turbulence increases, spectral broadening of the Doppler waveform becomes a clear indicator of turbulent flow seen in the post-stenotic region. The post-stenotic waveform is dampened with a delayed upstroke (see Fig. 12-3). If no post-stenotic turbulence can be identified, inappropriate angle alignment or a tortuous vessel should be suspected.

Power (or amplitude) Doppler is a complementary imaging technique that displays the total strength or amplitude of the returning Doppler signal.[15] In comparison with conventional color-flow imaging, color-flow sensitivity is increased by a factor of 3 to 5 times with power Doppler. This enhanced dynamic range can depict very slow flow in the area of a subtotal occlusion that may not be detected by conventional color-flow Doppler. Contrast agents can also help differentiate between occlusion and high-grade stenosis in carotid and renal arteries, especially in cases where multiple renal arteries are present.[16]

Carotid Duplex Ultrasound

The standard carotid duplex examination includes assessment of the carotid arteries as well as the vertebral, subclavian, and brachiocephalic arteries. Indications for this test include a bruit, transient ischemic attack (TIA), amaurosis fugax, stroke, and surveillance after revascularization.[17] The examination begins with a gray-scale survey of the extracranial carotid arteries in transverse and longitudinal views. The operator images the region from the clavicle to the angle of the jaw, in both anterolateral and posterolateral views.[18] The common carotid artery (CCA) is typically medial to the internal jugular vein, and the bifurcation is often located near the cricoid cartilage. The ICA is usually posterolateral, with a diameter at its origin greater than that of the anteromedially located external carotid artery (ECA).

Carotid artery stenosis can be focal, and flow patterns can normalize within a short distance. Therefore, the pulse-wave sample volume should be methodically advanced along the length of the vessel; color Doppler may be used for guidance in delineating areas of abnormal flow requiring change in position of the sample volume (Fig. 12-7). Representative velocity measurements should be recorded from the proximal, mid- and distal CCA. The CCA spectral waveform is a combination of the ECA and ICA waveforms, with greater diastolic flow than the ECA but less than the ICA. Atherosclerosis, when present, is usually most evident at the ICA origin, whereas fibromuscular dysplasia may be more evident distally. Using spectral Doppler, the sample volume is advanced throughout the entire ICA. At a minimum, PSV and EDV from the proximal, mid-, and distal ICA segments should be recorded. The vertebral artery is then located posterior to the carotid artery. The vertebral artery and vein lie between the spinous processes. The vertebral artery is followed as far cephalad as possible, sampling the spectral Doppler in the accessible portions of the vertebral artery.

FIGURE 12-6 Aliasing at the site of arterial stenosis. There is an abrupt change from low-velocity laminar flow **(A)** to high-velocity flow with aliasing **(B)** as velocity exceeds Nyquist limits. An echolucent (dark) plaque is evident at site of stenosis within superficial femoral artery (SFA) stent.

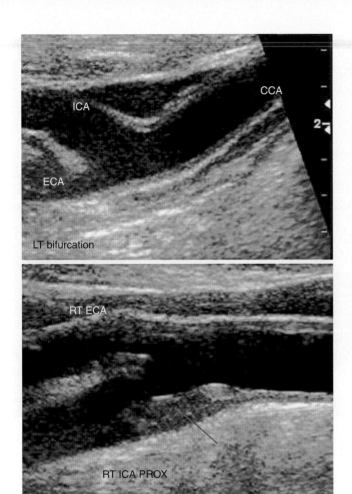

FIGURE 12-7 Gray-scale image of right and left carotid bifurcation. Internal carotid artery *(ICA)* in each is slightly wider at the origin than external carotid artery *(ECA)*. Red arrow indicates plaque in proximal right ICA. A branch is evident arising from left ECA. In the absence of identified branches, waveforms are necessary to distinguish the ICA from the ECA. CCA, common carotid artery.

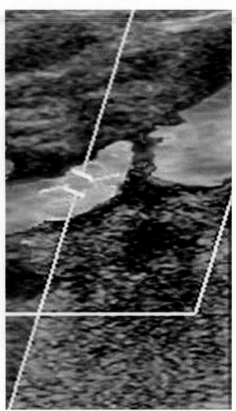

FIGURE 12-8   Color Doppler of internal carotid artery (ICA). Color Doppler is added to gray-scale picture of right ICA seen in Figure 12-7. Color aliasing identifies an area of high velocity adjacent to the plaque. This guides placement of spectral Doppler sample volume, identified by parallel white lines.

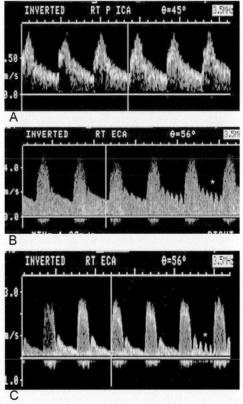

FIGURE 12-9   Spectral waveforms of internal and external carotid arteries *(ICA, ECA)* **during intermittent tapping of ipsilateral temporal artery. A,** No clear "tapping" pattern, and therefore likely ICA. **B,** High peak systolic velocity (PSV) of 400 cm/sec. Tapping *(asterisk)* clearly identified in diastolic component of waveform identifies the artery as ECA and indicates that the high PSV represents ECA stenosis. **C,** Typical ECA waveform is high resistance with low PSV and obvious tapping pattern of temporal artery during diastole.

Distinguishing between the ICA and ECA is critical to the examination (Fig. 12-8). The ECA is usually smaller, more anteromedial, and has less diastolic flow than the ICA. The ECA will also have branches in the cervical region, whereas the ICA will not. Direct comparison of the waveforms from the two vessels is critical. A velocity waveform obtained from the proximal vessel or the site of maximal velocity should be obtained while intermittently tapping on the preauricular branch of the temporal artery. The intermittent tapping is reflected clearly in the diastolic portion of the ECA waveform, but not in the ICA waveform (Fig. 12-9).

Interpretation of the spectral waveforms is based on parameters such as PSV, EDV, shape, and extent of spectral broadening[19] (Fig. 12-10). A number of criteria have been proposed, each having their own strengths and weaknesses (Table 12-1). Peak systolic velocity criteria for ICA stenosis have identified a cut point of 230 cm/sec as the threshold for detecting greater than 70% stenosis, and 125 cm/sec as the cut point for identifying greater than 50% stenosis. Criteria that include EDV use a cut point of greater than 140 cm/sec to identify greater than 80% stenosis. The ratio of peak ICA systolic velocity to mid-CCA velocity may be particularly useful in determining the presence of stenosis in the hemodynamic setting of low cardiac output or critical aortic stenosis. At a minimum, velocity criteria must distinguish less than 50% stenosis, 50% to 69% stenosis, and greater than 70% stenosis. Selection of criteria for use in an individual laboratory requires review of the published parameters and selection of those appropriate to laboratory practice. Individual vascular laboratories must validate the results of their own criteria for stenosis against a suitable standard such as arteriography.

FIGURE 12-10 Internal carotid artery (ICA) stenosis. Pulsed-wave sample volume is placed at the site of aliasing. There is marked spectral broadening. Waveform resembles that in Figure 12-9C.

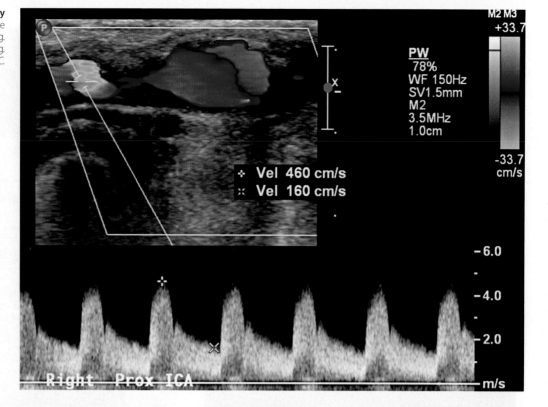

TABLE 12-1 Criteria for Internal Carotid Artery Stenosis

STENOSIS	ICA PSV	LUMEN PLAQUE	ICA/CCA PSV	ICA EDV*
0	<125	0	<2	<40
1-49	<125	+	<2	<40
50-69	>125	+	2-4	40-100
>70	>230	+	>4	>100
SUBTOTAL	VAR.	+++	VAR.	>0
TOTAL	0	+++	0	0

This table summarizes multiple criteria including PSV alone, PSV and EDV, and ICA/CCA ratio.

+, presence of plaque; CCA, common carotid artery; EDV, end-diastolic volume; ICA, internal carotid artery; PSV, peak systolic velocity; VAR, variable.

*From Grant EG, Benson CB, Moneta GL, et al: Carotid artery stenosis: gray-scale and Doppler US diagnosis—Society of Radiologists in Ultrasound Consensus Conference. Radiology 229:340, 2003.[19]

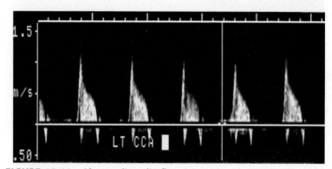

FIGURE 12-11 Absent diastolic flow in common carotid artery *(CCA)* suggesting presence of total occlusion of the ipsilateral internal carotid artery *(ICA)*.

Waveform analysis depends on evaluation of acceleration, diastolic flow, direction of flow, and comparison to the contralateral vessel. If the ICA is totally occluded, there will be absent or severely diminished diastolic flow in the ipsilateral CCA (Fig. 12-11). A delay in the upstroke suggests more proximal stenosis. For example, severe stenosis of the brachiocephalic artery will result in dampened right CCA waveforms. A step-up in systolic velocity in the cervical portion of the CCA indicates stenosis, with doubling indicating at least 50% stenosis and tripling indicating at least 75% stenosis.

Waveform evaluation is particularly valuable in the vertebral artery because the segments within the bone cannot be directly evaluated with ultrasound. Specific velocity criteria have not been developed for vertebral artery stenosis. Velocities greater than 125 cm/sec and dampened waveforms are two indicators of vertebral artery stenosis. Absent flow in the vertebral artery is confirmed when flow is detected in the vertebral vein, but not in the vertebral artery. Retrograde flow in the vertebral artery is referred to as *subclavian steal* (i.e., the subclavian circulation is stealing from the cerebral circulation). Reverse flow is confirmed

by comparing the direction of vertebral artery flow with that of the carotid artery (Fig. 12-12). Reverse flow typically will have a diminished diastolic component because flow is into the high-resistance bed of the subclavian artery (Fig. 12-13). If flow is cephalad but notching is evident in the systolic portion of the wave, subclavian steal can be elicited by reexamining flow after arm exercise or following deflation of a blood pressure cuff that had been inflated to suprasystolic pressures on the ipsilateral arm. These maneuvers will increase demand in the subclavian bed, and vertebral flow will completely reverse in the setting of subclavian stenosis proximal to the vertebral origin. The vast majority of these patients with subclavian stenosis are asymptomatic.

The subclavian artery is evaluated as close to the origin as possible. The probe is placed longitudinally above the clavicle and angled to obtain a scanning plane below the clavicle. Color Doppler surveillance is used to detect nonlaminar flow. The Doppler spectrum is obtained throughout the vessel.[20] Doubling of PSV is consistent with 50% or greater stenosis.

Plaque and Arterial Wall Characterization

Gray-scale imaging is used to evaluate carotid plaque and arterial wall characteristics. Atherosclerotic plaque is evident on ultrasound examination as material that thickens the intima and

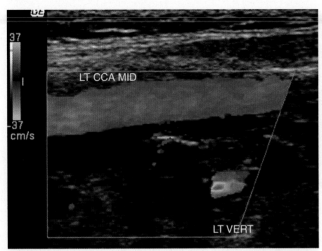

FIGURE 12-12 Color Doppler of common carotid artery *(CCA)* and vertebral arteries *(VERT)*, demonstrating flow in two different directions, antegrade carotid artery flow and retrograde vertebral artery flow.

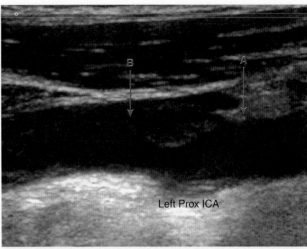

FIGURE 12-14 Gray-scale image of atherosclerotic plaque. Echolucent plaque is indicated *(arrow A)* adjacent to more echobright plaque *(arrow B)* in gray-scale image of this internal carotid artery (ICA).

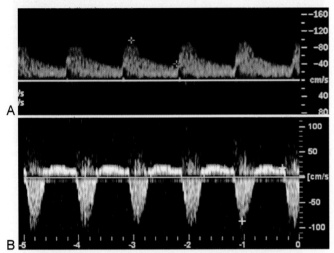

FIGURE 12-13 A, Spectral waveform of normal antegrade vertebral flow with low-resistance waveform. **B,** Reversed retrograde vertebral flow with high-resistance waveform.

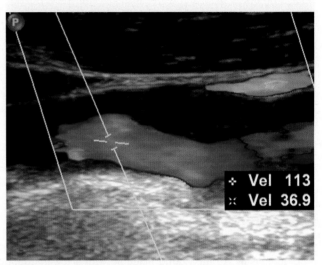

FIGURE 12-15 Duplex imaging of atherosclerotic plaque. Echolucent plaque is now clearly evident with addition of color Doppler.

protrudes into the arterial lumen. Plaque surface and echo characteristics can be determined and described. *Ulceration* refers to an excavation within the plaque containing flow. *Echolucent plaque* is characterized as plaque that is less echogenic than surrounding muscle (Fig. 12-14) and is often first detected by the presence of abnormal color flow (Fig. 12-15). The volume of plaque is appreciated best in the transverse view and with three-dimensional (3D) reconstruction.

Another potential technique to characterize plaque content and activity is contrast-enhanced ultrasound to detect ulceration and inflammation. Activated leukocytes attached to the inflamed vessel wall may bind the shells of lipid microbubbles, which are detectable by ultrasound.[21] Contrast also can be used to define the wall/lumen interface (Fig. 12-16A). Plaque thickness can be severely overestimated or underestimated in the longitudinal image, and is best evaluated in transverse images.

Ultrasound can also evaluate findings such as edema (Fig. 12-16B) and dissection of the carotid wall (Fig. 12-16C). Dissection can originate in the ICA or extend from the arch into the CCA. A flap separates the true and false lumen. The flap may be apparent on gray-scale imaging but generally requires color or contrast for elucidation. A flutter is occasionally identified in the downslope of the waveform on the affected side. Evaluation

should identify both the proximal and distal extent of dissection, and flow velocities in the true lumen.

Carotid Intima Media Thickness

Carotid ultrasonography has traditionally been used to evaluate the presence of obstructive atherosclerosis in the setting of symptomatic cerebrovascular disease or asymptomatic carotid bruit. More recently, carotid ultrasonography has been performed in epidemiological studies to detect nonobstructive plaque and intima media thickness (IMT).[22] *Intima media thickness* refers to the distance from the intima lumen interface to the media adventitia border. Protocols have measured ICA, CCA, ICA plus CCA, and carotid bulb IMT. Yield and reproducibility appear to be greatest for the far-wall CCA IMT measurement. Intima media thickness measurement is most commonly made from longitudinal images, with the assistance of semiautomated edge-detection software (Fig. 12-17). There is variability in this measurement from systole to diastole, and by age and gender. A single threshold value for abnormal IMT has not been determined. Ideally, threshold values derived from large population-based studies should be used in evaluation of IMT. Both plaque and IMT correlate with cardiovascular morbidity and mortality.[22] Indeed, the presence of carotid plaque resulting in 50% stenosis is included in the Adult Treatment Panel III guidelines as a coronary heart disease equivalent.

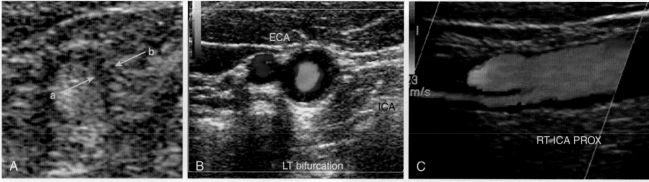

FIGURE 12-16   Arterial wall characteristics. A, Contrast is used to identify lumen/wall interface. Wall thickening is evident between intima lumen interface *(a)* and media adventitia interface *(b).* **B,** Power Doppler is used to identify lumen/wall interface. Thickened echolucent wall suggests presence of arteritis. **C,** Dissection of internal carotid artery *(ICA)* with flow evident in both true and false lumen.

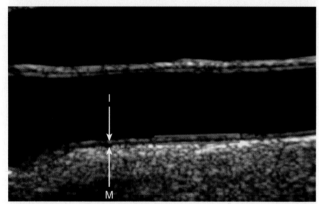

FIGURE 12-17   Intima media thickness (IMT). *I* indicates intima lumen border, and *M* indicates media adventitia border. Distance between intima lumen border and media adventitia border is determined with automated edge-detection program that averages thickness of wall over region, identified by blue lines laid over these borders.

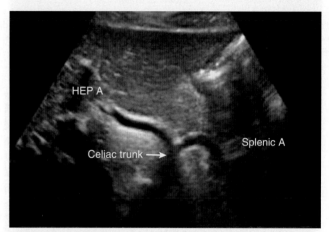

FIGURE 12-18   Transverse gray-scale image of splenic and hepatic arteries arising from celiac trunk. Celiac trunk is first branch from abdominal aorta.

Abdominal Aorta Evaluation

Abdominal ultrasound is used to diagnose and follow abdominal aortic aneurysms. An ultrasound machine with a low-frequency transducer (e.g., 2.5 MHz) is used to determine aneurysm size, shape, location (infrarenal or suprarenal), and distance from other arterial segments. The patient is required to fast prior to the study because bowel gas will obscure imaging. Aortic ultrasound scanning begins with the patient supine and the transducer placed in a subxiphoid position. The aorta is located slightly left of midline. The abdominal aorta from the diaphragm to the bifurcation is evaluated using three sonographic views: the sagittal plane (anteroposterior [AP] diameter), transverse plane (AP diameter and transverse diameters), and coronal plane (longitudinal and transverse diameters). Diameter is measured from outer wall to outer wall. If overlying bowel gas obstructs the aorta from view, patients are instructed to lie in the decubitus position, and the aorta is visualized via the coronal plane through either flank.[23] As the transducer is moved caudally, the celiac trunk will be evident branching into the common hepatic and splenic arteries (Fig. 12-18). The superior mesenteric artery (SMA) originates approximately 1 cm distal to the celiac trunk (Fig. 12-19). Next, the right renal artery may be seen emerging from the aorta and traveling under the inferior vena cava. The left renal vein then crosses over the aorta, and the left renal artery will be seen posterior to the vein. The inferior mesenteric artery (IMA) is the final branch arising from the aorta before it bifurcates into the iliac vessels. Spectral Doppler evaluation of the celiac and mesenteric vessels will demonstrate low-resistance waveforms following a meal and high resistance waveforms in the normal fasting patient (Fig. 12-20). In contrast, evaluation of the normal renal arteries always demonstrates low-resistance waveforms.

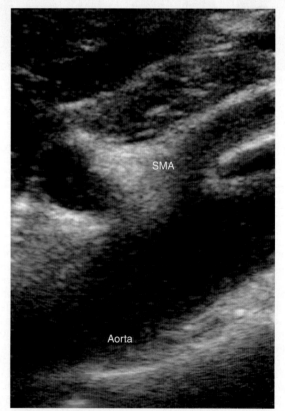

FIGURE 12-19   Longitudinal gray-scale image of aorta. Superior mesenteric artery *(SMA)* is second branch of abdominal aorta and is seen running parallel to aorta in this longitudinal image of abdominal aorta.

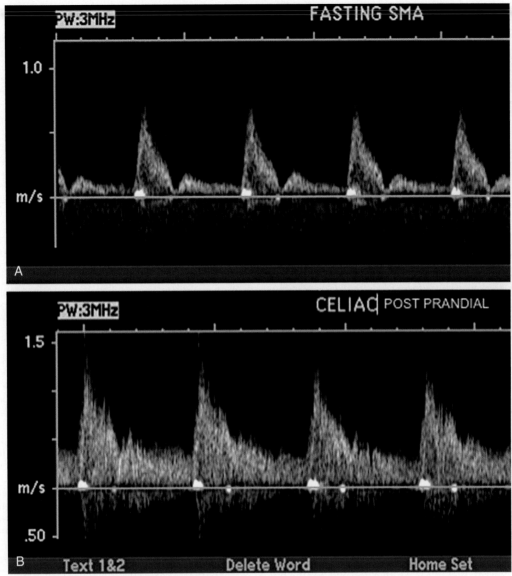

FIGURE 12-20   A, Fasting spectral waveform in superior mesenteric artery (SMA). B, Postprandial spectral waveform in celiac trunk.

An *abdominal aortic aneurysm* is defined as an aortic diameter of at least 1.5 times the adjacent normal segment, or a distal aorta diameter of greater than 3.0 cm (Fig. 12-21). Normal abdominal aortic diameters range from 1.4 to 3.0 cm.[24] The shape of the abdominal aortic aneurysm is described as *saccular, fusiform*, or

![Figure 12-21 image]

FIGURE 12-21   Gray-scale image from an abdominal aortic aneurysm screening examination. This transverse image of abdominal aorta has a maximum diameter of more than 5.6 cm, indicating aneurysm.

cylindrical. The majority of abdominal aortic aneurysms are fusiform in shape, located below the renal arteries, and involve one or both of the iliac arteries. Atherosclerotic plaque, mural thrombus, and dissection can be detected in the wall of the aneurysm.[25]

Ultrasound evaluation is also performed after endograft repair of abdominal aortic aneurysm. Flow within the graft is evaluated with longitudinal and transverse imaging. Endoleak is diagnosed when there is flow outside the graft but within the aneurysm. Dissection, pseudoaneurysm, and thrombus within the graft are other potential complications[26] that can be detected using ultrasound evaluation.

Renal Artery Duplex Ultrasonography

Atherosclerotic renal artery stenosis is recognized as a cause of hypertension and may contribute to decline in renal function (see Chapter 22). Duplex ultrasound of the renal arteries includes spectral Doppler evaluations of the aorta, the renal arteries and renal parenchyma, and B-mode determination of kidney size (also see Chapter 41). Abdominal obesity and bowel gas are barriers to adequate renal artery duplex examination.

A longitudinal view of the aorta is obtained with the patient in the supine position. The origins of the celiac artery and SMA are seen on the anterior aspect of the aorta cephalad to the renal arteries. Peak systolic velocity in the aorta is then recorded using a 60-degree Doppler angle. The probe is turned

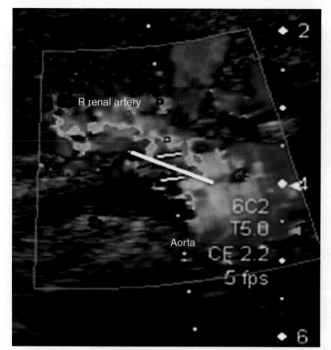

FIGURE 12-22 **Doppler image of origin of right renal artery.** Turbulent flow is evident in the renal artery origin, suggesting presence of atherosclerotic plaque and possibility of stenosis.

transverse to localize the renal arteries. The Doppler cursor is "walked" from the aorta into the ostium of the renal artery (Fig. 12-22). The right renal artery is generally seen most easily. It is followed from the origin to the hilum of the kidney. The left lateral decubitus position can also be used for examination of the right renal artery. The left renal artery is best evaluated in the right lateral decubitus position using a posterolateral transducer position. Ideally, the renal arteries are evaluated from two views to ensure that stenosis is not missed. Kidney length is measured from pole to pole with the patient in the decubitus position.

Color and spectral Doppler are obtained throughout the course of each renal artery. A low-velocity range and a low wall filter setting are used in spectral Doppler evaluations of the segmental renal arteries and hilar flow. The renal artery normally has a low-resistance waveform.[27] A 60% or more renal artery stenosis is characterized by a renal-to-aortic PSV ratio of greater than 3.5, combined with a PSV within the stenosis of greater than 200 cm/sec. Elevated EDV 150 cm/sec or more suggests 80% or greater stenosis (Fig. 12-23). The same criteria are used in native and stented renal arteries.[28] Low systolic flow, post-stenotic turbulence, and a color mosaic appearance indicate subtotal occlusion of the renal artery. Low parenchymal Doppler velocities support the diagnosis of an occluded renal artery in those cases where no flow can be detected in the renal artery. In addition, the ipsilateral kidney is often small, less than 9 cm in length. Overall sensitivity of duplex ultrasonography for renal artery stenosis is 98%, and specificity is 98% compared with arteriography.[29]

Measurement of the resistive index (RI) is used to evaluate renal parenchymal disease. Spectral Doppler waveforms are obtained from at least three regions of each kidney. The RI is calculated using the formula: $RI = [1 - (V_{min} \div V_{max})] \times 100$, where V_{min} denotes end-diastolic velocity, and V_{max} denotes peak systolic velocity. In severe renal artery stenosis where there is significant renal parenchymal disease, the EDV is often low. An RI above 0.80 suggests significant parenchymal renal disease[30] and may have implications regarding the outcome of therapy. Similarly, the PSV and EDV can be used to monitor renal transplants.[31]

Peripheral Arterial Ultrasonography

Ultrasound of the lower extremities is used to diagnose PAD in the setting of claudication, limb pain, or ulcers.[12] It is also indicated following lower-extremity revascularization and in planning therapy for known PAD. The goal of the examination is to elucidate the location and severity of limb arterial stenoses.[32] The study is tailored to individual requirements and can be limited to a given arterial segment, extended to evaluate both lower extremities in their entirety, or to evaluate the upper extremity.

Color Doppler is used initially to detect normal or abnormal flow states throughout the arterial segments or bypass grafts being evaluated.[33] Laminar flow is visible in the absence of disease (Fig. 12-24A), whereas turbulence and aliasing are present at the sites of disease. When an abnormal flow pattern is detected by color Doppler, pulsed (spectral) Doppler sampling is used to characterize the degree of stenosis. The pulse Doppler signal is acquired throughout the arterial segments. Peak systolic velocity determination and waveform analyses are the primary parameters used to quantify and localize disease. Peak systolic velocity measurements are obtained at the level of the lesion and from vascular segments proximal and distal to the lesion. Aneurysmal dilation is another etiology for abnormal color flow. Velocities will decrease as diameter doubles at the site of the aneurysm. The iliac, superficial femoral, and popliteal arteries are all sites of aneurysm (Fig. 12-25).

Peripheral arterial stenosis is categorized by pulsed-wave Doppler examination as percentage reduction of luminal diameter that is mild (0%-19%), moderate (20%-49%), or severe (≥50%).[12] With mild stenosis, there is some spectral broadening and a slight increase in PSV. With moderate stenosis, there is increased spectral broadening and a rise in PSV less than double that of the proximally sampled segment. Pulsed Doppler interrogation at the level of a severe stenosis reveals marked spectral broadening and a monophasic waveform. The waveform loses its normal diastolic reverse flow component, and flow is forward throughout the cardiac cycle. Also, the PSV is more than double the velocity measured in the proximal segment. An occlusion is present when flow is absent within an arterial segment. If there are no collateral vessels, high-resistance waveforms are present in the artery proximal to the occlusion. Antegrade diastolic flow is present in the proximal artery if there are collateral vessels. The reconstituted distal artery will have the characteristic post-stenotic *tardus et parvus waveform*. This Doppler waveform is particularly important to recognize because it signifies a proximal high-grade lesion.

Duplex ultrasound examination is accurate for diagnosing PAD. The comparison of duplex ultrasound evaluation with arteriography to detect significant stenoses in patients with symptomatic aortoiliac and femoropopliteal disease reveals high sensitivity (82%) and specificity (92%) for identifying significant stenoses.[33] Ratios of PSV between the stenosis and the proximal artery are preferred over absolute PSV measurements for classification of peripheral arterial stenosis because a wide range of absolute PSV measurements is obtained in normal and abnormal patients. There is a stronger correlation between PSV ratio and degree of stenosis than between absolute PSV and degree of stenosis. Peak systolic velocity ratios of 2 and 7 correspond to stenoses of 50% or more and 90% or more, respectively. There are conflicting data regarding precision of duplex ultrasound examination in determining stenosis severity when serial stenoses are present.

Extremity Arterial Ultrasound Following Revascularization

Ultrasound evaluation following endovascular procedures is performed to detect recurrence of stenoses at sites of intervention. The concept is similar to that for graft surveillance (i.e., early detection of lesions assists in identifying the need for reintervention

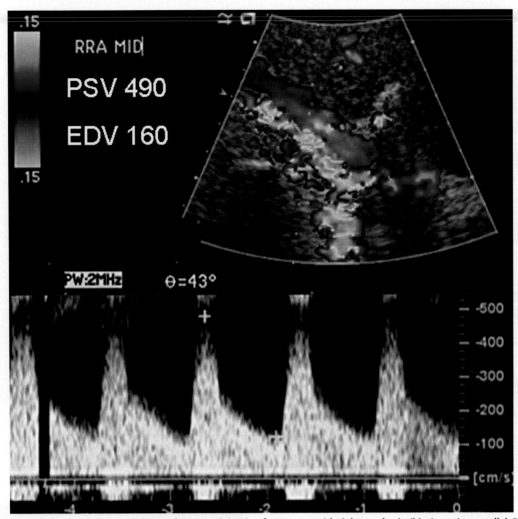

FIGURE 12-23 **Color Doppler demonstrates right renal artery originating from aorta, with right renal vein *(blue)* running parallel.** Elevated systolic and diastolic velocities in spectral Doppler are consistent with renal artery stenosis.

to maintain arterial patency).[33,34] Duplex ultrasonography is performed following the intervention, prior to discharge; 1, 3, and 6 months postintervention; then yearly. The color Doppler and pulsed-wave Doppler evaluations focus on the vessel proximal to the site of intervention, at the site of intervention, and distal to the site of intervention. Waveform analysis is used to categorize stenosis in a manner similar to that used in native vessels.[35] A doubling of PSV is consistent with hemodynamically significant stenosis (see Fig. 12-24B). Increases in velocity measurements and change in waveform shape from triphasic to monophasic on serial examinations suggest developing stenosis and warrant close-interval follow-up and consideration for revision.

Graft surveillance is extremely useful in efforts to preserve patency of peripheral arterial bypass grafts.[36] Graft failure in the first month is usually caused by technical factors. Between 1 month and 2 years postoperatively, it is often due to intimal hyperplasia. Graft failure after 2 years is likely the result of progression of atherosclerotic disease. The 5-year primary patency rate for an infrainguinal vein bypass graft ranges from 60% to 85%. Surgical revision of these stenoses identified with ultrasound surveillance improves the 5-year patency rate to 82% to 93%. By contrast, segmental pressure measurements have not proved useful to predict bypass graft thrombosis. To detect graft abnormalities before frank graft failure, standard graft surveillance protocols recommend duplex ultrasound evaluation at 1, 3, and 6 months during the first postoperative year, and 12 months thereafter.[37]

Location and type of graft are identified before performing ultrasound examination. Scanning techniques in the supine patient

are similar to native arterial examinations. Color Doppler is used initially to scan the entire graft. Color pulse repetition frequency is adjusted so focal stenoses or AVF appear as regions of aliasing, persistence, or bruit color flash artifact. Based on color Doppler findings, pulsed Doppler interrogation is used to determine the PSV. Sampling is done routinely at the proximal native artery, proximal anastomosis, throughout the graft, distal anastomosis, distal native vessel, and throughout sites of flow disturbance. These measurements are used also for serial comparison during subsequent examinations.

Pulsed Doppler is used to determine PSV ratios within the graft, similar to its use in the native arterial examination (Fig. 12-26). A segment distal (rather than proximal) to the lesion may be chosen for the ratio when there is a diameter mismatch in the graft or there are tandem lesions proximal to the flow disturbance. Doubling of the velocity ratio indicates a significant graft stenosis (>50% diameter reduction) with a sensitivity of 95% and specificity of 100%. Vein graft lesions also have been classified using PSV: (1) a minimal stenosis (<20%) has PSV ratio up to 1.4 with a PSV of less than 125 cm/sec; (2) a moderate stenosis (20%-50%) has a PSV ratio of 1.5 to 2.4 with a PSV up to 180 cm/sec; (3) a severe stenosis (50%-75%) has a PSV ratio of 2.5 to 4 with a PSV of more than 180 cm/sec; and (4) a high-grade stenosis (>75%) has a PSV ratio greater than 4 with a PSV greater than 300 cm/sec. Intervention is recommended for lesions categorized as severe or high grade.[38] Detection of low-flow velocities within the graft with pulsed Doppler suggests either proximal or distal stenosis. Low velocity flow can also be caused by large graft diameter or

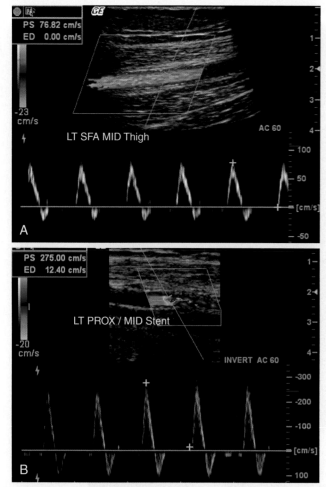

FIGURE 12-24 Duplex ultrasound of a superficial femoral artery *(SFA)* stent. **A,** Laminar flow is evident in longitudinal image of proximal stent. **B,** Color aliasing and elevated velocity are present at site of stenosis within distal SFA stent.

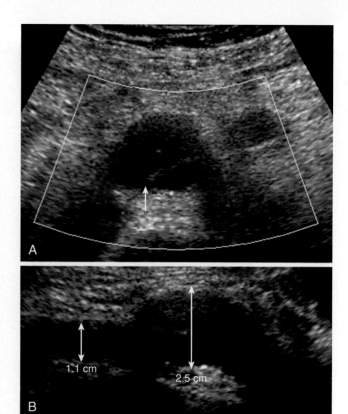

FIGURE 12-25 **A,** Transverse gray-scale image of right common iliac artery (CIA) aneurysm with dissection. Arrow indicates dissection flap. **B,** Longitudinal gray-scale image of right CIA aneurysm. Aneurysm is defined by a 1.5× or greater increase in arterial diameter compared with proximal segment. Thrombus develops in these aneurysms and can result in occlusion or distal embolization.

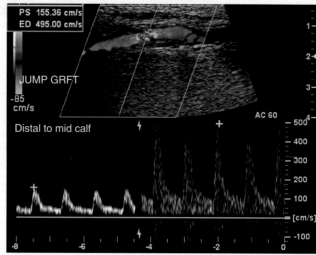

FIGURE 12-26 Duplex ultrasound of peripheral bypass graft. Proximal velocity is 155 cm/sec and increases to 495 cm/sec at site of stenosis. Aliasing of the Doppler is also evident at site of stenosis.

poor arterial inflow. Nonetheless, velocities within a functioning graft that are less than 45 cm/sec indicate that subsequent graft failure is likely to occur. Other worrisome findings are a significant decrease or increase in PSV on serial examination.

Pseudoaneurysm

A *pseudoaneurysm* is a contained arterial rupture. A hole through all layers of the arterial wall results in extravasation of blood, which is then enclosed by surrounding soft tissues.[39] Any patient who has undergone an arterial puncture for arteriography and experiences sudden pain at the access site, or is found to have pulsatile mass or a bruit on auscultation over the access site, should be evaluated for the presence of pseudoaneurysm.

Ultrasound evaluation is performed in the region of the puncture. Spectral waveforms are obtained in the native artery proximal and distal to the site of puncture, and in the femoral vein proximal and distal to the site of puncture. Color Doppler evaluation should focus on detecting an extravascular collection of flowing blood, most commonly anterior to the native artery (Fig. 12-27A-B). Posterior extravasation is less common. The neck is the connection between the native artery and the pseudoaneurysm sac. The neck is identified by a "to-and-fro" pattern of the Doppler waveform that is pathognomonic for pseudoaneurysm (Fig. 12-27C). This waveform results from systolic flow out of the native artery into the contained rupture, and diastolic flow back into the native artery. In addition to the to-and-fro signal in the neck, the segment of native artery proximal to the origin of the pseudoaneurysm may have a lower-resistance waveform when compared with that found in the artery distal to the pseudoaneurysm.

There are several options for treatment of pseudoaneurysms, including observation, surgical repair, manual compression, ultrasound-guided compression, or thrombin injection.[40] Ultrasound-guided compression is performed with visualization of the pseudoaneurysm neck while compressing until flow is absent in the neck. Pressure is applied for 20 minutes and may have to be maintained for much longer before thrombosis of the pseudoaneurysm sac is achieved. Reported success rate of compression varies from 60% to 80%. Ultrasound-guided thrombin injection is best suited for those pseudoaneurysms with a long, narrow

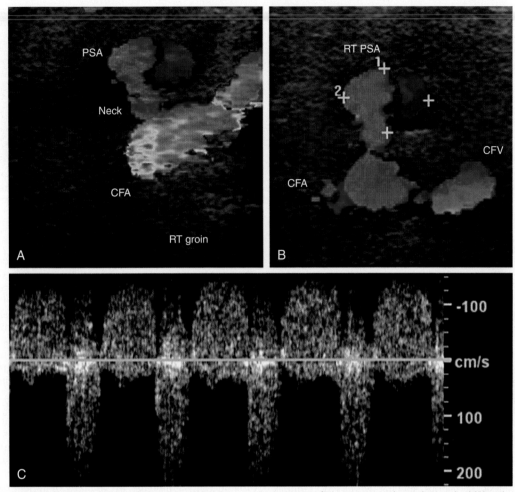

FIGURE 12-27 **Doppler evaluations of a pseudoaneurysm** *(PSA).* "Yin-yang" appearance of PSA cavity is evident in longitudinal **(A)** and transverse **(B)** images. Whereas artery lengthens in longitudinal image, the contained PSA rupture sac retains its saccular shape. **C,** Pulsed Doppler placed in neck of pseudoaneurysm demonstrates pathognomonic "to-and-fro" pattern of bidirectional flow into and out of the contained rupture.

neck.[41,42] Thrombin injection is contraindicated in those with allergy to bovine thrombin, those with overlying skin infections, in the presence of ipsilateral AVF, and in those with active limb ischemia. The injection is performed under sterile conditions using a syringe equipped with a three-way stopcock. The needle is placed into the sac while drawing back gently on the syringe. The tip of the needle is seen in the cavity, and blood return is noted. The stopcock is then switched to a position open to the thrombin, and 0.1 to 0.2 mL of thrombin are injected. The duplex ultrasound examination should include final pictures documenting thrombosis of the pseudoaneurysm and a patent artery of origin. Complications of thrombin injection include limb ischemia (if thrombin enters the native artery and causes a thrombus to form) and anaphylaxis.

Arteriovenous Fistulae

Arteriovenous fistulae occur secondary to trauma, including catheterization,[43] or are created intentionally for dialysis.[44] Duplex ultrasound findings include turbulent and pulsatile venous flow. Turbulence may result in a "color bruit" adjacent to the vein, caused by vibration of the surrounding soft tissue. Arterial flow proximal to the fistula will have a low-resistance pattern, rather than the typical high-resistance peripheral waveform (Fig. 12-28). Arterial flow distal to the fistula will have a high-resistance waveform. Venous flow pattern at the connection will resemble an arterial waveform.

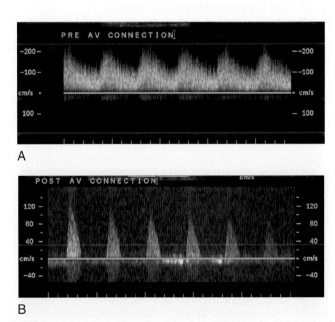

FIGURE 12-28 **Spectral Doppler evaluation of peripheral artery proximal (A) and distal (B) to an arteriovenous** *(AV)* **connection.** Low-resistance pattern in **A** occurs because artery is flowing into high-capacitance venous bed.

The actual arteriovenous connection may be too small to be seen in postcatheterization AVF.

Evaluation of dialysis fistulae use specific criteria for the Doppler spectra obtained from arterial inflow and venous outflow.[45,46] Peak systolic velocity is recorded throughout the native system and the graft. The arterial limb should demonstrate high velocities and continuous forward flow with a low-resistance waveform. The venous limb is expected to have slightly lower velocities. The normal PSV at the anastomosis is 300 cm/sec. The normal outflow vein has a PSV greater than 180 cm/sec and appears distended. Peak systolic velocity less than 150 cm/sec indicates a fistula in jeopardy of failure. The fistula may result in arterial steal from the distal circulation. If this is suspected, direction of distal flow should be evaluated before and after compression of the AVF.

Venous Duplex Ultrasound

Duplex examination of the extremity veins enables accurate noninvasive evaluation for deep vein thrombosis (DVT).[47] Normal veins have thin walls and an echo-free lumen. The vein lumen can be obliterated (compressed) with a small amount of extrinsic pressure (Fig. 12-29). The walls do not co-apt, however, when the lumen contains thrombus, even when enough pressure is applied to distort the shape of an adjacent artery. Vein compressibility is best tested in an image plane transverse to the vein axis. Veins are characterized by anatomical location as deep or superficial, and as proximal or distal. The major veins of the thigh and arm are larger in diameter than the corresponding arteries. Extremity veins have valves that permit only cephalad flow, and these increase in number from proximal to distal. Valve sinuses are widened areas of the lumen that accommodate the valve cusps.

Doppler evaluation of flow in normal veins has four important characteristics: (1) respirophasic variation, (2) augmentation with distal compression, (3) unidirectional flow toward the heart, (4) and abrogation of flow in the lower extremities by the Valsalva maneuver. Complete analysis of venous spectral waveforms requires comparison of the waveforms from both right and left limbs. Presence of a flattened, unvarying waveform (loss of respirophasic variation in flow) on one side compared with the other suggests the presence of more proximal obstruction of venous return proximal to the site of the Doppler interrogation.

Neck and Upper-Extremity Venous Duplex Ultrasound

Neck and upper-extremity duplex evaluation includes assessments of the internal jugular, subclavian, axillary, brachial, cephalic, and basilic veins.[48] The innominate veins and the superior vena cava cannot be evaluated with duplex ultrasound because of their location within the bony thorax. Examination begins with evaluation of the internal jugular (Fig. 12-30) and subclavian veins. The subclavian vein can be imaged from a supraclavicular or

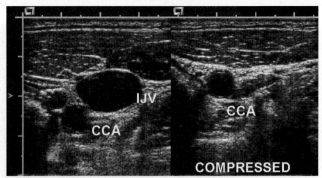

FIGURE 12-30 Transverse gray-scale imaging of internal jugular vein *(IJV)* and common carotid artery *(CCA)* without compression *(left)* and with gentle compression *(right)* obliterating vein lumen.

subclavicular approach. The arm is extended in a comfortable position for the evaluation of the axillary vein, paired brachial veins, basilic vein (medial), and cephalic vein (lateral). Examination includes color and spectral Doppler evaluation of flow in all these veins. Loss of respirophasic variation in the waveform in the subclavian or axillary veins suggests the presence of more proximal venous obstruction (due to thrombosis or extrinsic compression) (Fig. 12-31). The subclavian vein cannot be compressed where it lies directly below the clavicle, and venous thrombosis is suspected when flow is absent or echogenic material is seen within the lumen.

Loss of compressibility is the pathognomonic feature of venous thrombosis. As the thrombus progresses from acute to chronic, there is increased echogenicity of the thrombus and decreased diameter of the vein. Over time, collateral veins may develop and recanalization may occur in the thrombosed vessel. In the upper arm, both superficial and deep venous systems have a significant role in venous drainage. The majority of upper-extremity DVTs are secondary to indwelling venous catheters, pacemaker leads, or hypercoagulability. Primary upper-extremity DVT is a rare disorder that is idiopathic, attributed to effort thrombosis (Paget-Schrötter's syndrome), or related to thoracic outlet obstruction.[49] An unusual etiology of noncompressible veins is intravascular tumor. This is suspected when the echogenic material within the lumen appears to extend through the vessel wall and may contain arterial flow signals.

Lower-Extremity Venous Duplex Ultrasound

The venous ultrasound examination to evaluate the presence or absence of leg DVT begins at the inguinal ligament with identification of the common femoral vein and extends to the calf.[50] The proximal deep veins evaluated include the common femoral, femoral (previously known as *superficial femoral*), and popliteal veins. The deep calf veins include posterior tibial, peroneal, gastrocnemius (sural), and soleal veins. Special attention is given

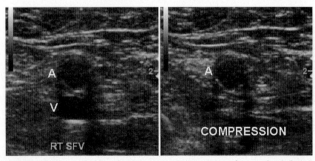

FIGURE 12-29 *Left,* Transverse gray-scale imaging of superficial femoral artery (SFA) *(A)* and vein *(V). Right,* With gentle compression, artery is unchanged and vein is obliterated.

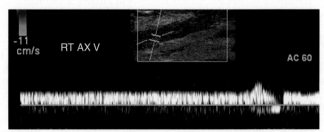

FIGURE 12-31 Spectral Doppler evaluation of axillary vein *(AX)* demonstrating loss of phasic variation in flow with respiration. This finding suggests more proximal venous obstruction. Increase in flow on right results from compression of forearm (augmenting venous return).

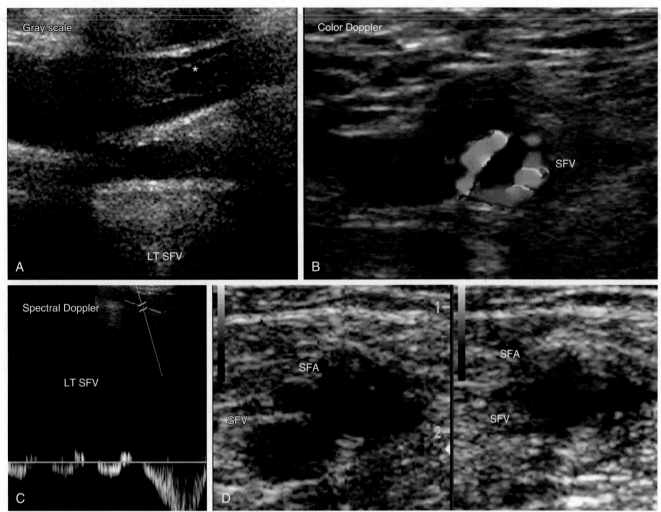

FIGURE 12-32 **Ultrasound evaluation of femoral vein thrombosis. A,** Gray-scale imaging with echogenic material *(asterisk)* seen within lumen of superficial femoral vein *(SFV)*. **B,** Doppler in SFV shows a flow void within lumen. **C,** Spectral Doppler demonstrates diminished flow with respirophasic variation. **D,** Superficial femoral artery *(SFA)* and SFV without *(left)* and with *(right)* compression; vein is only partially obliterated due to thrombus.

to the saphenofemoral and saphenopopliteal junctions because thrombus in the superficial veins of these regions deserve more aggressive treatment than thrombus limited to other parts of the superficial venous system. Examination includes color and spectral Doppler evaluation of flow in all these veins [51,52] (Fig. 12-32). Loss of respirophasic variation in the waveform of the common femoral vein suggests presence of obstruction proximal to the site of Doppler interrogation that is preventing venous return. Augmentation of flow with calf compression is not prevented by proximal venous obstruction. Proximal obstruction may be caused by extrinsic compression or venous thrombosis.

Bright-mode transverse images are used to determine compressibility along the entire course of the veins examined. Normally the vein walls fully coapt with gentle pressure. Lack of compressibility, which occurs because of a thrombosis in the vein, is the most reliable finding for determining venous thrombosis. With acute thrombosis, there is low echogenicity of the intraluminal thrombus, and the vein is dilated. As the thrombus ages, it becomes more echogenic and less central within the lumen. Vein diameter decreases as the thrombus retracts. Recanalization occurs, and flow can be detected by pulsed or color Doppler. The thrombus often appears eccentric and adjacent to the vein wall. When image quality is poor because of significant soft-tissue edema, it is not possible to exclude the presence of small nonocclusive thrombi. Sensitivity for detection of common femoral vein thrombosis is 91%, and for both the femoral and popliteal veins is 94%.

Duplex ultrasound is accurate for diagnosing deep calf vein thrombosis in symptomatic patients, so long as the calf veins

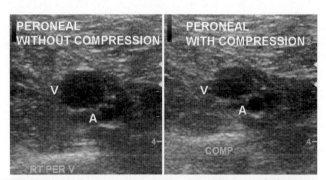

FIGURE 12-33 **Transverse gray-scale imaging of peroneal (deep) veins of calf.** Vein appears dilated in noncompression image on left. Vein lumen is not obliterated by gentle compression, indicating presence of calf vein thrombosis. A, artery; V, vein.

can be seen clearly (Fig. 12-33). When compared with angiography, sensitivity of compression ultrasound for deep calf vein thrombosis is 94% and specificity is 100%. Small calf veins cannot be visualized well in all patients. However, specificity and positive predictive value are high even when individuals with poor calf vein images are included in the evaluation. Thus, the diagnosis of DVT is made when calf veins are seen and cannot be compressed.

Lower-extremity venous ultrasound testing is often ordered when a patient is undergoing evaluation for pulmonary embolism (PE).

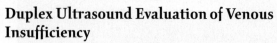

This test will provide information about presence or absence of venous thrombosis, but will not determine whether or not someone has had a PE.

Duplex Ultrasound Evaluation of Venous Insufficiency

Use of duplex ultrasound has been extended to detect reflux or obstruction and determine the anatomical extent of venous disease in patients with chronic venous insufficiency.[53] This development has been facilitated by color Doppler imaging to provide instant determination of the direction of blood flow. A 4- to 7-MHz linear array transducer is used. The saphenofemoral junction is examined first with the patient standing, and then in the supine reverse-Trendelenburg position. Compressibility is determined in transverse views of the veins. A longitudinal view of the saphenofemoral junction is then obtained.

One of two maneuvers can be used to elicit reflux. The first is the Valsalva maneuver. Intraabdominal pressure increases as the patient bears down, and venous outflow from the legs decreases. Venous return from the legs increases with release of the maneuver.[54] The second is thigh cuff inflation and deflation. Venous return is stopped with inflation of a cuff, typically to a level approximating arterial diastolic pressure. There is a transient increase in venous return that accompanies cuff deflation. Color flow is evaluated before and after one of these two maneuvers to elicit reflux. Baseline antegrade flow is displayed by blue color Doppler. Red color after the maneuver indicates retrograde flow. Reflux is present if red color persists for more than 0.5 seconds after either maneuver. Spectral Doppler can also be used to evaluate reflux. The Doppler cursor is placed midstream with an angle of 60 degrees with respect to the wall. Reverse flow over 0.5 seconds in duration is consistent with reflux (Fig. 12-34). Ideally, the remainder of the examination is performed with the patient standing with the weight on the leg not being examined.

The extent of reflux can be determined by repeating this assessment throughout the deep and superficial veins of the leg. For evaluation of the small saphenous and popliteal veins, the patient sits on the edge of the examination table with his/her foot resting on a stool. The probe is placed over the popliteal fossa. The gastrocnemius veins can be seen between the popliteal (which is deep) and small saphenous (which is superficial) vein. Compressibility and reflux following a Valsalva maneuver are determined in these veins. The posterior tibial and peroneal veins are assessed for reflux using the posteromedial and anterolateral views.

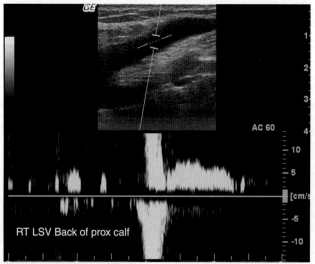

FIGURE 12-34 Spectral Doppler of venous insufficiency. Lesser saphenous vein is imaged at saphenopopliteal junction. Spectral Doppler demonstrates prolonged retrograde flow at this site.

Perforating veins are vessels connecting superficial and deep veins. Incompetent perforating veins are identified by sliding the transducer up and down dilated superficial varicose veins.[55] Color Doppler is then used while distal compression of the superficial vein is performed. The presence of different colors during compression and release indicates that the direction of venous flow changes with compression and relief. This finding is diagnostic of reflux in the perforator veins.

Plethysmographic Evaluation of Venous Reflux

Duplex ultrasound identifies reflux in individual veins, and plethysmographic methods evaluate the volume of venous reflux in the limb.[56] Air or strain gauge plethysmography is a simple screening test that has the potential to provide a complete analysis of venous hemodynamics (also see Chapter 55). The air chamber is filled with air to 6 mmHg and connected to a pressure transducer and recorder. Changes in the volume of the leg as a result of emptying or filling veins produce changes in the pressure of the air chamber. Recordings are made with the patient supine, and the leg elevated at a 45-degree angle. The patient then stands with the leg flexed slightly and bearing weight on the nonstudy leg. Venous filling time and venous volume are determined. The time until the volume plateaus after the raised limb is dropped is the venous filling time. Venous volumes of 80 to 150 mL are normal. The venous filling index (VFI) correlates best with the clinical severity of reflux.

$$VFI = .90 \, (\text{venous volume}) \div .9 \, (\text{venous filling time})$$

Values less than 2 mL/sec indicate the absence of significant reflux, whereas values over 10 mL/sec indicate high risks of edema, skin changes, and ulceration.[57]

Post-exercise plethysmography can be used to evaluate the ejecting capacity of the calf muscle pump. Venous volume is measured at rest, and again post-exercise. Rest volume minus post-exercise volume equals ejected volume. Ejection fraction is the ejected volume/rest volume × 100. Calf ejection fractions below 40% indicate patients most likely to benefit from deep vein reconstruction.

Vascular Laboratory Accreditation

Laboratory accreditation is obtained through organizations such as the Intersocietal Commission for the Accreditation of Vascular Laboratories (www.icavl.org) and the American College of Radiology (www.acr.org). The accreditation process reviews the educational credentials of the interpreting physicians and sonographers, as well as laboratory procedures. It provides excellent standards for setting up examination protocols and quality assurance programs.

REFERENCES

1. Boyajian RA, Otis SM: Integration and added value of the modern noninvasive vascular laboratory in vascular diseases management, *J Neuroimaging* 12:148, 2002.
2. Kupinski AM: Segmental pressure measurement and plethysmography, *J Vasc Technol* 26:32–38, 2002.
3. Rooke TW, Hirsch AT, Misra S et al: 2011 ACCF/AHA Focused Update of the Guideline for the Management of patients with peripheral artery disease (Updating the 2005 Guideline): a report of the American College of Cardiology Foundation/American Heart Association Task Force on practice guidelines. *Circulation* 124:2020–2045, 2011.
4. Aboyans V, Criqui M, Abraham P, et al: The measurement and interpretation of the ankle brachial index, *Circulation* In press.
5. Carter SA, Tate RB: The value of toe pulse waves in determination of risks for limb amputation and death in patients with peripheral arterial disease and skin ulcers or gangrene, *J Vasc Surg* 33:708–714, 2001.
6. Stein R, Hrilajac I, Halperin J, et al: Limitation of resting ankle brachial index in symptomatic patients with peripheral artery disease, *Vasc Med* 11:29–33, 2006.
7. Anderson CA: Noninvasive assessment of lower extremity hemodynamics in individuals with diabetes mellitus, *J Vasc Surg* 128:77S, 2010.
8. Feldman MK, Katyal S, Blackwood MS: US artifacts, *Radiographics* 4:1179–1189, 2009.
9. Grenier N, Basseau F, Rey MC, et al: Interpretation of Doppler signals, *Eur Radiol* 8:1295–1307, 2001.

10. Logason K, Barlin T, Jonsson M, et al: The importance of Doppler angle of insonation on differentiation between 50-69% and 70-99% carotid artery stenosis, *Eur J Endovasc Surg* 21:311, 2001.

11. Wood MM, Romine LE, Richman KM, et al: Spectral Doppler signature waveforms in ultrasonography: a review of normal and abnormal waveforms, *Ultrasound Q* 26:83–99, 2010.

12. Pellerito JS: Current approach to peripheral arterial sonography, *Radiol Clin North Am* 39:553–567, 2001.

13. Needham TN: Review of pressure and flow in the arterial system, 26:27, 2002.

14. Phillips GW: Review of vascular ultrasound, *World J Surg* 24:232–248, 2000.

15. Rubin JM: Power Doppler, *Eur J Radiol* 9:318S–322S, 1999.

16. Bokor D: Diagnostic efficacy of SonoVue, *Am J Cardiol* 86:19G–24G, 2000.

17. Brott TG, Halperin JL, Abbara S, et al: 2011 ASA/ACCF/AHA/AANN/AANS /ACR/ASNR/CNS/ SAIP/SCAI/SIR/SNIS/SVM/SVS guideline on the management of patients with extracranial carotid and vertebral artery disease: a report of the American College of Cardiology Foundation/American Heart Association Task Force on Practice Guidelines, and the American Stroke Association, American Association of Neuroscience Nurses, American Association of Neurological Surgeons, American College of Radiology, American Society of Neuroradiology, Congress of Neurological Surgeons, Society of Atherosclerosis Imaging and Prevention, Society for Cardiovascular Angiography and Interventions, Society of Interventional Radiology, Society of NeuroInterventional Surgery, Society for Vascular Medicine, and Society for Vascular Surgery, *Stroke* 42:e420–e463, 2011.

18. Gerhard-Herman M, Gardin JM, Jaff M, et al: Guidelines for noninvasive vascular laboratory testing. American Society of Echocardiography; Society for Vascular Medicine and Biology, *Vasc Med* 11:183–200, 2006.

19. Grant EG, Benson CB, Moneta GL, et al: Carotid artery stenosis: gray-scale and Doppler US diagnosis—Society of Radiologists in Ultrasound Consensus Conference, *Radiology* 229:340, 2003.

20. Ochoa VM, Yeghezarians Y: Subclavian artery stenosis: a review for the vascular medicine practitioner, *Vasc Med* 16:29–34, 2011.

21. Staub D, Schinkel AF, Coll B, et al: Contrast-enhanced ultrasound imaging of the vasa vasorum: from early atherosclerosis to the identification of unstable plaques, *J Am Coll Cardiol Cardiovasc Imaging* 3:761–771, 2010.

22. Polak JF, Pencina MJ, Pencina KM, et al: Carotid-wall intima-media thickness and cardiovascular events, *N Engl J Med* 365:213–221, 2011.

23. Hirsch AT, Haskal ZJ, Hertzer NR, et al: ACC/AHA 2005 Practice Guidelines for the management of patients with peripheral arterial disease (lower extremity, renal, mesenteric, and abdominal aortic): a collaborative report from the American Association for Vascular Surgery/Society for Vascular Surgery, Society for Cardiovascular Angiography and Interventions, Society for Vascular Medicine and Biology, Society of Interventional Radiology, and the ACC/AHA Task Force on Practice Guidelines (Writing Committee to Develop Guidelines for the Management of Patients With Peripheral Arterial Disease): endorsed by the American Association of Cardiovascular and Pulmonary Rehabilitation; National Heart, Lung, and Blood Institute; Society for Vascular Nursing; TransAtlantic Inter-Society Consensus; and Vascular Disease Foundation, *Circulation* 113:e463–e654, 2006.

24. Beales L, Wolstenholme S, Evans JA, et al: Reproducibility of ultrasound measurement of the abdominal aorta, *Br J Surg* 98:1517–1525, 2011.

25. Hong H, Yang Y, Liu B, et al: Imaging of the abdominal aortic aneurysm: the present and the future, *Curr Vasc Pharmacol* 8:808–819, 2010.

26. Cao P, De Rango P, Verzini F, et al: Endoleak after endovascular aortic repair: classification, diagnosis and management, *J Cardiovasc Surg (Torino)* 51:53–69, 2010.

27. Hedayati N, Del Pizzo DJ, Harris SE, et al: Predictors of diagnostic success with renal artery duplex sonography, *Ann Vasc Surg* 25:515–519, 2011.

28. Fleming SH, Davis RP, Cravens TE, et al: Accuracy of duplex sonography scans after renal artery stenting, *J Vasc Surg* 52:953–957, 2010.

29. Ciccone MM, Cortese F, Fiorella S, et al: The clinical role of contrast enhanced ultrasound in the evaluation of renal artery stenosis and diagnosis compared to traditional echo color Doppler flow imaging, *Int Angiol* 30:135–139, 2011.

30. Radermacher J, Chavan A, Bleck J, et al: Use of Doppler ultrasonography to predict the outcome of therapy for renal-artery stenosis, *N Engl J Med* 344:410, 2001.

31. Gao J, Rubin JM, Xiang DY, et al: Doppler parameters in renal transplant dysfunction, *J Ultrasound Med* 30:169–175, 2011.

32. Collins R, Cranny G, Burch J, et al: A systematic review of duplex ultrasound, magnetic resonance angiography and computed tomography angiography for the diagnosis and assessment of symptomatic, lower limb peripheral arterial disease, *Health Technol Assess* 11:1–184, 2007.

33. Begelman S, Jaff M: Noninvasive diagnostic strategies for peripheral arterial disease, *Cleve Clin J Med* 73:22–29, 2006.

34. Roth SM, Bandyk DF: Duplex imaging of lower extremity bypasses, angioplasties and stents, *Semin Vasc Surg* 12:275–284, 1999.

35. Shrikhande GV, Graham AR, Aparjita R, et al: Determining criteria for predicting stenosis with ultrasound duplex after endovascular intervention in infrainguinal lesions, *Ann Vasc Surg* 25:454–460, 2011.

36. Slim H, Tiwari A, Ritter JC, et al: Outcome of infrainguinal bypass grafts using vein conduit less than 3 mm in diameter in critical limb ischemia, *J Vasc Surg* 53:421–425, 2011.

37. Tinder CN, Bandyk DF: Detection of imminent graft occlusion: what is the optimal surveillance program? *Semin Vasc Surg* 22:252–260, 2009.

38. Tinder CN, Chavapun JP, Bandyk DF, et al: Efficacy of duplex ultrasound surveillance after infrainguinal vein bypass may be enhanced by identification of characteristics predicting stenosis development, *J Vasc Surg* 43:613–618, 2008.

39. Kapoor BS, Haddad HL, Saddekni S, et al: Diagnosis and treatment of pseudoaneurysms, *Curr Probl Diagn Radiol* 38:170–188, 2009.

40. Kang SS, Labropoulos N, Mansour MA, et al: Expanded indications for ultrasound-guided thrombin injection of pseudoaneurysms, *J Vasc Surg* 31:289, 2000.

41. Mohler ER III, Mitchell ME, Carpenter JP, et al: Therapeutic thrombin injection of pseudoaneurysms: a multicenter experience, *Vasc Med* 6:241, 2001.

42. La Perna L, Olin JW, Goines D, et al: Ultrasound-guided thrombin injection for the treatment of postcatheterization pseudo-aneurysms, *Circulation* 102:2391, 2000.

43. Seay T, Soares G, Dawson D: Postcatheterization arteriovenous fistula: CT, ultrasound and arteriographic findings, *Emerg Radiol* 9:269–299, 2002.

44. Rose SC: Noninvasive vascular laboratory for evaluation of peripheral arterial occlusive disease. Part III—clinical applications: nonatherosclerotic lower extremity arterial conditions and upper extremity arterial disease, *J Vasc Interv Radiol* 12:11, 2001.

45. Polkinghorne KR, McMahon LP, Becker GJ: Pharmacokinetic studies of dalteparin (Fragmin), enoxaparin (Clexane), and danaparoid sodium (Orgaran) in stable chronic hemodialysis patients, *Am J Kidney Dis* 40:990, 2002.

46. Gonzalez SB, Busquets JC, Figueiras RG, et al: Imaging arteriovenous fistulas, *AJR Am J Roentgenol* 31:1425–1433, 2009.

47. Tan M, van Rooden CJ, Westerbeek RE, et al: Diagnostic management of clinically suspected acute deep vein thrombosis, *Br J Haematol* 146:347–360, 2009.

48. Kucher N: Clinical practice: deep vein thrombosis of the upper extremities, *N Engl J Med* 3:861–869, 2011.

49. Joffe HV, Goldhaber SZ: Upper-extremity deep vein thrombosis, *Circulation* 106:1874, 2002.

50. Bounameaux H, Perrier A, Righini M: Diagnosis of venous thromboembolism: an update, *Vasc Med* 15:399–406, 2010.

51. Vogel P, Laing FC, Jeffrey RB Jr, et al: Deep venous thrombosis of the lower extremity: US evaluation, *Radiology* 163:747, 1987.

52. Elliot CG, Lovelace TD, Brown LM, et al: Diagnosis: imaging techniques, *Clin Chest Med* 4:641–657, 2010.

53. Kalodiki E, Nicolaides AN: Out of a recent CVI consensus: some features of a basic statement, *Int Angiol* 21:2, 2002.

54. Min RJ, Khilnani NM, Golia P: Duplex ultrasound evaluation of lower extremity venous insufficiency, *J Vasc Interv Radiol* 14:1233–1241, 2000.

55. Stuart WP, Adam DJ, Allan PL, et al: The relationship between the number, competence, and diameter of medial calf perforating veins and the clinical status in healthy subjects and patients with lower-limb venous disease, *J Vasc Surg* 32:138–143, 2000.

56. Miyazaki K, Nishibe T, Kudo F, et al: Hemodynamic changes in stripping operation or saphenofemoral ligation of the greater saphenous vein for primary varicose veins, *Ann Vasc Surg* 18:465–469, 2004.

57. Nicolaides AN: Investigation of chronic venous insufficiency: a consensus statement. Cardiovascular Disease Educational and Research Trust; European Society of Vascular Surgery; The International Angiology Scientific Activity Congress Organization; International Union of Angiology; Union Internationale de Phlebologie at the Abbaye des Vaux de Cernay, *Circulation* 102:E126–E163, 2000.

CHAPTER 13

Magnetic Resonance Imaging

Cihan Duran, Piotr S. Sobieszczyk, Frank J. Rybicki

Magnetic resonance angiography (MRA) is widely accepted for the majority of vascular imaging applications and is the modality of choice for many of them, particularly peripheral and renal arteriography.[1-3] Gadolinium-based contrast-enhanced (CE) MRA yields high-quality spatial resolution images with relatively short acquisition times. Detailed comparison with other imaging technologies is beyond the scope of this chapter, but general advantages and disadvantages appear in Table 13-1. These become important for many applications such as aortography, where multiple modalities (e.g., computed tomography [CT] and MRA) are routinely diagnostic and capable of providing images for planning most interventions.

Basic Principles

Magnetic resonance imaging (MRI) relies upon the inherent magnetic properties of human tissue and the ability to use these properties to produce tissue contrast. Magnetic resonance imaging detects the magnetic moment created by single protons in omnipresent hydrogen atoms. Because any moving electric charge produces a magnetic field, spinning protons produce small magnetic fields and can be thought of as little magnets or "spins." When a patient is placed in the bore of a large magnet (i.e., MRI scanner), hydrogen protons align with the externally applied static magnetic field (B_0) to create a net magnetization vector. On a quantum level, most protons will distribute randomly, either with or against the scanner's B_0. However, a slight excess of spins aligns with the field, causing net tissue magnetization. The time required for this alignment is denoted by the longitudinal relaxation time, T1. T1 variations between tissues is used to provide contrast.

Spinning protons wobble or "precess" about the axis of B_0. The frequency of the wobble is proportional to the strength of B_0. If a radiofrequency (RF) pulse is applied at the resonance frequency of the wobble, protons can absorb energy and jump to a higher energy state. This RF pulse deflects the protons, creating a new net magnetization vector distinct from the major axis of the applied magnetic field. The net magnetization vector tips from the longitudinal to the transverse plane (transverse magnetization). The protons are "flipped" by the RF pulse, and the net magnetization vector is defined by a "flip angle." The stronger the RF pulse applied, the greater the angle of deflection for the magnetization. Common flip angles for spin echo are 90° and 180°. For gradient echo (GRE) MRI, flip angles typically range between 10° and 70°. After the RF pulse tips the spinning protons out of alignment with the main magnetic field, new protons begin to align with the main magnetic field at a rate determined by the T1 relaxation time.

Energy is given off as the spins move from high to low energy states. The absorbed RF energy is retransmitted at the resonance frequency and can be detected with RF antennas or "coils" placed around the patient. These signals are compiled, and after mathematical processes become the MR images. Proton excitation with an externally applied RF field is repeated at short intervals to obtain signals. This MR parameter is referred to as *repetition time* (TR). For conventional MRI, TR is typically 0.5 to 2 seconds, whereas for MRA, TR ranges from 30 to less than 5 milliseconds. When the spins are tipped to the transverse plane, they all precess in phase. The speed of wobbling depends on the strength of the magnetic field each proton experiences. Some protons spin faster while others spin slower, and they quickly get out of phase relative to one another. Throughout the dephasing process, the MR signal decays. This loss of phase is termed *T2 relaxation time* or *transverse relaxation*. T2, like T1, is unique among tissues and is used for image contrast. In addition to the intrinsic T2 of tissue, inhomogeneity of B_0 results in rapid loss of transverse magnetization. The relaxation time that reflects the sum of these random defects with tissue T2 is called *T2**. To obtain an MRI signal, these spins must be brought back in phase and produce a signal or echo. The time at which it happens is referred to as *echo time* (TE). In spin echo imaging technique, the echo is obtained by using a refocusing 180° RF pulse, after which the spins begin to dephase. Another 180° RF pulse can be applied to generate a second echo and so on. Signal loss at longer echo times reflects tissue T2. In GRE imaging, the echo is obtained by gradient reversal rather than RF pulse. Because this includes effects from tissue homogeneity, TE-dependent signal loss reflects T2*. Recently, GRE sequences (balanced GRE steady-state free precession [SSFP]) have been developed that are insensitive to magnet field inhomogeneities and reflective of actual tissue T2.

Longitudinal and transverse magnetizations occur simultaneously but are two different processes that reflect properties of various tissues in the body. Since T1 measures signal recovery, tissues with short T1 are bright, whereas tissues with long T1 are dark. Fat has a very short T1. In contrast, T2 is a measure of signal loss. Therefore, tissues with short T2 are dark, and those with long T2 are bright. Simple fluids, such as cerebrospinal fluid and urine, have long T2. To differentiate between the tissues based on these relaxation times, MR images can be designed to be T1-weighted, T2-weighted, or proton-density weighted. Exogenous contrast such as gadolinium-based agents are routinely used to alter tissue conspicuity. Spatial encoding of signals obtained from tissues is required for imaging. Additional external time-varying magnetic fields are applied to spatially encode the MR signal. Spatially dependent gradients are used to locate the MR signal in space. In two-dimensional (2D) MRI, these are slice-selection, frequency-encoding, and phase-encoding gradients. In three-dimensional (3D) MRI, the slice-selection gradient is replaced by a second phase-encoding gradient.

Magnetic resonance echoes are digitized and stored in "k-space" composed of either two axes (for 2D imaging) or three axes (for 3D imaging). K-space represents frequency data and is related to image space by Fourier transformation. An important feature of k-space is that tissue contrast is determined by the center of k-space (central phase encoding lines), whereas the periphery of the k-space encodes the image detail. The order in which k-space lines are collected can be varied, strongly influencing tissue contrast. For example, in CE-MRA, the central contrast-defining portion of k-space may be acquired early in the scan (centric acquisition) during peak intraarterial contrast concentration to maximize arterial contrast. In addition to simple line-by-line k-space acquisition schemes, more complex schemes have been described. In spiral imaging, data acquisition begins at the center of k-space and spirals to the periphery. Slice-selective gradients applied along the z-axis will form axial images. Those along the y-axis will yield coronal images, and the x-axis gradients will provide sagittal images. An oblique slice can be selected by a combination of two or more gradients.

Magnetic Resonance Angiography Techniques

Magnetic resonance imaging relies on selective imaging of moving blood where signals from blood vessels are maximized, whereas signals from the stationary tissues are suppressed. Algorithms then enable reformatted images similar to those found in conventional x-ray angiography (Table 13-2).

Magnetic resonance angiography methods can depict blood as either black or white. For those "black-blood" methods that use standard spin echo (SE) sequences (Fig. 13-1A), the excitation RF pulse is applied at 90° and followed by a refocusing pulse at 180°. If the imaging slice cuts across a vessel, then depending on the flow

TABLE 13-1   Advantages and Disadvantages of Vascular Imaging Methods

METHOD	ADVANTAGES	DISADVANTAGES
MR	No ionizing radiation	Expensive hardware Acquisition requires technical expertise
CE	High signal from gadolinium-based agents Less nephrotoxic than comparable iodine-based imaging (CT)	Nephrogenic systemic fibrosis can occur rarely in patients with severe renal insufficiency
Non-contrast	Eliminates toxicity concern	Longer acquisition times compared to CE protocol Increased risk of artifacts that are largely mitigated with CE-MRA
CT	Rapid, high signal, high-quality image acquisition Less technical expertise required compared to MR	Ionizing radiation Nephrotoxicity of iodine
DSA	Intervention can be performed at time of diagnosis Highest spatial resolution	Invasive Nephrotoxicity of iodine Projectional data may be inferior to volumetric acquisitions (CT, MR) that can be viewed in any plane
Sonography	No ionizing radiation Less expensive Flow information readily obtained Portable	Better for superficial imaging Limited by artifacts from bone, air, and sonographic interfaces Lower CNR, SNR compared to CT and MRI Operator-dependent

CE, contrast-enhanced; CNR, contrast-to-noise ratio; CT, computed tomography; DSA, digital subtraction angiography; MRA, magnetic resonance angiography; MRI, magnetic resonance imaging; SNR, signal-to-noise ratio.

TABLE 13-2   Types of Magnetic Resonance Angiography Sequences

NAME OF SEQUENCE	DESCRIPTION	2D OR 3D	GATING USEFUL	FLOW QUANTIFICATION POSSIBLE	APPLICATIONS
TOF	Bright vessels produced by inflow of blood with full magnetization into a slice or volume where magnetization has been reduced by RF saturation	Both	Occasionally	No	Intracranial, carotid, pedal
PC	Bright vessels produced by application of flow encoding radiofrequency pulses that produce a phase image where intensity is proportional to velocity	Both	Occasionally	Yes	None in current practice
Dynamic CE	Bright vessels produced by rapid infusion of gadolinium contrast, with timing of scan to arterial and/or venous transit; mask subtraction may be used	3D	No	No	Carotid, chest, abdomen, extremity runoff
Postcontrast	Bright vessels produced by equilibrium enhancement of gadolinium contrast with fat saturation	Both	No	No	Veins, aorta
Black blood	Dark vessels produced by use of an inversion prepulse to null the signal of blood, based on its T1 recovery time	2D	Necessary	No	Plaque imaging

2D, two-dimensional; 3D, three-dimensional; CE, contrast-enhanced; PC, phase-contrast; RF, radiofrequency; TOF, time-of-flight.

velocity and time interval between the pulses, the blood volume originally excited by the first pulse may not "see" the second pulse. This results in a black-appearing signal void in the vessel lumen. The use of thin sections or long echo times can further emphasize this flow void. This technique allows detailed examination of arterial wall morphology. Fast spin echo (FSE) sequences, in which a long train of echoes is obtained by use of repeated 180° pulses, produce images more rapidly. The double inversion recovery (DIR) FSE offers a new approach to enhance black-blood sequences. The technique uses two consecutive inversion pulses: the first nulls or blackens the blood everywhere in the coil, and the second restores magnetization in the slice being imaged. Between these pulses and image production, blood within the slice is replaced by nulled blood from outside. This produces more reliable black blood than conventional approaches, making this sequence ideal for examining wall thickness, dissection flaps, and the presence of mural thrombus or inflammation.[4] This provides a clear advantage over traditional x-ray angiography.

"Bright blood" MRA techniques use GRE sequences and are generally divided into those measuring signal amplitude (time-of-flight [TOF]) and those based on phase effects (phase-contrast [PC]). In each GRE sequence, a single RF pulse is applied in short time intervals, eliminating signal loss due to flow void. The stationary protons occupying a given tissue slice do not have sufficient time to relax to their equilibrium state.

TOF-MRA techniques depend on the inflow of unsaturated protons in blood from outside the field of view (FOV) into the stationary tissue within a section already saturated by its exposure to repeated RF pulses. These "saturated" protons are unable to contribute signal to the image. The signals in the stationary tissues of GRE images used in MRA are therefore typically low. The "unsaturated" protons in blood flowing into the imaging plane have not experienced the RF pulses and yield maximum signal. The unsaturated blood appears bright compared to background tissue (Fig. 13-1B). The time required for blood to flow through an image slice and its effect on the resulting signal is known as *TOF*.

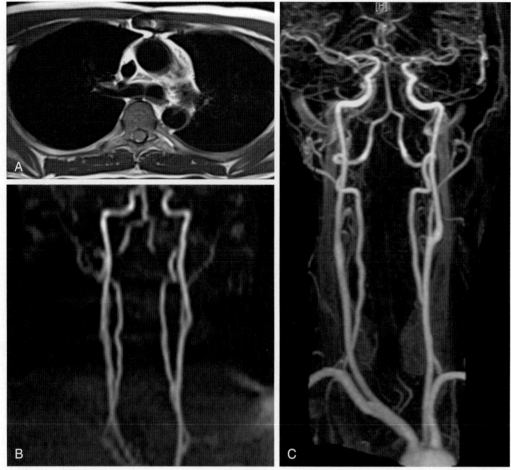

FIGURE 13-1 "Black-blood" and "bright-blood" imaging techniques. **A,** Cross-sectional T1-weighted image of ascending and descending aorta; lumen appears black. **B,** Time-of-flight (TOF) image of carotid-vertebral system. **C,** Maximum-intensity projection (MIP) reconstruction of arterial phase of contrast-enhanced magnetic resonance angiography (CE-MRA) images in same patient shows normal carotid-vertebral arteries at higher spatial resolution than corresponding TOF acquisition.

Saturation of signals can occur in vessels with slow-moving blood as a result of repeated RF excitation in the acquisition plane. This can create artifacts in vessels with stenotic lesions or reduced blood flow.

Time-of-flight techniques can be obtained in 2D or 3D. The 2D TOF utilizes multiple sequentially acquired, overlapping thin slices to form an image. The patient is instructed to hold his/her breath to minimize motion artifact. However, spatial misregistration may occur if patients cannot hold their breath at the same level each time. Thus, only one or two slices are typically acquired per breath-hold. 2D TOF has good sensitivity for identifying vessels with slow flow because blood must move only 3 to 5 mm to refresh a slice. 3D TOF consists of GRE acquisition of a volume into which blood is flowing. The advantage of this technique is higher signal-to-noise ratio (SNR) and improved resolution. The thick volumes of tissue imaged require rapid flow to fully refresh signals within the arteries. The technique is flow dependent and superior in vessels with rapid steady flow without respiratory motion. Additional saturation pulses can be applied to eliminate signal from veins. Segmented GRE sequence with cardiac triggering can be used to eliminate arterial pulsation artifacts.

A successful TOF image requires the section to be thin enough to allow for sufficient inflow between RF pulse repetitions, but thick enough to ensure adequate SNR and anatomical coverage. Section thickness of 3 to 4 mm is used for large vessels, and 1 to 2 mm for smaller vessels. Spatial presaturation pulses are applied above or below the imaged slice or volume to eliminate unwanted signal from arteries or veins, depending on which part of the vascular tree is being imaged. Optimal TR for TOF is 20 to 50 milliseconds. Short TR keeps background tissues saturated, but it must be long enough to allow for satisfactory inflow of unsaturated blood between successive repetitions. The best flip angle is usually 30° to 60°. With phasic flow in the extremities, systolic flow signal may be increased (because of greater transverse magnetization created), and distal flow may be decreased, creating view-to-view intensity changes and phase artifacts from pulsatile variations. This pulsation artifact is greatest at higher flip angles. Cardiac gating can be used to minimize these artifacts at the expense of increased imaging time.

Whereas TOF uses differences in signal amplitude to differentiate between stationary and flowing spins, the PC technique observes the phase shifts of signals. Moving spins experience different phase shifts in the presence of the applied magnetic fields used in MRA. Strength and orientation of the applied magnetic field are varied to encode different phase shifts for flowing protons relative to stationary protons. The faster the spins are moving, the greater their phase shift, and protons of flowing blood may be discriminated from stationary protons. The phase shifts result in a contrast between moving and stationary tissues and form the basis for PC imaging. Pairs of images are acquired that have different sensitivities to flow and are then subtracted to cancel background signal, leaving only the signal from flowing blood. Phase shift is proportional to velocity, allowing flow quantification with this modality. Phase-contrast acquisitions may be acquired in two or three dimensions; although used rarely in angiography today, Phase-contrast offers a reliable way to quantify amount and direction of flow. It requires long imaging times: two data sets in each direction are acquired by using flow-encoding gradients of opposite polarity, and up to three measurements in the orthogonal planes are needed to image flow in all directions.

Visualization of the arterial system with PC and TOF is adequate[5] but has limitations. Acquisition times can be long and prevent imaging within the time span of a single breath-hold. This increases the chance of movement artifacts. Some of the limitations are caused by flow-related artifacts such as in-plane saturation and phase dispersion. Flow-based imaging also has limits in areas of slow flow, such as aneurysms. Overgrading of stenotic lesions is most commonly a manifestation of signal loss in the areas of complex flow. Undergrading is a matter of inadequate spatial resolution. Complex turbulent flow patterns in areas of stenoses can create signal loss and mimic a critical lesion. This is due to "intravoxel dephasing." An accelerated flow across a stenosis consists of a wide distribution of velocities and thus a large distribution of proton phases. In the smallest volume element, a "voxel" of the image, this distribution of phases can result in cancellation rather than coherent addition of signals, accounting for the presence of signal voids at the site of stenosis. A short TE minimizes flow-phase dispersion artifacts. Phase dispersion is further decreased when voxel size is minimized using thin sections. Small voxels and short TE are most easily obtained with 3D TOF methods. The biggest drawback of the thick volumes used with 3D techniques is that slow or recirculating flow can become saturated. The MOTSA (multiple overlapping thin-slab acquisitions) technique of sequential 3D TOF gives better flow enhancement than single-slab 3D TOF techniques and less dephasing than 2D techniques. However, the need for substantial overlap of adjacent slabs increases acquisition time.

Contrast-Enhanced Magnetic Resonance Angiography

The introduction of CE-MRA has revolutionized MRA.[6,7] This technique overcomes many of the limitations of traditional bright blood modalities: respiratory motion artifacts, poor SNR, and flow and saturation-related artifacts (Fig. 13-1C). Gadolinium increases the signal intensity of blood on contrast-enhanced 3D T1-weighted (spoiled) GRE images. Blood contrast is not flow dependent. It is determined by the concentration of contrast agent within the arterial system while imaging data are being collected. Reliable images can be acquired irrespective of whether flow is laminar, turbulent, or stagnant. This technique acquires large-volume data sets in coronal or sagittal orientation within a single breath-hold during the first pass of the contrast material. The contrast agent, gadolinium, is a heavy metal but becomes inert when bound to a chelator. Intravenous (IV) administration of gadolinium-diethylenetriamine pentaacetic acid (DTPA) results in a marked reduction of the T1 or longitudinal relaxation time of blood, therefore reducing the effects of spin saturation. Signal reduction is also problematic in 3D TOF sequences. Moreover, the very short TE reduces spin dephasing and allows accurate evaluation of vascular stenoses.

Multiple refinements have resulted in a technique that is much faster than TOF-MRA. The development of high-performance gradient systems with ultra-short repetition TR and TE has shortened acquisition time in CE-MRA to allow imaging within a single breath-hold and minimize motion artifacts. Administration of agents shortening T1 allows selective visualization of contrast-containing structures and better visualization of circuitous collaterals. Digital subtraction, spoiling, and fat saturation techniques suppress background signal and enhance signal from the contrast agent in the vessels. The subtracted data sets can be postprocessed to provide 3D projectional images. CE-MRA still provides a luminogram, and conventional or FSE images are needed for a complete study so that true lumen diameter and presence of thrombus can be established.

Optimal images are generated when gadolinium concentration is highest in the vessel of interest. To make blood bright compared to background tissues, the gadolinium bolus must be administered in a way that ensures the majority of the contrast to be present in the arterial tree. This requires exact timing of the arrival of the gadolinium bolus. Acquisition prior to contrast arrival creates a "ringing" artifact, whereas late acquisition creates venous and tissue enhancement, contaminating the arterial signal. This is especially problematic in MRA of the extremities, where the images are obtained in multiple segments. Contrast transit time can be affected by low cardiac output, valvular regurgitation, large abdominal aneurysms, and flow-limiting stenoses. Proper timing can be achieved by empirical estimation of transit time or a test bolus in the anatomical field of interest. Alternatively, with automated triggering, a pulse sequence can be designed to sense the arrival of contrast and automatically trigger image acquisition. Magnetic resonance fluoroscopy allows the user to visualize arrival of the contrast bolus directly on the image and manually trigger the start of the scan. Areas that require higher spatial resolution, such as the lower extremities, also need larger doses of contrast for longer acquisition times.

Imaging during the arterial phase of gadolinium infusion takes advantage of higher arterial SNR and eliminates overlapping venous enhancement. This is a brief moment in time, but several methods allow slower MR image acquisition to capture that moment. The phase reordering (mapping k-space) technique acquires central k-space data (i.e., the low spatial frequency data) when contrast concentration is high in arteries but lower in veins. This allows a relatively long MR acquisition to achieve the image contrast associated with the shorter arterial phase of the contrast bolus. It is critical to time the contrast bolus to achieve maximum arterial gadolinium concentration during acquisition of central k-space data.

CE-MRA is limited by venous and soft-tissue enhancement. Contrast media not only passes into venous structures, dependent on the arteriovenous transit time of the tissue, but also rapidly leaks out of the vascular compartment, creating significant tissue enhancement. New "blood pool" agents, which are currently undergoing clinical trials, are retained within blood vessels and selectively enhance the blood pool on T1-weighted MR images. These use either gadolinium compounds that bind to albumin, or are large enough to stay within the vascular space or ultra-small iron particle. Another agent, gadobenate, has a higher T1 relaxation time because of its capacity for weak and transient interaction with serum albumin. This may enhance vascular signal intensity and thus increase diagnostic efficacy at doses comparable to those used for current gadolinium agents. It is approved for imaging use in Europe but is under clinical investigation in the United States. It provides a higher and longer-lasting vascular signal enhancement in the abdominal aorta compared with gadolinium, which does not interact with proteins.[8]

Gadolinium-based contrast has a very favorable safety profile. However, gadolinium is nephrotoxic. For patients with underlying chronic renal insufficiency, gadolinium chelates can cause acute renal failure. Nephrogenic systemic fibrosis (NSF) is linked to gadolinium-based contrast agents[9] and largely involves the skin, though it may also affect the muscle, joints, or internal organs such as the lungs, liver, and heart in patients with renal failure. Nephrogenic systemic fibrosis occurs in patients with severe renal disease who are exposed to high doses of gadolinium agents, or in patients who receive multiple standard doses of contrast agents in a short period of time. The reported prevalence of NSF among patients with glomerular filtration rate (GFR) less than 30 mL/min is 3% to 5%.[10] Therefore, the MR protocol should aim to minimize contrast volume, especially in patients with moderate to severe renal failure.[11]

Metal objects, such as surgical clips, lead to susceptibility artifacts in MRA. The increasing use of stents has important implications for MRA. Cavagna et al. evaluated CE-MRA of seven stent types in the aortic, iliac, and popliteal positions.[12] Few of the commonly used stents permitted visualization of the lumen. Susceptibility artifact results in significant signal loss that can preclude proper visualization of the stent lumen even with gadolinium-enhanced MRA. Some nitinol, tantalum, or polytetrafluoroethylene (PTFE)-based devices, on the other hand, cause less artifact on CE-MRA.

Postprocessing Techniques

Magnetic resonance data can be viewed as source images or be displayed in projections with any orientation. Image postprocessing allows reformation in any desired plane to improve conspicuity of overlapping vessels (Table 13-3). The origins of the left common carotid artery (CCA) and left subclavian artery, for example, can overlap in coronal projections, whereas the origins of the right subclavian artery and right CCA can overlap in some oblique views. The renal ostia are usually best seen in either coronal or slightly oblique view. The celiac axis and superior mesenteric artery (SMA) are best depicted on sagittal projections. One advantage of MR versus digital subtraction angiography (DSA) is that the latter may require multiple injections to assess the origins of these vessels. The details of image interpretation are beyond the scope of this review, but source image data, multiplanar reconstruction (MPR), maximum-intensity projection (MIP), and volume rendering (VR) are used (Fig. 13-2). Source images are the initial reconstructions and should be used for problem solving and to confirm

TABLE 13-3   Types of Postprocessing Techniques

TECHNIQUE	DESCRIPTION
MPR	Production of cross-sectional images in planes different from acquisition plane
MIP projection	Production of full- or partial-volume images along any desired axis from a stack of image slices
Volume rendering	Manipulation of MRI slices to produce full volumetric images; structures segmented for viewing by application of intensity thresholds and removal of unwanted structures

MIP, maximum intensity projection; MPR, multiplanar reconstruction; MRI, magnetic resonance imaging.

findings. Interpretation often begins with a vascular survey using MPR and MIP data sets. Multiplanar reconstructions are very useful in volumetric acquisitions because the desired imaging plane

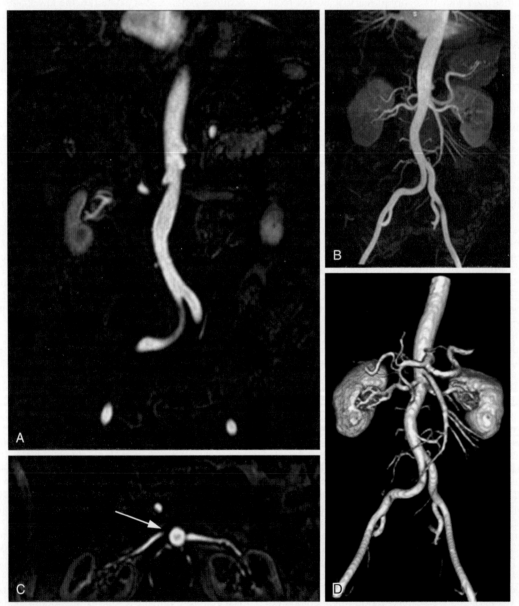

FIGURE 13-2   Postprocessing techniques; contrast-enhanced magnetic resonance angiography (CE-MRA) of abdominal aorta and branches. **A,** Coronal thin-section image of abdominal aorta. Summation of these images, projected with maximum intensity, is used for **(B)** coronal maximum-intensity projection (MIP) that includes normal renal and mesenteric arteries. **C,** Axial multiplanar reconstruction (MPR) image at level of left renal ostium does not include entire extent of both renal arteries, giving false impression of a proximal right renal artery occlusion *(arrow)*. **D,** Three-dimensional volume-rendered (3D-VR) image shows entire course of abdominal aorta and its branches.

can be prescribed to enhance vascular separations. Subtracted MIPs are routinely created from CE-MRA. The noncontrast (mask) images are subtracted from the enhanced images, and resulting high SNR data sets undergo projection of maximum intensity. By performing the projections of all angles around the z-axis of the patient, the data sets can be viewed *in cine*. These projections are referred to as *rotating MIPs*.

Clinical Applications

Extracranial Carotid and Vertebral Arteries

Atherosclerosis, dissection, and inflammatory diseases affect the extracranial carotid and vertebral arteries. Time-of-flight methods (2D and 3D) have been largely replaced by CE-MRA because CE-MRA allows imaging of the entire course of these vessels (Fig. 13-3). A problem with TOF imaging is turbulent flow at or near the carotid bifurcation where most of the lesions occur; this may lead to overestimation of lesion severity. Gadolinium-enhanced MRA has greater SNR than noncontrast imaging, is less sensitive to intravoxel dephasing from turbulence, and does not have signal loss from saturation effects. Phase-contrast sequences can supplement anatomical data for flow direction or quantification.

Transcranial flow has a rapid arteriovenous transit time, and thus venous contamination can limit image quality; therefore, time-resolved imaging may be required. Assessing the test characteristics of carotid MRA is challenging because technologies evolve, and the patients and methods are both heterogeneous. In a 41-study meta-analysis, carotid CE-MRA had high sensitivity (94%) and high specificity (93%) for diagnosis of severe (70%-99 %) carotid artery stenosis.[13] The sensitivity and specificity of CE-MRA for ostial stenosis also is very high.[14]

The intimal flap of CCA dissection can be visualized with either CT or MRA. For a patient with poor or uncertain hemodynamic stability, CT is the preferred modality because it is more rapid and has better patient monitoring capabilities. However, MR is preferred for stable patients, since it does not impart ionizing radiation to the thyroid gland for either initial or follow-up studies.

For vertebral artery dissection, MRA can detect the level of stenosis or obstruction and distinguish residual flow from intramural hematoma.

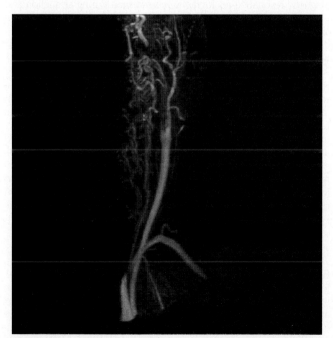

FIGURE 13-3 Carotid artery disease. Left internal carotid artery (ICA) dissection resulted in a thrombotic occlusion of proximal vessel. Internal carotid artery reconstitutes more distally.

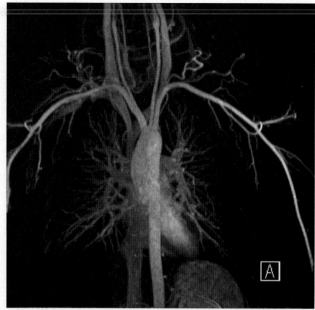

FIGURE 13-4 Maximum-intensity projection (MIP) image shows normal thoracic aorta and origin and course of supraaortic vessels.

Thoracic Aorta and Its Branches

Both CT and MRI provide comprehensive imaging of the aorta. Single breath-hold 3D CE-MRA imaging of the thoracic aorta (Fig. 13-4) is typically performed with electrocardiographic (ECG) gating to eliminate pulsation artifact.

AORTIC DISSECTION

A properly performed modern MRA is 100% sensitive for dissection and intramural hematoma.[15] The true and false lumens, location and extent of the intimal tear, and the relationship of the tear to the branch vessels are readily tracked in multiple planes. Cine images of the proximal aorta can identify aortic regurgitation complicating type A dissection (Fig. 13-5). Delayed phase images allow identification of intramural hematoma, ulceration, and complications including rupture. On T1-weighted SE sequences, intramural hematoma is seen as a concentric thickening of the wall, with increased intramural signal intensity.[16] Inflammatory changes are seen as arterial wall thickening and enhancement. When used with clinical parameters and other testing (e.g., blood pressure changes), MRA is useful to triage patients into either medical or surgical management options.[17]

THORACIC AORTIC ANEURYSM

Aneurysm imaging should consider slow blood flow through the lesion. Magnetic resonance angiography can demonstrate the location and size of an aneurysm, presence of a mural thrombus, and the relationship of the aneurysm to the branch vessels. Because MIP images from 3D CE-MRA are designed to highlight the lumen of the aorta, the source (including noncontrast) images should be evaluated to determine the extent of mural thrombus and the actual aneurysm size for accurate measurements. Time-resolved imaging shows delayed enhancement from slower flow.[18] Patients with a clinically suspected dissection and contraindication to gadolinium (e.g., severe allergy, acute renal failure) can undergo DIR imaging or often noncontrast techniques to evaluate the thoracic aorta.[19]

ARCH VESSEL DISEASE

Occlusive disease of the great vessels is usually due to atherosclerosis. Vasculitis, fibromuscular dysplasia (FMD), and radiation arteriopathy also can cause branch vessel stenoses. CE-MRA is an established tool for rapid and accurate definition of brachiocephalic

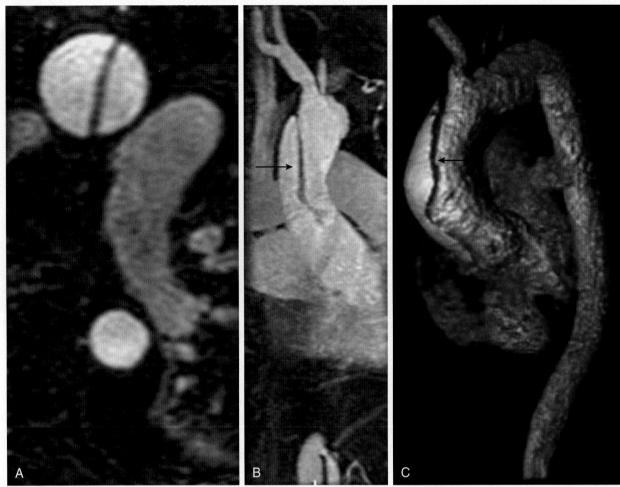

FIGURE 13-5 **Stanford type A dissection. A,** Axial multiplanar reconstruction (MPR) image. **B,** Coronal maximum-intensity projection (MIP). **C,** Three-dimensional volume-rendered (3D-VR) image shows intimal flap in ascending aorta *(arrow)*.

and subclavian arterio-occlusive disease[20] (Fig. 13-6). Rotating MIPs enable precise evaluation of the branch vessel origin without confounding signals from overlying vessels.

CONGENITAL ANOMALIES

Congenital lesions are well depicted with MRA. Aortic coarctation appears as a discrete narrowing of the aorta distal to the left subclavian artery (Fig. 13-7). Magnetic resonance angiography depicts the stenosis, tortuosity of the aorta, and associated collateral vessels.[21] Collateral flow assessment with MR velocity mapping can accurately evaluate the hemodynamic significance of a coarctation.[22] Cine-MR imaging also permits diagnosis of a concomitant bicuspid valve and possible aortic stenosis. Magnetic resonance angiography is used after intervention to exclude complications such as stenosis or aneurysm formation.[23]

Magnetic resonance angiography also can distinguish between coarctation and pseudocoarctation. Pseudocoarctation is a rare asymptomatic anomaly in the descending thoracic aorta and is characterized by an elongated redundant thoracic aorta with buckling distal to the origin of the left subclavian artery. There is no pressure gradient across the buckled segment. It is regarded as a benign condition, although several reports demonstrate that complications may occur.[24]

THORACIC OUTLET SYNDROME

Thoracic outlet syndrome results from compression of the neurovascular bundle (subclavian artery and vein plus the brachial plexus) at the thoracic inlet. Symptoms are typically from nerve compression; the brachial plexus is involved in up to 98% of cases. Magnetic

resonance imaging can demonstrate obstruction/compression of the fat surrounding the brachial plexus, and of the subclavian vein and artery. Magnetic resonance angiography is performed during abduction and adduction maneuvers of the arm to simulate physiological compression of the veins and/or arteries to confirm the diagnosis (Fig. 13-8).

Pulmonary Vessels

Radiofrequency ablation for atrial fibrillation has increased the role of noninvasive pulmonary vein mapping before intervention and for postprocedural surveillance for complications.[25] Magnetic resonance angiography enables comprehensive planning of electrophysiological procedures with respect to number, location, and size of the pulmonary veins (Fig. 13-9). Multidetector CT is the reference standard for pulmonary embolism (PE),[26] although pulmonary MRA can be performed in patients with severe allergy to iodinated contrast media (Fig. 13-10). Time-resolved MRA can be used to minimize venous contamination.[27] Pulmonary artery aneurysms and stenoses can also be characterized with MRA.

Coronary Arteries

Because of its superior soft-tissue contrast, MRI provides excellent cardiac morphology and function data. The coronary arteries, however, remain elusive because of their small caliber, motion, and tortuosity (Fig. 13-11). The modality that can best image the coronary arteries noninvasively in routine clinical practice is computed tomographic angiography (CTA).[28] Coronary MRA is only appropriate for coronary anomalies,[29] but CT is superior for this purpose and can be performed with less than 1 mSv of radiation.

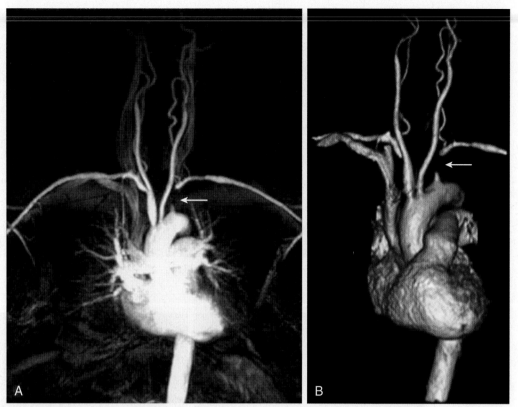

FIGURE 13-6 **Thoracic magnetic resonance angiography (MRA). A,** Coronal maximum-intensity projection (MIP). **B,** Three-dimensional volume-rendered (3D-VR) image shows proximal left subclavian artery occlusion *(arrow)* and subclavian steal syndrome.

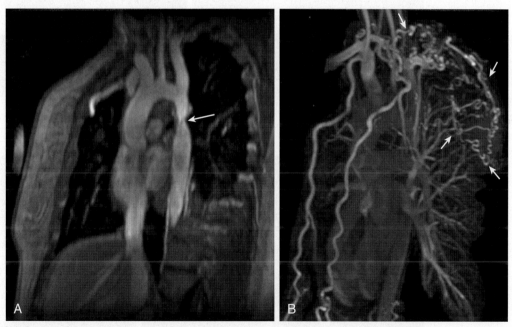

FIGURE 13-7 **A,** Oblique sagittal maximum-intensity projection (MIP) image shows aortic coarctation *(arrow)*. **B,** Three-dimensional volume-rendered (3D-VR) image shows larger field of view; extensive collaterals are evident *(arrows)*.

Peripheral Artery Disease of the Lower and Upper Extremities

Most peripheral artery disease (PAD) is due to atherosclerosis. Other conditions altering arterial flow to the legs include peripheral artery aneurysms, popliteal artery entrapment, cystic adventitial disease, thromboangiitis obliterans (TAO), giant cell and Takayasu's arteritis, and (rarely) FMD.

Magnetic resonance angiography evaluation of lower-extremity PAD typically extends from the aortic bifurcation to the level of the ankle and foot (Fig. 13-12). Magnetic resonance angiography is often used to evaluate vascular anatomy in patients with PAD to plan revascularization procedures. This enables identification and characterization of all occlusive lesions, plus an evaluation of inflow and outflow vessels.

Black-blood MRA images can assess the presence of wall thickening, thrombi, intramural hematoma, atherosclerotic plaques, and

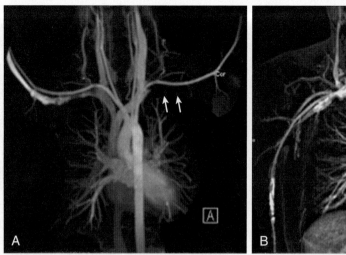

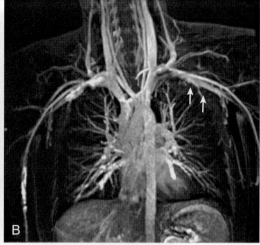

FIGURE 13-8 **Thoracic outlet syndrome. A,** Severe compression of left subclavian vein with arms up *(arrows)*. **B,** Left subclavian vein becomes widely patent *(arrows)* with arms down; no evidence of thrombosis.

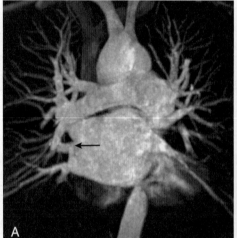

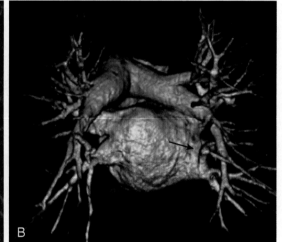

FIGURE 13-9 **A,** Coronal maximum-intensity projection (MIP) image. **B,** Posterior aspect of three-dimensional volume-rendered (3D-VR) image shows pulmonary arteries, left atrium and pulmonary veins, and separate opening of right middle lobe vein to left atrium *(arrow)*.

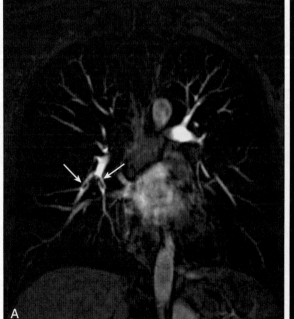

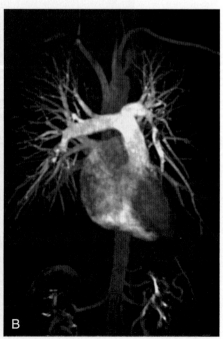

FIGURE 13-10 **A,** Coronal multiplanar reconstructed (MPR) image shows embolic filling defects in right lower lobe pulmonary artery branches *(arrows)*. **B,** Coronal maximum-intensity projection (MIP) image shows whole branching pattern of pulmonary arteries but hides details. Embolic filling defects in right lower lobe pulmonary artery cannot be seen clearly.

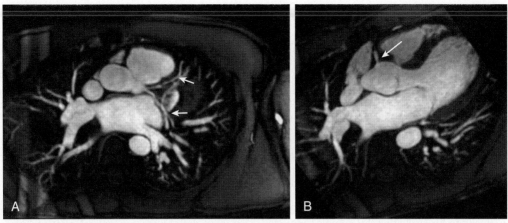

FIGURE 13-11 Contrast-enhanced magnetic resonance angiography (CE-MRA) of coronary arteries shows **(A)** normal origin of the left system *(arrows)* and **(B)** right coronary artery *(arrow)*.

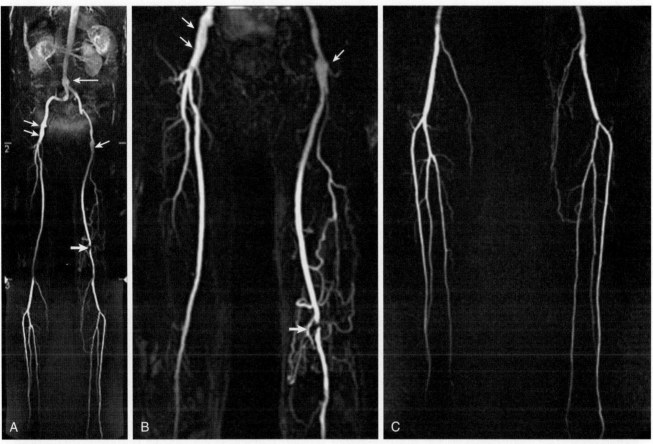

FIGURE 13-12 **A-C,** Abdominal aorta and bilateral lower-extremity runoff. Maximum-intensity projection (MIP) images show fusiform ectasia of infrarenal abdominal aorta *(arrow)*, mild ectasia of distal external iliac artery and proximal common femoral artery (CFA) *(short arrows)*, short-segment moderate to severe stenosis in left popliteal artery *(thick arrow)*, and collateral vascularization. Normal three-vessel runoff is seen in each calf.

penetrating atherosclerotic ulcers.[30] Black-blood MRA sequences are rarely used in current runoff protocols, largely because of long acquisition times.

The standard MR runoff uses 3D CE-MRA[6,31] for accurate and detailed assessment of the peripheral arteries. A recent meta-analysis of 32 studies from 1998 to 2009 shows a pooled sensitivity of 94.7% and specificity of 95.6% for diagnosing segmental steno-occlusive lesions in peripheral arteries.[32] The fundamental challenge in peripheral CE-MRA is balancing accurate imaging throughout the length of the vascular tree against the imaging capabilities of the system. In general, the craniocaudal FOV requires acquisition from the juxtarenal abdominal aorta to the foot in three or four overlapping stages. In one approach, the timing of the gadolinium bolus is optimized for the superior station (abdomen and pelvis), then imaging is performed as rapidly as possible to keep up with the flow of contrast material down the distal arteries. Image quality in the first stage is excellent but often suboptimal in the third stage as gadolinium enters the venous system, with resulting venous contamination of the image. This is especially true in patients with a short arteriovenous transit time, such as those with severely ischemic limbs, where precise definition of the tibial arteries is critical. On average, contrast reaches the common femoral artery (CFA) in 24 seconds, with only an additional 5 and 7 seconds needed to reach the popliteal artery and ankle, respectively.[33] Contrast travel time to the femoral arteries correlates with increasing age, male gender, history of myocardial infarction (MI), and diabetes, and is increased in the presence of aortic aneurysm. So-called moving table technology can be used to chase a single bolus of contrast agent in its distal progression.[34]

Goals of peripheral MRA are higher spatial resolution to better visualize smaller distal vessels, and faster scanning to lessen the negative impact of venous enhancement. Newer acquisitions and 3-tesla (3T) scanners provide technological advances. Parallel imaging with multichannel phased-array coils are used to reduce imaging time.[35] Full-length dedicated peripheral multichannel vascular surface coils improve signal. Time-resolved acquisitions can be used in standard protocols and may be particularly useful in the calves. To reduce venous contamination, subsystolic midfemoral venous compression can be applied.[36]

Hybrid injection protocols overcome some technical limitations and are more accurate for evaluating the popliteal trifurcation and foot vessels.[37,38] Initial precontrast low-resolution axial 2D TOF sequences are obtained to optimize prescription of the 3D slabs. The first injection is used to acquire high–spatial resolution MRA of the calf and foot to minimize venous contamination; 3D time-resolved MRA for this stage can eliminate the need for bolus timing and decrease the total contrast load. The second injection is used for acquisition of both the aortoiliac and femoral station. Complementary TOF sequences are used to assess the ankle and foot. A typical dose is 0.2 mmol/kg of gadolinium-based contrast administered at a flow rate of 1.5 to 2 mL/sec, followed by 20 mL of saline. Accurate synchronization of the peak contrast material in the vascular bed and central k-space acquisition is essential for high image quality. Timing can include a test bolus or bolus tracking. For patients with asymmetrical flow to the legs, optimal arterial opacification in the more symptomatic leg (i.e., slower flow) can be challenging. Time-resolved sequences can determine peak arterial and venous enhancement of both legs so timing can be adjusted for the more symptomatic leg.[31]

Magnetic resonance angiography can also be used to evaluate patients after endovascular intervention.[39] Following bypass surgery, CE-MRA can evaluate graft location, patency, and stenosis of the proximal and distal anastomosis, even for small distal grafts. However, magnetic susceptibility created by metallic clips is problematic even when source images are used for the evaluation.

Blood pool contrast agents show promise to decrease gadolinium doses and provide a much longer time window for data acquisition, based on prolonged relaxivity in comparison to conventional gadolinium agents.[40] Venous contamination and SNR loss from less pronounced T1 shortening are some challenges in blood pool MRA.[31] Newer noncontrast MRA techniques that use acquisitions in systole and diastole to produce contrast[41] are promising for runoff exams in patients with impaired renal function. Dedicated evaluation of the pedal arteries (Fig. 13-13) is comparable to selective DSA.[42]

Magnetic resonance angiography is used to evaluate patients with clinically suspected popliteal artery entrapment syndrome (Fig. 13-14) and cystic adventitial disease. Popliteal artery entrapment is an uncommon peripheral arterial disorder resulting from an anomalous relationship between the popliteal artery and the medial head of the gastrocnemius muscle. Magnetic resonance imaging defines the anatomical relationships, and MRA allows accurate evaluation of vascular compromise during provocative plantar flexion and at rest.[43,44] Cystic adventitial disease accounts for 1 in 1200 cases of calf claudication. A mucin-containing cyst in the popliteal artery wall compromises arterial flow and causes claudication. Water signal makes the cyst appear hyperintense on T2-weighted images, and MRA reveals popliteal artery stenosis.[43,45]

Upper-extremity vascular disease affecting the subclavian artery includes stenosis, aneurysm, or compression due to thoracic outlet syndrome. Imaging of the forearm and hand may be indicated to evaluate vasculitis or ischemia secondary to trauma (Fig. 13-15). The spatial resolution of MRA is inferior to DSA, although it is useful as a noninvasive technique.[46] The acquisition window is restricted to the few seconds between full enhancement of the arteries and the beginning of venous contamination. Blood pressure cuff inflation proximal to the imaged area can extend imaging time and enhance image quality of the palmar, metacarpal, and digital arteries.[47]

Abdominal Vessels

Both CT and MR provide excellent imaging of the abdominal aorta and its branches. Magnetic resonance angiography is indicated to evaluate renal artery stenosis (RAS), mesenteric artery disease, and abdominal aortic aneurysm (AAA), dissection, or occlusion. Single breath-hold CE-MRA permits high contrast between vessels and

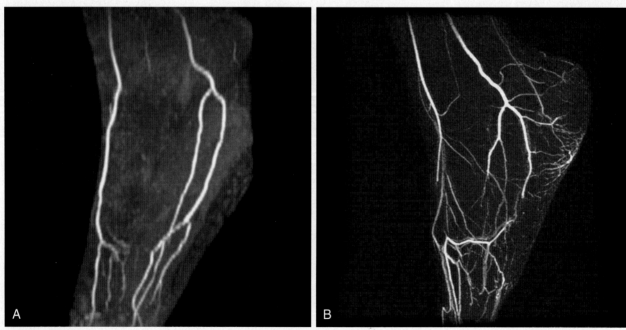

FIGURE 13-13 **A,** Time of flight (TOF) image of normal pedal arteries. **B,** Contrast-enhanced magnetic resonance angiography (CE-MRA) maximum intensity projection (MIP) reconstruction of pedal arteries in patient with cryoglobulinemia and small-vessel vasculitis. Arteries of pedal arch are occluded. Moderate venous enhancement is present.

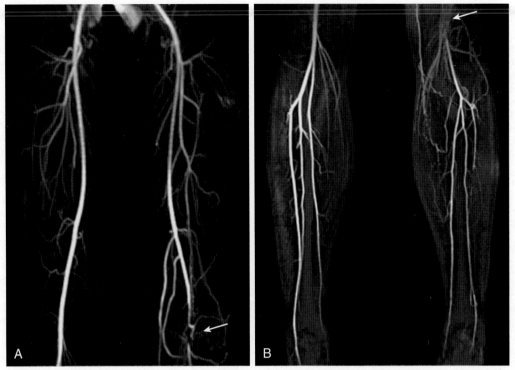

FIGURE 13-14   A-B, Arterial-phase maximum-intensity projection (MIP) images of leg show left popliteal artery entrapment *(arrows)*.

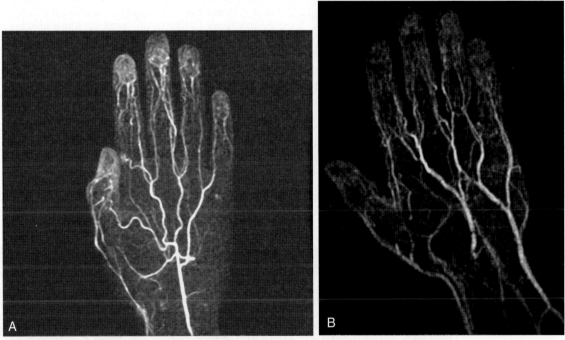

FIGURE 13-15   Contrast-enhanced magnetic resonance angiography (CE-MRA) of hand. A, Dominant ulnar supply to hand in patient with absent radial artery. **B,** Radial aspect of superficial palmar branch, showing stenosis (hypothenar hammer syndrome).

surrounding organs. Technical advances such as time-resolved and parallel imaging can be incorporated into clinical protocols. For detailed spatial measurements, black-blood (e.g., DIR) images are optimal for measurement of the lumen and vessel diameter and assessment of the aorta wall. Volumetric mask imaging will ensure that the 3D volume is appropriately placed. After contrast injection, at least two data sets (arterial and delayed phase) are acquired. This strategy does not significantly prolong the study and can provide valuable information, especially regarding venous structures. It can also be very useful for slow flow in large aneurysms,

or imaging a false lumen where the initial acquisition does not provide adequate enhancement. Contrast doses of 20 mL, administered at 2 mL/s, are usually sufficient.

RENAL ARTERY IMAGING

The most common cause of RAS is atherosclerosis, which often involves the ostia or proximal 1 to 2 cm of the renal arteries. Fibromuscular dysplasia is the second most common cause of RAS and typically affects the distal two thirds of the main renal artery.

Contrast-enhanced MR is the modality of choice for patients with hypertension and clinically suspected RAS.[48] Coronal imaging is prescribed to minimize acquisition time (i.e., fewer phase-encoding steps). Parallel imaging can be used to minimize craniocaudal motion in the distal renal arteries.[49] The advantage of MRA over CT is that dense calcification causes CT artifacts that obscure the lumen and cause overestimation of stenosis severity. Calcium deposits accumulate at or near the ostium where stenosis detection is critical. Three-dimensional CE-MRA with subtracted MIPs has less artifact at the ostium, and PC techniques can add information regarding hemodynamic significance. Secondary findings such as poststenotic dilation and delayed renal parenchymal enhancement are also important.

Magnetic resonance angiography can be used for clinically suspected FMD, but the presence of alternating webs and dilation may not be captured by the spatial resolution of MRA, particularly in the distal renal arteries. Thus, a negative MRA cannot entirely exclude the diagnosis.

ABDOMINAL AORTA IMAGING

Abdominal aortic aneurysms associated with atherosclerosis are typically fusiform; a saccular configuration should raise the possibility of a mycotic aneurysm. Aneurysm evaluation includes the proximal and distal extent of the aneurysm, as well as its relationship to visceral branch vessels. Three-dimensional MRA can identify the main and any supernumerary renal arteries (Fig. 13-16) and mesenteric arteries.

Multidetector CT is the preferred modality for planning endovascular repair of AAAs and surveillance of stent grafts. Magnetic resonance angiography does not image calcification.[50] Magnetic resonance angiography is safe for nonferromagnetic stents and does not induce heating or stent deflection.[51,52]

Susceptibility artifact from stents limit postprocedural studies. However, nitinol and PTFE devices have minimal MR artifact, and early data suggest that MRA can be used in patients with nitinol grafts.[53] Contrast-enhanced MRA is also accurate in the depiction of endoleaks. Time-resolved MRA is also an attractive method to characterize endoleaks because contrast passage into the aneurysm sac can be visualized as a cine loop.[54]

ABDOMINAL AORTIC DISSECTION

Magnetic resonance angiography is used to detect propagation of aortic dissection into the abdominal aorta. It can identify the proximal and distal flap as well as involvement of the visceral branches. The celiac trunk and SMA usually arise from the true lumen, but extension of the flap into the celiac trunk, thrombosis of the false lumen, or compression of the true lumen can lead to hepatic or splenic infarcts. Magnetic resonance angiography reliably depicts the true and false lumen. For 3D acquisitions, postprocessing enables selective viewing of branch vessels. Delayed imaging can be used to characterize slow flow into the false lumen.

AORTIC OCCLUSION

Distal aortic occlusion is most commonly due to thromboembolic disease. Thrombus may be superimposed on severe atherosclerosis of the distal aorta and common iliac arteries. Magnetic resonance angiography is used to evaluate not only the occlusion but also the collateral circulation and distal reconstitution.

MESENTERIC ARTERIES

Chronic mesenteric ischemia (CMI) is most commonly a consequence of atherosclerosis in the proximal visceral arteries, but can also be a sequela to dissection, median arcuate ligament syndrome (Fig. 13-17), visceral artery dissection, vasculitides, and connective tissue disorders.

Most patients do not develop symptoms of CMI unless two of the three mesenteric arteries are occluded. Magnetic resonance angiography is highly accurate for evaluating mesenteric origins, where the majority of stenoses develop (Fig. 13-18). High accuracy is maintained to the level of second-order branches. Qualitative and quantitative flow measurements with cine–phase contrast MRI from the SMA and vein can be performed.[55]

Patients who present with severe abdominal pain and clinical suspicion for acute mesenteric ischemia require urgent imaging because of the risk of irreversible bowel damage. Major causes of acute mesenteric ischemia are SMA emboli (30%-50%), SMA thrombosis (15%-30%), acute mesenteric vein thrombosis (5%-10%), and nonocclusive mesenteric vasoconstriction (20%-30%).[56] Multidetector CT is typically used for initial imaging, since it has more widespread availability, less motion artifact in patients who are acutely ill, and the risk of bowel ischemia/infarction outweighs potential concerns for iodine-induced nephrotoxicity. However, in patients who do not require immediate intervention, MRA can be used for follow-up to characterize chronic atherosclerosis, mesenteric occlusion, aneurysm formation, and vasculitis. Characteristics of vasculitis include findings of wall thickening and increased gadolinium enhancement (Fig. 13-19).

Transplantation

Magnetic resonance angiography is used in pre- and postoperative transplant patients. Detailed knowledge of vascular anatomy is essential to ensure safe and successful transplantation surgery.

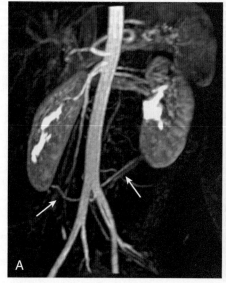
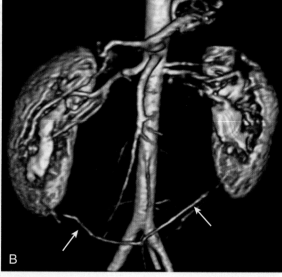

FIGURE 13-16 **A,** Coronal maximum-intensity projection (MIP) image. **B,** Three-dimensional volume-rendered (3D-VR) images show bilateral accessory inferior renal artery originating from left common iliac artery (CIA) *(arrows).*

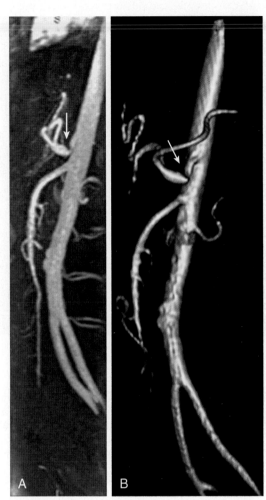

FIGURE 13-17 **Median arcuate ligament syndrome. A,** Sagittal maximum-intensity projection (MIP). **B,** Three-dimensional volume-rendered (3D-VR) images obtained from arterial phase of contrast-enhanced magnetic resonance angiography (CE-MRA) show stenosis due to median arcuate ligament compression in origin of celiac trunk *(arrow).*

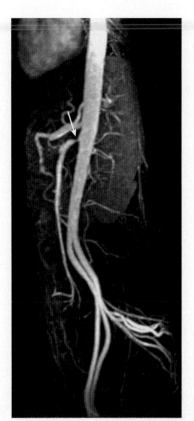

FIGURE 13-18 Sagittal maximum-intensity projection (MIP) image shows severe stenosis of superior mesenteric artery (SMA) *(arrow).*

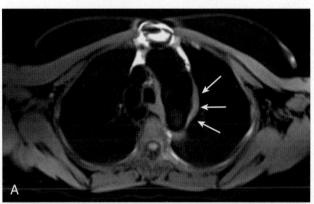

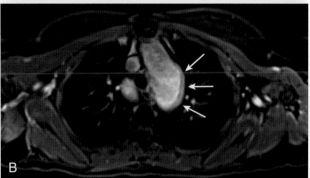

FIGURE 13-19 Axial precontrast **(A)** and postcontrast **(B)** T1-weighted images show aneurysmatic dilation, thickening, and contrast enhancement of aortic arch, consistent with aortitis *(arrows)* in patient with Takayasu's arteritis.

Magnetic resonance angiography is used in presurgical evaluation of the recipient and living donors[57,58] and in follow-up of patients after transplantation of the liver, kidney (Fig. 13-20), or pancreas, particularly in cases of suspected vascular complications.

In living donor liver transplantation, MRA provides a complete evaluation of the hepatic vascular anatomy in the presurgical phase. It provides information regarding biliary anatomy and assessment of hepatic parenchyma for diffuse and focal abnormalities.[59] Magnetic resonance angiography has high sensitivity and excellent negative predictive value for detection of clinically significant vascular stenosis in liver transplantation.[60]

After renal transplantation, MRA can be used for suspected vascular complications to identify patients who would benefit from angioplasty.[61] In pancreas transplantation, MRA identifies arterial and venous complications.[62] Accurate maps of rectus and gluteal muscle perforator arteries can also be obtained for preoperative planning of breast reconstruction.[63]

Inflammatory Diseases of the Arterial Wall

Magnetic resonance imaging is the primary technology for diagnosis and follow-up of patients with large vessel vasculitis, based on identification of vessel wall edema and thickening that can be seen before lumen changes. Black-blood DIR imaging is preferred for wall morphology, and postcontrast imaging can be used to demonstrate mural enhancement. Other wall abnormalities seen in vasculitis include ulceration, dissection, stenosis, occlusion, and aneurysm.

Takayasu's arteritis is an inflammatory disease that typically affects young women, and early diagnosis can be difficult because of its nonspecific symptoms and serological markers. Diagnosis and identification of disease activity with MRA is important to

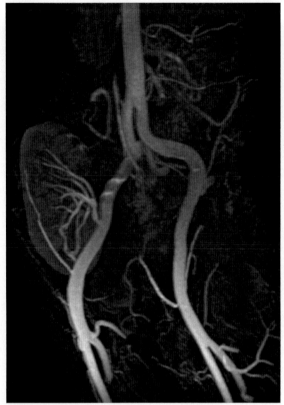

FIGURE 13-20 Oblique coronal maximum-intensity projection (MIP) reconstruction shows patency of renal artery anastomosis of transplanted kidney.

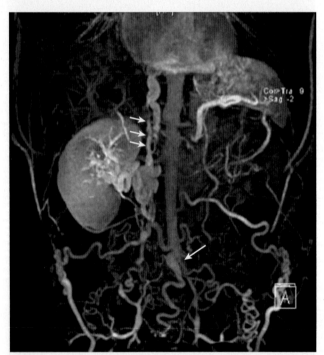

FIGURE 13-21 Coronal maximum-intensity projection (MIP) image shows occlusion of distal abdominal aorta in region of bifurcation *(arrow)*, intrahepatic inferior vena cava (IVC) thrombosis *(short arrows)*, and occlusion of bilateral common iliac vein, with extensive lumbar, epigastric, and azygos collateral veins in same patient.

guide adequate therapy because severe stenoses, occlusion, or aneurysm are late irreversible manifestations. MRA findings suggestive of Takayasu's arteritis include stenoses of the aorta and its major branches (Fig. 13-21). Involvement of the pulmonary

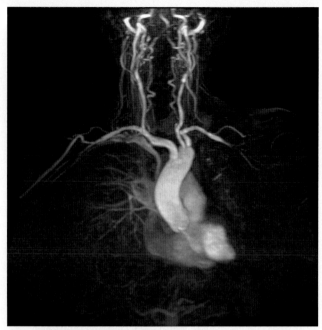

FIGURE 13-22 Giant cell arteritis (GCA). Both subclavian arteries have smooth, tapered stenoses in mid- to distal segments.

arteries is seen in 70% of patients and increases diagnostic confidence.[64] Biomarkers are less reliable, whereas MRA shows early changes and evaluates disease activity. Findings include arterial wall thickening and enhancement in the active phase, mural thrombi, fusiform vascular dilations, and multifocal stenosis, and then thickened aortic valvular cusps in the chronic phase.[65]

Giant cell arteritis (GCA) is a large-vessel inflammatory disease affecting primarily older patients. Magnetic resonance angiography is used to diagnose associated thoracic aortic aneurysms and evaluates involvement of large peripheral arteries such as the subclavian arteries (Fig. 13-22).

Magnetic Resonance Venography

Magnetic resonance venography (MRV) protocols differ from arterial imaging because of the differences in flow and disease patterns. As with arterial studies, noncontrast MRI such as TOF has been largely replaced with CE-MRV, even though 2D TOF can cover large volumes and detect slow flow.

The problems of flow-based techniques and the relatively long acquisition times are overcome by the rapid 3D sequences used for arteriography. Subtraction data sets can limit signal from arteries to produce high-quality venograms.[66]

Thrombus has relatively high T1 signal from the formation of methemoglobin. Blood products have characteristic MR signal changes that are used in the evaluation of very early to late hemorrhage.[67] Inflammatory changes from acute deep vein thrombosis (DVT) are characteristic. After contrast enhancement, mural enhancement of the vessel wall is seen around an acutely thrombosed vein, appearing as a bull's eye. In conjunction with the inflammatory changes and organization of the thrombus, this finding helps differentiate acute from chronic thrombosis.

Deep Vein Thrombosis

When the vein in question can be accessed by sonography, ultrasound is the first-line modality for DVT. Magnetic resonance venography is a second-line modality and used when ultrasound is limited by patient body habitus, limited acoustic window, or for other reasons. Gadolinium is typically used, and 3D sequences routinely identify filling defects diagnostic for DVT (Fig. 13-23). There is no role for DSA

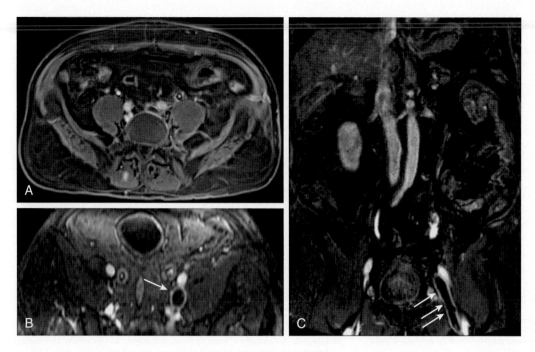

FIGURE 13-23 Axial (A-B) and coronal (C) postcontrast venous phase images show left common iliac, external iliac, and common femoral vein thromboses *(arrows)*.

in diagnosis, although percutaneous access can be used for therapy. Computed tomography venography can also be performed. Many early studies have established 2D TOF accuracy for thrombosis[68,69] in the large central veins, although contrast is beneficial for better characterization of more superficial and perforating veins with slow flow and retrograde flow.[70] Newer noncontrast MRA techniques have been used for DVT, but their utility requires more comprehensive studies. Magnetic resonance venography is also useful for patients with suspected renal vein thrombosis and can show enhancement of tumor thrombus.[71] Delayed-phase MRA also provides an evaluation of the inferior vena cava (IVC) and hepatic and portal veins.

Occlusive diseases of central thoracic veins (Fig. 13-24) are commonly seen in patients with malignancy or coagulopathy or long-term use of central venous catheters for hemodialysis,

hyperalimentation, or chemotherapy. Magnetic resonance venography is very helpful for vascular mapping in patients who have chronic venous occlusion but require central venous catheter placement. Magnetic resonance venography is the best modality for compression and occlusion of the abdomen and pelvis. The IVC (Fig. 13-25) and iliac veins, lymph nodes, tumors, and large organs can be identified. Finally, MRV delineates congenital venous anomalies and can be used to assess patency.

Vessel Wall Imaging

Sudden catastrophic adverse events such as stroke, MI, and limb ischemia do not necessarily correlate with lumen stenosis and may be better predicted by plaque characterization. Thus, vessel

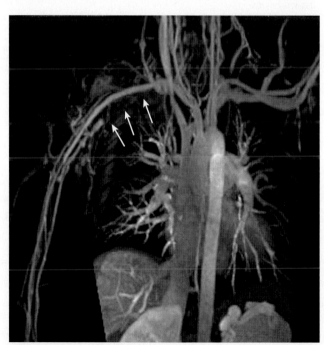

FIGURE 13-24 Coronal maximum-intensity projection (MIP) image shows right subclavian vein thrombotic occlusion *(arrows)* and patent left venous system.

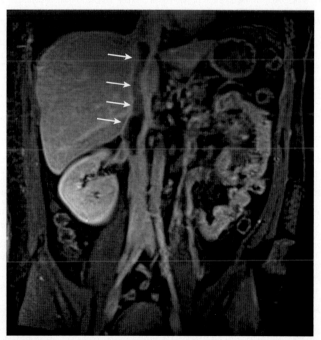

FIGURE 13-25 Abdominal magnetic resonance venography (MRV). Coronal maximum-intensity projection (MIP) image; large hypointense filling defect due to thrombosis seen in inferior vena cava (IVC) lumen *(arrows)*.

wall imaging will become a critical component of a comprehensive vascular study. Moreover, because of the multicontrast capabilities, MRI is well poised for wall component imaging, including the separation of wall layers[72] and imaging the lipid necrotic core and fibrous matrix. Noncontrast techniques have achieved spatial resolution to image segments of an arterial tree,[41] and contrast enhancement over time can quantify the size of the lipid necrotic core and evaluate plaque inflammation.[73] Sophisticated contrast agents, such as ultra-small superparamagnetic iron oxides that accumulate in predominantly ruptured or rupture prone atherosclerotic plaques, can potentially identify high-risk lesions.[74] Novel implantable contrast agents[75] may enable more accurate vessel wall planimetry for longitudinal studies of vessel walls. Delayed and dynamic contrast-enhanced studies have been used to study plaque neovascularization.[76] Finally, evaluation of wall-thickness changes in lower-extremity peripheral vein bypass grafts has been demonstrated.[72,77]

REFERENCES

1. Ho VB, Corse WR: MR angiography of the abdominal aorta and peripheral vessels, Radiol Clin North Am 41:115–144, 2003.
2. Levy RA, Prince MR: Arterial-phase three-dimensional contrast-enhanced MR angiography of the carotid arteries, AJR Am J Roentgenol 167:211–215, 1996.
3. Vogt FM, Goyen M, Debatin JF: MR angiography of the chest, Radiol Clin North Am 41:29–41, 2003.
4. Toussaint JF, LaMuraglia GM, Southern JF, et al: Magnetic resonance images lipid, fibrous, calcified, hemorrhagic, and thrombotic components of human atherosclerosis in vivo, Circulation 94:932–938, 1996.
5. Yucel EK, Anderson CM, Edelman RR, et al: AHA scientific statement. Magnetic resonance angiography: update on applications for extracranial arteries, Circulation 100:2284–2301, 1999.
6. Prince MR, Yucel EK, Kaufman JA, et al: Dynamic gadolinium-enhanced three-dimensional abdominal MR arteriography, J Magn Reson Imaging 3:877–881, 1993.
7. Prince MR: Gadolinium-enhanced MR aortography, Radiology 191:155–164, 1994.
8. Kroencke TJ, Wasser MN, Pattynama PM, et al: Gadobenate dimeglumine-enhanced MR angiography of the abdominal aorta and renal arteries, AJR Am J Roentgenol 179:1573–1582, 2002.
9. Cowper SE, Robin HS, Steinberg SM, et al: Scleromyxoedema-like cutaneous diseases in renal-dialysis patients, Lancet 356:1000–1001, 2000.
10. Sadowski EA, Bennett LK, Chan MR, et al: Nephrogenic systemic fibrosis: risk factors and incidence estimation, Radiology 243:148–157, 2007.
11. Ersoy H, Rybicki FJ: Biochemical safety profiles of gadolinium-based extracellular contrast agents and nephrogenic systemic fibrosis, J Magn Reson Imaging 26:1190–1197, 2007.
12. Cavagna E, Berletti R, Schiavon F: In vivo evaluation of intravascular stents at three-dimensional MR angiography, Eur Radiol 11:2531–2535, 2001.
13. Wardlaw JM, Chappell FM, Best JJ, et al: Non-invasive imaging compared with intra-arterial angiography in the diagnosis of symptomatic carotid stenosis: a meta-analysis, Lancet 367:1503–1512, 2006.
14. Randoux B, Marro B, Koskas F, et al: Proximal great vessels of aortic arch: comparison of three-dimensional gadolinium-enhanced MR angiography and digital subtraction angiography, Radiology 229:697–702, 2003.
15. Moore AG, Eagle KA, Bruckman D, et al: Choice of computed tomography, transesophageal echocardiography, magnetic resonance imaging, and aortography in acute aortic dissection: International Registry of Acute Aortic Dissection (IRAD), Am J Cardiol 89:1235–1238, 2002.
16. Buckley O, Rybicki FJ, Gerson DS, et al: Imaging features of intramural hematoma of the aorta, Int J Cardiovasc Imaging 26:65–76, 2010.
17. Hayashi H, Matsuoka Y, Sakamoto I, et al: Penetrating atherosclerotic ulcer of the aorta: imaging features and disease concept, Radiographics 20:995–1005, 2000.
18. Lohan DG, Krishnam M, Tomasian A, et al: Time-resolved MR angiography of the thorax, Magn Reson Imaging Clin N Am 16:235–248, viii, 2008.
19. Krishnam MS, Tomasian A, Malik S, et al: Image quality and diagnostic accuracy of unenhanced SSFP MR angiography compared with conventional contrast-enhanced MR angiography for the assessment of thoracic aortic diseases, Eur Radiol 20:1311–1320, 2010.
20. Cosottini M, Zampa V, Petruzzi P, et al: Contrast-enhanced three-dimensional MR angiography in the assessment of subclavian artery diseases, Eur Radiol 10:1737–1744, 2000.
21. Godart F, Labrot G, Devos P, et al: Coarctation of the aorta: comparison of aortic dimensions between conventional MR imaging, 3D MR angiography, and conventional angiography, Eur Radiol 12:2034–2039, 2002.
22. Holmqvist C, Stahlberg F, Hanseus K, et al: Collateral flow in coarctation of the aorta with magnetic resonance velocity mapping: correlation to morphological imaging of collateral vessels, J Magn Reson Imaging 15:39–46, 2002.
23. Bogaert J, Kuzo R, Dymarkowski S, et al: Follow-up of patients with previous treatment for coarctation of the thoracic aorta: comparison between contrast-enhanced MR angiography and fast spin-echo MR imaging, Eur Radiol 10:1847–1854, 2000.
24. Taneja K, Kawlra S, Sharma S, et al: Pseudocoarctation of the aorta: complementary findings on plain film radiography, CT, DSA, and MRA, Cardiovasc Intervent Radiol 21:439–441, 1998.
25. Kato R, Lickfett L, Meininger G, Dickfeld T, et al: Pulmonary vein anatomy in patients undergoing catheter ablation of atrial fibrillation: lessons learned by use of magnetic resonance imaging, Circulation 107:2004–2010, 2003.
26. Hunsaker AR, Lu MT, Goldhaber SZ, et al: Imaging in acute pulmonary embolism with special clinical scenarios, Circ Cardiovasc Imaging 3:491–500, 2010.
27. Ersoy H, Goldhaber SZ, Cai T, et al: Time-resolved MR angiography: a primary screening examination of patients with suspected pulmonary embolism and contraindications to administration of iodinated contrast material, AJR Am J Roentgenol 188:1246–1254, 2007.
28. Otero HJ, Steigner ML, Rybicki FJ: The "post-64" era of coronary CT angiography: understanding new technology from physical principles, Radiol Clin North Am 47:79–90, 2009.
29. Gharib AM, Ho VB, Rosing DR, et al: Coronary artery anomalies and variants: technical feasibility of assessment with coronary MR angiography at 3T, Radiology 247:220–227, 2008.
30. Tatli S, Lipton MJ, Davison BD, et al: From the RSNA refresher courses: MR imaging of aortic and peripheral vascular disease, Radiographics 23 Spec No:S59–S78, 2003.
31. Ersoy H, Rybicki FJ: MR angiography of the lower extremities, AJR Am J Roentgenol 190:1675–1684, 2008.
32. Menke J, Larsen J: Meta-analysis: accuracy of contrast-enhanced magnetic resonance angiography for assessing steno-occlusions in peripheral arterial disease, Ann Intern Med 153:325–334, 2010.
33. Prince MR, Chabra SG, Watts R, et al: Contrast material travel times in patients undergoing peripheral MR angiography, Radiology 224:55–61, 2002.
34. Meaney JF, Ridgway JP, Chakraverty S, et al: Stepping-table gadolinium-enhanced digital subtraction MR angiography of the aorta and lower extremity arteries: preliminary experience, Radiology 211:59–67, 1999.
35. Maki JH, Wilson GJ, Eubank WB, et al: Utilizing SENSE to achieve lower station sub-millimeter isotropic resolution and minimal venous enhancement in peripheral MR angiography, J Magn Reson Imaging 15:484–491, 2002.
36. Zhang HL, Ho BY, Chao M, et al: Decreased venous contamination on 3D gadolinium-enhanced bolus chase peripheral MR angiography using thigh compression, AJR Am J Roentgenol 183:1041–1047, 2004.
37. von Kalle T, Gerlach A, Hatopp A, et al: Contrast-enhanced MR angiography (CEMRA) in peripheral arterial occlusive disease (PAOD): conventional moving table technique versus hybrid technique, Rofo 176:62–69, 2004.
38. Tongdee R, Narra VR, McNeal G, et al: Hybrid peripheral 3D contrast-enhanced MR angiography of calf and foot vasculature, AJR Am J Roentgenol 186:1746–1753, 2006.
39. Rybicki FJ, Nallamshetty L, Yucel EK, et al: ACR appropriateness criteria on recurrent symptoms following lower-extremity angioplasty, J Am Coll Radiol 5:1176–1180, 2008.
40. Nikolaou K, Kramer H, Grosse C, et al: High-spatial-resolution multistation MR angiography with parallel imaging and blood pool contrast agent: Initial experience, Radiology 241:861–872, 2006.
41. Miyazaki M, Lee VS: Nonenhanced MR angiography, Radiology 248:20–43, 2008.
42. Kreitner KF, Kunz RP, Herber S, et al: MR angiography of the pedal arteries with gadobenate dimeglumine, a contrast agent with increased relaxivity, and comparison with selective intraarterial DSA, J Magn Reson Imaging 27:78–85, 2008.
43. Elias DA, White LM, Rubenstein JD, et al: Clinical evaluation and MR imaging features of popliteal artery entrapment and cystic adventitial disease, AJR Am J Roentgenol 180:627–632, 2003.
44. Atilla S, Ilgit ET, Akpek S, et al: MR imaging and MR angiography in popliteal artery entrapment syndrome, Eur Radiol 8:1025–1029, 1998.
45. Crolla RM, Steyling JF, Hennipman A, et al: A case of cystic adventitial disease of the popliteal artery demonstrated by magnetic resonance imaging, J Vasc Surg 18:1052–1055, 1993.
46. Krause U, Pabst T, Kenn W, et al: High resolution contrast enhanced MR-angiography of the hand arteries: preliminary experiences, Vasa 31:179–184, 2002.
47. Wentz KU, Frohlich JM, von Weymarn C, et al: High-resolution magnetic resonance angiography of hands with timed arterial compression (tac-MRA), Lancet 361:49–50, 2003.
48. Vasbinder GB, Nelemans PJ, Kessels AG, et al: Diagnostic tests for renal artery stenosis in patients suspected of having renovascular hypertension: a meta-analysis, Ann Intern Med 135:401–411, 2001.
49. Vasbinder GB, Maki JH, Nijenhuis RJ, et al: Motion of the distal renal artery during three-dimensional contrast-enhanced breath-hold MRA, J Magn Reson Imaging 16:685–696, 2002.
50. Lutz AM, Willmann JK, Pfammatter T, et al: Evaluation of aortoiliac aneurysm before endovascular repair: comparison of contrast-enhanced magnetic resonance angiography with multidetector row computed tomographic angiography with an automated analysis software tool, J Vasc Surg 37:619–627, 2003.
51. Shellock FG, Shellock VJ: Metallic stents: evaluation of MR imaging safety, AJR Am J Roentgenol 173:543–547, 1999.
52. Engellau L, Olsrud J, Brockstedt S, et al: MR evaluation ex vivo and in vivo of a covered stent-graft for abdominal aortic aneurysms: ferromagnetism, heating, artifacts, and velocity mapping, J Magn Reson Imaging 12:112–121, 2000.
53. Cejna M, Loewe C, Schoder M, et al: MR angiography vs CT angiography in the follow-up of nitinol stent grafts in endoluminally treated aortic aneurysms, Eur Radiol 12:2443–2450, 2002.
54. Stavropoulos SW, Charagundla SR: Imaging techniques for detection and management of endoleaks after endovascular aortic aneurysm repair, Radiology 243:641–655, 2007.
55. Ersoy H: The role of noninvasive vascular imaging in splanchnic and mesenteric pathology, Clin Gastroenterol Hepatol 7:270–278, 2009.
56. Fleischmann D: Multiple detector-row CT angiography of the renal and mesenteric vessels, Eur J Radiol 45(Suppl 1):S79–S87, 2003.
57. Vosshenrich R, Fischer U: Contrast-enhanced MR angiography of abdominal vessels: is there still a role for angiography? Eur Radiol 12:218–230, 2002.
58. Laissy JP, Trillaud H, Douek P: MR angiography: noninvasive vascular imaging of the abdomen, Abdom Imaging 27:488–506, 2002.
59. Sahani D, Mehta A, Blake M, et al: Preoperative hepatic vascular evaluation with CT and MR angiography: implications for surgery, Radiographics 24:1367–1380, 2004.
60. Kim BS, Kim TK, Jung DJ, et al: Vascular complications after living related liver transplantation: evaluation with gadolinium-enhanced three-dimensional MR angiography, AJR Am J Roentgenol 181:467–474, 2003.
61. Hohenwalter MD, Skowlund CJ, Erickson SJ, et al: Renal transplant evaluation with MR angiography and MR imaging, Radiographics 21:1505–1517, 2001.
62. Hagspiel KD, Nandalur K, Pruett TL, et al: Evaluation of vascular complications of pancreas transplantation with high-spatial-resolution contrast-enhanced MR angiography, Radiology 242:590–599, 2007.

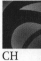

63. Newman TM, Vasile J, Levine JL, et al: Perforator flap magnetic resonance angiography for reconstructive breast surgery: a review of 25 deep inferior epigastric and gluteal perforator artery flap patients, *J Magn Reson Imaging* 31:1176–1184, 2010.
64. Yamada I, Nakagawa T, Himeno Y, et al: Takayasu arteritis: diagnosis with breath-hold contrast-enhanced three-dimensional MR angiography, *J Magn Reson Imaging* 11:481–487, 2000.
65. Choe YH, Han BK, Koh EM, et al: Takayasu's arteritis: assessment of disease activity with contrast-enhanced MR imaging, *AJR Am J Roentgenol* 175:505–511, 2000.
66. Lebowitz JA, Rofsky NM, Krinsky GA, et al: Gadolinium-enhanced body MR venography with subtraction technique, *AJR Am J Roentgenol* 169:755–758, 1997.
67. Bradley WG Jr: MR appearance of hemorrhage in the brain, *Radiology* 189:15–26, 1993.
68. Spritzer CE, Arata MA, Freed KS: Isolated pelvic deep venous thrombosis: relative frequency as detected with MR imaging, *Radiology* 219:521–525, 2001.
69. Carpenter JP, Holland GA, Baum RA, et al: Magnetic resonance venography for the detection of deep venous thrombosis: comparison with contrast venography and duplex Doppler ultrasonography, *J Vasc Surg* 18:734–741, 1993.
70. Ruehm SG, Zimny K, Debatin JF: Direct contrast-enhanced 3D MR venography, *Eur Radiol* 11:102–112, 2001.
71. Laissy JP, Menegazzo D, Debray MP, et al: Renal carcinoma: diagnosis of venous invasion with Gd-enhanced MR venography, *Eur Radiol* 10:1138–1143, 2000.
72. Mitsouras D, Owens CD, Conte MS, et al: *In vivo* differentiation of two vessel wall layers in lower extremity peripheral vein bypass grafts: application of high-resolution inner-volume black blood 3D FSE, *Magn Reson Med* 62:607–615, 2009.
73. Saam T, Hatsukami TS, Takaya N, et al: The vulnerable, or high-risk, atherosclerotic plaque: noninvasive MR imaging for characterization and assessment, *Radiology* 244:64–77, 2007.
74. Kooi ME, Cappendijk VC, Cleutjens KB, et al: Accumulation of ultrasmall superparamagnetic particles of iron oxide in human atherosclerotic plaques can be detected by *in vivo* magnetic resonance imaging, *Circulation* 107:2453–2458, 2003.
75. Mitsouras D, Vemula PK, Yu P, et al: Immobilized contrast-enhanced MRI: gadolinium-based long-term MR contrast enhancement of the vein graft vessel wall, *Magn Reson Med* 2010.
76. Calcagno C, Mani V, Ramachandran S, et al: Dynamic contrast enhanced (DCE) magnetic resonance imaging (MRI) of atherosclerotic plaque angiogenesis, *Angiogenesis* 13:87–99, 2010.
77. Rybicki FJ, Mitsouras D, Owens CD, et al: Lower-extremity peripheral vein bypass graft wall thickness changes demonstrated at 1 and 6 months after surgery with ultra-high spatial resolution black blood inner volume three-dimensional fast spin echo magnetic resonance imaging, *Int J Cardiovasc Imaging* 24:529–533, 2008.

CHAPTER 14

Computed Tomographic Angiography

Michael C. Walls, Sanjay Rajagopalan

Volumetric data acquisition with multidetector computed tomography (MDCT) has enabled the development of computed tomographic angiography (CTA), a diagnostic modality that has clearly revolutionized the diagnosis of vascular disorders. Adequate imaging of the peripheral vascular system during a single acquisition and a single injection of contrast medium became feasible with the introduction of a 4-slice computed tomography (CT) system with a 0.5-second gantry rotation (thinnest collimation 4 × 2.5 mm) in 1998.[1] The introduction of 8-slice CT in 2000 enabled shorter scan times, but did not yet provide improved longitudinal resolution (thinnest collimation 8 × 1.25 mm). The introduction of 16-slice CT made it possible to routinely acquire substantial anatomical volumes with isotropic sub-millimeter spatial resolution.[2] Computed tomographic angiography scans of the peripheral vasculature could now be routinely acquired with 16 × 0.625 mm or 16 × 0.75 mm collimation, which provided the level of resolution required to investigate small-vessel involvement (<1 mm).

The 64-slice CT systems introduced in 2004 were the next major advance, when two different scanner concepts were introduced by different vendors. The *volume concept* pursued by General Electric, Philips, and Toshiba aimed at a further increase in volume coverage speed by using 64 detector rows instead of 16, without changing the physical parameters of the scanner compared to the 16-slice version. The *resolution concept* pursued by Siemens used 32 physical detector rows in combination with *double z-sampling*, a refined z-sampling technique enabled by a periodic motion of the focal spot in the z-direction to simultaneously acquire 64 overlapping slices. The goal was pitch-independent increase of longitudinal resolution and reduction of spiral artifacts.

With the most recent generation of CT systems, further increases in detector arrays allow increases in volume coverage and acquisition of large volumes in single heartbeats. Although clearly advantageous in coronary imaging, these have also provided advantages for vascular imaging, including arterial phase imaging and diagnosis of vascular disorders such as dissection and arteriovenous malformations (AVMs).

This chapter discusses the basic principles of MDCT and provides an overview of its application in vascular diseases. Image interpretation methods have also evolved, with routine postprocessing methods for image display, analysis, and quantitation. These methods will be discussed, as well as the strengths and weaknesses of CTA, including radiation dose concerns.

Fundamentals of Computed Tomography Imaging

Major Components of a Computed Tomography Scanner

The major components of a CT scanner are an x-ray tube and generator, a collimator, and photon detectors. These components are mounted on a rotating gantry where the x-ray tube produces the x-rays necessary for imaging. The pre-detector collimator helps shape the x-ray beams that emanate from the x-ray tube in order to cut out unnecessary radiation. The detectors consist of multiple rows of detector elements (>900 elements per row in current scanners) that receive x-ray photons that have traversed through the patient, with the post-detector collimators preventing backscatter, which degrades image quality. Newer scanners have as many as 320 detector rows, and the width of each detector ("detector collimation") has decreased from 2.5 mm in 4-slice systems to 0.5 mm. The most important benefit of increasing the detector rows is increased coverage per gantry rotation (a 320-row detector CT with a detector width of 0.5 mm will have 160 mm z-axis coverage). The submillimeter detector width improves spatial resolution in the z-axis, while increased coverage shortens scan time. Each detector element contains radiation-sensitive solid state material (e.g., cadmium tungstate, gadolinium oxide, gadolinium oxysulfide) that converts the absorbed x-rays into visible light.[3] The light is then detected by a silicone photodiode, amplified, and converted into a digital signal.

Gantry rotation time determines the temporal resolution of the images, with older scanners having a rotation time of 0.75 seconds, and more contemporary scanners a rotation time of 0.33 seconds.[2] The temporal resolution of a single source scanner, one x-ray generator mounted on the gantry, is slightly higher than half the time it takes for the gantry to rotate 360 degrees. Thus a 0.33-second gantry rotation will effectively provide a temporal resolution of 0.17 seconds. With a dual-source scanner, two x-ray generators mounted on the gantry, the temporal resolution will improve by a factor of two.

Computed Tomography Attenuation Data for Image Reconstruction

Computed tomography measures the local x-ray attenuation coefficients of the tissue volume elements, or *voxels*, in an axial slice of the patient's anatomy. The attenuation coefficients are then translated into grayscale values (CT value) of the corresponding picture elements (*pixels*) in the displayed two-dimensional (2D) image of the slice. The numerical CT value is normalized to the attenuation properties of water and is reported as *Hounsfield units* (HU). Pixel values are stored as integers, in the range −1024 HU to 3071 HU, corresponding to 4096 different grayscale values. By convention, water = 0 HU, and air = −1000 HU and is independent of the x-ray spectrum. The CT values of human tissue, however, depend on the x-ray spectrum. In general, lung and fat have negative CT values, muscle has a positive HU, and bone has rather large CT values up to 2000 HU. Administration of iodine contrast agent increases the CT value, with contrast-filled vessels typically having CT values in the range 200 HU to 600 HU. In most cases, contrast-filled vessels can be easily differentiated from the surrounding tissue, which does not exceed a CT value of 100 HU, with the exception of bone.

This easy threshold-based differentiation is the basis for CTA and related image postprocessing techniques. The gantry rotates around the patient, collecting attenuation data from different angles. The attenuation coefficient also varies depending on the energy of the photons (measured in kiloelectron volts [keV]) that pass through them. The measured intensity of photons at the CT detector is related to the photon flux (number of photons) coming through the x-ray tube and that detected at the detector elements. Consequently, as the attenuation of the tissue increases, the fraction of photons detected at the detector element decreases. Photon energy (keV) and photon flux (milliamperes [mA]) are variables set by the user. Increasing tube current (mA) will improve image quality at the expense of increasing radiation dose. Certain manufacturers have introduced an "effective mAs" concept for spiral/helical scanning that incorporates the amount of time the tube current is being generated. Tube voltage (kilovolts [kV]) determines the energy of the x-ray beam or the hardness of the x-ray. High kV results in a smaller fraction of the x-ray beam being absorbed (reduced attenuation) but will result in improvements in contrast.

Scanning Modes

The two scanning modes used in CT are the axial mode and the spiral/helical mode. The major differences between these modes include (1) differences in table movement during image acquisition, (2) differences in assignment of data to each channel, and (3) need for interpolation for data reconstruction. Each mode has its benefits, but the mode used for vascular CTA is the spiral/helical mode. For coronary CTA, there has been a shift toward using axial mode for its benefit in significantly reducing radiation exposure.

SPIRAL/HELICAL MODE

During spiral scanning, there is continuous table movement while x-rays are generated the entire time; however, the tube current can be made to fluctuate. Since the table is moving during acquisition, the detector channels are not dedicated to a slice position of the patient, so data is received from multiple contiguous slices of the patient. An interpolation algorithm is necessary to reconstruct "virtual" axial slices, with some loss in image quality. Spiral imaging is fast and can provide infinite reconstruction of data, but at the cost of higher radiation.

Beam Pitch

Pitch is an expression of the relationship between the table distance moved per gantry rotation and the coverage of the scanner. Pitch = [table feed per gantry rotation (mm) / coverage (mm)]. If the pitch is 1, there would be no gaps between the data set. However, if the pitch is greater than 1, gaps would be present, and if the pitch is less than 1, there would be overlap in the data acquisition. The pitch for electrocardiographic (ECG)-gated cardiac scanning is typically 0.2 to 0.3, whereas for vascular CT, pitch ranges between 0.5 and 1.2.

General Acquisition Parameters

Selection of specific acquisition parameters for imaging depends on the employed scanner model, the patient's body habitus, and the clinical question. The two main adjustable parameters are the tube voltage and current. Voltage is typically set at 120 kV, although 100 kV provides acceptable images with significantly reduced radiation and can be employed for vascular imaging in most individuals who are not obese. Tube current is usually 200 to 300 mA and can be adjusted upward if the patient is very large. To reduce motion artifact, breath holding is required for chest and abdominal CTA acquisitions. In MDCT spiral scans, the volume coverage speed (v, cm/s) can be estimated by the following formula:

$$v = \frac{Ms_{coll}p}{t_{rot}}$$

where M = number of simultaneous acquired slices, s_{coll} = collimated slice width, p = pitch, and t_{rot} = gantry rotation time. Although current-generation scanners offer improved spatial resolution, their increased coverage and rotation speeds pose the risk of "out-running" the bolus of contrast in CTA applications. Accordingly, adjustments in both pitch and gantry rotation speed must be made to achieve a table translation speed of no more than 30 to 32 mm/s for CTA applications. In a 64-slice scanner, this usually is achieved by a reduction in t_{rot} to 0.5 seconds and a decrease in pitch to 0.8 or less.

Electrocardiographic Gating

Electrocardiographic gating is a method of gating imaging events to portions in the cardiac cycle where motion may be minimal, namely diastole. Electrocardiographic gating is indispensable for coronary imaging and vascular structures that are prone to cardiac motion artifact, such as the ascending aorta. The two most common ECG gating methods are retrospective and prospective gating. With traditional spiral scanning, ECG gating is performed retrospectively, where the data and ECG information are acquired, and subsequent reconstructions can be performed at various time points in the R-R interval.[4] Compared to prospective ECG gating, which is the method used for axial scanning, the scan is triggered at the R wave, and image acquisition occurs at a fixed point in the cardiac cycle. However, with recent advances in CT imaging, it is now possible to perform a prospectively ECG-triggered helical scan using high pitch with extremely low radiation exposure.[5] These have been referred to as *flash scans* and are gaining significant popularity for coronary imaging.

Contrast Administration

All angiographic x-ray contrast remains in the extracellular space and rapidly distributes between the intravascular and extravascular spaces immediately after intravenous (IV) administration.[6] It is the process during the early phase of rapid contrast distribution and redistribution that determines vascular enhancement. Vascular enhancement differs significantly from parenchymal (soft tissue) enhancement characteristics. The two key components that determine arterial enhancement are the amount of contrast per unit time (mL/s) and the duration of administration (seconds). The resulting product of the two is the volume of contrast (flow rate × duration). For example, 100 mL of contrast media given at 5 mL/s will require 20 seconds to deliver. The relationship between flow rate, volume of contrast, and duration of administration is the most important concept to understanding injection protocols for vascular imaging.

Currently, low or isoosmolar nonionic contrast agents are the most commonly used for CTA. It is imperative to assess renal function prior to administration of contrast so decisions can be made in regard to prophylactic measures, type of contrast used, and whether the study should be cancelled. Contrast is given IV using a power injector. Since contrast arrival time to the region of interest may vary, appropriate timing must be determined by using a test bolus or automated bolus tracking technique.[7] The less common technique of using a test bolus is performed by giving a small dose of contrast material and determining the time it takes for the region of interest to opacify. More commonly, a triggered or automated bolus tracking technique is used, where a region of interest is drawn on the aorta closest to the area of interest. A repetitive low-dose acquisition is acquired 5 to 10 seconds after contrast administration until a given HU threshold is achieved (typically 110 HU). The actual CTA will be acquired once this threshold is obtained. The typical volume of contrast used is 100 to 120 mL, with an iodine concentration between 320 and 370 mg/mL, administered at a rate of 4 mL/s and followed by a saline flush.

CONTRAST CONSIDERATIONS

Although MD-CTA uses substantially lower contrast volumes, the inherent nephrotoxicity of contrast media must be considered, especially in individuals with preexisting renal dysfunction (e.g., chronic kidney disease, diabetes mellitus). For these individuals, except in emergency situations, creatinine (Cr) clearance should be determined before scheduling the patient. An allergy to iodinated contrast material is a major contraindication for performing contrast CT studies. However, based on the severity of previous contrast reactions, an assessment may be made as to whether the study can be safely performed after premedication with oral steroids and antihistamines. Fasting is not mandatory except for patients with previous contrast-induced gastrointestinal reactions.

Image Reconstruction at the Scanner Console

Various image reconstruction filters are offered by each manufacturer. Filters are referred to as *sharp* or *soft*. Sharper reconstruction filters will provide more details but also more noise and are best for assessment of stents and areas of calcification. Softer reconstruction filters provide less image detail but less noise as well. Soft to medium filters are usually used for most CTA applications. Image reconstruction can also be performed at different cardiac phases of cardiac-gated acquisitions. It may be important in assessment of coronary anatomy in cases of thoracic aortic dissection and thoracic aortic aneurysms.[8] This is most important for cardiac CTA where coronary anatomy may have to be assessed at different phases to ensure accurate delineation of coronary stenosis. When ECG-gated thoracic aortic imaging is performed, various phases can be reconstructed to assess the aorta.

Slice width and slice increment used for image reconstruction at the scanner console depend on the anatomy being assessed and scanner capabilities. Reconstruction thickness for vascular imaging can be performed at the same width (thin) or several times the detector width (thick) to reduce noise. Thinner slices are associated with higher image noise compared to thicker slices, and take longer to review. A slice increment of approximately 50% of the slice thickness is typically used.

Image Postprocessing

Similar to vascular magnetic resonance angiography (MRA) (see Chapter 13), multiple postprocessing techniques can be used in vascular CTA to assess the hundreds to thousands of images generated. Usually two data sets are reconstructed: thick and thin sets. The thick set (5.0 mm) is used for general assessment, whereas the thin set (0.5-0.75 mm) is better suited for detailed evaluation. Image formats used for evaluation include (1) multiplanar reformats (MPR), (2) maximal intensity projections (MIP), (3) curved planer reformats (CPR), (4) volume rendering (VR), and (5) shaded surface display (SSD). Please refer to Chapter 13 for a description of these techniques.

For CTA, evaluation of the data set begins with review of the axial images to assess gross anatomy and scan quality. Maximal intensity projection format is used to view the vascular structure of interest in the traditional projections as well as in oblique orientations. A major caveat is the presence of calcium when viewing MIP images, since it can overestimate the severity of stenosis. For detailed evaluation, especially when calcium and stents are present, raw MPR images must be reviewed. Curved planar reconstruction is a unique technique that makes it possible to follow the course of any single vessel and displays it in a nontraditional plane, where the entire vessel can be seen in a single image. Three-dimensional (3D) VR images can also be reviewed to get a general appreciation of the anatomical variations if necessary. Each of these reconstruction methods has its pitfalls; it is important to develop a systematic process to identify and evaluate an abnormality.

Radiation Exposure and Radiation Dose Reduction

Radiation exposure of the patient during CT and the resulting potential radiation hazards has recently gained considerable attention from both the public and the scientific literature.[9-12] *Radiation exposure* is defined as the total charge of ions produced in a unit of dry air by a given amount of x-ray or γ-ray irradiation. In the International System of Units (SI), exposure is measured in terms of coulombs (C)/kg or amperes (A) ·s/kg. Exposure is also commonly measured in units of roentgens (R), where 1 R equals 2.58×10^{-4} C/kg. *Absorbed dose* is the energy imparted to a volume of matter by ionizing radiation, divided by the mass of the matter. The SI unit of absorbed dose is the gray (Gy), where 1 Gy equals 1 joule (J)/kg. The traditional unit is the *rad*, short for radiation absorbed dose, which equals 1 cGy or 10^{-2} Gy. Although absorbed dose is a useful concept, the biological effect of a given absorbed dose varies depending on the type and quality of radiation emitted. A dimensionless radiation weighting factor is used to normalize for this effect, where the weighting factor ranges from 1 for photons (including

x-rays and γ-rays) and electrons to 20 for α particles. The sievert (Sv), a special SI unit to represent *equivalent dose*, was adopted to avoid confusion with absorbed dose. One Sv equals 1 J/kg. The traditional unit for equivalent dose is the *rem*, short for roentgen equivalent man. One rem equals 1 cSv, or 10^{-2} Sv. Equivalent dose multiplied by the tissue-weighting factor is often termed *weighted equivalent dose*, properly measured in Sv or rem. The sum of the weighted equivalent dose over all organs or tissues in an individual is termed the *effective dose* (E).[13]

Computed Tomography–Specific Dosimetry

In addition to the nomenclature for radiation dosimetry described above, a particular set of terms has been developed for CT.[14] The dose profile (D[z]) for a CT scanner is a mathematical description of the dose as a function of position on the z axis (perpendicular to the tomographic plane). The CT dose index (CTDI), measured in Gy, is the area under the radiation dose profile for a single rotation and fixed table position along the axial direction of the scanner, divided by the total nominal scan width or beam collimation. CTDI is difficult to measure and therefore not commonly reported; instead, the $CTDI_{100}$ is measured. $CTDI_{100}$ represents the integrated radiation exposure from acquiring a single scan over a length of 100 mm. To estimate the average radiation dose to a cross-section of a patient's body, a weighted CTDI ($CTDI_w$) is calculated. This is determined by the equation:

$$CTDI_w = \tfrac{2}{3}\ CTDI_{100}\ \text{at periphery} + \tfrac{1}{3}\ CTDI_{100}\ \text{at center}$$

$CTDI_w$, given in mGy, is always measured in an axial scan mode and depends on scanner geometry, slice collimation, and beam prefiltration, as well as x-ray tube voltage, tube current (mA), and gantry rotation time (t_{rot}). The product of mA and t_{rot} is the mAs value of the scan. To obtain a parameter characteristic for the scanner used, it is helpful to eliminate the mAs dependence and introduce a normalized $(CTDI_w)_n$ given in mGy per mAs:

$$CTDI_w = mA \times t_{rot} \times \left(CTDI_w\right)_n = mAs \times \left(CTDI_w\right)_n$$

The important CT-specific dosimetry term is the *volume-weighted CTDI*, or $CTDI_{vol}$. This quantity represents the average radiation dose over the volume scanned in a helical or sequential sequence. It is determined from the $CTDI_w$ by the equation:

$$CTDI_{vol} = CTDI_w/pitch = CTDI_w \cdot \text{total nominal scan width}/ \text{distance between scans}$$

$CTDI_{vol}$ is used to determine the dose-length product (DLP), measured in units of mGy · cm. DLP reflects the integrated radiation dose for a complete CT examination and is calculated by:

$$DLP = CTDI_{vol} \cdot \text{length irradiated}$$

Many CT scanner consoles report the $CTDI_{vol}$ and DLP for a study. DLP can be related to E by the formula:

$$E = E_{DLP} \cdot DLP$$

where E_{DLP}, measured in units of mSv / (mGy · cm), is a body region–specific conversion factor. The most commonly used E_{DLP} values are reported in the 2004 CT Quality Criteria.[15] These E_{DLP} values are determined using Monte Carlo methods averaged for multiple scanners.

Dose Reduction Techniques

There are several ways to lower the dose delivered to a patient.[14,16] These methods can be used either in isolation or combined to exponentially lower exposure. Reducing tube current will lead to a direct reduction in radiation dose to a patient. However, a conscious decision must be made as to whether the tradeoff in radiation reduction outweighs image quality. This becomes very important in obese patients, where reduction in tube current may result in rather poor images. The contrast-to-noise ratio increases with decreasing x-ray tube voltage.[5] As a consequence, to obtain the adequate contrast-to-noise ratio, the dose to the patient may be reduced by lowering the kV setting. There is nearly a 50% reduction in radiation exposure when using 80 kV instead of 120 kV when performing CTA. A recent study recommends 100 kV as the standard mode for aortoiliac CTA, and reports dose savings of 30% without loss of diagnostic information.[17]

Electrocardiographic-controlled dose modulation is a method employed during continuous imaging with retrospective studies. Typically the output is kept at its nominal value during a user-defined phase (in general, the mid- to end-diastolic phase), while during the rest of the cardiac cycle, the tube output is reduced to 20% of its nominal value to allow for image reconstruction throughout the entire cardiac cycle. Using this technique, dose reduction of 30% to 50% has been demonstrated in clinical studies.[18–22]

Anatomical tube current modulation is a technique adapted to the patient's geometry during each rotation of the gantry. Tube output is modulated on the basis of the tissue attenuation characteristics of the localizer scan or determined online by evaluating the signal of a detector row. By employing such a technique, dose can be reduced by 15% to 35% without degrading image quality, depending on the body region.[23] A more sophisticated variation of anatomical tube current modulation varies tube output according to patient geometry in the longitudinal direction so as to maintain an adequate dose when moving to different body regions—for instance, from thorax to abdomen (automatic exposure control).[23] Automatic adaptation of the tube current to patient size prevents both over- and under-irradiation, considerably simplifies the clinical workflow for the technician, and eliminates the need to look up tables of patient weight and size for adjusting the mAs settings.

Clinical Applications for Computed Tomographic Angiography in Vascular Disease

Computed Tomographic Angiography of the Neurovascular Circulation

TECHNICAL CONSIDERATIONS

Computed tomographic angiography is comparable to digital subtraction angiography (DSA) for the measurement of residual carotid artery stenosis and is the preferred method of assessment at many institutions.[24–26] To perform CTA of the head and neck arteries, the patient is placed in the supine position with the arms along the sides of the body. The topogram is used to assist planning of the imaging volume, which should start from the aortic arch and end at the level of the circle of Willis. A submillimeter detector collimation is required for images, with the greatest spatial resolution in the z axis. A test bolus or bolus tracking algorithm can be used to determine the start of the scan. The pitch can range from 0.5 and 1.0, depending on the vendor and the number of detector rows. Breath-holding and cessation of swallowing is critical to eliminate motion artifacts. For assessment of carotid circulation, reconstruction is typically performed with smooth reconstruction kernels (e.g., Siemens B20f) using a slice thickness between 0.6 and 1.0 mm and a 50% to 80% reconstruction increment.

Attention to appropriate window settings will have significant impact on measured variances in luminal contrast density. Differences in the measured residual lumen and beam-hardening from calcified plaque will overestimate the degree of stenosis. To avoid this problem, a simple formula may be used to calculate the optimal window settings for carotid stenosis assessment with CTA.[27] The window width used is the product of the intraluminal HU × 2.07, and the widow level is the product

of the intraluminal HU × 0.72. The degree of stenosis should be reported in terms of percent stenosis or residual luminal area. *Percent stenosis* is defined as the ratio of the maximal luminal narrowing to the normal internal carotid artery (ICA) distal to the bulb, as was described in the North American Symptomatic Carotid Endarterectomy Trial (NASCET).[28] However, the segment of normal ICA measurement can range from 5 to 8 mm, which will affect the calculated degree of stenosis. This can be averted by using the residual luminal diameter instead of the percent stenosis,[29–33] or using a simple visual estimation of the degree of stenosis rather than using a caliper-based method.[34] The current standard uses the percent stenosis measurement based on NASCET, but there are papers describing the use of residual lumen diameter, where 1.5 mm is used as the cutoff for hemodynamically significant stenosis, which correlates with an ultrasound peak systolic velocity of greater than 250 cm/s and a NASCET measurement of more than 70% stenosis.[35]

If the clinical question is whether there is a total or subtotal internal carotid occlusion, an immediate delayed acquisition through the neck is helpful to detect slow opacification through a residual lumen. It is important to be aware that sometimes the ascending pharyngeal artery may mimic a subtotally occluded ICA. This is easily differentiated by the fact that the ascending pharyngeal artery does not reach the skull base, whereas the ICA does. Accurate distinction is critically important; a subtotally stenosed ICA may be amenable to revascularization.[36–38]

Computed Tomographic Angiography in Atherosclerotic and Nonatherosclerotic Disease

Technical advances in CTA from the last decade have allowed unprecedented imaging for a number of neurovascular applications, including evaluation for carotid artery stenosis, acute ischemic and hemorrhagic stroke, intracranial vascular anomalies, and craniocervical trauma. By far the most common indication for CTA of the extracranial circulation is for suspected carotid artery stenosis due to atherosclerosis (Fig. 14-1). Computed tomographic angiography is also part of the comprehensive evaluation of the patient with an acute stoke, where nonenhanced brain CT, vascular angiography, and perfusion imaging can be acquired during the comprehensive CT examination. Nonatherosclerotic diseases such as fibromuscular dysplasia (FMD), aneurysms or pseudoaneurysms, or dissections can also be imaged with high spatial resolution (Fig. 14-2). Additionally, CTA has a unique role in follow-up after carotid artery stenting procedures (see Fig. 14-1) instead of using MRA, which typically has significant susceptibility artifacts.

DIAGNOSIS OF CAROTID DISEASE

MDCT has shown a 100% correlation with invasive angiography for locating significant stenosis. The interobserver agreement in evaluating total versus subtotal occlusion, stenosis length, retrograde ICA flow, and location of the stenotic site is 1.0, 0.94, 0.86, and 0.89, respectively.[24,39] MDCT is also helpful in identifying underlying etiology such as dissection, atherosclerosis, or thrombosis. Berg et al. studied 35 consecutive symptomatic patients with cerebrovascular disorders (e.g., minor stroke, transient ischemic attack (TIA), amaurosis fugax, dizziness) and performed MD-CTA.[24] The main focus of the study was comparing MD-CTA to conventional x-ray DSA and rotational DSA as reference standards. In this study, the degree of stenosis was slightly underestimated with CTA, with mean differences (± standard deviation) per observer of 6.9 ± 17.6% and 10.7 ± 16.1% for cross-sectional, and 2.8 ± 19.2% and 9.1 ± 16.8% for oblique sagittal MPRs, compared with x-ray and rotational angiography, respectively. Computed tomographic angiography was somewhat inaccurate for measuring the absolute minimal diameter of subtotally occluded carotid arteries. For symptomatic lesions, interactive CTA interpretation combined with MPR measurements of

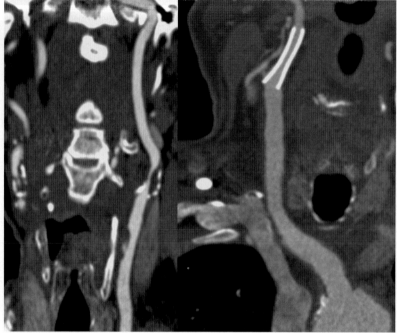

FIGURE 14-1 Carotid artery atherosclerosis. Curved planar reformation (CPR) from left carotid artery shows significant stenosis and noncalcified plaque, with minor calcifications at bifurcation and hemodynamically insignificant but ulcerated plaque at common carotid artery (CCA) *(left)*, and a widely patent right carotid artery stent *(right)*. *(Adapted with permission from Berg M et al: CT angiography of the extracranial and intracranial circulation with imaging protocols. In Mukherjee D, Rajagopalan S, editors: CT and MR angiography of the peripheral circulation: practical approach with clinical protocols, London, 2007, Informa UK Ltd., p. 67.)*

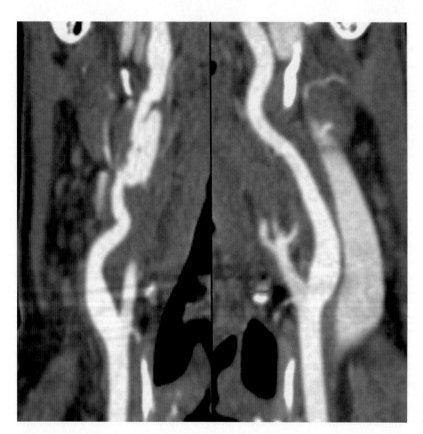

FIGURE 14-2 Carotid artery pseudoaneurysm. Curved planar reformation (CPR) of right carotid artery shows large pseudoaneurysm *(left)* of right internal carotid, with normal-appearing left common and internal carotid arteries *(right)*.

lesions with a visual estimate of 50% or greater diameter narrowing had a sensitivity of 95% and specificity of 93% for detection of carotid stenosis compared with DSA. Based on these data, it can be concluded that CTA is sensitive for detecting significant carotid artery stenosis.

Although MD-CTA is a very effective noninvasive means of assessing cervicocranial circulation, there are multiple limitations that may occasionally restrict its usefulness. Computed tomographic angiography does not include flow dynamics. Blooming artifact due to calcification in segments can obscure the lumen and lead to overestimation of stenosis severity. Surgical clips can also preclude accurate assessment. The radiation dose of neurovascular CTA is between 1.7 and 3.0 mSv, depending on the imaged volume, type of scanner, and use of radiation reduction algorithms. There may be overlapping veins that prevent detection of small cerebral artery aneurysms.

Computed Tomographic Angiography of the Thorax

PULMONARY ARTERIES

Technical Considerations and Clinical Applications

Pulmonary embolism (PE) is the third most common cause of cardiovascular death in the United States after ischemic heart disease and stroke, with an estimated annual incidence of 300,000 to 600,000 cases per year.[40] Even though there is a high prevalence of PE, it continues to be underdiagnosed, with only 43 to 53 patients per 100,000 being accurately identified.[41]

Computed tomography of the pulmonary arteries (CTPA) is the current diagnostic test of choice for assessing pulmonary thromboembolic disease. In the PIOPED-II study,[42] CTPA was principally performed on 4-slice CT with a slice thickness of 1 to 1.25 mm. In this study, the overall positive predictive value in diagnosing PE was 86% (97% for proximal, 68% for segmental, and 25% for subsegmental thrombus), and the negative predictive value was 95%. The value of CTPA varied with the clinical pretest probability of PE: in patients with high or intermediate clinical probability, the positive predictive value for PE was 96%. However, in the face of low clinical pretest likelihood, 42% of patients had a false-positive CTPA result. Therefore, a positive CTPA that was discordant with clinical data had little diagnostic value, at least on the basis of this study. There are randomized controlled studies using later-generation CT scanners that have addressed the issue of their superiority over the 4-slice systems used in PIOPED-II.[43–45] The expectation is that thinner detectors and larger detector assembly would allow rapid imaging of the pulmonary artery and branches in a few seconds, avoiding motion artifact.

To perform CTPA, the patient is placed supine with the hands above the head. Following the topogram, the field of view is prescribed to include the adrenals to the lung apices. The goal is to acquire the study with the thinnest slice collimation with a single short breath-hold in full-suspended respiration. The voltage, current, and pitch will vary depending on vendor and patient characteristics. There are two main methods for image acquisition: timing bolus and bolus tracking techniques. In the timing bolus technique, a region of interest is placed in the pulmonary trunk, and repeated scans are acquired at the same level every 2 to 4 seconds. A time density curve is obtained, allowing for calculation of the scan delay. The alternate approach is using an automated bolus tracking technique, where a region of interest is placed over the pulmonary trunk, and the image acquisition initiates once a specified attenuation threshold is achieved. The pulmonary arteries are imaged with the first pass of IV contrast, and the pelvis and lower-extremity veins can be imaged later with a scan delay of 2.5 to 3.5 minutes.

CTPA images can be reconstructed using several techniques; however, one suggested method is using a 1.25-mm slice thickness with a 50% to 60% slice increment. Larger slice thickness is used for reconstruction of the pelvis and lower-extremity veins. There are multiple artifacts that can limit detection of true PEs, so careful scrutiny of the acquired images with active scrolling in and out of each main, lobar, segmental, and subsegmental artery is necessary to avoid overcalling or missing PEs. Similarly, CT venography of the proximal lower extremities is difficult to interpret and suffers from several technical limitations, such as flow artifacts from suboptimal timing of contrast, arterial inflow contamination, streak artifacts from orthopedic hardware, arterial calcification, or dense contrast within the bladder.

The CTPA findings of acute PE can be divided into arterial findings and ancillary findings. Intraluminal filling defects may partially or completely occlude a pulmonary artery and typically cause significant dilation of the vessel. Acute emboli appear as adherent intravascular filling defects that form acute angles to the vessel wall, whereas chronic thrombi have the appearance of mural adherent thrombi contiguous with the vessel wall. Acute PEs that straddle the bifurcation of the left and right pulmonary arteries are referred to as *saddle emboli* (Fig. 14-3). Lung infarcts, atelectasis, and oligemia of the affected territory are common lung parenchymal findings with a PE.

CTPA examinations should have optimized window settings, where the window width is equal to the mean attenuation of the pulmonary artery plus 2 standard deviations, and the window level should be half this value. Active scrolling in and out each main, lobar, segmental, and subsegmental artery avoids confusion with veins or mucous-filled bronchi. Multiplanar reformats and MIPs of the pulmonary arteries can be used to improve reader confidence for subtle or questionable findings, but improved diagnostic accuracy has not been proven.[46,47] An important fact to keep in mind while interpreting a CTPA study is that most PEs are larger than 1 or 2 mm. Therefore, filling defects seen on only one 1.25-mm image are more likely to be artifact rather than true emboli. Pulmonary emboli typically originate from the pelvic and lower-extremity deep venous anatomy. Less commonly, the source of emboli will be from the thorax, such as the superior vena cava or brachiocephalic veins, likely as a complication of indwelling catheters.

Computed Tomographic Venography for Acute Deep Venous Thrombosis

The usual findings of a pelvic or proximal lower-extremity deep venous thrombosis (DVT) is a partial or complete IV filling defect. Commonly there is associated generalized leg and perivenous edema seen on the acquired images.[48]

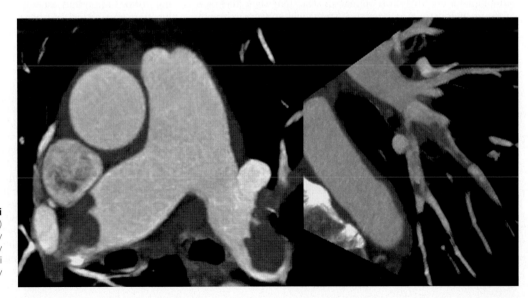

FIGURE 14-3 Pulmonary emboli (PEs). Maximal intensity projection (MIP) images showing large central pulmonary emboli of left and right main pulmonary artery *(left)*, and subsegmental emboli involving branches of left pulmonary artery *(right)*.

Predictors of Patient Outcome

There are many CTPA findings that give powerful prognostic information. These include the presence of right ventricular (RV) dilation, interventricular septal flattening suggesting significant RV pressure overload, and reflux of contrast into the inferior vena cava, all of which may result from a massive acute PE. A short-axis diameter ratio of the right to left ventricles of 1 to 1.5 or greater is an indicator for severe RV strain and carries a poor prognosis.[49] A right-to-left ventricular diameter ratio of greater than 0.9 in a 4-chamber view is associated with increased 30-day mortality, cardiopulmonary resuscitation, ventilator support, and the use of vasopressors.[50]

Other clinical applications of CTPA include assessment of pulmonary artery aneurysms and pseudoaneurysms, congenital anomalies such as pulmonary artery atresia, palliative shunts, AVMs, and pre-procedure planning for percutaneous pulmonary valve replacement or stenting of branch pulmonary artery stenosis.

THORACIC AORTA

Technical Considerations

Development of 16-slice MD-CTA and beyond has made it possible to acquire nearly isotropic submillimeter images within seconds. Standard protocol for acute aortic pathology should include precontrast CT to assess whether intramural hematoma (IMH) is present or if there is blood, which is high density, within the pericardium, pleural space, or mediastinum, indicating aortic rupture. Precontrast CT is performed with a low-dose technique using 1.5-mm collimation to reduce the total radiation dose.[51,52] The scan range of the precontrast CT should be restricted to an area from the lung apex to the upper abdomen, but the contrast-enhanced (CE) CT portion should cover the thoracic inlet to the femoral head.[53] There is no standard iodine concentration for a dedicated aortic protocol. Normally, a body weight–adapted iodine concentration accounting for flow rates of 1.0 to 1.6 g/s is sufficient to opacify the entire aorta.[54,55] An iodine concentration of 3 to 4 mL of 300 mg I/mL/s (0.9-1.2 g/s) may be adequate for most patients, whereas obese patients may require 5 mL of 300 mg I/mL/s (1.5 g/s) to obtain adequate opacification of the aorta. A bolus tracking method using 100 HU with a scan delay of 5 to 7 seconds, followed by a saline chaser to minimize venous contamination, is the ideal method to obtain CE-CTA images.[52]

Adequate opacification of the entire aorta is achieved by administering the contrast material at least as long as the scan time plus the delay time. For example, if the scan time and scan delay time are 15 and 5 seconds, respectively, a 20-second injection of contrast material followed by a 50-mL saline chaser would be sufficient. With 64-slice MDCT, it is possible to scan the entire aorta with submillimeter collimation (collimation, 0.625 mm; slice thickness, 0.625 mm; reconstruction interval, 0.3 mm) within a single breath-hold, thus making high-resolution 3D displays possible. Cardiac motion may simulate an intimal flap resembling aortic root dissection, which can be eliminated using ECG-gated acquisition.[54,56] This will substantially increase the amount of radiation received by the patient, but will lend improved ability to not only evaluate the aortic root but also the coronary arteries.

Clinical Applications

ACUTE AORTIC SYNDROMES

Computed tomographic angiography plays an important role in the assessment of acute aortic syndromes. These entities comprise penetrating aortic ulcerations (PAU), IMH, and acute aortic dissection (AAD) (see Chapter 34). Dissection presents with severe chest and/or back pain of sudden onset that is often described as "ripping" or "tearing." This is typically associated with hypertension and older age. However, there are other strong associations with inherited collagen disorders including Marfan's and Ehlers-Danlos' syndromes. MDCT is the imaging modality of choice for evaluating the presence of AAD. The major advantage of MDCT is its ability to visualize the entire aorta and the branch vessels, and

its rapid through-put. With MDCT, it is important to discern potential artifacts caused by motion of the aortic root and which may simulate an intimal flap. With ECG gating, motion artifact can be eliminated. This may be important in cases when also assessing coronary patency and left ventricular (LV) wall motion.

Penetrating aortic ulceration is the protrusion of plaque through the intima and internal elastic membrane of the aorta. Penetrating aortic ulceration can be seen when the lumen is filled with contrast. It appears as a focal contrast outpouching that may enhance the aortic wall. The most common site of PAU is the middle or lower descending thoracic aorta.[57] Penetrating aortic ulceration has to be differentiated from a nonpenetrating atheromatous ulcer, where the ulceration is confined within the intimal layer. The location of intimal calcification can be helpful in this situation.[58] Atheromatous ulcers overlie the aortic contour and calcified intima, whereas PAU extends beyond this margin.[51,58,59] However, differentiating a calcified mural thrombus, IMH, and PAU can be quite challenging.[60] The natural history of PAU can vary depending on the location.[61–64] Attenuation of the aortic wall on precontrast images can help distinguish acute IMH or PAU with some mural hemorrhage from chronic IMH. Typically, acute IMH has high attenuation (50-70 HU), in contrast to lower attenuation with chronic IMH. The size of a PAU has influence on its natural history.[65] Penetrating aortic ulceration depth and diameter greater than 10 mm and 20 mm, respectively, were independent predictors of extension of IMH or dissection and rupture in one study.[64] In another study, however, no predictors of adverse outcomes were acknowledged except for overt rupture upon presentation.[66] The interval change in diameter on follow-up CT may be more important than the size of the PAU on the initial CT exam to determine treatment options or patient prognosis.[57]

The pathogenesis of IMH is not well understood, but hypertension is the major predisposing factor. The two pathophysiological mechanisms of IMH are spontaneous bleeding into the media from the vasa vasorum and intimal tear with complete thrombosis of the false lumen. More recent studies suggest that most IMHs result from an entry tear similar to aortic dissection.[60,67–69] Identification of an intimal tear is often underappreciated on preoperative CT but is seen intraoperatively.[60] An IMH is visualized as a crescent or ring-shaped region of the aortic wall, with characteristic high attenuation.[51,70] In the International Registry of Aortic Dissection (IRAD), location of the IMH was associated with adverse outcome.[71] A recent publication from Korea, however, contradicted the IRAD findings.[72] New ulceration on follow-up CT and progression of IMH to a thickness greater than 11 mm are associated with progression to overt aortic dissection.[73,74]

Acute aortic dissection is easily detected by MDCT, a first-line imaging study for evaluating patients[59] (Fig. 14-4). Stanford classification is based on extent of the intimal flap, where type A dissection involves the ascending aorta, and type B only involves the descending aorta.[75] Important aspects of the evaluation of AAD include location and extent, site of entry/exit, side branch involvement, presence of aortic rupture, patency of false lumen, and associated complications. An inward displacement of intimal calcification can be a sign of aortic dissection on precontrast MDCT. Identifying the location of the entry tear is extremely important because this may affect endovascular treatment options. Likewise, reentry tears can be visualized in the descending and abdominal aorta or iliac arteries.[76] Differentiating between the true and false lumen is extremely important because the major side branches originating from the false lumen may be occluded after stent-graft placement.[59] The dissection flap may directly extend into or obstruct the ostium of an affected side branch vessel. A simple method to differentiate true from false lumen is to identify the communication with uninvolved aortic segment. The larger lumen is typically the false lumen because the pressure in the false lumen is higher than that of the true lumen.[51,59,70] Typically, the true lumen has greater opacification with contrast because of the higher velocity of blood compared to the false lumen.[51,59] The false lumen may also show a *beak sign*, which is the acute angle between the intimal flap and outer false lumen on axial images.[51,59,70] Intraluminal thrombus is much more commonly seen within the false lumen, owing to the slower flow of

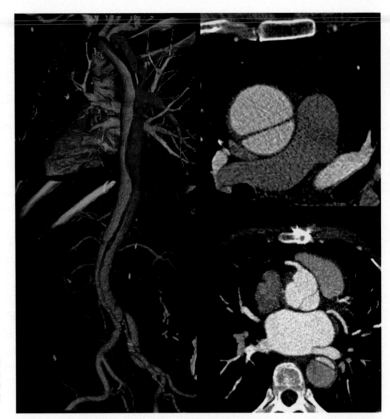

FIGURE 14-4   Aortic dissection. Three-dimensional (3D) computed tomographic angiography (CTA) volume-rendered image showing an extensive aortic dissection *(left)* and maximal intensity projection (MIP) images in the axial projection depicting ascending *(upper right)* and descending *(lower right)* dissection propagation.

blood. Less commonly seen are strands of incompletely torn connective tissue of the aortic media, known as the *cobweb sign.*[77]

THORACIC AORTIC ANEURYSMS
A true aortic aneurysm is a dilation of the aorta greater than 50% comprising the intima, media, and adventitial layers. The aortic root and ascending aorta are affected in nearly 60% of patients with a thoracic aneurysm, the aortic arch in 10%, the descending thoracic aorta in 40%, and the thoracoabdominal aorta in 10% of cases.[78] MDCT can determine the extent, location, and size of the aneurysm. The diameter of the aneurysm should be measured in the true aortic short axis. MDCT also can detect complications such as rupture, infection, and fistulas.

CONGENITAL ANOMALIES OF THE THORACIC AORTA
Computed tomographic angiography can be used to assess congenital anomalies such as aortic coarctation and anomalous origin of the head and neck vessels (see Chapter 63). Magnetic resonance angiography however, is more useful in this circumstance, because it provides additional hemodynamic data not possible with CTA. Computed tomography has a unique role in assessing the relationship of vascular structures such as the main pulmonary artery, ascending aorta, and mammary arteries to the sternum.

AORTITIS
Computed tomographic angiography can also be used for assessment of inflammatory diseases that involve the aorta and its proximal branches (e.g., giant cell arteritis [GCA], Takayasu's arteritis). Wall thickness can be easily assessed, and arterial-phase wall enhancement has at times been used as a marker of ongoing inflammatory disease activity.

Computed Tomographic Angiography of the Abdominal Aorta

TECHNICAL CONSIDERATIONS

Computed tomographic angiography has an important role in abdominal aortic imaging because of its ability to assess intrinsic vessel pathology and branches such as the renal and mesenteric arteries with a high degree of accuracy. Protocols for image acquisition vary significantly based on the clinical question and the CT scanner used for imaging. The patient is placed in the supine position, with imaging collimation placed at the lowest possible setting by the scanner. Scanning volume can range from the upper edge of the 12th rib superiorly to the femoral heads or the iliac crest inferiorly. Scanning is performed in the craniocaudal direction without cardiac gating. Breath-holding will improve image quality, especially of the upper abdominal vessels, and is recommended whenever possible. A noncontrast study may be performed using larger collimation to assess for hemorrhage or aortic hematoma. This is followed by a contrast study with triggering at the diaphragmatic or supraceliac aorta. A postcontrast study may be performed to evaluate venous anatomy, renal perfusion, or slow bleeding. Images can be reconstructed using a softer filter at submillimeter slice thickness with 50% slice increments.

CLINICAL APPLICATIONS

Abdominal Aortic Dissection

The most common cause for dissection of the abdominal aorta and iliac arteries is propagation of a thoracoabdominal aortic dissection. Focal dissection of the abdominal aorta is rare, occurring in only 1.3% of all aortic dissections.[79] A focal dissection is usually associated with hypertension, smoking, diabetes, previous aneurysm surgery, and hyperlipidemia.[80] In addition to assessing the vasculature, CTA can also provide information on soft-tissue structures, including complications such as hemorrhage. A noncontrast study may illustrate acute hemorrhage or IMH within an aortic dissection plane and may reveal complications. In addition, a precontrast study in conjunction with a postcontrast study may allow for comparison of subtle changes in thrombus opacification, suggesting a slow bleed. An additional delayed acquisition 1 to 2 minutes post contrast can help identify slow hemorrhage and venous abnormalities.

Abdominal Aortic Aneurysm

An abdominal aortic aneurysm (AAA) is defined by a greater than 50% enlargement of the abdominal aorta compared to a normal

CH
14

aortic segment. A less than 50% dilation of the aorta is referred to as *ectasia*.[81,82] Although ultrasound is the preferred screening modality for AAA, CTA is often required to assess the extent and complications of an AAA and to plan treatment.[81] Regardless of the indication for a CTA exam, true short- and long-axis measurements of the aneurysm must be reported. The distance between the lowermost renal artery and the superior border of the aneurysm, referred to as the *neck*, provides a standardized description of its location. Computed tomographic angiography can assess the shape and angulation of the neck, measure the maximum diameter of the AAA, and provide a thorough assessment of the iliac and femoral arteries. These determinations are important, especially when consideration is being made for endovascular aneurysm repair (EVAR; Fig. 14-5). Computed tomographic angiography can visualize mural thrombus and calcification within the aneurysm, which have important implications for EVAR (Fig. 14-6). Identifying the number and location of the renal arteries, the presence of a retroaortic left renal vein, and assessment of the mesenteric and hypogastric arteries also are important for operative planning.

SURVEILLANCE FOLLOWING ENDOVASCULAR ANEURYSM REPAIR

Computed tomographic angiography is the modality of choice for surveillance of patients who have undergone EVAR because it assesses potential complications, including endoleaks. A post–stent-graft examination consists of precontrast dynamic first circulation imaging, and immediate delayed postcontrast imaging. The precontrast study allows identification of calcification so that it is not confused with endoleak. The immediate delayed postcontrast study may identify a slow endoleak that might be missed on the dynamic first circulation study.[83] Computed tomographic angiography is used to measure the maximum external dimensions of the aneurysm sac, the lumen of the aortic stent-graft along with its two limbs, the distance between the proximal margin of the stent-graft and the inferior margin of the most inferior renal artery, and the lower margin of the stent-graft and the iliac artery bifurcation of each side.

Endoleaks cause increased pressure within the aneurysm sac and thereby increase the potential for continued aneurysm growth and rupture. A type I endoleak is either a proximal or distal attachment site endoleak, and is usually discovered during implantation. Delayed type I endoleak may be related to changes in tortuosity of the aorta secondary to aneurysm reshaping and should be suspected on CT when acute hemorrhage or contrast pooling is found in the aneurysm sac adjacent to the device attachment site.[84] Type II endoleak, the most common form of endoleak, is caused by continued blood flow into the aneurysm sac through a small arterial branch that is excluded by the stent-graft. This type of endoleak resolves spontaneously in most instances and is seen as a small area of contrast opacification within the aneurysm. It is often located at a distance from the graft.[85] Type III endoleak is caused by mechanical disruption of the material of an endograft or by separation of an iliac extender from the main graft. This type of endoleak is considered high pressure and carries a high risk for rupture. It appears as a large central collection of contrast distant from the landing zone of the graft.[86] A type IV endoleak is due to graft porosity, which is often detected near the time of implantation prior to endothelialization of the graft conduit. This type of endoleak is self-healing and resolves with cessation of anticoagulation. A type V endoleak is result of endotension from arterial pressurization within the aneurysm sac and is without an identifiable cause. This is a diagnosis of exclusion after CTA and invasive angiography fail to identify an alternative type of endoleak.[84]

Vasculitis

In the abdomen, CTA also has a role in assessing vascular wall and branch vessel changes associated with large-vessel and medium-vessel vasculitis, such as Takayasu arteritis and polyarteritis nodosa, respectively. There are four subtypes of Takayasu's arteritis (see Chapter 42): type 1 is confined to the aortic arch and branches, type 2 involves the descending thoracic and abdominal aorta, type 3 includes type 1 and 2 components, and type 4 combines type 1, 2, and 3 with pulmonary artery involvement. In patients in the acute stage of vasculitis, CTA findings include thickening and enhancement of the vessel wall. In the chronic form of the disease, there may be arterial stenosis, occlusion, or aneurysm formation.[87]

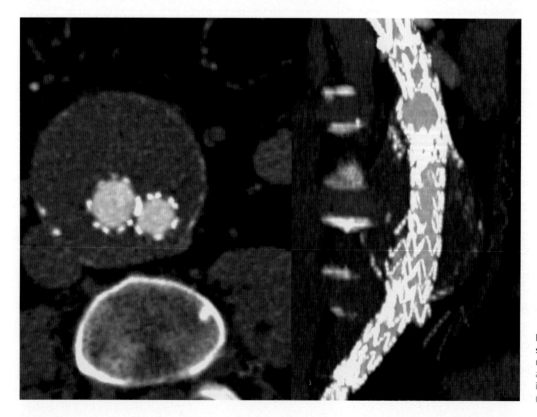

FIGURE 14-5   Aortoiliac composite stent-graft. Multiplanar projection reformation images depicting usual appearance of an aortoiliac stent-graft in axial *(left)* and sagittal oblique views *(right)*.

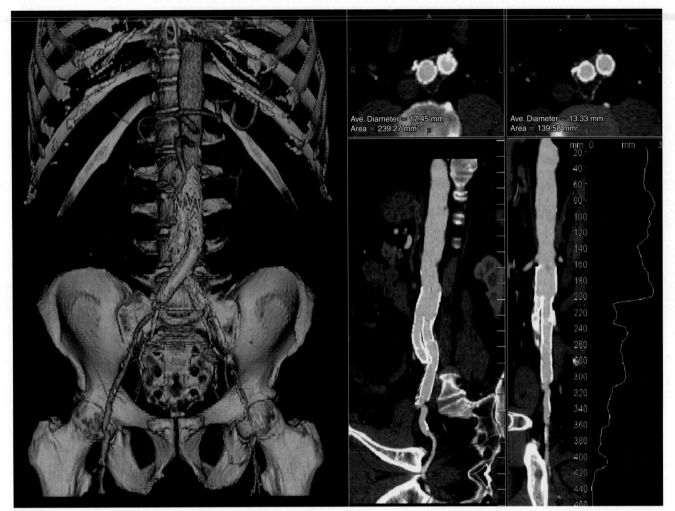

FIGURE 14-6   Aortoiliac composite stent-graft. Three-dimensional (3D) computed tomographic angiography (CTA) volume-rendered image *(left)* and curved planar reformation (CPR) *(right)* showing an aortoiliac stent-graft.

Other Applications of Computed Tomographic Angiography

RENAL ARTERY DISEASE

The superb isotropic spatial resolution ($0.5 \times 0.5 \times 0.5$ mm) of CTA enables assessment of the renal arteries that is unsurpassed by other imaging modalities. There are approximately 6 seconds between initial renal arterial and venous opacification because of the rapid transit time within the kidney.[88] This requires acquiring images with a very high temporal resolution to decrease the degree of venous contamination. Common applications for CTA of the renal arteries include renal artery stenosis (RAS) either from atherosclerosis or FMD, acute renal artery occlusion, and renal artery aneurysms. Atherosclerotic renal artery disease manifests as a stenosis occurring at the vessel origin or proximal segment (typically within 2 cm of the ostium).[89] Fibromuscular dysplasia often involves the mid- to distal renal artery and appears as multiple sequential stenoses ("string of pearls") and possibly renal artery aneurysm.[90] Acute renal artery occlusion may rapidly lead to renal infarction.[89] The CTA appearance includes occlusion of a renal artery with or without an intimal flap, the former indicting propagation of dissection. Renal artery infarction manifests as wedge-shaped or global perfusion abnormalities. Renal artery aneurysms are rare and are most commonly detected incidentally (Fig. 14-7). The most common cause of renal artery aneurysms is associated with atherosclerosis but may also be related to FMD, connective tissue disease, mycotic infection, or vasculitis (e.g., Behçet's syndrome, polyarteritis nodosa).[89,91] Computed tomographic

angiography also has a role in surveillance of patients after renal artery stenting. The biggest limitation of CTA use is that a large proportion of patients with renal artery disease also have advanced renal dysfunction, precluding a CE-CTA study.

MESENTERIC ARTERY DISEASE

Computed tomographic angiography is useful in the assessment of mesenteric artery disease, including mesenteric artery aneurysms, dissection, vasculitis, and FMD (Fig. 14-8). Mesenteric artery aneurysms involve the splenic (60%), hepatic (20%), superior mesenteric (5.5%), celiac (4%), pancreatic (2%), and gastroduodenal arteries (1.5%).[92,93] Traditionally, these types of aneurysms were diagnosed by invasive angiography. With the increased speed and resolution of CTA, they are increasingly detected noninvasively. Usually, celiac artery and superior mesenteric artery (SMA) dissections result from propagation of aortic dissection. On CTA, the dissection flap may be visualized in the proximal vessel and may cause complete occlusion. Rarely, spontaneous dissections of the SMA may occur. These have a relatively high mortality rate.[94,95] Stenosis of the celiac axis may be due to a fibrous band that unites the crura on both sides of the aortic hiatus. This is termed *median arcuate ligament syndrome.* Typically, the ligament crosses superior to the origin of the celiac axis, but in some people there is a variant in which it crosses inferiorly and can cause compression of the proximal portion of the celiac axis.[96] This diagnosis is suggested by CTA when there is focal narrowing with a "hook-like" appearance in the proximal celiac axis.

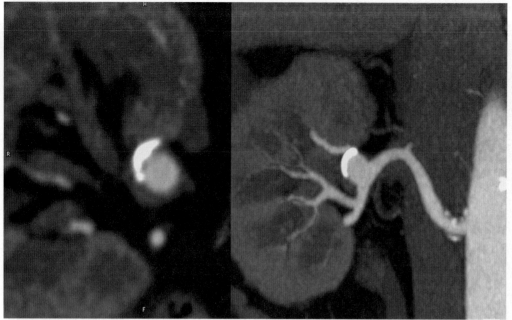

FIGURE 14-7 Renal artery aneurysm. Maximal intensity projection (MIP) images of a distal right renal artery aneurysm with peripheral calcification.

PERIPHERAL ARTERY DISEASE

Technical Considerations

Contemporary MDCT scanners are capable of assessing the distal vessels in lower extremities. To image vessels smaller than 1 mm in diameter, as is the case in pedal vessels, submillimeter detector collimation is necessary. Patients are placed in a supine position on the scanner table in a feet-first orientation. The typical field-of-view (FOV) should extend from the diaphragm to the toes, with an average scan length of 110 to 130 cm. The scanning protocol begins with a scout image of the entire FOV, followed by a test bolus or bolus triggering acquisition. Breath-holding may be necessary for the more proximal abdominal station, but not for the distal stations. This is followed by a CE angiographic acquisition during the arterial contrast phase. With newer scanners, care must be taken to set the gantry rotation times and pitch appropriately to avoid the risk of "outrunning" the contrast bolus. A second late acquisition of the calf vessels can be obtained in the event of inadequate pedal opacification during the arterial phase. For most CTA applications, 100 to 140 mL of contrast (with an iodine concentration between 350-370 mg/mL) is administered at a rate of 4 mL/s and followed by a saline flush.[97] Recently a fixed time strategy has been recommended to image peripheral artery disease (PAD)[98] (Table 14-1). In this strategy, the pitch is varied to accomplish a fixed scan time of 40 seconds in all patients. A biphasic injection protocol is used to provide sustained opacification of the arterial system. This approach standardizes PAD imaging protocols and consistently enables good-quality scans. Images are reconstructed using a smooth kernel into one data set of thicker slices at 5.0-mm slice thickness for general assessment, and another data set of thinner slices of 0.6 to 0.75 mm, incorporating a 25% to 50% overlap. When stenosis is present, the determination of severity is typically by visual estimation rather than a computer-based technique. The combination of MIP, CPR, and axial plane imaging will allow the experienced reader to discern mild (0%-50%), moderate (50%-70%), and severe (>70%) stenosis.[99,100]

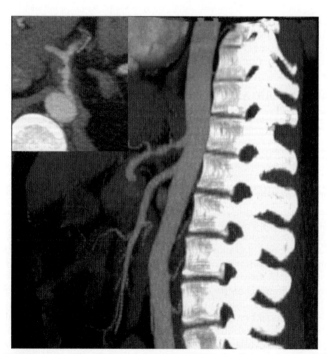

FIGURE 14-8 **Fibromuscular dysplasia (FMD) of celiac artery.** Maximal intensity projection (MIP) images show proximal FMD of celiac artery in lateral oblique and axial *(upper left)* orientations.

TABLE 14-1	Biphasic Injection Protocol for Peripheral Artery Disease Imaging
	Suggested Injection Protocol
Contrast agent	Low-osmolar nonionic, 350-370 mg/mL
Scan time	Fixed at 40 s
Injection duration	35 s
Pitch	Variable and adjusted to scan time of 40 s
Delay	Bolus trigger to occur on reaching threshold of 150-200 HU
Weight-based biphasic injection rate	< 55 kg: 20 mL (4 mL/s) + 96 mL (3.2 mL/s)
	56-65 kg: 23 mL (4.5 mL/s) + 108 mL (3.6 mL/s)
	66-85 kg: 25 mL (5.0 mL/s) + 120 mL (4.0 mL/s)
	86-95 kg: 28 mL (5.5 mL/s) + 132 mL (4.4 mL/s)
	> 95 kg: 30 mL (6.0 mL/s) + 144 mL (4.8 mL/s)

HU, Hounsfield unit; s, second.

Atherosclerotic Peripheral Artery Disease

The major indication for CTA in the evaluation of PAD is in the diagnosis and preinterventional evaluation of symptomatic patients (Fig. 14-9). Findings from CTA can assist the decision to use open surgical or endovascular therapy for revascularization.[101] Computed tomographic angiography is less useful in patients with tibioperoneal atherosclerotic disease, since these patients are typically diabetic and have heavily calcified vessels that may preclude accurate assessment of the degree of stenosis. A meta-analysis of CTA in PAD including mostly 4-slice systems reported a pooled sensitivity and specificity for detecting a stenosis of greater than 50% per segment of 92% (95% confidence interval [CI], 89%-95%) and 93% (95% CI, 91%-95%), respectively. The diagnostic performance of CTA in the infrapopliteal tract was lower, but not significantly different from that in the aortoiliac and femoropopliteal levels.[102–104]

At least one study has evaluated the comparative effectiveness of various imaging approaches in PAD. The outcome measures included clinical utility, functional patient outcomes, quality of life, and diagnostic and therapeutic costs related to the initial imaging test during 6 months of follow-up. Higher confidence and less additional imaging were found for MRA and CTA compared with duplex sonography, and at lower costs.[105]

Peripheral Artery Aneurysm

Approximately 10% of patients with AAAs have femoral and/or popliteal artery aneurysms (Fig. 14-10). Popliteal artery aneurysm is defined as arterial diameter greater than 7 mm, and femoral artery aneurysm is defined as arterial diameter greater than 10 mm.[106,107] Computed tomographic angiography has great utility in diagnosing concomitant aneurysms and also helps distinguish popliteal artery aneurysm from Baker cyst or cystic adventitial disease of the popliteal artery. In the case of femoral artery aneurysm, CTA is appropriate to define the presence of iliac and native femoral vessel disease and plan revascularization strategies.[108]

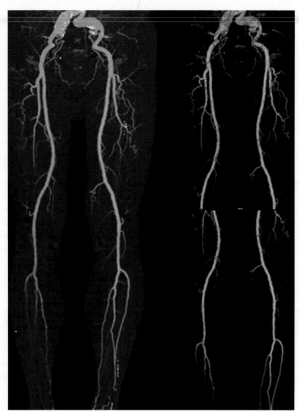

FIGURE 14-9 **Abdominal computed tomographic angiography (CTA) with runoff.** Maximal intensity projection (MIP) *(left)* and three-dimensional (3D) CTA volume-rendered images showing bilateral common iliac aneurysms with distal runoff disease of right lower extremity. *(Adapted from Cohen E, Doshi A, Lookstein R: CT angiography of the lower extremity circulation with protocols. In Mukherjee D, Rajagopalan S, editors: CT and MR angiography of the peripheral circulation: practical approach with clinical protocols, London, 2007, Informa UK Ltd., p. 140.)[97]*

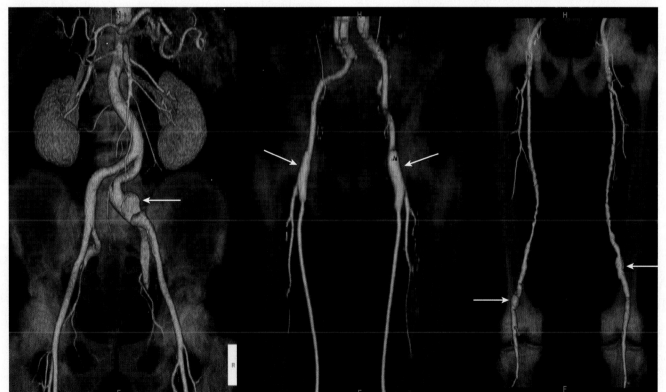

FIGURE 14-10 **Peripheral arterial aneurysms.** Three-dimensional (3D) computed tomographic angiography (CTA) volume-rendered images showing a focal aneurysmal dilation of distal portion of left common iliac artery (CIA) *(left)*, aneurysms of common femoral arteries (CFAs) bilaterally *(middle)* extending to origins of superficial femoral arteries, (SFAs) and focal aneurysmal dilation of bilateral popliteal arteries *(right)*. *(Adapted from Cohen E, Doshi A, Lookstein R: CT angiography of the lower extremity circulation with protocols. In Mukherjee D, Rajagopalan S, editors: CT and MR angiography of the peripheral circulation: practical approach with clinical protocols, London, 2007, Informa UK Ltd., p. 140.)[97]*

Vasculitis

The two most common types of arteritis affecting the lower extremity are thromboangiitis obliterans (TAO) (Buerger's disease) and Takayasu's arteritis (see Chapters 42 and 44 and Fig. 14-10). Thromboangiitis obliterans typically affects the small to medium-sized arteries of the extremities, and primarily affects young male smokers. The distal nature of the disease may favor the use of CTA over MRA in light of the submillimeter resolution of the technique, which permits imaging of femoropopliteal occlusive disease extending into the tibioperoneal circuit. The angiographic appearance is one of abrupt vessel occlusion or focal high-grade concentric stenoses associated with extensive collateral circulation, resulting in a "corkscrew" appearance. Takayasu's arteritis mostly involves the thoracic aorta and brachiocephalic vessels, with less frequent involvement of the abdominal aorta and visceral branches.[109] Other forms of arteritis may affect the peripheral circulation but are uncommon. These include polyarteritis nodosa, Behçet's disease, and Kawasaki disease. As seen on CTA, the patterns and types of vessels involved are useful in distinguishing these entities.

Endovascular Stent Evaluation

Computed tomographic angiography may be used for evaluation of in-stent restenosis, particularly in proximal vessels such as the iliac and femoral arteries. This may require reconstruction with alternate kernels and adjustment of window levels. There are only limited data comparing CT to other modalities for evaluating peripheral stents,[110] but there are emerging data for other circulatory beds that are similar or even smaller than lower-extremity vessels. For instance, a recent prospective study assessed renal in-stent restenosis in 86 patients (95 stents).[111] CTA had a negative predictive value of 100%, specificity of 99%, and positive predictive value of 90%. For renal artery in-stent restenosis, computed tomographic angiography was reported to have a specificity of 95% and positive predictive value of 56%. In the coronary circulation, sensitivity and specificity using 64-slice systems exceed 90%.[112] In practice, these rates may be lower owing to significant publication bias in these reports.

Computed tomographic angiography is used to evaluate patients who have aortoiliac, aortofemoral, or axillofemoral bypass grafts.[113] Surveillance of grafts is important and is primarily performed by duplex ultrasound evaluation. Recent studies, however, suggest that CTA may be superior to duplex ultrasound evaluation.[114] Attention must be paid to the cumulative radiation dose and the use of contrast agents. Assessment of the graft should include careful evaluation of the proximal anastomotic area to exclude stenosis or aneurysm, the body of the graft, and the touch-down site of the graft.

OTHER INDICATIONS

A variety of other conditions represent less common indications for the use of peripheral CTA. These include persistent sciatic artery, popliteal entrapment, and cystic medial adventitial disease (Fig. 14-11). Arteriovenous malformations and fistulas may be well delineated by acquiring images during the arterial and venous phase. Computed tomographic angiography imaging may be used to characterize congenital vascular anomalies.

Artifacts and Pitfalls of Computed Tomographic Angiography

There are several artifacts that can been seen with CT imaging. Artifacts include those that are patient related, procedure related, or reconstruction related. Three of the most common artifacts include motion artifact, beam hardening, and partial volume effects. Motion artifacts are due to patients' body motion during scanning or inability to hold their breath. Beam-hardening artifacts are due to the passage of photons through structures such as pacemaker leads, metal clips, or calcium, resulting in lower-energy photons being filtered out. As a consequence, dark areas are created next to these structures, which can affect assessment of lumen

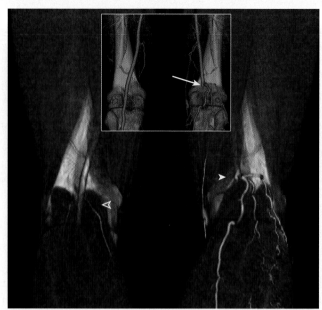

FIGURE 14-11 Popliteal artery entrapment. Three-dimensional (3D) computed tomographic angiography (CTA) volume-rendered (VR) image (posteroanterior view) of a young patient with right calf pain on exertion. Medial head of right gastrocnemius muscle demonstrates an abnormal origin lateral to popliteal artery *(closed arrowhead)*. Inset image shows complete occlusion of right popliteal artery *(arrow)* and multiple superficial collateral arteries originating just proximal to this level. Normal origin of medial head of left gastrocnemius medial to popliteal artery *(open arrowhead)* is shown for comparison. *(Adapted from Cohen E, Doshi A, Lookstein R: CT angiography of the lower extremity circulation with protocols. In Mukherjee D, Rajagopalan S, editors: CT and MR angiography of the peripheral circulation: practical approach with clinical protocols, London, 2007, Informa UK Ltd., p. 143.)[97]*

patency. Partial volume effects occur when parts of the voxel of a structure are affected by other structures with different attenuation properties. This results in averaging of the CT values for that voxel. As a consequence, the image appears distorted.

The most frequent artifacts that affect interpretation of CTA are deviations due to vascular segments affected by moderate to severe calcification or occupied by a stent. Selection of the adequate windowing set (≈1500 window width) may reduce the unavoidable blooming effect caused by structures with high signal attenuation. Cross-sectional MPR images of the vessel of interest are helpful in visualizing, at least in part, the underlying lumen in the presence of intense calcification or a stent. Other interpretation pitfalls such as pseudo-stenoses or pseudo-occlusions may potentially be generated by inadequate image postprocessing (e.g., partial or total vessel removal during MIP image editing, inaccurate centerline definition in CPR images).

Summary

With recent advances in CT technology, CT has moved to the forefront for the diagnosis and assessment of vascular disease. Understanding CT technology is critical to applying the correct technique for evaluation of the vascular system. Although artifacts from severe vessel calcification and stents are potential limitations, the high spatial resolution and rapid throughput of CTA has enabled its widespread acceptance as a modality of choice in evaluating vascular diseases.

REFERENCES

1. Ligon BL: Biography: history of developments in imaging techniques: Egas Moniz and angiography, *Semin Pediatr Infect Dis* 14:173–181, 2003.
2. Fleischmann D: Present and future trends in multiple detector-row CT applications: CT angiography, *Eur Radiol* 12(Suppl 2):S11–S15, 2002.
3. Kalender WA: Technical foundations of spiral CT, *Semin Ultrasound CT MR* 15:81–89, 1994.
4. Kalender WA, Seissler W, Klotz E, et al: Spiral volumetric CT with single-breath-hold technique, continuous transport, and continuous scanner rotation, *Radiology* 176:181–183, 1990.

5. Petersilka M, Bruder H, Krauss B, et al: Technical principles of dual source CT, *Eur J Radiol* 68:362–368, 2008.

6. Dawson P, Blomley MJ: Contrast media as extracellular fluid space markers: adaptation of the central volume theorem, *Br J Radiol* 69:717–722, 1996.

7. van Hoe L, Marchal G, Baert AL, et al: Determination of scan delay time in spiral CT-angiography: utility of a test bolus injection, *J Comput Assist Tomogr* 19:216–220, 1995.

8. Leschka S, Wildermuth S, Boehm T, et al: Noninvasive coronary angiography with 64-section CT: effect of average heart rate and heart rate variability on image quality, *Radiology* 241:378–385, 2006.

9. Einstein AJ, Henzlova MJ, Rajagopalan S: Estimating risk of cancer associated with radiation exposure from 64-slice computed tomography coronary angiography, *JAMA* 298:317–323, 2007.

10. Fazel R, Krumholz HM, Wang Y, et al: Exposure to low-dose ionizing radiation from medical imaging procedures, *N Engl J Med* 361:849–857, 2009.

11. Ron E: Cancer risks from medical radiation, *Health Phys* 85:47–59, 2003.

12. Einstein AJ, Moser KW, Thompson RC, et al: Radiation dose to patients from cardiac diagnostic imaging, *Circulation* 116:1290–1305, 2007.

13. Martin CJ: The application of effective dose to medical exposures, *Radiat Prot Dosimetry* 128:1–4, 2008.

14. Martin CJ: Radiation dosimetry for diagnostic medical exposures, *Radiat Prot Dosimetry* 128:389–412, 2008.

15. Bongartz G, Golding SJ, Jurik AG, et al: European guidelines for multislice computed tomography, 2004 Funded By The European Commission. Contract Number FIGM-CT2000-20078-CT-TIP. March 2004.

16. Blankstein R, Shah A, Pale R, et al: Radiation dose and image quality of prospective triggering with dual-source cardiac computed tomography, *Am J Cardiol* 103:1168–1173, 2009.

17. Wintersperger B, Jakobs T, Herzog P, et al: Aorto-iliac multidetector-row CT angiography with low kV settings: improved vessel enhancement and simultaneous reduction of radiation dose, *Eur Radiol* 15:334–341, 2005.

18. Lee EJ, Lee SK, Agid R, et al: Comparison of image quality and radiation dose between fixed tube current and combined automatic tube current modulation in craniocervical CT angiography, *AJNR Am J Neuroradiol* 30:1754–1759, 2009.

19. Arnoldi E, Johnson TR, Rist C, et al: Adequate image quality with reduced radiation dose in prospectively triggered coronary CTA compared with retrospective techniques, *Eur Radiol* 19:2147–2155, 2009.

20. Hurwitz LM, Yoshizumi TT, Goodman PC: v: Radiation dose savings for adult pulmonary embolus 64-MDCT using bismuth breast shields, lower peak kilovoltage, and automatic tube current modulation, *AJR Am J Roentgenol* 192:244–253, 2009.

21. Hausleiter J, Meyer T, Hadamitzky M, et al: Radiation dose estimates from cardiac multislice computed tomography in daily practice: impact of different scanning protocols on effective dose estimates, *Circulation* 113:1305–1310, 2006.

22. Raff GL, Chinnaiyan KM, Share DA, et al: Radiation dose from cardiac computed tomography before and after implementation of radiation dose-reduction techniques, *JAMA* 301:2340–2348, 2009.

23. Meeson S, Alvey CM, Golding SJ: The *in vivo* relationship between cross-sectional area and CT dose index in abdominal multidetector CT with automatic exposure control, *J Radiol Prot* 30:139–147.

24. Berg M, Zhang Z, Ikonen A, et al: Multi-detector row CT angiography in the assessment of carotid artery disease in symptomatic patients: comparison with rotational angiography and digital subtraction angiography, *AJNR Am J Neuroradiol* 26:1022–1034, 2005.

25. Josephson SA, Bryant SO, Mak HK, et al: Evaluation of carotid stenosis using CT angiography in the initial evaluation of stroke and TIA, *Neurology* 63:457–460, 2004.

26. Zhang Z, Berg MH, Ikonen AE, et al: Carotid artery stenosis: reproducibility of automated 3D CT angiography analysis method, *Eur Radiol* 14:665–672, 2004.

27. Saba L, Mallarin G: Window settings for the study of calcified carotid plaques with multidetector CT angiography, *AJNR Am J Neuroradiol* 30:1445–1450, 2009.

28. Fisher M, Martin A, Cosgrove M, et al: The NASCET-ACAS plaque project. North American Symptomatic Carotid Endarterectomy Trial. Asymptomatic Carotid Atherosclerosis Study, *Stroke* 24:I24–25, 1993 discussion I31–22.

29. Zhang Z, Berg M, Ikonen A, et al: Carotid stenosis degree in CT angiography: assessment based on luminal area versus luminal diameter measurements, *Eur Radiol* 15:2359–2365, 2005.

30. Bartlett ES, Walters TD, Symons SP, et al: Quantification of carotid stenosis on CT angiography, *AJNR Am J Neuroradiol* 27:13–19, 2006.

31. Bartlett ES, Walters TD, Symons SP, et al: Carotid stenosis index revisited with direct CT angiography measurement of carotid arteries to quantify carotid stenosis, *Stroke* 38:286–291, 2007.

32. Bartlett ES, Symons SP, Fox AJ: Correlation of carotid stenosis diameter and cross-sectional areas with CT angiography, *AJNR Am J Neuroradiol* 27:638–642, 2006.

33. Bartlett ES, Walters TD, Symons SP, et al: Classification of carotid stenosis by millimeter CT angiography measures: effects of prevalence and gender, *AJNR Am J Neuroradiol* 29:1677–1683, 2008.

34. Waaijer A, Weber M, van Leeuwen MS, et al: Grading of carotid artery stenosis with multidetector-row CT angiography: visual estimation or caliper measurements? *Eur Radiol* 19:2809–2818, 2009.

35. Suwanwela N, Can U, Furie KL, et al: Carotid Doppler ultrasound criteria for internal carotid artery stenosis based on residual lumen diameter calculated from en bloc carotid endarterectomy specimens, *Stroke* 27:1965–1969, 1996.

36. Lev MH, Romero JM, Goodman DN, et al: Total occlusion versus hairline residual lumen of the internal carotid arteries: accuracy of single section helical CT angiography, *AJNR Am J Neuroradiol* 24:1123–1129, 2003.

37. Chen CJ, Lee TH, Hsu HL, et al: Multi-Slice CT angiography in diagnosing total versus near occlusions of the internal carotid artery: comparison with catheter angiography, *Stroke* 35:83–85, 2004.

38. Bartlett ES, Walters TD, Symons SP, et al: Diagnosing carotid stenosis near-occlusion by using CT angiography, *AJNR Am J Neuroradiol* 27:632–637, 2006.

39. Delgado Almandoz JE, Romero JM, Pomerantz SR, et al: Computed tomography angiography of the carotid and cerebral circulation, *Radiol Clin North Am* 48:265–281, vii–viii, 2010.

40. Goldhaber SZ, Morpurgo M: Diagnosis, treatment, and prevention of pulmonary embolism. Report of the WHO/International Society and Federation of Cardiology Task Force, *JAMA* 268:1727–1733, 1992.

41. Stein PD, Beemath A, Olson RE: Trends in the incidence of pulmonary embolism and deep venous thrombosis in hospitalized patients, *Am J Cardiol* 95:1525–1526, 2005.

42. Stein PD, Fowler SE, Goodman LR, et al: Multidetector computed tomography for acute pulmonary embolism, *N Engl J Med* 354:2317–2327, 2006.

43. Coche E, Verschuren F, Keyeux A, et al: Diagnosis of acute pulmonary embolism in outpatients: comparison of thin-collimation multi-detector row spiral CT and planar ventilation-perfusion scintigraphy, *Radiology* 229:757–765, 2003.

44. Qanadli SD, Hajjam ME, Mesurolle B, et al: Pulmonary embolism detection: prospective evaluation of dual-section helical CT versus selective pulmonary arteriography in 157 patients, *Radiology* 217:447–455, 2000.

45. Winer-Muram HT, Rydberg J, Johnson MS, et al: Suspected acute pulmonary embolism: evaluation with multi-detector row CT versus digital subtraction pulmonary arteriography, *Radiology* 233:806–815, 2004.

46. Brader P, Schoellnast H, Deutschmann HA, et al: Acute pulmonary embolism: comparison of standard axial MDCT with paddlewheel technique, *Eur J Radiol* 66:31–36, 2008.

47. Chiang EE, Boiselle PM, Raptopoulos V, et al: Detection of pulmonary embolism: comparison of paddlewheel and coronal CT reformations–initial experience, *Radiology* 228:577–582, 2003.

48. Coche EE, Hamoir XL, Hammer FD, et al: Using dual-detector helical CT angiography to detect deep venous thrombosis in patients with suspicion of pulmonary embolism: diagnostic value and additional findings, *AJR Am J Roentgenol* 176:1035–1039, 2001.

49. Reid JH, Murchison JT: Acute right ventricular dilatation: a new helical CT sign of massive pulmonary embolism, *Clin Radiol* 53:694–698, 1998.

50. Quiroz R, Kucher N, Schoepf UJ, et al: Right ventricular enlargement on chest computed tomography: prognostic role in acute pulmonary embolism, *Circulation* 109:2401–2404, 2004.

51. Bhalla S, West OC: CT of nontraumatic thoracic aortic emergencies, *Semin Ultrasound CT MR* 26:281–304, 2005.

52. Salvolini L, Renda P, Fiore D, et al: Acute aortic syndromes: role of multi-detector row CT, *Eur J Radiol* 65:350–358, 2008.

53. Batra P, Bigoni B, Manning J, et al: Pitfalls in the diagnosis of thoracic aortic dissection at CT angiography, *Radiographics* 20:309–320, 2000.

54. Manghat NE, Morgan-Hughes GJ, Roobottom CA: Multi-detector row computed tomography: imaging in acute aortic syndrome, *Clin Radiol* 60:1256–1267, 2005.

55. Johnson TR, Nikolaou K, Wintersperger BJ, et al: Optimization of contrast material administration for electrocardiogram-gated computed tomographic angiography of the chest, *J Comput Assist Tomogr* 31:265–271, 2007.

56. Roos JE, Willmann JK, Weishaupt D, et al: Thoracic aorta: motion artifact reduction with retrospective and prospective electrocardiography-assisted multi-detector row CT, *Radiology* 222:271–277, 2002.

57. Hayashi H, Matsuoka Y, Sakamoto I, et al: Penetrating atherosclerotic ulcer of the aorta: imaging features and disease concept, *Radiographics* 20:995–1005, 2000.

58. Macura KJ, Corl FM, Fishman EK, et al: Pathogenesis in acute aortic syndromes: aortic dissection, intramural hematoma, and penetrating atherosclerotic aortic ulcer, *AJR Am J Roentgenol* 181:309–316, 2003.

59. Chiles C, Carr JJ: Vascular diseases of the thorax: evaluation with multidetector CT, *Radiol Clin North Am* 43:543–569, viii, 2005.

60. Park KH, Lim C, Choi JH, et al: Prevalence of aortic intimal defect in surgically treated acute type A intramural hematoma, *Ann Thorac Surg* 86:1494–1500, 2008.

61. Quint LE, Williams DM, Francis IR, et al: Ulcerlike lesions of the aorta: imaging features and natural history, *Radiology* 218:719–723, 2001.

62. Harris JA, Bis KG, Glover JL, et al: Penetrating atherosclerotic ulcers of the aorta, *J Vasc Surg* 19:90–98, 1994 discussion 98–99.

63. Coady MA, Rizzo JA, Hammond GL, et al: Penetrating ulcer of the thoracic aorta: what is it? How do we recognize it? How do we manage it? *J Vasc Surg* 27:1006–1015, 1998 discussion 1015–1006.

64. Ganaha F, Miller DC, Sugimoto K, et al: Prognosis of aortic intramural hematoma with and without penetrating atherosclerotic ulcer: a clinical and radiological analysis, *Circulation* 106:342–348, 2002.

65. Jeudy J, Waite S, White CS: Nontraumatic thoracic emergencies, *Radiol Clin North Am* 44:273–293, ix, 2006.

66. Cho KR, Stanson AW, Potter DD, et al: Penetrating atherosclerotic ulcer of the descending thoracic aorta and arch, *J Thorac Cardiovasc Surg* 127:1393–1399, 2004 discussion 1399–1401.

67. Beauchesne LM, Veinot JP, Brais MP, et al: Acute aortic intimal tear without a mobile flap mimicking an intramural hematoma, *J Am Soc Echocardiogr* 16:285–288, 2003.

68. Berdat PA, Carrel T: Aortic dissection limited to the ascending aorta mimicking intramural hematoma, *Eur J Cardiothorac Surg* 15:108–109, 1999.

69. Neri E, Capannini G, Carone E, et al: Evolution toward dissection of an intramural hematoma of the ascending aorta, *Ann Thorac Surg* 68:1855–1856, 1999.

70. Castaner E, Andreu M, Gallardo X, et al: CT in nontraumatic acute thoracic aortic disease: typical and atypical features and complications, *Radiographics* 23:Spec No:S93–S110, 2003.

71. Hagan PG, Nienaber CA, Isselbacher EM, et al: The International Registry of Acute Aortic Dissection (IRAD): new insights into an old disease, *JAMA* 283:897–903, 2000.

72. Song JK, Kim HS, Song JM, et al: Outcomes of medically treated patients with aortic intramural hematoma, *Am J Med* 113:181–187, 2002.

73. Sueyoshi E, Matsuoka Y, Imada T, et al: New development of an ulcerlike projection in aortic intramural hematoma: CT evaluation, *Radiology* 224:536–541, 2002.

74. Song MO, Kim KJ, Chung SI, et al: Distribution of human group a rotavirus VP7 and VP4 types circulating in Seoul, Korea between 1998 and 2000, *J Med Virol* 70:324–328, 2003.

75. Roberts WC: Aortic dissection: anatomy, consequences, and causes, *Am Heart J* 101:195–214, 1981.

76. Manghat NE, Walsh M, Roobottom CA, et al: Can the "vortex sign" be used as an imaging indicator of the false lumen in acute aortic dissection? *Clin Radiol* 60:1037–1038, 2005.

77. Williams DM, Joshi A, Dake MD, et al: Aortic cobwebs: an anatomic marker identifying the false lumen in aortic dissection--imaging and pathologic correlation, *Radiology* 190:167–174, 1994.

78. Isselbacher EM: Thoracic and abdominal aortic aneurysms, *Circulation* 111:816–828, 2005.

79. Trimarchi S, Tsai T, Eagle KA, et al: Acute abdominal aortic dissection: insight from the International Registry of Acute Aortic Dissection (IRAD), *J Vasc Surg* 46:913–919, 2007.

80. Jonker FH, Schlosser FJ, Moll FL, et al: Dissection of the abdominal aorta. Current evidence and implications for treatment strategies: a review and meta-analysis of 92 patients, *Endovasc Ther* 16:71–80, 2009.

81. Pande RL, Beckman JA: Abdominal aortic aneurysm: populations at risk and how to screen, *J Vasc Interv Radiol* 19:S2–S8, 2008.

82. Annambhotla S, Bourgeois S, Wang X, et al: Recent advances in molecular mechanisms of abdominal aortic aneurysm formation, *World J Surg* 32:976–986, 2008.

83. Rozenblit AM, Patlas M, Rosenbaum AT, et al: Detection of endoleaks after endovascular repair of abdominal aortic aneurysm: value of unenhanced and delayed helical CT acquisitions, *Radiology* 227:426–433, 2003.

84. Bashir MR, Ferral H, Jacobs C, et al: Endoleaks after endovascular abdominal aortic aneurysm repair: management strategies according to CT findings, *AJR Am J Roentgenol* 192:W178–W186, 2009.

85. Tolia AJ, Landis R, Lamparello P, et al: Type II endoleaks after endovascular repair of abdominal aortic aneurysms: natural history, *Radiology* 235:683–686, 2005.

86. Gorich J, Rilinger N, Sokiranski R, et al: Leakages after endovascular repair of aortic aneurysms: classification based on findings at CT, angiography, and radiography, *Radiology* 213:767–772, 1999.

87. Gotway MB, Araoz PA, Macedo TA, et al: Imaging findings in Takayasu's arteritis, *AJR Am J Roentgenol* 184:1945–1950, 2005.

88. Foley WD: Special focus session: multidetector CT: abdominal visceral imaging, *Radiographics* 22:701–719, 2002.

89. Kawashima A, Sandler CM, Ernst RD, et al: CT evaluation of renovascular disease, *Radiographics* 20:1321–1340, 2000.

90. Beregi JP, Louvegny S, Gautier C, et al: Fibromuscular dysplasia of the renal arteries: comparison of helical CT angiography and arteriography, *AJR Am J Roentgenol* 172:27–34, 1999.

91. Sabharwal R, Vladica P, Law WP, et al: Multidetector spiral CT renal angiography in the diagnosis of giant renal artery aneurysms, *Abdom Imaging* 31:374–378, 2006.

92. Chiesa R, Astore D, Guzzo G, et al: Visceral artery aneurysms, *Ann Vasc Surg* 19:42–48, 2005.

93. Rokke O, Sondenaa K, Amundsen S, et al: The diagnosis and management of splanchnic artery aneurysms, *Scand J Gastroenterol* 31:737–743, 1996.

94. Barmeir E, Halachmi S, Croitoru S, et al: CT angiography diagnosis of spontaneous dissection of the superior mesenteric artery, *AJR Am J Roentgenol* 171:1429–1430, 1998.

95. Krupski WC, Effeney DJ, Ehrenfeld WK: Spontaneous dissection of the superior mesenteric artery, *J Vasc Surg* 2:731–734, 1985.

96. Lindner HH, Kemprud E: A clinicoanatomical study of the arcuate ligament of the diaphragm, *Arch Surg* 103:600–605, 1971.

97. Cohen EI, Doshi A, Lookstein RA: CT angiography of the lower-extremity circulation with protocols. In Mukherjee D, Rajagopalan S, editors: *CT and MR angiography of the peripheral circulation: practical approach with clinical protocols*, London, 2007, Informa UK Ltd., pp 133–146.

98. Fleischmann D: CT angiography: injection and acquisition technique, *Radiol Clin North Am* 48:237–247, vii, 2010.

99. Catalano C, Fraioli F, Laghi A, et al: Infrarenal aortic and lower-extremity arterial disease: diagnostic performance of multi-detector row CT angiography, *Radiology* 231:555–563, 2004.

100. Schernthaner R, Stadler A, Lomoschitz F, et al: Multidetector CT angiography in the assessment of peripheral arterial occlusive disease: accuracy in detecting the severity, number, and length of stenoses, *Eur Radiol* 18:665–671, 2008.

101. Norgren L, Hiatt WR, Dormandy JA, et al: Inter-Society Consensus for the Management of Peripheral Arterial Disease (TASC II), *Eur J Vasc Endovasc Surg* 33(Suppl 1):S1–S75, 2007.

102. Heijenbrok-Kal MH, Kock MC, Hunink MG: Lower extremity arterial disease: multidetector CT angiography meta-analysis, *Radiology* 245:433–439, 2007.

103. Schernthaner R, Fleischmann D, Lomoschitz F, et al: Effect of MDCT angiographic findings on the management of intermittent claudication, *AJR Am J Roentgenol* 189:1215–1222, 2007.

104. Dellegrottaglie S, Sanz J, Macaluso F, et al: Technology insight: magnetic resonance angiography for the evaluation of patients with peripheral artery disease, *Nat Clin Pract Cardiovasc Med* 4:677–687, 2007.

105. Ouwendijk R, de Vries M, Stijnen T, et al: Multicenter randomized controlled trial of the costs and effects of noninvasive diagnostic imaging in patients with peripheral arterial disease: the DIPAD trial, *AJR Am J Roentgenol* 190:1349–1357, 2008.

106. Wright LB, Matchett WJ, Cruz CP, et al: Popliteal artery disease: diagnosis and treatment, *Radiographics* 24:467–479, 2004.

107. Diwan A, Sarkar R, Stanley JC, et al: Incidence of femoral and popliteal artery aneurysms in patients with abdominal aortic aneurysms, *J Vasc Surg* 31:863–869, 2000.

108. Lopera JE, Trimmer CK, Josephs SG, et al: Multidetector CT angiography of infrainguinal arterial bypass, *Radiographics* 28:529–548, 2008 discussion 549.

109. Chung JW, Kim HC, Choi YH, et al: Patterns of aortic involvement in Takayasu arteritis and its clinical implications: evaluation with spiral computed tomography angiography, *J Vasc Surg* 45:906–914, 2007.

110. Blum MB, Schmook M, Schernthaner R, et al: Quantification and detectability of in-stent stenosis with CT angiography and MR angiography in arterial stents *in vitro*, *AJR Am J Roentgenol* 189:1238–1242, 2007.

111. Steinwender C, Schutzenberger W, Fellner F, et al: 64-Detector CT angiography in renal artery stent evaluation: prospective comparison with selective catheter angiography, *Radiology* 252:299–305, 2009.

112. Sun Z, Almutairi AM: Diagnostic accuracy of 64 multislice CT angiography in the assessment of coronary in-stent restenosis: a meta-analysis, *Eur J Radiol* 73:266–273, 2009.

113. Foley WD, Stonely T: CT angiography of the lower extremities, *Radiol Clin North Am* 48:367–396, ix, 2010.

114. Willmann JK, Mayer D, Banyai M, et al: Evaluation of peripheral arterial bypass grafts with multi-detector row CT angiography: comparison with duplex US and digital subtraction angiography, *Radiology* 229:465–474, 2003.

CHAPTER 15 Catheter-Based Peripheral Angiography

Christopher J. White

Catheter-based invasive contrast angiography is the standard method for diagnosing peripheral artery disease (PAD), and against which all other methods are compared for accuracy. Angiography provides the "road map" on which therapeutic decisions are based. Knowledge of the vascular anatomy and its normal variations is a core element in the skill set required to safely perform peripheral vascular angiography and intervention.

Imaging Equipment

There are many radiographic equipment vendors and many different room layout schemes suitable for performing peripheral vascular angiography. However, if both cardiac and noncardiac types of peripheral vascular angiography are to be performed in the same room, equipment options become much more limited. One angiographic suite designed to perform both coronary and peripheral vascular angiography is a *dual-plane system* (Fig. 15-1). A dual-plane system encompasses a layout with two independent C-arm image intensifiers operated by a single x-ray generator and one computer. A dual-plane system is not synonymous with a biplane system, which is the simultaneous operation of an anteroposterior (AP) and lateral (LAT) image acquisition system. In a dual-plane system, the cardiac C-arm is a three-mode flat-panel image intensifier, and the noncardiac C-arm should be as large as possible, usually a 15- or 16-inch flat-panel image intensifier. For peripheral vascular imaging, particularly bilateral lower-extremity runoff angiography, an image intensifier smaller than 15 inches may not be able to include both legs in the same field. The noncardiac C-arm must be capable of head-to-toe digital imaging.

Ability to angulate the image intensifier is necessary to resolve bifurcation lesions and optimally image aorto-ostial branch lesions. Of the many imaging options available, those most often used include digital subtraction angiography (DSA), roadmapping, and a stepping table for lower-extremity (digital subtraction) runoff angiography.

Radiographic Contrast

Ionic low-osmolar or nonionic iodinated radiographic contrast is preferred for angiography of the peripheral vessels to avoid patient discomfort. Low-osmolar contrast agents produce fewer side effects (e.g., nausea, vomiting, local pain) and offer better patient tolerability. In addition, low-osmolar agents deliver a lesser osmotic load and thereby a lower intravascular volume, which may be important in patients with impaired left ventricular or renal function. Digital subtraction angiography is often preferred because nonvascular structures are removed and less contrast is required.

Alternatives to iodine-based radiographic contrast include carbon dioxide (CO_2) and gadolinium (gadopentetate dimeglumine).[1,2] To minimize the risk of distal embolization and stroke, it is recommended that CO_2 not be used for angiograms above the diaphragm.[3] Gadolinium, traditionally used with magnetic resonance imaging (MRI), is relatively nontoxic in patients with adequate renal function at a recommended dose not exceeding 0.4 mmol/kg.[4]

Imaging Technique

Many of the technical aspects of diagnostic cardiac imaging also apply to performing angiography of the aorta and peripheral vasculature. The basic principle of vascular angiography is not only to visualize the target lesion but also demonstrate the inflow and outflow vascular segments. Inflow anatomy constitutes the vascular segment preceding the target lesion, and outflow constitutes the vascular segment immediately distal to the target vessel and includes the runoff bed. For example, the inflow segment for the common iliac artery (CIA) is the infrarenal aorta, and the outflow segment is the external iliac and femoral vessels. The runoff bed would be the tibioperoneal vessels.

When performing selective arterial imaging, it is important for patients' safety that a coronary manifold with pressure measurement

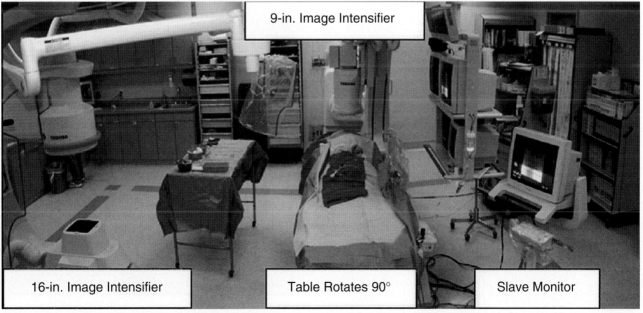

FIGURE 15-1 Dual-plane catheterization laboratory. Note two C-arm image intensifiers (9- and 16-inch), with catheterization table able to rotate 90°.

be used to monitor hemodynamic status and ensure that damping of the catheter has not occurred prior to injecting contrast. Use of pressure monitoring during selective angiography can prevent a myriad of complications—including the creation of dissections and air injection.

Angiography may be performed using a "bolus chase" cineangiographic method or with a digital subtraction stepping mode. The bolus chase technique involves injecting a bolus of contrast at the inflow of the territory, then "panning" or manually moving the image intensifier to follow the bolus of contrast through the target lesion and into the run-off segment. In digital subtraction stepping mode, the patient lies motionless on the angiographic table. A "mask" of the segments to be imaged is taken, and then contrast is injected. The table moves in steps to image the contrast-filled vessels, from which the mask is then subtracted, leaving only the contrast-filled vascular structures.

Obtaining Vascular Access

Vascular access for noncardiac diagnostic angiography is most commonly achieved at the common femoral artery (CFA), with alternative upper-extremity sites at the radial, brachial, or axillary artery.[5] The most common complications of angiographic procedures occur at vascular access sites.

A thorough understanding of the relationship of the CFA to anatomical landmarks is necessary to ensure safe CFA puncture (Fig. 15-2). The femoral artery and vein lie below the inguinal ligament, which is a band of dense fibrous tissue connecting the anterior superior iliac spine to the pubic tubercle. The inguinal skin crease, which is variable in location, is shown as a dotted line in the figure. Current recommendations are to use fluoroscopic guidance to image the femoral head to guide CFA puncture.[6]

The most important landmark for femoral access is the head of the femur. In a morphological study using CT images, there was not a single case in which a puncture would have passed cranial to the inguinal ligament or caudal to the femoral artery bifurcation if the CFA were entered at the level of the center of the femoral head.[7] Caudal to the femoral head, the CFA is encased in the femoral sheath and bifurcates into the superficial femoral artery (SFA) medially and the deep femoral artery (DFA) laterally. With these anatomical observations in mind, the importance of osseous support and entry of the needle into the CFA at the center of the femoral head is obvious.

Anatomical landmarks are initially identified by palpation of the anterior superior iliac spine and pubic tubercle to locate the inguinal ligament; position of the femoral head is confirmed fluoroscopically. Depending on the amount of subcutaneous fat, a skin incision should be made 1 to 2 cm caudal to the level of the center of the femoral head. The needle is directed in an oblique direction while palpating the CFA over the center of the femoral head. Once the CFA has been entered and brisk blood flow returns through the needle, a soft guidewire is advanced into the iliac artery, and a vascular sheath is inserted to secure vascular access.

Complications of CFA puncture are most commonly related to arterial entry that is either too high or too low. When the puncture is too high, a retroperitoneal hemorrhage may occur.[8] Presence of loose connective tissue in the retroperitoneal space can lead to large hematomas. Lack of osseous support and presence of a tense inguinal ligament at the arterial puncture site make manual compression difficult. Low punctures may be complicated by formation of arteriovenous fistulas (AVFs), false aneurysms, and hematomas.

Abdominal Aortography and Lower-Extremity Runoff

For abdominal aortography, vascular access with a 4F to 6F catheter is obtained in the CFA, although brachial or radial access may also be used. The angiographic catheter (e.g., pigtail, tennis racquet, omni flush) is positioned in the abdominal aorta such that the tip of the catheter reaches the level of the last rib. A power injector is used to deliver 20 to 30 mL of contrast at 15 mL/sec for digital subtraction (Fig. 15-3). Either biplane angiography may be obtained or, if needed, two separate angiograms with single-plane systems. Three visceral (mesenteric) arterial branches, the celiac trunk, superior mesenteric artery (SMA), and inferior mesenteric artery (IMA), arise from the anterior surface of the abdominal aorta (Fig. 15-4). The renal arteries originate from the lateral aspect of the abdominal aorta at the level of L1 to L2. The AP projection allows visualization of the aorta, renal arteries, and iliac artery bifurcation, whereas the LAT view demonstrates the origin of the celiac trunk and mesenteric arteries. Commonly in the AP view, the proximal portion of the SMA obscures the origin of the right renal artery. When this occurs, selective angiography of the renal artery may be required to visualize the origin of this vessel.

Generally, a nonselective abdominal aortogram is obtained before selective renal angiography, using a large format (9- to

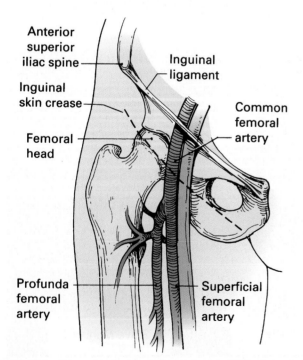

FIGURE 15-2 Schematic of common femoral artery (CFA) anatomical landmarks.

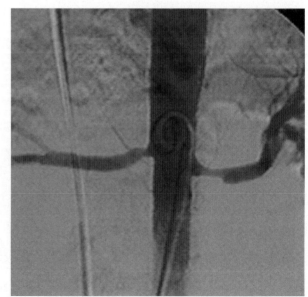

FIGURE 15-3 Femoral access. Pigtail catheter contrast injection of 20 mL/sec for 30 mL (5° left anterior oblique [LAO]) using a digital subtraction angiography (DSA) technique. Note bilateral renal artery stenosis.

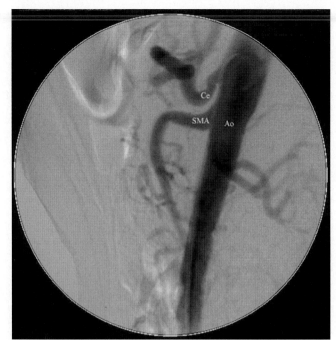

FIGURE 15-4   Femoral access. Lateral (LAT) aortogram. Aorta *(Ao)*, with celiac trunk *(Ce)* and superior mesenteric artery *(SMA)* arising from anterior aortic surface.

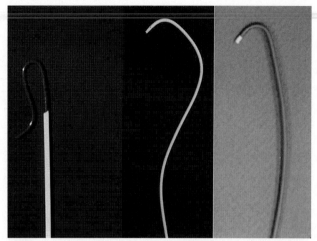

FIGURE 15-5   Selective renal angiographic catheters. *Left,* Sos. *Middle,* Cobra. *Right,* Internal mammary artery (IMA) catheter.

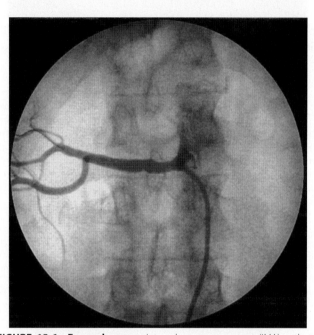

FIGURE 15-6   Femoral access. Internal mammary artery (IMA) catheter selectively engaged in right renal artery.

16-inch) image intensifier with digital subtraction imaging. The nonselective aortogram demonstrates the level at which the renal arteries arise, presence of any accessory renal arteries and their location, severity and location of aortoiliac pathology, and presence of significant renal artery stenosis. To optimize viewing of the renal arteries, the angiographic catheter should be placed below the origin of the SMA, and the image intensifier should be positioned such that the superior, inferior, and lateral borders of both kidneys are visualized. The ostia of the renal arteries are often better seen with slight rotation of the image intensifier, usually into left anterior oblique (LAO) position.

Selective Renal Angiography

Selective renal angiography is indicated to identify suspected renovascular disease. Selective renal artery engagement allows measurement of pressure gradients, particularly if ostial lesions are suspected. When measuring pressure gradients across lesions, it is important to use the smallest catheter possible (i.e., ≤4 F) to avoid creating an artificial gradient. The 0.014-inch pressure wire (RADI) is the optimal method of pressure gradient measurement. Usually, selective renal angiography is performed with 4 F to 6 F diagnostic catheters (Fig. 15-5) and a 9-inch image intensifier. Selective renal angiography is performed using hand injections with shallow oblique angulations to optimize visualization of the renal ostia (Figs. 15-6 and 15-7). Caudal or cranial angulation (15° to 20°) may occasionally be necessary for better visualization of some ostial lesions. An optimal image will reveal the ostial portion of the renal artery and distal branches at the cortex of the kidney.

Selective Mesenteric Angiography

As is the case for the renal arteries, nonselective aortography (AP and LAT) generally precedes selective angiography of the mesenteric arteries. Once the origin of the mesenteric vessel has been identified, selective angiography may be carried out in the LAT and oblique views using 4 F to 6 F catheters (Fig. 15-8). The celiac trunk, SMA, and IMA arteries arise from the anterior surface of the aorta. There commonly are collaterals between the mesenteric vessels, and it is uncommon for stenosis or occlusion of a single branch to cause clinical symptoms.

The mesenteric arteries often arise at an inferior (caudal) angle from the abdominal aorta, for which a shepherd's crook catheter via femoral artery access is helpful for selective engagement. Alternatively, upper-extremity vascular access allows the mesenteric arteries to be engaged with a multipurpose-shaped catheter. Analogous to the renal arteries, selective engagement of the mesenteric arteries also allows measurement of the pressure gradient. Selective angiographic images in multiple views are obtained with hand injections of contrast.

Aortoiliac and Lower-Extremity Angiography

The abdominal aorta bifurcates into the common iliac arteries (CIA), which bifurcate into the internal (IIA) and external (EIA) iliac arteries (Fig. 15-9). The IIA is often referred to as the *hypogastric artery* because this vessel commonly provides collateral circulation to the viscera. The EIA emerges from the pelvis just posterior to the inguinal ligament. At the level of the inguinal ligament, two small branches originate from the EIA: the inferior epigastric artery, which follows a medial direction, and the deep iliac circumflex artery, which takes a LAT and superior direction.

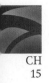

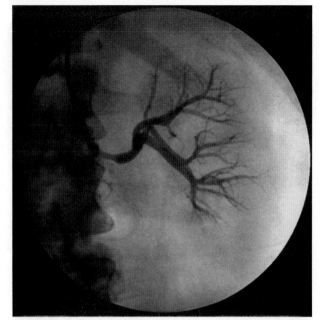

FIGURE 15-7 Upper-extremity access. Selective left renal artery engagement with multipurpose catheter.

On crossing the inguinal ligament, the EIA becomes the CFA, which lies over the femoral head. When it reaches the lower third of the femoral head, the CFA divides into the SFA and profunda femoris, or DFA. The DFA runs posterolaterally along the femur. The SFA continues down the anteromedial thigh, and in its distal portion dives deeper to enter Hunter's (adductor) canal and emerges as the popliteal artery (Fig. 15-10).

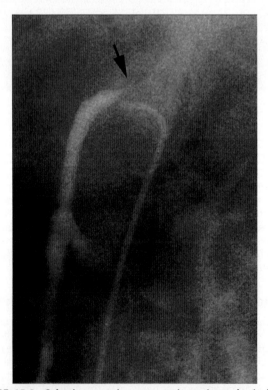

FIGURE 15-8 Selective superior mesenteric angiography in lateral (LAT) projection, with internal mammary artery (IMA) catheter. Note ostial stenosis *(arrow)*.

Below the knee, the popliteal artery bifurcates into the anterior tibial (AT) artery and tibioperoneal trunk (TPT). The AT artery runs laterally and anterior to the tibia toward the foot and continues onto the foot as the dorsalis pedis (DP) artery. The TPT bifurcates into the posterior tibial (PT) and peroneal arteries (Fig. 15-11). The PT artery courses posteriorly and medially in the calf, whereas the peroneal artery runs near the fibula between the AT and PT arteries. On the dorsum of the foot, the DP artery has lateral and medial tarsal branches. After the PT artery passes behind the medial malleus, it divides into medial and lateral plantar arteries. The lateral plantar and distal DP arteries join to form the plantar arch.

Vascular access for diagnostic aortoiliac and lower-extremity angiography is obtained in the CFA, preferentially in the least symptomatic extremity, although upper-extremity access (axillary, brachial, or radial) may also be used. A 4 F to 6 F pigtail catheter is positioned above the aortic bifurcation. The preferred technique is to use DSA with a stepping table and a large (15- or 16-inch) format image intensifier so that both legs are imaged together. A single bolus of contrast is injected from the catheter at the aortic bifurcation at 8 to 12 mL/sec for 8 to 10 seconds, and sequential images are obtained from the aorta to the feet.

Selective angiograms performed in angulated views of a particular artery or arterial segments are useful when clarification of a potential stenosis is needed. One option is to place a diagnostic catheter at different levels in the iliac, femoral, or popliteal artery for a more detailed examination of a particular arterial segment. If access has been obtained in the CFA and the arterial segment in question is located in the contralateral extremity, a 4 F internal mammary catheter is positioned at the level of the aortic bifurcation, with the tip of the catheter selectively engaged in the contralateral CIA (Fig. 15-12). An angled guidewire is advanced to the CFA, and the diagnostic catheter is advanced over the guidewire to the area of interest.

Several angiographic views are important to mention because they help clarify anatomical detail. In the AP view, there is often overlapping of the origin of the external and internal iliac arteries, and ostial stenoses in either or both vessels may be missed. The contralateral oblique view (20°) with 20° of caudal angulation is very useful to separate these vessels (Fig. 15-13).

Overlap at the origin of the SFA and DFA arteries commonly occurs in the AP projection and can be improved with a 20° to 30° LAT oblique view.[9] Another common source of artifact may occur when the tibial arteries overlie the relatively radiodense bony periosteum of the tibia or fibula. In that case, slight angulation will move the artery in question off the bony density to allow better visualization.

Aortic Arch and Brachiocephalic Vessels

The aortic arch includes portions of the ascending, transverse, and descending aorta (Fig. 15-14). The thoracic aorta gives rise to the brachiocephalic trunk in the proximal portion of the arch, the left common carotid artery in the mid-portion, and the left subclavian artery in the distal portion. In 10% to 20% of cases, the left common carotid artery originates from the brachiocephalic trunk, an anatomical variation known as a *bovine arch* (Fig. 15-15). Other common variations include the left vertebral artery originating directly from the aortic arch, between the left common carotid artery and left subclavian artery, and the right subclavian artery originating from the aortic arch distal to the origin of the left subclavian artery.

Thoracic aortography is commonly performed to diagnose pathological entities such as stenoses of the origin of the great vessels, aneurysms, aortic dissection, coarctation of the aorta, patent ductus arteriosus, and vascular rings, and to evaluate vascular injuries caused by blunt or penetrating chest trauma.[10] Vascular access is most often obtained at the CFA, although the brachial or radial approaches are also useful. A pigtail catheter is advanced into the ascending aorta and positioned proximal to the brachiocephalic trunk. Using a power injector, radiographic contrast material is injected at 15 to 20 mL/sec for a total of 2 to 3 seconds. The LAO

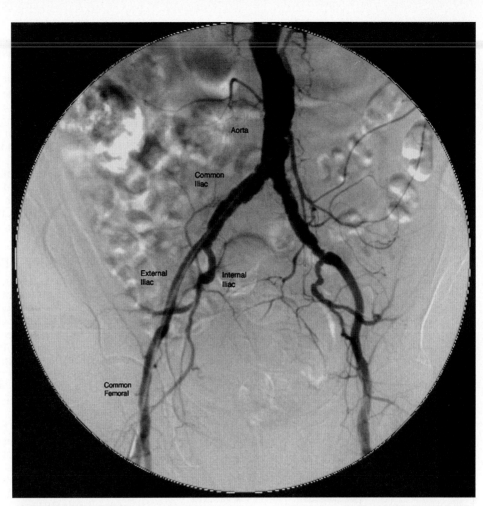

FIGURE 15-9 Aortoiliac angiography.
Pigtail catheter contrast injection of 20 mL/sec
for a total of 30 mL.

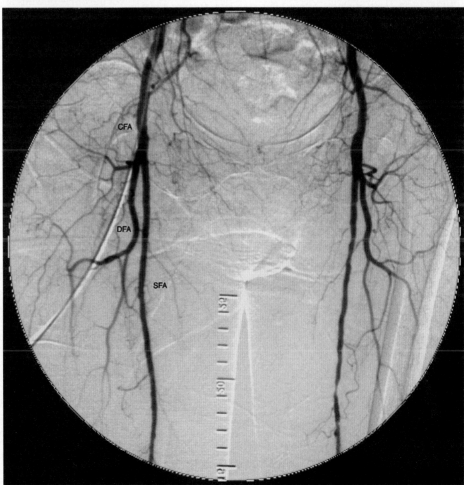

FIGURE 15-10 Common femoral arteries
(CFA) **branching into deep femoral artery**
(DFA) **and superficial femoral artery** *(SFA).*

CH
15

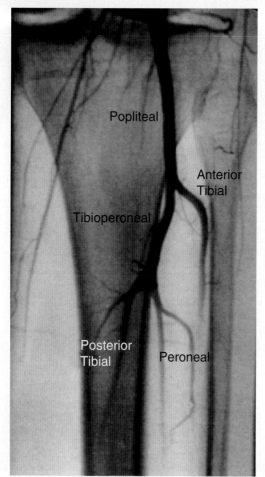

Popliteal

Anterior
Tibial

Tibioperoneal

Posterior
Tibial   Peroneal

FIGURE 15-11 Left popliteal artery bifurcates into anterior tibial (lateral) and tibioperoneal trunk, which then divides into posterior tibial (medial) and peroneal arteries.

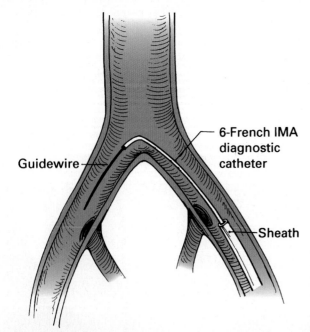

Guidewire

6-French IMA
diagnostic
catheter

Sheath

FIGURE 15-12 Drawing illustrating contralateral iliac access for selective angiography.

projection (30° to 60°) separates the ascending from the descending aorta and allows good visualization of the origin of the great vessels (see Fig. 15-14).

The brachiocephalic trunk, left common carotid artery, and subclavian arteries originate from the transverse thoracic aorta. The brachiocephalic trunk or innominate artery divides into the right common carotid artery and the right subclavian artery. The common carotid arteries run lateral to the vertebral bodies and bifurcate into the external and the internal carotid arteries at about the level of the fourth cervical vertebra (Fig. 15-16). In its extracranial portion, the internal carotid artery has no branches. On entering the skull, the internal carotid artery makes a sharp turn at the carotid siphon and thereafter divides into the middle (MCA) and anterior (ACA) cerebral arteries, from which the anterior communicating artery forms the anterior portion of the circle of Willis (Fig. 15-17).

Carotid Angiography

Selective carotid angiography is usually performed after obtaining an aortic arch aortogram in the LAO view, which allows the operator to visualize the origin of the brachiocephalic trunk and left common carotid artery. Using that same LAO angle, the brachiocephalic trunk is engaged with a diagnostic catheter (Fig. 15-18).

Once the origin of the common carotid artery has been engaged with a guidewire, the catheter is advanced into the common carotid artery over the wire. Care must be taken to clear the catheters and manifold of air and debris before injecting into the carotid artery. Carotid angiograms are obtained in the AP, oblique, and LAT views.

Because of the dense bony structure of the skull, it is preferable to use digital subtraction techniques for diagnostic images of the intracranial vascular anatomy. A 12-inch or larger image intensifier is optimal for intracranial angiography. It is important to emphasize using DSA for the intracranial portion of the internal carotid artery and its branches in the AP and LAT views. This enables assessment of the circle of Willis and demonstrates the presence of any collateral circulation.

Subclavian Angiography

Important branches of the subclavian artery include the vertebral (superior) and internal mammary (inferior) arteries (Fig. 15-19). The vertebral artery, the first and usually largest branch of the subclavian artery, arises from the superior and posterior surface of the subclavian. The AP view will disclose stenosis in the proximal subclavian artery (the left subclavian artery is affected three to four times as frequently as the right subclavian artery). In patients with a tortuous proximal left subclavian artery, a steep right anterior oblique (RAO) view with caudal angulation may help elucidate a proximal stenosis. If the proximal portion of the right subclavian artery is suspected of having a lesion, the AP view may not show the stenosis because of overlap with the origin of the right common carotid artery. A steep RAO caudal view (40°-60° RAO and 15°-20° caudal) will usually separate the ostia of these two vessels (Fig. 15-20).

Vertebral Angiography

The vertebral arteries are identified on the aortic arch aortogram. Often, a nonselective injection of contrast in the subclavian artery near the origin of the vertebral artery is performed to view ostial lesions. Cranial angulation (30°-40°) with shallow oblique views (RAO or LAO), may be necessary to view the origin (see Fig. 15-19). Nonselective angiography is preferred to avoid trauma when engaging the ostium of the vertebral artery with an angled catheter (Judkins right coronary, Berenstein, Cobra, or internal mammary artery catheter). Typically the catheter is placed very near the ostium, and hand injections of contrast are made to visualize the vertebral artery.

The vertebral artery runs cranially through the foramina of the transverse processes of the cervical vertebrae to the base of the skull

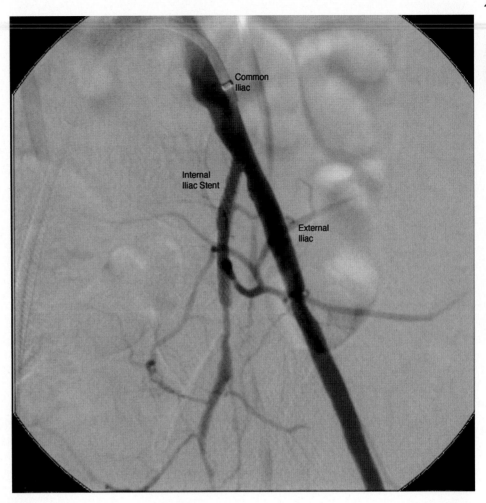

FIGURE 15-13 Selective left common iliac angiography (20° left anterior oblique [LAO] and 20° caudal view) demonstrating origin of internal iliac artery (IIA) (ostial stent present) and external iliac artery (EIA).

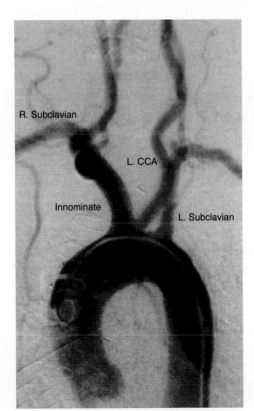

FIGURE 15-14 Aortic arch and brachiocephalic vessels. Digital subtraction angiogram injection of 15 mL per second of contrast material for 3 seconds, with image obtained at 30° left anterior oblique (LAO). CCA, common carotid artery.

(Fig. 15-21). After penetrating the foramen of the atlas, it enters the cranial cavity through the foramen magnum. The first branch of the vertebral artery, located in its V4 segment, is the posterior inferior cerebellar artery (PICA). The vertebral artery joins with the contralateral vertebral artery to form the basilar artery (Fig. 15-22).

Nonselective angiography is performed with hand injections, using a coronary manifold with pressure monitoring, analogous to selective coronary angiography. Anteroposterior and LAT views of the extracranial and intracranial course of the vertebral and basilar arteries should be performed with a DSA technique. Similar to views of the anterior cerebral circulation, it is important to determine the contribution of the posterior circulation to the circle of Willis.

Complications of Peripheral Vascular Angiography

Complications of peripheral vascular angiography may lead to significant morbidity or even mortality.[5] Complications may be thought of in three categories: (1) access site related, (2) systemic, or (3) catheter induced.[11] The best strategy to minimize these complications is to anticipate and avoid them.

Access Site–Related Complications

Vascular access site–related complications include hematoma formation, retroperitoneal hemorrhage, pseudoaneurysm formation, AVF creation, and infection. Access site bleeding is the most frequent complication following femoral arterial access.[12] It is important to note that femoral closure devices shorten time to ambulation but also add cost without reducing complications.[13] Management of access site bleeding depends on the severity and hemodynamic

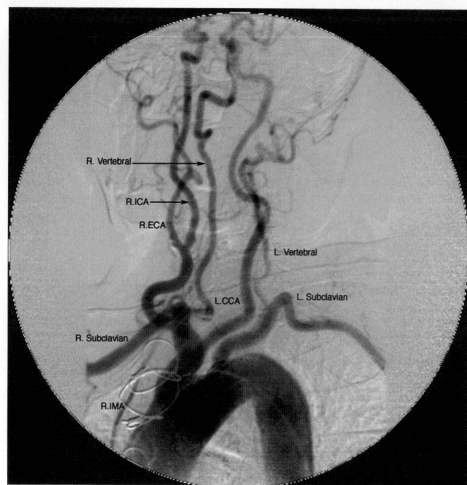

FIGURE 15-15 Bovine aortic arch angiogram injection of 15 mL of contrast per second for 3 seconds (total 45 mL contrast) at 45° left anterior oblique (LAO). L.CCA, left common carotid artery; R.ECA, right external carotid artery; R.ICA, right internal carotid artery; R.IMA, right internal mammary artery.

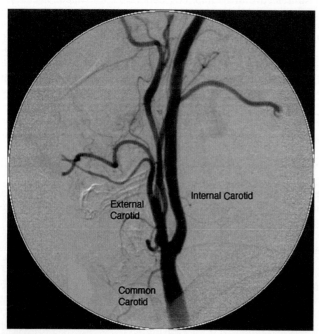

FIGURE 15-16 Common carotid bifurcation. External carotid artery is marked by presence of branch vessels.

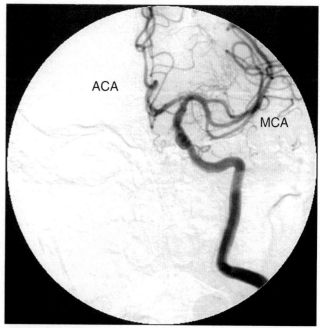

FIGURE 15-17 Intracranial carotid arteries (anteroposterior [AP] view). Internal carotid artery branches into middle cerebral artery (MCA) and anterior cerebral artery (ACA).

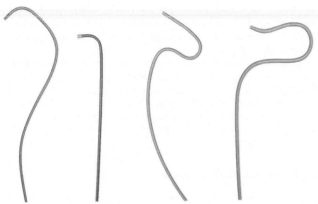

FIGURE 15-18 Commonly used brachiocephalic and carotid angiographic catheters.

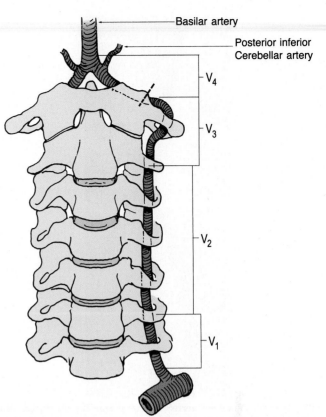

FIGURE 15-21 Drawing of vertebral artery, divided into four anatomical segments that course through cervical spine foramina.

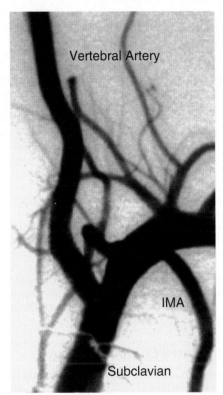

FIGURE 15-19 Left subclavian angiogram showing vertebral artery arising superiorly and internal mammary artery *(IMA)* arising inferiorly.

consequences of bleeding. In general, access site bleeding may be controlled by manual or mechanical compression and reversal of anticoagulation. If bleeding continues despite these steps, more aggressive therapies—including percutaneous intervention or surgical therapy—may be considered.[14]

Signs and symptoms of retroperitoneal bleeding include hypotension, abdominal distention or fullness, and pain. Diagnosis of retroperitoneal bleeding may be confirmed by computed tomography (CT) or abdominal/pelvic ultrasound. If retroperitoneal bleeding is suspected, anticoagulation should be reversed and discontinued. Volume resuscitation with crystalloid solutions and/or blood products should be administered if volume depletion is clinically evident. If bleeding causes hemodynamic embarrassment (hypotension), emergency angiography from the contralateral femoral artery access site should be performed to identify the bleeding site. Once the bleeding site has been identified, tamponade of bleeding with balloon occlusion will stabilize

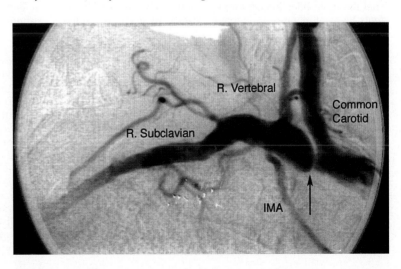

FIGURE 15-20 Proximal right subclavian stenosis *(arrow)*, seen best at 40° right anterior oblique (RAO) and 20° of caudal angulation. IMA, interior mammary artery.

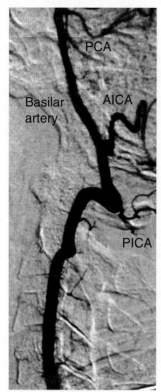

FIGURE 15-22 Proximal vertebral artery segment visualized with subclavian angiography. AICA, anterior inferior cerebellar artery; PCA, posterior cerebral artery; PICA, posterior inferior cerebellar artery.

the patient. If prolonged balloon inflation is not effective in stopping blood loss, consideration may be given to placing a covered stent to seal the leak. Open surgical repair may also be an option to consider.[14]

A pseudoaneurysm occurs when a hematoma communicates with the arterial lumen. Low arterial punctures (SFA or profunda femoris artery entry) are associated with pseudoaneurysm formation. Other risk factors include female sex, age older than 70 years, diabetes mellitus, and obesity.

Patients with pseudoaneurysms often present with pain at the access site several days following the intervention. On physical examination, a pulsatile hematoma may be present with a systolic bruit. Management of a femoral pseudoaneurysm is dependent on its size, severity of symptoms, and need for continued anticoagulation. A small pseudoaneurysm (<2 cm) may be observed and often will resolve spontaneously. Larger pseudoaneurysms may be treated with ultrasound-guided compression, percutaneous off-label thrombin injection, endovascular coil insertion, or covered stents. Surgical repair of pseudoaneurysms is usually reserved for failure of less invasive approaches.[14]

An AVF complicates vascular access when the needle punctures the femoral artery and nearby vein, creating a fistulous communication when the sheath is removed. The risk of creating an AVF is increased by either a high or low femoral puncture, multiple puncture attempts, or prolonged clotting times. Fistulae may not be clinically evident for several days following the procedure. An AVF is characterized by a continuous to-and-fro murmur over the access site. In some cases, there may be a swollen and tender extremity due to venous dilation, and in severe circumstances, arterial insufficiency (steal syndrome) may occur. Diagnosis of an AVF can be confirmed by color flow Doppler ultrasound.

Most AVFs following femoral access are small, not hemodynamically significant, and close spontaneously. Symptomatic AVFs require closure to prevent increased shunting and distal swelling and tenderness.[15] Surgical repair, traditional therapy

for closure of catheterization-related AVFs when necessary, has been replaced by percutaneous methods in most circumstances. Surgical correction is reserved for those patients who fail a less invasive approach.

Vascular access closure devices are designed to facilitate hemostasis, reduce time to ambulation, and decrease length of hospital stay. All devices currently approved by the U.S. Food and Drug Administration (FDA) have shown favorable results. However, these devices are prone to specific complications and have not been demonstrated to reduce access site complications.[16]

Systemic Complications

Systemic complications relate to allergic and anaphylactic reactions, as well as nephrotoxicity caused by iodinated contrast agents. Allergic or anaphylactic reactions occur in fewer than 3% of cases, and fewer than 1% require hospitalization.

Nonoliguric creatinine elevation, which peaks within 2 to 3 days and returns to baseline by 7 days, is the usual clinical scenario of contrast-induced nephrotoxicity. Patients at risk for contrast-induced nephropathy are those with baseline chronic renal insufficiency, diabetes mellitus, multiple myeloma, and those who are receiving other nephrotoxic drugs (e.g., aminoglycosides). All patients in general, but those at risk to develop contrast-induced nephropathy in particular, should be well hydrated before and after the procedure, and the amount of contrast volume should be minimized. One randomized trial reported that in patients with renal insufficiency, Iodopaque (iso-osmolar, nonionic) is less nephrotoxic than Omnipaque (low osmolar, nonionic) contrast, but there are conflicting studies.[17] Mucomyst (N-acetylcysteine) has shown mixed results in preventing contrast nephropathy.[18,19] The Acetylcysteine for the Prevention of Contrast-Induced Nephropathy (ACT) trial, a pragmatic multicenter randomized trial that evaluated acetylcysteine in patients undergoing coronary and vascular angiography was the largest randomized trial conducted to date. However, it demonstrated that acetylcysteine was ineffective in preventing contrast-induced nephropathy.[20]

Diuretics do not protect against contrast-induced nephrotoxicity. Hydration with half-normal saline for 12 hours before and after the procedure provides better protection against creatinine rise than the combination of hydration and diuretics. Two prospective trials have demonstrated that mannitol does not reduce contrast nephropathy.

Catheter Related Complications

Catheters may disrupt atherosclerotic plaque and cause atheroemboli (also see Chapter 47). When catheters are manipulated in the aorta or brachiocephalic vessels during a thoracic aortogram, stroke is a rare but potentially devastating complication.[5,21,22] In general, asymptomatic patients have a lower risk, whereas patients who undergo angiography in the setting of transient ischemic events have a slightly higher complication rate. Patients who develop a neurological complication should have an immediate neurological assessment, and angiography of the culprit vessel should be obtained prior to an emergency CT scan. If an embolic stroke has occurred, one option is to perform catheter-directed thrombolysis and/or angioplasty. In the presence of intracerebral hemorrhage, anticoagulants and antiplatelet agents should be reversed.

Atheroembolism is another cause of renal insufficiency following angiography. Unlike contrast-induced nephropathy, renal dysfunction after atheroembolization usually develops slowly (weeks to months) and some of these patients progress to renal failure. Diagnosis is confirmed by tissue examination (biopsy), and treatment is supportive. Systemic manifestations of atheroembolism include livedo reticularis, abdominal or foot pain, and purple toes associated with systemic eosinophilia (blue toe syndrome).

REFERENCES

1. Spinosa D, Angle J, Hagspiel K, et al: Feasibility of gadodiamide compared with dilute iodinated contrast material for imaging of the abdominal aorta and renal arteries, *J Vasc Interv Radiol* 11:733, 2000.
2. Diaz L, Pabon I, Garcia J, et al: Assessment of CO_2 arteriography in arterial occlusive disease of the lower extremities, *J Vasc Interv Radiol* 11:163, 2000.
3. Huber PR, Leimbach ME, Lewis WL, et al: CO_2 angiography, *Catheter Cardiovasc Interv* 55:398–403, 2002.
4. Ledneva E, Karie S, Launay-Vacher V, et al: Renal safety of gadolinium-based contrast media in patients with chronic renal insufficiency, *Radiology* 250:618–628, 2009.
5. Armstrong P, Han D, Baxter J, et al: Complication rates of percutaneous brachial artery access in peripheral vascular angiography, *Ann Vasc Surg* 17:107, 2003.
6. Fitts J, Ver Lee P, Hofmaster P, et al, for the Northern New England Cardiovascular Study G: fluoroscopy-guided femoral artery puncture reduces the risk of PCI-related vascular complications, *J Interv Cardiol* 21:273–278, 2008.
7. Abu-Fadel MS, Sparling JM, Zacharias SJ, et al: Fluoroscopy vs. traditional guided femoral arterial access and the use of closure devices: a randomized controlled trial, *Catheter Cardiovasc Interv* 74:533–539, 2009.
8. Dotter CT, Judkins MP: Transluminal treatment of arteriosclerotic obstruction: description of a new technic and a preliminary report of its application, *Circulation* 30:654, 1964.
9. Beales J, Adcock F, Frawley J, et al: The radiological assessment of disease of the profunda femoris artery, *Br J Radiol* 44:854, 1971.
10. Schainfield R, Jaff M: Angiography of the aorta and peripheral arteries. In Baim D, Grossman W, editors: *Grossman's cardiac catheterization, angiography and intervention*, Philadelphia, 2000, Lippincott Williams & Wilkins, pp 293.
11. Singh H, Cardella J, Cole P, et al: Quality improvement guidelines for diagnostic arteriography, *J Vasc Interv Radiol* 13:1, 2002.
12. Jolly SS, Amlani S, Hamon M, et al: Radial versus femoral access for coronary angiography or intervention and the impact on major bleeding and ischemic events: a systematic review and meta-analysis of randomized trials, *Am Heart J* 157(1):132–140, 2009.
13. Arora N, Matheny ME, Sepke C, et al: A propensity analysis of the risk of vascular complications after cardiac catheterization procedures with the use of vascular closure devices, *Am Heart J* 153(4):606–611, 2007.
14. Samal AK, White CJ: Percutaneous management of access site complications, *Catheter Cardiovasc Interv* 57:12, 2002.
15. Waigand J, Uhlich F, Gross C, et al: Percutaneous treatment of pseudoaneurysms and atriovenous fistulas after invasive vascular procedures, *Catheter Cardiovasc Interv* 47:157, 1999.
16. Toursarkissian B, Mejia A, Smilanich R, et al: Changing patterns of access site complications with the use of percutaneous closure devices, *Vasc Surg* 35:203, 2001.
17. Aspelin P, Aubry P, Fransson S, et al: Nephrotoxic effects in high-risk patients undergoing angiography, *N Engl J Med* 348:491, 2003.
18. Chow W, Chan T, Lo S, et al: Acetylcysteine for prevention of acute deterioration of renal function following elective coronary angiography and intervention: a randomized controlled trial, *JAMA* 289:553, 2003.
19. Ferrario F, Barone MT, Landoni G, et al: Acetylcysteine and non-ionic isoosmolar contrast-induced nephropathy: a randomized controlled study, *Nephrol Dial Transplant* 24:3103–3107, 2009.
20. Berwanger O, for the ACT Investigators: Acetylcysteine for the prevention of contrast-induced nephropathy (ACT) trial: a pragmatic multicenter randomized trial to evaluate the efficacy of acetylcysteine for the prevention of renal outcomes in patients undergoing coronary and vascular angiography, *Circulation* 122:2219, 2010.
21. Willinsky R, Taylor S, Terbrugge K, et al: Neurologic complications of cerebral angiography: prospective analysis of 2,899 procedures and review of the literature, *Radiology* 227:522, 2003.
22. Fayed A, White C, Ramee S, et al: Carotid and cerebral angiography performed by cardiologists: cerebrovascular complications, *Catheter Cardiovasc Interv* 55:277, 2002.

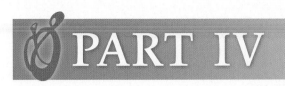

PART IV

PERIPHERAL ARTERY DISEASE

CHAPTER 16 | # The Epidemiology of Peripheral Artery Disease

Michael H. Criqui

Peripheral artery disease (PAD) is generally defined as partial or complete obstruction of one or more peripheral arteries due to atherosclerosis. Although the term *PAD* is sometimes inclusive of all peripheral arteries, in this chapter *PAD* refers to atherosclerotic occlusive disease of the lower extremities. Peripheral artery disease is associated with many of the same risk factors as atherosclerotic cardiovascular and cerebrovascular diseases, and is very common among the elderly. Peripheral artery disease that exhibits typical symptomatology, usually in the form of leg pain brought about by walking, has been conservatively estimated to reduce quality of life in at least 2 million Americans, and in some cases leads to a need for surgical revascularization or amputation.[1] Six million more Americans have measurable asymptomatic disease or disease with atypical symptoms.[2] Both symptomatic and asymptomatic PAD have been shown to be associated with a sharply elevated risk of mortality due to coronary and cerebrovascular disease.[3]

Symptoms and Measures of Peripheral Artery Disease in Epidemiology

It was recognized as long ago as the 18th century that insufficient blood supply to the legs could cause pain and dysfunction in the same way deficient coronary circulation could lead to angina. This type of pain is known as *intermittent claudication* and is characterized as leg pain or discomfort associated with walking and relieved by rest. Intermittent claudication is generally indicative of exercise-induced ischemic leg pain, primarily in the calf, caused by PAD.

Early studies of PAD focused primarily on claudication as the chief symptomatic manifestation of PAD. A number of patient questionnaires have been developed to uniformly identify claudication and distinguish it from other types of leg pain. The first of these was the *Rose questionnaire*, also referred to as the *World Health Organization questionnaire*.[4] The San Diego Claudication Questionnaire (SDCQ) is a modification of the Rose questionnaire that additionally captures information on the laterality of symptoms.[5] Recently we completed an evidence-based shortened revision of the SDCQ that is shown in Table 16-1.

Ankle-Brachial Index

Although intermittent claudication is an important manifestation of PAD, it is not pathognomonic. Atherosclerosis may have been developing for many years before claudication begins, and the extent to which it occurs is influenced by factors other than disease per se, such as the patient's level of activity.[6] Furthermore, the definitional distinctions used to separate claudication from other leg pain make claudication more specific to arterial disease but less sensitive to other types of pain that may in some cases be related to arterial disease. Spinal stenosis can cause leg pain similar to claudication during exercise.

For these reasons, another method of diagnosing PAD was needed. Low blood pressure at the ankle was proposed as a test for PAD as early as 1950[7] and led to development of a simple measure called the *ankle-brachial index* (ABI). The ABI is the ratio of the systolic blood pressure at the ankle to that in the arm. An abnormally low ABI is indicative of atherosclerosis of the lower extremities. The ABI has been shown to have good receiver operating curve characteristics as a test for PAD. Although there is no definitive cut point above which disease is always absent and below which disease is always present, an ABI of 0.9 or less is commonly used in both clinical practice and epidemiological research to diagnose PAD. The ABI is also sometimes referred to as the *ankle-brachial pressure index* (ABPI)[8] and the *ankle-arm index* (AAI).[9]

As a test for ABI-based PAD, claudication has been shown to have very high specificity but very low sensitivity. For example, in the Rotterdam Study, 99.4% of subjects with ABI 0.9 or greater did not have claudication, but only 6.3% of subjects with ABI of less than 0.9 had claudication.[10] In a study of elderly women in the United States, the percentages were 93.3% and 18.3%, respectively.[6] Peripheral artery disease based on ABI criteria is much more common than claudication in the general population, and large numbers of patients without claudication can be shown to have either atypical or no symptoms in the presence of PAD based on ABI.

To validate the ABI and the huge burden of previously unrecognized asymptomatic disease it implied, early studies compared the ABI-based diagnosis with angiography, which was considered the gold standard for visualizing atherosclerosis in the legs. Two such studies often cited reported the sensitivity and specificity of the ABI in the 97% to 100% range.[11,12] However, because angiography presents some risk to patients, it was not ethical to perform angiography on patients not suspected to have PAD, so these studies involved comparisons of patients with angiographically confirmed PAD with young healthy patients assumed not to have PAD. The sensitivities and specificities calculated are therefore based on the ability of the ABI to discriminate between extremes of disease and wellness. If measured among patients seen in routine clinical practice or the population in general, the specificity of the ABI remains in the 97% + range, but the sensitivity is somewhat less—closer to 80%[13]—in part due to some PAD patients with stiff peripheral arteries and false-negative ABIs.[14]

The ABI has been demonstrated to have strong associations with cardiovascular disease risk factors and disease outcomes. In the Cardiovascular Health Study (CHS) cohort, a dose-response relationship was demonstrated between ABI and cardiovascular disease risk factors, as well as both clinical and subclinical cardiovascular disease.[15] In a study in Edinburgh, asymptomatic patients with an ABI of less than 0.9 were shown to have a higher risk of developing claudication and higher mortality.[16] In a clinical study, patients with an ABI of less than 0.9 who did not have exertional leg pain were shown to have poorer lower-extremity functioning even after adjustment for

TABLE 16-1   San Diego Claudication Questionnaire (Brief Version)

Circle Answer

1. Do you get pain or discomfort in either leg on walking? (If no, stop.)	Right leg	Yes No	
	Left leg	Yes No	
2. Does this pain ever begin when you are standing still or sitting?	Right leg	Yes No	
	Left leg	Yes No	
3. Does this pain include your calf/calves?	Right leg	Yes No	
	Left leg	Yes No	
4. Do you get it when you walk at an ordinary pace on the level?	Right leg	Yes No	
	Left leg	Yes No	
5. What do you do if you get it when you are walking?	Right leg	Stop or slow down Continue on	
	Left leg	Stop or slow down Continue on	
6. What happens to it if you stand still?	Right leg	Lessened or relieved Unchanged	
	Left leg	Lessened or relieved Unchanged	

Determine pain category separately for each leg as follows:
1. No pain: 1 = no
2. Pain at rest: 1 = yes and 2 = yes
3. Non-calf: 1 = yes and 2 = no and 3 = no
4. Classic: 1 = yes and 2 = no and 3 = yes and 4 = yes and 5 = stop or slow down and 6 = lessened or relieved
5. Atypical calf: 1 = yes and 2 = no and 3 = yes and not classic

traditional risk factors and comorbidities.[17] The ABI correlates with ability to exercise as measured on an accelerometer,[18] and an ABI of less than 0.6 is related to development of walking impairment.[19] Thus, even aside from its association with claudication, the ABI is related to the types of functional outcomes, risk factors, and associated diseases that one would expect of a measure of PAD. The ABI has also been shown to have high intra- and inter-rater reliability.[20]

In practice, the ABI is measured using a blood pressure cuff, a standard sphygmomanometer, and a Doppler instrument to detect pulses. Pressure measurements are made with the patient at rest in a supine position for 5 minutes prior to measurement. Ankle pressure is measured in both legs at the dorsalis pedis and posterior tibial arteries. The higher pressure measurement in each ankle has traditionally been used as the numerator of the ABI for that ankle. Using the lower or average pressure can substantially change estimates of PAD prevalence; one study reported 47% prevalence based on the higher pressure versus 59% based on the lower.[20] Results of two recent studies support the use of the average of dorsalis pedis and posterior tibial pressures as the ankle pressure for each leg, based on superior reproducibility in repeated tests and closer statistical association with leg function.[20,21] However, the relative predictive value of the higher versus the average (or perhaps the lower) of the two ankle pressures for clinical events has not yet been evaluated. Practice also differs as to the brachial pressure used as the denominator of the ABI; the same brachial pressure is usually used for both left and right ABIs in the same patient, but that pressure may be the right arm, the average of both arms, or the highest of both arms. A recent study supports use of the average of the left and right arms, based on superior reproducibility,[21] but another study shows a strong correlation between PAD and subclavian stenosis, suggesting the highest arm pressure should be used in the ABI calculation.[22] Another issue is that the first arm pressure measured is typically higher because of the "white coat" effect, and a repeat of the first arm pressure after the other pressures are complete will often give a more accurate reading. Based on the numerators and denominators described, separate ABIs are calculated for the left and right legs of each subject. In epidemiological analyses, the unit of analysis is either the leg, with appropriate statistical adjustments for intrasubject correlation, or the subject, with disease status classified based on the "worst" limb (i.e., the limb with the lowest ABI).

The ABI has several limitations as a measure of PAD. Occlusive disease distal to the ankle is not detected by the ABI; other measures, such as pressure ratios using pressures measured in the toe, are required for detecting such distal disease. The ABI is also sensitive to the height of the patient, with taller patients having slightly higher ABIs; it is unlikely these differences are related to real differences in PAD.[23,24] Similarly, it has been noted in several studies that the ABI of the left leg tends to be slightly lower on average than the ABI of the right leg.[23,24] Recent data also document that ABIs in normal subjects, on average, are slightly lower in women and African Americans.[25]

Arterial calcification (medial calcinosis) can make the arteries of the ankle incompressible and lead to artificially high ABI values. This is particularly common in patients with diabetes.[26,27] Ankle-brachial index values above 1.5 are often excluded in epidemiological analyses and should be viewed with suspicion clinically.[6,15,28–30] In two large population-based studies in the United States, the proportion of patients with such elevated values was around 0.5%.[15,30] Some investigators use the more conservative cut point of 1.3. New evidence suggests 1.4 may be a good compromise.[31,32]

Incidence and Prevalence of Peripheral Artery Disease

Although uncommon among younger people, the prevalence of PAD rises sharply with age to include a substantial proportion of the elderly population. Figure 16-1 shows some ABI-based estimates of PAD prevalence by age from six large studies.[10,15,33–36] In four of the studies, the standard ABI of less than 0.9 criterion was used; in the Limburg Study, PAD was diagnosed based on two ABI measurements of less than 0.95,[35] whereas in the Rancho Bernardo Study, a combination of a conservative ABI cut point of 0.8 and other noninvasive tests was used.[33] Although estimates vary, prevalence appears to be well under 5% before age 50, around 10% by age 65 and in excess of 25% in patients 80 years of age or older. All studies show this stronger-than-linear relationship of prevalence to age, although there is some variability in the age at which prevalence begins to increase most dramatically.

Estimates of PAD incidence are reported somewhat less frequently in the literature, with more data based on claudication incidence than on ABI. With respect to claudication, data from the Framingham Study show claudication in men rising from less than 0.4 per 1000 per year in men aged 35 to 45 years to more than 6 per 1000 per year in men aged 65 years and older.[37] Incidence among women ranged from 40% to 60% lower by age, although

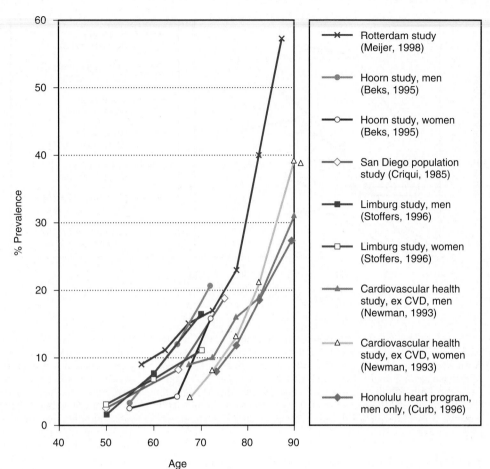

Legend:
- Rotterdam study (Meijer, 1998)
- Hoorn study, men (Beks, 1995)
- Hoorn study, women (Beks, 1995)
- San Diego population study (Criqui, 1985)
- Limburg study, men (Stoffers, 1996)
- Limburg study, women (Stoffers, 1996)
- Cardiovascular health study, ex CVD, men (Newman, 1993)
- Cardiovascular health study, ex CVD, women (Newman, 1993)
- Honolulu heart program, men only, (Curb, 1996)

FIGURE 16-1 Peripheral artery disease (PAD) prevalence. Estimates based on ankle-brachial index (ABI) from six large studies.

estimates in men and women were similar by age 65 to 74. In a group of Israeli men, incidence of claudication ranged from 6.3 per 1000 per year at ages 40 to 49 to 10.5 per 1000 at age 60 and greater.[1] In a study of 4570 men from Quebec, claudication incidence rose from 0.7 per 1000 per year at ages 35 to 44, to 3 per 1000 per year at ages 45 to 54, 7 per 1000 per year at ages 55 to 63, and 9 per 1000 at age 65 and greater.[38] In the Speedwell Study that followed English men aged 45 to 63 years for 10 years, claudication incidence per 1000 per year ranged from 3.1 in the youngest to 4.9 in the oldest age group, based on age at baseline examination.[39] A higher incidence of 15.5 per 1000 per year was reported among men and women aged 55 to 74 in the Edinburgh Artery Study; however, this study did not apply strict Rose criteria for probable claudication.[40]

In the Reykjavik Study, Ingolfsson et al. used Poisson regression techniques to conclude that intermittent claudication rates among Icelandic men dropped significantly between 1968 and 1986. Among 50-year-old men, their estimate of the rate of claudication dropped from 1.7 per 1000 per year in 1970 to 0.6 per 1000 per year in 1984, whereas in 70-year olds, the rate of claudication dropped from 6.0 to 2.0.[41] The authors attributed this to decreased smoking and cholesterol levels. The design and duration of this study were uniquely suited to estimating long-term trends in disease incidence; comparable studies for other populations are unavailable. The potential for trends of this magnitude should be considered in reviewing results of other studies. Figure 16-2 shows incidence rates by age for various studies identifying PAD based on claudication.[1,37–39,41]

There are very few ABI-based studies of PAD incidence, given the time and resources required to periodically retest study subjects for incident disease. In the Limburg PAOD Study, incidence rates for PAD were based on two ABI measurements of less than 0.95. Among men, annual incidence was 1.7 per 1000 at ages 40 to 54; 1.5 per 1000 at ages 55 to 64; and 17.8 per 1000 at ages 65 and greater.

Annual incidence in women was higher: 5.9, 9.1, and 22.9 per 1000, respectively, for the same age groups.[42]

Sex differences in incidence and prevalence of PAD are less clear than those in other cardiovascular diseases.

Claudication incidence and prevalence have usually been found to be higher in men than women. For example, in the Framingham Study, annual claudication incidence for all ages combined was 7.1 per 1000 in men versus 3.6 per 1000 in women, for a male-to-female ratio of 1.97.[37] In the Framingham Offspring Study, claudication prevalence was 1.9% in men versus 0.8% in women (ratio = 2.38), whereas in the Rotterdam Study it was 2.2% in men versus 1.2% in women (ratio = 1.83).[10,30] However, the Edinburgh Artery Study and the Limburg PAOD Study found much lower male-to-female ratios of claudication prevalence of 1.11 and 1.2, respectively.[23,35]

The case for an excess of disease among males is even weaker for PAD diagnosed based on ABI. This is true even in those studies finding a clear male excess with respect to claudication. For example, in the Framingham Offspring Study mentioned earlier, PAD based on ABI was found in 3.9% of men and 3.3% of women, for a ratio of 1.18.[30] In the Rotterdam Study, ABI-based PAD was actually lower in men than in women, with prevalences of 16.9% and 20.5% for a ratio of 0.82.[10] The Limburg PAOD Study, which reported a low male-to-female ratio for claudication, reported a similarly low ratio of 1.1 for ABI-based PAD.[35] A population-based study from Southern Italy found prevalences of PAD based on ABI of less than 0.9 to be very similar in men and women, with male to female ratios by age of .89 to .99.[43] In the CHS, ABI of less than 0.9 was somewhat more prevalent in men than women (13.8% vs. 11.4%; ratio = 1.21), but the association of disease with sex was not significant after adjustment for age and cardiovascular disease status.[15] In the Atherosclerosis Risk in Communities (ARIC) Study, PAD prevalence based on ABI was actually lower in men than women among both African Americans (3.3% vs. 4.0%) and whites (2.3% vs. 3.3%).[44]

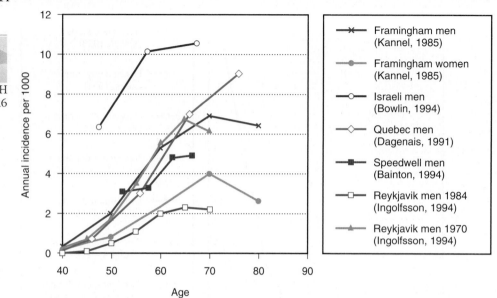

FIGURE 16-2 Peripheral artery disease (PAD) incidence. Estimates based on claudication from five large studies.

The greater male excess observed for symptomatic versus ABI-diagnosed disease may be related to severity of disease. A prevalence study in Southern California found that the excess of disease among males increased with severity of PAD.[33] A report from the Multi-Ethnic Study of Atherosclerosis (MESA) showed PAD prevalence (ABI of less than 0.90) was the same in men and women (3.7%), but borderline values of ABI (0.90-0.99) were much higher in women (10.6% vs. 4.3%).[45]

Peripheral Artery Disease Risk Factors

The section that follows reviews existing evidence for the association of various possible risk factors with PAD. It begins with a discussion of traditional risk factors long implicated in atherosclerotic processes underlying coronary heart and cerebrovascular disease, and then moves on to a discussion of emerging or "novel" risk factors. Where applicable, information on interaction between risk factors and the impact of risk factors on the natural history of disease are also provided.

The study of PAD epidemiology raises a number of methodological issues that should be kept in mind while reviewing the literature. As discussed earlier, the definition of disease has evolved over time, with earlier studies focusing more on claudication as measured using Rose and other criteria, and later studies using the ABI with a value of 0.9 or less, now widely used to define disease. These different potential definitions are noted throughout.

Methodologically, the strongest epidemiological evidence for a causal relationship between disease and putative risk factors comes from studies of incident disease. Such studies usually involve measurement of risk factors at a baseline examination, with subsequent tracking of incident disease among the subjects. Acute events such as myocardial infarction (MI) and stroke lend themselves to such study because the date of onset of disease is generally documented in the records of healthcare providers and recalled by subjects. Conversely, the onset of PAD as defined by ABI is often asymptomatic, and in any case is unlikely to be documented other than through periodic reexamination of all the subjects, which involves substantial time and expense. For that reason, many studies of PAD risk factors are based on cross-sectional associations; that is, the association between current disease status and current risk factor measurements. Although such studies are potentially informative, reported associations cannot conclusively prove causation because it is not known whether the risk factor preceded the disease or vice versa. Caution should therefore be exercised in reviewing results of such cross-sectional studies, particularly where reverse causation is plausible. For example, low physical activity

might cause claudication, but claudication might just as plausibly cause low physical activity.

It is necessary to adjust for multiple potential risk factors in a single statistical model to accurately estimate the unique contribution of any single risk factor because the potential risk factors for PAD are themselves interrelated in various ways. Estimates presented subsequently are based on such multiple adjustment for all traditional PAD risk factors except as noted. Null findings may indicate lack of a real association but may also be based on insufficient sample size. Most of the null findings discussed are based on failure of the risk factor of interest to remain statistically significant in stepwise regression models, which vary as to their algorithms for variable selection.

The following discussion of risk factors focuses on the results from five large epidemiological studies referred to as *index studies* (Table 16-2). These studies each had over 3000 subjects drawn from the general population and included both men and women. The studies are similar enough in their selection and manner of measuring risk factors and in their statistical analyses to allow reasonable comparisons for most of the common risk factors. Although the discussion draws on data from many other studies (see Table 16-2 for a partial list), data are presented from these five studies across all the conventional cardiovascular disease risk factors to provide some consistency and comparability for the reader, and as a check against potential biases that might be introduced by selecting all the studies to present for each risk factor in a more ad hoc fashion.

Smoking

Smoking is one of the strongest risk factors for PAD in virtually all studies. Studies vary as to their measurement of smoking, often combining a categorical assessment of smoking status (current, past, or never) with some measure of current or historical volume of smoking; these multiple approaches to measurement make comparisons difficult. However, even with some type of additional adjustment for volume of smoking, current smoking versus nonsmoking has been shown to at least double the odds of PAD in most studies, with some estimates as high as a four times greater risk among smokers than others. Among the index studies, current smoking (vs. never or former/never) resulted in 2.0 to 3.4 times higher odds of PAD in the three studies using such categorization; however, in two of these studies, the models also included pack-years of smoking as a significant variable. The Rotterdam study included only current packs/day, showing a doubling of the odds of PAD for each pack a day smoked (Table 16-3). All the large population-based studies reviewed found a significant independent association between PAD and smoking.

TABLE 16-2 Population-Based Studies of Peripheral Artery Disease

STUDY NAME	FIRST AUTHOR, YEAR*	NO. OF SUBJECTS	COUNTRY	POPULATION CHARACTERISTICS	STUDY DESIGN	PAD ENDPOINT
Index Studies						
Framingham Study	Murabito, 1997	5209	United States		Cross-sectional	IC
Framingham Offspring Study	Murabito, 2002	3313	United States		Longitudinal	ABI < 0.9
Cardiovascular Health Study	Newman, 1993	5084	United States	Ages 65+	Cross-sectional	ABI < 0.9
Rotterdam Study	Meijer, 2000	6450	Netherlands		Cross-sectional	ABI < 0.9 (<.7 also studied)
Multi-Ethnic Study of Atherosclerosis	Allison, 2006	6653	United States		Cross-sectional	ABI ≤ 0.9
Other Large Studies						
Honolulu Heart Program	Curb, 1996	3450	United States	Japanese American men	Cross-sectional and longitudinal	ABI < 0.9
Edinburgh Artery Study	Fowkes, 1992	1592	Scotland		Cross-sectional	ABI and reactive hyperemia
Limburg PAOD Study	Hooi, 2001	2327	Netherlands		Longitudinal	ABI < 0.95
Israeli Ischemic Heart Disease	Bowlin, 1994	10,059	Israel	Middle-aged men	Longitudinal	IC projected
Reykjavik Study	Ingolfsson, 1994	9141	Iceland	Men only	Longitudinal	IC
Quebec Cardiovascular Study	Dagenais, 1991	4570	Canada	Men only	Longitudinal	IC
Physicians' Health Study	Ridker, 2001	14,916	United States	Male physicians	Nested case-control	IC or PAD surgery
San Diego Population Study	Criqui, 2005	2343	United States	Multiethnic	Cross-sectional	ABI ≤ 0.9, abnormal waveform, PAD revascularization

*Where multiple papers were published, this refers to the paper most frequently referenced herein.
ABI, ankle-brachial index; IC, intermittent claudication, PAD, peripheral artery disease.

TABLE 16-3 Smoking as a Peripheral Artery Disease Risk Factor

STUDY	VARIABLE	ODDS RATIO	95% CI LOW	95% CI HIGH
Framingham Study	Current packs/day	1.96	1.69	2.25
Framingham Offspring Study	Current smoker (vs. former or never)	2.00	1.10	3.40
	Pack-years of smoking	1.03	1.02	1.03
Cardiovascular Health Study	Current smoker (vs. former or never)	2.55	1.76	3.68
	Pack-years of smoking	1.01	1.01	1.02
Rotterdam Study	Current smoker (vs. never)	2.69	1.67	4.33
	Former smoker (vs. never)	1.15	0.75	1.78
Multi-Ethnic Study of Atherosclerosis	Current smoker (vs. never)	3.42	2.48	4.73

Cessation of smoking among patients with claudication has been shown to improve various functional and physiological measures related to PAD, as well as reducing mortality.[46–48] However, because symptomatic PAD patients have long been advised to quit smoking, it is possible that observational comparisons of patients who quit smoking with those who do not are confounded by other differences in compliance with medical advice between the two groups. Randomized trials of this question would raise ethical issues, but substantial bias is unlikely, given the large effect size for cigarette smoking.

Aside from the large increase in risk associated with it, smoking is the traditional risk factor for which the best case can be made for a more important role in PAD than in other atherosclerotic diseases. In a comparison of risk factors conducted in the same large cohort, Fowkes et al. found smoking to be associated with a significantly higher relative risk for PAD compared to other cardiovascular diseases. Smoking was the only traditional cardiovascular disease risk factor for which the odds ratio differed significantly between PAD and other cardiovascular diseases.[49]

Diabetes

Diabetes is strongly associated with an elevated risk of PAD, although the evidence for an independent role in multivariable analysis is not entirely consistent. Four of the five index studies found diabetes, dichotomized based on different criteria, to be associated with PAD after multivariable adjustment, with odds ratios ranging from 1.89 to 4.05.[9,15,50,51] The Framingham Offspring Study found such an association on an age- and sex-adjusted basis, but not in multivariable models.[30]

Among other large population-based studies, multivariable logistic regression models have often shown a relationship to diabetes as a categorical variable,[1,34,36,42,52] or various blood sugar measures as linear variables.[39] Other null findings for diabetes or blood sugar measures were seen in the Edinburgh Artery Study[49] and the Reykjavik Study.[41]

More severe and/or long-standing diabetes appears to be more strongly related to PAD. In the Hoorn Study, it was shown that known diabetes was associated with PAD in multivariable analysis, whereas newly diagnosed diabetes was only of borderline significance, and impaired glucose tolerance was not associated with PAD.[34] In that study, after excluding known diabetics, none of the common glycemic indices that were tested were significantly associated with PAD based on ABI, although significant associations were observed when the PAD criteria were broadened to include patients with additional criteria. Studies conducted in patients with diabetes have shown that duration of diabetes and use of insulin are associated with PAD.[53–55]

Outcomes of PAD in diabetic patients have been shown to be worse. In one study, diabetic patients with PAD were five times more likely to have an amputation than other PAD patients; they also had more than three times the odds of mortality.[56] There is also some evidence to support a somewhat different anatomical distribution of disease, with more disease in arteries distal to the knee in diabetic than nondiabetic persons.[56,57]

Lipids

As is the case in cardiovascular disease epidemiology, the challenge of defining the roles of various lipid fractions in PAD lies in identifying the strongest independent risk factors from among multiple correlated measures. In recent studies, recognition that the ratio of total cholesterol to high-density lipoprotein (HDL) cholesterol is the best lipid measure of risk,[58] along with increasing use of medication, has led to analyses that employ both these variables in the same model[52] or combine the ratio with medication use in a single variable (e.g., "dyslipidemia").[51] Results from the index studies appear in Table 16-4.

Total cholesterol was the first lipid measure examined as a potential risk factor for PAD and has been the most widely studied. Total cholesterol was examined as a potential risk factor in four of the index studies, and was significantly associated with PAD in multivariable analysis in three. In the remaining study, total cholesterol was significant in univariate analysis but dropped out of multivariable models that considered other lipid measures.[30] Similarly, in other studies total cholesterol has usually been found to be associated with PAD,[1,36,41,49] with occasional null findings in multivariable analyses where other lipid measures are considered.[39,59] One of the few null findings for total cholesterol as the sole lipid measure was an analysis of the Quebec Cardiovascular Study cohort.[38]

High-density lipoprotein cholesterol (HDL-C) has been shown to be protective against PAD in most studies where it was evaluated, usually in models that also considered total cholesterol. High-density lipoprotein cholesterol was included among potential risk factors in three of the five index studies and in the TC/HDL-C ratio in a fourth, and was significantly associated with PAD in multivariable analysis in all four. In two studies, both HDL-C and total cholesterol were significant in multivariable analysis, whereas in one study HDL-C but not total cholesterol was significant. Other studies have also shown a protective effect of HDL-C.[36,59]

Bowlin et al. found that non-HDL cholesterol (total cholesterol minus HDL cholesterol) was significantly associated with incident claudication in a large cohort of Israeli men. Neither total cholesterol nor HDL cholesterol were significantly associated with disease in models that included non-HDL cholesterol.[1] In a comparison of incident cases of claudication with healthy controls in the Physician's Health Study, Ridker et al. found that the ratio of total to HDL cholesterol was the lipid measure most strongly associated with disease, with patients in the highest quartile having 3.9 times the claudication risk of patients in the lowest quartile. Screening for other lipid fractions was judged to have little clinical usefulness beyond measurement of this ratio.[60]

Evidence for high triglycerides as an independent risk factor for PAD is fragmentary. Early case-control studies showed a very consistent relationship between triglycerides and PAD, suggesting a uniquely strong relationship with PAD, but large population-based cohort studies employing multivariable modeling later called this into question.[49,61] Among the index studies, only two included triglycerides among the potential risk factors evaluated. In both cases, triglycerides were significant in univariate analysis but dropped out of multivariable models based on stepwise logistic regression.[15,30] Similarly, in the Edinburgh Artery Study cohort and in a large study of geriatric patients in the United States, triglycerides were not significantly associated with PAD after adjustment for other lipid meaures.[49,59] However, other studies have shown triglycerides to be significantly and independently associated with PAD in multivariable analysis.[39,53,62] There is also some evidence suggesting that elevated triglycerides may have a special role in disease progression or more severe PAD.[49,63]

In summary, although total cholesterol, HDL-C, and triglycerides all appear to be associated with PAD on a univariate basis, in multivariable analysis triglycerides frequently drop out as an independent risk factor. Although it has been the most extensively studied, it is not clear that total cholesterol is the strongest independent risk factor for PAD; in one comparison of PAD patients with healthy controls, it was found that mean total cholesterol did not differ significantly, whereas triglycerides, very low-density lipoprotein (VLDL) cholesterol, low-density lipoprotein (LDL) cholesterol, HDL cholesterol, and the total-to-HDL cholesterol ratio all did.[64]

Total and HDL cholesterol seem to provide distinct information and lend themselves to summarization in a single ratio. Because many early studies considered only total cholesterol, full resolution of the question of *which* lipid measures are most strongly and independently related to PAD awaits completion of additional large-scale studies that assess all relevant lipid risk factors. Irrespective of results from multivariable analysis, simple descriptive statistics and clinical observation both suggest that PAD patients are frequently diabetic or insulin resistant, with the typical dyslipidemia of insulin resistance (i.e., low HDL and high triglycerides).

Hypertension and Blood Pressure

The association of hypertension with PAD has been demonstrated in most studies in which blood pressure was studied. All five of the index studies reported a significant association between hypertension as a categorical variable and PAD. The lowest reported odds ratio was 1.32 as reported in the Rotterdam Study; this is somewhat understated relative to the others, since it was based on a model that included both a categorical hypertension variable and an adjustment for systolic blood pressure level that was also significant.[9] Other than this, odds ratios for hypertension ranged from 1.50 to 2.20. Most other large population-based studies have also found a significant independent association of hypertension or systolic blood pressures with PAD.[38,39,42,49,52]

Where both systolic and diastolic pressures were considered, systolic pressure was usually found to be associated with PAD,

TABLE 16-4 Lipid Measures as Peripheral Artery Disease Risk Factors

STUDY	VARIABLE	ODDS RATIO	95% CI	
			LOW	HIGH
Framingham Study*	Total cholesterol (10 mg/dL)	1.05	1.02	1.07
Framingham Offspring Study†	HDL cholesterol (5 mg/dL)	0.90	0.80	1.00
Cardiovascular Health Study‡	Total cholesterol (10 mg/dL)	1.10	1.06	1.14
	HDL cholesterol (5 mg/dL)	0.95	0.90	1.00
Rotterdam Study§	Total cholesterol (10 mg/dL)	1.05	1.01	1.08
	HDL cholesterol (5 mg/dL)	0.93	0.87	1.00
Multi-Ethnic Study of Atherosclerosis‖	Dyslipidemia (yes/no)	1.58	1.22	2.05

*Only total cholesterol was tested.
†Hypercholesterolemia (≥240 mg/dL or medication) and triglycerides dropped out of stepwise logistic regression model.
‡Triglycerides dropped out of stepwise logistic regression model.
§Triglycerides not tested.
‖Total/HDL cholesterol ratio > 5.0 or lipid medication use.
HDL, high-density lipoprotein.

whereas diastolic pressure was not significantly associated[9,15,65] or had a nonlinear relationship with PAD.[36] Two large studies found no relationship of blood pressure with PAD. In the Israeli Ischemic Heart Disease Project cohort, neither systolic nor diastolic blood pressure was associated with claudication,[1] whereas in the Reykjavik Study, systolic and diastolic blood pressures were significantly associated with claudication in cross-sectional but not longitudinal models.[41] It is interesting to note that both of these studies appear to have used blood pressure as a linear term in their models. Most other recent large studies have used a categorization of subjects into normotensive and hypertensive groups based on systolic and diastolic pressures as well as hypertension medication use.

Both of the null findings also come from studies in which claudication was the outcome of interest. It has been speculated that elevated central perfusion pressure as indicated by (axial) blood pressure will sometimes delay onset of claudication by increasing blood pressure in the lower extremities, which—if true—would obscure the relationship of hypertension with underlying disease processes.[66] However, randomized trials of blood pressure lowering in PAD patients generally do not report worsened claudication.

Although the relative risks associated with hypertension are modest in some studies, its high prevalence, particularly among older patients, make it a significant contributor to the total burden of PAD in the population. For example, in one large study from the Netherlands, the odds ratio for hypertension was 1.32, but its attributable risk (a measure of the proportion of PAD due to hypertension in the population) was 17.0%, second only to current smoking in this group.[9] In the Framingham Study, 30% of the risk of claudication in the population was attributable to blood pressure in excess of 160/100.[50]

Obesity

To date, the preponderance of evidence fails to support a consistent independent positive association between obesity and PAD. In one of the few large studies with a positive finding, Bowlin et al. estimated an odds ratio of 1.24 (95% confidence interval [CI], 1.05-1.46) for incident claudication related to a 5.0 kg/m^2 difference in body mass index (BMI) in a study of 10,059 Israeli men.[1]

Three of the index studies and a number of other large population-based studies have failed to find a significant association between obesity and PAD or claudication after multivariable adjustment.[9,30,41,42,51,59] There have also been many studies, including the other two index studies, in which higher relative weight or BMI was actually shown to be protective against PAD. In the Framingham Study, claudication was significantly inversely related to relative weight in men in multivariable analysis, and appeared to have a "U-shaped" nonlinear relationship with relative weight in women.[37] In an analysis from the Edinburgh Artery Study, BMI was significantly associated with less disease in preliminary multivariable analysis, although BMI was excluded from the paper's final multivariable model because it "suggested a counterintuitive effect."[49] The CHS found higher BMI to be significantly protective against PAD after multivariable adjustment in a large sample of Medicare beneficiaries.[15] Body mass index was significantly protective against PAD (defined based on a combination of ABI, Doppler flow curves, and history of surgery) in the Hoorn Study.[34] Similarly, the odds of PAD among subjects in the highest quintile of BMI compared with the lowest quintile were found to be significantly reduced in a cross-sectional analysis of elderly Japanese American men.[36] Subjects with higher BMI were again shown to be at significantly lower risk of PAD in a study of Taiwanese subjects with diabetes.[67] Finally, the multiethnic San Diego Population Study (SDPS) reported a significant inverse association for BMI and PAD.[52]

Obesity has been implicated in the etiology of other risk factors for PAD, such as hypertension, type II diabetes, and dyslipidemia. In epidemiology, adjusting for factors that are on the causal pathway between a risk factor and disease is known to attenuate the observed strength of that risk factor. Therefore, estimates of risks related to obesity in multivariable models are estimates of the risk of obesity that artificially ignore most of the mechanisms by which obesity might reasonably cause PAD. In a few cases, unadjusted models or models adjusted only for age and sex show a significant association with PAD, even though obesity was nonsignificant or protective after multivariable adjustment.[30,49,59] However, in other studies, obesity was found to be either protective or nonsignificant even in unadjusted models or models adjusted only for age and sex.[9,15,36,37,39] Thus, the failure to find more cases of positive association between PAD and obesity is not simply an artifact of adjusting for factors on the causal pathway in multivariable modeling, but seems to suggest a real lack of consistent evidence that such a relationship exists at all.

Unaccounted for in the multivariable analyses just cited is possible residual confounding by cigarette smoking, which is strongly associated with both PAD and lower BMI. In addition, chronic illness in older persons, including PAD, may lead to weight loss and allow for a spurious inverse correlation between obesity and PAD.

As in coronary heart disease (CHD) epidemiology, there is some evidence to suggest that central adiposity, rather than obesity per se, may be more closely related to an increased risk of PAD. Vogt et al. found that after adjustment for BMI, higher waist/hip ratio was associated with significantly higher risk of PAD.[6] In a group of patients with diabetes, it was shown that waist/hip ratio, but not BMI or body fat percentage, was associated with PAD.[53]

Alcohol Consumption

Evidence for a protective effect of light to moderate alcohol consumption, as seen in CHD, is less consistent for PAD. Two of the five index studies considered alcohol intake; neither showed alcohol to be significantly associated with PAD in either age- and sex-adjusted or multivariable models.[9,30] However, in a later analysis of data from one of these studies, a significant protective effect was found in women but not men.[68] Conversely, a protective effect of alcohol was seen in men but not women in the Edinburgh Artery Study, but this association disappeared after adjustment for social class.[69] In Native Americans, a protective effect of alcohol was seen in multivariable analysis,[70] but in elderly Japanese American men, alcohol intake was found to increase rather than decrease the risk of incident PAD.[36] Data from the Physician's Health Study suggest that a protective effect related to moderate alcohol consumption may exist.[71] In that study, there was no univariate association between alcohol and claudication incidence, but adjustment for cigarette smoking "unmasked" a significant protective association, reflecting the positive correlation of alcohol consumption with smoking, a strong risk factor for PAD. Based on this, it seems possible that incomplete adjustment for smoking in other studies might allow residual confounding that could obscure any protective effect of alcohol, despite multivariable adjustment.

Race and Ethnicity

Data on the association of race with PAD are limited because many large studies of PAD have been conducted in non-Hispanic white groups. A 2003 review of ethnicity and PAD concluded that there were "no large population-based studies assessing the prevalence of PAD in non-Caucasians."[72]

Several studies suggest a higher risk of PAD among blacks. The CHS, a study of 5084 Medicare beneficiaries in the United States, found that nonwhite (mostly black) race was associated with an odds ratio of 2.12 for PAD after adjustment for traditional risk factors.[15] A study of 933 women aged 65 and older found a higher percentage of black subjects among the PAD (36.3%) versus non-PAD (24.8%) groups.[17] In the ARIC Study, Zheng et al. found that PAD prevalence was higher in African Americans than whites in both men (3.3% vs. 2.3%) and women (4.0% vs. 3.3%).[44] The MESA reported a multivariable odds ratio of 1.67 for blacks versus non-Hispanic whites.[51] The SDPS reported an odds ratio of 2.34 for blacks versus non-Hispanic whites after adjustment for hypertension and diabetes,[52] and additional analyses also showed no evidence of a greater sensitivity of blacks to traditional cardiovascular disease risk factors. Finally, a synthesis of three studies addressing this question reported odds ratios of 2.3 to 3.1 for blacks versus non-Hispanic whites adjusted for age and gender; odds ratios of 1.7 to 2.9 after adjustment for traditional risk factors; and odds ratios of 1.5 to 2.0 after further adjustment for novel risk factors including inflammatory risk factors.[73] Thus, this association is in part explained by traditional risk factors and in part by novel risk factors, but there is an unexplained residual difference. Interestingly, hospital-based studies suggest that anatomical distribution of disease may differ in blacks, with a higher percentage of distal disease in black subjects, even after adjustment for diabetes and other cardiovascular risk factors.[72]

Data on other races and ethnic groups are limited. In a study in Honolulu, Hawaii, Asians were reported to have lower PAD prevalence than comparable non-Hispanic white subjects.[36] Both the MESA and the SDPS data suggest somewhat lower rates of PAD in Asians and Hispanics than in non-Hispanic whites.[51,52] A study of Native Americans suggested PAD prevalence comparable with that in non-Hispanic whites.[70]

Homocysteine

The association of homocysteine with PAD has been examined in a number of studies, with conflicting results. A 1995 meta-analysis of early case-control studies conducted in the late 1980s and early 1990s suggested an odds ratio of 6.8 for a 5 μmol/L difference in fasting total homocysteine (tHcy).[74] To put this in perspective, the differences between the 25th and 75th percentiles of tHcy among controls in the Physician's Health Study and a study of women in the Netherlands were between 3.5 and 4.0 μmol/L.[60,75] The 5 μmol/L difference noted is therefore not unreasonable as the difference between low and high tHcy levels in the population. In that light, an odds ratio of 6.8 might make homocysteine the single most powerful risk factor for PAD. Interestingly, the odds ratio for PAD in the meta-analysis was strikingly higher than the odds ratios for coronary artery disease (CAD) and cerebrovascular disease, which were below 2 in the same study.

However, more recent studies have produced much lower and frequently nonsignificant estimates of the PAD risk associated with homocysteine. In a large European case-control study, Graham et al. estimated an odds ratio of 1.7 for subjects in the top quintile of homocysteine for their control group versus all other subjects—a result of only borderline statistical significance.[76] One population-based study from the Netherlands found a 1.44 odds ratio for a 5 μmol/L difference in fasting tHcy, based on an extreme definition of PAD involving surgery or an ABI of less than 0.5.[77] However, an analysis of a subset of the Rotterdam Study cohort found no significant relationship between tHcy and PAD, based either on the conventional 0.9 ABI cut-off or on a 0.7 ABI cut-off for severe disease.[9] The MESA reported a significant association for homocysteine after multivariable adjustment for traditional risk factors, but the association just missed significance after adjustment for other novel risk factors.[51] A nested case-control study using the Physician's Health Study cohort failed to find any association between quartiles of fasting tHcy and claudication.[60] A recent case-control study of young women in the Netherlands also failed to find any significant association between fasting homocysteine and symptomatic PAD.[75] Among patients with PAD, disease progression based on ABI was not significantly different in patients with the highest and lowest 20% of homocysteine levels.[78]

At this point, although it is still possible that homocysteine may be an independent risk factor for PAD, it appears that the early results summarized in the 1995 meta-analysis may have overstated the importance of homocysteine. This may be related to the quality of the studies included in the meta-analysis, which included primarily small case-control studies.[74]

C-Reactive Protein and Fibrinogen

C-reactive protein (CRP) and fibrinogen are two inflammatory markers that have been shown to be associated with PAD in a number of studies. In an analysis from the Physician's Health Study, each was found to be significantly associated with PAD in multivariable

models, with odds ratios for the upper versus lower population quartiles of 2.2 for fibrinogen and 2.8 for CRP.[60] However, adding both variables to risk prediction models did not improve the accuracy of prediction because they are significantly intercorrelated. Of the index studies, CRP was studied only in the MESA, and it was not significant in multivariable analysis.[51] However, fibrinogen was included in four of the five studies and was significantly associated with PAD in multivariable analysis in three of them.[9,30,51] Other studies have also reported significant and independent associations of PAD with CRP[75] and fibrinogen.[36,78]

Other Risk Factors

A variety of other potential risk factors for PAD have been examined. In several studies, various measures of oral health have been shown to be independently associated with PAD, possibly based on common inflammatory pathways.[79] A study in young women found that self-reported history of various types of infectious diseases, such as chicken pox, shingles, mumps, pneumonia, chronic bronchitis, or peptic ulcer, was independently and significantly related to PAD.[75] Another study found that a history of arthritis was associated with PAD as diagnosed by ABI.[6]

Psychosocial factors were found to be associated with PAD in one large cohort in Scotland,[80] whereas in a large study of Israeli men, anxiety, job-related stress, and manner of coping with job-related conflicts were all significantly related to incident claudication even after adjustment for traditional risk factors.[1] Among patients with PAD, depressive symptoms were found to be associated with poorer lower-extremity functioning.[81]

Genetic factors appear to have a role in PAD, but data are limited. In a study of fraternal and identical twins, Carmelli et al. estimated that 48% of the variability in ABI could be explained by additive genetic effects.[82] It has also been shown that familial hypercholesterolemia, a genetic disorder, is related to a higher prevalence of PAD.[83]

Other possible risk factors for which some supporting data exist include antiphospholipid antibodies,[84,85] hypothyroidism,[86] and sedentary lifestyle.[87] Possible protective effects have been reported for hormone replacement therapy,[88] but the Women's Health Initiative randomized clinical trial of combined estrogen/progestin therapy showed no effect on the incidence of PAD.[89]

Interaction and Risk Factor Comparisons

Some research has been conducted into potential variations in the significance and strength of various risk factors as they are estimated in different subgroups and for different PAD-related outcomes.

Differences in the relative strength and significance of risk factors in men and women have been examined in several studies. Many of these studies have concluded that risk factors do not differ substantially in men and women. In the Rotterdam Study, separate models for men and women were compared and failed to reveal differences in risk factors for PAD.[9] In the large Framingham and Framingham Offspring cohorts, testing for statistical interactions between sex and risk factors failed to provide any evidence of such interactions.[30,50] One study of Medicare beneficiaries in the United States (age 65 and older) found similar risk factor associations with ABI in men and in women, the exceptions being total and LDL cholesterol levels, which were related to ABI in women but not in men.[15]

Meijer et al. looked at whether severe PAD, diagnosed based on ABI of less than 0.7, had different risk factors than ABI diagnosed based on the traditional cut-point of 0.9.[9] In their analysis, the direction and magnitude of odds ratios were similar for most risk factors under the two criteria. Point estimates suggested that age and current smoking were greater risk factors for conventionally defined PAD, whereas diabetes was more important for severe PAD; however, the 95% CIs overlapped in all cases.

Many risk factors that have been studied for their relationship to PAD were originally identified as risk factors for ischemic heart disease. In the most formal comparison of the relative significance and strength of risk factors for PAD versus ischemic heart disease, the same risk factors were analyzed for their association with the two diseases in the Edinburgh Artery Study cohort.[49] In that study, only the association with smoking was significantly different for PAD versus ischemic heart disease, with a higher association with PAD. Especially strong or consistent relationships to PAD that were suggested for triglycerides and homocysteine were generally not borne out in later studies, as described earlier. In general among risk factors, only smoking and possibly more severe diabetes seem to show stronger associations with PAD than with ischemic heart disease.

Progression of Peripheral Artery Disease

Little is known about the early natural history of PAD, particularly the progression from asymptomatic to early symptomatic disease. Average annual change in ABI has been estimated as 0.01 and 0.02 in various groups,[90,91] but these figures may be somewhat misleading because an average change in ABI masks a variety of changes of different directions and magnitudes.

A more meaningful approach may be to look at the percentage of the population achieving some categorically defined measure of change. The CHS, a population-based study, found that over 6 years of follow-up, 9.5% of persons showed incident PAD, defined as an ABI drop of more than 0.15 to a level of 0.9 or lower.[92] Nicoloff et al. found that in 5 years, 37% of patients experienced a significant (≥0.15) worsening of ABI, whereas 22% of patients experienced clinical progression of PAD based on a change in symptoms or a need for surgical intervention.[93] Among 415 English smokers with PAD referred for a surgical opinion, about half experienced a significant (≥0.14) drop in ABI over the following 48 months.[63] In a group of German PAD patients, PAD was reported to progress in 18.6% of patients during an average follow-up of 64 months, based on a variety of criteria including change in ABI.[94] Bird et al. defined a ranked series of six categories of PAD defined based on ABI and other tests; in a study of patients referred to a vascular laboratory, 30.2% of limbs progressed to a more serious category of PAD over an average follow-up time of 4.6 years, but 22.8% of limbs regressed to a less severe category during the same period.[90]

In a study based on angiography, 9.1% of patients annually were found to have evidence of progression of PAD.[95] In a study using development of rest pain or gangrene as the criteria for PAD progression, PAD progressed in 2.5% of patients annually.[87] In the latter study, it was noted that PAD progressed at a rate approximately three times greater in the first year following diagnosis than in subsequent years.[96] Because many studies of PAD progression have used subjects whose recruitment is linked to the referral for diagnostic testing, estimates of progression from such studies may be appropriate only for newly diagnosed populations, particularly if follow-up time is short.

Data on risk factors associated with progression of PAD are relatively sparse. In the CHS, significant independent predictors of decline were age, cigarette smoking, diabetes, and dyslipidemia.[92] One report showed age, diabetes, classic claudication, previous intervention, and PAD in the contralateral leg to be independently predictive of PAD progression.[90] One study of English smokers with PAD identified hypertriglyceridemia as the most important independent risk factor for progression of PAD and onset of critical ischemia.[63] Hemorheological factors have been shown to be associated with an increased risk of need for vascular intervention.[97] Patients with premature PAD (onset of symptoms at or before age 45) appear to have more rapid progression of disease and generally poorer outcomes.[98-102] Recent data suggest that while PAD progression in large arteries was related to smoking, the TC/HDL-C ratio, lipoprotein(a) (lp[a]), and high-sensitivity CRP assay (hs-CRP), only diabetes was associated with progression in smaller arteries.[103]

Co-Prevalence of Peripheral Artery Disease and Other Atherosclerotic Disease

Given the common risk factors for PAD and other cardiovascular and cerebrovascular diseases, it is not surprising that cross-sectionally, people with PAD are more likely to have these other disorders,

and vice versa. Among 5084 Medicare beneficiaries in the CHS, prevalence of history of MI was 2.5 times as high in subjects with PAD (based on ABI < 0.9) than those without. For angina, congestive heart failure (CHF), stroke, and transient ischemic attack (TIA), the prevalences were 1.9, 3.3, 3.1, and 2.3 times as high, respectively.[15] Conversely, prevalence of PAD was 2.1 times as high in patients with a history of MI than in those without. Corresponding ratios for angina, CHF, stroke, and TIA were 1.7, 2.6, 2.4, and 2.1, respectively.[15] Other studies have found similar cross-sectional correlations.[44,104,105] Subjects with PAD have also been shown to have an elevated prevalence of carotid artery stenosis,[106,107] and a modest but significant correlation between severities of the two diseases has been demonstrated.[108]

Peripheral Artery Disease as a Predictor of Mortality and Morbidity

Going beyond the cross-sectional associations discussed earlier, it has been shown that PAD is prospectively related to morbidity or mortality from other types of atherosclerotic disease, even after adjustment for known common risk factors. Although PAD seems unlikely to directly cause these other diseases, presence of PAD may serve as a marker for underlying atherosclerotic processes or susceptibilities affecting other vascular beds. These prospective relationships are clinically important to the extent that PAD has prognostic value independent of other known risk factors.

Attempts to elucidate this association epidemiologically began with studies of patients having symptomatic PAD in the form of intermittent claudication. Elevated mortality rates among subjects with claudication were reported in the 1970s and 1980s in the Framingham cohort, although this excess risk was markedly attenuated when subjects with baseline cerebrovascular and CHD were excluded.[37,109,110] Similarly, a 1982 Finnish study failed to find an association between claudication and total or cardiovascular mortality in men after adjustment for cardiovascular risk factors and baseline cardiovascular disease.[111] Other studies demonstrated increased mortality risk among claudicants but did not fully adjust for the conventional cardiovascular risk factors.[38,95,112] However, in a large and methodologically rigorous study, data from the 18,403 men in the Whitehall cohort were used to show that after adjusting for cardiovascular risk factors, claudication was a significant predictor of cardiovascular disease mortality even after excluding subjects with baseline disease.[113]

Development of the ABI and other noninvasive measures of PAD permitted further investigation into the association between PAD and cardiovascular disease. In 1985, it was first demonstrated that a combination of noninvasive measures, including ABI, were prospectively related to all-cause mortality even after adjustment for cardiovascular risk factors and exclusion of subjects with baseline cardiovascular disease.[114] Relative risks in this study were in the range of 4 to 5; a later reanalysis of the same cohort with additional mortality follow-up demonstrated elevated relative risks for cardiovascular disease and CHD in particular, with no significant increase in noncardiovascular death.[3]

In the 1990s, a number of other prospective studies confirmed that ABI was related to cardiovascular disease, based on either mortality or combined mortality and morbidity. This was found to be true in a variety of populations: vascular laboratory patients,[28,115] elderly patients with hypertension,[116] elderly women,[117] an employment-based cohort from Belgium,[118] the Edinburgh Artery Study cohort from Scotland,[16] and the CHS cohort.[29] Most of these studies controlled for various known cardiovascular disease risk factors and presence of cardiovascular disease at baseline. Relative risks reported ranged from roughly 2 to 5. Many of these studies also found PAD to be significantly associated with incident CHD in particular, although the very large CHS failed to find such associations for either total MI or angina.[29]

Data regarding the association of PAD with cerebrovascular disease are less conclusive. A 1991 study showed a strong association between multiple noninvasive measures of PAD and cerebrovascular disease morbidity and mortality, with risk ratios of 3.3 for men and 9.0 for women after multivariable adjustment.[119] Data from the Edinburgh Artery Study also showed such an association based on ABI, although after multivariable adjustment, the association persisted for nonfatal but not fatal stroke.[16] However, data from the CHS failed to show a relationship between low ABI and incident stroke.[29] Another large study, the ARIC Study, showed a significant association between ABI as a continuous variable and ischemic stroke after multivariable adjustment, but failed to show such association when ABI was categorized based on a 0.8 cut-point.[120]

Population studies suggest a high ABI (>1.4), is also associated with elevated risk of cardiovascular disease.[32] Such high ABIs are caused by stiff, often calcified, ankle arteries that may mask underlying PAD.[14] Recently, the MESA reported that both "low" (<1.00)

and "high" (>1.40) ABI were associated with increased risk of incident cardiovascular disease events, even after adjustment for traditional and novel risk factors.[121] Interestingly, high ABI showed a stronger association for stroke than low ABI. Also, this was the first report to show that the ABI predicted events independent of other measures of extant atherosclerosis—specifically, coronary artery calcium, carotid intima media thickness, and major electrocardiographic abnormalities. Recent evidence also indicates that independent of baseline ABI, a more rapid deterioration in ABI carries a worse prognosis.[122]

Table 16-5 provides a summary of studies of the association of PAD with various mortality and morbidity outcomes. The table is limited to studies using a noninvasive measure of PAD (usually ABI at various cut-points), and logistic or proportional hazards

TABLE 16-5   Peripheral Artery Disease as a Predictor of Coronary Heart and Cerebrovascular Disease Morbidity and Mortality

STUDY	PERIPHERAL ARTERY DISEASE MEASUREMENT	HAZARD RATIO	95% CI LOWER	95% CI UPPER	MODEL SPECIFICATIONS
Total Mortality					
Criqui, 1992	Large-vessel PAD	3.10	1.80	5.30	Adjusted for conventional risk factors; excludes subjects with baseline angina, MI, stroke (multiple criteria)
Newman, 1993	ABI < 0.9	3.40	1.60	7.10	Adjusted for conventional risk factors; excludes subjects with baseline cardiovascular disease
Vogt, 1993	ABI < 0.9	3.10	1.50	6.70	Adjusted for conventional risk factors; excludes subjects with baseline cardiovascular disease
Kornitzer, 1995	ABI < 0.9	2.07	0.90	4.77	Adjusted for conventional risk factors other than blood pressure; excludes baseline CHD
Jager, 1999	ABI < 0.9	1.50	0.79	2.84	Adjusted for conventional risk factors
Newman, 1999	ABI < 0.9	1.62	1.24	2.12	Adjusted for conventional risk factors; excludes subjects with baseline cardiovascular disease
Hooi, 2002	ABI < 0.7 (vs. > 0.95)	2.10	1.60	2.80	Adjusted for conventional risk factors
Cardiovascular Disease Mortality					
Criqui, 1992	Large-vessel PAD	6.30	2.60	15.00	Adjusted for conventional risk factors; excludes subjects with baseline angina, MI, stroke (multiple criteria)
Vogt, 1993	ABI < 0.9	4.50	1.50	6.70	Adjusted for conventional risk factors; excludes subjects with baseline cardiovascular disease
Kornitzer, 1995	ABI < 0.9	3.29	1.02	10.57	Adjusted for conventional risk factors other than blood pressure; excludes baseline CHD
Jager, 1999	ABI < 0.9	2.36	0.92	6.09	Adjusted for conventional risk factors
Newman, 1999	ABI < 0.9	2.03	1.22	3.37	Adjusted for conventional risk factors; excludes subjects with baseline cardiovascular disease
Hooi, 2002	ABI < 0.7 (vs. > 0.95)	2.30	1.70	3.10	Adjusted for conventional risk factors
Coronary Heart Disease Mortality					
Criqui, 1992	Large-vessel PAD	4.30	1.40	12.80	Adjusted for conventional risk factors; excludes subjects with baseline angina, MI, stroke (multiple criteria)
Kornitzer, 1995	ABI < 0.9	3.63	1.11	11.84	Adjusted for conventional risk factors other than blood pressure; excludes baseline CHD
Cardiovascular Morbidity					
Newman, 1993	ABI < 0.9	2.10	1.10	4.10	Adjusted for conventional risk factors
Hooi, 2002	ABI < 0.7 (vs. > 0.95)	1.70	1.30	2.40	Adjusted for conventional risk factors
Myocardial Infarction					
Newman, 1999	ABI < 0.9	1.40	0.90	2.17	Adjusted for conventional risk factors; excludes subjects with baseline cardiovascular disease
Stroke					
Newman, 1999	ABI < 0.9	1.12	0.74	1.70	Adjusted for conventional risk factors; excludes subjects with baseline cardiovascular disease
All Coronary Heart Disease Morbidity and Mortality					
Criqui, 2010	ABI <1.0	1.87	1.30	2.68	Adjusted for conventional risk factors; excludes subjects with baseline cardiovascular disease
	ABI >1.4	2.15	1.09	4.24	
All Stroke Morbidity and Mortality					
Criqui, 2010	ABI < 1.0	1.56	0.92	2.96	Adjusted for conventional risk factors; excludes subjects with baseline cardiovascular disease
	ABI > 1.4	2.69	0.97	7.55	

ABI, ankle-brachial index; CHD, coronary heart disease; MI, myocardial infarction; PAD, peripheral artery disease.

regression models with multivariable adjustment for conventional cardiovascular risk factors. Results are shown with multivariable adjustment and after exclusion of subjects with baseline cardiovascular disease, where such exclusion was attempted.

Summary and Conclusions

Peripheral artery disease is atherosclerotic obstruction of the arteries of the lower extremities. The most common symptom of PAD is intermittent claudication, which is pain in the legs associated with walking that is relieved by rest. However, noninvasive measures such as the ABI show that asymptomatic PAD is several times more common in the population than intermittent claudication. Peripheral artery disease prevalence is sharply age related, rising to more than 10% among patients in their 60s and 70s. Prevalence appears to be higher among men than women for moderate to severe disease. Major risk factors for PAD are similar to those for cardiovascular and cerebrovascular disease, with some differences in the relative importance of factors. Smoking is a particularly strong risk factor for PAD, as is diabetes. Peripheral artery disease is cross-sectionally associated with cardiovascular and cerebrovascular disease. After adjustment for known cardiovascular disease risk factors, PAD is associated with an increased risk of cardiovascular and cerebrovascular disease, morbidity, and mortality.

With general aging of the population, it seems likely that PAD will be increasingly common in the future. Diagnosis and treatment of PAD in its asymptomatic stage may prove highly beneficial, particularly with respect to interventions aimed at ameliorating risk factors common to atherosclerotic disease of the several vascular beds.

REFERENCES

1. Bowlin SJ, Medalie JH, Flocke SA, et al: Epidemiology of intermittent claudication in middle-aged men, *Am J Epidemiol* 140:418, 1994.
2. Allison MA, Ho E, Denenberg JO, et al: Ethnic-specific prevalence of peripheral arterial disease in the United States, *Am J Prev Med* 32:328, 2007.
3. Criqui MH, Langer RD, Fronek A, et al: Mortality over a period of 10 years in patients with peripheral arterial disease, *N Engl J Med* 326:381, 1992.
4. Rose GA: The diagnosis of ischaemic heart pain and intermittent claudication in field surveys, *Bull World Health Organ* 27:645, 1962.
5. Criqui MH, Denenberg JO, Bird CE, et al: The correlation between symptoms and non-invasive test results in patients referred for peripheral arterial disease testing, *Vasc Med* 1:65, 1996.
6. Vogt MT, Cauley JA, Kuller LH, et al: Prevalence and correlates of lower-extremity arterial disease in elderly women, *Am J Epidemiol* 137:559, 1993.
7. Winsor T: Influence of arterial disease on the systolic blood pressure gradients of the extremity, *Am J Med Sci* 220:117, 1950.
8. Hooi JD, Stoffers HE, Kester AD, et al: Peripheral arterial occlusive disease: prognostic value of signs, symptoms, and the ankle-brachial pressure index, *Med Decis Making* 22:99, 2002.
9. Meijer WT, Grobbee DE, Hunink MG, et al: Determinants of peripheral arterial disease in the elderly: the Rotterdam study, *Arch Intern Med* 160:2934, 2000.
10. Meijer WT, Hoes AW, Rutgers D, et al: Peripheral arterial disease in the elderly: the Rotterdam study, *Arterioscler Thromb Vasc Biol* 18:185, 1998.
11. Yao ST, Hobbs JT, Irvine WT: Ankle systolic pressure measurements in arterial disease affecting the lower extremities, *Br J Surg* 56:676, 1969.
12. Ouriel K, McDonnell AE, Metz CE, et al: Critical evaluation of stress testing in the diagnosis of peripheral vascular disease, *Surgery* 91:686, 1982.
13. Lijmer JG, Hunink MG, van den Dungen JJ, et al: ROC analysis of noninvasive tests for peripheral arterial disease, *J Ultrasound Med Biol* 22:391, 1996.
14. Aboyans V, Ho E, Denenberg JO, et al: The association between elevated ankle systolic pressures and peripheral occlusive arterial disease in diabetic and non-diabetic subjects, *J Vasc Surg* 48:1197, 2008.
15. Newman AB, Siscovick DS, Manolio TA, et al: Ankle-arm index as a marker of atherosclerosis in the Cardiovascular Health Study. Cardiovascular Heart Study (CHS) Collaborative Research Group, *Circulation* 88:837, 1993.
16. Leng GC, Fowkes FG, Lee AJ, et al: Use of ankle-brachial pressure index to predict cardiovascular events and death: a cohort study, *BMJ* 313:1440, 1996.
17. McDermott MM, Fried L, Simonsick E, et al: Asymptomatic peripheral arterial disease is independently associated with impaired lower extremity functioning: the Women's Health and Aging Study, *Circulation* 101:1007, 2000.
18. McDermott MM, Liu K, O'Brien E, et al: Measuring physical activity in peripheral arterial disease: a comparison of two physical activity questionnaires with an accelerometer, *Angiology* 51:91, 2000.
19. McDermott MM, Ferrucci L, Simonsick EM, et al: The ankle-brachial index and change in lower-extremity functioning over time: the Women's Health and Aging Study, *J Am Geriatr Soc* 50:238, 2002.
20. McDermott MM, Criqui MH, Liu K, et al: Lower ankle-brachial index, as calculated by averaging the dorsalis pedis and posterior tibial arterial pressures, and association with leg functioning in peripheral arterial disease, *J Vasc Surg* 32:116, 2000.

21. Aboyans V, Lacroix P, Lebourdon A, et al: The intra- and interobserver variability of ankle-arm blood pressure index according to its mode of calculation, *J Clin Epidemiol* 56:215, 2003.
22. Shadman R, Criqui MH, Bundens WP, et al: Subclavian artery stenosis: prevalence, risk factors, and association with cardiovascular diseases, *J Am Coll Cardiol* 44:618, 2004.
23. Fowkes FG, Housley E, Cawood EH, et al: Edinburgh Artery Study: Prevalence of asymptomatic and symptomatic peripheral arterial disease in the general population, *Int J Epidemiol* 20:384, 1991.
24. Hiatt WR, Hoag S, Hamman RF: Effect of diagnostic criteria on the prevalence of peripheral arterial disease: the San Luis Valley Diabetes Study, *Circulation* 91:1472, 1995.
25. Aboyans V, Criqui MH, McClelland RL, et al: Intrinsic contribution of gender and ethnicity to normal ankle-brachial index values: the Multi-Ethnic Study of Atherosclerosis (MESA), *J Vasc Surg* 45:319, 2007.
26. Kreines K, Johnson E, Albrink M, et al: The course of peripheral vascular disease in non-insulin-dependent diabetes, *Diabetes Care* 8:235, 1985.
27. Orchard TJ, Strandness DE Jr.: Assessment of peripheral vascular disease in diabetes. Report and recommendations of an international workshop sponsored by the American Heart Association and the American Diabetes Association, 18-20 September 1992, New Orleans, Louisiana, *Diabetes Care* 16:1199, 1993.
28. McKenna M, Wolfson S, Kuller L: The ratio of ankle and arm arterial pressure as an independent predictor of mortality, *Atherosclerosis* 87:119, 1991.
29. Newman AB, Shemanski L, Manolio TA, et al: Ankle-arm index as a predictor of cardiovascular disease and mortality in the Cardiovascular Health Study. The Cardiovascular Health Study Group, *Arterioscler Thromb Vasc Biol* 19:538, 1999.
30. Murabito JM, Evans JC, Nieto K, et al: Prevalence and clinical correlates of peripheral arterial disease in the Framingham Offspring Study, *Am Heart J* 143:961, 2002.
31. Wang JC, Criqui MH, Denenberg JO, et al: Exertional leg pain in patients with and without peripheral arterial disease, *Circulation* 112:3501, 2005.
32. Ankle Brachial Index Collaboration: Ankle brachial index combined with Framingham risk score to predict cardiovascular events and mortality. A meta-analysis, *JAMA* 300:197, 2008.
33. Criqui MH, Fronek A, Barrett-Connor E, et al: The prevalence of peripheral arterial disease in a defined population, *Circulation* 71:510, 1985.
34. Beks PJ, Mackaay AJ, de Neeling JN, et al: Peripheral arterial disease in relation to glycaemic level in an elderly Caucasian population: the Hoorn study, *Diabetologia* 38:86, 1995.
35. Stoffers HE, Rinkens PE, Kester AD, et al: The prevalence of asymptomatic and unrecognized peripheral arterial occlusive disease, *Int J Epidemiol* 25:282, 1996.
36. Curb JD, Masaki K, Rodriguez BL, et al: Peripheral artery disease and cardiovascular risk factors in the elderly. The Honolulu Heart Program, *Arterioscler Thromb Vasc Biol* 16:1495, 1996.
37. Kannel WB, McGee DL: Update on some epidemiologic features of intermittent claudication: the Framingham Study, *J Am Geriatr Soc* 33:13, 1985.
38. Dagenais GR, Maurice S, Robitaille NM, et al: Intermittent claudication in Quebec men from 1974-1986: the Quebec Cardiovascular Study, *Clin Invest Med* 14:93, 1991.
39. Bainton D, Sweetnam P, Baker I, et al: Peripheral vascular disease: consequence for survival and association with risk factors in the Speedwell prospective heart disease study, *Br Heart J* 72:128, 1994.
40. Leng GC, Lee AJ, Fowkes FG, et al: Incidence, natural history and cardiovascular events in symptomatic and asymptomatic peripheral arterial disease in the general population, *Int J Epidemiol* 25:1172, 1996.
41. Ingolfsson IO, Sigurdsson G, Sigvaldason H, et al: A marked decline in the prevalence and incidence of intermittent claudication in Icelandic men 1968-1986: a strong relationship to smoking and serum cholesterol—the Reykjavik Study, *J Clin Epidemiol* 47:1237, 1994.
42. Hooi JD, Kester AD, Stoffers HE, et al: Incidence of and risk factors for asymptomatic peripheral arterial occlusive disease: a longitudinal study, *Am J Epidemiol* 153:666, 2001.
43. Gallotta G, Iazzetta N, Milan G, et al: Prevalence of peripheral arterial disease in an elderly rural population of southern Italy, *Gerontology* 43:289, 1997.
44. Zheng ZJ, Sharrett AR, Chambless LE, et al: Associations of ankle-brachial index with clinical coronary heart disease, stroke and preclinical carotid and popliteal atherosclerosis: the Atherosclerosis Risk in Communities (ARIC) Study, *Atherosclerosis* 131:115, 1997.
45. McDermott MM, Liu K, Criqui MH, et al: The ankle brachial index and subclinical cardiac and carotid disease: the Multi-Ethnic Study of Atherosclerosis, *Am J Epidemiol* 162:33, 2005.
46. Faulkner KW, House AK, Castleden WM: The effect of cessation of smoking on the accumulative survival rates of patients with symptomatic peripheral vascular disease, *Med J Aust* 1:217, 1983.
47. Quick CR, Cotton LT: The measured effect of stopping smoking on intermittent claudication, *Br J Surg* 69(Suppl):S24, 1982.
48. Jonason T, Bergstrom R: Cessation of smoking in patients with intermittent claudication: effects on the risk of peripheral vascular complications, myocardial infarction and mortality, *Acta Med Scand* 221:253, 1987.
49. Fowkes FG, Housley E, Riemersma RA, et al: Smoking, lipids, glucose intolerance, and blood pressure as risk factors for peripheral atherosclerosis compared with ischemic heart disease in the Edinburgh Artery Study, *Am J Epidemiol* 135:331, 1992.
50. Murabito JM, D'Agostino RB, Silbershatz H, et al: Intermittent claudication: a risk profile from The Framingham Heart Study, *Circulation* 96:44, 1997.
51. Allison MA, Criqui MH, McClelland RL, et al: the effect of novel cardiovascular risk factors on the ethnic-specific odds for peripheral arterial disease in the Multi-Ethnic Study of Atherosclerosis (MESA), *J Am Coll Cardiol* 48:1190, 2006.
52. Criqui MH, Vargas V, Denenberg JO, et al: Ethnicity and peripheral arterial disease: the San Diego Population Study, *Circulation* 112:2703, 2005.
53. Katsilambros NL, Tsapogas PC, Arvanitis MP, et al: Risk factors for lower extremity arterial disease in non-insulin-dependent diabetic persons, *Diabet Med* 13:243, 1996.
54. Tseng CH: Prevalence and risk factors of peripheral arterial obstructive disease in Taiwanese type 2 diabetic patients, *Angiology* 54:331, 2003.
55. Kallio M, Forsblom C, Groop PH, et al: Development of new peripheral arterial occlusive disease in patients with type 2 diabetes during a mean follow-up of 11 years, *Diabetes Care* 26:1241, 2003.
56. Jude EB, Oyibo SO, Chalmers N, et al: Peripheral arterial disease in diabetic and nondiabetic patients: a comparison of severity and outcome, *Diabetes Care* 24:1433, 2001.

57. Haltmayer M, Mueller T, Horvath W, et al: Impact of atherosclerotic risk factors on the anatomical distribution of peripheral arterial disease, *Int Angiol* 20:200, 2001.

58. Natarajan S, Glick H, Criqui M, et al: Cholesterol measures to identify and treat individuals at risk for coronary disease, *Am J Prev Med* 25:50, 2003.

59. Ness J, Aronow WS, Ahn C: Risk factors for symptomatic peripheral arterial disease in older persons in an academic hospital-based geriatrics practice, *J Am Geriatr Soc* 48:312, 2000.

60. Ridker PM, Stampfer MJ, Rifai N: Novel risk factors for systemic atherosclerosis: a comparison of C-reactive protein, fibrinogen, homocysteine, lipoprotein(a), and standard cholesterol screening as predictors of peripheral arterial disease, *JAMA* 285:2481, 2001.

61. Fowkes FG: Epidemiology of atherosclerotic arterial disease in the lower limbs, *Eur J Vasc Surg* 2:2831, 1988.

62. Cheng SW, Ting AC, Wong J: Fasting total plasma homocysteine and atherosclerotic peripheral vascular disease, *Ann Vasc Surg* 11:217, 1997.

63. Smith I, Franks PJ, Greenhalgh RM, et al: The influence of smoking cessation and hypertriglyceridaemia on the progression of peripheral arterial disease and the onset of critical ischaemia, *Eur J Vasc Endovasc Surg* 11:402, 1996.

64. Mowat BF, Skinner ER, Wilson HM, et al: Alterations in plasma lipids, lipoproteins and high density lipoprotein subfractions in peripheral arterial disease, *Atherosclerosis* 131:161, 1997.

65. Criqui MH, Denenberg JO, Langer RD, et al: Peripheral arterial disease and hypertension. In Izzo JL, Black HR, editors: *Hypertension primer*, Dallas, 2003, American Heart Association, 250.

66. Dormandy J, Heeck L, Vig S: Predictors of early disease in the lower limbs, *Semin Vasc Surg* 12:109, 1999.

67. Tseng CH: Prevalence and risk factors of peripheral arterial obstructive disease in Taiwanese type 2 diabetic patients, *Angiology* 54:331, 2003.

68. Vliegenthart R, Geleijnse JM, Hofman A, et al: Alcohol consumption and risk of peripheral arterial disease: the Rotterdam Study, *Am J Epidemiol* 155:332, 2002.

69. Jepson RG, Fowkes FG, Donnan PT, et al: Alcohol intake as a risk factor for peripheral arterial disease in the general population in the Edinburgh Artery Study, *Eur J Epidemiol* 11:9, 1995.

70. Fabsitz RR, Sidawy AN, Go O, et al: Prevalence of peripheral arterial disease and associated risk factors in American Indians: the Strong Heart Study, *Am J Epidemiol* 149:330, 1999.

71. Camargo CA Jr., Stampfer MJ, Glynn RJ, et al: Prospective study of moderate alcohol consumption and risk of peripheral arterial disease in U.S. male physicians, *Circulation* 95:577, 1997.

72. Hobbs SD, Wilmink AB, Bradbury AW: Ethnicity and peripheral arterial disease, *Eur J Vasc Endovasc Surg* 25:505, 2003.

73. Ix JH, Allison MA, Denenberg JO, et al: Novel cardiovascular risk factors do not completely explain the higher prevalence of peripheral arterial disease among African Americans. The San Diego Population Study, *J Am Coll Cardiol* 51:2347, 2008.

74. Boushey CJ, Beresford SA, Omenn GS, et al: A quantitative assessment of plasma homocysteine as a risk factor for vascular disease. Probable benefits of increasing folic acid intakes, *JAMA* 274:1049, 1995.

75. Bloemenkamp DG, van den Bosch MA, Mali WP, et al: Novel risk factors for peripheral arterial disease in young women, *Am J Med* 113:462, 2002.

76. Graham IM, Daly LE, Refsum HM, et al: Plasma homocysteine as a risk factor for vascular disease. The European Concerted Action Project, *JAMA* 277:1775, 1997.

77. Hoogeveen EK, Kostense PJ, Beks PJ, et al: Hyperhomocysteinemia is associated with an increased risk of cardiovascular disease, especially in non-insulin-dependent diabetes mellitus: a population-based study, *Arterioscler Thromb Vasc Biol* 18:133, 1998.

78. Taylor LM Jr., Moneta GL, Sexton GJ, et al: Prospective blinded study of the relationship between plasma homocysteine and progression of symptomatic peripheral arterial disease, *J Vasc Surg* 29:8, 1999.

79. Hung HC, Willett W, Merchant A, et al: Oral health and peripheral arterial disease, *Circulation* 107:1152, 2003.

80. Whiteman MC, Deary IJ, Fowkes FG: Personality and social predictors of atherosclerotic progression: Edinburgh Artery Study, *Psychosom Med* 62:703, 2000.

81. McDermott MM, Greenland P, Guralnik JM, et al: Depressive symptoms and lower extremity functioning in men and women with peripheral arterial disease, *J Gen Intern Med* 18:461, 2003.

82. Carmelli D, Fabsitz RR, Swan GE, et al: Contribution of genetic and environmental influences to ankle-brachial blood pressure index in the NHLBI Twin Study. National Heart, Lung, and Blood Institute, *Am J Epidemiol* 151:452, 2000.

83. Kroon AA, Ajubi N, van Asten WN, et al: The prevalence of peripheral vascular disease in familial hypercholesterolaemia, *J Intern Med* 238:451, 1995.

84. Taylor LM Jr., Chitwood RW, Dalman RL, et al: Antiphospholipid antibodies in vascular surgery patients: a cross-sectional study, *Ann Surg* 220:544, 1994.

85. Lam EY, Taylor LM Jr., Landry GJ, et al: Relationship between antiphospholipid antibodies and progression of lower extremity arterial occlusive disease after lower extremity bypass operations, *J Vasc Surg* 33:976, 2001.

86. Mya MM, Aronow WS: Increased prevalence of peripheral arterial disease in older men and women with subclinical hypothyroidism, *J Gerontol A Biol Sci Med Sci* 58:68, 2003.

87. Asgeirsdottir LP, Agnarsson U, Jonsson GS: Lower extremity blood flow in healthy men: effect of smoking, cholesterol, and physical activity—a Doppler study, *Angiology* 52:437, 2001.

88. Westendorp IC, in't Veld BA, Grobbee DE, et al: Hormone replacement therapy and peripheral arterial disease: the Rotterdam Study, *Arch Intern Med* 160:2498, 2000.

89. Hsia J, Criqui MH, Rodabough R, et al: Estrogen plus progestin and the risk of peripheral arterial disease: the Women's Health Initiative, *Circulation* 109:620, 2004.

90. Bird CE, Criqui MH, Fronek A, et al: Quantitative and qualitative progression of peripheral arterial disease by non-invasive testing, *Vasc Med* 4:15, 1999.

91. Fowkes FG, Lowe GD, Housley E, et al: Cross-linked fibrin degradation products, progression of peripheral arterial disease, and risk of coronary heart disease, *Lancet* 342:84, 1993.

92. Kennedy M, Solomon C, Manolio TA, et al: Risk factors for declining ankle-brachial index in men and women 65 years or older: the Cardiovascular Health Study, *Arch Intern Med* 165:1896, 2005.

93. Nicoloff AD, Taylor LM Jr., Sexton GJ, et al: Relationship between site of initial symptoms and subsequent progression of disease in a prospective study of atherosclerosis progression in patients receiving long-term treatment for symptomatic peripheral arterial disease, *J Vasc Surg* 35:38, 2002.

94. Taute BM, Gläser C, Taute R, et al: Progression of atherosclerosis in patients with peripheral arterial disease as a function of angiotensin-converting enzyme gene insertion/deletion polymorphism, *Angiology* 53:375, 2002.

95. Walsh DB, Gilbertson JJ, Zwolak RM, et al: The natural history of superficial femoral artery stenoses, *J Vasc Surg* 14:299, 1991.

96. Jelnes R, Gaardsting O, Hougaard Jensen K, et al: Fate in intermittent claudication: outcome and risk factors, *Br Med J (Clin Res Ed)* 293:1137, 1986.

97. Smith FB, Lowe GD, Lee AJ, et al: Smoking, hemorheologic factors, and progression of peripheral arterial disease in patients with claudication, *J Vasc Surg* 28:129, 1998.

98. McCready RA, Vincent AE, Schwartz RW, et al: Atherosclerosis in the young: a virulent disease, *Surgery* 96:863, 1984.

99. Pairolero PC, Joyce JW, Skinner CR, et al: Lower limb ischemia in young adults: prognostic implications, *J Vasc Surg* 1:459, 1984.

100. Hallett JW Jr., Greenwood LH, Robison JG: Lower extremity arterial disease in young adults: a systematic approach to early diagnosis, *Ann Surg* 202:647, 1985.

101. Valentine RJ, MacGillivray DC, DeNobile JW, et al: Intermittent claudication caused by atherosclerosis in patients aged forty years and younger, *Surgery* 107:560, 1990.

102. Levy PJ, Hornung CA, Haynes JL, et al: Lower extremity ischemia in adults younger than forty years of age: a community-wide survey of premature atherosclerotic arterial disease, *J Vasc Surg* 19:873, 1994.

103. Aboyans V, Criqui MH, Denenberg JO, et al: Risk factors for progression of peripheral arterial disease in large and small vessels, *Circulation* 113:2623, 2006.

104. Criqui MH, Denenberg JO, Langer RD, et al: The epidemiology of peripheral arterial disease: importance of identifying the population at risk, *Vasc Med* 2:221, 1997.

105. Ness J, Aronow WS: Prevalence of coexistence of coronary artery disease, ischemic stroke, and peripheral arterial disease in older persons, mean age 80 years, in an academic hospital-based geriatrics practice, *J Am Geriatr Soc* 47:1255, 1999.

106. Alexandrova NA, Gibson WC, Norris JW, et al: Carotid artery stenosis in peripheral vascular disease, *J Vasc Surg* 23:645, 1996.

107. Pilcher JM, Danaher J, Khaw KT: The prevalence of asymptomatic carotid artery disease in patients with peripheral vascular disease, *Clin Radiol* 55:56, 2000.

108. Long TH, Criqui MH, Vasilevskis EE, et al: The correlation between the severity of peripheral arterial disease and carotid occlusive disease, *Vasc Med* 4:135, 1999.

109. Kannel WB, Skinner JJ Jr., Schwartz MJ, et al: Intermittent claudication: incidence in the Framingham Study, *Circulation* 41:875, 1970.

110. Kannel WB, Shurtleff D: The natural history of arteriosclerosis obliterans, *Cardiovasc Clin* 3:37, 1971.

111. Reunanen A, Takkunen H, Aromaa A: Prevalence of intermittent claudication and its effect on mortality, *Acta Med Scand* 211:249, 1982.

112. Kallero KS: Mortality and morbidity in patients with intermittent claudication as defined by venous occlusion plethysmography: a ten-year follow-up study, *J Chronic Dis* 34:455, 1981.

113. Smith GD, Shipley MJ, Rose G: Intermittent claudication, heart disease risk factors, and mortality: the Whitehall Study, *Circulation* 82:1925, 1990.

114. Criqui MH, Coughlin SS, Fronek A: Noninvasively diagnosed peripheral arterial disease as a predictor of mortality: results from a prospective study, *Circulation* 72:768, 1985.

115. McDermott MM, Feinglass J, Slavensky R, et al: The ankle-brachial index as a predictor of survival in patients with peripheral vascular disease, *J Gen Intern Med* 9:445, 1994.

116. Newman AB, Sutton-Tyrrell K, Vogt MT, et al: Morbidity and mortality in hypertensive adults with a low ankle/arm blood pressure index, *JAMA* 270:487, 1993.

117. Vogt MT, Cauley JA, Newman AB, et al: Decreased ankle/arm blood pressure index and mortality in elderly women, *JAMA* 270:465, 1993.

118. Kornitzer M, Dramaix M, Sobolski J, et al: Ankle/arm pressure index in asymptomatic middle-aged males: an independent predictor of ten-year coronary heart disease mortality, *Angiology* 46:211, 1995.

119. Criqui MH, Langer RD, Fronek A, et al: Coronary disease and stroke in patients with large-vessel peripheral arterial disease, *Drugs* 42(Suppl 5):16, 1991.

120. Tsai AW, Folsom AR, Rosamond WD, et al: Ankle-brachial index and 7-year ischemic stroke incidence: the ARIC study, *Stroke* 32:1721, 2001.

121. Criqui MH, McClelland RL, McDermott MM, et al: The ankle-brachial index and incident cardiovascular events in the MESA (Multi-Ethnic Study of Atherosclerosis), *J Am Coll Cardiol* 56:1506, 2010.

122. Criqui MH, Ninomiya JK, Wingard DL, et al: Progression of peripheral arterial disease predicts cardiovascular disease morbidity and mortality, *J Am Coll Cardiol* 52:1736, 2008.

CHAPTER 17

Pathophysiology of Peripheral Artery Disease, Intermittent Claudication, and Critical Limb Ischemia

William R. Hiatt, Eric P. Brass

Peripheral artery disease (PAD) is a manifestation of systemic atherosclerosis that commonly coexists with coronary and carotid artery disease. This places the patient with PAD at high risk of cardiovascular events, including myocardial infarction (MI), ischemic stroke, and death.[1,2] The pathobiology of atherosclerosis and atherothrombosis has been described previously (see Chapter 8).[3,4] The focus of this chapter is on the pathophysiology of atherosclerotic disease in the arteries of the lower extremity that leads to the symptomatic manifestations of PAD, including claudication and critical limb ischemia (CLI). Understanding the pathophysiological mechanisms that underlie the development and progression of limb atherosclerosis and ischemic symptoms is critical in the overall management of the patient with PAD and for the development of potential new therapies. Table 17-1 summarizes the major pathophysiological mechanisms contributing to intermittent claudication and CLI that are reviewed in this chapter.

Clinical Manifestations of Peripheral Artery Disease

The pathophysiology of PAD begins with progressive atherosclerosis, resulting in stenosis and occlusion of the major arteries supplying the lower extremities. Compared with the often acute nature of coronary and carotid atherothrombosis, clinical manifestations of PAD tend to be more chronic and progressive, with primarily functional consequences. Diagnosis of PAD can readily be established through noninvasive hemodynamic assessments. As noted in Chapter 16, the ankle-brachial index (ABI) is the ratio of the systolic blood pressure in the ankle to that in the arm. An ABI of 0.9 take all ABI values to second decimal place, i.e. 0.90 not 0.9 or less establishes a diagnosis of PAD with high sensitivity and specificity when compared with imaging modalities.[5]

Exercise Limitation and Systemic Risk

Patients with PAD suffer from exercise limitation secondary to impaired hemodynamics. The classic symptom of intermittent claudication is an exercise-induced discomfort in the calf associated with reversible muscle ischemia and relieved by rest. The term *claudication* is derived from the Latin word *claudicato*, meaning "to limp," which is typical of the gait pattern of the patient who experiences claudication when walking. Claudication is characterized by a cramping and aching in the affected muscle. Discomfort develops only during exercise, steadily increases during walking activity to a point where the patient has to stop, and then is quickly relieved by rest without change of position. This sequence of exercise-induced progression and complete relief with rest are important clinical differentiators of claudication from other lower-extremity musculoskeletal conditions. Patients with claudication have severe limitations in exercise performance and walking ability. Compared to healthy individuals of the same age, patients with claudication have a 50% to 60% reduction in peak treadmill performance, reflecting a disability similar to that of patients with severe congestive heart failure (CHF).[6] This exercise impairment is associated with a marked decrease in ambulatory activity and the physical dimension of several quality-of-life instruments.[7]

Although classic claudication symptoms occur in less than a third of patients with PAD, all patients with PAD have reductions in ambulatory activity and daily functional capacity.[8] Even "asymptomatic" patients with PAD have a marked reduction in quality of life.[9] Thus, major goals of treatment in ambulatory PAD patients are to prevent progression of systemic atherosclerosis and relieve the symptoms of claudication and enhance quality of life.

In addition to physical disability, PAD is a marker of systemic atherosclerotic disease and associated risk. Peripheral artery disease is associated with a three- to sixfold increased risk of coronary artery disease (CAD) and events, cerebral artery disease and stroke, and cardiovascular death.[1,10] Thus, consensus guidelines recommend that patients with PAD be considered to have established atherosclerotic disease, and secondary prevention standards are applicable.[11,12]

Critical Limb Ischemia

Critical limb ischemia is the most severe of the limb manifestations of PAD. Critical limb ischemia is defined by chronic ischemic pain at rest and/or presence of ischemic skin lesions (gangrene or ulcerations). Although its epidemiology is not well known, a recent population study of 8000 individuals between 60 and 90 years of age found the prevalence of CLI to be 1.2%, and more women than men were affected.[13] Prognosis for patients with CLI is poor.[14,15] In clinical trials enrolling patients with CLI and an ischemic foot ulcer, the annualized risk of death or major amputation ranges from 33% to 50%.[15] Independent predictors of worse outcomes include diabetes, end-stage renal disease, and cardiac dysfunction.[16,17] Patients with CLI have more severe hemodynamic compromise than patients with claudication, owing to multiple and more distal levels of arterial occlusions. Tibial vessels are most often affected in CLI, usually in combination with disease in the popliteal and superficial femoral arteries (and other more proximal vessels), which leads to a severe compromise of blood flow and oxygen delivery to distal tissues.[18] In CLI, ankle pressures typically are less than 50 mmHg. As CLI progresses, skin breakdown to ulceration and gangrene is inevitable. Resting energy expenditure is reduced in CLI compared to intermittent claudication, probably reflecting the fact that these patients become more inactive and sedentary.[19] Revascularization to directly address the hemodynamic compromise in CLI remains the primary therapeutic approach.

Hemodynamics in Peripheral Artery Disease

Skeletal Muscle Oxygen Consumption

Muscle oxygen consumption both at rest and during exercise involves oxygen delivery (pulmonary oxygen uptake, oxygen content of hemoglobin (Hb), and regional blood flow) and oxygen extraction by skeletal muscle mitochondria. In healthy persons, maximal muscle oxygen consumption is determined primarily by maximal oxygen delivery, rather than mitochondrial metabolic rate.[20] Muscle mitochondrial oxidative capacity remains tightly coupled with maximal exercise capacity and increases with exercise

TABLE 17-1	Abnormalities Observed in Peripheral Artery Disease	
CHANGES IN PAD	**POSSIBLE CONSEQUENCES**
Hemodynamic	
Arterial stenosis/occlusion	Pressure drop across stenosis
	Inability to increase flow relative to demand
Collateral formation	Partial compensation for arterial stenosis
Increased blood viscosity	Reduced flow
Endothelial dysfunction	Altered arteriolar regulation of flow
Muscle capillary supply	Increased oxygen diffusion
Oxidant Stress	
Free radical generation	Endothelial and muscle injury
White cell activation	Contributes to oxidant injury
Mitochondrial DNA deletions	Indication of mitochondrial injury
Structural	
Distal axonal denervation	Muscle weakness
Reinnervation	Partial compensation
Type II fiber loss	Decreased muscle mass/strength
Metabolic	
Increased oxidative enzymes	Compensation for reduced oxygen delivery
Increased short-chain acylcarnitine	Reflects altered oxidative metabolism
Decreased electron transport	Accumulation related to performance
Chain activity	Reduced ATP production

ATP, adenosine triphosphate; DNA, deoxyribonucleic acid; PAD peripheral artery disease.

training.[21] At the onset of submaximal exercise, skeletal muscle rapidly extracts oxygen from Hb, producing deoxyhemoglobin.[22] The kinetics of the changes in tissue oxygen uptake are coupled to systemic oxygen consumption to maintain a balance between oxygen delivery and oxygen utilization.

Determinants of Limb Blood Flow in Healthy Individuals

At any given systemic blood pressure, the major determinant of blood flow in normal regional circulation is the peripheral resistance of the vascular bed supplied by major conduit vessels. This basic relationship can be expressed as:

$$Blood flow = Pressure \div Vascular resistance$$

In healthy persons, exercise is a major stimulus for vasodilation, causing a decrease in peripheral resistance, which when combined with an increase in systemic pressure results in a large increase in arterial flow to skeletal muscle. Normal arteries have the capacity to support large volumetric increases in blood flow without a significant drop in pressure across the large and medium conduit vessels (Fig. 17-1).

Hemodynamic Abnormalities in Peripheral Artery Disease

The arterial occlusive disease process results in fixed-resistance elements in the circulation, and thus initiates multiple pathophysiological processes that manifest clinically as claudication, ischemic rest pain, or ulceration (see Fig. 17-1). Major factors that determine the pressure drop across an arterial stenosis include blood flow velocity and the resistance caused by the stenosis, which in turn is defined by the length and internal radius of the stenosis and blood viscosity. These parameters have been classically described by the Poiseuille equation, which defines the relationships between resistance, pressure, and flow:

$$Pressure drop across stenosis = Blood flow [8L\eta] \div \pi r^4$$

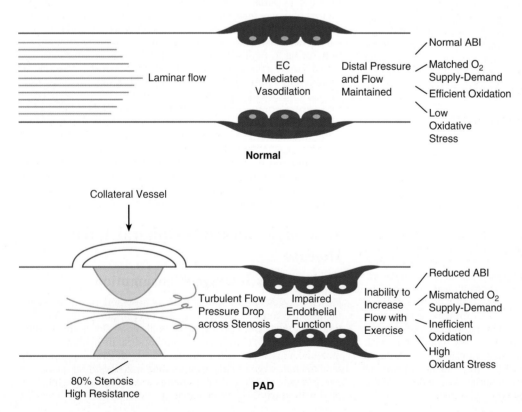

FIGURE 17-1 Normal arterial function. In healthy arteries *(top)* flow is laminar, and endothelial function is normal. Therefore, blood flow and oxygen delivery match muscle metabolic demand at rest and exercise. Muscle metabolism is efficient, resulting in low oxidative stress. In contrast, in peripheral artery disease *(bottom)* arterial stenosis results in turbulent flow. Increased resistance associated with stenosis and loss of kinetic energy results in pressure drop across stenosis. Collateral vessels only partially compensate for arterial stenosis. In addition, endothelial function is impaired, resulting in further loss of vascular function. These changes limit blood flow response to exercise, resulting in mismatch of oxygen delivery to muscle metabolic demand. Changes in skeletal muscle metabolism further compromise efficient generation of high-energy phosphates. Oxidant stress—the result of inefficient oxidation—further impairs endothelial function and muscle metabolism. ABI, ankle-brachial index; EC, endothelial cell; PAD, peripheral artery disease.

where L is length of stenosis, r is internal radius of the artery, and η is viscosity.

This equation makes clear that the radius or cross-sectional area of the stenosis is the primary factor in determining the drop in pressure and flow across a stenosis; a 50% reduction in cross-sectional diameter of the vessel results in a 16-fold increase in resistance. This relationship indicates that as a stenosis worsens, perfusion pressure (and thus the potential pressure that can be dissipated across the stenosis) and the maximal achieved blood flow will decrease dramatically. The dissipation of energy that occurs as blood flow traverses a stenosis is determined in part by the morphology of the stenosis and blood viscosity.[23] Pressure drop across the stenosis manifests as reduced limb systolic pressure and decreased ABI as discussed earlier. In patients with PAD, arterial occlusions limit increase in blood flow to exercising muscle. Resting blood flow is usually preserved because of the pressure of arterial collaterals in most patients. In patients with CLI, however, even resting flow may be reduced below normal levels.

A common angiographic finding is multilevel occlusive disease, particularly in patients with severe symptoms of PAD. A patient with mild claudication may have stenosis at only a single site, such as the iliac artery, but a patient with moderate or severe claudication could have occlusive disease at multiple sites, including the iliac, femoral, and popliteal arteries. Patients with CLI often have diffuse disease affecting multiple arterial segments, such as the iliac, femoral, and tibial arteries. Tibial disease is quite common in CLI and predictive of a higher risk of ischemic ulceration and risk of amputation. Progression of the disease from intermittent claudication to chronic CLI is modulated by collateral vessel development and other compensatory mechanisms.

Based on the Poiseuille equation, the length of an individual stenosis has only mild impact on blood flow and the pressure gradient. Nevertheless, the hemodynamic effect of two equivalent lesions in series is double that of a single lesion.[24] Thus, individual noncritical stenoses may become hemodynamically significant when combined in series in the same limb.[25] In CLI, patients typically have disease in the inflow vessels (aorta, iliac arteries) and outflow vessels (superficial femoral, popliteal and tibial arteries).[18] These lesions in series create more hemodynamic compromise than is typically seen in claudication.

Critical Artery Stenosis

The hemodynamic significance of an arterial stenosis is not only a function of the percent stenosis, but also linear flow velocity across the lesion, as reflected in the Poiseuille equation.[26,27] The term critical artery stenosis is defined as the degree of stenosis that causes a decrease in distal blood flow. The concept integrates the relationship of a stenotic narrowing in an artery with arterial flow velocity and the resultant volumetric flow distal to the stenosis. Importantly, a critical artery stenosis may differ between resting and exercising states because flow velocity in these two conditions is different. Because the pressure gradient across any given stenosis is proportional to the flow velocity, states of higher flow velocity, as occurs with exercise, may result in a decrease in distal perfusion pressure, whereas states of lower velocity, as occurs at rest, may not. For example, resting blood flow velocity in the femoral artery may be only 10 to 20 cm/s, corresponding to a downstream calf blood flow of 1 to 2 mL/100 mL of tissue/min.[28] When a large-vessel stenosis of 50% is imposed on the system at this resting flow velocity, loss of kinetic energy across the stenosis may cause no or only a minimal decrease in distal perfusion pressure. Distal flow will be maintained, since the mild reduction in perfusion pressure will be compensated by a reduction in downstream peripheral resistance. Once the stenosis becomes greater than 90%, there is a greater pressure gradient and fall in distal perfusion pressure, and changes in peripheral resistance can no longer compensate. Thus distal flow decreases. In this example, the critical arterial stenosis needed to reduce distal blood flow at rest is 90%.

During walking exercise, blood flow velocity increases—for example, to 150 cm/s. An exercise-induced increase in flow velocity across a 50% stenosis could significantly increase the pressure gradient and reduce distal perfusion pressure. The associated fall in peripheral resistance would be insufficient to compensate for the fall in pressure, and distal blood flow would decrease. Thus the critical arterial stenosis needed to reduce distal blood flow during exercise may be only 50%.[28] The concept of critical arterial stenosis has clinical significance. In a patient with a single iliac artery stenosis of 50%, the calf blood flow, pedal pulse examination, and ABI may be normal at rest. However, when flow velocity increases with exercise, the same iliac artery lesion becomes hemodynamically significant, resulting in a loss of pedal pulses due to the decrease in ankle pressure distal to the stenosis.

As in patients with CAD, the concept of fractional flow reserve describes the ratio of the blood flow through a diseased coronary artery to the maximal hyperemic flow through that artery in the absence of disease.[29,30] This approach is applicable to PAD and provides a functional interpretation of any degree of percent stenosis and the associated critical arterial stenosis. For example, a functional flow reserve of 0.80 indicates a 20% reduction in maximal hyperemic blood flow due to a stenotic lesion. However, minimal luminal area (MLA, or degree of stenosis) correlates poorly with functional flow reserve until the artery disease results in a large reduction in MLA. Thus anatomy per se may not provide sufficient evidence of the functional significance of a particular degree of arterial stenosis.

Blood Flow Response to Exercise in Intermittent Claudication

Most patients with PAD have no limb symptoms at rest (with the exception of those with CLI). This is because resting blood flow is sufficient to meet the relatively low metabolic needs of the tissue, and therefore there is no mismatch between supply and demand to maintain leg oxygen consumption.[31,32] At the onset of leg exercise, patients with PAD have an initial rise in leg blood flow and leg oxygen consumption that is delayed.[33] With a graded increase in exercise intensity, there is an initial linear increase in flow. However, as exercise intensity increases in PAD, blood flow reaches a plateau because of the limitation imposed by arterial obstructions. This plateau reflects dissipation of energy across the stenotic lesions, removing any additional driving force for increase in flow. Severity of arterial disease (defined by the ABI) correlates inversely with the maximal increase in flow.[34] With cessation of exercise, the hyperemic phase (increased flow over resting levels) is prolonged in patients with PAD relative to healthy controls. Despite the plateau in oxygen delivery during exercise, further increases in oxidative work output are supported by increases in muscle oxygen extraction.[35] Nonoxidative adenosine triphosphate (ATP) production also contributes to muscle energy metabolism.[36] Importantly, muscle ischemia is not simply due to lack of increase in blood flow. The resultant mismatch between the demands for bioenergetics and the flow supply also contribute (see Fig. 17-1).

Other Contributors to Altered Blood Flow in Peripheral Artery Disease

Although arterial flow limitations are of critical importance in the pathophysiology of claudication, the hemodynamic status of the limb correlates poorly with exercise performance. Most studies have shown that resting ankle blood pressure (or ABI) and exercise blood flow do not predict treadmill walking time,[37] whereas some studies have shown a weak positive correlation.[38,39] This lack of consistent relationship between ABI and claudication-limited exercise capacity is surprising, especially given the relationship between ABI and exercise-induced peak blood flow. Thus, factors distal to the arterial obstruction likely contribute to functional limitations in PAD.

Endothelial Regulation of Flow

Blood flow and its distribution within skeletal muscle beds are determined by endothelial and microcirculatory factors (see Fig. 17-1). Endothelium-derived nitric oxide (NO) is central to the physiological regulation of arteriolar tone. Nitric oxide and prostaglandins (PGs) are major autocrine and paracrine mediators of local vascular resistance during exercise in normal individuals.[40-42] Patients with atherosclerosis have a systemic abnormality in endothelial function that is associated with impaired vasodilation and enhanced platelet aggregation.[43] A primary mediator of endothelial dysfunction is felt to be oxidant stress from the generation of superoxide anion.[44] Consistent with the above, abnormalities in endothelium-dependent vasodilation have been observed in PAD.[45] Amputation of an ischemic limb in CLI is associated with improvement of some markers of endothelial function, suggesting local generation of oxidative stress from an ischemic segment of limb.[46] Thus, altered oxygen delivery to exercising skeletal muscle in PAD is related not only to the large-vessel occlusive process but also to endothelial dysfunction and impaired vasodilation.

Hemorheology in Peripheral Artery Disease

Peripheral artery disease is associated with altered hemorheology (flow properties of blood and its cellular components) that result in increased viscosity and altered flow as described by the Poiseuille equation (see earlier discussion). Patients with PAD have increased blood concentrations of fibrinogen, von Willebrand factor (vWF), and plasminogen activator inhibitor (PAI), as well as increased fibrin turnover.[47] These changes also may affect blood flow characteristics in the microcirculation, but none of these factors has been directly correlated with claudication-limited exercise performance. Previous reports have noted that PAD patients have higher blood viscosity than age-matched controls; according to the Poiseuille law, this could be a contributing factor for exercise-induced ischemia.[48] Red cell flexibility is reduced in patients with intermittent claudication, and thus the passage of erythrocytes through nutritive capillaries might be compromised by microcirculatory vessel plugging.[49]

Microcirculatory, Hemorheological, and Thrombophilic Abnormalities in Critical Limb Ischemia

A prominent feature of CLI is formation of cellular plugs and microthrombi in the microcirculation. Erythrocyte fluidity and erythrocyte volume fraction are reduced in patients with CLI compared with controls.[50] These flow properties improve after amputation, suggesting that limb ischemia per se contributes to changes in red blood cell fluidity.[51]

In patients with CLI, a high peripheral white blood cell (WBC) count is associated with future amputation.[52] However, it is unclear whether the increase in leukocytes is causative or simply reflects infection or other inflammatory process that predisposes to amputation. Leukocytes may play an important role in ischemic disease via formation of microemboli and induction of oxidative damage. Leukocyte adhesion is also increased in CLI.[53] This may be due to increased endothelial expression of the adhesion molecules vascular cell adhesion molecule (VCAM)-1 and E-selectin. Adherent cells may further decrease lumen diameter in the microcirculation. Activated neutrophils may adhere to other leukocytes and blood cells, further narrowing the vessel lumen and, through release of mediators, increasing vessel wall damage. Activated leukocytes found in many vascular diseases are abnormally rigid, potentially exacerbating microvascular occlusion in CLI.

Platelet number and platelet activation also are increased in CLI.[54] Activated platelets interact with endothelial receptors, releasing the potent vasoconstrictor thromboxane, further promoting vasoconstriction and platelet activation. In one study, P-selectin expression was significantly increased in patients with intermittent claudication and critical ischemia compared to controls.[54]

The vascular bed in PAD may be under increased vasoconstrictor tone. Decrease in the vasodilators NO and PGs was already discussed, as was increased exposure to the vasoconstrictor thromboxane. In CLI skeletal muscle resistance arterioles, α_1- and α_2-adrenergic receptor responses are increased.[55] This finding has been confirmed in other studies, although the functional significance is unclear.[56,57] Similarly, increases in endothelin messenger ribonucleic acid (mRNA) expression in CLI may cause vasoconstriction of the microcirculation.[58]

Edema in Critical Limb Ischemia

Microcirculatory abnormalities in CLI also predispose the patient to pedal edema.[59] In a study of the rate of fluid filtration through the capillary wall of patients with CLI, the capillary filtration coefficient was increased compared with nonischemic and control limbs. These observations suggest a mechanism to explain the propensity to develop edema in CLI.[60] Restoration of blood flow by surgical bypass grafting or angioplasty generates an increase in distal limb pressure, with associated increases in capillary hydrostatic pressure. This may lead to extravasation of fluid initially and tissue edema in patients who underwent revascularization for CLI.[61]

Inflammation and Oxidative Injury in Peripheral Artery Disease

In claudication, exercise is associated with an increase in plasma levels of thiobarbituric acid–reactive compounds, thromboxane, interleukin (IL)-8, soluble intercellular adhesion molecule (sICAM)-1, VCAM-1, vWF, E-selectin, and thrombomodulin.[62-67] These observations suggest an acute inflammatory response to muscle ischemia during exercise (possibly reflecting reperfusion injury during recovery). After exercise-induced claudication, total neutrophil number and the proportion of activated neutrophils are higher in venous blood draining from the affected leg than in arterial blood.[68] These venous-arterial differences are not observed in the circulation of the contralateral PAD-unaffected exercising leg. Furthermore, activated leukocytes release thromboxane A_2 (TxA_2), which is a vasoconstrictor and promotes platelet aggregation.[69] In claudicants, P-selectin, which mediates platelet-endothelium interaction, may also contribute to platelet alterations in the microcirculation.[70-72] Activated neutrophils also release elastase, which has been shown to exert harmful effects on the endothelium in vitro.[73] Circulating elastase activities increase progressively from healthy individuals, to asymptomatic PAD patients, to symptomatic claudication.[74] Furthermore, in patients with claudication, elastase activity increases further with exercise.[75] These inflammatory responses to exercise may mediate adverse interactions with the microcirculation and skeletal muscle metabolism, which could further compromise exercise performance. Thus the generation of free radicals and oxidative stress can be mediators of tissue injury.

Oxidative Injury in Peripheral Artery Disease

Animal models have shown that both ischemia and ischemia-reperfusion are associated with oxidative stress due to production of free radicals.[76,77] Patients with claudication do not deliver sufficient oxygen to exercising muscle and have a prolonged hyperemic oxygen-rich phase during recovery from exercise.[78] Muscle ischemia during exercise and reperfusion after claudication-limited exercise are associated with an increase in oxidant stress.[79,80] Blood levels of malondialdehyde (a marker of free radical generation) are elevated at rest in PAD and increase further with exercise.[80] Peripheral artery disease patients also have systemic evidence of neutrophil and platelet activation and endothelial injury.[62]

The oxidative stress observed in PAD may be part of a broad spectrum of inflammatory responses to systemic atherosclerosis that is enhanced by exercise.[66] Production of oxygen free radicals may be a unifying mechanism of skeletal muscle injury in PAD

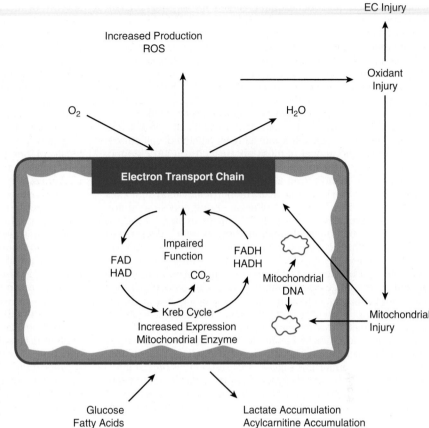

FIGURE 17-2 Alterations in muscle metabolism in peripheral artery disease (PAD). Oxidant stress results in endothelial and mitochondrial injuries that cause mitochondrial deoxyribonucleic acid (DNA) deletions and impairment of electron transport chain function. Sequelae are increase in expression of mitochondrial enzymes and accumulation of lactate and acylcarnitines. EC, endothelial cell.

(Fig. 17-2). Repeated episodes of ischemia during exercise and reperfusion during recovery may promote oxidant injury to endothelial cells (ECs), muscle mitochondria, muscle fibers, and distal motor axons. Oxidative injury to these tissues may in turn promote chronic changes in muscle structure and metabolism, leading to loss of function in PAD that cannot be explained simply by a reduction in blood flow and oxygen delivery. Mitochondria are the major source of free radicals within the cell, so mitochondrial deoxyribonucleic acid (DNA) may be a useful marker of oxidant injury.[81]

Muscle mitochondrial oxidative damage in patients with PAD is readily demonstrated as accumulation of somatic mutations in mitochondrial DNA. For example, patients with PAD have an increased frequency of a mitochondrial DNA 4977 bp deletion mutation.[82] This is a common finding in other tissues under conditions of oxidative stress. More importantly, muscle mitochondria from patients with PAD have specific defects in key steps of the electron transport chain (see Fig. 17-2). These steps have been previously identified as targets of oxidative injury in myocardial perfusion-reperfusion models.[83] Mitochondrial oxidative injury may represent a positive feedback system because electron transport chain impairment increases mitochondrial free radical production, which results in more electron transport dysfunction. Such mechanisms may eventually result in cell loss due to apoptosis.[84,85]

Strategies to reduce or modulate oxidant stress may be important to prevent not only atherosclerotic disease progression, but also to protect skeletal muscle from oxidant injury. Supplementation with the antioxidant vitamin C improves endothelial function in patients with diabetes.[86] However, long-term administration of vitamins C and E does not improve endothelial function in patients with cardiovascular disease.[87] In an animal model, ischemia-reperfusion injury of skeletal muscle microcirculation (defined as microvascular vasoconstriction and plugging and inhibition of NO production) is prevented by a combination of antioxidant vitamins and L-arginine.[88] Important challenges remain concerning

the development of antioxidant therapy. A relevant antioxidant should target specific subcellular locations (e.g., mitochondria) and not be capable of propagating oxidative injury. Thus it remains unclear how oxidant stress can be optimally modulated in PAD, or if antioxidants will favorably alter the pathophysiology of claudication.

Muscle Structure and Function in Peripheral Artery Disease

In healthy humans, exercise requires coordinated recruitment of appropriate muscle fiber types to meet the demands of specific exercise conditions. There is recruitment of type I oxidative slow-twitch fibers that have high mitochondrial content with low-intensity repetitive contractions. Depending on the exercise intensity of these contractions, the fuel is a balance of fat and carbohydrate oxidation. In contrast, rapid forceful muscle contractions require recruitment of type II glycolytic fast-twitch fibers. These fibers have fewer mitochondria than type I fibers and have easy fatigability. Type II fibers include two subtypes: type IIa fibers have intermediate oxidative and contractile properties, and type IIb fibers have the greatest capacity for force generation.

Patients with PAD develop several histological abnormalities in their skeletal muscle. These changes reflect a complex combination of changes associated with disuse due to exercise limitation and direct injury from ischemia, ischemia-reperfusion, and chronic inflammatory mechanisms. Muscle biopsy studies have shown a decrease in type II fast-twitch fiber area that is associated with muscle weakness.[89] These observations have been extended to patients with CLI, where decreases in skeletal muscle myosin isoforms of types IIa and IIb fibers were observed.[90] Various morphological alterations have been identified in the skeletal muscle of PAD patients, including muscle apoptosis and atrophy, increased fiber type switching from oxidative type I fibers to glycolytic type

II fibers, muscle fiber denervation, altered myosin heavy chain expression, and mitochondrial DNA injury.[82,89,91–93] Increasing evidence indicates that inflammatory mediators play an important role in skeletal muscle wasting and fatigue. Tumor necrosis factor (TNF)-α and IL-6, which are increased in PAD, induce skeletal muscle protein breakdown in rats and are negatively related to muscle mass and muscle strength in elderly individuals.[66,94–96] Furthermore, TNF-α may provoke apoptosis in skeletal myocytes.[97] McDermott et al. found that in PAD, higher levels of inflammatory markers (CRP, IL-6, and sVCAM-1) were associated with a small calf area. IL-6 and sVCAM-1 also were associated with a higher percent of calf muscle fat.[98] However, the impact of these observations on muscle function and exercise performance in PAD has not been established.

Patients with claudication also demonstrate extensive skeletal muscle denervation by histological criteria. Denervation injury has been confirmed by electrophysiological testing, and these abnormalities are progressive over time.[99] Changes in skeletal muscle fiber type and neurological function correlate with a decrease in muscle strength.[89] Sensory nerve function is impaired in PAD, particularly in patients with CLI.[100] Neuropathic symptoms are often obscured by the effects of ischemia on other tissues. The neurophysiological changes suggest that the underlying pathophysiology is a distal axonopathy affecting nerve fibers of all sizes. Measures of blood flow in the leg correlate with neurological symptom scores, examination scores, and electrophysiological testing.[101]

In addition to changes in muscle fibers, muscle capillarity is increased in skeletal muscle from patients with PAD.[102] If capillary architecture is normal, this suggests that distal diffusion distances are not a limiting factor for oxygen delivery in PAD. Increased capillarity may be in compensation for the reduction in large-vessel blood flow, and these changes in peripheral diffusion (higher conductance) may have functional relevance.[103]

Several gait abnormalities also have been described in claudication.[104] The findings are primarily slowed walking speed due to decreased step length and cadence. Gait stability is favored over walking speed. Whether these gait abnormalities are related to muscle denervation and weakness or are adaptations to minimize development of pain is unknown.[105] These observations may explain in part why the reduced exercise performance of a patient with claudication cannot be entirely explained by alterations in limb blood flow and pressure.

Alterations in Skeletal Muscle Metabolism

When patients with PAD exercise, skeletal muscle blood flow is insufficient to meet metabolic demand, as described earlier in this chapter. This limitation in the blood flow response to exercise has metabolic consequences. In patients with PAD, muscle oxygen saturation and phosphocreatine levels are normal at rest. At the onset of exercise, however, there is a marked delay in systemic uptake of oxygen that parallels a slowed response in skeletal muscle uptake of oxygen.[6,106] Phosphocreatine is used preferentially for energy creation in patients with PAD compared with control subjects at equivalent exercise work loads.[78] These observations would suggest that a block occurs in early utilization of oxygen at the onset of exercise and prior to limitation of oxygen delivery due to large-vessel occlusions.

Patients with PAD also have changes in oxidative metabolism that appear intrinsic to skeletal muscle. A potential site of impairment of oxidative metabolism in PAD is the electron transport chain, which is vulnerable to free radical injury, as noted earlier.[107] Skeletal muscle from legs affected by PAD has reduced activity of mitochondrial NADH dehydrogenase of complex I and ubiquinol–cytochrome C oxidoreductase (complex III).[108] These observations suggest that electron transport chain activity is impaired, likely secondary to ischemia-reperfusion injury, and may contribute to metabolic dysfunction in PAD.

Altered mitochondrial respiration may have functional consequences. For example, pulmonary oxygen uptake kinetics are slowed at the onset of exercise in patients with PAD, as described earlier. The kinetic changes are independent of the hemodynamic severity of the vascular disease and may thus relate to muscle metabolic abnormalities. Consistent with slowed ventilatory oxygen kinetics, patients with PAD have altered mitochondrial respiration. A number of investigators have used phosphorus-31 (^{31}P) magnetic resonance spectroscopy (MRS) to evaluate mitochondrial respiration in the muscle of control subjects and patients with PAD.[109] Using muscle adenosine diphosphate (ADP) concentration as a marker of the state of mitochondrial respiration, mitochondrial function in PAD is characterized by an increased level of ADP to maintain cellular respiration. An altered ADP–respiratory control relationship is unusual in human chronic diseases, but is characteristic of inherited disorders of the electron transport chain. Given these observations, PAD muscle energetics cannot entirely be explained by reduced blood flow.

Muscle mitochondrial content and mitochondrial enzyme activities reflect the functional state of the individual. Skeletal muscle mitochondrial oxidative enzyme activities increase with exercise training and decrease with prolonged bed rest or inactivity.[110] In healthy individuals, muscle mitochondrial content is positively correlated with peak oxygen uptake, indicating the importance of muscle oxidative capacity in determining exercise performance.[111] In PAD, marked limitation in walking activity and resultant sedentary behavior would be expected to result in a decrease in muscle mitochondrial enzyme content and activity (detraining). In contrast, several studies have shown an increased mitochondrial content in muscle of patients with PAD.[112,113] This increased mitochondrial expression appears to be a direct consequence of, and is proportionate to, the severity of occlusive disease as assessed by leg hemodynamics.[114] Thus, alterations in skeletal muscle mitochondria in PAD appear to reflect the severity of the underlying occlusive disease process. An increased mitochondrial content might improve oxygen extraction under ischemic conditions and could reflect a compensatory mechanism for any intrinsic abnormality in mitochondrial oxidative capacity. Interestingly, increased mitochondrial expression is also associated with inherited disorders of mitochondrial electron transport, suggesting a mechanistic and functional link with the acquired disorder in PAD discussed earlier.

During normal metabolic conditions, fuel substrates such as fatty acids, protein, and carbohydrates are converted to acyl-coenzyme A (CoA) intermediates for oxidative metabolism in the Krebs cycle. These coA–coupled intermediates are linked to the cellular carnitine pool through reversible transfer of acyl groups between carnitine and CoA.[115] One of the functions of carnitine is to serve as a buffer for the acyl-CoA pool by the formation of acylcarnitines. Thus, during conditions of metabolic stress, incomplete oxidation or utilization of an acyl-CoA will lead to their accumulation. Transfer of the acyl group to carnitine will result in accumulation of the corresponding acylcarnitine.

Patients with PAD have alterations in carnitine metabolism, as evidenced by accumulation of short-chain acylcarnitines in plasma and skeletal muscle from the legs affected by arterial disease.[116,117] This accumulation of acylcarnitines implies that acyl-CoA is not being efficiently oxidized, given that the acyl-CoA pool is in equilibrium with the acylcarnitine pool. Importantly, acylcarnitine accumulation may have functional significance in that patients with the greatest accumulation have the most reduced treadmill exercise performance. The degree of metabolic abnormality (as defined by acylcarnitine accumulation) is a better predictor of treadmill exercise performance than the ABI, emphasizing the importance of altered skeletal muscle metabolism in the pathophysiology of claudication.

Conclusions

Patients with PAD and claudication have profound limitation in their exercise performance. Large-vessel obstruction impairs delivery of oxygenated blood to skeletal muscle during exercise, resulting in a supply/demand mismatch. Arterial hemodynamics and large-vessel blood flow, however, do not fully account for the exercise limitations observed in patients with claudication.

Changes in microcirculation and skeletal muscle structure and metabolic function significantly contribute to disease pathophysiology. Understanding these multiple components of exercise limitation provides insight into treatment approaches that address the spectrum of abnormalities seen in patients with claudication.

Critical limb ischemia is a state characterized by severe impairment of blood flow to the limb whereby the metabolic requirements of the tissue at rest are not met. Multiple occlusive lesions of the limb arteries, coupled with functional and structural changes in the microcirculation, are responsible for inadequate tissue perfusion and formation of skin ulcers and necrosis. Age, smoking, and diabetes are major risk factors for CLI. Inflammatory mediators and endogenous procoagulants contribute to development and progression of CLI. Blood components such as red cells, white cells, and platelets aggregate and perturb blood flow in the microcirculation.

Revascularization procedures are the mainstay of treatment for CLI. Further understanding of the pathophysiological disturbances that occur in CLI may lead to additional strategies to preserve limb viability and improve symptoms.

REFERENCES

1. Criqui MH, Langer RD, Fronek A, et al: Mortality over a period of 10 years in patients with peripheral arterial disease, *N Engl J Med* 326:381–386, 1992.
2. Pande RL, Perlstein TS, Beckman JA, et al: Secondary prevention and mortality in peripheral artery disease: National Health and Nutrition Examination Study, 1999 to 2004, *Circulation* 124:17–23, 2011.
3. Libby P, Ridker PM, Hansson GK: Progress and challenges in translating the biology of atherosclerosis, *Nature* 473:317–325, 2011.
4. Rocha VZ, Libby P: Obesity, inflammation, and atherosclerosis, *Nat Rev Cardiol* 6:399–409, 2009.
5. Dachun X, Jue L, Liling Z, et al: Sensitivity and specificity of the ankle-brachial index to diagnose peripheral artery disease: a structured review, *Vasc Med* 15:361–369, 2010.
6. Bauer TA, Regensteiner JG, Brass EP, et al: Oxygen uptake kinetics during exercise are slowed in patients with peripheral arterial disease, *J Appl Physiol* 87:809–816, 1999.
7. McDermott MM, Greenland P, Liu K, et al: Leg symptoms in peripheral arterial disease: associated clinical characteristics and functional impairment, *JAMA* 286:1599–1606, 2001.
8. McDermott MM, Mehta S, Liu K, et al: Leg symptoms, the ankle-brachial index, and walking ability in patients with peripheral arterial disease, *J Gen Intern Med* 14:173–181, 1999.
9. Vogt MT, Cauley JA, Kuller LH, et al: Functional status and mobility among elderly women with lower extremity arterial disease: the study of osteoporotic fractures, *J Am Geriatr Soc* 42:923–929, 1994.
10. Fowkes FG, Murray GD, Butcher I, et al: Ankle brachial index combined with Framingham Risk Score to predict cardiovascular events and mortality: a meta-analysis, *JAMA* 300: 197–208, 2008.
11. Hirsch AT, Haskal ZJ, Hertzer NR, et al: ACC/AHA 2005 guidelines for the management of patients with peripheral arterial disease (lower extremity, renal, mesenteric, and abdominal aortic): executive summary a collaborative report from the American Association for Vascular Surgery/Society for Vascular Surgery, Society for Cardiovascular Angiography and Interventions, Society for Vascular Medicine and Biology, Society of Interventional Radiology, and the ACC/AHA Task Force on Practice Guidelines (Writing Committee to Develop Guidelines for the Management of Patients With Peripheral Arterial Disease) endorsed by the American Association of Cardiovascular and Pulmonary Rehabilitation; National Heart, Lung, and Blood Institute; Society for Vascular Nursing; TransAtlantic Inter-Society Consensus; and Vascular Disease Foundation, *J Am Coll Cardiol* 47:1239–1312, 2006.
12. Norgren L, Hiatt WR, Dormandy JA, et al: Inter-society consensus for the management of peripheral arterial disease (TASC II), *J Vasc Surg* 45:S5–S67, 2007.
13. Sigvant B, Wiberg-Hedman K, Bergqvist D, et al: A population-based study of peripheral arterial disease prevalence with special focus on critical limb ischemia and sex differences, *J Vasc Surg* 45:1185–1191, 2007.
14. Dormandy J, Mahir M, Ascady G, et al: Fate of the patient with chronic leg ischaemia. A review article, *J Cardiovasc Surg (Torino)* 30:50–57, 1989.
15. Belch J, Hiatt WR, Baumgartner I, et al: Effect of fibroblast growth factor NV1FGF on amputation and death: a randomised placebo-controlled trial of gene therapy in critical limb ischaemia, *Lancet* 377:1929–1937, 2011.
16. Gray BH, Grant AA, Kalbaugh CA, et al: The impact of isolated tibial disease on outcomes in the critical limb ischemic population, *Ann Vasc Surg* 24:349–359, 2010.
17. Faglia E, Clerici G, Clerissi J, et al: Long-term prognosis of diabetic patients with critical limb ischemia: a population-based cohort study, *Diabetes Care* 32:822–827, 2009.
18. Van BE, Nikol S, Norgren L, et al: Insights on the role of diabetes and geographic variation in patients with critical limb ischaemia, *Eur J Vasc Endovasc Surg* 42:365–373, 2011.
19. Gardner AW, Montgomery PS: Resting energy expenditure in patients with intermittent claudication and critical limb ischemia, *J Vasc Surg* 51:1436–1441, 2010.
20. Richardson RS, Grassi B, Gavin TP, et al: Evidence of O2 supply-dependent VO2 max in the exercise-trained human quadriceps, *J Appl Physiol* 86:1048–1053, 1999.
21. Richardson RS, Leigh JS, Wagner PD, et al: Cellular PO2 as a determinant of maximal mitochondrial O(2) consumption in trained human skeletal muscle, *J Appl Physiol* 87: 325–331, 1999.
22. Grassi B, Pogliaghi S, Rampichini S, et al: Muscle oxygenation and pulmonary gas exchange kinetics during cycling exercise on-transitions in humans, *J Appl Physiol* 95: 149–158, 2003.
23. Young DF, Tsai FY: Flow characteristics in models of arterial stenoses. II. Unsteady flow, *J Biomech* 6:547–559, 1973.
24. Flanigan DP, Tullis JP, Streeter VL, et al: Multiple subcritical arterial stenoses: effect on poststenotic pressure and flow, *Ann Surg* 186:663–668, 1977.
25. Karayannacos PE, Talukder N, Nerem RM, et al: The role of multiple noncritical arterial stenoses in the pathogenesis of ischemia, *J Thorac Cardiovasc Surg* 73:458–469, 1977.
26. Young DF, Cholvin NR, Kirkeeide RL, et al: Hemodynamics of arterial stenoses at elevated flow rates, *Circ Res* 41:99–107, 1977.
27. Demer L, Gould KL, Kirkeeide R: Assessing stenosis severity: coronary flow reserve, collateral function, quantitative coronary arteriography, positron imaging, and digital subtraction angiography. A review and analysis, *Prog Cardiovasc Dis* 30:307–322, 1988.
28. Lewis P, Psaila JV, Morgan RH, et al: Common femoral artery volume flow in peripheral vascular disease, *Br J Surg* 77:183–187, 1990.
29. Park SJ, Ahn JM, Kang SJ: Paradigm shift to functional angioplasty: new insights for fractional flow reserve- and intravascular ultrasound-guided percutaneous coronary intervention, *Circulation* 124:951–957, 2011.
30. Pijls NH, Van Gelder B, Van der Voort P, et al: Fractional flow reserve. A useful index to evaluate the influence of an epicardial coronary stenosis on myocardial blood flow, *Circulation* 92:3183–3193, 1995.
31. Pentecost BL: The effect of exercise on the external iliac vein blood flow and local oxygen consumption in normal subjects, and in those with occlusive arterial disease, *Clin Sci* 27:437–445, 1964.
32. Hillestad LK: The peripheral blood flow in intermittent claudication IV. The significance of the claudication distance, *Acta Med Scand* 173:467–478, 1963.
33. Bauer TA, Brass EP, Hiatt WR: Impaired muscle oxygen use at onset of exercise in peripheral arterial disease, *J Vasc Surg* 40:488–493, 2004.
34. Sumner DS, Strandness DE Jr.: The relationship between calf blood flow and ankle blood pressure in patients with intermittent claudication, *Surgery* 65:763–771, 1969.
35. Maass U, Alexander K: Effect of treadmill exercise on blood gases and acid-base balance in patients with intermittent claudication, *Z Kardiol* 72:537–542, 1983.
36. Hansen JE, Sue DY, Oren A, et al: Relation of oxygen uptake to work rate in normal men and men with circulatory disorders, *Am J Cardiol* 59:669–674, 1987.
37. Szuba A, Oka RK, Harada R, et al: Limb hemodynamics are not predictive of functional capacity in patients with PAD, *Vasc Med* 11:155–163, 2006.
38. Gardner AW, Ricci MA, Case TD, et al: Practical equations to predict claudication pain distances from a graded treadmill test, *Vasc Med* 1:91–96, 1996.
39. Gardner AW, Skinner JS, Cantwell BW, et al: Prediction of claudication pain from clinical measurements obtained at rest, *Med Sci Sports Exerc* 24:163–170, 1992.
40. Gordon MB, Jain R, Beckman JA, et al: The contribution of nitric oxide to exercise hyperemia in the human forearm, *Vasc Med* 7:163–168, 2002.
41. Kinlay S, Creager MA, Fukumoto M, et al: Endothelium-derived nitric oxide regulates arterial elasticity in human arteries *in vivo*, *Hypertension* 38:1049–1053, 2001.
42. Boushel R, Langberg H, Gemmer C, et al: Combined inhibition of nitric oxide and prostaglandins reduces human skeletal muscle blood flow during exercise, *J Physiol* 543:691–698, 2002.
43. Anderson TJ, Gerhard MD, Meredith IT, et al: Systemic nature of endothelial dysfunction in atherosclerosis, *Am J Cardiol* 75:71B–74B, 1995.
44. Tsao PS, Buitrago R, Chang H, et al: Effects of diabetes on monocyte-endothelial interactions and endothelial superoxide production in fructose-induced insulin-resistant and hypertensive rats, *Circulation* 92:A2666, 1995.
45. Liao JK, Bettmann MA, Sandor T, et al: Differential impairment of vasodilator responsiveness of peripheral resistance and conduit vessels in humans with atherosclerosis, *Circ Res* 68:1027–1034, 1991.
46. Newton DJ, Khan F, Kennedy G, et al: Improvement in systemic endothelial condition following amputation in patients with critical limb ischemia, *Int Angiol* 27:408–412, 2008.
47. Woodburn KR, Lowe GD, Rumley A, et al: Relation of haemostatic, fibrinolytic, and rheological variables to the angiographic extent of peripheral arterial occlusive disease, *Int Angiol* 14:346–352, 1995.
48. Dormandy JA, Hoare E, Colley J, et al: Clinical, haemodynamic, rheological, and biochemical findings in 126 patients with intermittent claudication, *Br Med J* 4:576–581, 1973.
49. Reid HL, Dormandy JA, Barnes AJ, et al: Impaired red cell deformability in peripheral vascular disease, *Lancet* 1:666–668, 1976.
50. Holmberg A, Sandhagen B, Bergqvist D: Hemorheologic variables in critical limb ischemia before and after infrainguinal reconstruction, *J Vasc Surg* 31:691–695, 2000.
51. Nash GB, Thomas PR, Dormandy JA: Abnormal flow properties of white blood cells in patients with severe ischaemia of the leg, *Br Med J (Clin Res Ed)* 296:1699–1701, 1988.
52. Belch JJ, Sohngen M, Robb R, et al: Neutrophil count and amputation in critical limb ischaemia, *Int Angiol* 18:140–144, 1999.
53. Anderson SI, Shiner R, Brown MD, et al: ICAM-1 expression and leukocyte behavior in the microcirculation of chronically ischemic rat skeletal muscles, *Microvasc Res* 71:205–211, 2006.
54. Cassar K, Bachoo P, Ford I, et al: Platelet activation is increased in peripheral arterial disease, *J Vasc Surg* 38:99–103, 2003.
55. Jarajapu YP, Coats P, McGrath JC, et al: Increased alpha(1)- and alpha(2)-adrenoceptor-mediated contractile responses of human skeletal muscle resistance arteries in chronic limb ischemia, *Cardiovasc Res* 49:218–225, 2001.
56. Coats P, Hillier C: Differential responses in human subcutaneous and skeletal muscle vascular beds to critical limb ischaemia, *Eur J Vasc Endovasc Surg* 19:387–395, 2000.
57. Jarajapu YP, McGrath JC, Hillier C, et al: The alpha 1-adrenoceptor profile in human skeletal muscle resistance arteries in critical limb ischaemia, *Cardiovasc Res* 57:554–562, 2003.
58. Tsui JC, Baker DM, Biecker E, et al: Evidence for the involvement of endothelin-1 but not urotensin-II in chronic lower limb ischaemia in man, *Eur J Vasc Endovasc Surg* 25:443–450, 2003.
59. Jacobs MJ, Ubbink DT, Kitslaar PJ, et al: Assessment of the microcirculation provides additional information in critical limb ischaemia, *Eur J Vasc Surg* 6:135–141, 1992.

60. Anvar MD, Khiabani HZ, Kroese AJ, et al: Alterations in capillary permeability in the lower limb of patients with chronic critical limb ischaemia and oedema, *Vasa* 29:106–111, 2000.

61. Coats P, Wadsworth R: Marriage of resistance and conduit arteries breeds critical limb ischemia, *Am J Physiol Heart Circ Physiol* 288:H1044–H1050, 2005.

62. Edwards AT, Blann AD, Suarez-Mendez VJ, et al: Systemic responses in patients with intermittent claudication after treadmill exercise, *Br J Surg* 81:1738–1741, 1994.

63. Belch JJ, McLaren M, Khan F, et al: The inflammatory process in intermittent claudication, *Eur Heart J* 4:B31–B34, 2002.

64. Belch JJ, Mackay IR, Hill A, et al: Oxidative stress is present in atherosclerotic peripheral arterial disease and further increased by diabetes mellitus, *Int Angiol* 14:385–388, 1995.

65. Brevetti G, De Caterina M, Martone VD, et al: Exercise increases soluble adhesion molecules ICAM-1 and VCAM-1 in patients with intermittent claudication, *Clin Hemorheol Microcirc* 24:193–199, 2001.

66. Signorelli SS, Mazzarino MC, Di Pino L, et al: High circulating levels of cytokines (IL-6 and TNFalpha), adhesion molecules (VCAM-1 and ICAM-1) and selectins in patients with peripheral arterial disease at rest and after a treadmill test, *Vasc Med* 8:15–19, 2003.

67. Blann AD, Dobrotova M, Kubisz P, et al: von Willebrand factor, soluble P-selectin, tissue plasminogen activator and plasminogen activator inhibitor in atherosclerosis, *Thromb Haemost* 74:626–630, 1995.

68. Neumann FJ, Waas W, Diehm C, et al: Activation and decreased deformability of neutrophils after intermittent claudication, *Circulation* 82:922–929, 1990.

69. Paul BZ, Jin J, Kunapuli SP: Molecular mechanism of thromboxane A(2)-induced platelet aggregation. Essential role for p2t(ac) and alpha(2a) receptors, *J Biol Chem* 274:29108–29114, 1999.

70. Kirkpatrick UJ, Mossa M, Blann AD, et al: Repeated exercise induces release of soluble P-selectin in patients with intermittent claudication, *Thromb Haemost* 78:1338–1342, 1997.

71. Cassar K, Bachoo P, Ford I, et al: Platelet activation is increased in peripheral arterial disease, *J Vasc Surg* 38:99–103, 2003.

72. Hope SA, Meredith IT: Cellular adhesion molecules and cardiovascular disease. Part I. Their expression and role in atherogenesis, *Intern Med J* 33:380–386, 2003.

73. Mehta J, Dinerman J, Mehta P, et al: Neutrophil function in ischemic heart disease, *Circulation* 79:549–556, 1989.

74. Lowe GDO, Fowkes FGR, Dawes J, et al: Blood viscosity, fibrinogen, and activation of coagulation and leukocytes in peripheral arterial disease and the normal population in the Edinburgh Artery Study, *Circulation* 87:1915–1920, 1993.

75. Turton EP, Coughlin PA, Kester RC, et al: Exercise training reduces the acute inflammatory response associated with claudication, *Eur J Vasc Endovasc Surg* 23:309–316, 2002.

76. Karmazyn M: Ischemic and reperfusion injury in the heart: cellular mechanisms and pharmacologic interventions, *Can J Physiol Pharmacol* 69:719–730, 1991.

77. Turrens JF, Beconi M, Barilla J, et al: Mitochondrial generation of oxygen radicals during reoxygenation of ischemic tissues, *Free Radic Res Commun* 12–13(Pt 2):681–689, 1991.

78. Kemp GJ, Roberts N, Bimson WE, et al: Mitochondrial function and oxygen supply in normal and in chronically ischemic muscle: a combined 31P magnetic resonance spectroscopy and near infrared spectroscopy study *in vivo*, *J Vasc Surg* 34:1103–1110, 2001.

79. Hickman P, Harrison DK, Hill A, et al: Exercise in patients with intermittent claudication results in the generation of oxygen derived free radicals and endothelial damage, *Adv Exp Med Biol* 361:565–570, 1994.

80. Ciuffetti G, Mercuri M, Mannarino E, et al: Free radical production in peripheral vascular disease. A risk for critical ischaemia? *Int Angiol* 10:81–87, 1991.

81. Melov S, Shoffner JM, Kaufman A, et al: Marked increase in the number and variety of mitochondrial DNA rearrangements in aging human skeletal muscle, *Nucleic Acids Res* 23:4122–4126, 1995.

82. Bhat HK, Hiatt WR, Hoppel CL, et al: Skeletal muscle mitochondrial DNA injury in patients with unilateral peripheral arterial disease, *Circulation* 99:807–812, 1999.

83. Rouslin W, Ranganathan S: Impaired function of mitochondrial electron transfer complex I in canine myocardial ischemia: loss of flavin mononucleotide, *J Mol Cell Cardiol* 15:537–542, 1983.

84. Kumar D, Jugdutt BI: Apoptosis and oxidants in the heart, *J Lab Clin Med* 142:288–297, 2003.

85. Sastre J, Pallardo FV, Vina J: The role of mitochondrial oxidative stress in aging, *Free Radic Biol Med* 35:1–8, 2003.

86. Ting HH, Timimi FK, Boles KS, et al: Vitamin C improves endothelium-dependent vasodilation in patients with non-insulin-dependent diabetes mellitus, *J Clin Invest* 97:22–28, 1996.

87. Kinlay S, Behrendt D, Fang JC, et al: Long-term effect of combined vitamins E and C on coronary and peripheral endothelial function, *J Am Coll Cardiol* 43:629–634, 2004.

88. Nanobashvili J, Neumayer C, Fuegl A, et al: Combined L-arginine and antioxidative vitamin treatment mollifies ischemia-reperfusion injury of skeletal muscle, *J Vasc Surg* 39:868–877, 2004.

89. Regensteiner JG, Wolfel EE, Brass EP, et al: Chronic changes in skeletal muscle histology and function in peripheral arterial disease, *Circulation* 87:413–421, 1993.

90. Steinacker JM, Opitz-Gress A, Baur S, et al: Expression of myosin heavy chain isoforms in skeletal muscle of patients with peripheral arterial occlusive disease, *J Vasc Surg* 31:443–449, 2000.

91. Askew CD, Green S, Walker PJ, et al: Skeletal muscle phenotype is associated with exercise tolerance in patients with peripheral arterial disease, *J Vasc Surg* 41:802–807, 2005.

92. McGuigan MR, Bronks R, Newton RU, et al: Muscle fiber characteristics in patients with peripheral arterial disease, *Med Sci Sports Exerc* 33:2016–2021, 2001.

93. Mitchell RG, Duscha BD, Robbins JL, et al: Increased levels of apoptosis in gastrocnemius skeletal muscle in patients with peripheral arterial disease, *Vasc Med* 12:285–290, 2007.

94. Goodman MN: Tumor necrosis factor induces skeletal muscle protein breakdown in rats, *Am J Physiol* 260:E727–E730, 1991.

95. Goodman MN: Interleukin-6 induces skeletal muscle protein breakdown in rats, *Proc Soc Exp Biol Med* 205:182–185, 1994.

96. Visser M, Pahor M, Taaffe DR, et al: Relationship of interleukin-6 and tumor necrosis factor-alpha with muscle mass and muscle strength in elderly men and women: the Health ABC Study, *J Gerontol A Biol Sci Med Sci* 57:M326–M332, 2002.

97. Meadows KA, Holly JM, Stewart CE: Tumor necrosis factor-alpha-induced apoptosis is associated with suppression of insulin-like growth factor binding protein-5 secretion in differentiating murine skeletal myoblasts, *J Cell Physiol* 183:330–337, 2000.

98. McDermott MM, Ferrucci L, Guralnik JM, et al: Elevated levels of inflammation, D-dimer, and homocysteine are associated with adverse calf muscle characteristics and reduced calf strength in peripheral arterial disease, *J Am Coll Cardiol* 50:897–905, 2007.

99. England JD, Ferguson MA, Hiatt WR, et al: Progression of neuropathy in peripheral arterial disease, *Muscle Nerve* 18:380–387, 1995.

100. Laghi PF, Pastorelli M, Beermann U, et al: Peripheral neuropathy associated with ischemic vascular disease of the lower limbs, *Angiology* 47:569–577, 1996.

101. Weinberg DH, Simovic D, Isner J, et al: Chronic ischemic monomelic neuropathy from critical limb ischemia, *Neurology* 57:1008–1012, 2001.

102. McGuigan MR, Bronks R, Newton RU, et al: Muscle fiber characteristics in patients with peripheral arterial disease, *Med Sci Sports Exerc* 33:2016–2021, 2001.

103. Sala E, Noyszewski EA, Campistol JM, et al: Impaired muscle oxygen transfer in patients with chronic renal failure, *Am J Physiol Regul Integr Comp Physiol* 280:R1240–R1248, 2001.

104. Scherer SA, Bainbridge JS, Hiatt WR, et al: Gait characteristics of patients with claudication, *Arch Phys Med Rehabil* 79:529–531, 1998.

105. Scherer SA, Hiatt WR, Regensteiner JG: Lack of relationship between gait parameters and physical function in peripheral arterial disease, *J Vasc Surg* 44:782–788, 2006.

106. Bauer TA, Brass EP, Barstow TJ, et al: Skeletal muscle StO(2) kinetics are slowed during low work rate calf exercise in peripheral arterial disease, *Eur J Appl Physiol* 100:143–151, 2007.

107. Rouslin W: Mitochondrial complexes I, II, III, IV, and V in myocardial ischemia and autolysis, *Am J Physiol* 244:H743–H748, 1983.

108. Brass EP, Hiatt WR, Gardner AW, et al: Decreased NADH dehydrogenase and ubiquinol-cytochrome c oxidoreductase in peripheral arterial disease, *Am J Physiol* 280:H603–H609, 2001.

109. Kemp GJ, Taylor DJ, Thompson CH, et al: Quantitative analysis by 31P magnetic resonance spectroscopy of abnormal mitochondrial oxidation in skeletal muscle during recovery from exercise, *NMR Biomed* 6:302–310, 1993.

110. Wibom R, Hultman E, Johansson M, et al: Adaptation of mitochondrial ATP production in human skeletal muscle to endurance training and detraining, *J Appl Physiol* 73:2004–2010, 1992.

111. Wang H, Hiatt WR, Barstow TJ, et al: Relationships between muscle mitochondrial DNA content, mitochondrial enzyme activity and oxidative capacity in man: Alterations with disease, *Eur J Appl Physiol* 80:22–27, 1999.

112. Lundgren F, Dahllof AG, Schersten T, et al: Muscle enzyme adaptation in patients with peripheral arterial insufficiency: Spontaneous adaptation, effect of different treatments and consequences on walking performance, *Clin Sci* 77:485–493, 1989.

113. Hiatt WR, Regensteiner JG, Wolfel EE, et al: Effect of exercise training on skeletal muscle histology and metabolism in peripheral arterial disease, *J Appl Physiol* 81:780–788, 1996.

114. Jansson E, Johansson J, Sylven C, et al: Calf muscle adaptation in intermittent claudication. Side-differences in muscle metabolic characteristics in patients with unilateral arterial disease, *Clin Physiol* 8:17–29, 1988.

115. Brass EP, Hoppel CL: Relationship between acid-soluble carnitine and coenzyme A pools in vivo, *Biochem J* 190:495–504, 1980.

116. Hiatt WR, Nawaz D, Brass EP: Carnitine metabolism during exercise in patients with peripheral vascular disease, *J Appl Physiol* 62:2383–2387, 1987.

117. Hiatt WR, Wolfel EE, Regensteiner JG, et al: Skeletal muscle carnitine metabolism in patients with unilateral peripheral arterial disease, *J Appl Physiol* 73:346–353, 1992.

CHAPTER 18

Peripheral Artery Disease: Clinical Evaluation

Joshua A. Beckman, Mark A. Creager

The least often recognized of the commonly occurring manifestations of atherosclerosis is peripheral artery disease (PAD). Epidemiological studies suggest that approximately 7.1 million people in the United States have PAD.[1] Among 7458 participants aged 40 years and older from the 1999 to 2004 National Health and Nutrition Examination Survey (NHANES), prevalence of PAD was 5.9%.[1,2] Despite its relative frequency, predictable patient population, and prognostic implications for life and limb, many cardiovascular physicians do not undertake clinical evaluation of PAD. This chapter will focus on the history, physical examination, and diagnostic tests important to management of limb atherosclerosis.

Patient History

Diagnosis of PAD begins with clinical suspicion in the typical patient population. This includes avid questioning and seeking to elicit historical evidence of limb and systemic atherosclerosis. Clinical suspicion should be heightened in older persons, in those with coronary or cerebral atherosclerosis, and in patients with atherosclerotic risk factors such as diabetes or tobacco use, as well as renal failure (see Chapter 16). Peripheral artery disease is uncommon before the age of 40 years. In the German Epidemiological Trial on Ankle Brachial Index (getABI) of 6990 unselected patients aged 65 years or older, prevalence of PAD in men and women was 20% and 17%, respectively.[3] In the PAD Awareness, Risk, and Treatment: New Resources for Survival (PARTNERS) program, a study of 6979 patients in 350 primary care practices across the United States, ankle-brachial index (ABI) screening was performed in subjects older than age 70, or older than age 50 if they were smokers or had diabetes.[4] In this primary care population, 29% of those screened with an ABI met the criteria for PAD.

Despite the relative frequency of disease, diagnosis of PAD is not often considered because the majority of patients with PAD are asymptomatic. In the PARTNERS program, only 11% of PAD patients had classic symptoms.[5] Similar data have been reported in other large cross-sectional studies (see Chapter 16). Even in high-risk subgroups with a higher population frequency of PAD, the diagnosis may be missed because PAD is often asymptomatic. The decision to look for PAD in the outpatient should be predicated on the pretest probability of finding it. Application of the PARTNERS criteria, for example, demonstrated the importance of risk factors in enriching the population with PAD to make ABI screening worthwhile. Thus, the presence of risk factors for atherosclerosis should lower the threshold for routine screening.

Symptoms of Peripheral Artery Disease

The most commonly ascribed symptom that develops as a result of PAD is intermittent claudication. The word *claudication* derives from the Latin word *claudicatio*, which was used to describe the limp gait of a lame horse. As defined in the Rose questionnaire,[6] claudication is development of an ischemic muscular pain on exertion. The pain can be characterized as aching, burning, heaviness, feeling leaden, tightness, or cramping. Pain should originate in a muscular bed, such as the calf, thigh, hip, or buttock, and not localize to a joint. The area of the worst blood flow limitation usually subtends the site of muscular discomfort. For example, patients who develop hip or buttock discomfort with walking most likely have distal aorta or iliac artery occlusive disease, whereas patients with calf claudication likely have superficial femoral or popliteal arterial stenoses or occlusions. Reduction of muscular work on

activity cessation rebalances available blood supply with muscle demand and quickly resolves the pain.

Both time of activity to pain onset and time to pain resolution should be consistent and predictable. The distance walked to the onset of leg discomfort is called the *initial claudication distance*, and the maximal distance the patient can walk without stopping because of leg discomfort is called the *absolute claudication distance*. Several classification schemes are used to categorize the severity of claudication, including the Fontaine (Table 18-1) and Rutherford classifications (Table 18-2).[7] When the interview is complete, the physician should have insight into the nature of discomfort, how long it has been present, the typical duration of exercise required to cause the discomfort, and the amount of rest necessary to relieve the symptoms.

Classic symptoms of claudication do not occur in all patients with PAD, including those with functional limitations. The application of questionnaires for claudication, such as the World Health Organization (WHO)/Rose questionnaire or the Walking Impairment Questionnaire,[6,8] may underestimate PAD prevalence by 50%. Data from McDermott et al. indicate that complaints other than claudication are common.[9] They evaluated functional tolerance across a range of symptoms in cross-sectional analyses of patients with and without PAD.[5,10] Peripheral artery disease patients demonstrated several types of leg discomfort, including leg pain at rest and with walking, pain with walking alone requiring cessation of activity, and pain patients could "walk through." This variety of presentations would be missed with questioning only for classic symptoms. Moreover, the type of discomfort predicted function. Patients with pain at rest and with walking had worse functional capacity than those whose pain occurred with walking and stopped with walking cessation, and those who were able to "walk through" the pain. Quality of leg pain, whether it is atypical or classic, does not predict severity of reduction in limb perfusion pressure as measured by the ABI.[11]

Presence of intermittent claudication has important prognostic implications regarding functional capacity and mortality. Three quarters of patients with intermittent claudication will have stable symptoms over the next 10 years; approximately 25% will progress to more disabling claudication or critical limb ischemia requiring revascularization or culminating in amputation.[6] Moreover, they will suffer a mortality more than twice that of the general population, approximating 30% at 5 years.[12]

Differential Diagnosis of Claudication

Once exercise-related discomfort has been established, several alternate vascular and nonvascular diagnoses should be considered (Box 18-1). Vascular disorders include popliteal artery entrapment (see Chapter 62), compartment syndrome, fibromuscular dysplasia, venous insufficiency (see Chapter 55), and vasculitis (see Chapters 41 through 45). Popliteal artery entrapment typically occurs in very active persons or athletes. Because of an abnormal origin of the medial (or less commonly, lateral) head of the gastrocnemius muscle, the popliteal artery may be compressed with walking and yield symptoms of claudication. Endofibrosis of the external iliac artery (EIA), a relatively rare occurrence in highly trained cyclists and other endurance athletes, may cause claudication.

Fibromuscular dysplasia is a noninflammatory arterial occlusive disease that most commonly affects the renal and carotid arteries but may involve other arterial beds (see Chapter 63).[13] Any of the

CH
18

TABLE 18-1   Fontaine Classification

STAGE	DESCRIPTION
I	Asymptomatic, ABI < 0.9
II	Intermittent claudication
III	Daily rest pain
IV	Focal tissue necrosis

ABI, ankle-brachial index.

TABLE 18-2   Rutherford Classification

GRADE	CATEGORY	DESCRIPTION
0	0	Asymptomatic
I	1	Mild claudication
I	2	Moderate claudication
I	3	Severe claudication
II	4	Ischemic rest pain
III	5	Minor tissue loss
IV	6	Major tissue loss

Box 18-1   Nonatherosclerotic Causes of Exertional Leg Pain

Nonatherosclerotic arterial disease
Atheroembolism
Vasculitis
Extravascular compression
Popliteal artery entrapment
Adventitial cysts
Fibromuscular dysplasia
Endofibrosis of the internal iliac artery
Venous claudication
Compartment syndrome
Lumbar radiculopathy
Spinal stenosis
Hip/knee arthritis
Myositis

arteries in the lower extremities may be affected, but the iliac arteries are the most common. Fibroplasias may involve the intima, media, or adventitial layer of the artery. The most common variety is medial fibroplasia. It can be diagnosed from the "string of beads" appearance on angiography and by its predilection for the nonbranching points of vessels. The etiology of fibromuscular dysplasia remains unknown.

Increased calf muscle size with exercise may inhibit venous outflow, cause exertional compartment syndrome—in which tissue pressure is increased and microvascular flow is impeded—and bring about complaints of calf pain or tightness with exertion. Symptoms improve with leg elevation after exercise cessation. Venous claudication may occur as a result of iliofemoral thrombosis with poor collateral vein formation. When venous outflow is impaired, the increase in arterial inflow with exercise increases venous pressure markedly and causes a severe tightness or bursting sensation in the limb. Patients may report improvement in symptoms with leg elevation following exercise cessation. These patients frequently have leg edema. Vasculitides such as Takayasu's arteritis, giant-cell arteritis (GCA), and thromboangiitis obliterans (TAO) are infrequent causes of claudication.

Nonvascular causes of exertional leg pain include lumbar radiculopathy, hip and knee arthritis, and myositis. Perhaps the most common nonvascular diagnosis is lumbar radiculopathy

causing nerve-based pain. Patients may complain of leg pain or paresthesias as a result of compression of the lumbar nerve roots from disc herniation or degenerative osteophytes. The paresthesias or pain tend to affect the posterior aspect of the leg and occur with specific positions such as standing or develop at the beginning of ambulation. These symptoms may improve with continued walking or when leaning forward because pressure on the nerve roots is reduced.

Osteoarthritis of the hip or knee may cause pain associated with walking. The pain may be confused with intermittent claudication because it typically occurs with exercise. The discomfort, however, is usually referable to a joint such as the hip or knee. It can be distinguished from claudication in that the level of activity required to precipitate symptoms varies and does not resolve rapidly with activity cessation.

Critical Limb Ischemia

Critical limb ischemia (CLI) is the most debilitating manifestation of PAD (Fig. 18-1). The TransAtlantic Inter-Society Consensus (TASC) Working Group estimates that the incidence of CLI is between 300 and 1000 persons per million per year.[6] Across the globe, frequency of amputation varies from 28 per million people per year in Madrid to 439 amputations per million people per year among Navajo Americans.[14] Prevalence of CLI was 1.2% and affected more women than men in a population study of 8000 persons between 60 and 90 years of age.[15]

Diabetes and smoking increase the risk of developing CLI. Diabetes is the cause of most nontraumatic lower-extremity amputations in the United States.[16] Diabetes increases the risk of amputation nearly fourfold, even with similar levels of blood flow limitation as in nondiabetic patients.[17] Cigarette smoking also increases the risk that PAD will progress to CLI. In a study of 343 consecutive patients with intermittent claudication, 16% of those who continued to smoke developed CLI, compared to none in those who were able to stop smoking.[18] In 190 patients undergoing lower-extremity revascularization followed for 3 years, those who smoked more than 15 cigarettes a day had a 10-fold higher risk (21%) of amputation compared to those who smoked fewer than 15 cigarettes a day (2%).[19] Critical limb ischemia occurs as a consequence of tissue ischemia at rest, and it manifests as foot pain, nonhealing ulcers, or tissue gangrene. The pain is often severe and unremitting and localized to the acral portion of the foot or toes, notably at the site of ulceration or gangrene. Blood flow limitation is so severe that the gravitational effects of leg position may affect symptoms. Patients commonly report that leg elevation worsens pain. This is typically worse at night when the patient is in bed and the leg, now at heart level, no longer benefits from the dependent position. Placing the foot on the floor beside the bed is a common action used by patients to reduce pain. Inability to use the leg and chronically placing the leg in a dependent position may cause

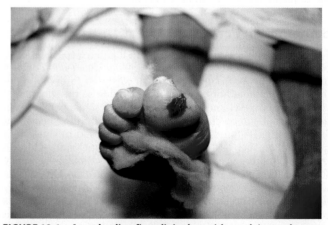

FIGURE 18-1   A nonhealing first-digit ulcer with overlying eschar.

peripheral edema, a finding occasionally mistaken for venous disease in these patients. With severe ischemia, any skin perturbation, including bedclothes or blankets, may cause pain; in ischemic neuropathy, this causes a lancinating pain in the foot. Other symptoms of CLI include hypesthesia, cold intolerance, muscular weakness, and joint stiffness of the affected limb. Severity of CLI is categorized in both the Fontaine and Rutherford classification schemes (see Tables 18-1 and 18-2).

Differential Diagnosis of Critical Limb Ischemia

Differential diagnosis of CLI includes vascular and nonvascular diseases (Box 18-2). Atheroembolism, or *blue toe syndrome*, occurs when components of large-vessel atherosclerotic plaque embolize to distal vessels (Fig. 18-2) (see Chapter 47). The embolized material is composed of fibroplatelet debris and cholesterol crystals. A common cause of atheroembolism is iatrogenic disturbance of the vessel, whether from catheterization or surgery. Several features may help in differentiating atheroembolism from traditional CLI. Patients typically have pulses palpable down into the feet, because the emboli require a patent pathway to distal portions of the extremities. Other clinical clues include new renal insufficiency and blood eosinophilia. On examination, the patient will have areas of cyanosis or violaceous discoloration of the toes or portions of the feet and areas of livedo reticularis.

Acute limb ischemia may occur from thrombosis *in situ* or from thromboemboli of large fibroplatelet accumulations that originate in the heart or large arteries and occlude conduit arteries (see Chapter 46). These patients have an accelerated course and may present with the "five Ps" of acute ischemia: pain, pallor, poikilothermia, paresthesia, and paralysis. Other causes of limb ischemia include vasospasm, TAO, other vasculitides, and connective tissue disorders (see Chapters 41, 44, and 48). Other causes of ulcers include neuropathy, venous disease, and trauma (see Chapter 61).

Nonvascular causes of foot pain include neuropathy, arthritides such as gout, fasciitis, and trauma (see Box 18-1).

Box 18-2 Differential Diagnosis of Critical Limb Ischemia

Ischemia
Atherosclerosis
Atheroemboli
Acute arterial occlusion:
  In situ thrombosis
  Emboli

Vasculitis
TAO
Scleroderma
SLE
MCTD
Cryoglobulinemia

Vasospasm
Raynaud phenomenon
Acrocyanosis

Ulcers
Neuropathy
Venous insufficiency
Trauma

Pain
Neuropathy

Arthritis
Gout
Rheumatoid arthritis
Fasciitis
Trauma

MCTD, mixed connective tissue disease; SLE, systemic lupus erythematosus; TAO, thromboangiitis obliterans.

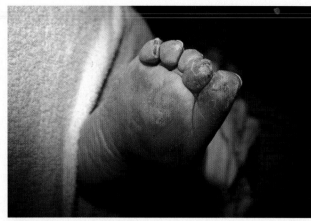

FIGURE 18-2 Atheroembolism after catheterization. Note areas of cyanosis and surrounding livedo reticularis. This patient had a palpable dorsalis pedis pulse.

Physical Examination

A comprehensive physical examination that includes general appearance of the patient, integument, heart, lungs, abdomen, and limbs should be performed during the initial patient encounter to elucidate evidence of systemic disease and provide insight into cause and manifestation of the patient's vascular disease. The entire vascular system should be examined. Blood pressure is measured in each arm. A blood pressure difference of 10 mmHg or more may be indicative of innominate, subclavian, axillary, or brachial artery stenosis. The carotid, brachial, radial, ulnar, femoral, popliteal, dorsalis pedis, and posterior tibial pulses should be palpated in every patient (Fig. 18-3). Several pulse-descriptive schemes have been promulgated. One is to grade the pulses as 0 (absent), 1 (diminished), and 2 (normal). A very prominent or forceful pulse may occur in patients with aortic regurgitation or high cardiac output states. Absence of any pulse in the lower extremity, except in the dorsalis pedis, increases the likelihood of PAD.[20] The dorsalis pedis pulse is not palpable in approximately 8% of healthy patients.[20] Absence of a peripheral pulse may indicate a significant stenosis between the present and absent pulse. Occasionally, pulses may be palpable below the level of a significant stenosis. This most commonly occurs in the setting of iliac artery disease when there may be sufficient collateral vessels to maintain perfusion to distal arteries.

The abdominal aorta should also be palpitated if permitted by body habitus to elicit evidence of aortic aneurysm. A widened pulse in the abdomen or over a peripheral artery (e.g., the popliteal artery) may be indicative of an aneurysm. Once palpated, the abdomen and several peripheral vessels also should be auscultated. Palpation of an expansile or pulsatile periumbilical mass is indicative of an abdominal aortic aneurysm. Proper auscultation of normal vessels with a stethoscope should reveal no sound. Bruits should be sought over the carotid and subclavian arteries, in the abdomen, in the lower back, and over the femoral arteries. Presence of a bruit, indicative of turbulent blood flow, typically occurs as a result of arterial stenosis, but may indicate extrinsic compression or arteriovenous malformation. Vessels with no flow, resulting from complete occlusion, do not convey bruits.

A skin examination should be performed, looking for alterations in temperature, edema, signs of active or healed lesions, or signs of chronic ischemia—including thin shiny skin, thickened yellow nails, and loss of hair. Foot or toe cyanosis or pallor may be a forerunner of ulceration. Inspection of the skin may reveal trophic signs of chronic ischemia, including sympathetic denervation (impaired hair growth or impaired sweating) and sensorimotor neuropathy (lack of vibratory sense). Critical limb ischemia may cause muscle and subcutaneous tissue atrophy,

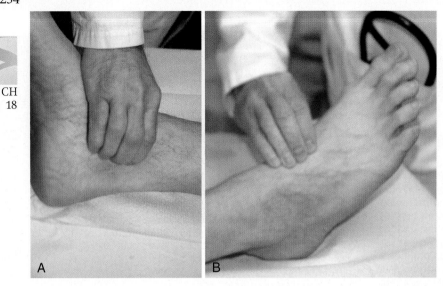

FIGURE 18-3 Palpation of pedal pulses. A, Palpation of posterior tibial (PT) pulse. Examiner should place his/her fingers in the curve below the malleolus with light pressure and reposition as needed. Application of passive foot dorsiflexion occasionally makes PT palpation easier. **B,** Dorsalis pedis pulse is typically appreciated within 1 cm of the dorsum, most prominent near navicular bone.

hair loss, petechiae, and thin or encrusted skin. In CLI, the toes and foot are cool and pallor may be present when the foot is in the neutral (or horizontal) position.

Changes in skin appearance with elevation and dependency may provide a gauge for PAD severity. The leg should be elevated to 45 to 60 degrees for 1 minute. If pallor develops quickly (within 10-15 seconds), severe PAD is likely. After 1 minute, the patient sits up and the leg is placed in a dependent position. The time to pedal vein refill should be recorded. Ischemic-induced arteriolar and venular dilation may lead to development of a violaceous appearance of the foot with dependency, called *dependent rubor* (Fig. 18-4). Normal refill occurs rapidly, typically within 10 to 15 seconds. Prolongation of venous filling or the development of numbness beyond 1 minute suggests severe PAD.

Arterial fissures most commonly develop in the heel, toes, in the web space between the toes, or in segments subjected to pressure (the ball of the foot). Arterial ulcers are circumscribed, tender, and prone to infection. The base of the ulcer is usually pale. The ulcers, in contrast to venous ulcers, are dry; however, the devitalized tissue is prone to infection, which may generate a purulent exudate. The ulcer may be covered by an eschar. In CLI, gangrene most commonly occurs in the digits but may occur on the ball of the foot or heel. In the absence of infection, gangrene tends to be dry, and the skin is mummified.

Two classification schemes are used to categorize the clinical assessment of patients with PAD: the Fontaine Stage Classification of PAD and the Rutherford Categorical Classification of PAD. In the system described by Fontaine, the severity of PAD is classified into 1 of 4 stages ranging from asymptomatic in stage 1, intermittent claudication in stage 2, daily rest pain in stage 3, and focal tissue necrosis in stage 4 (see Table 18-1). The Rutherford system employs seven categories, dividing severity of claudication into three categories (mild, moderate, and severe) and CLI into three categories (rest pain, minor tissue loss, and major tissue loss) (see Table 18-2).

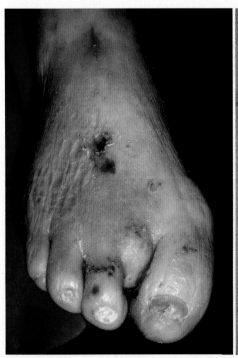
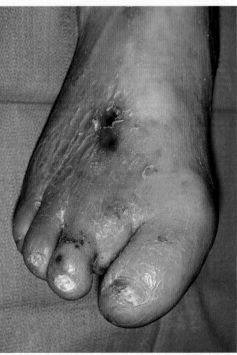

FIGURE 18-4 Dependent rubor. This patient with severe peripheral artery disease (PAD) (note previously amputated second digit) develops a ruborous appearance of the forefoot with dependent positioning as a result of arteriolar and venular dilation.

Diagnostic Testing

Office-Based Ankle-Brachial Index

Measurement of the ABI is a simple method employed to corroborate the historical and physical findings of PAD. The ABI is the ratio of the systolic blood pressure at the ankle and brachial artery. The latter is an estimate of central aortic pressure. Brachial artery systolic blood pressure is measured in both arms and ankles using a handheld 5- or 10-MHz Doppler ultrasound device and sphygmomanometric cuff. The cuffs are placed on each arm above the antecubital fossa and above each ankle. The cuffs are sequentially inflated above systolic pressure and then are slowly depressurized. The Doppler probe, placed over the brachial artery and the dorsalis pedis and posterior tibial arteries, monitors the pressure (Fig. 18-5). As the cuff is slowly deflated, reappearance of a Doppler signal indicates the systolic pressure at the level of the cuff.

Brachial artery pressures must be measured in both arms because atherosclerosis may occur in subclavian and axillary arteries. The higher of the two brachial systolic blood pressures is used for reference in the ABI calculation. Hence, the ABI is the

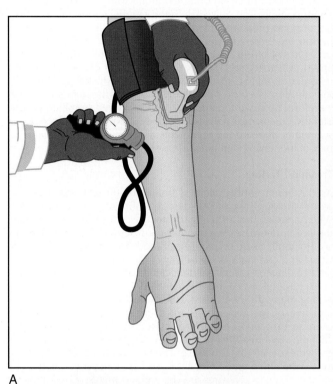

A

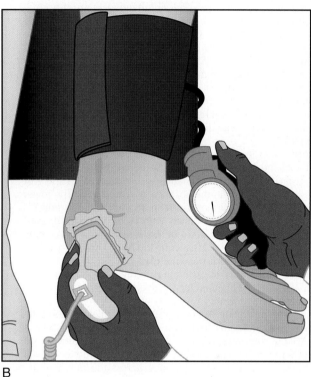

B

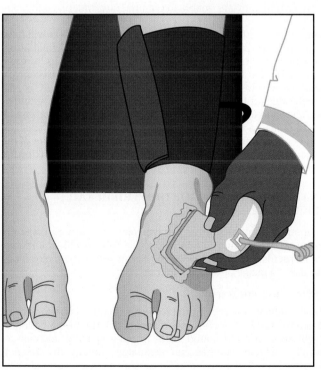

C

FIGURE 18-5 Measurement of the ankle-brachial index (ABI). Brachial artery systolic blood pressure is determined in both arms and both ankles using a handheld 5- or 10-MHz Doppler ultrasound and sphygmomanometric cuff. Because atherosclerosis may occur in subclavian and axillary arteries, brachial artery pressures must be measured in both arms **(A)**. The higher of the two brachial systolic blood pressures is used as the reference pressure in ABI calculation. In each ankle, pressure should be measured at dorsalis pedis **(B)** and posterior tibial pulse **(C)**. ABI is the quotient of the highest systolic pressure at each ankle divided by the highest pressure of the two brachial artery pressures.

systolic pressure at each ankle divided by the higher pressure of the two brachial artery pressures; an ABI may be generated for each leg. When assessing foot perfusion, the ABI uses the highest of the pedal pressures in each leg.[21] Both pedal pressures (dorsalis pedis and posterior tibial artery) are considered when seeking evidence of atherosclerosis. Some have suggested that ankle pressure used to calculate ABI should be an average of the two pedal pressures.[22]

Normal systolic pressure at the ankle should be at least the same as in the arm, yielding an ABI of 1.0 or greater. As a result of reflected arterial pressure waves, healthy persons tend to have an ABI ranging from 1.0 to 1.43. Recognizing an intrinsic (up to 10%) variability of blood pressure when measured sequentially, since ankle pressures are not measured simultaneously, an abnormal ABI consistent with the diagnosis of PAD is categorized as 0.9 or less, whereas an ABI above 0.9 to 1.0 is borderline abnormal.[23] The ABI is a reliable determinant of PAD, with a sensitivity for ABI 0.9 or less ranging from 79% to 95% and specificity of 96% to 100%.[21,24] An ABI of 0.4 or less is extremely abnormal and typically present in patients with CLI. Arterial calcification may introduce a false elevation in ABI, typically greater than 1.4, as a result of noncompressible vessels at the ankle. Arterial calcification occurs more commonly in patients with diabetes or end-stage renal disease and in the elderly.[25,26]

The ABI provides prognostic information because it is a barometer of the burden of systemic atherosclerosis. In the ABI Collaboration, the incidence of adverse events rose as the ABI dropped below 1.0, even in the absence of symptoms.[27] The lower the ABI, the greater the cardiovascular morbidity and mortality.[28,29] An ABI of 0.8 or less is associated with twice the age-adjusted 10-year mortality, and an ABI of 0.4 or less, is associated with a fourfold increase in mortality.[21,27] Measuring the ABI provides an assessment of both PAD and cardiovascular risk.

There are limitations to ABI measurement. The correlation between ABI, functional capacity, and symptoms is weak. Resting ABI is occasionally normal in patients with PAD; this may occur in patients with aortoiliac stenoses and a well-collateralized arterial system that maintains perfusion pressure. In patients with a normal ABI but a strong suspicion of significant PAD, office-based exercise testing may be performed. Exercise accentuates arterial gradients by increasing the turbulence across the flow-limiting lesion and decreasing muscular arteriolar resistance to significantly attenuate lower-extremity perfusion pressure. In fact, arterial pressure at the ankle may reach zero in patients who develop claudication and recover more than 10 minutes after exercise cessation. In the office, stair climbing or active pedal plantar flexion[30] may be used to elicit symptoms and document a decrease in ankle pressure (and ABI) to confirm the diagnosis of intermittent claudication.

Noninvasive Laboratory Testing for Peripheral Artery Disease

For patients in whom revascularization is considered, such as those with CLI or disabling claudication, location and severity of disease should be evaluated by additional noninvasive testing. There are two general formats of noninvasive testing to discern location and severity of PAD: physiological testing and anatomical imaging.

PHYSIOLOGICAL TESTING

Physiological or functional testing most commonly occurs in a noninvasive vascular laboratory (see Chapter 12). Measurement of limb segmental systolic pressures employs methods similar to ABI measurement (Fig. 18-6). Sphygmomanometric cuffs are placed on the proximal thigh, distal thigh, calf, and ankle. The cuffs are inflated sequentially to suprasystolic pressure and then deflated to determine systolic pressure at each site. A Doppler probe is placed on the posterior tibial or dorsalis pedis artery.

Arterial stenosis or occlusion will decrease the perfusion pressure. Arterial pressure gradients of more than 20 mmHg between thigh cuffs and 10 mmHg between cuffs below the knee indicate presence of a stenosis. As with the ABI, the most common source of error for the test is vascular calcification. In the setting of vascular calcification, a toe brachial index may be obtained. Pressures in the toe may be measured with strain gauge photoplethysmography. Pressure is measured in the toes and a ratio of toe pressure to brachial artery pressure is generated; a value of 0.7 or less is consistent with PAD.

Pulse volume recordings (PVRs) or segmental pneumatic plethysmography determines the relative change in limb volume with each pulse and can be obtained along with segmental pressure measurements. The pulse-volume waveform represents the product of pulse pressure and vascular wall compliance. In a healthy person, the pulse-volume waveform is similar to a normal arterial pressure waveform and includes rapid upstroke, dicrotic notch, and downstroke (see Fig. 18-6). The waveform changes when it is recorded distal to a significant stenosis as perfusion pressure falls. Initially, there is a loss of the dicrotic notch. As the stenosis worsens, waveform upstroke (anacrotic slope) is delayed, amplitude is less, and the downstroke (catacrotic slope) is slower. Combined use of segmental pressure measurements and PVRs improves the accuracy of identifying significant stenosis.

Treadmill Testing

As described earlier, eliciting symptoms through exercise may permit the diagnosis of PAD, despite a normal or near-normal ABI. When a vessel has a significant stenosis, increasing flow through the lesion decreases energy delivered beyond the area of stenosis. Treadmill exercise increases blood flow through a stenosed vessel and can increase sensitivity of the ABI. In the vascular laboratory, a diagnosis of intermittent claudication and a quantification of exercise tolerance may be obtained through treadmill exercise testing. Many protocols exist to test walking ability, but each falls into one of two types: constant or graded exercise. In constant exercise protocols (e.g., Carter protocol), a specific speed (1.5-2.0 mph) and treadmill grade (0%-12%) is chosen, whereas in the graded exercise protocols (e.g., Hiatt or Gardner protocol), speed and/or treadmill grade may increase.[31] In both protocols, the brachial and ankle pressures are determined pretest at rest, patients exercise until they are unable to continue, and brachial and ankle pressures are redetermined within 1 minute of exercise cessation. Patients with PAD as a cause of exercise limitation will have an attenuated rise in ankle pressure compared to brachial artery pressure or, more commonly, a fall in ankle pressure, thus lowering the ABI. The fall in ankle pressure is directly related to severity of arterial occlusive disease. Analogously, length of recovery is also directly related to disease severity. Two parameters are recorded in addition to the ABI: the time claudication begins (initial claudication time), and the time until exhaustion or cessation (absolute claudication time). Variability of walking distance is greater in the constant exercise protocols than the graded protocols, making the latter more commonly used.

ANATOMICAL IMAGING OF THE PERIPHERAL CIRCULATION

Defining arterial anatomy is not typically necessary to make the diagnosis of PAD but is required for patients who will be undergoing revascularization. Following is a discussion of the major methods used to image peripheral arteries.

Duplex Ultrasonography

Duplex ultrasonography of the lower extremities is performed in most vascular laboratories (see Chapter 12). The combination of bright (B)-mode ultrasound, color Doppler imaging, and pulsed-Doppler velocity analysis can accurately identify the location and severity of atherosclerotic lesions in the legs. Normally, flow through each arterial segment should be laminar, with a uniform

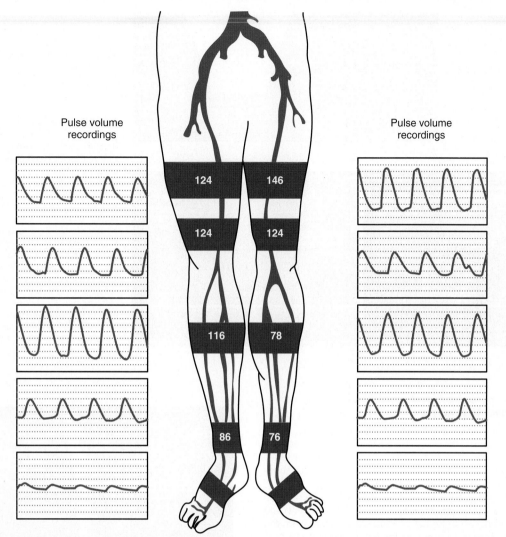

Pulse volume recordings

Pulse volume recordings

FIGURE 18-6   Segmental pressure measurements. Sequential Doppler pressures are measured by placing sphygmomanometric cuffs on the proximal thigh, distal thigh, calf, and ankle. Cuffs are inflated above systolic pressure and then slowly depressurized. Simultaneously, a Doppler probe placed over the dorsalis pedis or posterior tibial artery monitors pressure. As the cuff is slowly deflated, reappearance of Doppler signal indicates systolic pressure at the level of the cuff which permits blood flow. Arterial stenosis or occlusion will decrease perfusion pressure. Arterial pressure gradients between cuffs indicate presence of a stenosis. In this example, arterial pressures (mmHg) are noted in the location of each sphygmomanometric cuff. Patient has evidence of a systolic gradient between both upper thigh cuffs, suggestive of right iliac and/or common femoral arterial occlusive disease, and a gradient between right calf and ankle suggestive of arterial occlusive disease in the infrapopliteal arteries. A significant gradient between the left lower thigh cuff and calf cuff is indicative of distal superficial femoral artery and/or popliteal artery occlusive disease.

homogeneous color appearance. Blood flow becomes turbulent and velocity increases at sites of sclerosis, creating areas of color discordance. Pulsed Doppler measurements in the area of stenosis demonstrate increased flow velocity and spectral broadening.

Applying the concepts of the Poiseuille law regarding movement of incompressible viscous fluids through a tube, the ratio of peak systolic velocity in the area of a stenosis is compared with the normal area of artery proximal to the stenosis. A ratio of 2 or greater is consistent with stenosis of 50% or more (Fig. 18-7). In one meta-analysis of seven studies, the sensitivity and specificity of duplex ultrasound to detect 50% or greater stenosis or occlusion were 88% and 96%, respectively, and to detect complete occlusion were 90% and 99%, respectively.[32] In another meta-analysis of 14 studies, the sensitivity and specificity of duplex ultrasound with and without color-guided Doppler analysis to detect 50% or greater stenosis or occlusion was 93% and 95%, respectively.[33] Duplex ultrasonography is less accurate at the site of calcified plaque because of the acoustic shadowing caused by the dense calcium. Serial stenoses are more difficult to diagnose because ultrasound diagnosis relies on comparing peak arterial velocities between adjacent segments, and there are altered hemodynamics between sequential stenoses. Single-center studies have found that ultrasound may be used alone in planning both percutaneous and surgical peripheral revascularization.[34–37]

Duplex ultrasonography is also used in the postoperative surveillance of arterial bypass grafts. A program of routine ultrasound surveillance is more likely to diagnose significant bypass graft stenoses than history, physical examination, or ABI. Clinical trials have evaluated the efficacy of ultrasound surveillance as a strategy to identify graft stenosis and prompt repair before graft occlusion occurs.[38] One study randomized 156 patients to serial ultrasonography or ABI. Patients were referred for angiography and then corrective revascularization if 50% or greater stenosis was identified by ultrasound, or if the ABI decreased by 0.15 compared with the postoperative baseline.[39] Assisted primary cumulative vein graft patency in the ultrasound group was 78% compared with 53% in the ABI group after 3 years. In other randomized studies, however, no benefit was found for ultrasound compared with ABI 1 year after surgery.[40,41] The data for surveillance for synthetic bypass grafts[39,42,43] and after angioplasty[44] are less robust than for vein grafts.

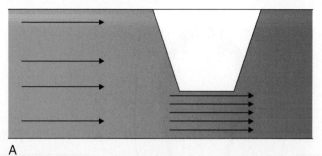

A

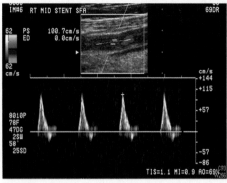

B

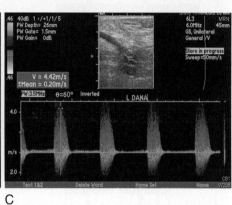

C

FIGURE 18-7 A, Poiseuille law defines movement of an incompressible viscous fluid through a tube. Fluid entry into tube must equal its exit; thus, the ratio of peak-systolic velocity in the area of stenosis is proportional to the segment of normal vessel proximal to stenosis. When the ratio is greater than 2, stenosis of more than 50% is diagnosed. Sensitivity and specificity of duplex ultrasound evaluation in determination of stenoses of 50% or greater range from 90% to 95%. Normal arterial flow velocity is approximately 100 cm/s. **B,** Doppler ultrasound is passed through a recently placed superficial femoral artery (SFA) stent, demonstrating normal flow velocity. This is indicative of a patent stent without evidence of restenosis. **C,** Doppler ultrasound is passed through distal anastomosis of a femoral-popliteal bypass graft, demonstrating a flow velocity of 4.4 m/s. This is consistent with greater than 75% stenosis. Velocity in proximal normal segment is 1.3 m/s (not shown).

Magnetic Resonance Angiography

Magnetic resonance angiography (MRA) is an accurate imaging modality to diagnose PAD, visualize peripheral arteries, and determine the location of stenoses (see Chapter 13). Techniques used to image the arterial tree include black blood, phase contrast, time of flight (TOF), and contrast-enhanced MRA.[45] The application of two magnetic pulses to suppress signal in the vessel lumen yields a dark appearance of flowing blood, with the vessel wall remaining white. Selective removal of blood from the image causes the lumen to appear black, and the technique is therefore called *black blood*. When the phase shift of moving electron spins in flowing blood is compared with surrounding stable tissue, blood volume and velocity can be measured to permit assessment of blood flow. Application of electrocardiographic gating while interrogating the flow-related enhancement of spins into a partially saturated area provides a time of flight angiogram.[46,47] Limitations of a flow-based TOF MRA include lengthy acquisition types, turbulence, nonlinear vascular structures, and retrograde flow.[48]

Most MRAs are performed using contrast, most commonly gadolinium. Contrast-enhanced MRA provides a high-resolution angiogram. Contrast-enhanced TOF MRA is useful as a noninvasive imaging test to define lower-extremity vascular anatomy. In a meta-analysis comparing contrast-enhanced MRA with TOF MRA, the contrast-enhanced study had a much greater diagnostic accuracy.[48] Use of contrast has improved scan quality and efficiency and enhanced vessel visualization and identification, especially in distal vessels[49] (Fig. 18-8). Magnetic resonance angiography can identify the presence of stenoses and reveal distal vessels suitable for bypass not demonstrated by contrast angiography.[50,51] In a meta-analysis of 32 studies of contrast-enhanced MRA and intraarterial digital subtraction angiography (DSA), the pooled sensitivity of MRA was 95%, and specificity was 96%.[52]

One potential limitation is a tendency for MRA to overestimate lesion severity.[53] Similar benefits and limitations exist in the imaging of bypass grafts. Magnetic resonance angiography has a sensitivity as high as 91% for identification of arterial bypass graft stenoses[54] but overestimates lesion severity in up to 30% of stenoses.[55,56] A sound strategy may involve use of MRA initially because

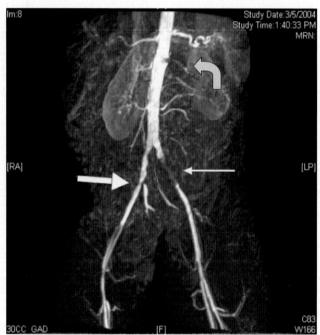

FIGURE 18-8 Gadolinium-enhanced magnetic resonance angiogram (MRA). This MRA was performed in a patient with Takayasu's arteritis. Several findings are notable. Patient has an occluded left renal artery, and right internal iliac artery has severe stenosis *(thick arrow).* At the thin arrow is an area of dropout due to image interference by a previously placed stent. Curved arrow indicates occluded left upper renal artery.

of the noninvasive nature of the test and its superior identification of bypass vessels, reserving DSA for cases requiring greater definition.[57] Technological advancement is rapid in MRA, improving detection and identification of arterial occlusive disease. As imaging protocols and techniques, such as three-dimensional (3D) MRA imaging, gain acceptance and are made commonly available, MRA may ultimately be used as a stand-alone evaluation prior to revascularization.[58–60]

Computed Tomographic Angiography

Computed tomographic angiography (CTA) has recently undergone rapid improvements in technology and imaging, allowing its entry into peripheral vascular imaging (see Chapter 14). Much of this advance results from development of multidetector-row CT scanners and improved resolution of arteries. Availability of higher resolution to scanners is particularly relevant for smaller and more distal arteries.

In meta-analyses of studies mostly using multidetector CT scanners, pooled sensitivity and specificity for detecting stenoses of 50% or greater in leg arteries were 91% to 92% and 91% to 93%, respectively.[32,61] As scanner number increases, newer CT scanners should have even greater accuracy.

Computed tomography angiography is commonly presented using a maximal intensity projection (MIP) or with a volume rendering technique (Fig. 18-9). The MIP algorithm displays only the pixel with the highest intensity along a ray perpendicular to the plane of projection. This algorithm creates a two-dimensional (2D) projectional image similar in appearance to MRA or contrast angiography. Volume rendering applies shades of gray to pixels of varying density.[62] Fourier transfer functions allow modification of the relative contribution of various pixel values. Volume rendering considers pixels that are only partially filled with contrast material. Arterial calcification limits imaging with both CT techniques. Optimal techniques used for postprocessing are being developed.[63] As resolution improves,

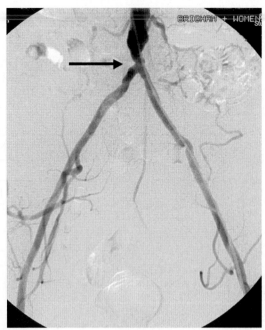

FIGURE 18-10 Contrast abdominal angiogram demonstrating significant aortic stenosis just proximal to bifurcation into iliac arteries (arrow).

CTA may become a regular instrument in the diagnostic armamentarium because of its rapid study time (typically <1 minute) or because of the 75% reduction in ionizing radiation compared with angiography.

Contrast Angiography

Contrast angiography is the most venerable and widely available method for imaging arterial anatomy (see Chapter 15). Angiography commonly serves as the standard for determining the sensitivity and specificity of newer techniques and is an excellent method to clarify arterial anatomical queries (Fig. 18-10). Technical improvements in equipment, including smaller catheters, image resolution, and digital subtraction, have enhanced the capability of angiography. Digital subtraction eliminates bony and soft-tissue shadows from the angiographic image, enhancing angiographic detail. Despite wide acceptance of angiography as a reliable method for defining arterial anatomy, its invasive nature, requirement for contrast, nephrotoxicity, risk of atheroembolism, and risk of pseudoaneurysms or arteriovenous fistula (AVF) continue to foster development of alternative angiographic methods.

Summary

An algorithm for evaluating the patient with PAD is depicted in Figure 18-11. Diagnosis and evaluation of PAD is required in patients predisposed to develop PAD because of age or the presence of atherosclerotic risk factors and in patients whose history or examination are suggestive of PAD. An office evaluation should include measurement of ABI. An exercise test with measurement of the ABI after exercise is appropriate if resting ABI is normal, yet clinical suspicion remains high. Patients with noncompressible ankle vessels should be referred to a vascular laboratory for additional testing, including segmental pressure measurements, pulse-volume recordings, and/or duplex ultrasonography. Symptomatic patients, particularly those with CLI who are being treated for revascularization, should undergo anatomical imaging with CT, MRA, or conventional carotid angiography.

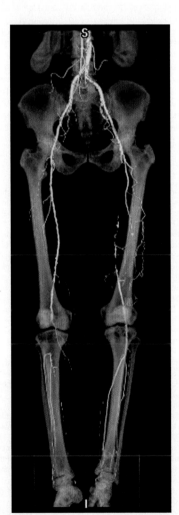

FIGURE 18-9 Volume-rendered computed tomographic (CT) angiogram of the lower extremities. Note superficial femoral artery (SFA) occlusion and collateral formation depicted by this study. *(Image courtesy Dr. Joseph Schoepf.)*

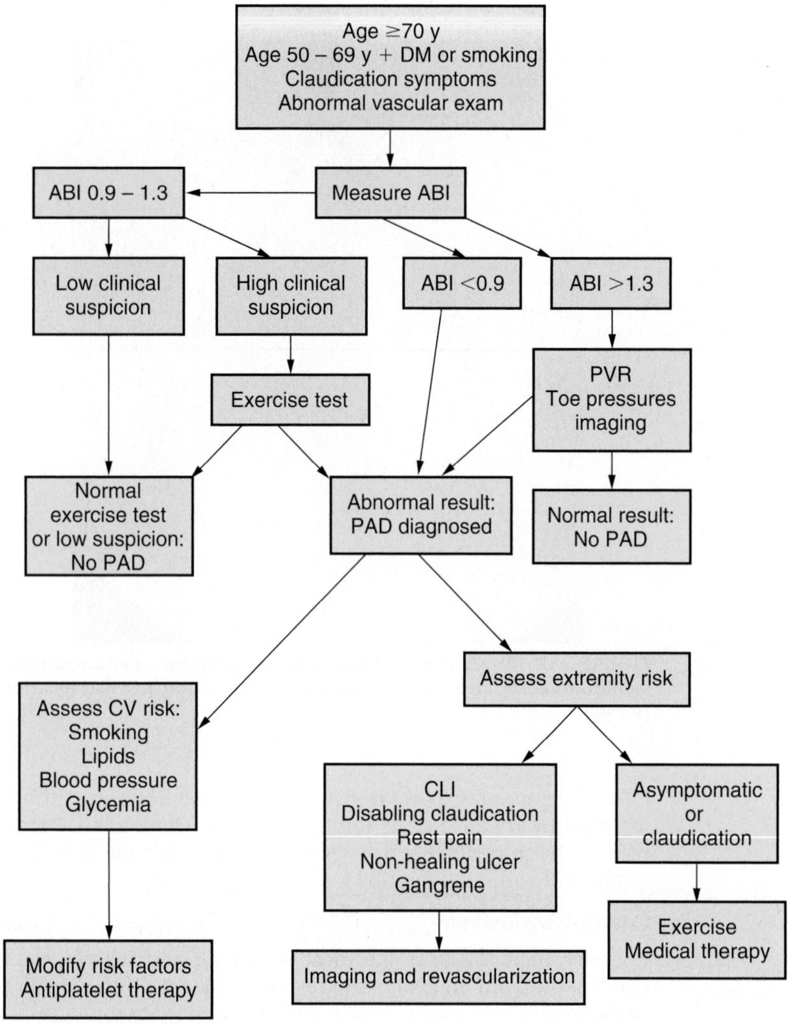

FIGURE 18-11 **Algorithm for peripheral artery disease (PAD) evaluation.** History, physical examination, and ankle-brachial index (ABI) make the diagnosis of PAD in majority of cases. Treadmill exercise testing is performed in conjunction with measurement of ABI performed prior to and immediately following exercise. Segmental pressure measurements, pulse volume recordings (PVR), toe pressures, and arterial duplex ultrasound imaging are noninvasive vascular tests used to consider and assess severity of PAD. Anatomical imaging by duplex ultrasonography, computed tomography angiography (CTA), magnetic resonance angiography (MRA), or conventional contrast angiography is used to assess symptomatic patients who require revascularization. Patients with PAD require risk factor assessment and treatment. The physician should more aggressively inquire about leg symptoms and inspect feet for evidence of critical limb ischemia (CLI). CV, cardiovascular; DM, diabetes mellitus.

REFERENCES

1. Pande RL, Perlstein TS, Beckman JA, et al: Secondary prevention and mortality in peripheral artery disease: National Health and Nutrition Examination Study, 1999 to 2004, *Circulation* 124:17–23, 2011.
2. Selvin E, Erlinger TP: Prevalence of and risk factors for peripheral arterial disease in the United States: Results from the National Health and Nutrition Examination Survey, 1999-2000, *Circulation* 110:738–743, 2004.
3. Diehm C, Schuster A, Allenberg JR, et al: High prevalence of peripheral arterial disease and co-morbidity in 6880 primary care patients: cross-sectional study, *Atherosclerosis* 172:95–105, 2004.
4. Hirsch AT, Criqui MH, Treat-Jacobson D, et al: Peripheral arterial disease detection, awareness, and treatment in primary care, *JAMA* 286:1317–1324, 2001.
5. McDermott MM, Greenland P, Liu K, et al: Leg symptoms in peripheral arterial disease: associated clinical characteristics and functional impairment, *JAMA* 286:1599–1606, 2001.
6. Rose GA: The diagnosis of ischaemic heart pain and intermittent claudication in field surveys, *Bull World Health Organ* 27:645–658, 1962.
7. Norgren L, Hiatt WR, Dormandy JA, et al: Inter-Society Consensus for the Management of Peripheral Arterial Disease (TASC II), *J Vasc Surg* 45(Suppl S):S5–S67, 2007.
8. Regensteiner JG, Steiner JF, Panzer RJ, et al: Evaluation of walking impairment by questionnaire in patients with peripheral arterial disease, *J Vasc Med Biol* 2:142, 1990.
9. McDermott MM, Mehta S, Greenland P: Exertional leg symptoms other than intermittent claudication are common in peripheral arterial disease, *Arch Intern Med* 159:387–392, 1999.
10. McDermott MM, Ferrucci L, et al: The ankle-brachial index is associated with the magnitude of impaired walking endurance among men and women with peripheral arterial disease, *Vasc Med* 15:251–257, 2010.
11. McDermott MM, Mehta S, Liu K, et al: Leg symptoms, the ankle-brachial index, and walking ability in patients with peripheral arterial disease, *J Gen Intern Med* 14:173–181, 1999.
12. Hirsch AT, Haskal ZJ, Hertzer NR, et al: ACC/AHA 2005 practice guidelines for the management of patients with peripheral arterial disease (lower extremity, renal, mesenteric, and abdominal aortic): a collaborative report from the American Association for Vascular Surgery/Society for Vascular Surgery, Society for Cardiovascular Angiography and Interventions, Society for Vascular Medicine and Biology, Society of Interventional Radiology, and the ACC/AHA Task Force on Practice Guidelines (Writing Committee to Develop Guidelines for the Management of Patients with Peripheral Arterial Disease): endorsed by the American Association of Cardiovascular and Pulmonary Rehabilitation; National Heart, Lung, and Blood Institute; Society for Vascular Nursing; Transatlantic Inter-Society Consensus; and Vascular Disease Foundation, *Circulation* 113:e463–e654, 2006.
13. Slovut DP, Olin JW: Fibromuscular dysplasia, *N Engl J Med* 350:1862–1871, 2004.
14. Epidemiology of lower extremity amputation in centres in Europe, North America and East Asia. The Global Lower Extremity Amputation Study Group, *Br J Surg* 87:328–337, 2000.
15. Sigvant B, Wiberg-Hedman K, Bergqvist D, et al: A population-based study of peripheral arterial disease prevalence with special focus on critical limb ischemia and sex differences, *J Vasc Surg* 45:1185–1191, 2007.
16. Diabetes-related amputations of lower extremities in the Medicare population--Minnesota, 1993-1995, *MMWR Morb Mortal Wkly Rep* 47:649–652, 1998.
17. Jude EB, Oyibo SO, Chalmers N, et al: Peripheral arterial disease in diabetic and nondiabetic patients: a comparison of severity and outcome, *Diabetes Care* 24:1433–1437, 2001.
18. Jonason T, Bergstrom R: Cessation of smoking in patients with intermittent claudication. Effects on the risk of peripheral vascular complications, myocardial infarction and mortality, *Acta Med Scand* 221:253–260, 1987.
19. Lassila R, Lepantalo M: Cigarette smoking and the outcome after lower limb arterial surgery, *Acta Chir Scand* 154:635–640, 1988.
20. Khan NA, Rahim SA, Anand SS, et al: Does the clinical examination predict lower extremity peripheral arterial disease? *JAMA* 295:536–546, 2006.
21. Aboyans V: ABI scientific statement, *Circulation* In press.
22. McDermott MM, Criqui MH, Liu K, et al: Lower ankle/brachial index, as calculated by averaging the dorsalis pedis and posterior tibial arterial pressures, and association with leg functioning in peripheral arterial disease, *J Vasc Surg* 32:1164–1171, 2000.
23. ACCF/AHA Focused Update of the Guideline for the Management of patients with peripheral artery disease (Updating the 2005 Guideline): a report of the American College of Cardiology Foundation/American Heart Association Task Force on practice guidelines. Circulation;124:2020–2045, 2011.
24. Lijmer JG, Hunink MG, van den Dungen JJ, et al: Roc analysis of noninvasive tests for peripheral arterial disease, *Ultrasound Med Biol* 22:391–398, 1996.
25. Leskinen Y, Salenius JP, Lehtimaki T, et al: The prevalence of peripheral arterial disease and medial arterial calcification in patients with chronic renal failure: requirements for diagnostics, *Am J Kidney Dis* 40:472–479, 2002.
26. Ishimura E, Okuno S, Kitatani K, et al: Different risk factors for peripheral vascular calcification between diabetic and non-diabetic haemodialysis patients–importance of glycaemic control, *Diabetologia* 45:1446–1448, 2002.

27. Fowkes FG, Murray GD, Butcher I, et al: Ankle brachial index combined with Framingham risk score to predict cardiovascular events and mortality: a meta-analysis, *JAMA* 300:197–208, 2008.

28. Vogt MT, McKenna M, Anderson SJ, et al: The relationship between ankle-arm index and mortality in older men and women, *J Am Geriatr Soc* 41:523–530, 1993.

29. Sikkink CJ, van Asten WN, van't Hof MA, et al: Decreased ankle/brachial indices in relation to morbidity and mortality in patients with peripheral arterial disease, *Vasc Med* 2:169–173, 1997.

30. McPhail IR, Spittell PC, Weston SA, et al: Intermittent claudication: an objective office-based assessment, *J Am Coll Cardiol* 37:1381–1385, 2001.

31. Hiatt WR, Hirsch AT, Regensteiner JG, et al: Clinical trials for claudication. Assessment of exercise performance, functional status, and clinical end points. Vascular Clinical Trialists, *Circulation* 92:614–621, 1995.

32. Collins R, Burch J, Cranny G, et al: Duplex ultrasonography, magnetic resonance angiography, and computed tomography angiography for diagnosis and assessment of symptomatic, lower limb peripheral arterial disease: systematic review, *BMJ* 334:1257, 2007.

33. de Vries SO, Hunink MG, Polak JF: Summary receiver operating characteristic curves as a technique for meta-analysis of the diagnostic performance of duplex ultrasonography in peripheral arterial disease, *Acad Radiol* 3:361–369, 1996.

34. Proia RR, Walsh DB, Nelson PR, et al: Early results of infragenicular revascularization based solely on duplex arteriography, *J Vasc Surg* 33:1165–1170, 2001.

35. Ascher E, Mazzariol F, Hingorani A, et al: The use of duplex ultrasound arterial mapping as an alternative to conventional arteriography for primary and secondary infrapopliteal bypasses, *Am J Surg* 178:162–165, 1999.

36. Lofberg AM, Karacagil S, Hellberg A, et al: The role of duplex scanning in the selection of patients with critical lower-limb ischemia for infrainguinal percutaneous transluminal angioplasty, *Cardiovasc Intervent Radiol* 24:229–232, 2001.

37. Mandolfino T, Canciglia A, D'Alfonso M, et al: Infrainguinal revascularization based on duplex ultrasound arterial mapping, *Int Angiol* 25:256–260, 2006.

38. Westerband A, Mills JL, Kistler S, et al: Prospective validation of threshold criteria for intervention in infrainguinal vein grafts undergoing duplex surveillance, *Ann Vasc Surg* 11:44–48, 1997.

39. Lundell A, Lindblad B, Bergqvist D, et al: Femoropopliteal-crural graft patency is improved by an intensive surveillance program: A prospective randomized study, *J Vasc Surg* 21:26–33, discussion 33–24, 1995.

40. Ihlberg L, Luther M, Alback A, et al: Does a completely accomplished duplex-based surveillance prevent vein-graft failure? *Eur J Vasc Endovasc Surg* 18:395–400, 1999.

41. Ihlberg L, Luther M, Tierala E, et al: The utility of duplex scanning in infrainguinal vein graft surveillance: results from a randomised controlled study, *Eur J Vasc Endovasc Surg* 16:19–27, 1998.

42. Tinder CN, Chavanpun JP, Bandyk DF, et al: Efficacy of duplex ultrasound surveillance after infrainguinal vein bypass may be enhanced by identification of characteristics predictive of graft stenosis development, *J Vasc Surg* 48:613–618, 2008.

43. Brumberg RS, Back MR, Armstrong PA, et al: The relative importance of graft surveillance and warfarin therapy in infrainguinal prosthetic bypass failure, *J Vasc Surg* 46:1160–1166, 2007.

44. Connors G, Todoran TM, Engelson BA, et al: Percutaneous revascularization of long femoral artery lesions for claudication: patency over 2.5 years and impact of systematic surveillance, *Catheter Cardiovasc Interv* 77:1055–1062, 2011.

45. Tatli S, Lipton MJ, Davison BD, et al: From the RSNA refresher courses: MR imaging of aortic and peripheral vascular disease, *Radiographics* 23 Spec No:S59–S78, 2003.

46. Steffens JC, Link J, Schwarzenberg H, et al: Lower extremity occlusive disease: diagnostic imaging with a combination of cardiac-gated 2D phase-contrast and cardiac-gated 2D time-of-flight MRA, *J Comput Assist Tomogr* 23:7–12, 1999.

47. Quinn SF, Sheley RC, Semonsen KG, et al: Aortic and lower-extremity arterial disease: evaluation with MR angiography versus conventional angiography, *Radiology* 206:693–701, 1998.

48. Nelemans PJ, Leiner T, de Vet HC, et al: Peripheral arterial disease: meta-analysis of the diagnostic performance of MR angiography, *Radiology* 217:105–114, 2000.

49. Dellegrottaglie S, Sanz J, Macaluso F, et al: Technology insight: magnetic resonance angiography for the evaluation of patients with peripheral artery disease, *Nat Clin Pract Cardiovasc Med* 4:677–687, 2007.

50. Dorweiler B, Neufang A, Kreitner KF, et al: Magnetic resonance angiography unmasks reliable target vessels for pedal bypass grafting in patients with diabetes mellitus, *J Vasc Surg* 35:766–772, 2002.

51. Kreitner KF, Kalden P, Neufang A, et al: Diabetes and peripheral arterial occlusive disease: prospective comparison of contrast-enhanced three-dimensional MR angiography with conventional digital subtraction angiography, *AJR Am J Roentgenol* 174:171–179, 2000.

52. Menke J, Larsen J: Meta-analysis: accuracy of contrast-enhanced magnetic resonance angiography for assessing steno-occlusions in peripheral arterial disease, *Ann Intern Med* 153:325–334, 2010.

53. Winterer JT, Schaefer O, Uhrmeister P, et al: Contrast enhanced MR angiography in the assessment of relevant stenoses in occlusive disease of the pelvic and lower limb arteries: diagnostic value of a two-step examination protocol in comparison to conventional DSA, *Eur J Radiol* 41:153–160, 2002.

54. Bendib K, Berthezene Y, Croisille P, et al: Assessment of complicated arterial bypass grafts: value of contrast-enhanced subtraction magnetic resonance angiography, *J Vasc Surg* 26:1036–1042, 1997.

55. Dorenbeck U, Seitz J, Volk M, et al: Evaluation of arterial bypass grafts of the pelvic and lower extremities with gadolinium-enhanced magnetic resonance angiography: comparison with digital subtraction angiography, *Invest Radiol* 37:60–64, 2002.

56. Loewe C, Cejna M, Schoder M, et al: Contrast material-enhanced, moving-table MR angiography versus digital subtraction angiography for surveillance of peripheral arterial bypass grafts, *J Vasc Interv Radiol* 14:1129–1137, 2003.

57. Brillet PY, Vayssairat M, Tassart M, et al: Gadolinium-enhanced MR angiography as first-line preoperative imaging in high-risk patients with lower limb ischemia, *J Vasc Interv Radiol* 14:1139–1145, 2003.

58. Cronberg CN, Sjoberg S, Albrechtsson U, et al: Peripheral arterial disease. Contrast-enhanced 3D MR angiography of the lower leg and foot compared with conventional angiography, *Acta Radiol* 44:59–66, 2003.

59. Bezooijen R, van den Bosch HC, Tielbeek AV, et al: Peripheral arterial disease: sensitivity-encoded multiposition MR angiography compared with intraarterial angiography and conventional multiposition MR angiography, *Radiology* 231:263–271, 2004.

60. Steffens JC, Schafer FK, Oberscheid B, et al: Bolus-chasing contrast-enhanced 3D MRA of the lower extremity. Comparison with intraarterial DSA, *Acta Radiol* 44:185–192, 2003.

61. Heijenbrok-Kal MH, Kock MC, Hunink MG: Lower extremity arterial disease: multidetector CT angiography meta-analysis, *Radiology* 245:433–439, 2007.

62. Lawler LP, Fishman EK: Multi-detector row CT of thoracic disease with emphasis on 3D volume rendering and CT angiography, *Radiographics* 21:1257–1273, 2001.

63. Becker CR, Wintersperger B, Jakobs TF: Multi-detector-row CT angiography of peripheral arteries, *Semin Ultrasound CT MR* 24:268–279, 2003.

CHAPTER 19

Medical Treatment of Peripheral Artery Disease

Heather L. Gornik, Mark A. Creager

Treatment of patients with peripheral artery disease (PAD) must take into consideration the risk of adverse cardiovascular events related to systemic atherosclerosis (myocardial infarction [MI], stroke, death) and limb-related symptoms and prognosis (functional capacity, quality of life, limb viability). The risk of MI, stroke, or death related to cardiovascular disease is increased three- to sixfold in patients with PAD (see Chapter 16). Functional limitations imposed by PAD, including symptoms of limb claudication, impaired walking ability, and critical limb ischemia (CLI), adversely affect quality of life and restrict patients' abilities to participate in many basic vocational and recreational activities. In addition, patients with PAD are at increased risk of lower-extremity ulceration and amputation, and thus foot care represents an important component of management of these patients. Medical management of the patient with PAD has three central goals: (1) prevention of cardiovascular events, (2) improvement of quality of life and functional capacity, and (3) protection and care of the limb (Fig. 19-1). In this chapter, we review the evidence to support aggressive risk factor modification and antiplatelet therapy for patients with PAD to reduce adverse cardiovascular events. We also review the physical and medical therapies used to treat patients with intermittent claudication and CLI to improve lower-extremity function and ameliorate symptoms. Foot care for PAD is briefly discussed. Catheter-based revascularization for PAD is reviewed in Chapter 20, and surgical revascularization for PAD is reviewed in Chapter 21. Multisocietal consensus guidelines for management of the patient with PAD are available and may be helpful in clinical practice.[1,2]

Risk Factor Modification and Antiplatelet Therapy for Prevention of Cardiovascular Events

Smoking Cessation

Tobacco smoking is strongly associated with development and progression of PAD, with the risk of PAD among smokers as high as threefold that of nonsmokers (see Chapter 16). Smoking cessation is a critical component of risk factor modification for patients with PAD. Epidemiological studies have established that smoking cessation improves both cardiovascular and limb-related outcomes among patients with PAD. Given the established hazards of cigarette smoking, it would be unethical to conduct a randomized clinical trial of smoking cessation.

Smoking cessation has salutary effects on claudication symptoms, exercise physiology, and limb-related outcomes in patients with symptomatic PAD. Patients with intermittent claudication who quit smoking have longer pain-free walking times and maximal walking times compared with patients who continue to smoke.[3] In a prospective study of patients with intermittent claudication followed with serial noninvasive vascular testing over a period of 10 months, patients who quit smoking had significant improvements in maximal treadmill walking distance and postexercise ankle pressure, whereas ongoing smokers had no changes in these parameters.[4] Smoking cessation is also associated with improved clinical outcomes in patients with PAD. In a Swedish study, patients with intermittent claudication who were active smokers or who had quit within 6 months were followed

prospectively for development of limb-related and cardiovascular outcomes.[5] At 7 years of follow-up, ongoing tobacco smoking was associated with development of CLI and was also an independent predictor of the need for surgical revascularization. Indeed, only patients who continued to smoke developed rest pain during the follow-up period. Ongoing smoking was also associated with development of MI and a trend toward decreased overall survival at 10 years of follow-up.

Continued cigarette smoking is associated with adverse outcome among patients with PAD referred for vascular surgery. In a prospective study of patients referred for femoropopliteal arterial bypass grafting, ongoing tobacco use was associated with a significant reduction in the 1-year cumulative patency rate of both venous and prosthetic lower-extremity bypass grafts.[6] In an Australian study of patients who underwent lumbar sympathectomy or lower-extremity bypass grafting for symptomatic PAD, patients who quit smoking following surgery had dramatically improved 5-year survival rates compared to patients who continued to smoke.[7] The majority of deaths that occurred in the postoperative patients were due to a major vascular event, whereas the remaining deaths were due to other smoking-related illnesses, principally chronic obstructive pulmonary disease (COPD) and lung cancer.

Degree of ongoing tobacco use following revascularization may also be predictive of adverse events. In a registry study of patients who underwent their first arterial revascularization procedure, patients categorized as heavy smokers (>15 cigarettes/day) had significantly reduced overall survival compared to moderate smokers (<15 cigarettes/day).[8] In addition, there was a 10-fold higher amputation rate among heavy smokers compared with moderate smokers at 3 years' follow-up.

Despite the multiple benefits of smoking cessation in patients with PAD, it is an extremely difficult goal to accomplish, and initial success rates are low. The efficacy of physician advice in achieving smoking cessation is less than 5%.[9] The success rate is at least 10-fold higher when smoking cessation advice and encouragement are given to patients at risk for MI, or patients who have survived an MI. Intensive counseling customized to PAD patients who continue to smoke is associated with a significant improvement in confirmed tobacco abstinence at 6 months of follow-up, compared to standard clinical smoking cessation advice.[10] Smoking cessation programs may be more successful when coupled with pharmacological therapy, including both nicotine and non-nicotine agents. The antidepressant bupropion has been demonstrated to improve tobacco abstinence rates at 12 months relative to placebo when used alone or in combination with the nicotine patch.[11] Recently, varenicline, a novel partial agonist of the nicotinic acetylcholine receptor (nAchR) $\alpha 4\beta$, has been shown to improve tobacco abstinence rates among subjects both with and without cardiovascular disease, including patients with PAD.[12,13] Among those with cardiovascular disease, varenicline was associated with a threefold likelihood of abstinence at 1-year follow-up compared with placebo, although the absolute abstinence rate was only 19.2%.[13] Side effects of varenicline include sleep abnormalities, nausea, and flatulence.[13,14] Both varenicline and bupropion are associated with an increased risk of neuropsychiatric side effects. Package labeling for both agents includes a black box warning recommending observation for changes in behavior or mood or development of suicidal ideation while receiving these agents for smoking cessation treatment.[14,15]

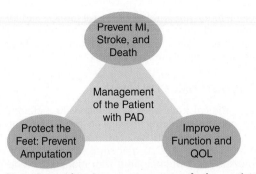

FIGURE 19-1 Comprehensive management of the patient with peripheral artery disease (PAD) must include three important components of care: prevention of adverse cardiovascular events, foot care, and improvement of functional capacity and quality of life (QOL). MI, myocardial infarction. *(Reproduced with permission from Cleveland Clinic Foundation.)*

RECOMMENDATIONS

Smoking cessation advice and encouragement of cessation efforts should be key components of each office visit. For patients motivated to quit smoking, treatment with nicotine replacement therapy, bupropion, or varenicline should be considered. These efforts may be incorporated into a formal smoking cessation program that includes longitudinal counseling on an individual basis or in a small group.

Lipid-Lowering Therapy

Dyslipidemia is a well-established risk factor for development of atherosclerotic vascular disease, including coronary artery disease (CAD) and cerebrovascular disease (CVD). In addition, epidemiological studies have established dyslipidemia—specifically high total and low-density lipoprotein (LDL) cholesterol—as a risk factor for development of atherosclerosis in the peripheral circulation[16–18] (see Chapter 16). There is a less established association between low levels of high density lipoprotein (HDL) cholesterol and development of claudication.[16,19,20] The association, if any, between elevated triglycerides and PAD is controversial.[19,20] The association of dyslipidemia with vascular disease has led to extensive investigation of lipid-lowering therapy as a clinical strategy to prevent myocardial ischemia, stroke, and death in patients with systemic atherosclerosis. Some of these studies specifically addressed the use of lipid-lowering therapy in patients with PAD.

Given convincing epidemiological evidence that dyslipidemia is a risk factor for development of atherosclerosis and subsequent cardiovascular events, multiple randomized clinical trials investigated the use of lipid-lowering agents for prevention of death and other major cardiovascular events in high-risk patients. Development of highly effective and safe agents, particularly HMG-CoA reductase inhibitors ("statins"), has led to widespread application of lipid-lowering therapy for patients with hyperlipidemia and atherosclerotic vascular disease. In recent decades, multiple large randomized controlled trials established the role of lipid-lowering pharmacotherapy, primarily with statins, in secondary prevention of cardiovascular events among patients with CAD.[21–24] Although these studies were not designed to specifically investigate the long-term benefit of lipid-lowering therapy in patients with PAD, the findings are of relevance in these patients because most patients with PAD have either symptomatic or asymptomatic coronary atherosclerosis.[25–27]

The Scandinavian Simvastatin Survival Study (4S) was the first major clinical trial to demonstrate the survival benefit of aggressive lipid-lowering therapy with statins in hypercholesterolemic patients with CAD.[22] In secondary analyses, the 4S investigators examined the effect of simvastatin on development of symptoms and signs of atherosclerotic vascular disease, including claudication and the appearance of a vascular bruit, during semiannual physical examinations of the study participants.[28] There was no significant difference in detection of new or worsening femoral bruits, although this endpoint was likely limited by interobserver variability and the limited sensitivity of the physical examination. There was a 38% reduction in the incidence of intermittent claudication and a 30% reduction in cerebrovascular events among patients randomized to simvastatin.[22,28] Similar findings have been confirmed in subsequent studies of the use of HMG-CoA reductase inhibitors for treatment of symptomatic claudication, discussed later in this chapter.

The Heart Protection Study extended use of statins to secondary prevention of cardiovascular events in patients with atherosclerosis in any major vascular bed, and to primary prevention of cardiovascular events in high-risk patients, particularly diabetics.[27,29] Patients were randomized to simvastatin or placebo and followed for a mean of 5 years. Eligible patients included those with documented CAD, CVD, or PAD, or patients without documented atherosclerotic vascular disease believed to be at high risk of a major vascular event due to diabetes or multiple cardiac risk factors. Patients enrolled in the study on the basis of PAD had intermittent claudication, had undergone lower-extremity revascularization, or had objective evidence of "leg artery stenosis." The majority of patients randomized in the study had a history of CAD (65%); of these, 30% had PAD. There was a 13% reduction in the relative risk of all-cause mortality among patients randomized to simvastatin, due largely to a 17% reduction in the risk of vascular death. There was a 24% reduction in the first occurrence of any major vascular event among patients randomized to simvastatin. Patients enrolled on the basis of PAD alone, with no documented CAD, had a 19% reduction in incidence of first major vascular event if randomized to simvastatin. In a subsequent subset analysis of the 4588 subjects with PAD, randomization to simvastatin was associated with a 20% reduction in noncoronary revascularization procedures compared to placebo.[30] There was no significant benefit of simvastatin on the incidence of lower-extremity amputation.

Non-LDL cholesterol, particularly low HDL cholesterol, has been identified as an independent risk factor for development of CAD.[31,32] Pharmacological agents that raise HDL cholesterol (e.g., fibric acid derivatives, niacin) have not been as widely studied as agents that lower total and LDL cholesterol (i.e., statins) for secondary prevention of cardiovascular events in patients with atherosclerotic vascular disease, and specifically for PAD. The Veterans Affairs High-Density Lipoprotein Cholesterol Intervention Trial (VA-HIT) investigators randomized men with documented CAD and low HDL cholesterol to gemfibrozil or placebo and found a 22% reduction in the primary composite endpoint of death from CAD or nonfatal MI in the gemfibrozil cohort after a median of 5.1 years of follow-up.[21] The incidence of peripheral vascular surgery, the only PAD endpoint studied, was not significantly different within the treatment groups. Cardiovascular benefit has not been found in subsequent studies of other fibrates. The Bezafibrate Infarction Prevention (BIP) study was a randomized study of bezafibrate or placebo in patients with a previous MI or stable angina.[33] Bezafibrate did not significantly affect the primary endpoint of fatal or nonfatal MI or sudden death. The Fenofibrate Intervention and Event Lowering in Diabetes (FIELD) study was a randomized study of fenofibrate or placebo in patients with diabetes.[34] Fenofibrate did not significantly affect the primary outcome of fatal coronary heart disease (CHD) and nonfatal MI, but did decrease secondary endpoints such as nonfatal MI and coronary and peripheral revascularization. Given these limited data, the role of therapies to target non-LDL cholesterol in the management of patients with PAD is uncertain.

RECOMMENDATIONS

The American College of Cardiology/American Heart Association (ACC/AHA) PAD guidelines recommend treatment of patients with PAD with an HMG-CoA reductase inhibitor to an LDL goal of less than 100 mg/dL (class I). A lower LDL goal of less than 70 mg/dL is recommended as a more aggressive option for those patients at very high risk of an ischemic event (class IIa).[1] Statins should be prescribed for all patients with PAD regardless of whether or not they have documented CAD. To date, no clinical trial has investigated the role of combination therapy (i.e., statin plus fibrate, statin plus ezetimibe) specifically among patients with PAD.

Treatment of Hypertension

Control of hypertension is critical for preventing stroke, MI, and congestive heart failure (CHF). Blood pressure control can be achieved with a number of pharmacological agents, either individually or in combination. Large randomized clinical trials have demonstrated the benefits of pharmacotherapy on clinical outcomes, including death.[35,36] Although patients with hypertension and PAD are at increased risk of serious vascular events, few studies have specifically addressed the benefit of blood pressure lowering in this population.

EFFECT OF BLOOD PRESSURE LOWERING ON CLAUDICATION

Conventional medical wisdom and small clinical trials have alleged that intensive blood pressure lowering, particularly with β-adrenergic blockers, may worsen symptoms in patients with claudication and PAD.[37-41] The safety of blood pressure–lowering therapy, specifically with β-adrenergic blockers, in patients with PAD and claudication is of great importance. A substantial percentage of patients with PAD have concomitant CAD. In these patients—in particular, those who have had an MI—treatment with a β-adrenergic blocker has been demonstrated to be lifesaving therapy in large multicenter randomized clinical trials.[42,43] β-Adrenergic blockers are also crucial for management of symptomatic angina pectoris in patients with CAD and patients with left ventricular (LV) dysfunction. In addition, β-adrenergic blockers are a key component of perioperative management of patients with PAD and claudication undergoing lower-extremity revascularization surgery.[44,45]

In a meta-analysis of small randomized controlled clinical trials of the use of β-blockers in patients with PAD and intermittent claudication, there was no significant effect on pain-free or maximal walking distance among patients treated with β-blockers.[46] Of the 11 studies included in the analysis, only one study of 20 patients demonstrated an adverse effect of β-blockers on leg symptoms.[40] Recently there has been interest in the potential for the β-blocker nebivolol to improve claudication symptoms.[47,48] In one study of 128 patients with intermittent claudication randomized to nebivolol or metoprolol for a 48-week treatment period, there was no significant difference in pain-free or maximal walking distance between the two β-blocker groups. There were modest improvements in initial (for nebivolol) and absolute (both nebivolol and metoprolol) claudication distance compared to baseline, but in the absence of a placebo-treated control group, interpretation of these findings is limited.[47]

Demonstration of the safety of angiotensin-converting enzyme (ACE) inhibitors in the majority of patients with claudication is very important, particularly given the findings of recent trials that have established the importance of this class of agents in preventing cardiovascular events.[49] The effect of blood pressure–lowering therapy for 6 weeks with the ACE inhibitor perindopril was studied in patients with hypertension and one of many comorbidities, including PAD.[50] A subgroup of patients had significant symptomatic PAD, defined as a pain-free walking distance of 80 to 200 meters (Fontaine IIb) and an imaging study that demonstrated evidence of iliac or femoral arterial occlusive disease. Among the patients with PAD, there was no difference in the pain-free or maximal walking distance between the perindopril and placebo groups, although walking distance increased modestly in both groups above baseline. None of the PAD patients reported worsening claudication. More recently, Ahimastos et al. reported a beneficial effect of the ACE inhibitor ramipril.[51] In a pilot study of 40 patients with

superficial femoral artery (SFA) occlusive disease and intermittent claudication, without diabetes mellitus or hypertension, there was significant improvement in maximal walking time among patients randomized to ramipril compared with placebo.

CLINICAL OUTCOMES TRIALS

Two major clinical trials have investigated the potential benefits of blood pressure–lowering therapy in preventing cardiovascular events in patients with PAD. The Appropriate Blood Pressure Control in Diabetes (ABCD) trial studied the effect of intensive blood pressure control compared with moderate blood pressure control on the occurrence of cardiovascular events and renal insufficiency in diabetic patients.[52,53] Normotensive (diastolic blood pressure 80-90 mm Hg) and hypertensive (diastolic blood pressure > 90 mm Hg) diabetic patients were enrolled. The hypertensive patients were randomized to receive either enalapril or nisoldipine as first-line therapy. The normotensive patients were randomized to either intensive blood pressure treatment (with further randomization to one of the two study drugs) to achieve a reduction in diastolic pressure of 10 mm Hg, or standard therapy, in which case they received a placebo. Patients were followed for a mean of 5 years. In a substudy of the diabetic patients in the normotensive cohort, the effect of intensive blood pressure treatment among patients with PAD was investigated.[53] Among the 220 normotensive patients randomized to intensive blood pressure treatment, there was a 65% reduction in the relative risk of MI, stroke, or cardiovascular death. There was a strong inverse relationship between baseline ankle-brachial index (ABI) and risk of a cardiovascular event. Intensive blood pressure control negated this relationship and normalized the odds of a cardiovascular event toward that of patients with a normal ABI (Fig. 19-2). The benefit of intensive blood pressure control was evident even in patients with a severely decreased ABI, a subset of patients that had been excluded from prior studies.[50] There were too few patients with PAD to analyze data for enalapril and nisoldipine separately. The findings of the ABCD trial emphasize the importance of intensive blood pressure control in diabetic patients with PAD.

The Heart Outcomes Prevention Evaluation (HOPE) investigators tested the efficacy of the ACE inhibitor ramipril for primary and secondary prevention of cardiovascular events in high-risk patients.[49] Patients were enrolled on the basis of established

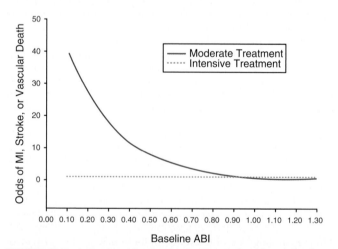

FIGURE 19-2 Intensive blood pressure control with enalapril or nisoldipine decreases the odds of a major vascular event among diabetic patients with peripheral artery disease (PAD). Results from the Appropriate Blood Pressure Control in Diabetics (ABCD) Trial. The inverse correlation of ankle-brachial index *(ABI)* and odds of a major vascular event are not present among patients randomized to the intensive blood pressure control group. MI, myocardial infarction. *(Reproduced with permission from Mehler PS, Coll JR, Estacio R, et al: Intensive blood pressure control reduces the risk of cardiovascular events in patients with peripheral arterial disease and type 2 diabetes. Circulation 107:753–756, 2003.)[53]*

atherosclerotic vascular disease (CAD, prior stroke, or PAD) or diabetes mellitus with additional cardiac risk factors. Some 44% of patients randomized had evidence of PAD, as manifested by a history of claudication with an abnormal ABI of less than 0.8, limb revascularization procedure, amputation, or angiographic evidence of arterial stenosis.[54] Patients were randomized to receive ramipril or placebo. At a mean of 5 years of follow-up, there was a 22% reduction in the primary composite endpoint of MI, stroke, or cardiovascular death among patients randomized to ramipril (Fig. 19-3). In subgroup analysis, the benefit of ramipril was present regardless of baseline blood pressure. The benefit of ramipril on the composite endpoint was present among the subgroup of patients with PAD. The benefit of ramipril was likely due to cardiovascular benefits other than its blood pressure–lowering properties because the mean decrease in blood pressure among patients randomized to active therapy was very small. The findings of the HOPE trial indicate that patients with PAD should be treated with an ACE inhibitor, regardless of baseline blood pressure or the presence or absence of diabetes.

For patients with PAD who are intolerant of ACE inhibitors (e.g., development of cough), an angiotensin receptor blocker (ARB) is an acceptable alternative agent for cardiovascular risk reduction. In the Ongoing Telmisartan Alone and in Combination with Ramipril Global Endpoint (ONTARGET) Trial, 25,620 patients at high risk for cardiovascular events, a population similar to the HOPE trial, were randomized to receive ramipril, the ARB telmisartan, or a combination of the two agents.[55] The ONTARGET population included 2468 patients with symptomatic PAD. After a median follow-up of 56 months, the primary cardiovascular event rates in the ramipril, telmisartan, and combination therapy groups were statistically the same (≈6.5%). The combination of ramipril and telmisartan, however, was associated with higher rates of renal insufficiency and hypotension than either agent alone.

RECOMMENDATIONS

Blood pressure control is an important component of cardiovascular risk reduction among patients with PAD, and all patients with PAD should routinely undergo blood pressure assessment. Blood pressure should be measured at least once in both upper extremities to exclude the possibility of occult subclavian stenosis leading to inaccurate blood pressure assessment in one of the arms. Any class of antihypertensive agents, including β-blockers, can be safely prescribed for blood pressure lowering, although ACE inhibitors or ARBs should be considered as first-line therapies. Caution should be exercised when managing the patient with CLI because

aggressive blood pressure lowering may be detrimental in this small subset of patients. Even normotensive patients with PAD may benefit from ACE inhibitor or ARB therapy. Aggressive blood pressure control is particularly important for diabetic patients with PAD. According to the ACC/AHA PAD guidelines, target blood pressure for patients with PAD is below 140/90 mm Hg for nondiabetic and below 130/80 for diabetic patients (class I recommendation).[1]

Control of Diabetes Mellitus

Multiple epidemiological studies have established a strong association between diabetes mellitus and PAD[16,17,56,57] (see Chapter 16). The relative risk of PAD is two to four times that of nondiabetic patients. Presence of diabetes is associated with adverse limb-related outcomes among patients with documented PAD, including the need for amputation.[58,59] In the Strong Heart Study, worsening glycemic control (determined by hemoglobin A_{1c} [HbA_{1c}] level) was associated with increased incidence of lower-extremity amputation among diabetic Native Americans with and without PAD.[60] In addition, diabetes is associated with a markedly increased risk of a major cardiovascular event, including myocardial ischemia, stroke, and death. Therapeutic options for achieving glycemic control in diabetic patients include insulin, sulfonylureas, metformin, the thiazolidinediones ("glitazones"), and novel agents that modify carbohydrate absorption and breakdown into glucose (α-glucosidase inhibitors) or increase insulin bioavailability through differing mechanisms (e.g., repaglinide, nateglinide, sitagliptin).[61] Whereas clinical trials have established the vital importance of rigorous glycemic control for preventing microvascular complications in diabetic patients, the benefits of glycemic control for prevention of major cardiovascular events has not been definitively established. In addition, recent randomized controlled trials have indicated that certain high-risk patients may be more likely to experience adverse effects with very intensive glycemic control.[62]

CLINICAL OUTCOMES TRIALS

The Diabetes Control and Complications Trial (DCCT) Research Group investigated whether intensive glycemic control could improve clinical outcomes in diabetic patients.[63] A total of 1441 young patients (aged 13-39 years) with type 1 diabetes mellitus, with and without retinopathy, were randomized to one of two glycemic control strategies: (1) intensive therapy with an insulin pump or frequent injections to maintain blood sugar as close to normal as possible, or (2) conventional therapy with once- or twice-daily insulin injections. Development or progression of retinopathy was the primary endpoint of the study, and the low cardiovascular risk profile of the study population reflected this goal. Peripheral artery disease endpoints included development of claudication, persistent loss of a pedal pulse, and need for a revascularization procedure or limb amputation. Patients were followed for a mean of 6.5 years. Among patients randomized to intensive glycemic control, there were significant reductions in development and progression of retinopathy and proteinuria and development of sensorimotor neuropathy compared to patients treated with conventional glycemic control. Owing to the young average age of the patient population, there were few deaths or major macrovascular events in either treatment group. Nonetheless, randomization to intensive glycemic control was associated with a nonsignificant 42% reduction in peripheral vascular and coronary events.[64] Perhaps more importantly, however, randomization to intensive glycemic control was protective against development of elevated total and LDL cholesterol—risk factors for future development of cardiovascular events in this young patient population. Long-term follow-up data from the DCCT study were recently published.[65] Additional observational follow-up data were available for 93% of patients enrolled in the original trial in the Epidemiology of Diabetes Interventions and Complications study. At a mean follow-up of 17 years, randomization to intensive glycemic control showed a persistent 42% reduction in risk for a major cardiovascular event.

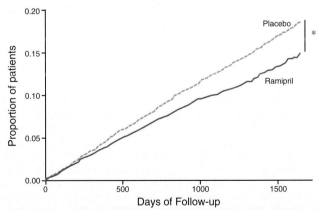

FIGURE 19-3 Ramipril reduces the incidence of myocardial infarction (MI), stroke, or cardiovascular death among high-risk patients with atherosclerotic vascular disease or diabetes mellitus. *, P <0.001. *(Reproduced with permission from Yusuf S, Sleight P, Pogue J, et al: Effects of an angiotensin-converting enzyme inhibitor, ramipril, on cardiovascular events in high-risk patients. The Heart Outcomes Prevention Evaluation Study Investigators. N Engl J Med 342:145–153, 2000.)[49]*

The United Kingdom Prospective Diabetes Study 33 (UKPDS 33) was designed to complement the findings of the DCCT by investigating the effect of intensive glycemic control (with sulfonylureas or insulin) on the incidence of macrovascular events in type 2 diabetic patients.[66] An earlier study of glycemic control strategies in type 2 diabetic persons found no cardiovascular benefit of intensive therapy with insulin and an excess of cardiovascular deaths among patients treated with the sulfonylurea tolbutamide.[67] This early finding generated concern regarding the safety and potential cardiovascular toxicity of sulfonylureas with prolonged use in diabetic patients. In the UKPDS 33, patients were randomized to intensive therapy with insulin or one of three sulfonylureas, or to conventional treatment with a prescribed diabetic diet; they were followed for a median of 10 years.[66] Although there were no differences in the treatment groups with regard to total mortality, cardiac mortality, or diabetes-related mortality, there was a 16% reduction in the relative risk of MI in the group randomized to intensive therapy. There was also a 39% reduction in relative risk of amputation in the intensive therapy group, which did not achieve statistical significance. There were too few deaths attributable to PAD to allow for comparison. Consistent with the findings of the DCCT, there was a highly significant 25% reduction in relative risk of microvascular complications among patients randomized to intensive glycemic control, including the need for retinal surgery.

A follow-up study evaluated a subset of participants from UKPDS 33 annually, either with clinical office visits or questionnaires, for up to 10 years after completion of the trial.[68] During this period of follow-up, patients were managed at the discretion of their physicians rather than per trial protocol, and differences in HbA_{1c} levels between the intensive and conventional treatment groups equalized. Despite this finding, the significant risk reduction in microvascular events among patients initially randomized to intensive therapy persisted (24% reduction). More importantly, there were statistically significant gains in terms of demonstration of delayed cardiovascular benefit of intensive therapy of diabetes, with reductions in all-cause mortality (27% reduction) and risk of MI (33% reduction). There was no significant reduction in risk of stroke or peripheral vascular outcomes.

Both the DCCT and UKPDS 33 trials established the importance of glycemic control in the prevention of microvascular complications in diabetic patients. The post-trial follow-up cohort studies for each of these trials have shown a sustained benefit of glycemic control on risk of microvascular complications and have also contributed data to support the possibility that intensive glycemic control (target $HbA_{1c} \approx 7\,g/dL$) in these trials may prevent macrovascular events, particularly MI.

There has been great interest in use of the insulin-sensitizing agents, metformin and the thiazolidinediones (glitazones), for prevention of cardiovascular events in diabetic patients. In a substudy of the UKPDS (UKPDS 34), newly diagnosed, overweight, type 2 diabetic patients were randomized to intensive therapy with metformin or a prescribed diabetic diet.[69] Patients were followed for a median of 10.7 years. In contrast to the sulfonylurea arm of the study, there was a significant 42% reduction in diabetes-related mortality and a 36% reduction in all-cause mortality among patients randomized to metformin therapy compared with patients randomized to diet. There was no difference in the incidence of PAD endpoints between the two groups, although the total number of clinical events related to PAD was small.

Use of thiazolidinediones for glycemic control and prevention of cardiovascular events among diabetic patients has been an area of recent study and significant controversy. In the Prospective Pioglitazone Clinical Trial in Macrovascular Events (PROactive) study, 5238 type 2 diabetic patients with established macrovascular (atherosclerotic) disease, including CAD, prior stroke, or PAD as defined by history of intermittent claudication (with abnormal ABI or toe-brachial index [TBI]) or prior major amputation were randomized to receive pioglitazone or placebo atop their established diabetes medical regimen and followed for incident cardiovascular events.[70] At a mean follow-up of nearly 6 years, there was no

significant difference between pioglitazone- and placebo-treated patients in the primary composite endpoint of all-cause mortality, nonfatal MI, stroke, acute coronary syndrome (ACS), coronary or leg endovascular or surgical revascularization, and amputation above the ankle. There was a 16% reduction in the secondary composite endpoint of death, nonfatal MI, or stroke in patients randomized to pioglitazone.

Recently, there have been safety concerns related to the safety of rosiglitazone, another thiazolidinedione, including risk of MI and congestive heart failure.[71] The RECORD (Rosiglitazone Evaluated for Cardiovascular Outcomes in Oral Agent Combination Therapy for Type 2 Diabetes) trial randomized type 2 diabetic patients on sulfonylurea or metformin therapy with adequate glycemic control to receive added rosiglitazone therapy or added sulfonylurea and metformin in an open-label design.[72] After a mean of follow-up of 5.5 years, there was no significant difference in the composite endpoint of cardiovascular death or hospitalization between the rosiglitazone and sulfonylurea/metformin combination therapy groups. There was, however, a more than twofold increase in risk of significant CHF (requiring hospitalization or leading to death) among rosiglitazone-treated patients. On the basis of previous meta-analyses and the findings of the RECORD trial, there is now a black box warning on the rosiglitazone label regarding adverse cardiovascular effects, and prescriptive access to this medication is restricted by the drug manufacturer.[73]

Three randomized controlled trials that have investigated the benefit of very intensive glycemic control (target HbA_{1c} 6%-6.5% or normoglycemia) versus modern standard glycemic control (target HbA_{1c} <7%-7.5%) among patients with type 2 diabetes.[74-76] In the Action and Diabetes and Vascular Disease: Preterax and Diamicron Modified Release Controlled Evaluation (ADVANCE) trial, there was a 14% reduction in microvascular events among patients randomized to highly intensive therapy, but there was no significant reduction in macrovascular events, including risk of death, MI, or stroke.[76] In the Action to Control Cardiovascular Risk in Diabetes (ACCORD) study, not only was there no benefit of highly intensive glycemic control on a composite endpoint of cardiovascular death or nonfatal MI or stroke, but there was also an increased risk of death from any cause (22%) or cardiovascular death (35%) among individuals randomized to highly intensive therapy.[74] There was a marked increase in hypoglycemic episodes requiring medical assistance (10.5% vs. 3.5%) among patients randomized to highly intensive therapy. The ACCORD trial was terminated early at the recommendation of its data safety and monitoring board based upon these findings. Finally, the Veterans Affairs Diabetes Trial (VADT) randomized type 2 diabetes patients to either standard therapy or highly intensive glycemic control (goal HbA_{1c} <6%) using rosiglitazone plus either glimepiride or metformin, based upon body mass index (BMI; metformin for patients with BMI $\geq$ 27 kg/m^2).[75] In this trial, there was no benefit of intensive glycemic control on the risk of macrovascular, or surprisingly microvascular, complications during 5.6 years of follow-up.

RECOMMENDATIONS

The American Diabetes Association has published guidelines for the medical care of diabetic patients with and without PAD.[77,78] The ACC/AHA PAD guidelines also address care of the diabetic patient with PAD.[1] In response to the findings of ACCORD, ADVANCE, and VADT, updated multisocietal guidelines for glycemic control have been published.[79] The standard target HbA_{1c} of less than 7% stands as a recommendation for most patients. However, it is recommended that less stringent glycemic control be considered for patients with prior history of severe hypoglycemic reaction, for those with extensive micro- and macrovascular disease, and for those with limited life expectancy. A more stringent target (e.g., HbA_{1c} <6%-6.5%) is recommended as a target for healthier patients with a long life expectancy and no major cardiovascular disease.

In addition to glycemic control, periodic foot examination by healthcare providers and patient education regarding preventive foot care is critical for diabetic patients with PAD, particularly given the prevalence of peripheral neuropathy. The American Diabetic Association and the ACC/AHA recommend ABI measurement for all diabetic persons older than 50 years of age and for some younger patients with additional risk factors.[1,77]

Treatment of Hyperhomocysteinemia

Hyperhomocysteinemia is a disorder associated with derangements of the metabolic pathway involved in metabolism of the essential amino acid methionine.[80] Hyperhomocysteinemia is due to an inherited defect of one of the enzymes involved in transsulfuration or remethylation of homocysteine, or can also occur as a result of malnutrition and deficiency of key cofactors for these enzymatic reactions (i.e., folic acid, vitamins B_6 and B_{12}). Hyperhomocysteinemia is associated with end-stage renal disease, although the mechanism by which this occurs is not well established.[80] Inherited homocystinuria, the most striking form of hyperhomocysteinemia, is due to homozygous deficiency of the enzyme cystathionine β-synthase, a critical enzyme of the transsulfuration pathway of homocysteine. Homocystinuria is associated with mental retardation, ectopia lentis, and premature coronary and peripheral atherosclerosis. Among heterozygotes for cystathionine β-synthase deficiency, homocysteine levels are significantly lower (on the order of 20-40 μmol/L vs. up to 400 μmol/L for homozygotes), although there is also a predisposition to premature atherosclerosis.[80] Multiple epidemiological studies have established an association between elevated plasma homocysteine levels and development and progression of CAD and CVD. Extensive epidemiological evidence has also established hyperhomocysteinemia as an independent risk factor for asymptomatic PAD and the clinical progression of symptomatic PAD.[81-84] In addition to premature atherosclerosis, elevated levels of homocysteine are associated with a hypercoagulable state characterized by a tendency toward venous and arterial thrombosis.[80,85]

Because elevated plasma homocysteine levels are associated with low levels of the enzymatic cofactors folic acid, vitamin B_6, and vitamin B_{12}, vitamin supplementation is an obvious therapeutic consideration for treating hyperhomocysteinemia. One small trial of healthy siblings of patients with hyperhomocysteinemia and premature atherosclerotic vascular disease (PAD, CAD, or CVD before age 56) randomized siblings to combination vitamin therapy with 5 mg folic acid and 250 mg vitamin B_6 or placebo.[86] Siblings with and without evidence of hyperhomocysteinemia were enrolled. Subjects continued therapy for a period of 2 years and were followed for development of CAD (abnormal stress test), PAD (abnormal ABI or lower-extremity arterial duplex scan), and CVD (abnormal carotid artery duplex scan). Among patients randomized to vitamins, fasting plasma homocysteine levels fell from 14.7 to 7.4 μmol/L (a nearly 50% decline); there was an 18% decline in the placebo group. There was no significant difference in the development of PAD or asymptomatic CVD among the two groups. Among the patients randomized to aggressive vitamin therapy, there was a decrease in the incidence of an abnormal stress test.

Although the effectiveness of supplementation with folic acid and vitamin B_{12} for lowering plasma homocysteine levels has been established, few data show a benefit of vitamin supplementation to prevent vascular events in patients with hyperhomocysteinemia or established vascular disease. In the second Heart Outcomes and Prevention Evaluation (HOPE-2) trial, patients with atherosclerotic vascular disease were randomized to receive folic acid, vitamin B_6 and B_{12}, or placebo and followed for incident cardiovascular events.[87,88] Less than 10% of patients in the study population of 5522 had known symptomatic PAD, defined as intermittent claudication or a history of bypass surgery or lower-extremity angioplasty.[88] After 5 years of follow-up and despite a mean reduction in plasma homocysteine of 2.4 μmol/L in the vitamin-treated group (compared to an increase of 0.8 μmol/L in the placebo group), there was no benefit of vitamin therapy on the primary composite outcome of fatal or nonfatal MI or stroke.

In the Norwegian Vitamin Trial (NORVIT), patients with acute MI within the preceding 7 days were randomized to one of four arms in a factorial design (placebo, vitamin B_6, folic acid + vitamin B_{12}, or combination-therapy folic acid and vitamins B_6 and B_{12}).[89] There was a 27% reduction in plasma homocysteine levels among individuals who received folic acid and vitamin B_{12}. However, with a median follow-up of 40 months, there was no benefit of folic acid plus vitamin B_{12} therapy, with or without vitamin B_6, on the composite cardiovascular endpoint. Indeed, there was a trend toward increased risk of a fatal or nonfatal cardiovascular event among individuals randomized to triple-vitamin therapy compared to placebo. The Study of the Effectiveness of Additional Reductions in Cholesterol and Homocysteine (SEARCH) trial assessed the effect of folic acid and vitamin B_{12} on vascular outcomes in 12,064 survivors of MI.[90] Treatment with these vitamins reduced homocysteine by 3.8 μmol/L (28%) but did not affect the primary outcome of first major vascular event, defined as a major coronary event, fatal or nonfatal stroke, or noncoronary revascularization.

RECOMMENDATIONS

To date, there have been no large clinical outcome randomized controlled trials that have specifically investigated treatment of hyperhomocysteinemia in a PAD population. In the absence of such studies, and given the findings of the HOPE-2, NORVIT, and SEARCH trials in patients with coronary and other atherosclerotic vascular disease, use of folic acid and vitamin B_6 and B_{12} supplementation to prevent cardiovascular events among PAD patients is not recommended.

Antiplatelet Therapy

The pivotal role of antiplatelet agents, particularly aspirin, in the secondary prevention of death and MI in patients with CAD has been established by large randomized clinical trials.[91,92] The role of antiplatelet therapy in the management of patients with PAD continues to evolve, with important new data gleaned from recent large clinical trials directed primarily at the prevention of cardiovascular events in patients with and without CAD.

A recent meta-analysis of six primary prevention trials of 95,000 individuals at low to average cardiovascular risk (representing 660,000 person-years) found that aspirin reduced the risk of any vascular event by 12%.[93] This was due primarily to a decrease in the risk of nonfatal MI, but not stroke or vascular mortality. This meta-analysis also included 16 secondary prevention trials of 17,000 individuals at high-average risk, representing 43,000 person-years. In the secondary prevention trials, aspirin reduced serious vascular events by 29%, including total stroke and coronary events, and was associated with a borderline nonsignificant 9% reduction in vascular mortality.

In 2002, the Antithrombotic Trialists' Collaboration updated the 1994 meta-analysis of the evidence supporting the use of antiplatelet agents in the management of high-risk patients with atherosclerotic vascular disease.[91] Studies with different antiplatelet agents (e.g., aspirin, dipyridamole, picotamide, ticlopidine) were included. The initial meta-analysis determined that antiplatelet therapy significantly reduced the odds of a major vascular event among high-risk patients with atherosclerosis by 27%.[92] Also, antiplatelet therapy was effective for preventing both coronary and peripheral artery bypass graft occlusion, with a reduction in relative risk of graft occlusion of approximately one third.[94] In the updated analysis, a total of 287 randomized trials with more than 200,000 patients were included.[91] Confirming the original findings, there was a 22% reduction in the odds of a serious vascular event (vascular death, nonfatal MI, or nonfatal stroke) among high-risk patients treated with antiplatelet agents. The benefit appeared to be greatest among studies that enrolled patients on the basis of high-risk criteria such as prior or acute MI, PAD, or atrial fibrillation. Among the 42 studies that enrolled 9214 high-risk patients on the basis of PAD, there was a 23% reduction in the odds of a major vascular event among patients randomized to antiplatelet therapy. The benefit of antiplatelet therapy was consistent across all PAD enrollment criteria, including intermittent claudication and surgical lower-extremity revascularization. Of note, 2304 patients in this category were enrolled in a study that randomized PAD patients to treatment with a nonaspirin antiplatelet agent, picotamide, or placebo.[95] Picotamide is an antiplatelet agent that both inhibits thromboxane A_2 (TxA_2) synthase and antagonizes the TxA_2 receptor of platelets. It is also noteworthy that none of the trials in this meta-analysis investigated the benefit of aspirin alone (i.e., not in combination with dipyridamole) in standard clinical dosage (81-325 mg daily) versus placebo, a fact that was highlighted by an updated meta-analysis of aspirin therapy for PAD by Berger et al. in 2009 (discussed later).[96]

The Critical Limb Ischaemia Prevention Study (CLIPS) randomized patients with ABI less than 0.85 or TBI less than 0.6 who were asymptomatic or had stable leg claudication (Fontaine stage I/II) to aspirin 100 mg daily or placebo.[97] Although an initial sample size of 2000 patients was planned, the trial was terminated early because of poor enrollment, and only 366 patients were randomized, with a minority followed for more than 2 years. Aspirin was associated with a 64% reduction in the relative risk of fatal and nonfatal vascular events and a 58% reduction in fatal and nonfatal vascular events or critical limb ischemia.

In contrast to the CLIPS trial, which included patients with clinically significant PAD (claudication or asymptomatic PAD with low ABI), there have been two large randomized clinical trials that investigated the efficacy of aspirin in low-risk asymptomatic PAD patients. The Prevention of Progression of Arterial Disease and Diabetes (POPADAD) trial randomized 1276 patients older than 40 years of age who had type 1 or 2 diabetes mellitus and an "abnormal" ABI of less than 1.0, but who had no known cardiovascular disease and no symptoms of PAD.[98] Subjects were randomized to aspirin 100 mg daily or placebo, as well as antioxidant vitamins, in a 2 × 2 factorial design. It is important to note that this was a population that was not only asymptomatic in terms of PAD but also had relatively mild disease, with a median ABI in the study population of 0.9, barely at the lower limit of normal. After a median follow-up of 6.7 years, there was no difference between the aspirin and placebo groups in the rate of fatal or nonfatal vascular events or amputation. In subset analysis, there was a nonsignificant trend toward benefit of aspirin among patients with ABI less than 0.9.

The largest trial of aspirin therapy for prevention of cardiovascular events among patients with PAD to date was the Aspirin for Asymptomatic Atherosclerosis (AAA) Trial.[99] In this trial, nearly 29,000 Scottish patients between the ages of 50 and 75 years who had no cardiovascular disease were offered a screening ABI examination. A total of 3350 individuals with ABI below 0.95 were randomized to receive 100 mg aspirin daily or placebo and followed for an average of 8.2 years. In this study, the lower of two ankle pressures was used for calculating the ABI. There was no statistically significant difference in occurrence of the primary composite endpoint of fatal and nonfatal coronary events, stroke, or revascularization between aspirin- and placebo-treated patients (Fig. 19-4).

Berger et al. performed a meta-analysis of 18 trials comprising 5269 patients with PAD that evaluated the efficacy of aspirin (± dipyridamole) for prevention of cardiovascular events including nonfatal MI, nonfatal stroke, and cardiovascular death.[96] This meta-analysis included the trials incorporated into the Antithrombotic Trialists' Collaboration 2002 meta-analysis, as well as new data from the POPADAD trial and CLIPS; the AAA study was not included. Aspirin therapy, with or without dipyridamole, did not significantly reduce the rate of cardiovascular events. In subset analyses, aspirin was associated with a significant reduction in the incidence of nonfatal stroke, but not cardiovascular mortality, MI, or major bleeding.

Large multicenter randomized clinical trials have investigated the use of the antiplatelet agent clopidogrel for secondary prevention of cardiovascular events. Clopidogrel is a thienopyridine derivative that inhibits platelet aggregation by antagonism of the adenosine

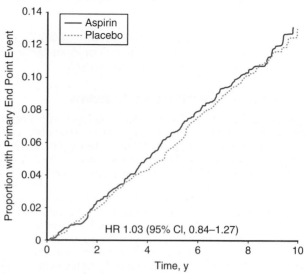

FIGURE 19-4 **Aspirin therapy does not reduce the incidence of major vascular events among asymptomatic individuals with ankle-brachial index (ABI) <0.95.** Results from the Aspirin for Asymptomatic Atherosclerosis (AAA) trial. There was no statistically significant difference in the primary composite outcome of fatal and nonfatal myocardial infarction (MI) or stroke or revascularization between the two groups. y, year. *(Reproduced with permission from Fowkes, FG, Price JF, Stewart, MC, et al. Aspirin for prevention of cardiovascular events in a general population screened for a low ankle-brachial index: a randomized controlled trial. JAMA 303:841–848, 2010.)[99]*

diphosphate receptor.[100] Clopidogrel is less likely to cause serious adverse hematological side effects, particularly neutropenia and thrombotic thrombocytopenic purpura, than its analog ticlopidine. Pooled analysis of early clinical trials suggested a trend toward a marginal benefit of ticlopidine over aspirin in the prevention of MI, stroke, or vascular death.[92]

The Clopidogrel versus Aspirin in Patients at Risk of Ischaemic Events (CAPRIE) study built on this finding and investigated the benefit of clopidogrel versus aspirin in the secondary prevention of cardiovascular events.[101] Patients with recent MI (within 35 days), ischemic stroke (within 6 months), or symptomatic PAD were randomized to clopidogrel (75 mg daily) or aspirin (325 mg daily). Patients enrolled on the basis of PAD had intermittent claudication and an abnormal ABI (ABI ≤0.85) or had undergone leg amputation or revascularization. A total of 19,185 randomized patients were followed for development of the primary composite endpoint of first occurrence of ischemic stroke, MI, or vascular death. After a mean 1.9 years of follow-up, there was an 8.7% relative risk reduction in the annual event rate of the primary endpoint among patients randomized to clopidogrel. The benefit of clopidogrel over aspirin was greatest among the subgroup of patients enrolled on the basis of symptomatic PAD, with a relative risk reduction of the composite endpoint of 23.8% (Fig. 19-5). There was no increase in minor or major bleeding episodes associated with clopidogrel, although there was an increased incidence of gastrointestinal hemorrhage among patients randomized to aspirin.

Dual antiplatelet therapy, namely the combination of aspirin and clopidogrel, reduced the rate of cardiovascular events among patients with ACS in the Clopidogrel in Unstable Angina to Prevent Recurrent Events (CURE) trial.[102] The role of dual antiplatelet therapy for secondary prevention of cardiovascular events among patients with stable atherosclerotic vascular disease was studied in the Clopidogrel and Aspirin versus Aspirin Alone for the Prevention of Atherothrombotic Events (CHARISMA) trial.[103] In this trial, 15,603 patients with symptomatic atherosclerotic vascular disease or multiple high risk features (e.g., diabetes mellitus, asymptomatic abnormal ABI) were randomized to receive either aspirin (75 to 162 mg) plus clopidogrel or aspirin plus placebo and followed for incident cardiovascular events. After a median 28 months of follow-up, there was no statistically significant difference in the primary endpoint, which was the rate of first fatal or nonfatal MI, stroke,

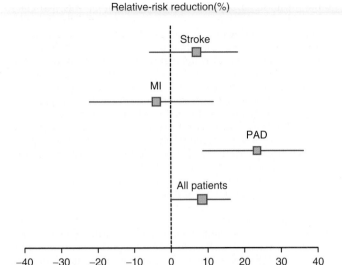

Relative-risk reduction(%)

FIGURE 19-5 Clopidogrel decreases the risk of the composite endpoint of stroke, myocardial infarction (MI), or vascular death relative to aspirin among high-risk patients with atherosclerotic vascular disease. Relative risk reduction for each subgroup of patients is displayed with 95% confidence intervals. The benefit of clopidogrel is particularly pronounced among the subset of patients with peripheral artery disease (PAD). (Adapted and reproduced with permission from the CAPRIE Steering Committee: A randomised, blinded trial of clopidogrel versus aspirin in patients at risk of ischaemic events [CAPRIE]. Lancet 348:1329–1339, 1996.)[101]

or cardiovascular death between the two groups. Dual antiplatelet therapy increased the rate of moderate bleeding (i.e., requiring blood transfusion) but did not increase the rate of fatal bleeding or intracranial hemorrhage. A number of subset analyses were performed, including a post hoc subset analysis of patients with either symptomatic or asymptomatic PAD (N = 3096).[104] Among PAD patients in CHARISMA, there was no significant difference in the primary composite cardiovascular endpoint, although there was a significant 37% reduction in the rate of MI among patients randomized to dual antiplatelet therapy.

In the Clopidogrel and Acetylsalicylic Acid in Bypass Surgery for Peripheral Arterial Disease (CASPAR) trial, 551 patients undergoing lower-extremity bypass surgery for claudication or CLI were randomized to dual antiplatelet therapy with aspirin (75 to 100 mg daily) plus clopidogrel (75 mg daily) or to aspirin plus placebo and followed for limb-related events (graft occlusion, repeat revascularization, major amputation) and cardiovascular events, including death, over a period of up to 2 years.[105] Compared to aspirin alone, dual antiplatelet therapy did not reduce the risk of clinical cardiovascular or limb-related events. In a post hoc analysis, dual antiplatelet therapy was associated with lower rates of graft occlusion and lower-extremity amputation among patients who had prosthetic (vs. venous) bypass grafting.

RECOMMENDATIONS

In light of the 20% to 25% reduction in serious vascular events attributable to antiplatelet therapy among patients with atherosclerotic vascular disease, all patients with PAD, regardless of concomitant CAD or CVD, should receive antiplatelet therapy. Antiplatelet therapy for patients with lower-extremity PAD is given a class I recommendation in the 2005 ACC/AHA PAD guidelines.[1,2] The evidence base in support of antiplatelet therapy is strongest for patients with symptomatic PAD. Given the constraints of the available evidence, aspirin remains a reasonable first-line agent for PAD and should be prescribed at a dose of 81 to 325 mg daily. Aspirin therapy is particularly important among patients undergoing surgical or percutaneous revascularization procedures, and should be continued perioperatively—or initiated as soon as possible postoperatively—if it had not been prescribed previously.

Clopidogrel is a therapeutic alternative among patients intolerant of aspirin (e.g., gastrointestinal distress, allergy, bronchospasm), and can also be considered as the initial choice for patients with PAD. With the exception of patients with recent ACS or those undergoing percutaneous coronary or peripheral interventions, there is currently insufficient evidence to support dual antiplatelet therapy with aspirin and clopidogrel for the secondary prevention of cardiovascular events.

Anticoagulant Therapy

Several clinical trials have addressed the role of anticoagulant therapy, typically with the vitamin K antagonist warfarin, in the management of patients with PAD. These include several small studies that explored the potential effect of oral anticoagulation on limb-related outcomes. A review of three small trials found that oral anticoagulation therapy had no benefit on walking capacity or limb-related outcomes, nor on cardiovascular outcomes among patients with intermittent claudication.[106] Another trial, the Dutch Bypass Oral Anticoagulants or Aspirin investigators compared the efficacy of high-intensity warfarin (target international normalized ratio [INR] 3.0-4.5) with aspirin (80 mg daily) therapy on graft occlusion in patients following infrainguinal bypass grafting.[107] After a mean 21 months of follow-up, there was no significant difference in the rate of graft occlusion between the warfarin and aspirin groups. Subset analyses, however, demonstrated a significant reduction (31%) in the rate of graft occlusion of venous conduit bypass grafts, but not prosthetic grafts, among patients randomized to warfarin.

The Warfarin Antiplatelet Vascular Evaluation (WAVE) trial studied the potential benefit of oral anticoagulation therapy in addition to aspirin for patients with noncoronary atherosclerotic vascular disease.[108] The study included 2161 patients with atherosclerotic vascular disease (symptomatic lower-extremity PAD, symptomatic or asymptomatic carotid artery disease (CAD), or subclavian artery stenosis) who were randomized to receive aspirin (dose 81-325 mg) or aspirin plus warfarin (INR goal of 2-3). More than 80% of patients enrolled had lower-extremity PAD. The co-primary endpoints of the trial were: (1) cardiovascular death, nonfatal MI, and nonfatal stroke, and (2) the above plus need for urgent coronary or peripheral revascularization. Over a follow-up period of 35 months, there was no significant benefit of oral anticoagulation therapy in either of the two co-primary endpoints. There was 3.4-fold relative risk of life-threatening bleeding, and a 15.2-fold relative risk for hemorrhagic stroke among patients randomized to oral anticoagulation therapy.

RECOMMENDATIONS

Based on the lack of compelling efficacy data for warfarin and the associated risk of bleeding, both the American College of Chest Physicians Conference on Antithrombotic and Thrombolytic Therapy and the ACC/AHA PAD guidelines have issued recommendations opposing routine use of oral anticoagulant therapy in patients with PAD.[1,2,109] Anticoagulation therapy may be considered following an episode of acute limb ischemia that had been treated with thrombolytic therapy, or may be warranted when there is a comorbid condition associated with increased risk for thromboembolism (e.g., atrial fibrillation, mechanical heart valve, prior venous thromboembolism [VTE]). In such cases involving patients with PAD, oral anticoagulation should be combined with low-dose aspirin.

Care and Protection of the Feet

Careful attention to foot care is indicated to reduce the likelihood of skin breakdown and infection, and is particularly important in diabetic persons with vascular disease and in patients with critical limb ischemia. Treatment of lower-extremity ulcers is discussed in Chapter 60. The feet of patients with PAD should be kept clean, and moisturizing lotion applied to prevent drying and fissuring.

Stockings should be made of absorbent natural fibers. Well-fitted shoes are recommended to reduce the risk of pressure-induced necrosis. In some patients, customized footwear or orthotic devices (e.g., for the patient with excessive callous formation or bony deformities) are indicated. The patient is advised to inspect the skin of the feet frequently so minor abrasions can be addressed promptly. High-grade graduated elastic stockings should generally be avoided because they can restrict cutaneous blood flow.

In patients with ischemia at rest, conservative measures include placing the affected limb in a dependent position (i.e., below heart level) to increase perfusion pressure and oxygen tension in ischemic tissues. If there is edema, which may impair healing, the limb is kept horizontal instead. Sheepskin should be placed beneath the heels of the feet to prevent skin breakdown at these sites. A footboard should be used to cradle the blankets over the feet in a fashion that minimizes frictional trauma. Alternatively, protective boots may be used. Wisps of cotton or lambswool inserted between the toes help protect the digits from intertriginous friction and moisture. Gentle warmth is recommended to minimize vasoconstriction, but excessive heat should be avoided. Tinea pedis should be treated with appropriate antimicrobial preparations to reduce the risk of cutaneous breakdown leading to bacterial superinfection. Caution is advised in the use of topical medications because of the possibility of local inflammatory reactions. Open sores should be kept clean, and deep cultures should be obtained (also see Chapter 60). Antibiotic medications are not always effective, in part because of impaired delivery to ischemic tissue. Plain roentgenographic examinations or magnetic resonance imaging (MRI) of underlying bone may be helpful in assessing the possibility of osteomyelitis, for which antibiotic therapy generally is given.

Improvement of Function and Quality of Life

Treatment of Intermittent Claudication and Critical Limb Ischemia

Physical and pharmacological therapies should be considered in the treatment plan of patients with symptomatic PAD. These include supervised exercise rehabilitation and pharmacotherapy. Drugs available for the treatment of intermittent claudication include cilostazol and pentoxifylline. Investigative pharmacotherapies include prostaglandins (PGs), metabolic agents, angiogenic growth factors, stem cell therapy, and statins. The evidence supporting and refuting the efficacy of drug therapy for intermittent claudication and CLI is reviewed subsequently. Endovascular and surgical reconstructions for the treatment of disabling claudication are reviewed in Chapters 20 and 21.

Exercise Training

Supervised exercise training programs improve walking duration, speed, and walking distance in patients with intermittent claudication. Although supervised exercise therapy has been shown to be highly cost-effective compared to catheter-based revascularization for treatment of lower-extremity claudication, it is not widely available owing to a lack of reimbursement by most third-party payers in the United States.[110,111] Two separate meta-analyses have supported the efficacy of supervised exercise training. One meta-analysis of 21 randomized and nonrandomized trials found that pain-free walking distance and maximal walking distance increased by 180% and 120%, respectively.[112] Another meta-analysis that included 10 randomized trials found that supervised exercise training improved maximal walking distance by 150%.[113] Strength or resistance training is not as effective as treadmill training in improving walking distances in patients with claudication.[114] In the recently published Claudication: Exercise Versus Endoluminal Revascularization (CLEVER) study,

randomization to supervised exercise training was associated with improved maximal walking time at 6 months follow-up compared to endovascular therapy or optimal medical therapy among patients with aortoiliac occlusive disease[115]. Supervised exercise training has also been shown to improve quality of life among patients with PAD and either claudication or atypical leg symptoms.[114] Unsupervised exercise training programs are not as effective as supervised programs.[116,117] Most comparative studies have found that home-based unsupervised exercise is not as effective as supervised exercise training. A recent study, however, did observe comparable improvement in walking time between home-based exercise coupled with activity monitoring and supervised exercise training.[116]

Several mechanisms have been proposed to explain the improvement in walking distance that results from exercise training. These include collateral blood vessel development, enhancement in endothelium-dependent nitric oxide (NO)-mediated vasodilation of the microcirculation, improved hemorrheology, increased oxidative capacity of calf skeletal muscle, and better walking biomechanics.[119] Exercise training has been found to improve collateral blood flow in animal models of hindlimb ischemia, as well as capillary density in humans.[120–122] Exercise-induced angiogenesis has been attributed to up-regulation of angiogenic growth factors such as vascular endothelial growth factor (VEGF).[123,124] Increased expression and activity of endothelial nitric oxide synthase (eNOS) and production of NO may contribute to angiogenesis.[121,123,125,126] In humans, several studies have found that exercise training improves maximal calf blood flow following exercise.[127,128] Similarly, exercise training improves calf blood flow during reactive hyperemia following an ischemic stimulus. There was no effect of exercise training on resting calf blood flow in these studies. Exercise training enhances endothelium-dependent vasodilation in peripheral conduit arteries, and thereby may contribute to improved blood flow and walking time in claudicants.[114,129,130] Improvement in skeletal muscle metabolic function, and specifically oxidative capacity, occurs with exercise training and may be relevant to the improvement in walking capacity experienced by patients with intermittent claudication.[131,132] Also, exercise training may improve walking distance by altering biomechanics and adapting patterns of walking that are more efficient, engaging skeletal muscle less affected by ischemia, and improving gait stability.[133]

A number of novel approaches to exercise training for improvement of functional capacity for patients with PAD are currently under investigation, including supervised interval training, home-based monitored exercise programs, and arm ergometry.[118,134–137]

RECOMMENDATIONS

In the ACC/AHA PAD guidelines, a program of supervised exercise training is recommended as an initial treatment modality for patients with intermittent claudication (class I).[1] Exercise programs should use a treadmill or a track and take place in sessions of 45 to 60 minutes at least 3 times a week for a minimum of 12 weeks. Prior to beginning exercise rehabilitation, patients should undergo a comprehensive cardiovascular risk assessment that includes a history, physical examination, and ascertainment of all relevant atherosclerotic risk factors. An electrocardiogram (ECG)-monitored exercise tolerance test tailored to the patient's symptoms and ability should be performed to assess development of any exercise-induced cardiac symptoms, heart rate and blood pressure responses, ST-segment depression, and arrhythmias. It also may serve as a baseline evaluation of the time to onset of claudication, and maximal walking time tolerated on the treadmill. During the training session, patients should be encouraged to walk until symptoms of moderate severity develop. Following a rest period and resolution of symptoms, walking should resume until symptoms recur. This cycle should be repeated as many times as needed during the 45- to 60-minute period. For patients unable to participate in a supervised exercise training program, a home-based walking program is recommended.

Vasodilator Drugs

Vasodilator drugs have undergone extensive investigation for treatment of patients with claudication and critical limb ischemia. It is tempting to assume that treatment with a medication that reduces arteriolar resistance would be as effective for patients with PAD as nitrates and calcium channel blockers are for patients with angina. In general, however, vasodilator drug therapy has been disappointing for relief of intermittent claudication. Differences in the pathophysiology of limb and myocardial ischemia may promote insight into the disparate efficiency of vasodilator drugs. Vasodilator therapy may decrease myocardial oxygen demand, but is not likely to affect skeletal muscle oxygen demand. Therefore, to be effective, vasodilators would have to improve the blood supply to exercising muscle.

When an obstructive arterial lesion produces critical stenosis, distal perfusion pressure is reduced (see Chapter 17). Intramuscular (IM) arterioles normally dilate in response to the metabolic demands of limb exercise, but flow augmentation is blunted in patients with proximal stenotic disease. Also, distal pressure falls during exercise, leading to accumulation of the ischemic metabolites believed to mediate the symptom of claudication. These substances potentiate local vasodilation and perfusion pressure falls, no longer balancing the extravascular compressive force exerted by exercising muscle within the tissue compartment. The distal vasculature virtually collapses under these circumstances, and this mechanism may not be mitigated by vasodilator therapy. Indeed, vasodilator drugs, including β-adrenergic agonists (isoproterenol, nylidrin), α-adrenergic antagonists (reserpine, guanethidine, tolazoline), calcium channel blockers, nitrates, and others (isoxsuprine, cyclandelate) have been evaluated in clinical trials. None increases blood flow in exercising skeletal muscle subtended by significant arterial obstructive lesions, nor do any of these improve symptoms of intermittent claudication or objective measures of exercise capacity. Nonetheless, one drug with vasodilator properties, cilostazol, has been reported to improve walking distance in patients with claudication.

CILOSTAZOL

Cilostazol was approved by the U.S. Food and Drug Administration (FDA) in 1999 for use in patients with intermittent claudication. As a phosphodiesterase (PDE) III inhibitor, cilostazol increases cyclic adenosine monophosphate (cAMP), causes vasodilation, and inhibits platelet aggregation.[138–141] The precise mechanism of action whereby cilostazol may improve symptoms of claudication, however, is not known. In a pooled analysis of 2491 patients in nine trials, cilostazol (100 mg twice daily) increased maximal walking distance by approximately 50% compared to 24% for placebo, corresponding to an absolute improvement of 42 meters more than the improvement with placebo[142] (Fig. 19-6). The efficacy of cilostazol compared to placebo among patients with CLI has not been evaluated, although observational studies have reported improvements in lower-extremity microcirculation and amputation-free survival among cilostazol-treated patients.[143,144]

Cilostazol is primarily metabolized in the liver by the CYP3A4 and CYP2C19 isoenzymes. Prescription of low-dose (50 mg twice daily) cilostazol is recommended for patients who concurrently take medications that are known to inhibit CYP3A4 or CYP2C19, including diltiazem, fluoxetine, fluconazole, erythromycin, and other macrolide antibiotics (CYP3A4), as well as omeprazole (CYP2C19).[145] Side effects of cilostazol are relatively common and include headache in approximately 25%, palpitations in approximately 15%, and diarrhea or abnormal stool in 15% to 20%.[146] The FDA has advised that cilostazol not be administered to patients with CHF of any severity.[145] The reason for this advisory is that when studied in patients with congestive heart failure, other PDE III inhibitors, such as milrinone or vesnarinone, were associated with increased mortality.[147,148] Cilostazol has not been associated with increased mortality rates, but it has not been studied in a heart failure population.

In the Cilostazol: A Study in Long-Term Effects (CASTLE) trial, 1435 patients with claudication were randomized to receive cilostazol (100 mg twice daily) or placebo and followed for adverse events.[149] At approximately 3 years of follow-up, there was no excess of death or serious bleeding events among those randomized to cilostazol compared to placebo. Importantly, the discontinuation rate of study medication was very high in this trial (>60%), perhaps reflective of the side effect profile of cilostazol.

Recommendations

Cilostazol is an effective therapy to improve walking distance in patients with intermittent claudication, and a therapeutic trial of cilostazol is recommended in the ACC/AHA PAD guidelines (class I).[1] Physicians should be aware of the side effect profile of this drug and are advised not to administer this medication to patients with congestive heart failure.

PROSTAGLANDINS

Vasodilator PGs have undergone somewhat extensive investigation for the treatment of patients with intermittent claudication or critical limb ischemia. This class of drugs includes prostaglandin E_1 (PGE1), prostacyclin (PGI_2), and its analogs beraprost and

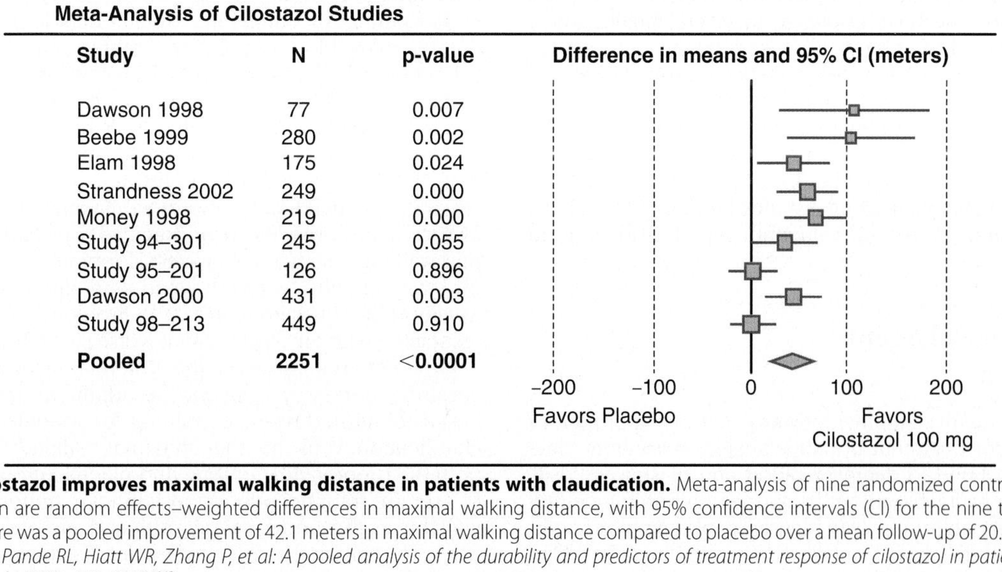

Meta-Analysis of Cilostazol Studies

Study	N	p-value	Difference in means and 95% CI (meters)
Dawson 1998	77	0.007	
Beebe 1999	280	0.002	
Elam 1998	175	0.024	
Strandness 2002	249	0.000	
Money 1998	219	0.000	
Study 94–301	245	0.055	
Study 95–201	126	0.896	
Dawson 2000	431	0.003	
Study 98–213	449	0.910	
Pooled	**2251**	**<0.0001**	

FIGURE 19-6 Cilostazol improves maximal walking distance in patients with claudication. Meta-analysis of nine randomized controlled trials including 1258 subjects. Shown are random effects–weighted differences in maximal walking distance, with 95% confidence intervals (CI) for the nine trials and the pooled treatment effect. There was a pooled improvement of 42.1 meters in maximal walking distance compared to placebo over a mean follow-up of 20.4 weeks. *(Reproduced with permission from Pande RL, Hiatt WR, Zhang P, et al: A pooled analysis of the durability and predictors of treatment response of cilostazol in patients with intermittent claudication. Vasc Med 15:181–188, 2010.)*[142]

iloprost. The efficacy of vasodilator PGs administered intraarterially (IA) or intravenously (IV) has been assessed in patients with intermittent claudication and in patients with critical limb ischemia. A systematic review of clinical trials of prostanoids for treatment of claudication found that short-term IA or IV administration of PGE1 to patients with intermittent claudication appeared to increase walking distance, whereas IV PGI$_2$ or its analog taprostene was found not to improve walking distance.[150] Two placebo-controlled trials of oral beraprost administered for 6 months had conflicting results, one showing improvement and one showing no change in pain-free or maximal walking distance.[151,152] In one multicenter placebo-controlled trial, iloprost administered for 6 months was no more effective than placebo in improving pain-free or maximal walking distance among patients with intermittent claudication.[153]

Short-term (i.e., 3-4 days) IA or IV administration of PGE1, iloprost, or ciprostene is not effective in ameliorating critical limb ischemia,[154] but when administered parenterally for longer periods of time (7-28 days) may reduce pain, ulcer size, or risk of amputation.[154] The Ischemia Cronica degli Arti Inferiori study assessed the efficacy of IV PGE1 or placebo in 1560 patients with critical limb ischemia. The relative risk of death, major amputation or persistence of critical limb ischemia, acute MI, or stroke was significantly reduced by 13% at the time of hospital discharge but not at 6 months. After 6 months of treatment, there was no difference between groups in death or amputation, but there was a greater chance of resolution of CLI in those survivors who did not have amputation.[155] Two randomized placebo-controlled studies assessed the effect of oral iloprost on critical limb ischemia.[156] There was no apparent benefit of iloprost in terms of reducing the risk of the primary endpoint of amputation or death, but there was a modest benefit in terms of resolution of ulcers and rest pain in those who survived without amputation. In a recent trial of patients with critical limb ischemia, twice-daily infusion of taprostene compared with placebo did not improve pain control, wound healing, or amputation rates.[157] Side effects of PGs include flushing, headache, and gastrointestinal distress.

Recommendations

The use of oral or IV vasodilator PGs, such as beraprost and iloprost, is not recommended to improve walking distance in patients with intermittent claudication.[1] In addition, these drugs are not effective therapy to reduce the risk of amputation or death in patients with critical limb ischemia.

CALCIUM CHANNEL BLOCKERS

The efficacy of calcium channel blockers in patients with intermittent claudication has been evaluated in several small clinical trials. Nifedipine failed to improve exercise tolerance as assessed by pedal ergometry in a randomized placebo-controlled trial.[158] In another placebo-controlled trial comparing nifedipine with atenolol, alone or in combination, nifedipine did not improve pain-free or absolute walking distance.[41] In one placebo-controlled dose-ranging crossover trial, verapamil improved pain-free walking distance by 29% and maximal walking distance by 49%.[159] There have been no subsequent trials with verapamil reported to confirm these findings.

Hemorrheological Agents

PENTOXIFYLLINE

Pentoxifylline is a methylxanthine derivative that was approved by the FDA in 1984 for treatment of patients with intermittent claudication. It is purported to decrease blood and plasma viscosity, improve red and white blood cell deformability, inhibit neutrophil adhesion and activation, and decrease plasma fibrinogen, although not all studies have confirmed these findings.[160–162] One meta-analysis of 11 trials comprising 612 patients found that pentoxifylline (600-1200 mg daily) improved pain-free walking distance by 29 meters and maximal claudication distance by 48 meters.[163] Another meta-analysis of six randomized double-blinded placebo-controlled trials found that pentoxifylline improved pain-free walking distance by 21 meters and maximal claudication distance by 44 meters.[164] The meta-analyses did not include a large randomized placebo-controlled trial of 698 patients with intermittent claudication, of whom 232 received pentoxifylline, 227 received cilostazol, and 239 received placebo.[146] In this trial, there was no difference in pain-free walking distance or maximal walking distance between the pentoxifylline- and placebo-treated groups after 24 weeks of treatment. Pain-free and maximal walking distance increased in the cilostazol group compared with both placebo and pentoxifylline. In a trial of iloprost versus pentoxifylline versus placebo among patients with intermittent claudication, there was a 14% improvement in maximal walking distance among patients randomized to pentoxifylline compared to placebo.[153]

The efficacy of pentoxifylline to improve CLI has been studied in two placebo-controlled trials.[165,166] In one study, patients with CLI were randomized to treatment with IV pentoxifylline (600 mg twice daily) or placebo for up to 21 days. Severity of rest pain was significantly reduced in patients treated with pentoxifylline compared with those who received a placebo.[165] Yet, in another placebo-controlled trial in which pentoxifylline (600 mg intravenously) was administered to patients with critical limb ischemia, there was no significant difference in pain relief between the placebo and pentoxifylline treatment groups.[166] It is not known whether pentoxifylline facilitates ulcer healing or reduces risk of amputation in patients with critical limb ischemia. Side effects of pentoxifylline include dyspepsia, nausea, vomiting, eructation, flatus, bloating, and dizziness. Side effects requiring discontinuation of the drug occur in up to 9.6% of patients.

Recommendations

The clinical efficacy of pentoxifylline for intermittent claudication is not well established. Improvement in claudication distance is very modest at best, and falls within a range that may not be clinically recognized by the patient. Nonetheless, pentoxifylline may be considered as a second-line alternative to cilostazol in the ACC/AHA PAD guidelines for treating intermittent claudication (class IIb) and is the only other FDA-approved agent for this indication.[1] Pentoxifylline is not useful in the treatment of critical limb ischemia.

Metabolic Agents

Symptoms of intermittent claudication may be related in part to abnormalities in skeletal muscle metabolism (see Chapter 17). Therefore, drugs that favorably affect oxidative metabolism may confer benefit by enhancing skeletal muscle function even without improving blood supply. For example, L-carnitine and its derivative propionyl-L-carnitine enhance glucose oxidation and oxidative metabolism via the Krebs cycle by providing a source of carnitine.[167] Three placebo-controlled trials have assessed the efficacy of propionyl-L-carnitine in patients with intermittent claudication.[168–170] In these studies, propionyl-L-carnitine administered as a 1-g oral dose twice daily improved maximal walking distance by 54% to 73%, whereas those randomized to placebo increased maximal walking distance 25% to 46%. Propionyl-L-carnitine improved physical function, walking speed, and distance as assessed by quality-of-life questionnaires.[168,171] Propionyl-L-carnitine was not associated with any significant adverse side effects.

A recent trial assessed the potential benefit of propionyl-L-carnitine therapy (vs. placebo) as adjunctive treatment to home-based monitored exercise training for patients with intermittent claudication.[172] In this trial, maximal walking time increased in both the propionyl-L-carnitine and placebo groups after 6 months of exercise training, with a nonsignificant trend toward improved walking in the propionyl-L-carnitine group. Propionyl-L-carnitine has potential merit for treating intermittent claudication, but should be considered investigational at this time.

Ranolazine is a piperazine derivative that inhibits fatty acid oxidation, activates pyruvate dehydrogenase, and shifts metabolism toward carbohydrate oxidation, thereby increasing efficiency of oxygen utilization.[173] Ranolazine improves exercise capacity and decreases angina frequency in patients with CAD and was associated with improvement in pain-free walking time (vs. placebo) among patients with intermittent claudication in a single-center pilot study.[174–176]

Angiogenic Growth Factors

Angiogenic growth factors have undergone investigation for treatment of PAD. This class of drugs includes VEGF, fibroblast growth factor (FGF), hepatocyte growth factor (HGF), and hypoxia-inducible factor-1α (HIF-1α). They may be administered as recombinant proteins or by gene transfer using plasmid deoxyribonucleic acid (DNA) or an adenoviral vector that encodes the angiogenic growth factor.[177] Vascular endothelial growth factor, FGF, and HIF-1α increase collateral blood vessels and improve blood flow in animal models of hindlimb ischemia.[178–181] Therefore, angiogenic growth factors have the potential to promote collateral blood vessel formation and thereby increase blood flow to the ischemic limbs of patients with PAD.

VASCULAR ENDOTHELIAL GROWTH FACTOR

Several nonrandomized open-label studies found that IA gene transfer therapy of $pHVEGF_{165}$ increased collateral blood vessels, as assessed by MRI or digital subtraction angiography (DSA) in patients with PAD.[182,183] Also, $pHVEGF_{165}$ administration improved blood flow and increased ABI in some patients who participated in these trials.[182] A randomized placebo-controlled trial of IM $VEGF_{121}$ was conducted (DSA) in patients with unilateral intermittent claudication. There was no significant improvement in pain-free or maximal walking distance after 12 or 26 weeks.[184]

FIBROBLAST GROWTH FACTOR

Recombinant FGF2 administered directly into the femoral artery was evaluated in a placebo-controlled study.[185] Patients were randomized to receive FGF2 on one occasion only, on two occasions 30 days apart, or placebo. One-time administration of FGF2 increased peak walking time at 90 days by 34% compared with 14% for placebo. Yet, there was no significant improvement in peak walking time compared with placebo when FGF2 was administered on two occasions. A nonrandomized study of patients with CLI observed that IM injection of plasmid DNA encoding FGF1 reduced pain and ulcer size and increased the ABI.[186] In a phase 2 placebo-controlled study of patients with critical limb ischemia, IM administration of FGF1 using a plasmid vector did not improve ulcer healing, the primary endpoint, but did decrease secondary endpoints including all amputations and the composite of major amputation and death.[187] However, in a follow-up phase 3 study of patients with critical limb IM, FGF1 did not decrease amputation-free survival.[188]

OTHER ANGIOGENIC GROWTH FACTORS

Hepatocyte growth factor using a plasmid vector and given as an IM injection increased $TcPO_2$ but did not improve pain, heal ulcers, or decrease amputations in a placebo-controlled trial of patients with critical limb ischemia.[189]

Hypoxia-inducible factor-1α is an inducible transcriptional regulatory factor. In conditions of low oxygen tension, HIF-1α binds to hypoxia-responsive elements in the promoter/enhancer region of target genes, inducing those encoding VEGF-A, platelet-derived growth factor (PDGF), angiotensin-1, and inducible nitric oxide synthase (iNOS).[190–192] In a phase 1 study, 34 patients with CLI with no revascularization options received an IM injection of an adenovirus encoding HIF-1α. The injections were well tolerated and

associated with complete wound healing in 5 of 18 patients in 1 year.[193] A subsequent trial randomized patients with intermittent claudication to placebo or one of three doses of the adenovirus encoding HIF-1α and found no benefit of HIF-1α on peak walking time, claudication onset time, or ABI up to 1 year after randomization.[194]

Stem Cell Therapy

Infusion of endothelial progenitor cells into mice in an experiment model of hindlimb ischemia has been shown to improve blood flow and capillary density in the ischemic hindlimb and reduce the rate of limb loss.[195] Bone marrow mononuclear cells include endothelial progenitor cells. Intramuscular injection of autologous bone marrow–derived mononuclear cells improved collateral blood vessel formation in animal models of myocardial and hindlimb ischemia.[196,197] Consequently, the effect of autologous implantation of bone marrow–derived mononuclear cells was studied in patients with PAD manifested as limb ischemia.[198] Injection of bone marrow mononuclear cells, compared with peripheral blood mononuclear cells, reduced rest pain and improved pain-free walking time. The improvement was sustained for 24 weeks. Angiographic evidence of collateral blood vessel formation was present in many of the patients who received bone marrow–derived mononuclear cells. Additional data supporting potential angiogenic benefit of IM injection or IA infusion of bone marrow–derived mononuclear cells or bone marrow–derived mesenchymal cells for patients with CLI and limited revascularization options have been reported in multiple small single-center early phase trials.[199–204] Many of these studies reported noninvasive testing (e.g., ABI, TBI, plethysmography) rather than angiography to document evidence of angiogenesis.

Several trials are planned or are in progress. The Use of Vascular Repair Cells in Patients with Peripheral Arterial Disease to Treat Critical Limb Ischemia (RESTORE-CLI) trial has randomized 86 patients to stem and progenitor cell therapy with lower-extremity (IM injection) versus a sham control procedure (injection of an electrolyte solution) at 18 U.S. centers.[205] In a published interim analysis, stem cell therapy was associated with improved amputation-free survival, and the results of the completed study are awaited. The Rejuvenating Endothelial Progenitor Cells via Transcutaneous Intraarterial Supplementation (JUVENTAS) trial is another multicenter randomized controlled trial of stem cell therapy in CLI that is currently underway.[206] In JUVENTAS, bone marrow–derived mononuclear cells (vs. placebo) will be administered to the lower extremities through IA infusion, and patients will be followed for the primary endpoint of lower-extremity amputation at 6 months.

Statins

As discussed earlier in this chapter, lipid-lowering therapy with statins reduces the risk of adverse cardiovascular events in patients with atherosclerosis, including those with PAD. Post hoc analysis of the 4S found that simvastatin reduced the risk of new or worsening claudication.[28] Several prospective studies found that statin therapy improved symptoms of claudication in patients with intermittent claudication. One placebo-controlled trial found that atorvastatin (80 mg/day) for 12 months improved pain-free walking time by 63%, compared with 38% in the placebo group[207] (Fig. 19-7). In other studies, 6 and 12 months of treatment with simvastatin (40 mg/day) improved pain-free and maximal walking distance.[208,209] The efficacy of lipid lowering therapy on walking time was not demonstrated, however, in another trial of patients with claudication who were randomized to lovastatin (40 mg) plus niacin 2000 mg daily, lovastatin plus niacin 1000 mg daily, or diet intervention.[210] After 28 weeks of follow-up, there was no significant difference in treadmill walking times among the three treatment groups.

There are several potential mechanisms whereby statin therapy may improve symptoms of claudication. These include

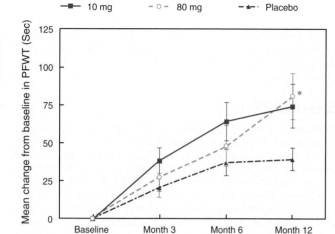

FIGURE 19-7   Atorvastatin improves pain-free walking time *(PFWT)* in patients with intermittent claudication. *, $P = 0.025$ for 80-mg dose at 12 months. *(Reproduced with permission from Mohler ER 3 rd, Hiatt WR, Creager MA: Cholesterol reduction with atorvastatin improves walking distance in patients with peripheral arterial disease. Circulation 108:1481–1486, 2003.)[207]*

reduction in plaque size, improvement in vasomotor regulation of blood flow (particularly in the microcirculation), promotion of angiogenesis, and increased skeletal muscle metabolic function. It is not likely that reduction of plaque size accounts for the improvement in symptoms. This is because angiographic studies have shown that treatment with statins induces only very mild changes in vascular lumen size, and these are unlikely to affect blood flow through a stenotic artery.[211] In the studies that have examined the effect of statins on patients with claudication, there have been no, or only very minor, changes in the ABI.[207,209] Endothelial function, particularly in the peripheral resistance vessels, is impaired in patients with atherosclerosis, including those with PAD.[212] Statin therapy has been shown to improve endothelial function in patients with CAD.[213,214] Therefore, statin therapy may improve blood flow to the microcirculation and thereby ameliorate symptoms of claudication. Animal studies have found that hypercholesterolemia inhibits angiogenesis.[215] This inhibition may be reduced when cholesterol concentration is reduced by statin therapy, enabling collateral formation to occur. In addition, statins have been shown to increase circulating endothelial progenitor cells independent of cholesterol reduction, and thereby may have a proangiogenic effect.[216] Favorable effects on metabolic function are not likely to account for the observed effects on walking time. Therapy with simvastatin, alone or in combination with ezetimibe, did not improve phosphocreatine recovery time, as assessed by phosphorus-31 magnetic resonance spectroscopy (MRS).[217]

Miscellaneous Pharmacological Agents

A number of additional pharmacological agents have been studied as potential therapies for intermittent claudication in recent clinical trials, but unfortunately none has yielded a consistently positive efficacy signal. Multiple serotonin receptor antagonists have been studied with mixed, and largely negative, clinical results to date.[218,219] The antichlamydial antibiotic rifalazil had no significant effect on treadmill walking times or quality-of-life parameters compared to placebo.[220]

Nutraceuticals and Alternative Therapies

Dietary supplements with nutrients, herbs, and vitamins such as L-arginine, ginkgo biloba, and vitamin E, as well as ethylenediaminetetraacetic acid (EDTA), have been studied as complementary therapeutic strategies to improve functional capacity in patients with intermittent claudication. The available evidence supporting

and refuting these holistic therapies is reviewed here because vascular specialists are frequently queried by their patients about these remedies.

L-ARGININE

Endothelium-derived NO is synthesized from its precursor, L-arginine, by eNOS.[221] Endothelium-dependent vasodilation, mediated by NO, contributes to the physiological regulation of blood flow at rest and during exercise.[222–224] Nitric oxide activates guanylyl cyclase on subjacent vascular smooth muscle and increases cyclic guanosine monophosphate (cGMP) and thereby causes vasodilation. Endothelium-dependent vasodilation is abnormal in conduit and resistance vessels in patients with PAD.[212]

In one study, L-arginine administered IV at a dose of 8 g twice daily for 3 weeks improved pain-free walking distance by 230% and maximal walking distance by 155%.[225] Another study examined the effect of a food bar containing L-arginine (3.3 g) and B-complex and antioxidant vitamins on walking distance in patients with intermittent claudication.[226] Pain-free and maximal walking distance improved by 66% and 23%, respectively, following 2 weeks of therapy in patients eating two bars per day. In a larger placebo-controlled trial, 80 patients with intermittent claudication were randomized to one of four daily L-arginine doses (0, 3, 6, or 9 g) administered in thrice-daily divided doses over a 12-week period.[227] There was less of a beneficial trend of L-arginine therapy on maximal walking distance among the patients randomized to the 6-g and 9-g treatment arms. The subsequent Nitric Oxide in Peripheral Arterial Insufficiency (NO-PAIN) randomized 133 claudicants to placebo versus 3 grams daily of oral L-arginine therapy that was continued for 6 months.[228] The findings of this trial were dramatic: not only was this a negative study, but randomization L-arginine treatment was associated with less brachial artery flow-mediated vasodilation and less improvement in treadmill walking distance than in the placebo group. In light of these data, long-term L-arginine supplementation is not recommended for patients with intermittent claudication.

VITAMIN E

Vitamin E (α-tocopherol) is a lipid-soluble antioxidant that has undergone evaluation in patients with intermittent claudication. It inhibits oxidation of polyunsaturated fatty acid. Vitamin E may improve erythrocyte deformability and improve blood flow through the microcirculation because polyunsaturated fatty acids are incorporated into the erythrocyte membrane. A Cochrane systematic review evaluated five placebo-controlled trials of vitamin E in patients with intermittent claudication.[229] The trials, conducted between 1953 and 1975, were small and measured different outcomes, precluding any conclusions regarding the efficacy of vitamin E for intermittent claudication. Both the Heart Protection Study (HPS) and the HOPE study failed to demonstrate any efficacy of vitamin E on adverse cardiovascular events in patients with atherosclerosis, including those with PAD.[27,49] Therefore, vitamin E is not recommended as therapy for patients with PAD, including those with intermittent claudication.

GINKGO BILOBA

Ginkgo biloba is an herb whose major constituents include flavonoids and terpene lactones, such as ginkgolides and bilobalide. Ginkgo may have antioxidant, antiplatelet, and hemorrheological actions.[230] It is one of the top-selling herbal medicinal products in the United States.

A meta-analysis of eight randomized placebo-controlled trials found that in recipients of ginkgo, the pain-free claudication distance was 34 meters more than in patients receiving placebo.[231] In the largest trial, 24 weeks of ginkgo treatment improved pain-free and maximal walking distance by 45 and 61 meters, respectively, whereas placebo improved these by 21 and 25 meters, respectively.[232] Doses employed in clinical trials range from 120 to 320 mg/day. The most common dosage is 40 mg 3 times daily. Potential adverse effects of ginkgo include gastro-intestinal symptoms, headache, nausea, vomiting, bleeding, or allergic skin reactions.[230] *Ginkgo biloba* is also associated with adverse interactions with many common prescription medications. It has been associated with cerebral hemorrhage in case reports.[233] *Ginkgo biloba* may be considered as an alternative therapy for treatment of claudication, but its efficacy is probably of marginal clinical importance.

DISODIUM ETHYLENEDIAMINETETRAACETIC ACID (EDTA)

EDTA combines with polyvalent cations, including calcium ions, to form a soluble nonionic complex that can be excreted. It requires IV administration and is usually administered two or more times a week. The rationale for using EDTA in patients with atherosclerosis, including those with PAD, is to leech calcium out of atherosclerotic plaque, induce plaque regression, and reduce the severity of stenosis. Also, EDTA may decrease metal ion-dependent formation of reactive oxygen species (ROS) and metal ion-dependent lipid peroxidation.[234] There is limited biological evidence to support its efficacy in atherosclerosis.[235]

The Program to Assess Alternative Treatment Strategies to Achieve Health (PATCH) assessed the effect of EDTA on endothelium-dependent vasodilation in patients with CAD. Up to 33 treatments of IV EDTA over a 6-month period caused no changes in peripheral endothelial function.[236] One clinical trial found no effect of EDTA on the severity of atherosclerosis in patients with PAD.[237] Two systematic reviews evaluated four placebo-controlled trials that assessed the efficacy of EDTA in patients with intermittent claudication.[238,239] These reviews found no evidence that EDTA improves pain-free or maximal walking distance in patients with intermittent claudication.

Potential serious adverse effects of EDTA include hypocalcemia, renal insufficiency, and proteinuria. Additional side effects include gastrointestinal and musculoskeletal symptoms, hypertension, tachycardia, and fever. Based on lack of efficacy as well as safety concerns, EDTA should not be used to treat patients with intermittent claudication.

Conclusions

Patients with PAD are at increased risk for adverse cardiovascular events such as MI, stroke, and death and have impaired functional capacity and qualify of life. In severe circumstances, limb viability is threatened. Comprehensive care of the PAD patient must address all aspects of care: prevention of cardiovascular events, foot care, and therapies to improve leg symptoms. Risk factor modification and antiplatelet therapy are critical components of the management of all patients with PAD. Supervised exercise rehabilitation and the PDE inhibitor cilostazol improve walking distance in patients with claudication. Unfortunately, the pharmacological armamentarium for treatment of claudication is limited. Available medical therapies are not effective in preserving limb viability for patients with critical limb ischemia, so these patients should be considered for revascularization, as reviewed in the next two chapters. Promising new therapies for claudication and critical limb ischemia, particularly stem cell therapy, are undergoing extensive clinical investigation.

REFERENCES

1. Hirsch AT, Haskal ZJ, Hertzer NR, et al: ACC/AHA 2005 practice guidelines for the management of patients with peripheral arterial disease (lower extremity, renal, mesenteric, and abdominal aortic): a collaborative report from the American Association for Vascular Surgery/Society for Vascular Surgery, Society for Cardiovascular Angiography and Interventions, Society for Vascular Medicine and Biology, Society of Interventional Radiology, and the ACC/AHA Task Force on Practice Guidelines (Writing Committee to Develop Guidelines for the Management of Patients With Peripheral Arterial Disease): endorsed by the American Association of Cardiovascular and Pulmonary Rehabilitation; National Heart, Lung, and Blood Institute; Society for Vascular Nursing; TransAtlantic Inter-Society Consensus; and Vascular Disease Foundation, Circulation 113:e463–e654, 2006.
2. Rooke TW, Hirsch AT, Misra S, et al: 2011 ACCF/AHA focused update of the guideline for the management of patients with peripheral artery disease (updating the 2005 guideline): a report of the American College of Cardiology Foundation/American Heart Association Task Force on Practice Guidelines, Circulation 124:2020–2045, 2011.
3. Gardner AW: The effect of cigarette smoking on exercise capacity in patients with intermittent claudication, Vasc Med 1:181–186, 1996.
4. Quick CR, Cotton LT: The measured effect of stopping smoking on intermittent claudication, Br J Surg 69(Suppl):S24–S26, 1982.
5. Jonason T, Bergstrom R: Cessation of smoking in patients with intermittent claudication. Effects on the risk of peripheral vascular complications, myocardial infarction and mortality, Acta Med Scand 221:253–260, 1987.
6. Powell JT, Greenhalgh RM: Changing the smoking habit and its influence on the management of vascular disease, Acta Chir Scand Suppl 555:99–103, 1990.
7. Faulkner KW, House AK, Castleden WM: The effect of cessation of smoking on the accumulative survival rates of patients with symptomatic peripheral vascular disease, Med J Aust 1:217–219, 1983.
8. Lassila R, Lepantalo M: Cigarette smoking and the outcome after lower limb arterial surgery, Acta Chir Scand 154:635–640, 1988.
9. Law M, Tang JL: An analysis of the effectiveness of interventions intended to help people stop smoking, Arch Intern Med 155:1933–1941, 1995.
10. Hennrikus D, Joseph AM, Lando HA, et al: Effectiveness of a smoking cessation program for peripheral artery disease patients: a randomized controlled trial, J Am Coll Cardiol 56:2105–2112, 2010.
11. Jorenby DE, Leischow SJ, Nides MA, et al: A controlled trial of sustained-release bupropion, a nicotine patch, or both for smoking cessation, N Engl J Med 340:685–691, 1999.
12. Jorenby DE, Hays JT, Rigotti NA, et al: Efficacy of varenicline, an alpha4beta2 nicotinic acetylcholine receptor partial agonist, vs. placebo or sustained-release bupropion for smoking cessation: a randomized controlled trial, JAMA 296:56–63, 2006.
13. Rigotti NA, Pipe AL, Benowitz NL, et al: Efficacy and safety of varenicline for smoking cessation in patients with cardiovascular disease: a randomized trial, Circulation 121:221–229, 2011.
14. Varenicline package insert, 2011Pfizer, Inc.
15. Bupropion (Zyban) package insert, 2011GlaxoSmithKline.
16. Bowlin SJ, Medalie JH, Flocke SA, et al: Epidemiology of intermittent claudication in middle-aged men, Am J Epidemiol 140:418–430, 1994.
17. Newman AB, Siscovick DS, Manolio TA, et al: Ankle-arm index as a marker of atherosclerosis in the Cardiovascular Health Study. Cardiovascular Heart Study (CHS) Collaborative Research Group, Circulation 88:837–845, 1993.
18. Murabito JM, D'Agostino RB, Silbershatz H, et al: Intermittent claudication. A risk profile from the Framingham Heart Study, Circulation 96:44–49, 1997.
19. Fowkes FG, Housley E, Riemersma RA, et al: Smoking, lipids, glucose intolerance, and blood pressure as risk factors for peripheral atherosclerosis compared with ischemic heart disease in the Edinburgh Artery Study, Am J Epidemiol 135:331–340, 1992.
20. Mowat BF, Skinner ER, Wilson HM, et al: Alterations in plasma lipids, lipoproteins and high density lipoprotein subfractions in peripheral arterial disease, Atherosclerosis 131: 161–166, 1997.
21. Rubins HB, Robins SJ, Collins D, et al: Gemfibrozil for the secondary prevention of coronary heart disease in men with low levels of high-density lipoprotein cholesterol. Veterans Affairs High-Density Lipoprotein Cholesterol Intervention Trial Study Group, N Engl J Med 341:410–418, 1999.
22. Randomised trial of cholesterol lowering in 4444 patients with coronary heart disease: the Scandinavian Simvastatin Survival Study (4S), Lancet 344:1383–1389, 1994.
23. Sacks FM, Pfeffer MA, Moye LA, et al: The effect of pravastatin on coronary events after myocardial infarction in patients with average cholesterol levels. Cholesterol and Recurrent Events Trial investigators, N Engl J Med 335:1001–1009, 1996.
24. Prevention of cardiovascular events and death with pravastatin in patients with coronary heart disease and a broad range of initial cholesterol levels. The Long-Term Intervention with Pravastatin in Ischaemic Disease (LIPID) Study Group, N Engl J Med 339:1349–1357, 1998.
25. Hirsch AT, Criqui MH, Treat-Jacobson D, et al: Peripheral arterial disease detection, awareness, and treatment in primary care, JAMA 286:1317–1324, 2001.
26. Zheng ZJ, Sharrett AR, Chambless LE, et al: Associations of ankle-brachial index with clinical coronary heart disease, stroke and preclinical carotid and popliteal atherosclerosis: the Atherosclerosis Risk in Communities (ARIC) Study, Atherosclerosis 131:115–125, 1997.
27. Heart Protection Study Collaborative Group: MRC/BHF Heart Protection Study of cholesterol lowering with simvastatin in 20,536 high-risk individuals: a randomised placebo-controlled trial, Lancet 360:7–22, 2002.
28. Pedersen TR, Kjekshus J, Pyorala K, et al: Effect of simvastatin on ischemic signs and symptoms in the Scandinavian simvastatin survival study (4S), Am J Cardiol 81:333–335, 1998.
29. MRC/BHF Heart Protection Study of cholesterol-lowering therapy and of antioxidant vitamin supplementation in a wide range of patients at increased risk of coronary heart disease death: early safety and efficacy experience, Eur Heart J 20:725–741, 1999.
30. Heart Protection Study Collaborative Group: Randomized trial of the effects of cholesterol-lowering with simvastatin on peripheral vascular and other major vascular outcomes in 20,536 people with peripheral arterial disease and other high-risk conditions, J Vasc Surg 45:645–654, 2007 discussion 653–644.
31. Goldbourt U, Yaari S, Medalie JH: Isolated low HDL cholesterol as a risk factor for coronary heart disease mortality. A 21-year follow-up of 8000 men, Arterioscler Thromb Vasc Biol 17:107–113, 1997.
32. Gordon DJ, Rifkind BM: High-density lipoprotein–the clinical implications of recent studies, N Engl J Med 321:1311–1316, 1989.
33. Secondary prevention by raising HDL cholesterol and reducing triglycerides in patients with coronary artery disease: the Bezafibrate Infarction Prevention (BIP) study, Circulation 102:21–27, 2000.

34. Keech A, Simes RJ, Barter P, et al: Effects of long-term fenofibrate therapy on cardiovascular events in 9795 people with type 2 diabetes mellitus (the FIELD study): randomised controlled trial, *Lancet* 366:1849–1861, 2005.

35. Psaty BM, Lumley T, Furberg CD, et al: Health outcomes associated with various antihypertensive therapies used as first-line agents: a network meta-analysis, *JAMA* 289:2534–2544, 2003.

36. Major outcomes in high-risk hypertensive patients randomized to angiotensin-converting enzyme inhibitor or calcium channel blocker vs. diuretic: the Antihypertensive and Lipid-Lowering Treatment to Prevent Heart Attack Trial (ALLHAT), *JAMA* 288:2981–2997, 2002.

37. Lip GY, Makin AJ: Treatment of hypertension in peripheral arterial disease, *Cochrane Database Syst Rev* 2003 CD003075.

38. Frishman WH: Beta-adrenergic receptor blockers. Adverse effects and drug interactions, *Hypertension* 11:II21–II29, 1988.

39. Rodger JC, Sheldon CD, Lerski RA, et al: Intermittent claudication complicating beta-blockade, *BMJ* 1:1125, 1976.

40. Roberts DH, Tsao Y, McLoughlin GA, et al: Placebo-controlled comparison of captopril, atenolol, labetalol, and pindolol in hypertension complicated by intermittent claudication, *Lancet* 2:650–653, 1987.

41. Solomon SA, Ramsay LE, Yeo WW, et al: Beta blockade and intermittent claudication: placebo controlled trial of atenolol and nifedipine and their combination, *BMJ* 303:1100–1104, 1991.

42. Timolol-induced reduction in mortality and reinfarction in patients surviving acute myocardial infarction, *N Engl J Med* 304:801–807, 1981.

43. A randomized trial of propranolol in patients with acute myocardial infarction. I. Mortality results, *JAMA* 247:1707–1714, 1982.

44. Mangano DT, Layug EL, Wallace A, et al: Effect of atenolol on mortality and cardiovascular morbidity after noncardiac surgery. Multicenter Study of Perioperative Ischemia Research Group, *N Engl J Med* 335:1713–1720, 1996.

45. Poldermans D, Boersma E, Bax JJ, et al: The effect of bisoprolol on perioperative mortality and myocardial infarction in high-risk patients undergoing vascular surgery. Dutch Echocardiographic Cardiac Risk Evaluation Applying Stress Echocardiography Study Group, *N Engl J Med* 341:1789–1794, 1999.

46. Radack K, Deck C: Beta-adrenergic blocker therapy does not worsen intermittent claudication in subjects with peripheral arterial disease. A meta-analysis of randomized controlled trials, *Arch Intern Med* 151:1769–1776, 1991.

47. Espinola-Klein C, Weisser G, Jagodzinski A, et al: Beta-blockers in patients with intermittent claudication and arterial hypertension: results from the nebivolol or metoprolol in arterial occlusive disease trial, *Hypertension* 58:148–154, 2011.

48. Diehm C, Pittrow D, Lawall H: Effect of nebivolol vs. hydrochlorothiazide on the walking capacity in hypertensive patients with intermittent claudication, *J Hypertens* 29:1448–1456, 2011.

49. Yusuf S, Sleight P, Pogue J, et al: Effects of an angiotensin-converting-enzyme inhibitor, ramipril, on cardiovascular events in high-risk patients. The Heart Outcomes Prevention Evaluation Study Investigators, *N Engl J Med* 342:145–153, 2000.

50. Overlack A, Adamczak M, Bachmann W, et al: ACE-inhibition with perindopril in essential hypertensive patients with concomitant diseases. The Perindopril Therapeutic Safety Collaborative Research Group, *Am J Med* 97:126–134, 1994.

51. Ahimastos AA, Lawler A, Reid CM, et al: Brief communication: ramipril markedly improves walking ability in patients with peripheral arterial disease: a randomized trial, *Ann Intern Med* 144:660–664, 2006.

52. Estacio RO, Jeffers BW, Hiatt WR, et al: The effect of nisoldipine as compared with enalapril on cardiovascular outcomes in patients with non-insulin-dependent diabetes and hypertension, *N Engl J Med* 338:645–652, 1998.

53. Mehler PS, Coll JR, Estacio R, et al: Intensive blood pressure control reduces the risk of cardiovascular events in patients with peripheral arterial disease and type 2 diabetes, *Circulation* 107:753–756, 2003.

54. The HOPE (Heart Outcomes Prevention Evaluation) Study: the design of a large, simple randomized trial of an angiotensin-converting enzyme inhibitor (ramipril) and vitamin E in patients at high risk of cardiovascular events. The HOPE Study Investigators, *Can J Cardiol* 12:127–137, 1996.

55. Yusuf S, Teo KK, Pogue J, et al: Telmisartan, ramipril, or both in patients at high risk for vascular events, *N Engl J Med* 358:1547–1559, 2008.

56. Adler AI, Stevens RJ, Neil A, et al: UKPDS 59: hyperglycemia and other potentially modifiable risk factors for peripheral vascular disease in type 2 diabetes, *Diabetes Care* 25:894–899, 2002.

57. Meijer WT, Hoes AW, Rutgers D, et al: Peripheral arterial disease in the elderly: the Rotterdam Study, *Arterioscler Thromb Vasc Biol* 18:185–192, 1998.

58. Jude EB, Oyibo SO, Chalmers N, et al: Peripheral arterial disease in diabetic and nondiabetic patients: a comparison of severity and outcome, *Diabetes Care* 24:1433–1437, 2001.

59. Bowers BL, Valentine RJ, Myers SI, et al: The natural history of patients with claudication with toe pressures of 40 mmHg or less, *J Vasc Surg* 18:506–511, 1993.

60. Resnick HE, Carter EA, Sosenko JM, et al: Incidence of lower-extremity amputation in American Indians: the Strong Heart Study, *Diabetes Care* 27:1885–1891, 2004.

61. Tahrani AA, Bailey CJ, Del Prato S, et al: Management of type 2 diabetes: new and future developments in treatment, *Lancet* 378:182–197, 2011.

62. Dluhy RG, McMahon GT: Intensive glycemic control in the ACCORD and ADVANCE trials, *N Engl J Med* 358:2630–2633, 2008.

63. The effect of intensive treatment of diabetes on the development and progression of long-term complications in insulin-dependent diabetes mellitus. The Diabetes Control and Complications Trial Research Group, *N Engl J Med* 329:977–986, 1993.

64. Effect of intensive diabetes management on macrovascular events and risk factors in the Diabetes Control and Complications Trial, *Am J Cardiol* 75:894–903, 1995.

65. Nathan DM, Cleary PA, Backlund JY, et al: Intensive diabetes treatment and cardiovascular disease in patients with type 1 diabetes, *N Engl J Med* 353:2643–2653, 2005.

66. Intensive blood-glucose control with sulphonylureas or insulin compared with conventional treatment and risk of complications in patients with type 2 diabetes (UKPDS 33). UK Prospective Diabetes Study (UKPDS) Group, *Lancet* 352:837–853, 1998.

67. Knatterud GL, Klimt CR, Levin ME, et al: Effects of hypoglycemic agents on vascular complications in patients with adult-onset diabetes. VII. Mortality and selected nonfatal events with insulin treatment, *JAMA* 240:37–42, 1978.

68. Holman RR, Paul SK, Bethel MA, et al: 10-year follow-up of intensive glucose control in type 2 diabetes, *N Engl J Med* 359:1577–1589, 2008.

69. Effect of intensive blood-glucose control with metformin on complications in overweight patients with type 2 diabetes (UKPDS 34). UK Prospective Diabetes Study (UKPDS) Group, *Lancet* 352:854–865, 1998.

70. Dormandy JA, Charbonnel B, Eckland DJ, et al: Secondary prevention of macrovascular events in patients with type 2 diabetes in the PROactive Study (PROspective pioglitAzone Clinical Trial In macroVascular Events): a randomised controlled trial, *Lancet* 366:1279–1289, 2005.

71. Nissen SE, Wolski K: Effect of rosiglitazone on the risk of myocardial infarction and death from cardiovascular causes, *N Engl J Med* 356:2457–2471, 2007.

72. Home PD, Pocock SJ, Beck-Nielsen H, et al: Rosiglitazone evaluated for cardiovascular outcomes in oral agent combination therapy for type 2 diabetes (RECORD): a multicentre, randomised, open-label trial, *Lancet* 373:2125–2135, 2009.

73. *Rosiglitazone maleate package insert*, 2011.

74. Gerstein HC, Miller ME, Byington RP, et al: Effects of intensive glucose lowering in type 2 diabetes, *N Engl J Med* 358:2545–2559, 2008.

75. Duckworth W, Abraira C, Moritz T, et al: Glucose control and vascular complications in veterans with type 2 diabetes, *N Engl J Med* 360:129–139, 2009.

76. Patel A, MacMahon S, Chalmers J, et al: Intensive blood glucose control and vascular outcomes in patients with type 2 diabetes, *N Engl J Med* 358:2560–2572, 2008.

77. Peripheral arterial disease in people with diabetes, *Diabetes Care* 26:3333–3341, 2003.

78. Standards of medical care for patients with diabetes mellitus, *Diabetes Care* (Suppl 1):S33–S50, 2003.

79. Skyler JS, Bergenstal R, Bonow RO, et al: Intensive glycemic control and the prevention of cardiovascular events: implications of the ACCORD, ADVANCE, and VA Diabetes Trials: a position statement of the American Diabetes Association and a Scientific Statement of the American College of Cardiology Foundation and the American Heart Association, *J Am Coll Cardiol* 53:298–304, 2009.

80. Welch GN, Loscalzo J: Homocysteine and atherothrombosis, *N Engl J Med* 338:1042–1050, 1998.

81. van den Bosch MA, Bloemenkamp DG, Mali WP, et al: Hyperhomocysteinemia and risk for peripheral arterial occlusive disease in young women, *J Vasc Surg* 38:772–778, 2003.

82. Malinow MR, Kang SS, Taylor LM, et al: Prevalence of hyperhomocysteinemia in patients with peripheral arterial occlusive disease, *Circulation* 79:1180–1188, 1989.

83. Darius H, Pittrow D, Haberl R, et al: Are elevated homocysteine plasma levels related to peripheral arterial disease? Results from a cross-sectional study of 6880 primary care patients, *Eur J Clin Invest* 33:751–757, 2003.

84. Taylor LM Jr, DeFrang RD, Harris EJ Jr, et al: The association of elevated plasma homocysteine with progression of symptomatic peripheral arterial disease, *J Vasc Surg* 13:128–136, 1991.

85. den Heijer M, Koster T, Blom HJ, et al: Hyperhomocysteinemia as a risk factor for deep-vein thrombosis, *N Engl J Med* 334:759–762, 1996.

86. Vermeulen EG, Stehouwer CD, Twisk JW, et al: Effect of homocysteine-lowering treatment with folic acid plus vitamin B6 on progression of subclinical atherosclerosis: a randomised, placebo-controlled trial, *Lancet* 355:517–522, 2000.

87. Lonn E, Yusuf S, Arnold MJ, et al: Homocysteine lowering with folic acid and B vitamins in vascular disease, *N Engl J Med* 354:1567–1577, 2006.

88. Lonn E, Held C, Arnold JM, et al: Rationale, design and baseline characteristics of a large, simple, randomized trial of combined folic acid and vitamins B6 and B12 in high-risk patients: the Heart Outcomes Prevention Evaluation (HOPE)-2 trial, *Can J Cardiol* 22:47–53, 2006.

89. Bonaa KH, Njolstad I, Ueland PM, et al: Homocysteine lowering and cardiovascular events after acute myocardial infarction, *N Engl J Med* 354:1578–1588, 2006.

90. Armitage JM, Bowman L, Clarke RJ, et al: Effects of homocysteine-lowering with folic acid plus vitamin B12 vs. placebo on mortality and major morbidity in myocardial infarction survivors: a randomized trial, *JAMA* 303:2486–2494, 2010.

91. Antithrombotic Trialists Collaboration: Collaborative meta-analysis of randomised trials of antiplatelet therapy for prevention of death, myocardial infarction, and stroke in high risk patients, *BMJ* 324:71, 2002.

92. Collaborative overview of randomised trials of antiplatelet therapy–I: prevention of death, myocardial infarction, and stroke by prolonged antiplatelet therapy in various categories of patients. Antiplatelet Trialists' Collaboration, *BMJ* 308:81–106, 1994.

93. Baigent C, Blackwell L, Collins R, et al: Aspirin in the primary and secondary prevention of vascular disease: collaborative meta-analysis of individual participant data from randomised trials, *Lancet* 373:1849–1860, 2009.

94. Collaborative overview of randomised trials of antiplatelet therapy–II: maintenance of vascular graft or arterial patency by antiplatelet therapy. Antiplatelet Trialists' Collaboration, *BMJ* 308:159–168, 1994.

95. Balsano F, Violi F: Effect of picotamide on the clinical progression of peripheral vascular disease. A double-blind placebo-controlled study. The ADEP Group, *Circulation* 87:1563–1569, 1993.

96. Berger JS, Krantz MJ, Kittelson JM, et al: Aspirin for the prevention of cardiovascular events in patients with peripheral artery disease: a meta-analysis of randomized trials, *JAMA* 301:1909–1919, 2009.

97. Catalano M, Born G, Peto R: Prevention of serious vascular events by aspirin amongst patients with peripheral arterial disease: randomized, double-blind trial, *J Intern Med* 261:276–284, 2007.

98. Belch J, MacCuish A, Campbell I, et al: The prevention of progression of arterial disease and diabetes (POPADAD) trial: factorial randomised placebo controlled trial of aspirin and antioxidants in patients with diabetes and asymptomatic peripheral arterial disease, *BMJ* 337:a1840, 2008.

99. Fowkes FG, Price JF, Stewart MC, et al: Aspirin for prevention of cardiovascular events in a general population screened for a low ankle brachial index: a randomized controlled trial, *JAMA* 303:841–848, 2010.

100. *Drugs for the heart*, ed 5, Philadelphia, 2001, WB Saunders.

101. A randomised, blinded, trial of clopidogrel versus aspirin in patients at risk of ischaemic events (CAPRIE). CAPRIE Steering Committee, *Lancet* 348:1329–1339, 1996.

102. Yusuf S, Zhao F, Mehta SR, et al: Effects of clopidogrel in addition to aspirin in patients with acute coronary syndromes without ST-segment elevation, *N Engl J Med* 345:494–502, 2001.

103. Bhatt DL, Fox KA, Hacke W, et al: Clopidogrel and aspirin versus aspirin alone for the prevention of atherothrombotic events, *N Engl J Med* 354:1706–1717, 2006.

104. Cacoub PP, Bhatt DL, Steg PG, et al: Patients with peripheral arterial disease in the CHARISMA trial, *Eur Heart J* 30:192–201, 2009.

105. Belch JJ, Dormandy J, Biasi GM, et al: Results of the randomized, placebo-controlled clopidogrel and acetylsalicylic acid in bypass surgery for peripheral arterial disease (CASPAR) trial, *J Vasc Surg* 52:825–833, 833 e821–833 e822, 2010.

106. Cosmi B, Conti E, Coccheri S: Anticoagulants (heparin, low molecular weight heparin and oral anticoagulants) for intermittent claudication, *Cochrane Database Syst Rev* 2001 CD001999.

107. Efficacy of oral anticoagulants compared with aspirin after infrainguinal bypass surgery (the Dutch Bypass Oral Anticoagulants or Aspirin Study): a randomised trial, *Lancet* 355:346–351, 2000.

108. Anand S, Yusuf S, Xie C, et al: Oral anticoagulant and antiplatelet therapy and peripheral arterial disease, *N Engl J Med* 357:217–227, 2007.

109. Sobel M, Verhaeghe R: Antithrombotic therapy for peripheral artery occlusive disease: American College of Chest Physicians Evidence-Based Clinical Practice Guidelines (8th edition), *Chest* 133:815S–843S, 2008.

110. O'Brien-Irr MS, Harris LM, Dosluoglu HH, et al: Endovascular intervention for treatment of claudication: is it cost-effective? *Ann Vasc Surg* 24:833–840, 2010.

111. Treesak C, Kasemsup V, Treat-Jacobson D, et al: Cost-effectiveness of exercise training to improve claudication symptoms in patients with peripheral arterial disease, *Vasc Med* 9:279–285, 2004.

112. Gardner AW, Poehlman ET: Exercise rehabilitation programs for the treatment of claudication pain. A meta-analysis, *JAMA* 274:975–980, 1995.

113. Leng GC, Fowler B, Ernst E: Exercise for intermittent claudication, *Cochrane Database Syst Rev* 2000 CD000990.

114. McDermott MM, Ades P, Guralnik JM, et al: Treadmill exercise and resistance training in patients with peripheral arterial disease with and without intermittent claudication: a randomized controlled trial, *JAMA* 301:165–174, 2009.

115. Murphy TP, Cutlip DE, Regensteiner JG, et al: CLEVER Study Investigators: Supervised exercise versus primary stenting for claudication resulting from aortoiliac peripheral artery disease: six-month outcomes from the claudication: exercise versus endoluminal revascularization (CLEVER) study, *Circulation* 125:130–139, 2012.

116. Regensteiner JG, Meyer TJ, Krupski WC, et al: Hospital vs. home-based exercise rehabilitation for patients with peripheral arterial occlusive disease, *Angiology* 48:291–300, 1997.

117. Degischer S, Labs KH, Hochstrasser J, et al: Physical training for intermittent claudication: a comparison of structured rehabilitation versus home-based training, *Vasc Med* 7:109–115, 2002.

118. Gardner AW, Parker DE, Montgomery PS, et al: Efficacy of quantified home-based exercise and supervised exercise in patients with intermittent claudication: a randomized controlled trial, *Circulation* 123:491–498, 2011.

119. Stewart KJ, Hiatt WR, Regensteiner JG, et al: Exercise training for claudication, *N Engl J Med* 347:1941–1951, 2002.

120. Duscha BD, Robbins JL, Jones WS, et al: Angiogenesis in skeletal muscle precede improvements in peak oxygen uptake in peripheral artery disease patients, *Arterioscler Thromb Vasc Biol* 31:2742–2748, 2011.

121. Lloyd PG, Yang HT, Terjung RL: Arteriogenesis and angiogenesis in rat ischemic hindlimb: role of nitric oxide, *Am J Physiol Heart Circ Physiol* 281:H2528–H2538, 2001.

122. Mathien GM, Terjung RL: Muscle blood flow in trained rats with peripheral arterial insufficiency, *Am J Physiol* 258:H759–H765, 1990.

123. Laufs U, Werner N, Link A, et al: Physical training increases endothelial progenitor cells, inhibits neointima formation, and enhances angiogenesis, *Circulation* 109:220–226, 2004.

124. Prior BM, Yang HT, Terjung RL: What makes vessels grow with exercise training? *J Appl Physiol* 97:1119–1128, 2004.

125. Niebauer J, Maxwell AJ, Lin PS, et al: Impaired aerobic capacity in hypercholesterolemic mice: partial reversal by exercise training, *Am J Physiol* 276:H1346–H1354, 1999.

126. Buckwalter JB, Curtis VC, Valic Z, et al: Endogenous vascular remodeling in ischemic skeletal muscle: a role for nitric oxide, *J Appl Physiol* 94:935–940, 2003.

127. Gardner AW, Katzel LI, Sorkin JD, et al: Exercise rehabilitation improves functional outcomes and peripheral circulation in patients with intermittent claudication: a randomized controlled trial, *J Am Geriatr Soc* 49:755–762, 2001.

128. Hiatt WR, Regensteiner JG, Hargarten ME, et al: Benefit of exercise conditioning for patients with peripheral arterial disease, *Circulation* 81:602–609, 1990.

129. Gokce N, Vita JA, Bader DS, et al: Effect of exercise on upper and lower extremity endothelial function in patients with coronary artery disease, *Am J Cardiol* 90:124–127, 2002.

130. Brendle DC, Joseph LJ, Corretti MC, et al: Effects of exercise rehabilitation on endothelial reactivity in older patients with peripheral arterial disease, *Am J Cardiol* 87:324–329, 2001.

131. Brass EP: Skeletal muscle metabolism as a target for drug therapy in peripheral arterial disease, *Vasc Med* 1:55–59, 1996.

132. Hiatt WR, Regensteiner JG, Wolfel EE, et al: Effect of exercise training on skeletal muscle histology and metabolism in peripheral arterial disease, *J Appl Physiol* 81:780–788, 1996.

133. Gardner AW, Forrester L, Smith GV: Altered gait profile in subjects with peripheral arterial disease, *Vasc Med* 6:31–34, 2001.

134. Collins TC, Lunos S, Carlson T, et al: Effects of a home-based walking intervention on mobility and quality of life in people with diabetes and peripheral arterial disease: a randomized, controlled trial, *Diabetes Care* 34:2174–2179, 2011.

135. Villemur B, Marquer A, Gailledrat E, et al: New rehabilitation program for intermittent claudication: interval training with active recovery. Pilot study, *Ann Phys Rehabil Med* 54:275–281, 2011.

136. Bronas UG, Treat-Jacobson D, Leon AS: Comparison of the effect of upper body-ergometry aerobic training vs. treadmill training on central cardiorespiratory improvement and walking distance in patients with claudication, *J Vasc Surg* 53:1557–1564, 2011.

137. Saxton JM, Zwierska I, Blagojevic M, et al: Upper- versus lower-limb aerobic exercise training on health-related quality of life in patients with symptomatic peripheral arterial disease, *J Vasc Surg* 53:1265–1273, 2011.

138. Oida K, Ebata K, Kanehara H, et al: Effect of cilostazol on impaired vasodilatory response of the brachial artery to ischemia in smokers, *J Atheroscler Thromb* 10:93–98, 2003.

139. Tanaka T, Ishikawa T, Hagiwara M, et al: Effects of cilostazol, a selective cAMP phosphodiesterase inhibitor on the contraction of vascular smooth muscle, *Pharmacology* 36:313–320, 1988.

140. Woo SK, Kang WK, Kwon KI: Pharmacokinetic and pharmacodynamic modeling of the antiplatelet and cardiovascular effects of cilostazol in healthy humans, *Clin Pharmacol Ther* 71:246–252, 2002.

141. Igawa T, Tani T, Chijiwa T, et al: Potentiation of anti-platelet aggregating activity of cilostazol with vascular endothelial cells, *Thromb Res* 57:617–623, 1990.

142. Pande RL, Hiatt WR, Zhang P, et al: A pooled analysis of the durability and predictors of treatment response of cilostazol in patients with intermittent claudication, *Vasc Med* 15:181–188, 2010.

143. Soga Y, Iida O, Hirano K, et al: Impact of cilostazol after endovascular treatment for infrainguinal disease in patients with critical limb ischemia, *J Vasc Surg* 54:1659–1667, 2011.

144. Miyashita Y, Saito S, Miyamoto A, et al: Cilostazol increases skin perfusion pressure in severely ischemic limbs, *Angiology* 62:15–17, 2011.

145. *Cilostazol package insert*, 2011.

146. Dawson DL, Cutler BS, Hiatt WR, et al: A comparison of cilostazol and pentoxifylline for treating intermittent claudication, *Am J Med* 109:523–530, 2000.

147. Cohn JN, Goldstein SO, Greenberg BH, et al: A dose-dependent increase in mortality with vesnarinone among patients with severe heart failure. Vesnarinone Trial Investigators, *N Engl J Med* 339:1810–1816, 1998.

148. Packer M, Carver JR, Rodeheffer RJ, et al: Effect of oral milrinone on mortality in severe chronic heart failure. THE PROMISE Study Research Group, *N Engl J Med* 325:1468–1475, 1991.

149. Hiatt WR, Money SR, Brass EP: Long-term safety of cilostazol in patients with peripheral artery disease: the CASTLE study (Cilostazol: A Study in Long-term Effects), *J Vasc Surg* 47:330–336, 2008.

150. Reiter M, Bucek RA, Stumpflen A, et al: Prostanoids for intermittent claudication, *Cochrane Database Syst Rev* 2004 CD000986.

151. Mohler ER 3rd, Hiatt WR, Olin JW, et al: Treatment of intermittent claudication with beraprost sodium, an orally active prostaglandin I2 analogue: a double-blinded, randomized, controlled trial, *J Am Coll Cardiol* 41:1679–1686, 2003.

152. Lievre M, Morand S, Besse B, et al: Oral beraprost sodium, a prostaglandin I(2) analogue, for intermittent claudication: a double-blind, randomized, multicenter controlled trial. Beraprost et Claudication Intermittente (BERCI) Research Group, *Circulation* 102:426–431, 2000.

153. Creager MA, Pande RL, Hiatt WR: A randomized trial of iloprost in patients with intermittent claudication, *Vasc Med* 13:5–13, 2008.

154. Second European Consensus Document on chronic critical leg ischemia, *Circulation* 84:IV1–IV26, 1991.

155. Prostanoids for chronic critical leg ischemia. A randomized, controlled, open-label trial with prostaglandin E1. The ICAI Study Group. Ischemia Cronica degli Arti Inferiori, *Ann Intern Med* 130:412–421, 1999.

156. Two randomised and placebo-controlled studies of an oral prostacyclin analogue (iloprost) in severe leg ischaemia. The Oral Iloprost in severe Leg Ischaemia Study Group, *Eur J Vasc Endovasc Surg* 20:358–362, 2000.

157. Belch JJ, Ray S, Rajput-Ray M, et al: The Scottish-Finnish-Swedish PARTNER study of taprostene versus placebo treatment in patients with critical limb ischemia, *Int Angiol* 30:150–155, 2011.

158. Lewis P, Psaila JV, Davies WT, et al: Nifedipine in patients with peripheral vascular disease, *Eur J Vasc Surg* 3:159–164, 1989.

159. Bagger JP, Helligsoe P, Randsbaek F, et al: Effect of verapamil in intermittent claudication A randomized, double-blind, placebo-controlled, cross-over study after individual dose-response assessment, *Circulation* 95:411–414, 1997.

160. Dawson DL, Zheng Q, Worthy SA, et al: Failure of pentoxifylline or cilostazol to improve blood and plasma viscosity, fibrinogen, and erythrocyte deformability in claudication, *Angiology* 53:509–520, 2002.

161. Schratzberger P, Dunzendorfer S, Reinisch N, et al: Mediator-dependent effects of pentoxifylline on endothelium for transmigration of neutrophils, *Immunopharmacology* 41:65–75, 1999.

162. Rao KM, Simel DL, Cohen HJ, et al: Effects of pentoxifylline administration on blood viscosity and leukocyte cytoskeletal function in patients with intermittent claudication, *J Lab Clin Med* 115:738–744, 1990.

163. Hood SC, Moher D, Barber GG: Management of intermittent claudication with pentoxifylline: meta-analysis of randomized controlled trials, *CMAJ* 155:1053–1059, 1996.

164. Girolami B, Bernardi E, Prins MH, et al: Treatment of intermittent claudication with physical training, smoking cessation, pentoxifylline, or nafronyl: a meta-analysis, *Arch Intern Med* 159:337–345, 1999.

165. Intravenous pentoxifylline for the treatment of chronic critical limb ischaemia. The European Study Group, *Eur J Vasc Endovasc Surg* 9:426–436, 1995.

166. Efficacy and clinical tolerance of parenteral pentoxifylline in the treatment of critical lower limb ischemia. A placebo controlled multicenter study. Norwegian Pentoxifylline Multicenter Trial Group, *Int Angiol* 15:75–80, 1996.

167. Broderick TL, Quinney HA, Lopaschuk GD: Carnitine stimulation of glucose oxidation in the fatty acid perfused isolated working rat heart, *J Biol Chem* 267:3758–3763, 1992.

168. Hiatt WR, Regensteiner JG, Creager MA, et al: Propionyl-L-carnitine improves exercise performance and functional status in patients with claudication, *Am J Med* 110:616–622, 2001.

169. Brevetti G, Diehm C, Lambert D: European multicenter study on propionyl-L-carnitine in intermittent claudication, *J Am Coll Cardiol* 34:1618–1624, 1999.

170. Brevetti G, Perna S, Sabba C, et al: Propionyl-L-carnitine in intermittent claudication: double-blind, placebo-controlled, dose titration, multicenter study, *J Am Coll Cardiol* 26:1411–1416, 1995.

171. Brevetti G, Perna S, Sabba C, et al: Effect of propionyl-L-carnitine on quality of life in intermittent claudication, *Am J Cardiol* 79:777–780, 1997.

172. Hiatt WR, Creager MA, Amato A, et al: Effect of propionyl-L-carnitine on a background of monitored exercise in patients with claudication secondary to peripheral artery disease, *J Cardiopulm Rehabil Prev* 31:125–132, 2011.

173. Stanley WC: Myocardial energy metabolism during ischemia and the mechanisms of metabolic therapies, *J Cardiovasc Pharmacol Ther* 9(Suppl 1):S31–S45, 2004.

174. Ma A, Garland WT, Smith WB, et al: A pilot study of ranolazine in patients with intermittent claudication, *Int Angiol* 25:361–369, 2006.

175. Chaitman BR, Skettino SL, Parker JO: v: Anti-ischemic effects and long-term survival during ranolazine monotherapy in patients with chronic severe angina, *J Am Coll Cardiol* 43:1375–1382, 2004.

176. Chaitman BR, Pepine CJ, Parker JO, et al: Effects of ranolazine with atenolol, amlodipine, or diltiazem on exercise tolerance and angina frequency in patients with severe chronic angina: a randomized controlled trial, *JAMA* 291:309–316, 2004.

177. Isner JM, Asahara T: Angiogenesis and vasculogenesis as therapeutic strategies for postnatal neovascularization, *J Clin Invest* 103:1231–1236, 1999.

178. Vincent KA, Shyu KG, Luo Y, et al: Angiogenesis is induced in a rabbit model of hindlimb ischemia by naked DNA encoding an HIF-1alpha/VP16 hybrid transcription factor, *Circulation* 102:2255–2261, 2000.

179. Takeshita S, Zheng LP, Brogi E, et al: Therapeutic angiogenesis. A single intraarterial bolus of vascular endothelial growth factor augments revascularization in a rabbit ischemic hind limb model, *J Clin Invest* 93:662–670, 1994.

180. Yang HT, Deschenes MR, Ogilvie RW, et al: Basic fibroblast growth factor increases collateral blood flow in rats with femoral arterial ligation, *Circ Res* 79:62–69, 1996.

181. Tsurumi Y, Takeshita S, Chen D, et al: Direct intramuscular gene transfer of naked DNA encoding vascular endothelial growth factor augments collateral development and tissue perfusion, *Circulation* 94:3281–3290, 1996.

182. Isner JM, Baumgartner I, Rauh G, et al: Treatment of thromboangiitis obliterans (Buerger's disease) by intramuscular gene transfer of vascular endothelial growth factor: preliminary clinical results, *J Vasc Surg* 28:964–973, 1998 discussion 973–965.

183. Baumgartner I, Pieczek A, Manor O, et al: Constitutive expression of phVEGF165 after intramuscular gene transfer promotes collateral vessel development in patients with critical limb ischemia, *Circulation* 97:1114–1123, 1998.

184. Rajagopalan S, Mohler ER 3rd, Lederman RJ, et al: Regional angiogenesis with vascular endothelial growth factor in peripheral arterial disease: a phase II randomized, double-blind, controlled study of adenoviral delivery of vascular endothelial growth factor 121 in patients with disabling intermittent claudication, *Circulation* 108:1933–1938, 2003.

185. Lederman RJ, Mendelsohn FO, Anderson RD, et al: Therapeutic angiogenesis with recombinant fibroblast growth factor-2 for intermittent claudication (the TRAFFIC study): a randomised trial, *Lancet* 359:2053–2058, 2002.

186. Comerota AJ, Throm RC, Miller KA, et al: Naked plasmid DNA encoding fibroblast growth factor type 1 for the treatment of end-stage unreconstructible lower extremity ischemia: preliminary results of a phase I trial, *J Vasc Surg* 35:930–936, 2002.

187. Nikol S, Baumgartner I, Van Belle E, et al: Therapeutic angiogenesis with intramuscular NV1FGF improves amputation-free survival in patients with critical limb ischemia, *Mol Ther* 16:972–978, 2008.

188. Belch J, Hiatt WR, Baumgartner I, et al: Effect of fibroblast growth factor NV1FGF on amputation and death: a randomised placebo-controlled trial of gene therapy in critical limb ischaemia, *Lancet* 377:1929–1937, 2011.

189. Powell RJ, Simons M, Mendelsohn FO, et al: Results of a double-blind, placebo-controlled study to assess the safety of intramuscular injection of hepatocyte growth factor plasmid to improve limb perfusion in patients with critical limb ischemia, *Circulation* 118:58–65, 2008.

190. Wang GL, Jiang BH, Rue EA, et al: Hypoxia-inducible factor 1 is a basic-helix-loop-helix-PAS heterodimer regulated by cellular O2 tension, *Proc Natl Acad Sci U S A* 92:5510–5514, 1995.

191. Guillemin K, Krasnow MA: The hypoxic response: huffing and HIFing, *Cell* 89:9–12, 1997.

192. Wenger RH, Gassmann M: Oxygen(es) and the hypoxia-inducible factor-1, *Biol Chem* 378:609–616, 1997.

193. Rajagopalan S, Olin J, Deitcher S, et al: Use of a constitutively active hypoxia-inducible factor-1alpha transgene as a therapeutic strategy in no-option critical limb ischemia patients: phase I dose-escalation experience, *Circulation* 115:1234–1243, 2007.

194. Creager MA, Olin JW, Belch JJ, et al: Effect of hypoxia-inducible factor-1{alpha} gene therapy on walking performance in patients with intermittent claudication, *Circulation* 124:1765–1773, 2011.

195. Kalka C, Masuda H, Takahashi T, et al: Transplantation of *ex vivo* expanded endothelial progenitor cells for therapeutic neovascularization, *Proc Natl Acad Sci U S A* 97:3422–3427, 2000.

196. Kamihata H, Matsubara H, Nishiue T, et al: Implantation of bone marrow mononuclear cells into ischemic myocardium enhances collateral perfusion and regional function via side supply of angioblasts, angiogenic ligands, and cytokines, *Circulation* 104:1046–1052, 2001.

197. Shintani S, Murohara T, Ikeda H, et al: Augmentation of postnatal neovascularization with autologous bone marrow transplantation, *Circulation* 103:897–903, 2001.

198. Tateishi-Yuyama E, Matsubara H, Murohara T, et al: Therapeutic angiogenesis for patients with limb ischaemia by autologous transplantation of bone-marrow cells: a pilot study and a randomised controlled trial, *Lancet* 360:427–435, 2002.

199. Forbes TL: Rationale and design of the JUVENTAS trial for repeated intra-arterial infusion of autologous bone marrow-derived mononuclear cells in patients with critical limb ischemia. Commentary, *J Vasc Surg* 51:1568, 2010.

200. Walter DH, Krankenberg H, Balzer JO, et al: Intraarterial administration of bone marrow mononuclear cells in patients with critical limb ischemia: a randomized-start, placebo-controlled pilot trial (PROVASA), *Circ Cardiovasc Interv* 4:26–37, 2011.

201. Wester T, Jorgensen JJ, Stranden E, et al: Treatment with autologous bone marrow mononuclear cells in patients with critical lower limb ischaemia. A pilot study, *Scand J Surg* 97:56–62, 2008.

202. Lara-Hernandez R, Lozano-Vilardell P, Blanes P, et al: Safety and efficacy of therapeutic angiogenesis as a novel treatment in patients with critical limb ischemia, *Ann Vasc Surg* 24:287–294, 2010.

203. Lu D, Chen B, Liang Z, et al: Comparison of bone marrow mesenchymal stem cells with bone marrow-derived mononuclear cells for treatment of diabetic critical limb ischemia and foot ulcer: a double-blind, randomized, controlled trial, *Diabetes Res Clin Pract* 92:26–36, 2011.

204. Perin EC, Silva G, Gahremanpour A, et al: A randomized, controlled study of autologous therapy with bone marrow-derived aldehyde dehydrogenase bright cells in patients with critical limb ischemia, *Catheter Cardiovasc Interv* 78:1060–1067, 2011.

205. Powell RJ, Comerota AJ, Berceli SA, et al: Interim analysis results from the RESTORE-CLI, a randomized, double-blind multicenter phase II trial comparing expanded autologous bone marrow-derived tissue repair cells and placebo in patients with critical limb ischemia, *J Vasc Surg* 54:1032–1041, 2011.

206. Sprengers RW, Moll FL, Teraa M, et al: Rationale and design of the JUVENTAS trial for repeated intra-arterial infusion of autologous bone marrow-derived mononuclear cells in patients with critical limb ischemia, *J Vasc Surg* 51:1564–1568, 2010.

207. Mohler ER 3rd, Hiatt WR, Creager MA: Cholesterol reduction with atorvastatin improves walking distance in patients with peripheral arterial disease, *Circulation* 108:1481–1486, 2003.

208. Aronow WS, Nayak D, Woodworth S, et al: Effect of simvastatin versus placebo on treadmill exercise time until the onset of intermittent claudication in older patients with peripheral arterial disease at six months and at one year after treatment, *Am J Cardiol* 92:711–712, 2003.

209. Mondillo S, Ballo P, Barbati R, et al: Effects of simvastatin on walking performance and symptoms of intermittent claudication in hypercholesterolemic patients with peripheral vascular disease, *Am J Med* 114:359–364, 2003.

210. Hiatt WR, Hirsch AT, Creager MA, et al: Effect of niacin ER/lovastatin on claudication symptoms in patients with peripheral artery disease, *Vasc Med* 15:171–179, 2010.

211. Brown BG, Zhao XQ, Sacco DE, et al: Lipid lowering and plaque regression. New insights into prevention of plaque disruption and clinical events in coronary disease, *Circulation* 87:1781–1791, 1993.

212. Liao JK, Bettmann MA, Sandor T, et al: Differential impairment of vasodilator responsiveness of peripheral resistance and conduit vessels in humans with atherosclerosis, *Circ Res* 68:1027–1034, 1991.

213. Anderson TJ, Meredith IT, Yeung AC, et al: The effect of cholesterol-lowering and antioxidant therapy on endothelium-dependent coronary vasomotion, *N Engl J Med* 332:488–493, 1995.

214. Treasure CB, Klein JL, Weintraub WS, et al: Beneficial effects of cholesterol-lowering therapy on the coronary endothelium in patients with coronary artery disease, *N Engl J Med* 332:481–487, 1995.

215. Van Belle E, Rivard A, Chen D, et al: Hypercholesterolemia attenuates angiogenesis but does not preclude augmentation by angiogenic cytokines, *Circulation* 96:2667–2674, 1997.

216. Vasa M, Fichtlscherer S, Adler K, et al: Increase in circulating endothelial progenitor cells by statin therapy in patients with stable coronary artery disease, *Circulation* 103:2885–2890, 2001.

217. West AM, Anderson JD, Epstein FH, et al: Low-density lipoprotein lowering does not improve calf muscle perfusion, energetics, or exercise performance in peripheral arterial disease, *J Am Coll Cardiol* 58:1068–1076, 2011.

218. Norgren L, Jawien A, Matyas L, et al: Sarpogrelate, a 5-hT2A receptor antagonist in intermittent claudication. A phase II European study, *Vasc Med* 11:75–83, 2006.

219. Hiatt WR, Hirsch AT, Cooke JP, et al: Randomized trial of AT-1015 for treatment of intermittent claudication. A novel 5-hydroxytryptamine antagonist with no evidence of efficacy, *Vasc Med* 9:18–25, 2004.

220. Jaff MR, Dale RA, Creager MA, et al: Anti-chlamydial antibiotic therapy for symptom improvement in peripheral artery disease: prospective evaluation of rifalazil effect on vascular symptoms of intermittent claudication and other endpoints in *Chlamydia pneumoniae* seropositive patients (PROVIDENCE-1), *Circulation* 119:452–458, 2009.

221. Gornik HL, Creager MA: Arginine and endothelial and vascular health, *J Nutr* 134:2880S–2887S, 2004; discussion 2895 S.

222. Maxwell AJ, Schauble E, Bernstein D, et al: Limb blood flow during exercise is dependent on nitric oxide, *Circulation* 98:369–374, 1998.

223. Duffy SJ, New G, Tran BT, et al: Relative contribution of vasodilator prostanoids and NO to metabolic vasodilation in the human forearm, *Am J Physiol* 276:H663–H670, 1999.

224. Gordon MB, Jain R, Beckman JA, et al: The contribution of nitric oxide to exercise hyperemia in the human forearm, *Vasc Med* 7:163–168, 2002.

225. Boger RH, Bode-Boger SM, Thiele W, et al: Restoring vascular nitric oxide formation by L-arginine improves the symptoms of intermittent claudication in patients with peripheral arterial occlusive disease, *J Am Coll Cardiol* 32:1336–1344, 1998.

226. Maxwell AJ, Anderson BE, Cooke JP: Nutritional therapy for peripheral arterial disease: a double-blind, placebo-controlled, randomized trial of HeartBar, *Vasc Med* 5:11–19, 2000.

227. Oka RK, Szuba A, Giacomini JC, et al: A pilot study of L-arginine supplementation on functional capacity in peripheral arterial disease, *Vasc Med* 10:265–274, 2005.

228. Wilson AM, Harada R, Nair N, et al: L-arginine supplementation in peripheral arterial disease: no benefit and possible harm, *Circulation* 116:188–195, 2007.

229. Kleijnen J, Mackerras D: Vitamin E for intermittent claudication, *Cochrane Database Syst Rev* 2000 CD000987.

230. Ernst E: The risk-benefit profile of commonly used herbal therapies: Ginkgo, St. John's wort, ginseng, echinacea, saw palmetto, and kava, *Ann Intern Med* 136:42–53, 2002.

231. Pittler MH, Ernst E: Ginkgo biloba extract for the treatment of intermittent claudication: a meta-analysis of randomized trials, *Am J Med* 108:276–281, 2000.

232. Peters H, Kieser M, Holscher U: Demonstration of the efficacy of ginkgo biloba special extract EGb 761 on intermittent claudication–a placebo-controlled, double-blind multicenter trial, *Vasa* 27:106–110, 1998.

233. De Smet PA: Herbal remedies, *N Engl J Med* 347:2046–2056, 2002.

234. Lamas GA, Ackermann A: Clinical evaluation of chelation therapy: is there any wheat amidst the chaff? *Am Heart J* 140:4–5, 2000.

235. Evans DA, Tariq M, Sujata B, et al: The effects of magnesium sulphate and EDTA in the hypercholesterolaemic rabbit, *Diabetes Obes Metab* 3:417–422, 2001.

236. Anderson TJ, Hubacek J, Wyse DG, et al: Effect of chelation therapy on endothelial function in patients with coronary artery disease: PATCH substudy, *J Am Coll Cardiol* 41:420–425, 2003.

237. Sloth-Nielsen J, Guldager B, Mouritzen C, et al: Arteriographic findings in EDTA chelation therapy on peripheral arteriosclerosis, *Am J Surg* 162:122–125, 1991.

238. Villarruz MV, Dans A, Tan F: Chelation therapy for atherosclerotic cardiovascular disease, *Cochrane Database Syst Rev* 2002 CD002785.

239. Ernst E: Chelation therapy for peripheral arterial occlusive disease: a systematic review, *Circulation* 96:1031–1033, 1997.

CHAPTER 20 # Endovascular Treatment of Peripheral Artery Disease

Christopher J. White

The concept of nonsurgical catheter-based peripheral vascular revascularization was first described by Charles Dotter[1] and further advanced with the development of balloon dilation catheters by Andreas Gruentzig.[2] Catheter-based revascularization has largely replaced conventional open surgery as the treatment of first choice in selected patients treated for lower-extremity ischemia.[3]

No single specialty program (cardiology, radiology, or surgery) offered training that satisfied the entire skill set needed to perform peripheral endovascular intervention (Table 20-1). Recognition of this unmet need for a trained cadre of clinicians to care for patients with peripheral artery disease (PAD) prompted the development of a core cardiology training symposium (COCATS-11) to codify the necessary cardiology fellowship training.[4]

Patient and Lesion Selection Criteria

Indications

ANATOMICAL AND FUNCTIONAL CRITERIA

Patient selection for catheter-based vascular intervention depends upon both anatomical and functional criteria (Table 20-2). Anatomical lesion criteria include ability to gain vascular access, a reasonable likelihood of crossing the lesion with a guidewire, and the expectation that a therapeutic catheter can be advanced across the target lesion (Fig. 20-1). A strategy of "provisional" (bail-out) stenting, or use of a stent for a failed balloon dilation attempt (in contrast to "primary" stenting, in which stents are placed with or without balloon predilation), has become the standard of practice for shorter, more discrete lesions. Longer lesions and occlusions are better treated with primary stent placement.[3,5–8]

Availability of endovascular stents (balloon expandable and self-expanding) has significantly extended the anatomical subset of patients who may be considered candidates for peripheral vascular intervention, particularly for longer stenotic lesions and occlusions. The rate-limiting step for nonsurgical revascularization of the aortoiliac vessels is the ability to pass a guidewire across the lesion. Regardless of the balloon dilation result, the option of stent placement offers a reliable and reproducible method to recanalize these large vessels.[9]

Vascular access site complications following catheter-based procedures often can be treated with percutaneous therapy[10] (Fig. 20-2). Patients with hypotension and a high suspicion of bleeding after common femoral artery (CFA) access require urgent diagnostic angiography from the contralateral femoral artery to determine the bleeding site. Rapid identification of the bleeding site may provide an opportunity for lifesaving hemostasis with balloon tamponade.

Functional criteria to select patients for peripheral endovascular revascularization typically include lifestyle- or vocational-limiting symptoms of claudication, critical limb ischemia (CLI; rest pain, nonhealing ulcers, or gangrene), or acute limb ischemia. Asymptomatic patients with anatomically suitable iliac artery lesions may be considered candidates for peripheral vascular intervention to facilitate vascular access, such as for intraaortic counterpulsation balloon placement or for vascular access to perform coronary intervention.

Patients with lifestyle-limiting symptoms of classical claudication or atypical claudication should first have an attempt at pharmacological therapy with cilostazol and supervised exercise training before endovascular intervention is attempted. If exercise training and pharmacotherapy are not effective, if patients are intolerant of cilostazol or cannot be treated with the drug because of heart failure (black box warning), or if a supervised exercise program is unavailable, an attempt at endovascular intervention is appropriate. In general, patients with claudication progress to limb loss at a rate of well under 5% per year, so endovascular revascularization is reserved for those patients with favorable anatomy who either fail conservative therapy and have lifestyle-limiting symptoms or have vocational-limiting symptoms. Therapeutic goals for claudicants are symptom relief, increased walking distance, and improved functionality and quality of life. For this reason, durability of the procedure becomes important; recurrent ischemic symptoms require repeated procedures.

Patients with CLI or limb-threatening ischemia (gangrene, non-healing ulcer, or rest pain) are candidates for urgent revascularization. When considering a patient with CLI for revascularization, it is important to remember that multilevel disease (iliac, femoral, and tibial) is likely to be present and that simply improving "inflow" without addressing the more distal vascular lesions or runoff vessels may fail to solve the clinical problem. Patients with CLI (rest pain, nonhealing ulcers, or gangrene) typically have more extensive disease than claudicants and require urgent revascularization to prevent tissue loss[3,11] (see Table 20-2).

Prognosis for patients presenting with CLI is poor.[12] Those with tobacco abuse and/or diabetes are 10 times more likely to require amputation. Patients with CLI tend to be older, with almost 50% of patients older than 80 years undergoing amputations. Within 3 months of presentation, 12% will require an amputation, and 9% will die; 1-year mortality rate is 22%. Anatomy suitable for endovascular therapy is often present in one or more below-knee vessels. Therapy should be designed to restore pulsatile straight-line flow to the distal part of the limb, with as low a procedural morbidity as possible. The guiding principle is that less blood flow is required to maintain tissue integrity than to heal a wound, so restenosis does not usually result in recurrent CLI unless there has been repeated injury to the limb. Therefore, the emphasis is less on long-term vessel patency and more on amputation-free survival.

The Bypass versus Angioplasty in Severe Ischaemia of the Leg (BASIL) trial was a multicenter randomized trial comparing an initial strategy of balloon angioplasty to open surgery in 452 patients with CLI.[13] The primary outcome was time to amputation or death (amputation-free survival). After 6 months, the two treatment strategies did not differ significantly in amputation-free survival. There was no difference between the groups for quality-of-life outcomes, but for the first year of follow-up, costs associated with a surgery-first strategy were higher than for angioplasty. For this reason, the authors concluded that a percutaneous-first strategy was the treatment of choice in patients who are candidates for either surgery or endovascular intervention.

Contraindications

Relative contraindications to catheter-based peripheral vascular intervention include (1) lesions likely to generate atheroemboli and (2) lesions that are not dilatable. Other relative contraindications include any other instances in which risks of the procedure seem to outweigh potential benefits. For example, the risk of contrast-induced nephropathy in a patient with severe renal impairment must be weighed against expected functional improvement.

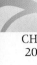

TABLE 20-1	Required Skill Elements for Optimal Peripheral Vascular Intervention
SKILL ELEMENT	DESCRIPTION
Cognitive	Extensive knowledge of vascular disease, including natural history, pathophysiology, diagnostic methods, and treatment alternatives
Technical	Competence in both diagnostic angiography and interventional techniques, such as use and selection of balloons, guidewires, stents, and emboli protection devices
Clinical	Ability to manage inpatients, interpret laboratory tests, obtain informed consent, assess risk/benefit ratio, and admitting privileges

Technical and Procedural Considerations

Preprocedure

GENERAL MEASURES

Prior to performing peripheral endovascular intervention, the patient should have a complete cardiovascular evaluation, with specific attention directed to the status of atherosclerotic risk factors. Atherosclerosis is a systemic disease, and appropriate risk-factor modification (tobacco-cessation counseling, treatment of lipids to target values), screening tests for cardiovascular diseases, and optimization of medical therapy should be performed.

Prior to performing lower-extremity endovascular intervention, it is necessary to objectively determine the patient's functional status. A history, physical examination, and appropriate noninvasive testing should be obtained prior to planning peripheral endovascular revascularization. If the patient is ambulatory, a rest and exercise ankle-brachial index (ABI) should be measured, and pulse volume recordings (PVR) should be performed. Other noninvasive modalities, such as vascular ultrasound, or alternative imaging modalities, such as magnetic resonance angiography (MRA) or computed tomographic angiography (CTA), may be helpful to resolve conflicting data and are used at the discretion of the physician (Fig. 20-3). When planning lower-extremity revascularization, status of the inflow and outflow vessels relative to the target lesion must be visualized angiographically. This is usually done with invasive diagnostic angiography, but in selected patients, MRA or CTA may be very useful.

PREMEDICATION

The only premedication requirement for peripheral endovascular intervention is aspirin therapy (81-325 mg daily). Use of other antiplatelet agents is optional, since there is no evidence that their use improves procedural success or decreases complications. If the patient is intolerant to aspirin, a thienopyridine drug would be appropriate. There is no evidence supporting use of dual antiplatelet therapy after peripheral endovascular intervention or following peripheral vascular stent placement.

TABLE 20-2 Classification of Peripheral Arterial Disease: Fontaine's Stages and Rutherford's Categories

Fontaine			Rutherford	
STAGE	CLINICAL	GRADE	CATEGORY	CLINICAL
I	Asymptomatic	0	0	Asymptomatic
IIa	Mild claudication	I	1	Mild claudication
IIb	Moderate to severe claudication	I	2	Moderate claudication
		I	3	Severe claudication
III	Rest pain	II	4	Rest pain
IV	Ulceration or gangrene	III	5	Minor tissue loss
		IV	6	Ulceration or gangrene

From Norgren L, Hiatt WR, Dormandy JA, et al: Inter-Society Consensus for the management of peripheral arterial disease (TASC II). J Vasc Surg 45 Suppl S:S5–S67, 2007[11].

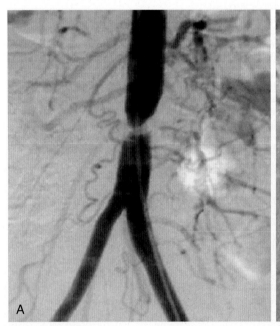

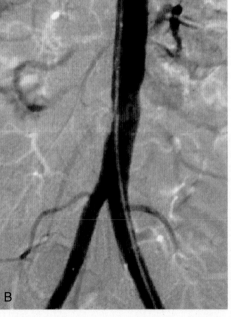

FIGURE 20-1 A, Tight stenosis of infrarenal aorta amenable to angioplasty. **B,** Final postangioplasty result.

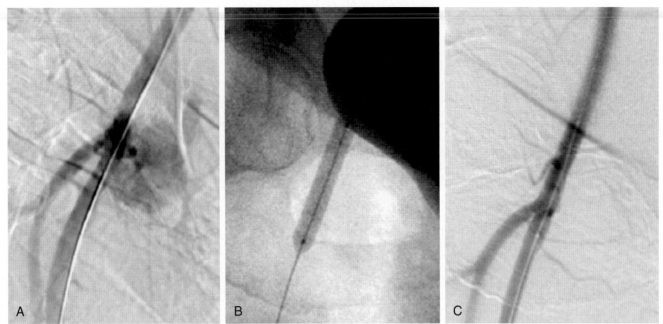

FIGURE 20-2 **Access site complication with bleeding (A) successfully tamponaded with balloon inflation (B), and final angiogram showing hemostasis.**

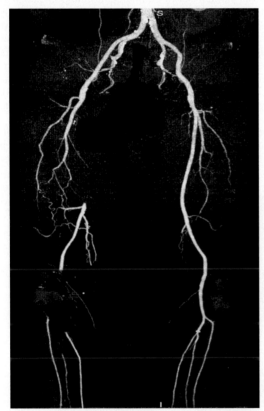

FIGURE 20-3 Computed tomographic angiogram (CTA) of lower-extremity vasculature. There is occlusion of arterial segments of the right femoral, popliteal, and tibial segments.

Procedure

ANTICOAGULATION

There is no standard for anticoagulation therapy, except to state that intravenous unfractionated heparin (UFH), in a dose up to 5000 International Units, is commonly used to achieve an activated clotting time (ACT) of 250 to 300 seconds. At present, there is no evidence that use of glycoprotein (GP)-IIb/IIIa platelet receptor antagonists, low-molecular-weight heparins, or antithrombins improve procedural efficacy or safety for peripheral vascular intervention.

VASCULAR ACCESS

The first step to ensure a successful procedure is to plan appropriate vascular access. The majority of peripheral endovascular intervention can be performed from multiple arterial access sites (i.e., radial, brachial, femoral, or popliteal arteries). However, cases occasionally require a specific access to achieve a successful result. Consequently, familiarity with a variety of vascular access sites and techniques is one of the most important components of the basic skill set. Ability to gain both retrograde and antegrade common femoral access is a required skill for the interventionalist. An infrapopliteal target lesion may be best approached with antegrade femoral access, whereas a proximal superficial femoral artery lesion may require a contralateral retrograde femoral approach. Occasionally, bilateral retrograde femoral artery access is desirable—for example, when treating a common iliac bifurcation lesion.

Equipment Choices

GUIDEWIRES

Trade-offs include smaller catheters with crossing lower profiles, smaller sheath sizes, and increased flexibility for the smallest 0.014-inch systems, which must be balanced against the increased support and pushability of the larger-profile 0.035-inch systems. It is most common that 0.014-inch systems are used for below-knee intervention where the vessels are smaller, compared to the usual 0.035-inch systems used for the larger balloons and stents placed in the iliac vessels. It is recommended that the interventional laboratory be stocked with several redundant lines of equipment to allow for flexibility in the approach to difficult or complex lesions. In general, the lowest profile system within the smallest vascular access sheath should be used.

Use of coated "glidewires" should be carefully restricted to instances when their unique properties are necessary because these wires are more difficult to control than conventional guidewires and are prone to vascular perforation. Their lack of a "transition point" makes them ideal for negotiating abrupt angles and crossing occlusions. Ideally, once they have crossed the occlusion, it is wise to exchange this potentially dangerous wire for a safer and more controllable wire.

BALLOON CATHETERS

A wide variety of monorail and over-the-wire balloon catheters are available that are suitable for dilating lower-extremity lesions. They come in a variety of diameters, with balloon lengths up to 15 cm. A pressure manometer is recommended to monitor balloon inflation pressure. Although no optimal inflation pressure or duration has been determined, it is generally recommended that the balloon be inflated with adequate pressure to ensure full expansion of the lesion.

STENTS

The two categories of stents are balloon expandable and self-expanding. Both types may be covered with material. Balloon expandable stents are intended for use within the axial skeleton to protect them from external compression. This generally limits their use to the iliac arteries, but coronary balloon expandable stents are used to salvage failed angioplasty results in below-knee vessels.[14,15]

Balloon expandable stents can be deployed with more precision than self-expanding stents, although there is some shortening associated with their expansion. Self-expanding stents resist permanent deformation and are elastic. Their flexible nature allows them to delivered in longer lengths, and they will fit themselves to a tapering artery. Self-expanding stents may be made of nitinol or a stainless steel alloy. At this time, there is no evidence that either material is associated with any safety or efficacy advantage.[16,17]

ADJUNCTIVE DEVICES

Other adjunctive devices, such as laser catheters, atherectomy catheters (rotational and directional), brachytherapy catheters, cryotherapy balloons, and cutting balloons have been developed, tested, and aggressively marketed. With the possible exception of the brachytherapy devices, there is no comparative evidence that these adjunctive devices bring any added value, efficacy, or increased safety over balloons and stents when treating lower extremities.

Clinical Outcomes

Aortoiliac Vessels

The current best practice, in experienced hands, for aorto-iliac lesions favors an endovascular strategy (Fig. 20-4). This recommendation is based upon the morbidity and mortality associated with major vascular surgery in patients with significant comorbidity, and the excellent outcomes available with current endovascular techniques. In a large single-center registry of 505 iliac stent procedures, the technical success rate was 98%, 8-year primary stent patency rate was 74%, and secondary patency rate was 84%.[18] In a 10-year iliac stent patency study, there was no effect of age, diabetes, tobacco smoking, or hypertension on patency.[19] Common iliac artery (CIA) lesions had greater long-term patency than external iliac artery (EIA) lesions. Outcomes from another series of 89 consecutive patients with symptomatic occluded iliac arteries demonstrated a 92% success rate for endovascular treatment.[20] Increasing severity and complexity of lesions did not significantly alter iliac artery patency rates.

An observational study compared nonrandomized results of iliac artery stenting with surgery in patients with moderately complex lesions.[21] There was no difference regarding limb salvage or patient survival out to 5 years, but vessel patency was reduced in limbs treated with stents compared to surgery. A nonrandomized retrospective comparison of endovascular intervention compared to open surgery for complex aortoiliac occlusive lesions found a shorter hospital stay, fewer postprocedural complications, and lower primary patency rates but equivalent secondary patency rates for the endovascular arm.[22]

There is debate regarding the most efficacious method of endovascular therapy between "provisional stent placement," which is selective use of stents only when balloon dilation has failed or is

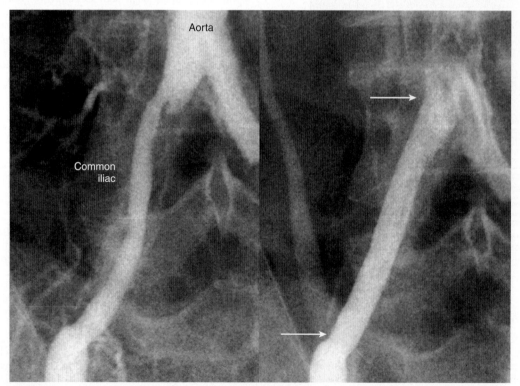

FIGURE 20-4 *Left,* Baseline angiogram of right common iliac stenosis. *Right,* Angiogram after angioplasty and self-expanding stent *(arrows).*

suboptimal, and "primary stent placement," which is the practice of deploying a stent regardless of the balloon result. The Dutch Iliac Stent Trial demonstrated that selective iliac artery stenting achieved an equivalent hemodynamic result compared to primary stenting. Translesional pressure gradients after primary stent placement (5.8 ± 4.7 mmHg) were significantly lower than after balloon angioplasty alone (8.9 ± 6.8 mmHg), but not after provisional stenting (5.9 ± 3.6 mmHg) in the percutaneous transluminal angioplasty (PTA) group.[23] The procedural success rate, defined as a postprocedural gradient less than 10 mmHg, revealed no difference between the two treatment strategies, (primary stenting = 81% vs. PTA plus provisional stenting = 89%). By employing a provisional stenting strategy in the iliac artery, stent placement was avoided in 63% of lesions. After 5 years of follow-up, the selective stent placement strategy had greater symptomatic improvement compared with primary stent placement, but there was no difference in patency rates, ABI, and quality of life between groups.[24,25]

Preferred clinical practice, however, is primary stent placement, and this is supported by a meta-analysis which looked at more than 2000 patients.[26] Procedural success was higher in the primary stent group, and there was a 43% reduction in 4-year failures for aortoiliac stent placement compared to balloon angioplasty alone. Advantages of primary stent placement include efficient and reliable vascular reconstruction, minimizing concern over abrupt occlusion. Direct stenting minimizes the technical challenges of determining translesional pressure gradients and the need to administer vasodilator medications. The current American College of Cardiology/American Heart Association (ACC/AHA) guideline document supports primary stenting of the common and EIAs with a class I recommendation (Level of Evidence B).[3]

Femoral-Popliteal Vessels

ANGIOPLASTY AND STENT PLACEMENT

Comparative outcomes data in femoral-popliteal artery disease are available for medical therapy, PTA, stent placement, brachytherapy, and laser angioplasty. Self-expanding stents are preferred in this location because of the risk of stent compression from external trauma. Notably absent despite their prominent position in the marketplace are comparative data for debulking atherectomy, cutting balloons, or cryoplasty.

A meta-analysis comparing angioplasty to exercise therapy in patients with intermittent claudication reported that ABI improved more with endovascular therapy than with exercise, but quality-of-life outcomes at 3 and 6 months were similar.[27] A cost-effectiveness study suggested that cost-effectiveness for quality-adjusted life-year was greater with percutaneous therapy than exercise alone.[28]

A matched cohort study of 526 patients with intermittent claudication found significant advantages for a revascularization strategy (surgery or PTA) compared to medical therapy.[29] Revascularization was more effective than medical therapy for improvement in physical function, bodily pain, and walking distance. Patients with the greatest improvement in their ABI results had the most clinical improvement.

A recently published trial from the United Kingdom randomized 178 patients with claudication into three groups: supervised exercise, balloon angioplasty, and both if they had suitable lesions for angioplasty of the femoral-popliteal arteries.[30] The study demonstrated that combining supervised exercise with angioplasty produced superior clinical outcomes, but that there was no significant difference among the three groups for quality-of-life outcomes. Two main limitations of this trial were use of balloon-only treatment and the fact that the exercise time was capped at 207 meters, which may have underestimated the degree of improvement from revascularization (Fig. 20-5).

Clinical success in patients with femoral artery lesions depends upon a durable long-lasting procedure. A meta-analysis demonstrated superior patency at 3 years for stents compared to PTA in the most severely affected patients, who were those with occlusions and CLI.[31] There have been three randomized controlled

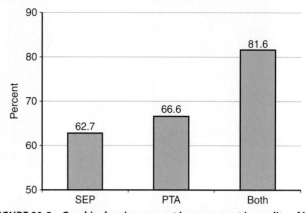

Quality of Life Improvement

FIGURE 20-5 **Graphic showing percent improvement in quality of life (QOL) for three randomized groups of claudicators: supervised exercise program (SEP), percutaneous transluminal angioplasty (PTA), and both.** *(From Mazari FA, Gulati S, Rahman MN, et al: Early outcomes from a randomized, controlled trial of supervised exercise, angioplasty, and combined therapy in intermittent claudication. Ann Vasc Surg 24:69–79, 2010.)[30]*

trials comparing primary stenting to balloon angioplasty with bailout stenting (provisional stenting).[6-8] Lesion length and complexity accounted for restenosis rates for balloon angioplasty, but not for stent placement (Fig. 20-6). Synthesizing these results, the data suggest that longer femoral-popliteal lesions (≥7 cm) are better approached with a strategy of primary stenting, whereas more discrete lesions (<4 cm) do well with a provisional stenting strategy in which balloon angioplasty is given an opportunity to stand alone (Table 20-3).

Stent fractures have been associated with restenosis of femoral artery lesions.[32] There are differences regarding stent fracture among femoral artery stents, presumably related to their composition and architecture. Fracture rates are 28% for the SMART stent (Cordis, Miami Lakes, Fla.), 19% for the Wallstent (Boston Scientific, Natick, Mass.), and 2% for the Dynalink/Absolute (Abbott Vascular, Santa Clara, Calif.).[33]

COVERED STENTS

Covered stents are used effectively to treat vascular perforations and exclude aneurysms in the peripheral vascular circulation. The Viabahn stent graft (W.L. Gore, Flagstaff, Ariz.) has a 1-year femoral artery patency rate of 62%. In one study, patients randomized to the Viabahn stent graft had about twice as many major adverse events (8.2%) as patients randomized to PTA (4.0%). The theoretical benefit for the Viabahn stent graft is that ingrowth of tissue between the stent struts, which plagues femoral stents, is prevented. However, edge restenosis may not be avoided, and concerns about stent thrombosis must be addressed. In one study of 60 limbs treated with a covered stent, two patients had major procedural complications requiring surgical correction. Thrombotic occlusion of the covered stent occurred in 10% of patients within 30 days, and the 1-year primary patency rate was 67%.[34] Late occlusion was presumed to represent edge restenosis and thrombosis. In another study, 86 patients were randomized to bypass surgery or endovascular therapy with a covered stent graft. No significant difference was observed for primary or secondary patency, but there was a trend favoring surgery for more complex lesions.[35,36]

DRUG-ELUTING BALLOONS AND STENTS

A clinical trial of a small number of patients randomized to either a bare metal self-expanding stent or a drug-eluting (sirolimus) self-expanding stent (Smart, Cordis, Miami Lakes, Fla.) found no difference in severity of restenosis.[17,37] A recently completed Cook Zilver PTX trial randomized 420 patients has not reported results; however, the registry data have shown some promise.[38] There have been two small randomized trials of drug-coated (paclitaxel) balloons

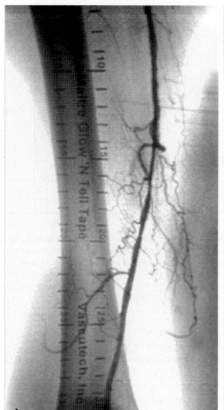
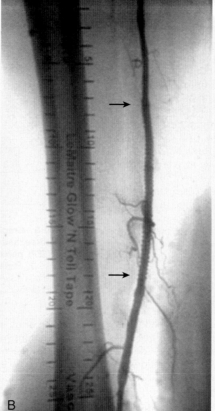
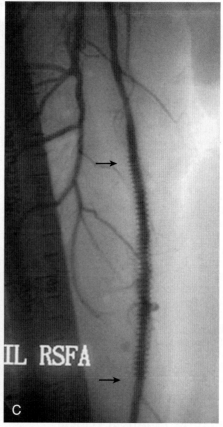

FIGURE 20-6 **A,** Baseline angiogram of distal superficial femoral artery (SFA) stenosis. **B,** Post-stent placement *(between arrows).* **C,** Six-month follow-up with patent SFA stent segment.

TABLE 20-3	Comparison of Primary and Provisional Femoral-Popliteal Stenting	
	SCHILLINGER	**KRANKENBERG**
Stent	Guidant	Bard
Lesion length	101 mm	45 mm
Stent restenosis	36.7%	31.7%
PTA restenosis	63.5%	38.6%*

*P = 0.004
PTA, percutaneous transluminal angioplasty.
From Schillinger M, Sabeti S, Loewe C, et al: Balloon angioplasty versus implantation of nitinol stents in the superficial femoral artery. N Engl J Med 354:1879–1888, 2006; and Krankenberg H, Schluter M, Steinkamp HJ, et al: Nitinol stent implantation versus percutaneous transluminal angioplasty in superficial femoral artery lesions up to 10 cm in length: the Femoral Artery Stenting Trial (FAST). Circulation 116:285–292, 2007.[5,6]

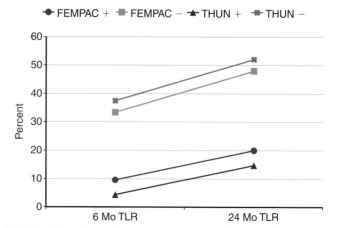

FIGURE 20-7 **Comparison of drug-coated balloon studies showing 6- and 24-month target lesion revascularization rates for drug-coated balloons (FEMPAC + and THUN+) versus control balloons (FEMPAC – and THUN–).** TLR, target lesion revascularization. *(From Tepe G, Zeller T, Albrecht T, et al: Local delivery of paclitaxel to inhibit restenosis during angioplasty of the leg. N Engl J Med 358:689–699, 2008; and Werk M, Langner S, Reinkensmeier B, et al: Inhibition of restenosis in femoropopliteal arteries: paclitaxel-coated versus uncoated balloon: Femoral Paclitaxel Randomized Pilot Trial. Circulation 118:1358–1365, 2008.)[39,40]*

for femoral disease that have shown positive results.[39,40] These trials found that lumen loss, restenosis, and target lesion revascularization were less after treatment with coated balloons than with uncoated balloons (Fig. 20-7). Reasons for failure of drug-eluting stents (DES) and early success for balloons in the femoral artery may be related to stent fracture and the ongoing irritant related to the metal stent against the vessel wall.[41]

BRACHYTHERAPY

Adjunctive endovascular brachytherapy (EBT) with an iridium-192 source, with a prescribed dose of 12 to 14 Gy, compared to PTA alone for treatment of de novo long-segment stenoses of the femoral artery has a delaying effect on the occurrence of restenosis.[42,43] In one study, there appeared to be an early restenosis benefit for the EBT plus PTA group; however, at 5-year follow-up, there was "catch-up," and the recurrence rate was equal (72.5%) in both groups.[43] Brachytherapy has greater efficacy in restenotic lesions compared

with de novo lesions.[44,45] A novel approach has been to deliver external beam irradiation to de novo femoral artery lesions after PTA. At the 1-year follow-up of one trial, there was a significant benefit for patients treated with 14 Gy in a single treatment session, compared with a control group and a group who received lower Gy doses.[46]

ATHERECTOMY

There had been expectation that by "debulking" atherosclerotic plaque, primary patency of femoral artery interventions could be improved.[47] Yet, successive generations of atherectomy catheters have failed to demonstrate any benefit over less-expensive conventional therapies.[48,49] Comparative studies are lacking, and the data supporting the use of devices are derived from self-reported registries and subject to bias. Also, there are safety concerns regarding the incidence of distal embolization and perforation.[50–52]

LASER-ASSISTED ANGIOPLASTY

Laser-assisted angioplasty does not appear to add any benefit to conventional endovascular therapy for peripheral arterial recanalization.[53,54] The Peripheral Excimer Laser Angioplasty (PELA) trial randomized 251 patients to either PTA or laser-assisted PTA in patients with claudication and a total femoral occlusion. There was no difference in clinical events or patency rates at 1 year of follow-up.

CUTTING BALLOON

The cutting balloon is used in coronary arteries for "undilatable" lesions. There is limited evidence that would support extending the indications for this device beyond peripheral arteries,[55] and there is no evidence that a cutting balloon is an efficacious treatment for in-stent restenosis.

CRYOPLASTY

Clinical trials have failed to demonstrate any advantage for cryoplasty over conventional angioplasty in peripheral arterial intervention.[56] In a diabetic population with femoral-popliteal artery lesions, cryoplasty was associated with lower primary patency rates and more clinically driven repeat procedures after long-term follow-up than conventional balloon angioplasty.[57]

Infrapopliteal Intervention

TIBIOPERONEAL ANGIOPLASTY

Below-knee angioplasty has generally been reserved for treatment of CLI and threatened limbs because of the technical difficulty of using conventional peripheral angioplasty equipment in these vessels and the fear of limb loss should a complication occur (Fig. 20-8). Experience with PTA demonstrated the feasibility of a percutaneous approach with procedural success rates better than 80% for tibioperoneal angioplasty.[58,59] Replacement of bulkier

0.035-inch equipment with the 0.014-inch devices used in coronary angioplasty improved results of below-knee intervention. In 111 patients treated with tibioperoneal angioplasty for treatment of claudication, tissue loss, or rest pain, Dorros et al.[60] reported a primary success rate of 90% for all lesions, including a 99% success rate for stenoses and a 65% success rate for occlusions. At the time of hospital discharge, 95% of patients were symptomatically improved.

Two clinical trials have demonstrated the efficacy and attractiveness of an initial percutaneous approach to selected patients with CLI and below-knee vascular disease.[58,61] The limb salvage rate in these patients treated with PTA ranged from 85% to 91% after 2 to 5 years. This evidence supports the contention that angioplasty of the tibioperoneal vessels should not necessarily be reserved for limb salvage situations. However, caution is still advised in patient selection, since the surgical options are limited if angioplasty fails.

Optimal treatment of infrapopliteal disease requires appropriate patient and lesion selection for treatment. Focal stenoses have the best outcomes, and vessels with fewer than five separate lesions are associated with a higher success rate. Anatomically, the goal is to open as many tibial artery stenoses as possible to increase the degree of revascularization and improve clinical outcomes.[62] Treatment success is measured by relief of rest pain, healing of ulcers, and avoiding amputation, not necessarily by long-term vessel patency. When trying to heal ischemic ulcers, the basic principle is that it takes more oxygenated blood flow to heal a wound than to maintain tissue integrity.[58] Percutaneous therapy can result in long-term limb salvage in more than 80% of patients and should be considered the current standard of treatment in patients with limb-threatening ischemia who are candidates for endovascular intervention.

TIBIOPERONEAL STENTS

The role of provisional versus primary stent placement in tibial arteries is unsettled.[63] A recent small randomized trial of PTA compared to PTA with a bare metal stent (BMS) demonstrated no significant differences for 1-year outcomes, including patency rates, limb salvage, or survival[64] (Fig. 20-9). Preliminary results of the use of balloon expandable coronary DES in tibial vessels have been reported.[14,15,65,66] Smaller series have shown excellent patency when comparing below-knee BMS to DES.[67,68] The largest published series is a nonrandomized report of 106 patients (118 limbs) with CLI treated with below-knee DES.[15] The 3-year cumulative incidence of amputation was only 6%, and amputation-free survival was 68%.

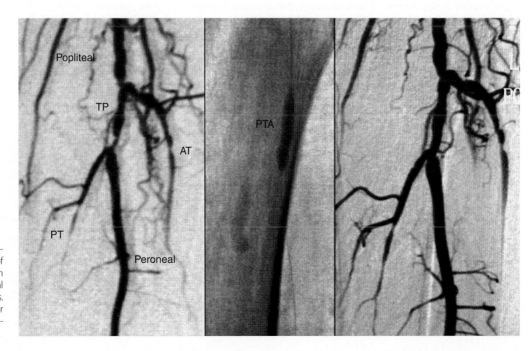

FIGURE 20-8 *Left,* Baseline angiogram of severe stenosis (70%) of tibioperoneal *(TP)* artery. *Middle,* Balloon angioplasty of TP trunk. *Right,* Final angiogram with less than 30% stenosis. AT, anterior tibial artery; PT, posterior tibial artery; PTA, percutaneous transluminal angioplasty.

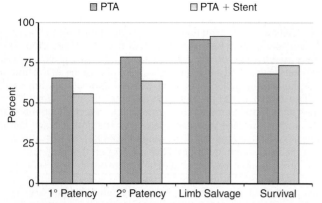

FIGURE 20-9 Bar graph of 12-month patency rates comparing infrapopliteal percutaneous transluminal angioplasty (PTA) alone to PTA with bare metal stent (BMS) placement in 38 limbs with critical limb ischemia (CLI). *(From Randon C, Jacobs B, De Ryck F, Vermassen F: Angioplasty or primary stenting for infrapopliteal lesions: results of a prospective randomized trial. Cardiovasc Intervent Radiol 33:260–269, 2010.)*[64]

ANGIOGENESIS

Not infrequently, the severity of infrapopliteal disease abolishes most if not all of the named vasculature, and percutaneous mechanical revascularization is not possible. Therapeutic angiogenesis using growth factors as agents (e.g., vascular endothelial growth factor [VEGF], fibroblast growth factor [FGF]), genes, and cellular therapies have been proposed as a means of maintaining limb viability.[69–71] At present, there have been no clinical breakthroughs, but much ongoing basic science activity appears to be promising.[72]

Conclusions

Percutaneous revascularization therapies are rapidly replacing open surgery as the treatment of choice for lower-extremity PAD. Stents appear to improve outcomes for iliac and femoral-popliteal artery lesions. Their role in infrainguinal revascularization, however, is not established so their use should be limited to bailout situations after failed or failing angioplasty. Adjunctive high-cost niche devices, such as atherectomy, lasers, cryotherapy, and cutting balloons, have a very limited role if any in the treatment of lower-extremity ischemic lesions.

Successful development of antirestenosis therapies, including DES and drug-coated balloons for peripheral arteries, will launch a new era of percutaneous revascularization, with efficacy and durability similar to that seen for coronary DES. The primacy of endovascular therapy for treatment of PAD will be established if antirestenosis therapies prove as effective in preserving late patency as they have in coronary arteries.

REFERENCES

1. Dotter CT, Judkins MP: Transluminal treatment of arteriosclerotic obstruction. Description of a new technique and a preliminary report of its application, *Circulation* 30:654–670, 1964.
2. Gruntzig A, Hopff H: Percutaneous recanalization after chronic arterial occlusion with new dilator-catheter (modification of the Dotter technique) (author's transl), *Dtsch Med Wochenschr* 99:2502–2510, 1974.
3. Hirsch AT, Haskal ZJ, Hertzer NR, et al: ACC/AHA 2005 guidelines for the management of patients with peripheral arterial disease (lower extremity, renal, mesenteric, and abdominal aortic): executive summary of a collaborative report from the American Association for Vascular Surgery/Society for Vascular Surgery, Society for Cardiovascular Angiography and Interventions, Society for Vascular Medicine and Biology, Society of Interventional Radiology, and the ACC/AHA Task Force on Practice Guidelines (Writing Committee to Develop Guidelines for the Management of Patients with Peripheral Arterial Disease) endorsed by the American Association of Cardiovascular and Pulmonary Rehabilitation; National Heart, Lung, and Blood Institute; Society for Vascular Nursing; TransAtlantic Inter-Society Consensus; and Vascular Disease Foundation, *J Am Coll Cardiol* 47:1239–1312, 2006.
4. Creager MA, Cooke JP, Olin JW, et al: Task force 11: training in vascular medicine and peripheral vascular catheter-based interventions endorsed by the Society for Cardiovascular Angiography and Interventions and the Society for Vascular Medicine, *J Am Coll Cardiol* 51:398–404, 2008.
5. AbuRahma AF, Hayes JD, Flaherty SK, et al: Primary iliac stenting versus transluminal angioplasty with selective stenting, *J Vasc Surg* 46:965–970, 2007.
6. Schillinger M, Sabeti S, Loewe C, et al: Balloon angioplasty versus implantation of nitinol stents in the superficial femoral artery, *N Engl J Med* 354:1879–1888, 2006.
7. Krankenberg H, Schluter M, Steinkamp HJ, et al: Nitinol stent implantation versus percutaneous transluminal angioplasty in superficial femoral artery lesions up to 10 cm in length: The Femoral Artery Stenting Trial (FAST), *Circulation* 116:285–292, 2007.
8. Laird JR, Katzen BT, Scheinert D, et al: Nitinol stent implantation versus balloon angioplasty for lesions in the superficial femoral artery and proximal popliteal artery: twelve-month results from the RESILIENT randomized trial, *Circ Cardiovasc Interv* 3:267–276, 2010.
9. Scheinert D, Schroder M, Ludwig J, et al: Stent-supported recanalization of chronic iliac artery occlusions, *Am J Med* 110:708–715, 2001.
10. Samal AK, White CJ: Percutaneous management of access site complications, *Catheter Cardiovasc Interv* 57:12–23, 2002.
11. Norgren L, Hiatt WR, Dormandy JA, et al: Inter-Society Consensus for the management of peripheral arterial disease (TASC II), *J Vasc Surg* 45(Suppl S):S5–S67, 2007.
12. Jamsen T, Manninen H, Tulla H, et al: The final outcome of primary infrainguinal percutaneous transluminal angioplasty in 100 consecutive patients with chronic critical limb ischemia, *J Vasc Interv Radiol* 13:455–463, 2002.
13. Adam DJ, Beard JD, Cleveland T, et al: Bypass versus Angioplasty in Severe Ischaemia of the Leg (BASIL): multicentre, randomised controlled trial, *Lancet* 366:1925–1934, 2005.
14. Grant AG, White CJ, Collins TJ, et al: Infrapopliteal drug-eluting stents for chronic limb ischemia, *Catheter Cardiovasc Interv* 71:108–111, 2008.
15. Feiring AJ, Krahn M, Nelson L, et al: Preventing leg amputations in critical limb ischemia with below-the-knee drug-eluting stents: the PaRADISE (PReventing Amputations using Drug eluting StEnts) trial, *J Am Coll Cardiol* 55:1580–1589, 2010.
16. Ponec D, Jaff MR, Swischuk J, et al: The Nitinol SMART stent vs. Wallstent for suboptimal iliac artery angioplasty: CRISP-US trial results, *J Vasc Interv Radiol* 15:911–918, 2004.
17. Duda SH, Bosiers M, Lammer J, et al: Drug-eluting and bare nitinol stents for the treatment of atherosclerotic lesions in the superficial femoral artery: long-term results from the SIROCCO trial, *J Endovasc Ther* 13:701–710, 2006.
18. Murphy TP, Ariaratnam NS, Carney WI Jr., et al: Aortoiliac insufficiency: long-term experience with stent placement for treatment, *Radiology* 231:243–249, 2004.
19. Park KB, Do YS, Kim JH, et al: Stent placement for chronic iliac arterial occlusive disease: the results of 10 years experience in a single institution, *Korean J Radiol* 6:256–266, 2005.
20. Leville CD, Kashyap VS, Clair DG, et al: Endovascular management of iliac artery occlusions: extending treatment to TransAtlantic Inter-Society Consensus class C and D patients, *J Vasc Surg* 43:32–39, 2006.
21. Timaran CH, Prault TL, Stevens SL, et al: Iliac artery stenting versus surgical reconstruction for TASC (TransAtlantic Inter-Society Consensus) type B and type C iliac lesions, *J Vasc Surg* 38:272–278, 2003.
22. Hans SS, DeSantis D, Siddiqui R, et al: Results of endovascular therapy and aortobifemoral grafting for Transatlantic Inter-Society type C and D aortoiliac occlusive disease, *Surgery* 144:583–589, 2008 discussion 589–590.
23. Tetteroo E, Haaring C, van der Graaf Y, et al: Intraarterial pressure gradients after randomized angioplasty or stenting of iliac artery lesions. Dutch Iliac Stent Trial Study Group, *Cardiovasc Intervent Radiol* 19:411–417, 1996.
24. Klein WM, van der Graaf Y, Seegers J, et al: Long-term cardiovascular morbidity, mortality, and reintervention after endovascular treatment in patients with iliac artery disease: the Dutch Iliac Stent Trial Study, *Radiology* 232:491–498, 2004.
25. Klein WM, van der Graaf Y, Seegers J, et al: Dutch iliac stent trial: long-term results in patients randomized for primary or selective stent placement, *Radiology* 238:734–744, 2006.
26. Bosch JL, Hunink MG: Meta-analysis of the results of percutaneous transluminal angioplasty and stent placement for aortoiliac occlusive disease, *Radiology* 204:87–96, 1997.
27. Spronk S, Bosch JL, Veen HF, et al: Intermittent claudication: functional capacity and quality of life after exercise training or percutaneous transluminal angioplasty–systematic review, *Radiology* 235:833–842, 2005.
28. de Vries SO, Visser K, de Vries JA, et al: Intermittent claudication: cost-effectiveness of revascularization versus exercise therapy, *Radiology* 222:25–36, 2002.
29. Feinglass J, McCarthy WJ, Slavensky R, et al: Functional status and walking ability after lower extremity bypass grafting or angioplasty for intermittent claudication: results from a prospective outcomes study, *J Vasc Surg* 31:93–103, 2000.
30. Mazari FAK, Gulati S, Rahman MNA, et al: Early outcomes from a randomized, controlled trial of supervised exercise, angioplasty, and combined therapy in intermittent claudication, *Ann Vasc Surg* 24:69–79, 2010.
31. Muradin GS, Bosch JL, Stijnen T, et al: Balloon dilation and stent implantation for treatment of femoropopliteal arterial disease: meta-analysis, *Radiology* 221:137–145, 2001.
32. Scheinert D, Scheinert S, Sax J, et al: Prevalence and clinical impact of stent fractures after femoropopliteal stenting, *J Am Coll Cardiol* 45:312–315, 2005.
33. Schlager O, Dick P, Sabeti S, et al: Long-segment SFA stenting–the dark sides: in-stent restenosis, clinical deterioration, and stent fractures, *J Endovasc Ther* 12:676–684, 2005.
34. Fischer M, Schwabe C, Schulte KL: Value of the Hemobahn/Viabahn endoprosthesis in the treatment of long chronic lesions of the superficial femoral artery: 6 years of experience, *J Endovasc Ther* 13:281–290, 2006.
35. McQuade K, Gable D, Hohman S, et al: Randomized comparison of ePTFE/nitinol self-expanding stent graft vs. prosthetic femoral-popliteal bypass in the treatment of superficial femoral artery occlusive disease, *J Vasc Surg* 49:109–115, 116 e1–e9, 2009; discussion 116.
36. McQuade K, Gable D, Pearl G, et al: Four-year randomized prospective comparison of percutaneous ePTFE/nitinol self-expanding stent graft versus prosthetic femoral-popliteal bypass in the treatment of superficial femoral artery occlusive disease, *J Vasc Surg* 52:584–590, 2010.
37. Duda SH, Pusich B, Richter G, et al: Sirolimus-eluting stents for the treatment of obstructive superficial femoral artery disease: six-month results, *Circulation* 106:1505–1509, 2002.
38. Dake MD, Van Alstine WG, Zhou Q, et al: Polymer-free paclitaxel-coated Zilver PTX Stents–evaluation of pharmacokinetics and comparative safety in porcine arteries, *J Vasc Interv Radiol* 22:603–610, 2011.
39. Tepe G, Zeller T, Albrecht T, et al: Local delivery of paclitaxel to inhibit restenosis during angioplasty of the leg, *N Engl J Med* 358:689–699, 2008.

40. Werk M, Langner S, Reinkensmeier B, et al: Inhibition of restenosis in femoropopliteal arteries: paclitaxel-coated versus uncoated balloon: femoral paclitaxel randomized pilot trial, *Circulation* 118:1358–1365, 2008.

41. Gray WA, Granada JF: Drug-coated balloons for the prevention of vascular restenosis, *Circulation* 121:2672–2680, 2010.

42. Diehm N, Silvestro A, Do DD, et al: Endovascular brachytherapy after femoropopliteal balloon angioplasty fails to show robust clinical benefit over time, *J Endovasc Ther* 12:723–730, 2005.

43. Wolfram RM, Budinsky AC, Pokrajac B, et al: Endovascular brachytherapy for prophylaxis of restenosis after femoropopliteal angioplasty: five-year follow-up–prospective randomized study, *Radiology* 240:878–884, 2006.

44. Wolfram RM, Budinsky AC, Pokrajac B, et al: Endovascular brachytherapy: restenosis in de novo versus recurrent lesions of femoropopliteal artery–the Vienna experience, *Radiology* 236:338–342, 2005.

45. Pokrajac B, Kirisits C, Rainer S, et al: Beta endovascular brachytherapy using CO2-filled centering catheter for treatment of recurrent superficial femoropopliteal artery disease, *Cardiovasc Revasc Med* 10:162–165, 2009.

46. Therasse E, Donath D, Lesperance J, et al: External beam radiation to prevent restenosis after superficial femoral artery balloon angioplasty, *Circulation* 111:3310–3315, 2005.

47. Reekers J: Challenging a myth: directional atherectomy, *Cardiovasc Intervent Radiol* 32:203–204, 2009.

48. Vroegindeweij D, Tielbeek AV, Buth J, et al: Directional atherectomy versus balloon angioplasty in segmental femoropopliteal artery disease: two-year follow-up with color-flow duplex scanning, *J Vasc Surg* 21:255–268, 1995 discussion 268–9.

49. Indes JE, Shah HJ, Jonker FHW, et al: Subintimal angioplasty is superior to Silverhawk atherectomy for the treatment of occlusive lesions of the lower extremities, *J Endovasc Ther* 17:243–250, 2010.

50. Zeller T, Rastan A, Schwarzwalder U, et al: Percutaneous peripheral atherectomy of femoropopliteal stenoses using a new-generation device: six-month results from a single-center experience, *J Endovasc Ther* 11:676–685, 2004.

51. Suri R, Wholey MH, Postoak D, et al: Distal embolic protection during femoropopliteal atherectomy, *Catheter Cardiovasc Interv* 67:417–422, 2006.

52. Zeller T, Rastan A, Sixt S, et al: Long-term results after directional atherectomy of femoropopliteal lesions, *J Am Coll Cardiol* 48:1573–1578, 2006.

53. Scheinert D, Laird JR Jr., Schroder M, et al: Excimer laser-assisted recanalization of long, chronic superficial femoral artery occlusions, *J Endovasc Ther* 8:156–166, 2001.

54. Steinkamp HJ, Rademaker J, Wissgott C, et al: Percutaneous transluminal laser angioplasty versus balloon dilation for treatment of popliteal artery occlusions, *J Endovasc Ther* 9:882–888, 2002.

55. Engelke C, Sandhu C, Morgan RA, et al: Using 6-mm cutting balloon angioplasty in patients with resistant peripheral artery stenosis: preliminary results, *AJR Am J Roentgenol* 179:619–623, 2002.

56. Wildgruber M, Berger H: Cryoplasty for the prevention of arterial restenosis, *Cardiovasc Intervent Radiol* 31:1050–1058, 2008.

57. Spiliopoulos S, Katsanos K, Karnabatidis D, et al: Cryoplasty versus conventional balloon angioplasty of the femoropopliteal artery in diabetic patients: long-term results from a prospective randomized single-center controlled trial, *Cardiovasc Intervent Radiol*, 33: 929–938, 2010.

58. Dorros G, Jaff MR, Dorros AM, et al: Tibioperoneal (outflow lesion) angioplasty can be used as primary treatment in 235 patients with critical limb ischemia: five-year follow-up, *Circulation* 104:2057–2062, 2001.

59. Krankenberg H, Sorge I, Zeller T, et al: Percutaneous transluminal angioplasty of infrapopliteal arteries in patients with intermittent claudication: acute and one-year results, *Catheter Cardiovasc Interv* 64:12–17, 2005.

60. Dorros G, Lewin RF, Jamnadas P, et al: Below-the-knee angioplasty: tibioperoneal vessels, the acute outcome, *Cathet Cardiovasc Diagn* 19:170–178, 1990.

61. Soder HK, Manninen HI, Jaakkola P, et al: Prospective trial of infrapopliteal artery balloon angioplasty for critical limb ischemia: angiographic and clinical results, *J Vasc Interv Radiol* 11:1021–1031, 2000.

62. Peregrin J, Kožnar B, Kováč J, et al: PTA of infrapopliteal arteries: long-term clinical follow-up and analysis of factors influencing clinical outcome, *Cardiovasc Intervent Radiol* 33:720–725, 2010.

63. Feiring AJ, Wesolowski AA, Lade S: Primary stent-supported angioplasty for treatment of below-knee critical limb ischemia and severe claudication: early and one-year outcomes, *J Am Coll Cardiol* 44:2307–2314, 2004.

64. Randon C, Jacobs B, De Ryck F, et al: Angioplasty or primary stenting for infrapopliteal lesions: results of a prospective randomized trial, *Cardiovasc Intervent Radiol* 33:260–269, 2010.

65. Siablis D, Karnabatidis D, Katsanos K, et al: Infrapopliteal application of sirolimus-eluting versus bare metal stents for critical limb ischemia: analysis of long-term angiographic and clinical outcome, *J Vasc Interv Radiol* 20:1141–1150, 2009.

66. Biondi-Zoccai GG, Sangiorgi G, Lotrionte M, et al: Infragenicular stent implantation for below-the-knee atherosclerotic disease: clinical evidence from an international collaborative meta-analysis on 640 patients, *J Endovasc Ther* 16:251–260, 2009.

67. Scheinert D, Ulrich M, Scheinert S, et al: Comparison of sirolimus-eluting vs. bare-metal stents for the treatment of infrapopliteal obstructions, *EuroIntervention* 2:169–174, 2006.

68. Siablis D, Kraniotis P, Karnabatidis D, et al: Sirolimus-eluting versus bare stents for bailout after suboptimal infrapopliteal angioplasty for critical limb ischemia: 6-month angiographic results from a nonrandomized prospective single-center study, *J Endovasc Ther* 12:685–695, 2005.

69. Lederman RJ, Mendelsohn FO, Anderson RD, et al: Therapeutic Angiogenesis with Recombinant Fibroblast Growth Factor-2 for Intermittent Claudication (the TRAFFIC study): a randomised trial, *Lancet* 359:2053–2058, 2002.

70. Rajagopalan S, Mohler ER 3rd, Lederman RJ, et al: Regional angiogenesis with vascular endothelial growth factor in peripheral arterial disease: a phase II randomized, double-blind, controlled study of adenoviral delivery of vascular endothelial growth factor 121 in patients with disabling intermittent claudication, *Circulation* 108:1933–1938, 2003.

71. Henry TD, Annex BH, McKendall GR, et al: The VIVA Trial: Vascular Endothelial Growth Factor in Ischemia for Vascular Angiogenesis, *Circulation* 107:1359–1365, 2003.

72. Tongers J, Roncalli JG, Losordo DW: Therapeutic angiogenesis for critical limb ischemia: microvascular therapies coming of age, *Circulation* 118:9–16, 2008.

ENDOVASCULAR TREATMENT OF PERIPHERAL ARTERY DISEASE

CHAPTER 21

Reconstructive Surgery for Peripheral Artery Disease

Matthew T. Menard, James T. McPhee, Michael Belkin

The clinical manifestations and complications of atherosclerosis are the most common therapeutic challenge encountered by vascular surgeons. The tendency for lesions to develop at specific anatomical sites and follow recognizable patterns of progression was appreciated as long ago as the late 1700s by the extraordinary British anatomist and surgeon John Hunter. Considered one of the forefathers of vascular surgery, his dissections of atherosclerotic aortic bifurcations remain on view at the Hunterian museum in London and presage the disease process Leriche would give a name to 150 years later.[1]

The modern era of surgical reconstruction for complex atherosclerotic occlusive disease began in earnest in 1947 when the Portuguese surgeon J. Cid dos Santos successfully endarterectomized a heavily diseased common femoral artery (CFA).[2] Four years later in San Francisco, Wylie et al. extended this new technique to the aortoiliac level.[3] At the same time, and building on the pioneering work of Alexis Carrel,[4] Kunlin[5] would report the first long-segment vein bypass in the lower extremity. It would be another 10 years before synthetic grafts were being regularly used for aortic bypass grafting and the first efforts to extend vein grafting to the tibial level were described by McCaughan.[6] Tremendous advances in our understanding of atherosclerosis biology and ability to percutaneously treat arterial occlusive disease have dramatically affected treatment algorithms for arterial insufficiency in recent years. This chapter will review the current role for surgical management of aortoiliac and infrainguinal arterial occlusive disease.

Aortoiliac Occlusive Disease

Chronic obliterative atherosclerosis of the distal aorta and iliac arteries commonly manifests as symptomatic arterial insufficiency of the lower extremities. Disease in this location is seen often in combination with occlusive disease of the femoropopliteal arteries, producing a range of symptoms from mild claudication to more severe levels of tissue loss and critical ischemia. Patients with hemodynamic impairment limited to the aortoiliac system may have intermittent claudication of the calf muscles alone or involvement of the thigh, hip, and/or buttocks. If disease distribution also targets the hypogastric vessels, patients may additionally suffer from difficulty in achieving and maintaining an erection due to inadequate perfusion of the internal pudendal arteries. The equivalent impact of impaired pelvic perfusion in women remains poorly understood but has attracted investigative attention.[7] A well-characterized constellation of symptoms and signs known as *Leriche's syndrome*, associated with aortoiliac occlusive disease in men, includes thigh, hip, or buttock claudication, leg muscle atrophy, impotence, and reduced femoral pulses.[8]

Although atherosclerotic disease limited to the aortoiliac region commonly gives rise to claudication of varying degrees, it is rarely associated with lower-extremity ischemic rest pain or ischemic tissue loss. This is largely the result of adequate collateralization around the point of obstruction via lumbar, sacral, and circumflex iliac vessels that serves to reconstitute the infrainguinal system with enough well-perfused arterial blood to ensure sufficient resting tissue perfusion (Fig. 21-1). A well-recognized exception to this general observation arises in the situation of embolic disease. *Blue toe syndrome* represents a situation where atherosclerotic debris breaks free from an aortic or iliac plaque and embolizes to distal vessels.[9,10] Wire manipulation during coronary or peripheral angiographic procedures and cross-clamping across a calcific aortic plaque during cardiac surgery are common sources of such

emboli. The terminal target of the microembolic particles, be they cholesterol crystals, calcified plaque, thrombus, or platelet aggregates, is typically the small vessels of the toes.

If aortoiliac occlusive disease is found in combination with femoropopliteal occlusive disease, ischemic rest pain or even more severe perfusion impairment leading to ischemic tissue loss or gangrene is not uncommon.[11] Such progressive disease affecting multiple levels of the peripheral vasculature tree is most frequently encountered in the elderly. Approximately a third of patients operated on for symptomatic aortoiliac occlusive disease have orificial profunda femoris occlusive disease, and more than 40% have superficial femoral artery (SFA) occlusions. Aortoiliac disease typically begins at the distal aorta and common iliac artery (CIA) origins, and slowly progresses proximally and distally over time.[12] This progression is quite variable but may ultimately extend to the level of the renal arteries or result in total aortic occlusion.

A particularly virulent form of atherosclerotic arterial disease is often found in young women smokers.[13] Radiographic imaging in this subset of patients typically reveals atretic narrowed vasculature with diffusely calcific atherosclerotic changes. Frequently, a focal stenosis is found posteriorly near the aortic bifurcation. This particular distribution of disease and the characteristic patient profile have been referred to as *small aorta syndrome*[14] (Fig. 21-2). Such patients invariably have an extensive smoking history, with or without other typical factors for atherosclerosis. Given the diminutive size of the aorta and iliac vessels, the durability of endovascular intervention is generally inferior in these patients, particularly in the face of continued cigarette use.

The diagnosis of aortoiliac occlusive disease is generally made based on patient symptomatology, physical examination, and noninvasive tests such as segmental pressure measurements and pulse volume recordings (PVRs) (see Chapters 11 and 12). Following diagnosis of aortoiliac disease and the decision to pursue intervention, further imaging is warranted. In many centers, magnetic resonance angiography (MRA) and computed tomographic angiography (CTA) have supplanted contrast angiography as the initial imaging studies of choice. Advances have solved many of the technical limitations of earlier studies, and reliable roadmaps to guide operative planning are now reproducibly obtainable. Both MRA and CTA allow for a comprehensive view of the vascular tree with three-dimensional (3D) reconstructions (see Chapters 13 and 14). Computed tomographic angiography has the additional benefit of evaluating vessel morphology beyond the flow lumen, and allows for appreciation of degree of vessel calcification as well as anatomical localization based on surrounding structures. Angiographic findings of CTA compare favorably to standard digital subtraction angiography (DSA).[15] Should a lesion amenable to percutaneous therapy be identified on MRA or CTA, formal angiography is then pursued. In cases in which a good-quality roadmap is obtained with MRA or CTA, and the clinical situation or anatomical pattern is unfavorable to a percutaneous approach, surgery can in most instances be planned directly, obviating the need for traditional subtraction angiography.[16]

In the minority of cases necessitating DSA for preoperative planning, a retrograde femoral approach is typically used, whereas the transbrachial approach serves as a useful alternative in patients with particularly challenging anatomy.[17] Additional lateral and oblique views of the abdominal aorta are advised if concomitant mesenteric or renal occlusive disease is present, and multiple projections of the iliac and femoral bifurcations are essential in clarifying the extent of disease in these regions (see Chapter 15). Finally,

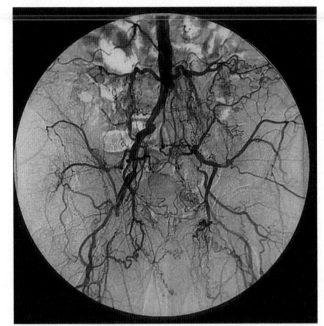

FIGURE 21-1 Aortoiliac occlusive disease results in a variable degree of collateralization. Here, left hypogastric artery is reconstituted via prominent distal lumbar collaterals and right hypogastric artery. Hypogastric collaterals are in turn perfusing femoral circumflex vessels.

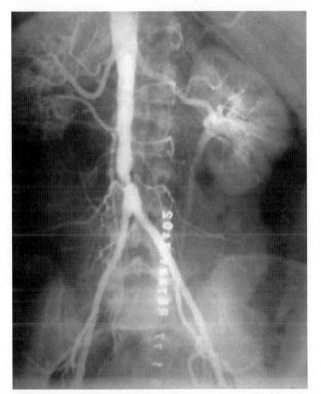

FIGURE 21-2 Aortoiliac occlusive disease may consist of a short-segment stenosis localized to distal aorta, a lesion particularly common in young female smokers. Such a lesion may be amenable to endarterectomy.

full runoff views of the lower extremities are needed to assess the presence or absence of femoropopliteal or crural disease. In ambiguous cases, pullback pressure measurements, both before and after administration of a systemic vasodilator such as papaverine or nitroglycerine, or application of a tourniquet to induce reactive hyperemia can be useful in documenting the hemodynamic significance of a particular stenotic zone.[18]

Management

Risk factor modification remains a cornerstone of management of aortoiliac occlusive disease (see Chapter 19). Smoking cessation, blood pressure control, and aggressive efforts at cholesterol lowering should be addressed with every patient with atherosclerotic disease. Strong evidence exists supporting the benefit of a structured walking program[19] in increasing walking distance of patients with claudication. The benefit of walking outside of a structured regimen with close follow-up is more debatable.[20] Medical management with cilostazol has benefit in a subset of patients and is a reasonable first-line approach to improving claudication symptoms.[21]

A considerable change in the management approach to claudication has taken place in recent years. Patients suffering from disabling claudication, rest pain, or ischemia-related tissue loss warrant serious consideration for arteriography and either percutaneous or surgical intervention. Previously, however, such aggressive treatment would have been considered inappropriate for claudication that was not clearly disabling. As percutaneous treatment has become increasingly safer and more effective, however, and its application spread to increasingly more arterial beds, indications for endovascular revascularization have correspondingly increased (see Chapter 20). Such a sea change in the overall management approach to aortoiliac disease has had a dramatic impact on the numbers of patients now proceeding to open surgery. Just as escalating use of renal angioplasty and stenting for renal occlusive disease has led to a considerable drop in open surgical renal artery reconstructions, the rising popularity and success of aortic and iliac balloon angioplasty and stenting as first-line therapy has noticeably reduced the volume of aortoiliac reconstructive procedures performed in this country.

When medical therapy or percutaneous treatment has proven to be inadequate or is technically inadvisable, open surgical revascularization remains indicated for those patients with aortoiliac disease and disabling claudication, ischemic rest pain, and ischemic ulceration or gangrene. Patients with nighttime foot rest pain or tissue loss usually have multisegment disease, and the decision whether to perform both supra- and infrainguinal revascularization procedures or to perform only an inflow procedure is guided by severity of the ischemia.[11,22–24] In general, patients presenting with significant tissue loss or gangrene are much more likely to require simultaneous or staged inflow and outflow procedures.

The numerous surgical options available to the trained vascular surgeon allow tailoring of the approach to the particular overall and anatomical situation of each patient. Historically, reconstructive options for aortoiliac occlusive disease include aortoiliac endarterectomy, aortobifemoral bypass, and so-called extra-anatomical revascularization in the form of iliofemoral, femorofemoral, or axillofemoral grafting.

ENDARTERECTOMY

Aortic endarterectomy was commonly performed in the early era of aortoiliac reconstruction.[25,26] Although it is particularly suited to localized disease limited to the distal aorta or proximal iliac arteries, it has proven to be less reliable for disease involving the entire infrarenal aorta and extending into the external iliac arteries (EIAs).[27,28] The obvious benefit of endarterectomy is elimination of the need for a prosthetic graft, removing the possibility of myriad late graft-related complications. Long-term patency of limited endarterectomy is excellent and on par with bypass procedures.[29] However, the number of patients suitable for this reconstructive approach is small and continues to diminish in the era of endoluminal reconstruction. Experience with endarterectomy during one's training or early surgical career is another important factor influencing the choice of therapy offered because significant technical expertise is required, and many surgeons in the current era have limited familiarity with this approach.

AORTOBIFEMORAL BYPASS

Aortobifemoral bypass remains the mainstay of operative treatment for aortoiliac occlusive disease. During the last 20 years, the procedure has supplanted both aortic endarterectomy and aortoiliac bypass procedures. In the latter case, this change was largely driven by recognition of subsequent graft failure due to progression of native iliac arterial disease.[27,30] Early experience with aortobifemoral grafting in the 1970s was associated with a 5% to 8% 30-day operative mortality rate.[28,29,31,32] Over recent decades, mortality rates of 1% have been reported, on par with those of elective abdominal aortic aneurysm repair.[33,34]

Typically, half of patients proceeding to surgery for aortoiliac occlusive disease will have significant coronary artery disease, (CAD) even more will have hypertension, and almost 80% will be current or earlier cigarette smokers.[33] The reduced mortality and morbidity seen in recent years are in large part due to advances in management of concomitant coronary disease. Specifically, the importance and benefit of better preoperative identification of patients in need of initial coronary revascularization, awareness of the benefit of waiting an interval period following coronary stenting before proceeding with major noncoronary vascular surgery, improved perioperative pharmacological management of patients with impaired myocardium, and more focused efforts to tailor operative and postoperative fluid administration to the individual patient's myocardial reserve are all well recognized.[35,36] General advances in postoperative intensive care unit management, including pulmonary care, infection control, and blood product utilization, have further contributed to the progress seen.

Current early patency rates for aortobifemoral bypass grafting are excellent, approaching 100% in many reporting institutions. Five-year patency rates are greater than 80%,[29,31–33,37] whereas 10-year rates are near 75%.[29] There are multiple reasons for the improved patency. The current graft material used by most surgeons for aortoiliac reconstruction is a knitted Dacron prosthesis with enhanced hemostatic properties; it tends to have a more stable pseudointima than earlier-used woven grafts.[38,39] More attention is paid to avoiding graft redundancy and ensuring a good size match between the graft and the recipient vessels. Grafts are more routinely extended beyond the iliac level to the femoral vessels, which not only improves exposure and makes for a technically easier distal anastomosis but is also associated with less graft thrombosis from unanticipated progression of atherosclerotic disease in the external iliac vessels.[30] With meticulous skin preparation, close attention to draping, careful surgical technique, and judicious use of a short course of intravenous antibiotic therapy, the feared higher rate of graft infection from placing the distal dissection at the groins has not materialized.[40] An exception to this general practice is recommended in certain circumstances, however. For example, patients with hostile groin creases from prior surgery or radiation therapy, or obese diabetic patients with an intertriginous rash at the inguinal crease, will all likely be better served by performing the distal anastomosis at the external iliac level if their anatomy for such is suitable.

Increased awareness of the critical role played by the deep femoral artery (DFA) in preserving long-term patency of aortobifemoral grafts[29,32,41,42] has also undoubtedly contributed to the better results seen. This awareness parallels a better overall appreciation for the importance of establishing adequate outflow at the femoral level in achieving higher early and late graft patency rates and sustained symptom relief. The true impact of concomitant SFA disease is unclear from the literature. Some reports have indicated similar patency rates between those patients with and without SFA occlusion,[22,23] whereas others have suggested late patency rates are reduced in this setting.[40,43] What has definitely been shown is the benefit of a profundaplasty in the presence of significant superficial and profunda femoral occlusive disease.[44,45] Some authors have even recommended that a profundaplasty should be carried out in every case of superficial artery occlusion, even in the absence of orificial profunda disease, arguing that a "functional" obstruction on the order of 50% stenosis is present in these patients.[46] Although

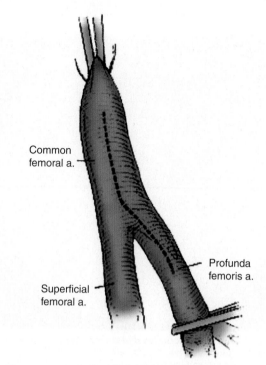

FIGURE 21-3 In the setting of superficial femoral artery (SFA) and orificial profunda femoral artery disease, extending common femoral arteriotomy into origin of profunda and performing a profundaplasty prior to completing distal anastomosis of aortobifemoral bypass will improve outflow and maximize graft patency.

this position has not been universally adopted, it is now common practice to extend the hood of the distal anastomosis over the origin of the profunda femoral artery to enhance the graft outflow, especially in situations in which the SFA is occluded or severely diseased. In the presence of significant common femoral or profunda femoral origin plaque, an extensive endarterectomy and/or profundaplasty is indicated (Fig. 21-3). In these circumstances, it is preferable to close the endarterectomized recipient bed with a vein, bovine pericardial patch, or Dacron patch onto which the distal anastomosis can then be attached, rather than creating a long femoris patch with the graft limb.[41]

Several technical considerations related to aortobifemoral bypass grafting are the subject of considerable and passionate debate. The first involves the manner of the proximal anastomotic creation. Advocates of an end-to-end configuration claim that it facilitates a more comprehensive thromboendarterectomy of the proximal stump and allows for a direct, more inline flow pattern with less turbulence and more favorable flow characteristics.[47] Obviation of competitive flow through the excluded iliac vessels with this approach is likely more of theoretical rather than real benefit. Certainly, with concomitant aneurysmal disease or complete aortic occlusion extending up to the level of the renal arteries, end-to-end grafting is indicated. Creation of an end-to-side anastomosis can at times be technically challenging in a heavily diseased aorta partially occluded by a side-biting clamp. A lower rate of proximal suture line pseudoaneurysms and better long-term patency rates have been found in some series.[48] Stapling or oversewing of the distal aorta with the end-to-end technique minimizes the immediate risk of clamp-induced emboli to the lower extremities following release of the distal clamp. Finally, those in favor of this approach claim that ability to more effectively close the retroperitoneum, particularly after resection of a short segment of the infrarenal aorta, results in lower rates of late graft infection and aortoenteric fistulae, although there is no direct evidence to support this assertion.

There are certain circumstances when an end-to-side proximal anastomotic configuration is advantageous. The most common indication involves those patients with occluded external iliac arteries, in whom interruption of forward aortic flow may result in loss of perfusion to an important hypogastric or inferior mesenteric artery (IMA) and consequent significant pelvic ischemia. Colon ischemia (1%-2%),[49] or even more rarely, paraplegia secondary to cauda equina syndrome (<1%),[50] are additional complications that can be avoided by an end-to-side configuration. Although advocated by some,[51] routine preservation of a patent IMA is not universally practiced.

Operative Management

The operative procedure is performed under general endotracheal anesthesia, with an epidural catheter placed for postoperative pain control. The patient is sterilely prepped and draped from the mid-chest to the mid-thighs. The femoral vessels are first exposed through bilateral longitudinal oblique incisions, thereby reducing the time in which the abdomen is open and the viscera exposed. Extent of exposure of the femoral vessels is dictated by severity of disease and level of reconstruction planned for the CFA and its bifurcation. Next, the inferior aspect of the retroperoneal tunnel through which the graft will course to reach the femoral region is begun with digital manipulation posterior to the inguinal ligament and tracking along the anterior aspect of the external iliac artery. Antibiotic-soaked sponges are then placed in the groin wounds, and attention is turned to the aortic dissection.

The proximal reconstruction is performed via a midline laparotomy. In general, aortic dissection is limited to the region between the renal arteries and the inferior mesenteric artery. This allows avoidance of extensive dissection anterior to the aortic bifurcation, where the autonomic nerve plexus regulating erection and ejaculation in men sweeps over the aorta. An intriguing recent survey indicated no significant differences in the rate of sexual dysfunction with open compared with endovascular repair of abdominal

aortic aneurysms, suggesting the effects of aortic dissection in this area are perhaps less important than typically believed.[52]

In situations where significant aortic calcification extends up to the level of the renal arteries, it may be necessary to continue aortic dissection to the suprarenal or even supraceliac level to allow for safe proximal clamp placement. Alternatively, proximal control may be obtained by intraluminal balloon deployment. If end-to-side repair is planned, circumferential dissection of the aortic segment to be clamped is recommended; gaining control of any lumbar or accessory renal vessels encountered prior to performing the aortotomy helps avoid troublesome backbleeding. The superior aspect of the graft limb tunnels are then completed, taking care to maintain a course anterior to the common iliac vessels but posterior to the ureters. Between 5000 and 7000 units of heparin are then administered, with additional heparin given throughout the procedure to maintain the activated clotting time near the target range of 250 to 300 seconds. After allowing sufficient time for the heparin to circulate, atraumatic vascular clamps are placed above the IMA and just below the renal arteries. The distal clamp is applied first to avoid any distal embolization of plaque dislodged with placement of the proximal clamp. If an end-to-end anastomosis is planned, the aorta is transected 1 to 2 cm below the proximal clamp, and a short segment of the distal aortic cuff is excised (Fig. 21-4A). This results in better exposure of the aortic neck and a more precise proximal reconstruction, and also allows the graft to lie flat against the vertebral column rather than anteriorly oriented, facilitating later retroperitoneal coverage. If necessary, a thromboendarterectomy of the infrarenal neck is carried out at this point (Fig. 21-4B). Anastomosis is performed with a running suture of 3-0 polypropylene (Fig. 21-4C). The distal aorta is then oversewn with two layers of a running monofilament suture or stapled with a surgical stapler. If an end-to-side anastomosis is performed, an anterior longitudinal arteriotomy is carried out after placement of proximal and distal transaortic clamps. If necessary,

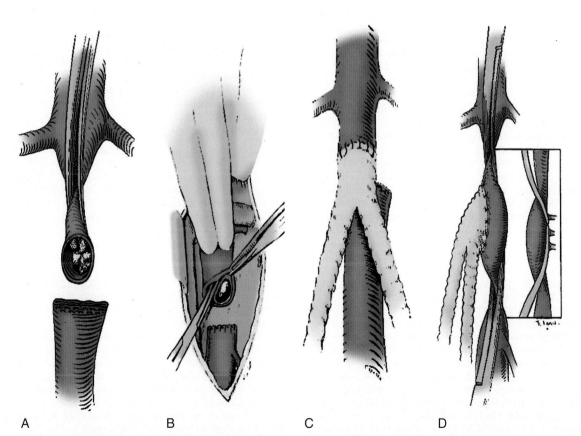

A   B   C   D

FIGURE 21-4   End-to-end proximal anastomosis for aortofemoral reconstruction is initiated with infrarenal aorta cross-clamp placed in anterior/ posterior direction as close to origin of renal arteries as possible. Aorta is transected 1 to 2 cm below proximal clamp. A short segment of distal aortic cuff is excised, and aorta is stapled or oversewn just proximal to origin of inferior mesenteric artery (IMA) **(A)**. If necessary, a thromboendarterectomy of the aortic cuff is carried out **(B)**. End-to-end configuration allows graft to lie flat against vertebral column and results in less turbulent flow **(C)**. End-to-side configuration is required to preserve antegrade pelvic perfusion in situations where retrograde flow would be compromised due to heavily diseased or occluded external iliac arteries (EIAs) **(D)**.

an endarterectomy is performed and anastomosis carried out after the graft is beveled appropriately (Fig. 21-4D). If minimal plaque is present, the distal anastomosis is performed to the common femoral artery, and individual dissection of the superficial femoral and profunda femoral arteries is not necessary.

Another point of some debate concerns optimal management of patients with multilevel occlusive disease. The question frequently arises as to whether or under what circumstances a concomitant or staged outflow procedure should be performed. It is generally believed that up to 80% of patients with both inflow and outflow disease will be substantially improved following aorto-femoral bypass grafting.[11,22] Other reports, however, have suggested that as many as a quarter to a third of such patients will not have significant symptomatic relief with an inflow procedure alone.[23] Although no single parameter exists to reliably guide the surgeon to know in which circumstances a combined procedure is optimal, severity of distal ischemia is probably the most important factor to be considered. Overall medical condition of patients and their ability to tolerate a prolonged operative procedure is also clearly important. Finally, the status of the profunda femoral artery must be taken into consideration. In the presence of SFA occlusion, a profunda that is atretic or extensively diseased may well be unable to provide sufficient collateral runoff to the foot.

If on the one hand, the bypass procedure is undertaken for claudication alone or mild rest pain, restoring adequate inflow may provide sufficient and relatively durable symptomatic relief. If on the other hand, significant tissue loss is present, a combined inflow and outflow procedure is likely warranted if limb salvage is to be achieved. If several operating teams are used, performing both procedures at the same time can be done in an acceptably timely fashion and has been found to be safe. Indeed, several recent reports found no significant differences in operative mortality or perioperative morbidity in patients undergoing concurrent inflow and outflow procedures compared with those having major inflow reconstruction alone.[53,54] Although staged revascularization may be preferable in certain circumstances, both the risk of wound and graft infection resulting from redissection in the groin and the risk of progressive tissue loss during the initial recuperative period must be considered with this approach.

Results

Aortobifemoral bypass grafting is associated with patency rates that are among the highest reported for any major arterial reconstruction. As indicated earlier, 5-year primary patency rates of 70% to 88%[29,31,32] and 10-year rates of 66% to 78%[29] have been described. Better rates have been realized in those patients with good infrainguinal outflow operated on for claudication, compared with those with limb-threatening ischemia and associated infrainguinal occlusive disease. In general, patients with disease limited to the aortoiliac region have excellent relief of symptoms following aortobifemoral grafting, whereas those with multilevel disease have less complete levels of symptom diminution. Perioperative mortality rates average 4%, whereas 5-year survival rates between 70% and 75% have been reported.[31,55,56] This latter rate is notably less than the 5-year survival rate of age-matched control population but on par with that typically seen for claudicants in general.

Although the early and late mortality rates are similar across different age groups, the 5-year primary and secondary patency rates are significantly increased with each increase in age group.[33] Reed et al. reported that primary patency rates were 66%, 87%, and 96%, and secondary patency rates were 79%, 91%, and 98% (Fig. 21-5), respectively, for those younger than 50, 50 to 59, and older than 60 years of age.[33] It seems prudent, based on these findings, to apply caution in the application of aortobifemoral bypass grafting for younger patients with virulent aortoiliac disease. The potential impact of graft failure and need for subsequent complex interventions should be considered, especially given the longer life expectancy of younger patients. Full utilization of all medical and endovascular options appears to be the best first-line option for younger patients with severe aortoiliac occlusive disease.

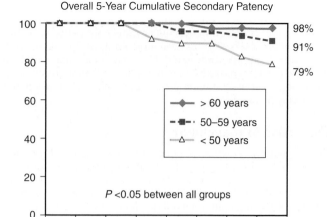

FIGURE 21-5 **Overall 5-year cumulative secondary patency rates in a recent cohort of patients undergoing aortobifemoral bypass grafting, indicating an inverse relationship between age and graft patency.** *(From Reed AB, Conte MS, Donaldson MC, et al: The impact of patient age and aortic size on the results of aortobifemoral bypass grafting, J Vasc Surg 37:1219, 2003.)*

EXTRA-ANATOMICAL BYPASS

When comorbid disease renders a patient with aortoiliac occlusive disease particularly unsuitable for major vascular surgery and aortic cross-clamping, or when sepsis, prior surgery, or the presence of a stoma presents a hostile surgical environment for abdominal exploration, several alternatives are available to the vascular surgeon. Reconstructive options in which the thoracic aorta, axillary, iliac, or femoral arteries serve as donor vessels are generally referred to as *extra-anatomical* to distinguish them from the inline flow represented by an aortobifemoral procedure. The concept of extra-anatomical arterial reconstruction emerged in the 1950s during a time of many new developments in the field of vascular surgery. Freeman and Leeds provided one of the first descriptions in 1952 in their report of the use of the SFA as the conduit for a crossover femorofemoral bypass graft.[57] These approaches are also called on in desperate situations represented by infection of a previously placed aortic graft.

AXILLOBIFEMORAL BYPASS

Axillobifemoral bypass grafting was introduced by Blaisdell[58] in the early 1960s and has since enjoyed increasing popularity as an alternative to aortobifemoral bypass. This is largely due to the reliability of the axillary artery as a donor vessel and the minimal morbidity incurred, making it a particularly appealing option for patients with significant operative risk from comorbid disease. It is also appropriate in patients with significant aortoiliac occlusive disease of the distal aorta and the iliac arteries in the setting of intraabdominal sepsis, a history of multiple prior abdominal operations, intraabdominal adhesions, or prior pelvic irradiation. Of note, LoGerfo et al.[59] have shown that axillobifemoral grafting has improved long-term patency compared with axillo-unifemoral grafting, presumably owing to the increased flow afforded by the second outflow limb.

Although usually performed under general anesthesia, it is possible to carry out the procedure using a combination of local anesthesia and intravenous conscious sedation. In the event that one arm has a higher blood pressure or a stronger pulse, that side should be selected as the donor site. If both sides are equal, the right axillary artery is chosen because evidence suggests there is a lower risk of arterial occlusive disease developing in the right subclavian artery compared with the left.

The axillary artery is exposed through a short infraclavicular incision parallel to the clavicle in the deltopectoral groove. The pectoralis major muscle is then bluntly separated between the clavicular and sternal heads, and the pectoralis minor muscle is identified and typically divided, enhancing exposure and allowing more space for the graft as it courses from the axilla to the subcutaneous space. The axillary artery medial to the pectoralis minor is then isolated because the proximal anastomosis is optimally placed as close to the chest as possible to minimize the risk of kinking or graft avulsion during rotational shoulder movement. Avoiding more lateral dissection further reduces the risk of injuring the medial and lateral cords of the brachial plexus as they emerge anteriorly to form the median nerve. A tunnel is created between the axillary and femoral arteries in the subcutaneous space, tracking deep to the pectoralis major muscle and inferiorly along the midaxillary line before coursing medial to the anterior superior iliac spine; this latter orientation is important to avoid kinking of the conduit in the sitting position. Long, rigid tunneling devices with a removable central obturator are specifically designed for this step and have helped lower the incidence of graft infection by obviating the need for counterincisions.

The CFAs are then dissected through standard bilateral short groin incisions, and a second subcutaneous tunnel is fashioned between them in an extrafascial suprapubic plane. A Dacron or polytetrafluoroethylene (PTFE) graft, typically 8 mm in diameter, is then drawn through the tunnel. Although there is no convincing evidence that one graft material is superior to the other, several reports support the common practice of using an externally reinforced graft.[60,61] Newer grafts are available that are prefigured in an axillobifemoral configuration, thereby reducing from four to three the number of anastomoses needed. As in aortobifemoral bypass grafting, unrestricted outflow should be ensured by carrying the hood of the femoral grafts down over the profunda orifice and performing an endarterectomy or profundaplasty when necessary. If a prefigured graft is unavailable, the origin of the cross-femoral graft can be tailored to the body habitus of the patient. In most cases, the graft is taken off the distal hood of the descending axillofemoral graft. In particularly obese individuals, however, it may be preferable to move the takeoff more proximally to prevent kinking at the level of the inguinal ligament. Orienting the takeoff of the crossover graft at an acute angle to give an S-shaped final configuration has been associated with higher patency rates in some studies.[62]

Many of the complications following axillofemoral grafting are directly related to the graft and potentially avoidable. Disruption of the proximal anastomosis, or *axillary pullout syndrome*, can be minimized by proper orientation of the proximal hood and ensuring that the descending limb of the graft is free from undue tension.[63] Kinking and subsequent thrombosis of the graft can be reduced by strict attention to tunnel position and use of a reinforced conduit. Given the minimal physiological insult, most patients undergoing axillofemoral grafting are ambulatory and able to tolerate a regular diet on the first postoperative day.

Reported long-term patency rates of axillofemoral grafts have varied significantly, ranging from as low as 29% to as high as 85%.[60,64–66] Favorable results were reported by Passman et al.,[67] who achieved 5-year patency rates of 74% and a long-term limb salvage rate of 89%, and who are vocal advocates of a wider use for this approach. In general, axillobifemoral grafting should be reserved for high-risk patients with significant tissue loss and in danger of limb loss, and not be used for treating claudication.

FEMOROFEMORAL BYPASS

Femorofemoral bypass grafts are ideally suited to patients with preserved flow in both the aorta and one iliac branch, but occlusion or severe stenosis of the contralateral iliac not amenable to percutaneous treatment (Figs. 21-6 and 21-7A-B). Although possible to perform under local anesthesia in high-risk patients, it is best carried out under regional or general anesthesia. On occasion, it has been performed in an intensive care unit setting in the particular instance of a leg rendered acutely ischemic by placement of

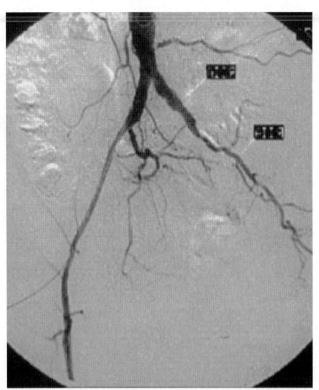

FIGURE 21-6 **Oblique-view digital subtraction angiogram indicating a long-segment total occlusion of left external iliac artery (EIA).** Extraanatomical left-to-right femorofemoral or iliofemoral bypass grafting would be appropriate options for this anatomical disease distribution (see also Fig. 21-7).

an intraaortic balloon pump. Technical details are identical to those of the crossover component of the axillobifemoral grafting discussed earlier. The suprapubic tunnel is created in a gentle C curve just superficial to the deep fascia, and can in most instances be completed by blunt finger dissection approaching from both groin incisions. Although some surgeons advocate placement of the tunnel beneath the rectus sheath, this is a minority view. Again, if warranted by the presence of significant concomitant femoral disease, an endarterectomy or profundaplasty is indicated prior to completion of the proximal or distal anastomosis.

Graft failure due to progression of inflow disease following femorofemoral grafting is less problematic than one might predict. Some investigators have argued that the increased flow through the donor iliac artery following restoration of bilateral outflow, in essence shifting the aortic bifurcation to a more distal point, serves to impede further development of atherosclerotic disease. Animal studies correlating blood flow and shear stress with intimal hyperplasia lend support to this explanation.[68] Maini and Mannick reported a 5-year cumulative patency rate of 80%.[69] This is similar to other reports in the literature[70–72] and compares favorably with the 85% rate seen with conventional aortobifemoral bypass grafting.[33]

With its high patency rates and low associated morbidity, cross-femoral grafting is an excellent option in patients with favorable anatomy. Given the risk of late graft failure from progression of inflow disease and the potential need to reintervene on previously dissected femoral beds should a later aortobifemoral graft be needed, however, it has traditionally been advised to proceed directly to aortobifemoral grafting in good-risk patients with any evidence of atherosclerotic disease in the aorta or patent iliac vessels. In the current era, aortic or iliac angioplasty and/or stenting in combination with cross-femoral grafting is a viable alternative in this setting, particularly for those patients at increased operative risk.

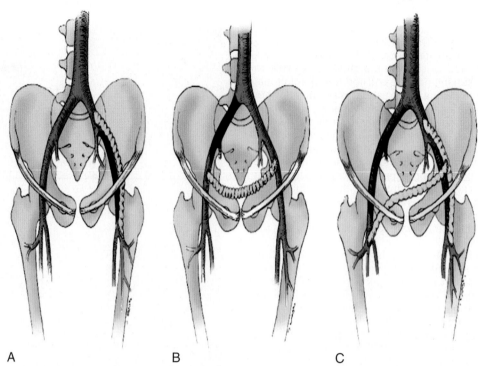

FIGURE 21-7 **Patent common or external iliac artery (EIA) may be used as donor vessel for (A) iliofemoral, (B) ilioiliac, or (C) iliobifemoral bypass grafts depicted.** Lesions depicted in **A** and **B** would also be appropriate for femorofemoral grafts, whereas lesion in **C** would be appropriate for aortobifemoral or axillobifemoral grafting.

ILIOFEMORAL BYPASS

Iliofemoral grafting is another alternative to aortobifemoral grafting for a selected group of patients with hemodynamically significant disease limited to the EIA (see Fig. 21-6). Currently, most patients with this anatomical pattern of disease would typically undergo an attempt at percutaneous recanalization of a tightly stenotic or long-segment external iliac occlusion. Indeed, as the success rates with such efforts increase, the number of iliofemoral bypass grafts performed has continued to fall. However, if the percutaneous approach is unsuccessful, an iliofemoral bypass remains an excellent surgical option because it can be performed with minimal morbidity and cardiopulmonary insult and avoids the long, descending limb necessitated by an axillofemoral graft (see Fig. 21-7). Because the grafts are situated within the pelvis, they are also better protected from kinking, infection, and thrombosis than either axillofemoral or femorofemoral grafts. Less disturbance of inguinal lymph nodes and lymphatic channels typically occurs with the more limited dissection necessary.

Either the ipsilateral common iliac or proximal EIA can serve as the donor site, and if need be, a bifurcated graft can be used and taken to both femoral vessels. Alternatively, bilateral iliofemoral grafts or an ilioiliac graft can be fashioned as appropriate. Iliac exposure can be achieved through an oblique suprainguinal "transplant" incision and development of the retroperitoneal plane, which affords excellent proximal exposure even in the obese patient. Care must be taken in isolating the donor vessel and tunneling the graft to avoid injury to the ureter coursing over the iliac bifurcation. If a crossover graft is used, it can be tunneled retroperitoneally in the iliac fossa or across the properitoneum deep to the rectus sheath.

In early experience with iliac origin grafts reported by Couch et al., there were no operative deaths and a 77% 4-year patency rate.[73] Nearly half of these patients were operated on for limb salvage in the face of critical ischemia. In patients undergoing revascularization with bilateral iliofemoral grafts, the 4-year patency rates were 92%, whereas an 85% patency rate was seen if both the superficial and deep femoral vessels were patent.[73] Other reported series of iliofemoral bypass grafting have indicated similar patency rates.[71,74]

THORACIC AORTA–TO–FEMORAL ARTERY BYPASS

As early as 1961, Blaisdell et al. reported on a novel extra-anatomical bypass from the descending thoracic aorta to the femoral artery, followed by a femorofemoral bypass.[75] Although carried out in the setting of sepsis after a ruptured aneurysm repair and not for occlusive disease, it provided a new alternative when the infrarenal aorta was inaccessible or inappropriate as a donor vessel. The procedure is performed through a thoracotomy incision, typically entering the chest through the eighth or ninth interspace. A muscle-sparing technique in which the latissimus dorsi muscle is not divided aids in postoperative pain management. The distal descending thoracic aorta is circumferentially dissected enough to allow for clamp control, with care taken to avoid injury to the adjacently positioned esophagus. A tunnel is fashioned by separating the diaphragm from the posterior chest wall over a distance of two finger breadths. In 1994, Criado and Keagy[76] reviewed the literature and summarized 193 reconstructions taken off the descending thoracic aorta. Not unexpectedly, the majority were performed for thrombosis or infection of a previously placed aortic graft, although some primary procedures undertaken in the setting of a "hostile" abdomen were included. Cumulative 5-year primary and secondary patency rates of 73% and 83%, respectively, were obtained, and the operative mortality rate was 6%.[76]

LAPAROSCOPIC REVASCULARIZATION

There is an increasing interest in applying laparoscopic techniques to the treatment of aortic occlusive disease, reflected in a small but growing body of literature of individual case series.[77,78] Some surgeons have favored a more limited approach using hand-assisted techniques and smaller incisions,[79] whereas others have championed the use of complete laparoscopic or robot-assisted revascularization.[77,80,81] The purported benefits of shorter hospital stays, less perioperative pain, and fewer postoperative complications are balanced against longer operative times and lack of long-term data to support the durability of this alternative approach. It remains at present an extremely technically challenging procedure with a significant learning curve. As the technology advances and improvement is seen with anastomotic devices and instrumentation, the role of aortofemoral bypass will likely expand and become more defined. At present, however, it has failed to gain widespread acceptance and is routinely undertaken in only a limited number of centers.

Infrainguinal Arterial Occlusive Disease

Infrainguinal arterial occlusive disease is the most prevalent manifestation of chronic arterial occlusive disease encountered and treated by the vascular surgeon. Isolated disease of the SFA typically manifests as calf muscle claudication, whereas patients with multilevel disease involving the superficial femoral, popliteal, and tibial arteries generally have rest pain or ischemic tissue loss. The ischemia ulcerations usually begin as small, dry ulcers of the toes or heel area and progress to frankly gangrenous changes of the forefoot or heel, with greater degrees of arterial insufficiency. Several identifiable patterns of disease are recognized, with smokers typically having disease limited to the SFA and corresponding symptoms of claudication. Diabetes most often targets the popliteal and tibial vessels, and patients may present with frank tissue necrosis with no history of claudication.

Infrainguinal reconstruction for treatment of peripheral vascular occlusive disease has been increasingly successful for both long-term palliation of intermittent claudication and for salvage of limbs threatened by critical ischemia. There are times when primary amputation represents the safest and most advisable solution in the face of irreversible ischemia, particularly in cases where extensive infection or tissue necrosis is present. In addition, certain patient populations may have a combination of risk factors that may be predictive of a prohibitively poor outcome. This may include patients of advanced age or those in a dependent living situation on hemodialysis.[82] Otherwise, an attempt at reconstruction is almost always indicated when a limb is threatened by severe ischemia. Improvements in perioperative management and surgical technique have allowed progressively more distal reconstructions to be successfully completed in an older, sicker, and more challenging patient population. In general, high rates of relief for claudication and up to an 80% to 90% limb salvage rate may be anticipated for patients with critical ischemia at institutions devoted to peripheral bypass surgery.

A large prospective randomized double-blinded multicenter trial, the Project of Ex Vivo Graft Engineering via Transfection III (PREVENT III), was recently conducted to evaluate the efficacy of edifoligide in preventing autogenous vein graft failure in lower extremity revascularization for critical limb ischemia (CLI).[83] Although the trial failed to show any significant primary patency or limb salvage benefit of the studied medication, it did provide valuable contemporary information regarding infrainguinal bypass outcomes. In the study cohort of 1404 patients from 83 North American sites, the 30-day operative mortality rate was 2.7%. Assisted primary patency, limb salvage, and survival at 1 year were 77%, 88%, and 84%, respectively.[83] A validated risk score subsequently created to allow stratification of patient risk factors in the setting of limb-threatening ischemia demonstrated that amputation-free survival was negatively associated with dialysis dependence, tissue loss, age older than 75, anemia, and coronary artery disease.[84] The PREVENT III dataset additionally provided one of the first comprehensive evaluations of patient quality of life before and after surgical revascularization. Notably, patients undergoing successful surgical revascularization reported a significant quality-of-life improvement at 1 year compared to baseline levels.[85]

The two major indications for surgical intervention of infrainguinal arterial occlusive disease are claudication and limb-threatening critical ischemia. Claudication is a relative indication, given the natural history of the disease; of patients with claudication, only 1% per year will ultimately progress to limb loss.[86,87] As such, it remains a subjective assessment on the parts of both patient and surgeon as to the relative degree of disability a given level of claudication pain represents.

Role of Percutaneous Transluminal Angioplasty

Of relevance in this regard is the significant shift in the indications for percutaneous intervention for infrainguinal occlusive disease witnessed in recent years. As the associated risks of balloon angioplasty and stenting have fallen and relative success rates have risen, the threshold for offering endovascular treatment to claudicants has decreased considerably. Patients once considered appropriate only for risk factor modification, exercise therapy, and medical treatment are now increasingly being offered percutaneous revascularization as a secondary or even primary treatment option (see Chapter 20). The relative merits of early intervention as opposed to traditional risk factor modification and exercise therapy for individuals with claudication remains controversial.[88] Some authors have found no improvement in quality-of-life outcomes following percutaneous treatment for claudication over and above supervised exercise training programs and have also demonstrated endovascular therapy to be cost-ineffective for this indication.[89] Others have noted an additive benefit when combining percutaneous intervention with supervised exercise programs and optimal medical management, as indicated by improved quality-of-life indices.[90,91]

In terms of patients with severe limb ischemia secondary to infrainguinal occlusive disease, the awaited long-term results of the Bypass versus Angioplasty in Severe Ischaemia of the Leg (BASIL) trial recently became available.[92] The BASIL trial was a randomized controlled trial performed in 27 U.K. centers from 1999-2004. This seminal work was designed to compare a strategy of open surgical revascularization first to that of percutaneous angioplasty first in a population of patients with severe limb ischemia, and represents the only level-I evidence comparing these treatment modalities to date. The initial analysis published in 2005[93] found no difference in the primary endpoints of overall or amputation-free survival for open surgery vs. angioplasty, though it did find that surgery was more costly in the short term. The more recently published longer-term follow-up results also indicated the two study arms had equivalent amputation-free and overall survival by intention to treat analysis.[94] However, for patients who survived beyond 2 years (representing 70% of the total cohort), open surgical bypass conferred improved overall survival and a trend toward improved amputation-free survival. The trialists concluded that for patients with available autologous vein and a life expectancy exceeding 2 years, the preferred method of revascularization is open bypass surgery. They further noted that when percutaneous angioplasty was employed as the primary intervention, it had a significantly negative impact on the outcome of future surgical revascularization attempts.

Occlusive disease of the tibial vessels, once thought to be the exclusive domain of operative bypass, is increasingly being treated percutaneously. The impact of these trends on the natural history of the disease, and to what extent the expanding reach of percutaneous therapy will affect subsequent operative management in a given patient, remains to be seen. Certainly, as enthusiasm for less invasive options has spread to include the infrapopliteal level, the relative roles of surgical and percutaneous intervention are being further redefined. Newer-generation atherectomy devices, drug-eluting balloon angioplasty, and flexible stents designed to withstand the unique torsional forces of the leg or with drug-eluting capability may significantly improve the patency and durability rates currently seen.[95,96] Until the efficacy of infrainguinal percutaneous intervention is better defined, however, surgical revascularization remains the standard for any patient with critical limb ischemia. For patients with favorable anatomy and significant operative risk, and for treatment of claudication in general, percutaneous therapy has assumed a more primary role.

Duplex ultrasonography, MRA, and CTA are increasingly used as first-line modalities in the assessment of patients with infrainguinal occlusive disease (see Chapters 12, 13, and 14). Although a growing body of literature supports use of duplex scanning as a stand-alone preoperative mapping modality,[97] this requires a highly dedicated vascular laboratory and, to date, has not gained wide acceptance. Magnetic resonance angiography and CTA are particularly useful as noninvasive screening tests to determine patient suitability for percutaneous therapy. In some instances, operative planning may be based solely on such noninvasive radiographic information, but many surgeons are reluctant to undertake surgical reconstruction without the confirmation afforded by standard contrast angiography. This is particularly true if the distal target is at the tibial or pedal level, where CTA and MRA technology remains more limited.

Operative Management

Infrainguinal bypass can be performed under general anesthesia or, in the appropriate patient, under regional, spinal, or epidural anesthesia. The multiple sites of dissection and the harvesting of saphenous vein or an alternative vein conduit make these procedures particularly suited to a two-team approach. The time saved, particularly in cases involving potentially more tedious arm vein or lesser saphenous vein harvesting, has direct benefit in minimizing the total anesthetic load and physiological insult to the patient. Typically, the site proposed for the distal anastomosis is explored first to ascertain whether the preoperative imaging was accurate in predicting the suitability of the target vessel. On occasion, the operation is begun with an on-table angiogram to clarify the anatomy if preoperative imaging was deferred or ambiguous.

The above-knee popliteal vessel is easily exposed through a medial thigh incision, with subsequent posterolateral retraction of the sartorius muscle. The popliteal artery, with its accompanying vein and nerve, is found just posterior to the femur. The vessel is palpated to determine the presence of atherosclerotic plaque, which will guide the extent of dissection and the optimal bypass target site. The below-knee popliteal artery is also exposed through a medial incision in the proximal calf (Fig. 21-8). If the saphenous vein is to be harvested, the incision is made directly over the vein to minimize creation of devascularized skin flaps. With the exposed vein carefully protected, the incision is carried through the deep muscular fascia, and the medial head of the gastrocnemius is reflected posterolaterally to expose the below-knee popliteal fossa. The distal popliteal artery is then dissected free from the adjacent tibial nerve posteriorly and popliteal vein medially. If the distal target is the tibioperoneal trunk, the dissection is continued along the anteromedial surface of the distal popliteal artery after dividing the origin of the soleus muscle from the tibia (Fig. 21-9). In instances in which the below-knee popliteal artery has previously been exposed or where sepsis is involved, a lateral approach with excision of a segment of proximal fibula is a useful alternative approach to the below-knee popliteal artery.

Although exposure of the proximal posterior and peroneal vessels can be gained by extending the tibioperoneal trunk dissection distally, more distal exposure of these vessels is best gained through targeted medial incisions. The posterior tibial artery is found more medially on the reflected soleus muscle, whereas the peroneal artery is deeper and more lateral. The posterior tibial artery at the level of the ankle is a relatively easier target given the proximity of the vessel to the skin surface. The initial incision is made just posterior to the medial malleolus, and the artery is exposed by division of the overlying retinaculum. Further distal dissection allows access to the bifurcation and medial and lateral plantar branches.[98] The anterior tibial artery is typically approached from the anterolateral aspect of the calf (see Fig. 21-9) and is found deep within the anterior compartment with the adjacent deep peroneal nerve and anterior tibial veins. The dorsalis pedis artery is easily exposed through an axial incision on the dorsum of the foot just lateral to the extensor hallucis longus tendon (see Fig. 21-9).

Following exposure of the distal anastomotic target vessel, the site of the proximal anastomosis is dissected. For patients with SFA disease, this will most commonly be at the level of the common femoral artery. The artery is mobilized as already described, from the level of the inguinal ligament to its terminal bifurcation. The distal extent of this dissection is dictated by the presence of concomitant femoral plaque. Lymphatic tissue overlying the femoral vessels is best ligated and divided to prevent postoperative development of lymph fistulas or lymphoceles. If an extensive endarterectomy or profundaplasty is required, the proximal profunda femoral artery is dissected along its proximal length accordingly.

If all or part of the SFA is spared of significant atherosclerotic involvement, the proximal anastomosis can be moved distally as dictated by the particular anatomical pattern of disease, and a

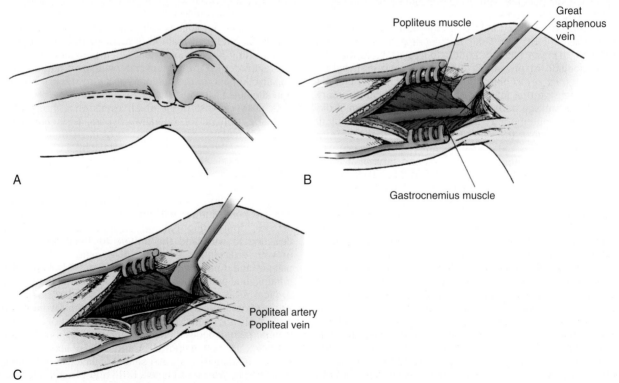

FIGURE 21-8 Exposure of popliteal artery below knee. Medial incision is made **(A)** directly overlying course of great saphenous vein **(B)**. After posterior reflection of the gastrocnemius muscle the tibial nerve, popliteal vein, and popliteal artery are encountered in the deep posterior compartment.

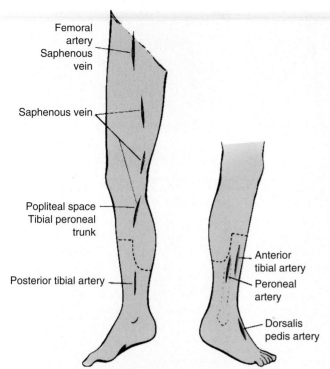

Femoral
artery
Saphenous
vein

Saphenous vein

Popliteal space
Tibial peroneal
trunk

Posterior tibial artery

Anterior
tibial artery

Peroneal
artery

Dorsalis
pedis artery

FIGURE 21-9 Placement of incisions for femoropopliteal and femorotibial bypass and for greater saphenous vein harvest. These should avoid the incision lines for a below-knee amputation.

so-called distal origin graft can be fashioned[99] (Fig. 21-10). This situation is particularly applicable to the diabetic population, where infrapopliteal disease is the rule, and sparing of the superficial femoral and popliteal arteries is not uncommon. It is also used in situations where conduit is sparse and a moderately diseased proximal vessel is accepted as an inflow source for a more distal origin bypass graft in the interests of performing a fully autologous vein graft rather than using prosthetic material. An increasingly popular approach when only limited conduit is available is to combine, either concurrently in the operating room or as a staged preoperative procedure, catheter-based treatment of the superficial femoral or popliteal artery inflow with more distal bypass.[99]

AUTOGENOUS VEIN BYPASS

In general, infrainguinal bypass surgery is best performed with autogenous vein conduit, preferably the ipsilateral greater saphenous vein if available.[100] This is particularly true for grafts extending below the knee, where prosthetic conduits of Dacron or PTFE have significantly poorer patency rates. The first report of a femoropopliteal bypass graft using autogenous greater saphenous vein in a reversed orientation was by Kunlin in 1951.[5] Given the orientation of the vein valves, the vein is reversed such that the distal end of the vein is sewn to the proximal inflow artery, and the larger proximal end of the vein is sewn to the distal outflow artery. The vein is harvested through a long incision overlying the course of the vein or by more tedious but less invasive sequential skip incisions with intervening cutaneous skin bridges (see Fig. 21-9). All side branches are ligated, and after harvest, the vein is cannulated and gently dilated with a solution containing heparin and papaverine to assess its suitability. Veins with chronic fibrosis or that fail to dilate to a diameter of 3 mm or greater will likely have poor long-term function.

For prosthetic grafts, a tunnel is usually fashioned through the subsartorial plane between the groin incision and the above-knee popliteal space in the interests of protecting the graft from subsequent infection. For vein conduits, it remains the surgeon's preference as to whether the graft is tunneled deeply or

in a superficial location in the subcutaneous space. The more superficial configuration greatly facilitates ongoing clinical examination and ultrasonographic surveillance as well as later surgical revision, but it carries a risk of graft exposure should there be wound-healing problems. Occlusion from trauma to grafts placed superficially has been of theoretical but not practical concern.

The order of anastomoses is surgeon dependent, with strong feelings expressed in each camp. Before occluding the target vessel, the patient is systemically anticoagulated with 5000 to 10,000 units of heparin. The artery is then clamped proximally and distally and incised, the vein spatulated, and a beveled anastomosis is carried out. Typically, a 5-0 monofilament suture of Prolene is used for the femoral anastomosis, a 6-0 suture is used at the popliteal level, and a very fine 7-0 suture is used at the tibial or pedal level. If the target tibial vessel is deep within the calf and visibility is challenging, a technique of "parachuting" the heel of the distal anastomosis is often employed. After completing the first anastomosis, the graft is carefully marked to ensure against mechanical twisting or kinking of the graft during the tunneling process. One of the benefits of performing the proximal anastomosis first is that following release of the clamps, adequacy of flow through the graft can be assessed.

Occasionally, such extensive calcification of the target vessel is encountered that the risk of a significant injury from clamping, even with the minimally traumatic clamps in use today, is prohibitively high. In such cases, proximal inflow and distal artery backbleeding can be controlled by occlusion balloons placed intraluminally. For distal anastomoses at the knee or more distal level, another alternative technique is use of a proximally placed sterile pneumatic tourniquet. This is particularly advantageous when sewing to diminutive distal tibial or pedal targets, where the impact of a crush injury or plaque dislodgment on graft function could be considerable. Removing the need for clamps by using the tourniquet has two more advantages. First, it improves operative visibility. Second, and more importantly, given that less longitudinal and circumferential dissection are needed, the degrees of vessel spasm and venous bleeding that frequently accompany vessel exposure at this level are kept to a minimum.

Flow through the graft and outflow arteries is assessed with continuous-wave Doppler ultrasound following completion of the bypass. Ideally, a contrast angiogram is also performed after directly cannulating the proximal graft (Fig. 21-11). This allows for immediate repair of any technical defects—for example, intraluminal thrombus, twisting or kinking of the graft, or retained valve cusps, that are identified[101] (Fig. 21-12). Intraoperative completion duplex ultrasonography is a sensitive screen for hemodynamically significant abnormalities within the graft.[102,103]

Current reports of the 5-year results of reversed saphenous vein graft using modern techniques have been excellent, with primary and secondary patency rates of 75% and 80%, respectively, and limb salvage rates of 90%.[104,105]

IN SITU GRAFTING

There has been ongoing enthusiasm in some circles for *in situ* vein bypass grafting, whereby except for its proximal and distal extent, the greater saphenous vein is left undisturbed in its native bed. This technique was first described in 1962[106] but was later popularized by Leather and Karmody in the late 1970s.[107] Recent reports of *in situ* saphenous vein grafting have indicated 5-year graft patency rates approaching 80% and limb salvage rates of 84% to 90%.[105,108–110]

The approach minimizes trauma to the vein during excision and handling, and in theory enhances preservation of the vasa vasorum and endothelium. It further lowers the considerable risk of wound healing complications seen with traditional vein harvesting and facilitates creation of more technically precise anastomoses because the proximal and distal vein diameters are more closely matched to those of the inflow and outflow target vessels (Fig. 21-13). Extent of proximal vein mobilization is dictated by location of the saphenofemoral junction relative to the

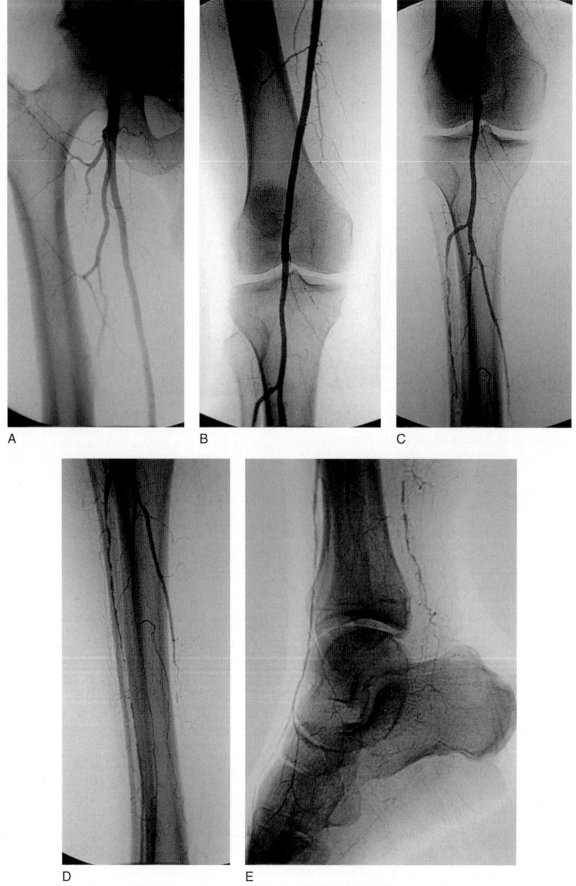

A

B

C

D

E

FIGURE 21-10 **A-E,** Arteriogram indicating preservation of superficial femoral artery (SFA) and popliteal arteries with mid-calf occlusions of all three infrageniculate vessels. This anatomical pattern of disease is amenable to "distal origin" vein grafting from below-knee popliteal or proximal posterior tibial artery to dorsalis pedis artery.

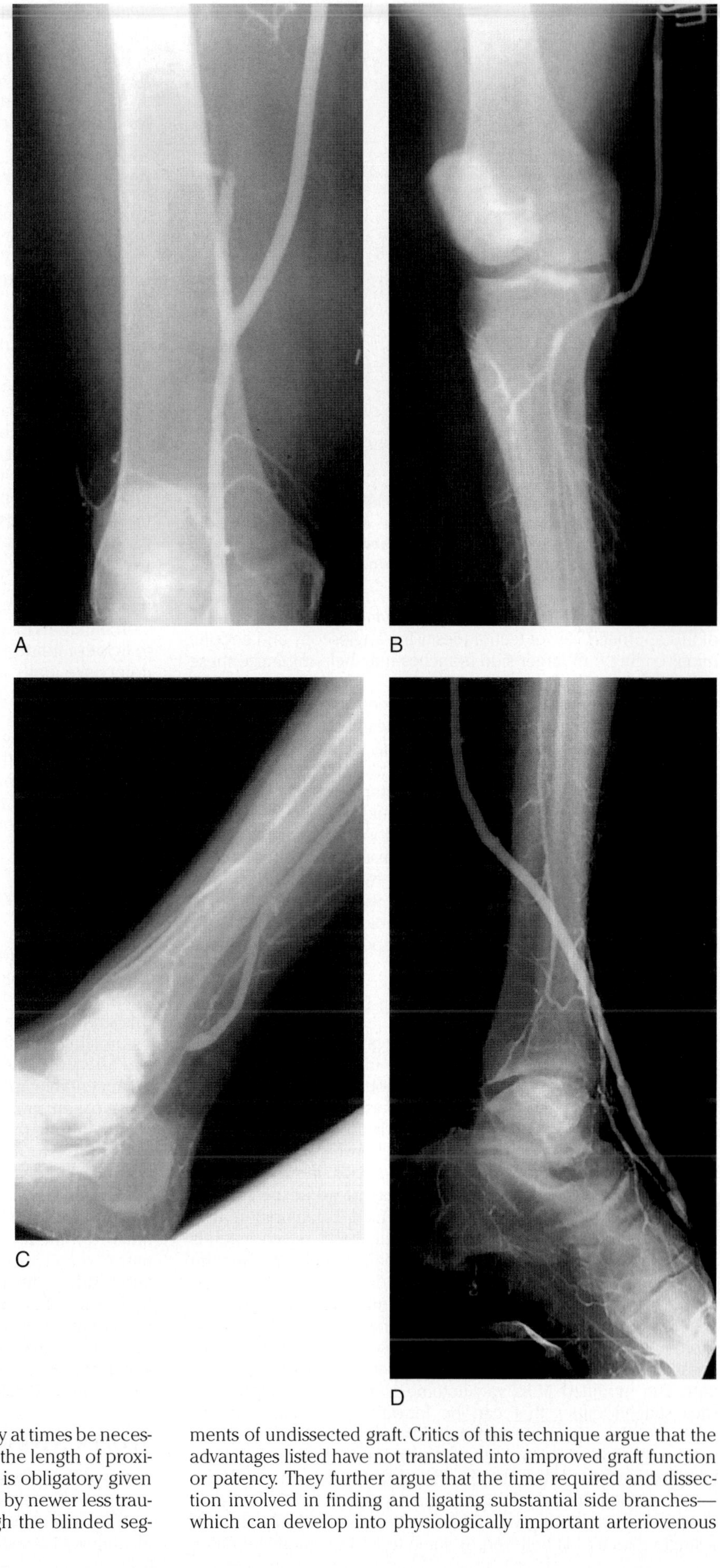

FIGURE 21-11 Intraoperative completion arteriograms of distal anastomoses to above-knee popliteal (A), below-knee popliteal (B), distal posterior tibial (C), and dorsalis pedis (D) arteries.

proposed site of the proximal anastomosis. It may at times be necessary to perform an endarterectomy of the SFA if the length of proximal vein is insufficient. Lysis of the valve cusps is obligatory given the nonreversed configuration, and is facilitated by newer less traumatic valvulotomes that function safely through the blinded seg-

ments of undissected graft. Critics of this technique argue that the advantages listed have not translated into improved graft function or patency. They further argue that the time required and dissection involved in finding and ligating substantial side branches—which can develop into physiologically important arteriovenous

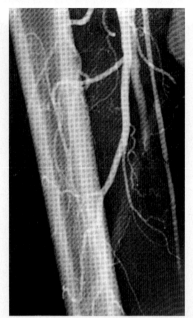

FIGURE 21-12 Intraoperative completion arteriogram of *in situ* femoropopliteal vein graft indicating retained valve, visualized as a filling defect in graft, and persistent arteriovenous fistula (AVF).

fistulae (AVF) that "steal" distal flow—obviates the stated benefits of this approach. Newer techniques using angioscopy and endoluminal coiling[111] of larger side branches may help minimize these concerns.

Angioscopic-assisted valve lysis has been employed for more than a decade but has not gained widespread favor. Although there is a significant learning curve with this technology, and operative times—at least initially—are significantly prolonged, advocates cite fewer wound complications, shorter hospital stays, and decreased recuperative periods as potential benefits. Proponents of routine angioscopy for direct visualization of valve lysis stress its particular utility in demonstrating such unsuspected endoluminal venous pathology as phlebitic strictures, webs, and fibrotic valve cusps.[112] This adjunct may be particularly useful in cases in which arm vein is used, when endoluminal pathology is more frequently encountered and is presumably partly responsible for suboptimal results.[113]

NONREVERSED SAPHENOUS VEIN GRAFTS

Recognizing the many practical advantages inherent to the *in situ* technique, Belkin et al. and others have modified the approach to infrainguinal bypass grafting with venous conduit to incorporate several of the same principles.[114] In particular, if the harvested vein is tapered to any significant extent, it is used in a nonreversed fashion. By optimizing the size matching between the artery and vein at both the proximal and distal anastomosis sites as discussed earlier, one can often use smaller veins than would be suitable for reversed vein grafting. The nonreversed configuration also allows preservation of the saphenous vein hood, which extends the available conduit length and is especially beneficial when the femoral artery is thick walled and diseased.

The vein is harvested and dilated in a similar fashion to reversed vein grafts, and the cusps of the proximal valve of the greater saphenous vein are excised under direct vision with fine Potts scissors. There are currently two main types of valvulotomes available. The modified Mills valvulotome is a short, metal, hockey stick–shaped cutter that can be introduced through the distal end of the vein or through the side branches. After the proximal anastomosis is performed, and with the perfused conduit on gentle stretch, the valves are carefully lysed in a sequential fashion by pulling the valvulotome inferiorly. An alternative recently designed self-centering valvulotome allows lysis of all valves in a single pass and is believed by some to be less traumatic. Once

acceptable pulsatile flow is ensured, the distal anastomosis is performed in the standard fashion.

It is important to note that similar patency rates have consistently been demonstrated regardless of which technique is applied,[109,110] so surgeon preference and comfort level are acceptable reasons for choosing one method over another.

ALTERNATIVE VEIN SOURCES

The ipsilateral greater saphenous vein (GSV) remains the conduit of choice for infrainguinal arterial reconstructions. However, the ipsilateral GSV may be unusable or absent in as many as 20% to 40% of patients requiring surgical revascularization.[115,116] In patients without adequate ipsilateral GSV, alternative vein sources include the contralateral GSV, the small saphenous vein, and the cephalic and basilic arm veins. Some groups advocate preserving the contralateral GSV and preferentially utilize upper-extremity veins as the most appealing ectopic autologous conduit,[117] but the majority of vascular surgeons, the present authors included, favor the use of contralateral GSV in this setting, citing quite favorable patency and morbidity profiles.[115] Regardless of the strategy employed, the quality of the vein conduit chosen is of paramount importance. Preoperative duplex ultrasound surveillance can be used to reliably assess the presence of available venous conduit, as well as the relative quality with regard to wall thickness, compressibility, and diameter. The ultimate viability of the vein, however, is determined intraoperatively following cannulation and gentle dilation with heparinized saline.[118]

In situations in which an adequate single length of vein necessary to achieve inline pulsatile flow to the ischemic limb is unavailable, composite grafts whereby shorter usable vein lengths are spliced together in an end-to-end fashion can be used. Graft patency and limb salvage rates of such composite grafts are reduced compared to results with single-segment saphenous vein but have historically been better than those of prosthetic grafts (see Reoperative Bypass Surgery).[118] Cryopreserved cadaver vein allografts (CVG) remain a conduit of last resort, reserved for highly selective cases given their extremely poor patency rates in comparison to other conduit choices.[119]

PROSTHETIC BYPASS

As stated, it is recommended that infrainguinal bypass surgery be performed with saphenous vein or an autologous substitute whenever feasible, given the clearly demonstrated enhanced patency rates.[100,120] Despite the ample published data supporting this strategy, some institutions and surgeons more frequently rely on prosthetic grafts. When the distal target is the above-knee popliteal artery and the tibial outflow is relatively well preserved, this is an acceptable approach; patency rates in this situation approach those of vein grafts.[121] A variety of surgical adjunctive procedures, from patching the distal anastomotic target vessel, to creation of a distal AVF, to use of various autogenous vein cuffs interposed between the distal prosthetic and the target artery have all been attempted as a means of improving patency rates of grafts extending below the knee.[122] More recently, flared grafts designed to minimize turbulence and shear stress between the prosthetic and the native vessel have gained some popularity. Polyester (Dacron) and PTFE grafts are the two main types of prosthetics available, and as in other anatomical positions, available data show generally equal results with either choice. The entire procedure is carried out through two small proximal and distal incisions between which the graft is tunneled anatomically. The selection of a 6- or 8-mm graft is dictated by the size of the native vessels.

REOPERATIVE BYPASS SURGERY

As the patient population treated by vascular surgeons has increased in age, and more and more challenging cases are accepted for primary treatment, there has been a corresponding increase in the incidence of reoperative bypass surgery performed for infrainguinal

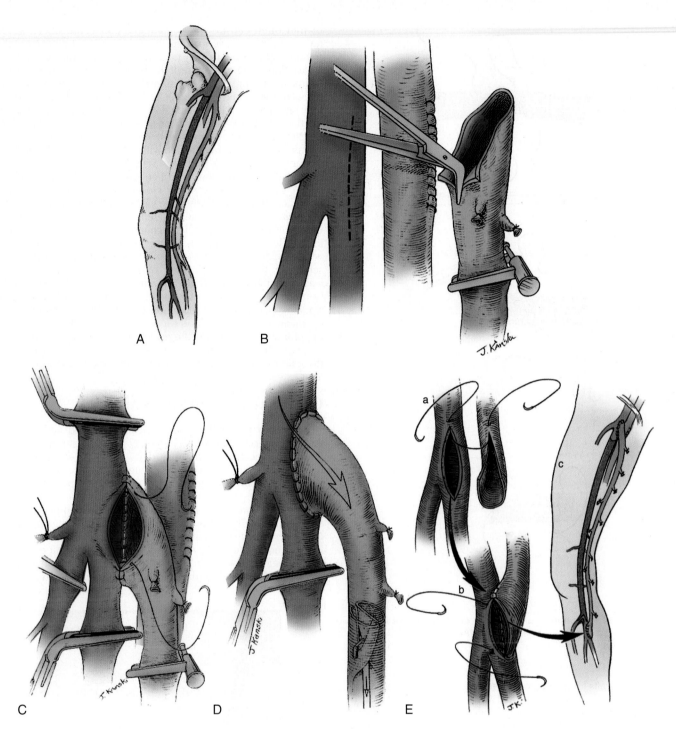

FIGURE 21-13 *In situ* **method of infrainguinal reconstruction.** Saphenous vein is left undisturbed in its native bed, except at proximal and distal anastomotic sites—in this case, common femoral artery (CFA) and tibioperoneal trunk, respectively (**A**). Saphenofemoral junction is transected in groin, venotomy in femoral vein is oversewn, and proximal end of saphenous vein is spatulated in preparation for anastomosis (**B**). After first venous valve is excised under direct vision, graft is anastomosed end-to-side to femoral artery (**C**). Flow is then restored through vein graft, and valvulotome passed from distal end to lyse residual valves (**D**) before distal anastomosis is performed (**E**).

arterial occlusive disease. Such reoperative procedures are particularly challenging, both because of the scarring present at the inflow and outflow target sites and because there is typically a lack of ipsilateral greater saphenous vein. Whenever possible, the first problem is addressed by choosing anastomotic sites just above or below the previous touchdown points, thereby avoiding dissection through often densely scarred tissue planes. When ipsilateral greater saphenous vein is absent due to prior infrainguinal or coronary artery bypass surgery or prior saphenous vein stripping, there are a number of alternative conduit sites available, as already mentioned. Chew et al. studied the consequence of using the contralateral greater saphenous vein in these situations and found it to be the

optimal conduit. Despite the presumably high incidence of contralateral lower extremity as well as coronary occlusive disease in this population, short- and long-term impacts were found to be minimal.[115]

Use of arm veins, in general, can be extremely technically challenging and for that reason has not been universally adopted. Often the arm veins distal to the antecubital crease are scarred and of small caliber, but their more proximal counterparts are often of excellent size and quality. Dissection of the basilic vein can be particularly tedious because it has multiple side branches and lies adjacent to several important nerves. Because arm veins are often relatively short, a venovenostomy is often required to create

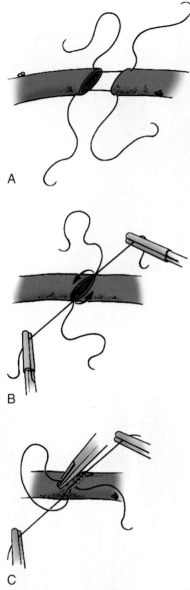

FIGURE 21-14 Creation of a composite graft by venovenostomy.
A widely spatulated venovenostomy is optimal **(A)**. The posterior wall **(B)** and anterior wall **(C)** are aligned with separate strands of suture to avoid a "purse string" effect on the suture line.

composite grafts long enough to complete the arterial reconstruction (Fig. 21-14). This is performed with generous spatulation of each vein hood to create a widely patent vein-to-vein anastomosis. Given their thin-walled nature, arm vein grafts are also quite prone to twisting and kinking, and special care must be taken during the tunneling process to avoid these problems. The more proximal arm veins can be relatively large, and it is often advantageous to use one or more of the segments in a nonreversed fashion to better match the graft to the inflow vessel size.

Not surprisingly, the results of reoperative infrainguinal bypass surgery do not match those of primary reconstruction. With autogenous vein, 5-year patency rates of 60% and limb salvage rates of 70% to 80% have been reported.[115,123] Coumadin is often used postoperatively in patients with compromised outflow or in whom the conduit was of marginal quality and has been associated with improved long-term patency.[124]

Post-Reconstruction Management

Many patients undergoing surgical reconstruction for arterial insufficiency will require one or more adjunctive operative procedures of their foot. Small uninfected ulcerations of the toe

or foot often can be safely managed conservatively. However, larger gangrenous lesions of the toe, forefoot, or heel usually require débridement of all necrotic tissue at completion of the revascularization procedure. If the ischemia is particularly severe or infection is present, toe or transmetatarsal amputation may be necessary to achieve a margin of healthy tissue. This is particularly important in patients with diabetes or end-stage renal disease, in whom persistent infection or necrosis can result in limb loss despite the presence of a well-revascularized extremity. Wounds are usually left open and treated with saline wet-to-dry dressings or newer vacuum sponge dressings. Serial débridements on the ward or in the operating room are often necessary for larger wounds, which can then be surgically closed after an interval healing period or allowed to slowly close via secondary intention.

Unless otherwise contraindicated, all patients are maintained indefinitely on an antiplatelet regimen with either aspirin or clopidogrel following surgical bypass. As stated earlier, in cases in which a graft is at increased risk of failure, such as in the redo setting or when compromised outflow or a marginal conduit was accepted, the antiplatelet agent may be supplemented with Coumadin.[124] Aggressive risk factor modification in the form of smoking cessation, lipid reduction, exercise, blood pressure management, and diabetic blood sugar control is of further paramount importance in minimizing the risk of disease progression or recurrence.[125] More immediately, aggressive rehabilitation maximizes the chances of and shortens the time to a return to full function after extensive reconstructive surgery.

Graft Failure and Surveillance

Postoperative graft failures are typically classified according to the time interval from surgery as early, intermediate, or late. Graft thrombosis occurring within 30 days, so-called early graft failures, are generally believed to be due to technical or judgment errors by the surgeon. Included in this list would be such technical errors as twists, kinks, incompletely lysed valves, or anastomotic defects, as well as judgment errors in using a poor-quality vein or targeting an outflow vessel with inadequate runoff to support the graft. Intermediate graft failures include those between 30 days and 2 years and are generally attributed to the proliferation of intimal hyperplasia at the anastomoses or prior valve sites within the graft (Fig. 21-15). Randomized trials are currently underway to determine

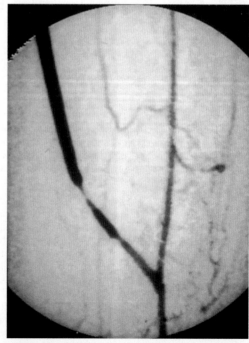

FIGURE 21-15 Arteriogram demonstrating severe stenosis of distal graft from intimal hyperplasia, likely at prior valve site.

the impact of genetic modulation of vein grafts on the development of intimal hyperplasia, and hold some promise in reducing or minimizing this significant cause of vein graft failure.[126] Late graft failures occurring beyond 2 years are typically due to progression of atherosclerotic occlusive disease within the inflow or outflow arteries.

Given the known incidence of graft failure and the potentially dire consequence in terms of limb salvage or preservation of limb function in a patient with limited options for secondary or tertiary bypass, the ability to maintain graft patency through early identification and prompt correction of graft stenoses is of paramount importance.[127] Serial postoperative surveillance scanning with a duplex ultrasound has proved an excellent means of accurately identifying hemodynamically significant stenoses within the vein graft that threaten the graft patency.[128] Subsequent confirmation by angiography and prophylactic treatment by percutaneous cutting balloon angioplasty, surgical patch angioplasty, or interposition grafting of significant lesions minimizes the risk of graft thrombosis and ensures optimal long-term graft patency.

REFERENCES

1. Gray EA: *Portrait of a surgeon: a biography of John Hunter*, London, 1952, Robert Hale.
2. dos Santos JC: *Sur la desobstion des thromboses arterielles anciennes, Mem Acad Chir (Paris)* 73:409, 1947.
3. Wylie EJ, Kerr E, Davies O: Experimental and clinical experiences with the use of fascia lata applied as a graft about major arteries after thromboendarterectomy and aneurysmorrhaphy, *Surg Gynecol Obstet* 93:257, 1951.
4. Carrel A: The surgery of blood vessels, etc, *John Hopkins Hosp Bull* 190:18, 1907.
5. Kunlin J: Le traitement de l'ischemie arteritique par la greffe veineuse longue, *Rev Chir* 70:206, 1951.
6. McCaughan JJ Jr.: Surgical exposure of the distal popliteal artery, *Surgery* 44:536, 1958.
7. Berman JR, Berman LA, Goldstein I: Female sexual dysfunction: incidence, pathophysiology, evaluation and treatment options, *Urology* 54:385, 1999.
8. Leriche R, Morel A: The syndrome of thrombotic obliteration of the aortic bifurcation, *Ann Surg* 127:193, 1948.
9. Wingo JP, Nix ML, Greenfield LJ, et al: The blue toe syndrome: hemodynamic and therapeutic correlates of outcome, *J Vasc Surg* 3:475, 1986.
10. Karmody AM, Powers SR, Monaco VJ, et al: "Blue toe" syndrome, *Arch Surg* 111:1263, 1976.
11. Brewster DC, Perler BA, Robison JG, et al: Aortofemoral graft for multilevel occlusive disease: predictors of success and need for distal bypass, *Arch Surg* 117:1593, 1982.
12. Imparata AM, Kim G, Davidson T, et al: Intermittent claudication: its natural course, *Surgery* 78:795, 1975.
13. Cronenwett JL, Davis JT, Gooch JB, et al: Aortoiliac occlusive disease in women, *Surgery* 88:775, 1980.
14. Caes F, Cham B, Van den Brande P, et al: Small artery syndrome in women, *Surg Gynecol Obstet* 161:165, 1985.
15. Shareghi S, Gopal A, Gul K, et al: Diagnostic accuracy of 64 multidetector computed tomography angiography in peripheral vascular disease, *Catheter Cardiovasc Intervent* 75:23–31, 2010.
16. Carpenter JP, Owen RS, Holland GA, et al: Magnetic resonance angiography of the aorta, iliac and femoral arteries, *Surgery* 116:17, 1994.
17. Seldinger SE: Catheter replacement of needle in percutaneous arteriography: new technique, *Acta Radiol* 39:368, 1953.
18. Udoff EJ, Barth KH, Harrington DP, et al: Hemodynamic significance of iliac artery stenosis: pressure measurements during angiography, *Radiology* 132:289, 1979.
19. Nehler MR, Hiatt WR: Exercise therapy for claudication, *Ann Vasc Surg* 13:109, 1999.
20. Regensteiner JG, Meyer TJ, Krupski WC: Hospital versus home-based exercise rehabilitation for patients with peripheral arterial occlusive disease, *Angiology* 48:291, 1997.
21. Dawson DL, Cutler BS, Hiatt WR, et al: A comparison of cilostazol and pentoxifylline for treating intermittent claudication, *Am J Med* 109:523, 2000.
22. Martinez BD, Hertzer NR, Beven EG: Influence of distal arterial occlusive disease on prognosis following aortobifemoral bypass, *Surgery* 88:795, 1980.
23. Hill DA, McGrath MA, Lord RSA, et al: The effect of superficial femoral artery occlusion on the outcome of aortofemoral bypass for intermittent claudication, *Surgery* 87:133, 1980.
24. Harris PL, Cave-Bigley DJ, McSweeney L: Aortofemoral bypass and the role of concomitant femorodistal reconstruction, *Br J Surg* 72:317, 1985.
25. Darling RC, Linton RR: Aortoiliofemoral endarterectomy for atherosclerotic occlusive disease, *Surgery* 110:1458, 1975.
26. Barker WF, Cannon JA: An evaluation of endarterectomy, *Arch Surg* 66:488, 1953.
27. Crawford ES, Manning LG, Kelly TF: "Redo" surgery after operations for aneurysm and occlusion of the abdominal aorta, *Surgery* 81:41, 1977.
28. Perdue GD, Long WD, Smith RB III, et al: Perspective concerning aortofemoral arterial reconstruction, *Ann Surg* 173:940, 1971.
29. Brewster DC, Darling RC: Optimal methods of aortoiliac reconstruction, *Surgery* 84:739, 1978.
30. Baird RJ, Feldman P, Miles JT, et al: Subsequent downstream repair after aorta-iliac and aorta-femoral bypass operations, *Surgery* 82:785, 1977.
31. Crawford ES, Bomberger RA, Glaeser DH, et al: Aortoiliac occlusive disease: factors influencing survival and function following reconstructive operation over a twenty-five year period, *Surgery* 90:1055, 1981.
32. Malone JM, Moore WS, Goldstone J: The natural history of bilateral aortofemoral bypass grafts for ischemia of the lower extremities, *Arch Surg* 110:1300, 1975.
33. Reed AB, Conte MS, Donaldson MC, et al: The impact of patient age and aortic size on the results of aortobifemoral bypass grafting, *J Vasc Surg* 37:1219, 2003.
34. Menard MT, Chew DK, Chan RK, et al: Outcome in patients at high risk after open surgical repair of abdominal aortic aneurysm, *J Vasc Surg* 37:285, 2003.
35. Whittemore AD, Clowes AW, Hechtman HB, et al: Aortic aneurysm repair: reduced operative mortality associated with maintenance of optimal cardiac performance, *Ann Surg* 173:940, 1971.
36. Kaluza GL, Joseph J, Lee JR, et al: Catastrophic outcomes of noncardiac surgery soon after coronary stenting, *J Am Coll Cardiol* 35:1288, 2000.
37. Mozersky DJ, Summer DS, Strandness DE: Long-term results of reconstructive aortoiliac surgery, *Am J Surg* 123:503, 1972.
38. Cooley DA, Wukasch DC, Bennett JG, et al: *Double velour knitted Dacron grafts for aortoiliac vascular replacements*, Paper presented at Vascular Graft Symposium, Bethesda, Md, November 5, 1976, National Institutes of Health.
39. Yates SG, Barros D'Sa AA, Berger K, et al: The preclotting of porous arterial prosthesis, *Ann Surg* 188:611, 1978.
40. Nevelsteen A, Wouters L, Suy R: Aorto-femoral Dacron reconstruction for aortoiliac occlusive disease: a 25-year survey, *Eur J Vasc Surg* 5:179, 1991.
41. Malone JM, Goldstone J, Moore WS: Autogenous profundaplasty: the key to long-term patency in secondary repair of aortofemoral graft occlusion, *Ann Surg* 188:817, 1978.
42. Morris GC Jr., Edwards W, Cooley DA, et al: Surgical importance of profunda femoris artery, *Arch Surg* 82:32, 1961.
43. Rutherford RB, Jones DN, Martin MS, et al: Serial hemodynamic assessment of aortobifemoral bypass, *J Vasc Surg* 4:428, 1986.
44. Bernhard VM, Ray LI, Militello JP: The role of angioplasty in the profunda femoris artery in revascularization of the ischemic limb, *Surg Gynecol Obstet* 142:840, 1976.
45. Malone JM, Goldstone J, Moore WS: Autogenous profundaplasty: the key to long-term success and need for distal bypass, *Arch Surg* 117:1593, 1982.
46. Berguer R, Higgins RF, Cotton LT: Geometry, blood flow, and reconstruction of the deep femoral artery, *Am J Surg* 130:68, 1975.
47. Juleff RS, Brown OW, McKain MM, et al: The influence of competitive flow on graft patency, *J Cardiovasc Surg* 33:415, 1992.
48. Pierce GE, Turrentine M, Stringfield S, et al: Evaluation of end-to-side vs. end-to-end proximal anastomosis in aortobifemoral bypass, *Arch Surg* 117:1580, 1982.
49. Brewster DC, Franklin DP, Cambria RP, et al: Intestinal ischemia complicating abdominal aortic surgery, *Surgery* 109:447, 1991.
50. Gloviczki P, Cross SA, Stanson AW, et al: Ischemic injury to the spinal cord or lumbosacral plexus after aorto-iliac reconstruction, *Am J Surg* 162:131, 1991.
51. Seegar JM, Coe DA, Kaelin LD, et al: Routine reimplantation of patent inferior mesenteric arteries limits colon infarction after aortic reconstructions, *J Vasc Surg* 15:635, 1992.
52. Prinssen M, Buskens E, Blankensteijn JD: *Sexual dysfunction after conventional or endovascular AAA repair: results of a randomized trial*. Paper presented at 17th International Congress of Endovascular Interventions, Phoenix, February 12, 2004.
53. Nypaver TJ, Ellenby MI, Mendoza O, et al: A comparison of operative approaches and parameters of success in multilevel arterial occlusive disease, *J Am Coll Surg* 179:449, 1994.
54. Dalman RL, Taylor LM Jr., Moneta GL, et al: Simultaneous operative repair of multilevel lower extremity occlusive disease, *J Vasc Surg* 13:211, 1991.
55. Malone JM, Moore WS, Goldstone J: Life expectancy following aortofemoral arterial grafting, *Surgery* 81:551, 1977.
56. Szilagyi DE, Hageman JH, Smith RF, et al: A thirty-year survey of the reconstructive surgical treatment of aortoiliac occlusive disease, *J Vasc Surg* 3:421, 1986.
57. Freeman NE, Leeds FH: Operations on large arteries, *Calif Med* 77:229, 1952.
58. Blaisdell FW, Hall AD: Axillary-femoral artery bypass for lower extremity ischemia, *Surgery* 54:563, 1963.
59. LoGerfo FW, Johnson WC, Carson JD, et al: A comparison of the late patency rates of axillo-bilateral femoral and axillo-unilateral femoral grafts, *Surgery* 81:33, 1977.
60. Harris EJ, Taylor LM, McConnell DB, et al: Clinical results of axillobifemoral bypass using externally supported polytetrafluoroethylene, *J Vasc Surg* 12:416, 1990.
61. El-Massry S, Saad E, Sauvage LR, et al: Axillofemoral bypass using externally-supported, knitted Dacron grafts: a follow-up through twelve years, *J Vasc Surg* 17:107, 1993.
62. Broome A, Christenson JT, Ekloff B, et al: Axillofemoral bypass reconstructions in sixty-one patients with leg ischemia, *Surgery* 88:673, 1980.
63. Taylor LM, Park TC, Edwards JM, et al: Acute disruption of polytetrafluoroethylene grafts adjacent to axillary anastomoses: a complication of axillofemoral grafting, *J Vasc Surg* 20:520, 1994.
64. Donaldson MC, Louras JC, Buckman CA: Axillofemoral bypass: a tool with a limited role, *J Vasc Surg* 3:757, 1986.
65. Ascer E, Veith FJ, Gupta SK, et al: Comparison of axillounifemoral and axillobifemoral bypass operations, *Surgery* 97:169, 1985.
66. Rutherford RB, Patt A, Pearce WH: Extra-anatomic bypass: a closer look, *J Vasc Surg* 6:437, 1987.
67. Passman MA, Taylor LM, Moneta GL, et al: Comparison of axillofemoral and aortofemoral bypass for aortoiliac occlusive disease, *J Vasc Surg* 23:263, 1996.
68. Berguer R, Higgins RJ, Reddy DJ: Intimal hyperplasia: an experimental study, *Arch Surg* 115:332, 1980.
69. Maini BS, Mannick JA: Effect of arterial reconstruction on limb salvage, *Arch Surg* 113:1297, 1978.
70. Plecha FR, Plecha FM: Femorofemoral bypass grafts: ten years experience, *J Vasc Surg* 1:555, 1984.
71. Harrington ME, Harrington EB, Haimov M, et al: Iliofemoral versus femorofemoral bypass: the case for an individualized approach, *J Vasc Surg* 16:841, 1992.
72. Schneider JR, Besso SR, Walsh DB, et al: Femorofemoral versus aortobifemoral bypass: outcome and hemodynamic results, *J Vasc Surg* 19:43, 1994.
73. Couch NP, Clowes AW, Whittemore AD, et al: The iliac-origin graft arterial graft: a useful alternative for iliac occlusive disease, *Surgery* 97:183, 1985.
74. Kalman PG, Hosang M, Johnston KW, et al: Unilateral iliac disease: the role of iliofemoral bypass, *J Vasc Surg* 6:139, 1987.
75. Blaisdell FW, DeMattei GA, Gauder PG: Extraperitoneal thoracic aorta to femoral bypass grafts as replacement for an infected aortic bifurcation prosthesis, *Am J Surg* 102:583, 1961.
76. Criado E, Keagy BA: Use of the descending thoracic aorta as an inflow source in aortoiliac reconstruction: indications and long-term results, *Ann Vasc Surg* 8:38, 1994.

77. Dion YM, Gracia CR: A new technique for laparoscopic aortobifemoral grafting in occlusive aortoiliac disease, *J Vasc Surg* 26:685, 1997.

78. Ahn SS, Hiyama DT, Rudkin GH, et al: Laparoscopic aortobifemoral bypass, *J Vasc Surg* 26:128, 1997.

79. Kelly JJ, Kercher KW, Gallagher KA, et al: Hand-assisted laparoscopic aortobifemoral bypass versus open bypass for occlusive disease, *J Laparoendosc Adv Surg Tech A* 12:339, 2002.

80. Wisselink W, Cuesta MA, Gracia C, et al: Robot-assisted laparoscopic aortobifemoral bypass for aortoiliac occlusive disease: a report of two cases, *J Vasc Surg* 36:1079, 2002.

81. Stadler P, Dvoracek L, Vitasek P, et al: Is robotic surgery appropriate for vascular procedures? Report of 100 aortoiliac cases, *Eur J Vasc Endovasc Surg* 36:405–406, 2008.

82. Crawford RS, Cambria RP, Abularrage CJ, et al: Preoperative functional status predicts perioperative outcomes after infrainguinal bypass surgery, *J Vasc Surg* 51:351–358, 2010.

83. Conte MS, Bandyk DF, Clowes AW, et al: Results of PREVENT III: a multicenter, randomized trial of edifoligide for the prevention of vein graft failure in lower extremity bypass surgery, *J Vasc Surg* 43:742–751, 2006.

84. Schanzer A, Mega J, Meadows J, et al: Risk stratification in critical limb ischemia: derivation and validation of a model to predict amputation-free survival using multicenter surgical outcomes data, *J Vasc Surg* 48:1464–1471, 2008.

85. Nguyen LL, Moneta G, Conte MS, et al: Prospective multicenter study of quality of life before and after lower extremity vein bypass in 1404 patients with critical limb ischemia, *J Vasc Surg* 44:977–984, 2006.

86. McAllister FF: The fate of patients with intermittent claudication managed non-operatively, *Am J Surg* 132:593, 1976.

87. Walsh DB, Gilbertson JJ, Zwolak RM, et al: The natural history of superficial femoral artery stenoses, *J Vasc Surg* 14:299, 1991.

88. Murphy TP, Hirsch AT, Ricotta JJ, et al: The Claudication: Exercise Vs. Endoluminal Revascularization (CLEVER) study: rationale and methods, *J Vasc Surg* 47:1356–1363, 2008.

89. Spronk S, Bosch JL, den Hoed PT, et al: Cost-effectiveness of endovascular revascularization compared to supervised hospital-based exercise training in patients with intermittent claudication: a randomized controlled trial, *J Vasc Surg* 48:1472–1480, 2008.

90. Greenhalgh RM, Belch JJ, Brown LC, et al: The adjuvant benefit of angioplasty in patients with mild to moderate intermittent claudication (MIMIC) managed by supervised exercise, smoking cessation advice and best medical therapy: results from two randomized trials for stenotic femoropopliteal and aortoiliac arterial disease, *Eur J Vasc Endovasc Surg* 36:680–688, 2008.

91. Nylaende M, Abdelnoor M, Stranden E, et al: The Oslo balloon angioplasty versus conservative treatment study (OBACT)—the 2 years results of a single centre, prospective, randomised study in patients with intermittent claudication, *Eur J Vasc Endovasc Surg* 33:3–12, 2007.

92. Bradbury AW, Adam DJ, Bell J, et al: Bypass versus Angioplasty in Severe Ischaemia of the Leg (BASIL) trial: analysis of amputation free and overall survival by treatment received, *J Vasc Surg* 51:18S–31S, 2010.

93. Adam DJ, Beard JD, Cleveland T, et al: Bypass versus Angioplasty in Severe Limb Ischemia of the Leg (BASIL) trial: multicentre, randomised controlled trial, *Lancet* 366:1925–1934, 2005.

94. Bradbury AW, Adam DJ, Bell J, et al: Bypass versus Angioplasty in Severe Ischaemia of the Leg (BASIL) trial: an intention-to-treat analysis of amputation-free and overall survival in patients randomized to a bypass surgery-first or a balloon angioplasty-first revascularization strategy, *J Vasc Surg* 51:5S–17S, 2010.

95. Faries PF, Morrisey NJ, Teodorescu V, et al: Recent advances in peripheral angioplasty and stenting, *Angiology* 53:617, 2002.

96. Duda SH, Poerner TC, Wiesenger B, et al: Drug-eluting stents: potential applications for peripheral arterial occlusive disease, *J Vasc Interv Radiol* 14:291, 2003.

97. Grassbaugh JA, Nelson PR, Rzucidlo EM, et al: Blinded comparison of preoperative duplex ultrasound scanning and contrast arteriography for planning revascularization at the level of the tibia, *J Vasc Surg* 37:1186, 2003.

98. Ascher E, Veith FJ, Gupta SK: Bypasses to plantar arteries and other tibial branches: an extended approach to limb salvage, *J Vasc Surg* 8:434, 1988.

99. Reed AB, Conte MS, Belkin M, et al: Usefulness of autogenous bypass grafts originating distal to the groin, *J Vasc Surg* 35:48, 2002.

100. Veith FJ, Gupta SK, Ascer E, et al: Six-year prospective multicenter randomized comparison of autologous saphenous vein and expanded polytetrafluoroethylene graft in infrainguinal arterial reconstruction, *J Vasc Surg* 3:104, 1986.

101. Baxter BT, Rizzo RJ, Flinn WR, et al: A comparative study of intraoperative angioscopy and completion arteriography following femorodistal bypass, *Arch Surg* 125:997, 1990.

102. Gilbertson JJ, Walsh DB, Zwolak RM, et al: A blinded comparison of angiography, angioscopy, and duplex scanning in the intraoperative evaluation of *in situ* saphenous vein bypass grafts, *J Vasc Surg* 15:121, 1992.

103. Bandyk D, Johnson B, Gupta A, et al: Nature and management of duplex abnormalities encountered during infrainguinal vein bypass grafting, *J Vasc Surg* 24:430, 1996.

104. Taylor LM, Edwards JM, Porter JM: Present status of reversed vein bypass grafting: five-year results of a modern series, *J Vasc Surg* 11:193, 1990.

105. Fogle MA, Whittemore AD, Couch NP, et al: A comparison of *in situ* and reversed saphenous vein grafts for infrainguinal reconstruction, *J Vasc Surg* 5:46, 1987.

106. Hall KV: The great saphenous vein used "*in situ*" as an arterial shunt after extirpation of vein valves, *Surgery* 51:492, 1962.

107. Leather RP, Powers SR, Karmody AM: A reappraisal of the *in situ* saphenous vein arterial bypass: its use in limb salvage, *Surgery* 86:453, 1979.

108. Donaldson MC, Mannick JA, Whittemore AD: Femoral-distal bypass with *in situ* greater saphenous vein: long-term results using Mills valvulotome, *Ann Surg* 213:457, 1991.

109. Moody AP, Edwards PR, Harris PL: *In situ* versus reversed femoropopliteal vein grafts: long-term follow-up of a prospective, randomized trial, *Br J Surg* 79:750, 1992.

110. Wengerter KR, Veith FJ, Gupta SK, et al: Prospective randomized multicenter comparison of *in situ* and reversed vein infrapopliteal bypasses, *J Vasc Surg* 13:189, 1991.

111. Rosenthal D, Dickson C, Rodriquez F, et al: Infrainguinal endovascular *in situ* saphenous vein bypass: ongoing results, *J Vasc Surg* 20:389, 1994.

112. Panetta Tf, Marin ML, Veith FJ, et al: Unsuspected pre-existing saphenous vein pathology: an unrecognized cause of vein bypass failure, *J Vasc Surg* 15:102, 1992.

113. Marcaccio EJ, Miller A, Tannenbaum GA, et al: Angioscopically directed interventions improve arm vein bypass grafts, *J Vasc Surg* 17:994, 1993.

114. Belkin M, Knox J, Donaldson MC, et al: Infrainguinal arterial reconstruction with nonreversed greater saphenous vein, *J Vasc Surg* 24:957, 1996.

115. Chew DK, Owens CD, Belkin M, et al: Bypass in the absence of ipsilateral greater saphenous vein: safety and superiority of the contralateral greater saphenous vein, *J Vasc Surg* 35:1085–1092, 2002.

116. Taylor LM, Edwards JM, Brant B: Autogenous reversed vein bypass for lower extremity ischemia in patients with absent or inadequate greater saphenous vein, *Am J Surg* 153:505–510, 1987.

117. Holzenbein TJ, Pomposelli FB Jr., Miller A: Results of a policy with arm veins used as the first alternative to an unavailable ipsilateral greater saphenous vein for infrainguinal bypass, *J Vasc Surg* 23:130–140, 1996.

118. Chew DK, Contes MS, Donaldson MC, et al: Autogenous composite vein bypass graft for infrainguinal arterial reconstruction, *J Vasc Surg* 33:259–265, 2001.

119. Bannazadeh M, Sarac TP, Bena J: Reoperative lower extremity revascularization with cadaver vein for limb salvage, *Ann Vasc Surg* 23:24–31, 2009.

120. Whittemore AD, Kent KC, Donaldson MC, et al: What is the proper role of polytetrafluoroethylene grafts in infrainguinal reconstruction? *J Vasc Surg* 10:299, 1989.

121. Quinones-Baldrich WJ, Prego AA, Ucelay-Gomez R, et al: Long-term results of infrainguinal revascularization with polytetrafluoroethylene: a ten-year experience, *J Vasc Surg* 16:209, 1992.

122. Miller JH, Foreman RK, Ferguson L, et al: Interposition vein cuff for anastomosis of prosthesis to small artery, *Aust N Z J Surg* 54:283, 1984.

123. Belkin M, Conte MS, Donaldson MC, et al: Preferred strategies for secondary infrainguinal bypass: lessons learned from 300 consecutive reoperations, *J Vasc Surg* 21:282, 1995.

124. Sarac TP, Huber TS, Back MR, et al: Warfarin improves the outcome of infrainguinal vein bypass grafting at high risk for failure, *J Vasc Surg* 28:446, 1998.

125. Creager MA: Medical management of peripheral arterial disease, *Cardiol Rev* 9:238, 2001.

126. Mann MJ, Whittemore AD, Donaldson MC, et al: Ex-vivo gene therapy of human vascular bypass grafts with E2F: the PREVENT single-centre, randomized, controlled trial, *Lancet* 354:1493, 1999.

127. Veith FJ, Weiser RK, Gupta SK, et al: Diagnosis and management of failing lower extremity arterial reconstructions prior to graft occlusion, *J Cardiovasc Surg* 25:381, 1984.

128. Bandyk DF, Schmitt DD, Seabrook GR, et al: Monitoring functional patency of *in situ* saphenous vein bypasses: the impact of a surveillance protocol and elective revision, *J Vasc Surg* 9:286, 1989.

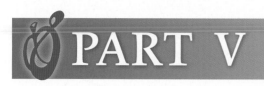

RENAL ARTERY DISEASE

CHAPTER 22 **Pathophysiology of Renal Artery Disease**

Stephen C. Textor

Vascular disease affecting the renal arteries presents complex challenges to clinicians. Thanks to recent advances in vascular imaging, more patients than ever before are being identified with some degree of atherosclerotic or fibromuscular renovascular disease. Many of these lesions are of minor hemodynamic importance at the time of detection. Some reach a degree at which perfusion pressures and intrarenal hemodynamics are altered, leading to changes in blood pressure regulation and renal function. These can produce a variety of recognizable clinical syndromes illustrated in Figure 22-1. These range from modest changes in systemic arterial pressure to impaired volume control associated with congestive heart failure (CHF) to threatened viability of the kidney, sometimes designated *ischemic nephropathy*. Understanding the pathways by which renovascular disease affects cardiovascular and renal disease is important for both diagnosis and for defining optimal management using tools both to block the renin-angiotensin system and to restore the circulation.

Most renovascular lesions are the result of atherosclerosis. With the aging of the U.S. and other Western populations and reduced mortality from stroke and coronary disease, the prevalence of vascular disease in other vascular beds reaching clinically critical levels appears to be increasing.[1] Understanding the variety of clinical manifestations of these lesions, the potential for disease progression, and the benefits and limitations of vascular repair are essential for vascular medicine specialists. This chapter will examine the pathophysiology of renovascular lesions regarding blood pressure control, ischemic nephropathy, and clinical syndromes such as flash pulmonary edema. Specific issues regarding diagnostic evaluation and management are addressed elsewhere (see Chapter 23).

A wide range of lesions can affect the renal blood supply, some of which are summarized in Box 22-1. Historically, recognition of renovascular disease resulted from searching for underlying causes of hypertension. This followed the seminal observations of Goldblatt more than 70 years ago[2] that renal artery constriction produced a rise in arterial pressure in the dog. These studies were among the first to establish a primary role of the kidney in overall blood pressure regulation. Renovascular hypertension produced by a "clipped" renal artery remains among the most widely studied experimental forms of angiotensin-dependent hypertension.[3,4]

Epidemiology of Renal Artery Disease

Fibromuscular disease may be identified in 1% to 3% of normal kidney donors subjected to angiography before donor nephrectomy.[5] Of those developing clinical hypertension and referred for revascularization, more than 85% are females with a predilection for disease in the right renal artery.[6] The location of these lesions is most commonly in the midportion and distal segments of the renal artery. A variety of fibromuscular lesions have been described, but the most common is medial fibroplasia. Occasionally, such lesions may be found in the carotid and other vascular beds, but most commonly they are limited to the renal arteries. Most do not progress to impair renal function, although some lead to arterial dissection and/or thrombosis with loss of the kidney.

Atherosclerosis is the most common cause of renal artery disease. Its presence and severity are related to age and the presence of other atherosclerotic disease of the descending aorta and lower extremities. Population-based series, such as one from North Carolina, indicate that among 834 subjects older than 65 years, significant *renal artery stenosis* (RAS; defined as Doppler peak systolic velocity (PSV) above 1.8 m/s) can be identified in 6.8% of the general population, regardless of race.[7] Recent series of carotid, coronary, and peripheral angiography indicate that the prevalence of renovascular disease corresponds to overall atherosclerotic burden. Incidental renal artery occlusive disease (>50% stenosis) has been reported in 11% to 18% of patients with coronary artery disease (CAD), particularly when significant hypertension is present.[8] Peripheral vascular and aortic disease is associated with higher prevalence (25%-33%). As expected, risk factors predicting the presence of RAS include smoking, hyperlipidemia, hypertension, and diabetes. A corollary observation is that renovascular hypertension resulting from these lesions is now most commonly superimposed gradually upon preexisting essential hypertension. Hence, the blood pressure response and "cure" rates after successful restoration of blood flows to the kidney are limited by preexisting conditions.

Pathophysiological Consequences of Renovascular Disease

Under basal conditions, renal blood flow is among the highest of all organs. This feature reflects the kidney's filtration function, and less than 10% of delivered oxygen is sufficient to maintain renal metabolic needs. Importantly, a fall in renal blood flow is accompanied by decreased oxygen consumption, partly due to reduced metabolic demands of filtration and tubular solute reabsorption. Reduced renal blood flow can be sustained without measurable change in total kidney oxygen levels (as assessed by renal vein oxygen tension),[9] stimulation of erythropoietin release,[10] or reduced medullary and cortical tissue oxygenation as measured in human subjects using blood oxygen level–dependent (BOLD) magnetic resonance (MR).[11] These observations argue against an overall lack of oxygen as a primary stimulus for either hypertension or renal tissue injury and cast some doubt on the term *ischemic nephropathy*. Alternative terms proposed included *azotemic renovascular disease* and *hypoperfusion injury*.[12] Nonetheless, severe vascular stenosis leading to diminished renal perfusion eventually does lead to renal tissue injury and interstitial fibrosis.

Syndromes of Renovascular Disease

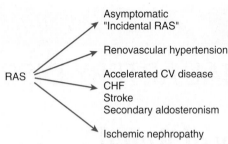

FIGURE 22-1 **Renal artery stenosis (RAS) produces a broad range of manifestations, ranging from "incidental" disease with no hemodynamic effect to deteriorating kidney function and accelerating cardiovascular morbidity.** CHF, congestive heart failure; CV, cardiovascular. *(Modified with permission from Garovic V, Textor SC: Renovascular hypertension and ischemic nephropathy. Circulation 112:1362–1374, 2005.)*[89]

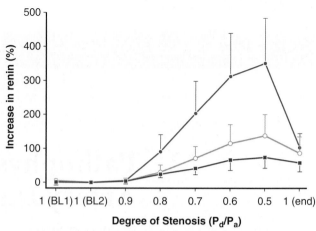

FIGURE 22-2 **Relationship between developed pressure gradient between aorta *(Pa)* and distal renal artery *(Pd)* and activation of renin-angiotensin system in humans.** Progressive gradients were developed by expanding a catheter balloon. Data indicate that activation of renal venous renin activity from stenotic kidney *(closed circles)*, nonstenotic kidney *(open circles)*, and aorta *(closed squares)* occurred only after a translesional gradient between 10 and 20 mmHg was created. Such a gradient usually requires advanced occlusive disease, usually more than 70% lumen occlusion. *(Reproduced with permission from De Bruyne B, Manoharan G, Pijls NH, et al: Assessment of renal artery stenosis severity by pressure gradient measurements. J Am Coll Cardiol 48:1851–1855, 2006.)*[16]

 Box 22-1   Vascular Lesions That Produce Renal Hypoperfusion and Renovascular Hypertension Syndrome

Unilateral Disease (Analogous to Two-Kidney, One-Clip [2K1C] Hypertension)
Unilateral atherosclerotic renal artery stenosis (RAS)
Unilateral fibromuscular dysplasia (FMD)
  Medial fibroplasia
  Perimedial fibroplasia
  Intimal fibroplasia
  Medial hyperplasia
Renal artery aneurysm
Arterial embolus
Arteriovenous fistula (AVF) (congenital/traumatic)
Segmental arterial occlusion (posttraumatic)
Extrinsic compression of renal artery (e.g., pheochromocytoma)
Renal compression (e.g., metastatic tumor)

Bilateral Disease or Solitary Functioning Kidney (Analogous to One-Kidney, One-Clip [1K1C] Model)
Stenosis to a solitary functioning kidney
Bilateral RAS
Aortic coarctation
Systemic vasculitis (e.g., Takayasu's arteritis, polyarteritis)
Atheroembolic disease
Vascular occlusion due to endovascular aortic stent graft

Subcritical Levels of Stenosis

The majority of renal artery lesions that compromise renal function are caused by gradually developing atherosclerosis of the renal vascular bed. As noted earlier, some patients undergoing cardiac catheterization have "incidental" renal lesions producing more than 50% cross-sectional stenosis,[13] for whom the presence of RAS is a strong independent predictor of mortality. Moreover, nonobstructive RAS (20%-50% decrease in renal arterial luminal diameter) can be found in an additional 28% of patients undergoing cardiac catheterization[13] and 48% of patients undergoing aortography for peripheral vascular disease.[14] A recent systematic analysis of these reports including more than 15,000 subjects confirmed this overall range of disease prevalence and the rise with increasing atherosclerotic burden.[8] Although lesions producing less than 50% in arterial luminal diameter are not considered hemodynamically significant, the relationships between resting pressure gradients and angiographic degree of stenosis are curvilinear and only approximate at best. As a predictor of mortality, even low-grade atherosclerotic lesions denote a hazard nearly equal to more advanced disease.[15] Estimating severity of vascular occlusion from angiographic images is notoriously unreliable. It should be emphasized that activation of pressor mechanisms depends upon the presence of a pressure gradient between the aorta and distal renal vasculature[16] (Fig. 22-2). There is a general relationship between estimated diameter stenosis and peak

translesional pressure gradients, but the relationship is not linear. In some instances, an abrupt fall in poststenotic pressure develops beyond a subcritical range of stenosis.[17] Even moderate stenosis, especially when superimposed on intrarenal microvascular disease, may contribute to adverse renal outcomes. Kidneys with a baseline renal artery disease classification of less than 60% stenosis have 11.7% 2-year cumulative incidence of renal atrophy (defined radiologically as a loss of kidney size)[18] and 28% cumulative incidence of renal artery disease progression, although progression to total renal artery occlusion is uncommon.[19] Increased severity of RAS in patients undergoing cardiac catheterization has an adverse effect on survival, with the 4-year adjusted survival for patients with a 50% stenosis decreasing to 70%, compared to 89% in patients without RAS.[20] Therefore, even relatively minor stenosis in the renal artery might have long-term functional implications, especially in the presence of additional risk factors or coexisting renal disease.

RENAL MICROVASCULAR DISEASE

Lesions in the main renal artery may be superimposed upon or confused with other causes for ischemic renal injury. Intrarenal vascular lesions are commonly observed in the course of various nephropathies, many of which have an ischemic component.[21] Risk factors including diabetes, hypertension, atherosclerosis, and aging elicit vasoconstriction or structural changes leading to intrarenal small-vessel disease and ischemic injury similar to that observed in large-vessel disease. Loss of microvessels and impaired capillary repair correlate with development of glomerular and tubulointerstitial scarring,[22,23] and may lead to end-stage renal failure. Renal microvascular disease distal to a stenosis in the renal artery may perpetuate and exacerbate renal parenchymal injury and may blunt renal recovery. The presence of small microvessel injury is difficult to verify but may account for changes in diastolic blood flow such as that producing changes in renal resistance index. Elevations of renal resistance index have been proposed to predict poor outcomes in many renal diseases, including renovascular disease.[24]

Critical Renal Artery Stenosis

High-grade vascular stenosis eventually leads to a decrease in renal perfusion pressure. *Critical stenosis* is identified when it produces a fall in renal blood flow and glomerular filtration rate (GFR).

During experimental renal artery occlusion, the kidney sustains autoregulation of blood flow through a range of perfusion pressures from 200 mmHg to approximately 80 mmHg. Mechanisms underlying autoregulation include myogenic responses to changes in wall tension, release of vasoactive substances, and the tubuloglomerular feedback. The latter responds to decreased renal perfusion pressure and salt delivery by decreasing vascular resistance distal to the obstruction. In addition, during a fall in renal perfusion pressure, the kidney activates multiple pathways that elevate systemic blood pressure, an effect that tends to restore renal perfusion pressure and sustain renal blood flow at the expense of arterial hypertension (Fig. 22-3). Consequently, as long as systemic arterial pressure is allowed to rise, a fall in renal blood flow does not occur until renal arterial diameter is reduced by 65% to 75%. Recent clinical studies suggest that noninvasive radiological imaging commonly overstates the degree of stenosis. Measurement of physiological stimuli, such as the release of renin, indicate that a translesion gradient of at least 10% to 20% reduction is necessary for biological responses to occur in humans.[16] To achieve such a gradient, luminal occlusion may need to exceed 80% stenosis. Under some conditions, gradients above 20 mmHg that develop during intrarenal hyperemic challenge with dopamine may disclose hemodynamic significance of lesions under 60% in severity.[25]

When renal perfusion pressure falls gradually, additional mechanisms are recruited that protect the kidney from the functional and morphological consequences observed after acute ischemic injury. These include development of collateral vessels and redistribution of intrarenal blood flow from the cortex to the medulla. Renal cortical blood flow autoregulates more efficiently than the outer medulla, which is continuously on the verge of anoxia. During chronic reduction of renal blood flow, medullary perfusion and oxygenation are relatively maintained by adaptive mechanisms at the expense of cortical blood flow.[26] When poststenotic renal artery pressures eventually fall further, either due to progressive vascular occlusion or reduction of systemic blood pressures by drug therapy, renal volume decreases.

In clinical terms, *renal atrophy* can be defined as a loss of renal length by at least 1 centimeter, and a difference in size between the two kidneys is suggestive of unilateral RAS (or a higher grade of stenosis in one of the kidneys). A decrease in renal volume results from a decrease in filling pressure, filtrate, and blood content of the kidney, as well as structural atrophy of the renal tubules due to apoptosis and necrosis. Apoptosis is an active, pre-programmed

form of cell death that is intricately regulated and distinct from cellular necrosis and likely serves as a protective mechanism to allow renal "hibernation." These changes may be reversible, since tubular cells show vigorous potential for regeneration. Loss of intrarenal microvessels that accompanies the ongoing scarring process may also contribute to renal shrinkage[27] (Fig. 22-4), but might be partly reversible upon enhancement of angiogenic signaling.[28] However, if a blood flow deficit persists, permanent damage to the kidney may occur. As mentioned, decreased renal blood flow is often accompanied by a decline in GFR and inhibition of tubular epithelial transport that limit renal oxygen consumption and maintain oxygen saturation. Hence, the kidney does not actually develop "ischemia" until an extreme decrease in renal blood flow develops.

RENOVASCULAR HYPERTENSION

Goldblatt et al and Loesch were the first to show in the 1930s that obstruction of the renal artery is followed by an increase in systemic blood pressure.[2,29] The characteristics of renovascular hypertension depend to a large extent on the status of the kidneys. Unilateral RAS may be present with an intact contralateral renal artery (the experimental form is termed *two-kidney, one-clip*, or *2K1C*). This model is characterized by counterregulatory processes in the contralateral kidney leading to sodium excretion in response to elevated arterial pressure (pressure natriuresis; Fig. 22-5A-B). Alternatively, RAS may affect a solitary kidney (*one-kidney, one-clip*, or *1K1C*; Fig. 22-6 A-B). Bilateral RAS and 1K1C lead to more severe renovascular hypertension, although bilateral RAS may behave similarly to 2K1C if one kidney is significantly less ischemic than the other. Patients with this constellation of findings have higher mortality, are more prone to circulatory congestion, and are more likely to experience deterioration of kidney function during administration of antihypertensive agents, including angiotensin-converting enzyme (ACE) inhibitors or angiotensin II (Ang II) receptor blockers (ARBs).

The exact mechanisms responsible for renovascular hypertension have long been debated. The immediate increase in blood pressure in RAS results from release of renin from the stenotic kidney. This leads to increased formation of Ang II, which increases peripheral vascular resistance, plasma aldosterone, sodium retention, extracellular volume, and cardiac output (Fig. 22-7). Early studies using ACE inhibitors[30] and more recent studies in an AT1A receptor knockout mouse model of 2K1C confirm the essential role of Ang II in mediating Goldblatt hypertension during its initial phase.[31] Experiments with kidney transplantation in these knockout strains indicate that both renal and extrarenal angiotensin receptors participate in regulation of blood pressure.[4] Blockade of angiotensin action in experimental models prevents the initial series of events and delays the development of renovascular hypertension indefinitely. Activation of the sympathetic nervous system also plays an important role in the pathogenesis of renovascular hypertension[32] primarily via the renal afferent nerves. Both the peripheral and central aspects of the autonomic system are also under the influence of Ang II. If the increase in pressure restores renal perfusion pressure distal to the stenosis, most of these alterations return to baseline levels, with the exception of peripheral vascular resistance.

After the initial rise in activity from the renin-angiotensin system, maintenance of renovascular hypertension in 1K1C models depends mainly on volume expansion. In 2K1C, the interplay between plasma renin activity and extracellular volume is more complex. The contralateral kidney responds to the elevated systemic pressure by increasing sodium excretion (pressure natriuresis), an effect that tends to drive blood pressure down and decrease perfusion pressure of the stenotic kidney. This effect again leads to an increase in renin release, which in turn elevates systemic blood pressure, and so forth. In high-grade RAS, this cycle of events may induce extracellular volume depletion and renal failure. Although these features are consistently demonstrated in

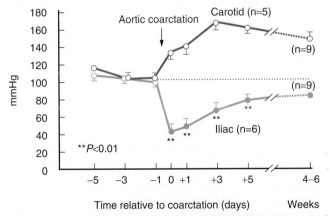

FIGURE 22-3 Development of arterial hypertension after placement of renal artery clip lesion in conscious rat aortic coarctation model. Poststenotic pressures (iliac artery) rise to near-baseline levels at the expense of systemic arterial pressures (carotid). Despite significant pressure gradient, renal perfusion is maintained. Reduction of systemic pressures, however, lowers renal perfusion and activates pressor systems, including renin-angiotensin system (see text). *(Reproduced with permission from Textor SC, Smith-Powell L: Post-stenotic arterial pressure, renal haemodynamics and sodium excretion during graded pressure reduction in conscious rats with one- and two-kidney coarctation hypertension. J Hypertens 6:311–319, 1988.)[90]*

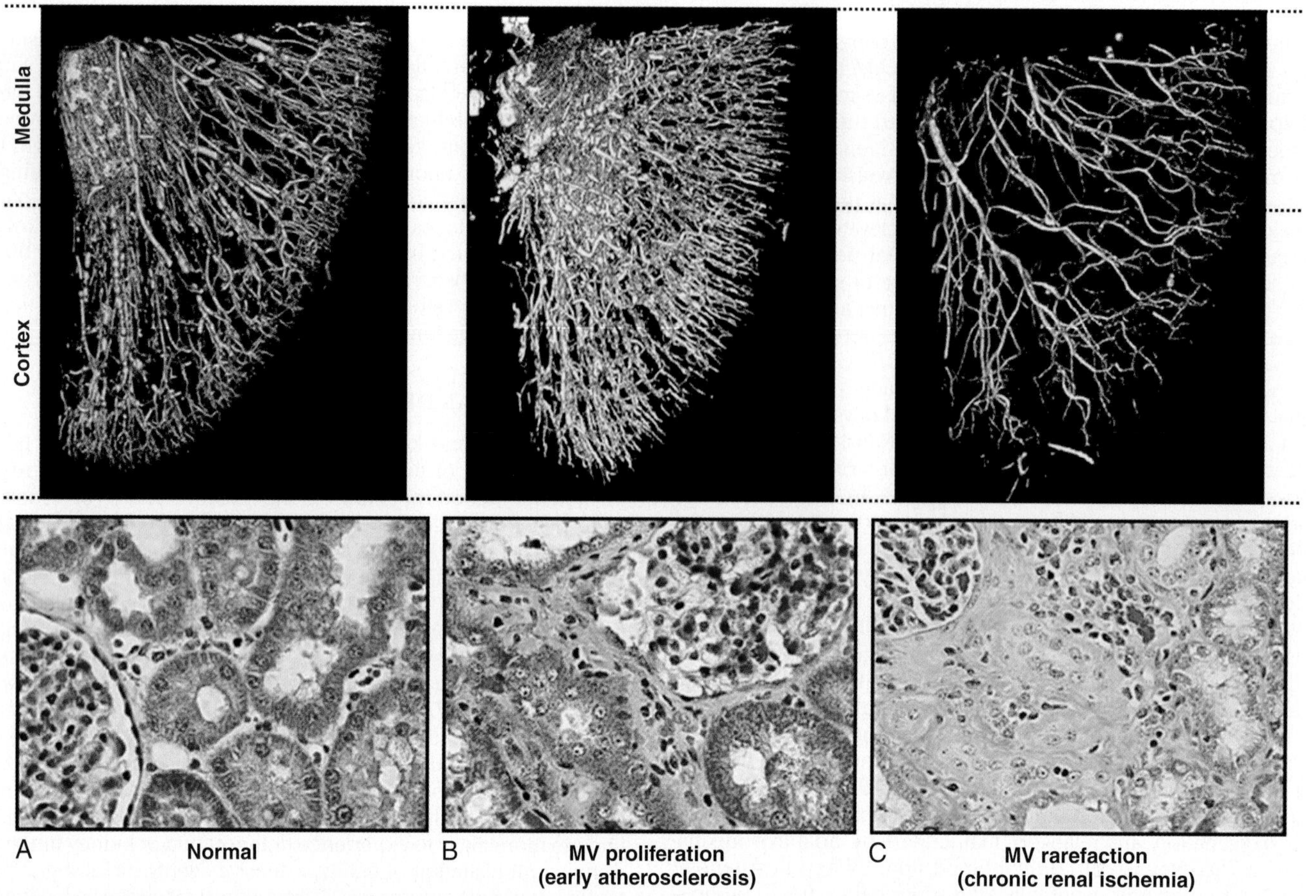

FIGURE 22-4 **Microcomputed tomography imaging of vascular structures in kidney cortex and medulla in a swine model. A,** Normal vascular density. **B,** Microvascular (MV) proliferation observed after cholesterol feeding. **C,** MV rarefaction and interstitial fibrosis observed beyond a high-grade renal artery stenosis (RAS). *(Reproduced with permission from Lerman LO, Chade AR: Angiogenesis in the kidney: a new therapeutic target? Curr Opin Nephrol Hypertens 18:160–165, 2009.)*[91]

experimental models, human renovascular hypertension frequently has elements of both 1K and 2K pathophysiology, particularly when the function of the contralateral kidney is compromised.

It is important to recognize that activation of the systemic renin-angiotensin system is temporary in renovascular hypertension. After a period of time, circulating levels of plasma renin activity and angiotensin fall despite sustained elevation of peripheral vascular resistance. This may be the result of both (1) a slow response to Ang II, through which low levels of angiotensin have pressor actions, and (2) recruitment of additional mechanisms of vasoconstriction. The latter include activation of vasoconstrictor lipoxygenase products, oxidative stress, and endothelin. Additional rise in pressure results from an imbalance between vasoconstrictors and vasodilators, such as that derived from decreased bioavailability of nitric oxide (NO). An important role is ascribed to dissociation between systemic blood pressure, extracellular volume, and inappropriate levels of Ang II.[33] The complexity of these relationships partly explains the failure of measuring any single pathway to predict blood pressure responses to renal revascularization.[34]

ACCELERATED HYPERTENSION AND PULMONARY EDEMA

Series of patients referred for renal revascularization in the last decade have included older patients with more widespread atherosclerotic disease than ever before.[35,36] This reflects both improved medical care leading to better blood pressure control and reduced mortality from coronary and cerebrovascular disease. Patient demographics commonly include more women than men and a high prevalence of coronary disease, CHF, and

known cerebrovascular disease. In some cases, suspicion arises regarding RAS because of rapid acceleration of these processes, particularly the rapid rise in arterial pressure in a previously stable patient. When untreated, a cycle of malignant-phase hypertension and hyponatremia (attributed to the dipsogenic action of Ang II) may ensue. In other cases, presenting symptoms include recent progression of hypertension followed by neurological symptoms of an acute stroke.

Some patients develop cycles of worsening CHF out of proportion to left ventricular (LV) dysfunction. This sometimes has been designated *flash pulmonary edema*.[37] Many of these patients have bilateral disease or stenosis to a solitary functioning kidney. When volume expanded, renal function may improve slightly at the price of hypertension and circulatory congestion. Sudden pulmonary edema partly reflects diastolic dysfunction precipitated by a rapid rise in afterload[38] in addition to impaired sodium excretion as a result of renal hypoperfusion. During volume depletion, serum creatinine commonly rises with evidence of *prerenal azotemia*. This condition warrants recognition because several series indicate that cycles of symptomatic exacerbation and hospitalization can be improved with successful renal revascularization.[39,40]

RENAL HYPOPERFUSION INJURY: ISCHEMIC NEPHROPATHY

The precise mechanisms responsible for irreversible renal scarring in so-called ischemic nephropathy in the absence of true ischemia have not been fully elucidated. They are likely related to interaction among several systems activated in the kidney, the most prominent of which is the renin-angiotensin system.

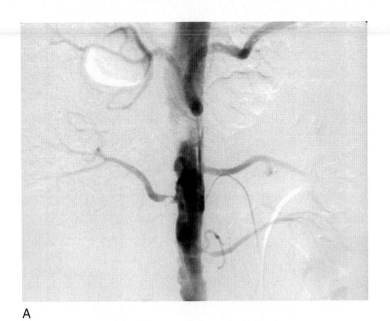

A

Unilateral Renal Artery Stenosis

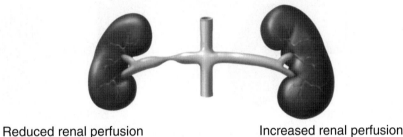

Reduced renal perfusion   Increased renal perfusion

↑ Renin-angiotensin system (RAS)   Suppressed RAS   Increased Na+ excretion
↑ Renin   (pressure natriuresis)
↑ Ang II
↑ Aldosterone

Ang II-dependent hypertension

Effect of blockade of RAS
Reduced arterial pressure
Enhanced lateralization of diagnostic tests
GFR in stenotic kidney may fall

Diagnostic tests
Plasma renin activity elevated
Lateralized features (e.g., renin levels in renal veins, captopril-enhanced renography)

B

FIGURE 22-5   A, Angiogram of unilateral renal arterial stenosis with well-preserved vascular supply to contralateral kidney. **B,** Schematic illustrating pathophysiology of unilateral renovascular hypertension (two-kidney, one-clip [2K1C]). Stenotic kidney responds to reduced perfusion with activation of renin-angiotensin system, producing widespread effects that include rise in arterial pressure. Elevated pressures subject nonstenotic kidney to so-called pressure natriuresis, leading to asymmetrical sodium excretion, fall in blood pressure, and continued stimuli to stenotic kidney. Such asymmetry is the basis for diagnostic testing such as captopril renography and renal vein renin measurements. Ang, angiotension; GFR, glomerular filtration rate.

Renal Vasoactive Hormonal Systems

ANGIOTENSIN II

Renal hypoperfusion is accompanied by activation of the renin-angiotensin system, a mechanism normally designed to regulate volume homeostasis and maintain GFR during a transient decrease in renal perfusion pressure. Angiotensin II maintains glomerular capillary pressure and GFR by way of its predominant vasoconstrictor effect on the efferent arteriole. The importance of Ang II for preserving GFR is most evident under conditions of reduced preglomerular arterial pressures, particularly under conditions of volume depletion.[41] This feature underlies the fall in

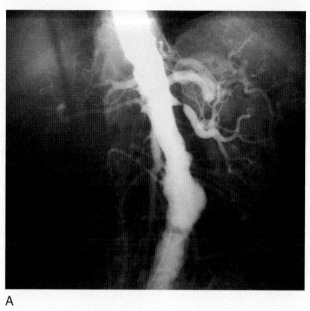

A

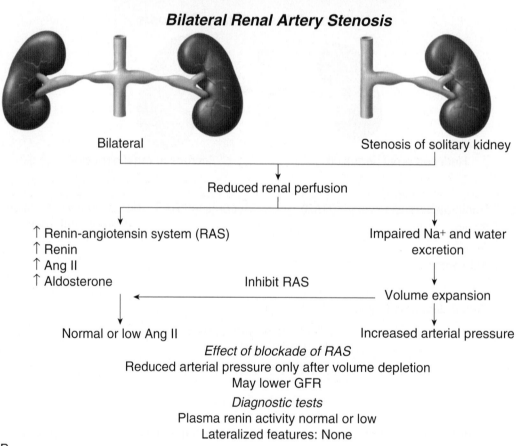

Bilateral Renal Artery Stenosis

Bilateral

Stenosis of solitary kidney

Reduced renal perfusion

↑ Renin-angiotensin system (RAS)
↑ Renin
↑ Ang II
↑ Aldosterone

Impaired Na⁺ and water excretion

Inhibit RAS

Volume expansion

Normal or low Ang II

Increased arterial pressure

Effect of blockade of RAS
Reduced arterial pressure only after volume depletion
May lower GFR

Diagnostic tests
Plasma renin activity normal or low
Lateralized features: None

B

FIGURE 22-6   A, Angiogram illustrating renal artery stenosis affecting entire renal mass, in this case a solitary functioning kidney. Contralateral kidney is occluded. **B,** Schematic illustrating pathophysiology of renovascular hypertension in which stenosis affects entire renal mass. In the absence of a normal contralateral kidney, sodium retention occurs, and hypertension is heavily dependent upon volume mechanisms. Ang, angiotension; GFR, glomerular filtration rate.

GFR sometimes observed following administration of ACE inhibitors to patients with RAS, particularly when the entire renal mass is affected.

Angiotensin II effects in the kidney include induction of cell hypertrophy and hyperplasia, and stimulation of hormone synthesis and ion transport. It also seems to contribute to the pathogenesis of renal fibrosis by recruiting bone marrow–derived fibrocytes, circulating cells that contribute to the pathogenesis of

fibrotic diseases.[42] Its renal actions are mediated primarily through AT1 receptors expressed on endothelial, epithelial, and vascular smooth muscle cells (VSMCs). Chronic activation of AT1 receptors in renal ischemic injury may elicit local inflammatory and fibrogenic responses. Angiotensin II has been implicated in stimulation of vascular smooth muscle and mesangial cell growth, platelet aggregation, generation of superoxide, activation of adhesion molecules and macrophages, infiltration of inflammatory cells,

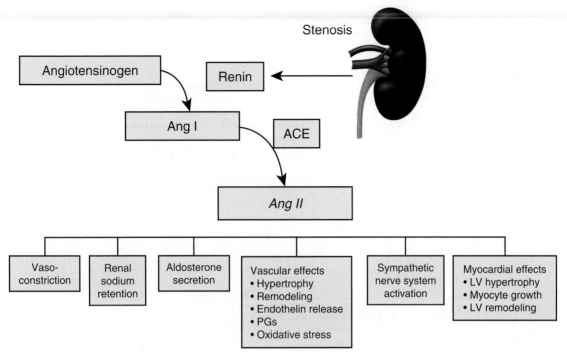

FIGURE 22-7   Actions of angiotensin II (Ang II) in generation of renovascular hypertension. In addition to direct effects on vascular tone and sodium homeostasis, Ang II modulates and induces vasoconstriction by several independent mechanisms, including oxidative stress. Induction of "slow pressor" responses are associated with reduction of circulating levels of plasma renin activity and loss of demonstrable pressure dependence upon Ang II (see text). ACE, angiotensin-converting enzyme; Ang, angiotensin; LV, left ventricular; PF, prostaglandin.

increased expression of extracellular matrix (ECM) proteins, and induction of proto-oncogenes.

The intrarenal effects of Ang II during renal ischemia are modulated by interactions with other humoral systems (Fig. 22-8). Vasodilator prostaglandins (PGs) attenuate vasoconstriction caused by Ang II and may limit ischemia due to elevated levels of this hormone.[43] Nitric oxide negates many actions of Ang II, modulates the effects of Ang II on the afferent arteriole and the proximal tubule, and down-regulates ACE and AT1 gene expression.[44] On the other hand, endothelin-1 (ET-1) regulates renal ACE expression, mediates some of the vascular effects of Ang II and amplifies its pressor effects, and activates a similar signal transduction pathway for growth- and differentiation-related genes. Thromboxane A_2, TxA_2, a vasoconstrictor metabolite of arachidonic acid, is also released within the kidney by Ang II and mediates much of the pressor and renal hemodynamic responses to Ang II.[45]

Therefore, Ang II is involved in short-term renal adaptive response to ischemia, but long-term activation of the renin-angiotensin system and its interaction with other humoral systems can lead to progressive destruction of renal tissue.

NITRIC OXIDE

Nitric oxide is synthesized from L-arginine within the kidney by a family of nitric oxide synthases (NOS) and plays a crucial role in the regulation of renal hemodynamics and excretory function. Differential expression, localization, and regulation of three isoforms of NOS expressed in the kidney—neuronal (nNOS), inducible (iNOS), and endothelial (eNOS)—contribute to diverse intrarenal actions.[46] Consequently, NO reduces vascular tone, increases sodium excretion, modulates tubuloglomerular feedback, has antithrombotic protection, inhibits growth-related responses to injury, and modulates the aforementioned renal actions of Ang II. Nitric oxide further buffers many processes implicated in the pathogenesis of tissue injury in renovascular disease, including growth of (VSMCs), mesangial cell hypertrophy and hyperplasia, and synthesis of ECM. However, regulation of renal blood flow becomes less dependent on eNOS-derived NO and more dependent on PGs as RAS progresses[47] because of

a decrease in renal perfusion pressure and vascular shear stress distal to the stenosis, which are primary stimuli to eNOS. On the other hand, the contralateral kidney continues to rely on NO to negate the actions of Ang II.[48]

The role of NO in renal tissue ischemia is complex, however. The iNOS isoform is up-regulated during renal ischemia[49] and generates NO that can be cytotoxic to renal epithelial cells and contributes to tubular injury, both by decreasing activity of the eNOS isoform and by formation of the oxidant peroxynitrite.

ENDOTHELINS

The endothelin peptides comprise a family of peptides produced and released from endothelial cells (ECs), which have potent and long-lasting vasoconstrictor effects on the renal microcirculation and modify tubular function. Endothelin release can be stimulated by Ang II, thrombin, transforming growth factor (TGF)-β, and other cytokines (e.g., tumor necrosis factor [TNF]-α, interleukin [IL]-1β). Tissue levels of ET-1 are increased in the stenotic kidney,[50] and in fact in most forms of renal failure, and may persist for days after resolution of the initial injury. Its involvement in renal ischemic injury is underscored by the observation that ET-1 blockade is more efficient in improving the early course of postischemic renal injury than inhibition of Ang II.[51] Chronic blockade of the endothelin-A receptor directly inhibits cellular growth and gene expression, and in ischemic acute renal failure provides long-term functional and morphological benefits. These effects are greater than those observed during simultaneous blockade of both the A and B receptor,[52] likely because of the role of the latter in eliminating salt, although the endothelin-B receptor has also been implicated in inflammation and fibrosis in progressive renal injury.[53]

PROSTAGLANDINS

Prostaglandins are cyclooxygenase (COX) derivatives of arachidonic acid that have important roles in maintaining renal blood flow and glomerular filtration. Biosynthesis of vasodilator PGs like prostacyclin (PGI_2) and prostaglandin E_2 protects the kidney against the effects of prolonged ischemia and Ang II[43]

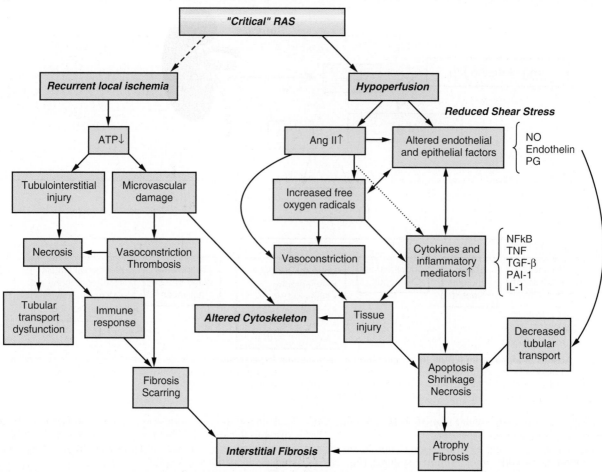

FIGURE 22-8 **Proposed pathways by which renal hypoperfusion activates fibrogenic mechanisms within kidney and ultimately produce irreversible parenchymal injury and interstitial fibrosis.** Both intermittent local ischemia *(left)* and vasoconstrictor-mediated cytokine-mediated pathways *(right)* participate in this process. Ang, angiotensin; ATP, adenosine triphosphate; IL-1, interleukin 1; NO, nitric oxide; NF-κB, nuclear factor kappa B; PAI-1, plasminogen activator inhibitor 1; PG, prostaglandin; RAS, renal artery stenosis; TGF-β, transforming growth factor beta; TNF, tumor necrosis factor. *(Modified with permission from Lerman L, Textor SC: Pathophysiology of ischemic nephropathy. Urol Clin North Am 28:793–803, 2001.)*[92]

and prevents hypoxic tissue injury. In RAS, they selectively prevent preglomerular constriction and thus limit a fall in GFR in the stenotic kidney,[54] potentially through regulatory interactions with NO. Conversely, TxA_2 is an endothelium-derived vasoconstrictor PG that is up-regulated in kidneys with renovascular disease.[55] It is released within the kidney by reactive oxygen species (ROS) or Ang II, modulates some of the deleterious effects of Ang II and ET-1, and contributes to kidney disease. Blockade of TxA_2 receptors thus improves urine volume, GFR, and renal plasma flow in ischemic kidneys and exerts a variety of beneficial effects that reduce the severity of ischemic damage. Furthermore, vascular expression of COX-2 is up-regulated in kidneys with arterial stenosis,[56] and COX-2-derived prostaglandin I_2 regulates renin release and renovascular hypertension in severe and moderate RAS.

Oxidative Stress

A growing body of evidence implicates increased generation of reactive radical species in the mechanisms of renal injury in renovascular disease.[3,57] Angiotensin II is a potent stimulus for superoxide production via the membrane NADH/NADPH oxidase system, and xanthine oxidase is an important source of oxygen free radicals during renal ischemia. Increased oxidative stress can promote formation of a variety of vasoactive mediators including ET-1, leukotrienes, and prostaglandin $F_{2\alpha}$ isoprostanes, endogenous products of lipid peroxidation. In addition, a chemical reaction between superoxide anion and NO not only decreases bioavailability of NO but also leads to production of toxic species (e.g., peroxynitrite [$ONOO^-$]). Functionally, ROS

have been implicated in decreasing stenotic kidney blood flow and sustaining renovascular hypertension.[58,59]

Furthermore, oxidative stress contributes to progressive tissue damage in the stenotic kidney. In mesangial cells, superoxide promotes hypertrophy and ECM production by both interaction with NO and by acting as an intracellular signal for growth-related responses, which may lead to microvascular and tissue remodeling.[60] In addition, ROS are implicated in the pathogenesis of ischemic renal injury by causing lipid peroxidation of cell and organelle membranes and disrupting the structural integrity and capacity for cell transport and energy production, especially in the proximal tubule. Activation of growth factors and cytokines like nuclear factor (NF)-κB[61] may also play an important role in the mechanism of action of Ang II and ROS. Studies in humans confirm that oxidative stress contributes to the impairment in endothelium-dependent vasodilation observed in patients with renovascular hypertension, which can be reversed with successful renal revascularization.[62]

The fibrogenic factors TGF-β, tissue inhibitor of matrix metalloproteinases (TIMP)-1, and plasminogen activator inhibitor (PAI)-1, which are up-regulated in stenotic kidneys,[61] are important mediators of ECM synthesis that characterizes progression of renal tissue injury. Early induction of TGF-β via the AT1 receptor plays a major role in tissue fibrosis[63] by increasing type IV collagen deposition and may play a role in interstitial scarring observed in chronic renal injury characterized by increased activity of intrarenal Ang II.[64] It interacts with endothelin and several growth factors and cytokines in promoting progressive interstitial fibrosis, primarily via its downstream effectors from the Smad family, but also participates in postischemic renal healing.

Tubular Cells

Acute ischemic renal failure is characterized by a rapid decline in adenosine triphosphate (ATP) that leads to secondary cascades of cellular injury, including increases in intracellular calcium, activation of phospholipases, and generation of oxygen radicals, which cause significant surface membrane damage.[65] The susceptible proximal tubule cells are primarily responsible for the pathophysiological and clinical aspects of ischemic acute renal failure. Of central importance is disruption and dissociation of the actin cytoskeleton and associated surface membrane structures that occur rapidly and are dependent on the severity and duration of ischemic injury.[66] These alterations may be secondary to activation and relocation of the actin-associated protein actin depolymerizing factor/cofilin and β_1-integrin to the apical membrane. Adenosine triphosphate depletion also induces necrotic cell death[67] by opening a plasma membrane "death channel" normally kept closed in ischemic tissue by tissue glycine and decreased pH. The epithelial brush border may disappear in association with apical membrane blebbing, interruption of cell-to-cell junctions, and subsequently epithelial desquamation. Detachment of tubule cells and microvilli contributes to backleak of glomerular filtrate and formation of intraluminal aggregations of exfoliated cells, proteins, and glycoproteins (GPs) such as fibronectin (FN), resulting in tubular obstruction. The functional ramifications of these changes are substantial in terms of tubular reabsorption, function of the intercellular tight junction, impaired cell substrate adhesion, and integral membrane protein function.

Tubulointerstitial Injury

In patients with atherosclerotic RAS, the severity of pathological tissue damage is an important determinant and predictor of renal functional outcome.[68] The earliest and most prominent pathological feature in renal ischemia is tubulointerstitial injury, which is considered to be the best prognostic factor in all nephropathies and may subsequently contribute to development of hypertension. The early phase of tubulointerstitial injury involves cellular activation, migration of mononuclear cells into the interstitium, leukocyte-endothelial interactions, and release of inflammatory products by myofibroblasts/activated fibroblasts. Altered antigenic profile of the tubular epithelium may initiate a cell-mediated immune response and be accompanied by interstitial inflammatory infiltrates composed of B lymphocytes, T-helper lymphocytes, and macrophages.[69] Subsequently, immunosuppressive regulatory T cells (Tregs) promote repair during the healing process, possibly by regulating proinflammatory cytokine production of other T-cell subsets.[70] Although the tubular lesions are initially reversible, tubulointerstitial injury may lead to irreversible fibrosis. A plethora of fibrogenic factors have been implicated in development of renal fibrosis following ischemic injury, such as TGF-β1, PAI-1, TIMP-1, α-1(IV) collagen, fibronectin-EIIIA (FN-EIIIA), tissue transglutaminase,[71] and others, which may increase synthesis of ECM. Recent evidence suggests that in the context of atherosclerosis, matrix degradation is also impaired so that the overall matrix turnover balance favors fibrosis.

Glomerulosclerosis

In human atherosclerotic RAS, glomerulosclerosis is a relatively late sequela and is exacerbated by long duration, preexisting renal injury, and comorbid clinical conditions. In experimental models of chronic moderate RAS, glomerular lesions are initially minimal. Ischemia may elicit global or focal segmental glomerulosclerosis, manifested as segmental collapse or sclerosis, with or without reactive podocyte hypertrophy and proliferation. Initiation of glomerular cell apoptosis, thickening of the basement membrane, and expansion of the mesangial ECM involve progression of glomerulosclerosis.[72] Presence of glomeruli that are not connected to normal tubule segments correlates with the concomitant decrease in GFR.

Cellular Death and Repair

Reactive oxygen species produced in renal proximal tubule epithelium under conditions of ischemia/reperfusion or hypoxia/reoxygenation are partly responsible for the apoptotic death of these cells.[73] This process is partly mitigated by autophagy, a process of degradation and recycling of cytoplasmic constituents that may either contribute to cell death or ameliorate further cellular damage. During hypoxic and ischemic renal injury, autophagy seems to provide a protective mechanism and enhance cell survival.[74]

Despite various defense mechanisms that are activated during an ischemic insult, cell loss by apoptosis or necrosis does occur when renal hypoxia is severe. For reconstitution of its function, successful repair of the kidney requires rapid replacement of injured cells.[75] Cell loss during kidney injury is followed by dedifferentiation and proliferation of adjacent surviving tubular cells, which are the chief contributors to tubular repair, and to a lesser degree interstitial kidney stem cells are stimulated to divide, migrate, and undergo phenotypical changes that allow them to replace lost cells. Bone marrow–derived cells likely contribute relatively little to this process.[76] Nevertheless, exogenous administration of progenitor cells has been shown to improve renal function and attenuate renal damage in the chronic RAS in swine[28,77] and ischemia/reperfusion injury in mice,[78] suggesting a potential therapeutic utility for this experimental approach to preserve the ischemic kidney.

Renal Artery Disease and Mortality

Role of Disease Progression

Follow-up studies of patients with incidentally identified renal artery disease[20] indicate that RAS independently predicts subsequent mortality. Rarely is this risk due to progressive renal disease alone, but more commonly to associated cardiovascular events. Mortality is remarkably similar in those treated with either medical management or renal revascularization.[79-81] Data from recent prospective randomized trials with atherosclerotic RAS indicate that progression of renal dysfunction is relatively uncommon.[82] Death is most commonly related to cardiovascular events, and only infrequently is progressive renal failure the primary cause of death.[79,81] Some authors suggest that atherosclerotic disease affecting the kidney is a general marker of the degree of atherosclerotic burden. Others argue that renovascular disease augments these conditions and directly accelerates cardiovascular mortality.[83] Available data do not support a direct role for renal revascularization to improve overall survival,[84] although observational series indicate that patients experiencing an improvement in GFR after successful revascularization do in fact have reduced cardiovascular mortality over several years of follow-up.[85,86]

Survival is reduced in patients with bilateral renal artery disease or stenosis to a solitary functioning kidney. Prospective studies using Doppler ultrasound indicate that atherosclerotic lesions can progress in severity over periods of 3 to 5 years.[87] Risks of progression are related to initial severity of the stenotic lesion and systolic blood pressure levels. It must be emphasized that clinical manifestations of renal artery disease within an individual patient may change over time. It is important that clinicians identify these transitions to consider interventions timed to when they are most likely to be effective.[88]

Specific decisions regarding management of patients with renovascular disease depend heavily upon recognizing the clinical syndromes developing as a result of these lesions. As with many other forms of peripheral vascular disease, the opportunity to benefit patients is greatest in those with overt clinical manifestations of the disease. It is our hope that understanding the pathophysiology underlying the clinical syndromes identified here will assist the clinician in choosing patients most likely to benefit from intervention.

REFERENCES

1. Fatica RA, Port FK, Young EW: Incidence trends and mortality in end-stage renal disease attributed to renovascular disease in the United States, *Am J Kidney Dis* 37:1184–1190, 2001.
2. Goldblatt H, Lynch J, Hanzal RE, et al: Studies on experimental hypertension I: the production of persistent elevation of systolic blood pressure by means of renal ischemia, *J Exp Med* 59:347–379, 1934.
3. Welch WJ, Mendonca M, Aslam S, et al: Roles of oxidative stress and AT1 receptors in renal hemodynamics and oxygenation in the postclipped 2K,1C kidney, *Hypertension* 41:692–696, 2003.
4. Crowley SD, Gurley SB, Oliverio MI, et al: Distinct roles for the kidney and systemic tissues in blood pressure regulation by the renin-angiotensin system, *J Clin Invest* 115(4):1092–1099, 2005.
5. Lorenz EC, Vrtiska TJ, Lieske JC, et al: Prevalence of renal artery and kidney abnormalities by computed tomography among healthy adults, *Clin J Am Soc Nephrol* 5:431–438, 2010.
6. Slovut DP, Olin JW: Current concepts: fibromuscular dysplasia, *N Engl J Med* 350:1862–1871, 2004.
7. Hansen KJ, Edwards MS, Craven TE, et al: Prevalence of renovascular disease in the elderly: a population based study, *J Vasc Surg* 36:443–451, 2002.
8. de Mast Q, Beutler JJ: The prevalence of atherosclerotic renal artery stenosis in risk groups: a systematic literature review, *J Hypertens* 27:1333–1340, 2009.
9. Gloviczki ML, Glockner JF, Lerman LO, et al: Preserved oxygenation despite reduced blood flow in poststenotic kidneys in human atherosclerotic renal artery stenosis, *Hypertension* 55:961–966, 2010.
10. Wiecek A, Kokot F, Kuczera M, et al: Plasma erythropoietin concentration in renal venous blood of patients with unilateral renovascular hypertension, *Nephrol Dial Transplant* 7:221–224, 1992.
11. Textor SC, Glockner JF, Lerman LO, et al: The use of magnetic resonance to evaluate tissue oxygenation in renal artery stenosis, *J Am Soc Nephrol* 19:780–788, 2008.
12. Textor SC, Wilcox CS: Renal artery stenosis: a common, treatable cause of renal failure? *Annu Rev Med* 52:421–442, 2001.
13. Rihal CS, Textor SC, Breen JF, et al: Incidental renal artery stenosis among a prospective cohort of hypertensive patients undergoing coronary angiography, *Mayo Clin Proc* 77:309–316, 2002.
14. Iglesias JI, Hamburger RJ, Feldman L, et al: The natural history of incidental renal artery stenosis in patients with aortoiliac vascular disease, *Am J Med* 109:642–647, 2000.
15. Dechering DG, Kruis HM, Adiyaman A, et al: Clinical significance of low-grade renal artery stenosis, *J Intern Med* 267:305–315, 2010.
16. De Bruyne B, Manoharan G, Pijls NHJ, et al: Assessment of renal artery stenosis severity by pressure gradient measurements, *J Am Coll Cardiol* 48:1851–1855, 2006.
17. Gross CM, Kramer J, Weingartner O, et al: Determination of renal arterial stenosis severity: comparison of pressure gradient and vessel diameter, *Radiology* 220:751–756, 2001.
18. Caps MT, Zierler RE, Polissar NL, et al: Risk of atrophy in kidneys with atherosclerotic renal artery stenosis, *Kidney Int* 53:735–742, 1998.
19. Pearce JD, Craven BL, Craven TE, et al: Progression of atherosclerotic renovascular disease: a prospective, population-based study, *J Vasc Surg* 44:955–963, 2006.
20. Conlon PJ, Little MA, Pieper K, et al: Severity of renal vascular disease predicts mortality in patients undergoing coronary angiography, *Kidney Int* 60:1490–1497, 2001.
21. Meyrier A, Hill GW, Simon P: Ischemic renal diseases: new insights into old entities, *Kidney Int* 54:2–13, 1998.
22. Kang DH, Kanellis J, Hugo C, et al: Role of the microvascular endothelium in progressive renal disease, *J Am Soc Nephrol* 13:806–816, 2002.
23. Urbieta-Caceres VH, Lavi R, Zhu XY, et al: Early atherosclerosis aggravates the effect of renal artery stenosis on the swine kidney, *Am J Physiol Renal Physiol* 299:F135–F140, 2010.
24. Radermacher J, Chavan A, Bleck J, et al: Use of Doppler ultrasonography to predict the outcome of therapy for renal-artery stenosis, *N Engl J Med* 344:410–417, 2001.
25. Mangiacapra F, Trana C, Sarno G, et al: Translesional pressure gradients to predict blood pressure response after renal artery stenting in patients with renovascular hypertension, *Circ Cardiovasc Interven* 99:999, 2010.
26. Evans RG, Gardiner BS, Smith DW, et al: Intrarenal oxygenation: unique challenges and the biophysical basis of homeostasis, *Am J Physiol Renal Physiol* 295:F1259–F1270, 2008.
27. Zhu XY, Chade AR, Rodriquez-Porcel M, et al: Cortical microvascular remodeling in the stenotic kidney. Role of increased oxidative stress, *Arterioscler Thromb Vasc Biol* 24:1854–1859, 2004.
28. Chade AR, Zhu X, Lavi R, et al: Endothelial progenitor cells restore renal function in chronic experimental renovascular disease, *Circulation* 119:547–557, 2009.
29. Loesch J: Ein Beitrag zur experimentellen Nephritis und zum arteriellen Hochdruck I. Die Veranderungen im Blutdruck II. Die Veranderungen in der Blutchemie, *Zentralblatt fur Innere Medizin* 7:144–169, 1933.
30. DeForrest JM, Knappenberger RC, Antonaccio MJ, et al: Angiotensin II is a necessary component for the development of hypertension in the two-kidney, one clip rat, *Am J Cardiol* 49:1515–1517, 1982.
31. Cervenka L, Horacek V, Vaneckova I, et al: Essential role of AT1-A receptor in the development of 2K1C hypertension, *Hypertension* 40:735–741, 2002.
32. Grisk O, Rettig R: Interactions between the sympathetic nervous system and the kidneys in arterial hypertension, *Cardiovasc Res* 61:238–246, 2004.
33. Reckelhoff JF, Romero JC: Role of oxidative stress in angiotensin-induced hypertension, *Am J Physiol* 284:R893–R912, 2003.
34. Safian RD, Textor SC: Medical progress: renal artery stenosis, *N Engl J Med* 344:431–442, 2001.
35. Conlon PJ, O'Riordan E, Kalra PA: Epidemiology and clinical manifestations of atherosclerotic renal artery stenosis, *Am J Kidney Dis* 35:573–587, 2000.
36. Textor SC, McKusick M: Renovascular hypertension and ischemic nephropathy: angioplasty and stenting. In Brady HR, Wilcox CS, editors: *Therapy in nephrology and hypertension*, London, 2003, WB Saunders, pp 599–609.
37. Messina LM, Zelenock GB, Yao KA, et al: Renal revascularization for recurrent pulmonary edema in patients with poorly controlled hypertension and renal insufficiency: a distinct subgroup of patients with arteriosclerotic renal artery occlusive disease, *J Vasc Surg* 15:73–82, 1992.
38. Gandhi SK, Powers JC, Nomeir AM, et al: The pathogenesis of acute pulmonary edema associated with hypertension, *N Engl J Med* 344:17–22, 2001.
39. Missouris CG, Belli AM, MacGregor Ga: "Apparent" heart failure: a syndrome caused by renal artery stenoses, *Heart* 83:152–155, 2000.
40. Pickering TG, Herman L, Devereux RB, et al: Recurrent pulmonary oedema in hypertension due to bilateral renal artery stenosis: treatment by angioplasty or surgical revascularisation, *Lancet* 2:551–552, 1988.
41. Hall JE: Renal function in one-kidney, one-clip hypertension and low renin essential hypertension, *Am J Hypertens* 4:523s–533s, 1991.
42. Sakai N, Wada T, Matsushima K, et al: The renin-angiotensin system contributes to renal fibrosis through regulation of fibrocytes, *J Hypertens* 26:780–790, 2008.
43. Stebbins CL, Symons JD, Hageman KS, et al: Endogenous prostaglandins limit angiotensin-II induced regional vasoconstriction in conscious rats, *J Cardiovasc Pharmacol* 42:10–16, 2003.
44. Singh P, Deng A, Weir MR, et al: The balance of angiotensin II and nitric oxide in kidney diseases, *Curr Opin Nephrol Hypertens* 17:51–56, 2010.
45. Wilcox CS, Welch WJ: Angiotensin II and thromboxane in the regulation of blood pressure and renal function, *Kidney Int* 38:S81–S83, 1990.
46. Kone BC, Baylis C: Biosynthesis and homeostatic roles of nitric oxide in the normal kidney, *Am J Physiol* 272:F561–F578, 1997.
47. Tokuyama H, Hayashi K, Matsuda H, et al: Stenosis-dependent role of nitric oxide and prostaglandins in chronic renal ischemia, *Am J Physiol* 282:F859–F865, 2002.
48. Helle F, Hultstrom M, Skogstrand T, et al: Angiotensin II induced contraction is attenuated by nitric oxide in afferent arterioles from the non-clipped kidney in 2K1C, *Am J Physiol Renal Physiol* 296:F78–F86, 2010.
49. Chade AR, Rodriguez-Porcel M, Grande JP, et al: Distinct renal injury in early atherosclerosis and renovascular disease, *Circulation* 106:1165–1171, 2002.
50. Firth JD, Ratcliffe PJ: Organ distribution of the three rat endothelin messenger RNAs and the effects of ischemia on renal gene expression, *J Clin Invest* 90:1023–1031, 1992.
51. Jerkic M, Miloradovic Z, Jovovic D, et al: Relative roles of endothelin-1 and angiotensin II in experimental post-ischaemic acute renal failure, *Nephrol Dial Transplant* 19:83–94, 2004.
52. Forbes JM, Hewitson TD, Becker GJ, et al: Simultaneous blockade of endothelin A and B receptors in ischemic acute renal failure is detrimental to long-term kidney function, *Kidney Int* 59:1333–1341, 2001.
53. Neuhofer W, Pittrow D: Role of endothelin and endothelin receptor antagonists in renal disease, *Eur J Clin Invest* 36(Suppl 3):78–88, 2006.
54. Milot A, Lambert R, Lebel M, et al: Prostaglandins and renal function in hypertensive patients with unilateral renal artery stenosis and patients with essential hypertension, *J Hypertens* 14:765–771, 1996.
55. Welch WJ, Patel K, Modlinger P, et al: Roles of vasoconstrictor prostaglandins, COX-1 and -2, and AT1, AT2, and TP receptors in a rat model of early 2K,1C hypertension, *Am J Physiol Heart Circ Physiol* 293:H2633–H2699, 2007.
56. Therland KL, Stubbe J, Thiesson HC, et al: Cycloxygenase-2 is expressed in vasculature of normal and ischemic adult human kidney and is co-localized with vascular prostaglandin E2 EP4 receptors, *J Am Soc Nephrol* 15:1189–1198, 2004.
57. Lerman LO, Nath KA, Rodriguez-Porcel M, et al: Increased oxidative stress in experimental renovascular hypertension, *Hypertension* 37:541–546, 2001.
58. Chade AR, Krier JD, Rodgriguez-Porcel M, et al: Comparison of acute and chronic antioxidant interventions in experimental renovascular disease, *Am J Physiol* 286:F1079–F1086, 2004.
59. Palm F, Onozato M, Welch WJ, et al: Blood pressure, blood flow, and oxygenation in the clipped kidney of chronic 2-kidney, 1-Clip rats: effects of tempol and angiotensin blockade, *Hypertension* 55:298–304, 2010.
60. Carlstrom M, Lai EY, Ma Z, et al: Superoxide dismutase 1 limits renal microvascular remodeling and attenuates arteriole and blood pressure responses to angiotensin II via modulation of nitric oxide bioavailability, *Hypertension* 56:907–913, 2010.
61. Chade AR, Rodriguez-Porcel M, Grande JP, et al: Mechanisms of renal structural alterations in combined hypercholesterolemia and renal artery stenosis, *Arterioscler Thromb Vasc Biol* 23:1295–1301, 2003.
62. Higashi Y, Sasaki S, Nakagawa K, et al: Endothelial function and oxidative stress in renovascular hypertension, *N Engl J Med* 346:1954–1962, 2002.
63. Leask A: Potential therapeutic targets for cardiac fibrosis: TGF beta, angiotensin, endothelin, CCN2, and PDGF: partners in fibroblast activation, *Circ Res* 106:1675–1680, 2010.
64. Yang F, Chung AC, Huang XR, et al: Angiotensin II induces connective tissue growth factor and collagen I expression via transforming growth factor beta-dependent and -independent Smad pathways: the role of Smad3, *Hypertension* 54:877–884, 2009.
65. Kellerman PS: Cellular and metabolic consequences of chronic ischemia on kidney function, *Semin Nephrol* 16:33–42, 1996.
66. Sutton TA, Molitoris BA: Mechanisms of cellular injury in ischemic acute renal failure, *Semin Nephrol* 18:490–497, 1998.
67. Bonventre JV, Weinberg JM: Recent advances in the pathophysiology of ischemic acute renal failure, *J Am Soc Nephrol* 14:199–2210, 2003.
68. Wright JR, Duggal A, Thomas R, et al: Clinicopathological correlation in biopsy-proven atherosclerotic nephropathy: implications for renal functional outcome in atherosclerotic renovascular disease, *Nephrol Dial Transplant* 16:765–770, 2001.
69. Truong LD, Farhood A, Tasby J, et al: Experimental chronic renal ischemia: morphologic and immunologic studies, *Kidney Int* 41:1676–1689, 1992.
70. Gandolfo MT, Jang HR, Bagnasco SM, et al: Foxp3+ regulatory T-cells participate in repair of ischemic acute kidney injury, *Kidney Int* 76:717–729, 2009.
71. Johnson TS, El-Koriaie AF, Skill NJ, et al: Tissue transglutaminase and the progression of human renal scarring, *J Am Soc Nephrol* 14:2052–2062, 2003.
72. Makino H, Sugiyama H, Kashihara N: Apoptosis and extracellular matrix-cell interactions in kidney disease, *Kidney Int* 77(Supplement):S67–S75, 2000.

73. Chien CT, Lee PH, Chen CF, et al: De novo demonstration and co-localization of free radical production and apoptosis formation in rat kidney subjected to ischemia/reperfusion, *J Am Soc Nephrol* 12:973–982, 2001.

74. Jiang M, Liu K, Luo J, et al: Autophagy is a renoprotective mechanism during *in-vitro* hypoxia and *in-vivo* ischemia-reperfusion injury, *Am J Pathol* 176:1181–1190, 2010.

75. Guo JK, Cantley LG: Cellular maintenance and repair of the kidney, *Annu Rev Physiol* 72:357–376, 2010.

76. Lin F, Moran A, Igarashi P: Intrarenal cells, not bone marrow-derived cells, are the major source for regeneration in postischemic kidney, *J Clin Invest* 115:1756–1764, 2005.

77. Chade AR, Zhu XY, Krier JD, et al: Endothelial progenitor cells homing and renal repair in experimental renovascular disease, *Stem Cells* 28:1039–1047, 2010.

78. Li B, Cohen A, Hudson TE, et al: Mobilized human hematopoietic stem/progenitor cells promote kidney repair after ischemia/reperfusion injury, *Circulation* 121:2211–2220, 2010.

79. Chabova V, Schirger A, Stanson AW, et al: Outcomes of atherosclerotic renal artery stenosis managed without revascularization, *Mayo Clin Proc* 75:437–444, 2000.

80. Dorros G, Jaff M, Mathiak L, et al: Multicenter Palmaz stent renal artery stenosis revascularization registry report: four-year follow-up of 1,058 successful patients, *Catheter Cardiovasc Interv* 55:182–188, 2002.

81. Uzzo RG, Novick AC, Goormastic M, et al: Medical versus surgical management of atherosclerotic renal artery stenosis, *Transplant Proc* 34:723–725, 2002.

82. The ASTRAL Investigators: Revascularization versus medical therapy for renal-artery stenosis, *N Engl J Med* 361:1953–1962, 2009.

83. Rimmer JM, Plante DA, Madias NE: Therapeutic decision making in renal vascular hypertension. In Novick AC, Scoble J, Hamilton G, editors: *Renal vascular disease*, London, 1996, W.B. Saunders, pp 245–266.

84. Textor SC, Lerman L, McKusick M: The uncertain value of renal artery interventions: where are we now? *J Am Coll Cardiol Cardiovasc Interv* 2:175–182, 2009.

85. Kennedy DJ, Colyer WR, Brewster PS, et al: Renal insufficiency as a predictor of adverse events and mortality after renal artery stent placement, *Am J Kidney Dis* 14:926–935, 2003.

86. Kalra PA, Chrysochou C, Green D, et al: The benefit of renal artery stenting in patients with atheromatous renovascular disease and advanced chronic kidney disease, *Catheter Cardiovasc Interv* 75:1–10, 2010.

87. Caps MT, Perissinotto C, Zierler RE, et al: Prospective study of atherosclerotic disease progression in the renal artery, *Circulation* 98:2866–2872, 1998.

88. Textor SC: Progressive hypertension in a patient with "incidental" renal artery stenosis, *Hypertension* 40:595–600, 2002.

89. Garovic V, Textor SC: Renovascular hypertension and ischemic nephropathy, *Circulation* 112:1362–1374, 2005.

90. Textor SC, Smith-Powell L: Post-stenotic arterial pressure, renal haemodynamics and sodium excretion during graded pressure reduction in conscious rats with one- and two-kidney coarctation hypertension, *J Hypertens* 6:311–319, 1988.

91. Lerman LO, Chade AR: Angiogenesis in the kidney: a new therapeutic target? *Curr Opin Nephrol Hypertens* 18:160–165, 2009.

92. Lerman L, Textor SC: Pathophysiology of ischemic nephropathy, *Urol Clin North Am* 28:793–803, 2001.

CH 22

PATHOPHYSIOLOGY OF RENAL ARTERY DISEASE

CHAPTER 23

Clinical Evaluation of Renal Artery Disease

Joe F. Lau, Jeffrey W. Olin

Data from the National Health and Nutrition Examination Survey (NHANES) 2005 to 2008, extrapolated to 2008, estimated that approximately 76,400,000 adults 20 years of age or older have essential (primary) hypertension.[1] Renovascular disease and renal parenchymal disease are the most common secondary causes of hypertension after obesity, excess alcohol ingestion, drug abuse, and oral contraceptive use are excluded.

The presence of anatomical renal artery stenosis (RAS) does not necessarily establish that the hypertension or renal failure is due to RAS. Incidentally discovered RAS is quite common, whereas renovascular hypertension only occurs in 1% to 5% of all patients with hypertension.[2,3] Approximately 90% of all renovascular disease is caused by atherosclerosis.[4,5] Fibromuscular dysplasia (FMD) is the second most common cause of RAS.[6] Patients with atherosclerotic RAS are typically older than age 55 and have the usual risk factors for atherosclerosis, but FMD is more common in younger women. The predominant clinical manifestation of FMD is hypertension; atherosclerotic RAS may present with hypertension, renal failure (ischemic nephropathy), and/or recurrent episodes of congestive heart failure (CHF) and "flash" pulmonary edema.[7] Whereas atherosclerotic RAS most often occurs at the ostium or proximal portion of the renal artery, FMD usually occurs in the mid- to distal renal artery and its primary branches (Figs. 23-1 and 23-2).

The effects of atherosclerosis on the coronary and carotid arteries are well recognized, but involvement of the renal arteries is frequently overlooked. In addition to the sequelae of RAS (hypertension, renal failure), patients with atherosclerotic RAS succumb prematurely from myocardial infarction (MI) and stroke.[8-11] Thus, early diagnosis and treatment is important to avoid the consequences of RAS.

When considering the diagnosis of RAS, it is useful to think in terms of the circumstances in which RAS is likely to occur (Box 23-1).

Hypertension

Individuals who develop hypertension between the ages of 30 and 55 usually have primary (essential) hypertension. If the initial diagnosis of hypertension is made before the age of 30, it is usually due to FMD if other known secondary causes (obesity, oral contraceptive use, drug abuse, and parenchymal renal disease) have been excluded. Since atherosclerosis occurs in older individuals, it is usually the cause of RAS after the age of 55. In one population-based study of Medicare patients aged 65 or older, the prevalence of atherosclerotic RAS was 6.8%.[12] In this cohort, RAS was found in nearly twice as many men as women (9.1% vs. 5.5%; $P = 0.053$); no significant differences were identified between Caucasians and African American subjects (6.9% vs. 6.7%; $P = 0.933$).[12] Although RAS can be associated with both systolic and diastolic hypertension, the diagnosis of RAS should be seriously considered in individuals who present with new-onset diastolic hypertension after the age of 55, primarily because diastolic blood pressure usually declines after age 55 in normal individuals. It is not uncommon for patients to have primary hypertension for many years, and as they age, develop atherosclerotic RAS. This cohort of patients may have had well-controlled blood pressure that suddenly becomes more difficult to control.

Patients may have anatomically significant RAS and no hypertension at all. Dustan and colleagues reviewed 149 aortograms and found that approximately half of patients with 50% or more RAS did *not* have hypertension.[13] Moreover, in a recent systematic review of 40 studies that evaluated a total of 15,879 patients, the mean prevalence of RAS among patients with suspected renovascular hypertension was 14.1%.[11] On further analysis of the patients who were incidentally found to have RAS on imaging studies, 65.5% were hypertensive and 27.5% had renal failure.[11] Therefore, the mere presence of RAS and hypertension does not necessarily mean that one is causing the other.

Accelerated or malignant hypertension also has been associated with a very high prevalence of RAS.[14] *Resistant hypertension* is defined as failure to normalize blood pressure to less than 140/90 mmHg following an optimal medical regimen consisting of at least three drugs with different mechanisms of action, including a diuretic.[15] The diagnosis of renovascular disease should be strongly considered in patients with true drug-resistant hypertension.

Renal Abnormalities

Gifford et al. found that 71% of patients (53 of 75 patients) with an atrophic kidney had severe stenosis or complete occlusion of the renal artery supplying the small kidney.[16] Three studies have shown that if there is a discrepancy in size between the two kidneys or if one kidney is atrophic, the contralateral renal artery (normal-sized kidney) is severely stenotic about 60% of the time.[2,16,17] Therefore, the presence of an atrophic kidney or a discrepancy in size between the two kidneys demands a thorough investigation for the presence of renovascular disease.

Numerous reports suggest that patients who develop azotemia while receiving angiotensin-converting enzyme (ACE) inhibitors or angiotensin II receptor blocking (ARB) agents have bilateral RAS, RAS to a solitary functioning kidney, or decompensated CHF in the sodium-depleted state.[18-22] These clinical scenarios are absolute indications for investigation, since they usually reflect the presence of severe RAS to the entire functioning renal mass, thus placing the patient in jeopardy of renal failure. The mechanisms of acute and chronic renal failure in patients with RAS are discussed in detail in Chapter 22.

There are no prospective studies evaluating how often atherosclerotic renovascular disease leads to end-stage renal disease (ESRD). Scoble et al. found that atherosclerotic renovascular disease was the cause of ESRD in 14% of patients starting dialysis therapy.[23,24] In a retrospective review over a 20-year period in 683 patients, 83 (12%) patients had documented RAS as a cause of ESRD. Since arteriography was only performed in patients with suspected RAS, it is entirely possible that the true incidence of RAS as a cause of ESRD was underestimated. De Mast and Beutler reported that 41% of patients with ESRD had at least one renal artery with more than 50% stenosis.[11] Renal artery stenosis must be excluded in every patient starting dialysis if a clear-cut etiology for the ESRD is not known because the mortality in this patient population is extremely high. In the series by Mailloux et al., median survival in patients with ESRD secondary to RAS was 25 months, while 2-, 5-, and 10-year survival was 56%, 18%, and 5%, respectively.[9,10]

Effects of Renal Artery Stenosis on the Heart

Recurrent CHF and flash pulmonary edema unrelated to ischemic heart disease can result from bilateral RAS (or unilateral RAS to a single functioning kidney). In one renal artery stent series, 39 patients (19% of all patients undergoing renal artery

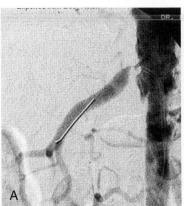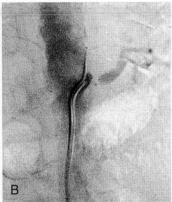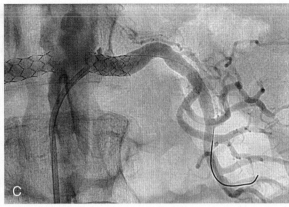

FIGURE 23-1 **A-B,** Digital subtraction angiogram (DSA) showing typical features of atherosclerotic renal artery stenosis (RAS). There is severe bilateral ostial RAS. **C,** Angiogram after stents were placed in right and left renal arteries.

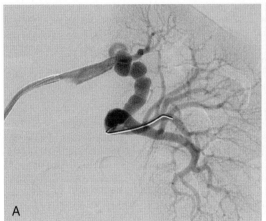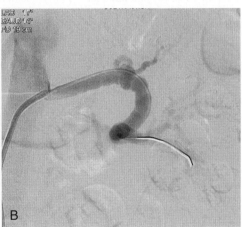

FIGURE 23-2 **A,** Digital subtraction angiogram (DSA) demonstrating medial fibroplasia located in mid- to distal part of left renal artery. Note "beading," with beads larger than normal caliber of artery, typical of medial fibroplasia. **B,** Angiogram of left renal artery after percutaneous balloon angioplasty. Angiographic appearance is improved, and there was resolution of pressure gradient.

Box 23-1   Clinical Clues That Suggest Presence of Renal Artery Stenosis

Hypertension
Hypertension onset age <30 or >55 years
Malignant or accelerated hypertension
Resistant hypertension (blood pressure >140/90 mmHg despite appropriate three-drug regimen, including a diuretic)
Loss of blood pressure control in a previously well-controlled patient

Renal Abnormalities
Acute renal failure precipitated by an angiotensin-converting enzyme (ACE) inhibitor or angiotensin receptor blocking (ARB) agent
Unexplained azotemia
Patient receiving renal replacement therapy (dialysis) without a definite known cause of end-stage renal disease (ESRD)
Atrophic or small kidney

Cardiac Disease
Recurrent congestive heart failure (CHF) or flash pulmonary edema
Angina disproportionate to coronary anatomy

Presence of Atherosclerosis in Other Vascular Beds
Peripheral artery disease (PAD)
Aortoiliac occlusive disease
Aortic aneurysm
Multivessel coronary artery disease (CAD)

stent implantation from 1991–1997) had recurrent episodes of CHF or flash pulmonary edema as the primary indication for renal artery stenting.[25] Nineteen of 39 patients had moderate to severe left ventricular (LV) systolic function. Although not completely understood, the mechanism of CHF may be related in part to the inability to use ACE inhibitors or ARBs to the direct adverse effects of angiotensin II (Ang II) on myocardial function, or to the inability to control volume adequately. If coronary ischemia has been excluded as a cause of CHF, renal revascularization (percutaneous stenting or surgical) is a very effective method of treatment in these individuals.[25–27]

One retrospective study demonstrated improvement in anginal symptoms in patients undergoing renal artery stent implantation. The mechanism of such improvement is not clearly delineated, but 88% of these patients had improved blood pressure control after stenting. This effect may account at least in part for decreased anginal symptoms.[28]

Presence of Atherosclerosis in Other Vascular Beds

Several series have examined the prevalence of renovascular disease in patients who have atherosclerotic disease elsewhere. To determine the prevalence of atherosclerotic RAS, Olin et al. studied 395 consecutive patients who had undergone arteriography as part of an evaluation for either an abdominal aortic aneurysm, aortoiliac occlusive disease, or peripheral artery disease (PAD)[2] (Table 23-1). These patients did not have the usual clinical clues to suggest RAS. High-grade bilateral renal artery disease was present in approximately 13% of patients. In addition, 76 patients had an aortogram performed for suspected RAS, and RAS was present in 70% of these subjects. Other studies have shown that 22% to 59% of patients with PAD have significant RAS.[29]

It has also been established that RAS is common in patients with coronary artery disease (CAD). Of 7758 patients undergoing cardiac catheterization during a 78-month period of time, 3987 underwent aortography at the time of catheterization to screen for RAS[30];

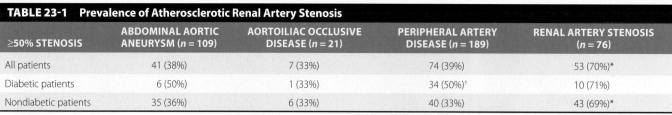

TABLE 23-1 Prevalence of Atherosclerotic Renal Artery Stenosis

≥50% STENOSIS	ABDOMINAL AORTIC ANEURYSM (n = 109)	AORTOILIAC OCCLUSIVE DISEASE (n = 21)	PERIPHERAL ARTERY DISEASE (n = 189)	RENAL ARTERY STENOSIS (n = 76)
All patients	41 (38%)	7 (33%)	74 (39%)	53 (70%)*
Diabetic patients	6 (50%)	1 (33%)	34 (50%)†	10 (71%)
Nondiabetic patients	35 (36%)	6 (33%)	40 (33%)	43 (69%)*

*P < 0.001
†P < 0.02

From Olin JW, Melia M, Young JR, et al: Prevalence of atherosclerotic renal artery stenosis in patients with atherosclerosis elsewhere. *Am J Med* 88:46 N–51 N, 1990.[2]

191 (4.8%) had more than 75% RAS, and 0.8% had severe bilateral disease. In a Mayo Clinic series, renal arteries were studied at the time of cardiac catheterization in patients with hypertension.[31] Ninety percent of the renal arteries were adequately visualized, and no complications occurred from the aortogram. More than 50% RAS was present in 19.2%, more than 70% stenosis in 7%, and bilateral RAS was present in 3.7% of patients. The likelihood of significant RAS is markedly increased in patients with two or more coronary artery lesions.[32] A prospective study of the long-term natural history of patients undergoing cardiac catheterization and renal angiography is needed to determine whether diagnosing RAS in this setting improves patient outcome measures. Renal artery disease is also associated with atherosclerotic disease in the carotid arteries. Louie et al. demonstrated that 46% of patients with more than 60% RAS also had more than 50% carotid stenosis.[33] All of these studies support the fact that atherosclerotic RAS is a manifestation of systemic atherosclerosis and reinforce the concept of treating the entire patient, not just the circulatory bed involved at a given point in time.

The presence of RAS even prior to development of ESRD portends a poor prognosis. Patient survival decreases as the severity of RAS increases, with 2-year survival rates of 96% in patients with unilateral RAS, 74% in patients with bilateral RAS, and 47% in patients with stenosis or occlusion to a solitary functioning kidney.[34] Dorros et al. demonstrated that as serum creatinine increases, survival decreases in patients with atherosclerotic RAS.[35] The 3-year probability of survival was 92 ± 4% for patients with a serum creatinine below 1.4 mg/dL, 74 ± 8% for patients with a serum creatinine of 1.5 to 1.9 mg/dL, and 51 ± 8% for patients with a serum creatinine 2.0 mg/dL or higher.

Long-term survival was investigated in a cohort of 1235 patients who underwent abdominal aortography at the time of cardiac catheterization. The 4-year survival rate of patients without RAS was 88% versus 57% for those with RAS.[34]

Physical Examination

The physical examination is generally not helpful in the diagnosis of RAS. Evidence of coronary, cerebral, or PAD is associated with a higher likelihood of renal artery disease because of the systemic nature of atherosclerosis. A systolic abdominal bruit is common and nonspecific, but the presence of both a systolic *and* diastolic bruit auscultated over the epigastrium may point to underlying renal artery disease.[36] Presence of a diastolic component to the bruit indicates that the degree of narrowing of the artery is severe, since there is continued flow during diastole.[37] An abdominal bruit with a systolic and diastolic component occurs more often in patients with FMD (53%) than in patients who have atherosclerotic disease (12.5%).[36] Presence of a bruit is helpful, but absence does not exclude the diagnosis of either atherosclerotic renovascular disease or FMD.

Diagnosis of Renovascular Disease

In the past, indirect methods of assessing the renal arteries were commonly used to diagnose RAS. Intravenous urography is obsolete as a screening tool, owing to its poor sensitivity and specificity.[38] Plasma renin activity as a stand-alone screening test is not reliable for diagnosing or excluding renal artery disease. Elevated plasma renin activity may be present in approximately 15% of patients with essential hypertension. In addition, patients with bilateral disease or disease to a solitary functioning kidney may have normal or low plasma renin activity due to extracellular volume expansion, position of the patient during the test, or medication use. The test is less accurate in azotemic patients and in African American patients.[39] The captopril test (plasma renin measurement before and after administration of captopril) is not an ideal screening test and is rarely used. Renal vein renin measurement is not a useful test to screen for RAS; in addition, it has little value in determining who will benefit from revascularization. Except under unusual circumstances, this test is rarely used to make clinical decisions.

Captopril Scintigraphy

Radionuclide imaging techniques are a noninvasive and safe way of evaluating renal blood flow and excretory function, but the renal flow scan has unacceptably high false-positive and false-negative rates for diagnosing RAS.[40] When an ACE inhibitor such as captopril is added to isotope renography, sensitivity and specificity of the test improve considerably, especially for patients with unilateral RAS. In most instances of unilateral RAS, the glomerular filtration rate (GFR) of the stenotic kidney falls by approximately 30% after captopril administration.[41,42] In contrast, the contralateral normal kidney exhibits an increase in GFR, urine flow, and salt excretion despite a reduction in systemic blood pressure. These expected physiological changes within the stenotic and contralateral kidneys are the basis of the asymmetry of renal function following ACE inhibition detected by renal scintigraphy (see Chapter 22).[43-45]

In patients with normal renal function and unilateral disease, captopril renography has a sensitivity of around 85% to 90% (range 45-94) and specificity around 93% to 98% (range 81-100).[46] However, the presence of significant azotemia or bilateral RAS may adversely affect the accuracy of captopril renography. Many investigators have excluded patients with a serum creatinine exceeding 2.5 to 3.0 mg/dL.[47] Although the captopril renogram was once the noninvasive diagnostic test of choice for patients with RAS, it is now rarely used because the quality of the images of duplex ultrasound, magnetic resonance angiography (MRA), and computed tomographic angiography (CTA) are excellent, as discussed later.

Imaging Modalities to Detect Renal Artery Stenosis

Although catheter-based renal angiography with pressure gradient measurements is the definitive gold standard of RAS assessment, several noninvasive imaging modalities such as duplex ultrasound, CTA, and MRA, have become more practical first-line tests for the diagnosis of RAS. Imaging has become so sophisticated and accurate, it is seldom necessary to perform catheter-based angiography for the *diagnosis* of renal artery disease, and it usually is reserved for imaging at the time of percutaneous revascularization. The ideal imaging procedure should[48]:

1. Identify the main renal arteries as well as accessory or polar vessels.
2. Localize the site of stenosis or disease.

3. Determine the type of disease present (e.g., atherosclerosis, FMD).
4. Provide evidence for the hemodynamic significance of the lesion.
5. Determine the likelihood of a favorable response to revascularization.
6. Identify associated pathology (i.e., abdominal aortic aneurysm, renal mass, etc.) that may have an impact on the treatment of the renal artery disease.
7. Detect restenosis after percutaneous or surgical revascularization.

Duplex ultrasonography, CTA, and MRA do not by themselves fulfill all these criteria. Local expertise and availability, as well as economic costs, often dictate the preferred imaging modality used (Fig. 23-3). Factors that may play a role in determining the optimal screening test include the patient's renal function, body habitus, and personal preference (e.g., claustrophobia).

DUPLEX ULTRASONOGRAPHY

Duplex ultrasonography (also see Chapter 12), which is composed of real-time brightness (B-mode/gray scale) imaging and color pulsed-wave Doppler, has the advantages of being noninvasive, the least expensive of the imaging modalities, and provides both anatomical and functional information about the arterial segments being evaluated. Duplex ultrasonography also does not require the use of potentially nephrotoxic agents.

Overall, when compared to angiography, duplex ultrasonography has a sensitivity and specificity of 84% to 98% and 62% to 99%, respectively, when used to diagnose RAS.[49-55] In a prospective blinded study, there was a very good correlation between duplex ultrasonography and angiography (Table 23-2). In addition, it was determined that if the end-diastolic velocity (EDV) was 150 cm/s or greater, the degree of stenosis was likely to be 80% or more.[56]

Renal artery ultrasound should be performed from both an anterior and oblique (or posterior [flank]) approach (Fig. 23-4). In the longitudinal view, the peak systolic flow velocity in the aorta is recorded at the level of the renal arteries. The renal-to-aortic ratio (RAR), which is the ratio of the highest peak systolic value (PSV) in the renal arteries to the PSV in the aorta, can then be calculated to help classify the degree of stenosis (see Table 23-3).[54,56]

The renal arteries are best visualized in a transverse (short-axis) view. Using the B-mode image and a 60-degree angle of insonance, the arteries are interrogated with pulsed wave Doppler. The Doppler should be swept through the artery from its origin to the renal hilum, which will allow the examiner to survey the artery for velocity shifts along the entire course of the renal artery. Velocities should be recorded at the origin, proximal, mid-, and distal arterial segments. From an oblique approach, the renal artery can be visualized at the renal hilum and followed to the aorta. By studying the patient from an anterior and an oblique approach, Doppler velocity measurements are obtained in two views, assuring that a focal stenosis is not missed and that the angle of insonation is correct. Since medial fibroplasia most often occurs in the mid- to distal renal artery, the oblique approach is particularly good for detecting this type of stenosis. It is important to note that segmental Doppler interrogation (spot-checking) of the renal artery velocities is inadequate and often leads to an inaccurate result.[54,56,57] When there is a discrepancy in kidney size of 1.5 cm or greater, the ultrasonographer should search very carefully for the presence of RAS or an occluded renal artery.

A three-category classification scheme based on the PSV within the proximal segment of the renal arteries is commonly used: 0% to 59% stenosis; 60% to 99% stenosis, and total occlusion. If the PSV is greater than 200 cm/s and turbulence is present in color Doppler flow, the stenosis would be classified as 60% to 99%. In the presence of a severe stenosis, there may be characteristic spectral broadening of the Doppler arterial waveform or parvus-tardus waveform just distal to the lesion. In addition to the PSV, the RAR is also used to help classify the degree of stenosis (Table 23-2). The caveat is that the RAR is not an accurate representation of the degree of stenosis when the aortic velocity is less than 40 cm/s or greater than 100 cm/s, or when an abdominal aortic aneurysm, or aortic stent graft is present.

Indirect assessment using the acceleration time (AT), acceleration index (AI), and resistance index (RI) have been used by some

TABLE 23-2	Comparison of Duplex Ultrasound with Arteriography				
STENOSIS BY ULTRASOUND	*Stenosis by Arteriography*				
	0%-59%	**60%-79%**	**80%-99%**	**100%**	**TOTAL**
0%-59%	62	0	1	1	64
60%-99%	1	31	67	0	99
100%	0	1	1	22	24
TOTAL	63	32	69	23	187
Sensitivity	0.98				
Specificity	0.98				
Positive predictive value	0.99				
Negative predictive value	0.97				

From Olin JW, Piedmonte MR, Young JR, et al: The utility of duplex ultrasound scanning of the renal arteries for diagnosing significant renal artery stenosis. *Ann Intern Med* 122:833–838, 1995.[56]

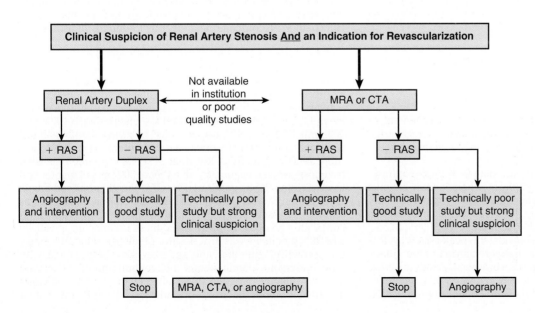

FIGURE 23-3 Algorithm for diagnosis of renal artery stenosis (RAS). CTA, computed tomographic angiography; MRA, magnetic resonance angiography. *(Adapted from Carman T, Olin JW: Diagnosis of renal artery stenosis: what is the optimal diagnostic test? Curr Interv Cardiol Rep 2:111–118, 2000.)*[48]

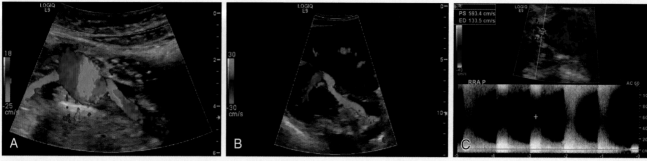

FIGURE 23-4 **A,** Color duplex ultrasound of renal arteries from an anterior approach. The right renal artery takes off at approximately 9-10 o'clock and the left renal artery at 3-4 o'clock. **B,** Color duplex ultrasound from oblique view imaging from kidney to proximal renal artery. Note how entire renal artery is visualized from this approach. **C,** Duplex ultrasound from anterior view. There is turbulence to flow on color Doppler and markedly increased velocities of blood flow (peak systolic velocity [PSV] 593 cm/sec and end-diastolic velocity [EDV] 134 cm/sec), indicating severe stenosis.

TABLE 23-3	Duplex Criteria for Diagnosis of Renal Artery Stenosis	
RAR <3.5 and PSV <200 cm/s		0%-59%
RAR ≥3.5 and PSV >200 cm/s		60%-99%
RAR >3.5 and EDV ≥150 cm/s		80%-99%
Absent flow, low-amplitude parenchymal signal		Occluded

EDV, end-diastolic velocity; PSV, peak systolic velocity; RAR, renal-to-aortic ratio.

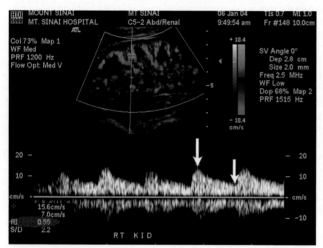

FIGURE 23-5 Measurement of resistance index (RI) {[1-(end-diastolic velocity/peak systolic velocity)] × 100}. Parenchyma of the kidney is visualized. Note blood flow within kidney. Doppler angle is zero degrees to optimize Doppler waveform. Color velocity scale is set low to optimize color flow. By measuring peak systolic velocity (PSV) *(arrow)* and end-diastolic velocity (EDV) *(arrow)*, ultrasound machine calculates RI (shown in the gray area at bottom left portion of this image). RI = 0.55 × 100 = 55.

investigators to *diagnose* RAS. However, direct measurement of blood flow velocities in the visualized segments of the renal arteries is the most accurate method of determining whether significant RAS is present.

There are two other important advantages of duplex ultrasonography. First, duplex ultrasonography may help identify patients who will have a favorable clinical outcome after surgical or catheter-based renal revascularization.[58] The RI is calculated as follows: [1-(end-diastolic velocity/peak systolic velocity)] × 100 (Fig. 23-5). Using a zero-degree angle of insonation, the peak systolic velocity and EDV are measured within the parenchyma of the kidney. Two studies help support use of the RI. A prospective study followed 138 patients with more than 50% RAS who underwent renal artery angioplasty or surgery for blood pressure control or preservation

of renal function. A renal RI of 80 or greater identified patients in whom angioplasty or surgery was not associated with improved blood pressure, renal function, or kidney survival. Ninety-seven percent of patients with an increased renal RI demonstrated no improvement in blood pressure, and 80% had no improvement in renal function. The authors suggested that the increased RI identifies structural abnormalities in the small vessels of the kidney. Such small-vessel disease is typical of long-standing hypertension associated with nephrosclerosis or glomerulosclerosis.[59] Similar conclusions were drawn from a more recent study that retrospectively evaluated the significance of associating preprocedural RI with postintervention outcomes (endovascular or open surgical repair for RAS treatment). Crutchley et al. found that a preprocedural RI of 0.8 or higher was highly associated with a postprocedural decline in renal function, and that the RI was also highly predictive of all-cause mortality.[60] However, not all investigators believe RI is an accurate predictor of response to renal artery revascularization. A prospective study of renal stent placement in 241 patients demonstrated that individuals with an elevated RI (>80) achieved a favorable blood pressure response and renal functional improvement a year after renal arterial intervention.[61,62] Zeller et al. demonstrated that patients with the most abnormal RI values experienced the greatest magnitude of benefit.[61] Until more information becomes available, an elevated RI should not be considered a contraindication to performing renal artery revascularization.[63]

The second major advantage of duplex ultrasonography is its ability to detect restenosis after percutaneous therapy or surgical bypass[64–66] (Fig. 23-6). Unlike MRA (which may be affected by artifact or scatter produced by the stent), ultrasound transmission through the stent is not a problem. Computed tomographic angiography has not been adequately studied in this respect. Hudspeth et al. compared angiography to duplex ultrasound for follow-up of RAS after angioplasty and demonstrated a sensitivity and specificity of 69% and 98%, respectively, for detecting stenosis greater than 60%.[65] In a more contemporary series, Bakker et al. showed that duplex ultrasonography was an excellent technique to detect restenosis after stent implantation. In 33 consecutive patients using threshold values of 226 cm/s for peak systolic velocity and 2.7 for RAR, sensitivities and specificities were 100% and 90%, and 100% and 84%, respectively.[66] In a series of 134 patients with renal artery stents, velocity-derived criteria were developed. All patients with a PSV of less than 241 cm/s were free of in-stent restenosis, while all patients with a PSV of 300 cm/s or greater had in-stent restenosis as confirmed by CTA or catheter-based angiogram. If the PSV was between 241 and 299 cm/s, a judgment was required assessing the degree of turbulence and appearance on gray scale and color Doppler. Using these criteria, the sensitivity was 91%, specificity was 97%, positive predictive value 91%, negative predictive value 96%, and accuracy 95%.[67] All patients who have undergone percutaneous intervention should be placed in a surveillance program in an attempt to identify restenosis and treat it before the artery occludes. Following PTA and stent

CLINICAL EVALUATION OF RENAL ARTERY DISEASE

CH 23

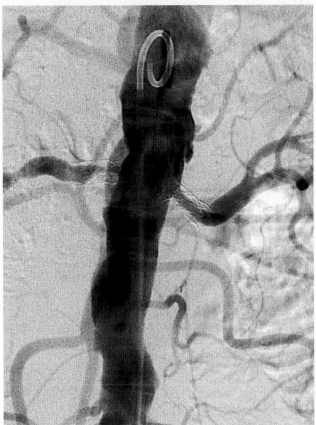

A

B

FIGURE 23-6 **A,** Duplex ultrasound demonstrating severe stenosis on first surveillance ultrasound 6 months after bilateral renal artery stent implantation. There is turbulence on color image. Peak systolic velocity (PSV) in right renal artery is 444 cm/s, and end-diastolic velocity (EDV) is 265 cm/s, with a renal-to-aortic ratio of 7.4. This is consistent with an 80%-99% stenosis. **B,** Digital subtraction angiogram (DSA) of same patient demonstrating severe bilateral in-stent restenosis, right more severe than left.

implantation, a renal artery duplex should be obtained at the first office visit, 6 months, 12 months, and yearly thereafter.[7,68]

There are several limitations of duplex ultrasonography. It is technically demanding, there is a steep learning curve, and it is particularly challenging in the obese individual. The sensitivity of identifying accessory renal arteries is only about 67%.[49] In addition, approximately 5% of renal artery ultrasound studies are of suboptimal quality because of the presence of too much bowel gas. It is highly recommended that these patients return to be studied at a later date after having not eaten in the previous 12 hours.

Magnetic resonance angiography (also see Chapter 13) of the renal arteries can be performed rapidly with excellent image quality, does not involve ionizing radiation, and allows for direct visualization of the aorta and renal arteries. Furthermore, MRA can provide functional assessment of blood flow via absolute blood flow rate and GFR measurements.[69] There is recent evidence that functional renal perfusion can be assessed by MRA.[70,71]

Compared to conventional catheter angiography as the reference standard, three-dimensional (3D) contrast-enhanced gadolinium MRA has a mean sensitivity of 96% and mean specificity of 93%[72-83] (Table 23-4). Magnetic resonance angiography techniques that do not use gadolinium contrast agents have improved significantly and can be comparable to contrast-enhanced MRA in diagnostic quality.[84] These gadolinium-free techniques, such as 3D time-of-flight (TOF) and inversion-recovery steady-state free precession (SSFP), have similar sensitivities (≈92%) and specificities (94%) for detecting RAS[84-88] (Table 23-5 and Fig. 23-7).

Contrast-enhanced 3D MRA has become a commonly used modality for renal artery imaging because of its ability to produce 3D angiographic images with excellent image quality and improved speed of acquisition.[57,70,89,90] Contrast-enhanced 3D MRA exploits the T1-shortening effects of gadolinium-based contrast agents. Blood appears bright, and stationary tissues have a dark appearance. Use of gadolinium shortens image acquisition times, significantly limiting artifact due to patient movement and respiration.[91] Because signal intensity with gadolinium is concentration dependent and not flow based, low-flow related artifacts are reduced, and visualization of small vessels is improved compared to other MRI techniques.[92] Contrast-enhanced MRA is performed using fast 3D gradient echo pulse sequences. These pulse sequences are available primarily at higher magnetic field strengths (1.0 and 1.5 Tesla). Because hundreds of images are acquired, 3D image processing is subsequently performed to project vessels in views of high diagnostic interest.

Kidneys, adrenal glands, and surrounding soft tissues are evaluated by T1- and T2-weighted image acquisition. Time-of-flight (high-velocity jet within stenosis appears black owing to signal loss), phase contrast (gadolinium injection allows phase shift difference detection and rendering of renal arterial blood flow), and maximal intensity projection are the most widely applied MRA

TABLE 23-4	Accuracy of Three-Dimensional Gadolinium Magnetic Resonance Angiography for Renal Artery Stenosis			
AUTHOR	YEAR	PATIENTS	SENSITIVITY	SPECIFICITY
Snidow[80]	1996	47	100	89
Hany[78]	1997	39	93	98
De Cobelli[76]	1997	55	100	97
Rieumont[79]	1997	30	100	71
Bakker[72]	1998	54	97	92
Schoenberg[73]	1999	50	94	100
Hahn[74]	1999	22	91	79
Fain[77]	2001	25	97	92
Hood[126]	2002	21	100	74
Willmann[109]	2003	46	93	100
Patel[127]	2005	68	87	69
Eklof[128]	2005	58	93	91
Bicakci[81]	2006	84	69-100	86-96
Rountas[82]	2007	58	90	94
Stacul[83]	2008	35	83	73-78

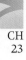

TABLE 23-5   Accuracy of Magnetic Resonance Angiography without Contrast for Renal Artery Stenosis

AUTHOR	YEAR	PATIENTS	TECHNIQUE	SENSITIVITY	SPECIFICITY
Tello[129]	2003	16	T2 dark blood	96	92
Maki[86]	2007	40	Nav SSFP	100	84
Wyttenbach[88]	2007	53	SSFP	100	93
Utsunomiya[87]	2008	26	Time SLIP SSFP	78	91
Korpraphong[85]	2009	114	B-FFE	57-62	92-94

B-FFE, balanced fast-field echo; SLIP, time-spatial labeling inversion; SSFP, steady-state free precession.

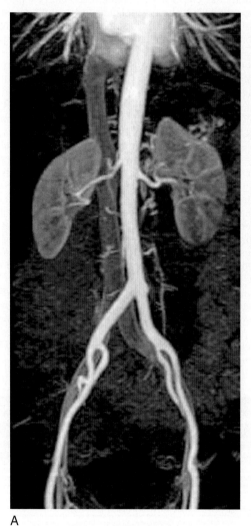

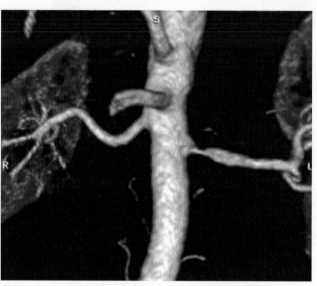

FIGURE 23-7   A, Three-dimensional (3D) gadolinium-enhanced magnetic resonance angiogram (MRA) demonstrating normal renal arteries bilaterally. There is an excellent view of aorta from diaphragm to inguinal ligament. By imaging a large field of view, one can be certain not to miss an accessory renal artery. Kidneys are also well seen with this technology. Inferior vena cava can be seen in background. **B,** Severe atherosclerotic renal artery stenosis (RAS) of left renal artery. Right renal artery was normal.

imaging techniques. After 20 minutes of source image acquisition, additional time is required for reformatting. As with CTA, software allows for both two dimensional (2D) and 3D reconstruction, which increases diagnostic yield. Proper equipment, software, and technical expertise are critical for optimal renal MRA and account for significant variability of study quality between institutions.

Despite recent advances, MRA is still limited by several factors, including high cost and imaging artifacts, such as those attributed to patient movement, and difficulty resolving highly tortuous vessels and the smaller accessory renal arteries. Magnetic resonance angiography acquisition times are longer than those for CTA, and patients must therefore be able to remain motionless for minutes at

a time. Moreover, MRA may not be possible for patients with claustrophobia and those with metal clips, pacemakers, or other metallic devices. For these reasons, MRA is most useful in patients after inconclusive preliminary workup for RAS or in those with a high clinical suspicion for renovascular hypertension or with contraindications to other imaging modalities. Magnetic resonance angiography is also not useful for monitoring patients after renal artery angioplasty and stenting because of artifact produced by the stent. It also has a tendency to overestimate stenosis severity and may miss accessory renal arteries if the field of view is too narrow.

Exposure to gadolinium-based contrast agents in the setting of renal failure has been associated with nephrogenic systemic fibrosis (NSF), an exceedingly rare condition that involves fibrosis of the skin, joints, eyes, and internal organs.[93-95] Current recommendations advise against administering gadolinium contrast to individuals with a GFR below 30 mL/min/1.73m² or those with acute renal failure or acute deterioration of chronic renal failure.[95]

COMPUTED TOMOGRAPHIC ANGIOGRAPHY

Computed tomographic angiography (also see Chapter 14) can be performed rapidly and safely for assessment of renal artery disease. Multidetector-row CTA provides excellent image quality with higher resolution than could be obtained previously with single-detector-row technology. Most clinical imaging centers currently use 64- to 256-multidetector-row scanners, with 320-multidetector-row scanners currently reserved mostly for research applications or for studying the coronary arteries and bypass grafts.[96,97] Advantages of CTA over catheter-based angiography are[98-103]: volumetric acquisition, demonstrating better visualization of the anatomy from multiple angles and in multiple planes after a single acquisition; improved visualization of soft tissues and other adjacent anatomical structures; less invasive and thus fewer complications; and lower cost.

Computed tomographic angiography has several advantages over MRA, such as higher spatial and temporal resolution, absence of flow-related phenomena that may distort MRA images, and capability to visualize calcification and metallic implants such as endovascular stents or stent grafts. Computed tomographic angiography also involves markedly decreased total examination time, with most 64-multidetector scanners currently performing a complete vascular examination of the abdominal aorta, mesenteric, renal, and iliac arteries in 5 to 10 seconds with submillimeter spatial resolution. When exposure to ionizing radiation is a concern (e.g., in younger patients), MRA may be the preferred imaging modality.

The increased speed of acquisitions coupled with subsecond gantry rotations obtained with multidetector-row CTA allows for greater longitudinal coverage for a given scan duration and greater spatial resolution.[104] This may not be of as much importance for assessing renal artery disease, but it has great advantages when assessing the thoracoabdominal, aortoiliac, and lower-extremity inflow and runoff, which may require up to 1400 mm of coverage.[105] Rapid acquisition of images allows for reduction in the amount of iodinated contrast material needed while maintaining excellent and uniform vascular enhancement.[98,101-103,106]

Thin beam collimation (<1 mm), rotational speed of the tube, and rate of table feed are key parameters in determining imaging protocols. The first set of images produced are sequential or overlapping axial images, which should be interpreted with full attention to all nonvascular structures including bones, bowel, visceral organs, and lung. To create angiographic representations, post-processing of the volumetric data is necessary. The best post-processed images are created from overlapping submillimeter reconstructed images (Fig. 23-8). In the absence of overlap, the angiographic images may have a marked stair-step appearance.

Over the past several years, more complex post-processing algorithms have been formulated to display volumetric data, including maximum intensity projection (MIP), shaded surface display (SSD), and volumetric rendering (VR).[106-108] These techniques allow manipulation of raw data so as to optimize visualization of relevant lesions or disease processes. An important common pitfall is selective visualization of the maximally opacified vascular lumen. Both automated and manual creation of post-processed images risk inadvertent rejection of critical vascular and nonvascular information. Post-processed images alone should never be used for interpretation of CT angiography.[105]

The sensitivity of CTA for RAS ranges from 89% to 100% and specificity from 82% to 100%[77,103,105,109-113] (Table 23-6). The area of acquisition should include the area from just proximal to the celiac artery to and including the iliac arteries. This will ensure that accessory renal arteries are detected and associated aortic and visceral artery pathology is not overlooked.

Results obtained using duplex ultrasound, MRA, or CTA are not nearly as good for assessing RAS secondary to FMD; catheter-based angiography remains the imaging modality of choice if FMD is suspected.[6,114]

CATHETER-BASED ANGIOGRAPHY

Although duplex ultrasonography, MRA, and CTA have replaced catheter-based angiography for the diagnosis of RAS in most circumstances, catheter-based angiography remains the gold standard. It is the most accurate test to diagnose RAS secondary to both atherosclerosis and FMD. It can clearly visualize branch vessels and cortical blood flow and is excellent for identifying accessory renal arteries.

Digital subtraction angiography (DSA) has replaced screen-film angiography in the majority of institutions for vascular applications. The resolution of DSA is less than that of screen film but can approach three to four line pairs per millimeter with current equipment (see Fig. 23-1). The standard imaging matrix is now 1024 × 1024, with image intensifiers that range up to 16 inches in diameter. Flat-panel image intensifiers will soon become available. It is important to recognize that the renal arteries often come off

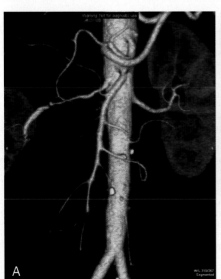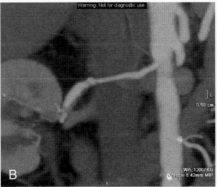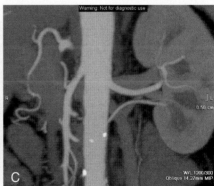

FIGURE 23-8   Three-dimensional (3D) computed tomographic angiogram (CTA) of renal arteries with 250 multidetector CT scanner. Volume rendering **(A)** and maximal intensity projection (MIP) **(B-C)** demonstrating a dissection and severe focal stenosis of right renal artery and a normal left renal artery.

TABLE 23-6		Accuracy of Computed Tomographic Angiography for Assessment of Visceral and Renal Artery Stenosis		
AUTHOR	YEAR	PATIENTS	SENSITIVITY (%)	SPECIFICITY (%)
Kaatee[112]	1997	71	92-100	96-100
Kim[111]	1998	50	90-100	97
Johnson[113]	1999	25	89-94	87-99
Qanadli[110]	2000	47	91	100
Willmann[109]	2003	46	91-92	99
Vasbinder[130]	2004	402	64	92
Eklof[128]	2005	58	94	62
Rountas[82]	2007	58	94	93

of the aorta posteriorly, and therefore oblique views of the aorta may be needed to adequately visualize the origin of the renal arteries. Pressure gradients should also be obtained to confirm the physiological significance of a given lesion.

New developments in hardware and software have led to greater diagnostic accuracy and better safety. Bolus chasing, rapid image acquisition, vessel diameter analysis, regional pixel shifting, image stacking, 3D reconstructions from rotational angiograms, and angioscopic representations of DSA data are now routinely available from manufacturers.[105,115–119]

Carbon dioxide (CO_2) angiography provides an alternative to conventional angiography or DSA using iodinated contrast agents. This may be particularly useful in patients with renal insufficiency in whom contrast exposure may accelerate the decline of renal function. When compared to conventional angiography, CO_2 angiography has a sensitivity of 83% and a specificity of 99%.[120,121]

Advantages of DSA are the high resolution compared to current cross-sectional imaging techniques, ability to selectively evaluate individual vessels, access direct physiological information such as pressure gradients, and utilization as a platform for intervention. Disadvantages are exposure to ionizing radiation, use of iodinated contrast agents (contrast-induced nephropathy), and risks related to vascular access (pseudoaneurysm, hematoma, retroperitoneal bleed) and catheterization (atheromatous embolization). Nevertheless, until an alternative platform is developed for intervention or completely MR-compatible devices become available, DSA will continue to have a central role in the management of patients with vascular disease.

RENAL ANGIOGRAPHY AT THE TIME OF CARDIAC CATHETERIZATION

This controversial subject has led to numerous debates over the most appropriate management strategy for patients with CAD and possible RAS. It has been demonstrated that patients with CAD have a higher prevalence of RAS than the general population. In addition, patients with RAS have a markedly increased mortality from cardiovascular disease. Conlon et al. reported that the 4-year survival for patients with no RAS detected at the time of cardiac catheterization was 90% compared to survival rates of 70% for 50% to 75% stenosis, 68% for 75% to 95% stenosis, and 48% for more than 95% stenosis.[30,122] Proponents of angiography at the time of catheterization state that the procedure can be performed accurately with no added risk and provide the cardiologist with knowledge that the patient has RAS so that the patient can then be followed serially and treated with optimal secondary preventive measures.[31] Those against routine angiography claim that knowing that the patient has RAS adds nothing to the patient's overall management other than to tempt the angiographer to stent the stenotic lesion in the absence of accepted clinical indications.[46,123] This has been termed the *renal oculosten(t)otic reflex*.[124]

It is appropriate to perform renal angiography at the time of cardiac catheterization if acceptable indications for renal artery intervention are present.[125] Further prospective natural history studies in this asymptomatic population are needed, however, to answer the question of whether routine screening should be performed at the time of cardiac catheterization.

REFERENCES

1. Pleis JR, Lucas JW, Ward BW: Summary health statistics for U.S. adults: National Health Interview Survey, 2008, *Vital Health Stat* 10(242):1–157, 2009.
2. Olin JW, Melia M, Young JR, et al: Prevalence of atherosclerotic renal artery stenosis in patients with atherosclerosis elsewhere, *Am J Med* 88(1N):46N–51N, 1990.
3. Harding MB, Smith LR, Himmelstein SI, et al: Renal artery stenosis: prevalence and associated risk factors in patients undergoing routine cardiac catheterization, *J Am Soc Nephrol* 2(11):1608–1616, 1992.
4. Safian RD, Textor SC: Renal-artery stenosis, *N Engl J Med* 344(6):431–442, 2001.
5. Dworkin LD, Cooper CJ: Clinical practice. Renal-artery stenosis, *N Engl J Med* 361(20):1972–1978, 2009.
6. Olin JW, Sealove BA: Diagnosis, management, and future developments of fibromuscular dysplasia, *J Vasc Surg* 53(3):826–836, 2011.
7. Olin JW: Atherosclerotic renal artery disease, *Cardiol Clin* 20(4):547–562, 2002.
8. Connolly JO, Higgins RM, Walters HL, et al: Presentation, clinical features and outcome in different patterns of atherosclerotic renovascular disease, *QJM* 87(7):413–421, 1994.
9. Mailloux LU, Napolitano B, Bellucci AG, et al: Renal vascular disease causing end-stage renal disease, incidence, clinical correlates, and outcomes: a 20-year clinical experience, *Am J Kidney Dis* 24(4):622–629, 1994.
10. Mailloux LU, Bellucci AG, Napolitano B, et al: Survival estimates for 683 patients starting dialysis from 1970 through 1989: identification of risk factors for survival, *Clin Nephrol* 42(2):127–135, 1994.
11. de Mast Q, Beutler JJ: The prevalence of atherosclerotic renal artery stenosis in risk groups: a systematic literature review, *J Hypertens* 27(7):1333–1340, 2009.
12. Hansen KJ, Edwards MS, Craven TE, et al: Prevalence of renovascular disease in the elderly: a population-based study, *J Vasc Surg* 36(3):443–451, 2002.
13. Dustan HP, Humphries AW, DeWolfe VG: Normal arterial pressure in patients with renal arterial stenosis, *JAMA* 187:1028–1029, 1964.
14. Davis BA, Crook JE, Vestas RE, et al: Prevalence of renovascular hypertension in patients with grade III or IV hypertensive retinopathy, *N Engl J Med* 301:1273–1276, 1979.
15. Chobanian AV, Bakris GL, Black HR, et al: The Seventh Report of the Joint National Committee on Prevention, Detection, Evaluation, and Treatment of High Blood Pressure: the JNC 7 Report, *JAMA* 289(19):2560–2571, 2003.
16. Gifford RW Jr, McCormack LJ, Poutasse EF: The atrophic kidney: its role in hypertension, *Mayo Clin Proc* 40(834):852, 1965.
17. Lawrie GM, Morris GC Jr, Glaeser DH, et al: Renovascular reconstruction: factors affecting long-term prognosis in 919 patients followed up to 31 years, *Am J Cardiol* 63(15):1085–1092, 1989.
18. Textor SC, Tarazi RC, Novick AC, et al: Regulation of renal hemodynamics and glomerular filtration in patients with renovascular hypertension during converting enzyme inhibition with captopril, *Am J Med* 76(5B):29–37, 1984.
19. Textor SC, Novick AC, Steinmuller DR, et al: Renal failure limiting antihypertensive therapy as an indication for renal revascularization. A case report, *Arch Intern Med* 143(11):2208–2211, 1983.
20. Silas JH, Klenka Z, Solomon SA, et al: Captopril induced reversible renal failure: a marker of renal artery stenosis affecting a solitary kidney, *BMJ* 286(6379):1702–1703, 1983.
21. Packer M, Lee WH, Medina N, et al: Functional renal insufficiency during long-term therapy with captopril and enalapril in severe chronic heart failure, *Ann Intern Med* 106:346–354, 1987.
22. Textor SC: Renal failure related to ACE inhibitors, *Semin Nephrol* 17:67–76, 1997.
23. Scoble JE, Maher ER, Hamilton G: Atherosclerotic renovascular disease causing renal impairment–a case for treatment, *Clin Nephrol* 31:119–122, 1989.
24. Scoble JE: Renal artery stenosis as a cause of renal impairment: implications for treatment of hypertension and congestive heart failure, *J R Soc Med* 92(10):505–510, 1999.
25. Gray BH, Olin JW, Childs MB, et al: Clinical benefit of renal artery angioplasty with stenting for the control of recurrent and refractory congestive heart failure, *Vasc Med* 7(4):275–279, 2002.
26. Pickering TG, Herman L, Devereux RB, et al: Recurrent pulmonary oedema in hypertension due to bilateral renal artery stenosis: treatment by angioplasty or surgical revascularisation, *Lancet* 2(8610):551–552, 1988.
27. Diamond JR: Flash pulmonary edema and the diagnostic suspicion of occult renal artery stenosis, *Am J Kidney Dis* 21(3):328–330, 1993.
28. Khosla S, Kunjummen B, Manda R, et al: Prevalence of renal artery stenosis requiring revascularization in patients initially referred for coronary angiography, *Catheter Cardiovasc Interv* 58(3):400–403, 2003.
29. Scobel JE: The epidemiology and clinical presentation of atherosclerotic renal artery disease. In Novick AC, Scoble JE, Halmilton G, editors: *Renal vascular disease*, London, 1996, WB Saunders Co, Ltd, pp 303–314.
30. Conlon PJ, Little MA, Pieper K, et al: Severity of renal vascular disease predicts mortality in patients undergoing coronary angiography, *Kidney Int* 60(4):1490–1497, 2001.
31. Rihal CS, Textor SC, Breen JF, et al: Incidental renal artery stenosis among a prospective cohort of hypertensive patients undergoing coronary angiography, *Mayo Clin Proc* 77(4):309–316, 2002.
32. Weber-Mzell D, Kotanko P, Schumacher M, et al: Coronary anatomy predicts presence or absence of renal artery stenosis. A prospective study in patients undergoing cardiac catheterization for suspected coronary artery disease, *Eur Heart J* 23(21):1684–1691, 2002.
33. Louie J, Isaacson JA, Zierler RE, et al: Prevalence of carotid and lower extremity arterial disease in patients with renal artery stenosis, *Am J Hypertens* 7(5):436–439, 1994.

34. Conlon P, O'Riordan E, Kalra P: New insights into the epidemiologic and clinical manifestations of atherosclerotic renovascular disease, *Am J Kidney Dis* 35(4):573–587, 2000.

35. Dorros G, Jaff M, Mathiak L, et al: Four-year follow-up of Palmaz-Schatz stent revascularization as treatment for atherosclerotic renal artery stenosis, *Circulation* 98(7):642–647, 1998.

36. Eipper DF, Gifford RW Jr, Stewart B, et al: Abdominal bruits in renovascular hypertension, *Am J Cardiol* 37:48–52, 1976.

37. Olin JW: Evaluation of the peripheral circulation. In Izzo JL, Sicca DA, Black HR, editors: *Hypertension primer*, ed 4, Dallas, 2007, American Heart Association, pp 374–378.

38. Canzanello VJ, Textor SC: Noninvasive diagnosis of renovascular disease, *Mayo Clin Proc* 69(12):1172–1181, 1994.

39. Emovon OE, Klotman PE, Dunnick NR, et al: Renovascular hypertension in blacks, *Am J Hypertens* 9(1):18–23, 1996.

40. Maxwell MH, Lupu AN, Taplin GV: Radioisotope renogram in renal arterial hypertension, *J Urol* 100(4):376–383, 1968.

41. Ploth DW: Angiotensin-dependent renal mechanisms in two-kidney, one-clip renal vascular hypertension, *Am J Physiol* 245(2):F131–F141, 1983.

42. Nally JV, Barton DP: Contemporary approach to diagnosis and evaluation of renovascular hypertension, *Urol Clin North Am* 28(4):781–791, 2001.

43. Black HR, Bourgoignie JJ, Pickering T, et al: Report of the Working Party Group for Patient Selection and Preparation, *Am J Hypertens* 4(12 Pt 2):745S–746S, 1991.

44. Setaro JF, Chen CC, Hoffer PB, et al: Captopril renography in the diagnosis of renal artery stenosis and the prediction of improvement with revascularization. The Yale Vascular Center experience, *Am J Hypertens* 4(12 Pt 2):698S–705S, 1991.

45. Setaro JF, Saddler MC, Chen CC, et al: Simplified captopril renography in diagnosis and treatment of renal artery stenosis, *Hypertension* 18(3):289–298, 1991.

46. Olin JW, Begelman SM: Renal artery disease. In Topol E, editor: *Textbook of Cardiovascular medicine*, ed 2, Philadelphia, 2002, Lippincott Raven, pp 2139–2159.

47. Fommei E, Ghione S, Hilson AJ, et al: Captopril radionuclide test in renovascular hypertension: a European multicentre study. European Multicentre Study Group, *Eur J Nucl Med* 20(7):617–623, 1993.

48. Carman TL, Olin JW: Diagnosis of renal artery stenosis: what is the optimal diagnostic test? *Curr Interv Cardiol Rep* 2(2):111–118, 2000.

49. Hansen KJ, Tribble RW, Reavis SW, et al: Renal duplex sonography: evaluation of clinical utility, *J Vasc Surg* 12(3):227–236, 1990.

50. Hoffmann U, Edwards JM, Carter S, et al: Role of duplex scanning for the detection of atherosclerotic renal artery disease, *Kidney Int* 39(6):1232–1239, 1991.

51. Kohler TR, Zierler RE, Martin RL, et al: Noninvasive diagnosis of renal artery stenosis by ultrasonic duplex scanning, *J Vasc Surg* 4(5):450–456, 1986.

52. Malatino LS, Polizzi G, Garozzo M, et al: Diagnosis of renovascular disease by extra- and intrarenal Doppler parameters, *Angiology* 49(9):707–721, 1998.

53. Miralles M, Cairols M, Cotillas J, et al: Value of Doppler parameters in the diagnosis of renal artery stenosis, *J Vasc Surg* 23(3):428–435, 1996.

54. Olin JW: Role of duplex ultrasonography in screening for significant renal artery disease, *Urol Clin North Am* 21(2):215–226, 1994.

55. Williams GJ, Macaskill P, Chan SF, et al: Comparative accuracy of renal duplex sonographic parameters in the diagnosis of renal artery stenosis: paired and unpaired analysis, *AJR Am J Roentgenol* 188(3):798–811, 2007.

56. Olin JW, Piedmonte MR, Young JR, et al: The utility of duplex ultrasound scanning of the renal arteries for diagnosing significant renal artery stenosis, *Ann Intern Med* 122(11):833–838, 1995.

57. Carman TL, Olin JW, Czum J: Noninvasive imaging of the renal arteries, *Urol Clin North Am* 28(4):815–826, 2001.

58. Radermacher J, Chavan A, Bleck J, et al: Use of Doppler ultrasonography to predict the outcome of therapy for renal-artery stenosis, *N Engl J Med* 344(6):410–417, 2001.

59. Soulez G, Therasse E, Qanadli SD, et al: Prediction of clinical response after renal angioplasty: respective value of renal Doppler sonography and scintigraphy, *AJR Am J Roentgenol* 181(4):1029–1035, 2003.

60. Crutchley TA, Pearce JD, Craven TE, et al: Clinical utility of the resistive index in atherosclerotic renovascular disease, *J Vasc Surg* 49(1):148–155, 2009 .

61. Zeller T, Muller C, Frank U, et al: Stent angioplasty of severe atherosclerotic ostial renal artery stenosis in patients with diabetes mellitus and nephrosclerosis, *Catheter Cardiovasc Interv* 58(4):510–515, 2003.

62. Zeller T, Frank U, Muller C, et al: Predictors of improved renal function after percutaneous stent-supported angioplasty of severe atherosclerotic ostial renal artery stenosis, *Circulation* 108(18):2244–2249, 2003.

63. Hirsch AT, Haskal ZJ, Hertzer NR, et al: ACC/AHA 2005 guidelines for the management of patients with peripheral arterial disease (lower extremity, renal, mesenteric, and abdominal aortic): executive summary a collaborative report from the American Association for Vascular Surgery/Society for Vascular Surgery, Society for Cardiovascular Angiography and Interventions, Society for Vascular Medicine and Biology, Society of Interventional Radiology, and the ACC/AHA Task Force on Practice Guidelines (Writing Committee to Develop Guidelines for the Management of Patients With Peripheral Arterial Disease) endorsed by the American Association of Cardiovascular and Pulmonary Rehabilitation; National Heart, Lung, and Blood Institute; Society for Vascular Nursing; TransAtlantic Inter-Society Consensus; and Vascular Disease Foundation, *J Am Coll Cardiol* 47(6):1239–1312, 2006.

64. Taylor DC, Moneta GL, Strandness DE Jr: Follow-up of renal artery stenosis by duplex ultrasound, *J Vasc Surg* 9(3):410–415, 1989.

65. Hudspeth DA, Hansen KJ, Reavis SW, et al: Renal duplex sonography after treatment of renovascular disease, *J Vasc Surg* 18(3):381–388, 1993.

66. Bakker J, Beutler JJ, Elgersma OE, et al: Duplex ultrasonography in assessing restenosis of renal artery stents, *Cardiovasc Intervent Radiol* 22:475–480, 1999.

67. Galin I, Trost B, Kang K, et al: Validation of renal duplex ultrasound in detecting renal artery stenosis post stenting, *J Am Coll Cardiol* 51(Suppl I) (10):A317, 2008.

68. White CJ, Olin JW: Diagnosis and management of atherosclerotic renal artery stenosis: improving patient selection and outcomes, *Nat Clin Pract Cardiovasc Med* 6(3):176–190, 2009.

69. Soulez G, Oliva VL, Turpin S, et al: Imaging of renovascular hypertension: respective values of renal scintigraphy, renal Doppler US, and MR angiography, *Radiographics* 20(5):1355–1368, 2000.

70. Schoenberg SO, Knopp MV, Londy F, et al: Morphologic and functional magnetic resonance imaging of renal artery stenosis: a multireader tricenter study, *J Am Soc Nephrol* 13(1):158–169, 2002.

71. Aumann S, Schoenberg SO, Just A, et al: Quantification of renal perfusion using an intravascular contrast agent (part 1): results in a canine model, *Magn Reson Med* 49(2):276–287, 2003.

72. Bakker J, Beek FJ, Beutler JJ, et al: Renal artery stenosis and accessory renal arteries: accuracy of detection and visualization with gadolinium-enhanced breath-hold MR angiography, *Radiology* 207(2):497–504, 1998.

73. Schoenberg SO, Essig M, Bock M, et al: Comprehensive MR evaluation of renovascular disease in five breath holds, *J Magn Reson Imaging* 10(3):347–356, 1999.

74. Hahn U, Miller S, Nagele T, et al: Renal MR angiography at 1.0 T: three-dimensional (3D) phase-contrast techniques versus gadolinium-enhanced 3D fast low-angle shot breath-hold imaging, *AJR Am J Roentgenol* 172(6):1501–1508, 1999.

75. Tan KT, van Beek EJ, Brown PW, et al: Magnetic resonance angiography for the diagnosis of renal artery stenosis: a meta-analysis, *Clin Radiol* 57(7):617–624, 2002.

76. De Cobelli F, Vanzulli A, Sironi S, et al: Renal artery stenosis: evaluation with breath-hold, three-dimensional, dynamic, gadolinium-enhanced versus three-dimensional, phase-contrast MR angiography, *Radiology* 205(3):689–695, 1997.

77. Fain SB, King BF, Breen JF, et al: High-spatial-resolution contrast-enhanced MR angiography of the renal arteries: a prospective comparison with digital subtraction angiography, *Radiology* 218(2):481–490, 2001.

78. Hany TF, Debatin JF, Leung DA, et al: Evaluation of the aortoiliac and renal arteries: comparison of breath-hold, contrast-enhanced, three-dimensional MR angiography with conventional catheter angiography, *Radiology* 204(2):357–362, 1997.

79. Rieumont MJ, Kaufman JA, Geller SC, et al: Evaluation of renal artery stenosis with dynamic gadolinium-enhanced MR angiography, *AJR Am J Roentgenol* 169(1):39–44, 1997.

80. Snidow JJ, Johnson MS, Harris VJ, et al: Three-dimensional gadolinium-enhanced MR angiography for aortoiliac inflow assessment plus renal artery screening in a single breath hold, *Radiology* 198(3):725–732, 1996.

81. Bicakci K, Soker G, Binokay F, et al: Estimation of the ratio of renal artery stenosis with magnetic resonance angiography using parallel imaging technique in suspected renovascular hypertension, *Nephron Clin Pract* 104(4):c169–c175, 2006.

82. Rountas C, Vlychou M, Vassiou K, et al: Imaging modalities for renal artery stenosis in suspected renovascular hypertension: prospective intraindividual comparison of color Doppler US, CT angiography, GD-enhanced MR angiography, and digital subtraction angiography, *Ren Fail* 29(3):295–302, 2007.

83. Stacul F, Gava S, Belgrano M, et al: Renal artery stenosis: comparative evaluation of gadolinium-enhanced MRA and DSA, *Radiol Med* 113(4):529–546, 2008.

84. Glockner JF, Takahashi N, Kawashima A, et al: Non-contrast renal artery MRA using an inflow inversion recovery steady state free precession technique (Inhance): comparison with 3D contrast-enhanced MRA, *J Magn Reson Imaging* 31(6):1411–1418, 2010.

85. Korpraphong P, Tovanabutra P, Muangsomboon K: Renal artery stenosis: diagnostic performance of balanced fast field gradient echo MRA, *J Med Assoc Thai* 92(8):1077–1083, 2009.

86. Maki JH, Wilson GJ, Eubank WB, et al: Navigator-gated MR angiography of the renal arteries: a potential screening tool for renal artery stenosis, *AJR Am J Roentgenol* 188(6):W540–W546, 2007.

87. Utsunomiya D, Miyazaki M, Nomitsu Y, et al: Clinical role of non-contrast magnetic resonance angiography for evaluation of renal artery stenosis, *Circ J* 72(10):1627–1630, 2008.

88. Wyttenbach R, Braghetti A, Wyss M, et al: Renal artery assessment with nonenhanced steady-state free precession versus contrast-enhanced MR angiography, *Radiology* 245(1):186–195, 2007.

89. Prince MR, Chenevert TL, Foo TK, et al: Contrast-enhanced abdominal MR angiography: optimization of imaging delay time by automating the detection of contrast material arrival in the aorta, *Radiology* 203(1):109–114, 1997.

90. Zhang J, Pedrosa I, Rofsky NM: MR techniques for renal imaging, *Radiol Clin North Am* 41(5):877–907, 2003.

91. Saloner D: Determinants of image appearance in contrast-enhanced magnetic resonance angiography: a review, *Invest Radiol* 33:488–495, 1998.

92. Thornton J, O'Callaghan J, Walshe J, et al: Comparison of digital subtraction angiography with gadolinium-enhanced magnetic resonance angiography in the diagnosis of renal artery stenosis, *Eur Radiol* 9(5):930–934, 1999.

93. Kribben A, Witzke O, Hillen U, et al: Nephrogenic systemic fibrosis: pathogenesis, diagnosis, and therapy, *J Am Coll Cardiol* 53(18):1621–1628, 2009.

94. Perazella MA: Advanced kidney disease, gadolinium and nephrogenic systemic fibrosis: the perfect storm, *Curr Opin Nephrol Hypertens* 18(6):519–525, 2009.

95. Prince MR, Zhang HL, Roditi GH, et al: Risk factors for NSF: a literature review, *J Magn Reson Imaging* 30(6):1298–1308, 2009.

96. de Graaf FR, van Velzen JE, Witkowska AJ, et al: Diagnostic performance of 320-slice multidetector computed tomography coronary angiography in patients after coronary artery bypass grafting, *Eur Radiol* 21(11):2285–2296, 2011.

97. van Velzen JE, de Graaf FR, Kroft LJ, et al: Performance and efficacy of 320-row computed tomography coronary angiography in patients presenting with acute chest pain: results from a clinical registry, *Int J Cardiovasc Imaging* 2011. May 26. [Epub ahead of print] DOI 10.1007/s10554-011-9889-z

98. Rubin GD: Three-dimensional helical CT angiography, *Radiographics* 14(4):905–912, 1994.

99. Rubin GD: MDCT imaging of the aorta and peripheral vessels, *Eur J Radiol* 45(Suppl 1):S42–S49, 2003.

100. Rubin GD: 3-D imaging with MDCT, *Eur J Radiol* 45(Suppl 1):S37–S41, 2003.

101. Rubin GD: Techniques for performing multidetector-row computed tomographic angiography, *Tech Vasc Interv Radiol* 4(1):2–14, 2001.

102. Bluemke DA, Chambers TP: Spiral CT angiography: an alternative to conventional angiography, *Radiology* 195(2):317–319, 1995.

103. Liu PS, Platt JF: CT angiography of the renal circulation, *Radiol Clin North Am* 48(2):347–365, 2010.

104. Bluemke DA, Soyer PA, Chan BW, et al: Spiral CT during arterial portography: technique and applications, *Radiographics* 15(3):623–637, 1995.

105. Olin JW, Kaufman JA, Bluemke DA, et al: Atherosclerotic Vascular Disease Conference. American Heart Association, Imaging, Writing Group IV, *Circulation* 109:2626–2633, 2004.

106. Zeman RK, Silverman PM, Vieco PT, et al: CT angiography, *AJR Am J Roentgenol* 165(5):1079–1088, 1995.

107. Ibukuro K, Charnsangavej C, Chasen MH, et al: Helical CT angiography with multiplanar reformation: techniques and clinical applications, *Radiographics* 15(3):671–682, 1995.

108. Addis KA, Hopper KD, Iyriboz TA, et al: CT angiography: *in vitro* comparison of five reconstruction methods, *AJR Am J Roentgenol* 177(5):1171–1176, 2001.

109. Willmann JK, Wildermuth S, Pfammatter T, et al: Aortoiliac and renal arteries: prospective intraindividual comparison of contrast-enhanced three-dimensional MR angiography and multi-detector row CT angiography, *Radiology* 226(3):798–811, 2003.

110. Qanadli SD, Mesurolle B, Coggia M, et al: Abdominal aortic aneurysm: pretherapy assessment with dual-slice helical CT angiography, *AJR Am J Roentgenol* 174(1):181–187, 2000.

111. Kim TS, Chung JW, Park JH, et al: Renal artery evaluation: comparison of spiral CT angiography to intra-arterial DSA, *J Vasc Interv Radiol* 9(4):553–559, 1998.

112. Kaatee R, Beek FJ, de Lange EE, et al: Renal artery stenosis: detection and quantification with spiral CT angiography versus optimized digital subtraction angiography, *Radiology* 205(1):121–127, 1997.

113. Johnson PT, Halpern EJ, Kuszyk BS, et al: Renal artery stenosis: CT angiography–comparison of real-time volume-rendering and maximum intensity projection algorithms, *Radiology* 211(2):337–343, 1999.

114. Slovut DP, Olin JW: Fibromuscular dysplasia, *N Engl J Med* 350(18):1862–1871, 2004.

115. Bosanac Z, Miller RJ, Jain M: Rotational digital subtraction carotid angiography: technique and comparison with static digital subtraction angiography, *Clin Radiol* 53(9):682–687, 1998.

116. Seymour HR, Matson MB, Belli AM, et al: Rotational digital subtraction angiography of the renal arteries: technique and evaluation in the study of native and transplant renal arteries, *Br J Radiol* 74(878):134–141, 2001.

117. Meijering EH, Niessen WJ, Bakker J, et al: Reduction of patient motion artifacts in digital subtraction angiography: evaluation of a fast and fully automatic technique, *Radiology* 219(1):288–293, 2001.

118. Meijering EH, Niesssen WJ, Viergever MA: Retrospective motion correction in digital subtraction angiography: a review, *IEEE Trans Med Imaging* 18(1):2–21, 1999.

119. Ashleigh RJ, Hufton AP, Razzaq R, et al: A comparison of bolus chasing and static digital subtraction arteriography in peripheral vascular disease, *Br J Radiol* 73(872):819–824, 2000.

120. Schreier DZ, Weaver FA, Frankhouse J, et al: A prospective study of carbon dioxide-digital subtraction vs standard contrast arteriography in the evaluation of the renal arteries, *Arch Surg* 131(5):503–507, 1996.

121. Hawkins IF Jr, Wilcox CS, Kerns SR, et al: CO2 digital angiography: a safer contrast agent for renal vascular imaging? *Am J Kidney Dis* 24(4):685–694, 1994.

122. Conlon PJ, Athirakul K, Kovalik E, et al: Survival in renal vascular disease, *J Am Soc Nephrol* 9(2):252–256, 1998.

123. Textor SC: Progressive hypertension in a patient with "incidental" renal artery stenosis, *Hypertension* 40(5):595–600, 2002.

124. White CJ: The renal oculosten(t)otic reflex, *Cathet Cardiovasc Diagn* 37(3):251, 1996.

125. White CJ, Jaff MR, Haskal ZJ, et al: Indications for renal arteriography at the time of coronary arteriography: a science advisory from the American Heart Association Committee on Diagnostic and Interventional Cardiac Catheterization, Council on Clinical Cardiology, and the Councils on Cardiovascular Radiology and Intervention and on Kidney in Cardiovascular Disease, *Circulation* 114(17):1892–1895, 2006.

126. Hood MN, Ho VB, Corse WR: Three-dimensional phase-contrast magnetic resonance angiography: a useful clinical adjunct to gadolinium-enhanced three-dimensional renal magnetic resonance angiography? *Mil Med* 167(4):343–349, 2002.

127. Patel ST, Mills JL Sr, Tynan-Cuisinier G, et al: The limitations of magnetic resonance angiography in the diagnosis of renal artery stenosis: comparative analysis with conventional arteriography, *J Vasc Surg* 41(3):462–468, 2005.

128. Eklof H, Ahlstrom H, Bostrom A, et al: Renal artery stenosis evaluated with 3D-Gd-magnetic resonance angiography using transstenotic pressure gradient as the standard of reference. A multireader study, *Acta Radiol* 46(8):802–809, 2005.

129. Tello R, Mitchell PJ, Witte DJ, et al: T2 dark blood MRA for renal artery stenosis detection: preliminary observations, *Comput Med Imaging Graph* 27(1):11–16, 2003.

130. Vasbinder GB, Nelemans PJ, Kessels AG, et al: Accuracy of computed tomographic angiography and magnetic resonance angiography for diagnosing renal artery stenosis, *Ann Intern Med* 141(9):674–682, 2004.

CHAPTER 24

Medical and Endovascular Treatment of Renal Artery Disease

Robert D. Safian, Ryan D. Madder

The clinical diagnosis of renal artery stenosis (RAS) relies on a high index of suspicion and confirmation by noninvasive and invasive imaging modalities (see Chapter 23). There are interrelated syndromes associated with RAS, including renovascular (renin-dependent) hypertension, essential hypertension, reversible ischemic renal dysfunction, and irreversible ischemic nephropathy. Clinical features that heighten suspicion for RAS include abrupt-onset or accelerated hypertension at any age, unexplained acute or chronic azotemia, azotemia induced by angiotensin-converting enzyme inhibitors (ACEIs), asymmetrical renal dimensions, and sudden pulmonary edema in the setting of normal left ventricular (LV) systolic function. Therapeutic considerations, alone or in combination, include medical therapy, percutaneous revascularization with angioplasty (PTA) or stenting, and surgical revascularization with bypass surgery or endarterectomy (Table 24-1). Revascularization of RAS with the goal of improving renal function and blood pressure remains controversial, so patient selection is extremely important (Fig. 24-1).

General Considerations for Treatment

Atherosclerosis accounts for more than 90% of cases of RAS, whereas the remaining 10% are associated with fibromuscular dysplasia (FMD) or inflammatory diseases of the renal arterial circulation. Whereas FMD is typically a disease of young and middle-aged females and usually involves the distal two thirds of the renal artery and its branches, atherosclerotic RAS (ARAS) is a disease of the elderly, particularly those with diabetes, aortoiliac occlusive disease, coronary artery disease (CAD), and hypertension. Atherosclerotic RAS usually involves the ostium and proximal one third of the renal artery, and it is a common manifestation of progressive atherosclerosis.[1]

Despite the prevalence and progressive nature of ARAS, it is likely many cases are never detected. Most patients with ARAS are identified during evaluation for refractory hypertension or progressive renal failure, or fortuitously as part of angiographic evaluation for aneurysmal or occlusive diseases of the aorta and lower-extremity arterial circulation. In general, decisions about treatment of patients with ARAS are usually based on blood pressure control, preservation of renal excretory function, and modification of risk factors for atherosclerosis.[2]

Identification of Renovascular Syndromes

There are five interrelated renovascular syndromes associated with RAS that can be broadly classified as *anatomical RAS*, *renin-dependent hypertension*, *essential hypertension*, *reversible renal ischemic dysfunction*, and *irreversible ischemic nephropathy*. These syndromes may occur alone or in combination with each other and with other nonvascular renal diseases. Furthermore, although the type of RAS (FMD, ARAS) is influenced by age, gender, and other patient-related risk factors for atherosclerosis, clinical manifestations (regarding effects on the kidney, heart, and brain) may be similar. Renin-dependent hypertension is much more likely to be caused by FMD in young patients, whereas ARAS in elderly patients is more likely to be associated with essential hypertension. Although both FMD and ARAS can be associated with similar manifestations of injury to the kidneys, heart, and brain (Table 24-2), renal revascularization is more likely to cure hypertension in FMD patients, whereas ARAS patients are likely to require lifelong antihypertensive medical therapy, despite

revascularization. The key point is that patients with anatomical RAS without other clinical manifestations may be treated conservatively without revascularization. Prior to revascularization, patients with RAS and other clinical manifestations should undergo assessment of renal perfusion and the extent of parenchymal disease to determine the likelihood of clinical benefit.[2]

Evaluation of Renal Perfusion

As is true in the coronary circulation, there is poor correlation between angiographic RAS severity and hemodynamic significance, even when quantitative angiography is used.[3] As a result, angiography alone is insufficient to establish the presence of renal hypoperfusion, regardless of stenosis severity. Several noninvasive and invasive methods are available to assess the physiological impact of ARAS and identify renal hypoperfusion (Box 24-1; also see Chapter 23). Nuclear scintigraphy and direct glomerular filtration rate (GFR) measurements can assess single- and total-kidney blood flow; diminished renal blood flow ipsilateral to a stenotic renal artery provides reliable evidence of renal hypoperfusion.[4-6] Invasively, renal hypoperfusion can be identified with fractional flow reserve or translesional pressure gradients.[3,7,8]

In patients with FMD, angiography alone is nearly useless for assessment of stenosis severity before or after revascularization, or for assessment of renal perfusion. In FMD patients, translesional pressure gradients are extremely useful for localizing the site of critical stenosis and assessing results after intervention (Fig. 24-2). Intravascular ultrasound (IVUS) can also be used to assess intraluminal and vessel dimensions, which are nearly impossible to assess by angiography alone.

Evaluation of Nephropathy

Assessment of baseline parenchymal disease is essential in selecting patients for renal revascularization (Table 24-3), since the presence of parenchymal disease prior to intervention is the most important predictor of adverse outcome. Even if renal hypoperfusion is present, identification of advanced parenchymal disease suggests that renal dysfunction maybe irreversible regardless of revascularization.[9] The exception is the patient with advanced parenchymal disease, bilateral RAS, and recent dialysis, in whom a small increase in renal blood flow may permit separation from dialysis.[2,10]

Initial clinical evaluation of parenchymal disease includes serum creatinine (Cr), urinalysis for proteinuria, and renal duplex ultrasound to measure renal resistive index (RRI) and kidney dimensions. When evaluating baseline renal function in patients with ARAS, it is important to realize that serum creatinine–based GFR estimates demonstrate good sensitivity but only modest specificity for identifying a measured GFR below $60\,mL/min/1.73\,m^2$ in individuals with ARAS.[11] As a result, additional testing besides serum Cr should be performed to evaluate the presence of underlying nephropathy. Renal resistive index is obtained by averaging values obtained in the upper, middle, and lower intrarenal segmental arteries according to the formula $100 \times [1 - (EDV/PSV)]$, where *EDV* and *PSV* are Doppler-derived end-diastolic and peak-systolic velocities, respectively. Compared to patients with RRI less than 80, those with RRI above 80 are older and have more extensive atherosclerosis and worse baseline renal function, consistent with more parenchymal disease. Additionally, baseline RRI greater than 80 is associated with inadequate blood pressure control, worsening Cr clearance, more frequent progression to dialysis, and higher mortality after

TABLE 24-1 **Therapeutic Options for Patients with Renal Artery Stenosis**

TREATMENT	IMPACT ON HYPERTENSION	IMPACT ON NEPHROPATHY	COMMENTS
Medical therapy	Effective for control of hypertension, but most patients require ≥2 medications; resistant hypertension is common	No confirmed benefit for reversing or stabilizing renal function	Mandatory for risk-factor modification (aspirin, lipid-lowering therapy, smoking cessation)
PTA	Effective for refractory hypertension in patients with FMD; not superior to medical therapy in patients with ARAS	Uncertain role; complex relationship between revascularization vs. complications (distal embolization, contrast nephropathy)	Not useful for ostial ARAS because of suboptimal results
Stents	Not evaluated in patients with FMD; effective for achieving "statistical" improvement in blood pressure; not clearly superior to medical therapy	Same as for PTA; anecdotal experience suggests benefit if patient does not have advanced nephropathy	Treatment of choice in most patients with ARAS if revascularization is needed
Bypass surgery	Not employed for FMD; not clearly useful in patients with ARAS	Anecdotal experience suggests possible benefit in the absence of advanced renal dysfunction	Rarely used; perioperative mortality rate 2%-6%

ARAS, atherosclerotic renal artery stenosis; FMD, fibromuscular dysplasia; PTA, percutaneous transluminal angioplasty.

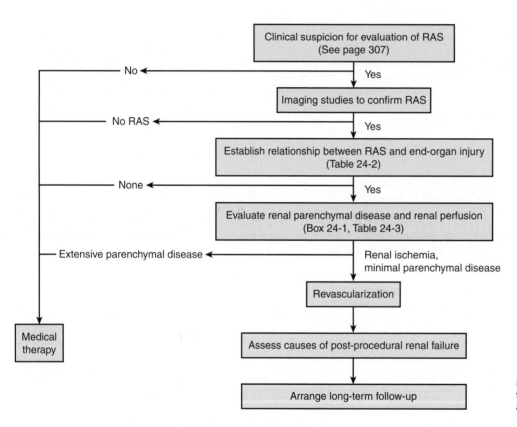

FIGURE 24-1 Management algorithm for patients with atherosclerotic renal artery stenosis *(RAS)*.

TABLE 24-2	**Vital Organ Injury That May Be Caused by Hemodynamically Significant Renal Artery Stenosis**
ORGAN SYSTEM	**INJURY**
Renal	Ischemia/hypoperfusion
Cardiovascular	Hypertensive crisis ACS Unexplained pulmonary edema Aortic dissection
Cerebrovascular	Hypertensive crisis TIA Stroke ICH Severe retinopathy

ACS, acute coronary syndrome; ICH, intracerebral hemorrhage; TIA, transient ischemic attack.

Box 24-1 Clinical Evaluation of Renal Artery Stenosis and Renal Hypoperfusion

Noninvasive Assessment of Renal Blood Flow
^{125}I-iothalamate GFR (total GFR)
^{99M}Tc-DTPA (split renal function and single-kidney GFR)

Invasive Assessment of Significance of Renal Artery Stenosis
Percent diameter stenosis by visual estimates or quantitative angiography
Translesional pressure gradient
Fractional flow reserve
IVUS
Renal frame counts
Renal blush score

GFR, glomerular filtration rate; ^{125}I-iothalamate, iodine 125—labeled iothalamate; IVUS, intravascular ultrasound; ^{99M}Tc-DTPA, technetium-labeled diethylene-triamine-pentacetate.
Adapted from Safian RD, Madder RD: Refining the approach to renal artery revascularization. JACC Cardiovasc Interv 2:161—174, 2009.[2]

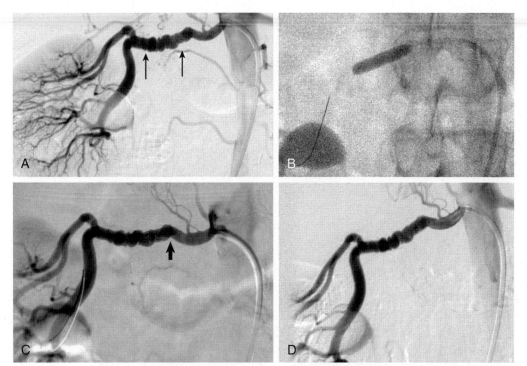

FIGURE 24-2   A 71-year-old female with refractory hypertension was found to have right renal artery stenosis (RAS) by noninvasive imaging. Selective renal angiography demonstrated fibromuscular dysplasia (FMD) of the right renal artery, but stenosis severity was difficult to assess **(A)**. Intravascular ultrasound (IVUS) revealed complex intraluminal webs (not shown), and the translesional pressure gradient across the diseased segment *(black arrows)* was 15 mmHg at rest and 20 mmHg after administration of intrarenal dopamine. Angioplasty of the right renal artery **(B)** did not result in a significant change in appearance by angiography **(C)** or (IVUS). After initial balloon angioplasty, the hyperemic translesional pressure gradient remained 20 mmHg. A guidewire pullback revealed a pressure gradient limited to a focal segment of FMD at the leading edge *(black arrowhead)*. Repeat angioplasty in the proximal right renal artery did not alter the appearance of the artery by angiography **(D)**, but resulted in complete resolution of the translesional pressure gradient.

TABLE 24-3	Clinical Evaluation of Renal Parenchymal Disease
FACTOR	**COMMENT**
Serum Cr	Easy to measure and inexpensive. Relatively insensitive to degree of renal dysfunction and not reliable for differentiating nephropathy from renal ischemia.
Proteinuria	Easy to measure and inexpensive. Proteinuria ≥1 g/24 h is a good indication of nephropathy, but lesser degrees of proteinuria are less reliable.
Renal dimensions	Renal length 10-12 cm is generally favorable. Renal length ≤6 cm indicates irreversible renal injury (atrophic kidney).
RRI	RRI <70 is a good measure of reversibility. Although RRI >80 indicates parenchymal disease, it should not be used as the sole indicator of irreversible renal dysfunction.
Renal arteriogram	Preservation of cortical blood flow and absence of intrarenal arteriolar disease are indicators of reversible renal dysfunction. Poor cortical blood flow and severe diffuse intrarenal arteriolar disease are markers of advanced nephropathy.
Renal biopsy	Reliable for histological confirmation of nephropathy, but not practical for most patients.

Cr, creatinine; RRI, renal resistive index.
Adapted from Safian RD, Madder RD: Refining the approach to renal artery revascularization. JACC Cardiovasc Interv 2:161–174, 2009.[2]

renal revascularization.[9] Several factors (renal dimensions, serum creatinine, presence of collaterals, and intact glomeruli by renal biopsy) have been proposed to suggest reversible renal failure, but the predictive value of these factors has not been validated, and renal biopsy is rarely employed for this purpose. Factors that identify irreversible dysfunction include severe diffuse intrarenal arteriopathy, proteinuria greater than 1 g/24 h (especially in a diabetic patient), and marked atrophy of the renal cortex.[2]

The nephrogram is often overlooked during selective renal arteriography, since many operators tend to focus on the renal artery itself. However, there are several arteriographic features that can indicate the presence of nephropathy, including intrarenal arteriolar narrowing, pruning (cut-off) of interlobar arterioles, and diminished cortical blood flow (Fig. 24-3). It is important to understand that it is best to use *all* the variables discussed to obtain a "nephropathy profile" because individual variables alone are not sufficiently reliable to assess the degree of nephropathy.[2]

In the process of evaluating patients, the goal is to differentiate the impact of ARAS on reversible kidney dysfunction from other causes of irreversible parenchymal disease, such as diabetic and hypertensive nephropathy. If renal hypoperfusion is absent, renal dysfunction is not attributable to ARAS and is more likely due to intrinsic nephropathy. Also, a patient with unilateral ARAS and serum Cr over 2 mg/dL is likely to have significant parenchymal disease, and revascularization of such patients may not improve renal function, especially in the absence of renal hypoperfusion.

Medical Therapy for Renal Artery Disease

The risk of cardiovascular events in hypertensive adults is most dependent on the degree of hypertension rather than its cause. True renovascular hypertension (i.e., renin-dependent hypertension) is much more likely in young patients with FMD than in elderly patients with ARAS. In fact, most hypertensive patients with ARAS have essential hypertension, whereas those with accelerated or malignant hypertension may have a renovascular component superimposed on a background of essential hypertension.[2]

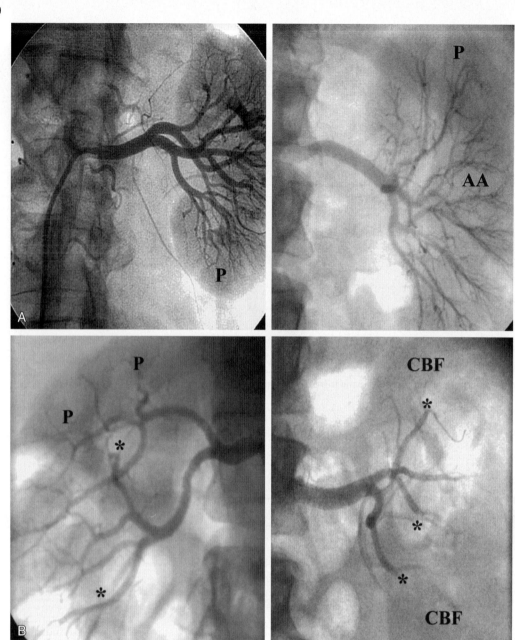

FIGURE24-3 Arteriographic patterns of progressive hypertensive nephropathy. A, Normal renal arteriogram and nephrogram *(left)*, showing excellent cortical blood flow extending into renal pyramids. In mild hypertensive nephropathy *(right)*, cortical blood flow into renal pyramids is preserved, but there is diffuse intrarenal arteriolar narrowing *(AA)*. **B,** This is a more advanced stage of hypertensive nephropathy *(left)* characterized by diminished cortical blood flow, some circulation to renal pyramids *(P)*, and pruning *(*)* of several lobar arteries. In end-stage hypertensive nephropathy *(right)*, cortical blood flow is absent *(CBF)*, and there is generalized pruning *(*)* of most lobar vessels.

Patients with FMD rarely have excretory dysfunction, and hypertension generally responds to ACEIs. In contrast, there are a number of issues concerning medical management of patients with ARAS. First, although never specifically studied in patients with ARAS, it is reasonable to treat all patients with aggressive risk-factor modification to limit atherosclerosis. These measures include aspirin, lipid-lowering therapy, smoking cessation, and aggressive treatment of diabetes mellitus to limit diabetic nephropathy.[12] Second, medical therapy for hypertensive patients with ARAS is similar to that for patients with essential hypertension. Even after renal artery revascularization, antihypertensive medical therapy is necessary in most ARAS patients, since revascularization cures hypertension (i.e., normal blood pressure off all medications) in less than 10% of patients.[13,14] Third, patients with ischemic renal dysfunction represent a particularly high-risk group with a poor prognosis, and there are no studies demonstrating benefit of medical therapy for reversing or stabilizing renal function. The impact of medical therapy on long-term renal function in ARAS is controversial. One study reported a rise in serum Cr concentration in 5% to 10% of patients,[15] whereas another showed a progressive rise in Cr despite excellent blood pressure control.[16]

Use of an ACEI or angiotensin receptor blocker (ARB) is controversial in hypertensive patients with ARAS. Important considerations relate to extent of RAS and degree of baseline renal impairment. Patients with hypertension, unilateral ARAS, and normal baseline renal function are good candidates for an ACEI or ARB. In fact, ACEIs appear to be more effective than other antihypertensive agents in this setting. In patients with hypertension, unilateral RAS, and abnormal baseline renal function, ACEIs exert a beneficial impact on survival without affecting renal function. In these patients, long-term renal function is influenced most by the degree of baseline renal dysfunction and proteinuria, not by pharmacological treatment. In diabetic patients with hypertension, unilateral renal artery stenosis, proteinuria, and normal or abnormal renal function, ACEIs and ARBs are effective antihypertensive agents, and drug-induced reduction of intraglomerular capillary pressure decreases proteinuria and renal injury.[17] It is interesting to speculate whether renal revascularization in this subgroup of patients could offset the benefit of ACEIs by increasing intraglomerular capillary pressure, proteinuria, and renal injury.

In contrast to patients with unilateral ARAS, patients with bilateral RAS (or stenosis in a single solitary kidney) may be especially sensitive to declines in intraglomerular pressure leading to progressive renal failure. Such changes in intraglomerular pressure may occur in association with ACEIs or ARBs (due to vasodilation of the efferent arterioles), reduction in intravascular volume (due to diuretics, dehydration, bleeding), or a decline in cardiac output due to congestive heart failure (CHF). In studies of thousands of patients with hypertension or CHF (many of whom may have had occult RAS), discontinuation of ACEI therapy owing to renal dysfunction was reported in only 0.5% of patients, although mild to moderate increases in serum Cr were reported in 0.1% to 10%. In contrast, discontinuation of ACEI therapy owing to renal dysfunction was necessary in 5% to 20% of patients with bilateral ARAS or stenosis of a solitary kidney.

Taken together, available data suggest that most patients with unilateral and bilateral ARAS and hypertension will benefit from an ACEI or ARB. For patients with bilateral ARAS (or stenosis of a solitary kidney), renal function and serum potassium levels should be monitored closely during initiation of therapy to identify those who may be intolerant.

Selecting Patients for Renal Artery Endovascular Revascularization

The major challenge in selecting patients for renal revascularization is the absence of compelling data supporting doing so. A review of worldwide studies of ARAS identified approximately 5000 studies of renal revascularization,[18] including only two randomized controlled trials (RCTs) of PTA (not stenting) versus medical therapy.[19,20] A subsequent review nearly led to withdrawal of Center for Medicare and Medicaid Services (CMS) reimbursement for renal stenting.[21] Those two RCTs, two subsequent RCTs,[22,23] and another comparative trial[24] reported no benefit of renal revascularization (PTA or stenting) compared to best medical therapy with respect to hypertension control and estimated GFR during 1- to 2-year follow-up. In contrast, numerous observational studies reported stabilization or improvement in renal function[4,25–27] and hypertension control[8,28,29] after renal stenting. There are several potential explanations for the negative results of RCTs and discrepant findings among studies, including treatment of patients with anatomical stenosis but normal renal perfusion (i.e., oculostenotic reflex), failure to differentiate reversible ischemic renal dysfunction from irreversible parenchymal disease (i.e., nephropathy), and unrealistic expectations that ARAS patients have renin-dependent (i.e., renovascular hypertension) rather than essential hypertension.[2] In addition, many RCTs have significant methodological flaws that limit their ability to measure changes in renal function,[11] raising doubts about the validity of their results and conclusions (Table 24-4). Finally, the medical literature is filled with ambiguous and inconsistent terminology regarding renovascular syndromes.[2]

The 2005 American College of Cardiology/American Heart Association (ACC/AHA) guidelines propose recommendations for renal artery revascularization,[12] even though the recommendations have not been established by any randomized clinical trials. In general, ACC/AHA revascularization guidelines are based on the assumption that the RAS is hemodynamically significant, and that revascularization will improve blood pressure control, preserve renal function, or have a favorable impact on cardiovascular manifestations of severe hypertension. Accordingly, patient selection can be enhanced by identification of clear clinical syndromes that link RAS to reversible injury to the heart, brain, or kidneys; by demonstration that RAS causes renal hypoperfusion; and by assessment of baseline renal parenchymal disease.

TABLE 24-4	Limitations of Randomized Controlled Trials of Renal Stenting		
LIMITATION	STAR	ASTRAL	CORAL
N	140	806	1080
Exclude beneficiaries	—	Yes*	Yes†
Assess perfusion	No	No	No
Assess parenchymal disease	No	No	No
Urine protein (mg/day)	140	550	500
RAS <70%	33%	40%	NA
Baseline Cr (mg/dL)	1.7	2.0	<3.0
Major renal endpoint	EGFR ↓ > 20%	1/Cr	2 × Cr

*Patients who were thought to benefit from renal revascularization were excluded.
†Patients with refractory hypertension and/or cardiovascular injury were excluded.
Cr, creatinine; EGFR, estimated glomerular filtration rate; NA = not available; RAS, renal artery stenosis.
From Bax L, Woittiez AJ, Kouwenberg HJ, et al: Stent placement in patients with atherosclerotic renal artery stenosis and impaired renal function: a randomized trial. Ann Intern Med 150:840–848, 2009; the ASTRAL Investigators: Revascularization versus medical therapy for renal artery stenosis. N Engl J Med 361:1953–1962, 2009; and Cooper CJ, Murphy TP, Matsumoto A, et al: Stent revascularization for the prevention of cardiovascular and renal events among patients with renal artery stenosis and systolic hypertension: rationale and design of the CORAL trial. Am Heart J 152:59–66, 2006.[36]

The best candidates for revascularization are patients with RAS, vital organ injury, renal hypoperfusion, and no underlying nephropathy. Conversely, the worst patients for revascularization are those with RAS, advanced nephropathy, and normal renal perfusion.[2] Vital organ injury includes functional impairment of the heart, brain, or kidneys attributable to renal artery stenosis; such manifestations include hypertensive crisis (nonischemic pulmonary edema, acute coronary syndrome (ACS), aortic dissection, or neurological impairment) and renal insufficiency (rising Cr due to ACEIs, bilateral ARAS and rising Cr or declining nuclear GFR, and unilateral ARAS and fractional GFR ≤40%).

Patients with Renal Artery Stenosis and Refractory Hypertension

In patients with ARAS, refractory hypertension, and normal renal perfusion, it is reasonable to intensify the antihypertensive regimen, seek alternative etiologies for refractory hypertension, and follow patients clinically for development of vital organ injury. For patients with unilateral or bilateral ARAS, refractory hypertension, and objective evidence of renal hypoperfusion, revascularization is reasonable if advanced baseline nephropathy is not present (Fig. 24-4). For patients with hypertension and renal FMD, PTA should be performed if patients do not respond to ACEIs or ARBs.[2] Additionally, such patients should undergo carotid duplex ultrasound and intracranial magnetic resonance angiography (MRA) or computed tomographic angiography (CTA), because carotid FMD and berry aneurysms of the circle of Willis are common.

Patients with Isolated Atherosclerotic Renal Artery Stenosis

In patients with unilateral or bilateral ARAS and no evidence of baseline nephropathy or cardiovascular injury, renal perfusion should be evaluated by noninvasive or invasive techniques. If renal perfusion is normal, revascularization is not indicated regardless of stenosis severity; such patients should be followed for development of vital organ injury. If renal hypoperfusion is documented, such patients may be considered to have "unilateral" renal injury. This form of renal injury is not mentioned in existing guidelines and has not been studied in randomized controlled trials, but we generally consider such patients candidates for renal revascularization to preserve renal function.[2,4]

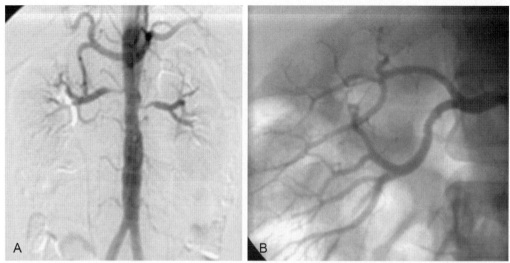

FIGURE 24-4   A 70-year-old man with persistent hypertension despite four antihypertensive medications was diagnosed with bilateral renal artery stenosis (RAS) (A). Serum creatinine (Cr) was 1.7 mg/dL, and estimated glomerular filtration rate (GFR) was 39 mL/min/1.73 m^2. Renal scan demonstrated symmetrical renal blood flow (49% to right kidney, 51% to left kidney), and measured GFR was 30 mL/min/1.73 m^2. Urine collection revealed 500 mg protein in 24 hours, and renal resistive index (RRI) was 82 bilaterally. Renal dimensions were 9.5 cm on the right and 10.0 cm on the left. Selective renal angiography showed extensive intrarenal arteriolar disease, including pruning of distal vessels, ill-defined renal pyramids, and poor cortical blood flow (B). Medical therapy was adjusted because of advanced parenchymal disease without renal intervention, and blood pressure normalized.

Patients with Atherosclerotic Renal Artery Stenosis and Chronic Kidney Disease

Decisions regarding revascularization of patients with ARAS and renal dysfunction are often challenging.[2] In general, patients without renal hypoperfusion should not be revascularized. For patients with unilateral ARAS, renal hypoperfusion, and underlying nephropathy, decisions regarding revascularization should be individualized; revascularization may not improve renal function but might be beneficial if other cardiovascular injury is present. Patients with renal dysfunction and bilateral ARAS or ARAS of a solitary kidney may have global renal ischemia; such patients should be considered for renal revascularization unless advanced parenchymal disease is identified (Fig. 24-5). In nondiabetic patients who have been on dialysis for less than 1 year, it is reasonable to perform diagnostic testing for bilateral ARAS, since some may benefit from renal revascularization and separate from dialysis.[2,10]

Type of Revascularization

Percutaneous revascularization is now widely accepted as the best technique for renal revascularization in most patients. For patients with refractory hypertension and FMD, PTA is preferred and results in renal artery patency rates of 90% at 10 years.[30] Although PTA achieves excellent results in patients with FMD, stenting is the endovascular procedure of choice in patients with ARAS. Stenting in ARAS can be accomplished with procedural success rates exceeding 95%, major complications in less than 5%, and restenosis in 10% to 15%.

Impact of Endovascular Revascularization on Hypertension

The impact of revascularization on hypertension depends on the type of RAS, presence of renal hypoperfusion, and degree of renal parenchymal disease.[2] Although numerous observational studies and two small randomized trials of PTA and medical therapy for ARAS demonstrated a significant decrease in blood pressure and fewer medications after PTA,[9,20] a more recent randomized trial in hypertensive patients with ARAS showed no difference in outcomes between PTA and medical therapy.[24] Published studies on the impact of renal revascularization on hypertension have numerous limitations including inclusion of patients with heterogeneous causes of hypertension, varying degrees of renal dysfunction, inconsistent techniques for revascularization, and ambiguous terminology and endpoints to assess clinical benefit. For example, hypertension has been classified as "cured" (i.e., blood pressure is normal without the need for medication),

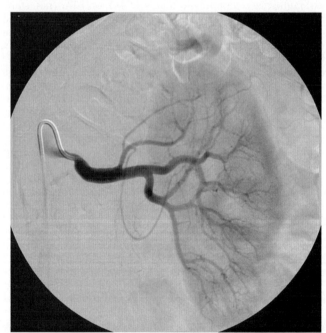

FIGURE 24-5   A 69-year-old man with persistent hypertension despite two antihypertensive medications was diagnosed with unilateral renal artery stenosis (RAS) by noninvasive imaging. Serum creatinine (Cr) was 1.1 mg/dL and estimated glomerular filtration rate (GFR) was 63.4 mL/min/1.73 m^2. Renal scan demonstrated abnormal renal perfusion (65% to right kidney, 35% to left kidney), and measured GFR was 80 mL/min/1.73 m^2. There was no proteinuria, renal dimensions were 12.2 cm on the right and 11.0 cm on the left, and renal resistive index (RRI) was 62 bilaterally. Selective left renal arteriography confirmed severe left RAS and a normal intrarenal arteriolar pattern. Left renal artery stenting was performed because of hypoperfusion of left kidney and absence of parenchymal disease. Two years later, measured GFR was 86 mL/min/1.73 m^2 (53% to right kidney, 47% to left kidney), consistent with sustained improvement in renal blood flow.

improved (number or dose of medications is reduced, blood pressure is better controlled, or both), or unchanged. Interpretation of data is limited by the uncertain clinical relevance of these classification groups. Furthermore, there are several potential reasons why renal artery revascularization for ARAS may not result in dramatic improvement or cure of hypertension. First, many patients with ARAS probably have essential, not renovascular hypertension. Experimental Goldblatt models demonstrate renin-angiotensin activation due to RAS, but hypertension in humans is more complex than indicated by these models.[31] Hypertension in ARAS may be confounded by the presence of sympathetic and cerebral nervous system activation, vasoactive oxygen species, abnormalities in endothelial-dependent relaxation, and ischemic and hypertensive intrarenal injury.[32] A more complex milieu than suggested by Goldblatt models is suggested by similar degrees of renin activation in hypertensive patients with and without ARAS and by the low cure rates demonstrated after successful revascularization. Second, many patients with hypertension have intrarenal parenchymal disease, leading to hypertensive nephropathy and self-perpetuating hypertension. In these patients, hypertension is sustained by intrarenal mechanisms including increased sympathetic nerve activity, renin-angiotensin system activity, and impaired sodium excretion regardless of patency of the proximal renal artery.

Despite these limitations, it is apparent that hypertension is more likely to be cured after revascularization in patients with FMD than in those with ARAS (75% vs. < 20%), regardless of the type of revascularization.[20,30] With respect to differences in unilateral and bilateral ARAS, one study suggested that improvement in hypertension after renal stenting was more likely in the presence of severe bilateral ARAS and severe baseline hypertension (mean arterial pressure >110 mmHg),[33] especially when parenchymal disease is absent.[9,34] A contemporary study reports substantial improvement in blood pressure when renal hypoperfusion was sought and corrected by renal stenting.[8]

Impact of Revascularization on Renal Function

Observational studies suggest that renal artery revascularization can stabilize or improve renal function (Fig. 24-6). Surgical revascularization results in significant improvement in postoperative total- and single-kidney nuclear GFR, a slower decline in GFR, and improvements in renal dimensions and hyperconcentration of urinary creatine. Improvement in renal function after stenting occurred in 8% to 22% of patients in a systematic review,[18] and 20 of 22 cohort studies reported improvement or stabilization of renal function.

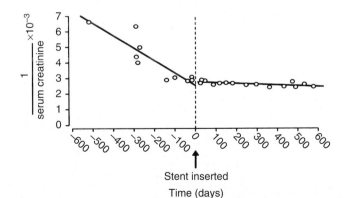

FIGURE 24-6 Relationship of reciprocal serum creatinine (Cr) concentration over time in patient with ischemic nephropathy treated by stenting. In the 600 days prior to revascularization, renal function deteriorated progressively. After stenting, the slope of the reciprocal Cr relationship is zero, suggesting stabilization of renal function. (*Reproduced with permission from Harden PN, MacLeod MJ, Rodger RS, et al: Effect of renal artery stenting on progression of renovascular renal failure. Lancet 349:1133, 1997.*)[26]

In contrast to these observational data, five prospective randomized trials of renal revascularization failed to demonstrate improvement in renal outcomes after intervention.[19,20,22-24] Interpretation of these studies is confounded by failure to assess renal perfusion and the extent of baseline nephropathy prior to revascularization. Additionally, these studies relied on reciprocal serum Cr or creatinine-based GFR estimates as major renal endpoints, which have been shown to be unreliable for serial assessment of renal function in ARAS patients.[11] Taken collectively, these studies suggest that patient selection for revascularization of ARAS that is based on the oculostenotic reflex, and without assessment of renal ischemia and parenchymal disease, is likely not beneficial.

Impact of Revascularization on Cardiovascular Outcome

Understanding the impact of renal revascularization on long-term outcome is hampered by selection bias and poorly designed randomized controlled trials. The survival of medically treated patients with renovascular disease has not been defined, but most late deaths are due to cardiovascular events rather than progressive renal failure. After revascularization, predictors of 5- and 10-year mortalities include age older than 60 years, CAD, baseline renal insufficiency, and persistent elevation of postoperative creatinine. Baseline Cr above 1.5 mg/dL is the strongest independent predictor of late mortality at 4 years (relative risk [RR] 5.0); is a stronger correlate of late mortality than diabetes (RR 2.5) or age older than 70 years (RR 1.9); and is associated with a greater risk of deterioration in renal function.[35] Together, these data suggest that elderly patients with advanced generalized atherosclerosis, manifested by occlusive diseases in multiple vascular beds and baseline renal insufficiency, have a worse prognosis than patients with limited atherosclerosis and normal renal function. These data also suggest that the outcomes of renal revascularization are better when revascularization is performed before the development of advanced parenchymal disease.

To address the impact of renal artery revascularization on overall cardiovascular outcomes, best medical therapy alone is being compared to medical therapy plus stenting in the CORAL trial (Cardiovascular Outcomes with Renal Atherosclerotic Lesions). Enrollment of approximately 1100 randomized patients is expected by 2012, and the primary endpoint is a composite of death, myocardial infarction (MI), stroke, hospitalization for congestive heart failure, need for renal replacement, and doubling of serum Cr at 5 years.[36]

Conclusions

Patients with true renin-dependent (renovascular) hypertension are typically young or middle-aged females with FMD. Initial therapy for renovascular hypertension associated with FMD is an ACEI; refractory hypertension responds readily to PTA without stenting. In contrast, ARAS is highly prevalent among elderly patients with other manifestations of atherosclerosis, and frequently results from in-growth of atherosclerotic plaque from the abdominal aorta, compromising the ostium of the renal artery. In elderly patients with generalized atherosclerosis and ARAS, hypertension is usually not renin-dependent (i.e., essential hypertension). Because renal revascularization rarely cures hypertension, these patients should be treated aggressively with antihypertensive medical therapy. Patients with ARAS, hypertension, and functional impairment of the heart, brain, or kidneys should be considered for renal revascularization. Patients with renal hypoperfusion should be treated before the development of advanced renal failure and ischemic nephropathy. The best candidates for revascularization are those with baseline serum Cr less than 2.0 mg/dL, bilateral ARAS, normal renal resistive indices, no proteinuria, and one or more manifestations of cardiac, cerebral, or renal functional impairment. In these patients, renal revascularization is best accomplished by stenting.

REFERENCES

1. Safian RD, Textor SC: Renal-artery stenosis, *N Engl J Med* 344:431, 2001.
2. Safian RD, Madder RD: Refining the approach to renal artery revascularization, *JACC Cardiovasc Interv* 2:161–174, 2009.
3. Subramanian R, White CJ, Rosenfield K, et al: Renal fractional flow reserve: a hemodynamic evaluation of moderate renal artery stenoses, *Catheter Cardiovasc Interv* 64:480–486, 2005.
4. Hanzel G, Balon H, Wong O, et al: Prospective evaluation of aggressive medical therapy for atherosclerotic renal artery stenosis, with renal artery stenting reserved for previously injured heart, brain, or kidney, *Am J Cardiol* 96:1322–1327, 2005.
5. Leertouwer TC, Derkx FH, Pattynama PM, et al: Functional effects of renal artery stent placement on treated and contralateral kidneys, *Kidney Int* 62:574–579, 2002.
6. La Batide-Alanore A, Azizi M, Froissart M, et al: Split renal function outcome after renal angioplasty in patients with unilateral renal artery stenosis, *J Am Soc Nephrol* 12:1235–1241, 2001.
7. Tonino PAL, De Bruyne B, Pijls NHJ, et al: Fractional flow reserve versus angiography for guiding percutaneous coronary intervention, *N Engl J Med* 360:213–224, 2009.
8. Mangiacappra F, Trana C, Sarno G, et al: Translesional pressure gradients to predict the blood pressure response after renal artery stenting in patients with renovascular hypertension, *Circ Cardiovasc Interv* 3:537–542, 2010.
9. Radermacher J, Chavan A, Bleck J, et al: Use of Doppler ultrasonography to predict the outcome of therapy for renal-artery stenosis, *N Engl J Med* 344:410–417, 2001.
10. Textor SC, Wilcox CS: Renal artery stenosis: a common treatable cause of renal failure, *Annu Rev Med* 52:421–442, 2001.
11. Madder RD, Hickman L, Crimmins GM, et al: Validity of estimated glomerular filtration rates for assessment of baseline and serial renal function in patients with atherosclerotic renal artery stenosis: implications for clinical trials of renal revascularization, *Circ Cardiovasc Interv* 4:219–225, 2011.
12. Hirsch AT, Haskal ZJ, Hertzer NR, et al: ACC/AHA 2005 Practice guidelines for the management of patients with peripheral arterial disease, *Circulation* 113:463–654, 2006.
13. Cooper CJ, Murphy TP: Is renal artery stenting the correct treatment of renal artery stenosis? the case for renal artery stenting for treatment of renal artery stenosis, *Circulation* 115:263–270, 2007.
14. Dworkin LD, Jamerson KA: Case against angioplasty and stenting of atherosclerotic renal artery stenosis, *Circulation* 115:271–276, 2007.
15. Caps MT, Zierler RE, Polissar NL, et al: Risk of atrophy in kidneys with atherosclerotic renal artery stenosis, *Kidney Int* 53:735, 1998.
16. Toto RD, Mitchell HC, Lee HC, et al: Reversible renal insufficiency due to angiotensin converting enzyme inhibitors in hypertensive nephrosclerosis, *Ann Intern Med* 115:513, 1991.
17. Remuzzi G, Bertani T: Pathophysiology of progressive nephropathies, *N Engl J Med* 339:1448, 1998.
18. Balk E, Raman G, Chung M, et al: Effectiveness of management strategies for renal artery stenosis: a systematic review, *Ann Intern Med* 145:901–912, 2006.
19. Webster J, Marshall F, Abdalla M, et al: Randomised comparison of percutaneous angioplasty vs. continued medical therapy for hypertensive patients with atheromatous renal artery stenosis, *J Hum Hypertens* 12:329–335, 1998.
20. Plouin PF, Chatellier G, Darne B, et al: Blood pressure outcome of angioplasty in atherosclerotic renal artery stenosis: a randomized trial, *Hypertension* 31:823–829, 1998.
21. Balk EM, Raman G: Comparative effectiveness of management strategies for renal artery stenosis: 2007 update, comparative effectiveness review no. 5 update. (Prepared by Tufts New England Medical Center under Contract No. 290-02-0022) Rockville, MD, 2007, Agency for Healthcare Research and Quality.
22. Bax L, Woittiez AJ, Kouwenberg HJ, et al: Stent placement in patients with atherosclerotic renal artery stenosis and impaired renal function: a randomized trial, *Ann Intern Med* 150:840–848, 2009.
23. The ASTRAL Investigators: Revascularization versus medical therapy for renal-artery stenosis, *N Engl J Med* 361:1953–1962, 2009.
24. Van Jaarsveld BC, Krijnen P, Pieterman H, et al: The effect of balloon angioplasty on hypertension in atherosclerotic renal-artery stenosis, *N Engl J Med* 342:1007–1014, 2000.
25. Muray S, Martín M, Amoedo ML, et al: Rapid decline in renal function reflects reversibility and predicts the outcome after angioplasty in renal artery stenosis, *Am J Kidney Dis* 39:60–66, 2002.
26. Harden PN, MacLeod MJ, Rodger RS, et al: Effect of renal-artery stenting on progression of renovascular renal failure, *Lancet* 349:1133–1136, 1997.
27. Watson PS, Hadjipetrou P, Cox SV, et al: Effect of renal artery stenting on renal function and size in patients with atherosclerotic renovascular disease, *Circulation* 102:1671–1677, 2000.
28. De Bruyne B, Manharan G, Pijls NHJ, et al: Assessment of renal artery stenosis severity by pressure gradient measurements, *J Am Coll Cardiol* 48:1851–1855, 2006.
29. Mahmud E, Smith TWR, Palakodeti V, et al: Renal frame count and renal blush grade: quantitative measures that predict the success of renal stenting in hypertensive patients with renal artery stenosis, *J Am Coll Cardiol Interv* 1:286–292, 2008.
30. Slovut DP, Olin JW: Fibromuscular dysplasia, *N Engl J Med* 350:1862–1871, 2004.
31. Krum H, Sobotka P, Mahfoud F, et al: Device-based antihypertensive therapy: therapeutic modulation of the autonomic nervous system, *Circulation* 123:209–215, 2011.
32. Higashi Y, Sasaki S, Nakagawa K, et al: Endothelial function and oxidative stress in renovascular hypertension, *N Engl J Med* 346:1954–1962, 2002.
33. Rocha-Singh KJ, Mishkel GJ, Katholi RE, et al: Clinical predictors of improved long-term blood pressure control after successful stenting of hypertensive patients with obstructive renal artery atherosclerosis, *Catheter Cardiovasc Interv* 47:167, 1999.
34. Zeller T, Ulrich F, Muller C, et al: Predictors of improved renal function after percutaneous stent-supported angioplasty of severe atherosclerotic ostial renal artery stenosis, *Circulation* 108:2244–2249, 2003.
35. Dorros G, Jaff M, Mathiak L, et al: Four-year follow-up of Palmaz-Schatz stent revascularization as treatment for atherosclerotic renal artery stenosis, *Circulation* 98:642, 1998.
36. Cooper CJ, Murphy TP, Matsumoto A, et al: Stent revascularization for the prevention of cardiovascular and renal events among patients with renal artery stenosis and systolic hypertension: rationale and design of the CORAL trial, *Am Heart J* 152:59–66, 2006.

CH
24

CHAPTER 25

Surgical Management of Atherosclerotic Renal Artery Disease

Billy G. Chacko, William B. Newton III, Kimberley J. Hansen

The introduction of new, more potent antihypertensive agents and percutaneous endovascular techniques has influenced surgical intervention for atherosclerotic renal artery disease (ARAS).[1] Many physicians currently limit surgical intervention to severe hypertension despite maximal medical therapy, or disease patterns not amenable to percutaneous transluminal renal artery angioplasty (PTRA), or renovascular disease associated with excretory renal insufficiency (i.e., ischemic nephropathy). As a result, the patient population selected for operative management is often characterized by bilateral ostial renal artery stenosis (RAS) or occlusion (85%) superimposed on diffuse extrarenal atherosclerotic disease (91%) in combination with renal insufficiency (60%).[1-3]

Although there are several operative methods that can correct ARAS, no single technique is clearly superior. Optimal methods of operative renal reconstruction vary with the patient, pattern of renal artery disease, and clinical significance of associated aortic lesions.

Prevalence, Evaluation, and Diagnosis

Prevalence

As discussed in Chapter 23, it has long been recognized that anatomical renal artery disease may be clinically silent. Conversely, the disease may account for 3% of hypertension within the general population. Of patients presenting for chronic renal replacement therapy, 10% to 20% have renal artery disease.[4-6] Although its prevalence in patients with mild hypertension is low, renovascular disease is frequently present in patients with severe hypertension. Dietch et al. found that 50% of patients aged 60 years or older with diastolic blood pressure 104 mmHg or higher demonstrated significant RAS or occlusion.[5] When these characteristics were associated with serum creatinine (SCr) greater than 2.0 mg/dL, the prevalence of renal artery disease increased to 70%. Half of these latter patients demonstrated bilateral renal artery disease.

These data suggest that the probability of finding clinically significant renal artery disease varies directly with the patient's age, severity of hypertension, and severity of renal insufficiency. With this in mind, we recommend evaluation for renovascular disease in all persons with severe hypertension, especially when severe hypertension is found in combination with excretory renal insufficiency.

Evaluation

Through continued improvements in software and probe design, renal duplex ultrasonography is an accurate and reliable method to identify hemodynamically significant renal atherosclerotic disease.[7,8] The examination poses no risk to residual excretory renal function, and overall accuracy is not affected by concomitant aortoiliac disease. In addition, preparation is minimal (an overnight fast), and there is no need to alter antihypertensive medications.

When evaluating for renovascular renal insufficiency, a negative renal duplex ultrasound examination effectively excludes ischemic nephropathy because the primary consideration is global renal ischemia based on main renal artery disease affecting both kidneys. When screening for renovascular hypertension, however, a negative duplex ultrasound examination does not reliably exclude surgical disease due to stenotic accessory arteries or branch renal artery disease.[7] Despite enhanced recognition of multiple arteries

by color Doppler flow, only 40% of these accessory renal vessels are currently identified by renal duplex ultrasound examination.

Aortography and renal angiography may be indicated after a positive duplex ultrasound study in selected patients. Patients with severe hypertension and negative or nondiagnostic duplex ultrasound examinations, especially children and young adults, should also undergo angiography. Diagnostic digital subtraction angiography (DSA) can be performed with minimal risk in an outpatient setting. In planning open operative therapy, imaging includes lateral aortography to evaluate the mesenteric vessels. Concurrent mesenteric artery disease was identified in 50% of patients with significant RAS in an angiographic case series of U.S. veterans.[9] In an elderly population-based cohort, the authors identified a significant and independent association of mesenteric artery stenosis with renal artery stenosis.[10] Concurrent mesenteric artery disease has bearing on the use of splanchnorenal reconstruction.

Diagnosis

When a unilateral renal artery lesion is confirmed in an adult patient with severe hypertension, its functional significance should be defined. Unfortunately, measurement of renal vein renin does not have great value when severe bilateral disease or disease to a solitary kidney is present. Therefore, the decision for empirical intervention is based on severity of the renal artery lesions, severity of hypertension, and degree of associated renal insufficiency. In the latter instance, issues determining recovery of excretory renal function in patients with ischemic nephropathy remain ill-defined. Our center's experience with over 240 patients with severe hypertension (mean, 201/104 mmHg) and a preoperative SCr of 1.8 mg/dL or greater has demonstrated a significant association between improved renal function after operative intervention and the site of renal artery disease, extent of renovascular repair, and rate of decline in preoperative renal function.[1,2,11-15] Complete renal artery repair after a rapid decline in excretory renal function is associated with the best opportunity for recovery of renal function.[11,12,14] Most importantly, improved renal function after operation is the primary determinant of dialysis-free survival among patients with preoperative ischemic nephropathy.[14]

Surgical repair of unilateral renal artery disease may be appropriate as a combined aortic procedure in the absence of functional studies (e.g., renal vein renin assay) when hypertension is severe, the patient does not have significant risk factors for operation, and the probability of technical success is certain (>99%). In these circumstances, correction of a renal artery lesion may be justified to eliminate all possible causes of hypertension and renal dysfunction. Because the probability of blood pressure benefit is lower in such a patient, morbidity from the procedure must also be predictably low.[3,16]

When a patient has bilateral RAS and hypertension, the surgical decision to intervene is based on severity of the renovascular lesions and degree of hypertension.[2,16] If the pattern of renal artery disease consists of severe stenosis on one side and only mild or moderate disease on the contralateral side, the patient is treated as though only a unilateral lesion exists. If both renal arteries have only moderately severe disease (65%-80% diameter-reducing stenosis), renal revascularization is undertaken only if hypertension is severe.

315

In contrast, if both renal artery lesions are severe (>80% stenosis) and the patient has resistant hypertension despite medical therapy, bilateral simultaneous renal revascularization is performed.

Furthermore, at least mild excretory renal insufficiency is often present. Because renal insufficiency usually parallels the severity of hypertension, a patient who presents with severe renal insufficiency but only mild to moderate hypertension usually has renal parenchymal disease. Characteristically, renovascular hypertension associated with severe renal insufficiency or dialysis dependence is associated with very severe bilateral stenoses or total renal artery occlusions.[2,14] When considering repair of renal artery disease, one should evaluate the clinical status with respect to this characteristic presentation.

Management Options

Management of renal artery disease discovered incidentally during evaluation of cardiac, aortoiliac, or infrainguinal disease is controversial. In this setting, the decision must address the need for additional diagnostic tests and the decision whether or not to perform combined intervention. Advocates for combined intervention frequently cite "natural history" data (Table 25-1) that suggest atherosclerotic lesions of the renal artery frequently progress and progression is associated with irretrievable decline in kidney size and function. Recent experience, however, disputes this view. In an 8-year follow-up study of Cardiovascular Health Study participants,[27] no individual with hemodynamically significant RAS at baseline demonstrated progression on follow-up. Renal artery stenosis at baseline was not associated with a decline in kidney size or function. In the absence of renovascular hypertension or insufficiency (i.e., ischemic nephropathy), these prospective data suggest that incidental renovascular disease should not be submitted to intervention by any method. This conclusion is supported by the retrospective experience reported by Williamson et al.[28]

No prospective randomized clinical trial compares medical management, percutaneous renal angioplasty with stent, and surgical reconstruction in patients with atherosclerotic renovascular disease (also see Chapter 24). In patients with functionally significant renal artery lesions and severe hypertension, contemporary results of operative management argue for a selective approach toward renal artery intervention.[1,2] Whether by open surgical repair or catheter-based methods, indications for intervention are the same. These include all patients with severe or difficult-to-control hypertension, especially when associated with renal insufficiency.

Patient age, type of lesion, medical comorbidity, and concomitant aortic disease must be considered in selecting patients for open surgical or endovascular management. In the complete absence of hypertension, renal artery intervention is not recommended by any method.

Operative Management
GENERAL ISSUES

The presence of severe hypertension is considered a prerequisite for renal artery intervention. In general, functional studies are used to guide management of unilateral lesions. Empirical renal artery repair is performed without functional studies when hypertension is severe and renal artery disease is bilateral or the patient has ischemic nephropathy.[1,12,14] Accordingly, prophylactic renal artery repair in the absence of hypertension, whether as an isolated operative or catheter-based procedure or combined with aortic reconstruction, is not recommended. With the exception of disease requiring bilateral *ex vivo* reconstructions that are staged, all hemodynamically significant renal artery disease is corrected in a single operation. Having observed beneficial blood pressure and renal function response regardless of kidney size or histological pattern on renal biopsy, nephrectomy is reserved for unreconstructible renal artery disease to a nonfunctioning kidney (i.e., <10% function by renography).[3,7,12,14] Direct aortorenal reconstructions are preferred over indirect methods because concomitant disease of the celiac axis is present in 40% to 50% of patients, and bilateral renal artery repair is required in 50%.[3,9] Failed surgical repair is associated with a significant and independent increased risk of eventual dialysis dependence.[3] To minimize these failures, intraoperative duplex ultrasound is used to evaluate the technical results of surgical repair.[29]

PREOPERATIVE PREPARATION

Antihypertensive medications are reduced during the preoperative period to the minimum necessary for blood pressure control. Patients requiring large doses of multiple medications will often have reduced requirements while hospitalized on bed rest. If continued therapy is required, vasodilators and selective β-adrenergic blocking agents are the drugs of choice. If an adult's diastolic blood pressure exceeds 120 mmHg, operative treatment is postponed until the pressure is brought under control. In this instance, intravenous (IV) therapy is administered in an intensive care setting.

TABLE 25-1   Natural History Studies of Atherosclerotic Renal Artery Stenosis

REFERENCE	YEAR	NO. OF PATIENTS	NO. OF RENAL ARTERIES	MEAN FOLLOW-UP (MONTHS)	ANATOMICAL PROGRESSION (% OF PATIENTS)	PROGRESSION TO OCCLUSION (% OF ARTERIES)	ANATOMICAL EVALUATION
Wollenweber[17]	1968	109	252	42	59	—	Angiography
Meaney[18]	1968	39	78	34	36	4	Angiography
Dean[19]	1981	41	—	44	17	12	Angiography
Schreiber[20]	1984	85	126	52	44	11	Angiography
Tollefson[21]	1991	48	—	54	53*	9*	Angiography
Zierler[22]	1996	76	132	32	20	7	Duplex ultrasound
Webster[23]	1998	30	—	—	13†	0†	Angiography
Crowley[24]	1998	1178	—	30	11	0.3	Angiography
Caps[25]	1998	170	295	33	31	3	Duplex ultrasound
van Jaarsveld[26]	2000	50	100	12	20	5	Angiography

*Percent of renal arteries with baseline stenosis or stenosis in follow-up.
†Of eight patients with serial angiography.
From Edwards MS, Hansen KJ: Combined aortorenal reconstruction. In Green RM, editor: Complex aortic surgery, New York, 2008, Informa Healthcare.

OPERATIVE TECHNIQUES

A variety of operative techniques have been used to treat renal artery atherosclerosis. From a practical standpoint, the three basic operations that have been most frequently used are *aortorenal bypass*, *renal artery thromboendarterectomy*, and *renal artery reimplantation*. Although each method may have its proponents, no single approach provides optimal repair for all types of renal artery disease. Aortorenal bypass, preferably with saphenous vein, is probably the most versatile technique. However, thromboendarterectomy is especially useful for ostial atherosclerosis involving multiple renal arteries. When the artery is sufficiently redundant, reimplantation is probably the simplest technique and one particularly appropriate for combined repairs of aortic and renal pathology.

Certain measures are used in almost all renal artery operations. Mannitol is administered IV in 12.5-g doses early, and repeated before and after periods of renal ischemia, up to a total dose of 1 g/kg patient body weight. Just prior to renal artery occlusion, a bolus of 100 units of heparin per kilogram body weight is given intravenously, and systemic anticoagulation is verified by activated clotting time. Unless required for hemostasis, protamine is not routinely administered for reversal of heparin at completion of the operation.

Aortorenal Bypass

The most common method of revascularization is aortorenal bypass (Fig. 25-1). Three types of material are available for conduit: autologous saphenous vein, autologous hypogastric artery, and prosthetic grafts. The choice of conduit depends on a number of factors. In adults, we preferentially use the saphenous vein. However, if the vein is small (<4 mm in diameter) or sclerotic, the hypogastric artery or a synthetic prosthetic graft may be preferable. A 6-mm, thin-walled polytetrafluoroethylene (PTFE) graft is satisfactory when the distal renal artery is of large caliber (≥4 mm) and provides long-term patency equivalent to that of saphenous vein.

Thromboendarterectomy

In cases of bilateral atherosclerosis of the renal artery origins, simultaneous bilateral endarterectomy may be the most appropriate procedure. Although endarterectomy may be performed in a transrenal fashion, the transaortic technique is used in the majority of instances. The transaortic method is particularly applicable in patients with multiple renal arteries that demonstrate orificial disease. Transaortic endarterectomy is performed through a longitudinal aortotomy, with sleeve endarterectomy of the aorta and eversion endarterectomies of the renal arteries (Fig. 25-2). When combined aortic replacement is planned, the transaortic endarterectomy is performed through the transected aorta (Fig. 25-3). When using the transaortic technique, it is important to mobilize the renal arteries extensively to allow eversion of the vessel into the aorta. This allows the distal endpoint to be completed under direct vision.

Renal Artery Reimplantation

After the renal artery has been dissected from the surrounding retroperitoneal tissue, the vessel may be somewhat redundant. When the RAS is orificial and there is sufficient vessel length, the renal artery can be transected and reimplanted into the aorta at a slightly lower level. The renal artery must be spatulated and a portion of the aortic wall removed, as in renal artery bypass.

Splanchnorenal Bypass

Splanchnorenal bypass and other indirect procedures are also used as alternative methods for renal revascularization.[30] In general, the authors do not believe these procedures demonstrate long-term patency equivalent to direct aortorenal reconstructions, but they are useful in a selected subgroup of high-risk patients. Subcostal incisions are used to perform splanchnorenal bypass.[30] The right and left renal arteries are exposed through medial visceral rotation. A great saphenous vein (GSV) graft is typically used to construct the bypass. Occasionally the gastroduodenal artery on the

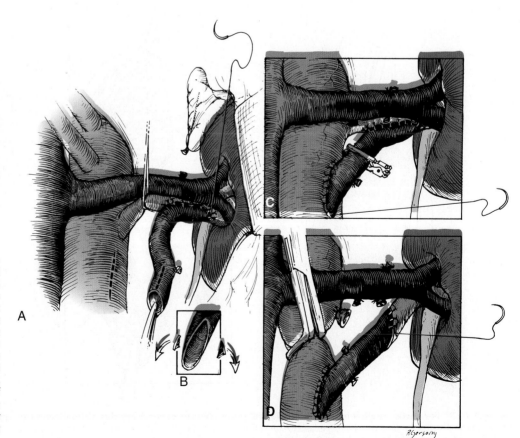

FIGURE 25-1 Technique for end-to-side (A-C) and end-to-end (D) aortorenal bypass grafting. Length of arteriotomy is at least three times diameter of artery to prevent recurrent anastomotic stenosis. For the anastomosis, 6-0 or 7-0 monofilament polypropylene sutures are used in continuous fashion under loupe magnification. If apex sutures are placed too deeply or with excess advancement, stenosis can be created, posing risk of late graft thrombosis. *(From Benjamin ME, Dean RH: Techniques in renal artery reconstruction: part I. Ann Vasc Surg 10:306–314, 1996.)*

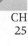

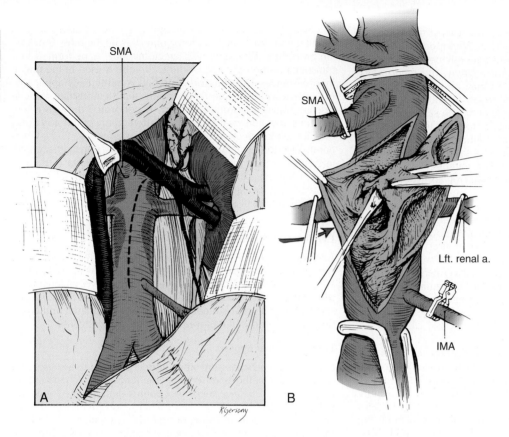

SMA

SMA

Lft. renal a.

IMA

R.Gersony

FIGURE 25-2 Exposure for longitudinal transaortic endarterectomy is through standard transperitoneal approach. Duodenum is mobilized from the aorta laterally in standard fashion or, for more complete exposure, ascending colon and small bowel are mobilized. **A,** Dotted line shows location of aortotomy. **B,** Plaque is transected proximally and distally, and with eversion of renal arteries, atherosclerotic plaque is removed from each renal ostium. Aortotomy is typically closed with a running 4-0 or 5-0 polypropylene suture. IMA, inferior mesenteric artery; SMA, superior mesenteric artery. *(From Benjamin ME, Dean RH: Techniques in renal artery reconstruction: part I. Ann Vasc Surg 10:306–314, 1996.)*

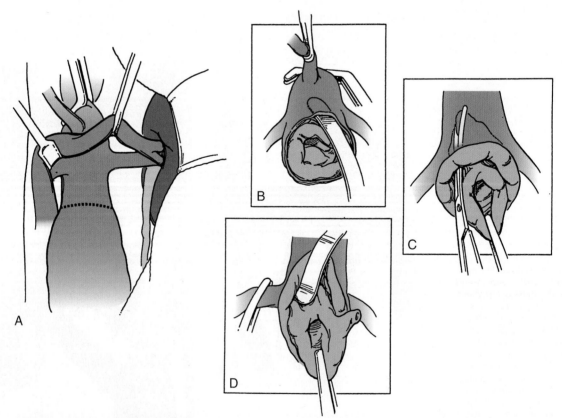

FIGURE 25-3   For aortic repair combined with bilateral ostial stenosis of renal arteries, thromboendarterectomy is most commonly performed through the divided aorta. *(With permission from Edwards MS, Cherr GS, Hansen KJ: Treatment of renovascular disease: surgical therapy. In Hallet JW, Mills JL, Earnshaw J, Reekers JA, editors: Comprehensive vascular and endovascular surgery, Edinburgh, 2004, Mosby.)*

right and splenic artery on the left can be transected and anastomosed directly to the renal artery.

Ex Vivo Reconstruction

Operative strategy for renal artery branch vessel repair is determined by the required exposure and anticipated period of renal ischemia. When reconstruction can be accomplished with less than 30 minutes of ischemia, an *in situ* repair is undertaken without special measures for renal preservation (Fig. 25-4). When longer periods of ischemia are anticipated, one of two techniques for hypothermic preservation of the kidney are considered. These techniques include renal mobilization without renal vein transection and *ex vivo* repair and anatomical replacement in the renal fossa. *Ex vivo* management is necessary when extensive exposure will be required for extended periods. For atherosclerotic renovascular disease, *ex vivo* techniques are most commonly required for branch renal artery repair after failed or complicated PTRA.

INTRAOPERATIVE DUPLEX ULTRASONOGRAPHY

Provided the best method of reconstruction is chosen for renal artery repair, the short course and high blood flow rates characteristic of renal reconstruction favor long-term patency. Consequently, flawless technical repair plays a dominant role in determining postoperative success. Intraoperative duplex ultrasonography provides a rapid, safe method of verifying technically flawless repair.[29] Because the ultrasound probe can be placed immediately adjacent to the vascular repair, high carrying frequencies may be used that provide excellent B-scan detail sensitive to less than 1-mm anatomical defects. Once imaged, defects can be viewed in multiple projections during conditions of uninterrupted pulsatile blood flow. Intimal flaps not apparent during static conditions are easily imaged while avoiding the adverse effects of additional renal ischemia. In addition to excellent anatomical detail, important hemodynamic information is obtained from spectral analysis of the Doppler-shifted signal proximal and distal to the imaged defect.[29] Our technique of intraoperative

assessment with routine participation of a vascular technologist has yielded a scan time of 7 to 10 minutes and a 98% study completion rate.[31]

We have studied more than 800 renal artery repairs with anatomical follow-up evaluation and reported on a subgroup of 249 repairs.[32] Intraoperative assessment was normal in 157, whereas 84 repairs (35%) demonstrated one or more defects by ultrasound imaging. Twenty-five of these defects (10%) had focal increases in peak systolic velocity (PSV) of 2.0 ms or greater with turbulent distal waveform and were defined as major. Each major defect prompted immediate operative revision, and in each case a significant defect was discovered. Ultrasound defects defined as minor were not repaired. At 12-month follow-up, renal artery patency free of critical stenosis was demonstrated in 97% of normal studies, 100% of minor defects, and 88% of revised major defects, providing an overall patency of 97%. Among the five failures with normal ultrasound studies, three occurred after *ex vivo* branch renal artery repair.

Results of Surgical Management

Marone et al. reported on operative management for ischemic nephropathy due to ARAS.[33] Ninety-six patients underwent 104 renal artery revascularizations between 1990 and 2001. Perioperative mortality was 4.1%. Perioperative morbidity occurred in 5% of patients. After open surgical repair, 42% of their patients demonstrated improved early renal function (defined as ≥20% decrease in SCr), 17% experienced a 20% or more increase in SCr, and the remaining 41% exhibited no significant change. Improved renal function was durable among surgical survivors at a mean follow-up of 46 months, whereas 28% developed worsened function, and 39% remained unchanged. These authors noted that early renal function response was an accurate predictor of long-term survival.

The results of Marone et al. are similar to those from the authors' center. From January 1987 through December 1999, 626 patients

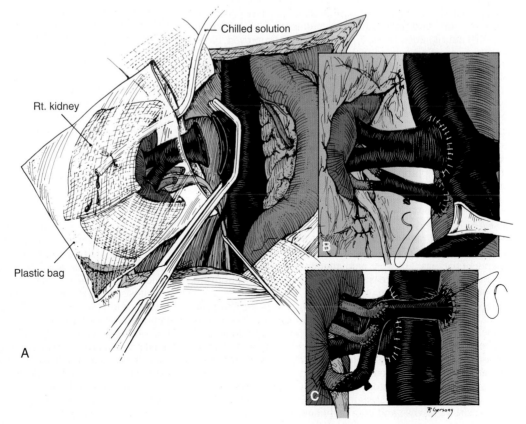

FIGURE 25-4 **A,** An ellipse of vena cava containing renal vein origin is excised by placement of a large, partially occluding clamp. After *ex vivo* branch repair, renal vein can then be reattached without risk of anastomotic stricture. **B,** Kidney is repositioned in its native bed after *ex vivo* repair. Gerota fascia is reattached to provide stability to replaced kidney. Arterial reconstruction can be accomplished via end-to-end anastomoses (as here) or occasionally with a combination of end-to-end and end-to-side anastomoses **(C)**. *(From Benjamin ME, Dean RH: Techniques in renal artery reconstruction: part II. Ann Vasc Surg 10:409–414, 1996.)*

had operative renal artery repair at our center.[2] Overall, 254 women and 246 men (mean age, 65 ± 9 years) underwent repair for atherosclerotic renovascular disease. Their mean blood pressure was 200 ± 35/104 ± 21 mmHg, with a mean duration of hypertension of 10 years. Preoperative mean and median SCr was 2.6 mg/dL and 1.7 mg/dL, respectively, with a mean estimated glomerular filtration rate (EGFR) of 40.5 ± 23.2 mL/min/m[2]. As a group, patients with atherosclerosis had widespread extrarenal disease, with 70% demonstrating at least one manifestation of cardiac disease, and 32% a history of cerebrovascular disease. Overall, 90% of patients exhibited some clinical manifestation of extrarenal atherosclerosis. Evidenced by SCr 1.8 mg/dL or greater, 49% were considered to have ischemic nephropathy, including 40 patients who were dialysis dependent.

Among 720 renal artery reconstructions, aortorenal bypass was performed in 384 instances, with 204 vein grafts, 159 PTFE grafts, and 21 Dacron prosthetic grafts. Splanchnorenal bypass was performed in 13 instances. Renal artery reimplantation was performed in 56 instances, whereas renal artery thromboendarterectomy was performed in 267 instances. Revascularization was combined with aortic or mesenteric reconstruction in 41% of patients. Of the 776 kidneys that were operated on, 56 required nephrectomy.

Perioperative mortality, defined as in-hospital death or death within 30 days of surgery, occurred in 23 patients (4.6%). This figure was comparable to reports from other centers with a large experience in renovascular disease.[34] All but one death occurred following bilateral renal artery reconstruction or renal reconstruction combined with simultaneous aortic or mesenteric artery repair. Mortality following isolated renal artery repair (0.8%) differed significantly from mortality following combined or bilateral repair (6.9%). Perioperative mortality was significantly and independently associated with advanced age and congestive heart failure (CHF).

Blood pressure measurements and medication requirements at least 1 month after operative intervention were used to define blood pressure response.[3] Among all surgical survivors, 85% were cured or improved, and 15% were considered failed. When compared with blood pressure improved or failed, blood pressure cure was significantly and independently associated with an improved dialysis-free survival. Although improved blood pressure was associated with significant postoperative decreases in mean blood pressure and medication requirements (205/107 mmHg vs. 147/81 mmHg, and 2.8 vs. 1.7 medications), improved blood pressure was not associated with increased dialysis-free survival. Product-limit estimates of dialysis-free survival according to postoperative blood pressure response are depicted in Figure 25-5.

Considering all surgical survivors, renal function increased significantly after operation (preoperative vs. postoperative mean EGFR, 41.1 ± 23.9 mL/min/m[2] vs. 48.2 ± 25.5 mL/min/m[2] [P <0.0001]). For individual patients, a significant change in excretory renal function was defined as a change in EGFR of 20% or more obtained at least 3 weeks after repair. Some 58% of patients with ischemic nephropathy (preoperative SCr ≥1.8 mg/dL) were improved, including 28 patients who were removed permanently from dialysis; 35% remained unchanged; and 7% had worsened renal function.[2,14,31] When patients were selected for surgery based on severe hypertension and rapidly deteriorating renal function, the proportion of patients who improved increased with increasing severity of preoperative renal dysfunction. Among dialysis-dependent patients, 70% were permanently removed from dialysis. This association with increased preoperative SCr and improved postoperative renal function was significant (P <0.0001).

Success after renal artery intervention is measured by survival free of dialysis dependence. Freedom from death or dialysis was significantly and independently associated with cured compared with improved or unchanged hypertension. Freedom from dialysis was also significantly and independently associated with improved compared with unchanged or worsened postoperative renal function. Preoperative factors significantly and independently associated with death or dialysis included diabetes mellitus, severe aortic occlusive disease, and poor preoperative renal function.

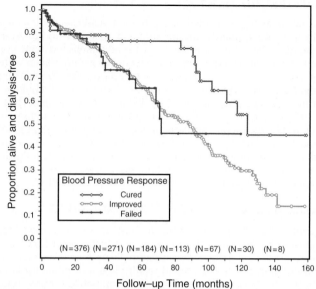

FIGURE 25-5 Product-limit estimates of time to death or dialysis according to blood pressure response to operation. *(From Cherr GS, Hansen KJ, Craven TE, et al: Surgical management of atherosclerotic renovascular disease. J Vasc Surg 35:236–245, 2002.)*

The relationship between each category of renal function response and dialysis-free survival demonstrated significant interactions with preoperative renal function. An increased risk of death or dialysis was observed for all patients if there was no improvement in postoperative renal function (Fig. 25-6A).[2] For patients with unchanged renal function following surgery, an increased risk of death or dialysis was significantly associated with a preoperative renal function at the 25th percentile of EGFR or less (i.e., with ischemic nephropathy). These relationships are shown for predicted dialysis-free survival for 25th percentile and median values of preoperative EGFR according to postoperative renal function response (see Fig. 25-6).[2]

These associations between renal function response and dialysis-free survival suggest that the designation of renal function unchanged after intervention as "preserved" may be misleading. Patients with ischemic nephropathy unchanged after open surgical repair remain at increased risk for death or dialysis. Similar data relating renal function response and survival free from dialysis after catheter-based intervention are not currently available.

Consequences of Operative Failures

Renal artery repairs failed in approximately 4% of patients during follow-up.[3] Blood pressure response after secondary operative intervention was equivalent to that observed after primary operative intervention. However, patients requiring secondary renal artery intervention had a significant and independent risk of eventual dialysis dependence (35% vs. 4%).[3] To date, no peer-reviewed report has examined the dialysis risk associated with restenosis after catheter-based interventions.

Our experience with failed renal artery repairs reinforces two important issues. First, the irretrievable loss of excretory renal function observed after failed renal artery repair supports the view that renal revascularization should be performed for clear clinical indications, not as a "prophylactic" procedure in the absence of either hypertension or renal insufficiency.[2,13,16] Second, direct aortorenal reconstructions in these patients are characterized by prolonged patency. Early failures of repair reflect errors in surgical technique or operative judgment.

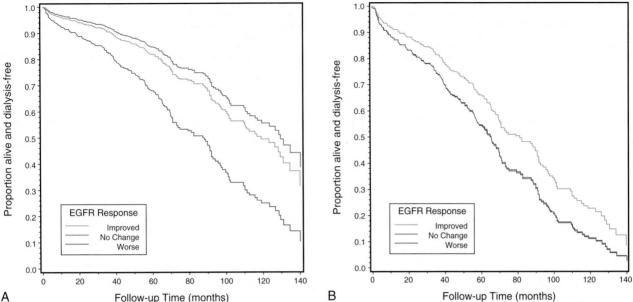

FIGURE 25-6 A-B, Predicted dialysis-free survival according to postoperative renal function response for patients with a preoperative estimated glomerular filtration rate (EGFR) of 25 mL/min/m² (25th percentile) or 38 mL/min/m² (median value). Interaction between preoperative EGFR and renal function response for dialysis-free survival was significant and independent. *(From Cherr GS, Hansen KJ, Craven TE, et al: Surgical management of atherosclerotic renovascular disease. J Vasc Surg 35:236–245, 2002.)*

Surgery After Failed Percutaneous Transluminal Renal Artery Angioplasty

Our experience with 29 atherosclerotic patients repaired after a failed PTRA has been reported.[35] We examined the influence of failure of PTRA on methods of secondary surgical management, and blood pressure and excretory renal function response to operation.

Secondary operative repair was considered complicated in more than half of these patients. In all, four nephrectomies were required. Branch renal artery reconstruction was required in two thirds of patients. Hypertension after operative repair for failed PTRA was cured in 7%, improved in 50%, and considered unchanged in 43%. Compared with patients treated by operative repair only, operative management following failed PTRA was associated with blood pressure benefit (57% vs. 89% benefited [P <0.001]).

Summary

With proper patient selection, operative repair of atherosclerotic renovascular disease results in both improved blood pressure and renal function. Improvement in renal function is associated with a significant increase in dialysis-free survival independent of all other covariates. The application of intraoperative duplex ultrasonography to assess renal artery reconstruction results in long-term primary patency exceeding 96%. However, when failure of operative repair occurs, eventual renal function is worsened, culminating in an increased risk of dialysis dependence and death.

Percutaneous transluminal angioplasty with or without stenting offers blood pressure benefit similar to operative repair for non-ostial atherosclerotic lesions of the main renal artery. However, cumulative data for ostial lesions associated with ischemic nephropathy suggest that PTRA with or without endoluminal stenting yields inferior renal function benefit. The common practice of reporting unchanged renal function as "preserved" or "stabilized" after renal artery intervention may be misleading. Patients with ischemic nephropathy unchanged after open surgical repair

remain at increased risk for eventual dialysis dependence and death.[2,12,14] For these reasons, the authors recommend open operative repair of bilateral ostial atherosclerosis and renal artery occlusion associated with severe hypertension and renal insufficiency in good-risk patients.

REFERENCES

1. Hansen KJ, Starr SM, Sands RE, et al: Contemporary surgical management of renovascular disease, *J Vasc Surg* 16:319, 1992.
2. Cherr GS, Hansen KJ, Craven TE, et al: Surgical management of atherosclerotic renovascular disease, *J Vasc Surg* 35:236, 2002.
3. Hansen KJ, Deitch JS, Oskin TC, et al: Renal artery repair: consequence of operative failures, *Ann Surg* 227:678, 1998.
4. Appel RG, Bleyer AJ, Reavis S, et al: Renovascular disease in older patients beginning renal replacement therapy, *Kidney Int* 48:171, 1995.
5. Deitch JS, Hansen KJ, Craven TE, et al: Renal artery repair in African-Americans, *J Vasc Surg* 26:465, 1997.
6. Mailloux LU, Bellucci AG, Mossey RT, et al: Predictors of survival in patients undergoing dialysis, *Am J Med* 84:855, 1988.
7. Hansen KJ, Tribble RW, Reavis SW, et al: Renal duplex sonography: evaluation of clinical utility, *J Vasc Surg* 12:227, 1990.
8. Motew SJ, Cherr GS, Craven TE, et al: Renal duplex sonography: main renal artery versus hilar analysis, *J Vasc Surg* 32:462, 2000.
9. Valentine RJ, Martin JD, Myers SI, et al: Asymptomatic celiac and superior mesenteric artery stenoses are more prevalent among patients with unsuspected renal artery stenoses, *J Vasc Surg* 14:195, 1991.
10. Hansen KJ, Wilson DB, Craven TE, et al: Mesenteric artery disease in the elderly, *J Vasc Surg* 40:45, 2004.
11. Dean RH, Tribble RW, Hansen KJ, et al: Evolution of renal insufficiency in ischemic nephropathy, *Ann Surg* 213:446, 1991.
12. Hansen KJ, Thomason RB, Craven TE, et al: Surgical management of dialysis-dependent ischemic nephropathy, *J Vasc Surg* 21:197, 1995.
13. Hansen KJ, Benjamin ME, Appel RG, et al: Renovascular hypertension in the elderly: results of surgical management, *Geriatr Nephrol Urol* 6:3, 1996.
14. Hansen KJ, Cherr GS, Craven TE, et al: Management of ischemic nephropathy: dialysis-free survival after surgical repair, *J Vasc Surg* 32:472, 2000.
15. Fergany A, Kolettis P, Novick AC: The contemporary role of extra-anatomical surgical renal revascularization in patients with atherosclerotic renal artery disease, *J Urol* 153(6):1798–1801, 1995.
16. Dean RH, Benjamin ME, Hansen KJ: Surgical management of renovascular hypertension, *Curr Probl Surg* 34:209, 1997.
17. Wollenweber J, Sheps SG, Davis GD: Clinical course of atherosclerotic renovascular disease, *Am J Cardiol* 21:60, 1968.
18. Meaney TF, Dustan HP, McCormack LJ: Natural history of renal arterial disease, *Radiology* 91:881, 1968.

19. Dean RH, Kieffer RW, Smith BM, et al: Renovascular hypertension: anatomic and renal function changes during drug therapy, *Arch Surg* 116:1408, 1981.

20. Schreiber MJ, Pohl MA, Novick AC: The natural history of atherosclerotic and fibrous renal artery disease, *Urol Clin North Am* 11:383, 1984.

21. Tollefson DF, Ernst CB: Natural history of atherosclerotic renal artery stenosis associated with aortic disease, *J Vasc Surg* 14:327, 1991.

22. Zierler RE, Bergelin RO, Davidson RC, et al: A prospective study of disease progression in patients with atherosclerotic renal artery stenosis, *Am J Hypertens* 9:1055, 1996.

23. Webster J, Marshall F, Abdalla M, et al: Randomised comparison of percutaneous angioplasty vs. continued medical therapy for hypertensive patients with atheromatous renal artery stenosis. Scottish and New Castle Renal Artery Stenosis Collaborative Group. *J Hum Hypertens* 12:329, 1998.

24. Crowley JJ, Santos RM, Peter RH, et al: Progression of renal artery stenosis in patients undergoing cardiac catheterization, *Am Heart J* 136:913, 1998.

25. Caps MT, Perissinotto C, Zierler RE, et al: Prospective study of atherosclerotic disease progression in the renal artery, *Circulation* 98:2866, 1998.

26. van Jaarsveld BC, Krijnen P, Pieterman H, et al: The effect of balloon angioplasty on hypertension in atherosclerotic renal-artery stenosis, *N Engl J Med* 342:1007, 2000.

27. Pearce JD, Craven BL, Craven TE, et al: Progression of atherosclerotic renovascular disease: a prospective population-based study, *J Vasc Surg* 44(5):955–962, 2006.

28. Williamson WK, Abou-Zamzam AM, Jr, Moneta GL, et al. Prophylactic repair of renal artery stenosis is not justified in patients who require infrarenal aortic reconstruction, *J Vasc Surg* 28:14–20, 1998.

29. Hansen KJ, O'Neil EA, Reavis SW, et al: Intraoperative duplex sonography during renal artery reconstruction, *J Vasc Surg* 14:364, 1991.

30. Moncure AC, Brewster DC, Darling RC, et al: Use of the splenic and hepatic arteries for renal revascularization, *J Vasc Surg* 3:196, 1986.

31. Messina LM: Operative evaluation of renal and visceral arterial reconstruction using duplex sonography. In Ernst CB, Stanley JC, editors: *Current Therapy in Vascular Surgery*, ed 4, Philadelphia, 2001, Mosby, pp 753–756.

32. Hansen KJ, Reavis SW, Dean RH: Duplex scanning in renovascular disease, *Geriatr Nephrol Urol* 6:89, 1996.

33. Marone LK, Clouse WD, Dorer DJ, et al: Preservation of renal function with surgical revascularization in patients with atherosclerotic renovascular disease, *J Vasc Surg* 39:322, 2004.

34. Stanley JC, David M: Hume memorial lecture: surgical treatment of renovascular hypertension, *Am J Surg* 174:102, 1997.

35. Wong JM, Hansen KJ, Oskin TC, et al: Surgery after failed percutaneous renal artery angioplasty, *J Vasc Surg* 30:468, 1999.

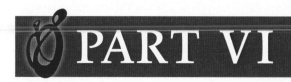

PART VI

MESENTERIC VASCULAR DISEASE

CHAPTER **26** **Epidemiology and Pathophysiology of Mesenteric Vascular Disease**

Rachel C. Danczyk, Gregory J. Landry, Gregory L. Moneta

Severe acute intestinal ischemia results from sudden symptomatic reduction in intestinal blood flow of sufficient magnitude to potentially result in intestinal infarction.[1] Acute ischemia of the small bowel and/or right colon may result from mesenteric arterial occlusion (embolus or thrombosis), mesenteric venous occlusion, and nonocclusive processes, especially vasospasm (Fig. 26-1). Isolated dissections of the superior mesenteric artery (SMA), either in association with cystic medial degeneration of the arteries or, more commonly, as progression of an existing dissection in the descending thoracic aorta into the SMA and celiac artery, may also result in acute intestinal ischemia.

Acute Arterial Occlusive Mesenteric Ischemia

Acute Mesenteric Arterial Embolism

Roughly 25% of all cases of acute mesenteric ischemia are due to emboli to the SMA, 25% of cases are due to thrombosis of preexisting atherosclerotic lesions, and the remaining 50% are due to a variety of other etiologies.[2] Mesenteric emboli can originate from left atrial or ventricular mural thrombi or from cardiac valvular lesions.[1] These thrombi are most often associated with cardiac dysrhythmias such as atrial fibrillation, global myocardial dysfunction with poor ejection fraction, or discrete hypokinetic regions produced by previous myocardial infarction (MI).[3] About 15% of emboli lodge at the origin of the SMA, but the majority lodge 3 to 10 cm distally in the tapered segment of the SMA just past the origin of the middle colic artery.[2] More than 20% of emboli to the SMA are associated with concurrent emboli to another arterial bed.[4] Intestinal ischemia due to embolic arterial occlusion can be compounded by reactive mesenteric vasospasm, further reducing collateral flow and exacerbating the ischemic insult.[2,5]

Acute Mesenteric Arterial Thrombosis

Thrombosis of the SMA or the celiac artery is usually associated with preexisting critical stenoses. Many of these patients have histories consistent with chronic mesenteric ischemia (CMI), including postprandial pain, weight loss, "food fear," and early satiety.[1,6] Superior mesenteric artery thrombosis can be regarded as a complication of untreated chronic intestinal ischemia.[1] The SMA plaque likely progresses slowly to a critical stenosis over years until thrombosis occurs.

Unlike embolic occlusions, thrombosis of the SMA generally occurs flush with the aortic origin of the vessel. Aortic dissection involving the visceral vessels, though rare, can cause acute mesenteric ischemia. The intimal flap of the dissection can extend into, compress, or exclude the mesenteric orifice.[5] Acute mesenteric ischemia is also an uncommon (< 1%) but serious complication of

cardiac surgery, with a reported mortality rate of greater than 50% in most series.[5,7] Presumably, the nonpulsatile perfusion delivered by most extracorporeal circuits allows severely stenotic visceral vessels to occlude during cardiopulmonary bypass. Identified risk factors for this complication include prolonged cross-clamp times, use of intraaortic balloon counterpulsation, low cardiac output syndromes, blood transfusion, triple-vessel disease, coronary artery disease (CAD), and peripheral artery disease (PAD).[7]

Pathophysiology of Occlusive Acute Mesenteric Ischemia

Acute mesenteric ischemia, whether the underlying cause is embolic or thrombotic, may eventually lead to intestinal infarction (Fig. 26-2). Hypoxia and hypercarbia that occur during flow interruption, and reperfusion injury once intestinal blood flow is restored, all contribute to tissue loss[8] (Fig. 26-3). Reperfusion injury is believed to be principally mediated by activation of the enzyme xanthine oxidase and recruitment and activation of circulating neutrophils (PMNs).[9] The mechanism of injury likely involves production of oxygen-derived free radicals by xanthine oxidase that then causes profound local tissue injury through lipid peroxidation, membrane disruption, and increased microvascular permeability.[5,9] The ischemic endothelium recruits PMNs in an autocrine and paracrine manner by secreting chemotactic cytokines (tumor necrosis factor [TNF]-α, interleukin [IL]-1, platelet-derived growth factor [PDGF]) that perpetuate further damage to the reperfused tissue. Once activated, PMNs degranulate, releasing myeloperoxidase, collagenases, and elastases that further injure already ischemic and vulnerable tissue.[5,10] Activation of this endogenous inflammatory cascade is not restricted to the injured organ and may also have deleterious systemic effects, with cardiac, pulmonary, and other organ system dysfunction.[5]

Natural History of Acute Mesenteric Arterial Occlusive Disease

The mortality rate for occlusive acute mesenteric ischemia exceeds 70% in most series.[1,2,5,11,12] Occlusive acute intestinal ischemia resulting from SMA embolism has a more favorable prognosis than that resulting from SMA thrombosis.[1] Survival following acute intestinal ischemia due to SMA thrombosis is rare. The more favorable prognosis associated with embolism is attributable to the fact that most emboli lodge distally in the SMA (beyond the origin of the middle colic artery), thus allowing perfusion of the proximal intestine via middle colic and jejunal artery branches.[1] Thrombotic occlusion of the SMA usually occurs proximal to the middle colic artery, and therefore completely interrupts mid-gut arterial perfusion in patients with poorly developed celiac artery or inferior mesenteric artery (IMA) collateral flow.[1,3,6]

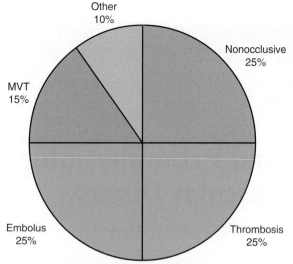

FIGURE 26-1 Etiology of acute mesenteric ischemia. MVT, mesenteric venous thrombosis.

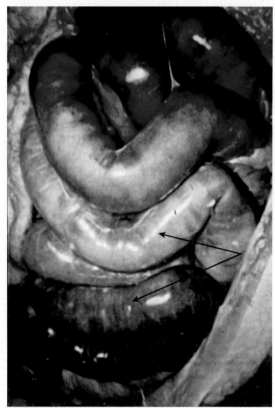

FIGURE 26-2 Ischemic bowel. Arrows indicate segments of clearly infarcted intestine.

Nonocclusive Mesenteric Ischemia

Epidemiology

Nonocclusive mesenteric ischemia (NOMI) accounts for 25% of all episodes of acute intestinal ischemia.[1,5,13,14] In NOMI, microscopic arterial blood flow is inadequate to supply perfusion to the bowel. The result is intestinal ischemia and infarction in the presence of a patent macroscopic vasculature.[15] Previous reports[15-17] have identified multiple risk factors for development of NOMI (Box 26-1). Mesenteric arterial vasospasm may occur following elective revascularization procedures for chronic SMA occlusion. In such cases, vasoconstriction of small and medium-sized vessels is precipitated by early enteral feeding.[18] Without prompt intervention, NOMI may

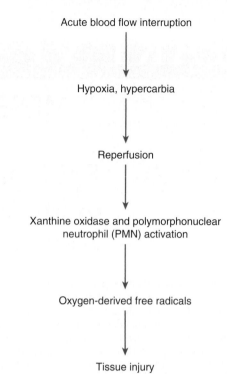

FIGURE 26-3 Pathophysiological mechanisms of acute occlusive mesenteric ischemia.

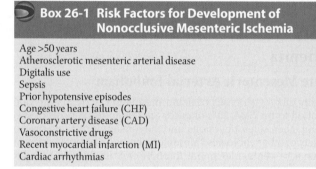

Box 26-1 Risk Factors for Development of Nonocclusive Mesenteric Ischemia

Age >50 years
Atherosclerotic mesenteric arterial disease
Digitalis use
Sepsis
Prior hypotensive episodes
Congestive heart failure (CHF)
Coronary artery disease (CAD)
Vasoconstrictive drugs
Recent myocardial infarction (MI)
Cardiac arrhythmias

progress from localized intestinal ischemia to transmural infarction, peritonitis, and death.[19,20] Mortality is high regardless of treatment, owing to the underlying medical conditions that precipitate NOMI and frequent delays in diagnosis.[5,13-15]

Pathophysiology

Nonocclusive mesenteric ischemia was first recognized in autopsies of patients with small-intestinal gangrene in the absence of arterial or venous occlusion.[21,22] Investigation of the regulatory mechanisms of mesenteric circulation has demonstrated that the pathophysiology of NOMI is multifactorial. Virtually all patients with NOMI have a severe coexisting illness, commonly severe cardiac failure.[23] It is postulated that hypoperfusion from cardiac failure, resulting in peripheral hypoxemia and splanchnic vasoconstriction, precipitates intestinal ischemia.[13,14] Mesenteric vasoconstriction, intestinal hypoxia, and ischemia-reperfusion injury all contribute to development of NOMI.

Mesenteric vasoconstriction, the hallmark of NOMI, represents an exaggerated homeostatic mechanism induced by excessive sympathetic activity during cardiogenic shock or hypovolemia. The body attempts to maintain cardiac and cerebral perfusion at the expense of splanchnic and peripheral circulations. Experimental evidence suggests that the mediators of this response are endothelin-1 (ET-1), nitric oxide (NO), vasopressin, and angiotensin (Ang).[24,25] Endothelin-1 is a potent vasoconstrictor secreted from endothelial cells (ECs); in concert with other vasoactive peptides, it regulates myogenic cells in the vascular wall. Nitric oxide can have paradoxical effects on vascular tone, depending on local concentration.[26] At low concentrations it acts as a vasodilator, whereas at higher concentrations it acts as an oxygen-derived free radical, impairing mitochondrial energy production.

The splanchnic autoregulatory system is affected by local arteriolar smooth muscle relaxation and vasodilation, as well as increased cellular oxygen extraction.[27] Adequate oxygen delivery may be maintained despite declining perfusion pressures until a critical threshold is reached. In experimental models, maximal extraction is reached at a pressure of 40 mmHg, but beyond this point, oxygen consumption declines, and ischemia ensues.[28] Neri et al. recently demonstrated that postoperative cardiac surgery patients who develop NOMI had persistent deficits between oxygen delivery (Do_2) and consumption (Vo_2) because of poor circulatory reserve. In contrast, postoperative cardiac patients who did not develop NOMI were able to normalize their Do_2:Vo_2 ratio by optimizing their cardiac output.[14] In the presence of impaired perfusion, blood flow is not evenly distributed in the bowel wall. The mucosa retains its perfusion at the expense of the serosal layers through mucosal production of NO, prostaglandins (PGs), and stimulation of dopamine-I receptors.[27] Histological damage is first observed at the villous tip and progresses to the deeper muscularis, submucosa, and mucosa within a few hours.

Once set in motion, mesenteric vasospasm may persist despite correction of the precipitating event.[13,14] The etiology of persistent vasoconstriction once adequate blood flow is restored is unknown, but it may respond to direct intraarterial papaverine infusion or other vasodilators, including iloprost.[29] This phenomenon of protracted vasoconstriction, however, plays an important role in development and maintenance of occlusive and nonocclusive intestinal ischemia, and may also complicate mesenteric revascularization.[18]

Use of vasoconstrictor agents and digitalis has been associated with the majority of cases of NOMI. Vasoactive agents, including α-adrenergic drugs and vasopressin, produce splanchnic vasoconstriction directly, whereas digoxin preparations alter mesenteric vasoreactivity by stimulating arterial and venous smooth muscle cell (SMC) contraction.[27,29] This may enhance mesenteric arteriolar vasoconstriction in the setting of acute venous hypertension.[29]

Restoration of blood flow to the ischemic intestine may be complicated by reperfusion injury. During critical ischemia, adenosine triphosphate (ATP) levels are depleted, causing distortion of ATP-dependent cell membrane systems. This results in loss of cellular homeostasis, with cellular swelling and electrolyte imbalances.[27] Reduction in ATP levels also generates large amounts of adenosine, a precursor of hypoxanthine. Within the swollen cells, calcium accumulates and triggers hydrolysis of the enzyme xanthine dehydrogenase into xanthine oxidase, which reacts with intracellular hypoxanthine to produce uric acid and toxic oxygen free radicals.[5,27] These free radicals exert direct damage to cellular membranes, causing capillary leak syndrome, and incite endogenous inflammatory cascades that cause widespread tissue injury. The deleterious effects of free radicals are usually limited by endogenous scavengers such as glutathione, catalase, superoxide dismutase, and NO.[27] However, in cases of prolonged ischemia, the capacity of this scavenger system to eliminate reactive oxygen species (ROS) is exceeded, and continued damage occurs. The degree of reperfusion injury is thus related to the frequency and duration of the ischemic episodes. Clark and Gewertz demonstrated that two short 15-minute periods of low flow followed by reperfusion resulted in a more severe histological injury than a single 30-minute period of ischemia.[30,31]

In NOMI, a similar scenario exists: hypoperfusion may be partial and occasionally repetitive. It is believed that episodic reperfusion creates a local environment replete with primed neutrophils within the ischemic bed that are capable of degranulating and releasing superoxide. This concept is substantiated by recent experimental evidence that reperfusion injury may be attenuated by reperfusion with leukodepleted blood or by blockade of EC surface receptors

for leukocyte adherence.[32] In addition, several compounds including *N*-acetylcysteine and vitamin E have been shown in animal models to reduce tissue damage caused by reactive oxygen species.[33] Application of these novel approaches in human NOMI awaits further study.

Mesenteric Venous Thrombosis

Mesenteric venous thrombosis (MVT) refers to thrombosis of the veins draining the intestine (inferior mesenteric, superior mesenteric, splenic, and portal veins). The obstruction in venous return leads to edema, distention, and in some cases, infarction of the affected segments.[1,5]

Epidemiology

Mesenteric venous thrombosis is a comparatively rare form of mesenteric ischemia. The presentation may vary from asymptomatic to fulminant with intestinal infarction and hemodynamic collapse. Mesenteric venous thrombosis was first described by Elliot in 1895 as "thrombosis of the portomesenteric venous system."[34] In 1935, Warren and Eberhard characterized MVT as a distinct clinical entity. These authors reported a 34% mortality rate following intestinal resection for venous thrombosis.[35]

Mesenteric venous thrombosis currently constitutes no more than 5% to 15% of all cases of acute mesenteric ischemia.[36] Only 372 patients with MVT were reported from 1911 to 1984,[37] and MVT accounted for only 6.2% of 1167 patients treated for mesenteric ischemia at the Mayo Clinic from 1972 to 1993.[38] Ottinger and Austen found that MVT represented 0.006% of hospital admissions.[39] It is estimated that intestinal infarction due to MVT is encountered in less than 1 in 1000 laparotomies for acute abdomen.[40]

Pathophysiology

Mesenteric venous thrombosis can be classified as primary or secondary. Primary MVT is defined as spontaneous idiopathic thrombosis of mesenteric veins not associated with any other disease or etiological factor.[1,5,36] The number of patients in this group has decreased substantially in the past decade because of increased recognition of inherited thrombotic disorders and hypercoagulable states.

Patients in whom an etiological factor can be identified are said to have secondary MVT. Currently, however, a causative factor can be identified in only 35% of patients with MVT.[36,38] Known causes of secondary MVT are shown in Box 26-2. Oral contraceptive use accounts for 9% to 18% of episodes of MVT in young women.[41] Protein C and protein S deficiency, antithrombin III deficiency, dysfibrinogenemia, abnormal plasminogen, polycythemia vera, thrombocytosis, sickle cell disease (SCD), and factor V Leiden mutation have all been associated with MVT.[1,5,36,41,42] Localized secondary MVT has also been reported, most commonly associated with volvulus, intussusception, or mechanical bowel strangulation.

Location of the thrombus may be predicted by etiology. Thrombosis due to an intraabdominal cause such as inflammatory

---

Box 26-2 Causes of Secondary Mesenteric Venous Thrombosis

Trauma
Surgery
Cancer
Cirrhosis
Portal hypertension
Inflammatory bowel disease
Oral contraceptive use
Splenomegaly
Pancreatitis
Dehydration
Infection
Diverticular disease
Hypercoagulable states

conditions or surgery starts in the larger vessels at the site of compression and propagates distally to involve the smaller venous arcades and arcuate channels.[41] In contrast, thrombosis due to an underlying hypercoagulable state usually begins in the small vessels and later involves the larger vessels.[36,41] Occlusion of the venae rectae and the intramural vessels interferes with adequate venous drainage, with eventual hemorrhagic infarction of the involved bowel segment. The transition from normal to ischemic bowel is usually gradual, unlike that seen with acute embolic or thrombotic occlusion.

Natural History

The natural history of MVT varies based on the etiology. In most cases, it usually does not result in gangrenous bowel.[1,5,41,42] Similarly, symptomatic manifestations are diverse. Patients may present with a benign abdominal examination and few symptoms or with profound hemodynamic collapse. Most patients have abdominal pain. Although it can be sudden in onset, most frequently it begins insidiously and worsens over time. Approximately 50% of patients have pain from 5 to 30 days before seeking medical attention, and 27% report abdominal pain for more than 1 month.[43] In a recent review, only 16% of patients had severe peritonitis, and 33% required bowel resection.[42] Despite improved diagnostic modalities and more aggressive treatment regimens, symptomatic acute MVT is an indicator of poor prognosis, with an approximate 10% to 20% 30-day mortality rate and a 3-year survival rate of 35%.[42,44] Patients with evidence of chronic thrombosis fare somewhat better because collateral venous channels form and thereby augment intestinal venous drainage.

Chronic Mesenteric Ischemia

Symptomatic chronic mesenteric arterial insufficiency is a well-described but infrequently encountered clinical problem. Although the earliest report of chronic intestinal ischemia was by Councilman in 1894,[45] in 1918, Goodman credited Baccelli as the first individual to correctly associate postprandial pain with CMI. Eighteen years later, Dunphy suggested that the abdominal pain associated with chronic mesenteric arterial occlusion was a possible precursor of later intestinal infarction.[46] Later, Shaw and Maynard performed the first successful endarterectomy for CMI.[47] Morris et al. described the technique of retrograde aortovisceral bypass in 1962.[48]

Epidemiology

Chronic mesenteric ischemia results from atherosclerosis in 90% of cases.[1,5,49–51] Nonatherosclerotic causes of CMI are listed in Box 26-3. Nonatherosclerotic etiologies have been described in young adults

Box 26-3 Nonatherosclerotic Conditions Associated with Chronic Mesenteric Ischemia

Neurofibromatosis
Middle aortic syndrome
Median arcuate ligament compression
Visceral artery dissection
Buerger's disease
Rheumatoid arthritis
Cocaine abuse
Systemic lupus erythematosus (SLE)
Thoracic aortic aneurysm (TAA)
Cogan's syndrome
Polyarteritis nodosa
Aortic coarctation repair
Radiation injury
Thrombosis associated with TAA repair
Mesenteric arteritis
Congenital afibrinogenemia
Ergot poisoning

and children as young as 30 months of age.[49–51] In general, Risk factors for atherosclerotic-associated CMI are similar to those of other atherosclerotic conditions, including a positive family history, sedentary lifestyle, hypertension, hypercholesterolemia, and smoking.[1,5,46–51] In contrast to other atherosclerotic vascular diseases, approximately 60% of patients with CMI are female, and nearly 50% of patients have a history of earlier cardiovascular surgery.[51] Symptomatic CMI generally manifests at a mean age of about 58 years.[1,5,46,52–56] More than one third of patients have hypertension, coronary artery disease, and/or cerebrovascular disease.[1,5,53–56] Nearly 20% have evidence of chronic renal insufficiency, and 10% have diabetes.[49,56]

Although there is a high prevalence of mesenteric atherosclerosis, the clinical syndrome of symptomatic mesenteric ischemia is uncommon.[1,54,55] An autopsy series of unselected patients found significant stenoses in approximately 50% of celiac arteries, 30% of SMAs, and 30% of IMAs.[52] In a more recent series of 120 consecutive autopsies, however, rates of significant stenoses in the celiac, SMA, and IMA were not quite as high, with 22%, 16%, and 10% incidence, respectively.[55] The prevalence of potentially flow-limiting stenosis within the mesenteric vessels increases with age, with up to 67% of those older than 80 years of age having more than 50% stenosis in some mesenteric artery.[55] Aortograms performed for aortic aneurysmal or occlusive disease demonstrate significant stenosis of the celiac artery in 33% of cases and SMA lesions in nearly 20%.[54–56]

Pathophysiology and Natural History

Chronic mesenteric ischemia occurs when the blood supply is insufficient to meet the metabolic demands of the bowel, resulting from increased motility, secretion, and absorption after meals.[57] The infrequent occurrence of symptomatic disease may be explained in part by the extensive mesenteric collateral circulation, which includes both viscerovisceral (celiac artery-SMA-IMA), and parietovisceral (hypogastric-IMA) blood flow.[1,5,55–57] The slow development of a chronic high-grade stenosis or occlusion of one or more of the major mesenteric vessels may thus be fully compensated by collateral blood flow. In addition, recent evidence suggests that preexisting significant stenoses in even remote arterial beds may provide protective effects through the mechanism of ischemic preconditioning.[58–60]

It has been proposed that the pathophysiology of symptomatic CMI involves a regional vascular steal phenomenon.[61] Investigators have used tonometric assessment of splanchnic blood flow in dogs with 50% stenoses of both the celiac artery and SMA to show that food intake reduced intestinal perfusion by 50%. This reduction was associated with a significant decrease in intestinal intramural pH that was attributed to steal from the intestinal to the gastric circulation stimulated by a food bolus within the stomach.[61]

Rarely, single-vessel disease of the SMA may produce symptoms characteristic of CMI. The vast majority of patients who present with symptomatic CMI, however, have arteriographic evidence of multivessel visceral artery disease.[1,5,49–52,55,56]

A variety of pain syndromes characterize patients with CMI. In general, the symptoms consist of upper abdominal cramping or aching pain beginning 20 to 30 minutes after eating. At first the pain may be of short duration, but later it may become more persistent and last for 3 to 4 hours after eating. As the disease progresses, the amount of food that precipitates abdominal pain may decrease. Patients avoid eating to prevent the resulting abdominal pain. Most patients with CMI suffer weight loss secondary to diminished nutritional intake; malabsorption is not the primary mechanism of weight loss.[57]

No form of bowel activity is "classic" for CMI. Patients may have diarrhea (which can potentially exacerbate their nutritional depletion), constipation, or normal bowel habits. Without intervention, such patients develop severe protein-calorie malnutrition, and CMI can progress to visceral infarction.[49,50,55–57]

Most fatal cases of CMI occur in patients with a prolonged history of chronic abdominal complaints.[1,49–51,55–57] Such cases are frequently characterized by months of abdominal complaints and multiple negative endoscopies, CT scans, and other diagnostic tests. In retrospect, the diagnosis is usually obvious. A high index of suspicion and prompt intervention are clearly indicated in cases of unexplained abdominal pain and weight loss. Early diagnosis may prevent acute thrombosis of stenotic vessels and the often fatal complication of intestinal infarction.[1,49–51,55–57]

REFERENCES

1. Moneta G: Acute mesenteric ischemia. In Rutherford RB, editor: *Diagnosis of intestinal ischemia*, Philadelphia, 2000, WB Saunders, p 2508.
2. McKinsey J, Gewertz BL: Acute mesenteric ischemia, *Surg Clin North Am* 77:307, 1997.
3. Park WM, Gloviczki P, Cherry KJ: Contemporary management of acute mesenteric ischemia: factors associated with survival, *J Vasc Surg* 35:445, 2002.
4. Kaleya RN, Sammartano RJ, Boley SJ: Aggressive approach to acute mesenteric ischemia, *Surg Clin North Am* 72:157, 1992.
5. Schwartz LB, McKinsey JF, Gewertz BL: Visceral ischemic syndromes. In Moore WS, editor: *Vascular surgery: a comprehensive review*, ed 6, Philadelphia, 2002, WB Saunders, p 572.
6. Sreenarasimhaiah J: Diagnosis and management of intestinal ischemic disorders, *BMJ* 326:1372, 2003.
7. Ghosh S, Roberts N, Firmin RK, et al: Risk factors for intestinal ischemia in cardiac surgical patients, *Eur J Cardiothorac Surg* 21:411, 2002.
8. Wyers MC: Acute mesenteric ischemia: diagnostic approach and surgical treatment, *Semin Vasc Surg* 23:9–20, 2010.
9. Kozuch PL, Brandt LJ: Review article: diagnosis and management of mesenteric ischaemia with an emphasis on pharmacotherapy, *Aliment Pharmacol Ther* 21:201–215, 2005.
10. Korthius RJ, Anderson DC, Granger DN: Role of neutrophil-endothelial cell adhesion in inflammatory disorders, *J Crit Care* 9:47, 1994.
11. Lock G: Acute mesenteric ischemia: classification, evaluation and therapy, *Acta Gastroenterol Belg* 65:220, 2002.
12. Edwards MS, Cherr GS, Craven TE, et al: Acute occlusive mesenteric ischemia: surgical management and outcomes, *Ann Vasc Surg* 17:72, 2003.
13. Trompeter M, Brazda T, Remy CT, et al: Non-occlusive mesenteric ischemia: etiology, diagnosis, and interventional therapy, *Eur Radiol* 12:1179, 2001.
14. Neri E, Sassi C, Massetti M, et al: Nonocclusive mesenteric ischemia in patients with acute aortic dissection, *J Vasc Surg* 36:738, 2002.
15. Howard TJ, Plaskon LA, Wiebke EA, et al: Nonocclusive mesenteric ischemia remains a diagnostic dilemma, *Am J Surg* 171:405, 1996.
16. Lock G, Scholmerich J: Non-occlusive mesenteric ischemia, *Hepatogastroenterology* 42:234, 1995.
17. Wilcox MG, Howard TJ, Plakson LA, et al: Current theories of pathogenesis and treatment of nonocclusive mesenteric ischemia, *Dig Dis Sci* 40:709, 1995.
18. Gewertz BL, Zarins CK: Postoperative vasospasm after antegrade mesenteric revascularization: a report of three cases, *J Vasc Surg* 14:382, 1991.
19. Patel A, Kaleya RN, Sammartano RJ: Pathophysiology of mesenteric ischemia, *Surg Clin North Am* 72:31, 1992.
20. Williams LF, Anastasia LF, Hasiotis CA, et al: Non-occlusive mesenteric infarction, *Am J Surg* 114:376, 1967.
21. Case records of the Massachusetts General Hospital (Case 35082), *N Engl J Med* 240:308, 1949.
22. Haglund U, Lundgren O: Nonocclusive acute intestinal vascular failure, *Br J Surg* 66:155, 1979.
23. Trompeter M, Brazda T, Remy CT, et al: Non-occlusive mesenteric ischemia: etiology, diagnosis, and interventional therapy, *Eur Radiol* 12:1179–1187, 2002.
24. Mitsuyoshi A, Obama K, Shinkura N, et al: Survival in nonocclusive mesenteric ischemia: early diagnosis by multidetector row computed tomography and early treatment with continuous intravenous high-dose prostaglandin E1, *Ann Surg* 246:229–235, 2007.
25. Luckner G, Jochberger S, Mayr VD, et al: Vasopressin as adjunct vasopressor for vasodilatory shock due to non-occlusive mesenteric ischemia, *Anaesthesist* 55:283–286, 2006.
26. Lamarque D, Whittle BJ: Increase in gastric intramucosal hydrogen ion concentration following endotoxin challenge in the rat and the actions of nitric oxide synthase inhibitors, *Clin Exp Pharmacol Physiol* 28:164, 2001.
27. Kolkman JJ, Mensink PB: Non-occlusive mesenteric ischemia: a common disorder in gastroenterology and intensive care, *Best Pract Res Clin Gastroenterol* 17:457, 2003.
28. Mesh CL, Gewertz BL: The effect of hemodilution on blood flow regulation in normal and postischemic intestine, *J Surg Res* 48:183, 1990.
29. Char D, Hines G: Chronic mesenteric ischemia: diagnosis and treatment, *Heart Dis* 3:231, 2001.
30. Kim EH, Gewertz BL: Chronic digitalis administration alters mesenteric vascular reactivity, *J Vasc Surg* 5:382, 1987.
31. Clark ET, Gewertz BL: Intermittent ischemia potentiates intestinal reperfusion injury, *J Vasc Surg* 13:606, 1991.
32. Toledo-Pereyra LH: Leukocyte depletion, ischemic injury and organ preservation, *J Surg Res* 169:188–189, 2011.
33. Dimakakos PB, Kotsis T, Kondi-Pafiti A, et al: Oxygen free radicals in abdominal aortic surgery: an experimental study, *J Cardiovasc Surg (Torino)* 43:77, 2002.
34. Elliot JW: The operative relief of gangrene of intestine due to occlusion of the mesenteric vessels, *Ann Surg* 21:9, 1895.
35. Warren S, Eberhard TP: Mesenteric venous thrombosis, *Surg Gynecol Obstet* 61:102, 1935.
36. Rhee RY, Gloviczki P: Mesenteric venous thrombosis, *Surg Clin North Am* 77:327, 1997.
37. Abdu R, Zakhour BJ, Dallis DJ: Mesenteric venous thrombosis—1911–1984, *Surgery* 101:383, 1987.
38. Rhee RY, Glovickzi P, Medonca CT, et al: Mesenteric venous thrombosis: still a lethal disease in the 1990s, *J Vasc Surg* 20:688, 1994.
39. Ottinger LW, Austen WG: A study of 136 patients with mesenteric infarction, *Surg Gynecol Obstet* 124:251, 1967.
40. Kazmers A: Intestinal ischemia caused by venous thrombosis. In: *Vascular Surgery*, Philadelphia, 1995, WB Saunders, p 526.
41. Kumar S, Sarr MG, Kamath PS: Mesenteric venous thrombosis, *N Engl J Med* 345:686, 2001.
42. Harward TR, Green D, Bergan JJ, et al: Mesenteric venous thrombosis, *J Vasc Surg* 9:328, 1989.
43. Morasch MD, Ebaugh JL, Chiou AC, et al: Mesenteric venous thrombosis: a changing clinical entity, *J Vasc Surg* 34:680, 2001.
44. Harnik IG, Brandt LJ: Mesenteric venous thrombosis, *Vasc Med* 15:407–418, 2010.
45. Councilman WT: Three cases of occlusion of the superior mesenteric artery, *Boston Med Surg J* 130:410, 1894.
46. Taylor LM, Porter JM: Treatment of chronic intestinal ischemia, *Semin Vasc Surg* 3:186, 1990.
47. Shaw RS, Maynard EP III: Acute and chronic thrombosis of the mesenteric arteries associated with malabsorption: a report of two cases successfully treated with thromboendarterectomy, *N Engl J Med* 258:874, 1958.
48. Morris GC, Crawford ES, Cooley DA, et al: Revascularization of the celiac and superior mesenteric arteries, *Arch Surg* 84:113, 1962.
49. White CJ: Chronic mesenteric ischemia: diagnosis and management, *Prog Cardiovasc Dis* 54:36–40, 2011.
50. Sanders BM, Dalsing MC: Mesenteric ischemia affects young adults with predisposition, *Ann Vasc Surg* 17:270, 2003.
51. Zeller T, Rastan A, Sixt S: Chronic atherosclerotic mesenteric ischemia, *Vasc Med* 15:333–338, 2010.
52. Crawford ES, Morris GC, Myhre HO, et al: Celiac axis, superior mesenteric artery, and inferior mesenteric artery occlusion: surgical considerations, *Surgery* 82:856, 1977.
53. Shanley CJ, Ozaki CK, Zelenock GB: Bypass grafting for chronic mesenteric ischemia, *Surg Clin North Am* 77:381, 1997.
54. Cleveland TJ, Nawaz S, Gaines PA: Mesenteric arterial ischemia: diagnosis and therapeutic options, *Vasc Med* 7:311, 2002.
55. Chang JB, Stein T: Mesenteric ischemia: acute and chronic, *Ann Vasc Surg* 17:323, 2003.
56. Chang JB, Stein TA: Mesenteric ischemia, *Asian J Surg* 26:55, 2003.
57. van Bockel JH, Geelkerken RH, Wasser MN: Chronic splanchnic ischemia, *Best Pract Res Clin Gastroenterol* 15:99, 2001.
58. Heusch G, Schulz R: Remote preconditioning, *J Mol Cell Cardiol* 34:1279, 2002.
59. Cinel I, Avlan D, Cinel L, et al: Ischemic preconditioning reduces intestinal apoptosis in rats, *Shock* 19:588, 2003.
60. Asoyek S, Cinel I, Avlan D, et al: Intestinal ischemic preconditioning protects the intestine and reduces bacterial translocation, *Shock* 18:476, 2002.
61. Poole JW, Sammartano RJ, Boley SJ: Hemodynamic basis of the pain of chronic mesenteric ischemia, *Am J Surg* 153:171, 1987.

CHAPTER 27

Clinical Evaluation and Treatment of Mesenteric Vascular Disease

Rachel C. Danczyk, Gregory L. Moneta

Evaluation

Clinical evaluation of possible mesenteric ischemia begins with a careful history and physical examination and—above all—an appropriate index of suspicion for the diagnosis. The major etiologies of mesenteric ischemia include *mesenteric venous thrombosis* (MVT), *acute mesenteric ischemia*, *nonocclusive mesenteric ischemia* (NOMI), and *chronic mesenteric ischemia* (CMI). These differ in their underlying pathologies and the clinical settings in which they occur, but there may be significant overlap in their clinical presentation. The most crucial point is to understand the variety of clinical settings in which intestinal ischemia can occur and to include mesenteric ischemia in the differential diagnosis of patients presenting with abdominal pain. The goal is to achieve a diagnosis prior to the onset of bowel infarction. Without consideration of intestinal ischemia, the appropriate diagnostic evaluation is unlikely to be obtained, resulting in needless additional morbidity and mortality.

Acute Occlusive Mesenteric Ischemia

SIGNS AND SYMPTOMS

Acute occlusive mesenteric ischemia is caused by embolism to the superior mesenteric artery (SMA) or acute thrombotic occlusion of an atherosclerotic SMA. Mortality exceeds 60%.[1]

Thrombotic occlusion of the SMA carries a worse prognosis than embolism to the SMA because with thrombotic occlusion, the SMA occludes proximal to the middle colic artery and interrupts arterial flow to the entire small intestine. Emboli, which usually originate from the heart, typically lodge in the SMA distal to the origin of the middle colic artery, thereby maintaining some perfusion to the small intestine via the middle colic and jejunal artery branches.

Abdominal pain is the most common presenting symptom in patients with occlusive acute mesenteric ischemia, and physical findings can range from nonspecific tenderness to an acute abdomen. Distention, rigidity, and rebound tenderness occur, particularly when the diagnosis of acute mesenteric ischemia is delayed. The classic presentation is sudden onset of acute abdominal pain out of proportion to the physical findings. This reflects profound intestinal ischemia without associated bowel perforation and peritonitis. Vomiting, fever, and diarrhea are present in one third of patients with acute mesenteric ischemia. Patients with embolism tend to present with an acute onset of abdominal pain, whereas patients with thrombosis of a stenotic SMA may have a more delayed presentation.

Laboratory values are typically nonspecific. The majority of patients will have moderate to marked leukocytosis, but about 10% of patients will have a normal white blood cell (WBC) count. Elevated serum amylase and metabolic acidosis may occur in patients with necrotic bowel, but an absence of these findings does not exclude bowel necrosis.

RADIOLOGICAL DIAGNOSIS

Ultrasound has a limited role in diagnosing acute occlusive mesenteric ischemia. Duplex ultrasonography in the setting of an acute abdomen is limited by abdominal distention, excessive bowel gas, and patient discomfort.

An abdominal computed tomography (CT) scan is often obtained during evaluation of a patient with abdominal pain. In addition to finding other abdominal pathologies causing abdominal pain, CT scans can detect late findings of acute mesenteric ischemia with a sensitivity of 90%, including bowel luminal dilation, bowel wall thickening, submucosal edema or hemorrhage, pneumatosis intestinalis, and portal venous gas.[2] These findings are associated with some degree of intestinal infarction. Emboli tend to lodge distally, and thus the sensitivity of CT scanning in detecting mesenteric arterial embolic occlusion is low and ranges from 37% to 80%[3] (Fig. 27-1). In patients with early ischemia, there may be minimal findings on CT scans. These patients benefit most from early diagnosis and definitive mesenteric revascularization before the onset of intestinal infarction. Therefore, a high index of suspicion and thorough physical examination is of the utmost importance in this population of patients.

Mesenteric angiography remains the gold standard for diagnosing vascular lesions associated with acute mesenteric ischemia, but its use is predicated on clinical judgment. In a patient with obvious peritoneal findings and suspected necrotic bowel, as evidenced by hypotension and acidosis, an urgent exploratory laparotomy is required to resect necrotic bowel and perform revascularization. In this emergent situation, preparation and performance of a mesenteric angiogram may delay definitive operative treatment and increase mortality.

In patients without peritoneal findings but clinically suspected to have mesenteric ischemia, angiography can be performed to make the definitive diagnosis and plan additional therapy. Abrupt occlusion of the SMA distal to the origin of the middle colic artery is typically seen in patients with an embolus (Figs. 27-2 through 27-4), whereas patients with thrombotic occlusion of a chronically stenotic SMA show signs of occlusion beginning at its origin from the aorta.

TREATMENT

Treatment of acute mesenteric occlusive ischemia is aimed at the etiology of the disease. With acute embolic disease, embolectomy can be performed. Thrombotic disease should generally be addressed with a bypass operation. Bypass as an option for acute mesenteric occlusive ischemia treatment is discussed later in the chapter.

Operative Embolectomy

Once angiography has identified embolic disease, the patient is taken to the operating room for abdominal exploration and embolectomy. When performing an SMA embolectomy, a midline incision in the abdomen is made, followed by a thorough examination of the abdominal contents. This may or may not reveal intestinal infarction. The transverse colon is then reflected superiorly, and the SMA is approached at the root of the small-bowel mesentery. The ligament of Treitz is divided and the proximal SMA mobilized. If the embolus is located more distally, the distal SMA may be exposed at the root of the small-bowel mesentery. Embolectomy is performed through a transverse arteriotomy using standard balloon catheters, and the embolus is extracted. The arteriotomy is then closed, and the intestines are again inspected for viability; any nonviable bowel is resected. A Doppler probe can be used to assess the antimesenteric border for intestinal arterial flow. If the bowel viability is equivocal, a "second look" operation can be planned in the following 24 to 48 hours to reassess the bowel and resect if necessary.[4]

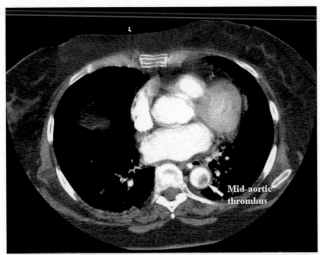

FIGURE 27-1 Axial computed tomography (CT) scan demonstrating a mid-aortic thrombus that caused embolic occlusion of superior mesenteric artery (SMA).

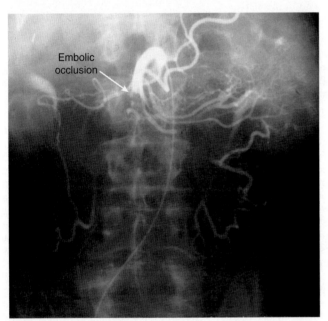

FIGURE 27-2 Anteroposterior angiogram demonstrating abrupt embolic occlusion of superior mesenteric artery (SMA).

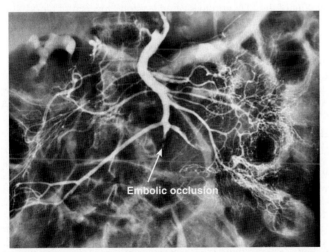

FIGURE 27-3 Anteroposterior angiogram of the superior mesenteric artery (SMA) demonstrating embolic occlusion of distal SMA.

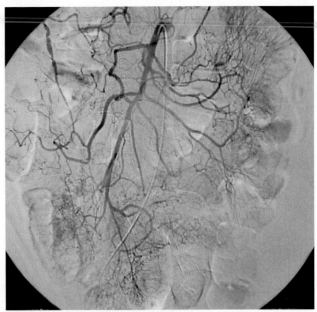

FIGURE 27-4 Anteroposterior angiogram of superior mesenteric artery (SMA) after operative embolectomy demonstrating filling of distal SMA.

Chronic Mesenteric Ischemia

SIGNS AND SYMPTOMS

Patients with CMI are typically women (3:1 female-to-male ratio) between the ages of 40 and 70 years, and a history of recurrent abdominal pain is the most critical factor in the diagnosis. The pain associated with CMI is mid-abdominal or epigastric in origin and is described as colicky or a dull intense ache that may radiate to the back. Pain is postprandial and generally begins 15 to 30 minutes after eating and lasts up to 4 hours. There are no signs of peritonitis, and the degree of pain may reflect the volume of the ingested meal.

Patients may ingest some meals without pain early in the course of CMI, so pain may be initially attributed to cholelithiasis, peptic ulcer disease, or malignancy. Patients often undergo extensive evaluation with endoscopy, CT, barium studies, and abdominal ultrasonography prior to reaching a diagnosis of CMI. As the disease progresses, patients begin to experience pain with each meal and may develop a fear of food. Weight loss, the hallmark of CMI, results from limited nutritional intake, not malabsorption; patients with CMI will have normal gastrointestinal absorption test results.

RADIOLOGICAL DIAGNOSIS

Mesenteric Angiography

Chronic mesenteric ischemia is a clinical diagnosis. There are no absolute confirmatory tests, but contrast mesenteric angiography is the standard to diagnose arterial lesions associated with CMI. Radiographs are obtained in the lateral and anteroposterior projections. Findings on angiography suggestive of CMI include stenosis or occlusion of the celiac artery (CA) and/or the SMA (Fig. 27-5). When the origins of the CA or SMA are occluded, the more distal vessels are often patent through filling by enlarged and easily visualized pancreaticoduodenal arterial collaterals. Occasionally, one can find mid-SMA stenosis with a normal proximal SMA (Fig. 27-6) or a "coral reef" aorta with associated SMA occlusion (Fig. 27-7). Not all patients with mesenteric artery obstruction, however, have mesenteric ischemia. It is vitally important to differentiate high-grade mesenteric artery stenosis from the clinical entity of CMI.

Duplex Ultrasonography

Duplex ultrasonography can serve as a valuable noninvasive screening test for splanchnic artery stenosis and for follow-up in patients with mesenteric artery reconstructions. Despite the

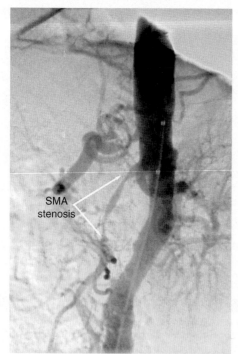

FIGURE 27-5 Lateral aortogram demonstrating long-segment stenosis of superior mesenteric artery *(SMA)*.

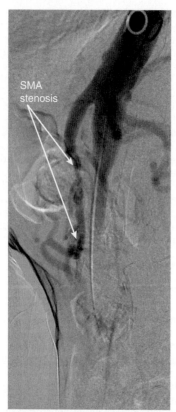

FIGURE 27-6 Lateral aortogram demonstrating long-segment stenosis of middle superior mesenteric artery *(SMA)*.

accuracy of duplex detection of mesenteric artery stenoses, an appropriate history and physical examination and angiographic confirmation of high-grade stenoses or occlusion of the splanchnic vessels are still required for the diagnosis of CMI. Duplex examination of the mesenteric arteries can be technically difficult and should be performed by vascular technologists with extensive experience in abdominal ultrasound techniques.

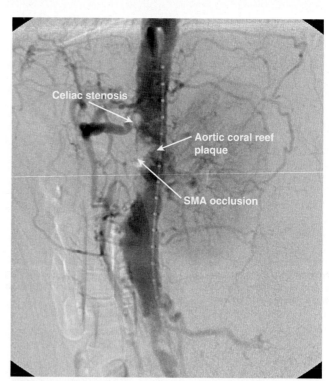

FIGURE 27-7 Lateral aortogram demonstrating "coral reef" atherosclerotic plaque in aorta, with associated superior mesenteric artery *(SMA)* occlusion and celiac artery *(CA)* stenosis.

In healthy individuals, fasting blood flow velocity waveforms differ between the SMA and the CA. Arterial waveforms reflect endorgan vascular resistance. The liver and spleen have relatively high constant metabolic requirements and are therefore low-resistance organs. As a result, CA waveforms are generally biphasic with a peak systolic component, no reversal of end-systolic flow, and a relatively high end-diastolic velocity (EDV). The normal fasting SMA velocity waveform is triphasic, reflecting the high vascular resistance of the intestinal tract at rest (Figs. 27-8 and 27-9). There is a peak systolic component, often an end-systolic reverse flow component, and a minimal diastolic flow component.

Changes in Doppler-derived arterial waveforms in response to feeding are different in the CA and SMA. Because the liver and spleen have fixed metabolic demands, there is no significant change in CA velocity waveform after eating. Blood flow in the SMA, however, increases markedly after a meal, reflecting a marked decrease in intestinal arterial resistance. Waveform changes in the SMA postprandially include a near doubling of systolic velocity, tripling of the EDV, and loss of end-systolic reversal of blood flow. In addition, there is a small but detectable increase in the diameter of the SMA postprandially. The diameter of the SMA has been shown to be 0.60 ± 0.09 cm in the fasting state and 0.67 ± 0.09 cm after a meal. These changes are maximal at 45 minutes after ingestion of a test meal[5] and are dependent on the composition of the meal ingested. Mixed composition meals produce the greatest flow increase in the SMA when compared with equal caloric meals composed solely of fat, glucose, or protein.[6]

DETECTION OF SPLANCHNIC ARTERIAL STENOSIS

Duplex ultrasound can detect hemodynamically significant stenoses in splanchnic vessels. In 1986, investigators at the University of Washington found that flow velocities in stenotic SMAs and CAs were significantly increased when compared with normal SMAs and CAs.[7] Quantitative criteria for splanchnic artery stenosis were first developed and validated at Oregon Health & Science University.[8]

In a blinded prospective study of 100 patients who underwent mesenteric artery duplex scanning and lateral aortography, a peak systolic velocity (PSV) in the SMA of 275 cm/s or more indicated 70% or greater SMA stenosis with a sensitivity of 92%, specificity of

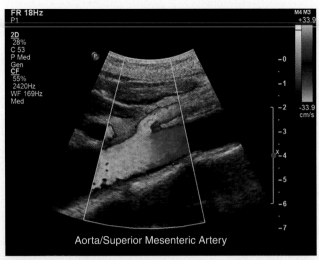

FIGURE 27-8 Duplex ultrasonography of aorta and superior mesenteric artery (SMA).

96%, positive predictive value of 80%, negative predictive value of 99%, and accuracy of 96%[9] (Fig. 27-10). In the same study, a PSV of 200 cm/s or higher identified 70% or greater angiographic CA stenosis with a sensitivity of 87%, specificity of 80%, positive predictive value of 63%, negative predictive value of 94%, and accuracy of 82% (Fig. 27-11).

Other duplex criteria for mesenteric artery stenoses are also in use. An SMA EDV greater than 45 cm/s correlates with 50% or greater SMA stenosis with 92% specificity and 100% sensitivity. A CA EDV of 55 cm/s or higher predicts 50% or greater CA stenosis with 93% sensitivity, 100% specificity, and 95% accuracy.[10,11]

Postprandial mesenteric duplex scanning has been used as an adjunct to fasting duplex scanning to aide in the diagnosis of mesenteric artery stenoses.[12] In patients with less than 70% SMA stenosis, postprandial SMA PSV increases by more than 20% over baseline velocity. The percent increase in SMA PSV is less in patients with 70% or greater SMA stenosis. Specificity for the combination of fasting SMA PSV and postprandial PSV, however, is marginally improved over that provided by a fasting duplex scan alone. Therefore, although theoretically attractive, postprandial duplex

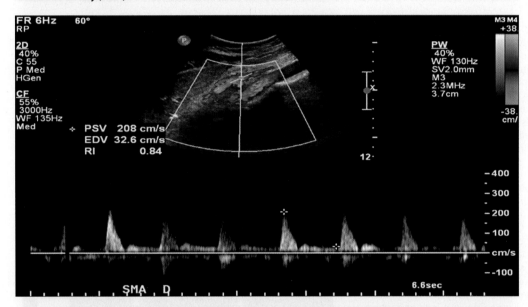

FIGURE 27-9 Duplex ultrasonography of superior mesenteric artery (SMA), with peak systolic velocity (PSV) of 208 cm/s signifying a normal SMA.

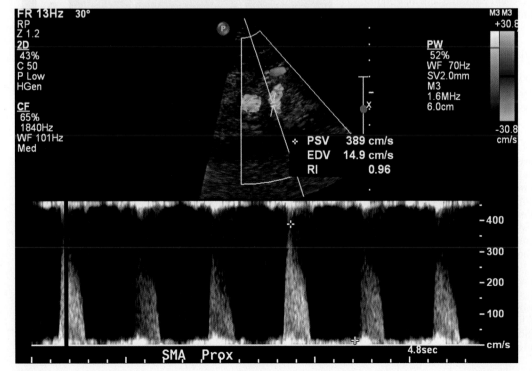

FIGURE 27-10 Duplex ultrasonography of superior mesenteric artery (SMA), with peak systolic velocity (PSV) of 389 cm/s signifying 70% or greater SMA stenosis.

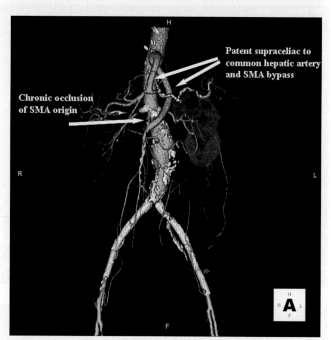

FIGURE 27-11 Duplex ultrasonography of celiac artery (CA), with peak systolic velocity (PSV) of 331 cm/s signifying 70% or greater CA stenosis.

scanning offers no significant improvement over fasting mesenteric duplex scanning; its routine use as part of ultrasound assessment of mesenteric artery stenosis is unnecessary. Postprandial examinations are occasionally useful in technically difficult ultrasound studies in that if there is a postprandial response, the insonated vessel can be confirmed as being the SMA.

Duplex ultrasonography is best used as an initial screening study to evaluate for visceral artery stenosis in patients with chronic abdominal pain that may be consistent with CMI. Angiography is required to establish a definitive diagnosis of mesenteric artery stenosis.

Computed Tomography

Standard CT imaging can be of some value in mesenteric artery stenosis evaluation (also see Chapter 14). Currently, however, no studies have compared the accuracy of spiral CT with angiography in assessing visceral artery stenoses. Computed tomography angiography can detect but not precisely quantify proximal stenosis of the CA and SMA, and it is limited by lower resolution and bowel motion artifact in its ability to detect lesions involving more distal branches.[13] Computed tomography scans are often obtained to evaluate abdominal pain. Findings suggestive of mesenteric artery stenosis include calcification at the origin of the CA and SMA and lack of contrast enhancement within the vessel lumen (Fig. 27-12).

Magnetic Resonance Imaging

Development of fast breath-hold three-dimensional gadolinium-enhanced magnetic resonance angiography (3D Gd-enhanced MRA) has improved the ability of MRA to detect proximal splanchnic artery lesions (also see Chapter 13). Magnetic resonance angiography is limited in its ability to image more distal visceral branches because of limited spatial resolution, peristaltic and respiratory motion, and chemical shift changes between the vessels and fat. The accuracy of 3D Gd-enhanced MRA in detecting visceral artery stenosis has been well studied. Overall sensitivity and specificity for detecting 75% or greater stenosis or occlusion of the CA, SMA, or inferior mesenteric artery (IMA) were 100% and 95%, respectively.[14]

In addition to providing anatomical details, magnetic resonance (MR) technology can quantify arterial flow using the phase-contrast magnetic resonance imaging (MRI) technique, which provides information about the presence, magnitude, and direction of blood flow and has been studied in patients with CMI.[15] Fasting and postprandial flow in the SMA have been compared in patients with documented atherosclerotic disease and normal volunteers. Mean fasting SMA blood flow has been shown to be higher in atherosclerotic patients than in normal individuals. This difference can be used to evaluate for CMI. The addition of MR oximetry technology, where increased oxygen extraction after a meal is seen in those with significant mesenteric vessel atherosclerosis, is promising with

FIGURE 27-12 Computed tomographic angiogram (CTA) demonstrating a patent supraceliac aorta to common hepatic artery, and superior mesenteric artery *(SMA)* bypass. Proximal SMA is occluded.

regard to diagnosing CMI.[15] Further validation studies correlating the degree of change in mesenteric blood flow and oxygenation with angiographic percentage of stenosis will be necessary before phase-contrast MRI and MR oximetry are universally adopted as routine noninvasive diagnostic methods for patients with CMI.

Treatment

Chronic and Acute Mesenteric Occlusive Disease

The available literature includes no randomized or controlled clinical trials of surgical intervention for treatment of mesenteric ischemia, and none are likely to be performed. Published clinical reports include varied recommendations for treatment, and many do not include descriptions of operative methods. Others describe technically demanding procedures requiring extensive dissections in difficult areas.[16,17] Only recently has objective determination of postoperative graft patency been included in clinical series.[18,19] For all these reasons, there is no current consensus regarding the surgical details of treatment for intestinal ischemia.

HISTORY

In 1936, Dunphy reviewed the medical records of 12 patients dying from intestinal ischemia and discovered that more than half (58%) had evidence of chronic abdominal pain.[20] This finding suggested that timely surgical intervention may have prevented progression to intestinal infarction and death. In 1957, Mikkelsen described the arteriographic appearance of typical orificial atherosclerotic lesions affecting the mesenteric arteries. That same year, the first successful surgical procedure (SMA endarterectomy) for treatment of chronic intestinal ischemia was performed by Maynard and Shaw.[21]

Since then, numerous techniques have been developed to revascularize the mesenteric arteries. One debated issue is the optimal number of vessels to revascularize. Proponents of multiple-vessel or "complete" revascularization have worried that although single-vessel bypass is effective in relieving symptoms initially, there may be a higher incidence of recurrent symptoms secondary to graft failure. With a few exceptions, as noted subsequently, surgery of some sort remains an integral part of the treatment of all etiologies of mesenteric ischemia.

MULTIPLE-VESSEL REVASCULARIZATION

Multiple-vessel revascularization implies repair or bypass of all diseased or occluded vessels, most often the CA and SMA. Most agree that bypass to the IMA is unnecessary for successful revascularization except in unusual cases. Grafts can be oriented antegrade from the supraceliac aorta or retrograde from the infrarenal aorta or an iliac artery.

An early report from the Mayo Clinic first suggested that "complete" revascularization resulted in decreased symptomatic recurrence.[22] A subsequent report including these patients and others indicated that graft patency and survival in patients with three-vessel revascularization were improved compared to single-vessel revascularization.[23] The authors speculated that this difference in outcome was a result of complete revascularization, which theoretically provides an additional measure of safety. These two studies, however, were limited to patients with chronic intestinal ischemia and did not use objective methods to determine postoperative graft patency. In the latter study, McAfee et al.[23] noted that symptoms of recurrent ischemia were an unreliable measure of graft patency because two of their three early occlusions were asymptomatic. Lack of symptoms may have resulted from the presence of additional patent grafts. Although these retrospective studies suggest that complete revascularization resulted in fewer recurrences and deaths, the results were not statistically significant.

Some believe that antegrade orientation provides better inflow than retrograde orientation because prograde flow is less turbulent, there may be less graft kinking, and the supraceliac aorta is usually less diseased than the infrarenal aorta or an iliac artery. In the Mayo Clinic series published in 1981, the symptomatic recurrence rate was 26%; none of these grafts were antegrade.[22] In more current studies in which the majority of grafts are positioned antegrade, the recurrence rate is lower.[24] Clearly, the reduction in recurrence is multifactorial and cannot be attributed solely to graft orientation.

More recent data suggest the rate of symptomatic recurrence is unaffected by the number of vessels revascularized or graft orientation. In a study of 91 patients treated for CMI with a bypass procedure, there were patients with both single- and multiple-vessel reconstructions and with grafts in either orientation. Survival was unaffected by number of vessels revascularized. Patients with retrograde grafts had decreased survival, but these patients were older than those with antegrade grafts.[24]

SINGLE-VESSEL REVASCULARIZATION

Proponents of single-vessel revascularization have reported long-term results similar to multiple-vessel revascularizations. Series from France have shown SMA reconstruction alone to be a durable form of treatment for intestinal ischemia. Kieny et al.[25] performed 60 direct or indirect (using a short prosthetic segment) reimplantations of the SMA (10% of patients had additional vessels reconstructed) in patients with atherosclerotic lesions of the visceral arteries. Mean follow-up was 8.5 years; five patients (8.3%) developed recurrences, and one patient died as a result. The 5-year actuarial survival was 69.6%.

Favorable results for single-vessel revascularization have also been reported in the United States.[26,27] Stanton et al.[26] performed 20 reconstructions in 17 patients, and at 60.9 months they found no symptomatic recurrences. One method of mesenteric revascularization is transaortic endarterectomy (TAE), with antegrade aortoceliac bypass reserved for older or poor-risk patients.[28] Transaortic endarterectomy usually involves revascularization of both the celiac axis and the SMA. Similar recurrence rates have been observed between the two techniques, with 86% of patients in both groups being asymptomatic at 5 years. Durable relief of symptoms did not appear to correlate with number of visceral arteries repaired.

At Oregon Health & Science University, the surgical approach to managing acute and CMI has changed in the last 2 decades. In 1994, Gentile et al.[27] reported 26 patients who had 29 isolated bypasses to the SMA for intestinal ischemia (23 chronic, 5 acute, 1 asymptomatic). Perioperative mortality was 10%. Mean follow-up was 40 months, and the life table–determined 4-year primary graft patency rate and survival rate were 89% and 82%, respectively. This compared favorably with contemporary reports in the literature. Based on this experience, revascularization of the SMA alone is recommended for most cases of intestinal ischemia.

Foley et al. recently reported a series of 50 SMA revascularizations, employing objective means to determine graft postoperative patency.[19] This series differed from others with respect to the larger number of patients with previous attempts at revascularization (24%), higher percentage of patients presenting with acute ischemia (42%), and higher percentage of patients requiring simultaneous bowel resection (28%). Overall perioperative mortality (12%), however, was comparable to other recent series. Perioperative mortality was 3% for patients operated on electively. The incidence of perioperative graft occlusions (6%) was similar to other recent series, only one of which contains a significant number of patients presenting with acute intestinal ischemia. Three graft occlusions occurred during long-term follow-up and resulted in death in two patients, accounting for 22% of late deaths. In this series, the number of symptomatic late graft occlusions, number of deaths attributable to recurrent ischemia, and life table–determined survival were comparable to other recent series employing more complete visceral revascularizations (Table 27-1).

Although acute mesenteric ischemia is accompanied by a higher perioperative mortality rate, McMillan et al.[29] found no differences in long-term patency of bypass grafts between patients with acute or chronic ischemia. Two of the three late occlusions in this series occurred in patients whose initial graft was placed for CMI, but one of these occluded in the perioperative period and was replaced. Revascularization of the SMA alone continues to compare favorably with more complete mesenteric revascularizations. Several authors have noted that symptoms are an insensitive measure of graft failure.[23,29] With improvements in duplex scanning, several studies have objective data for long-term graft patency.[29-31]

INDICATIONS FOR OPERATION

Revascularization is clearly indicated for symptomatic intestinal ischemia. Revascularization for asymptomatic high-grade SMA obstruction is recommended only in patients undergoing otherwise indicated aortic surgery for aneurysmal or occlusive disease. In this group of patients, acute intestinal ischemia following aortic surgery has been well documented, and SMA reconstruction seems prudent.[32]

TABLE 27-1   Recent Mesenteric Revascularization Outcomes

AUTHOR	PATIENTS (% ACUTE)	PERIOPERATIVE MORTALITY (%)	PERIOPERATIVE OCCLUSIONS (%)	LATE OCCLUSIONS*	% LATE DEATHS FROM ISCHEMIA	5-YEAR SURVIVAL† (%)
Foley 2000	50 (42)	12	6	3	22	61
Mateo 1999¶	85 (0)	8	3.5	16	21	64
Kihara 1999¶	42 (0)	10	0	4	33	70
Moawad 1997¶	24 (0)	4	4	2	25	71
McMillan 1995¶	25 (36)	12	4	0	0	N/A‡

*Symptomatic recurrences.
†Life-table determined.
‡Not available.
¶Included multiple-vessel revascularizations.
From Foley MI, Moneta GL, Abou-Zamzam AM, et al: Revascularization of the superior mesenteric artery alone for treatment of intestinal ischemia. J Vasc Surg 32:37, 2000; Mateo RB, O'Hara PJ, Hertzer NR, et al: Elective surgical treatment of symptomatic chronic mesenteric occlusive disease: early results and late outcomes. J Vasc Surg 29:821, 1999; Kihara TK, Blebea J, Anderson KM, et al: Risk factors and outcomes following revascularization for chronic mesenteric ischemia. Ann Vasc Surg 13:37, 1999; Moawad J, McKinsey JF, Wyble CW, et al: Current results of surgical therapy for chronic mesenteric ischemia. Arch Surg 132:613, 1997; and McMillan WD, McCarthy WJ, Bresticker M, et al: Mesenteric artery bypass: objective patency determination. J Vasc Surg 21:729, 1995.

TECHNIQUES OF SUPERIOR MESENTERIC ARTERY BYPASS

Retrograde Bypass

The distal infrarenal aorta as an origin for an SMA bypass graft has advantages and disadvantages. This exposure is familiar, and risks of dissection and clamping are less than with more proximal aortic exposures. In addition, the procedure can be readily combined with other intraabdominal vascular procedures. The primary disadvantage is that the infrarenal aorta and iliac arteries are frequently calcified, increasing the technical difficulty of the proximal anastomosis.

Prosthetic grafts are used most often in cases of mesenteric revascularization. Exceptions are cases complicated by bowel necrosis. For these patients, vein grafts are preferred to minimize the possibility of graft infection. Special attention to graft configuration must be paid to avoid graft kinking when the graft is placed in a retrograde configuration. A preference for the origin of the graft is from the area of the junction of the aorta and right common iliac artery (CIA), although any suitable site on the infrarenal aorta or either CIA is satisfactory. A single limb is cut from a bifurcation graft in the manner described by Wylie et al.; this provides a "flange" for sewing and prevents anastomotic stricture (Fig. 27-13). The ligament of Treitz is dissected. The proximal (inflow) anastomosis is completed first. The graft is then arranged first cephalad, then turning anteriorly and inferiorly a full 180 degrees to terminate in an antegrade anastomosis to the anterior wall of the SMA—just beyond the inferior border of the pancreas (Fig. 27-14). The graft is excluded from the peritoneal cavity by closing the mesenteric peritoneum, reapproximating the ligament of Treitz, and closing the posterior parietal peritoneum.

Antegrade Bypass

Antegrade bypasses originate from the anterior surface of the aorta proximal to the CA. The proximal aorta is exposed through the upper midline (Fig. 27-15) or, when the intraabdominal supraceliac aorta is calcified, using a low thoracoabdominal incision. Antegrade bypass provides prograde flow to the mesenteric vessels and is clearly the preferred approach in patients with contraindications to use of the infrarenal aorta or an iliac artery as a bypass origin. Visceral bypass grafts can be constructed to many supraceliac aortas with partial-occlusion clamping of the aorta, although in most cases the "partial" occlusion is near-total occlusion. Transient hepatic and renal ischemia is usually well tolerated but is a potential disadvantage to the antegrade approach. To minimize the risk associated with supraceliac aortic surgery, the procedure should be reserved for patients in whom this arterial segment is angiographically normal. Significantly diseased supraceliac aortas are dangerous origins for a visceral artery bypass.

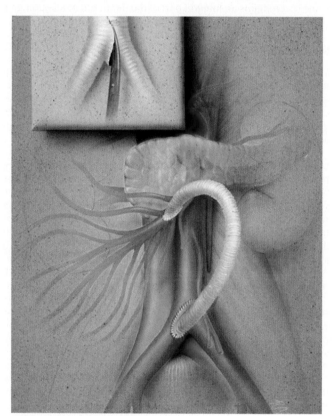

FIGURE 27-13   Artist's depiction of technique of infrarenal aorta–to–superior mesenteric artery (SMA) bypass. Graft is fashioned using one limb of a bifurcated graft.

Antegrade grafts to the SMA are normally tunneled behind the pancreas and anastomosed to the anterior wall of the SMA in end-to-side fashion (Fig. 27-16). A disadvantage of antegrade bypass is that the retropancreatic space is limited, and great care is necessary when tunneling the graft. Some surgeons advocate prepancreatic tunneling to avoid compression of the graft within the tunnel. A prepancreatic tunnel, however, places the graft in opposition to the posterior wall of the stomach and theoretically increases the possibility of graft infection. Occasionally, in the setting of very focal SMA origin disease and an easily mobilized pancreas, the antegrade bypass can be constructed entirely superior to the pancreas, obviating the need for a retropancreatic tunnel.

Postoperative Monitoring of Graft Patency

The authors use sterilized Doppler probes to confirm normal flow signals in visceral artery bypass grafts and in the native mesenteric arteries distal to the anastomotic sites after graft completion.

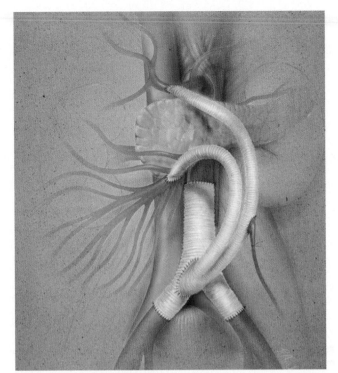

FIGURE 27-14 Artist's depiction of a retrograde mesenteric bypass to celiac and superior mesenteric arteries, with reimplantation of inferior mesenteric artery (IMA).

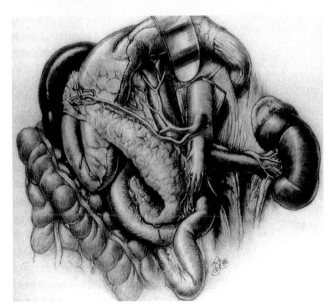

FIGURE 27-15 Artist's depiction of exposure of supraceliac aorta.

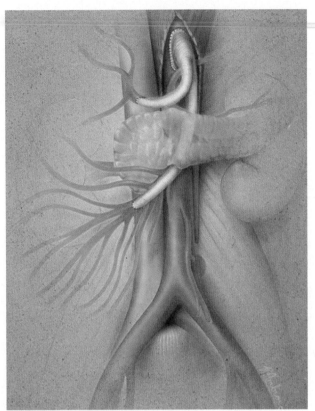

FIGURE 27-16 Artist's depiction of technique of antegrade bypass from supraceliac aorta to celiac and superior mesenteric arteries.

revascularization patency is prudent (Figs. 27-17 and 27-18). If the graft is occluded or otherwise unsatisfactory, reoperation is mandatory.

Postoperative Care

Patients with chronic visceral ischemia often have significant ischemic bowel injury that requires time for recovery. "Food fear" due to preoperative postprandial pain may persist at least temporarily.

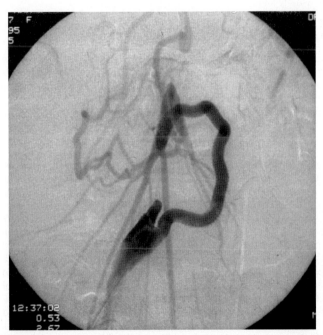

FIGURE 27-17 Postoperative arteriogram showing patent prosthetic graft from iliac artery to superior mesenteric artery (SMA).

Arterial Doppler signals should be easily detected on the antimesenteric border of the revascularized bowel as well. It is important to repeat Doppler insonation after all packs and retractors have been removed and after the viscera have been returned to the peritoneum. This approach helps minimize technical failures from graft kinking.

In contrast to the situation with other vascular repairs, continuous monitoring of the patency of visceral artery repairs is impossible in the postoperative period. Postoperative graft thrombosis may be asymptomatic or confused with other causes of postoperative pain. When symptoms do occur with resumption of oral intake, reoperation may be difficult or impossible because of postoperative inflammatory scarring. Thus, routine imaging of the reconstruction 5 to 7 days postoperatively to confirm visceral

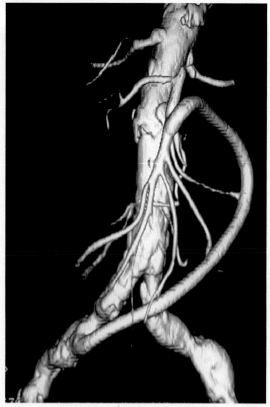

FIGURE 27-18 Postoperative computed tomographic angiogram (CTA) of a patent prosthetic graft from iliac artery to superior mesenteric artery (SMA).

Prolonged periods of inability to achieve adequate oral nutrition are frequent following visceral revascularization. For this reason, total parenteral nutrition is used liberally. Some patients with severe preoperative ischemia develop *postoperative revascularization syndrome*, which consists of abdominal pain, tachycardia, leukocytosis, and intestinal edema. It has been attributed to intestinal vasospasm after revascularization.[33] Any departure from a normal postoperative course should prompt arteriography, reexploration, or both. Delayed diagnosis of graft occlusion or intestinal necrosis is usually fatal.

ENDOVASCULAR THERAPY FOR MESENTERIC OCCLUSIVE DISEASE

Catheter-based therapy has become an accepted method for the treatment of mesenteric occlusive disease, especially in patients who are frail and unable to tolerate an operation, and those who have short-segment SMA disease. Whereas long-segment stenoses, heavily calcified arteries, or irregular plaques are generally more amenable to operative revascularization, short-segment SMA disease allows for angioplasty and stenting (Figs. 27-19 and 27-20) with good short-term and reasonable long-term results. Initial published series reported immediate technical success with endovascular therapy, but long-term success rates were disappointing early on and inferior to open surgery. Mortality and complication rates in these studies range from 0% to 6% and 0% to 32%, respectively.

In a study by Sharafuddin et al., 25 patients underwent angioplasty and stenting of the SMA or CA.[34] Primary patency determined by ultrasound was 92% at 6 months. Early series established that endovascular treatment of mesenteric artery stenosis is technically feasible, but no data were available with respect to long-term durability. More recently, Lee et al. showed a primary patency rate of 69% at 7 years, but freedom from recurrent symptoms was only 56%. Although endoluminal therapy for CMI carries low morbidity and mortality, long-term therapeutic benefit is not as reliably achieved; catheter-based treatment should be reserved for patients without a good surgical option.[35]

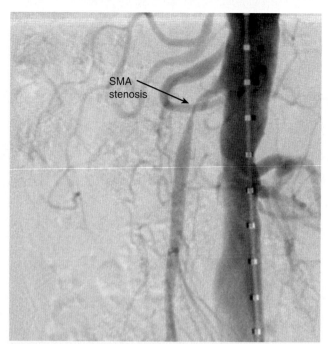

FIGURE 27-19 Lateral aortogram demonstrating stenosis of superior mesenteric artery *(SMA)* just prior to stent placement.

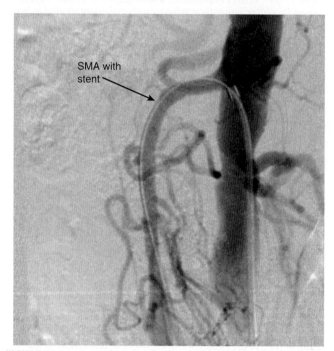

FIGURE 27-20 Lateral aortogram demonstrating patency of superior mesenteric artery *(SMA)* just after stent placement.

To date, there have been several studies, mostly retrospective, comparing the durability of endovascular revascularization for CMI with operative bypass. A comparison was made by Kasirajan et al.[36] where 28 patients were treated with percutaneous angioplasty (PTA) with and without stenting and compared to a previously reported series of 85 patients treated with a variety of operative procedures for CMI. Early complication rates and mortality rates were similar, but the rate of recurrent symptoms was higher in the PTA/stent group.[36] A second group, Sivamurthy et al.,[37] evaluated 60 patients treated with either operative reconstruction or angioplasty and stenting for CMI. Perioperative and 3-year mortality rates were similar between the groups, and overall patency rates were not statistically different. The major difference between these groups was the number of patients free from recurrent symptoms, which was worse in the angioplasty and stent group than in the operative group (46% vs. 71%, respectively).[37]

A recent paper by Davies et al.[38] confirms prior conclusions. Their group performed a retrospective review of 27 patients with 56 diseased vessels; 17 operative revascularizations were performed (38 vessels), and 15 endovascular reconstructions were performed (28 vessels). Both groups were similar in comorbidities and anatomy of disease. The primary patencies of the operative revascularizations and endovascular reconstructions groups was 83% and 54%, respectively. More patients in the operative revascularization group were free from symptoms at 1 and 2 years than in the endovascular repair group (100% vs. 73%, $P = 0.014$).[38] In another recent publication, Schermerhorn et al. looked at the Nationwide Inpatient Sample to compare mortality and complication rates between patients treated with PTA and stenting and patients treated with open surgery for mesenteric ischemia. This study included over 6000 patients undergoing PTA/stent and over 16,000 patients undergoing open surgery. Overall mortality rates were lower for those patients undergoing PTA/stent than after open surgery for both acute mesenteric ischemia (16% vs. 28%) and CMI (3.7% vs. 13%).[39]

Given these data, endovascular reconstruction for mesenteric ischemia is feasible and can be a good option, although long-term symptom recurrence is worse with angioplasty and stenting. Endovascular options, however, could be considered in patients requiring more time to improve nutritional status prior to undergoing elective bypass operations, or perhaps in those patients who have an expected short-term lifespan.

Summary

Symptomatic CMI remains uncommon. Recognition and treatment of CMI may avoid progression to acute ischemia, alleviate symptoms, and provide durable long-term relief. This may be accomplished by a number of techniques. Single-vessel bypass to the SMA compares favorably in terms of graft patency, death from recurrent ischemia, and survival to recent reports of intestinal revascularizations employing bypasses to multiple arteries.

With the small numbers of patients in previously published series, as well as differences in patient selection, it has been difficult to demonstrate a significant benefit of one technique over others. The technical issues involved in mesenteric revascularization are basic vascular surgical principles: choice of proximal anastomosis, distal target, and conduit. It is largely accepted that prosthetic grafts are effective for mesenteric revascularization. However, there has been considerable debate surrounding the choice of inflow vessel, number of vessels revascularized, and orientation of the graft. Surgeons should choose a revascularization procedure for CMI that fits the patient. It is not necessary to rigidly adhere to a single approach. If the operation is well planned and technically well performed, excellent results can be expected.

Acute Nonocclusive Mesenteric Ischemia

SIGNS AND SYMPTOMS

Acute NOMI occurs as a result of severe and prolonged mesenteric arterial vasospasm without evidence of arterial or venous obstruction and has been well documented. Twenty-five percent of patients with acute mesenteric ischemia have NOMI, and mortality rates between 30% and 90% have been reported.[40] Patients with NOMI are often critically ill with decreased cardiac output and episodes of hypotension. They also tend to have significant comorbidities that can result in decreased intestinal perfusion. Although a hypoperfusion state is present in most patients with NOMI, some have NOMI due to visceral vasoconstriction alone, as is the case with cocaine or ergot intoxication.[41,42] Early definitive diagnosis and treatment are essential for patient survival.

Recognition of factors associated with NOMI is critical to its prompt diagnosis. These include acute myocardial infarction (AMI), congestive heart failure (CHF), valvular heart disease, aortic dissection, cardiopulmonary bypass (CPB), renal failure requiring hemodialysis, sepsis, and the use of pharmacological agents such as vasopressors and digitalis.[43–45]

Findings on physical examination are varied and do not confirm or exclude the diagnosis of NOMI. Abdominal pain may be present and can vary widely in character, location, and intensity but is absent in 20% to 25% of patients with NOMI.[44] Abdominal distention with occult or frank gastrointestinal bleeding may be present. As in occlusive acute mesenteric ischemia, laboratory values are nonspecific.

RADIOLOGICAL DIAGNOSIS

Radiological evaluation of patients with NOMI is similar to that of patients with occlusive acute mesenteric ischemia. Plain abdominal films are obtained to rule out a perforated viscus. If technically feasible, duplex ultrasonography may detect persistent flow in the mesenteric arteries and exclude occlusive disease.

Patients suspected to have NOMI should undergo urgent mesenteric angiography to confirm the diagnosis. Significant mortality is associated with a delayed diagnosis. Images in the anteroposterior and lateral planes are obtained. Findings of NOMI include patent mesenteric arterial trunks, with tapered or spastic narrowing of visceral artery branches and impaired filling of intramural vessels.[44]

TREATMENT

The primary treatment of NOMI is correction of the systemic condition leading to generalized hypoperfusion. The largest percentage of patients with NOMI have severe cardiac failure.[46–53] Etiology of the cardiac failure is not as important as optimization of blood pressure and cardiac output with as little dependence as possible on agents that result in peripheral vasoconstriction.

In the past, digitalis was frequently used to treat congestive heart failure. Although digitalis is used much less frequently in modern practice, many patients remain on this drug or one of its derivatives. Patients treated with digitalis preparations are at risk for NOMI in the setting of worsening congestive heart failure.[50] Animal experiments indicate that baseline intestinal arterial resistance is not altered by digitalis, but compared with controls, arterial resistance in animals treated with digitalis *does* increase in response to intestinal venous hypertension.[54] Thus, patients who are treated with digitalis and have increases in portal pressure, such as occur with worsening heart failure, may be more susceptible to development of NOMI as a result of arterial mesenteric vasoconstriction. In patients with possible NOMI, digitalis preparations must be withdrawn and alternative medications used to treat underlying cardiac abnormalities.

In patients with peritonitis, an operation is required to adequately evaluate bowel viability. For this reason, catheter-based therapy alone is insufficient in patients with peritoneal findings. At operation, the bowel is inspected for viability and necrotic intestine removed. A handheld Doppler instrument is used to assess the mesenteric vessels proximally and distally.[55] Intravenous (IV) fluorescein is also used to evaluate areas of possible ischemia; absent, perivascular, or patchy fluorescein patterns represent areas of ischemia.[56] A "second look" procedure within 24 to 48 hours allows for reassessment of bowel viability, and additional bowel resection can be performed if necessary.

Mesenteric Venous Thrombosis

SIGNS AND SYMPTOMS

Patients with MVT present with a wide range of symptoms ranging from asymptomatic state to an acute abdomen with peritoneal signs on physical exam. Acute mesenteric ischemia occurs in approximately 25% of patients as a result of MVT.[57,58] Abdominal pain is the most common symptom and is present in approximately 80% of patients with documented MVT.[58] Typically, patients present with prolonged abdominal discomfort associated with abdominal distention related to increasing intestinal edema. With transmural bowel infarction, peritoneal findings may be present in addition to other symptoms such as nausea, vomiting, and/or gastrointestinal bleeding, which can be present in 20% to 30% of patients. Leukocytosis and metabolic acidosis may accompany MVT that has resulted in bowel infarction; these patients generally have reduced intravascular volume as a result of fluid third-spacing. In addition to urgent anticoagulation, they often need aggressive fluid resuscitation. Ileus is also present in these patients, and bowel rest and decompression with nasogastric suction is required.

Mesenteric venous thrombosis can be classified into primary or secondary thrombosis. Primary MVT is associated with hereditary or acquired hypercoagulation disorders including factor V Leiden and deficiencies of protein C, protein S, and antithrombin III. Secondary MVT can result from malignancy or inflammatory disorders, and is also associated with trauma, cirrhosis, portal hypertension, or oral contraceptives.

RADIOLOGICAL DIAGNOSIS

Plain abdominal radiographs are usually obtained in patients with abdominal pain. Free air suggestive of a perforated viscus should be ruled out. However, in most patients with MVT, plain abdominal radiographs show a nonspecific bowel gas pattern and are generally nondiagnostic.

In patients who have minimal abdominal pain or are asymptomatic, duplex ultrasonography may be used to evaluate patency of the mesenteric veins. The examination is performed after a period of fasting, and blood flow velocities within the aorta, inferior vena cava (IVC), hepatic veins, portal vein, hepatic artery, splenic vein, and superior mesenteric vein are evaluated. Additional information that can be obtained from duplex ultrasonography include the presence or absence of ascites, recanalized umbilical vein, and/or liver mass. Hepatopetal (toward the liver) or hepatofugal (away from the liver) flow within the portal vein can also be determined.

Duplex ultrasonography is limited in the evaluation of the mesenteric veins when there is severe ascites, recent surgery or liver biopsy, and obesity. Occasionally the liver is located high in the right upper quadrant and is obscured by ribs. In patients with peritoneal findings, duplex ultrasonography is difficult to perform because of patient discomfort and significant amounts of bowel gas.

Currently, contrast-enhanced abdominal CT scanning is the diagnostic study of choice in patients suspected of having MVT. In addition to MVT, CT scanning can accurately detect portal and ovarian vein thrombosis. Other suggestive findings include bowel-wall thickening, pneumatosis intestinalis, or mesenteric edema. In one series, contrast-enhanced abdominal CT scanning was diagnostic for MVT in 90% of patients.[58]

Arterioportography is indicated when associated arterial ischemia is suspected or when findings on abdominal CT scanning are equivocal. The mesenteric venous system cannot be directly punctured, but is visualized indirectly through catheter-directed contrast injections into the SMA and CA, followed by delayed filming (Fig. 27-21). Mesenteric venous thrombosis is demonstrated by a filling defect within the mesenteric veins.

TREATMENT

Urgent laparotomy is undertaken in patients with peritoneal findings. This is a minority of patients with MVT. Perioperative broad-spectrum antibiotics are administered. Findings at laparotomy consist of edema and cyanotic discoloration of the mesentery and bowel wall with thrombus involving the distal mesenteric veins. Complete thrombosis of the superior mesenteric vein is rare, occurring in only 12% of patients undergoing laparotomy for suspected MVT.[59] The arterial supply to the involved bowel is usually intact.

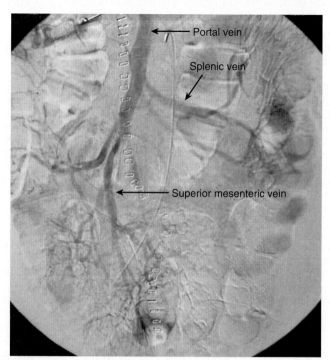

FIGURE 27-21 **Aortoportography demonstrating patent portal vein, superior mesenteric vein, and splenic vein.**

Nonviable bowel is resected and primary anastomosis performed. If viability of the remaining bowel is in question, a repeat "second look" operation is performed in 24 to 48 hours. Thrombolytic therapy or surgical thrombectomy of mesenteric veins is not required; these interventions are not usually technically successful.

In patients without peritoneal findings, anticoagulation with IV unfractionated heparin (UFH) is promptly initiated, and the patient is observed with serial abdominal examinations while maintaining bowel rest. Ileus may be prolonged, so hyperalimentation should be considered early. Once the patient's clinical status improves, oral intake can be cautiously introduced. A search for a predisposing primary or secondary hypercoagulable condition is required. In the interim, the patient is transitioned to oral anticoagulation over 3 to 4 days, once intestinal function has returned. Lifelong anticoagulation is usually maintained, especially in cases of idiopathic MVT or when an uncorrectable hypercoagulable state has been identified.

REFERENCES

1. Char DJ, Cuadra SA, Hines GL, et al: Surgical intervention for acute intestinal ischemia: experience in a community teaching hospital, *Vasc Endovascular Surg* 37:245, 2003.
2. Sreenarasimhaiah J: Diagnosis and management of intestinal ischemic disorders, *BMJ* 326:1372, 2003.
3. Menke J: Diagnostic accuracy of multidetector CT in acute mesenteric ischemia: systematic review and meta-analysis, *Radiology* 256:93–101, 2010.
4. Lin PH, Bush RL, Lumsden AB: Treatment of acute visceral artery occlusive disease. In Zelenock GB, Huber TS, Messina LM, et al, editors: *Mastery of vascular and endovascular surgery*, Philadelphia, 2006, Lippincott, Williams & Wilkins, p 295.
5. Jager K, Bollinger A, Valli C, et al: Measurement of mesenteric blood flow by duplex scanning, *J Vasc Surg* 3:462, 1986.
6. Moneta GL, Taylor DC, Helton WS, et al: Duplex ultrasound measurement of postprandial intestinal blood flow: effect of meal composition, *Gastroenterology* 95:1294, 1988.
7. Nicholls SC, Kohler TR, Martin RL, et al: Use of hemodynamic parameters in the diagnosis of mesenteric insufficiency, *J Vasc Surg* 3:507, 1986.
8. Moneta GL, Yeager RA, Dalman R, et al: Duplex ultrasound criteria for diagnosis of splanchnic artery stenosis or occlusion, *J Vasc Surg* 14:511, 1991.
9. Moneta GL, Lee RW, Yeager RA, et al: Mesenteric duplex scanning: a blinded prospective study, *J Vasc Surg* 17:79, 1993.
10. Bowersox JC, Zwolak RM, Walsh DB, et al: Duplex ultrasonography in the diagnosis of celiac and mesenteric artery occlusive disease, *J Vasc Surg* 14:780, 1991.
11. Zwolak RM, Fillinger MF, Walsh DB, et al: Mesenteric and celiac duplex scanning: a validation study, *J Vasc Surg* 27:1078, 1998.
12. Gentile AT, Moneta GL, Lee RW, et al: Usefulness of fasting and postprandial duplex ultrasound examinations for predicting high-grade superior mesenteric artery stenosis, *Am J Surg* 169:476, 1995.

13. Aschoff AJ, Stuber G, Becker BW, et al: Evaluation of acute mesenteric ischemia: accuracy of biphasic mesenteric multi-detector CT angiography, *Abdom Imaging* 34:345–357, 2008.

14. Shih MC, Hagspiel KD: CTA and MRA in mesenteric ischemia: part 1, role in diagnosis and differential diagnosis, *AJR Am J Roentgenol* 188:452–461, 2007.

15. Chow LC, Chan FP, Li KC: A comprehensive approach to MR imaging of mesenteric ischemia, *Abdom Imaging* 27:507–516, 2002.

16. Zeller T, Rastan A, Sixt S: Chronic atherosclerotic mesenteric ischemia, *Vasc Med* 15: 333–338, 2010.

17. Beebe HG, MacFarlane S, Raker EJ: Supraceliac aortomesenteric bypass for intestinal ischemia, *J Vasc Surg* 5:749, 1987.

18. Kruger AF, Walker PJ, Foster WJ, et al: Open surgery for atherosclerotic chronic mesenteric ischemia, *J Vasc Surg* 46:941–945, 2007.

19. Foley MI, Moneta GL, Abou-Zamzam AM, et al: Revascularization of the superior mesenteric artery alone for treatment of intestinal ischemia, *J Vasc Surg* 32:37, 2000.

20. Dunphy JE: Abdominal pain of vascular origin, *Am J Med Sci* 192:109, 1936.

21. Shaw RS, Maynard EP III: Acute and chronic thrombosis of the mesenteric arteries associated with malabsorption: a report of two cases successfully treated with thromboembolectomy, *N Engl J Med* 258:874, 1958.

22. Hollier LH, Bernatz PE, Pairolero PC, et al: Surgical management of chronic intestinal ischemia: a reappraisal, *Surgery* 90:940, 1991.

23. McAfee MK, Cherry KJ, Naessens JM, et al: Influence of complete revascularization on chronic mesenteric ischemia, *Am J Surg* 164:220, 1992.

24. Park WM, Cherry KJ Jr, Chua HK, et al: Current results of open revascularization for chronic mesenteric ischemia: a standard for comparison, *J Vasc Surg* 35:853, 2002.

25. Kieny R, Batellier J, Kretz J: Aortic reimplantation of the superior mesenteric artery for atherosclerotic lesions of the visceral arteries: sixty cases, *Ann Vasc Surg* 4:122, 1990.

26. White CJ: Chronic mesenteric ischemia: diagnosis and management, *Prog Cardiovasc Dis* 54:36–40, 2011.

27. Gentile AT, Moneta GL, Taylor LM Jr, et al: Isolated bypass to the superior mesenteric artery for intestinal ischemia, *Arch Surg* 129:926, 1994.

28. Rapp JH, Reilly LM, Qvarfordt PG, et al: Durability of endarterectomy and antegrade grafts in the treatment of chronic visceral ischemia, *J Vasc Surg* 3:799, 1986.

29. McMillan WD, McCarthy WJ, Bresticker M, et al: Mesenteric artery bypass: objective patency determination, *J Vasc Surg* 21:729, 1995.

30. Moneta GL: Screening for mesenteric vascular insufficiency and follow-up of mesenteric bypass procedures, *Semin Vasc Surg* 14:186, 2001.

31. Oderich GS, Malgor RD, Ricotta JJ: Open and endovascular revascularization for chronic mesenteric ischemia: tabular review of the literature, *Ann Vasc Surg* 23(5):700–712, 2009.

32. Connolly JE, Stemmer EA: Intestinal gangrene as the result of mesenteric arterial steal, *Am J Surg* 126:197, 1973.

33. Gewertz BL, Zarins CK: Postoperative vasospasm after antegrade mesenteric revascularization: a report of three cases, *J Vasc Surg* 14:382, 1991.

34. Sharafuddin MJ, Olson CH, Sun S, et al: Endovascular treatment of celiac and mesenteric arteries stenoses: applications and results, *J Vasc Surg* 38:692, 2003.

35. Lee RW, Bakken AM, Palchik E, et al: Long-term outcomes of endoluminal therapy for chronic atherosclerotic occlusive mesenteric disease, *Ann Vasc Surg* 22:541–546, 2008.

36. Kasirajan K, O'Hara PJ, Gray BH, et al: Chronic mesenteric ischemia: open surgery versus percutaneous angioplasty and stenting, *J Vasc Surg* 33:63–71, 2001.

37. Sivamurthy N, Rhodes JM, Lee D, et al: Endovascular versus open mesenteric revascularization: immediate benefits do not equate with short-term functional outcomes, *J Am Coll Surg* 202:859–867, 2006.

38. Davies R, Wall ML, Silverman SH, et al: Surgical versus endovascular reconstruction for chronic mesenteric ischemia: a contemporary UK series, *Vasc Endovascular Surg* 43(2): 157–164, 2009.

39. Schermerhorn ML, Giles KA, Hamdan AD, et al: Mesenteric revascularization: management and outcomes in the United States, 1988–2006, *J Vasc Surg* 50:341–348, 2009.

40. Klotz S, Vestring T, Rotker J, et al: Diagnosis and treatment of nonocclusive mesenteric ischemia after open heart surgery, *Ann Thorac Surg* 72:1583, 2001.

41. Green FL, Ariyan S, Stausel HC Jr: Mesenteric and peripheral vascular ischemia secondary to ergotism, *Surgery* 81:311, 1977.

42. Myers SI, Clagett GP, Valentine RJ, et al: Chronic intestinal ischemia caused by intravenous cocaine use: report of two cases and review of the literature, *J Vasc Surg* 23:724, 1996.

43. Diamond S, Emmett M, Henrich W: Bowel infarction as a cause of death in dialysis patients, *JAMA* 256:2545, 1986.

44. Bassiouny H: Nonocclusive mesenteric ischemia, *Surg Clin North Am* 77:319, 1997.

45. Valentine R, Whelan T, Meyers H: Non-occlusive mesenteric ischemia in renal patients: recognition and prevention of intestinal gangrene, *Am J Kidney Dis* 15:598, 1990.

46. Zeier M, Weisel M, Ritz E: Non-occlusive mesenteric infarction in dialysis patients: risk factors, diagnosis, intervention and outcome, *Int J Artif Organs* 15:387, 1992.

47. John A, Tuerff S, Kerstein M: Nonocclusive mesenteric infarction in hemodialysis patients, *J Am Coll Surg* 190:84, 2000.

48. Aldrete JS, Hansy SY, Laws HL, et al: Intestinal infarction complicating low cardiac output states, *Surg Gynecol Obstet* 144:371, 1977.

49. Williams LF, Anastasia LF, Hasiotis CA: Nonocclusive mesenteric infarction, *Am J Surg* 114:376, 1967.

50. Britt LG, Cheek RC: Nonocclusive mesenteric vascular disease: clinical and experimental observations, *Ann Surg* 169:704, 1969.

51. Garofalo M, Borioni R, Nardi P, et al: Early diagnosis of acute mesenteric ischemia after cardiopulmonary bypass, *J Card Surg* 43:455–459, 2002.

52. Venkateswaran RV, Charman SC, Goddard M, et al: Lethal mesenteric ischaemia after cardiopulmonary bypass: a common complication? *Eur J Cardiothorac Surg* 22: 534–538, 2002.

53. Landreueau RJ, Fry WJ: The right colon as a target organ of nonocclusive mesenteric ischemia, *Arch Surg* 125:591, 1990.

54. Kim EH, Gewertz BL: Chronic digitalis administration alters mesenteric vascular reactivity, *J Vasc Surg* 5:382, 1987.

55. Hobson RW II, Wright CB, Rich NM, et al: Assessment of colonic ischemia during aortic surgery by Doppler ultrasound, *J Surg Res* 20:231, 1976.

56. Gloviczki P, Bergman RT, Stanson AW, et al: The role of intravenous fluorescein in the detection of colon ischemia during aortic reconstruction, *Int Angiol* 11:281, 1992.

57. Rhee RY, Gloviczki P, Jost C, et al: Acute mesenteric venous thrombosis. In Gloviczki P, Yao JST, editors: *Handbook of venous disorders*, New York, 2001, Arnold, p 321.

58. Morasch MD, Ebaugh JL, Chiou AC, et al: Mesenteric venous thrombosis: a changing clinical entity, *J Vasc Surg* 34:680, 2001.

59. Rhee RY, Gloviczki P, Mendonca CT, et al: Mesenteric venous thrombosis: still a lethal disease in the 1990s, *J Vasc Surg* 20:688, 1994.

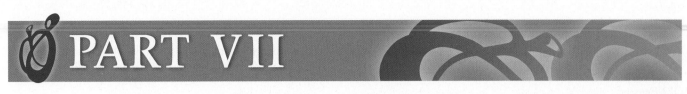

PART VII

VASCULOGENIC ERECTILE DYSFUNCTION

CHAPTER **28** # Vasculogenic Erectile Dysfunction

Kirk A. Keegan, David F. Penson

Introduction

The first historical descriptions of erectile dysfunction (ED) date back to Egyptian papyrus nearly 4000 years ago. Egyptian scholars described two types of ED: a "natural" form in which the man was incapable of performing the sex act, and a "supernatural" form rooted in evil charms and spells.[1] Ancient thinkers such as Hippocrates and Aristotle also theorized on the etiology of ED. However, the first accurate depiction of penile anatomy and rudimentary analysis of erection was not published until 1585, when Ambroise Paré described it in his *Ten Books on Surgery* and the *Book of Reproduction*.[2] In these texts, Paré portrayed the penis as a tube with concentric coats of nerves, veins, arteries, two "ligaments" composed of the corpora cavernosa, and the urinary tract.

Over the succeeding centuries, there has been considerable investigation into the hemodynamic and anatomical mechanisms of male erection. Modern understanding of erectile physiology has been delineated only in the last 30 years. Central to our current theories of erectile physiology is the role of smooth muscle in control of arterial and venous flow, the architecture of the tunica albuginea, the role of nitric oxide (NO) as the principal neurotransmitter regulating tumescence, and the function of phosphodiesterases (PDEs) for detumescence. Recent research on the role of endothelial regulation of smooth muscle, the influence of ion channels, and the integral function of endothelial gap junctions has furthered our understanding. This chapter will review these findings, as well as the prevalence, clinical evaluation, diagnostic testing, medical and surgical management, clinical outcomes, and current guidelines regarding vasculogenic ED in detail.

Definition and Classifications

In 1992, the National Institutes of Health convened a Consensus Development Conference on Impotence. The group renamed impotence as *male erectile dysfunction* and defined it as "the inability to achieve or maintain an erection sufficient for satisfactory sexual performance."[3] Furthermore, they noted that *erectile dysfunction* represents the most appropriate term, given that sexual desire, orgasm, and ejaculation may be intact despite inability to achieve or maintain erection.

Multiple schema have been proposed to classify the different types of ED. Broadly, ED can be described in terms of organic and psychogenic dysfunction (Box 28-1). The main thrust of this chapter will center on vasculogenic ED, which comprises impaired endothelial function, arterial occlusive disease, veno-occlusive dysfunction, and structural changes to the corpora cavernosa.

Prevalence and Incidence

Erectile dysfunction is quite common, affecting approximately 30 million men in the United States.[4] Several population-based studies have been performed to address male sexual function and specifically the prevalence and incidence of ED in the American male population.

The 1992 National Health Social and Life Survey (NHSLS) was a national survey of 1410 American men between the ages of 18 and 59. In the study group, the prevalence of ED in men aged 18 to 29 years was 7%, aged 30 to 39 was 9%, aged 40 to 49 was 11%, and aged 50 to 59 was 18%.[5] The Massachusetts Male Aging Study (MMAS), a longitudinal population-based study, evaluated 1709 men between the ages of 40 and 70 who returned questionnaires about a broad range of physiological measures, demographic information, and self-reported sexual function. Participants were surveyed between the years 1987 and 1989 and then reevaluated between 1995 and 1997. In this series, the age-adjusted prevalence of significant ED was 39% in men with coronary artery disease (CAD), 25% in men with diabetes mellitus, and 15% in men with hypertension. Incidence of ED on reevaluation was 25.9 cases per 1000 men per year (95% confidence interval [CI], 22.5-29.9).[6] Using these data, it was estimated that for Caucasian men, 617,715 new cases of ED would present in the 40 to 69 age group each year.[7] Data from European and Brazilian researchers suggest a similar incidence of ED in their respective countries.[8,9]

Functional Anatomy

The functional anatomy of the human penis is composed of several key components. Principally, these are three cylindrical structures—two corpora cavernosa surrounded by a tough tunica albuginea, and the solitary corpus spongiosum which contains the urethra. Vascular components include arteries and arterioles, highly compliant sinusoids within the corpora cavernosa, and compressible venules and veins.

Corporal Bodies, Sinusoids, and Glans

The corpora cavernosa are paired spongy cylinders that lie on the superior aspect of the penis. They are enveloped by the tunica albuginea. The proximal ends of the corpora are separate structures anchored at the ischial ramus. The corpora then fuse underneath the pubic ramus and share a common septum distally towards the glans.

Within the corpora, interconnected sinusoids are enveloped by trabeculae of smooth muscle, collagen, and elastin (Fig. 28-1). The sinusoidal smooth muscle is in intimate association with the cavernous nerves and helicine arteries within the penis. The sinusoids are tonically constricted during the flaccid state. Arterial blood flow diffuses through larger central sinusoids to smaller peripheral sinusoids. In the flaccid state, this slow diffusion of arterial blood results in blood gas values similar to venous blood. During sexual stimulation, release of neurotransmitters causes the smooth muscle around the sinusoids to relax. This results in rapid influx of arterial blood, subsequent entrapment of blood within these expanding sinusoids, and occlusion of veins traversing the tunica albuginea. Subsequent tumescence results in pressure increases of several hundred mmHg and blood gas values approaching arterial levels.[10]

Box 28-1 International Society of Impotence Research Classification of Erectile Dysfunction

Organic
I. Vasculogenic
II. Neurogenic
III. Anatomic
IV. Endocrine

Psychogenic
I. Generalized
  A. Lack of Response
  B. Inhibition
II. Situational
  A. Partner related
  B. Performance related
  C. Distress related

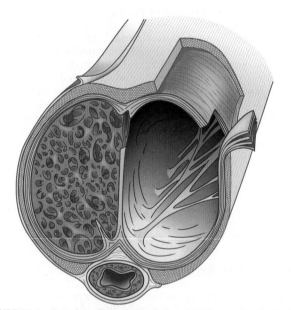

FIGURE 28-1 Drawing of three-dimensional anatomy of human penis, demonstrating inner circular layers and outer longitudinal layers of the tunica albuginea, intervening supports, sinusoidal tissue in corpora cavernosa, corpus spongiosum, and urethra.

The interior of the glans and corpus spongiosum share a similar sinusoidal architecture as the corpora cavernosa. However, the tunica surrounding the spongiosum is thinner and is completely absent around the glans. The corpus spongiosum is a highly compliant body that houses the urethra and facilitates expulsion of semen. The glans is exquisitely sensitive, conical in shape, eases intromission, and forms a cushion for the rigid corporal bodies. These areas engorge in a similar fashion as the corpora cavernosa but to a lesser degree, largely owing to an absence of the tunica albuginea and diminished venous trapping.

Tunica Albuginea

The tunica albuginea is composed primarily of tough type I collagen with a minority component of more flexible type III collagen and elastin. It is arranged in a bilayer, with inner circular layers and outer longitudinal layers (see Fig. 28-1). Intervening struts traverse the body of the corpora cavernosa and provide further support.[11] The longitudinal layers of the tunica are present from the glans to the proximal crura, where each corporal body inserts into its ischial ramus to form a foundation for support of the erect penis. Emissary veins (Fig. 28-2) pierce the tunica albuginea. During engorgement, these veins become compressed and allow entrapment of blood within the penis.

Arterial System

The internal pudendal artery, a branch of the internal iliac artery (IIA), is the principal source of blood flow to the penis. Up to 70% of men may have accessory pudendal branches that originate from the external iliac, obturator, or vesical arteries.[12] The internal pudendal artery gives rise to the penile artery, which in turn branches in to the dorsal, bulbourethral, and cavernous arteries (Fig. 28-3). The cavernous artery supplies the corpus cavernosum via helicine arteries, which lie in close approximation to the sinusoidal tissue. During erection, these vessels dilate, resulting in engorgement.

Venous System

Venous drainage originates from the three corporal bodies. Venules interdigitate through the cavernosal sinusoids and coalesce below the tunica albuginea into a subtunical plexus. The plexi then form emissary veins that penetrate the tunica albuginea. From there, numerous subcutaneous veins course along the shaft of the penis to form the superficial dorsal vein and a deep dorsal venous system, which in turn drain into the saphenous vein and retropubic venous plexus, respectively[13] (Fig. 28-4; also see Fig. 28-2).

Nervous System

Penile innervation occurs via both autonomic (parasympathetic and sympathetic) and somatic (motor and sensory) pathways. Erection and detumescence are largely regulated via the autonomic system. Sympathetic and parasympathetic nerves coalesce to form the cavernous nerve, which penetrates the corpora cavernosa to exert its effect on erection (Fig. 28-5). Sensation and contraction of penile musculature occurs via the somatic nerves.

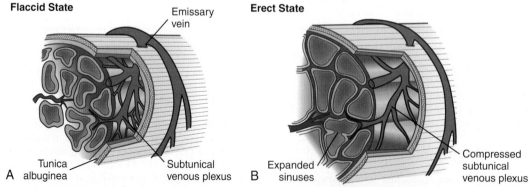

FIGURE 28-2 **Penile erection. A,** When flaccid, the corpora cavernosa, including arterioles, sinusoids, and arteries, are contracted. This allows free flow of blood through intervening sinusoidal spaces. Blood exits the corpora cavernosa via emissary veins. **B,** During erection, arterioles, sinusoids, and arteries relax. This constricts venules and veins and effectively compresses emissary veins under the tunica albuginea. Vascular inflow exceeds outflow, effectively creating an erection.

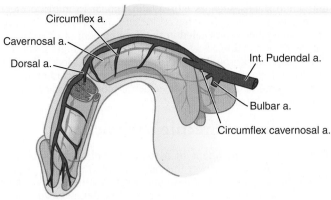

FIGURE 28-3   Penile arterial supply.

AUTONOMIC PATHWAYS

Between the T11 and L2 spinal segments, the sympathetic trunk begins. These fibers then form the sympathetic chain ganglia, which continue caudally to the inferior mesenteric and superior hypogastric plexi. Further sympathetic fibers exit to form the hypogastric nerves, and ultimately the sympathetic portions of the pelvic plexus.[14]

Between the S2-S4 spinal cord segments, the parasympathetic pathway originates. These fibers also continue caudally to the pelvic plexus (see Fig. 28-5), where they join the aforementioned sympathetic nerves. Together, these nerves then join to form a network of nervous tissue that passes along the lateral and posterior aspect of the prostate to create the cavernous nerves.[15] Stimulation of the sympathetic trunk via the cavernous nerves results in detumescence. Excitation of the parasympathetic aspects of the pelvic plexus and cavernous nerves is responsible for erection. To avoid iatrogenic ED, clear understanding of the location of these nerves is critical during pelvic surgery such as radical prostatectomy or abdominal perineal resection.

SOMATIC PATHWAYS

Sensory receptors in the penile skin and glans are unique in the human body.[16] They are composed of free nerve endings comprising unmyelinated C fibers and thin myelinated A-delta fibers. These coalesce into the dorsal nerve of the penis, which ultimately forms the pudendal nerve. The pudendal nerve then enters the S2-S4 nerve roots at the spinal cord. Via spinothalamic and spinoreticular pathways, sensations such as touch, pain, and temperature are

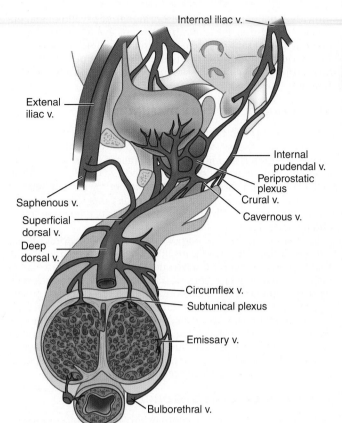

FIGURE 28-4   Penile venous drainage.

perceived.[17] Interestingly, research by Burnett et al.[18] suggests that the dorsal nerve of the penis carries both autonomic and somatic signals, and therefore contributes to penile sensation, erection, and ejaculation.

Pathophysiology of Erectile Dysfunction

Vasculogenic Erectile Dysfunction

As noted in Box 28-1, ED often represents a multifactorial disease state. Although the focus of this chapter is on the vasculogenic determinants of ED, it is worth noting that within an

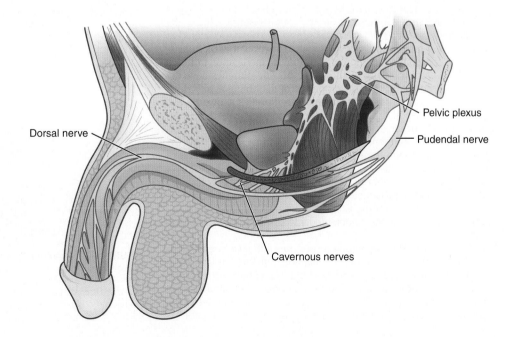

FIGURE 28-5   Penile nerves.

individual patient, neurological, hormonal, or psychological etiologies of ED may be of contributory or even primary importance. With that said, it is clear the vascular system is responsible for providing blood flow to the erectile tissues of the penis, so any dysfunction within the vascular system may affect erectile function.

ARTERIOGENIC ERECTILE DYSFUNCTION

Arteriogenic ED can be due to atherosclerotic or traumatic arterial occlusive disease. Michal and Ruzbarsky[19] noted impaired penile perfusion is an indicator of generalized atherosclerotic disease, and that the age of onset of ED and CAD is often similar. In fact, ED has been shown to be a bellwether for development of CAD in asymptomatic men,[20] and both diseases share the same risk factors—specifically smoking, diabetes, hypercholesterolemia, and hypertension.[21]

In arteriogenic ED, the corpora cavernosa demonstrate lower oxygen tension,[22] which may result in a decreased volume of sinusoidal smooth muscle and subsequent venous leak.[23] In an experimental animal model, rabbits with iatrogenic iliac atherosclerotic disease demonstrated alterations in their downstream penile arteries and a reduction in cavernosal smooth muscle content.[24] These alterations were associated with decreased nitric oxide synthase (NOS)- and NO-mediated relaxation of corpora cavernosal tissue.[25] Erectile dysfunction due to traumatic stenosis of cavernous or pudendal arteries has been noted in young men with pelvic trauma[26] and in long-distance cyclists.[27]

VENOGENIC ERECTILE DYSFUNCTION

Not only can diabetes, hypertension, hypercholesterolemia, and penile injury result in penile arterial disease, these disorders can also result in loss of elastic fibers within the cavernosal venules and sinusoids. This loss of compliance results in diminished venous trapping and subsequent veno-occlusive dysfunction.[28] In fact, diminished venous occlusion may represent the most common form of vasculogenic ED.[29] Loss of smooth muscle relaxation due to heightened adrenergic tone or decreased NO release may exacerbate already poor compliance in these fibrotic sinusoids.[30] Finally, fibrosis leading to increased collagen deposition between cell membranes may abolish critical signaling and intercellular transmission via disrupted gap junctions.[31]

Drug-Induced (Iatrogenic) Erectile Dysfunction

The data are clear that diabetes, hypercholesterolemia, and hypertension have strong influences on ED. Not surprisingly, some of the medications used to treat these disorders have been implicated as contributing factors in its development. However, it is often difficult to ascertain the direction of causation in medication-induced ED. Of the cardiovascular medications, thiazide diuretics have the strongest association with development of ED. Chang et al.[32] demonstrated that men treated with thiazide diuretics showed a significant increase in ED relative to those men prescribed placebo medication. Further evidence of the role of thiazides in ED was noted in the Treatment of Mild Hypertension Study (TOMHS), which demonstrated the prevalence of ED was twofold higher in men taking a thiazide versus placebo or other agent.[33] Curiously, after 4 years of treatment in this study, prevalence of ED within the placebo group approached that of those receiving thiazide. The significance of this finding is unclear but may be related to early unmasking of clinically undetected ED in those men receiving thiazides.

Nonselective β-blockers such as propranolol have been shown to inhibit erection compared to placebo, but this has not been demonstrated in selective β_1-antagonists.[34] In clinical series, there does not appear to be a deleterious influence of either angiotensin-converting enzyme (ACE) inhibitors or calcium channel blockers on erection.[33,35] Interestingly, angiotensin receptor antagonists

and some statins, such as atorvastatin, appear to improve erectile function.[36,37] Of note, some α-blockers, such as terazosin, have occasionally been implicated in the development of priapism, or pathological erection, likely related to the α-adrenergic blockade of the sympathetic outflow necessary for detumescence.[38] Other medications implicated in the development of ED include spironolactone, some antipsychotics, selective serotonin reuptake inhibitors, opiates, and antiandrogens.[39]

Evaluation of Erectile Dysfunction

Evaluation and treatment of a man presenting with ED has changed considerably over the last 30 years. This shift is largely due to the influence of oral therapies for treatment and a transition to a more patient-centered and evidence-based treatment plan. Evaluation should begin with an in-person and detailed medical, sexual, and psychosocial history (Fig. 28-6). Additionally, the use of a quantifiable questionnaire such as the International Index of Erectile Function (IIEF)[40] may be useful to establish baseline sexual function and to assess future treatment efficacy.

History

The history should begin with a thorough discussion of the patient's medical history, with particular attention to medical comorbidities. As previously mentioned, ED is an early marker for systemic atherosclerotic disease, and all patients should be questioned about their cardiovascular health.[41] In particular, a detailed discussion regarding any chest pain, palpitations, dyspnea, and limb pain may reveal occult CAD, congestive heart failure, or peripheral artery disease. Querying the patient about his medication use may elucidate agents that contribute to ED or may be contraindications to oral PDE therapy (e.g., nitrates). A sexual history should focus on timing, duration, and severity

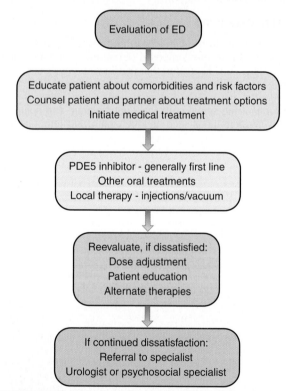

FIGURE 28-6 **Algorithm for evaluation of erectile dysfunction (ED).** PDE, phosphodiesterase 5. (*Adapted from Lue TF, Giuliano F, Montorsi F, et al: Summary of the Recommendations on sexual dysfunctions in men, J Sex Med 1:6–23, 2004, and Lue, TF, Broderick, GA: Evaluation and nonsurgical management of erectile dysfunction and premature ejaculation. In Wein AJ, Kavoussi LR, Nocik AC, et al, editors: Campbell-Walsh Urology, ed 9, Philadelphia, 2007, Saunders, pp 751–752.*)

of the patient's ED, as well as the occurrence of other associated problems, such as premature ejaculation, desire, or anorgasmia. To complete the sexual history, a psychosocial evaluation may be relevant; sexual dysfunction may affect self-esteem and coping. Both depression and treatment for depression may be associated with ED.

Physical Examination

Physical examination may be equally revealing. The patient's general appearance may alert the physician to serious underlying cardiovascular disease if the patient is cyanotic, dyspneic, emaciated, or plethoric. Additional pertinent findings on physical examination include general body habitus, secondary sex characteristics, staining of fingers associated with smoking, nail clubbing, lower-extremity ulcers, or edema. A thorough cardiopulmonary examination is required. Finally, an examination of the genitalia may demonstrate chordee, Peyronie disease, or signs of hypogonadism such as Kallmann's or Klinefelter's syndromes.

Laboratory Assessments

Laboratory testing for men with sexual dysfunction may include fasting glucose, lipid levels, sex hormone values (including morning free and total testosterone levels), and other endocrine tests, such as thyroid function tests and prolactin levels. Again, this testing may reveal comorbid conditions such as diabetes, hyperlipidemia, or hypogonadism that may contribute to ED. Prostate-specific antigen (PSA) testing may be considered in men over 40, men with a strong family history of prostate cancer, or men in whom testosterone replacement is being considered, although this is a point of debate in some circles.[42] The optimal laboratory test panel for the evaluation of ED has yet to be determined.

Education and Referral

At this point in the medical interview, it is important to review with the patient the likely etiologies, pertinent anatomy and physiology, and potential treatment options. This refocusing lies at the center of the patient-centered approach and shared decision making. Additionally, the opportunity for patient education provides a chance to address modifiable risk factors, such as diet, exercise, smoking, alcohol abuse, and medication use, that may contribute to ED.

With the advent of oral PDE inhibitors, the majority of initial ED consultations now occur in the primary care physician's office. However, based upon the findings of the history, physical examination, laboratory testing, or on initial oral drug treatment failure, it may be beneficial to refer the patient to a specialist (endocrinologist, cardiologist, urologist). Particularly germane to the urologist will be further evaluation of the penile vascular system via injection of vasodilators such as papaverine, phentolamine, or alprostadil.

Although rarely performed in 2010 and usually only after an empirical trial of oral PDE5 inhibitors, first-line urological evaluation of penile blood flow consists of a combined intracavernous injection of a single or combination of vasodilators and some form of penile stimulation. This testing allows the urologist to evaluate the specific mechanics of the erectile response and avoid the confounding influence of neurological or hormonal factors. Second-line urological evaluation includes intracavernous injection of a vasodilator and blood flow measurement with duplex ultrasonography, possibly Doppler waveform analysis, and peak systolic velocity calculations. Third-line evaluations may include calculations of cavernous arterial systolic occlusion pressures (CASOP), pharmacological arteriography, pharmacological cavernosometry, or cavernosography.[43] These increasingly invasive procedures are often reserved for young men with traumatic pelvic or penile arterial injuries who may be candidates for arterial revascularization.

Treatment

As noted previously, the initial step in penile tumescence is arousal and subsequent release of NO into vascular and cavernous smooth muscle cells (SMCs). This causes stimulation of guanylyl cyclase, with a concomitant rise in cyclic guanosine monophosphate (cGMP) and resultant reduction of cytoplasmic calcium. This leads to smooth muscle relaxation, increased arterial inflow, venous trapping, and subsequent erection.[44] With the discovery that PDE inhibitors prevent breakdown of cGMP[45] and ensuing FDA approval of sildenafil in 1998, a new era in ED treatment was born.

Oral Agents

Sildenafil was the first specific PDE inhibitor approved for treatment of ED. Vardenafil and tadalafil have since followed suit. Multiple PDE subtypes have been identified, but PDE5 is present in high concentrations in corpora cavernosal tissues. As such, sildenafil, vardenafil, and tadalafil represent specific PDE5 inhibitors. These three medications appear to have equivalent efficacy and are generally well tolerated. Primary side effects include visual disturbances, flushing, and dyspepsia. Vardenafil should be avoided in patients who take type 1A antiarrhythmics such as quinidine or procainamide, type 3 antiarrhythmics such as sotalol or amiodarone, or in patients with congenital prolonged QT syndrome. Sildenafil, vardenafil, and tadalafil should all be avoided in patients taking nitrates. Each medication requires about 15 minutes to 1 hour to be effective. The half-lives of sildenafil and vardenafil are shorter, at approximately 5 hours, while the half-life of tadalafil is about 18 hours. For those patients who do not respond to oral treatment or are not candidates for oral PDE5 inhibitors, a number of other options are available, although all are more invasive.

Alprostadil (Prostaglandin E₁)

Prostaglandin E₁ (PGE1) mediates relaxation of corporal cavernosal tissue by activating prostaglandin (PG) receptors and subsequently increasing cyclic adenosine monophosphate (cAMP) levels in the corporal smooth muscle. Elevated cAMP results in reduction of cytosolic calcium and relaxation of smooth muscle. Alprostadil is formulated for both intraurethral placement and intracavernosal injection. Intraurethral administration involves insertion of a pellet approximately 3 mm in size, 2 to 3 cm within the distal urethra. Alprostadil is absorbed via the urethral mucosa, passes through the corpus spongiosum, and then via the emissary veins. The medication passes into the corpora cavernosa to exert its vasodilatory effects. Efficacy of intraurethral alprostadil is about 66% in office placement and about 50% in home placement.[46] Penile pain is often a significant side effect of alprostadil treatment.

Intracavernous injection of alprostadil works by the same mechanism as intraurethral placement. Researchers have noted higher efficacy with intracavernosal placement. However, alprostadil is still limited by pain during erections in 16.8% of patients, penile fibrosis in 2%, hematoma at the injection site in 1.5%, and priapism in 1.3% of patients.[47] Alprostadil is formulated in a powder and must be reconstituted and refrigerated.

Papaverine and Phentolamine

Other injectable agents include papaverine and phentolamine. Papaverine exerts its effect on penile erectile tissue by an inhibitory action on PDE, resulting in increased cAMP and cGMP as well as inhibition of voltage-gated calcium channels. These mechanisms each result in cavernosal smooth muscle relaxation and subsequent erection. Papaverine's efficacy is approximately 50%, though it has not been expressly approved by the FDA for use in ED therapy. The incidence of priapism may be as high as 33% in patients receiving solitary papaverine treatment, and the incidence of penile fibrosis with this form of treatment is high.[43]

Phentolamine is also used for injection therapy but works by a different mechanism; it functions as a competitive α-adrenergic antagonist. It is postulated to induce erection by releasing sympathetic tone and thereby increasing corporal blood flow. Systemic hypotension, reflex tachycardia, and nasal congestion are its principal side effects.[48]

Typically these drugs are used in two- or three-drug combinations that allow dose reductions of each medication, increased efficacy approaching 90%, and decreased rates of pain, fibrosis, and priapism. For men unwilling or unable to inject themselves to induce erections, several other options exist.

Vacuum Erection Devices

In 1917, Otto Lederer was awarded the first patent for a surgical device to induce and maintain erection.[49] Since then, the vacuum erection device (VED) has been modified and perfected, yet the principle remains the same. The VED consists of a cylinder and suction pump that induces erection by negative pressure and subsequent increased corporal flow. A compression band is then placed at the base of the penis to trap engorged blood (Fig. 28-7). The erection is different than a physiological erection in that girth is increased, the penis is cooler, and it is less rigid than a natural erection. However, success rates are good, and patient and partner satisfaction are high. Cookson et al. noted a 90% chance of achieving a good-quality erection with satisfaction rates over 80%.[50] For patients failing the treatments discussed, surgery is typically reserved as a final treatment option.

Surgery

In 1936, a Russian surgeon named Bogoraz was the first person to create a functional autologous penile implant. He used rib cartilage in an attempt to correct ED. Although innovative, his success with this treatment was largely limited by resorption of the cartilage.[51] In 1973, Scott ushered in the modern era of penile implantation with development of the three-piece inflatable penile prosthesis.[52] Penile prostheses are typically reserved for men with organic ED who have failed or rejected treatments such as oral medications, vacuum erection devices, intraurethral alprostadil, or injection therapy. Three classes of penile implants exist: malleable, semirigid, and inflatable. Malleable and semirigid prostheses are typically placed via a distal penile approach. The inflatable prosthesis comes either as a two-piece or three-piece model that is composed of inflatable cylinders, tubing, a pump mechanism, and a reservoir (Fig. 28-8). Typically these are placed under general

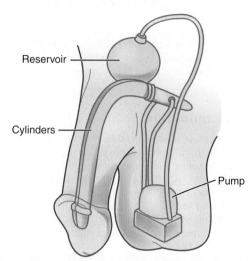

FIGURE 28-8 Surgically implanted inflatable penile prosthesis.

anesthetic, via a penoscrotal or infraumbilical incision. Infection rates vary from 3% to 8%.[53] Patient and partner satisfaction is over 90%, and freedom from mechanical failure ranges between 80% and 95% at 5 years.[54]

Vascular Surgery

During the 1970s and 1980s, surgery for arteriogenic ED was routinely performed. However, a more contemporary understanding of the pathophysiology of ED has limited the use of vascular surgery for ED. We now understand that ED often represents a systemic disruption of vascular smooth muscle. Currently, the only patient group in whom penile revascularization surgery is likely to be successful is in nonsmoking, non-diabetic young men who have no demonstrable venous leak, and have stenosis of the internal pudendal artery due to trauma or congenital causes. As noted previously, these patients should undergo dynamic infusion cavernosography and cavernosometry (DICC) to rule out veno-occlusive dysfunction before embarking on surgical treatment.

Longitudinal Psychological Outcomes

There is significant interplay between psychological health and ED, but the direction of that relationship is not always clear. Few studies have evaluated the psychological benefit from ED treatment or baseline psychological characteristics of men with ED. In 2006, we evaluated 153 men in an observational ED registry and collected clinical and psychosocial data at baseline and during follow-up. Of those patients who responded to treatment, these men reported significant improvements in sexual self-efficacy, while nonresponders reported small decrements. Surprisingly, nearly 42% of the patients describing ED were not offered treatment by their physicians.[55] Given the benefits in psychological health suggested by this study, and the high incidence of occult cardiovascular disease noted in previous studies, this should be a call to all healthcare providers to actively diagnose and treat ED in their patients.

Guidelines

In 2005, the American Urologic Association convened a consensus group of experts within the discipline of erectile dysfunction.[56] The committee created a set of guidelines to help clarify the standard of care, recommended treatments, and offered expert opinions on treatment of ED. The primary findings of these guidelines are presented in Box 28-2 and form the basis of current standard practice.

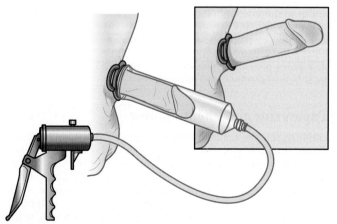

FIGURE 28-7 Vacuum erection device.

Box 28-2 American Urological Association Management Guidelines for Erectile Dysfunction

Standards of Care

Oral phosphodiesterase type 5 (PDE5) inhibitors, unless contraindicated, should be offered as first-line therapy for erectile dysfunction (ED).

PDE5 inhibitors are contraindicated in patients taking organic nitrates.

The initial trial dose of alprostadil intraurethral suppositories should be administered under healthcare provider supervision, owing to the risk of syncope.

The initial trial dose of intracavernous injection therapy should be administered under healthcare provider supervision.

Physicians who prescribe intracavernous injection therapy should (1) inform patients of the potential occurrence of prolonged erections, (2) have a plan for urgent treatment of prolonged erections, and (3) inform the patient of the plan.

The patient considering prosthesis implantation and, when possible, his partner should be informed of the following: types of prostheses available; possibility and consequences of infection and erosion, mechanical failure, and resulting reoperation; differences from the normal flaccid and erect penis, including penile shortening; and potential reduction of effectiveness of other therapies if the device is subsequently removed.

Prosthetic surgery should not be performed in the presence of systemic, cutaneous, or urinary tract infection.

Antibiotics providing gram-negative and gram-positive coverage should be administered preoperatively.

Recommendations

Monitoring of patients receiving continuing PDE5 inhibitor therapy should include a periodic follow-up of efficacy, side effects, and any significant change in health status, including medications.

Prior to proceeding to other therapies, patients reporting failure of PDE5 inhibitor therapy should be evaluated to determine whether the trial of PDE5 inhibition was adequate.

Patients who have failed a trial with PDE5 inhibitor therapy should be informed of the benefits and risks of other therapies, including use of a different PDE5 inhibitor, alprostadil intraurethral suppositories, intracavernous drug injection, vacuum constriction devices, and penile prostheses.

Only vacuum constriction devices containing a vacuum limiter should be used, whether purchased over the counter or procured with a prescription.

Use of trazodone in the treatment of ED is not recommended.

Testosterone therapy is not indicated for treatment of ED in the patient with a normal serum testosterone level.

Yohimbine is not recommended for treatment of ED.

Herbal therapies are not recommended for treatment of ED.

Surgeries performed with the intent to limit the venous outflow of the penis are not recommended.

Opinion

Arterial reconstructive surgery is a treatment option only in healthy individuals with recently acquired ED secondary to a focal arterial occlusion, and in the absence of any evidence of generalized vascular disease.

Modified from http://www.auanet.org/content/guidelines-and-quality-care/clinical-guidelines.cfm ?sub=ed. Accessed December 2010.

REFERENCES

1. Lue TF: Physiology of penile erection and pathophysiology of erectile dysfunction. In Wein AJ, Kavoussi LR, Novick AC, Partin AW, Peters CA, editors: *Campbell-Walsh urology*, ed 9, 2007.
2. Brenot P: Male impotence—a historical perspective, *L' Esprit du Temps* 1994.
3. Impotence: *NIH Consens Statement* 10:1, 1992.
4. Sun P, Cameron A, Seftel A, et al: Erectile dysfunction—an observable marker of diabetes mellitus? A large national epidemiological study, *J Urol* 176:1081–1085, 2006.
5. Laumann E, Paik A, Rosen R: Sexual dysfunction in the United States: prevalence and predictors, *JAMA* 281:537–544, 1999.
6. Johannes CB, Araujo AB, Feldman HA, et al: Incidence of erectile dysfunction in men 40 to 69 years old: longitudinal results from the Massachusetts Male Aging Study, *J Urol* 163:460–463, 2000.
7. Lewis RW, Hatzchistou D, Laumann E, et al: Epidemiology and natural history of erectile dysfunction: risk factors including iatrogenic and aging, In: *Proceedings of the First International Consultation on Erectile Dysfunction*, 2000, Health Publication, pp 21–51.
8. Schouten BW, Bosch JL, Bernsen RM, et al: Incidence rates of erectile dysfunction in the Dutch general population. Effects of definition, clinical relevance, and duration of follow-up in the Krimpen study, *Int J Impot Res* 17:58–62, 2005.
9. Moreira ED, Lbo CR, Diament A, et al: Incidence of erectile dysfunction in men 40-69 years old: results from a population based cohort in Brazil, *Urology* 61:431–436, 2003.
10. Sattar AA, Salpigidis G, Schulman CC, et al: Relationship between intrapenile O2 lever and quantity of intracavernous smooth muscle fibers: current physiopathological concept, *Acta Urol Belg* 63:53–59, 1995.
11. Hsu GL, Brock G, Martinez-Pineiro L, et al: The three dimensional structure of the human tunica albuginea: anatomical and ultrastructural levels, *Int J Impot Res* 4:117–129, 1992.
12. Droupy S, Benoit G, Giuliano F, et al: Penile arteries in humans, *Surg Radiol Anat* 19:161–167, 1997.
13. Hsu GL, Hsieh CH, Wen HS, et al: Penile venous anatomy: an additional description and its clinical implication, *J Androl* 24:921–927, 2003.
14. de Groat WC, Booth A: Neural control of penile erection. In Maggi CA, editor: *The autonomic nervous system*, London, 1993, Harwood, pp 465–513.
15. Walsh PC, Brendler CB, Chang T, et al: Preservation of sexual function in men during radical pelvic surgery, *Md Med J* 39:389–393, 1990.
16. Halata Z, Munger BL: The neuroanatomical basis for the protopathic sensibility of the human glans penis, *Brain Res* 371:205–230, 1986.
17. McKenna KE: Central control of penile erection, *Int J Impot Res* 10(Suppl):S25–S34, 1998.
18. Burnett AL, Tillman SL, Chang TS, et al: Immunohistochemical localization of nitric oxide synthase in the autonomic innervation of the human penis, *J Urol* 150:73–76, 1993.
19. Michal V, Ruzbarsky V: Histological changes in the penile arterial bed with aging and diabetes. In Zorgniotti AW, Rossi G, editors: *Vasculogenic impotence: proceedings of the First International Conference on Corpus Cavernosum Revascularization*, Springfield, Ill, 1980, pp 113–119.
20. Vlachopoulos C, Rokkas K, Ioakeimidis N, et al: Prevalence of asymptomatic coronary artery disease in men with vasculogenic erectile dysfunction: a prospective angiographic study, *Eur Urol* 48:996–1003, 2005.
21. Gratzke C, Angulo J, Chitaley K, et al: Anatomy, physiology, and pathophysiology of erectile dysfunction, *J Sex Med* 7:445–475, 2010.
22. Tarhan F, Kuyumcuoglu U, Kolsuz A, et al: Cavernous oxygen tension in the patients with erectile dysfunction, *Int J Impot Res* 9:149–153, 1997.
23. Nehra A, Azadoi KM, Moreland RB, et al: Cavernosal expandability is an erectile tissue mechanical property which predicts trabecular histology in an animal model of vasculogenic erectile dysfunction, *J Urol* 159:2229–2236, 1998.
24. Azadzoi KM, Park K, Andry C, et al: Relationship between cavernosal ischemia and corporal veno-occlusive dysfunction in an animal model, *J Urol* 157:1011–1017, 1997.
25. Azadzoi KM, Krane RJ, Saenz de Tejada I, et al: Endothelium-derived nitric oxide and cyclooxygenase products modulate corpus cavernosum smooth muscle tone, *J Urol* 147:220–225, 1992.
26. Levine FJ, Greenfield AJ, Goldstein I: Arteriographically determined occlusive disease within the hypogastric-cavernous bed in impotent patients following blunt perineal and pelvic trauma, *J Urol* 144:11147–11153, 1990.
27. Richiuti VS, Haas CA, Seftel AD, et al: Pudendal nerve injury associated with avid bicycling, *J Urol* 162:2099–2100, 1999.
28. Sattar AA, Wespes E, Schulman CC: Computerized measurement of penile elastic fibers in potent and impotent men, *Eur Urol* 25:142–144, 1994.
29. Rajfer J, Rosciszewski A, Mehringer M: Prevalence of corporeal venous leakage in impotent men, *J Urol* 140:69–71, 1988.
30. Christ GJ, Maayani S, Valcic M, et al: Pharmacological studies of human erectile tissue: characteristics of spontaneous contractions and alterations in alpha-adrenoreceptor responsiveness with age and disease in isolated tissues, *Br J Pharmacol* 101:375–381, 1990.
31. Christ GJ, Moreno AP, Parker ME, et al: Intercellular communication through gap junctions: a potential role in pharmacomechanical coupling and syncytial tissue contraction in vascular smooth muscle isolated from the human corpus cavernosum, *Life Sci* 49:PL195–PL200, 1991.
32. Chang SW, Fine R, Siegel D, et al: The impact of diuretic therapy on reported sexual function, *Arch Intern Med* 151:2402–2408, 1991.
33. Grimm RH Jr, Grandits GA, Prineas RJ, et al: Long term effects on sexual function of five anti-hypertensive drugs and nutritional hygienic treatment in hypertensive men and women. Treatment of Mild Hypertension Study (TOMHS), *Hypertension* 29:8–14, 1997.
34. Franzen D, Metha A, Seifert N, et al: Effects of beta-blockers on sexual performance in men with coronary artery disease. A prospective, randomized, and double blinded study, *Int J Impot Res* 13:348–351, 2001.
35. Fogari R, Zoppi A, Corradi L, et al: Sexual function in hypertensive males treated with lisinopril or atenolol: a crossover study, *Am J Hypertens* 11:1244–1247, 1998.
36. Llisteri JL, Lozano JV, Aznar VJ, et al: Sexual dysfunction in hypertensive patients treated with losartan, *Am J Med Sci* 321:336–341, 2001.
37. Salzman EA, Guay AT, Jacobson J: Improvement in erectile function in men with organic erectile dysfunction by correction of elevated cholesterol levels: a clinical observation, *J Urol* 172:255–258, 2004.
38. Sadeghi-Nejah H, Jackson I: New onset priapism associated with ingestion of terazosin in an otherwise healthy man, *J Sex Med* 6:1766–1768, 2007.
39. Gratzke C, Angulo J, Chitaley K, et al: Anatomy, physiology, and pathophysiology of erectile dysfunction, *J Sex Med* 7:445–475, 2010.
40. Rosen RC, Riley A, Wagner G, et al: The International Index of Erectile Function (IIEF): a multidimensional scale for assessment of erectile dysfunction, *Urology* 49:822–830, 1997.
41. Schwartz BG, Kloner RA: How to save a life during a clinic visit for erectile dysfunction by modifying cardiovascular risk factors, *Int J Impot Res* 21:327–335, 2009.

42. Green KL, Albertsen PC, Babaian RL, et al: AUA prostate specific antigen best practice guideline: 2009 update, *J Urol* 182:2232–2241, 2009.

43. Lue TF, Broderick GA: Evaluation and nonsurgical management of erectile dysfunction and premature ejaculation. In Wein AJ, Kavoussi LR, Novick AC, et al, editors: *Campbell-Walsh Urology*, ed 9, 2007.

44. Prieto D: Physiological regulation of penile arteries and veins, *Int J Impot Res* 20:17–29, 2008.

45. Francis SH, Lincoln TM, Corbin JD: Guanosine 3′-5′ cyclic monophosphate binding proteins in rat tissues, *Proc Natl Acad Sci U S A* 73:2559–2563, 1976.

46. Hellastrom WJ, Bennett AH, Gesundheit N, et al: A double blind, placebo controlled evaluation of the erectile response to transurethral alprostadil, *Urology* 48:851–856, 1996.

47. Linet OL, Neff LL: Intracavernous prostaglandin E1 in erectile dysfunction, *Clin Invest* 72:139–149, 1994.

48. Padma-Nathan J, Christ G, Adaikan G, et al: Pharmacotherapy for erectile dysfunction, *J Sex Med* 1:128–140, 2004.

49. Earle CM, Seah M, Coulden SE, et al: The use of the vacuum erection device in the management of erectile impotence, *Int J Impot Res* 8:237–240, 1996.

50. Cookson MS, Nadig PW: Long term results with vacuum constriction device, *J Urol* 149:290–294, 1993.

51. Mulcahy JJ, Austoni E, Barada JH, et al: The penile implant for erectile dysfunction, *J Sex Med* 1:98–109, 2004.

52. Subrini L: Subrini penile implants: surgical, sexual, and psychological results, *Eur Urol* 8:222–226, 1982.

53. Hellstrom JG, Montague DK, Moncada I, et al: Implants, mechanical devices, and vascular surgery for erectile dysfunction, *J Sex Med* 7:501–523, 2010.

54. Montorsi F, Rigatti P, Carmignani G, et al: AMS three-piece inflatable implants for erectile dysfunction: a long term multi-institutional study in 200 consecutive patients, *Eur Urol* 37:50–55, 2000.

55. Latini DM, Penson DF, Wallace KL, et al: Longitudinal differences in psychological outcomes for men with erectile dysfunction: Results from ExCEED, *J Sex Med* 3:1068–1076, 2006.

56. http://www.auanet.org/content/guidelines-and-quality-care/clinical-guidelines.cfm?sub=ed. Accessed December 2010.

CH
28

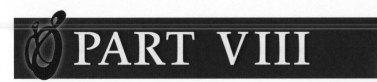

PART VIII

CEREBROVASCULAR ISCHEMIA

CHAPTER 29

Epidemiology of Cerebrovascular Disease

Larry B. Goldstein, Judith H. Lichtman

Overview

Stroke is the second leading cause of death worldwide, accounting for 4 million deaths in 2004.[1] Until recently, stroke ranked as the third leading cause of death in the United States.[2] Owing to a reclassification of respiratory diseases using the 10th version of the International Classification of Diseases (ICD-10), preliminary data from the Centers for Disease Control and Prevention (CDC) released on December 9, 2010, ranks cerebrovascular disease as the fourth most common cause of death in the country behind diseases of the heart, cancer, and chronic lower respiratory diseases. On average, every 40 seconds someone in the United States has a stroke, and every 4 minutes someone dies.[2] Stroke is also a leading cause of long-term disability in adults. There are a variety of nontreatable and treatable stroke risk factors (Box 29-1).

Stroke Burden

In the United States, an estimated 795,000 persons have a stroke each year, and 7 million individuals 20 years of age or older have had a stroke.[2] Ischemic strokes account for 87% of all strokes, with the remaining 13% due to intracranial hemorrhages. About three quarters of these strokes are first cerebrovascular events, and the remainder are recurrent.[2] The risk of first ischemic stroke varies by race-ethnicity, increasing from 88 per 100,000 in whites, to 149 per 100,000 in Hispanics/Latinos, to 191 per 100,000 in blacks.[2] There were over three quarters of a million hospital discharges for stroke in 2007, and approximately 3.7 million ambulatory care visits attributable to stroke in 2008.[3] Up to 70% of cerebrovascular events evaluated in hospitals are ischemic strokes, with 30% due to transient ischemic attacks (TIAs) and hemorrhagic strokes.[4] Two thirds of patients hospitalized for stroke are older than age 65; half are older than 70. Importantly, stroke is the second leading cause of death in persons aged 85 and over, who by 2050 will number approximately 20.9 million.[5] As measured by disability-adjusted life-years, the burden of stroke relative to other diseases is anticipated to continue to increase worldwide from sixth in 1990 to fourth in 2020.[6]

A TIA precedes approximately 15% to 23% of ischemic strokes and carries a 90-day stroke risk of 9% to 17%[7] and a 25% risk of death over the ensuing year.[8] About half of all patients who have a TIA fail to report their symptoms to a healthcare provider.[9] With an estimated 240,000 TIAs diagnosed annually in the United States, TIA represents an important target for secondary stroke prevention.

Mortality from stroke accounted for 1 of every 18 deaths in 2007, for a total of 135,952 deaths.[2] Mortality in the 5 years after stroke ranges from 27% to 61% across sex-age subgroups.[2] Current data on long-term survivorship following ischemic stroke reflects wide ranges of estimated mortality; 13% to 45% at 1 year, 36% to 69% at 5 years, and 31% to 87% at 10 years.[10–29] These estimates were primarily obtained from international studies or single regions within the United States and included a relatively small number of cases. Women and minority populations may have higher long-term mortality following stroke, although the evidence is limited, and more research is needed to investigate differences by patient characteristics.[13,23,25]

In addition to the relatively high mortality from stroke, its aftermath can be devastating. Twenty percent of stroke survivors require institutional care after 3 months, and 15% to 30% are permanently disabled.[30] Given the large number of stroke survivors in this country, effective rehabilitation and secondary prevention are important targets for public health intervention.

Cost

Stroke is among the 10 highest contributors to Medicare costs.[31] In 2007, the annual cost of stroke in the United States was estimated at $40.9 billion, with $25.2 billion in direct costs.[2] Total stroke-related costs were estimated at $68.9 billion in 2009.[4] These costs are projected to exceed $2.2 trillion through 2050.[32] The mean lifetime cost of ischemic stroke is now estimated at $140,048 in 1999 dollars.[33]

Regional Patterns of Stroke

Over the last 50 years, stroke mortality has varied regionally in the United States, with the highest mortality rates in the Southeast, a region of the country termed the "Stroke Belt."[34–38] The Stroke Belt is usually defined as including the eight southern states of North Carolina, South Carolina, Georgia, Tennessee, Mississippi, Alabama, Louisiana, and Arkansas. These geographic differences have been documented since at least 1940,[34] and despite some minor shifts[35] still persist.[36–38] The reason for the existence of the Stroke Belt remains uncertain. Within it, a "buckle" region along the coastal plain of North Carolina, South Carolina, and Georgia has been identified with even higher stroke mortality rates than other portions.[39] Overall average stroke mortality is about 20% higher in the Stroke Belt than in the rest of the nation and about 40% higher in the stroke buckle. Individuals living in the southeastern United States have a 50% greater risk of dying from a stroke than residents of other regions.[39]

Higher stroke mortality rates are now also noted in the Pacific Northwest.[40,41] Overall mortality reflects a combination of incidence and case-fatality rates. Stroke incidence is higher in the Southeast,[37,42,43] whereas case-fatality rates vary little across the country.[37] The CDC published an atlas showing geographic patterns in age-adjusted stroke hospitalization rates by county that are consistent with stroke mortality patterns (Figure 29-1).[44] There are also regional differences in recurrent stroke events within the year after stroke hospitalization, even after adjusting for common risk

Box 29-1 Stroke Risk Factors (Partial List)

Demographic Factors
Age
Sex
Race-ethnicity

Lifestyle Factors
Diet/nutrition
Physical inactivity
Overweight/obesity
Alcohol consumption

Environmental Factors
Air pollution
Cigarette smoking

Medically Treatable Risk Factors
Hypertension
Lipids
Diabetes
Atrial fibrillation
Sickle cell disease
Sleep-disordered breathing

Other Risk Factors
Fibrinogen, clotting factors, and inflammation
Blood homocysteine levels
Migraine

factors.[45,46] Causes for these shifts remain unclear, and contemporary national data are needed to monitor incident and prevalent stroke patterns over time, particularly by age, race-ethnicity, and sex subgroups.

Stroke Risk Factors

Demographic Factors

AGE

Stroke is rare in young children, occurring at a rate of 4.6 to 6.4 per 100,000 children in the United States.[2] The incidence of stroke in adults is strongly age dependent,[25] and the rate of adverse outcomes and complications associated with stroke increases with advanced age.[47] The mean age of stroke patients in this country is 70 years. The U.S. population is aging, and by the year 2050, the total number of people aged 65 and older will nearly triple, increasing from 34 million in 2000 to 90 million.[5,48,49] This means that by 2050, 20% of the population will be 65 years of age or older and at increased risk for stroke. A report released by the CDC in collaboration with the Center for Medicare & Medicaid Services (CMS), the *Atlas of Stroke Hospitalizations Among Medicare Beneficiaries*, found that 30-day stroke mortality rates varied by age: 9% in patients aged 65 to 74, 13.1% in those aged 74 to 84, and 23% in those aged 85 or older.[44] Because stroke is so strongly age dependent, understanding the

Medicare Beneficiaries Ages 65 and Older
1995–2002

Stroke Hospitalization Rates
Total Population

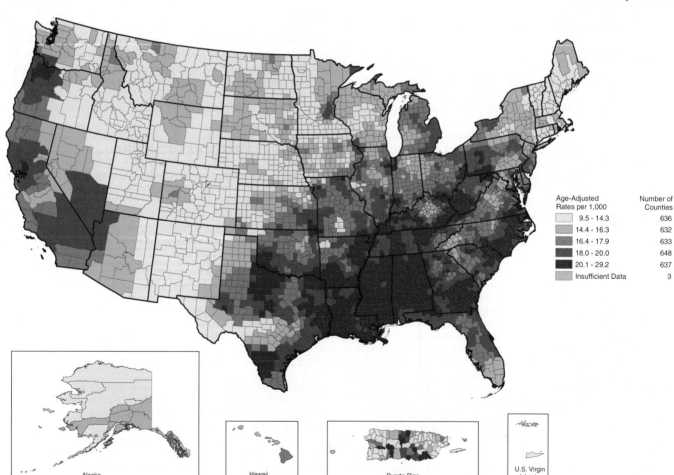

FIGURE 29-1   Geographic patterns of stroke hospitalization in the United States. *(From Casper M, Nwaise I, Croft J, Nilasena D: Atlas of stroke hospitalizations among Medicare beneficiaries, Atlanta, 2008, U.S. Department of Health and Human Services, Centers for Disease Control and Prevention.)*

epidemiology of stroke in the elderly is critical for both clinicians and policy makers.

SEX

Women are older at stroke onset compared with men (75 years vs. 71 years).[2] Overall, women have a lower age-adjusted stroke incidence than men, but sex-related differences in stroke risk are modified by age. Data from the Framingham Heart Study demonstrate that compared with white men, white women 45 to 84 years of age have lower stroke risk than men, but this association is reversed in women older than 85, whose risk is higher than men.[2] The absolute number of strokes in the population is, however, greater for women because of the increasing risk of stroke with advancing age, combined with women's longer life expectancy.

A focus on age-adjusted and age-specific stroke mortality rates conceal the greater total number of stroke deaths in women. The excess deaths in women result from the higher mortality in women and their disproportionate representation in the population. About 55% of all strokes occur in women, who have approximately 60% of stroke-related deaths. Not only do more strokes occur in women, the bulk occur in women over the age of 70, who are more likely to be socially isolated, live alone, have fiscal constraints, and higher rates of comorbid disease. The greater burden of stroke deaths in women is predicted to be even greater in the future, based on population projections; an excess of 32,000 stroke deaths in women in 2000 is anticipated to increase to nearly 68,000 excess deaths by 2050.[50]

The rate of stroke increases during pregnancy, with the majority occurring during the postpartum period. Pregnancy-related intracerebral hemorrhage (ICH) has the highest mortality and morbidity of all stroke types. Risk factors for stroke in pregnancy include advanced maternal age, African American race-ethnicity, migraines, preeclampsia, and gestational hypertension.[51] Meta-analyses summarizing over 30 years of studies show that oral contraceptive users have about a twofold increased risk of stroke compared with nonusers; hypertension, cigarette smoking, and migraine headaches further increase stroke risk in women taking oral contraceptives.[51] Women younger than 50 are generally considered to be at lower risk for stroke than men, although recent studies show that women aged 35 to 64 were almost three times more likely than men to report prior stroke, largely because of higher rates in 45- to 54-year-olds.[52] Prevalence of stroke increases as women reach the menopausal transition. Studies suggest that women are protected by endogenous estrogens, but clinical trials have not found a lower risk of either stroke or cardiac events in postmenopausal women treated with exogenous estrogen and progesterone.[50]

RACE-ETHNICITY

There are prominent stroke race-ethnic disparities. Blacks and Hispanic/Latinos have two to four times the rate of stroke, stroke recurrence, and stroke-related deaths as whites.[53-56] Although differences may be more prominent in younger age groups,[57] race-ethnic differences remain among older age groups.[56,58] Stroke incidence has been decreasing in U.S. whites, but not in U.S. blacks over the past decade, suggesting a worsening of racial disparity in stroke incidence.[59]

Lifestyle Factors

DIET/NUTRITION

Numerous studies implicate dietary factors in the risk for stroke. Aspects of diet that have received attention include individual dietary factors such as omega-3 fatty acids, vitamins C and E, potassium, calcium, fatty acids, homocysteine, and sodium, as well as food groups and dietary patterns such as consumption of fruits and vegetables, the Dietary Approaches to Stop Hypertension (DASH) diet, and the Mediterranean diet.[60] Intake of antioxidant vitamin supplements such as vitamin C and E do not lower stroke risk. Although some evidence suggests higher total fat intake increases

stroke risk,[61] higher fish consumption, a marker for omega-3 fatty acid intake, was associated with reduced stroke risk in the Nurses' Health Study and the Health Professionals' Follow-up Study.[62,63] Higher fruit and vegetable consumption has been associated with lower stroke risk in many studies[64-68] and was found to reduce the risk of stroke in a clinical trial.[69] A meta-analysis of cohort studies reported a 26% reduction in stroke risk associated with consumption of five or more servings a day of fruits and vegetables compared with consumption of less than three servings a day.[70]

Reduced sodium and increased potassium intake have also been associated with decreased stroke risk.[71-74] The proposed effects of sodium and potassium on stroke risk are likely in part due to their role in lowering blood pressure. The DASH diet, characterized by high intake of fruits and vegetables, consumption of low-fat dairy products, and low intake of saturated and total fat, effectively lowers blood pressure in clinical trials[75] and was associated with an 18% lower risk of stroke in the Nurses' Health Study (highest quintile vs. lowest quintile).[76] The Mediterranean style diet has also received considerable attention with regard to its favorable impact on cardiovascular health. Women in the Nurses' Health Study at the highest vs. lowest quintiles of the Alternate Mediterranean Diet Score had a lower risk of stroke (relative risk [RR] = 0.87; 95% CI, 0.73-1.02) after 20 years of follow-up.[77] Analyses in the same group of women evaluating consumption of a so-called prudent diet (high in vegetable, fruit, legume, fish, and whole grain intake) and a so-called Western diet (one high in red and processed meats, refined grains, sweets, and desserts) found a 58% increased risk of stroke in the highest vs. lowest quintile of a Western diet and a 22% lower risk of stroke in the highest vs. lowest quintile of a prudent diet.[78]

Current dietary guidelines for stroke prevention recommend reduced sodium intake and increased intake of potassium and fruits and vegetables. Unfortunately, according to national surveys conducted in 2005-2006, average adult consumption ranges from 1.1 to 1.8 servings a day of fruit and 1.2 to 2.1 servings a day of vegetables across race-ethnic groups,[4] whereas sodium intake exceeds recommendations for 90% of the adult U.S. population.[79] Low fruit and vegetable intake is estimated to account for 9% and 11% of stroke deaths in high-income and mid- to low-income countries, respectively.[80]

PHYSICAL INACTIVITY

Lack of regular physical activity is a well-established predictor of early mortality and cardiovascular disease, and regular exercise is associated with a lower risk of stroke in prospective and case-control studies.[81-88] The effects of physical activity are thought to be mediated through reductions in blood pressure, control of other cardiovascular risk factors, improvements in glucose tolerance and body weight, reductions in plasma fibrinogen and platelet activity, and elevations in high-density lipoprotein (HDL) cholesterol concentration.[88-94] Current guidelines recommend a minimum of 30 minutes per day of moderate-intensity physical activity most days of the week.[95,96] In the 2008 National Health and Nutrition Examination Survey (NHANES), only 32.5% of adults aged 18 and older reported they engaged in regular leisure time physical activity.[4] Physical inactivity accounts for 8% and 6% of stroke deaths worldwide in high-income and middle- to low-income countries, respectively.[80] Participants in the Physicians' Health Study engaging in vigorous exercise five or more times per week had a 14% lower risk of stroke compared with those engaging in vigorous activity less than 1 time per week.[94] The Framingham Heart Study and the Honolulu Heart Program have found similar effects in men.[81,82] Studies in women, including the Nurses' Health Study and the Copenhagen City Heart Study, also report reductions in stroke incidence with increased physical activity.[87,88] Among women aged 45 and older in the Women's Health Study, higher levels of physical activity (measured in kcal/wk) were associated with a 20% to 40% reduction in stroke risk.[97] Finally, in the Northern Manhattan Stroke Study, there was an overal 63% reduction in stroke risk associated with physical

352

CH
29

activity; this protective effect was found in all subgroups of age, sex, and race-ethnicity (white, black, Hispanic). There is some uncertainty as to the dose and intensity of physical activity required for adequate reduction in stroke risk, and comparison studies are limited. An analysis of the Northern Manhattan Study suggested that heavy physical activity was more beneficial than low to moderate activity.[86] Other evidence supports the beneficial effect of light exercise. The intensity of physical activity was not related to stroke risk among participants in the Women's Health Study, although walking time and pace were inversely related to stroke risk.[97]

OVERWEIGHT/OBESITY

Obesity likely increases stroke risk through multiple mechanisms including increased blood pressure, impaired glucose tolerance, and more frequent atherogenic serum lipid levels. Traditionally, weight categorization has been defined according to the body mass index (BMI; weight [kg] divided by the square of height [m]), with 25 and 30 kg/m^2 used as cut-points defining overweight and obesity, respectively. In the Framingham cohort, BMI was related to first cerebrovascular events after adjustment for traditional stroke risk factors.[98] Relative risks for stroke in an analysis of women aged 30 to 55 in the Nurses' Health Study ranged from 1.75 for a BMI of 27 to 28.9 kg/m^2 to 2.37 for a BMI above 32 kg/m^2, and were independent of other risk factors including age, smoking, hormone use, and menopausal status.[99]

Obesity was also identified as an independent stroke risk factor in the Honolulu Heart Study.[100] Abdominal obesity has emerged as an even stronger risk factor for stroke than BMI. In a study of 28,643 male health professionals, the relative risk of stroke was 2.3 times higher in the upper compared with the lower quintiles of waist-to-hip ratio.[101] Obesity is a major public health problem in the United States and worldwide. According to a national survey, 67% of U.S. adults are overweight, and 30% are obese.[102] As a population attributable risk factor, obesity accounts for an estimated 20% of stroke deaths in high-income countries and 15% in middle- to low-income countries, a risk that is likely to increase in the United States owing to the epidemic of obesity in the young.

Environmental Factors

Air pollution reflects a heterogenous amalgamation of gases, liquids, and particulate matter that has gained attention as a risk factor for stroke. A 2004 American Heart Association (AHA) Scientific Statement on the relationship between particulate matter (PM) air pollution and cardiovascular disease concluded that both short- and long-term exposure to ambient PM increases the risk of acute cardiovascular events.[103] With the proliferation of studies on this topic following this Scientific Statement, an update was published in 2010.[104] Indeed, most epidemiological studies have corroborated the initial conclusions, generally reporting an elevated risk of cardiovascular events associated with exposure to fine PM less than 2.5 μm in aerodynamic diameter (PM$_{2.5}$) for susceptible individuals (e.g., the elderly, those with existing cardiovascular conditions). Recent research also suggests a role for ultrafine particulates less than 0.1 μm, co-pollutants such as ozone and nitrogen oxides, and specific sources of pollution such as motor vehicle traffic.

Among the subcategories of cardiovascular disease, the strength of evidence for an association between air pollution and cerebrovascular disease is less than that for heart disease, but the literature is still growing.[104] Among more than 60,000 postmenopausal women initially free of cardiovascular disease in the Women's Health Initiative, each 10 μm/m^3 increase in annual PM$_{2.5}$ exposure was associated with a 28% increased risk of stroke, a 35% increased risk of stroke or fatal cerebrovascular disease, and an 83% increased risk of fatal cerebrovascular disease.[105] There was no association between fatal cerebrovascular and long-term PM$_{2.5}$ exposure in a cohort of over 300,000 adults derived from the American Cancer Society's Cancer Prevention Study-II.[106] Several studies have reported small but statistically significant associations

for short-term pollutant exposure. Daily time-series studies from Korea (Seoul),[107,108] China (Shanghai),[109] and Finland (Helsinki)[110] reported associations between elevated levels of air pollution and stroke mortality; however, the associations were found for ischemic but not hemorrhagic stroke mortality in one study,[109] and in the warm but not cold seasons in another.[110] A U.S. study of Medicare hospitalizations for stroke or cerebrovascular disease in nine cities found that several measures of air pollution within the 0 to 2 days before hospitalization were associated with ischemic but not hemorrhagic stroke. Additional studies using surveillance data from Dijon, France,[111] and Corpus Christi, Texas,[112] have also linked certain types of air pollutants with the risk of ischemic stroke and TIA.

In addition to acute cardiovascular events, air pollutants potentially contribute to numerous subclinical physiological changes including systemic inflammation and oxidative stress, coagulation/thrombosis, systemic and pulmonary arterial blood pressure, vascular function, atherosclerosis, heart rate variability, cardiac ischemia and repolarization abnormalities, epigenetic changes, and traditional cardiovascular risk factors.[104] Such associations provide further support for a relationship between cardiovascular disease and air pollution and provide insight into plausible mechanistic pathways. As a potentially avoidable risk factor, it may be prudent for those at high risk of cardiovascular disease and stroke to limit outdoor air exposure on high pollution days.

CIGARETTE SMOKING

Cigarette smoking is consistently identified as a major independent risk factor for ischemic stroke in epidemiological studies including the Framingham Heart Study,[113] Cardiovascular Health Study,[114] Honolulu Heart Study,[115] and INTERSTROKE,[116] among many others. In general, cigarette smoking leads to an approximate twofold increase in stroke risk.[117] Smoking is also associated with a two- to fourfold increase in risk of subarachnoid hemorrhage (SAH).[118–121] Data are inconclusive regarding a relationship between smoking and the risk of parenchymal ICH. Analyses of data from the Hemorrhagic Stroke Project,[122] Physicians' Health Study,[120] and the Women's Health Study[119] find an association between smoking and increased ICH risk, whereas analyses from other studies, including a pooled analysis of data from the Atherosclerosis Risk in Communities (ARIC) Study and the Cardiovascular Health Study, find no relationship.[123] One meta-analysis even reported a paradoxical protective effect of smoking for ICH risk,[124] although a more contemporary review found an approximate 30% increase in ICH risk associated with smoking.[125] Using data from the National Health Interview Survey and death certificates for 2000 to 2004, the CDC estimates that nearly 16,000 cerebrovascular deaths annually can be attributed to smoking, equating to approximately 13% of cerebrovascular deaths for men and 8% for women.[126]

Environmental tobacco smoke (also known as *passive* or *secondhand smoke*) is also thought to increase the risk of stroke for lifelong nonsmokers. A meta-analysis of 24 sex-specific estimates from 15 studies found an overall 25% (95% CI, 16%-36%) increased risk of stroke with current spousal exposure (or its nearest equivalent).[127] There was no heterogeneity by sex, publication year, or outcome, but risk estimates tended to be lower for prospective studies and those studies with U.S. or European cohorts. There was not an increased risk for SAH, and overall risk estimates were similar when using ever spousal exposure or total exposure rather than current spousal exposure. A 56% (95% CI, 34%-82%) increased risk of stroke was found for the highest level of spousal exposure.

Although data strongly support a relationship between smoking and stroke, the linearity of a dose effect remains uncertain. A number of studies suggest a nonlinear effect, with the stroke risk attributable to smoking increasing sharply at lower cigarette consumption levels and then leveling off as the number of cigarettes per day increases.[128] Similarities between stroke risk estimates and changes in biomarkers of cardiovascular risk for active and passive smokers further support a nonlinear effect of cigarette smoking, suggesting a low overall threshold of tobacco smoke exposure.[117,129,130]

Clinical and experimental studies indicate both acute and chronic effects of cigarette smoking that likely contribute to increased stroke risk.[128] Cigarette smoking causes endothelial injury and dysfunction in both the coronary and peripheral arteries. It increases the risk of thrombus generation in atherosclerotic arteries and creates a chronic state of inflammation associated with development of atherosclerosis. Smoking also leads to an atherogenic lipid profile (increased triglycerides and decreased HDL cholesterol), and it is thought to produce insulin resistance that, along with chronic inflammation, can accelerate macrovascular and microvascular complications such as nephropathy. Smoking even just one cigarette increases heart rate, mean blood pressure, and cardiac index and decreases arterial distensibility.[131,132] A number of studies also demonstrate a synergistic action of smoking with other cardiovascular risk factors in increasing stroke risk. Such factors include systolic blood pressure,[133] vital exhaustion,[134] and oral contraceptives[135,136] among others.

Smoking cessation is generally accepted as an essential component of primary and secondary stroke prevention.[117] Rapid reduction in stroke risk with smoking cessation is often observed, with considerable reductions apparent within 5 years.[124,137-141] Although stroke risk is greatly lower for former compared to current smokers, it remains unclear whether risk ever reverts to that of never smokers. The Framingham Study[139] and the Nurses' Health Study[137] show a near-complete loss of excess risk, whereas the Honolulu Heart Program,[140] British Regional Heart Study,[138] and others[124,141] report a slight excess risk for former compared to never smokers. Several studies suggest that this excess risk may be retained for up to 2 decades after quitting.[138,141] Heavy smokers may have more sustained excess risk compared with light smokers, whose risk falls more rapidly to the level of nonsmokers.[138,141] It is possible that past level of smoking rather than years since cessation or duration of smoking might be the determining factor in achieving risk equivalence.

Alcohol Consumption

The effects of alcohol intake on stroke risk appear to be dependent on both level of consumption and stroke type. In the Honolulu Heart Study, there was a very strong dose-response relationship between alcohol intake and intracranial and subarachnoid hemorrhage.[142] Alcohol intake also appears to confer risk for ischemic stroke, although effects at low to moderate levels are less clear, with most evidence suggesting a beneficial effect. A study following male health professionals reported increased risk of stroke with an intake of more than two drinks per day, but no clear association with lower levels of consumption.[143] Other studies support a J-shaped relationship between alcohol intake and the risk of ischemic stroke, such that low to moderate levels of intake are associated with reduced stroke risk, and heavy consumption is associated with increasingly higher risk.[144-150] A meta-analysis of the effects of alcohol (1 drink defined as 12 g of alcohol) and stroke risk reported a 20% to 28% reduced risk of stroke among those consuming fewer than 1 or 1 to 2 drinks a day relative to abstainers.[151] In contrast, heavy drinking (>5 drinks/day) was associated with a 69% increased risk. The population attributable risk associated with alcohol use for stroke mortality in high-income and middle- and low-income countries is estimated at 11% and 5%, respectively.[80] Heavy alcohol use may impact risk through increases in blood pressure, higher rates of atrial fibrillation and coagulation disorders, and reductions in cerebral blood flow. At moderate levels of intake, however, alcohol may have beneficial effects through reductions in platelet aggregation and plasma fibrinogen concentration, and improvements in HDL cholesterol levels and endothelial function. Current guidelines recommend moderate drinking of two or less drinks per day for men and one drink or less per day for nonpregnant women who consume alcohol.[152]

Medically Treatable Risk Factors

Hypertension

Hypertension, or high blood pressure—defined as systolic blood pressure 140 mmHg or greater, diastolic blood pressure 90 mmHg or greater, or requiring antihypertensive medication—occurs in one in three adults in the United States. Hypertension currently affects more than 76 million people in the country. Prevalence is particularly high in individuals older than 65, in whom it exceeds 67%.[153,154] Lifetime risk of hypertension in individuals aged 55 years is 90%. African Americans have one of the highest rates of hypertension in the world; prevalence in this group is 32.3%, compared with 23.0% for whites and 21.5% for Hispanics/Latinos. Despite the relative ease of diagnosis and effectiveness of treatment, approximately 20.4% of adults with hypertension are unaware of their condition, 29.1% are not being treated, and 52.2% do not have adequately controlled blood pressure. Control is lower in Mexican Americans (35.2%) compared with non-Hispanic whites (46.1%) and non-Hispanic blacks (46.5%).[2]

High blood pressure is one of the most important modifiable risk factors for both ischemic and hemorrhagic stroke. Individuals with blood pressures below 120/80 mmHg have approximately half the lifetime risk of stroke of those with hypertension.[4] There is a 38% increased relative risk of stroke for every 10 to 20 mmHg increase in systolic blood pressure, and a 34% increased relative risk for every 5 mmHg increase in diastolic blood pressure.[155] This increased risk is a graded response with no apparent threshold, even within the normal range. Lowering blood pressure reduces the incidence of stroke.[155]

Lifestyle changes can effectively lower blood pressure levels. Adherence to the DASH diet (low in sodium, high in potassium and low-fat dairy) lowers blood pressure.[69,75] Weight loss is strongly related with improved blood pressure; a meta-analysis found that a 5.1 kg loss of body weight was associated with an average lowering of systolic blood pressure by 4.4 mmHg and diastolic by 3.6 mmHg.[156] Treatment with β-blockers lowers the risk for stroke by 29% (RR = 0.71; 95% CI, 0.59-0.86), and diuretics are estimated to reduce the risk by 51% (RR = 0.49; 95% CI, 0.39-0.62).[157] Overall reduction in incident stroke with antihypertensive therapy is estimated at 35% to 44%.[158] Recent data suggest that reductions in stroke risk may be related to type of antihypertensive used, based on the agent's relative effects on blood pressure variability.[159]

Lipids

A clear linear relationship exists between serum cholesterol levels and coronary heart disease; the relationship between serum cholesterol and stroke is less certain. The totality of evidence from large epidemiological studies suggests, at best, a minimal association between increased total cholesterol levels and stroke risk.[117,160] A meta-analysis of 45 prospective cohorts involving 450,000 people and 13,000 incident strokes found no relationship between total cholesterol and stroke.[161] The cohorts upon which the analyses were based included many middle-aged participants, and stroke subtypes were not specified. Subsequent studies found a small association between higher total or low-density lipoprotein (LDL) cholesterol levels and increasing ischemic stroke risk; paradoxically, lower total or LDL cholesterol has generally been associated with an increased risk of hemorrhagic stroke.[117,160] These differing risks may in part explain the lack of a relationship between cholesterol levels and overall stroke rates.

An individual-data meta-analysis of nearly 900,000 patients from 61 studies worldwide found only a weak positive association between total cholesterol and total stroke mortality at ages 40 to 59, with no association at older ages.[162] A weak positive association was also found between total cholesterol and ischemic stroke, with a negative association with hemorrhagic stroke. For both total and ischemic stroke mortality, associations were larger at baseline systolic blood pressure below 145 mmHg.

High-density lipoprotein cholesterol protects against atherosclerosis through reverse cholesterol transport, improvement of endothelial function, and antioxidant, antiinflammatory, and antithrombotic effects.[163,164] Numerous large cohort studies have evaluated the relationship between serum HDL cholesterol and stroke risk.[164] Despite using different HDL cholesterol cut-points and including cohorts of different ages and geography, most of these studies find either a strong and statistically significant inverse relationship[165-169] or a trend towards such a relationship.[170,171] The risk of atherosclerotic stroke, in particular, may be most strongly related to low HDL cholesterol levels.[172-174] A recent large meta-analysis, however, found no evidence for a significant association between HDL cholesterol and stroke mortality, and only a weak positive association between the ratio of total to HDL cholesterol and stroke mortality for those aged 40 to 69.[162] There have been no studies showing that pharmacologically raising HDL cholesterol levels decreases stroke risk.

Findings about the relationship between triglycerides and ischemic stroke are conflicting. Fasting levels were not associated with ischemic stroke in the ARIC and other studies,[171] but a meta-analysis of prospective studies in the Asia-Pacific region showed a 50% increase in ischemic stroke risk for those with the highest vs. lowest fasting levels.[175] In the Copenhagen City Heart Study[176] and the Women's Health Study,[177] higher nonfasting triglycerides were associated with increased risk of ischemic stroke. The Women's Health Study also evaluated fasting triglycerides and found no association with ischemic stroke.[177]

Although no large consistent association between cholesterol and total stroke has been observed in epidemiological cohorts, data from randomized trials show that statin therapy reduces risk of stroke among patients with established coronary heart disease and in those at increased vascular risk.[178,179] One meta-analysis of data from 14 trials including more than 90,000 patients found an approximate 17% to 21% reduction in the relative risk of incident stroke per mmol/L decrease in LDL cholesterol.[178] A significant trend with greater proportional reductions in stroke was associated with greater mean absolute LDL cholesterol reductions. Another meta-analysis including nearly 166,000 participants in trials of statins in combination with other preventive efforts also found an approximate 21% decrease in stroke for each mmol/L decrease in LDL cholesterol.[179] Incidence of all strokes was reduced by 18%, and a reduction in the risk of recurrent stroke and major cardiovascular events among persons with noncardioembolic stroke was found, with a trend toward a lower incidence of fatal stroke.

Use of statin therapy to reduce cholesterol did not lead to increased risk of hemorrhagic stroke in primary stroke prevention populations. Among those with prior stroke or TIA, statins may be associated with an increased risk of hemorrhagic stroke that partially attenuates their overall benefit. Other lipid-modification therapies including niacin, fibric acid derivatives, bile acid sequestrants, and ezetimibe also have favorable effects on lipid parameters, but evidence in support of such strategies for stroke prevention is not well established.[117]

Diabetes

Diabetes is a complex metabolic condition with recognized microvascular and macrovascular complications. In 2007, the CDC estimated that 23.5 million Americans had diabetes, 6 million of whom were undiagnosed.[180] Prevalence of diabetes among those aged 20 years or older was estimated at 11%, and for those aged 60 years or older, 23%. Diabetes is overrepresented among patients who present with ischemic stroke, with prevalence estimates of 15% to 33%.[181] Diabetic patients are more susceptible to development of atherosclerosis and often have other cardiovascular risk factors such as hypertension, dyslipidemia, atrial fibrillation, heart failure, and prior myocardial infarction (MI). Epidemiological studies show the relationship between diabetes and stroke is independent of other such risk factors.

An individual-data meta-analysis based on 97 studies involving nearly 600,000 people worldwide without prior vascular disease found a more than twofold excess risk of incident fatal or first-ever nonfatal ischemic stroke among persons with diabetes, even after adjusting for other vascular risk factors.[182] The excess risk with diabetes was similar for unclassified stroke (84% increased risk) but slightly lower for hemorrhagic stroke (56% increased risk). Although diabetes was consistently associated with increased ischemic stroke risk across clinically relevant strata, risks tended to be higher for women, younger adults (age 40-59 years), and those within the highest tertile of BMI. Individual studies report variations in stroke risk by race-ethnicity among younger age groups.[117]

Much more moderate and nonlinear associations with stroke risk were observed for fasting blood glucose concentration in an individual data meta-analysis including 54 studies involving nearly 300,000 people. Moreover, among persons with no history of diabetes, neither fasting blood glucose concentration nor impaired fasting glucose status improved prediction of vascular disease beyond that of conventional risk factors.

Diabetes is a strong predictor of stroke outcomes[181]; it doubles the risk of recurrent stroke, and an estimated 9% of recurrent strokes can be attributed to diabetes. Diabetic patients have higher stroke mortality rates, greater residual disability, and slower recovery after stroke.[182,183]

Evidence that tight control of glycemic levels lowers stroke (or cardiovascular risk) is lacking.[117] Stroke risk, however, can be modified among diabetic patients.[117] A comprehensive cardiovascular program that includes hypertension control with an angiotensin-converting enzyme inhibitor (ACEI) or angiotensin receptor blocker (ARB) reduces stroke risk. Statin treatment, especially among diabetic patients with additional risk factors, decreases the risk of a first or a recurrent stroke. Monotherapy with a fibrate may be helpful in reducing stroke risk, but data are conflicting; addition of a fibrate to statin therapy has not been found to lower stroke risk among diabetic patients.

Atrial Fibrillation

Atrial fibrillation is a major risk factor for ischemic stroke. Prevalence of atrial fibrillation in the United States increases from 0.5% in those aged 50 to 59 years to 1.8% at 60 to 69 years, 4.8% at 70 to 79 years, and 8.8% at 80 to 89 years.[117] The population attributable stroke risk for atrial fibrillation increases from 1.5% to 2.8%, 9.9%, and 23.5%, respectively, over these same age groups. About 2.3 million Americans have atrial fibrillation. In a U.S. national biracial sample of adult men and women, among individuals with confirmed atrial fibrillation, blacks were approximately one third as likely to be aware as whites that they had the condition.[184]

In addition to age, a variety of other patient characteristics can affect atrial fibrillation–related stroke risk. A review of seven studies, including six independent cohorts, found the strongest, most consistent risk factors for stroke in persons with atrial fibrillation were a history of prior stroke or TIA (RR = 2.5; 95% CI, 1.8-3.5), increasing age (RR = 1.5 per decade; 95% CI, 1.3-1.7), history of hypertension (RR = 2.0; 95% CI, 1.6-2.5), and diabetes mellitus (RR = 1.7; 95% CI, 1.4-2.0).[185] Stroke rates for single independent risk factors were 1.5% to 3% per year for age older than 75, 6% to 9% per year for prior stroke/TIA, 1.5% to 3% per year for history of hypertension, and 2.0% to 3.5% per year for diabetes.

Several published schemes are available to stratify an individual patient's atrial fibrillation–related stroke risk. A comparison of 12 of these schemes found that they varied considerably.[186] Of these, seven were based on extant data and five on expert consensus. Factors most commonly included were previous stroke/TIA (all schemes), patient age (83%), hypertension (83%), and diabetes (83%), with eight additional variables included in one or more schemes. When applied to the same cohort, the fractions of patients categorized by the different schemes varied considerably (proportions of patients categorized) as low risk varied from 9% to 49%, and proportions categorized as high risk varied from 11% to 77%. These differences are not trivial and have important public health and clinical implications.

The so-called CHADS2 scheme is the most commonly used for stroke risk stratification in patients with atrial fibrillation.[187] One point is given for congestive heart failure (C), hypertension (H), age older than 75 years (A), and diabetes mellitus (D); and 2 points for a history of prior stroke or TIA. A validation study found that a score of 0 points reflected low risk (0.5%-1.7% per year); 1 point, moderate risk (1.2%-2.2% per year); and 2 points or more, high risk (1.9%-7.6% per year).[186] It should be noted, however, that a history of prior stroke or TIA in a patient with atrial fibrillation alone is associated with a high risk of recurrent cerebrovascular events (6%-10% per year).[185]

Patients with paroxysmal or chronic atrial fibrillation at moderate or high stroke risk are candidates for treatment with an anticoagulant for prevention of stroke. Treatment with adjusted-dose warfarin leads to a 64% (95% CI, 49%-74%) relative reduction in stroke risk vs. placebo, aspirin with 9% (95% CI, 1%-35%) relative reduction vs. placebo, and adjusted-dose warfarin a 39% (95% CI, 19%-53%) relative reduction vs. aspirin.[117] Yet many persons with atrial fibrillation who should be anticoagulated go untreated.[117] Novel anticoagulants including direct thrombin inhibitors (DTIs) and oral factor Xa inhibitors are now becoming available for treatment of this population of patients.[117]

Sickle Cell Disease

Prevalence of sickle cell disease (SCD), an autosomal recessive inherited disorder, is 0.25% in blacks and confers a 200- to 400-fold increased relative risk of stroke compared to black children without the condition.[117] Prevalence of stroke by age 20 years is approximately 11% in persons homozygous for SCD.[188] Transcranial Doppler (TCD) ultrasonography is useful in identifying children with SCD who are at high and low stroke risk. Children with a timed mean TCD velocity in the middle cerebral artery (MCA) greater than 200 cm/sec have a stroke rate in excess of 10% a year, whereas those with velocities below this level have stroke rates of about 1% a year.[189] Although a variety of treatments are available, regular red blood cell transfusion is the only preventive intervention proven in randomized trials to prevent stroke in children with SCD.[190] Transfusion therapy reduced the risk of stroke from 10% a year to less than 1%.

Sleep-Disordered Breathing

Sleep-disordered breathing (SDB) is highly prevalent in patients with established cardiovascular disease. Obstructive sleep apnea (OSA), one form of SDB, affects an estimated 15 million adult Americans and is present in a large proportion of patients with hypertension and those with other cardiovascular conditions including coronary artery disease (CAD), atrial fibrillation, and stroke.[191-197] Obstructive sleep apnea is characterized by repetitive interruption of ventilation during sleep caused by collapse of the pharyngeal airway. A meta-analysis suggests that nearly three fourths of stroke and TIA patients have SDB, with the predominate form being OSA.[195] In this review, SDB was more common among men and those with recurrent strokes or strokes of unknown etiology; SDB was less common among patients whose strokes were of cardioembolic etiology. An observational study of consecutive patients who underwent polysomnography, with subsequent verified events (strokes and deaths), found that even after adjusting for age, sex, race-ethnicity, and comorbid conditions, OSA syndrome significantly increased the risk of stroke or death from any cause (adjusted hazard ratio, 1.97; 95% CI, 1.12-3.48).[197]

In a trend analysis, increased severity of sleep apnea at baseline was associated with an increased risk of development of this composite end point.[197] Recent 10-year follow-up data of patients with stroke show an increased risk of death in patients with OSA (adjusted hazard ratio, 1.76; 95% CI, 1.05-2.95) that is independent of age, sex, and other common cardiovascular risk factors.[196] Application of noninvasive positive airway pressure ventilation offers patients with sleep apnea the opportunity to increase their rehabilitation potential after stroke, but can be limited by continuous positive airway pressure (CPAP) compliance. Whether patients with stroke and OSA benefit from treatment with CPAP remains to be determined.

Other Risk Factors

Fibrinogen, Clotting Factors, and Inflammation

Evidence supports a role for inflammation in the initiation, progression, and complications of atherosclerosis, as well as being a contributor to destabilization of atherosclerotic lesions.[198] A diverse set of proinflammatory factors have been evaluated as a means to add further prognostic information beyond that already provided by traditional risk factors. High-sensitivity C-reactive protein (CRP) is one of the most widely studied of these biomarkers. C-reactive protein is an acute-phase reactant released predominately by hepatocytes in response to inflammatory cytokine stimulation. It is also released in response to systemic inflammation, such as in connective tissue disease and in response to local infections. Despite lack of specificity for the origin of the inflammation, a multitude of epidemiological studies, including the Physicians' Health Study, the Women's Health Study, and Framingham, have demonstrated a significant association between elevated CRP and risk of incident and recurrent vascular events, including stroke.[117] Risks for those in the highest tertiles/quartiles of CRP concentration ranged between 1.5 and 2 times higher than those in the lowest tertiles/quartiles.

A meta-analysis of individual records from over 50 prospective studies involving over 160,000 participants without preexisting vascular disease found log-transformed CRP concentrations linearly related, with no apparent risk threshold to risk of ischemic stroke.[199] One standard deviation increase in log-transformed CRP concentration (threefold increase) was associated with 27% to 44% increased risk of ischemic stroke and 55% to 71% increased risk of vascular mortality, depending upon risk-adjustment factors. Although somewhat controversial, guidelines have tended to suggest that CRP measurement be limited to persons with intermediate cardiovascular risk (10%-20% 10-year risk based upon Framingham Risk Score) as a means to help guide clinical decision making.[117,200] The 2011 American Heart Association/American Stroke Association (AHA/ASA) Guidelines for the Primary Prevention of Stroke recommends consideration of a measurement of CRP in patients without cardiovascular disease as a means of identifying patients who may be at increased risk of stroke, although the Guidelines also notes that the usefulness in routine clinical practice is not well established.[117] Other markers of inflammation such as lipoprotein-associated protein A2 (LpPLA2) may also be useful.[117]

In addition to examining the relationship between inflammation and stroke via measurement of proinflammatory factors, studies have also evaluated the occurrence of vascular disease in those with systemic chronic inflammatory conditions, such as rheumatoid arthritis and systemic lupus erythematosus, generally finding an excess risk for cardiovascular events as well as stroke.[117] Chronic infection with *Helicobacter pylori* might promote atherosclerosis, but randomized trials of antibiotics have not shown a benefit for prevention of vascular events. Finally, acute infectious diseases have been studied under the hypothesis that they could trigger a TIA or stroke via possible induction of clotting factors such as fibrinogen or the destabilization of atherosclerotic plaques. Influenza has been associated with increased cardiovascular mortality, and antiviral treatment of influenza within a few days of onset decreases 6-month risk of stroke or TIA. A relationship between influenza vaccination and reduced risk for stroke has also been found.

Fibrinogen, a clotting factor thought to accelerate the thrombotic process, is another potentially useful marker of inflammation for use in vascular disease prediction and prevention.[201] An individual-data meta-analysis of 31 prospective studies involving over 150,000 participants without preexisting vascular disease found an approximate log-linear association of usual fibrinogen level and risk of first nonfatal or fatal stroke.[201] This association was present within each age group (40-59, 60-69, ≥70), with no risk threshold. In analyses adjusted for age, sex, and other established vascular risk factors, risk of stroke was nearly doubled with each 1 g/L increase in usual fibrinogen level. When stroke was categorized into subtypes, the magnitude of association with fibrinogen was present for ischemic stroke and stroke attributed to unspecified causes, but was somewhat lower for hemorrhagic stroke. The role of other abnormal clotting factors (e.g., factor V Leiden, prothrombin 20210A mutations, protein C and protein S deficiencies, lupus anticoagulants, anticardiolipin antibodies) as risk factors for ischemic stroke is unclear.[117]

Blood Homocysteine Levels

Homocysteine is an intermediary amino acid formed during metabolism of the essential amino acid methionine. Normal plasma levels of homocysteine are 5 to 15 µmol/L. Elevated homocysteine levels, or hyperhomocysteinemia, may result from genetic defects that reduce enzymatic activity in homocysteine metabolism (e.g., homozygosity for the thermolabile variant of methylene tetrahydrofolate reductase [MTHFR; TT genotype]), nutritional deficiencies in vitamin cofactors (e.g., vitamin B_6, vitamin B_{12}, folic acid), chronic medical conditions (e.g., chronic renal failure that retards renal clearance of homocysteine), certain medications (e.g., fibrates and nicotinic acid, which are used to treat hypercholesterolemia), or lifestyle behaviors (e.g., smoking).[117,202–206]

Numerous studies support a modest association between elevated homocysteine levels and atherosclerotic vascular diseases.[207–216] One meta-analysis involving 463 nonfatal or fatal stroke or TIA events from 12 prospective studies found that a 25% lower usual homocysteine level (≈3 µmol/L) was associated with a 19% (95% CI, 5%-31%) lower risk of stroke after adjustment for known cardiovascular risk factors and regression dilution bias.[207] Another meta-analysis that involved 676 stroke events from eight prospective studies and adjusted for similar factors found a 59% increased risk of stroke for a 5 µmol/L increase in homocysteine.[208] On this basis, a 3 µmol/L decrease in current homocysteine concentrations would be expected to reduce the risk of stroke by 24% (95% CI, 15%-33%). This meta-analysis did not find a statistically significant relationship of the MTHFR TT polymorphism (compared to wild-type CC) with stroke (odds ratio [OR] 1.65; 95% CI, 0.66-4.13), although the seven MTHFR studies included yielded relatively few data. More recent studies continue to report a relationship between hyperhomocysteinemia and stroke, recurrent stroke, and silent brain infarction.[210–216] In a larger and more contemporary meta-analysis of data from over 15,000 persons initially free of cardiovascular disease, homozygotes for the T allele of the MTHFR polymorphism had a greater mean homocysteine level and a 26% (95% CI, 1.14-1.40) greater risk of stroke.[209] Cohort restrictions by age, race, and geographic location yielded similar results.

Laboratory findings and genetic association studies support the biological plausibility of a causal role for elevated homocysteine in stroke pathogenesis, but results of randomized clinical trials have not established the efficacy of homocysteine-lowering therapies for reduction of stroke risk.[117] Clinical trials confirm that vitamins B_6, B_{12}, and folic acid lower homocysteine levels, but several large trials of supplementation with these vitamins as a means of lowering homocysteine levels in patients with established cardiovascular disease have generally found no reduction in major vascular events or death. The largest of such trials to date, Vitamins to Prevent Stroke (VITATOPS), was a double-blind placebo-controlled trial including over 8000 patients with recent TIA or stroke from 20 countries who were followed for a median duration of 3.4 years.[217] Although VITATOPS found daily administration of B vitamins was safe and lowered homocysteine levels, it was not more effective than placebo in reducing risk of the primary combined end point of stroke, MI, or vascular death (RR = 0.91; 95% CI, 0.82-1.00). Secondary analyses by outcome revealed similar results, except for a reduction in vascular death (RR = 0.86; 95% CI, 0.75-0.99). Results were generally consistent across subgroups, although B

vitamins may have a role in reducing risk of vascular events among patients with symptomatic small-vessel intracranial disease. When the VITATOPS findings were included in a meta-analysis with other randomized controlled trials of homocysteine-lowering therapy in patients with and without preexisting cardiovascular disease, trial results were corroborated, with B vitamins not significantly more effective than control for reducing risk of stroke (RR = 0.94; 95% CI, 0.86-1.01) or composite stroke, MI, or vascular death (RR = 0.99; 95% CI, 0.94-1.03).

Despite negative trial results for B vitamins in preventing stroke, a clinically beneficial effect of homocysteine-lowering therapies cannot be excluded. Interventions that are powered to detect smaller risk reductions, that can achieve and sustain larger reductions in homocysteine, or that are focused on certain subgroups such as those with lacunar infarction or ICH caused by small-vessel disease could produce clinically beneficial results. Several trials of B vitamins are ongoing, and a meta-analysis of individual data from these trials and all previous trials is planned as a means to provide more reliable estimates of the long-term effects of B-vitamin supplementation for stroke prevention.

Migraine

Accumulating evidence suggests a relationship between migraine headache and an increased risk of ischemic stroke. A meta-analysis of 14 studies published through June 2004 reported a pooled RR of 2.16 (95% CI, 1.89-2.48); results were similar for analyses restricted to persons younger than 45 years of age and were consistent among those having migraine with and without aura.[218] An updated meta-analysis incorporating nine studies published through January 2009 also reported an increased risk of ischemic stroke among persons with any type of migraine compared to those without migraine (pooled RR = 1.73; 95% CI, 1.31-2.29).[219] Stratification by migraine aura status, however, showed that the higher risk of stroke was largely confined to those having migraine with aura (pooled RR = 2.16; 95% CI, 1.53-3.03 for those with aura vs. pooled RR = 1.23; 95% CI, 0.90-1.69 for those without aura).

Additional stratified analyses suggested a greater risk of ischemic stroke for the following groups: women with migraine (pooled RR = 2.08; 95% CI, 1.13-3.84) but not men (pooled RR = 1.37; 95% CI, 0.89-2.11); persons aged younger than 45 years (pooled RR = 2.65; 95% CI, 1.41-4.97), particularly women (pooled RR = 3.65; 95% CI, 2.21-6.04); smokers (pooled RR = 9.03; 95% CI, 4.22-19.34); and women currently using oral contraceptives (pooled RR = 7.02; 95% CI, 1.51-32.68). Three studies each examined the relationship of any migraine to TIA and hemorrhagic stroke; higher risk was found for TIA (pooled RR = 2.34; 95% CI, 1.90-2.88) but not for hemorrhagic stroke (pooled RR = 1.18; 95% CI, 0.87-1.60). Several studies found an association between migraine headache and nonspecific white matter hyperintensities on magnetic resonance imaging (MRI), localized predominantly in the posterior circulation white matter or cerebellum.[220–223] The clinical significance of these MRI findings is uncertain. There is no evidence that migraine control lowers stroke risk, but as noted earlier, risk of migraine-associated stroke is higher among women who smoke and use oral contraceptives.

Awareness of Stroke Warning Signs and Acute Treatment

Studies indicate that recognition of stroke symptoms is higher in women than men, among whites versus blacks and Hispanics-Latinos, and among people with higher versus lower educational attainment.[224] Although awareness of stroke warning signs has improved over time, recognition of multiple warning signs remains low, as does people's ability to identify tissue-type plasminogen activator (tPA) as an available drug therapy, or the importance of presenting within a window of under 3 hours for treatment.[225] Symptoms associated with increased likelihood of calling 9-1-1 include weakness, confusion/decreased level of consciousness, speech/language deficits, and dizziness/coordination/vertigo; however, numbness and headache were not associated with the decision to call.[226] Administration of intravenous tissue plasminogen activator (IV-tPA) to selected ischemic stroke patients within 4.5 hours of symptom onset improves the likelihood that they will have an excellent outcome. Despite this benefit, only about 2% of ischemic stroke patients in the United States are treated with IV-tPA.[227]

Other potential or emerging risk factors not addressed in this chapter are available for review in the AHA Primary Stroke Guidelines.[117]

REFERENCES

1. World Health Organization: *World Health Report 2004*, Geneva (Switzerland), 2004.
2. Roger VL, Go AS, Lloyd-Jones DM, et al: Heart disease and stroke statistics–2011 update: a report from the American Heart Association, *Circulation* 123(4):e18–e209, 2011.
3. Centers for Disease Control and Prevention. National Center for Health Statistics: *2008 National Ambulatory Medical Care Survey and 2008 National Hospital Ambulatory Medical Care Survey*, 2008.
4. Lloyd-Jones D, Adams RJ, Brown TM, et al: Heart disease and stroke statistics–2010 update: a report from the American Heart Association, *Circulation* 121(7):e46–e215, 2010.
5. Department of Health and Human Services: *Administration of Aging. Statistics on the Aging Population*. Available at: http://www.aoa.gov/prof/Statistics/statistics.aspx. Accessed June 10, 2008.
6. Murray CJL, Lopez AD, Harvard School of Public Health, World Health Organization, World Bank: *The global burden of disease : a comprehensive assessment of mortality and disability from diseases, injuries, and risk factors in 1990 and projected to 2020*, Cambridge, MA, 1996, Published by the Harvard School of Public Health on behalf of the World Health Organization and the World Bank ; Distributed by Harvard University Press.
7. Wu CM, McLaughlin K, Lorenzetti DL, et al: Early risk of stroke after transient ischemic attack: a systematic review and meta-analysis, *Arch Intern Med* 167(22):2417–2422, 2007.
8. Kleindorfer D, Panagos P, Pancioli A, et al: Incidence and short-term prognosis of transient ischemic attack in a population-based study, *Stroke* 36(4):720–723, 2005.
9. Johnston SC, Fayad PB, Gorelick PB, et al: Prevalence and knowledge of transient ischemic attack among US adults, *Neurology* 60(9):1429–1434, 2003.
10. Bravata DM, Ho SY, Brass LM, et al: Long-term mortality in cerebrovascular disease, *Stroke* 34(3):699–704, 2003.
11. Bronnum-Hansen H, Davidsen M, Thorvaldsen P: Long-term survival and causes of death after stroke, *Stroke* 32(9):2131–2136, 2001.
12. Collins TC, Petersen NJ, Menke TJ, et al: Short-term, intermediate-term, and long-term mortality in patients hospitalized for stroke, *J Clin Epidemiol* 56(1):81–87, 2003.
13. Eriksson M, Norrving B, Terent A, et al: Functional outcome 3 months after stroke predicts long-term survival, *Cerebrovasc Dis* 25(5):423–429, 2008.
14. Hallstrom B, Jonsson AC, Nerbrand C, et al: Stroke incidence and survival in the beginning of the 21st century in southern Sweden: comparisons with the late 20th century and projections into the future, *Stroke* 39(1):10–15, 2008.
15. Hankey GJ, Jamrozik K, Broadhurst RJ, et al: Long-term risk of first recurrent stroke in the Perth Community Stroke Study, *Stroke* 29(12):2491–2500, 1998.
16. Hankey GJ, Jamrozik K, Broadhurst RJ, et al: Five-year survival after first-ever stroke and related prognostic factors in the Perth Community Stroke Study, *Stroke* 31(9):2080–2086, 2000.
17. Hardie K, Hankey GJ, Jamrozik K, et al: Ten-year survival after first-ever stroke in the Perth community stroke study, *Stroke* 34(8):1842–1846, 2003.
18. Hartmann A, Rundek T, Mast H, et al: Mortality and causes of death after first ischemic stroke: the Northern Manhattan Stroke Study, *Neurology* 57(11):2000–2005, 2001.
19. Kammersgaard LP, Olsen TS: Cardiovascular risk factors and 5-year mortality in the Copenhagen Stroke Study, *Cerebrovasc Dis* 21(3):187–193, 2006.
20. La Spina P, Savica R, Serra S, et al: Long-term survival and outcome after first stroke in the Sicilian Aeolian Island Archipelago population, *Neurol Sci* 29(3):153–156, 2008.
21. Lai SM, Alter M, Friday G, et al: Prognosis for survival after an initial stroke, *Stroke* 26(11):2011–2015, 1995.
22. Prencipe M, Culasso F, Rasura M, et al: Long-term prognosis after a minor stroke: 10-year mortality and major stroke recurrence rates in a hospital-based cohort, *Stroke* 29(1):126–132, 1998.
23. Qureshi AI, Suri MF, Zhou J, et al: African American women have poor long-term survival following ischemic stroke, *Neurology* 67(9):1623–1629, 2006.
24. Sacco RL, Shi T, Zamanillo MC, et al: Predictors of mortality and recurrence after hospitalized cerebral infarction in an urban community: the Northern Manhattan Stroke Study, *Neurology* 44(4):626–634, 1994.
25. Sacco RL, Wolf PA, Kannel WB, et al: Survival and recurrence following stroke. The Framingham Study, *Stroke* 13(3):290–295, 1982.
26. Terent A: Trends in stroke incidence and 10-year survival in Soderhamn, Sweden, 1975-2001, *Stroke* 34(6):1353–1358, 2003.
27. Tu JV, Gong Y: Trends in treatment and outcomes for acute stroke patients in Ontario, 1992-1998, *Arch Intern Med* 163(3):293–297, 2003.
28. von Arbin M, Britton M, de Faire U: Mortality and recurrences during eight years following stroke, *J Intern Med* 231(1):43–48, 1992.
29. Andersen KK, Olsen TS: One-month to 10-year survival in the Copenhagen stroke study: interactions between stroke severity and other prognostic indicators, *J Stroke Cerebrovasc Dis* 20(2):117–123, 2011.
30. Asplund K, Stegmayr B, Peltonen M: From the twentieth to the twenty-first century: a public health perspective on stroke. In Ginsberg MD, Bogousslavsky J, editors: *Cerebrovascular disease pathophysiology, diagnosis, and management*, vol 2, Malden, MA, 1998, Blackwell Science.
31. Andrews R, Elixhauser A: *The national hospital bill: growth trends and 2005 update on the most expensive conditions by payer. Healthcare cost and utilization project–statistical brief #42*, Washington, DC, 2007, Agency for Healthcare Research and Quality.
32. Brown DL, Boden-Albala B, Langa KM, et al: Projected costs of ischemic stroke in the United States, *Neurology* 67(8):1390–1395, 2006.
33. Taylor TN, Davis PH, Torner JC, et al: Lifetime cost of stroke in the United States, *Stroke* 27(9):1459–1466, 1996.
34. Borhani NO: Changes and geographic distribution of mortality from cerebrovascular disease, *Am J Public Health Nations Health* 55:673–681, 1965.
35. El-Saed A, Kuller LH, Newman AB, et al: Geographic variations in stroke incidence and mortality among older populations in four US communities, *Stroke* 37(8):1975–1979, 2006.
36. Lanska DJ: Geographic distribution of stroke mortality in the United States: 1939-1941 to 1979-1981, *Neurology* 43(9):1839–1851, 1993.
37. Lanska DJ, Kryscio R: Geographic distribution of hospitalization rates, case fatality, and mortality from stroke in the United States, *Neurology* 44(8):1541–1550, 1994.
38. Pickle LW, Mungiole M, Gillum RF: Geographic variation in stroke mortality in blacks and whites in the United States, *Stroke* 28(8):1639–1647, 1997.
39. Howard G: Why do we have a stroke belt in the southeastern United States? A review of unlikely and uninvestigated potential causes, *Am J Med Sci* 317(3):160–167, 1999.
40. Howard G, Evans GW, Pearce K, et al: Is the stroke belt disappearing? An analysis of racial, temporal, and age effects, *Stroke* 26(7):1153–1158, 1995.
41. Howard G, Howard VJ, Katholi C, et al: Decline in US stroke mortality: an analysis of temporal patterns by sex, race, and geographic region, *Stroke* 32(10):2213–2220, 2001.
42. Gillum RF, Ingram DD: Relation between residence in the southeast region of the United States and stroke incidence. The NHANES I Epidemiologic Followup Study, *Am J Epidemiol* 144(7):665–673, 1996.
43. Howard VJ, Kleindorfer DO, Judd SE, et al: Disparities in stroke incidence contributing to disparities in stroke mortality, *Ann Neurol* 69(4):619–627, 2011.
44. Casper M, Nwaise I, Croft J, et al: Atlas of stroke hospitalizations among medicare beneficiaries. In *U.S. Department of Health and Human Services Centers for Disease Control and Prevention*, Atlanta, 2008.
45. Allen NB, Holford TR, Bracken MB, et al: Geographic variation in one-year recurrent ischemic stroke rates for elderly Medicare beneficiaries in the USA, *Neuroepidemiology* 34(2):123–129, 2010.
46. Allen NB, Holford TR, Bracken MB, et al: Trends in one-year recurrent ischemic stroke among the elderly in the USA: 1994-2002, *Cerebrovasc Dis* 30(5):525–532, 2010.
47. Davenport RJ, Dennis MS, Wellwood I, et al: Complications after acute stroke, *Stroke* 27(3):415–420, 1996.
48. *2000-2050 Population projections of the United States by age, sex, race, Hispanic origin, and nativity: 1999-2100*, 2000. US Census Bureau. Available at: www.census.gov/population/www/projections/natproj.html.
49. Day JC: *Population projections of the United States by age, sex, race, and hispanic origin: 1995 to 2050*, Washington, DC, 1996, U.S. Bureau of the Census, Current, Population Reports, U.S. Government Printing Office.
50. Reeves MJ, Bushnell CD, Howard G, et al: Sex differences in stroke: epidemiology, clinical presentation, medical care, and outcomes, *Lancet Neurol* 7(10):915–926, 2008.
51. Bushnell CD: Stroke in women: risk and prevention throughout the lifespan, *Neurol Clin* 26(4):1161–1176, xi, 2008.
52. Towfighi A, Markovic D, Ovbiagele B: Persistent sex disparity in midlife stroke prevalence in the United States, *Cerebrovasc Dis* 31(4):322–328, 2011.
53. Sheinart KF, Tuhrim S, Horowitz DR, et al: Stroke recurrence is more frequent in blacks and Hispanics, *Neuroepidemiology* 17(4):188–198, 1998.
54. Gillum RF: Epidemiology of stroke in Hispanic Americans, *Stroke* 26(9):1707–1712, 1995.
55. Sacco RL, Hauser WA, Mohr JP, et al: One-year outcome after cerebral infarction in whites, blacks, and Hispanics, *Stroke* 22(3):305–311, 1991.
56. Bian J, Oddone EZ, Samsa GP, et al: Racial differences in survival post cerebral infarction among the elderly, *Neurology* 60(2):285–290, 2003.
57. Lackland DT, Bachman DL, Carter TD, et al: The geographic variation in stroke incidence in two areas of the southeastern stroke belt: the Anderson and Pee Dee Stroke Study, *Stroke* 29(10):2061–2068, 1998.
58. Matchar DB, Samsa GP: *Secondary and tertiary prevention of stroke. Patient Outcome Research Team (PORT) final report–phase 1*. Prepared by Duke University Medical Center under contract no. 290-91-0028. Rockville, MD, 2000, Agency for Healthcare Research and Quality.
59. Kleindorfer DO, Khoury J, Moomaw CJ, et al: Stroke incidence is decreasing in whites but not in blacks: a population-based estimate of temporal trends in stroke incidence from the Greater Cincinnati/Northern Kentucky Stroke Study, *Stroke* 41(7):1326–1331, 2010.
60. Boden-Albala B, Sacco RL: Lifestyle factors and stroke risk: exercise, alcohol, diet, obesity, smoking, drug use, and stress, *Curr Atheroscler Rep* 2(2):160–166, 2000.
61. Boden-Albala B, Elkind MS, White H, et al: Dietary total fat intake and ischemic stroke risk: the Northern Manhattan Study, *Neuroepidemiology* 32(4):296–301, 2009.
62. Iso H, Rexrode KM, Stampfer MJ, et al: Intake of fish and omega-3 fatty acids and risk of stroke in women, *JAMA* 285(3):304–312, 2001.
63. Gillum RF, Mussolino ME, Madans JH: The relationship between fish consumption and stroke incidence. The NHANES I Epidemiologic Follow-up Study (National Health and Nutrition Examination Survey), *Arch Intern Med* 156(5):537–542, 1996.
64. Bazzano LA, Serdula MK, Liu S: Dietary intake of fruits and vegetables and risk of cardiovascular disease, *Curr Atheroscler Rep* 5(6):492–499, 2003.
65. Johnsen SP, Overvad K, Stripp C, et al: Intake of fruit and vegetables and the risk of ischemic stroke in a cohort of Danish men and women, *Am J Clin Nutr* 78(1):57–64, 2003.
66. Sauvaget C, Nagano J, Allen N, et al: Vegetable and fruit intake and stroke mortality in the Hiroshima/Nagasaki Life Span Study, *Stroke* 34(10):2355–2360, 2003.
67. Steffen LM, Jacobs DR Jr, Stevens J, et al: Associations of whole-grain, refined-grain, and fruit and vegetable consumption with risks of all-cause mortality and incident coronary artery disease and ischemic stroke: the Atherosclerosis Risk in Communities (ARIC) Study, *Am J Clin Nutr* 78(3):383–390, 2003.

68. Joshipura KJ, Ascherio A, Manson JE, et al: Fruit and vegetable intake in relation to risk of ischemic stroke, *JAMA* 282(13):1233–1239, 1999.

69. John JH, Ziebland S, Yudkin P, et al: Effects of fruit and vegetable consumption on plasma antioxidant concentrations and blood pressure: a randomised controlled trial, *Lancet* 359(9322):1969–1974, 2002.

70. He FJ, Nowson CA, MacGregor GA: Fruit and vegetable consumption and stroke: meta-analysis of cohort studies, *Lancet* 367(9507):320–326, 2006.

71. He J, Ogden LG, Vupputuri S, et al: Dietary sodium intake and subsequent risk of cardiovascular disease in overweight adults, *JAMA* 282(21):2027–2034, 1999.

72. Nagata C, Takatsuka N, Shimizu N, et al: Sodium intake and risk of death from stroke in Japanese men and women, *Stroke* 35(7):1543–1547, 2004.

73. Khaw KT, Barrett-Connor E: Dietary potassium and stroke-associated mortality. A 12-year prospective population study, *N Engl J Med* 316(5):235–240, 1987.

74. Ascherio A, Rimm EB, Hernan MA, et al: Intake of potassium, magnesium, calcium, and fiber and risk of stroke among US men, *Circulation* 98(12):1198–1204, 1998.

75. Appel LJ, Moore TJ, Obarzanek E, et al: A clinical trial of the effects of dietary patterns on blood pressure. DASH Collaborative Research Group, *N Engl J Med* 336(16):1117–1124, 1997.

76. Fung TT, Chiuve SE, McCullough ML, et al: Adherence to a DASH-style diet and risk of coronary heart disease and stroke in women, *Arch Intern Med* 168(7):713–720, 2008.

77. Fung TT, Rexrode KM, Mantzoros CS, et al: Mediterranean diet and incidence of and mortality from coronary heart disease and stroke in women, *Circulation* 119(8):1093–1100, 2009.

78. Fung TT, Stampfer MJ, Manson JE, et al: Prospective study of major dietary patterns and stroke risk in women, *Stroke* 35(9):2014–2019, 2004.

79. Centers for Disease Control and Prevention: Sodium intake among adults - United States, 2005-2006, *MMWR Morb Mortal Wkly Rep* 59(24):746–749, 2010.

80. Ezzati M, Hoorn SV, Lopez AD, et al: Comparative quantification of mortality and burden of disease attributable to selected risk factors. In Lopez AD, Mathers CD, Ezzati M, et al, editors: *Global burden of disease and risk factors*, Washington DC, 2006, World Bank.

81. Abbott RD, Rodriguez BL, Burchfiel CM, et al: Physical activity in older middle-aged men and reduced risk of stroke: the Honolulu Heart Program, *Am J Epidemiol* 139(9):881–893, 1994.

82. Kiely DK, Wolf PA, Cupples LA, et al: Physical activity and stroke risk: the Framingham Study, *Am J Epidemiol* 140(7):608–620, 1994.

83. Haheim LL, Holme I, Hjermann I, et al: Risk factors of stroke incidence and mortality. A 12-year follow-up of the Oslo Study, *Stroke* 24(10):1484–1489, 1993.

84. Gillum RF, Mussolino ME, Ingram DD: Physical activity and stroke incidence in women and men. The NHANES I Epidemiologic Follow-up Study, *Am J Epidemiol* 143(9):860–869, 1996.

85. Wannamethee G, Shaper AG: Physical activity and stroke in British middle aged men, *BMJ* 304(6827):597–601, 1992.

86. Sacco RL, Gan R, Boden-Albala B, et al: Leisure-time physical activity and ischemic stroke risk: the Northern Manhattan Stroke Study, *Stroke* 29(2):380–387, 1998.

87. Lindenstrom E, Boysen G, Nyboe J: Lifestyle factors and risk of cerebrovascular disease in women. The Copenhagen City Heart Study, *Stroke* 24(10):1468–1472, 1993.

88. Manson JE, Colditz GA, Stampfer MJ, et al: A prospective study of maturity-onset diabetes mellitus and risk of coronary heart disease and stroke in women, *Arch Intern Med* 151(6):1141–1147, 1991.

89. Blair SN, Kampert JB, Kohl HW 3rd, et al: Influences of cardiorespiratory fitness and other precursors on cardiovascular disease and all-cause mortality in men and women, *JAMA* 276(3):205–210, 1996.

90. Kokkinos PF, Holland JC, Pittaras AE, et al: Cardiorespiratory fitness and coronary heart disease risk factor association in women, *J Am Coll Cardiol* 26(2):358–364, 1995.

91. Lakka TA, Salonen JT: Moderate to high intensity conditioning leisure time physical activity and high cardiorespiratory fitness are associated with reduced plasma fibrinogen in eastern Finnish men, *J Clin Epidemiol* 46(10):1119–1127, 1993.

92. Williams PT: High-density lipoprotein cholesterol and other risk factors for coronary heart disease in female runners, *N Engl J Med* 334(20):1298–1303, 1996.

93. Wang HY, Bashore TR, Friedman E: Exercise reduces age-dependent decrease in platelet protein kinase C activity and translocation, *J Gerontol A Biol Sci Med Sci* 1(6):M12–M16, 1995.

94. Lee IM, Hennekens CH, Berger K, et al: Exercise and risk of stroke in male physicians, *Stroke* 30(1):1–6, 1999.

95. Pate RR, Pratt M, Blair SN, et al: Physical activity and public health. A recommendation from the Centers for Disease Control and Prevention and the American College of Sports Medicine, *JAMA* 273(5):402–407, 1995.

96. Physical activity and cardiovascular health. NIH Consensus Development Panel on Physical Activity and Cardiovascular Health, *JAMA* 276(3):241–246, 1996.

97. Sattelmair JR, Kurth T, Buring JE, et al: Physical activity and risk of stroke in women, *Stroke* 41(6):1243–1250, 2010.

98. Wilson PW, Bozeman SR, Burton TM, et al: Prediction of first events of coronary heart disease and stroke with consideration of adiposity, *Circulation* 118(2):124–130, 2008.

99. Rexrode KM, Hennekens CH, Willett WC, et al: A prospective study of body mass index, weight change, and risk of stroke in women, *JAMA* 277(19):1539–1545, 1997.

100. Burchfiel CM, Curb JD, Arakaki R, et al: Cardiovascular risk factors and hyperinsulinemia in elderly men: the Honolulu Heart Program, *Ann Epidemiol* 6(6):490–497, 1996.

101. Walker SP, Rimm EB, Ascherio A, et al: Body size and fat distribution as predictors of stroke among US men, *Am J Epidemiol* 144(12):1143–1150, 1996.

102. Hedley AA, Ogden CL, Johnson CL, et al: Prevalence of overweight and obesity among US children, adolescents, and adults, 1999-2002, *JAMA* 291(23):2847–2850, 2004.

103. Brook RD, Franklin B, Cascio W, et al: Air pollution and cardiovascular disease: a statement for healthcare professionals from the expert panel on population and prevention science of the American Heart Association, *Circulation* 109(21):2655–2671, 2004.

104. Brook RD, Rajagopalan S, Pope CA, et al: Particulate matter air pollution and cardiovascular disease: an update to the scientific statement from the American Heart Association, *Circulation* 121(21):2331–2378, 2010.

105. Miller KA, Siscovick DS, Sheppard L, et al: Long-term exposure to air pollution and incidence of cardiovascular events in women, *N Engl J Med* 356(5):447–458, 2007.

106. Pope CA III, Burnett RT, Thurston GD, et al: Cardiovascular mortality and long-term exposure to particulate air pollution: epidemiological evidence of general pathophysiological pathways of disease, *Circulation* 109(1):71–77, 2004.

107. Hong Y-C, Lee J-T, Kim H, et al: Effects of air pollutants on acute stroke mortality, *Environ Health Perspect* 110(2):187–191, 2002.

108. Hong Y-C, Lee J-T, Kim H, et al: Air pollution: a new risk factor in ischemic stroke mortality, *Stroke* 33(9):2165–2169, 2002.

109. Kan H, Jia J, Chen B: Acute stroke mortality and air pollution: new evidence from shanghai, China, *J Occup Health* 45(5):321–323, 2003.

110. Kettunen J, Lanki T, Tiittanen P, et al: Associations of fine and ultrafine particulate air pollution with stroke mortality in an area of low air pollution levels, *Stroke* 38(3):918–922, 2007.

111. Henrotin JB, Besancenot JP, Bejot Y, et al: Short-term effects of ozone air pollution on ischaemic stroke occurrence: a case-crossover analysis from a 10-year population-based study in Dijon, France, *Occup Environ Med* 64(7):439–445, 2007.

112. Lisabeth LD, Escobar JD, Dvonch JT, et al: Ambient air pollution and risk for ischemic stroke and transient ischemic attack, *Ann Neurol* 64(1):53–59, 2008.

113. Wolf P, D'Agostino R, Belanger A, et al: Probability of stroke: a risk profile from the Framingham Study, *Stroke* 22(3):312–318, 1991.

114. Manolio TA, Kronmal RA, Burke GL, et al: Short-term predictors of incident stroke in older adults: the Cardiovascular Health Study, *Stroke* 27(9):1479–1486, 1996.

115. Rodriguez BL, D'Agostino R, Abbott RD, et al: Risk of hospitalized stroke in men enrolled in the Honolulu Heart Program and the Framingham Study: a comparison of incidence and risk factor effects, *Stroke* 33(1):230–236, 2002.

116. O'Donnell MJ, Xavier D, Liu L, et al: Risk factors for ischaemic and intracerebral haemorrhagic stroke in 22 countries (the INTERSTROKE study): a case-control study, *Lancet* 376(9735):112–123, 2010.

117. Goldstein LB, Bushnell CD, Adams RJ, et al: Guidelines for the primary prevention of stroke. A guideline for healthcare professionals From the American Heart Association/American Stroke Association, *Stroke* 42:517–584, 2011.

118. Feigin VL, Rinkel GJE, Lawes CMM, et al: Risk factors for subarachnoid hemorrhage: an updated systematic review of epidemiological studies, *Stroke* 36(12):2773–2780, 2005.

119. Kurth T, Kase CS, Berger K, et al: Smoking and risk of hemorrhagic stroke in women, *Stroke* 34(12):2792–2795, 2003.

120. Kurth T, Kase CS, Berger K, et al: Smoking and the risk of hemorrhagic stroke in men, *Stroke* 34(5):1151–1155, 2003.

121. Feigin V, Parag V, Lawes CMM, et al: Smoking and elevated blood pressure are the most important risk factors for subarachnoid hemorrhage in the Asia-Pacific region: an overview of 26 cohorts involving 306, 620 participants, *Stroke* 36(7):1360–1365, 2005.

122. Feldmann E, Broderick JP, Kernan WN, et al: Major risk factors for intracerebral hemorrhage in the young are modifiable, *Stroke* 36(9):1881–1885, 2005.

123. Sturgeon JD, Folsom AR, Longstreth WT Jr, et al: Risk factors for intracerebral hemorrhage in a pooled prospective study, *Stroke* 38(10):2718–2725, 2007.

124. Shinton R, Beevers G: Meta-analysis of relation between cigarette smoking and stroke, *BMJ* 298(6676):789–794, 1989.

125. Ariesen MJ, Claus SP, Rinkel GJE, et al: Risk factors for intracerebral hemorrhage in the general population: a systematic review, *Stroke* 34(8):2060–2065, 2003.

126. CDC: Smoking-attributable mortality, years of potential life lost, and productivity losses - United States, 2000-2004, *MMWR Morb Mortal Wkly Rep* 57(45):1226–1228, 2008.

127. Lee PN, Forey BA: Environmental tobacco smoke exposure and risk of stroke in nonsmokers: a review with meta-analysis, *J Stroke Cerebrovasc Dis* 15(5):190–201, 2006.

128. U.S. Department of Health and Human Services: *How tobacco smoke causes disease: the biology and behavioral basis for smoking-attributable disease: a report of the Surgeon General*, Atlanta, GA, 2010, Department of Health and Human Services, Centers for Disease Control and Prevention, National Center for Chronic Disease Prevention and Health Promotion, Office on Smoking and Health.

129. Ambrose JA, Barua RS: The pathophysiology of cigarette smoking and cardiovascular disease: an update, *J Am Coll Cardiol* 43(10):1731–1737, 2004.

130. Howard G, Thun MJ: Why is environmental tobacco smoke more strongly associated with coronary heart disease than expected? A review of potential biases and experimental data, *Environ Health Perspect* 107:853–858, 1999.

131. Kool M, Hoeks A, Struijker Boudier H, et al: Short- and long-term effects of smoking on arterial wall properties in habitual smokers, *J Am Coll Cardiol* 22(7):1881–1886, 1993.

132. Silvestrini M, Troisi E, Matteis M, et al: Effect of smoking on cerebrovascular reactivity, *J Cereb Blood Flow Metab* 16(4):746–749, 1996.

133. Nakamura K, Barzi F, Lam T-H, et al: Cigarette smoking, systolic blood pressure, and cardiovascular diseases in the Asia-Pacific region, *Stroke* 39(6):1694–1702, 2008.

134. Schwartz SW, Carlucci C, Chambless LE, et al: Synergism between smoking and vital exhaustion in the risk of ischemic stroke: evidence from the ARIC study, *Ann Epidemiol* 14(6):416–424, 2004.

135. WHO Collaborative Study of Cardiovascular Disease and Steroid Hormone Contraception: Ischaemic stroke and combined oral contraceptives: results of an international, multicentre, case-control study, *Lancet* 348(9026):498–505, 1996.

136. WHO Collaborative Study of Cardiovascular Disease and Steroid Hormone Contraception: Haemorrhagic stroke, overall stroke risk, and combined oral contraceptives: results of an international, multicentre, case-control study, *Lancet* 348(9026):505–510, 1996.

137. Kawachi I, Colditz GA, Stampfer MJ, et al: Smoking cessation and decreased risk of stroke in women, *JAMA* 269(2):232–236, 1993.

138. Wannamethee SG, Shaper AG, Whincup PH, et al: Smoking cessation and the risk of stroke in middle-aged men, *JAMA* 274(2):155–160, 1995.

139. Wolf PA, D'Agostino RB, Kannel WB, et al: Cigarette smoking as a risk factor for stroke, *JAMA* 259(7):1025–1029, 1988.

140. Abbott RD, Yin Y, Reed DM, et al: Risk of stroke in male cigarette smokers, *N Engl J Med* 315(12):717–720, 1986.

141. Shinton R: Lifelong exposures and the potential for stroke prevention: the contribution of cigarette smoking, exercise, and body fat, *J Epidemiol Community Health* 51(2):138–143, 1997.

142. Donahue RP, Abbott RD, Reed DM, et al: Alcohol and hemorrhagic stroke. The Honolulu Heart Program, *JAMA* 255(17):2311–2314, 1986.

143. Mukamal KJ, Ascherio A, Mittleman MA, et al: Alcohol and risk for ischemic stroke in men: the role of drinking patterns and usual beverage, *Ann Intern Med* 142(1):11–19, 2005.

144. Sacco RL, Elkind M, Boden-Albala B, et al: The protective effect of moderate alcohol consumption on ischemic stroke, *JAMA* 281(1):53–60, 1999.

145. Hillbom M, Numminen H, Juvela S: Recent heavy drinking of alcohol and embolic stroke, *Stroke* 30(11):2307–2312, 1999.

146. Gill JS, Zezulka AV, Shipley MJ, et al: Stroke and alcohol consumption, *N Engl J Med* 315(17):1041–1046, 1986.

147. Stampfer MJ, Colditz GA, Willett WC, et al: A prospective study of moderate alcohol consumption and the risk of coronary disease and stroke in women, *N Engl J Med* 319(5):267–273, 1988.

148. Berger K, Ajani UA, Kase CS, et al: Light-to-moderate alcohol consumption and risk of stroke among U.S. male physicians, *N Engl J Med* 341(21):1557–1564, 1999.

149. Iso H, Baba S, Mannami T, et al: Alcohol consumption and risk of stroke among middle-aged men: the JPHC Study Cohort I, *Stroke* 35(5):1124–1129, 2004.

150. Malarcher AM, Giles WH, Croft JB, et al: Alcohol intake, type of beverage, and the risk of cerebral infarction in young women, *Stroke* 32(1):77–83, 2001.

151. Reynolds K, Lewis B, Nolen JD, et al: Alcohol consumption and risk of stroke: a meta-analysis, *JAMA* 289(5):579–588, 2003.

152. Anonymous: Report of the Dietary Guidelines Advisory Committee Dietary Guidelines for Americans, 1995, *Nutr Rev* 53(12):376–379, 1995.

153. Fields LE, Burt VL, Cutler JA, et al: The burden of adult hypertension in the United States 1999 to 2000: a rising tide, *Hypertension* 44(4):398–404, 2004.

154. Chobanian AV, Bakris GL, Black HR, et al: The Seventh Report of the Joint National Committee on Prevention, Detection, Evaluation, and Treatment of High Blood Pressure: the JNC 7 report, *JAMA* 289(19):2560–2572, 2003.

155. Law M, Wald N, Morris J: Lowering blood pressure to prevent myocardial infarction and stroke: a new preventive strategy, *Health Technol Assess* 7(31):1–94, 2003.

156. Neter JE, Stam BE, Kok FJ, et al: Influence of weight reduction on blood pressure: a meta-analysis of randomized controlled trials, *Hypertension* 42(5):878–884, 2003.

157. Psaty BM, Smith NL, Siscovick DS, et al: Health outcomes associated with antihypertensive therapies used as first-line agents. A systematic review and meta-analysis, *JAMA* 277(9):739–745, 1997.

158. Neal B, MacMahon S, Chapman N: Effects of ACE inhibitors, calcium antagonists, and other blood-pressure-lowering drugs: results of prospectively designed overviews of randomised trials. Blood Pressure Lowering Treatment Trialists' Collaboration, *Lancet* 356(9246):1955–1964, 2000.

159. Webb AJ, Fischer U, Mehta Z, et al: Effects of antihypertensive-drug class on interindividual variation in blood pressure and risk of stroke: a systematic review and meta-analysis, *Lancet* 13;375(9718):906–915.

160. Amarenco P, Lavallée P, Touboul P-J: Stroke prevention, blood cholesterol, and statins, *Lancet Neurol* 3(5):271–278, 2004.

161. Prospective Studies Collaboration: Cholesterol, diastolic blood pressure, and stroke: 13,000 strokes in 450,000 people in 45 prospective cohorts, *Lancet* 346:1647–1653, 1995.

162. Prospective Studies Collaboration: Blood cholesterol and vascular mortality by age, sex, and blood pressure: a meta-analysis of individual data from 61 prospective studies with 55,000 vascular deaths, *Lancet* 370(9602):1829–1839, 2007.

163. Brewer HB: Increasing HDL cholesterol levels, *N Engl J Med* 350(15):1491–1494, 2004.

164. Sanossian N, Saver JL, Navab M, et al: High-density lipoprotein cholesterol: an emerging target for stroke treatment, *Stroke* 38(3):1104–1109, 2007.

165. Curb JD, Abbott RD, Rodriguez BL, et al: High density lipoprotein cholesterol and the risk of stroke in elderly men, *Am J Epidemiol* 160(2):150–157, 2004.

166. Soyama Y, Miura K, Morikawa Y, et al: High-density lipoprotein cholesterol and risk of stroke in Japanese men and women: the Oyabe Study, *Stroke* 34(4):863–868, 2003.

167. Simons LA, McCallum J, Friedlander Y, et al: Risk factors for ischemic stroke: Dubbo Study of the Elderly, *Stroke* 29(7):1341–1346, 1998.

168. Lindenstrom E, Boysen G, Nyboe J: Influence of total cholesterol, high density lipoprotein cholesterol, and triglycerides on risk of cerebrovascular disease: the Copenhagen city heart study, *BMJ* 309(6946):11–15, 1994.

169. Tanne D, Yaari S, Goldbourt U: High-density lipoprotein cholesterol and risk of ischemic stroke mortality: a 21-year follow-up of 8586 men from the Israeli Ischemic Heart Disease Study, *Stroke* 28(1):83–87, 1997.

170. Wannamethee SG, Shaper AG, Ebrahim S: HDL-cholesterol, total cholesterol, and the risk of stroke in middle-aged British men, *Stroke* 31(8):1882–1888, 2000.

171. Shahar E, Chambless LE, Rosamond WD, et al: Plasma lipid profile and incident ischemic stroke: the Atherosclerosis Risk in Communities (ARIC) Study, *Stroke* 34(3):623–631, 2003.

172. Sacco RL, Benson RT, Kargman DE, et al: High-density lipoprotein cholesterol and ischemic stroke in the elderly, *JAMA* 285(21):2729–2735, 2001.

173. Tirschwell DL, Smith NL, Heckbert SR, et al: Association of cholesterol with stroke risk varies in stroke subtypes and patient subgroups, *Neurology* 63(10):1868–1875, 2004.

174. Johnsen SH, Mathiesen EB, Fosse E, et al: Elevated high-density lipoprotein cholesterol levels are protective against plaque progression: a follow-up study of 1952 persons with carotid Atherosclerosis The Tromso Study, *Circulation* 112(4):498–504, 2005.

175. Asia Pacific Cohort Studies Collaboration: Serum triglycerides as a risk factor for cardiovascular diseases in the Asia-Pacific region, *Circulation* 110(17):2678–2686, 2004.

176. Freiberg JJ, Tybjærg-Hansen A, Jensen JS, et al: Nonfasting triglycerides and risk of ischemic stroke in the general population, *JAMA* 300(18):2142–2152, 2008.

177. Bansal S, Buring JE, Rifai N, et al: Fasting compared with nonfasting triglycerides and risk of cardiovascular events in women, *JAMA* 298(3):309–316, 2007.

178. Cholesterol Treatment Trialists' (CTT) Collaborators: Efficacy and safety of cholesterol-lowering treatment: prospective meta-analysis of data from 90,056 participants in 14 randomised trials of statins, *Lancet* 366(9493):1267–1278, 2005.

179. Amarenco P, Labreuche J: Lipid management in the prevention of stroke: review and updated meta-analysis of statins for stroke prevention, *Lancet Neurol* 8(5):453–463, 2009.

180. CDC: *National diabetes fact sheet, 2007.* Available at: http://www.cdc.gov/diabetes/pubs/pdf/ndfs_2007.pdf. Accessed December 22, 2010.

181. Furie KL, Kasner SE, Adams RJ, et al: Guidelines for the prevention of stroke in patients with stroke or transient ischemic attack: a guideline for healthcare professionals from the American Heart Association/American Stroke Association, *Stroke* 42(1):227–276, 2011.

182. The Emerging Risk Factors Collaboration: Diabetes mellitus, fasting blood glucose concentration, and risk of vascular disease: a collaborative meta-analysis of 102 prospective studies, *Lancet* 375(9733):2215–2222, 2010.

183. Mankovsky BN, Ziegler D: Stroke in patients with diabetes mellitus, *Diabetes Metab Res Rev* 20(4):268–287, 2004.

184. Meschia JF, Merrill P, Soliman EZ, et al: Racial disparities in awareness and treatment of atrial fibrillation: the REasons for Geographic and Racial Differences in Stroke (REGARDS) Study, *Stroke* 41(4):581–587, 2010.

185. Hart RG, Pearce LA, Albers GW, et al: Independent predictors of stroke in patients with atrial fibrillation: a systematic review, *Neurology* 69:546–554, 2007.

186. Hart RG, Pearce LA, Halperin JL, et al: Comparison of 12 risk stratification schemes to predict stroke in patients with nonvalvular atrial fibrillation, *Stroke* 39(6):1901–1910, 2008.

187. Gage BF, Waterman AD, Shannon W, et al: Validation of clinical classification schemes for predicting stroke: results from the National Registry of Atrial Fibrillation, *JAMA* 285:2864–2870, 2001.

188. Ohene-Frempong K, Weiner SJ, Sleeper LA, et al: Cerebrovascular accidents in sickle cell disease: rates and risk factors, *Blood* 91:288–294, 1998.

189. Adams RJ, McKie VC, Carl EM, et al: Long-term stroke risk in children with sickle cell disease screened with transcranial Doppler, *Ann Neurol* 42:699–704, 1997.

190. Adams RJ, McKie VC, Hsu L, et al: Prevention of a first stroke by transfusions in children with sickle cell anemia and abnormal results on transcranial Doppler ultrasonography, *N Engl J Med* 339:5–11, 1998.

191. Bagai K: Obstructive sleep apnea, stroke, and cardiovascular diseases, *Neurologist* 16(6):329–339, 2010.

192. Budhiraja R, Budhiraja P, Quan SF: Sleep-disordered breathing and cardiovascular disorders, *Respir Care* 55(10):1322–1330, 2010.

193. Dyken ME, Im KB: Obstructive sleep apnea and stroke, *Chest* 136(6):1668–1677, 2009.

194. Hermann DM, Bassetti CL: Sleep-related breathing and sleep-wake disturbances in ischemic stroke, *Neurology* 73(16):1313–1322, 2009.

195. Johnson KG, Johnson DC: Frequency of sleep apnea in stroke and TIA patients: a meta-analysis, *J Clin Sleep Med* 6(2):131–137, 2010.

196. Somers VK, White DP, Amin R, et al: Sleep apnea and cardiovascular disease: an American Heart Association/American College of Cardiology Foundation scientific statement from the American Heart Association Council for High Blood Pressure Research Professional Education Committee, Council on Clinical Cardiology, Stroke Council, and Council on Cardiovascular Nursing, *Circulation* 118(10):1080–1111, 2008.

197. Yaggi H, Mohsenin V: Sleep apnea and stroke: a risk factor or an association? *Sleep Med Clin* 2(4):583–591, 2007.

198. Libby P, Ridker PM: Inflammation and atherothrombosis: from population biology and bench research to clinical practice, *J Am Coll Cardiol* 48(9_Suppl_A):A33–A46, 2006.

199. The Emerging Risk Factors Collaboration: C-reactive protein concentration and risk of coronary heart disease, stroke, and mortality: an individual participant meta-analysis, *Lancet* 375(9709):132–140, 2010.

200. Pearson TA, Mensah GA, Alexander RW, et al: Markers of inflammation and cardiovascular disease: application to clinical and public health practice: a statement for healthcare professionals from the Centers for Disease Control and Prevention and the American Heart Association, *Circulation* 107(3):499–511, 2003.

201. Fibrinogen Studies Collaboration: Plasma fibrinogen level and the risk of major cardiovascular diseases and nonvascular mortality, *JAMA* 294(14):1799–1809, 2005.

202. Welch GN, Loscalzo J: Homocysteine and atherothrombosis, *N Engl J Med* 338(15):1042–1050, 1998.

203. Selhub J, Jacques PF, Wilson PWF, et al: Vitamin status and intake as primary determinants of homocysteinemia in an elderly population, *JAMA* 270(22):2693–2698, 1993.

204. Dierkes J, Westphal S, Luley C: The effect of fibrates and other lipid-lowering drugs on plasma homocysteine levels, *Expert Opin Drug Saf* 3(2):101–111, 2004.

205. Rosenson RS: Antiatherothrombotic effects of nicotinic acid, *Atherosclerosis* 171(1):87–96, 2003.

206. Bazzano LA, Jiang H, Munter P, et al: Relationship between cigarette smoking and novel risk factors for cardiovascular disease in the United States, *Ann Intern Med* 138(11):891, 2003.

207. Homocysteine Studies Collaboration: Homocysteine and risk of ischemic heart disease and stroke, *JAMA* 288(16):2015–2022, 2002.

208. Wald DS, Law M, Morris JK: Homocysteine and cardiovascular disease: evidence on causality from a meta-analysis, *BMJ* 325(7374):1202, 2002.

209. Casas JP, Bautista LE, Smeeth L, et al: Homocysteine and stroke: evidence on a causal link from mendelian randomisation, *Lancet* 365(9455):224–232, 2005.

210. Boysen G, Brander T, Christensen H, et al: Homocysteine and risk of recurrent stroke, *Stroke* 34(5):1258–1261, 2003.

211. Iso H, Moriyama Y, Sato S, et al: Serum total homocysteine concentrations and risk of stroke and its subtypes in Japanese, *Circulation* 109(22):2766–2772, 2004.

212. Kelly PJ, Rosand J, Kistler JP, et al: Homocysteine, MTHFR 677C→T polymorphism, and risk of ischemic stroke, *Neurology* 59(4):529–536, 2002.

213. Kim NK, Choi BO, Jung WS, et al: Hyperhomocysteinemia as an independent risk factor for silent brain infarction, *Neurology* 61(11):1595–1599, 2003.

214. Li Z, Sun L, Zhang H, et al: Elevated plasma homocysteine was associated with hemorrhagic and ischemic stroke, but methylenetetrahydrofolate reductase gene C677T polymorphism was a risk factor for thrombotic stroke: a multicenter case-control study in China, *Stroke* 34(9):2085–2090, 2003.

215. McIlroy SP, Dynan KB, Lawson JT, et al: Moderately elevated plasma homocysteine, methylenetetrahydrofolate reductase genotype, and risk for stroke, vascular dementia, and Alzheimer disease in Northern Ireland, *Stroke* 33(10):2351–2356, 2002.

216. Tanne D, Haim M, Goldbourt U, et al: Prospective study of serum homocysteine and risk of ischemic stroke among patients with preexisting coronary heart disease, *Stroke* 34(3):632–636, 2003.

217. The VITATOPS Trial Study Group: B vitamins in patients with recent transient ischaemic attack or stroke in the VITAmins TO Prevent Stroke (VITATOPS) trial: a randomised, double-blind, parallel, placebo-controlled trial, *Lancet Neurol* 9(9):855–865, 2010.

218. Etminan M, Takkouche B, Isorna F.C.o, et al: Risk of ischaemic stroke in people with migraine: systematic review and meta-analysis of observational studies, *BMJ* 330(7482):63, 2005.

219. Schürks M, Rist PM, Bigal ME, et al: Migraine and cardiovascular disease: systematic review and meta-analysis, *BMJ* 339, 2009.

220. Kruit MC, Launer LJ, Ferrari MD, et al: Infarcts in the posterior circulation territory in migraine. The population-based MRI CAMERA study, *Brain* 128(9):2068–2077, 2005.

221. Kruit MC, van Buchem MA, Hofman PAM, et al: Migraine as a risk factor for subclinical brain lesions, *JAMA* 291(4):427–434, 2004.

222. Scher AI, Gudmundsson LS, Sigurdsson S, et al: Migraine headache in middle age and late-life brain infarcts, *JAMA* 301(24):2563–2570, 2009.

223. Swartz RH, Kern RZ: Migraine is associated with magnetic resonance imaging white matter abnormalities: a meta-analysis, *Arch Neurol* 61(9):1366–1368, 2004.

224. Awareness of stroke warning symptoms--change to N dash. 13 States and the District of Columbia, 2005, *MMWR Morb Mortal Wkly Rep* 57(18):481–485, 2008.

225. Kleindorfer D, Khoury J, Broderick JP, et al: Temporal trends in public awareness of stroke: warning signs, risk factors, and treatment, *Stroke* 40(7):2502–2506, 2009.

226. Kleindorfer D, Lindsell CJ, Moomaw CJ, et al: Which stroke symptoms prompt a 911 call? A population-based study, *Am J Emerg Med* 28(5):607–612, 2010.

227. Kleindorfer D, Lindsell CJ, Brass L, et al: National US estimates of recombinant tissue plasminogen activator use: ICD-9 codes substantially underestimate, *Stroke* 39(3):924–928, 2008.

CHAPTER 30 Clinical Presentation and Diagnosis of Cerebrovascular Disease

Mark J. Alberts

Stroke is a common and serious disorder. Each year stroke affects almost 800,000 people in the United States and about 16 million people throughout the world.[1] Associated high morbidity and mortality provide impetus for improving diagnosis, acute management, and prevention of strokes. A full understanding of how patients with stroke and cerebrovascular disease come to medical attention, along with a logical approach for defining the mechanism of stroke, are needed for safe and effective implementation of acute therapies and prevention strategies. This chapter will focus on clinical manifestations of all types of cerebrovascular disease and how clinicians can approach diagnostic evaluation.

Overview of Clinical Stroke

Stroke and cerebrovascular disease are caused by some disturbance of the cerebral vessels in almost all cases. In simple terms, we can divide stroke into two major types: ischemic and hemorrhagic. Ischemic stroke is the most common variety and is responsible for 80% to 85% of all strokes; hemorrhagic stroke accounts for the remainder.[2] On occasion, an ischemic stroke can undergo secondary hemorrhagic transformation; likewise, a cerebral hemorrhage (particularly a subarachnoid hemorrhage [SAH]) can cause a secondary ischemic stroke via vasospasm.

Ischemic stroke occurs when a blood vessel in or around the brain becomes occluded or has a high-grade stenosis that reduces the perfusion of distal cerebral tissue. A variety of mechanisms and processes can lead to such occlusions and will be discussed later in more detail. On rare occasions, venous thrombosis can occlude a cerebral vein and lead to ischemic as well as hemorrhagic strokes (venous infarction).

Hemorrhagic stroke (intracerebral hemorrhage [ICH] and SAH) occurs when a blood vessel in or around the brain ruptures or leaks blood into the brain parenchyma (ICH) or into the subarachnoid space (SAH). It is not uncommon for there to be some overlap, such as an ICH also causing some degree of SAH and/or an intraventricular hemorrhage. Likewise, an SAH can produce some elements of an ICH if the aneurysmal rupture directs blood into the brain parenchyma. As with ischemic stroke, a variety of processes and lesions can produce ICH and SAH, but most affect integrity of the vessel wall in some way.

Clinical Manifestations of Stroke and Cerebrovascular Disease

Stroke is similar to real estate in that much of its presentation and prognosis depend on size and location. The area of brain involved dictates presenting symptoms. Blood vessels that supply different parts of the brain are affected by different types of cerebrovascular disease and have different mechanisms (pathophysiology) for the stroke. This concept greatly influences and defines the approach a vascular neurologist or neurosurgeon uses when assessing patients with a stroke or cerebrovascular disease.[3,4]

For example, a patient with evidence of involvement of the left hemispheric cortex (e.g., aphasia, visual field defect, weakness of contralateral face and arm) is likely to have a process involving the left middle cerebral artery (MCA). If head computed tomography (CT) does not show evidence of a hemorrhage, likely etiologies would include an embolic event from the heart (e.g., atrial fibrillation) or an artery-to-artery embolism (as might be seen with a high-grade lesion at the carotid bifurcation in the neck). Another patient with a pure motor hemiparesis but no other deficits is likely to have a lesion affecting the motor pathways in the internal capsule, often due to occlusion of a small penetrating artery (lenticulostriate vessel) deep in the brain. Most ischemic strokes will respect the vascular territory of one or more arteries.[5] Indeed, lesions that do not respect typical arterial territories lead to concern for a nonvascular process (e.g., tumor, infection). Common ischemic stroke syndromes can be found in Tables 30-1 and 30-2.

Evaluation of hemorrhagic stroke follows a similar logical assessment, but is further complicated by spread of the initial bleed, the effects of increased intracranial pressure, and other secondary effects that lead to neurological manifestations beyond the original injury. In this case, detailed cerebral imaging is vital for understanding the mechanism of the stroke and reasons for secondary worsening. The discussions that follow offer more detailed descriptions of common hemorrhagic stroke syndromes correlated with their likely anatomy and most likely pathophysiology.

Besides location of the stroke, the tempo of onset and progression of symptoms often provide valuable information about stroke etiology and mechanism. Stroke symptoms that progress in a casual manner with gradual onset and worsening over many minutes or longer often suggest a thrombotic process or hypoperfusion due to occlusion or stenosis of a larger proximal vessel. Such a leisurely progression can also be seen with stroke mimics such as complicated migraines or partial seizures. The converse is a stroke syndrome with sudden onset of maximal symptoms that remain stable; this suggests an embolic process such as a cardioembolic stroke due to atrial fibrillation.

Similar reasoning holds true for most cases of hemorrhagic stroke. Intracerebral hemorrhage often presents with abrupt onset of symptoms, but close questioning may reveal that symptoms actually progressed over 15 to 30 minutes as the hematoma grew and expanded.[6] Subarachnoid hemorrhage is often characterized by sudden onset of the worst headache of one's life, with significant nausea, vomiting, and stiff neck in many cases. The phrase "worst headache of my life" is so characteristic of SAH that a patient who presents to the physician or emergency department with that symptom complex is assumed to have SAH until proven otherwise.[7]

Transient Ischemic Attack

A transient ischemic attack (TIA) is often a prodrome to an ischemic stroke. Symptoms of a TIA are identical to those of a stroke, but with resolution within 24 hours (according to the old definition of a TIA). In reality, most TIA syndromes last just a few minutes, not many hours. In fact, modern brain imaging using magnetic resonance imaging (MRI) with diffusion-weighted sequences has now shown that 25% to 30% of patients with a TIA lasting 30 min to 2 hours will have a new diffusion-weighted imaging (DWI) lesion on MRI indicating a stroke based on a tissue definition.[8] Transient ischemic attack symptoms lasting 6 hours or longer have a 50% likelihood of having a new stroke on MRI with DWI techniques. Therefore the perceived distinction between a TIA and a stroke should be viewed more as a continuum from minor transient neuronal dysfunction to permanent brain infarction.

Although it was once thought that the risk of stroke after a TIA was low, new imaging studies as well as epidemiological studies have proven this is not the case. Based on purely clinical criteria (not MRI results), several recent studies have shown that after a TIA, 10% of patients will have a stroke within 3 months, and half

TABLE 30-1 Common Large-Vessel Ischemic Stroke Syndromes

SYNDROME	ANATOMY INVOLVED	MAJOR SYMPTOMS	VESSELS INVOLVED	ETIOLOGY
Left MCA	Left frontal/parietal cortex and subcortical structures	Aphasia, right visual field cut, right motor/sensory deficits; face > arm > leg weakness; left gaze preference	Left MCA or major branch; could also be left ICA or siphon	Emboli from heart or proximal lesion; intrinsic atherothrombosis
Right MCA	Right frontal/parietal cortex and subcortical structures	Neglect syndrome, agnosia, apraxia, left motor/sensory deficits, visual field deficit; right gaze preference	Right MCA or major branch; right ICA or siphon	Same as left MCA
Left ACA	Left frontal and parasagittal areas	Speech disturbance, behavioral changes, leg > arm weakness	Left ACA	Intrinsic atherothrombosis, embolic
Right ACA	Right frontal and parasagittal areas	Behavioral changes, leg > arm weakness	Right ACA	Same as left ACA
Brainstem	Pons, midbrain, medulla, cerebellum	Ophthalmoplegia, bilateral motor deficits, ataxia/dysmetria; nausea/vomiting/vertigo, coma/altered mentation	Basilar artery	Intrinsic atherothrombosis, embolism from heart or proximal vessel
PCA	Upper midbrain, occipital cortex/subcortex, thalamus, medial temporal lobes	Visual field cut, motor/sensory loss, seizures, gaze problems; 3rd nerve deficits	Posterior cerebral artery, thalamic perforators	Embolism from proximal lesion, intrinsic atherothrombosis

ACA, anterior cerebral artery; ICA, internal carotid artery; MCA, middle cerebral artery; PCA, posterior cerebral artery.

TABLE 30-2 Common Lacunar Stroke Syndromes

SYNDROME	VESSEL TYPICALLY INVOLVED	BRAIN LOCATION	SYMPTOMS
Pure motor hemiparesis	Lenticulostriate or basilar/pontine perforator	Internal capsule, pons	Unilateral weakness only
Mixed motor/sensory	Lenticulostriate or thalamic perforator or deep white matter vessel	Internal capsule, deep white matter, thalamus	Motor and sensory deficits
Pure sensory	Thalamic perforator	Posterior thalamus	Loss of contralateral sensory modalities
Ataxic hemiparesis	Lenticulostriate or basilar/pontine perforator	Internal capsule, basis pontis	Unilateral weakness with prominent ataxia, leg > arm
Dysarthria/clumsy hand	Lenticulostriate or deep white matter vessel	Internal capsule, deep white matter	Prominent dysarthria with isolated hand weakness

those strokes (5%) will occur within 48 hours of the initial TIA. About 25% of patients with a TIA will have a stroke, myocardial infarction (MI), death, recurrent TIA, or be hospitalized within the next 3 months.[9] Based on these poor outcomes, recently published guidelines recommend hospital admission for patients with a recent TIA.[8]

Further studies have attempted to better define those patients with a TIA who are at higher risk of having a stroke within the next 2 to 7 days. Several scoring systems have been developed (Table 30-3) that may be useful for assessing such risks. Of course, any such assessment tool must be tempered by good clinical judgment and consideration of all clinical factors.

TABLE 30-3 Transient Ischemic Attack Scoring Systems

ABCD	Age, blood pressure, clinical symptoms, duration
ABCD2	Age, blood pressure, clinical symptoms, duration, diabetes
ABCD2I	Age, blood pressure, clinical symptoms, duration, infarction

Age: 60 years or greater = 1 point
Blood pressure: systolic 140 mmHg or greater = 1 point or diastolic 90 mmHg or greater = 1 point
Clinical symptoms: unilateral weakness = 2 points; speech disturbance without weakness = 1 point
Duration: 60 minutes or more = 2 points; 10-59 minutes = 1 point
Diabetes: 1 point (on antidiabetic medications)
Infarction: evidence for acute ischemic stroke on CT or MRI

CT, computed tomography; MRI, magnetic resonance imaging.
From Johnston SC, Rothwell PM, Nguyen-Huynh MN, et al: Validation and refinement of scores to predict very early stroke risk after transient ischaemic attack. *Lancet* 369:283–292, 2007.[50]

Several types of TIAs deserve special mention because of their unique presentations. One is sudden blindness in one eye, which typically occurs as a "shade coming down" over the eye. Some patients report a graying out of vision in the eye, like looking through a gray haze or cloud. This type of TIA is often referred to as *amaurosis fugax*. This symptom complex typically resolves in a few minutes, although it can last for several hours. There is sometimes pain in or around the eye, but patients usually do not have any other focal neurological complaints. Some cases of amaurosis are due to emboli to the retinal circulation from an ulcerated plaque in or near the carotid bifurcation in the neck. Other cases can be due to local disease in the ophthalmic artery or in the posterior ciliary artery that supplies the optic nerve.[10]

The other unique type of TIA is the *limb-shaking TIA*. This typically involves the arm or leg on one side of the body. Patients report uncontrollable shaking of a limb that can be precipitated by movement. These spells can last seconds to minutes. They are not epileptic in origin; electroencephalogram (EEG) is unremarkable. These TIAs are associated with severe stenosis of the contralateral internal or common carotid artery.[11] Once the carotid artery is opened (usually with an endarterectomy), the spells cease.

Lastly is the topic of *crescendo TIAs*. This refers to a pattern where TIAs are recurrent, last longer, or are more severe in nature. This is a very worrisome type of TIA and is associated with a risk of stroke as high as 25% to 50% over the next few weeks.[12]

Some hemorrhagic strokes may also have a TIA equivalent, namely the *sentinel headache* before a SAH. The sentinel headache present as an acute headache that is unusual in terms of its nature, severity, and onset. It typically lasts more than an hour but does not have other impressive focal neurological findings and resolves prior to the definitive SAH presentation. Sentinel headaches occur in 25% to 50% of patients with a subsequent aneurysmal SAH and typically antedate the SAH by days to weeks (average 2 weeks).[13,14] It is thought that most of these headaches are due to either minor leakage from a fragile aneurysm or enlargement of the aneurysm, resulting in pressure on a nearby structure that produces pain.

Ischemic Stroke Syndromes

There are numerous manifestations of ischemic stroke, and they can be classified based on brain location involved, artery affected, or symptoms produced. Although advanced diagnostic techniques have altered some of the clinical rules of stroke symptoms and etiology, there are still some useful concepts that can guide us in terms of stroke location and mechanism. Tables 30-1 and 30-2 list some classic ischemic stroke syndromes with their major clinical manifestations, vascular territory, and underlying pathophysiology.[5]

Broadly speaking, ischemic strokes typically involve one or more vessels or vascular territories and produce a clinical picture of focal neurological deficit. Typically, clinicians look for unilateral weakness or sensory deficits, unilateral visual field abnormalities, speech disturbance (aphasia or dysarthria), neglect syndromes, unilateral ataxia, ophthalmoplegias, or gaze abnormalities as clues of a stroke. Symptoms such as vague diffuse weakness alone, headaches alone, memory loss, abnormal behavior, or isolated dizziness are rarely caused by an ischemic stroke. The appearance of a lesion in a typical vascular territory (based on brain imaging) is a key feature of almost all stroke syndromes.[4]

Presence of cortical deficits (aphasia, visual field cuts, neglect syndromes) often indicates involvement of a major cerebral vessel in the cerebral hemispheres. Presence of ataxia, bilateral motor or sensory deficits, Horner's syndrome, ophthalmoplegias, and crossed sensory findings (one side of the face and the other side of the body) often indicates a stroke in the posterior (vertebral-basilar) territory. There are specific syndromes that indicate small-vessel involvement deep in the brain. These so-called lacunar strokes are due to occlusion of small penetrating arteries that arise directly from larger parent vessels. Favored locations include the deep basal ganglia structures, thalamus, and brainstem (pons). A listing of large-vessel and lacunar syndromes appears in Tables 30-1 and 30-2.

Atherothrombosis accounts for the majority of ischemic strokes. These lesions can occur anywhere in the cerebral vasculature, but they tend to have a preference for specific locations such as the bifurcation of the carotid artery in the neck, intracranial carotid siphons, proximal portion of the middle cerebral artery, mid-portion of the basilar artery, and aortic arch. An atherosclerotic plaque forms over many years, then ruptures causing formation of a superimposed thrombus.[15] This atherothrombotic lesion can totally occlude the vessel, produce severe narrowing (leading to watershed ischemia), or be a source of embolic material that embolizes to more distal parts of the cerebral vasculature (artery-to-artery emboli).

Cardiac embolism accounts for 15% to 20% of all ischemic strokes. A variety of conditions such as atrial fibrillation, endocarditis, prior myocardial infarction, valvular disease, and cardiomyopathy often lead to formation of intracardiac thrombi that subsequently embolize to the brain (and other organs).[4,16] Most lacunar strokes are due to either lipohyalinosis or microatheromata occluding a small penetrating artery.

Special Cases

ISCHEMIC STROKE IN YOUNG ADULTS

All clinicians see young adults (often defined as ≤45 years of age) with ischemic strokes. Such cases often entail a special evaluation because of the unique processes and conditions that can produce strokes in this age group. Many case series have examined the diseases leading to ischemic strokes in the young, and in general they fall into a few major categories: (1) premature atherosclerosis, (2) unusual vascular pathologies, (3) cardiac etiology, (4) coagulopathy, and (5) other diseases.[17]

Premature atherosclerosis typically occurs in patients with risk factors for atherosclerosis; in some cases these have not been diagnosed or not properly treated. Examples include hypertension, hyperlipidemia, diabetes, smoking, and obesity. The types of uncommon vascular pathologies often seen in young adults with a stroke include dissection of a vessel (often not related to any obvious trauma), fibromuscular dysplasia, moyamoya disease, or a vasculitis related to an inflammatory condition or drug abuse.[17] Numerous cardiac processes can lead to strokes in the young, such as congenital heart disease, a patent foramen ovale (particularly with evidence of venous thrombi), valvular disease (infectious or inflammatory), cardiomyopathy, myxoma, papillary fibroelastoma, and many others. Myriad clotting disorders have been associated with strokes in young adults, the most common being lupus anticoagulants, anticardiolipin antibodies, and protein C and protein S deficiency.[18] In general, these coagulopathies are more likely to cause venous thrombosis than arterial thrombosis. Clotting disorders related to hematological malignancies can cause both ischemic and hemorrhagic strokes.[19] Various systemic diseases are also associated with hypercoagulable states such as inflammatory bowel disease, hemoglobinopathies, elevated homocysteine, and cancer.

The "other" category covers a host of conditions, some rare and some common, that cause strokes in young adults. Migraine headaches and pregnancy are the most common of these. Patients with complex or complicated migraines, prolonged auras, or taking contraceptives have a higher risk of stroke.[20] Pregnancy, particularly in the third trimester and up to 3 months postpartum is associated with increased stroke risk, particularly venous thrombosis and cerebral hemorrhage.[21,22] Drug abuse is another common cause of ischemic and hemorrhagic strokes in young adults.[23] Other rare conditions include CADASIL (cerebral autosomal dominant arteriopathy with subcortical infarcts and leukoencephalopathy), MELAS (mitochondrial encephalomyopathy, lactic acidosis, and stroke), isolated central nervous system (CNS) vasculitis, Sneddon syndrome (combination of a livedo reticular rash, antiphospholipid antibodies, and ischemic stroke), Marfan's syndrome, and a host of others (especially connective tissue disorders) have been known to cause strokes in this population.

STROKES RELATED TO SYSTEMIC DISEASE

Numerous systemic disorders are important and potent risk factors for stroke: hypertension, diabetes, hyperlipidemia, smoking, heart disease (atrial fibrillation, myocardial infarction, valvular disease, etc.), drug abuse, and others. These have been covered in other chapters of this book. Our focus here is on specific systemic disorders that lead to specific or unusual types of strokes.

There are a number of unique systemic disorders that cause strokes in patients of any age. Autoimmune diseases, such as lupus, can produce strokes through a variety of mechanisms that include advanced or premature atherosclerosis, vasculitis, hypercoagulable states, and cardioembolic events.[24] Sickle cell disease (SCD) also leads to ischemic strokes and hemorrhagic strokes due to myriad processes including a large-vessel arteriopathy, small-vessel occlusion, rupture of moyamoya vessels (producing ICH and/or SAH), and accelerated atherosclerosis due to hypertension and renal failure.[25,26]

Drug abuse, particularly cocaine, can produce ischemic strokes via a number of processes including vasospasm, cardiac emboli (due to cardiomyopathy), hypertension, and endocarditis.[27] Drug abuse can produce an ICH or SAH due to extreme hypertension and necrotizing vasculitis. It is a fallacy to assume that drug abuse only occurs in young patients or those from certain demographic groups. All patients admitted with a stroke should be tested for drug abuse with urine toxicology screens, not excluding those older than 50 years and white-collar professionals.

Human immunodeficiency virus/acquired immunodeficiency syndrome (HIV/AIDS) is now recognized as increasing the risk of stroke. This is partially because patients with HIV/AIDS are living longer, and some are having strokes as a result of accelerated development of typical stroke risk factors. It is also clear that modern drug therapy for AIDS can increase the risk of stroke (particularly ischemic stroke).[28,29]

Systemic cancer is a commonly overlooked cause of strokes. Sometimes the stroke diagnosis precedes diagnosis of the underlying cancer. Mechanisms for strokes related to cancer include a hypercoagulable state and nonbacterial thrombotic endocarditis. Oftentimes these strokes are multiple, variable in size, and in different vascular territories.[30,31] Such patients may also have deep venous thrombosis (DVT). Liver failure appears to increase risk of ischemic and hemorrhagic stroke.

Intracerebral Hemorrhage

In broad terms, ICH can be divided into traumatic and nontraumatic etiologies. This chapter will focus on nontraumatic ICH, since ICH related to trauma is not routinely considered a stroke. Intracerebral hemorrhage is typically caused by rupture of a blood vessel within the brain parenchyma. Patients typically develop a focal neurological deficit suddenly, but symptoms often evolve over 10 to 30 minutes as the hematoma gradually expands. Headache is commonly present, and the vast majority of patients have markedly elevated blood pressure (often in excess of 200 mmHg systolic) even without a prior history of hypertension. Nausea and vomiting can also occur, particularly with ICH that involves the brainstem and/or cerebellum.

Chronic or acute hypertension is the most common etiology for nontraumatic ICH, and this type of bleed typically occurs in specific brain locations (Table 30-4). As with ischemic stroke, location of the ICH is highly correlated with the type of symptoms produced. Recent studies using serial brain scans have shown that 30% to 40% of ICHs will expand over the first 24 hours after admission; such expansion is almost always associated with clinical worsening.[6,32] High blood pressure may be a risk factor for ICH expansion, although this association has not been mechanistically proven.

Another increasingly common etiology for ICH is cerebral amyloid angiopathy (CAA), which typically affects patients older than 70 years of age. Cerebral amyloid angiopathy is caused by deposition of one or more amyloid proteins within the wall of cerebral small arterioles. A typical CAA bleed occurs in a lobar region (junction of gray matter and white matter), most commonly in the parietal, temporal, and occipital lobes. Intracerebral hemorrhages due to CAA can be multiple and recurrent.[33-35] There is a clear asso-

ciation between CAA, ICH, and Alzhemier's disease. Sometimes an ischemic stroke can undergo hemorrhagic transformation and become an ICH. This occurs in up to 15% of cases of ischemic stroke and is associated with large strokes, cardioembolic strokes, and the use of anticoagulants and thrombolytic agents.

A variety of vascular malformations can cause an ICH, particularly arteriovenous malformations (AVMs) and cavernous malformations (less commonly, capillary telangiectasias and developmental venous anomalies). Arteriovenous malformations are the most common and serious type of vascular malformation that cause an ICH, and recurrent ICHs, as well as producing seizures and local neurological deficits.[36] The characteristics and hemorrhagic risk of each of these lesions is shown in Table 30-5.

Intracerebral hemorrhage can occur as a consequence of anticoagulation use, administration of thrombolytic therapy (either for a stroke or another systemic condition), other coagulopathies, hematological disorders, endocarditis, infections (fungal, bacterial, viral), drug abuse (cocaine, heroin, amphetamines), brain tumors (typically metastases), and venous thrombosis.[6] Iatrogenic causes of ICH deserve special mention, since there is now extensive use of powerful antiplatelet agents and anticoagulants for a variety of conditions. The use of tissue plasminogen activator (tPA) as well as endovascular therapies (thrombectomy, stenting) as therapies for acute ischemic stroke can lead to ICH (and less commonly SAH).[37]

TABLE 30-4	Location and Symptoms for Common Types of Intracerebral Hemorrhage	
ICH LOCATION	LIKELY ETIOLOGY	COMMON SYMPTOMS
Basal ganglia	Hypertension	Contralateral hemiparesis, speech changes, gaze deviation, altered mentation if large
Lobar	Hypertension, CAA	Cortical syndromes, weakness, visual field lesions, altered mentation if large
Thalamus	Hypertension	Altered mentation, sensory changes, gaze abnormalities
Pons	Hypertension	Coma, gaze and pupil abnormalities, quadriparesis
Cerebellum	Hypertension, AVM	Ipsilateral ataxia, dizziness, vertigo, nausea/vomiting
Hemispheric cortex	AVM, extreme hypertension, mycotic aneurysm	Headaches, seizures, cortical syndromes

AVM, arteriovenous malformation; CAA, cerebral amyloid angiopathy; ICH, intracerebral hemorrhage.

TABLE 30-5	Common Types of Central Nervous System Vascular Lesions That Lead to Cerebral Hemorrhage				
LESION TYPE	TYPICAL LOCATION	ANATOMY	PRESSURE CHARACTERISTICS	TYPICAL HEMORRHAGE TYPE	RISK OF BLEEDING/ OTHER EVENTS
Aneurysm	Arterial bifurcations around circle of Willis	Degeneration of parts of vessel wall leads to outpouching of vessel	High	SAH	Depends on size; about 1% or less in general population
AVM	Anywhere in CNS	Arteries draining directly into veins; abnormal intervening brain tissue	High	ICH and/or SAH	High; may also cause seizures
Cavernous angioma	Anywhere is CNS	Collection of enlarged capillaries; no intervening brain tissue	Low	ICH most common	Low in most cases; may cause seizures
Telangiectasia (capillary)	Anywhere; brainstem and white matter most common	Dilated capillaries with normal intervening brain	Low	Pontine ICH	Low
Venous angioma	Hemisphere, cerebellum	Collection of small veins; radial pattern; draining vein; normal brain tissue	Low	Deep white matter, cerebellum	Very low

AVM, arteriovenous malformation; CNS, central nervous system; ICH, intracerebral hemorrhage; SAH, subarachnoid hemorrhage.

Subarachnoid Hemorrhage

As noted earlier, most cases of nontraumatic SAH are due to rupture of a saccular aneurysm that typically occurs at the bifurcation of blood vessels around the circle of Willis at the base of the brain. However, using modern imaging techniques, we can now image aneurysms that occur more distally in the arterial tree. Such lesions are often due to an underlying infection (most commonly endocarditis), although they can be seen as a complication of vasculitis or inherited conditions (polycystic kidney disease, Marfan's syndrome).[38]

Subarachnoid hemorrhage typically produces a severe and sudden headache along with nausea/vomiting, nuchal rigidity, and elevated blood pressure. Depending on the location of the ruptured aneurysm, some patients may have additional focal neurological findings. For example, an aneurysm involving the posterior communicating artery can produce an ipsilateral third nerve palsy that involves the pupil. Rupture of an aneurysm of the anterior communicating artery can produce speech and behavioral changes. Aneurysmal rupture that leads to extensive bleeding around the brain and into the ventricles can lead to altered mental status, coma, and sometimes early or sudden death due to dramatic increases in intracranial pressure. A listing of common aneurysm locations and symptoms can be found in Table 30-6.

Following an aneurysmal SAH, patients are at high risk for a number of complications including rebleeding (if the aneurysm is not secured by surgery or coiling), vasospasm causing ischemic stroke, seizures, hydrocephalus, SIADH (syndrome of inappropriate antidiuretic hormone secretion), and central fever, among others.

An ICH or SAH that causes extensive hemorrhage into the ventricular system can produce an acute or subacute hydrocephalus syndrome with worsening headaches, nausea/vomiting, and altered mental status leading to coma in some cases. All strokes, but particularly ICH or SAH, can produce seizures, particularly if the blood involves parts of the cortex or epileptogenic deep structures such as the hippocampus. In the long term, such patients may develop dementia and personality changes.

Stroke Mimics

It is incumbent upon the clinician to ensure that a patient with a presumed stroke is having a real cerebrovascular event. Many medical conditions can present with stroke-like symptoms and even physical findings, but with a different etiology. This has obvious implications in terms of acute therapy, ongoing care, and secondary prevention. Table 30-7 lists some common stroke mimics and diagnostic tests that may be helpful for making the diagnosis.

Clinical Assessment Tools

History and Physical

Any assessment of a patient with suspected stroke or TIA begins with a focused history and physical. Factors of key concern include prior medical history with assessment of stroke risk factors (hypertension, diabetes, heart disease, etc.), as well as the presenting symptoms, their mode of onset, precipitating factors, and time course (stable, improving, getting worse). We are particularly concerned about symptoms such as disturbances of speech, language, and mentation; evidence of cranial nerve dysfunction (diplopia, vision loss in one eye or sector, dysarthria, dysphagia, facial weakness); focal motor weakness or coordination problems; gait abnormalities; and sensory symptoms. A particular challenge for stroke patients is that often their ability to sense or report these various symptoms may be affected by the very stroke causing the symptoms. This makes obtaining historical details from family, friends, or caregivers very important.

TABLE 30-6	Common Locations for Saccular Aneurysms and Related Symptoms in Subarachnoid Hemorrhage
LOCATION	**CLINICAL SYMPTOMS**
Anterior communicating artery	Leg weakness, speech disturbance, personality changes, seizures, memory loss
Posterior communicating artery/ internal carotid artery (ICA) junction	Ipsilateral 3rd nerve palsy
Bifurcation of middle cerebral artery (MCA)	Contralateral weakness, sensory changes, speech changes
Basilar artery tip	Altered mentation, pupil and gaze abnormalities

TABLE 30-7	Common Stroke Mimics: Diagnosis and Treatment		
STROKE MIMIC	**DIAGNOSTIC CLUES**	**CONFIRMATORY TESTS**	**TREATMENT**
Hypoglycemia/ hyperglycemia	Hx of diabetes, taking glycemic medications	Blood glucose; serial testing	Correct underlying disease
Electrolyte disturbance	Predisposing condition, taking medications	Electrolyte monitoring	Correct underlying condition
Migraine	Gradual Sx onset; prior Hx of headaches; family Hx of migraine	Rule out other conditions; identify precipitating factors	Avoid triggers; prophylactic medications if frequent migraines, discontinue hormone therapies
Seizures	Aura at beginning; preexisting illness; postictal lethargy	EEG; may require serial monitoring	Antiepileptic medications
Conversion reaction	Nonphysiological neurological examination; prior psychiatric events; secondary gain	Rule out other conditions; repeated examinations with inconsistent findings	Psychiatric evaluation
Demyelinating disease (MS)	Young age; gradual Sx onset	MRI findings; LP results	Treat MS with immunotherapy
CNS tumor	Lesion in nonvascular territory; risk factors for cancer	MRI findings; serial scans evaluate for systemic neoplasm	Treat tumor
Subdural hematoma	Head trauma; bleeding risk factors	Head CT or MRI	Correct coagulopathy; surgical drainage
Medication side effects	Sx associated with medication ingestion	Rule out other conditions	Change/discontinue medications
Infection	Fever, high white count	Brain imaging, LP, blood cultures	Antibiotics, antiviral medications

CT, computed tomography; EEG, electroencephalogram; Hx, history; LP, lumbar puncture; MRI, magnetic resonance imaging; MS, multiple sclerosis; Sx, symptom(s).

Another key aspect is time of onset of stroke symptoms, since this will determine whether the patient is a candidate for acute intervention (this is of particular importance for ischemic stroke). Time of stroke onset is often (and incorrectly) assumed to be when the patient is found with evidence of a stroke. The correct definition of time of onset is when stroke symptoms first began. If a patient has been under constant observation, the time of onset will be when the patient was first noticed to have stroke symptoms. But if a patient has been home alone and discovered with stroke symptoms by a family member, the time of onset has to be when the patient was last known to be normal (assuming the patient cannot determine the time of onset). Therefore, in the case of a patient who awakens in the morning unable to speak at 7 AM, time of onset is assumed to be when the patient went to bed normal the night before, unless there is clear documentation otherwise. This strict definition essentially rules out many patients with so-called wakeup strokes from receiving acute therapies such as tPA.[39]

Physical examination will provide valuable information about the likely location of the stroke and suggest the vascular territory and blood vessel or vessels most likely to be involved. As already noted, this is a key step in determining stroke mechanism and etiology. Besides vital signs and a thorough neurological examination, there are particular aspects of the general medical examination that provide important diagnostic information to the clinician. These include an assessment for cervical bruits, a complete cardiac examination, checking blood pressure and pulses in both arms, a skin examination, and evidence of trauma to the head and neck. Table 30-8 offers an outline of a neurological assessment for patients with known or suspected cerebrovascular disease.

Clinicians often use a variety of scales or scoring systems to assess severity of various types of stroke. These scoring systems can provide guidance about treatment options as well as overall prognosis. The National Institutes of Health Stroke Scale (NIHSS) is often used to assess patients with an ischemic stroke. The NIHSS is a formalized neurological examination, and scores can range form 0 to 42 (0 being normal, higher score being more severe). The Glasgow Coma Scale (GCS) is often used in patients with ICH and SAH. It measures a patient's responses to a variety of stimuli. The GCS can range from 0 to 15, with 15 being normal. The Hunt and Hess Scale is used to assess severity of SAH, with 1 being an asymptomatic headache and 5 being deep coma. The Fisher Grade is used to measure the amount of subarachnoid blood seen on the head CT. Scores range from 1 (no blood seen) to 4 (intraventricular or parenchymal blood).

Brain Imaging

Our ability to rapidly and accurately image the brain and cerebral vasculature has been an important step and driver in our capability to determine the type of stroke, its locations, and likely mechanism.[40] Almost every hospital in the United States is able to perform a head CT scan on patients in the emergency department. On-site personnel or remote radiology reading technologies and services can provide a reading within 30 to 60 minutes. The ability to rapidly perform and interpret brain imaging is a key component of a primary stroke center.[41]

A head CT scan can easily, rapidly, and safely be used to diagnose an acute stroke, especially if it is a hemorrhagic stroke. In some cases when a patient with an ischemic stroke is imaged very soon after symptom onset, the head CT may be negative or show only subtle changes. In such cases, a repeat head CT in 12 to 24 hours will almost certainly show changes indicative of a large or medium-sized ischemic stroke (Fig. 30-1). However, a head CT can miss small and acute strokes, particularly if they are in the brainstem or posterior fossa.

Head CT is very sensitive for imaging hemorrhagic strokes, particularly ICH. Intracerebral hemorrhages appear as white lesions in the brain parenchyma that represent the actual hematoma (Fig. 30-2A). Often there is early evidence of edema around the ICH, which can worsen over several hours and days. In 30% to 40% of ICH cases, the actual hematoma will expand and lead to clinical worsening. In patients with a large SAH, the head CT will show bright signal (blood) at the base of the brain and within some cortical sulci (Fig. 30-2B). However, a small SAH or sentinel bleed may be missed by CT and even MRI. Hence a lumbar puncture is needed to definitively rule out a small SAH.

Numerous studies as well as recent guidelines have supported use of brain MRI for assessment of patients with known or suspected strokes.[42] Magnetic resonance imaging using DWI techniques is extremely sensitive and accurate for diagnosing essentially all types of ischemic strokes (and some types of hemorrhagic stroke). Magnetic resonance imaging is particularly useful for imaging small strokes, acute strokes, and those in the posterior

TABLE 30-8	Typical Components of a Neurological Examination Pertinent to Stroke
TESTING DOMAIN	**SPECIFIC FUNCTIONS TESTED**
Mentation and cognition	Level of alertness, orientation, speech, naming/repetition, memory, personality, apraxia, agnosia, neglect syndromes
Cranial nerves	Testing of nerves II-XII typically performed, including visual acuity and funduscopic examination
Motor function	Tone, bulk, abnormal movements; strength, fine movements
Cerebellar function	Coordination, rapid movements, balance
Gait	Ability to walk, balance, tandem gait
Sensory	Pain/pin prick, light touch, vibration/proprioception
Reflexes	Deep tendon reflexes, plantar response (Babinski); cutaneous reflexes, primitive reflexes (snout, suck, grasp, palmomental)
Vascular system	Auscultation of neck and heart; blood pressure measurements in both arms; check pulses in hands and feet; consider ankle-brachial index (ABI)

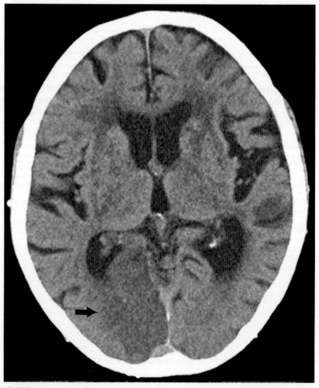

FIGURE 30-1   Head computed tomography (CT) scan without contrast. Arrow indicates a subacute stroke (*darker gray area*) in right occipital lobe in a patient with a new visual field deficit present for about 24 hours.

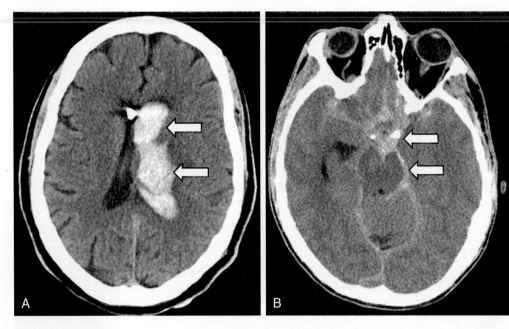

FIGURE 30-2 A, Head computed tomography (CT) scan without contrast. Arrows indicate a deep intracerebral hemorrhage (ICH) with rupture into the ventricular system *(white area)*. **B,** Head CT scan without contrast. Arrows indicate a subarachnoid hemorrhage (SAH) *(white areas)* at the base of the brain filling the basal cisterns.

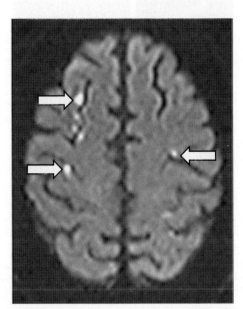

FIGURE 30-3 Magnetic resonance imaging (MRI) of brain with diffusion-weighted sequence. White dots *(arrows)* show areas of acute ischemic or infarction consistent with several acute strokes in a patient with atrial fibrillation.

fossa (Fig. 30-3). In addition to DWI sequences, use of gradient echo sequences allows detection of small amounts of blood. Using this technique, studies have shown that up to 40% of ischemic strokes may have microhemorrhages within the area of ischemia.[43]

Magnetic resonance imaging results will often provide invaluable information about stroke etiology, even if the patient's symptoms and presentation suggest an alternative etiology. For example, a patient may present with symptoms pointing to a small-vessel stroke deep in the brain. In the proper setting, this type of stroke might be caused by typical vascular risk factors such as hypertension or diabetes. However, if the MRI showed evidence of other small acute strokes in other vascular territories, this would shift focus away from an isolated small-vessel stroke to alternative mechanisms such as cardioembolic strokes due to atrial fibrillation, a hypercoagulable state, or even a vasculitis.

Another advantage of MRI is that it can accurately distinguish acute strokes from subacute strokes using lesion characteristics. An acute ischemic stroke will be bright on DWI, dark on apparent diffusion coefficients (ADC) and not show enhancement with gadolinium (Fig. 30-4A-B). A stroke that is 7 to 10 days old will be less bright on DWI, less dark on ADC, and show enhancement with gadolinium (Fig. 30-4C). A chronic stroke may be bright on DWI (due to T2 shine through), bright on ADC, and show no enhancement.

Advanced MRI techniques are now available that can identify potentially salvageable brain from infarcted brain based on comparing DWI lesions with magnetic resonance (MR) perfusion lesions (Fig. 30-5). Patients with an acute stroke who have a large area of

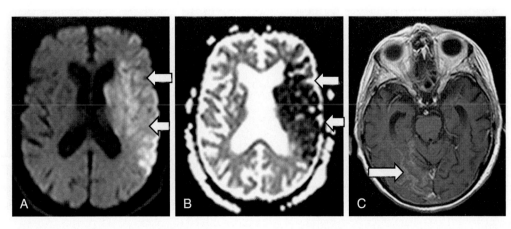

FIGURE 30-4 A, Magnetic resonance imaging (MRI) of the brain with diffusion-weighted sequences shows evidence of a large left hemispheric stroke *(white areas with arrows)*. **B,** Apparent diffusion coefficient (ADC) of same region; dark area is abnormal and indicates ischemia/infarction consistent with an acute stroke. **C,** Brain MRI after infusion of gadolinium showing enhancement of a right occipital stroke consistent with a subacute infarction (at least 5-7 days old).

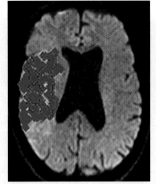

FIGURE 30-5 Magnetic resonance imaging (MRI) of brain with superimposed perfusion and diffusion images showing areas of "mismatch" indicating existence of an apparent ischemic penumbra. Perfusion defect is blue; infarcted brain is pink/purple.

perfusion abnormality on an MR perfusion study but a smaller area of ischemia (DWI lesion) may benefit from reperfusion therapy using lytic or endovascular therapies even 6 to 8 hours after stroke onset. Use of these advanced MRI techniques to select patients with an apparent "ischemic penumbra" is an area of active research.[42,44]

Magnetic resonance imaging of an ICH is more complex, owing to signal changes caused by metabolism of various blood constituents. About 48 to 72 hours after an ICH, the hemoglobin (Hb) in the hematoma is metabolized into intracellular methemoglobin, which appears bright on the MRI using T1 sequences and dark on T2 sequences. After a week or more, methemoglobin becomes extracellular and becomes bright on T1 and T2 sequences. Hemosiderin is then formed in the hematoma and produces a dark signal in gradient echo sequences[45] (Fig. 30-6).

Imaging Cerebral Vasculature

Of equal importance to imaging brain parenchyma is detailed imaging of the cerebral vasculature, both extracranial (aorta, carotid and vertebral arteries) and intracranial vessels.[40] Although in most cases we are focusing on the arterial vasculature, in certain cases it is also important to image the cerebral veins (so-called sinuses) to rule out a cerebral venous thrombosis.

There are several noninvasive modalities available for imaging the cerebral vessels, including magnetic resonance angiography (MRA) (see Chapter 13), computed tomographic angiography (CTA) (see Chapter 14), duplex Doppler ultrasound (see Chapter 12), and transcranial Doppler (TCD) (Figs. 30-7 and 30-8). Each method has certain advantages as well as some limitations (Table 30-9). We typically use either MRA or CTA because they are capable of imaging the entire cerebral vasculature (from the great vessels in the chest to

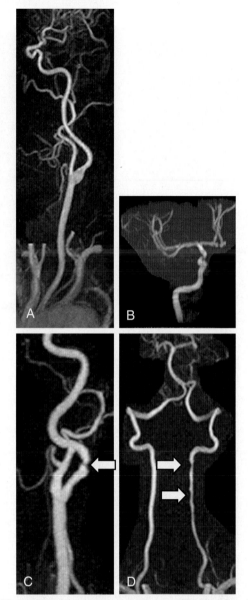

FIGURE 30-7 Magnetic resonance angiogram (MRA) with gadolinium, showing normal extracranial common, internal, and external carotid arteries (A) and intracranial vessels (B). **C,** Stenosis due to atherosclerosis in proximal internal carotid artery (ICA) *(arrow)*. **D,** MRA of vertebral-basilar system showing irregularity of left vertebral artery due to either fibromuscular dysplasia (FMD) or dissection *(arrows)*.

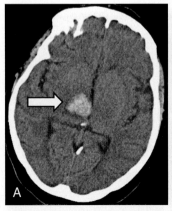
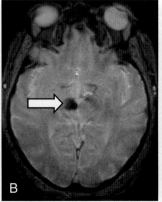
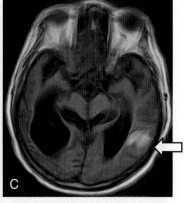

FIGURE 30-6 A, Head computed tomography (CT) showing right thalamic intracerebral hemorrhage (ICH) *(white area with arrow)*. **B,** Brain magnetic resonance imaging (MRI) with gradient echo sequences showing same stroke *(arrow)*. Dark area represents iron deposition caused by the bleed. **C,** Subacute ICH white area *(arrow)* is methemoglobin formed from a recent cerebral hemorrhage.

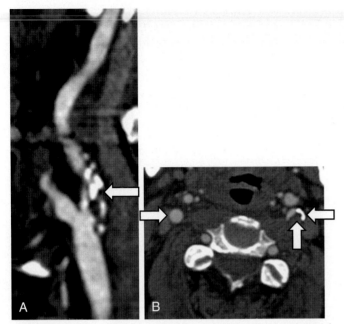

FIGURE 30-8 Computed tomographic angiogram (CT) of neck vessels. A, Side oblique view shows severe calcification of distal common carotid artery (CCA) and proximal internal carotid artery (ICA) *(arrow).* **B,** Axial images show a normal right carotid artery *(blue arrow)* and calcified left ICA. Calcified region is depicted with yellow area; soft plaque is shown by red arrow.

medium-sized intracranial vessels) at one time in only 5 to 10 minutes for CTA, and 25 to 30 minutes for MRA. Computed tomographic angiography requires intravenous contrast agents, whereas Magnetic resonance angiography can be done either with intravenous gadolinium or without (using a time-of-flight [TOF] protocol). Magnetic resonance angiography with contrast (vs. no contrast) provides better images, permitting visualization of small lesions such as dissections or a vasculitis. Computed tomographic angiography provides modestly more precise anatomical detail in terms of its ability to detect small aneurysms and small dissection flaps, and accurately determine the degree of arterial stenoses. However, CTA does expose patients to ionizing radiation.

Carotid duplex ultrasound is a safe and noninvasive method to image selected segments of the large vessels in the neck.

Transcranial Doppler is another safe and noninvasive technique to image segments of the intracranial vasculature. Both techniques can provide information about direction and velocity of blood flow. Carotid ultrasound can be performed serially over the course of months and years to assess changes in the degree of stenosis of a neck artery, and it can determine plaque size and composition. Transcranial Doppler is often performed daily after SAH to determine whether there is development of cerebral vasospasm that may cause an ischemic stroke.

The gold-standard imaging modality for cerebral vessels remains the digital subtraction angiogram (DSA). In cases where CTA and MRA show different degrees of stenosis, we may do a DSA to determine the exact degree of stenosis (often before doing a carotid endarterectomy or carotid artery stent). Besides offering precise imaging of small, medium, and large vessels, a DSA also provides invaluable information about cerebral hemodynamics. By injecting the various cerebral vessels, an angiogram can determine (in cases of a vessel stenosis or occlusion) exactly where the blood supply is coming from and going to. The angiogram can detect collateral vessels (or lack thereof) that may be supplying a region of brain thought to be poorly perfused due to occlusion of a proximal vessel. We have often seen patients with apparent lack of flow through a severely diseased basilar artery, only to find that abundant collaterals are supplying the brainstem with adequate perfusion. A DSA is also very important when planning surgical treatment for an AVM, aneurysm, and other vascular lesions.

Using computer reconstruction algorithms, images from all the above techniques can be assembled into three-dimensional (3D) pictures to provide a comprehensive view of the cerebral vessels. These images can be rotated and flipped as needed to aid the clinician in determining the type, location, and severity of the lesion (stenosis, aneurysm, etc.).

Laboratory Tests

All patients with a stroke (ischemic or hemorrhagic) require standard testing that should include a complete blood cell count (CBC), chemistry panel, coagulation studies, chest x-ray, electrocardiogram (ECG), urinalysis, and the brain imaging already detailed.[46] Again, *all* patients should undergo toxicology screening for drug use, since this is a common condition, and patients are often not forthcoming about drug abuse. The Centers for Disease Control and Prevention

TABLE 30-9	Vascular Imaging Techniques			
TEST NAME	**IMAGING TECHNIQUE**	**VASCULATURE IMAGED**	**ADVANTAGES**	**DISADVANTAGES**
Carotid Doppler	Ultrasound	Extracranial carotid and vertebral arteries	Safe, noninvasive, no radiation, inexpensive; provides some anatomical and physiological data	Limited to extracranial vasculature in the neck
TCD	Ultrasound	Intracranial arteries	Safe, noninvasive, no radiation, inexpensive; provides some physiological data	Limited to mostly intracranial vasculature; limited anatomical detail
MRA	Magnetic resonance	Large and medium extracranial and intracranial arteries and veins; great vessels in chest	Safe, noninvasive, no radiation; some anatomical details; can image most vessels; can evaluate cerebral perfusion; some aneurysm detection	Cannot be used with a pacemaker or metal; limited in severe claustrophobia; contrast often needed; expensive
CTA	X-ray	Extracranial and intracranial arteries and veins; great vessels in chest; can detect some small vessels	Significant anatomical detail; can evaluate cerebral perfusion; can image most vessels; accurate stenosis and aneurysm measurements	Radiation exposure; requires contrast; limited use with renal dysfunction; expensive
Digital cerebral angiography	X-ray	All arteries and veins, including small vessels	Significant anatomical detail; can evaluate cerebral perfusion and collateral flow; accurate stenosis and aneurysm measurement	Invasive procedure; radiation exposure; requires contrast; limited use with renal dysfunction; expensive

CTA, computed tomographic angiography; MRA, magnetic resonance angiography; TCD, transcranial Doppler.
Some data derived from Latchaw RE, Alberts MJ, Lev MH, et al: Recommendations for imaging of acute ischemic stroke: a scientific statement from the American Heart Association. *Stroke* 40:3646–3678, 2009.

TABLE 30-10   Suggested Laboratory Testing for Patients with Stroke

ROUTINE TESTS	TESTS FOR SPECIAL CASES*	COMMENTS (FOR SPECIAL TESTS)
CBC with differential	Hb electrophoresis	Useful if SCD or thalassemia suspected
Comprehensive chemistry profile	Vasculitis screen (ANA, rheumatoid factor, etc.)	Useful if arteries show beading
APTT, PT, INR	Hypercoagulable screen (lupus anticoagulant, anticardiolipin antibodies, protein C and S activity; factor V Leiden and prothrombin gene mutations; cryoglobulin screen; antithrombin III level	Useful for ischemic strokes in young adults; postpartum; cryptogenic strokes
Sedimentation rate	Fibrinogen, DIC screen	Detects ongoing thrombosis
Fasting lipid profile	CADASIL gene mutation	Characteristic MRI and positive family history
Hb A$_{1c}$	Apolipoprotein E genotype	CAA with recurrent ICH, dementia, MRI changes
Homocysteine	Fabry's disease test	Positive family history; skin changes; renal disease
Vitamins B$_{12}$ and folate	Blood cultures	Suspected endocarditis; multiple strokes
Thyroid panel	Assay of clotting factors	Recurrent cerebral hemorrhages
HIV	CT of chest/abdomen/pelvis	Look for cancer in patient with recurrent stroke
Urine toxicology screen (drug abuse)		
Platelet function tests†		

*Special cases refer to unusual or atypical presentations or stroke syndromes, including cryptogenic etiologies.
†Benefits of platelet function testing for improving efficacy and safety of stroke therapy remain experimental; however, such testing may be important for detecting platelet dysfunction in patients with hemorrhagic stroke.
ANA, antinuclear antibody; APTT, activated partial thromboplastin time; CAA, cerebral amyloid angiopathy; CADASIL, cerebral autosomal dominant arteriopathy with subcortical infarcts and leukoencephalopathy; (CBC), complete blood cell count; DIC, disseminated intravascular coagulopathy; Hb, hemoglobin; HIV, human immunodeficiency virus; ICH, intracerebral hemorrhage; INR, International Normalized Ratio; MRI, magnetic resonance imaging; PT, prothrombin time; SCD, sickle cell disease.

(CDC) recommends HIV testing for most adults who are hospitalized, and this would include patients with an acute stroke.[47] Table 30-10 lists routine laboratory testing for patients with ischemic stroke.

Special blood tests are warranted if a hypercoagulable state is suspected based on the patient's age, lack of other risk factors, or if another condition is suspected.[48] An elevated D-dimer may indicate ongoing thrombosis. Blood cultures may be obtained in patients with multiple embolic strokes to rule out endocarditis. In patients with suspected vasculitis or a possible autoimmune disorder, tests for inflammatory conditions, such as a sedimentation rate, antinuclear antibody (ANA) titers, and other serologies, may be performed. Hemoglobin electrophoresis can rule out SCD or trait, as well as thalassemia.

Since the heart can be the cause of up to 25% of all strokes, a thorough cardiac assessment is needed in most cases. Beyond the cardiac clinical examination and an electrocardiogram, all patients with an ischemic stroke should receive at least 48 hours of cardiac monitoring using computerized telemetry to detect rhythm changes that could cause a stroke (e.g., atrial fibrillation) as well as dysrhythmia that could indicate underlying coronary artery disease (CAD) or cardiomyopathy (e.g., ventricular tachycardia).[46] In some cases, more prolonged monitoring using the Holter device is warranted to further assess for paroxysmal atrial fibrillation. Cardiac imaging including a transthoracic echocardiogram (TTE) or a transesophageal echocardiogram (TEE) is often performed to evaluate cardiac function and assess for presence of a cardiac clot or other structural lesion. Typically we begin with a TTE, and if negative then proceed to the TEE.[49]

Monitoring a patient's respiratory status and oxygen saturation is important in the acute setting, since changes may indicate an increase in intracranial pressure or presence of obstructive sleep apnea (OSA) (which is an underrecognized risk factor for stroke).

Duplex ultrasound examination of the lower and upper extremities is commonly performed to detect DVT when this is considered a possible source of stroke (in patients with a patent foramen ovale) or a complication of stroke (in patients who are obese, sedentary, or were found down at home after many hours or days). Presence of DVT can also be an indicator of an underlying hypercoagulable state or cancer. A thorough evaluation for underlying malignancy should be considered in patients with a stroke and DVT, as well as patients with cryptogenic strokes.

A lumbar puncture is warranted in patients with suspected vasculitis or if a small SAH is suspected but not proven based on brain CT or MRI. Special genetic testing is performed in cases of suspected disorders such as CADASIL or Marfan's syndrome. Apolipoprotein E genotype analysis in patients with suspected CAA may be appropriate, since the e2 and e4 alleles are strongly associated with CAA-related ICH.

The utility of these tests is greatest in patients with strokes of unusual type, size, and location, particularly if there are no risk factors for atherothrombotic and cerebrovascular disease. A typical patient with one or more risk factors who has an uncomplicated ischemic stroke of known mechanism does not require the special testing listed (in most cases).

Conclusions

Stroke is a complex and heterogeneous disease that is the culmination of a variety of medical factors and cerebral vascular anatomy. Based on results of the history, physical, blood, and imaging tests, the clinician can make an accurate assessment as to the location, type, mechanism and cause of the stroke. Based upon this formulation, an approach for acute therapy can be planned, along with interventions to avoid secondary complications and prevent a recurrent stroke. A better understanding of the basics of stroke in terms of type, cause, presentation, and diagnosis will lead to improved therapies and increase the chance that the patient will have a better outcome.

REFERENCES

1. Lloyd-Jones D, Adams RJ, Brown TM, et al: Executive summary: heart disease and stroke statistics–2010 update: a report from the American Heart Association, *Circulation* 121:948–954, 2010.
2. Broderick J, Brott T, Kothari R, et al: The Greater Cincinnati/Northern Kentucky Stroke Study: preliminary first-ever and total incidence rates of stroke among blacks, *Stroke* 29:415–421, 1998.
3. Brott T, Bogousslavsky J: Treatment of acute ischemic stroke, *N Engl J Med* 343:710–722, 2000.
4. Caplan LR: Diagnosis and treatment of ischemic stroke, *JAMA* 266:2413–2418, 1991.
5. Kumar S, Caplan LR: Why identification of stroke syndromes is still important, *Curr Opin Neurol* 20:78–82, 2007.

6. Fewel ME, Thompson BG Jr, Hoff JT: Spontaneous intracerebral hemorrhage: a review, *Neurosurg Focus* 15:E1, 2003.

7. Suarez JI, Tarr RW, Selman WR: Aneurysmal subarachnoid hemorrhage, *N Engl J Med* 354:387–396, 2006.

8. Easton JD, Saver JL, Albers GW, et al: Definition and evaluation of transient ischemic attack: a scientific statement for healthcare professionals from the American Heart Association/American Stroke Association Stroke Council; Council on Cardiovascular Surgery and Anesthesia; Council on Cardiovascular Radiology and Intervention; Council on Cardiovascular Nursing; and the Interdisciplinary Council on Peripheral Vascular Disease. The American Academy of Neurology affirms the value of this statement as an educational tool for neurologists, *Stroke* 40:2276–2293, 2009.

9. Johnston SC, Gress DR, Browner WS, et al: Short-term prognosis after emergency department diagnosis of TIA, *JAMA* 284:2901–2906, 2000.

10. Adams HP Jr, Putman SF, Corbett JJ, et al: Amaurosis fugax: the results of arteriography in 59 patients, *Stroke* 14:742–744, 1983.

11. Baquis GD, Pessin MS, Scott RM: Limb shaking–a carotid TIA, *Stroke* 16:444–448, 1985.

12. Donnan GA, O'Malley HM, Quang L, et al: The capsular warning syndrome: pathogenesis and clinical features, *Neurology* 43:957–962, 1993.

13. Gorelick PB, Hier DB, Caplan LR, et al: Headache in acute cerebrovascular disease, *Neurology* 36:1445–1450, 1986.

14. de Falco F: Sentinel headache, *Neurol Sci* S215–S217, 2004.

15. Kannel WB, Wolf PA: Peripheral and cerebral atherothrombosis and cardiovascular events in different vascular territories: insights from the Framingham Study, *Curr Atheroscler Rep* 8:317–323, 2006.

16. White H, Boden-Albala B, Wang C, et al: Ischemic stroke subtype incidence among whites, blacks, and Hispanics: the Northern Manhattan Study, *Circulation* 111:1327–1331, 2005.

17. Adams HP Jr, Kappelle LJ, Biller J, et al: Ischemic stroke in young adults. Experience in 329 patients enrolled in the Iowa Registry of stroke in young adults, *Arch Neurol* 52:491–495, 1995.

18. Urbanus RT, Siegerink B, Roest M, et al: Antiphospholipid antibodies and risk of myocardial infarction and ischaemic stroke in young women in the RATIO study: a case-control study, *Lancet Neurol* 8:998–1005, 2009.

19. Hart RG, Kanter MC: Hematologic disorders and ischemic stroke. A selective review, *Stroke* 21:1111–1121, 1990.

20. Chen M: Stroke as a complication of medical disease, *Semin Neurol* 29:154–162, 2009.

21. Feske SK: Stroke in pregnancy, *Semin Neurol* 27:442–452, 2007.

22. Skidmore FM, Williams LS, Fradkin KD, et al: Presentation, etiology, and outcome of stroke in pregnancy and puerperium, *J Stroke Cerebrovasc Dis* 10:1–10, 2001.

23. Sloan MA: Illicit drug use/abuse and stroke, *Handb Clin Neurol* 93:823–840, 2009.

24. Kitagawa Y, Gotoh F, Koto A, et al: Stroke in systemic lupus erythematosus, *Stroke* 21:1533–1539, 1990.

25. Earley CJ, Kittner SJ, Feeser BR, et al: Stroke in children and sickle-cell disease: Baltimore-Washington Cooperative Young Stroke Study, *Neurology* 51:169–176, 1998.

26. Roach ES, Golomb MR, Adams R, et al: Management of stroke in infants and children: a scientific statement from a Special Writing Group of the American Heart Association Stroke Council and the Council on Cardiovascular Disease in the Young, *Stroke* 39:2644–2691, 2008.

27. Caplan LR, Hier DB, Banks G: Current concepts of cerebrovascular disease–stroke: stroke and drug abuse, *Stroke* 13:869–872, 1982.

28. Dobbs MR, Berger JR: Stroke in HIV infection and AIDS, *Expert Rev Cardiovasc Ther* 7:1263–1271, 2009.

29. Ortiz G, Koch S, Romano JG, et al: Mechanisms of ischemic stroke in HIV-infected patients, *Neurology* 68:1257–1261, 2007.

30. Cestari DM, Weine DM, Panageas KS, et al: Stroke in patients with cancer: incidence and etiology, *Neurology* 62:2025–2030, 2004.

31. Kwon HM, Kang BS, Yoon BW: Stroke as the first manifestation of concealed cancer, *J Neurol Sci* 258:80–83, 2007.

32. Broderick J, Connolly S, Feldmann E, et al: Guidelines for the management of spontaneous intracerebral hemorrhage in adults: 2007 update: a guideline from the American Heart Association/American Stroke Association Stroke Council, High Blood Pressure Research Council, and the Quality of Care and Outcomes in Research Interdisciplinary Working Group, *Stroke* 38:2001–2023, 2007.

33. Towfighi A, Greenberg SM, Rosand J: Treatment and prevention of primary intracerebral hemorrhage, *Semin Neurol* 25:445–452, 2005.

34. Smith EE, Gurol ME, Eng JA, et al: White matter lesions, cognition, and recurrent hemorrhage in lobar intracerebral hemorrhage, *Neurology* 63:1606–1612, 2004.

35. Greenberg SM, Eng JA, Ning M, et al: Hemorrhage burden predicts recurrent intracerebral hemorrhage after lobar hemorrhage, *Stroke* 35:1415–1420, 2004.

36. Wilkins RH: Natural history of intracranial vascular malformations: a review, *Neurosurgery* 16:421–430, 1985.

37. Flaherty ML, Woo D, Kissela B, et al: Combined IV and intra-arterial thrombolysis for acute ischemic stroke, *Neurology* 64:386–388, 2005.

38. Schuknecht B: High-concentration contrast media (HCCM) in CT angiography of the carotid system: impact on therapeutic decision making, *Neuroradiology* 49(Suppl 1):S15–S26, 2007.

39. Hills NK, Johnston SC: Why are eligible thrombolysis candidates left untreated? *Am J Prev Med* 31:S210–S216, 2006.

40. Latchaw RE, Alberts MJ, Lev MH, et al: Recommendations for imaging of acute ischemic stroke: a scientific statement from the American Heart Association, *Stroke* 40:3646–3678, 2009.

41. Alberts MJ, Hademenos G, Latchaw RE, et al: Recommendations for the establishment of primary stroke centers. Brain Attack Coalition, *JAMA* 283:3102–3109, 2000.

42. Schellinger PD, Bryan RN, Caplan LR, et al: Evidence-based guideline: The role of diffusion and perfusion MRI for the diagnosis of acute ischemic stroke: report of the Therapeutics and Technology Assessment Subcommittee of the American Academy of Neurology, *Neurology* 75:177–185, 2010.

43. Koennecke HC: Cerebral microbleeds on MRI: prevalence, associations, and potential clinical implications, *Neurology* 66:165–171, 2006.

44. Latchaw RE, Yonas H, Hunter GJ, et al: Guidelines and recommendations for perfusion imaging in cerebral ischemia: a scientific statement for healthcare professionals by the writing group on perfusion imaging, from the Council on Cardiovascular Radiology of the American Heart Association, *Stroke* 34:1084–1104, 2003.

45. Anzalone N, Scotti R, Riva R: Neuroradiologic differential diagnosis of cerebral intraparenchymal hemorrhage, *Neurol Sci* 25(Suppl 1):S3–S5, 2004.

46. Adams HP Jr, del Zoppo G, Alberts MJ, et al: Guidelines for the early management of adults with ischemic stroke: a guideline from the American Heart Association/American Stroke Association Stroke Council, Clinical Cardiology Council, Cardiovascular Radiology and Intervention Council, and the Atherosclerotic Peripheral Vascular Disease and Quality of Care Outcomes in Research Interdisciplinary Working Groups: the American Academy of Neurology affirms the value of this guideline as an educational tool for neurologists, *Circulation* 115:e478–e534, 2007.

47. Branson BM, Handsfield HH, Lampe MA, et al: Revised recommendations for HIV testing of adults, adolescents, and pregnant women in health-care settings, *MMWR Recomm Rep* 55:1–17, 2006 quiz CE11-CE14.

48. Bushnell CD, Goldstein LB: Diagnostic testing for coagulopathies in patients with ischemic stroke, *Stroke* 31:3067–3078, 2000.

49. de Bruijn SF, Agema WR, Lammers GJ, et al: Transesophageal echocardiography is superior to transthoracic echocardiography in management of patients of any age with transient ischemic attack or stroke, *Stroke* 37:2531–2534, 2006.

50. Johnston SC, Rothwell PM, Nguyen-Huynh MN, et al: Validation and refinement of scores to predict very early stroke risk after transient ischaemic attack, *Lancet* 369:283–292, 2007.

CHAPTER 31 Prevention and Treatment of Stroke

Marc Fisher, Mehmet Zülküf Önal

Medical management of stroke encompasses a wide range of therapies that include interventions directed at reducing the extent of acute injury, managing physiological parameters in the acute phase, and preventing recurrent strokes. Ischemic stroke is the most common form of cerebrovascular disease and will be the focus of this chapter, which will overview acute treatments and prevention measures. Only a brief mention of primary intracerebral hemorrhage (ICH) in regard to acute management and secondary prevention will be included.

Acute ischemic stroke (AIS) occurs after occlusion of an intracranial or extracranial vessel by a thrombus that in most cases has embolized from the heart or a more proximal vessel. Unlike acute myocardial infarction (AMI), *in situ* thrombosis is uncommon. As a consequence of acute vascular occlusion, a cascade of intracellular events (Fig. 31-1) is initiated; over varying periods of time, they lead to irreversible tissue injury such as infarction.[1] The temporal development of infarction within the ischemic brain region is quite variable, and portions of the ischemic brain tissue may not be irreversibly injured for many hours after the initial vascular occlusion.[2] Ischemic brain tissue that remains viable and potentially amenable to salvage with timely initiation of therapeutic interventions is called the *ischemic penumbra*, and this potentially salvageable tissue is the target of AIS therapies.[3,4] The basic concept underlying AIS therapy is that reducing the extent of brain infarction should translate into improved clinical outcome, as measured by commonly used outcome scales such as the modified Rankin Scale (mRS) or Barthel Index.[5]

The most important factor predisposing ischemic brain tissue to infarction is the severity of cerebral blood flow (CBF) decline.[6] Regions with little or no residual CBF will evolve into infarction rapidly and are not the target of AIS therapies because reperfusion cannot in most cases be performed rapidly enough to salvage this ischemic core region. In the ischemic penumbra, CBF decline is more modest, and this ischemic tissue progresses more slowly toward infarction, providing a time window for intervention that can salvage tissue to some extent. A variety of definitions for the ischemic penumbra were suggested over time and are outlined in Box 31-1. Besides the severity of CBF decline, other factors that affect evolution of ischemic injury include temperature, glucose, blood pressure, and other metabolic factors.[7,8] The implication of these factors that contribute to the evolution of ischemic injury is that individual AIS patients have quite variable therapeutic time windows for successful therapeutic intervention, and that the earlier a therapy is initiated, the more likely it is to be beneficial. Acute ischemic stroke therapy can be divided into two broad areas: (1) recanalization/reperfusion approaches directed at improving altered CBF within ischemic tissue and (2) neuroprotection designed to impede the cellular consequences of ischemic injury. The focus of this chapter will be on the former because no neuroprotection strategies have been demonstrated to be of significant benefit. Recanalization/reperfusion can be accomplished with intravenous (IV) or intraarterial (IA) thrombolytics as well as mechanical devices. These approaches comprise the currently available AIS treatments.

Prehospital and Emergency Department Management of Ischemic Stroke

Prehospital management and field treatment are critically important to increasing survival rates of stroke patients. This phase starts with the emergency medical services (EMS) call and continues in the hospital emergency department (ED; Table 31-1). The majority of ischemic stroke patients do not reach the hospital soon enough, owing to lack of local services, facilities, and social reasons. When first suspected to have a stroke, the patient should be rapidly transported to an appropriate facility for diagnostic evaluation and treatment initiation.[9] Stroke patients who present within 3 to 4.5 hours of symptom onset are eligible for IV thrombolysis.[10–14] Emergency medical services use is strongly associated with a decreased time to initial physician examination, initial computed tomography (CT) imaging, and neurological evaluation.[13,15–17] The benefits of EMS contact are superior to contacting the family physician or hospital directly, and were confirmed with several studies.[18,19] Stroke should be given a priority dispatch as for MI and trauma.[20] Patients who show signs and symptoms of hyperacute stroke must be treated as time-sensitive emergency cases and transported without delay to the closest institution that provides emergency stroke care.

To ease and facilitate this process, medical authorities and media sources should encourage the recognition of stroke signs by providing public education about this condition.[21] All members of the public should be able to recognize and identify the signs and symptoms of stroke, which include sudden localized weakness, difficulty speaking, loss of vision, headache, and dizziness.[22] Patient, family, and caregiver education is an integral part of stroke care that should be addressed at all stages across the continuum of stroke care for both adult and pediatric patients.[22] Currently, thrombolytic treatment with tissue plasminogen activator (tPA) is the only approved treatment option for AIS. The National Institute of Neurological Disorders and Stroke (NINDS) and Advanced Cardiac Life Support Resources (ACLSR) recommend the possible timing sequences shown in Table 31-2 for the potential thrombolysis candidate.

Data from the Thomas Lewis Latané (TLL) Temple Foundation Stroke Project controlled trial showed the benefits of educational interventions on stroke identification and management targeting patients, EMS, hospitals, and community physicians. This approach increased thrombolytic use in patients with ischemic stroke from 2.21% to 8.65% as compared with communities that did not have such programs, which saw only a 0.06% increase. For patients with ischemic stroke who were eligible for thrombolytic therapy, rates of tPA usage increased from 14% to 52% in intervention communities.[23,24] Prehospital delays continue to contribute the largest proportion of time to late initiation of therapy.[25]

Emergency medical services arrival starts the diagnostic and management processes. The EMS crew should transfer the patient to a medical center that can provide appropriate diagnostic and treatment modalities to stroke patients.[9] After the ambulance arrives on the scene, EMS providers should obtain a brief history and patient examination, stabilize vital signs, and rapidly transport the patient to the closest, most appropriate facility (Table 31-3). Prehospital evaluation is helpful for ED physicians and the inpatient care team for planning treatment options. The Los Angeles Prehospital Stroke Screen and Cincinnati Prehospital Stroke Scale are the most widely used and preferred prehospital evaluation instruments and facilitate evaluation of potential stroke patients. Critical medical interventions in the ED should focus on the need for intubation, blood pressure control, and determining risk/benefit for thrombolytic intervention.[26] General ED stroke care issues are outlined in Table 31-4.[27,28]

Acute stroke patients urgently need IV access and cardiac monitoring in the ED, preferably initiated in the transporting ambulance. These patients are at also risk for acute cardiac diseases such as arrhythmias and myocardial infarction (MI). In addition,

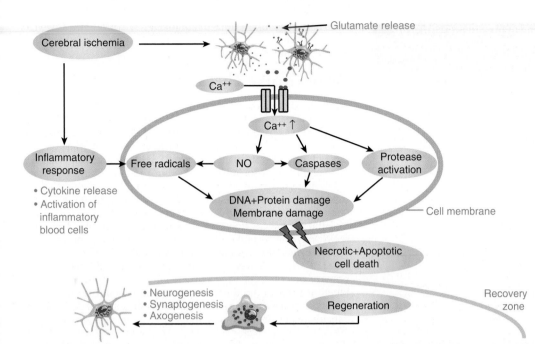

FIGURE 31-1 Depiction of the major events that encompass the ischemic cascade of cellular injury. DNA, deoxyribonucleic acid; NO, nitric oxide. *(Courtesy Dr. Wolf-Rudiger Schaebitz.)*

Box 31-1 Definitions of the Ischemic Penumbra Over Time

- A region of reduced CBF with absent electrical activity but preserved ion homeostasis and transmembrane electrical potentials
- A region with reduced CBF and preserved energy metabolism
- A region with impaired protein synthesis but preserved ATP levels
- A region that is potentially salvageable with timely intervention*

*This definition is the most clinically relevant one and relates directly to imaging identification.
ATP, adenosine triphosphate; CBF, cerebral blood flow.

TABLE 31-1 Stroke Chain of Survival

DETECTION	RECOGNITION OF STROKE SIGNS AND SYMPTOMS
Dispatch	Call 911 (emergency phone number) and priority EMS dispatch
Delivery	Prompt transport and prehospital notification to hospital
Door	Immediate ED triage
Data	ED evaluation, prompt laboratory studies, and CT imaging
Decision	Diagnosis and decision about appropriate therapy
Drug	Administration of appropriate drugs or other interventions

CT, computed tomography; ED, emergency department; EMS, emergency medical services.
Adapted from Adams HP Jr, del Zoppo G, Alberts MJ, et al: Guidelines for the early management of adults with ischemic stroke: a guideline from the American Heart Association/American Stroke Association Stroke Council, Clinical Cardiology Council, Cardiovascular Radiology and Intervention Council, and the Atherosclerotic Peripheral Vascular Disease and Quality of Care Outcomes in Research Interdisciplinary Working Groups: the American Academy of Neurology affirms the value of this guideline as an educational tool for neurologists. Stroke 38:1655–1711, 2007.[9]

TABLE 31-2 Stroke Evaluation Time Benchmarks for Potential Thrombolysis Candidate

TIME INTERVAL	TIME TARGET
Door to doctor	10 min
Access to neurological expertise	15 min
Door to CT scan completion	25 min
Door to CT scan interpretation	45 min
Door to treatment	60 min
Admission to monitored bed	3 h

CT, computed tomography.

TABLE 31-3 Guidelines for Emergency Medical Services Management of Patients with Suspected Stroke

RECOMMENDED	NOT RECOMMENDED
Manage ABCs	Dextrose-containing fluids in nonhypoglycemic patients
Cardiac monitoring	Hypotension/excessive blood pressure reduction
IV access	Excessive IV fluids
Oxygen (as required for O$_2$ saturation <92%)	
Assess for hypoglycemia	
Nil per os (NPO)	
Alert receiving emergency department	
Rapid transport to closest appropriate facility capable of treating acute stroke	

ABCs, airway, breathing, circulation; IV, intravenous.
Adapted from Adams HP Jr, del Zoppo G, Alberts MJ, et al: Guidelines for the early management of adults with ischemic stroke: a guideline from the American Heart Association/American Stroke Association Stroke Council, Clinical Cardiology Council, Cardiovascular Radiology and Intervention Council, and the Atherosclerotic Peripheral Vascular Disease and Quality of Care Outcomes in Research Interdisciplinary Working Groups: the American Academy of Neurology affirms the value of this guideline as an educational tool for neurologists. Stroke 38:1655–1711, 2007.[9]

---

atrial fibrillation may be associated with acute stroke as either the etiology (embolic disease) or as a result.[29,30] Acute stroke patient evaluation in the ED should include a detailed history, physical examination, neurological examination, and stroke scale scores (National Institutes of Health Stroke Scale [NIHSS] and appropriate diagnostic tests; Box 31-2).[9]

Patients presenting with compromised ventilation require emergent airway control via nasal oxygenation or rapid sequence intubation. Adequate tissue oxygenation is important in the acute

TABLE 31-4	General Management of Patients with Acute Stroke
BLOOD GLUCOSE	**TREAT HYPOGLYCEMIA WITH D₅₀**
Blood pressure	Evaluate recommendations for thrombolysis candidates and noncandidates
Cardiac monitor	Continuous monitoring for ischemic changes and atrial fibrillation
IV fluids	Avoid D₂W and excessive fluid administration; IV isotonic sodium chloride solution at 50 mL/h unless otherwise indicated
Oral intake	NPO initially; aspiration risk is great; avoid oral intake until swallowing assessed
Oxygen	Supplement if indicated (Sao₂ <93%, hypotensive, etc.)
Temperature	Avoid hyperthermia; oral or rectal acetaminophen and cooling blankets as needed

IV, intravenous; NPO, nil per os; Sao₂, arterial blood oxygen saturation.
Adapted from Krieger D, Hacke W: The intensive care of the stroke patient. In Barnett HJ, Mohr JP, Stein BM, editors: Stroke: pathophysiology, diagnosis and management, ed 3, New York, 1998, Churchill Livingstone; and SPORTIF Executive Steering Committee for the SPORTIF V Investigators: Ximelagatran vs. warfarin for stroke prevention in patients with nonvalvular atrial fibrillation: a randomized trial. JAMA 293:690–698, 2005.[27,28]

Box 31-2 Immediate Diagnostic Studies for Patients with Suspected Acute Ischemic Stroke*

All Patients
Noncontrast brain CT or brain MRI
Blood glucose
Serum electrolytes/renal function
ECG
Markers of cardiac ischemia
CBC, including platelet count
Prothrombin time/INR
APTT
Oxygen saturation

Selected Patients
Hepatic function tests
Toxicology screen
Blood alcohol level
Pregnancy test
Arterial blood gas tests (if hypoxia is suspected)
Chest radiography (if lung disease is suspected)
Lumbar puncture (if SAH is suspected and CT scan is negative for blood)
EEG (if seizures are suspected)

*Although it is desirable to know the results of these tests before giving rtPA, thrombolytic therapy should not be delayed while awaiting the results unless (1) there is clinical suspicion of a bleeding abnormality or thrombocytopenia, (2) the patient has received heparin or warfarin, or (3) use of anticoagulants is not known.
APTT, activated partial thromboplastin time; CBC, complete blood cell count; CT, computed tomography; ECG, electrocardiogram; EEG, electroencephalogram; INR, International Normalized Ratio; MRI, magnetic resonance imaging; SAH, subarachnoid hemorrhage.
Adapted from Adams HP Jr, del Zoppo G, Alberts MJ, et al: Guidelines for the early management of adults with ischemic stroke: a guideline from the American Heart Association/American Stroke Association Stroke Council, Clinical Cardiology Council, Cardiovascular Radiology and Intervention Council, and the Atherosclerotic Peripheral Vascular Disease and Quality of Care Outcomes in Research Interdisciplinary Working Groups: the American Academy of Neurology affirms the value of this guideline as an educational tool for neurologists. Stroke 38:1655–1711, 2007.[9]

management of acute cerebral ischemia to prevent hypoxia and further brain damage. The most common causes of hypoxia in the patient with acute stroke are partial airway obstruction, hypoventilation, atelectasis, or aspiration pneumonia.[9,26,27,31] Oxygen need should be monitored with pulse oximetry, with a target oxygen saturation level of 92% or better.[32] Endotracheal intubation, supplemental nasal oxygen, and hyperbaric oxygen are choices to augment oxygen intake. If brain herniation is present, hyperventilation using mechanical ventilation is an option to decrease intracranial pressure (ICP) by decreasing CBF, is recommended with an endpoint arterial partial pressure of carbon dioxide (Pco₂) of

32 to 36 mmHg. Intravenous mannitol can be considered as well to reduce increased intracranial pressure. Oxygen supplementation should be guided by a pulse oximeter.[26,27,31]

Acute Stroke Therapy

The only AIS treatment currently approved by regulatory agencies is IV tPA initiated within 3 hours after stroke onset. Approval of this treatment was based on results of the NINDS tPA trial that demonstrated a highly significant improvement in 90-day outcome on various outcome measures including mRS, Barthel Index, and NIHSS.[33] The benefit was observed in different stroke subtypes and in patients with various ranges of baseline stroke severity, ranging from relatively mild to fairly severe.[34] Despite a risk of 6.4% for symptomatic intracranial hemorrhage with IV tPA treatment observed in the NINDS trial, the overall treatment effect was highly significant. Following the NINDS trial, several other studies of IV tPA were performed that tried to extend the therapeutic time window to 6 hours from stroke onset.[35–37] None of these demonstrated a significant benefit on the primary outcome measure chosen for the trial. However, a combined analysis of the European Cooperative Acute Stroke Studies (ECASS) I and II as well as the ATLANTIS trial demonstrated a significant treatment effect with IV tPA out to 4.5 hours from stroke onset.[38] This observation suggested that the therapeutic time window for IV tPA could be extended and was evaluated in the ECASS III trial. The study evaluated AIS patients between 3 and 4.5 hours after onset and reflected the European license for tPA: excluding patients over 80, those with very severe strokes, history of prior stroke, diabetes, and use of anticoagulants prior to stroke.[39] The ECASS III study demonstrated that 52.4% of tPA-treated patients achieved a favorable outcome of 0 to 1 on the mRS, compared to 45.2% with placebo treatment (odds ratio [OR], 1.34; 95% confidence interval [CI], 1.02-1.76; $P = 0.04$). The results of ECASS III led to recommendations from the American Heart Association (AHA) and other groups that the use of IV tPA be extended to 4.5 hours in selected AIS patients.[40] Subgroup analysis of the ECASS III data suggested that patients older than 65 and those with more severe strokes had less benefit than younger patients or those with milder deficits[41] (Box 31-3). Unfortunately, only standard CT scans were employed in the ECASS III trial, so it is unclear how more modern imaging techniques such as diffusion/perfusion magnetic resonance imaging (MRI) or perfusion CT may contribute to identifying AIS patients more or less likely to benefit from IV tPA in this extended time window when ischemic penumbral survival tends to wane.

Currently, IA thrombolysis remains an unproven therapy for AIS patients, despite its widespread use at larger centers. The only phase III trial that evaluated this therapeutic approach was the PROACT-III trial that compared prourokinase ($n = 121$) to placebo ($n = 59$) in severely compromised patients with angiographically confirmed large-vessel occlusion treated up to 6 hours after stroke onset.[42] A prior safety trial demonstrated a reasonable safety profile. In the PROACT-II trial, 40% of treated patients achieved a favorable outcome,

---

Box 31-3 Subgroup Analysis of the ECASS III Trial of Intravenous tPA in the 3- to 4.5-Hour Time Window

Patient Characteristics Associated with Modest or No Benefit with tPA
- Females
- Age >65*
- Moderate baseline stroke severity*
- Diabetes mellitus
- Hypertension*
- Atrial fibrillation*

*Denotes patients with an increased risk for symptomatic intracerebral hemorrhage (ICH). tPA, tissue plasminogen activator.
Adapted from Bluhmki E, Chamorro A, Dávalos A, et al: Stroke treatment with alteplase given 3.0-4.5 h after onset of ischaemic stroke (ECASS III): additional outcomes and subgroup analysis of a randomised controlled trial. Lancet Neurol 8:1095–1102, 2009.[42]

defined as an mRS score of 0 to 2, compared to 25% in the placebo group (*P* = 0.04). The rates of partial or complete recanalization were 66% and 18%, respectively. Symptomatic ICH was increased in the prourokinase group, but not significantly. The trial showed that IA therapy could be beneficial up to 6 hours from stroke onset in patients with large intracranial vascular occlusions. Prourokinase was not approved by regulatory agencies based upon this one modestly sized trial, and a second confirmatory trial was never performed. Prourokinase is not available for clinical use.

Studies of the IA use of tPA are limited to combination trials with initial IV tPA use followed by subsequent IA treatment. In the IMS I trial, the combined use of tPA both IV and IA was observed to carry a similar risk for ICH as IV tPA alone in the NINDS IV trial.[43] In the IMS II trial, patients initially received IV tPA within 3 hours of stroke onset. An angiogram was then performed, and if a clot was observed, IA therapy was initiated either through a standard catheter or an EKOS microinfusion catheter.[44] Among 81 patients included in the trial, 26 received IV tPA alone, 33 IV plus IA tPA via the EKOS catheter, and 19 the combination IA via a standard catheter. There was no control group, but when compared to the placebo group in the NINDS trial, this combined treatment approach tended to have a more favorable outcome. IMS III, a much larger trial comparing IV tPA with various combined IV and IA therapies, is ongoing, but recruitment has lagged. A European study comparing IV versus IA tPA is also ongoing.

The use of urokinase given IA was studied in the Japanese MELT trial that randomized 114 patients with angiographically confirmed middle cerebral artery (MCA) occlusion to active therapy or standard medical therapy within 6 hours of stroke onset.[45] The IA urokinase group achieved a favorable outcome (mRS 0-2) in 49.1% of patients, compared to 38.6% in the control group, a nonsignificant trend toward benefit in an underpowered trial. A detailed analysis of the randomized IA thrombolytic trials concluded that there was no evidence of proven benefit with this treatment approach when compared with the expected rate in a prognostic model.[46]

Device recanalization was evaluated with both the MERCI retriever and PENUMBRA device. Both of these devices received U.S. Food and Drug Administration (FDA) clearance to remove clots in intracranial blood vessels but are not approved to treat AIS, a curious paradox when considering why a device would be used to remove a clot. Approval of the MERCI retriever was based upon an open nonrandomized trial in 141 AIS patients, most with anterior circulation occlusions, treated up to 8 hours after stroke onset who did not receive tPA.[47] These treated patients were then compared to historical controls, the placebo group from the PROACT-II trial. Partial or complete recanalization occurred in 48% of the patients treated with the MERCI retriever, but only 27.1% achieved an mRS score of 0 to 2 at 90 days, essentially the same as the 25% rate of mRS observed in the control group in the PROACT-II trial. Serious adverse events related to employment of the device occurred in 7.1% of the patients, but this did not include an additional 7.8% of patients who developed symptomatic ICH.

A second open-label study of a subsequent generation of the MERCI retriever, the Multi-MERCI study, was reported, but this study is difficult to interpret because concomitant use of IV and/or IA tPA was allowed and occurred in the majority of the patients in the study.[48] The partial or complete recanalization rate was slightly higher (57.3%), as was the rate of patients achieving a 90-day mRS score of 0 to 2 (36%). Symptomatic ICH occurred in 9.8% of patients, and serious adverse events occurred in 7.9%. The PENUMBRA device was also evaluated in an open trial and compared to historical controls from the PROACT II trial.[49] In this study, 125 patients were treated with the device up to 8 hours after stroke onset. Partial or complete recanalization occurred in 82% of the patients, device-related serious adverse events in 1.6%, and symptomatic ICH in 11.2%. At day 90, 25% of the patients achieved an mRS of 0 to 2, identical to the control group in the PROACT II trial.

Based on these two open studies that compared the device outcomes to historical controls from PROACT II, the devices both received clearance from the FDA for removal of intracranial clots.

The trials do demonstrate that both devices effectively induce partial/complete vessel recanalization when employed up to 8 hours after stroke onset. However, the recanalization was not associated with improved clinical outcome, insofar as both trials demonstrated clinical outcomes essentially identical to the control group of untreated patients in PROACT II, and the rate of symptomatic ICH was concerning.

Despite the lack of proven clinical benefit, both IA tPA and device clot removal are used in some centers up to 8 hours and beyond after stroke onset. The lack of clinical benefit is concerning because both therapeutic approaches clearly induce recanalization of occluded vessels in the majority of patients treated, and this should translate into clinical improvement based upon the earlier time window IV tPA trials. The implication is that despite successful opening of occluded vessels in many patients, clinical benefit was not derived because not enough ischemic tissue was salvaged at the late time points evaluated, especially in the two device trials. Additionally, the rate of symptomatic hemorrhage rate seen in the MERCI and PENUMBRA studies may have detracted from potential clinical improvements. The results suggest that late recanalization alone is not sufficient for inducing clinical benefit, and those other factors such as tissue salvage at such late time points must be considered to demonstrate clinical efficacy.

In addition to recanalization therapies that have demonstrated clear benefit when initiated within 4.5 hours of stroke onset, the only other acute intervention with a documented significant improvement in outcome is the use of specialized stroke care units. In acute coronary care, specialized units have a long-standing history and proven track record. For AIS, the development and use of specialized care units is much more recent, and efficacy was documented later than for coronary care units. Several studies found that admission of AIS patients to stroke care units reduces mortality and disability when compared to care on general medical units with stroke team consultation.[50,51] The precise reasons for these benefits are uncertain but likely relate to stricter adherence to care guidelines, better blood pressure and glucose management, and earlier mobilization.[52] Additionally, it is now apparent that management guidelines such as the AHA "Get with the Guidelines" recommendations reduce complications after AIS, and that these guidelines should be implemented both in stroke units and general hospital units if at all possible.[53]

The other approach to AIS treatment besides recanalization/ reperfusion is neuroprotection, or reduction of infarction by treatments targeting the manifold cellular consequences of focal brain ischemia, which has a long and undistinguished track record. In animal stroke models, many categories of neuroprotective drugs reduce infarct size, and some also improve functional outcome[54,55] (Box 31-4). The reduction of infarct size for many neuroprotective drugs occurred without reperfusion, implying that enough of the drug reached the ischemic penumbra in sufficient concentration

---

> **Box 31-4 Types of Neuroprotective Drugs That Have Been Evaluated as Potential Treatments for Acute Ischemic Stroke**
>
> - NMDA antagonists
> - AMPA antagonists
> - Free radical scavengers
> - Growth factors
> - Calcium channel antagonists
> - GABA agonists
> - Serotonin antagonists
> - Potassium channel activator
> - Antiinflammatory agents
>
> AMPA, α-amino-3-hydroxy-5-methyl-4-isoxazolepropionate; GABA, γ-aminobutyric acid; NMDA, N-methyl-D-aspartate.
> Adapted from Schabitz WR, Fisher M: Perspectives on neuroprotective stroke therapy. Biochem Soc Trans 34:1271–1276, 2006; and Donnan GA: A new road map for neuroprotection. Stroke 39:242–248, 2008.[55,56]

to impede development of infarction. This can occur because there is sufficient residual CBF in the penumbral region to deliver the neuroprotective drug and allow this tissue to survive.

Based on preclinical data of varying quality and extensiveness, many neuroprotective drugs went into clinical development, including phase III trials in some cases.[56] None of the neuroprotective drugs demonstrated significant efficacy, and currently no neuroprotective drug is available for AIS treatment. Many reasons for the multitude of neuroprotective drug development programs were proposed regarding both the preclinical assessment of these agents and the clinical development programs[57] (Box 31-5). Neuroprotection as an AIS treatment strategy remains appealing either as monotherapy or in combination with reperfusion.

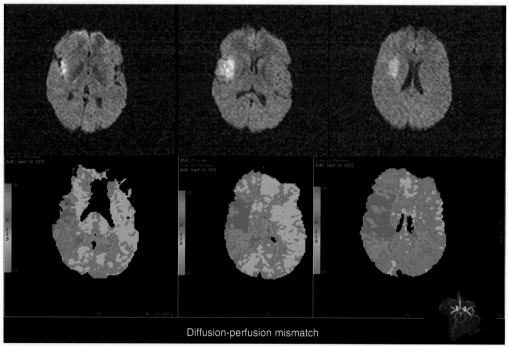

Box 31-5 Potential Preclinical and Clinical Trials Flaws That May Have Hampered Neuroprotective Drug Development

Preclinical Testing Flaws
- Inadequate sample sizes in treatment experiments
- Lack of adequate physiological monitoring
- Lack of blinding to treatment outcomes
- Not testing the drug in animals that were female, aged, or had relevant comorbidities
- Only testing the study drug in rodents
- Only evaluating histological endpoints and not behavioral outcomes
- Lack of determining effects on both ischemic gray and white matter

Clinical Trial Flaws
- Treating patients too long after stroke onset
- Including stroke subtypes not likely to respond to treatment, such as lacunar stroke patients
- Moving to phase III trials without adequate assessment of the study drug's pharmacology
- Side effects precluded reaching the therapeutic blood level shown to be effective in animals
- Inadequately powered phase III trials to detect a modest but clinically meaningful treatment effect
- Using an insensitive or flawed primary outcome measure

Adapted from Gladstone DJ, Black SE, Hakim AM: Toward wisdom from failure: lessons from neuroprotective stroke trials and new directions. Stroke 33:2123–2136, 2002.[58]

A safe and modestly effective neuroprotective drug with clear stand-alone efficacy for improving outcome after AIS could be widely used, especially in hospitals without the adequate infrastructure for giving even IV tPA. Combining neuroprotection with reperfusion therapy can be envisioned in several ways. Very early initiation of a neuroprotectant could potentially extend survival of the ischemic penumbra, allowing for later deployment of an IV or IA reperfusion therapy. In animals, both high-flow 100% oxygen delivery and granulocyte colony stimulating factor (GCSF) have the capability to extend penumbral survival, but this approach has not yet been tested in clinical trials.[58,59] Another potential combination of neuroprotection with reperfusion would be to use an appropriate agent to reduce potential deleterious tissue consequences of successful reperfusion (i.e., reperfusion injury).[60] Neuroprotective drugs that affect free radicals or reduce the recruitment of inflammatory white blood cells (WBCs) may be particularly suited to reduce reperfusion injury, and clinical development programs with such agents after successful reperfusion should be considered.

A final consideration for future neuroprotection development programs would be to use agents that reduce infarct size when given early after AIS, but also enhance the natural recovery processes that occurs weeks and months later.[61] This combination approach is appealing because both the reduction of infarct size engendered by the neuroprotective effect and the recovery-enhancing effect will contribute to improved stroke outcome. Current pessimism related to neuroprotection for AIS could be replaced by guarded optimism, but the organization and conduct of clinical trials will be more complex and difficult than in the past.

The most important future directions for AIS therapy are to extend the treatment window beyond the currently proven 4.5 hours from onset with IV tPA and to maximize the therapeutic benefit of this treatment within the currently documented time-to-treatment window. An attractive hypothesis for accomplishing both objectives is to use advanced imaging to identify AIS patients with extensive, persistent ischemic penumbra, the target of acute stroke therapy.[3] Two imaging modalities, diffusion- or perfusion-weighted MRI (DWI/PWI; Fig. 31-2) and perfusion CT (Fig. 31-3) may be appropriate for this task.[62,63] With DWI, regions of high-energy metabolism failure that developed cytotoxic edema

FIGURE 31-2 Example of a diffusion and perfusion mismatch on an acute magnetic resonance imaging (MRI) scan.

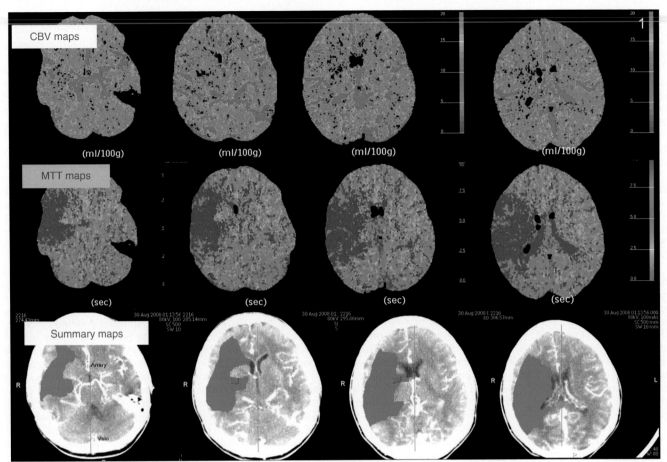

FIGURE 31-3 Perfusion computed tomography (CT) scan of an acute ischemic stroke (AIS) patient, demonstrating a very small basal ganglial abnormality on the cerebral blood volume map and a large area of hypoperfusion on the mean transit time map of brain perfusion.

can be readily identified and quantified as regions of hyperintensity that can be easily differentiated from normal brain regions. On PWI, various methods can be used to identify hypoperfused tissue, but approaches such as mean transit time mapping, time to peak mapping, and CBF mapping all have deficiencies in reliably differentiating among the ischemic core with very low CBF, the ischemic penumbra with moderate CBF, reductions, and oligemic tissue that is not destined for infarction.[64,65] Currently, it is suggested that Tmax mapping that corrects for the arterial input of contrast in normal brain contralateral to the ischemic region likely provides the best distinction among these three ischemic regions. The ischemic penumbra is thought to be represented by regions that are abnormal on PWI by Tmax thresholding but are normal on DWI, the so-called DWI/PWI mismatch.[66] Preliminary data support this concept because without therapy this DWI/PWI mismatch region is highly likely to demonstrate infarction on delayed T2 or fluid-attenuated inversion recovery (FLAIR) imaging. Magnetic resonance angiography (MRA) can also be acquired along with DWI and PWI and can depict the location of occlusion in large and medium-sized vessels.

The obvious application of the DWI/PWI mismatch would be to identify patients with substantial amounts of residual ischemic penumbra at various time points after stroke onset, and then to randomize such patients in clinical trials. In a large European case series, it was observed that patients with a DWI/PWI mismatch identified 3 to 6 hours after AIS stroke onset had essentially the same rate of favorable clinical outcome when treated with IV tPA as patients treated 0 to 3 hours after stroke onset.[67] Two early-phase clinical trials evaluated the utility of DWI/PWI in conjunction with IV tPA treatment in the 3- to 6-hour time window and demonstrated that patients more likely to respond to therapy can be identified.[68,69]

A third group of imaging-based trials used a different thrombolytic drug, desmoteplase, derived from bat saliva. Two small preliminary desmoteplase trials in which DWI/PWI and MRA were obtained at baseline demonstrated that reperfusion was greatly enhanced with this novel thrombolytic drug when compared to placebo, and that ischemic lesion growth tended to be reduced.[70,71] A third, larger desmoteplase trial did not demonstrate clinical efficacy despite using DWI/PWI in two thirds of patients and perfusion CT in the remainder.[72] It was observed that with DWI/PWI, patients who had a substantially larger mismatch tended to have a much better response to treatment than patients with a smaller mismatch. These preliminary studies that used DWI/PWI in conjunction with IV thrombolysis should be judged to be hypothesis generating. It is quite possible that DWI/PWI can be used to identify patients more likely to respond to treatment, and therefore reduce the sample size for future trials because the percentage of uninformative patients will be reduced.

General Medical Management of Acute Stroke Patients

Hypoglycemia should be corrected with rapid IV administration of concentrated glucose solution. Hypoglycemia is detrimental to the ischemic process. At the opposite end of the spectrum, a blood glucose of 200 mg/dL (10 mmol/L) or higher justifies immediate insulin administration. Hyperglycemia is found in nearly 20% to 50% of stroke patients.[73–75] Severe hyperglycemia is independently associated with stroke progression, increase in infarct size, and poor prognosis. Increased blood glucose causes reduced reperfusion in thrombolysis, as well as extension of the infarcted territory.[76–80] Glucose-containing IV fluids should not be given to normoglycemic stroke patients because this may lead to hyperglycemia and may worsen ischemic cerebral injury. Blood sugar control should be tightly maintained to establish normoglycemia (90-140 mg/dL).[9]

Core temperature is elevated in up to 50% of patients within 48 hours after stroke onset. High temperature is an alarming sign whether or not there is infection. Management of fever could notably have favorable or unfavorable consequences. Pyrogens can enhance the effects of interferons (molecules involved in the immune response), inhibit growth of some microorganisms, enhance the activity of white blood cells, and enhance tissue repair. The presence of fever has been found to correlate with poorer outcome in stroke, mostly because of increased metabolic demand, enhanced release of neurotransmitters, and increased free radical production.[35,81-85] Fever has been shown experimentally to increase infarct size, and high body temperature may favor stroke progression and poor long-term outcome.[86] Antipyretics are indicated for febrile stroke patients, since hyperthermia accelerates ischemic neuronal injury.

The Paracetamol (Acetaminophen) in Stroke (PAIS) trial assessed whether early treatment with paracetamol improves functional outcome in patients with acute stroke by reducing body temperature and preventing fever. Patients ($n = 1400$) were randomly assigned to receive acetaminophen (6 g daily) or placebo within 12 hours of symptom onset. After 3 months, improvement on the mRS with acetaminophen was not greater than expected. These results do not support routine use of high-dose acetaminophen in patients with acute stroke.[89] Antipyretics are recommended early in the management of acute stroke until the temperature is lowered to 37.5 °C. Antibiotics should be used early in cases of apparent bacterial infection.[79]

Hypothermia is currently being evaluated in clinical trials as a neuroprotective approach.[87,88] It has been shown to be neuroprotective in experimental and focal hypoxic brain injury models. Although strong experimental and clinical evidence indicates that induced hypothermia can protect the brain in the presence of hypoxia or ischemia, including after cardiac arrest, there is little data about the utility of induced hypothermia for treatment of patients with stroke.[90-95]

Cerebral perfusion pressure is high when patients are maintained in a supine position. However, lying flat may serve to increase ICP and thus is not recommended in cases of subarachnoid or other ICH. This information is applicable during transportation of stroke patients for enhancing favorable outcome.[96] Life-threatening space-occupying brain edema occurs in up to 10% of patients with supratentorial infarcts and is associated with an increased mortality rate of nearly 80%.[97] Stroke patients develop maximal cerebral edema 48 to 72 hours after onset.[9] Cerebral edema worsens ischemic stroke by increasing ICP and by its indirect effects. Hyperventilation and mannitol are used routinely to decrease ICP quickly and temporarily but are of uncertain long-term value. Both approaches require careful monitoring of blood chemistry. There is no evidence supporting the use of corticosteroids to decrease cerebral edema in AIS. Many patients who develop hemorrhagic transformation or progressive cerebral edema will demonstrate acute clinical decline. In cases of evolving large MCA infarction, early surgical decompression is now the "antiedema" therapy of first choice for patients younger than 60 years, independent of affected hemisphere. Whether this aggressive treatment is beneficial for elderly patients or when performed after 48 hours is currently being tested. Over the past decade, decompressive hemicraniectomy for malignant MCA infarction has been reported to lower mortality without increasing the number of severely disabled survivors in several uncontrolled case series.[98-103]

Maintaining electrolyte balance is also important during the acute stages of stroke, especially to avoid plasma volume contraction. Disturbance of fluid balance could worsen brain perfusion pressure. Patients should be adequately hydrated. All stroke patients should receive IV fluid therapy, with a slightly positive fluid balance according to the level of dehydration, as indicated by the hematocrit and serum osmolality. A careful approach should be employed in patients having possible cerebral edema. Therefore, all stroke patients need daily electrolyte monitoring.[79]

Although patients with heart disease are at high risk for ischemic stroke, both myocardial ischemia and cardiac arrhythmias are potential complications of acute cerebrovascular diseases.[30,104] The most common arrhythmia detected in the setting of stroke is atrial fibrillation, which may be either related to the cause of stroke or a complication.[9] Other potentially life-threatening cardiac arrhythmias are relatively uncommon, but sudden death may occur.[31,105] No clinical trials have tested the utility of cardiac monitoring for most patients with ischemic stroke, or the use of cardioprotective agents or medications to prevent serious cardiac arrhythmias. Still, a consensus exists that patients with AIS should have cardiac monitoring for at least the first 24 hours, and that any serious cardiac arrhythmia should be treated. The utility of prophylactic administration of medications to prevent cardiac arrhythmias among patients with stroke is unclear.[9]

Hypertension has a devastating effect on the brain and is a major risk factor for ischemic and hemorrhagic stroke. Hypertension alters the structure of cerebral blood vessels and disrupts intricate vasoregulatory mechanisms that ensure adequate blood supply to the brain. These alterations threaten cerebral blood supply and increase susceptibility of the brain to ischemic injury.[106] High blood pressure is often detected in the first hours after stroke. Blood pressure monitoring and treatment is one of the most critical issues in stroke treatment. Hypotension and hypertension are both dangerous for stroke patients because of the disturbed cerebral perfusion. Hypotension and abnormalities in cardiac rhythm must be corrected as quickly as possible to ensure adequate cerebral perfusion. However, elevated blood pressure should be managed according to suggested guidelines.[107,108] Aggressive efforts to lower blood pressure may decrease cerebral perfusion pressure and worsen the ischemic process.

Both elevated and low blood pressures are associated with poor outcomes in patients with acute stroke.[109,110] Blood pressure normalization may acutely reduce the hemorrhagic transformation risk of ischemic stroke and reduce the risk of stroke recurrence and brain edema. Aggressive antihypertensive therapy should be used in stroke patients with hypertensive encephalopathy, aortic dissection, acute renal failure, acute pulmonary edema, or AMI.[110,111] Unfortunately, aggressive treatment of blood pressure may lead to neurological worsening by reducing perfusion pressure to ischemic brain areas.[110,112,113] Excessive lowering of blood pressure acutely in ischemic stroke patients has been associated with neurological worsening. When the blood pressure must be lowered, titratable short-acting IV medication is preferred to minimize the risk of cerebral hypoperfusion.[114] Typically, during the first hours after stroke onset, but sometimes not until 24 hours later, blood pressure drops spontaneously, unrelated to any specific medication.[115]

Precise recommendations for control of hypertension in the setting of acute stroke are controversial owing to results of several studies related to acute blood pressure control.[110] Systolic blood pressure (SBP) greater than 185 mmHg or diastolic pressure of greater than 110 mmHg are contraindications to thrombolysis; emergency blood pressure control is indicated to allow for thrombolytic administration.[35] Outside of the consideration of thrombolytic administration, in the absence of hypertension-related complications, no data support administration of emergency antihypertensive drugs in acute stroke. The consensus recommendation is to lower blood pressure only if systolic pressure is in excess of 220 mmHg or if diastolic pressure is greater than 120 mmHg.[9] However, rapid reduction of blood pressure, no matter the degree of hypertension, may in fact be harmful.

Management of blood pressure in patients with AIS is divided into those who are candidates for thrombolytic therapy and those who are not. For patients who are not tPA candidates and whose SBP is less than 220 mmHg and diastolic blood pressure is less than 120 mmHg in the absence of evidence of end-organ involvement (i.e., pulmonary edema, aortic dissection, hypertensive encephalopathy), blood pressure should be monitored (without acute intervention), and stroke symptoms and complications should be treated (increased ICP, seizures). For patients with SBPs elevated above 220 mmHg or diastolic blood pressures between 120 and 140 mmHg, labetalol (10-20 mg IV for 1-2 min) should be the initial drug of choice unless a contraindication to its use exists.[113] Dosing may be repeated or doubled every 10 minutes to a maximum dose of 300 mg. Alternatively, nicardipine (5 mg/h IV initial infusion) titrated to effect via increasing 2.5 mg/h every 5 minutes to a maximum dose of 15 mg/h may be used for blood pressure control. Lastly, nitroprusside at 0.5 µg/kg/min IV infusion may be used in the setting of continuous blood pressure monitoring. The goal of intervention is a reduction of 10% to 15% of blood pressure.[9,26]

For patients who will be receiving tPA, SBP should be lower than 185 mmHg and diastolic blood pressure lower than 110 mmHg. Monitoring and control of blood pressure during and after thrombolytic administration are vital because uncontrolled hypertension is associated with hemorrhagic complications.[35] For the first 2 hours after IV thrombolysis, blood pressure should be checked every 15 minutes, then every 30 minutes for 6 hours, and finally every hour for 16 hours. If blood pressure levels are in the ranges of 180 to 230 mmHg systolic or 105 to 120 mmHg diastolic, it is appropriate to administer labetalol 10 mg IV over 1 to 2 minutes. This may be repeated every 10 to 20 minutes to a maximum dose of 300 mg. If blood pressure is not controlled, sodium nitroprusside should be considered[32,116] (Table 31-5).

Anticoagulation and Antiplatelet Therapy

Intravenous anticoagulation therapy is widely used, even though there are no data confirming its benefit. It is unknown whether IV heparin prevents recurrent cardioembolic stroke in the subacute phase, and it is unlikely this therapy inhibits progression of stroke deficits. Current guidelines do not recommend IV anticoagulation for any stroke subgroup.[117–122] Immobilized stroke patients who are not receiving anticoagulants (e.g., IV heparin, an oral anticoagulant) may benefit from low-dose subcutaneous unfractionated (UFH) or low-molecular-weight heparin (LMWH), which reduces the risk of deep vein thrombosis (DVT).[9] Multiple past studies of LMWH failed to show beneficial effects for AIS. Although trials of

anticoagulants in the treatment of AIS are ongoing, no data exist to support their use in AIS.[9]

Published guidelines for prevention of stroke in patients with ischemic stroke or transient ischemic attack (TIA) due to atrial fibrillation recommend anticoagulation with adjusted-dose warfarin for secondary prevention (target international normalized ratio [INR] 2.5, range 2.0-3.0).[116] Oral anticoagulation with warfarin is also recommended for patients with ischemic stroke due to AMI in whom left ventricular (LV) mural thrombus is identified, patients with dilated cardiomyopathy, and patients with valvular heart disease for secondary prevention.[116]

For patients with noncardioembolic ischemic stroke or TIA, including strokes caused by large-artery atherosclerosis, small penetrating artery disease, and cryptogenic infarcts, antiplatelet agents rather than oral anticoagulation are recommended to reduce the risk of recurrent stroke and other cardiovascular events.

Direct thrombin inhibitors, such as dabigatran etexilate, have recently been evaluated. For stroke prevention in patients with atrial fibrillation, dabigatran 110 mg given twice daily was associated with rates of stroke and systemic embolism similar to those associated with warfarin but lower rates of hemorrhagic side effects. Dabigatran 150 mg twice daily, compared with warfarin, was associated with lower rates of stroke and systemic embolism but similar rates of major hemorrhage.[123] However, even if drugs are proven superior to dose-adjusted warfarin, their benefits must be substantial (retaining high efficacy with added safety and convenience) to offset their increased cost.[124,125]

Heparin or LMWH in AIS are associated with increased risk of bleeding complications and symptomatic hemorrhagic transformation. Although antiplatelet agents were shown to be useful for preventing recurrent stroke or stroke after TIA, their use should be regarded as a preventive measure, not an acute stroke treatment.[26]

The International Stroke Trial (IST) and Chinese Acute Stroke Trial (CAST) demonstrated modest benefit of aspirin in the setting of AIS. CAST evaluated 21,106 patients and had a 4-week mortality reduction of 3.3% with aspirin, compared to 3.9% with placebo.[126] A separate study, IST, also found that the combination of aspirin and LMWH did not significantly improve outcomes.[127] IST randomized 20,000 patients within 24 hours of stroke onset to treatment with aspirin 325 mg, subcutaneous heparin in two different dose regimens, aspirin with heparin, and a placebo. The study found that aspirin therapy reduced the risk of early stroke recurrence.[127] The CAST and IST results suggest that the use of

TABLE 31-5 Blood Pressure Management in Patients with Stroke

PATIENT	BLOOD PRESSURE	TREATMENT
Candidates for fibrinolysis	Pretreatment: SBP >185 mmHg or DBP >110 mmHg	Labetalol 10-20 mg IVP 1-2 doses or Enalapril 1.25 mg IVP
	Posttreatment: DBP >140 mmHg SBP >230 mmHg or DBP 121-140 mmHg SBP 180-230 mmHg or DBP 105-120 mmHg	Sodium nitroprusside (0.5 µg/kg/min) Labetalol 10-20 mg IVP, and consider labetalol infusion at 1-2 mg/min or nicardipine 5 mg/h IV infusion and titrate Labetalol 10 mg IVP, may repeat and double every 10 min up to maximum dose of 150 mg
Noncandidates for fibrinolysis	DBP >140 mmHg	Sodium nitroprusside 0.5 µg/kg/min; may reduce approximately 10%-20%
	SBP >220 mmHg or DBP 121-140 mmHg or MAP >130 mmHg	Labetalol 10-20 mg IVP over 1-2 min; may repeat and double every 10 min up to maximum dose of 150 mg or Nicardipine 5 mg/h IV infusion and titrate
	SBP >220 mmHg or DBP 105-120 mmHg or MAP <130 mmHg	Antihypertensive therapy indicated only if AMI, aortic dissection, severe CHF, or hypertensive encephalopathy present

AMI, acute myocardial infarction; CHF, congestive heart failure; DBP, diastolic blood pressure; IV, intravenous; IVP, IV push; MAP, mean arterial pressure; SBP, systolic blood pressure.
Adapted from Krieger D, Hacke W: The intensive care of the stroke patient. In Barnett HJ, Mohr JP, Stein BM, editors: Stroke: pathophysiology, diagnosis and management, ed 3, New York, 1998, Churchill Livingstone; and Sacco RL, Adams R, Albers G, et al: Guidelines for prevention of stroke in patients with ischemic stroke or transient ischemic attack: a statement for healthcare professionals from the American Heart Association/American Stroke Association Council on Stroke: co-sponsored by the Council on Cardiovascular Radiology and Intervention: the American Academy of Neurology affirms the value of this guideline. Stroke 37:577–617, 2006.

aspirin started within 48 hours of stroke results in a 1% absolute reduction in risk of stroke and death over the first 2 weeks after stroke.[128] Early aspirin therapy is therefore recommended within 48 hours of the onset of symptoms, but should be delayed for at least 24 hours after rtPA administration. Aspirin should not be considered as an alternative to IV thrombolysis or other therapies aimed at improving outcomes after stroke.[9]

Other antiplatelet agents were evaluated for use in the acute phase of ischemic stroke. The platelet glycoprotein (GP) IIb/IIIa inhibitors were evaluated in the treatment of AIS because they may increase the rate of spontaneous recanalization and improve microvascular patency.[129,130] In a preliminary pilot study, abciximab was given within 6 hours to establish a safety profile. A trend toward improved outcome at 3 months for the treatment versus the placebo group was noted.[131] Treatment with abciximab showed a nonsignificant shift in favorable outcome as defined by mRS scores at 3 months, after adjustment for baseline severity of stroke, age, and interval from stroke.[131,132] The Abciximab in Emergent Stroke Treatment Trial (AbESTT) was a randomized double-blinded placebo-controlled phase IIb study that involved 400 patients with AIS who were treated 3 to 6 hours after symptom onset.[133] Results demonstrated significant improvements in outcomes of abciximab-treated patients, measured by mRS, Barthel Index, and NIHSS.[134] A subsequent phase III trial evaluating the safety and efficacy of abciximab in patients with AIS was halted because of an increased rate of bleeding and lack of efficacy.[133]

The use of ticlopidine, clopidogrel, or dipyridamole in the setting of AIS has not been evaluated.[135] Dipyridamole treatment following ischemic stroke or TIA was evaluated in 46 stroke units in Germany.[136] Patients presenting with an NIHSS score of 20 or below were randomly assigned to receive aspirin 25 mg plus extended-release dipyridamole 200 mg twice daily (early dipyridamole regimen) (n = 283), or aspirin monotherapy (100 mg once daily) for 7 days (n = 260). Therapy in either group was initiated within 24 hours of stroke onset. After 2 weeks, all patients received aspirin plus dipyridamole for up to 90 days. At day 90, 154 (56%) patients in the early dipyridamole group and 133 (52%) in the aspirin plus later dipyridamole group had no or mild disability (P = 0.45). The authors concluded that early initiation of aspirin plus extended-release dipyridamole is likely to be as safe and effective in preventing disability as later initiation after 7 days following stroke onset. Further clinical trials are necessary. For secondary stroke prevention, aspirin, clopidogrel, and extended-release dipyridamole/aspirin have all shown efficacy and are recommended by treatment guidelines.

Viscosity and Hemodilution

Acute ischemic stroke patients have a variety of abnormalities that may increase blood viscosity.[108–110] Accordingly, hemodilution could improve CBF to hyperperfuse potentially viable brain tissue supplied by leptomeningeal collaterals in an attempt to salvage the ischemic penumbra.[9,137–140] In all trials, and in the Multicenter Austrian Hemodilution Stroke Trial study in particular, hemodilution did not significantly reduce deaths within the first 4 weeks but did influence deaths within 3 to 6 months.[141] Hemodilution also had no significant influence on death, dependency, or institutionalization/long-term care. In several trials, hemodilution was associated with a tendency toward reduction in deep venous thrombosis (DVT) and pulmonary embolism (PE) at 3 to 6 months. Despite volume expansion and hemodilution, the risk of significant cardiac events did not increase.[9] Maintenance of a normal circulating blood volume with regulation of metabolic parameters within physiological ranges is desirable.[9]

Secondary Prevention of Ischemic Stroke

Secondary stroke prevention includes measures that prevent stroke in patients with TIAs and treatments that prevent recurrent stroke in patients who have had an ischemic stroke. A TIA

is defined as a transient episode of neurological dysfunction caused by focal ischemia, initially lasting up to 24 hours but now modified to 1 hour in duration.[142] The overall risk for stroke after a TIA is approximately 10% over the subsequent 90 days, with the greatest risk within the first week after the event.[143] Patients with a transient focal neurological deficit lasting less than 24 hours who have an ischemic lesion on DWI have higher risk for subsequent stroke than those who do not have this MRI abnormality, especially if they have evidence of vessel narrowing on MRA.[144] This substantial stroke risk with TIA is why TIA should be considered a medical emergency and requires urgent evaluation and treatment.[145] The history, physical, and laboratory examinations should help exclude less frequent causes of transient focal neurological symptoms, such as pressure-related or positionally related peripheral nerve or nerve root compression, peripheral vestibulopathy, and metabolic abnormalities (also see Chapter 30). The initial evaluation should also exclude other possible causes of focal neurological symptoms such as seizures, migraine auras, and syncope.[146]

Patients who have had a TIA should have an evaluation that includes basic blood work studies (e.g., electrolytes, glucose, complete blood cell count [CBC]), an electrocardiogram, brain imaging, and neurovascular imaging. Brain imaging can be performed with either CT or MRI scans, although the latter is preferable because DWI can detect abnormalities not seen on CT scans that can predict a higher risk of subsequent stroke. In the past, carotid ultrasound was the initial study employed to evaluate the carotid arteries. Currently, both CT and contrast-enhanced MRA have distinct advantages over carotid ultrasound. Both of these imaging modalities can accurately image the vessels in the neck and brain, providing information about the status of the vessels in both locations, as well as the presence of an occult aneurysm or vascular malformation. The accuracy of both CT and contrast-enhanced MRA allow for their use in planning a procedure such as carotid endarterectomy (CEA) or stenting. In rare cases, digital subtraction angiography (DSA) may be needed. If a cardiac source for the TIA is a consideration, echocardiography and electrocardiographic monitoring should be performed.

Treatment decisions should be made rapidly in TIA patients after information from the workup has been obtained. Evaluation and treatment of TIA patients can be performed in the hospital or an urgent-access outpatient clinic. Urgent-access TIA evaluation clinics were shown to substantially reduce the incidence of subsequent stroke, and highlight the appropriateness of considering TIA a medical emergency.[147] The basic consideration for deciding upon the treatment for a TIA patient is whether a procedure such as CEA or carotid stenting is appropriate, or whether the patient should be treated with medical therapy alone (also see Chapters 32 and 33). Carotid artery procedures are not appropriate for patients with TIA symptoms in the posterior circulation; such patients should receive appropriate medical therapy. For patients with anterior circulation TIA symptoms, the degree of carotid stenosis is the primary factor for deciding whether a procedure is needed. For symptomatic patients with greater than 70% stenosis of the proximal internal carotid artery (ICA), the North American Symptomatic Carotid Endarterectomy Trial (NASCET) demonstrated clear evidence that CEA was superior to medical therapy, and this procedure is recommended for most such patients.[148] For patients with 50% to 70% carotid artery stenosis, an extension of this trial demonstrated significant benefit of CEA for men but not for women overall, likely related to the lower subsequent stroke risk in women.[149] In women with 50% to 70% stenosis and a TIA, high-risk subgroups were shown to have significant benefit. Patients with less than 50% stenosis were not shown to benefit from CEA. In the NASCET trial, the degree of carotid artery stenosis was confirmed by DSA. Currently, this invasive procedure is performed infrequently, and decisions about the percent stenosis can be reliably made by computed tomographic angiography (CTA) or contrast MRA.

Another procedure for treating carotid artery stenosis is carotid stenting. The benefits and side effects of carotid artery stenting and CEA were compared directly in the Carotid Revascularization Endarterectomy versus Stenting Trial (CREST). No significant difference between the two procedures on the primary outcome measure of stroke, death, or nonfatal MI was observed.[150] However, the risk of periprocedural stroke was significantly lower in the CEA group, and the risk of MI was significantly lower in the stenting group. A relationship between age and the effects of treatment was observed, with patients younger than 65 years of age benefiting more from stenting, and those older than 65 doing better with CEA. The CREST trial included more asymptomatic patients with carotid stenosis than TIA patients, so generalizing the results to TIA patients is problematic. In choosing which procedure to recommend to patients, the clinician must be aware of complication rates of the operators who will be doing the procedure. It is our practice to recommend CEA to most patients and to reserve the use of stenting for high-risk patients, such as those with radiation-induced stenosis and after a failed prior CEA.

Risk factor modification and antiplatelet therapy for patients who have had a TIA or ischemic stroke is indicated. Underlying risk factors should be managed as in poststroke patients. Patients should be started on an antiplatelet agent; choices include aspirin, clopidogrel, or extended-release dipyridamole/low-dose aspirin. Low-dose aspirin (50-81 mg) is usually recommended as the initial approach. In patients who have a TIA on aspirin, one of the other antiplatelet drugs may be substituted, or they may be used initially in high-risk patients with multiple vascular risk factors. The combination of extended-release dipyridamole/low-dose aspirin was shown to be superior to aspirin in two large clinical trials, but when this combination was compared to clopidogrel, no significant difference in subsequent stroke outcome was observed.[151,152] The combination therapy group had a significantly greater risk for major bleeding side effects and drug discontinuation because of headaches. In addition, patients should be treated with statins to reduce low-density lipoprotein (LDL) cholesterol.[116,153,154]

The effect of risk factor modification in asymptomatic carotid disease has yet to be studied directly. The AHA/American Stroke Association guidelines for primary prevention of stroke suggest aggressive risk factor modification, as recommended for coronary heart disease (CHD), CHD risk equivalents, and diabetes mellitus.[155]

Antihypertensive therapy is also indicated to prevent recurrent stroke. A meta-analysis of 15,257 patients with previous stroke or TIA demonstrated that antihypertensive therapy with a variety of agents (β-adrenergic blockers, diuretics, angiotensin-converting enzyme [ACE] inhibitors) resulted in a 24% reduction in recurrent stroke.[156] In the Morbidity and Mortality After Stroke, Eprosartan Compared with Nitrendipine for Secondary Prevention (MOSES) study, 1405 subjects with a stroke or TIA and hypertension were randomized to the angiotensin receptor blocker (ARB) eprosartan, or the calcium channel blocker nitrendipine. Despite similar reductions in blood pressure, total strokes and TIAs were reduced by 25% among those randomized to eprosartan. It should be noted that the reduction in TIAs accounted for most of the cerebrovascular benefit, with no significant difference in ischemic strokes noted.[157] In the Perindopril Protection Against Recurrent Stroke (PROGRESS) Study of 6105 subjects with a history of stroke or TIA, those randomized to perindopril had a significant reduction in recurrent stroke.[158] In this trial, the thiazide diuretic indapamide could be used at the discretion of the treating physician. Patients treated with the combination of perindopril and indapamide had the greatest stroke reduction (43%). Interestingly, in the Prevention Regimen for Effectively Avoiding Second Strokes (PRoFESS) study of 20,332 patients with ischemic stroke, telmisartan did not significantly reduce the rate of stroke compared to placebo.[159] The negative findings have been ascribed to aggressive antihypertensive management in the placebo group and a minimal difference in blood pressure between groups.

Until the advent of the statin era, the impact of lipids on cerebrovascular disease was described as modest, with reductions in ischemic stroke offset by increases in hemorrhagic stroke with decreasing levels of LDL. In the Stroke Prevention by Aggressive Reduction in Cholesterol Levels (SPARCL) study, 4731 patients with stroke or TIA and LDL-C levels between 100 and 190 mg/dL were randomized to atorvastatin 80 mg or placebo.[160] Over 5 years of follow-up, there was a 16% risk reduction of recurrent stroke. The trial was positive, despite only a 78% adherence to trial-allocated therapies by the end of the trial. In a post hoc analysis of SPARCL, patients with the greatest reduction in LDL also enjoyed the most impressive stroke reduction.[153] Patients with a 50% or greater reduction in LDL saw a 31% reduction in stroke risk and a 33% decrease in ischemic stroke.

Primary Prevention of Ischemic Stroke

The management of patients with asymptomatic carotid stenosis is somewhat controversial. Two large earlier randomized trials that compared CEA to medical therapy in patients with more than 60% stenosis demonstrated a significant reduction in stroke occurrence with CEA. The absolute risk reduction was only about 1% per year.[161,162] With the improvement in medical management of patients with asymptomatic carotid stenosis, it has been suggested that in many cases the previously confirmed benefit for CEA may no longer be applicable.[163] It may be possible to identify higher- and lower-risk asymptomatic carotid stenosis patients based on a more sophisticated ultrasound evaluation of plaque characteristics and/or the detection of intracranial emboli on a transcranial Doppler (TCD) ultrasound study.[164] Based on results of the CREST trial, both CEA and carotid stenting could be considered if a procedure is deemed appropriate for an individual patient. The acceptable rate of periprocedural complications in asymptomatic patients undergoing a procedure is lower than for symptomatic patients because of the lower stroke risk in asymptomatic patients.

Management of Primary Intracerebral Hemorrhage

Extravasation of blood into the brain occurs when blood vessels within the parenchyma rupture, leading to the development of ICH. Intracerebral hemorrhage can also occur with use of oral or IV anticoagulants and is then termed *secondary to anticoagulant use*, although in many cases, blood vessel rupture is also the likely cause. Intracerebral hemorrhage accounts for 10% to 15% of the acute cerebrovascular events and is more common among Asians, African Americans, and Latin Americans than the U.S. Caucasian population.[165] The pathophysiology of tissue injury is distinctly different than observed with ischemic stroke. The developing hematoma causes local cellular injury by direct mechanical effects, but may also secondarily induce cellular injury by local effects on CBF, edema development, mitochondrial dysfunction, and neurotransmitter release.[166] It is now well established that the majority of ICH patients experience hematoma enlargement during the first few hours after onset, and that ICH growth is associated with a poorer prognosis[167] (Fig. 31-4). Modern imaging with MRI or CT can readily identify the presence of ICH and distinguish this condition from ischemic stroke.[168] In most ICH cases, either catheter angiography or MRA/CTA should be performed to look for the presence of an underlying arteriovenous malformation (AVM), aneurysm, or dural venous thrombosis.

Initial management of ICH includes airway assessment, blood pressure control, and treatment of elevated ICP if present. ICH patients with moderate to severe deficits should be managed in an intensive care unit (ICU) or specialized stroke care unit. Patients with respiratory compromise or at high risk for aspiration will require intubation, and intubated patients

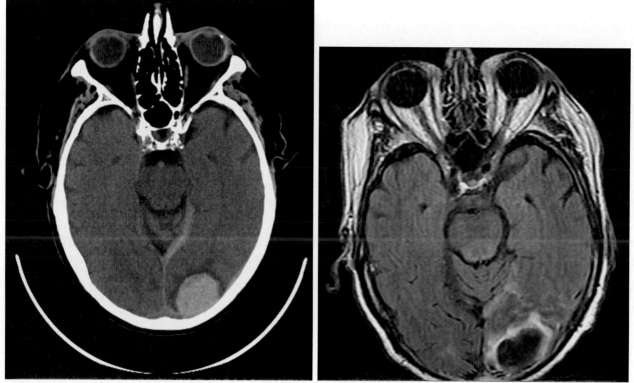

FIGURE 31-4 *Left,* **Acute intracerebral hemorrhage (ICH) in left occipital lobe on computed tomography (CT) scan.** *Right,* Same hemorrhage on T1-weighted magnetic resonance imaging (MRI). *(Courtesy Dr. Magdy Selim.)*

can more easily undergo induced hyperventilation, which may be useful in reducing elevated ICP.[169] Hyperventilation can rapidly reduce elevated ICP but may also reduce CBF, potentially exacerbating perihematomal injury. Many ICH patients have elevated blood pressure initially, and this may be a factor associated with hematoma expansion. The precise blood pressure target in ICH patients remains uncertain, but a 15% lowering of mean arterial pressure or a target of less than 160/90 mmHg may be reasonable based on recent guidelines. Many antihypertensive agents are used[169] (see Table 31-5). A recent modestly sized blood pressure–lowering trial suggested that aggressive treatment may be beneficial in reducing hematoma expansion but did not affect clinical outcome.[170] The optimal approach for treating elevated ICP in ICH patients remains contentious. The osmotic agent mannitol is widely used in ICH patients, but clear evidence of efficacy remains lacking.[171] Mannitol may induce hypovolemia and a hyperosmotic state, so when it is used, serum osmolality should be monitored regularly and maintained in the range of 300 to 320 mOsm/kg. Dexamethasone should be avoided because a trial demonstrated an increased risk of infection.[172] If the ICH patient is febrile, temperature should be lowered with parenteral acetaminophen to normothermia. It is unclear whether induction of hypothermia is beneficial. If clinical seizures occur, an anticonvulsant should be initiated, but anticonvulsant prophylaxis should probably be avoided.[169] Most ICH patients will be immobilized for a period of time and are at risk for developing DVT and PE. Intermittent pneumatic compression should be initiated at admission, and subcutaneous LMWH or UFH may be started several days later if the patient remains immobilized.[173] Gastric ulceration is common in ICH patients, and the prophylactic initiation of H2 blockers is warranted.

Approximately 20% of ICH patients are receiving an oral anticoagulant at the time of onset, and this cause of ICH is associated with a poorer prognosis than patients who are not receiving such treatment.[174] Early reversal of the anticoagulant effect should be initiated, and several options are available. The standard approach to oral anticoagulation–related ICH is to give IV vitamin K and fresh frozen plasma. This treatment approach may take a long time to reverse the anticoagulant effect, and the large fluid load associated with the use of fresh frozen plasma may be problematic. Two newer approaches to the reversal of oral anticoagulation are prothrombin complex concentrate and recombinant activated factor VII (rFVIIa). Both of these approaches can reverse the effects of oral anticoagulation more rapidly than vitamin K/fresh frozen plasma and appear to also reduce the rate of hematoma expansion but may be associated with an increased risk for thromboembolic events.[175–177]

No specific therapy directed at the underlying pathophysiology of ICH-induced injury is available. Since the appreciation of the role of hematoma expansion as a predictor of worse outcome, treatment directed at reducing this mechanism of injury was proposed. Recombinant FVIIa in nonanticoagulated ICH patients was tested in two clinical trials. In the phase II trial, three doses of rFVIIa (40, 80, or 160 μg/kg) or vehicle were given to ICH patients within 3 hours of onset.[178] Hematoma expansion was reduced, as was mortality with rFVIIa. In a phase III trial that used 20 or 80 μg/kg of rFVIIa compared to vehicle.[179] Hematoma expansion was again reduced with both rFVIIa doses, but no clinical benefit was observed. The 80 μg/kg dose had an increased risk of thrombotic events when compared to vehicle. A subsequent subgroup analysis suggested that patients younger than 70 with smaller ICH volumes may benefit.

Surgical evacuation of the hematoma has an inherent appeal for the treatment of ICH, but aside from cerebellar hemorrhages, remains of unproven value.[180] Many randomized trials comparing surgical evacuation of ICH to medical therapy were performed and failed to show benefit. Current treatment guidelines do not recommend routine surgical evacuation of the hematoma, but it should be considered early after onset for patients with lobar hemorrhages close to the surface who are in good neurological condition.[180] Early surgical evacuation is recommended for larger cerebellar hemorrhages, especially if neurological deterioration occurs or hydrocephalus is developing.

REFERENCES

1. Hossman KA: Pathophysiology and therapy of experimental stroke, *Cell Mol Neurobiol* 26:1055–1081, 2006.
2. Baron J: Mapping the ischaemic penumbra with PET: implications for acute stroke treatment, *Cerebrovasc Dis* 9:193–201, 1999.
3. Fisher M: The ischemic penumbra: a new opportunity for neuroprotection, *Cerebrovasc Dis* 21(Suppl 2):64–70, 2006.
4. Heiss W: Ischemic penumbra: evidence from functional imaging in man, *J Cereb Blood Flow Metab* 20:1276–1293, 2000.
5. Fisher M: Characterizing the target of acute stroke treatment, *Stroke* 28:866–872, 1997.
6. Bang OY, Saver JL, Buck BH, et al, UCLA Collateral Investigators: Impact of collateral flow on tissue fate in acute ischaemic stroke, *J Neurol Neurosurg Psychiatry* 79:625–629, 2008.
7. Martini SR, Kent TA: Hyperglycemia in acute ischemic stroke: a vascular perspective, *J Cereb Blood Flow Metab* 27:435–451, 2007.
8. Ntaios G, Bath P, Michel P: Blood pressure treatment in acute ischemic stroke: a review of studies and recommendations, *Curr Opin Neurol* 23:46–52, 2010.
9. Adams HP Jr, del Zoppo G, Alberts MJ, et al: Guidelines for the early management of adults with ischemic stroke: a guideline from the American Heart Association/American Stroke Association Stroke Council, Clinical Cardiology Council, Cardiovascular Radiology and Intervention Council, and the Atherosclerotic Peripheral Vascular Disease and Quality of Care Outcomes in Research Interdisciplinary Working Groups: the American Academy of Neurology affirms the value of this guideline as an educational tool for neurologists, *Stroke* 38:1655–1711, 2007.
10. Handschu R, Poppe R, Rauss J, et al: Emergency calls in acute stroke, *Stroke* 34:1005–1009, 2003.
11. Williams JE, Rosamond WD, Morris DL: Stroke symptom attribution and time to emergency department arrival: the delay in accessing stroke healthcare study, *Acad Emerg Med* 7:93–96, 2000.
12. Zweifler RM, Mendizabal JE, Cunningham S, et al: Hospital presentation after stroke in a community sample: the Mobile Stroke Project, *South Med J* 95:1263–1268, 2002.
13. Lacy CR, Suh DC, Bueno M, et al: Delay in presentation and evaluation for acute stroke: Stroke Time Registry for Outcomes Knowledge and Epidemiology (S.T.R.O.K.E.), *Stroke* 32:63–69, 2001.
14. De Luca A, Toni D, Lauria L, et al: An emergency clinical pathway for stroke patients – results of a cluster randomised trial (isrctn41456865) and the "IMPLementazione percorso clinico assistenziale ICtus Acuto (IMPLICA) study group, *BMC Health Serv Res* 9:14, 2009. http://www.biomedcentral.com/1472-6963/9/14.
15. Schroeder EB, Rosamond WD, Morris DL, et al: Determinants of use of emergency medical services in a population with stroke symptoms: the Second Delay in Accessing Stroke Healthcare (DASH II) Study, *Stroke* 31:2591–2596, 2000.
16. Morris DL, Rosamond WD, Hinn AR, et al: Time delays in accessing stroke care in the emergency department, *Acad Emerg Med* 6:218–223, 1999.
17. Menon SC, Pandey DK, Morgenstern LB: Critical factors determining access to acute stroke care, *Neurology* 51:427–432, 1998.
18. Barsan WG, Brott TG, Broderick JP, et al: Time of hospital presentation in patients with acute stroke, *Arch Intern Med* 153:2558–2561, 1993.
19. Wester P, Radberg J, Lundgren B, et al, Seek-Medical-Attention-in-Time Study Group: Factors associated with delayed admission to hospital and in-hospital delays in acute stroke and TIA: a prospective, multicenter study, *Stroke* 30:40–48, 1999.
20. American Heart Association Guidelines for Cardiopulmonary Resuscitation and Emergency Cardiovascular Care, *Circulation* 112(Suppl I):IV-1–IV-203, 2005.
21. Schwamm L, Fayad P, Acker JE 3rd, et al: Translating evidence into practice: a decade of efforts by the American Heart Association/American Stroke Association to reduce death and disability due to stroke: a presidential advisory from the American Heart Association/American Stroke Association, *Stroke* 41:1051–1065, 2010.
22. Lindsay P, Bayley M, Hellings C, et al (Canadian Stroke Strategy Best Practices and Standards Writing Group, on behalf of the Canadian Stroke Strategy, a joint initiative of the Canadian Stroke Network and the Heart and Stroke Foundation of Canada*): Canadian best practice recommendations for stroke care (updated 2008), *CMAJ* 179(12 Suppl):S1–S25, 2008.
23. Morgenstern LB, Bartholomew LK, Grotta JC, et al: Sustained benefit of a community and professional intervention to increase acute stroke therapy, *Arch Intern Med* 163:2198–2202, 2003.
24. Morgenstern LB, Staub L, Chan W, et al: Improving delivery of acute stroke therapy: the TLL Temple Foundation Stroke Project, *Stroke* 33:160–166, 2002.
25. Evenson KR, Foraker R, Morris DL, et al: A comprehensive review of prehospital and in-hospital delay times in acute stroke care, *Int J Stroke* 4:187–199, 2009.
26. Becker JU, Wira CR, Arnold JL: Stroke, ischemic. eMedicine Specialties > Emergency Medicine >, *Neurology* June 4 2010. http://emedicine.medscape.com/article/793904-overview.
27. Krieger D, Hacke W: The intensive care of the stroke patient. In Barnett HJ, Mohr JP, Stein BM, editors: *Stroke: pathophysiology, diagnosis and management*, ed 3, New York, 1998, Churchill Livingstone.
28. SPORTIF Executive Steering Committee for the SPORTIF V Investigators: Ximelagatran vs. warfarin for stroke prevention in patients with nonvalvular atrial fibrillation: a randomized trial, *JAMA* 293:690–698, 2005.
29. Oppenheimer SM, Hachinski VC: The cardiac consequences of stroke, *Neurol Clin* 10(1):167–176, 1992.
30. Kolin A, Norris JW: Myocardial damage from acute cerebral lesions, *Stroke* 15:990–993, 1984.
31. Milhaud D, Popp J, Thouvenot E, et al: Mechanical ventilation in ischemic stroke, *J Stroke Cerebrovasc Dis* 13:183–188, 2004.
32. Treib J, Grauer MT, Woessner R, et al: Treatment of stroke on an intensive stroke unit: a novel concept, *Intensive Care Med* 26:1598–1611, 2000.
33. The NINDS rt-PA Stroke Study Group: Tissue plasminogen activator for acute ischemic stroke. The National Institute of Neurological Disorders and Stroke rt-PA Stroke Study Group, *N Engl J Med* 333:1581–1587, 1995.
34. The National Institute of Neurological Disorders and Stroke rt-PA Stroke Study Group: Generalized efficacy of t-PA for acute stroke: subgroup analysis of the NINDS t-PA Stroke Trial, *Stroke* 28:2119–2125, 1997.
35. Hacke W, Kaste M, Fieschi C, et al: Intravenous thrombolysis with recombinant tissue plasminogen activator for acute hemispheric stroke. The European Cooperative Acute Stroke Study (ECASS), *JAMA* 274:1017–1025, 1995.
36. Hacke W, Kaste M, Fieschi C, et al: Randomised double-blind placebo-controlled trial of thrombolytic therapy with intravenous alteplase in acute ischaemic stroke (ECASS II). Second European-Australasian Acute Stroke Study Investigators, *Lancet* 352:1245–1251, 1998.
37. Clark WM, Wissman S, Albers GW, et al: Recombinant tissue type plasminogen activator (alteplase) for ischemic stroke 3 to 5 hours after symptom onset. The ATLANTIS Study: a randomized controlled trial, Alteplase Thrombolysis for Acute Noninterventional Therapy in Ischemic Stroke, *JAMA* 282:2019–2026, 1999.
38. Hacke W, Donnan G, Fieschi C, et al: Association of outcome with early stroke treatment: pooled analysis of ATLANTIS, ECASS, and NINDS rt-PA stroke trials, *Lancet* 363:768–774, 2004.
39. Hacke W, Kaste M, Bluhrnki E, et al: Thrombolysis with alteplase 3 to 4.5 hours after acute ischemic stroke, *N Engl J Med* 359:1317–1329, 2008.
40. Del Zoppo GJ, Saver JL, Jauch EC, et al, on behalf of the American Heart Association Stroke Council: Expansion of the time window for treatment of acute ischemic stroke with intravenous tissue plasminogen activator. A science advisory from the American Heart Association/American Stroke Association, *Stroke* 40:2945–2948, 2009.
41. Bluhmki E, Chamorro A, Dávalos A, et al: Stroke treatment with alteplase given 3.0–4.5 h after onset of ischaemic stroke (ECASS III): additional outcomes and subgroup analysis of a randomised controlled trial, *Lancet Neurol* 8:1095–1102, 2009.
42. Furlan A, Higashida R, Wechsler L, et al: Intra-arterial prourokinase for acute ischemic stroke. The PROACT II study: a randomized controlled trial. Prolyse in acute cerebral thromboembolism, *JAMA* 282:2003–2011, 1999.
43. IMS Study Investigators: Combined intravenous and intra-arterial recanalization for acute ischemic stroke: the Interventional Management of Stroke Study, *Stroke* 35:904–911, 2004.
44. The IMS II Trial Investigators: The Interventional Management of Stroke (IMS) Study, *Stroke* 38:2127–2135, 2007.
45. Ogawa A, Mori E, Minematsu K, et al: Randomized trial of intraarterial infusion of urokinase within 6 hours of middle cerebral artery stroke, *Stroke* 38:2633–2639, 2007.
46. Mandava P, Kent TA: Intra-arterial therapies for acute ischemic stroke, *Neurology* 68:2132–2139, 2007.
47. Smith WS, Sung G, Starkman S, et al: Safety and efficacy of mechanical embolectomy in acute ischemic stroke: results of the MERCI trial, *Stroke* 36:1432–1440, 2005.
48. Smith WS, Sung G, Saver J, et al: Mechanical thrombectomy for acute ischemic stroke: final results of the Multi MERCI trial, *Stroke* 39:1205–1211, 2008.
49. The Penumbra Pivotal Stroke Trial Investigators: The penumbra pivotal stroke trial: safety and effectiveness of a new generation of mechanical devices for clot removal in intracranial large vessel occlusion, *Stroke* 2661–2666, 2009.
50. Indredavik B, Bakke F, Slordahl SA, et al: Treatment in a combined acute and rehabilitation stroke unit: which aspects are most important? *Stroke* 30:917–923, 1999.
51. Gilligan AK, Thrift AG, Sturm JW, et al: Stroke units, tissue plasminogen activator, aspirin and neuroprotection: which stroke intervention could provide the greatest community benefit? *Cerebrovasc Dis* 20:239–244, 2005.
52. Cadilhac DA, Ibrahim J, Pearce DC, et al: Multicenter comparison of processes of care between stroke units and conventional care wards in Australia, *Stroke* 35:1035–1040, 2004.
53. Schwamm LH, Foranow GC, Reeves MJ, et al: Get with the guidelines-stroke is associated with sustained improvement in care for patients with stroke or transient ischemic attack, *Circulation* 119:107–115, 2009.
54. Schabitz WR, Fisher M: Perspectives on neuroprotective stroke therapy, *Biochem Soc Trans* 34:1271–1276, 2006.
55. Donnan GA: A new road map for neuroprotection, *Stroke* 39:242–248, 2008.
56. O'Collins VE, Macleod MR, Donnan GA, et al: 1,026 experimental treatments in acute stroke, *Ann Neurol* 59:467–477, 2006.
57. Gladstone DJ, Black SE, Hakim AM: Toward wisdom from failure: lessons from neuroprotective stroke trials and new directions, *Stroke* 33:2123–2136, 2002.
58. Henninger N, Bratane BT, Bastan B, et al: Normobaric hyperoxia and late tPA in a rat embolic stroke model, *J Cereb Blood Flow Metab* 29:119–129, 2009.
59. Bratane B, Bouley J, Schneider A, et al: Granulocyte colony stimulating factor delays mismatch evolution and reduces final infarct volume in permanent suture and embolic rat focal cerebral ischemia models, *Stroke* 40:3102–3106, 2009.
60. Warach SW, Latour LL: Evidence of reperfusion injury, exacerbated by thrombolytic therapy, in human focal brain ischemia using a novel imaging marker of early blood–brain barrier disruption, *Stroke* 35:2559–2661, 2004.
61. Fisher M: New approaches to neuroprotective drug development, *Stroke* 42:S24–S27, 2012.
62. Duong TQ, Fisher M: Applications of diffusion/perfusion MRI in experimental and clinical aspects of stroke, *Curr Atheroscler Rep* 6:257–263, 2004.
63. Pepper EM, Parsons MW, Bateman GA, et al: CT perfusion source images improve identification of early ischaemic change in hyperacute stroke, *J Clin Neurosci* 13:199–205, 2006.
64. Detre J, Duong T: Magnetic resonance imaging of ischemic penumbra: new techniques: c. arterial spin labeling. In Donnan G, et al, editors: *The ischemic penumbra*, New York, 2007, Taylor & Francis Inc, pp 234–240.
65. Kane I, Carpenter T, Chappell F, et al: Comparison of 10 different magnetic resonance perfusion imaging processing methods in acute ischemic stroke, *Stroke* 38:3158–3164, 2007.
66. Butcher KS, Parsons M, MacGregor L, et al: Refining the perfusion-diffusion mismatch hypothesis, *Stroke* 36:1153–1159, 2005.
67. Schellinger PD, Gotz T, Fiehler J, et al: MRI and CT-based thrombolytic therapy in acute stroke within and beyond established time windows, *Stroke* 38:2640–2645, 2007.
68. Albers GW, Thijs VN, Wechsler L, et al: Magnetic resonance imaging profiles predict clinical response to early reperfusion: the diffusion and perfusion imaging evaluation for understanding stroke evolution (DEFUSE) study, *Ann Neurol* 60:508–517, 2006.
69. Davis SM, Donnan GA, Parsons MW, et al: Effects of alteplase beyond 3h after stroke onset in the Echoplanar Imaging Thrombolytic Evaluation Trial (EPITHET): a placebo-controlled randomized trial, *Lancet Neurol* 7:299–399, 2008.

70. Hacke W, Albers GW, Al-Rawi Y, et al: The desmoteplase in acute ischemic stroke trial (DIAS): a phase II MRI-based 9-hour window acute stroke thrombolysis trial with intravenous desmoteplase, *Stroke* 36:66–73, 2005.
71. Furlan AJ, Eyding D, Albers GW, et al: Escalation of Desmoteplase for Acute Ischemic Stroke (DEDAS): evidence of safety and efficacy 3 to 9 hours after stroke onset, *Stroke* 37:1227–1231, 2006.
72. Hacke W, Furlan AJ, Al-Rawi Y, et al: Intravenous desmoteplase in patients with acute ischaemic stroke selected by MRI perfusion-diffusion weighted imaging or perfusion CT (DIAS-2): a prospective, randomized, double-blind, placebo controlled study, *Lancet Neurol* 8:141–150, 2009.
73. Williams LS, Rotich J, Qi R, et al: Effects of admission hyperglycemia on mortality and costs in acute ischemic stroke, *Neurology* 59:67–71, 2002.
74. Scott JF, Robinson GM, French JM, et al: Prevalence of admission hyperglycaemia across clinical subtypes of acute stroke, *Lancet* 353:376–377, 1999.
75. Baird TA, Parsons MW, Barber PA, et al: The influence of diabetes mellitus and hyperglycaemia on stroke incidence and outcome, *J Clin Neurosci* 9:618–626, 2002.
76. Baird TA, Parsons MW, Phanh T, et al: Persistent poststroke hyperglycemia is independently associated with infarct expansion and worse clinical outcome, *Stroke* 34:2208–2214, 2003.
77. Bruno A, Levine SR, Frankel MR, et al, NINDS rt-PA Stroke Study Group: Admission glucose level and clinical outcomes in the NINDS rt-PA Stroke Trial, *Neurology* 59:669–674, 2002.
78. Bruno A, Biller J, Adams HP Jr, et al, Trial of ORG 10172 in Acute Stroke Treatment (TOAST) Investigators: Acute blood glucose level and outcome from ischemic stroke, *Neurology* 52:280–284, 1999.
79. Toni D, Chamorro A, Kaste M, et al, EUSI Executive Committee, EUSI Writing Committee: Acute treatment of ischaemic stroke. European Stroke Initiative, *Cerebrovasc Dis* 17(Suppl 2):30–46, 2004.
80. Bruno A, Kent TA, Coull BM, et al: Treatment of Hyperglycemia In Ischemic Stroke (THIS), a randomized pilot trial, *Stroke* 39:384–389, 2008.
81. Azzimondi G, Bassein L, Nonino F, et al: Fever in acute stroke worsens prognosis: a prospective study, *Stroke* 26:2040–2043, 1995.
82. Castillo J, Davalos A, Marrugat J, et al: Timing for fever-related brain damage in acute ischemic stroke, *Stroke* 29:2455–2460, 1998.
83. Ginsberg MD, Busto R: Combating hyperthermia in acute stroke: a significant clinical concern, *Stroke* 29:529–534, 1998.
84. Wang Y, Lim LL, Levi C, et al: Influence of admission body temperature on stroke mortality, *Stroke* 31:404–409, 2000.
85. Kammersgaard LP, Jorgensen HS, Rungby JA, et al: Admission body temperature predicts long-term mortality after acute stroke: the Copenhagen Stroke Study, *Stroke* 33: 1759–1762, 2002.
86. Alberts MJ, Hademenos G, Latchaw RE, et al, Brain Attack Coalition: Recommendations for the establishment of primary stroke centers, *JAMA* 283:3102–3109, 2000.
87. Marion DW: Controlled normothermia in neurologic intensive care, *Crit Care Med* 32(Suppl):S43–S45, 2004.
88. Olsen TS, Weber UJ, Kammersgaard LP: Therapeutic hypothermia for acute stroke, *Lancet Neurol* 2:410–416, 2003.
89. den Hertog HM, van der Worp HB, et al, PAIS Investigators: The Paracetamol (Acetaminophen) In Stroke (PAIS) trial: a multicentre, randomised, placebo-controlled, phase III trial, *Lancet Neurol* 8:434–440, 2009.
90. Hammer MD, Krieger DW: Hypothermia for acute ischemic stroke: not just another neuroprotectant, *Neurologist* 9:280–289, 2003.
91. Georgiadis D, Schwarz S, Kollmar R, et al: Endovascular cooling for moderate hypothermia in patients with acute stroke: first results of a novel approach, *Stroke* 32:2550–2553, 2001.
92. Krieger DW, De Georgia MA, Abou-Chebl A, et al: Cooling for Acute Ischemic Brain Damage (COOL AID): an open pilot study of induced hypothermia in acute ischemic stroke, *Stroke* 32:1847–1854, 2001.
93. Slotboom J, Kiefer C, Brekenfeld C, et al: Locally induced hypothermia for treatment of acute ischaemic stroke: a physical feasibility study, *Neuroradiology* 46:923–934, 2004.
94. Milhaud D, Thouvenot E, Heroum C, et al: Prolonged moderate hypothermia in massive hemispheric infarction: clinical experience, *J Neurosurg Anesthesiol* 17:49–53, 2005.
95. Correia M, Silva M, Veloso M: Cooling therapy for acute stroke, *Cochrane Database Syst Rev* (2):CD001247, 2000.
96. Paula WK: Heads down: flat positioning improves blood flow velocity in acute ischemic stroke, *Neurology* 65:1514, 2005.
97. Bardutzky J, Schwab S: Section Editor: Fisher M. Antiedema therapy in ischemic stroke, *Stroke* 38:3084–3094, 2007.
98. Gupta R, Connolly ES, Mayer S, et al: Hemicraniectomy for massive middle cerebral artery territory infarction: a systematic review, *Stroke* 35:539–543, 2004.
99. Vahedi K, Hofmeijer J, Juettler E, et al: Early decompressive surgery in malignant infarction of the middle cerebral artery: a pooled analysis of three randomised controlled trials, *Lancet Neurol* 6:215–222, 2007.
100. Juttler E, Schwab S, Schmiedek P, et al: Destiny. Decompressive surgery for the treatment of malignant infarction of the middle cerebral artery—outcome results [abstract], *Int J Stroke* 1:s38, 2006.
101. Vahedi K, Vicaut E, Mateau J, et al: Decimal trial: a sequential design, multicenter, randomized, controlled trial of decompressive craniectomy in malignant middle cerebral artery (MCA) infarction [abstract], *Int J Stroke* 1:s38, 2006.
102. Hofmeijer J, Amelink GJ, Algra A, et al: Hemicraniectomy after middle cerebral artery infarction with life-threatening edema trial (HAMLET). Protocol for a randomised controlled trial of decompressive surgery in space-occupying hemispheric infarction, *Trials* 7:29, 2006.
103. Kocan MJ: Cardiovascular effects of acute stroke, *Prog Cardiovasc Nurs* 14:61–67, 1999.
104. Britton M, de Faire U, Helmers C, et al: Arrhythmias in patients with acute cerebrovascular disease, *Acta Med Scand* 205:425–428, 1979.
105. Iadecola C, Davsson RL: Hypertension and cerebrovascular dysfunction, *Cell Metab* 7: 476–484, 2008.
106. Hacke W, Watkins C, Riesgo LGC, et al: *Improving patient management and outcomes in acute stroke: a coordinated approach.* Act Now Expert Report, Act Now, 2006, Boehringer Ingelheim.
107. Bath FJ, Bath P: What is the correct management of blood pressure in acute stroke: the Blood Pressure in Acute Stroke Collaboration, *Cerebrovasc Dis* 7:205–213, 1997.
108. Castillo J, Leira R, Garcia MM, et al: Blood pressure decrease during the acute phase of ischemic stroke is associated with brain injury and poor stroke outcome, *Stroke* 35: 520–526, 2004.
109. Johnston KC, Mayer SA: Blood pressure reduction in ischemic stroke: a two-edged sword? *Neurology* 61:1030–1031, 2003.
110. Kaplan NM: Management of hypertensive emergencies, *Lancet* 344:1335–1338, 1994.
111. Powers WJ: Acute hypertension after stroke: the scientific basis for treatment decisions, *Neurology* 43(pt 1):461–467, 1993.
112. Goldstein LB: Blood pressure management in patients with acute ischemic stroke, *Hypertension* 43:137–141, 2004.
113. Adams HP Jr, Brott TG, Furlan AJ, et al: Guidelines for thrombolytic therapy for acute stroke: a supplement to the guidelines for the management of patients with acute ischemic stroke. A statement for healthcare professionals from a Special Writing Group of the Stroke Council, American Heart Association, *Circulation* 94:1167–1174, 1996.
114. Phillips SJ: Pathophysiology and management of hypertension in acute ischemic stroke, *Hypertension* 23:131–136, 1994.
115. Leonardi-Bee J, Bath PM, Phillips SJ, et al, IST Collaborative Group: Blood pressure and clinical outcomes in the International Stroke Trial, *Stroke* 33:1315–1320, 2002.
116. Sacco RL, Adams R, Albers G, et al: Guidelines for prevention of stroke in patients with ischemic stroke or transient ischemic attack: a statement for healthcare professionals from the American Heart Association/American Stroke Association Council on Stroke: co-sponsored by the Council on Cardiovascular Radiology and Intervention: the American Academy of Neurology affirms the value of this guideline, *Stroke* 37:577–617, 2006.
117. Al-Sadat A, Sunbulli M, Chaturvedi S: Use of intravenous heparin by North American neurologists: do the data matter? *Stroke* 33:1574–1577, 2002.
118. Adams HP Jr: Emergency use of anticoagulation for treatment of patients with ischemic stroke, *Stroke* 33:856–861, 2002.
119. Caplan LR: Resolved: heparin may be useful in selected patients with brain ischemia, *Stroke* 34:230–231, 2003.
120. Donnan GA, Davis SM: Heparin in stroke: not for most, but the controversy lingers, *Stroke* 34:232–233, 2003.
121. Moonis M, Fisher M: Considering the role of heparin and low molecular-weight heparins in acute ischemic stroke, *Stroke* 33:1927–1933, 2002.
122. Sandercock P: Full heparin anticoagulation should not be used in acute ischemic stroke, *Stroke* 34:231–232, 2003.
123. Maegdefessel L, Spin JM, Azuma J, et al: New options with dabigatran etexilate in anticoagulant therapy, *Vasc Health Risk Manag* 6:339–349, 2010.
124. Martí-Fàbregas J, Mateo J: Old and new anticoagulant agents for the prevention and treatment of patients with ischemic stroke, *Cerebrovasc Dis* 27(Suppl 1):111–119, 2009.
125. Agnelli G, Eriksson BI, Cohen AT, et al, EXTEND Study Group: Safety assessment of new antithrombotic agents: lessons from the EXTEND study on ximelagatran, *Thromb Res* 123:488–497, 2009.
126. CAST: randomised placebo-controlled trial of early aspirin use in 20,000 patients with acute ischaemic stroke. CAST (Chinese Acute Stroke Trial) Collaborative Group, *Lancet* 349:1641–1649, 1997.
127. The International Stroke Trial (IST): a randomised trial of aspirin, subcutaneous heparin, both, or neither among 19435 patients with acute ischaemic stroke. International Stroke Trial Collaborative Group, *Lancet* 349:1569–1581, 1997.
128. Tan LB: Interpretation of IST and CAST stroke trials. International Stroke Trial. Chinese Acute Stroke Trial, *Lancet* 9:350, 443, 1997.
129. Lapchak PA, Araujo DM: Therapeutic potential of platelet glycoprotein IIb/IIIa receptor antagonists in the management of ischemic stroke, *Am J Cardiovasc Drugs* 3:87–94, 2003.
130. Janardhan V, Qureshi AI: Mechanisms of ischemic brain injury, *Curr Cardiol Rep* 6:117–123, 2004.
131. Abciximab in acute ischemic stroke: a randomized, double-blind, placebo-controlled, dose-escalation study. The Abciximab in Ischemic Stroke Investigators, *Stroke* 31:601–609, 2000.
132. Abciximab Emergent Stroke Treatment Trial Investigators: Emergency administration of abciximab for treatment of patients with acute ischemic stroke: results of a randomized phase 2 trial, *Stroke* 36:880–890, 2005.
133. Mitsias PD, Lu M, Morris D, et al: Treatment of acute supratentorial ischemic stroke with abciximab is safe and may result in early neurological improvement. A preliminary report, *Cerebrovasc Dis* 18:249–250, 2004.
134. Adams HP Jr, Leclerc JR, Bluhmki E, et al: Measuring outcomes as a function of baseline severity of ischemic stroke, *Cerebrovasc Dis* 18:124–129, 2004.
135. Albers GW, Amarenco P, Easton JD, et al: Antithrombotic and thrombolytic therapy for ischemic stroke: the Seventh ACCP Conference on Antithrombotic and Thrombolytic Therapy, *Chest* 126(Suppl):483S–512S, 2004.
136. Dengler R, Diener H-C, Schwartz A, et al: Early treatment with aspirin plus extended release dipyridamole for transient ischaemic attacks or ischaemic stroke with 24 h of symptom onset (EARLY trial), *Lancet Neurol* 9:159–166, 2010.
137. Belayev L, Busto R, Zhao W, et al: Effect of delayed albumin hemodilution on infarction volume and brain edema after transient middle cerebral artery occlusion in rats, *J Neurosurg* 87:595–601, 1997.
138. Belayev L, Liu Y, Zhao W, et al: Human albumin therapy of acute ischemic stroke: marked neuroprotective efficacy at moderate doses and with a broad therapeutic window, *Stroke* 32:553–560, 2001.
139. Belayev L, Pinard E, Nallet H, et al: Albumin therapy of transient focal cerebral ischemia: *in vivo* analysis of dynamic microvascular responses, *Stroke* 33:1077–1084, 2002.
140. Stocchetti N, Maas AI, Chieregato A, et al: Hyperventilation in head injury, *Chest* 127: 1812–1827, 2005.
141. Aichner FT, Fazekas F, Brainin M, et al: Hypervolemic hemodilution in acute ischemic stroke: the Multicenter Austrian Hemodilution Stroke Trial (MAHST), *Stroke* 29:743–749, 1998.
142. Easton JD, Saver JL, Albers GW, et al: Definition and evaluation of transient ischemic attack: a scientific statement for healthcare professionals from the American Heart

Association/American Stroke Association Stroke Council; Council on Cardiovascular Surgery and Anesthesia; Council on Cardiovascular Radiology and Intervention; Council on Cardiovascular Nursing; and Interdisciplinary Council on Peripheral Vascular Disease. The American Academy of Neurology affirms the value of this statement as an educational tool for neurologists, *Stroke* 40:2276, 2009.

143. Kleindorfer D, Panagos P, Pancioli A, et al: Incidence and short-term prognosis of transient ischemic attack in a population-based study, *Stroke* 36:720–723, 2005.

144. Mlynash M, Olivot JM, Tong DC, et al: Yield of combined perfusion and diffusion MR imaging in hemispheric TIA, *Neurology* 72:1127, 2009.

145. Donnan GA, Davis SM, Hill MD, et al: Patients with transient ischemic attack or minor stroke should be admitted to hospital, *Stroke* 37:1137, 2006.

146. Johnston SC, Nguyen-Huynh MN, Schwarz ME, et al: National Stroke Association guidelines for the management of transient ischemic attacks, *Ann Neurol* 60:301, 2006.

147. Rothwell PM, Giles MF, Chandratheva A, et al: Early use of Existing Preventive Strategies for Stroke (EXPRESS) study: effect of urgent treatment on transient ischaemic attack and minor stroke on early recurrent stroke, *Lancet* 370:1432–1442, 2007.

148. The North American Symptomatic Carotid Endarterectomy Trialist's Collaborative group: Beneficial effects of carotid endarterectomy in symptomatic patients with high-grade carotid stenosis, *N Engl J Med* 325:445–452, 1991.

149. Barnett HJM, Taylor DW, Eliasziw M, et al: Benefit of carotid endarterectomy in symptomatic patients with moderate and severe stenosis, *N Engl J Med* 339:1415–1425, 1998.

150. Brott TG, Hobson RW, Howard G, et al: Stenting versus endarterectomy for treatment of carotid stenosis, *N Engl J Med* 363:11–23, 2010.

151. Sacco RL, Diener CH, Yusuf S, et al: Aspirin and extended-release dipyridamole versus clopidogrel for recurrent stroke, *N Engl J Med* 359:1238–1251, 2008.

152. The ESPRIT Study Group: Medium intensity oral anticoagulation versus aspirin after cerebral ischaemia of arterial origin, *Lancet Neurol* 6:115–124, 2007.

153. Amarenco P, Goldstein LB, Szarek M, et al: Effects of intense low-density lipoprotein cholesterol reduction in patients with stroke or transient ischemic attack: the Stroke Prevention by Aggressive Reduction in Cholesterol Levels (SPARCL) trial, *Stroke* 38:3198–3204, 2007.

154. Amarenco P, Labreuche J: Lipid management in the prevention of stroke: review and updated meta-analysis of statins for stroke prevention, *Lancet Neurol* 8:453–463, 2009.

155. Goldstein LB, Bushnell CD, Adams RJ, et al: Guidelines for the primary prevention of stroke: a guideline for healthcare professionals from the American Heart Association/American Stroke Association, *Stroke* 42:517–584, 2011.

156. Rashid P, Leonardi-Bee J, Bath P: Blood pressure reduction and secondary prevention of stroke and other vascular events: a systematic review, *Stroke* 34:2741–2748, 2003.

157. Schrader J, Luders S, Kulschewski A, et al: Morbidity and Mortality After Stroke, Eprosartan Compared with Nitrendipine for Secondary Prevention: principal results of a prospective randomized controlled study (MOSES), *Stroke* 36:1218–1226, 2005.

158. Randomised trial of a perindopril-based blood-pressure-lowering regimen among 6,105 individuals with previous stroke or transient ischaemic attack, *Lancet* 358:1033–1041, 2001.

159. Yusuf S, Diener HC, Sacco RL, et al: Telmisartan to prevent recurrent stroke and cardiovascular events, *N Engl J Med* 359:1225–1237, 2008.

160. Amarenco P, Bogousslavsky J, Callahan A 3rd, et al: High-dose atorvastatin after stroke or transient ischemic attack, *N Engl J Med* 355:549–559, 2006.

161. Executive Committee for the Asymptomatic Carotid Atherosclerosis Study: Endarterectomy for asymptomatic stenosis, *JAMA* 273:1421–1428, 1995.

162. Halliday A, Mansfield A, Marro J, et al: Prevention of disabling and fatal strokes by successful carotid endarterectomy in patients without recent neurological symptoms: randomized controlled trial, *Lancet* 363:1491–1502, 2004.

163. Spence JD, Coates V, Li H, et al: Effects of intensive medical therapy on microemboli and cardiovascular risk in asymptomatic carotid stenosis, *Arch Neurol* 67:180–186, 2010.

164. Madani A, Beletsky V, Tamayo A, et al: High-risk asymptomatic carotid stenosis: ulceration on 3D ultrasound versus TCD microemboli, *Neurology* 77:744–750, 2011.

165. Labovitz DL, Halim A, Boden-Albala B, et al: The incidence of deep and lobar intracerebral hemorrhage in whites, blacks and Hispanics, *Neurology* 65:518–522, 2005.

166. Manno EM, Atlkinson JL, Fulgham JR, et al: Emergency medical and surgical management strategies in the evaluation and treatment of intracerebral hemorrhage, *Mayo Clin Proc* 80:420–433, 2005.

167. Brott T, Broderick J, Kothari R, et al: Early hemorrhage growth in patients with intracerebral hemorrhage, *Stroke* 28:1–5, 1997.

168. Kidwell CS, Chalela JA, Saver JL, et al: Comparison of MRI and CT for detection of intracerebral hemorrhage, *JAMA* 292:1823–1830, 2004.

169. Broderick J, Connolly S, Feldmann E, et al: Guidelines for the management of spontaneous intracranial hemorrhage in adults, 2007 update, *Stroke* 38:2001–2023, 2007.

170. Anderson CS, Huang Y, Wang JG, et al: Intensive blood pressure reduction in acute cerebral hemorrhage trial (INTERACT): a randomized pilot trial, *Lancet Neurol* 7:391–399, 2008.

171. Misra UK, Kalita J, Ranjan P, et al: Mannitol in intracerebral hemorrhage: a randomized controlled study, *J Neurol Sci* 234:41–45, 2005.

172. Poungvarin N, Bhoopat W, Viriyavejakul A, et al: Effects of dexamethasone in primary spontaneous intracerebral hemorrhage, *N Engl J Med* 316:1229–1233, 1987.

173. Lacut K, Bressollee L, Le Gal G, et al: Prevention of venous thrombosis in patients with acute intracerebral hemorrhage, *Neurology* 65:865–869, 2005.

174. Flaherty ML, Kissela B, Woo D, et al: The increasing incidence of anticoagulation-associated intracerebral hemorrhage, *Neurology* 68:116–121, 2007.

175. Flibotte JJ, Hagan N, O'Donnell J, et al: Warfarin, hematoma expansion and outcome of intracerebral hemorrhage, *Neurology* 63:1059–1064, 2004.

176. Huttner HB, Schellinger PD, Hartmann M, et al: Hematoma growth and outcome in treated neurocritical care patients with intracerebral hemorrhage related to oral anticoagulant therapy: a comparison of acute treatment strategies using vitamin K, fresh frozen plasma and prothrombin complex concentrate, *Stroke* 37:1465–1470, 2006.

177. Brody DL, Aiyagari V, Shackleford AM, et al: Use of recombinant factor VIIa in patients with warfarin-associated intracranial hemorrhage, *Neurocrit Care* 2:263–267, 2005.

178. Mayer SA, Brunn NC, Begtrup K, et al: Recombinant activated factor VII for acute intracerebral hemorrhage, *N Engl J Med* 352:777–785, 2005.

179. Mayer SA, Brun NC, Begtrup K, et al: Efficacy and safety of recombinant activated factor VII for acute intracerebral hemorrhage, *N Engl J Med* 358:2127–2138, 2008.

180. Qureshi AI, Mendelow AD, Hanley DF: Intracerebral hemorrhage, *Lancet* 373:1632–1644, 2009.

CHAPTER 32 Carotid Artery Stenting

Sriram S. Iyer, Jonathon Habersberger, Jiri Vitek, Christina Brennan, Gary Roubin

On May 6th, 2011, the U.S. Food and Drug Administration (FDA) followed up on the January 2011 recommendation of the FDA Circulatory System Device Panel[1] and approved the RX Acculink carotid stent (Abbott Vascular, Santa Clara, Calif.) for use in conjunction with Abbott's embolic protection device (EPD), the Accunet filter. The expanded label as a result of the FDA's approval was for treatment of extracranial carotid stenosis in symptomatic and asymptomatic patients who would otherwise be considered standard risk for surgical carotid endarterectomy (CEA). This was a landmark event because for the first time, carotid stenting, at least in the United States, qualified as a standard-of-care treatment and was no longer investigational or experimental for the majority of patients with carotid artery disease. (Earlier in [2004], the FDA had approved carotid artery stenting [CAS] for high CEA risk patients). This chapter reviews historical aspects and development of CAS, discusses stenting technique in detail, and reviews clinical trial data that support current indications for this procedure.

Historical Perspective

Carotid Endarterectomy

Surgical treatment for carotid artery stenoses was introduced in the early 1950s.[2] Although early observational data suggested benefit for surgery over medical therapy, large prospective randomized trials investigating the beneficial effect of CEA on stroke reduction were not initiated until the late 1980s and early 1990s. Landmark studies including the North American Symptomatic Carotid Endarterectomy Trial (NASCET),[3–6] European Carotid Surgery Trial (ECST),[7] Asymptomatic Carotid Atherosclerosis Study (ACAS),[8] and Asymptomatic Carotid Surgery Trial (ACST)[9] confirmed the benefits of surgery over best available medical treatment for reducing the risk of stroke in both symptomatic (NASCET, ECST) and asymptomatic patients (ACAS, ACST). Carotid endarterectomy surgery is comprehensively discussed in Chapter 33.

Patients included in these surgical studies were carefully selected; specifically, subjects who were considered high CEA risk were excluded from participation. Thus, octogenarians, patients with recurrent stenosis following prior ipsilateral endarterectomy, intracranial stenosis that was more severe than the surgically accessible lesion in the neck, unstable angina pectoris, recent myocardial infarction (MI), contralateral CEA, patients on long-term anticoagulation therapy, and surgically inaccessible lesions were all excluded from these trials.[3,8]

Endovascular Approaches to Treat Carotid Stenosis

The mission to develop safer percutaneous endovascular solutions to treat arterial stenosis was pioneered by Dotter[10] and Gruntzig and Hopff[11] in the 1960s and 1970s. In 1977, Klaus Mathias, an interventional radiologist, described a catheter system that could be used for performing balloon angioplasty of cervical carotid stenosis,[12] and this was followed by a few case reports of successful carotid angioplasty performed in the surgical suite.[13,14] In 1984, Vitek and his neuroradiology colleagues from the University of Alabama at Birmingham (UAB)[15] reported angioplasty of the innominate artery aided by balloon occlusion protection of the common carotid artery (CCA). This early report represents the first percutaneous intervention performed with the benefit of distal embolic protection. During the 1980s, clinical reports of carotid angioplasty were sporadic and limited to small single-center series of patients.[16] Kachel et al. summarized the results of carotid angioplasty published in the literature through 1995 and noted that 503 of the 523 (96%) procedures were technically successful. There were no deaths, major strokes occurred in 2.1%, and minor complications were in the single digits (6.3%).[17] In 1985, Rabkin and Germashev began using early-generation nitinol (an alloy of nickel and titanium) stents as an endovascular prosthesis and subsequently reported their 5-year experience.[18]

Resistance to widespread acceptance and the slow progress of angioplasty involving the supraaortic vessels was largely due to two major concerns: (1) local vessel injury related to balloon inflation causing a flow-limiting dissection with a risk of acute vessel closure (present era), and (2) the risk of distal embolization. In later years, these key limitations would be overcome by the introduction and widespread adoption of stents and EPDs.

In March 1994, Iyer, Vitek, and Roubin initiated the carotid angioplasty program at UAB under carefully scrutinized institutional protocols.[19] Initial interventions were performed using stand-alone balloon angioplasty (no stents). To maximize the luminal result, a long inflation was performed using a 5-mm over-the-wire balloon; the center port of this balloon could accommodate a 0.035-inch guidewire. Once the balloon was in place, the wire was withdrawn, and oxygenated arterial blood withdrawn from the femoral artery was infused through the center port of the balloon with the help of a special pump device, permitting a long 10-minute balloon inflation. The first four patients were treated without complications. Patient #5, a woman with contralateral carotid occlusion, presented with a transient ischemic attack (TIA) related to a high-grade stenosis in the index carotid artery and underwent an uncomplicated balloon angioplasty procedure. Despite a perfectly acceptable angiographic result, approximately an hour after the procedure, there was acute closure of the angioplastied carotid artery. Although a technically successful, urgent reintervention with recanalization and stenting of the occluded vessel was performed, the patient did not recover from the major stroke related to the acute closure and subsequently expired. This case triggered the decision by the UAB group to perform elective carotid stenting—irrespective of the angiographic results of balloon angioplasty—and primary stenting became the intervention of choice for treatment of cervical carotid stenosis. The subsequent rapid adoption of this approach by interventional cardiologists in particular, and the endovascular interventional community in general, heralded the modern era of endovascular treatment for extracranial carotid bifurcation disease.[19–22]

Although balloon expandable stents were used in the first 100 patients, by the summer of 1995 (when the initial patients returned for their follow-up angiograms) it became clear that these stents were prone to deformation (stent crush) because of the superficial location of the carotid artery and the associated movements of the neck.[23] The Alabama group were the first to report this complication, seen in approximately 15% of patients at 6-month follow-up.[23] Fortunately, stent deformation was largely a cosmetic issue, with only one patient presenting with symptoms in this series. This observation, as well as the recognition that chances for regulatory approval for balloon expandable stents for treating extracranial carotid stenosis were slim, led to the rapid introduction, testing, and adoption of self-expanding stents. Stents have all but abolished acute carotid vessel closure, and in contemporary practice, primary carotid stenting is the norm. The reader should note that unlike in coronary arteries, the risk of acute stent thrombosis and instant restenosis, two major limitations of coronary stents, are nonissues when stents are deployed in the extracranial carotid location.

In 1996, Theron et al.[24] reported results from his seminal work using his triple coaxial catheter that incorporated distal balloon occlusion for providing embolic protection during carotid bifurcation angioplasty. Unfortunately, this early-generation distal protection balloon could only be used with balloon angioplasty (and not with stents). By 2000, the first investigational distal balloon occlusion EPD, the Percusurge Guardwire (Medtronic, Minneapolis, Minn.) was introduced into clinical trials in the United States. This was soon followed by a number of clinical trials, all of which included a filter as the distal EPD. Unlike Theron's distal occlusion balloon, the Percusurge balloon—as well as all such filters—can be used with both over-the-wire and monorail stent delivery systems. As increasing clinical data became available, use of distal protection devices was recognized and accepted by many (but not all[25]) as an integral if not mandatory part of carotid artery dilation and stenting.[26-31] In our opinion, EPDs, when selected and used appropriately, improve procedure safety by significantly reducing the risk of procedure related embolic major and fatal strokes.

The multicenter Carotid and Vertebral Artery Transluminal Angioplasty Study (CAVATAS-I)[9] was conducted between 1992 and 1997 in the United Kingdom during an era when stents were neither widely available nor perceived as integral. This prospective randomized trial compared outcomes of balloon angioplasty and CEA in 504 patients; only 55 patients (26%) within the group assigned to endovascular treatment received stents. Initially, stents were used only as a bailout treatment, with increased elective use toward the end of the study; distal protection devices were not used. Major event rates within 30 days after treatment did not differ significantly between endovascular treatment and surgery: disabling stroke or death (6.4% vs. 5.9%) and any major stroke lasting more than 7 days or death (10.0% vs. 9.9%). This study also demonstrated that endovascular techniques were superior to surgery when considering other risks related to the incision in the neck and use of general anesthesia. Cranial nerve injury was reported in 8.7% of surgical patients; no events occurred in patients undergoing endovascular procedures (P < 0.0001). Major groin or neck hematomas occurred less often after endovascular treatment than after surgery (1.2% vs. 6.7%, P < 0.0015). The results of this early clinical trial set the stage for investigation of carotid stenting.

Indications and Contraindications

The indications for carotid artery revascularization have been well delineated in the recent American Stroke Association/American College of Cardiology Foundation/American Heart Association (ASA/ACCF/AHA) et al. *Guideline on the Management of Patients with Extracranial Carotid and Vertebral Artery Disease*[32] and essentially depend on symptomatic status and severity (degree) of stenosis. Hence, before an informed decision on a treatment option can be made (surgery or percutaneous intervention), it is critically important for patients and physicians to have a good understanding of the operator as well as the center's procedural and 30-day experience and outcomes.

Symptomatic Patients

Symptomatic carotid stenosis refers to ischemia or infarction in the distribution of the internal carotid artery (ICA) causing neurological abnormalities that include but are not limited to contralateral motor and/or sensory events, speech, and/or visual problems (monocular blindness, field defects). *Amaurosis fugax* refers to transient monocular visual loss, typically described by the patient as a shade being drawn down or across the eye (*amaurosis*, Greek for "darkening," and *fugax*, Latin for "fleeting"). Dizziness and problems with balance are symptoms that typically result from ischemia or infarction in the vertebrobasilar system, and the presence of a carotid artery stenosis in a patient presenting with dizziness is almost always incidental i.e., the carotid stenosis is most often asymptomatic and NOT causally related to the symptoms. The culprit stenosis is considered symptomatic for 6 months beyond the

event. Additionally, the risk of recurrent stroke is lower in patients who present with amaurosis as the sole symptom in comparison to patients who present with a hemispheric TIA.

It is well accepted that revascularization should be offered to all symptomatic patients if the diameter of the ICA is reduced more than 70% as documented by noninvasive imaging, or more than 50% as documented by catheter angiography (Table 32-1). There is, however, one important caveat: the periprocedural risk of stroke or death related to the revascularization procedure (CEA or CAS) should be under 6%.[32] In symptomatic patients, there is a well-established correlation between increasing stenosis severity and stroke risk. The NASCET study[3] demonstrated the benefit of CEA over medical treatment for reducing the risk of future stroke in symptomatic patients with carotid stenosis between 70% and 99%. The NASCET results also showed that symptomatic patients with a lesser degree of stenosis (between 50% and 70%) benefit less. Revascularization is typically recommended in this group if there are additional unfavorable angiographic features (e.g., ulceration or other features associated with increased risk of vessel-to-vessel embolization).

An important, albeit controversial and unsettled, issue in the treatment of symptomatic patients relates to the timing of the revascularization procedure after the index symptomatic event.[33-37] Risk of a recurrent neurological event after a TIA or stroke is estimated to be between 15% and 20%, and this elevated risk persists for approximately 6 months after the initial event and underlies the rationale for the 6-month threshold for defining symptomatic patients. Proponents of early intervention i.e., within a few days of the symptomatic event. Argue that the highest risk of a recurrent event is during this early period and any delay in treatment will significantly diminish its therapeutic value, since a substantial portion of these patients would have already experienced a neurological event during the waiting period. A key reason underlying the reluctance of operators to perform revascularization (CEA or CAS) soon after a stroke (less so after a TIA) is the concern that

TABLE 32-1	Modified American Heart Association Recommendations for Carotid Artery Revascularization	
INDICATION LEVEL	SYMPTOMATIC STENOSIS*	ASYMPTOMATIC STENOSIS*
Proven	70%-99% stenosis	>80% stenosis
	Periprocedural complication risk <6%	Periprocedural complication risk <3%
		Life expectancy >5 years
Acceptable	50%-69% stenosis	>60% stenosis
	Periprocedural complication risk <3%	Periprocedural complication risk <3%
		Planned CABG
Unacceptable	<49% stenosis or	<60% stenosis or
	Periprocedural complication risk >6%	Periprocedural complication risk >5%

*Lesion severity is determined according to the North American Symptomatic Carotid Endarterectomy Trial (NASCET) methodology (i.e., the ratio between lumen diameter at the point of maximal stenosis and the lumen diameter of the non tapered segment of the distal internal carotid artery).[153]
CABG, coronary artery bypass graft surgery.
Modified from Brott TG, Halperin JL, Abbara S, et al: ASA/ACCF/AHA/AANN/AANS/ACR/ASNR/CNS/SAIP/SCAI/SIR/SNIS/SVM/SVS guideline on the management of patients with extracranial carotid and vertebral artery disease: executive summary. A Report of the American College of Cardiology Foundation/American Heart Association Task Force on Practice Guidelines, and the American Stroke Association, American Association of Neuroscience Nurses, American Association of Neurological Surgeons, American College of Radiology, American Society of Neuroradiology, Congress of Neurological Surgeons, Society of Atherosclerosis Imaging and Prevention, Society for Cardiovascular Angiography and Interventions, Society of Interventional Radiology, Society of NeuroInterventional Surgery, Society for Vascular Medicine, and Society for Vascular Surgery, developed in collaboration with the American Academy of Neurology and Society of Cardiovascular Computed Tomography. J Am Coll Cardiol 57:1002-1044, 2011; and Roubin GS, Iyer S, Halkin A, et al. Realizing the potential of carotid artery stenting: proposed paradigms for patient selection and procedural technique. Circulation 113:2021-2030, 2006.

early treatment increases the risk of hemorrhagic transformation of the culprit, (nonhemorrhagic) infarct. Although the increased risk of intracranial hemorrhage following early intervention has been challenged,[33] a recent retrospective analysis[38] of a large national inpatient database involving more than 57 million in-hospital admissions, conducted to determine the prevalence and risk factors of intracranial hemorrhage among patients undergoing CEA (N = 215,012) and CAS (N = 13,884), arrived at a different conclusion. Symptomatic presentations represented the minority of indications for CEA (n = 10,049 [5%]), as well as CAS (n = 1251 [10%]). Intracranial hemorrhage occurred significantly more frequently after CAS than CEA in both symptomatic (4.4% vs. 0.8%; P <0.0001) and asymptomatic presentations (0.5% vs. 0.06%; P <0.0001). Multivariate regression suggested that symptomatic presentations (vs. asymptomatic) and CAS procedures (vs. CEA) were both independently predictive of six- to sevenfold increases in the frequency of postoperative intracranial hemorrhage. The observations from this retrospective population-based analysis are at variance with observations from recent large prospective randomized trials involving symptomatic and asymptomatic patients, wherein the risk of mortality and major stroke was uniformly low in both CEA and CAS arms, and the higher incidence of neurological events in the CAS arm was a result of minor strokes (ischemic rather than hemorrhagic).[39–41] Pending resolution of this issue by future studies, the current approach of waiting a minimum of 3 weeks following the index event (longer for larger strokes) is likely to continue.

Asymptomatic Patients

Asymptomatic carotid disease refers to the presence of a stenosis resulting in a 60% or greater reduction of the luminal diameter of the extracranial ICA without symptoms of ipsilateral stroke, TIA, or amaurosis fugax. Treatment of patients with asymptomatic carotid artery stenosis has become extremely controversial, with two main issues fuelling this ongoing debate[42–44]:

1. Which asymptomatic patients (if any) are appropriate for intervention (CEA or CAS)? Current guidelines suggest that it is reasonable to refer asymptomatic patients for ICA revascularization in the setting of more than 80% stenosis and low periprocedural risk.[32]
2. What should be the choice of treatment? In the event revascularization is to be performed in an asymptomatic patient, should the patient be referred for CEA or CAS?

MEDICAL TREATMENT VS. INTERVENTION (CEA/CAS) FOR ASYMPTOMATIC CAROTID DISEASE

Despite publication of several guidelines that provide a best assessment of current research, considerable divergence of opinion regarding care of the carotid artery remains an issue among physicians worldwide.[45] One reason why enthusiasm for revascularization may be low is recognition that the annualized risk of a stroke in patients with asymptomatic carotid artery disease treated with contemporary medical treatment is low and dropping (Table 32-2). This reduction in stroke risk has been attributed to the benefits of risk-factor modification, use of antihypertensive medications,[46] antiplatelet agents,[47] smoking cessation, and statin therapy.[48,49]

The guidelines respond to this concern by limiting revascularization to those asymptomatic patients in whom periprocedural

TABLE 32-2	Annualized Stroke Risk in Asymptomatic Patients with Greater Than 50% Carotid Artery Stenosis Treated with Best Medical Therapy Available During Trial Period		
		Annualized Risk	
STUDY	YEAR	ANY STROKE	IPSILATERAL STROKE
ACAS[8]	1995	3.5%	2.2%
ACST[151]	2004	2.4%	1.1%
ACSRS[154]	2005	2.1%	1.7%
ASED[55]	2005	2.2%	1.0%

ACAS, Asymptomatic Carotid Atherosclerosis Study; ACSRS, Asymptomatic Carotid Stenosis and Risk of Stroke; ACST, Asymptomatic Carotid Surgery Trial; ASED, Asymptomatic Stenosis Embolus Detection.

risk of a stroke or death is expected to be below 3%.[32] Hence, some clinicians argue that there is an urgent need for a new three-arm randomized clinical trial for asymptomatic carotid disease that includes not only CEA and CAS but also has a medical treatment arm. A critical message from the asymptomatic CEA trials was that for surgical revascularization to be beneficial in reducing future stroke risk in asymptomatic patients (Table 32-3), the periprocedural risk of revascularization should not exceed 3%. If the risk breaches the 3% threshold, the difference in stroke risk between the medically treated arm and the surgical arm will not be significant (i.e., the benefit of stroke reduction from the surgery no longer accrues to the patient). The second Carotid Revascularization Endarterectomy versus Stenting Trial (CREST II) will be a three-arm study involving asymptomatic patients, and this protocol is currently under review for funding by the National Institutes of Health (NIH).

IDENTIFYING THE ASYMPTOMATIC PATIENT AT HIGH RISK FOR DEVELOPING A STROKE

Much of the controversy surrounding treatment of asymptomatic carotid stenosis could be resolved if physicians had a method of reliably identifying the asymptomatic patient at high risk for a future stroke; interventional treatment could then be selectively directed at these patients. Understandably, such an approach would greatly improve the yield and cost-effectiveness of prophylactic invasive treatment with either CEA or CAS.[50] Some of the metrics that have been proposed as predictors of increased risk of ipsilateral ischemic events in asymptomatic patients with carotid stenosis include higher grades of stenosis or substantial progression of carotid stenosis to a higher grade,[51,52] unfavorable plaque characteristics and composition, including plaque ulceration and echolucency,[53,54] or verifying the presence or absence of microemboli by using transcranial Doppler.[55–58] Other clinical and radiological markers for predicting an increased risk of stroke in asymptomatic patients include occult cerebral infarction on brain imaging studies,[59] contralateral carotid occlusion,[60] or detection of intraplaque hemorrhage by magnetic resonance imaging (MRI).[61] Nicolaides et al.[62] have suggested that combining clinical risk factors, such as diabetes and smoking, with high-risk ultrasound features (e.g., echolucent plaque) may help identify the high-risk asymptomatic patient. These are listed in Table 32-4.

TABLE 32-3	Event Rates from the Two Major Randomized Carotid Surgical Trials in Asymptomatic Patients					
				Five-Year Stroke Risk		
STUDY	N	YEAR	CEA	MEDICAL THERAPY	HAZARD RATIO (CEA VS. MEDICAL THERAPY)	
ACAS[8]	1662	1995	5.1%	11%	0.46	
ACST[151]	3120	2004	3.8%	11.0%	0.29	

ACAS, Asymptomatic Carotid Atherosclerosis Study; ACST, Asymptomatic Carotid Surgery Trial; CEA, carotid endarterectomy.

TABLE 32-4	Postulated Clinical/Investigative Features to Identify High Stroke Risk Patients with Asymptomatic Carotid Disease	
CRITERIA	**AUTHOR(S)/REFERENCE**	
Anatomical		
High-grade carotid stenosis with substantial progression	Bock,[51] Hirt[52]	
Contralateral carotid occlusion	AbuRahma[60]	
Plaque Characteristics		
Plaque composition, ulceration, or echolucency	Nicolaides,[53] Spence[54]	
Intraplaque hemorrhage	Altaf[61]	
Plaque composition and clinical risk factors	Nicolaides[62]	
Imaging		
Microembolization	Abbott,[55] Markus,[56] Spence[57,58]	
Occult cerebral infarction	Norris[59]	

Although one cannot dispute the clinical appeal and practical usefulness of being able to identify the asymptomatic patient at high risk for a stroke, none of the approaches outlined thus far have been validated to justify and provide clinically relevant recommendations. Hence, at present, degree of carotid diameter stenosis severity remains the predominant basis for clinically deciding whether or not to treat patients with asymptomatic carotid stenosis.

In contemporary practice, most clinicians will (should) only treat an angiographically confirmed 80% or greater, unilateral, incidentally discovered (i.e., diagnosed on routine duplex screening, following workup of a carotid bruit) asymptomatic carotid stenosis. Patients with stenosis less than 60% are managed medically, with periodic (usually annual) ultrasound surveillance to monitor stenosis progression. Although stenosis severity between 60% and 80% is typically managed with conservative medical treatment, this recommendation may have to be altered based on individual circumstances. Some examples include:

- Contralateral carotid occlusion and a stenosis between 60% and 80% in the index carotid artery that also supplies the territory of occluded carotid artery via collaterals.
- Bilateral greater than 70% but less than 80% stenosis.
- Magnetic resonance imaging or computed tomography (CT) findings of clinically silent (asymptomatic) prior ipsilateral stroke(s).
- Patients scheduled to undergo coronary artery bypass grafting (CABG) and/or valve surgery (especially if surgery will be performed on-pump).

In the absence of an established reliable method of identifying the asymptomatic patient with carotid stenosis at high risk for developing a future neurological event, the decision to treat is predominantly based on degree of stenosis, an approach supported by the large CEA clinical trials. The threshold for treating asymptomatic carotid stenosis is 80% or greater stenosis confirmed by angiography (NASCET criteria), with corresponding elevated duplex velocities. Although standard risk-factor modification approaches should be implemented in all these patients, there is no convincing evidence to date that risk-modifying measures by themselves will reduce stroke risk in patients with severe degrees of stenosis that cannot be further improved with revascularization when the periprocedural risk is 3% or less. This nonnegotiable low tolerance for periprocedural complications constitutes what the authors have framed as the *3% Rule of Carotid Stenting*.[63] How to avoid breaching this rule is central to the theme of patient selection for carotid stenting. The critical all-important task of identifying the standard-risk patient for carotid stenting (not CEA) is discussed later in the chapter.

Deciding on the type of intervention, CAS or CEA, is also discussed later.

Patient Selection for Carotid Stenting

Prior to recommending carotid stenting as a choice for therapeutic intervention, it is important for both physician and patient to understand the natural history of the condition without intervention, the procedure-related risks (which can immediately erode the benefits of a procedure done purely with the intent of future benefit), and the clinical durability of the stenting procedure.

Procedure-Related Risks

Over the past decade, one of the most important advances in the field of carotid stenting relates to our understanding of what constitutes "high stent risk." It is important to remember that CEA was first performed in the 1950s, and over the course of the next several years, surgeons identified both anatomical features and comorbidities that would increase the risk of endarterectomy (high–CEA risk group). Furthermore, these high–CEA risk patients were excluded from participating in the major randomized CEA trials.

EVOLUTION IN OUR UNDERSTANDING OF THE CONCEPT OF HIGH STENT RISK

To help the interventionist decide whether stenting is an appropriate treatment for a particular patient (and lesion), it is important for the operator to understand, recognize, and differentiate the standard-risk (Box 32-1) from the high-risk CAS patient. This determination, based on an individualized analysis, is the single most important element of the CAS risk stratification process and should be performed for every patient. The designation of *high stent risk* has evolved over time, and in retrospect was a critical component of the learning curve of the early adopters of the CAS treatment modality. Because the attributes that define high CEA risk (Box 32-2) are distinct from those that define high stent risk, a patient who is high risk for CEA does not automatically become suitable (i.e., standard risk) for CAS. The presence of high-risk features for stenting was unrecognized during the early clinical trials and the criteria for inclusion in these trials only specified "high–CEA risk patients," thus permitting unbalanced comparisons of technique. Hence, the high event rates observed in early high–CEA risk stent registries resulted in large part from the unwitting inclusion of high stent risk patients. With the more recent

> ### Box 32-1 Standard Risk for Carotid Stenting: Patient and Lesion Characteristics
>
> **Recognize the Ideal Patient for Carotid Stenting**
> - Male or female patient, <75 years of age
> - Preserved brain function (no compromise of brain reserve)
> - Asymptomatic carotid bruit
> - Good LV function, no aortic stenosis
> - Known coronary anatomy
> - Normal renal function
> - Duplex ultrasound PSV: 450 cm/s; EDV: 130 cm/s
>
> **Recognize Ideal Lesion and ICA Morphology for Carotid Stenting**
> - Angle between the ICA and ECA is <90 degrees
> - Minimal vessel tortuosity (i.e., no carotid redundancy)
> - Minimal calcification
> - No ulceration or obvious filling defects
> - Stenosis severity and whether plaque is concentric or eccentric are less important, as long as flow is normal (i.e. TIMI III)
> - Lesion located in a straight segment (as opposed to a bend) of the ICA
> - Artery cephalad to the stenosis is straight (minimal bends and vessel tortuosity)
> - ICA: 4-5 mm; CCA: 8-10 mm

CCA, common carotid artery; ECA, external carotid artery; EDV, end-diastolic velocity; ICA, internal carotid artery; LV, left ventricular; PSV, peak systolic velocity; TIMI, Thrombolysis in Myocardial Infarction.

Box 32-2 Anatomical Features and Comorbidities Associated with High Carotid Endarterectomy Risk

Anatomical

Surgically inaccessible lesions above C-2 or below the level of the clavicle
Contralateral carotid artery occlusion
Restenosis after a previous ipsilateral CEA
Previous head/neck radiation therapy or surgery that included the area of stenosis
Ipsilateral radical neck dissection for the treatment of cancer
Obese/short neck
Fibromuscular dysplasia
Spinal immobility of the neck due to cervical arthritis
Presence of laryngeal palsy
Presence of a tracheostoma

Comorbidities

Chronic Obstructive pulmonary disease (COPD) with a forced expiratory volume (FEV) 1 less than 30%
Requirement for staged and scheduled coronary artery bypass graft (CABG) or valve replacement procedures more than 30 days following the stent procedure
Age 80 years or more
Recent myocardial infarction more than 72 hours and less than 30 days
Severe lung disease
Two or more major diseased coronary arteries that require revascularization (70% or more)

CAD, coronary artery disease; CEA, carotid endarterectomy.

exclusion of high stent risk patients, a corresponding improvement in procedural outcomes has been noted. For example, by 2005 the concept of high stent risk was better established, and in the second half of the CREST study, many of these high-risk stent patients were generally excluded (since the CREST protocol written in the late 1990s did not specifically call out high stent risk exclusions).[39] The Asymptomatic Carotid Trial (ACT-I), a trial that specifically excludes high stent risk patients, is in progress (NCT00106938).

STANDARD STENT RISK

Although carotid stenting outcomes are not influenced by gender, age is a very important determinant. The concept of *brain reserve* is akin to cardiac reserve—a patient with poor left ventricular (LV) function is more likely to manifest and experience complications related to a percutaneous coronary intervention (PCI) or CABG procedure. Similarly, a patient with compromised brain function (diminished brain reserve) is more likely to clinically manifest neurological events related to periprocedural embolization. Embolization is a universal occurrence with all CAS procedures and happens despite the use of EPDs. Patients with prior large strokes, multiple small strokes, or lacunar infarcts and those with dementia are examples of patients with compromised brain reserve. Dementia in particular is a problem. Despite having a perfectly acceptable angiographic and clinical result (i.e., no procedure-related events) in the follow-up period, anecdotal reports suggest a marked deterioration in memory and other cognitive functions. The reason for this is unclear, but dementia should be considered at least a relative contraindication for CAS.

Close attention should be paid to the end-diastolic ultrasound flow velocity. If this value exceeds 100 cm/s (especially >120 cm/s), the angiographic stenosis severity will exceed 80% (as defined by the NASCET criteria; Fig. 32-1) and will meet the treatment threshold for treating asymptomatic lesions.

Figure 32-2 illustrates lesion and vessel features that are ideal for stenting using distal embolic protection. These features include:

- A narrow acute angle between the ICA and external carotid artery (ECA). The wider this bifurcation (i.e., the angle approaches 90 degrees or is frankly obtuse), the greater the technical difficulty in advancing a distal embolic protection filter device with a fixed-wire system (Fig. 32-3). The technical difficulty imparted by an open ICA/ECA angle is compounded if there is additional tortuosity in the ICA distal to the stenosis (Fig. 32-4).
- Minimal calcification and no ulceration. Some degree of calcification is nearly ubiquitous in a diseased carotid bifurcation, but heavy concentric calcification in association with a severe stenosis is a major problem. Although the demonstration of carotid calcification is straightforward and requires only fluoroscopy (Fig. 32-5), the distinction between deep

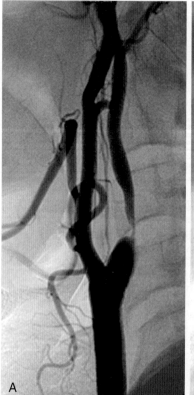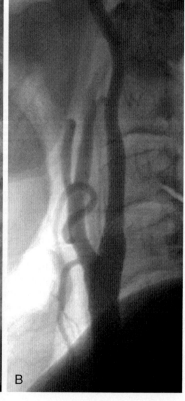

FIGURE 32-1   Ideal lesion and vessel morphology for carotid stenting. Ideal lesion **(A)** has high-grade (>80%) internal carotid artery (ICA) stenosis (enddiastolic velocity 124 cm/s). Note that ICA/external carotid artery angle is acute, and the artery cephalad to stenosis is free of significant bends. **B,** Same lesion following carotid stenting using a distal embolic protection device (EPD [filter]).

A   B

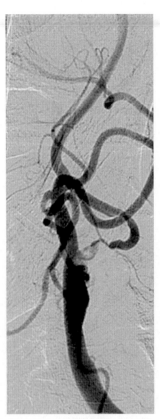

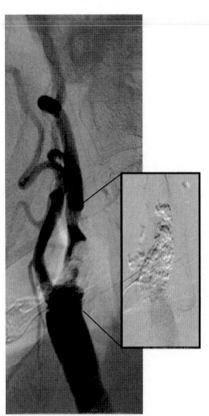

FIGURE 32-2   This lesion is unsuitable for carotid artery stenting. The high grade of stenosis, 90-degree angle between the internal carotid artery and external carotid artery, and proximal calcification make passage of wires and equipment hazardous.

FIGURE 32-4   Extensive circumferential calcification of the internal carotid artery makes this lesion unsuitable for carotid artery stenting. Subtraction imaging without contrast shows calcification of both the internal carotid artery and external carotid artery.

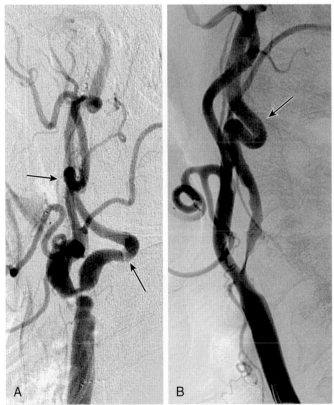

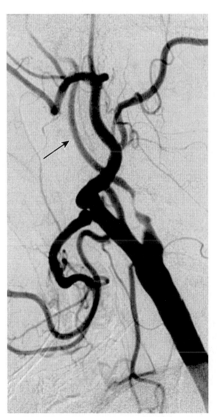

FIGURE 32-3   These lesions are unsuitable for carotid artery stenting using a distal embolic protection device. This is due to the high degree of tortuosity of the internal carotid artery distal to the lesion, preventing safe and effective positioning of a filter device.

FIGURE 32-5   This vessel demonstrates a string sign with high-grade stenosis and reduced cranial flow and internal carotid artery filling (arrow). Note the relatively complete filling of the external carotid artery vessels in comparison.

vessel wall calcium and superficial calcium encroaching on the vessel lumen may be difficult, and the decision to declare the case unsuitable for CAS is largely subjective. We arbitrarily define *heavy calcification* as calcification 3 mm or more in width, with *concentricity* defined by imaging in two orthogonal views. The unyielding nature of calcium, along with the stiffness it imparts to the involved vessel segment, makes it difficult to predilate and advance the EPD and stent delivery system through the lesion (especially the stent). Forcing these devices in an attempt to cross the stenosis not only increases the chances of prolapsing the sheath out of the CCA, it also increases the risk of embolization, spasm, and dissection. Inability to completely dilate and expand the deployed stent despite using larger and/or high-pressure balloons (resulting in a stent with an hourglass appearance) is an intraprocedural nightmare.

- The artery, especially cephalad to the stenosis, is free of any significant kinks or bends. Presence or absence of this key unfavorable feature is extremely important to note on preprocedure magnetic resonance angiography (MRA), computed tomographic angiography (CTA), or invasive angiography, since it increases the degree of difficulty when attempting to place a distal filter EPD. *Excessive vascular tortuosity* is defined as two or more bend points that are 90 degrees or greater (see Fig. 32-4). At times the tortuosity can be extreme and may impart a hairpin bend to the ICA (see Fig. 32-4). Worsening grades of tortuosity increase the difficulty when attempting to cross the stenosis and may make device delivery difficult or impossible. Straightening of the tortuous vessel segment by stiff wires or devices may result in vessel spasm and reduced antegrade flow. Thus, despite filter placement, the patient does not receive the benefit of brisk antegrade flow and may manifest ischemic symptoms in the absence of adequate collaterals. Additionally, slow flow increases the risk of fibrin deposition within the filter. The longer the dwell time of the EPD, the higher the risk of an iatrogenic thrombus. Iatrogenic tortuosity can also be introduced by placement of the sheath in a redundant carotid artery, so tortuosity should be assessed after the sheath is in place below the carotid bifurcation.

Stenosis severity and eccentricity/concentricity are not problems as long as the flow in the vessel is normal (Thrombolysis in Myocardial Infarction [TIMI] grade III). A severe stenosis in association with less than TIMI III flow (*string sign*, Fig. 32-6) and an occluded artery are contraindications (Fig. 32-7) for CAS. Ulceration is often noted, even on angiograms from asymptomatic patients, and although not a contraindication, operators should be aware that the risk of embolization might be higher, particularly during the phase of poststent balloon dilation. Angiographic filling defects that are consistent with a thrombus are a contraindication to CAS (Fig. 32-8). Note that both calcium and thrombus may appear as filling defects, and the differentiation is based on the clinical presentation. Whereas a filling defect in a symptomatic patient should be presumed to be thrombus (see Fig. 32-7), filling defects in asymptomatic patients are frequently a result of calcium encroaching on the vessel lumen (Fig. 32-9).

As a rule, unfavorable anatomical features (Figs. 32-10 and 32-11; also see Figs. 32-3 through 32-9) should be considered contraindications for CAS. Although special techniques (e.g., use of a heavy-gauge buddy wire to straighten tortuous vessel segments, use of cutting balloons to dilate unyielding lesions) may result in a satisfactory angiographic outcome, the risk of a procedure-related neurological event should be presumed to breach the accepted periprocedural complication threshold.

Durability of Carotid Artery Stenting

Durability is defined by the ability to reduce the risk of a future stroke (the reason why these procedures are performed) and by the frequency of in-stent restenosis (discussed later in this chapter.)

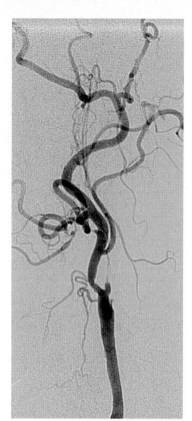

FIGURE 32-6 An occluded carotid artery is an absolute contraindication to stenting.

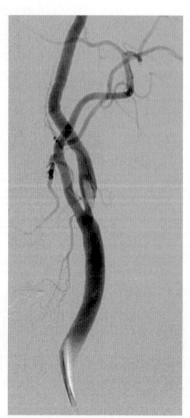

FIGURE 32-7 Thrombus located in proximal internal carotid artery in a patient with symptomatic carotid artery disease. This is identified by the hazy appearance and is only visible following contrast injection.

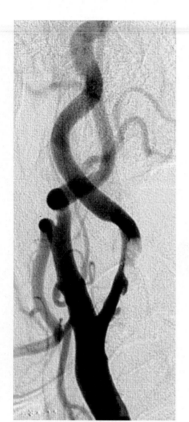

FIGURE 32-8 **This patient demonstrates eccentric calcification, which may at times closely resemble thrombus.** Fluoroscopy without contrast injection will typically reveal calcification, as also shown in Figure 32-5.

Procedural Considerations for Carotid Artery Stenting

Initial Evaluation

PATIENT INTERVIEW, CLINICAL EXAM, AND DIAGNOSTIC STUDIES

Except in rare instances, nearly all carotid revascularization procedures are elective, and there is no justification for an ad hoc carotid procedure (e.g., combining a carotid intervention with another scheduled invasive procedure such as coronary angiography). A comprehensive history and physical examination, including a detailed neurological exam, are mandatory first steps when evaluating a patient for a possible carotid intervention. Often, patients referred for treatment of "symptomatic" carotid artery stenosis have other reasons for their symptoms, including posterior circulation (vertebrobasilar) disease, cardiac arrhythmias, or a cardioembolic source (e.g., a patient with atrial fibrillation with a clot in the atrial appendage). These patients have incidental (i.e., asymptomatic) carotid disease; the risk assessment and approach to treatment of these patients are very different from the patient with true symptomatic carotid artery stenosis. A formal neurological consultation and additional diagnostic imaging are often helpful in sorting out these patients.

Another frequently encountered problem relates to suboptimal images that result in unreliable noninvasive diagnostic studies (carotid duplex ultrasound and MRA). Whereas quality and reliability of a duplex ultrasound study are very technician dependent, quality of the MRA study is influenced not only by the generation status of the equipment but also by the scanning protocol (with or without gadolinium), the correct timing sequence, and the skill and experience of the interpreting radiologist. It is critical that the ultrasound evaluation be performed in an Intersocietal Commission for

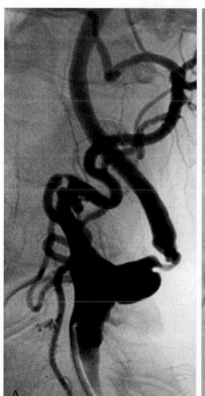
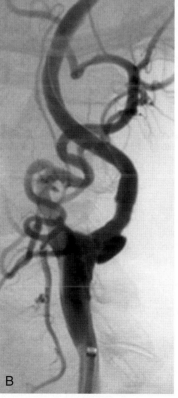

FIGURE 32-9 **Unfavorable vessel morphology for carotid stenting. A,** Unfavorable lesion. Note obtuse internal carotid artery/external carotid artery (ICA/ECA) angle, high-grade eccentric stenosis immediately distal to bifurcation, and ulcer proximal to stenosis near carotid bulb. Vessel distal to stenosis is straight. **B,** Result can be seen after treatment using an Emboshield (Abbott Vascular, Santa Clara, Calif.) filter. Wire is independent of filter, and negotiating the unfavorable bifurcation and severe eccentric stenosis is far easier with a wire uncoupled from the filter element. Pre-predilation may be needed. Open-cell stent was used to treat the lesion on the bend; this stent design does not introduce any additional bends in ICA post stenting. Care should be taken to place proximal end of stent flush with origin of ICA. If it hangs between ICA origin and common carotid artery (CCA), stent edge can cause problems in advancing postdilatation balloon as well as filter retrieval catheter. Note that ulcer is excluded, not obliterated, and no attempt should be made to obliterate ulcer by using larger balloons. Flow to ulcer crater will seal off in time.

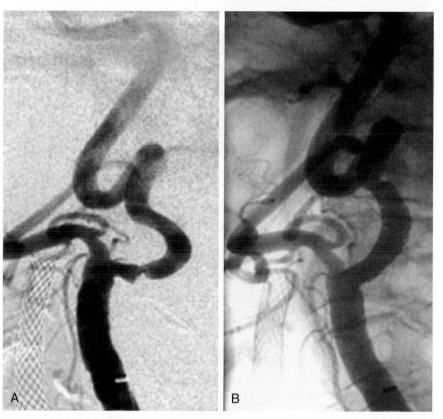

FIGURE 32-10 Unfavorable vessel morphology for carotid stenting. A, Complex lesion. There is an obtuse internal carotid artery/external carotid artery (ICA/ECA) angle as well extreme tortuosity of the ICA distal to the stenosis. Note the carotid stent in the contralateral carotid artery. **B,** Final result after carotid artery stenting. This lesion was treated using a Percusurge GuardWire (Medtronic, Minneapolis, Minn.) distal occlusion balloon for embolic protection and an open-cell stent. Distal filters are contraindicated. Proximal flow reversal is an option, provided the arch anatomy is favorable for placing larger French-size catheters in the carotid artery. This type of vessel morphology will be technically challenging and should be a contraindication for the beginner and low- and medium-volume operators.

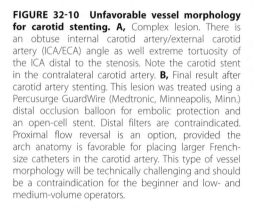

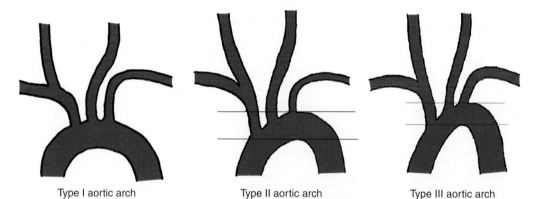

Type I aortic arch   Type II aortic arch   Type III aortic arch

FIGURE 32-11 Classification of the aortic arch. In the frontal projection, a horizontal line is drawn across the origin of the left subclavian artery. Type I: all the great vessels originate at same level and meet this line. Access to left carotid and innominate arteries is easiest with this aortic arch configuration. Type II and type III: as the aorta becomes more unfolded and elongated (a function of increasing age and hypertension), origin of great vessels becomes displaced more posteriorly, and on the frontal projection, origins are progressively displaced inferior to the horizontal line referenced above. Access becomes increasingly difficult because a catheter approaching from the descending aorta tends to prolapse into the ascending aorta.

the Accreditation Vascular Laboratories (ICAVL) certified laboratory. These considerations are especially important in the patient with asymptomatic carotid artery disease. We strongly recommend that a knowledgeable family member be present during the initial patient interview and subsequent interactions. Besides the science and rationale for the procedure, the discussion should also include regulatory approval and reimbursement status.

The goal of the clinical examination (history, physical including a neurological evaluation) and diagnostic testing (noninvasive as well as angiography) is to provide answers to the following questions/issues:

1. Is the patient symptomatic or asymptomatic?
2. If symptomatic, are symptoms referable to stenosis at the carotid bifurcation?
3. What is the severity of the stenosis (duplex ultrasound velocities, MRA, CTA, angiography, NASCET criteria)
4. Risk assessment:

- Is the patient suitable for CAS?
- Is the patient suitable for CEA?
- Overall recommendation: CAS, CEA or continued medical management?

Preprocedure Issues

Patients who consent to brachiocephalic angiography and possible stent placement should undergo a comprehensive clinical cardiovascular evaluation to assess for presence of coronary artery disease(CAD), aortic stenosis, and LV dysfunction. The presence of these comorbidities will impact a patient's tolerance of the hemodynamic effects of CAS. All patients should undergo evaluation of the preprocedure neurological status, and baseline NIH, Rankin, and Barthel Stroke Scales should be documented. All symptomatic patients, those with a prior history of stroke, and those with an abnormal neurological examination should have a CT or MRI scan of the brain to document baseline status.

Antiplatelet Agents and Anticoagulants

In the clinical protocol, great emphasis is placed on dual antiplatelet therapy before and after carotid stenting. The non-event of stent thrombosis and the low rates of peri- and postprocedural embolic events are predicated upon administration of the correct doses of adjunctive antiplatelet therapy. All patients should receive aspirin, 81 to 325 mg daily, and clopidogrel, 75 mg daily, prior to the procedure and for a minimum of 30 days after the procedure.[32] If a patient has not received both aspirin and clopidogrel on a daily basis, we suggest they receive a 600-mg loading dose of clopidogrel at least 4 hours prior to the procedure. If this is not possible, the procedure should be rescheduled. There is no experience using prasugrel in patients undergoing carotid stenting.

The approach to patients who are on chronic anticoagulation with warfarin should be individualized, with the acknowledgement that triple therapy with aspirin, clopidogrel, and warfarin increases the risk of bleeding. Discontinuing warfarin while the patient is on dual antiplatelet treatment may be acceptable in patients at low risk for systemic embolism. If the patient requires anticoagulant therapy because of a high risk of thromboembolism, such as a prosthetic mechanical valve, it is appropriate to discontinue warfarin for approximately 4 days prior to the scheduled invasive procedure, "bridge" the patient with heparin if appropriate, and then restart warfarin on the evening of the carotid stent procedure. In patients requiring warfarin in the poststent period, dual antiplatelet therapy should include 81 mg of aspirin together with 75 mg of clopidogrel. Dual antiplatelet medications maintained for 6 to 8 weeks after carotid stenting is optimal.

Antihypertensive and β-Blocker Medication

Blood pressure and/or heart rate–lowering medications are typically withheld the day of the procedure to avoid excessive bradycardia and hypotension resulting from procedure-related carotid baroreceptor stimulation. Postprocedure, blood pressure and heart rate should be followed closely and medications reintroduced as soon as the clinical situation permits. In patients with restenosis following prior CEA (denervated carotid bulb) or in cases where the location of the stenosis is such that balloon inflations and stent deployment are clearly cephalad to the carotid bifurcation, there may be no need to discontinue these medications. In these patients, postprocedural blood pressure requires careful management to minimize the risk and/or consequences of cerebral hyperperfusion syndrome (discussed later).

Technique of Carotid Stenting

The current technique of carotid angioplasty and stenting described here has been adopted (with minor modifications) by most high-volume carotid angioplasty centers. Angiography and stenting are performed under local anesthesia. Heart rate and rhythm, blood pressure, and neurological status should be closely monitored throughout the intervention.

Technical aspects of the procedure are discussed under the following headings:
- Vascular Access.
- Diagnostic Angiographic Evaluation.
- Carotid Sheath Placement.
- Embolic Protection Devices.
- Lesion Predilation.
- Stents.
- Postdilation.
- Final Angiographic Assessment.
- Embolic Protection Device and Sheath Removal and Access Site Hemostasis.
- Management of Hemodynamics.

Vascular Access

Femoral artery access is the preferred and recommended approach. Carotid interventions via brachial or radial artery approach have been described in patients with so-called hostile anatomy of the aortic arch. Direct percutaneous puncture of the carotid artery as a method of vascular access has, for the most part, been abandoned. The frequent need for general anesthesia, proximity of the access site to the site of the lesion, problems related to local hematoma including the risk of airway compromise, and difficulty in compressing a superficial stented vessel for securing hemostasis are some of the reasons why direct carotid artery catheter insertion is no longer used. Femoral venous access is unnecessary unless a reliable peripheral venous access is unavailable. Routine prophylactic placement of a temporary venous pacemaker is no longer recommended but should be readily available.

Diagnostic Angiographic Evaluation

It is mandatory to have a high-quality complete diagnostic cerebral and extracranial carotid angiogram prior to initiating the stenting procedure. Imaging of the aortic arch by angiography, MRA, or CTA may be helpful to define the arch type and anomalous origins of the vessels. The most common anomaly, seen in approximately 7% of patients, is independent origin of the left vertebral artery from the arch and origin of the left carotid artery from the innominate. Figure 32-12 shows classification of the aortic arch.

A complete cerebral angiogram requires anatomical definition of both intracranial and extracranial carotid arteries as well as the dominant vertebral artery. The decision to perform selective cannulation and angiography of the vertebral artery should be individualized. The vertebral arteries frequently have a tortuous course, and the vessel is prone to spasm—features that predispose to dissection with catastrophic sequelae. It is important for the operator to understand the collateral circulation to the brain hemisphere

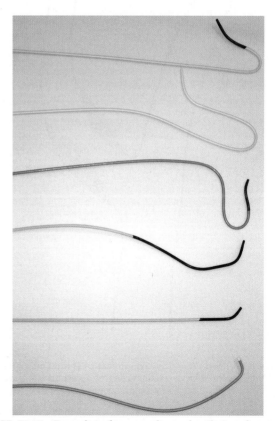

FIGURE 32-12 Examples of commonly used catheters for cervicocerebral angiography: the double-curved Vitek and Simmons catheters, JR4, Berenstein and Headhunter catheter.

of interest. Clear definition of the collateral circulation is especially important if a flow-arresting balloon occlusion–type EPD is being considered. Interrupting antegrade flow in the absence of good collateral circulation may cause the patient to have a seizure and require rapid premature deflation of the occlusion balloon. Interruption or even termination of the procedure under these circumstances increases the risk of periprocedural complications.

CATHETER SELECTION FOR DIAGNOSTIC ANGIOGRAPHY

A variety of catheters are available for diagnostic cerebral angiography, and selection is tied to operator familiarity and experience. Examples of diagnostic catheters are shown in Figure 32-13. It should be understood that catheters that require additional manipulations to reshape them within the ascending aorta increase the risk of embolization. Use of such catheters should be reserved for negotiating the difficult aortic arch anatomy (e.g., patients with extended, stiff, calcified aortas [see Fig. 32-12, type III arch]) when use of alternative preshaped catheters that require less manipulation have either failed or are expected to fail.

Diagnostic angiography involves injection of 2 to 3 mL of non-ionic contrast diluted with an equal amount of saline. Immediately prior to acquisition of the subtraction angiogram, patients are asked not to breathe, move, or swallow to minimize motion artifact. They are also warned that they may experience a funny taste and may see flashing or multicolored lights in the ipsilateral eye.

Diagnostic angiography consists of visualization of the origins of the innominate and left common carotid arteries from the aortic arch (by selective injections), both carotid bifurcations in orthogonal projections, and both vertebral arteries (usually by nonselective injections). Intracranial images of both carotid arteries are routinely acquired, and occasionally selective injection of one or both vertebral arteries is also performed. Brachiocephalic angiography has several advantages:

1. It is a reliable, reproducible method for precisely measuring the degree of carotid artery stenosis (see Fig. 32-1).
2. It demonstrates anatomical conditions that can be unfavorable for carotid stenting. Examples include dilated/extended aortic arch (see Fig. 32-12), marked vessel tortuosity, heavily calcified stenosis, and lesions with obvious filling defects (see Figs. 32-3 through 32-11).
3. It helps define the status of collateral circulation to the ipsilateral cerebral hemisphere (i.e., the one supplied by the stenotic carotid artery being evaluated for treatment). Knowledge of contralateral carotid stenosis or occlusion and status of the collateral supply influences the stenting technique: shorter balloon inflations, for example, and choice of protection device—flow interrupting (occlusion balloon) vs. flow preserving (filter devices). The term *isolated hemisphere* describes the anatomical situation where the cerebral hemisphere of interest is entirely dependent on the ipsilateral ICA for its blood supply, owing to absence of the anterior and posterior communicating arteries.
4. It reliably demonstrates significant flow-limiting stenosis distal to the carotid bifurcation. Although the bifurcation stenosis may be treatable, the ultimate benefit of stroke reduction may not accrue to the patient because of additional cephalad disease.
5. In the event there is an intraprocedural neurological event, the postevent intracranial angiograms can be compared with the baseline preprocedure pictures.

The main risks of invasive cerebral angiography relate to the use of contrast and the possibility of a neurological event. The typical sequence of acquisition and the usual angiographic views are listed in Box 32-3.

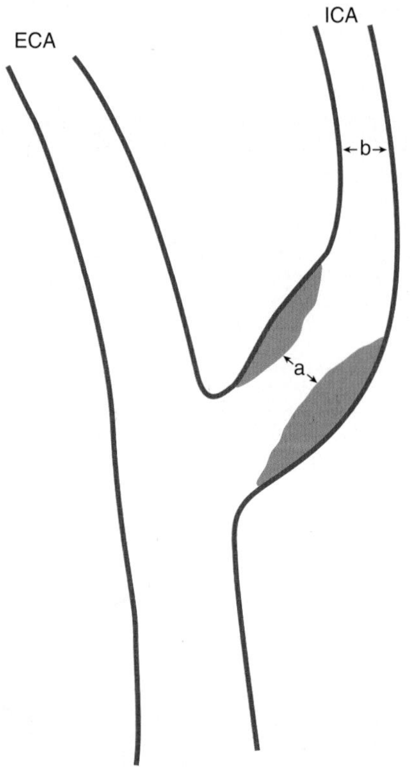

Carotid Sheath Placement

Once the diagnostic study is completed, the ICA with the target stenosis is identified, and there are no anatomical contraindications for stenting, a 90-cm long, 6 F sheath is advanced into the CCA using one of two techniques shown in Figure 32-14.

FIGURE 32-13 North American Symptomatic Carotid Endarterectomy Trial (NASCET) criteria for determining degree of carotid artery stenosis. Luminal diameter at site of greatest narrowing is recorded in three planes and used as the numerator (a). A reference diameter is taken across a plaque-free section of internal carotid artery distal to stenosis (b) and is used as the denominator. A percentage stenosis is then calculated. *(From North American Symptomatic Carotid Endarterectomy Trial. Methods, patient characteristics, and progress. Stroke 22:711–720, 1991.)*

Box 32-3 Overview of Carotid Angiography Acquisition Views

Left Subclavian Angiogram (PA View)
- The ostium of the left vertebral artery is usually seen well in the frontal projection; if not, the RAO-cranial projection should be tried.
- If a selective angiogram of the left vertebral artery is to be acquired, a roadmap to facilitate entry and selective placement of the catheter is recommended.
- Selective or nonselective intracranial views of the vertebrobasilar system are acquired in the lateral and steep AP cranial views.

Selective Left Carotid Angiograms
- The bifurcation is imaged in LAO 45-degree as well as lateral projections. If the bifurcation is "overrotated," an AP caudal view usually separates the external and internal carotid arteries very well.
- Intracranial images of the left carotid artery are acquired in the lateral and AP cranial (15- to 30-degree) views.

Innominate Angiogram in the RAO Caudal View
- Best for separating the carotid and the right subclavian arteries and hence very helpful for defining lesions involving the origin of the right subclavian artery.

Selective Right Carotid Angiograms
- Bifurcation is imaged in the RAO 45-degree as well as lateral projections.
- Intracranial images of the right carotid artery are acquired in the lateral and AP cranial (15- to 30-degree) views.

AP, anteroposterior; LAO, left anterior oblique; PA, posteroanterior; RAO, right anterior oblique.

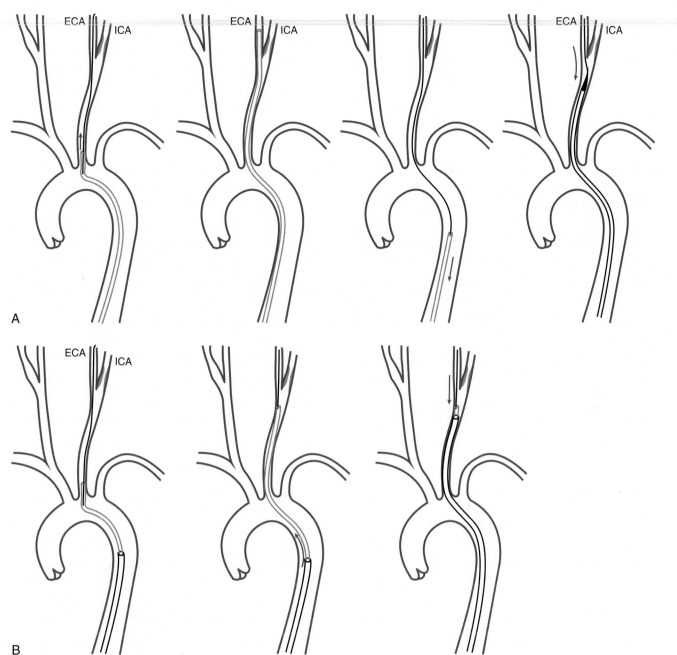

FIGURE 32-14　Carotid sheath placement. A, In the two-step approach using a diagnostic catheter, a Glidewire (Boston Scientific, Watertown, Mass.) is inserted into external carotid artery (ECA). Catheter is advanced to the ECA, and the Glidewire exchanged for a support wire such as a Supra Core (Abbott Vascular, Santa Clara, Calif.) wire. Catheter is then removed, and sheath with introducer is advanced over support wire to common carotid artery (CCA). Finally the introducer and wire are removed. **B,** In the single-step or telescoping approach, sheath is placed in descending aorta. A catheter is used to place a Glidewire in the ECA, and the catheter is advanced to the CCA. Glidewire and catheter are fixed in place and the sheath advanced over the two. With sheath in place, Glidewire and catheter are then removed.

TWO-STEP OVER-THE-WIRE APPROACH

The two-step over-the-wire approach is suitable in cases where the 100-cm 5 F diagnostic catheter is already in place in the CCA below the carotid bifurcation. A small quantity of diluted contrast is injected to produce a map of the bifurcation and the ipsilateral ECA. Once the origin and course of the ECA are defined, the 0.038-inch Glidewire (Boston Scientific, Watertown, Mass.) is reintroduced into the catheter and used to help direct the catheter into the ECA. The Glidewire is withdrawn and replaced with a 0.035-inch support wire, the catheter is withdrawn, and the sheath is advanced into the CCA over the exchange-length support wire, anchored as far distal as possible in the ECA. The main advantage of this approach is that the carotid artery need not be reengaged, reducing catheter manipulation in the aortic arch.

ONE-STEP (TELESCOPING) APPROACH

If diagnostic angiography has been performed in an earlier procedure, the stenting procedure begins with placement of the sheath into the descending thoracic aorta a short distance below the origin of the left subclavian artery. After withdrawing the inner dilator from the sheath, a 125-cm 5 F diagnostic catheter is inserted through the rotating valve of the Tuohy-Borst adaptor into the 6 F sheath. Using a 0.038-inch Glidewire and the catheter, the innominate or left CCA is engaged, and the catheter is then advanced into the carotid artery (road mapping is often helpful at this stage). The 6 F sheath is advanced over the diagnostic catheter into the CCA. If advancement of the sheath encounters resistance, the catheter is exchanged for the inner dilator of the sheath and then advanced into the CCA. If additional support is required, the 0.038-inch

Glidewire can be exchanged for stiffer 0.035- or 0.038-inch support guidewires. As soon as the sheath is placed into the arterial system, the patient is systemically anticoagulated with heparin (70 units/kg) to raise the activated clotting time (ACT) to between 225 and 250 seconds. Since the usual procedure time from this point is 20 minutes, further heparin administration is rarely required. Larger doses of heparin may increase the risk of catastrophic postperfusion hemorrhage. If bivalirudin is used, the standard bolus and infusion are a 0.75 mg/kg bolus and 1.75 mg/kg/h infusion, respectively. Reduced doses should be used for patients with significant renal impairment.

ADVANTAGES OF THE COAXIAL SHEATH TECHNIQUE

The coaxial sheath technique has a number of advantages:
1. It permits continuous access to the CCA once the sheath is in the CCA below the bifurcation.
2. Once the sheath is placed in a suitable spot below the bifurcation of the CCA, unfavorable anatomy (elongated arch, tortuosity of the CCA) will not impact the technical success of the procedure.
3. When passing the guidewire through the stenosis is difficult (eccentric stenosis, ulcerations, ICA kinks and tortuosity, or angulated takeoff of the ICA) or in the event of a complication (dissection, intracranial embolism), the coaxial configuration offers more support and allows easy introduction of other interventional tools.
4. The sheath carries a large-bore Tuohy-Borst adaptor that permits catheter or other device introduction with minimal blood loss and minimal risk of air trapping. The side arm allows intermittent or continuous flushing and contrast injection and also allows for continuous intraarterial (IA) blood pressure monitoring.
5. The integrated dilator provides a good fit and a smooth transition, features that facilitate advancement of the sheath in the two-step technique with minimal scraping of the plaque at the origin of the great vessels/aortic arch.

DISADVANTAGES OF THE COAXIAL SYSTEM (SHEATH OR GUIDING CATHETER)

There are also a few disadvantages to the coaxial system:
1. If the carotid artery is tortuous, placement of the sheath exaggerates existing kinks and redundancies, and the tortuosity, along with the carotid bifurcation, is frequently displaced cephalad. Although these disappear once the sheath is withdrawn, these iatrogenic problems can increase the complexity and technical difficulty of the stenting procedure.
2. Rarely, dissection of the innominate artery or CCA may result following advancement of the sheath over the 5 F diagnostic catheter (telescoping technique).
3. There is always the possibility of embolization during sheath placement, a part of the procedure that cannot be neuroprotected.

SHEATH VS. GUIDE CATHETER

A guide catheter sits fairly low in the carotid artery, since it only engages the origin and first few centimeters of the carotid artery. Hence, use of a guide catheter is preferred if there is significant tortuosity of the proximal segment of the CCA because placement of the sheath across this tortuous segment (assuming it will be possible to traverse the entire CCA and straighten the tortuosity) will result in the redundancy being displaced cephalad, with obvious disadvantages.

IMAGING FOLLOWING SHEATH PLACEMENT

Once the sheath is in position, baseline angiograms are acquired using appropriately angled views to help display the maximum severity of the stenosis. Note that the optimal angulations for performing the intervention need not be identical to the one needed for displaying the maximum severity of the stenosis. The working projection (i.e., the one used for the stenting procedure) should maximally separate the ICA and ECA and clearly display bony landmarks. The operator should have a clear idea about the stenosis location in relation to the bony landmarks, recognizing that placement of the sheath can alter the relationship by displacing loops and bends in the carotid artery cephalad.

Embolic Protection Devices

Although not all steps of the carotid intervention can be "emboli protected" because placement of the sheath occurs prior to deployment of the EPD. It is important to recognize, however, that the risk of embolization is highest during stent deployment and balloon dilation.[64]

A number of EPDs are available and can be broadly divided into *flow-interrupting* (occlusive) and *flow-preserving* (nonocclusive) devices (Fig. 32-15). Occlusion EPDs can be subdivided into *distal occlusion* and *proximal occlusion* types. An example of a flow-interrupting EPD that is deployed distal to the stenosis is the Percusurge GuardWire (Medtronic, Minneapolis, Minn.). Proximal occlusion devices include those developed by Gore (Flagstaff, Ariz.) and the MoMa device (Medtronic, Minneapolis, Minn.). Although flow-interrupting occlusive-type EPDs are intuitively appealing (no blood flow = no emboli), some issues with their use have arisen. For example, to permit occlusion and interruption of antegrade flow in the ipsilateral carotid artery, it is mandatory to demonstrate robust collateral circulation to the hemisphere being treated. Infrequent use of the GuardWire device, as well as occasional device failure (inadequate balloon inflation and suboptimal seal of the carotid artery and/or premature deflation), has resulted in virtual abandonment of this device for carotid intervention. The rationale for use of proximal occlusion devices is

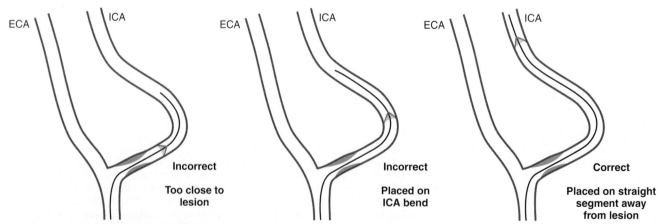

FIGURE 32-15 Correct placement of embolic protection device. Device is deployed cephalad to stenosis in a straight segment of the internal carotid artery (ICA) to ensure all antegrade flow passes through, not around, the filter. It must also be sufficiently distal to lesion to enable stent deployment and expansion. Filters must not be placed on curves of the ICA.

based not only on interruption of antegrade flow but also flow reversal in the ipsilateral ICA. This combination is achieved by balloon occlusion of both the CCA and ECA. Although procedural outcomes using these devices are favorable,[65,66] they are more in the category of a niche device, since the catheters are substantially larger. They are particularly useful in cases with tortuous distal ICA anatomies or lesions with filling defects that may embolize during wire passage *prior to* deployment of the distal EPD.

The nonocclusive flow-preserving devices are the filters. Depending on construction, the filter body can be supported with a nitinol frame or be unsupported and resemble a windsock. The underlying principles and rationale for use are the same for all filter EPDs: preserving antegrade flow while preventing passage of embolic debris. As may be expected, each of these EPDs has certain unique features, and familiarity with their construction and attributes will allow judicious selection of the device most appropriate for use with a particular anatomy.

EMBOLIC PROTECTION DEVICE DEPLOYMENT

The device has to be placed approximately 2 cm cephalad to the stenosis to provide adequate space (the "landing zone" for the EPD) to accommodate the tip of the stent delivery system and allow satisfactory coverage of the lesion with the stent (Fig. 32-16).

For severe subocclusive stenosis, "pre-predilation" using a low-profile coronary angioplasty balloon (2 or 2.5 mm diameter) is very helpful. Although this type of dilation is not protected, the risk of this approach should be counterbalanced with the problems of trying to force an EPD through a very severe stenosis. The tip of the wire relative to the EPD should be angiographically visible throughout all steps of the procedure, and the operator should ensure that the wire and EPD are stable with minimal or no movement, since excessive movement can lead to spasm and slow flow.

Lesion Predilation

Lesion predilation should be considered the default strategy because:
- Experimental studies using *ex vivo* models[67] have demonstrated that large amounts of embolic debris are released with primary stenting without predilation.
- Postdilation of the constricted stent can worsen the scissoring effect of the stent wires on the plaque, increasing risk of embolization.

- Predilation facilitates smoother passage of the 5 F or 6 F self-expanding stent delivery system.
- Without predilation, the operator may find it difficult to withdraw the distal tip of the stent delivery system through the narrowed constricted portion of the stent.
- The narrowed stent may present problems during balloon passage for stent postdilation.

Use of a 3 or 3.5 mm × 30 mm coronary balloon inflated to nominal pressure is recommended for predilation. The markers on the ends of the 30-mm-long balloon help the operator select the length of the stent (30 or 40 mm). Predilation is generally brief, and gradual deflation is recommended. On rare occasion when treating a heavily calcified lesion, the stent may not pass easily through the stenosis, despite adequate predilation. In this setting, a larger 4- or 5-mm balloon may be needed for additional predilations. Following predilation and immediately prior to stenting, an arteriogram is performed to once again establish the relationship of the stenosis to the bony landmarks.

Stents

To eliminate the risk of deformation and crushing[23] seen with balloon expandable stents, self-expanding stents are exclusively used for carotid stenting, with the following notable *exceptions*:

1. When treating an aorto-ostial stenosis of the CCA.
2. When the stenosis and treatment involve the distal portion of the cervical carotid artery (close to the skull base). There is minimal risk of stent deformation of a balloon expandable stent deployed at this level, and advancing the bulkier 5 F or 6 F self-expanding stent delivery systems to the distal ICA can be technically difficult.

Although the Elgiloy (a cobalt chromium alloy) tracheobronchial Wallstent, (Boston Scientific, Natick, Mass.) was initially used, most operators currently use self-expanding nitinol stents. The Wallstent, an example of a closed-cell stent (see later discussion), fell out of favor largely because of its unpredictable foreshortening. This feature makes precise positioning of the stent very difficult. Despite structural and technical differences between the Elgiloy Wallstent and nitinol stents, there was no significant difference in carotid stenting outcomes using the Wallstent approved for use in the carotid circulation on the basis of the Boston Scientific EPI: A Carotid Stenting Trial for High-Risk Surgical Patients (BEACH) trial.[68]

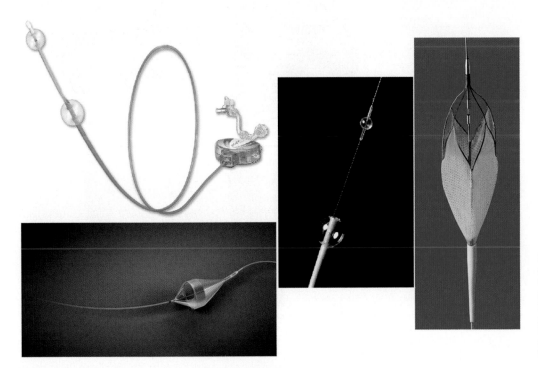

FIGURE 32-16 Examples of embolic protection devices. *Clockwise from Top Left,* MoMa proximal occlusion device (Medtronic, Minneapolis, Minn.) and Gore flow-reversal system (Gore, Flagstaff, Ariz.). Nonocclusive filters are the Accunet and Emboshield (both from Abbott Vascular, Santa Clara, Calif.).

The unconstrained diameter of the self-expanding stent should be at least 1 or 2 mm larger than the largest-diameter segment intended to be covered by the stent, almost always the CCA. For example, our preference in most cases is to use an 8- to 10-mm tapered stent; an 8-mm-diameter stent segment is deployed in the ICA, while the wider 10-mm end of the stent extends into the CCA. The stent is deployed slowly to minimize its tendency to jump forward. It is important to ensure that the caudal end of the stent is firmly anchored in the CCA. If not, the angulated proximal edge of the stent can cause difficulties in recrossing the stent with either the post-dilation balloon or the EPD retrieval sheath.

Tips in stent selection, deployment, and positioning include:

1. If the lesion is on a bend, an open-cell (Fig. 32-17A) stent design should be selected (instead of a closed-cell design). Open-cell stents conform to the bend in the artery; a more rigid closed-cell (Fig. 32-17B) stent straightens the bend. Since the carotid artery is fixed at the skull base (as well as at its origin from the aorta), kinks and bends in the artery, a con-

sequence of carotid redundancy resulting from elongation of the artery (seen with increasing frequency in the elderly hypertensive patient) cannot be eliminated by placing a stent in the kink. Instead, these kinks are displaced cephalad.

2. Deploying a closed-cell stent in a patient with significant tortuosity almost always results in a sharp angulation of the carotid artery immediately cephalad to the distal stent edge (Fig. 32-18). The stented portion of the artery appears as a straight segment.

3. An important technical point is to release the distal 3 to 5 mm of the stent and wait for the stent to expand fully and stabilize against the vessel wall before releasing the remainder of the stent. Nitinol stents have a tendency to jump distally if released too fast.

4. In our technique, the caudal end of the stent rests in the CCA, so a tapered stent with a diameter of 10 mm is preferred. Rarely, the stent is placed exclusively in the ICA. In this case, a 6- or 8-mm-diameter stent can be selected.

5. In almost all cases, the stent is placed across the bifurcation into the CCA and crosses the origin of the ECA. Covering the

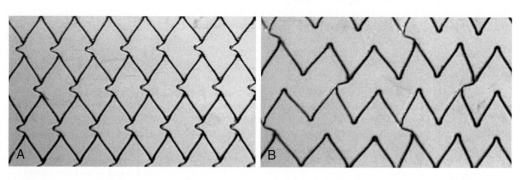

FIGURE 32-17 Comparison of open- and closed-cell stent designs. Operators should have one of each type available and be familiar with its use, enabling the correct choice to be made in each individual case.

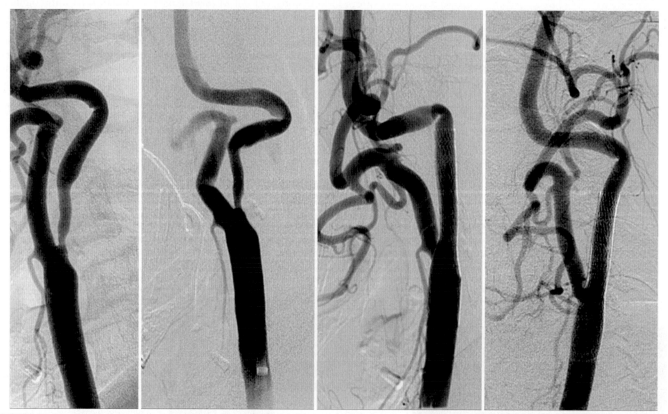

FIGURE 32-18 Angulation of cranial segment of internal carotid artery (ICA) due to catheter introduction and stent implantation. First panel demonstrates acute angulation of ICA distal to stenosis, with a 5 F diagnostic catheter in position. Introduction of a 6 F guide sheath further exacerbates this and induces a stenosis at the bend. Following stent implantation (open-cell) in third panel and almost complete withdrawal of sheath, stenosis and angulation significantly resolve. This lesion was not treated. Panel 4 shows same lesion at angiography 3 months later when patient returned for contralateral carotid artery stenting.

origin of the ECA with a stent rarely causes a lasting clinical problem. The ECA can be re-canalized if it becomes significantly stenosed or occluded after post-dilation of the stent, or if the patient is symptomatic (jaw or facial pain).

6. It is important to acquire an angiogram just prior to introducing the stent delivery system through the Touhey-Bourst adaptor. Stent deployment should be done using cervical spine bony landmarks as a guide (a road map can also be used to help guide stent deployment and positioning). Once the stent delivery system is in place across the carotid bifurcation, additional dye injections to help guide stent positioning are *contraindicated*. This is an important safety consideration because injecting dye with the stent delivery system in place (prior to releasing the stent) has been associated with an approximately 15% incidence of air embolism.

7. A closed-cell stent design (see Fig. 32-17), because of its smaller free cell area, gives the maximal and best circumferential wall coverage and a visually compelling angiographic result. Further, in our experience involving more than 2000 closed-cell nitinol stents, restenosis rates are very low. Some operators have proposed that the closed-cell structure can act as a barrier, preventing release of any additional embolic debris. Although open-cell stents (see Fig. 32-17) conform very well to the bends in the artery, there have been concerns that the stent struts projecting into the lumen of the artery may cause problems with recrossing the stent with the post-dilation balloon an d/or EPD retrieval catheter. There are theoretical advantages and disadvantages to each of the two stent designs. Some have proposed that use of closed-cell stents may be associated with lower stroke and death rates when compared to stenting with open-cell designs.[69,70] The issue is far from settled. Two recent publications showed no difference in either embolic load[71] or long-term outcomes[72] based on stent design. Additionally, there were no differences in outcomes in two large postapproval studies. The second phase of the Carotid RX Acculink/RX Accunet Post-Approval Trial to Uncover Unanticipated or Rare Events (CAPTURE 2; $n = 4175$) used the Acculink stent, an open-cell design from Abbott Vascular, Santa Clara, California, and the Emboshield and Xact Post-Approval Carotid Stent Trial (EXACT; $n = 2145$) used Abbott Vascular's Xact stent, a closed-cell design.[73]

Post-dilation

The size of the post-dilation balloon is matched to the diameter of the ICA at the site of the stenosis. Typically, the self-expanding stent is post-dilated with a 5-mm, 0.014-inch wire-compatible balloon. On occasion, high-pressure balloons may be needed to postdilate a stent deployed within a heavily calcified stenosis.

Post-dilation of the stent is a critical step:

1. It is possibly the time when the greatest number of emboli are released, and consequently the patient is at the greatest risk of stroke. The embolic load can be minimized by:
   - Using balloons that are no larger than 5.0 mm in diameter.
   - Inflating the postdilation balloon to nominal pressures.
   - Accepting a 10% to 20% residual stenosis. This degree of residual stenosis does not cause hemodynamic problems and does not impact the rate of restenosis. Self-expanding stents have a tendency for late progressive expansion.
   - Performing a SINGLE post-implantion dilation.

2. It is safer to underdilate than overdilate a self-expanding stent. Overdilation with a high-pressure balloon has the potential to squeeze the atherosclerotic material through the stent mesh, increasing the risk of distal embolization.

3. In some cases, a residual ulcer that is opacified by contrast flow through the stent struts is seen. No attempt should be made to obliterate this ulcer by using larger balloons or higher pressures in an effort to fill the ulcer crater with the stent. This communication (with the ulcer via the stent struts) will seal off and is of no clinical consequence.

Final Angiographic Assessment

CERVICAL INTERNAL CAROTID ARTERY

Following stent post-dilation, final angiograms are required in the same projections that demonstrated the maximum severity of the lesion in both digitally subtracted and regular formats. Particular attention must be directed to the ICA immediately cephalad to the stent and the site of the EPD placement. It is not unusual to encounter vessel spasm in this segment, particularly if the ICA is tortuous or there has been some movement of the distal EPD. A small dose of IA nitroglycerin should be judiciously used (as a consequence of the stretch of the carotid baroreceptors, most patients would be relatively hypotensive, limiting the use of nitroglycerin; see also discussion on hyperperfusion hemorrhage). Pulling back the sheath to the CCA origin relaxes the artery, helps relieve the spasm, and enables the operator to more accurately assess the status of the stented vessel. Distal linear edge dissections are unusual, and when present are short and for the most part inconsequential. Occasionally, such dissections may require treatment, and an additional stent may be necessary.

INTRACRANIAL VESSELS

Postprocedural intracranial angiograms are indicated if the patient has had any intraprocedural neurological deficit. Nearly all current carotid stenting investigational protocols call for repeat intracranial views, which should be acquired in the same projections as baseline.

Embolic Protection Device and Sheath Removal and Access Site Hemostasis

To be effective as an emboli trapping device, the size of the pores in the fabric of the filter have to be microns in diameter. Passage of blood through these small pores stimulates the deposition of fibrin within the filter, providing the perfect conditions for formation of a thrombus within the filter. The longer the dwell time, the greater the chances of formation of an iatrogenic thrombus. When using filter EPDs, it is important to minimize both the number of contrast injections and the *in vivo* dwell time; median time should not exceed 7 minutes, and consistent breach of this time limit is a quality concern. If the proximal edge of the stent is not well opposed to the wall of the CCA, either as a result of stent undersizing or improper positioning, it may be difficult to advance the EPD retrieval sheath (or postdilation balloons) through the stent. The best ways to overcome this difficulty are to (1) ask the patient to turn the head to one side or (2) advance the sheath into the stent. Some have recommended that only the proximal part of the filter should be captured, since pulling the filter completely into the capture sheath may squeeze out the emboli. Following withdrawal of the EPD, the Tuohy-Bourst adaptor should be fully opened and allowed to bleed back generously in case particles and atheromatous debris have been released into the guide catheter during withdrawal of the EPD device.

At the completion of the procedure, the sheath should be gently pulled back and out of the carotid artery and exchanged for a short sheath, which can be removed when hemostasis can be safely achieved. The vagal response to manual sheath removal and compression can compound the baroreflex effect of carotid stenting and lead to profound hypotension and bradycardia. In most patients, access-site hemostasis can be obtained using closure devices, although no improvement in outcomes has been demonstrated.[74] Finally, although low blood pressure is not unusual in the immediate postprocedure phase, other causes (e.g., retroperitoneal hemorrhage related to access-site bleeding) should be considered as reasons for unexplained persistent hypotension.

Patients are monitored in a telemetry bed overnight, and more than 95% will be ready for discharge approximately 24 hours following the procedure. All patients should have a postprocedural neurological exam and assessment of the NIH and Rankin Stroke

Box 32-4 Discharge Protocol

- Ambulate as tolerated next day.
- NIH Stroke Scale before discharge.
- Aspirin 325 mg PO daily for 1 month, then 81 mg PO indefinitely; clopidogrel 75 mg PO daily for a minimum of 4 weeks.
- Clinical evaluation at 1 month, 6 months, 12 months, and yearly thereafter.
- Carotid duplex ultrasound at 1 month, 6 months, 12 months, and yearly thereafter.
- Neurological evaluation at 1 month and 12 months.
- MRI (e.g., of cervical spine) is not contraindicated, since the stent is nonferromagnetic. However, follow-up MRA to evaluate stent status is contraindicated because there will be a dropout in the image within the stented segment (suggesting stent occlusion) related to the Faraday cage effect.
- Patients who have received radiation treatment to the neck for malignancy should be on lifelong dual antiplatelet therapy.
- At discharge, decision to restart β-blockers, diuretics, and other antihypertensive medications is dictated by the hemodynamics. Almost all patients will be back on the preprocedure doses of these medications within a few days of discharge.
- Maintain meticulous follow-up records and a database to enable tracking patient outcomes.

MRA, magnetic resonance angiography; MRI, magnetic resonance imaging; NIH, National Institutes of Health; PO, per os (orally).

Scales. Once patients are able to ambulate without difficulty, they can be discharged with instructions to return for follow-up in 4 weeks (Box 32-4).

Management of Hemodynamics

The carotid sinus baroreceptor, innervated by the glossopharyngeal nerve (cranial nerve IX), is located in the adventitia of the carotid artery and is activated by stretching of the blood vessel wall. The physiological role of this mechanoreceptor is to detect, respond, and regulate the systemic blood pressure. Stimulation of the carotid sinus baroreceptor (via stretching) stimulates the glossopharyngeal nerve, which in turn stimulates the vasomotor center in the medulla via the tractus solitarius, which then modulates the activity of the autonomic nervous system (suppresses sympathetic and stimulates parasympathetic output). The net effect of stimulation of the carotid baroreceptor is bradycardia (negative chronotropy), as well as some reduction in cardiac contractility. Additionally, the decreased sympathetic output results in vasodilation, causing hypotension. As might be expected, carotid sinus stimulation and the resultant hemodynamic perturbations are most profound when the lesion and the stretch from the postdilation balloon involve the carotid bifurcation, less so if the stenosis is cephalad to the bifurcation. These changes are not seen (or occur with much less intensity and frequency) in the postendarterectomy patient whose carotid bulb is denervated. The bradycardia and hypotension can be profound and are worse in younger patients and when treating highly calcified stenosis (where higher pressures are used for postdilating the stent). In anticipation of these hemodynamic changes:

1. Antihypertensive drugs, such as β-blockers and diuretics, are withheld on the morning of the procedure. The opening systolic pressure (i.e., pressure at the beginning of the procedure) may be elevated. Typically this is not treated; the first balloon inflation will reduce heart rate and blood pressure.
2. Ensure that the patient has adequate venous access for fluid administration. Prophylactic placement of a temporary venous pacer is no longer practiced.
3. All patients receive a prophylactic dose of atropine immediately prior to the predilation step.
4. Hypotension is primarily managed by hydration with 0.9% saline infusion. Patients with severe aortic stenosis and those with severe CAD do not tolerate hypotension and bradycardia. We consider placement of a temporary transvenous pacemaker, and occasionally placement of an intraaortic balloon

pump prior to the procedure in such cases. These can typically be removed at the conclusion of the procedure.
5. Pharmacological management of hypotension involves use of α-agonists like intravenous (IV) phenylephrine. If there has been significant reduction in blood pressure prior to the post-dilation step, it is a good strategy to administer phenylephrine prior to balloon dilation. This will temporarily elevate blood pressure, and hemodynamic issues will not prevent the operator from performing a single inflation with the balloon inflated to the appropriate pressure.
6. We do *not* advocate use of dopamine. Although blood pressure will improve, there are also unwanted side effects of tachycardia and/or provocation of arrhythmias, which can be a problem in patients with underlying coronary artery disease.

Close attention should be paid to both intra- and post-procedure blood pressure management. The hemodynamic effect of the atropine and α-agonists used during the procedure is short-lived. In the postprocedure phase, *hypotension* with systolic blood pressures as low as 70 to 80 mmHg is usually asymptomatic and may be managed expectantly. The systolic blood pressure will typically increase by 15 to 30 mmHg by next morning. Hypotension usually presents a problem in two settings: (1) patients with a periprocedural embolic event or a severe contralateral carotid stenosis can become symptomatic, and (2) patients with baseline renal insufficiency may have worsening kidney function as a result of the combination of low blood pressure and contrast exposure.

The risk of hyperperfusion syndrome (discussed later) is increased if blood pressure remains *elevated* following dilation (e.g., in the post-endarterectomy patient with severe post-CEA restenosis).

Management of Neurological Complications

The neurological status of the patient should be monitored at frequent intervals since every maneuver in the carotid artery has the potential to cause embolization. We ask the patient to squeeze a toy placed in the contralateral hand. Also, conversing with the patient and judging the speed and the appropriateness of the response to simple questions is very useful. Any departure from baseline status in an unsedated patient (including frequent yawning) are red flags indicating a possible neurological event (which at times can be very subtle).

The incidence of major stroke and any stroke in contemporary stenting practice is low. Major and fatal ischemic strokes are thought to be prevented by EPDs. Transient ischemic attacks and minor strokes continue to occur and may be due to embolic particles that evade the filters or embolization that occurs during unprotected phases of the procedure.

If the patient develops a neurological deficit during the procedure, the procedure should be completed, the EPD removed, and normal flow established. Patients should be hydrated with isotonic fluids, and adequate blood pressure should be maintained (both hypotension and relative dehydration worsen the effects of small emboli that otherwise may be clinically silent). At the conclusion of the procedure, the patient should be reassessed clinically, and intracranial angiograms should be repeated in views comparable to baseline projections. Angiograms may reveal:

1. Occlusion of a proximal vessel segment (e.g., M1 or M2 segment). Intervention is generally required, since these patients are unlikely to make a spontaneous recovery.
2. Distal occlusion of a single small branch—best managed with conservative measures.
3. Normal appearance, no loss of branches—good prognosis for full recovery of function.
4. Slow flow and/or appearance of emboli in multiple branches—prognosis is guarded, and chances for full recovery are generally poor.

If a neurovascular rescue intervention is required, it usually will involve mechanical recanalization (wires, balloons, snares) in an attempt to reestablish flow in the affected segment. In general, use of additional pharmacological agents like IA tissue plasminogen activator (tPA) or glycoprotein (GP) IIb/IIIa antagonists are contraindicated because of the prohibitive risk of intracranial bleeding and its attendant high mortality.

Rarely, a patient may develop ipsilateral partial or complete loss of vision due to retinal infarction. Unless there is spontaneous recovery of vision soon after the event, the prognosis for full recovery of vision is poor, despite immediate decompression of intraophthalmic pressure and attempts to move the occluding embolus distally to minimize the extent of retinal infarction.

In contemporary practice of carotid stenting, the overall risk of a clinically significant intracerebral hemorrhage (ICH) is small—around 0.5 to 1%. Chances of iatrogenic intracerebral bleeding can be minimized by using lower doses of anticoagulants during the procedure (ACT is maintained between 225 and 250 seconds), avoiding GP IIb/IIIa inhibitors, and careful wire control during the procedure.

Cerebral Hyperperfusion Syndrome

Cerebral hyperperfusion syndrome (CHS) is a rare but serious complication of carotid revascularization. Following successful carotid revascularization, there is an increase in ipsilateral blood flow to the affected cerebral hemisphere. Most often the patient remains asymptomatic[75]; however, in some patients this increase can overwhelm normal compensatory mechanisms, resulting in a marked increase in flow. *Cerebral hyperperfusion* is defined as an increase in blood flow of greater than 100% from baseline, and CHS is hyperperfusion associated with neurological deficit. Estimated incidence varies according to methodology and definitions, but most published studies report a rate less than 3%.[76]

The pathophysiology of CHS is not completely understood but is most likely due to a combination of factors. Patients with chronic cerebral hypoperfusion have maximal dilation of the intracranial arterioles, and normal autoregulation may not be restored for several days or weeks following revascularization. *Impaired autoregulation* refers to failure of the brain at the microcirculatory level to modulate blood flow and blood pressure such that sudden increase in flow and pressure is not transmitted to small blood vessels. Rather, pressure and flow are maintained within a narrow range. Impaired autoregulation of small-vessel cerebral blood flow (CBF) has been implicated in CHS in experimental models. This is either due to endothelial dysfunction resulting from free radical accumulation,[77] or neurogenic failure of smooth-muscle regulation.[78] Failure of the normal baroreceptor reflex is another possibility, with uncompensated postprocedural hypertension contributing to hyperperfusion.[79] Impairment of the trigeminovascular reflex may also contribute because it plays a role in maintaining normal cerebrovascular tone.[80] Hyperperfusion results in fluid entering the interstitial space and causing edema, predominantly in the posterior circulation.

Those with severe (>90%) subocclusive stenosis, with limited collateral supply (isolated hemisphere), are most at risk for hyperperfusion.[81] Baseline severe hypertension and persistence of increased blood pressure in the postprocedure period (not uncommon in patients postendarterectomy) can result in hyperperfusion lasting several days following a procedure.[81]

The most common clinical symptom of cerebral hyperperfusion is headache. Not uncommonly, patients report this symptom on the table soon after the procedure is completed. The headache may last a few days, is typically unilateral, and is associated with a nonfocal neurological exam. A more serious presentation, possibly related to cerebral edema, is seizure. Patients with CHS can present with a variety of neurological deficits, including isolated speech disturbance. In patients who develop neurological symptoms following carotid revascularization, other etiologies must be considered in the differential diagnosis. Differentiation must be made between procedure-related embolic complications with an ischemic infarct, manifestation of a low-flow state, and a high-flow state characteristic of CHS. The diagnosis of CHS is best confirmed with MRI.[76]

Treatment involves lowering blood pressure, reduction in cerebral edema, and anticonvulsant therapy. Because vasorelaxation may further increase cerebral blood flow, calcium antagonists and nitrates are contraindicated in the treatment of CHS. Hence, the operator must resist the urge to administer nitrates to relieve spasm (e.g., at the site of deployment of the EPD noted on the postprocedure angiogram); it will resolve gradually with time. Although nitrates will rapidly resolve spasm, they can also predispose to development of hyperperfusion. Owing to their ability to reduce cerebral perfusion pressure, labetalol and clonidine[76,82] are the preferred agents. Duration of therapy is not well defined; treatment may be needed for several days or months post procedure.[83] There is insufficient evidence to support the treatment of cerebral edema, although corticosteroids and barbiturates have been used to good effect. Prophylactic anticonvulsant treatment is not recommended but should be introduced if seizures occur.[76]

The relative infrequency of this condition and the heterogeneity of presentations make it hard to generalize outcomes following CHS. However, the limited data from the CEA literature suggest that a third of patients may remain disabled following CHS,[84] with others reporting mortality rates of up to 50%.[85] Therefore, although rare, the diagnosis should be considered in all patients who develop neurological symptoms following carotid revascularization.

Results of Carotid Stenting without Embolic Protection

As was the case with other arterial percutaneous interventions, the evolution and availability of arterial stents transformed the procedure. By the early 1990s, prospective observational studies of carotid stenting had been initiated.[21] From the outset, carotid stenting performed by experienced operators produced acceptable outcomes in terms of disabling stroke and death. Nondisabling neurological events were evident and clustered in patients with advanced age, complex aortic arch and ICA anatomies, and severe ICA stenoses.[22,86] Recognition of the importance of patient selection and continued refinement of the technique, largely made possible by the introduction of devices dedicated for use in the extracranial carotid arteries, helped improve outcomes by minimizing neurological complications.

Numerous case reports and clinical series of carotid stenting without embolic protection have been published.[20,22,87–93] An early report of 117 carotid stenting procedures by Diethrich et al.[89] documented a 6.4% rate of periprocedural neurological events; most of these were transient ischemic events or minor strokes with eventual full recovery. A high rate of local adverse events was related to direct common carotid cervical access, a technique that has largely been abandoned.

Following this, there were several encouraging reports of outcomes from other experienced centers.[20,22,87,88,90,91] These were mixed series of symptomatic and asymptomatic patients with varying degrees of arterial stenosis. Asymptomatic patients were generally required to have more severe stenosis or additional evidence of compromised cerebral circulation.[19,22,89] Some reports included CCA lesions, which are not easily accessible by surgical techniques.[22,89,94,95] These studies reported very high rates (>95%) of procedural and stenting success, with periprocedural minor stroke rates of 1.6% to 4.8% and major stroke/mortality rates between 1% and 1.5%.

Reviews of the status of carotid artery stent placement prior to the introduction of EPDs were published in 1998[96] and 2000.[87] These observational and unaudited data provided an overall perspective on the status of stenting at that time. Thirty-six centers participated in the survey, which included 5210 stenting procedures. These documented a technical success rate of 98.4%. The 30-day rates of TIAs, minor strokes, major strokes, and mortality were 2.6%, 2.5%, 1.4%, and 0.8%, respectively.[87] It was noted that technical failures were usually related to inability to access the CCA (2%-7% of patients), and prolonged procedural time was associated with increased morbidity.[96] These results in a large series of patients at high surgical risk were encouraging; rates of adverse outcomes were comparable to standard CEA risk patients treated with surgery.

Results of Carotid Stenting Using Embolic Protection

Periprocedural neurological events related to embolization during carotid arterial stent placement were not unexpected. In an effort to reduce the incidence of these adverse events, transcranial Doppler studies were performed to investigate which stages of the procedure were responsible for microemboli. Few particles are released during sheath placement, with a modest number during wire crossing and predilation. The majority of particles were found to be released from the atheromatous plaque during stent deployment and the postdilation procedure.[64] The fragments consisted of plaque debris, fibrin and platelet aggregates, lipid vacuoles, and calcium fragments.[31,97] These findings provided the basis for development and routine use of embolic protection systems during carotid stenting.

Carotid Stenting in High-Risk Carotid Endarterectomy Patients

In 1998, the Stroke Council of the AHA published a series of recommendations relating to the performance of CEA in patients with extracranial bifurcation carotid artery stenosis.[98] These recommendations were based largely on the results of ECST,[7] NASCET,[3] and ACAS.[80] These three large randomized clinical trials established the benefit of CEA over prevailing best medical treatment and have provided much of the evidence base for current treatment of carotid artery disease. The AHA Stroke Council recommended surgical revascularization in symptomatic (prior symptoms of a nondisabling stroke or TIA) patients with more than 70% carotid stenosis, provided the perioperative risk of stroke and death is less than 6%. In patients with more than 60% stenosis without prior symptoms (asymptomatic group), the recommendation for revascularization is valid provided the perioperative risk of stroke and death is less than 3% and the patient has a life expectancy of at least 5 years.

> ### Box 32-5   Clinical and Anatomical Characteristics Used to Define Patients at High Endarterectomy Risk in the NASCET and ACAS Trials
>
> **Anatomical**
> Significant lesion cranial to the body of the second cervical vertebrae
> Previous ipsilateral endarterectomy
>
> **Comorbidities**
> Age 80 years or older
> History of renal, cardiac, or hepatic failure
> Life expectancy less than 5 years

ACAS, Asymptomatic Carotid Atherosclerosis Study; NASCET, North American Symptomatic Carotid Endarterectomy Trial.

To minimize potential confounding variables, such as conditions known to increase the risk of operative treatment, patients in the NASCET and ACAS studies were carefully selected, and those who were regarded as high surgical (CEA) risk were excluded. Box 32-5 lists anatomical characteristics and comorbidities that were used to define high CEA risk. In the NASCET study, contralateral occlusion was not excluded, and 30-day risk of stroke and death in this cohort was 9.4% (≈2.2 times the risk without this problem).[6] Excluding the SAPPHIRE study (see below), surgical outcomes in high–CEA risk patients have never been tested in a large multicenter prospective trial with independent neurological assessment and event adjudication, rendering conclusions about benefit of the procedure in this population less clear.

During the initial investigation of CAS with embolic protection as a therapeutic alternative to CEA, the target population included patients who were high risk for CEA. These clinical trials were designed using a nonrandomized registry format. Since the FDA considers each carotid stent and embolic protection system as a unique device set, each with its own risk profile, as a condition of marketing (PMA) approval, every manufacturer was required to perform its own separate study. This regulatory requirement explains why so many "CEA high-risk registries"[73,99-103] were formed, all of which enrolled the same target population (Table 32-5). The study design, study hypothesis, and statistical approach were largely similar for all the registries. The goal was to determine whether outcomes in high-risk surgical patients treated with the particular sponsor's stent in conjunction with its EPD was less than or equal to that of objective performance criteria (OPC) derived from historical controls undergoing surgical intervention with CEA.

TABLE 32-5	Published Outcomes from High Carotid Endarterectomy Risk Registries*						
TRIAL	YEAR (LAST PATIENT ENROLLED)	SPONSOR	STENT	EMBOLIC PROTECTION DEVICE	DEATH/MAJOR STROKE RATE	DEATH/ STROKE/MI RATE	ASYMPTOMATIC
SAPPHIRE	2002	Cordis	Smart/Precise	Angioguard	NA	6.90%	71.2%
ARCHeR	2003	Abbott	Acculink	Accunet	2.90%	8.30%	76.2%
SECuRITY	2003	Abbott	Xact	Emboshield	3.00%	7.20%	NA
BEACH	2003	Boston	Wallstent	Filterwire EZ	2.50%	5.40%	76.7%
MAVErIC	2004	Medtronic	AVE	GuardWire	3.00%	5.40%	NA
CAPTURE	2006	Abbott	Acculink	Accunet	2.60%	6.10%	86.2%
EXACT	2007	Abbott	Xact	Emboshield	1.80%	4.60%	90.1%
EMPiRE	2008	Gore	Not specified	Gore Flow Reversal	1.60%	3.70%	68%
CAPTURE 2	2009	Abbott	Acculink	Accunet	1.40%	3.50%	86.9%
PROTECT	2009	Abbott	Xact	Emboshield	0.50%	2.30%	NA
CHOICE	Ongoing	Abbott	Xact/Acculink	Emboshield/Accunet	1.80%	3.90%	NA

*The first of these began enrolling patients in 2000 and were largely completed by 2008.
MI, myocardial infarction, NA, not available.

An OPC of 15% for patients with comorbidities and 11% for patients with anatomical risk factors was negotiated a priori and agreed to by the FDA.

The SAPPHIRE[101] study was the only one that included a randomized arm (CAS vs. stent). This multicenter noninferiority randomized study was conducted in 29 centers across the United States, and results were published in 2004.[101] The study enrolled symptomatic patients (≥50% stenosis on duplex ultrasound, 29% of the patient population) and asymptomatic patients (≥80% stenosis on duplex ultrasound), and the primary endpoint was defined as the cumulative incidence of death, stroke, and MI within 30 days of treatment, or death and ipsilateral stroke between day 31 and 1 year from the time of the procedure. Although the inclusion criteria included high–CEA risk patients, prior to randomization, all members of the investigative team (neurologist, vascular or neurosurgeon, and interventionalist) had to agree that the patient was a suitable candidate for either endarterectomy or stenting. If the surgeon assessing the patient concluded that endarterectomy could not be safely performed, but the interventional physician judged that stenting was feasible, the patient was not randomized, but instead was entered into a stent registry (n = 406). Likewise, if the surgeon deemed the patient suitable for surgery, but the interventional physician did not think stenting was feasible, the patient was entered into a surgical registry (n = 7).

Between August 2000 and July 2002, 747 patients were enrolled in the study, and 334 patients underwent randomization. Of the 167 patients randomly assigned to stenting, 159 received the assigned treatment. Of the 167 patients assigned to surgery, 151 received the assigned treatment. All 334 patients were followed. Patients undergoing CAS received the nitinol self-expanding Precise stent and the AngioGuard filter-type EPD (Cordis/Johnson & Johnson, Bridgewater, N.J.). In early 2002, the pace of enrollment abruptly slowed because several carotid stent registries (nonrandomized) had become available. The trial was therefore terminated because of the decrease in enrollment, and the primary endpoint was analyzed with respect to the noninferiority of CAS compared with CEA, using interval-censored survival data at 1 year.

By intention-to-treat analysis, the primary endpoint at 1 year occurred in 20 CAS patients (12.2%) and 32 CEA patients (20.1%); P = 0.05. Cranial nerve injuries were seen in 5% of the patients undergoing CEA. The investigators concluded that carotid stenting with embolic protection was not inferior to CEA in a high surgical risk population. The durability of carotid stenting in this patient group (*durability* refers to the procedure's ability to prevent stroke, not the need for repeat intervention due to restenosis) has been supported by the 3-year follow-up data, which demonstrated that there was no significant difference in long-term outcomes between patients who underwent CAS using an EPD and those who underwent endarterectomy.[104]

Post-approval Registries

As part of the condition for marketing approval of its devices (stents and EPDs), the sponsor, Abbott Vascular, agreed to perform FDA-mandated post-approval studies to assess the occurrence of rare and unanticipated device-related events. These post-approval studies have also provided an opportunity to assess the outcomes of carotid stenting in high–CEA risk patients in the non-trial setting (real world). In 2009, Gray et al.[73] reported the outcomes of two such prospective multicenter (280 U.S. sites, 672 operators) post-market surveillance studies involving CAS with distal embolic

protection using filters in high–CEA risk patients. These studies had pre- and postprocedure neurological evaluation and independent adjudication of neurological events. Results of these two studies, as well as the outcomes of an earlier large (n = 4225) post-approval study (CAPTURE),[102] are summarized in Table 32-6.

In summary, key outcomes from the CAPTURE 2 and EXACT data sets[73] are:

- 30-day death and stroke: 6.4% (95% confidence interval [CI], 4.8%-8.4%) in the combined symptomatic population and 3.2% (95% CI, 2.8%-3.7%) for the combined asymptomatic population.
- 30-day death and major stroke: 1.5% (95% CI, 1.2%-1.8%) for the combined population and 2.6% (95% CI, 1.6%-4.0%) and 1.3% (95% CI, 1.0%-1.6%) for the combined symptomatic and asymptomatic groups, respectively.
- In subjects with anatomical features unfavorable for surgery, independent of age:
  - Symptomatic (n = 60): 30-day death and stroke rate was 1.7% (95% CI, 0.0%-8.9%; the single stroke was adjudicated as major).
  - Asymptomatic (n = 371) 30-day death and stroke rate was 2.7% (95% CI, 1.3%-4.9%; 78% of strokes were minor).
- In the cohort of patients identified with physiological factors unfavorable for surgery, the combined 30-day rate of death and stroke for 574 symptomatic patients was 6.4% (95% CI, 4.6%-8.8%), and for the 4603 asymptomatic patients was 3.3% (95% CI, 2.8%-3.9%).

Operator Experience

In a recent publication, the CAPTURE 2 study investigators[105] analyzed the carotid stenting outcomes of 3388 patients (representing 64% of the total number of patients) to determine whether physician or site-related variables affected outcomes of CAS. Symptomatic patients and patients older than 80 years of age (two known predictors of adverse outcomes) were excluded. During a 3-year interval between March 2006 and January 2009, 459 operators treated the study population in 180 U.S. hospitals. The composite rates of death, stroke, and MI, and the composite rates of death and stroke at 30 days were 3.5% and 3.3%, respectively, for the full CAPTURE 2 study cohort and 2.9% and 2.7%, respectively, for the asymptomatic nonoctogenarian subgroup.

Two thirds of the sites (118 of 180 [66%]) had no death or stroke events. Within the remaining sites, an inverse relationship between adverse event rates and hospital patient volume as well as individual operator volume was observed. The death and stroke rates trended lower for interventional cardiologists compared with other specialties. Similar conclusions were drawn from a German registry analysis[106] and a recent meta-analysis of published studies.[107] The CAPTURE 2 study authors concluded that both site and operator volume were the most important determinants of perioperative events, and defined a threshold of 72 cases for consistently achieving a 30-day death and stroke rate of less than 3%. This 72 case number is higher than the entry threshold for operators participating in randomized trials like CREST or ACT I (Carotid Stenting vs. Surgery of Severe Carotid Artery Disease and Stroke Prevention in Asymptomatic Patients) trials.

Analysis and Critique

The analysis and critique that follows should be interpreted bearing in mind the limitations imposed by subset analysis and small numbers of patients within these subsets.

TABLE 32-6	Postapproval Surveillance Studies					
STUDY	ENROLLMENT	N	SYMPTOMATIC	ASYMPTOMATIC	STENT	EMBOLIC PROTECTION DEVICE
CAPTURE[102]	2004-2006	3500	483 (14%)	3017 (86%)	Acculink	Accunet
CAPTURE 2[73]	2006-enrolling	4175	548 (13%)	3627 (87%)	Acculink	Accunet
EXACT[73]	2005-2007	2145	213 (10%)	1931 (90%)	Xact	Emboshield

With the exception of SAPPHIRE, all other studies dealing with carotid stenting in high–CEA risk patients were registry studies. Despite the registry label, it should be noted that the high-risk CAS registries were performed under FDA-scrutinized clinical protocols, with prospective data collection and event adjudication. The importance of prospective independent clinical review was demonstrated by Rothwell and Warlow[108] investigating adverse event rates following CEA. They found a threefold difference in neurological events between operator self-reported and independent neurologist-assessed events. Both NASCET and ACAS used such prospective independent evaluations.

Individually and collectively, a large number of patients, mainly asymptomatic, have been studied within the context of these registry trials and provide a robust data set for analysis of high–CEA risk patients undergoing carotid stenting in the United States. Cumulatively, a total of more than 10,000 patients were included and analyzed in the three postmarketing studies (90% asymptomatic), and analysis of the data has helped provide answers to important questions concerning carotid stenting in a real-world setting.

Carotid stenting outcomes have shown a steady and continuous improvement since the initial introduction of these devices in U.S. trials (Fig. 32-19). For example, compared with outcomes in the ARCHeR and the original CAPTURE registries, the combined results of the CAPTURE 2 and EXACT studies showed improvement (30-day death and stroke: 6.9% vs. 5.7% vs. 3.6%, respectively), and these improved outcomes meet AHA guidelines in the younger than 80 years age group. As will be discussed later, in the CREST study, the majority of neurological events were minor strokes, with substantial if not complete resolution of the neurological deficits during the follow-up period.

Several factors contributed to the improvement in the results of carotid stenting. First is recognition of the clinical features that define the high–stent risk patient. This was not appreciated at the time when these registry studies were initiated. As operators became more experienced, these high–stent risk patients were excluded from studies initiated later in the decade with corresponding better outcomes.

Second, the pool of qualified experienced operators has expanded with time, with corresponding improvement in outcomes. Moreover, there have been improvements in the devices. For example, the profile of the EPDs has become smaller, and a variety of nitinol stents specifically for use at the carotid bifurcation have been developed. Improvements in technology, along with minor adjustments in the procedure protocol (e.g., limiting post inflation to a single inflation), have likely contributed to improved outcomes.

As a result, CAS outcomes in non-octogenarian, high–surgical risk patients, both symptomatic and asymptomatic, are within the acceptable thresholds of AHA standards. Additionally, in patients deemed high CEA risk due to unfavorable anatomical features, the outcomes meet AHA guidelines in both symptomatic and asymptomatic patients irrespective of age.

The higher event rates in the early (pre-2005) high risk CEA carotid stent registries (i.e., event rates that breached the AHA thresholds) is one likely explanation for lack of Centers for Medicare and Medicaid Services (CMS) reimbursement for asymptomatic patients undergoing carotid stenting, despite FDA approval for this indication in 2004. The outcomes of the CAPTURE 2 and the EXACT post-marketing registries are compelling because at least in the non-octogenarian high–CEA risk population, both symptomatic and asymptomatic (Table 32-7), the death and stroke outcomes were within the AHA guidelines.

The octogenarian and older population continues to be a challenge, and the decision to recommend and perform carotid stenting, especially in the asymptomatic patient older than 80 years of age, has to be individualized.

Carotid Stenting in Symptomatic Standard-Risk Patients

The introduction of CAS into clinical practice as an alternative to CEA has required the completion of randomized trials to evaluate its efficacy and safety. In patients with symptomatic carotid disease, there are four completed large, multicenter randomized controlled trials. These include the Endarterectomy versus Angioplasty in Patients with Symptomatic Severe Carotid Stenosis (EVA-3S) trial,[41] the Stent-Supported Percutaneous Angioplasty of the Carotid Artery versus Endarterectomy (SPACE) trial,[40] the International Carotid Stenting Study (ICSS),[109] and CREST.[39] Since the CREST study also included asymptomatic patients, it is discussed separately. Although the results from these individual trials remain a source of controversy, the results are broadly similar and have enabled the publication of guidelines by national societies.

EVA-3S,[41] a non-inferiority study, was conducted in 30 centers across France and recruited and randomized usual (standard-risk) CEA patients. These patients were within 120 days of either a TIA or

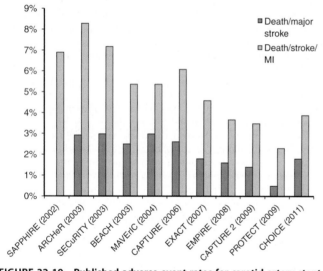

FIGURE 32-19 Published adverse event rates for carotid artery stent studies and registries over the past 10 years. Note progressive decline in events over time. The year in brackets is the time of last patient enrollment.

TABLE 32-7	Postapproval Surveillance Studies Outcomes		
STUDY	30-DAY: STROKE + DEATH (OVERALL)	30-DAY: STROKE + DEATH (<80 YEARS)	30-DAY: STROKE + DEATH (≥80 YEARS)
CAPTURE	Symptomatic 12.1% Asymptomatic 5.4%	4.8% (combined)*	9.0% (combined)*
CAPTURE 2	Symptomatic 6.2% Asymptomatic 3.0%	Symptomatic: 5.3%† Asymptomatic: 2.9%†	Symptomatic: 10.5%† Asymptomatic: 4.4%†
EXACT	Symptomatic 7.0% Asymptomatic 3.7%		

*Data from CAPTURE were not analyzed specifically for age by symptomatic status.
†Data from CAPTURE 2 and EXACT were pooled for the purposes of age-group analysis.

non-disabling stroke and had an ICA stenosis of 60% or greater in the index (symptomatic) carotid artery. Stenosis severity was verified by catheter angiography or duplex ultrasound and MRA. The primary endpoint was any stroke or death within 30 days of treatment. Although the enrollment target was 872 patients, the trial was stopped prematurely by the data safety monitoring board (DSMB) after 527 patients had been enrolled for reasons of safety and futility. The primary endpoint was seen in 9.6% of patients in the stenting group, compared to 3.9% in those undergoing endarterectomy (P = 0.01). Later analyses demonstrated that the difference between the two groups persisted out to 4 years.[110]

SPACE[40] was a multicenter (n = 35) multinational (German, Austrian, and Swiss participation) non-inferiority study. This trial recruited and randomized standard–CEA risk patients within 180 days of either a TIA or moderate stroke (Rankin score <4). Patients had a stenosis severity of 70% or greater (ECST criteria; ≥50% NASCET) in the index carotid artery. Stenosis severity was determined by catheter angiography or duplex ultrasound. The primary endpoint was ipsilateral stroke and death within 30 days of treatment. The trial was stopped after data from 1183 patients had been analyzed, which led to the conclusion that a larger sample size (almost 2500 patients) would be needed; however, further funding was not available. Event rates were 6.84% in the stenting group, compared with 6.34% in patients undergoing endarterectomy. Although the outcome rates were similar between the two groups, the trial failed to demonstrate the noninferiority of CAS (i.e., the study failed to prove that outcomes in patients undergoing stenting were no worse than outcomes of CEA).

ICSS,[109] a multicenter (n = 50) multinational (Europe, Australia, New Zealand, and Canada) equivalence study, recruited and randomized standard–CEA risk patients (n = 1713) to either CAS or CEA within 12 months of symptoms. Patients had a stenosis severity of 50% or greater (by NASCET criteria) in the index carotid artery. Stenosis severity and study entry eligibility were determined by duplex ultrasound or other noninvasive imaging of the carotid artery. The primary endpoint was long-term (3-year) incidence of death or disabling stroke in any territory and has not yet been reported. In 2010, an interim analysis reported the composite of stroke, death, and MI at 120 days, which was 72/857 (8.5%) for the CAS arm and 44/857 (5.2%) for the CEA arm (P = 0.006). No significant difference in the 120-day incidence of disabling stroke or death was noted: 34/857 (4.0%) in the CAS arm vs. 27/857 (3.2%) in the CEA group (P = NS). Following the interim analysis, the investigators concluded that pronouncement of efficacy of CAS in comparison to CEA should await the results of 3-year follow-up (2013), and until such time, CEA should remain the treatment of choice for symptomatic patients suitable for surgery.

Analysis and Critique

INCLUSION AND EXCLUSION CRITERIA

For the outcomes comparison between the two treatment strategies (CAS and CEA) to be valid, the two patient groups should be comparable. Specifically, for the patients enrolled in these studies, it should not matter whether they were in the CAS or CEA arms, since in a well-designed, adequately enrolled randomized clinical trial, this is not an issue. The process of randomization should cancel the noise and even out the imbalances between the two arms. However, despite randomization, an important imbalance continued to persist between the two treated groups related to the inclusion and exclusion criteria that handicapped the outcomes in the CAS arm. For example, in each one of these trials, patients with known anatomical characteristics that would render them high risk for CEA (tandem lesions, additional intracranial high-grade stenosis, "hostile necks" as a result of prior surgery or radiation) were all excluded from trial participation. On the other hand, the trial protocol did not specify exclusions for high stent risk. Additionally, when the trial protocol permits trial entry and randomization on the basis of duplex ultrasound imaging, anatomical features that

make stenting high risk (extended type III aortic arch, tortuous extra-cranial carotid anatomy, obvious lesion filling defect[s] due to a fresh, friable, loose thrombus) cannot be excluded. Inclusion of these patients made little or no difference to the outcomes for CEA, but may have negatively impacted CAS outcomes. The concept of high–stent risk patients is a recent one, however, and the EVA-3 S study recruited patients between the years 2000 and 2005, a time period during which the concept of high stent risk was neither well appreciated nor understood.

ANTIPLATELET REGIMEN

Contemporary carotid stent results are predicated on mandatory administration of adequate doses of dual antiplatelet medications in all patients prior to initiation of the stenting procedure and continuing them for at least 4 weeks post-CAS.[111,112] In all three of the above trials, dual antiplatelet agent use was recommended but not mandated. Approximately 20% of patients in the EVA-3 S and SPACE studies did not receive adequate antiplatelet medications.

INCONSISTENT USE OF EMBOLIC PROTECTION DEVICES

In EVA-3 S, during the first 3 years of enrollment (2000-2003), EPDs were used in approximately three quarters of the procedures. In 2003 after review of outcomes, the DSMB made use of EPDs mandatory. Analysis of the outcomes with and without use of EPDs reveals higher complication rates in the latter group. In SPACE, EPDs were used in only 27% of the cases. In ICSS, use of EPDs was recommended but not mandatory. Less than three quarters of the cases were performed using an EPD. Since the protocol was silent with respect to the need for familiarity with these devices prior to use within the trial, experience and expertise with the use of these devices was minimal if any. In contemporary carotid stenting practice, careful, critical analysis of the extracranial carotid artery anatomy is an important component of the risk stratification process. If the anatomy cephalad to the stenosis is markedly tortuous and/or there is no adequate landing zone (i.e., there is insufficient room between the caudal extent of the EPD and the area where the distal tip of the stent delivery system is expected to land), unless the case is suitable for a proximal (flow-reversal) EPD, the case should be considered high stent risk, and carotid stenting should not be performed (rather than proceeding with unprotected carotid stenting).

OPERATOR EXPERIENCE

Among practitioners of CAS, a major concern with all three of these studies has been the lack of experience of the investigators. Whereas the surgeons were experienced CEA operators and needed to have performed a minimum of 25 CEA surgeries in the year preceding study participation (EVA-3 S and SPACE), the entry barrier for CAS operators was much lower.[113–115] In EVA-3 S, for example, a total stenting experience of 12 CAS procedures or 5 CAS procedures plus 30 non-CAS supra-aortic stent procedures was sufficient for entry qualification.[114] Surprisingly, first-ever CAS cases in the presence of a proctor in the room were allowed within the trial. A disproportionately high number of patients underwent CAS using general anesthesia or conscious sedation, a reflection of operator inexperience and unfamiliarity with the CAS procedure and contrary to contemporary CAS practice. This has led many investigators[42,116] to question the validity of establishing clinical criteria and guidelines for CAS on the basis of these trials and explain the rationale requiring additional studies to clarify the issue.

Carotid Stenting in Symptomatic and Asymptomatic Standard-Risk Patients

The CREST study[39] conducted in 107 U.S. and 9 Canadian centers randomized standard-risk CEA patients to either CAS or CEA. The trial, which commenced in 2000, began by enrolling symptomatic patients who were within 6 months from the index event. In 2005,

CH
32

enrollment criteria were modified to include asymptomatic patients. Symptomatic patients needed to have a stenosis severity of 50% or greater on conventional angiography (NASCET criteria), or 70% or greater stenosis on duplex ultrasonography, CTA, or MRA in the index carotid artery. For asymptomatic patients, the stenosis eligibility criteria were 60% or greater on conventional angiography, 70% or greater by duplex ultrasonography, or 80% or greater stenosis on CTA or MRA. Trial sponsors included the NIH as well as a commercial partner, Abbott Vascular, whose devices (Accunet filter and Acculink stent) were used in the study.

The primary endpoint of the CREST study was the composite of any stroke, MI, or death from any cause during the periprocedural period or ipsilateral stroke within 4 years after randomization. The data were also analyzed using a composite endpoint that included any stroke, MI, and all death within 30 days of the procedure, plus ipsilateral stroke between day 31 and day 365. This endpoint was used by the industry sponsor for FDA submission for device approval. Secondary endpoints included all death, any stroke, or MI at 30 days (periprocedural), a 1-year composite endpoint stratified by symptomatic status and age (octogenarian status), acute procedural success, target lesion revascularization at 12 months, access site complications requiring treatment, cranial nerve injury unresolved at 1 and 6 months, and a prespecified interaction analyses involving gender and symptomatic status.

Data analysis was performed with four prespecified analysis populations: (1) intent-to-treat (ITT), (2) as-treated (AT), (3) modified as-treated (MAT), and (4) per protocol (PP). These four populations are defined in Figure 32-20.

The sample size of 2500 symptomatic patients in the initial proposal was based on a non-inferiority analysis for a study with 80% power and one-sided alpha of 0.05, assuming a composite endpoint rate of 7.48% and a non-inferiority margin of 2.6. When asymptomatic patients were added in 2005, the assumption was that 50% of the patient population would be asymptomatic. The assumed composite rate was ratcheted down to 6.76%, and the study power increased marginally to 82% with a one-sided alpha of 0.05.

Of the 2307 patients in the per-protocol population, 1219 (52.8%) were symptomatic, and 1088 (47.2%) were asymptomatic. The demographics of the two groups were well matched; approximately 9% of the patients were octogenarians, 30% had diabetes, and cardiovascular disease was present in about 45%.

The outcomes of the primary endpoints are shown in Table 32-8. Both analyses are consistent and complimentary, and CAS was shown to be non-inferior to CEA in both analyses (pre-specified non-inferiority margin of 2.6%).

During the peri-procedural period, there was a greater risk of stroke with stenting (4.1% vs. 2.3%; $P = 0.01$), but this difference was driven by the increased number of minor strokes in the CAS group (3.2% vs. 1.7%; $P = 0.01$). It is worth noting and emphasizing that for the endpoints of death and major stroke, not only was there no significant difference between the two groups, the event rates for these two key endpoints was low with both CEA and CAS (Table 32-9).

Minor Strokes

All interventions for extracranial carotid artery disease, CEA or CAS, are prophylactic, and the specific goal of the procedure is to reduce the patient's future risk of a stroke. Although survival free of a major stroke is the principal goal of the therapeutic intervention, minor strokes cannot be ignored. In fact, especially when treating asymptomatic patients, operators should have an extremely low tolerance for any procedure-related neurological event, be it major or minor stroke or cranial nerve injury. In the CREST study,

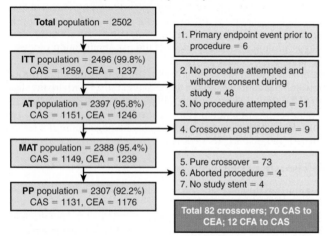

FIGURE 32-20 Prespecified analysis populations in the Carotid Revascularization Endarterectomy versus Stenting Trial (CREST). AT, as-treated; CAS, carotid artery stenting; CEA, carotid endarterectomy; ITT, intent-to-treat; MAT, modified as-treated; PP, per protocol.

TABLE 32-8	Primary Endpoint Analysis from the CREST Trial*			
	CAS	CEA	95% CL[†]	P_{NI}
Abbott PMA analysis: 1-year per-protocol	7.1%	6.6%	2.26%	0.0245
NIH analysis: 4-year ITT	7.2%	6.8%	2.26%	0.0259

*Two separate calculations were made, one by the trial sponsor Abbott and a second by the NIH. The noninferiority margin was reached in both groups using a margin of 2.6%.
[†]Prespecified noninferiority margin of 2.6%.
CAS, carotid artery stenting; CEA, carotid endarterectomy; CL, confidence limits; CREST, Carotid Revascularization Endarterectomy versus Stenting Trial; ITT, intent-to-treat; NIH, National Institutes of Health; PMA, premarket approval; P_{NI}, noninferiority P value.

TABLE 32-9	Periprocedural (30 days) Primary Endpoint and Endpoint Components According to Treatment Group			
	CAS N=1262 NO. OF PATIENTS (% ± SE)	CEA N=1240 NO. OF PATIENTS (% ± SE)	TREATMENT EFFECT (CAS VS. CEA) PERCENTAGE (95% CI)	UNADJUSTED P VALUE
Death/stroke/MI	66 (5.2 ± 0.6)	56 (4.5 ± 0.6)	0.7 (−1.0 to 2.4)	0.38
Death	9 (0.7 ± 0.2)	4 (0.3 ± 0.2)	0.4 (−0.2 to 1.0)	0.18
Any stroke	52 (4.1 ± 0.6)	29 (2.3 ± 0.4)	1.8 (0.4 to 3.2)	0.01
Major stroke	11 (0.9 ± 0.3)	8 (0.6 ± 0.2)	0.2 (−0.5 to 0.9)	0.52
Minor stroke	41 (3.2 ± 0.5)	21 (1.7 ± 0.4)	1.6 (0.3 to 2.8)	0.01
MI	14 (1.1 ± 0.3)	28 (2.3 ± 0.4)	−1.1 (−2.2 to −0.1)	0.03

CAS, carotid artery stenting; CEA, carotid endarterectomy; CI, confidence interval; MI, myocardial infarction; SE, standard error.
From Brott TG, Hobson RW 2nd, Howard G, et al: Stenting versus endarterectomy for treatment of carotid-artery stenosis. N Engl J Med 363:11–23, 2010.

an increased incidence of minor strokes contributed to the excess stroke hazard in the CAS arm. Analysis of the NIH Stroke Scale data of patients suffering a peri-procedural minor stroke reveals that although residual defects were disproportionately higher in the CAS arm at 1 month (1.10% vs. 0.60%), this difference was no longer evident at the 6-month time point (0.6% vs. 0.6%). A similar trend to equalization was noted when objective classification of the residual deficits was performed using the Rankin Scale. Importantly, the occurrence of a minor stroke did not negatively impact the patient's long-term survival. Thus, although there were more minor strokes in the CAS arm, the neurological impairment was minimal, and by 6 months both groups had similar outcomes.

Myocardial Infarction

In CREST, MI was defined by biomarker elevation (creatine kinase [CK]-MB or troponin > twice the upper limit of normal) plus either chest pain or electrocardiographic (ECG) evidence of ischemia (>1 mm ST elevation or depression in two contiguous leads). An additional pre-specified category included biomarker elevation without chest pain or ECG abnormality (biomarker positive only). When compared to patients without biomarker elevation, mortality was higher over 4 years for those with MI (HR 3.40; 95% CI, 1.67-6.92) or biomarker positive only (HR 3.57; 95% CI, 1.46-8.68). After adjustment of baseline risk factors, the occurrence of MI or elevation of biomarkers only remained independently associated with increased mortality.[117] In EVA-3-S, SPACE, and ICSS, cardiac biomarkers were not measured as part of the protocol.

The negative impact on survival in patients experiencing a peri-procedural MI is consistent with observations from other cardiac and non-cardiovascular procedures. It has repeatedly been shown that small peri-procedural elevations of cardiac enzymes were associated with increased future mortality.[118–121] How should one interpret these findings? The occurrence of a peri-procedural MI or biomarker elevation likely serves as a marker for more extensive underlying atherosclerotic disease. None of the other studies referenced in this section, including CREST, was able to positively conclude whether or not the occurrence of this procedure-related ischemic event in some way further adds to the baseline increased mortality risk. Thus, physicians have to factor in the occurrence as well as the consequences of MI when making treatment recommendations for an individual patient—especially the asymptomatic octogenarian.

Cranial Nerve Injuries and Their Sequelae

Cranial nerve injuries, a consistent complication of CEA (≈5%; Table 32-10) are rarely considered when discussing outcomes. Some of these deficits can be permanent and on occasion can be the source of major morbidity. For example, in the ICSS study, two of the cranial nerve injuries (out of 857 endarterectomies) were classified as disabling—both patients required gastrostomies. In the CREST study, more than 80% of the cranial nerve injuries were motor deficits, and 2% of the cranial nerve injuries were unresolved at 6-month follow-up. In future trials, consideration should be given

TABLE 32-10	Published Cranial Nerve Injury Rates from Large Randomized Trials*	
	Cranial Nerve Injuries	
	CEA	CAS
SAPPHIRE[101]	4.9%	0
EVA-3 S[41]	7.7%	1.1%
ICSS[109]	5.3%	0.1%
CREST[39]	5.3%	0

*The 1.1% rate seen in EVA-3 S was due to three events, two from patients who crossed over to CEA (intent-to-treat [ITT] analysis).
CAS, carotid artery stenting; CEA, carotid endarterectomy.

to the inclusion of cranial nerve injuries as part of a composite primary endpoint together with death, stroke, and MI.

Secondary Endpoints

Pre-specified interaction analysis showed symptom status and gender did not modify the treatment effect. However, age at treatment did have an influence, and the crossover was approximately 70 years. The impact of age on treatment selection is discussed later.

Clinical Durability of Carotid Stenting

Knowledge of the risk of an ipsilateral stroke after CAS during the follow-up period is vital to demonstrate the clinical durability of CAS. Clinical durability of CEA in both symptomatic and asymptomatic patients with extracranial carotid artery disease was established by NASCET[3] and ACAS.[8] The rates of ipsilateral stroke during the 4-year CREST follow-up period were low and similar in both treatment arms—2.0% for CAS and 2.4% for CEA. These results are similar to the rates in the EVA-3-S[110] and SPACE trials,[122] suggesting excellent durability for up to 4 years. The durable benefits of carotid stenting (i.e., freedom from ipsilateral stroke) in these large randomized studies reinforce the results published by the authors almost a decade ago.[22] To further investigate the long-term outcomes following carotid intervention, subject follow-up in the CREST study has been extended to 10 years and will provide additional information on this issue.

Restenosis Following Carotid Stenting

Restenosis rates have been documented following CAS in the large randomized trials and are approximately 10% at 2 years,[122,123] as measured by duplex ultrasonography. Although duplex ultrasound is an excellent method of following these patients, velocity criteria conventionally applied to diagnose stenosis in nonstented arteries may require modification because of mechanical changes in the carotid artery following stenting. It has been suggested that a peak systolic velocity greater than 300 cm/s be used to define a stenosis of 70%[124–126] in the stented patient. Other modalities also present challenges. Computed tomography angiography may be used as a complementary form of imaging,[127] but it requires contrast and radiation exposure. Magnetic resonance angiography is not useful in a stented patient.

Evaluating restenosis by tracking the need for target lesion revascularization is a commonly accepted method to define clinically relevant in-stent restenosis. At 1-year follow-up, both CAS and CEA had close to 99% freedom from target lesion revascularization,[39] with only 0.8% of patients requiring repeat revascularization. Furthermore, even in patients with evidence of in-stent restenosis, the event rate is low, suggesting restenosis is generally a benign condition.[123] These results, together with previously reported very low rates of carotid stent restenosis, support durability of the self-expanding stent for this indication. Since the stent is implanted within a superficial artery that is subject to a variety of torsional forces associated with neck movement, questions of stent fracture have been raised and are being addressed by follow-up fluoroscopy in some ongoing trials.[128] In the authors' experience, stent thrombosis, stent fractures, and in-stent restenosis are rare issues for stents placed in the extracranial cervical carotid location. The rate of stent fracture is currently under study.

Summary of CREST Results

1. In experienced hands, both CEA and CAS are excellent revascularization options for treatment of symptomatic and asymptomatic extracranial carotid stenosis in patients of either gender.
2. Both procedures were associated with similar rates of the primary composite outcome that included periprocedural stroke, MI, or death and subsequent ipsilateral stroke to 4 years.

3. Not only was there no significant difference between major disabling stroke and death between the CAS and CEA arms, the incidence of these major events was very low with either treatment option.
4. Minor non disabling strokes were greater with CAS than with CEA. Using the objective NIH Stroke Scale, at 6 months, the deficits in the stenting cohort had equalized with those in the CEA arm of the study. The occurrence of a minor stroke did not affect survival.
5. Myocardial infarction's were more frequently seen with CEA than CAS, and the occurrence of MI negatively impacted survival.
6. Cranial injuries were seen in approximately 5% of the CEA patients, the vast majority were motor deficits, and 2% of the injuries had persistent deficits at 6 months. There were no cranial injuries in the CAS patients.
7. At one year, stroke had a greater adverse effect than MI on a broad range of health status domains.[129]

Special Patient Groups

Carotid Stenosis Following Cervical Irradiation

Carotid artery stenosis is a delayed complication of neck irradiation (radiation arteritis).[130] Although stenosis following prior radiation is often seen at the carotid bifurcation, patients with prior neck radiation frequently have lesions that are high (at or above the C2 vertebra) or low (at or below the level of the clavicle). Stenosis at multiple locations within the same artery is not unusual. The typical interval between the radiation treatment and detection of stenosis is at least 10 years. In patients who had neck irradiation but also have multiple risk factors for atherosclerotic vascular disease and who present with an isolated bifurcation stenosis, it may be very difficult to determine the etiology of the carotid disease.

Surgical treatment of these patients is complicated by a number of factors. Many patients have had radical neck dissections in association with radiation therapy, resulting in fibrosis and scarring. There is an increased risk of stenosis of the CCA, its low position making surgical access more difficult. There is also an increase in postoperative necrosis, infections, wound breakdown, and cranial nerve palsies that have been observed post CEA in this population,[131] compared to patients without prior radiation. In contrast, none of these difficulties are faced by operators performing CAS, making it an appealing technique for this indication.

Owing to the infrequent nature of this presentation, there are no randomized studies; however, several case series have demonstrated that CAS is safe and efficacious in this setting.[132,133] Reported peri-procedural stroke and death rates have been low and have not exceeded those observed in general patient cohorts undergoing CAS. The only limitation of stenting in this group is the possible increased risk of in-stent restenosis following the procedure. Restenosis rates from 5%[132] to 41%[133] have been reported at intervals from 12 to 24 months. Although higher than that seen in patients without prior radiation, these events have not been associated with symptoms and restenotic lesions are amenable to repeat percutaneous intervention.

Despite the absence of randomized trial data apart from those patients enrolled in the SAPPHIRE study, the low peri-procedural complication rates with CAS makes this the preferred approach for this patient group and the authors support the level IIa recommendation of the multispecialty guidelines[32] in recommending the use of CAS for carotid stenosis following cervical radiotherapy. Patients should be closely followed by serial duplex ultrasound examinations after the procedure to monitor for restenosis. Because of problems of delayed healing and incomplete endothelialization of the stent struts, patients with prior neck radiation who undergo stenting are prescribed lifelong dual antiplatelet treatment.

Post–Carotid Endarterectomy Restenosis

Restenosis after CEA is a well-recognized phenomenon. Restenosis that occurs within the first 2 years after CEA has been attributed to intimal hyperplasia, whereas after 2 years, progressive atherosclerosis is thought to be responsible. Restenosis rates vary depending on the study and methodology and are reported from 5% at 1 year[123] to 36% during long-term follow-up.[134] Revision CEA is technically challenging and associated with higher complication rates than primary surgery, with increased rates of stroke (4.8% vs. 0.8%), TIA (4.0% vs. 1.1%), and cranial nerve injury (17.0% vs. 5.3%).[135] Carotid artery stenting is therefore an appealing technique in this setting.

There have been no randomized trials to assess which method is superior. Single-center studies evaluating the experience of CAS following prior CEA have demonstrated that low complication rates can be achieved. Thirty-day death/stroke rates ranging from 1%[136] to 4%[137] have been published and have compared favorably to endarterectomy.[136] Of note, these published figures are slightly superior to those seen in randomized trials of symptomatic patients.[39] The durability of CAS after previous CEA has not been well established; however, the limited data suggest that stent restenosis is not significantly higher than that seen in primary CAS.[137]

Given that the current literature demonstrates no particular increase in CAS risk following prior CEA but a significant increase in complications during revision CEA, CAS is the recommended approach in this setting.

Carotid Stenting in Women

Some authors have postulated a variance in outcomes dependent on the sex of the patient. Women typically have smaller-caliber arteries and aortic arches, potentially leading to increased technical difficulties and higher complication rates. Although individual trials have not had sufficient power to detect such differences, the Carotid Stenting Trialists Collaboration (CSTC) published a meta-analysis of three randomized controlled trials. This study revealed no significant difference in outcomes at 4 years between men and women, although there was a trend toward higher adverse event rates in men.[138] A separate review of the CREST study data found that women are more likely to have complications following CAS, and men more likely after CEA.[139] The authors suggested that the treatment strategy for carotid stenoses could be customized, with a preference for CEA in women and vice versa. If the data from this study are further pooled with the data from CSTC, there is no significant difference in outcomes.[140] Given the conflicting study data and absence of clear evidence, there is currently no basis for tailoring treatment approaches on the basis of gender.

Carotid Stenting in the Elderly

Elderly patients (generally interpreted to mean patients >80 years) with carotid stenosis pose several challenges for carotid revascularization. The association between older age and increased risk of adverse events after CAS was seen in the CREST lead-in cohort,[141] the SPACE trial,[40] and the ICSS.[109] Indeed, octogenarian patients are more likely to be excluded because they have one or more features deemed high risk for carotid stenting, as shown in Box 32-1. By carefully excluding patients with adverse features—decreased cerebral reserve, excessive tortuosity (2 bends >90 degrees after the origin of the CCA from the aortic arch or ICA from the carotid bifurcation), or heavy concentric calcification—it has been shown that adverse event rates comparable to those seen following CEA[142] can be achieved.

In the CREST study, an interaction between age and treatment efficacy was detected with a crossover at an age of approximately 70 years. This led the CREST investigators to conclude that "carotid-artery stenting tended to show greater efficacy at younger ages, and CEA at older ages."[39] Hence, treatment recommendation in the elderly patient with carotid stenosis must be highly individualized and take into account high-risk features that will make stenting or CEA (or both options) unsuitable.

Treatment of Carotid Stent Restenosis

On the rare occasion when treatment is deemed necessary, treatment of in-stent restenosis is usually performed by dilation with either a noncompliant or cutting balloon.[143] In some cases, vessel recoil makes an additional stent necessary. It has been speculated that the controlled trauma of a cutting balloon may result in lower occurrence of in-stent restenosis than a conventional angioplasty balloon, but this has not been studied systematically. Zhou et al. used cutting balloons in five of seven patients, and two required further stent implantation.[144] In theory, because restenotic lesions are generally fibrotic, the risk of periprocedural embolization in these lesions (in-stent restenosis or stenosis recurrence following endarterectomy) is thought to be low. However, in practice, use of a distal EPD is recommended even when intervening on these lesions. Rates of target lesion revascularization in the CREST study were very low, with only 0.8% of patients requiring repeat intervention during the 4-year follow-up period.[39] A comparable rate of 1.5% was obtained from the 4-year published data from EVA-3S.[110]

Treatment of Concomitant Carotid and Coronary Arterial Disease

The generalized nature of atherosclerosis makes concomitant coronary and carotid artery disease a common finding. The issue of treatment of carotid disease is of particular concern in the management of patients who require CABG. These patients have a high incidence of at least moderate carotid artery disease (15% of patients >70 years of age[145]) and perioperative stroke is associated with a 25% mortality.[146] Large meta-analyses of published studies have found that stroke as a complication of CABG occurs in 1.7% of all cases.[146,147] This risk is to 3% for patients with an asymptomatic 50% to 99% unilateral stenosis, 5% for those with bilateral 50% to 99% stenoses, and 7% to 11% for patients with a carotid artery occlusion.[146] However, pathological and radiological examination revealed that only 40% of such strokes could be attributed to the ipsilateral stenosis. Therefore, even if 100% effective at preventing ipsilateral ischemia, carotid intervention can only reduce peri-operative (CABG) stroke rates by less than half. This issue is further clouded because there are currently no randomized trial data to provide guidance as to the optimal management of these patients.

Observational studies have evaluated the outcomes of both CEA and CAS, either prior to or concurrently with CABG. A meta-analysis of published peri-operative stroke/death rates for combined CEA/CABG revealed a stroke/death rate of 8.7% for combined surgery and 6.1% for a staged CEA then CABG.[148] However, this reduction in stroke risk for a staged procedure comes at the cost of an increased MI rate, from 3.6% for the synchronous procedure to 6.5% for staged.[148] This is a significant concern because peri-procedural MI has been associated with an increased risk of mortality, as seen in the CREST study.[117] The SAPPHIRE study, which enrolled high-risk surgical patients (including those requiring CABG), showed that in high-risk patients, CAS was a safer alternative than CEA, with lower combined death and stroke rates at 1 year.[101] This finding has been further supported by a retrospective study comparing outcomes between CEA and CAS followed by CABG. Again there was both a numerical reduction in 30-day death/stroke rates (7.1% vs. 12.6%, respectively; $P = 0.28$) and MI (3.3 vs. 12.6%, respectively; $P = 0.06$). This has led to staged CAS followed by CABG at least 14 days later following cessation of at least one antiplatelet agent being adopted by many centers.[149] Single-center studies have reported periprocedural death/stroke rates of 4.8%.[150]

At present there are no randomized data to support either approach in asymptomatic patients. Patients with three-vessel CAD were not enrolled in the landmark studies for asymptomatic carotid disease[8,151]; the study findings may not necessarily be extrapolated to this high-risk population. Overall, the authors believe that patients with bilateral carotid artery disease or unilateral carotid stenosis plus a contralateral occlusion are most likely to benefit

from carotid revascularization prior to CABG, and that CAS is a safer alternative to CEA where feasible.

Current Recommendations and the Future of Carotid Artery Stenting

Stroke is the fourth leading cause of death in the United States[152] and the single most important cause of long-term physical and intellectual disability. Despite spectacular advances and progress in several areas of medicine, the treatment options for an established stroke are limited, and the expectation for reversibility or improvement of a neurological deficit is both guarded and unpredictable.

Given the high risk of recurrence after a symptomatic event, there is little controversy or argument that most if not all symptomatic patients with 70% or greater stenosis on angiography, and many symptomatic patients with a 50% to 70% stenosis, should be offered a definitive revascularization procedure—either CEA or CAS—unless the expected procedural risks breach the AHA recommendation threshold of 6%. Additionally, these patients should be on appropriate atherothrombotic risk-reduction measures.

For asymptomatic patients, however, the issue of which patient needs treatment is far from settled. It would be reasonable to offer revascularization for asymptomatic patients with 80% or greater stenosis. In certain situations (e.g., those requiring CABG), patients with less than 80% but more than 70% stenosis also may be offered treatment. Carotid stenting can be scientifically and ethically justified as a treatment option for asymptomatic patients only if operators and centers are experienced and have a verifiable peri-procedural risk of 3% or less. If the expected peri-procedural risk associated with revascularization (CEA or CAS) in an asymptomatic patient exceeds 3%, the patient should be managed conservatively.

Patient selection remains the single most important predictor of complications. Although EPDs are routinely used, no protection device can replace critical risk analysis and sound operator judgment. In general, it is reasonable to recommend CAS in symptomatic patients who are younger than 80 years of age. For patients older than 80, the decision must be individualized, and the recommendation for revascularization should be arrived at after a rigorous and critical analysis of the risks and benefits. Many of these patients may be best managed medically—no CAS or CEA.

For asymptomatic patients considered high risk for endarterectomy, CAS is a reasonable option with two important caveats: (1) high risk for endarterectomy does not automatically mean high risk for stroke (with conservative medical management), and (2) a proportion of high surgical risk patients will also be high risk for CAS—these patients should be treated conservatively.

The conventional approach for treatment of extracranial carotid artery disease involves revascularization on the basis of the presumed surgical risk (the conventional paradigm depicted in Fig. 32-21). In other words, if a patient requires treatment for carotid stenosis, the first question that has been traditionally posed is: Is the patient standard risk for CEA? Patients considered high risk for

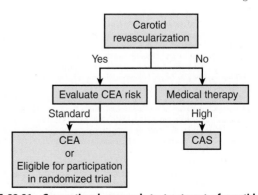

FIGURE 32-21 Conventional approach to treatment of carotid arterial disease has been based on the answer to the question: Is the patient suitable (standard risk) for carotid endarterectomy (CEA)? CAS, carotid artery stenting.

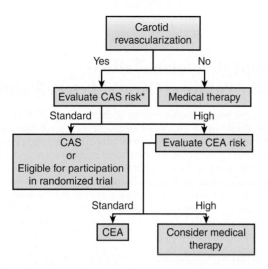

*Age, Cerebral reserve, Lesion, and Vessel morphology

FIGURE 32-22   In the future, we will see a paradigm shift, and the approach to carotid revascularization will be based on the answer to the question: Is the patient suitable (standard risk) for carotid artery stenting (CAS)? CEA, carotid endarterectomy.

CEA are often referred for carotid stenting, arbitrarily considered a low-risk intervention because little attention had been paid to defining what constituted high stent risk. However, the full clinical potential of carotid stenting can only be realized if there is a paradigm shift in the process of procedural risk stratification and selection of patients for revascularization. This applies to both everyday clinical practice and the design of randomized trials. Clinical decision making that incorporates this paradigm shift is depicted in the future approach shown in Figure 32-22, wherein the first question that should be asked is: Is the patient standard risk for stenting?

So, what can we expect in the future? A randomized trial to answer the question of the risk of stroke with contemporary medical treatment in asymptomatic patients is already underway (SPACE II), and another trial (CREST II) is awaiting funding. ACT I, a large prospective study involving asymptomatic patients is randomizing patients (3:1, CAS vs. CEA). Although this study does not include a medical arm, prior to randomization, patients have to be suitable (i.e., standard risk) for both CAS and CEA—an important strength of the trial design. Finally, in the future we can expect continued technical and device improvements to further improve the safety of carotid stenting.

REFERENCES

1. Department of Health & Human Services: *Summary of the Circulatory System Devices Panel Meeting*, Jan, 26th 2011. Available at: www.fda.gov/downloads/AdvisoryCommittees/CommitteesMeetingMaterials/MedicalDevices/MedicalDevicesAdvisoryCommittee/CirculatorySystemDevicesPanel/UCM241779.pdf.
2. Gurdjian ES: History of occlusive cerebrovascular disease. II. After Moniz, with special reference to surgical treatment, *Arch Neurol* 36:427–432, 1979.
3. Beneficial effect of carotid endarterectomy in symptomatic patients with high-grade carotid stenosis. North American Symptomatic Carotid Endarterectomy Trial Collaborators, *N Engl J Med* 325:445–453, 1991.
4. Clinical alert: benefit of carotid endarterectomy for patients with high-grade stenosis of the internal carotid artery. National Institute of Neurological Disorders and Stroke, Stroke and Trauma Division. North American Symptomatic Carotid Endarterectomy Trial (NASCET) investigators, *Stroke* 22:816–817, 1991.
5. Barnett HJ, Taylor DW, Eliasziw M, et al: Benefit of carotid endarterectomy in patients with symptomatic moderate or severe stenosis. North American Symptomatic Carotid Endarterectomy Trial Collaborators, *N Engl J Med* 339:1415–1425, 1998.
6. Ferguson GG, Eliasziw M, Barr HW, et al: The North American Symptomatic Carotid Endarterectomy Trial: surgical results in 1415 patients, *Stroke* 30:1751–1758, 1999.
7. Randomised trial of endarterectomy for recently symptomatic carotid stenosis: final results of the MRC European Carotid Surgery Trial (ECST), *Lancet* 351:1379–1387, 1998.
8. Endarterectomy for asymptomatic carotid artery stenosis. Executive Committee for the Asymptomatic Carotid Atherosclerosis Study, *JAMA* 273:1421–1428, 1995.
9. Endovascular versus surgical treatment in patients with carotid stenosis in the Carotid and Vertebral Artery Transluminal Angioplasty Study (CAVATAS): a randomised trial, *Lancet* 357:1729–1737, 2001.
10. Dotter CT: Transluminal angioplasty: a long view, *Radiology* 135:561–564, 1980.
11. Gruntzig A, Hopff H: Percutaneous recanalization after chronic arterial occlusion with a new dilator-catheter (modification of the Dotter technique) (author's transl), *Dtsch Med Wochenschr* 99:2502–2510, 2511, 1974.
12. Mathias K: A new catheter system for percutaneous transluminal angioplasty (PTA) of carotid artery stenoses, *Fortschr Med* 95:1007–1011, 1977.
13. Kerber CW, Cromwell LD, Loehden OL: Catheter dilatation of proximal carotid stenosis during distal bifurcation endarterectomy, *AJNR Am J Neuroradiol* 1:348–349, 1980.
14. Mullan S, Duda EE, Patronas NJ: Some examples of balloon technology in neurosurgery, *J Neurosurg* 52:321–329, 1980.
15. Vitek JJ, Raymon BC, Oh SJ: Innominate artery angioplasty, *AJNR Am J Neuroradiol* 5:113–114, 1984.
16. Theron J, Raymond J, Casasco A, et al: Percutaneous angioplasty of atherosclerotic and postsurgical stenosis of carotid arteries, *AJNR Am J Neuroradiol* 8:495–500, 1987.
17. Kachel R: Results of balloon angioplasty in the carotid arteries, *J Endovasc Surg* 3:22–30, 1996.
18. Rabkin I, Germashev VG: 5-year experience with roentgenologically controlled endovascular nitinol prosthesis, *Kardiologiia* 30:11–17, 1990.
19. Yadav JS, Roubin GS, Iyer S, et al: Elective stenting of the extracranial carotid arteries, *Circulation* 95:376–381, 1997.
20. Yadav JS, Roubin GS, King P, et al: Angioplasty and stenting for restenosis after carotid endarterectomy. Initial experience, *Stroke* 27:2075–2079, 1996.
21. Roubin GS, Yadav S, Iyer SS, et al: Carotid stent-supported angioplasty: a neurovascular intervention to prevent stroke, *Am J Cardiol* 78:8–12, 1996.
22. Roubin GS, New G, Iyer SS, et al: Immediate and late clinical outcomes of carotid artery stenting in patients with symptomatic and asymptomatic carotid artery stenosis: a 5-year prospective analysis, *Circulation* 103:532–537, 2001.
23. Mathur A, Dorros G, Iyer SS, et al: Palmaz stent compression in patients following carotid artery stenting, *Cathet Cardiovasc Diagn* 41:137–140, 1997.
24. Theron JG, Payelle GG, Coskun O, et al: Carotid artery stenosis: treatment with protected balloon angioplasty and stent placement, *Radiology* 201:627–636, 1996.
25. Baldi S, Zander T, Rabellino M, et al: Carotid artery stenting without angioplasty and cerebral protection: a single-center experience with up to 7 years' follow-up, *AJNR Am J Neuroradiol* 32:759–763, 2011.
26. Theron J, Courtheoux P, Alachkar F, et al: New triple coaxial catheter system for carotid angioplasty with cerebral protection, *AJNR Am J Neuroradiol* 11:869–874, 1990; discussion 875–867.
27. Henry M, Amor M, Henry I, et al: Carotid stenting with cerebral protection: first clinical experience using the PercuSurge GuardWire system, *J Endovasc Surg* 6:321–331, 1999.
28. Al-Mubarak N, Roubin GS, Vitek JJ, et al: Effect of the distal-balloon protection system on microembolization during carotid stenting, *Circulation* 104:1999–2002, 2001.
29. Henry M, Henry I, Klonaris C, et al: Benefits of cerebral protection during carotid stenting with the PercuSurge GuardWire system: midterm results, *J Endovasc Surg* 9:1–13, 2002.
30. Al-Mubarak N, Colombo A, Gaines PA, et al: Multicenter evaluation of carotid artery stenting with a filter protection system, *J Am Coll Cardiol* 39:841–846, 2002.
31. Whitlow PL, Lylyk P, Londero H, et al: Carotid artery stenting protected with an emboli containment system, *Stroke* 33:1308–1314, 2002.
32. Brott TG, Halperin JL, Abbara S, et al: ASA/ACCF/AHA/AANN/AANS/ACR/ASNR/CNS/SAIP/SCAI/SIR/SNIS/SVM/SVS guideline on the management of patients with extracranial carotid and vertebral artery disease: executive summary. A report of the American College of Cardiology Foundation/American Heart Association Task Force on Practice Guidelines, and the American Stroke Association, American Association of Neuroscience Nurses, American Association of Neurological Surgeons, American College of Radiology, American Society of Neuroradiology, Congress of Neurological Surgeons, Society of Atherosclerosis Imaging and Prevention, Society for Cardiovascular Angiography and Interventions, Society of Interventional Radiology, Society of NeuroInterventional Surgery, Society for Vascular Medicine, and Society for Vascular Surgery Developed in Collaboration With the American Academy of Neurology and Society of Cardiovascular Computed Tomography, *J Am Coll Cardiol* 57:1002–1044, 2011.
33. Naylor AR: Delay may reduce procedural risk, but at what price to the patient? *Eur J Vasc Endovasc Surg* 35:383–391, 2008.
34. Giles MF, Rothwell PM: Risk of stroke early after transient ischaemic attack: a systematic review and meta-analysis, *Lancet Neurol* 6:1063–1072, 2007.
35. Wu CM, McLaughlin K, Lorenzetti DL, et al: Early risk of stroke after transient ischemic attack: a systematic review and meta-analysis, *Arch Intern Med* 167:2417–2422, 2007.
36. Chandratheva A, Mehta Z, Geraghty OC, et al: Population-based study of risk and predictors of stroke in the first few hours after a TIA, *Neurology* 72:1941–1947, 2009.
37. Ois A, Cuadrado-Godia E, Rodriguez-Campello A, et al: High risk of early neurological recurrence in symptomatic carotid stenosis, *Stroke* 40:2727–2731, 2009.
38. McDonald RJ, Cloft HJ, Kallmes DF: Intracranial hemorrhage is much more common after carotid stenting than after endarterectomy: evidence from the National Inpatient Sample, *Stroke* 42:2782–2787, 2011.
39. Brott TG, Hobson RW 2nd: Howard G, et al: Stenting versus endarterectomy for treatment of carotid-artery stenosis, *N Engl J Med* 363:11–23, 2010.
40. Ringleb PA, Allenberg J, Bruckmann H, et al: 30 day results from the SPACE trial of Stent-Protected Angioplasty versus Carotid Endarterectomy in symptomatic patients: a randomised non-inferiority trial, *Lancet* 368:1239–1247, 2006.
41. Mas JL, Chatellier G, Beyssen B, et al: Endarterectomy versus stenting in patients with symptomatic severe carotid stenosis, *N Engl J Med* 355:1660–1671, 2006.
42. Fiehler J, Bakke SJ, Clifton A, et al: Plea of the defence-critical comments on the interpretation of EVA3S, SPACE and ICSS, *Neuroradiology* 52:601–610, 2010.
43. Spence JD: Asymptomatic carotid stenosis: mainly a medical condition, *Vascular* 18:123–126, 2010 discussion 127–129.
44. Naylor AR: What is the current status of invasive treatment of extracranial carotid artery disease? *Stroke* 42:2080–2085, 2011.
45. Klein A, Solomon CG, Hamel MB: Clinical decisions. Management of carotid stenosis-polling results, *N Engl J Med* 358:e23, 2008.

46. Whitworth JA: 2003 World Health Organization (WHO)/International Society of Hypertension (ISH) statement on management of hypertension, *J Hypertens* 21:1983–1992, 2003.

47. Diener HC, Weimar C, Weber R: Antiplatelet therapy in secondary stroke prevention–state of the art, *J Cell Mol Med* 14:2552–2560, 2010.

48. Amarenco P, Bogousslavsky J, Callahan A 3rd, et al: High-dose atorvastatin after stroke or transient ischemic attack, *N Engl J Med* 355:549–559, 2006.

49. Amarenco P: Atorvastatin in prevention of stroke and transient ischaemic attack, *Expert Opin Pharmacother* 8:2789–2797, 2007.

50. Lanzino G, Rabinstein AA, Brown RD Jr: Treatment of carotid artery stenosis: medical therapy, surgery, or stenting? *Mayo Clin Proc* 84:362–387, 2009 quiz 367–368.

51. Bock RW, Gray-Weale AC, Mock PA, et al: The natural history of asymptomatic carotid artery disease, *J Vasc Surg* 17:160–169, 1993 discussion 170–161.

52. Hirt LS: Progression rate and ipsilateral neurological events in asymptomatic carotid stenosis, *Stroke* 2011 published online ahead of print. doi: 10.1161/STROKEAHA.111.613711.

53. Nicolaides AN, Kakkos SK, Griffin M, et al: Effect of image normalization on carotid plaque classification and the risk of ipsilateral hemispheric ischemic events: results from the asymptomatic carotid stenosis and risk of stroke study, *Vascular* 13:211–221, 2005.

54. Spence JD: Cerebrovascular disease: identifying high-risk patients from carotid plaque composition, *Nature Reviews Cardiology* 7:426–428, 2010.

55. Abbott AL, Chambers BR, Stork JL, et al: Embolic signals and prediction of ipsilateral stroke or transient ischemic attack in asymptomatic carotid stenosis: a multicenter prospective cohort study, *Stroke* 36:1128–1133, 2005.

56. Markus HS, King A, Shipley M, et al: Asymptomatic embolisation for prediction of stroke in the Asymptomatic Carotid Emboli Study (ACES): a prospective observational study, *Lancet Neurol* 9:663–671, 2010.

57. Spence JD, Tamayo A, Lownie SP, et al: Absence of microemboli on transcranial Doppler identifies low-risk patients with asymptomatic carotid stenosis, *Stroke* 36:2373–2378, 2005.

58. Spence JD, Coates V, Li H, et al: Effects of intensive medical therapy on microemboli and cardiovascular risk in asymptomatic carotid stenosis, *Arch Neurol* 67:180–186, 2010.

59. Norris JW, Zhu CZ: Silent stroke and carotid stenosis, *Stroke* 23:483–485, 1992.

60. AbuRahma AF, Metz MJ, Robinson PA: Natural history of > or = 60% asymptomatic carotid stenosis in patients with contralateral carotid occlusion, *Ann Surg* 238:551–561, 2003; discussion 561–552.

61. Altaf N, Daniels L, Morgan PS, et al: Detection of intraplaque hemorrhage by magnetic resonance imaging in symptomatic patients with mild to moderate carotid stenosis predicts recurrent neurological events, *J Vasc Surg* 47:337–342, 2008.

62. Nicolaides AN, Kakkos SK, Kyriacou E, et al: Asymptomatic internal carotid artery stenosis and cerebrovascular risk stratification, *J Vasc Surg* 52:1486–1496, e1481–e1485, 2010.

63. Roubin GS, Iyer S, Halkin A, et al: Realizing the potential of carotid artery stenting: proposed paradigms for patient selection and procedural technique, *Circulation* 113:2021–2030, 2006.

64. Al-Mubarak N, Roubin GS, Vitek JJ, et al: Microembolization during carotid stenting with the distal-balloon antiemboli system, *Int Angiol* 21:344–348, 2002.

65. Leal JI, Orgaz A, Fontcuberta J, et al: A prospective evaluation of cerebral infarction following transcervical carotid stenting with carotid flow reversal, *Eur J Vasc Endovasc Surg* 39:661–666, 2010.

66. Criado E, Fontcuberta J, Orgaz A, et al: Transcervical carotid stenting with carotid artery flow reversal: 3-year follow-up of 103 stents, *J Vasc Surg* 46:864–869, 2007.

67. Ohki T, Roubin GS, Veith FJ, et al: Efficacy of a filter device in the prevention of embolic events during carotid angioplasty and stenting: an *ex vivo* analysis, *J Vasc Surg* 30:1034–1044, 1999.

68. Iyer SS, White CJ, Hopkins LN, et al: Carotid artery revascularization in high-surgical-risk patients using the Carotid WALLSTENT and FilterWire EX/EZ: 1-year outcomes in the BEACH Pivotal Group, *J Am Coll Cardiol* 51:427–434, 2008.

69. Bosiers M, de Donato G, Deloose K, et al: Does free cell area influence the outcome in carotid artery stenting? *Eur J Vasc Endovasc Surg* 33:135–141, 2007; discussion 142–133.

70. Hart JP, Peeters P, Verbist J, et al: Do device characteristics impact outcome in carotid artery stenting? *J Vasc Surg* 44:725–730, 2006; discussion 730–721.

71. Timaran CH, Rosero EB, Higuera A, et al: Randomized clinical trial of open-cell vs. closed-cell stents for carotid stenting and effects of stent design on cerebral embolization, *J Vasc Surg* 54:1310–1316 e1; discussion 6, 2011.

72. Jim J, Rubin BG, Landis GS, et al: Society for Vascular Surgery Vascular Registry evaluation of stent cell design on carotid artery stenting outcomes, *J Vasc Surg* 54:71–79, 2011.

73. Gray WA, Chaturvedi S, Verta P: Thirty-day outcomes for carotid artery stenting in 6320 patients from 2 prospective, multicenter, high-surgical-risk registries, *Circ Cardiovasc Interv* 2:159–166, 2009.

74. Schneider LM, Polena S, Roubin G, et al: Carotid stenting and bivalirudin with and without vascular closure: 3-year analysis of procedural outcomes, *Catheter Cardiovasc Interv* 75:420–426, 2010.

75. Ogasawara K, Yukawa H, Kobayashi M, et al: Prediction and monitoring of cerebral hyperperfusion after carotid endarterectomy by using single-photon emission computerized tomography scanning, *J Neurosurg* 99:504–510, 2003.

76. van Mook WN, Rennenberg RJ, Schurink GW, et al: Cerebral hyperperfusion syndrome, *Lancet Neurol* 4:877–888, 2005.

77. Holm J, Nilsson U, Waters N, et al: Production of free radicals measured by spin trapping during operations for stenosis of the carotid artery, *Eur J Surg* 167:4–9, 2001.

78. Skydell JL, Machleder HI, Baker JD, et al: Incidence and mechanism of post-carotid endarterectomy hypertension, *Arch Surg* 122:1153–1155, 1987.

79. Timmers HJ, Wieling W, Karemaker JM, et al: Baroreflex failure: a neglected type of secondary hypertension, *Neth J Med* 62:151–155, 2004.

80. Macfarlane R, Moskowitz MA, Sakas DE, et al: The role of neuroeffector mechanisms in cerebral hyperperfusion syndromes, *J Neurosurg* 75:845–855, 1991.

81. Hosoda K, Kawaguchi T, Ishii K, et al: Prediction of hyperperfusion after carotid endarterectomy by brain SPECT analysis with semiquantitative statistical mapping method, *Stroke* 34:1187–1193, 2003.

82. Muzzi DA, Black S, Losasso TJ, et al: Labetalol and esmolol in the control of hypertension after intracranial surgery, *Anesth Analg* 70:68–71, 1990.

83. Dalman JE, Beenakkers IC, Moll FL, et al: Transcranial Doppler monitoring during carotid endarterectomy helps to identify patients at risk of postoperative hyperperfusion, *Eur J Vasc Endovasc Surg* 18:222–227, 1999.

84. Meyers PM, Higashida RT, Phatouros CC, et al: Cerebral hyperperfusion syndrome after percutaneous transluminal stenting of the craniocervical arteries, *Neurosurgery* 47:335–343, 2000; discussion 343–335.

85. Piepgras DG, Morgan MK, Sundt TM Jr, et al: Intracerebral hemorrhage after carotid endarterectomy, *J Neurosurg* 68:532–536, 1988.

86. Mathur A, Roubin GS, Iyer SS, et al: Predictors of stroke complicating carotid artery stenting, *Circulation* 97:1239–1245, 1998.

87. Wholey M, Wholey M., Mathias K, et al: Global experience in cervical carotid artery stent placement, *Catheter Cardiovasc Interv* 50:160–167, 2000.

88. Henry M, Amor M, Klonaris C, et al: Angioplasty and stenting of the extracranial carotid arteries, *Tex Heart Inst J* 27:150–158, 2000.

89. Diethrich EB, Ndiaye M, Reid DB: Stenting in the carotid artery: initial experience in 110 patients, *J Endovasc Surg* 3:42–62, 1996.

90. Al-Mubarak N, Gomez CR, Vitek JJ, et al: Stenting of symptomatic stenosis of the intracranial internal carotid artery, *AJNR Am J Neuroradiol* 19:1949–1951, 1998.

91. Bergeron P, Becquemin JP, Jausseran JM, et al: Percutaneous stenting of the internal carotid artery: the European CAST I Study. Carotid Artery Stent Trial, *J Endovasc Surg* 6:155–159, 1999.

92. Qureshi AI, Luft AR, Janardhan V, et al: Identification of patients at risk for periprocedural neurological deficits associated with carotid angioplasty and stenting, *Stroke* 31:376–382, 2000.

93. Gupta A, Bhatia A, Ahuja A, et al: Carotid stenting in patients older than 65 years with inoperable carotid artery disease: a single-center experience, *Catheter Cardiovasc Interv* 50:1–8, 2000; discussion 9.

94. Wholey MH, Jarmolowski CR, Eles G, et al: Endovascular stents for carotid artery occlusive disease, *J Endovasc Surg* 4:326–338, 1997.

95. Shawl F, Kadro W, Domanski MJ, et al: Safety and efficacy of elective carotid artery stenting in high-risk patients, *J Am Coll Cardiol* 35:1721–1728, 2000.

96. Wholey M, Wholey M, Bergeron P, et al: Current global status of carotid artery stent placement, *Cathet Cardiovasc Diagn* 44:1–6, 1998.

97. Angelini A, Reimers B, Della Barbera M, et al: Cerebral protection during carotid artery stenting: collection and histopathologic analysis of embolized debris, *Stroke* 33:456–461, 2002.

98. Biller J, Feinberg WM, Castaldo JE, et al: Guidelines for carotid endarterectomy: a statement for healthcare professionals from a Special Writing Group of the Stroke Council, American Heart Association, *Circulation* 97:501–509, 1998.

99. Higashida RT, Popma JJ, Apruzzese P, et al: Evaluation of the Medtronic exponent self-expanding carotid stent system with the Medtronic GuardWire temporary occlusion and aspiration system in the treatment of carotid stenosis: combined from the MAVErIC (Medtronic AVE Self-expanding CaRotid Stent System with distal protection In the treatment of Carotid stenosis) I and MAVErIC II trials, *Stroke* 41:e102–e109, 2010.

100. Clair DG, Hopkins LN, Mehta M, et al: Neuroprotection during carotid artery stenting using the GORE flow reversal system: 30-day outcomes in the EMPiRE Clinical Study, *Catheter Cardiovasc Interv* 77:420–429, 2011.

101. Yadav JS, Wholey MH, Kuntz RE, et al: Protected carotid-artery stenting versus endarterectomy in high-risk patients, *N Engl J Med* 351:1493–1501, 2004.

102. Gray WA, Yadav JS, Verta P, et al: The CAPTURE registry: results of carotid stenting with embolic protection in the post approval setting, *Cathet Cardiovasc Interv* 69:341–348, 2007.

103. Gray WA, Hopkins LN, Yadav S, et al: Protected carotid stenting in high-surgical-risk patients: the ARCHeR results, *J Vasc Surg* 44:258–268, 2006.

104. Gurm HS, Yadav JS, Fayad P, et al: Long-term results of carotid stenting versus endarterectomy in high-risk patients, *N Engl J Med* 358:1572–1579, 2008.

105. Gray WA, Rosenfield KA, Jaff MR, et al: Influence of site and operator characteristics on carotid artery stent outcomes: analysis of the CAPTURE 2 (Carotid ACCULINK/ACCUNET Post Approval Trial to Uncover Rare Events) clinical study, *JACC Cardiovasc Interv* 4:235–246, 2011.

106. Theiss W, Hermanek P, Mathias K, et al: Predictors of death and stroke after carotid angioplasty and stenting: a subgroup analysis of the Pro-CAS data, *Stroke* 39:2325–2330, 2008.

107. Smout J, Macdonald S, Weir G, et al: Carotid artery stenting: relationship between experience and complication rate, *Int J Stroke* 5:477–482, 2010.

108. Rothwell PM, Slattery J, Warlow CP: A systematic review of the risks of stroke and death due to endarterectomy for symptomatic carotid stenosis, *Stroke* 27:260–265, 1996.

109. Ederle J, Dobson J, Featherstone RL, et al: Carotid artery stenting compared with endarterectomy in patients with symptomatic carotid stenosis (International Carotid Stenting Study): an interim analysis of a randomised controlled trial, *Lancet* 375:985–997, 2010.

110. Mas JL, Trinquart L, Leys D, et al: Endarterectomy versus Angioplasty in Patients with Symptomatic Severe Carotid Stenosis (EVA-3S) trial: results up to 4 years from a randomised, multicentre trial, *Lancet Neurol* 7:885–892, 2008.

111. McKevitt FM, Randall MS, Cleveland TJ, et al: The benefits of combined anti-platelet treatment in carotid artery stenting, *Eur J Vasc Endovasc Surg* 29:522–527, 2005.

112. Dalainas I, Nano G, Bianchi P, et al: Dual antiplatelet regime versus acetyl-acetic acid for carotid artery stenting, *Cardiovasc Intervent Radiol* 29:519–521, 2006.

113. Featherstone RL, Brown MM, Coward LJ: International carotid stenting study: protocol for a randomised clinical trial comparing carotid stenting with endarterectomy in symptomatic carotid artery stenosis, *Cerebrovasc Dis* 18:69–74, 2004.

114. Endarterectomy vs. Angioplasty in Patients with Symptomatic Severe Carotid Stenosis (EVA-3S) Trial, *Cerebrovasc Dis* 18:62–65, 2004.

115. Ringleb PA, Kunze A, Allenberg JR, et al: The Stent-Supported Percutaneous Angioplasty of the Carotid Artery vs. Endarterectomy Trial, *Cerebrovasc Dis* 18:66–68, 2004.

116. Roffi M, Sievert H, Gray WA, et al: Carotid artery stenting versus surgery: adequate comparisons? *Lancet Neurol* 9:339–341, 2010; author reply 341–332.

117. Blackshear JL, Cutlip DE, Roubin GS, et al: Myocardial infarction after carotid stenting and endarterectomy: results from the Carotid Revascularization Endarterectomy versus Stenting Trial, *Circulation* 123:2571–2578, 2011.

118. Kim LJ, Martinez EA, Faraday N, et al: Cardiac troponin I predicts short-term mortality in vascular surgery patients, *Circulation* 106:2366–2371, 2002.

119. Landesberg G, Shatz V, Akopnik I, et al: Association of cardiac troponin, CK-MB, and postoperative myocardial ischemia with long-term survival after major vascular surgery, *J Am Coll Cardiol* 42:1547–1554, 2003.

120. Chong CP, Lam QT, Ryan JE, et al: Incidence of post-operative troponin I rises and 1-year mortality after emergency orthopaedic surgery in older patients, *Age Ageing* 38:168–174, 2009.

121. Prasad A, Singh M, Lerman A, et al: Isolated elevation in troponin T after percutaneous coronary intervention is associated with higher long-term mortality, *J Am Coll Cardiol* 48:1765–1770, 2006.

122. Eckstein HH, Ringleb P, Allenberg JR, et al: Results of the Stent-Protected Angioplasty versus Carotid Endarterectomy (SPACE) study to treat symptomatic stenoses at 2 years: a multinational, prospective, randomised trial, *Lancet Neurol* 7:893–902, 2008.

123. Arquizan C, Trinquart L, Touboul PJ, et al: Restenosis is more frequent after carotid stenting than after endarterectomy: the EVA-3S study, *Stroke* 42:1015–1020, 2011.

124. Zhou W, Felkai DD, Evans M, et al: Ultrasound criteria for severe in-stent restenosis following carotid artery stenting, *J Vasc Surg* 47:74–80, 2008.

125. Lal BK, Hobson RW 2nd, Tofighi B, et al: Duplex ultrasound velocity criteria for the stented carotid artery, *J Vasc Surg* 47:63–73, 2008.

126. AbuRahma AF, Abu-Halimah S, Bensenhaver J, et al: Optimal carotid duplex velocity criteria for defining the severity of carotid in-stent restenosis, *J Vasc Surg* 48:589–594, 2008.

127. Nolz R, Wibmer A, Beitzke D, et al: Carotid artery stenting and follow-up: Value of 64-MSCT angiography as complementary imaging method to color-coded duplex sonography, *Eur J Radiol* 281:89–94, 2012.

128. Chang CK, Huded CP, Nolan BW, et al: Prevalence and clinical significance of stent fracture and deformation following carotid artery stenting, *J Vasc Surg* 54:685–690, 2011.

129. Cohen DJ, Stolker JM, Wang K, et al: Health-related quality of life after carotid stenting versus carotid endarterectomy results from CREST (Carotid Revascularization Endarterectomy versus Stenting Trial), *J Am Coll Cardiol* 58:1557–1565, 2011.

130. Brown PD, Foote RL, McLaughlin MP, et al: A historical prospective cohort study of carotid artery stenosis after radiotherapy for head and neck malignancies, *Int J Rad Onc Biol Phys* 63:1361–1367, 2005.

131. Tallarita T, Oderich GS, Lanzino G, et al: Outcomes of carotid artery stenting versus historical surgical controls for radiation-induced carotid stenosis, *J Vasc Surg* 53:629–636, e621–e625, 2011.

132. Sadek M, Cayne NS, Shin HJ, et al: Safety and efficacy of carotid angioplasty and stenting for radiation-associated carotid artery stenosis, *J Vasc Surg* 50:1308–1313, 2009.

133. Dorresteijn LD, Vogels OJ, de Leeuw FE, et al: Outcome of carotid artery stenting for radiation-induced stenosis, *Int J Rad Oncol Biol Phys* 77:1386–1390, 2010.

134. van Lammeren GW, Peeters W, de Vries JP, et al: Restenosis after carotid surgery: the importance of clinical presentation and preoperative timing, *Stroke* 42:965–971, 2011.

135. AbuRahma AF, Jennings TG, Wulu JT, et al: Redo carotid endarterectomy versus primary carotid endarterectomy, *Stroke* 32:2787–2792, 2001.

136. AbuRahma AF, Abu-Halimah S, Hass SM, et al: Carotid artery stenting outcomes are equivalent to carotid endarterectomy outcomes for patients with post-carotid endarterectomy stenosis, *J Vasc Surg* 52:1180–1187, 2010.

137. Counsell A, Ghosh J, McCollum CC, et al: Carotid stenting for restenosis after endarterectomy, *Cardiovasc Intervent Radiol* 34:488–492, 2011.

138. Bonati LH, Dobson J, Algra A, et al: Short-term outcome after stenting versus endarterectomy for symptomatic carotid stenosis: a preplanned meta-analysis of individual patient data, *Lancet* 376:1062–1073, 2010.

139. Howard VJ, Lutsep HL, Mackey A, et al: Influence of sex on outcomes of stenting versus endarterectomy: a subgroup analysis of the Carotid Revascularization Endarterectomy versus Stenting Trial (CREST), *Lancet Neurol* 10:530–537, 2011.

140. Brown MM, Raine R: Should sex influence the choice between carotid stenting and carotid endarterectomy? *Lancet Neurol* 10:494–497, 2011.

141. Hopkins LN, Roubin GS, Chakhtoura EY, et al: The Carotid Revascularization Endarterectomy versus Stenting Trial: credentialing of interventionalists and final results of lead-in phase, *J Stroke Cerebrovasc Dis* 19:153–162, 2010.

142. Chiam PT, Roubin GS, Iyer SS, et al: Carotid artery stenting in elderly patients: importance of case selection, *Catheter Cardiovasc Interv* 72:318–324, 2008.

143. Bendok BR, Hopkins LN: Cutting balloon angioplasty to treat carotid in-stent restenosis, *J Invasive Cardiol* 16:A16, 2004; discussion A16.

144. Zhou W, Lin PH, Bush RL, et al: Management of in-sent restenosis after carotid artery stenting in high-risk patients, *J Vasc Surg* 43:305–312, 2006.

145. Berens ES, Kouchoukos NT, Murphy SF, et al: Preoperative carotid artery screening in elderly patients undergoing cardiac surgery, *J Vasc Surg* 15:313–321, 1992; discussion 322–313.

146. Naylor AR, Mehta Z, Rothwell PM, et al: Carotid artery disease and stroke during coronary artery bypass: a critical review of the literature, *Eur J Vasc Endovasc Surg* 23:283–294, 2002.

147. Yan TD, Padang R, Poh C, et al: Drug-eluting stents versus coronary artery bypass grafting for the treatment of coronary artery disease: a meta-analysis of randomized and nonrandomized studies, *J Thorac Cardiovasc Surg* 141:1134–1144, 2011.

148. Naylor AR, Bell PR: Does the risk of post-CABG stroke merit staged or synchronous reconstruction in patients with asymptomatic carotid disease? *J Cardiovasc Surg* 44:383–394, 2003.

149. Aqel R, Dorfman TA: The brain first or the heart: the approach to revascularizing severe co-existing carotid and coronary artery disease, *Clin Cardiol* 32:418–425, 2009.

150. Van der Heyden J, Suttorp MJ, Bal ET, et al: Staged carotid angioplasty and stenting followed by cardiac surgery in patients with severe asymptomatic carotid artery stenosis: early and long-term results, *Circulation* 116:2036–2042, 2007.

151. Halliday A, Mansfield A, Marro J, et al: Prevention of disabling and fatal strokes by successful carotid endarterectomy in patients without recent neurological symptoms: randomised controlled trial, *Lancet* 363:1491–1502, 2004.

152. Roger VL, Go AS, Lloyd-Jones DM, et al: Heart disease and stroke statistics–2012 update: a report from the american heart association, *Circulation* 125:e2–e220, 2012.

153. Moneta GL, Edwards JM, Chitwood RW, et al: Correlation of North American Symptomatic Carotid Endarterectomy Trial (NASCET) angiographic definition of 70% to 99% internal carotid artery stenosis with duplex scanning, *J Vasc Surg* 17:152–157, 1993; discussion 157–159.

154. Nicolaides AN, Kakkos S, Griffin M, et al: Severity of asymptomatic carotid stenosis and risk of ipsilateral hemispheric ischaemic events: results from the ACSRS study, Nicolaides, et al: *EJVES* 30:275–284, 2005. *Eur J Vasc Endovasc Surg* 31:336, 2006.

CHAPTER 33 Carotid Endarterectomy

Wesley S. Moore

Historical Background

The development of surgery for carotid artery disease required three important advances: (1) recognition of the relationship between atherosclerotic disease of the carotid bifurcation and stroke, (2) premorbid identification of carotid bifurcation disease, and (3) the vascular surgical techniques necessary to remove carotid bifurcation atherosclerotic plaque.

For many years, the relationship between carotid artery disease and stroke was overlooked because autopsy protocol did not include harvesting the cervical vessels. Therefore, the only pathology observed in hemispheric stroke was thrombus in the intracranial vessels, most commonly the middle cerebral artery (MCA). One of the earliest observations of the relationship of cervical carotid artery disease with stroke was made in 1856 by Savory, who described a patient with left monocular blindness, right hemiplegia, right dysesthesia, and an occluded left internal carotid artery (ICA) at the carotid bifurcation.[1] A similar observation was made by Gowers in 1875.[2] It was not until 1914 that Hunt described the relationship between carotid artery disease, transient ischemic attacks (TIAs), and stroke.[3] The ability to identify carotid bifurcation disease prior to death awaited the work of Moniz, who in 1927 reported on the technique of carotid angiography. This, for the first time, provided the opportunity to identify carotid artery occlusive disease in the living patient.[4] In spite of this, clinicians solely used cerebral angiography to evaluate the intracranial circulation. In 1951, Fisher reemphasized the importance of the cervical carotid artery, pointing out that prior to occlusion, a stenosis was present that might be amenable to surgical correction.[5]

The surgical phase for treating carotid artery disease began in 1951. Carrea et al. from Buenos Aires resected the diseased segment of an ICA and restored flow by anastomosing the external carotid artery (ECA) to the distal ICA. They waited until 1955 for sufficient follow-up before reporting the case.[6] Probably the first successful carotid endarterectomy (CEA) was performed by DeBakey et al. in 1953, but it was not reported until 1959, with a long-term follow-up reported in 1975.[7] The publication that led to rapid incorporation of carotid artery surgery into clinical practice was the operation reported by Eastcott et al. in 1954. They described a case of a woman who was experiencing hemispheric TIAs, with an associated stenosis of the bulb of the carotid artery. They resected the carotid artery bifurcation and restored flow by a direct anastomosis between the common and distal ICAs with a successful outcome and cessation of symptoms. This report led to an explosion of interest in the treatment of carotid bifurcation disease.[8]

Pathology of Carotid Bifurcation Disease

The most common lesion of the carotid artery bifurcation is an atherosclerotic plaque involving the bulb of the ICA. This localization of plaque is predictable and provides the opportunity for treatment with CEA. The plaque can be calcific, fibrous, or composed of atherosclerotic elements of mixed consistency. Plaques can expand slowly or, with intraplaque hemorrhage, rapidly. Other pathological lesions causing carotid artery stenosis include fibromuscular dysplasia (FMD), Takayasu's arteritis (TA), radiation arteriopathy, and (rarely) aneurysms of the cervical ICA.

Pathogenetic Mechanisms of Stroke and Transient Ischemic Events

The pathogenetic mechanism for ischemic events is primarily thrombotic or atheroembolic (also see Chapter 30). If the occlusive plaque in the carotid bulb progresses to critical flow reduction, the ICA will proceed to thrombotic occlusion. The pace of the occlusive process is important. If this process occurs slowly, collateral circulation may develop from the contralateral carotid and vertebral arteries. In addition, the ipsilateral ECA can be a source of collateral blood flow by flow reversal through the ophthalmic artery to the siphon of the ICA. Under these circumstances, thrombosis of the ICA may be a silent event. On the other hand, if plaque expansion occurs rapidly or if collateral circulation is inadequate, there will be thrombotic propagation beyond the ophthalmic branch of the ICA into the middle cerebral artery, causing hemisphere infarction and neurological deficit.

In addition to thrombotic occlusion of the ICA, the more common mechanism for ischemic events is rupture of the intimal cover of the atherosclerotic plaque, permitting the discharge of soft atherosclerotic debris into the blood flow stream. These fragments are carried distally to the intracranial branches, fostering either permanent branch occlusion and cerebral infarction or, with fragmentation and thrombolysis of the embolus, a temporary and reversible neurological deficit or TIA. Following plaque rupture and a primary wave of embolization, a defect is left in the plaque that on angiographic inspection resembles an ulcer. This ulcer or plaque defect can be the source of continual embolization, or it can be the nidus for platelet aggregate and thrombotic material to reside. Since there is no attachment of this material within the ulcer crater, pulsatile blood flow can dislodge the material residing with the ulcer crater, leading to a secondary wave of embolization.

Clinical Evaluation

Clinical evaluation of patients with cerebrovascular disease (carotid artery disease) is discussed in Chapter 30.

Preoperative Imaging

The noninvasive examination of choice for patients with suspected carotid artery disease is a carotid duplex ultrasound scan using modern equipment in a validated vascular laboratory (also see Chapter 12). This study identifies lesions in the carotid artery, classifies the severity of stenosis, and provides information regarding plaque consistency. The opportunity to examine flow velocity and pulse wave velocity analysis provides information about other portions of the circulation, including proximal lesions at the level of the aortic arch and distal intracranial lesions. In many centers, the duplex scan serves as the definitive preoperative study.[9] Additional studies such as magnetic resonance imaging (MRI), magnetic resonance angiography (MRA), computed tomographic angiography (CTA), or catheter-based contrast angiography are reserved for special circumstances.[9] Use of MRA or CTA in conjunction with duplex ultrasound of the carotid artery is considered when the results of duplex ultrasonography are difficult to interpret or inconsistent with the clinical presentation.

Magnetic resonance angiography is used frequently because it does not require ionizing radiation. When contrast is added, the images are often clear and resemble those obtained via catheter-based intraarterial angiography, providing a sensitivity and specificity of 88% and 84%, respectively, for diagnosing a 70% to 99% stenosis.[9] Magnetic resonance angiography permits imaging of the intracranial vascular anatomy, and when combined with MRI, can identify areas of cerebral infarction or other intracranial pathology. The major limitation of MRA is that it tends to overestimate percent stenosis of lesions in the carotid bifurcation (also see Chapter 13). This phenomenon occurs because turbulent blood blow, such as occurs at carotid bulb stenosis, results in signal dropout and void, giving the impression of a high-grade carotid stenosis.

Computed tomography (CT) and CTA are also quite helpful in identifying intracranial lesions. Computed tomography angiography is accurate in identifying and quantifying intracranial and extracranial carotid stenosis (also see Chapter 14). The sensitivity and specificity of CTA for determination of carotid artery stenosis are 95% and 99%, respectively.[10] The major drawbacks of CT scanning are exposure to ionizing radiation and the requirement for a large volume of iodinated contrast material, which can be nephrotoxic or cause allergic reaction in patients sensitive to iodine.

Intraarterial contrast angiography is considered the gold standard for identifying and quantifying arterial stenoses. Major disadvantages of this invasive procedure include arterial injury, occlusion, and embolization resulting in cerebral infarction. In the Asymptomatic Carotid Artery Study (ACAS), angiography was associated with a 1% stroke rate.[11] In addition, it requires ionizing radiation and iodinated contrast material. This technique is now rarely indicated prior to carotid endarterectomies. It does have a role for preprocedure imaging as a part of carotid angioplasty/stenting.

Techniques of Carotid Endarterectomy

An arterial canula is placed for continuous blood pressure monitoring and periodic sampling of blood gases. Carotid endarterectomy can be performed under either local or general anesthesia. General anesthesia is more comfortable for the patient. It affords a quiet operative field and allows the surgeon to concentrate without distraction by patient movement or discomfort. It also allows optimal airway control, ventilation, and oxygenation.

The patient is positioned supine on the operating table. A cushion is placed under the shoulders to allow for mild neck extension, and the head is rotated away from the side of incision.

When the carotid artery is clamped for the endarterectomy procedure, the surgeon has several choices regarding the assurance of adequate blood flow to the ipsilateral cerebral hemisphere. About 90% of patients tolerate temporary clamping of the carotid artery because adequate collateral circulation is provided through the circle of Willis. For patients with inadequate collateral circulation, a temporary shunt is required to maintain adequate cerebral perfusion during endarterectomy to avoid periprocedural cerebral infarction. These observations have led to two forms of practice: routine shunting of all patients or selective shunting based upon intraoperative monitoring. The argument for routine shunting is that special monitoring is not required. The argument in favor of selective shunting is that there are complications unique to the use of an internal shunt. These include intimal damage with shunt placement and embolization of air or atheromatous debris through the shunt to the intracranial circulation, resulting in a cerebral infarction. In addition, when a shunt is in place, it is difficult to see the end of the endarterectomized segment, thus opening the possibility of leaving a residual intimal flap that can lead to thromboembolism and possibly postoperative carotid occlusion. Therefore, since only 10% of patients undergoing CEA require a shunt, there is little reason to expose the majority 90% who do not require a shunt to its potential complications.

There are several acceptable methods for monitoring the adequacy of cerebral perfusion. The first method that was described was measurement of ICA backpressure in patients undergoing CEA under local anesthesia. With clamping of the common carotid artery (CCA) and ECA, the residual pressure in the carotid artery determines the perfusion in the middle cerebral artery. One study found that the conscious response to clamping correlated with the ICA backpressure.[12] The minimum pressure associated with no neurological deficit was 25 mmHg. This observation was subsequently validated in patients undergoing operation with general anesthesia.[13,14] The next method, and one that is most commonly used today, is continuous electroencephalographic (EEG) monitoring. This method is sensitive, easy to use, and has the advantage of providing continuous monitoring rather than a single

observation. Other methods used to monitor cerebral perfusion include assessment of the somatosensory evoked response and transcranial Doppler (TCD) interrogation.

There are two possible incisions that can be used. Some surgeons use an oblique incision in a skin crease, with the thought that the resulting scar will be more cosmetic in appearance. More proximal or distal exposure, when required, is quite difficult to obtain with this incision. The alternative is an incision placed along a line connecting the suprasternal notch with the mastoid process. The surgeon can begin with a relatively short incision over the carotid bifurcation and extend it proximally or distally if necessary. The incision is deepened through the platysma layer. The sternocleidomastoid muscle is mobilized until the jugular vein is identified. The common facial vein and any accessory facial veins are divided between ligatures. The vein is allowed to retract laterally, and the carotid artery will be found immediately below the vein. Care must be taken to identify the vagus nerve because its relationship within the carotid sheath can be quite variable. The CCA is circumferentially mobilized within the perivascular plane of Leriche. Mobilization is continued distally until the carotid bifurcation, ICA, and ECA are fully mobilized. The ICA should be exposed far enough so that circumferentially normal artery is encountered. If additional exposure is required, the nerve to the carotid sinus can be divided. This will allow the carotid bifurcation to drop inferiorly and permit more distal mobilization of the ICA. In the case of a high carotid bifurcation or long extension of the plaque in the ICA, more extensive exposure of the ICA can be obtained by mobilizing or, if necessary, dividing the posterior belly of the digastric muscle. Finally, exposure of the ICA to the base of the skull can be obtained by dividing the styloid process. This is very rarely required.

Once the arteries are sufficiently mobilized, intravenous (IV) heparin is administered. The dose varies from 2500 units to 5000 units depending upon the size of the patient and the nature of preoperative antiplatelet agents administered. The internal, external, and common carotid arteries are then clamped. A longitudinal arteriotomy is made in the CCA and extended through the plaque distal to normal ICA. During this time, the EEG monitor is observed. If no EEG changes indicative of brain ischemia appear with clamping, the surgeon proceeds with the endarterectomy procedure. If there are EEG changes with clamping, an internal shunt is placed. The exception for selective shunting occurs in patients who have had a prior stroke on the side of operation; shunt placement can lessen the risk of stroke in the ischemic penumbra that surrounds the area of infarction.

Once the decision is made concerning the shunt, the surgeon proceeds with endarterectomy. Endarterectomy of the external carotid is blind. There should be a feathered endpoint in the ICA. The endarterectomy is carried to the clamp, which serves as the endpoint. The plaque should be cleared in the common carotid artery, and the proximal endpoint may require sharp division. Once the plaque is removed, the carotid artery is irrigated with heparinized saline, and any loose bits of medial debris are carefully removed. The segment between the ICA endarterectomy and normal intima is carefully inspected to ensure that the intima is adherent to the media at that level. If an intimal flap is present, it is carefully removed back to a point of adherence.

The arteriotomy is closed with a patch (typically Dacron) to prevent stenosis and accommodate any restriction from intimal hyperplasia that might occur with primary closure. Patch closure is associated with a lower incidence of postoperative thromboembolic complication and recurrent carotid stenosis.[15] Before the arteriotomy is completely closed, the vessels should be "backbled" and flushed to remove any debris. Upon completion of closure, flow is restored first to the ECA and then the ICA. At this time, it is important to verify the quality of the endarterectomy by intraoperative duplex ultrasound scanning or a completion angiogram. The latter permits accurate visualization of the carotid artery bifurcation and the intracranial portion of the repaired ICA to detect any anatomical problems or residual stenosis. If an intimal flap is seen in the ICA, the patch is removed and the arteriotomy extended beyond the flap, thereby reducing the risk of postoperative thromboembolism. A new patch is used to close the arteriotomy. More commonly, an endpoint problem is found in the ECA, which can lead to postoperative thrombosis of the ECA and then in retrograde propagation of thrombus to the ICA, embolism, and stroke.[16] When a problem is identified, the ECA is clamped both at its origin and distally. A transverse arteriotomy is made just distal to the residual lesion, and the remaining plaque is removed. The transverse arteriotomy is closed with interrupted polypropylene sutures, and flow is restored. The neck incision is then closed. Closure consists of a running absorbable suture in the platysma layer and a running absorbable subcuticular suture for cosmetic skin closure.

Postoperative Management

A brief postoperative neurological assessment is performed in the operating room following extubation. If no neurological deficits are noted, the patient is transferred to the recovery room for monitoring. Once the patient is fully awake, the blood pressure controlled, and the neck free of hematoma, the patient is transferred to a regular hospital room for overnight observation. Postoperative blood pressure monitoring and treatment is important. Patients often become hypertensive after awakening from anesthesia. Regulation of blood flow is impaired on the side of endarterectomy for approximately 3 to 6 weeks, so the ipsilateral cerebral hemisphere is vulnerable to elevated postoperative blood pressure. Uncontrolled hypertension can result in excessive perfusion pressure, the consequences of which range from headache to seizures and lead to intracerebral bleeding resulting in major stroke or death. Hypotension and bradycardia occur from baroreceptor activation caused by stimulation of the nerve to the carotid sinus. This can easily be treated by injecting the nerve with 1% lidocaine. Following recovery from anesthesia, hypotension is a rare occurrence.

If the patient is stable overnight and does not have a new neurological complication, he or she can be discharged the following morning. The patient is instructed to resume usual medications, including an antiplatelet agent.

The first postoperative visit should occur in approximately 3 weeks, at which time a carotid duplex ultrasound scan is performed to assess the result of endarterectomy and establish a new baseline for further follow-up. Additional carotid ultrasound examinations are recommended at 6 months and then 1 year from the time of operation.

Complications of Carotid Endarterectomy

The mortality rate reported in large surgical trials of CEA is approximately 1% and is usually cardiovascular in nature.[17] This mortality rate is similar to that observed in a general vascular surgical practice.[18] The risk of stroke is approximately 2.6%.[19] The principal etiology of postoperative stroke is embolism of thrombus or atheromatous debris.[20]

Cranial nerve injury occurs in up to 7% of patients, although permanent nerve palsy is noted in 1%.[21] Several cranial nerves lie within the operative field, including the vagus (X), hypoglossal (XII), and (less commonly) glossopharyngeal (IX). The mandibular branch of the facial nerve (VII) may be at risk if the surgical incision is made anterior to the ear instead of on a line connecting the mastoid process and the suprasternal notch.

Despite achieving hemostasis prior to wound closure, hematomas may develop. These are usually evident within the first 4 hours following operation. Patients with expanding hematomas should return to the operating room for evacuation and restitution of hemostasis. A bleeding source after hematoma evacuation usually is not found. Judicious use of heparin, particularly if the patient is on more than one antiplatelet agent, is important. Heparin reversal with protamine is associated with risk of anaphylaxis.

Prevention may be the best strategy. Irrigating the wound with a dilute antibiotic solution and observing for bleeding sites (to be controlled with ligature or electrocoagulation) may be the best strategy.

Wound infection is rare because patients undergoing CEA receive prophylactic antibiotics. If a wound infection occurs, the patient should be hospitalized and treated with an IV antibiotic therapy regimen. A deep wound infection may affect a prosthetic patch and threaten the integrity of the carotid artery.

Clinical Trials of Carotid Endarterectomy

Prospective randomized trials comparing CEA to medical management involve either symptomatic or asymptomatic patients. They serve as the basis for current CEA recommendations in appropriately selected patients.[21]

Symptomatic Carotid Endarterectomy Trials

The North American Symptomatic Carotid Endarterectomy Trial (NASCET) was a multicenter prospective randomized trial carried out in the United States and Canada. The trial was divided into two cohorts; one involved patients with carotid artery stenosis of 70% to 99%, and the other involved patients with stenosis of 50% to 69%. The high-grade (70%-99%) stenosis component of the study was stopped after only 18 months because stroke morbidity and mortality for CEA was 9%, compared with 26% for best medical management.[22] The second part of the study, for patients with moderate stenosis, went to completion. It demonstrated a 5-year event rate after CEA of 15.7%, vs. 22.2% for medical management.[23] The European Carotid Endarterectomy Trial (ECST) was conducted during the same time as NASCET. It recruited a population similar to the high-grade stenosis portion of NASCET, with similar findings. Stroke morbidity and mortality after CEA was 10.3%, vs. 16.8% for medical management.[24] The Veterans Administration Symptomatic Trial was started after the other two trials were ongoing. It was stopped after 189 patients were entered as the results of the North American and European trials were reported. Despite the small number of patients, the rate of stroke and crescendo TIA after only 12 months' follow-up was 7.7% for surgery and 19.4% for medical management.[25] Based on these trials, CEA is recommended for symptomatic patients with greater than 50% stenosis.[21]

Asymptomatic Carotid Endarterectomy Trials

The Veterans Affairs Asymptomatic Carotid Endarterectomy Trial enrolled 444 asymptomatic men with carotid artery stenoses greater than 50% as documented by angiography. These were randomized to CEA plus best medical management, or best medical management alone. At the end of 5 years, the primary event rate of TIA, stroke, and death was 8% for surgery, vs. 20.6% for medical management.[26] The ACAS trial was a multicenter prospective randomized trial that compared CEA plus best medical management to best medical management alone. At the end of 5 years, the primary event rate of stroke or death was 5.1% for CEA and 11% for medical management.[11] The Asymptomatic Carotid Stenosis Trial (ACST) randomized 1560 patients to immediate CEA and 1560 patients to medical management. At the end of 5 years, the primary event rate for immediate CEA was 6.4%, compared with 11.8% in patients randomized to medical management.[19] The American College of Cardiology/American Heart Association (ACC/AHA) guidelines give a class IIa recommendation for CEA for asymptomatic patients with carotid artery stenosis greater than 70%.

Carotid Endarterectomy Compared to Carotid Angioplasty/Stenting

Carotid artery angiography and stenting is described in detail in Chapter 32. Several clinical trials have compared CEA with carotid artery stenting (CAS).

The Stenting and Angioplasty with Protection in Patients at High Risk for Endarterectomy (SAPPHIRE) trial was a prospective multicenter randomized trial of symptomatic and asymptomatic patients considered high risk for surgery due to coexisting medical morbidity or a hostile neck; 156 patients were randomized to CAS, and 151 were randomized to CEA. The primary composite endpoint included death, stroke, and myocardial infarction (MI). The 30-day rates of death and stroke were no different between the two procedures, but with MI added to death and stroke, the composite endpoint rate for CAS was 5.8%, vs. 12.6% for CEA. These differences persisted for 1 year, but by 4 years, there was no difference between the two groups regarding event-free survival.[27,28]

The Endarterectomy versus Angioplasty in Patients with Symptomatic Severe Carotid Stenosis (EVA-3S) trial was a prospective multicenter trial carried out in France. A total of 527 patients with greater than 60% stenosis were randomized to CEA (262) or CAS (265). The study was stopped early because the death and stroke rate at 30 days was 3.9% for CEA and 9.6% for CAS. The study patients were followed for 4 years, at which time the death and stroke rates were 6.2% for those treated with CEA and 11.1% for those treated with CAS.[29,30]

The Stent-Protected Angioplasty versus Carotid Endarterectomy for Symptomatic Stenosis (SPACE) trial, carried out in Germany, Austria, and Switzerland, was a prospective multicenter randomized trial of symptomatic patients with high-grade carotid stenoses. The hypothesis was that CAS was not inferior to CEA. Twelve hundred patients were randomized, but the study was stopped because a futility analysis was performed indicating that the primary hypothesis could not be proved. At the time the study was stopped, the death and stroke rate for CAS was 7.7%, vs. 6.5% for CEA. Of note, by 2 years, the recurrent stenosis rate was 10.7% for CAS and 4.6% for CEA.[31]

The International Carotid Artery Stenting Study (ICSS) compared CEA with CAS. It involved 50 academic centers in the United Kingdom, Europe, Australia, New Zealand, and Canada. A total of 1713 patients with high-grade carotid stenoses were randomly allocated to CEA (858) or CAS (855). The primary outcomes were stroke, death, or procedural MI analyzed at 120 days following the procedure. The incidence of the combined endpoints of death, stroke, and MI in the CAS group was 8.5%, vs. 5.2% for CEA. Subgroup analyses of the patients who underwent pre- and post-procedure MRI found that 50% of the CAS group had at least one new area of cerebral infarction, vs. 17% of the CEA group.[32]

The Carotid Revascularization Endarterectomy versus Stenting (CREST) trial was a multicenter prospective randomized trial of symptomatic and asymptomatic patients with hemodynamically significant carotid stenoses; it was carried out in 108 centers in the United States and Canada. Between the years 2000 and 2008, 2502 patients were randomized; 47% were asymptomatic, and 53% were symptomatic. The initial analysis occurred after the last group of patients had at least 1 year of follow-up, and median follow-up was 2.5 years. The primary composite endpoint was periprocedural death, stroke in any distribution, and MI, which occurred in 4.5% of patients randomized to CEA and 5.2% randomized to CAS. The differences were not significant. The combined rate of death and stroke was 2.3% for CEA and 4.4% for CAS. There was a higher nonfatal MI rate in the CEA group. The study identified age as an important differentiating factor between CEA and CAS. Older patients did better with CEA, and younger patients did better with CAS. The inflection point occurred at age 70.[33] Based on these studies, the ACC/AHA guidelines give a class IIa recommendation for CEA over CAS for older patients.

REFERENCES

1. Savory WS: Case of a young woman in whom the main arteries of both upper extremities and of the left side of the neck were throughout completely obliterated, *Med Chir Trans* 39:205–219, 1856.
2. Gowers W: On a case of simultaneous embolism of central retinal and middle cerebral arteries, *Lancet* 2:794, 1875.
3. Hunt J: The role of the carotid arteries in the causation of vascular lesions of the brain, with remarks on certain special features of symptomatology, *Am J Med Sci* 147:704–713, 1914.
4. Moniz E: L'encephalographie arterielle: Son importance dans la localization des tumeurs cerebrale, *Rev Neurol (Paris)* 2:72–90, 1927.
5. Fisher M: Occlusion of the internal carotid artery, *AMA Arch Neurol Psychiatry* 65:346–377, 1951.
6. Carrea R, Molins M, Murphy G: Surgical treatment of spontaneous thrombosis of the internal carotid artery in the neck: carotid-carotidal anastomosis. Report of a case, *Acta Neurol Latinoam* 1:71–78, 1955.
7. DeBakey ME: Successful carotid endarterectomy for cerebrovascular insufficiency. Nineteen-year follow-up, *JAMA* 233:1083–1085, 1975.
8. Eastcott HH, Pickering GW, Rob CG: Reconstruction of internal carotid artery in a patient with intermittent attacks of hemiplegia, *Lancet* 267:994–996, 1954.
9. Ricotta JJ, Aburahma A, Ascher E, et al: Updated Society for Vascular Surgery guidelines for management of extracranial carotid disease, *J Vasc Surg* 54:e1–e31, 2011.
10. Anzidei M, Napoli A, Zaccagna F, et al: Diagnostic accuracy of colour Doppler ultrasonography, CT angiography and blood-pool-enhanced MR angiography in assessing carotid stenosis: a comparative study with DSA in 170 patients, *Radiol Med (Torino)* 117; 54–71, 2011.
11. Executive Committee for the Asymptomatic Carotid Atherosclerosis Study: Endarterectomy for asymptomatic carotid artery stenosis, *JAMA* 273:1421–1428, 1995.
12. Naylor AR, Whyman M, Wildsmith JA, et al: Immediate effects of carotid clamp release on middle cerebral artery blood flow velocity during carotid endarterectomy, *Eur J Vasc Surg* 7:308–316, 1993.
13. Moore WS, Hall AD: Carotid artery back pressure: a test of cerebral tolerance to temporary carotid occlusion, *Arch Surg* 99:702–710, 1969.
14. Moore WS, Yee JM, Hall AD: Collateral cerebral blood pressure. An index of tolerance to temporary carotid occlusion, *Arch Surg* 106:521–523, 1973.
15. AbuRahma AF, Robinson PA, Saiedy S, et al: Prospective randomized trial of bilateral carotid endarterectomies: primary closure versus patching, *Stroke* 30:1185–1189, 1999.
16. Moore WS, Martello JY, Quinones-Baldrich WJ, et al: Etiologic importance of the intimal flap of the external carotid artery in the development of post carotid endarterectomy stroke, *Stroke* 21:1497–1502, 1990.
17. Halliday A, Harrison M, Hayter E, et al: 10-year stroke prevention after successful carotid endarterectomy for asymptomatic stenosis (ACST-1): a multicentre randomised trial, *Lancet* 376:1074–1084, 2010.
18. Finks JF, Osborne NH, Birkmeyer JD: Trends in hospital volume and operative mortality for high-risk surgery, *N Engl J Med* 364:2128–2137, 2011.
19. Halliday A, Mansfield A, Marro J, et al: Prevention of disabling and fatal strokes by successful carotid endarterectomy in patients without recent neurological symptoms: randomised controlled trial, *Lancet* 363:1491–1502, 2004.
20. Spencer MP: Transcranial Doppler monitoring and causes of stroke from carotid endarterectomy, *Stroke* 28:685–691, 1997.
21. Brott TG, Halperin JL, Abbara S, et al: ASA/ACCF/AHA/AANN/AANS/ACR/ASNR/CNS/SAIP/SCAI/SIR/SNIS/SVM/SVS guideline on the management of patients with extracranial carotid and vertebral artery disease. A report of the American College of Cardiology Foundation/American Heart Association Task Force on Practice Guidelines, and the American Stroke Association, American Association of Neuroscience Nurses, American Association of Neurological Surgeons, American College of Radiology, American Society of Neuroradiology, Congress of Neurological Surgeons, Society of Atherosclerosis Imaging and Prevention, Society for Cardiovascular Angiography and Interventions, Society of Interventional Radiology, Society of NeuroInterventional Surgery, Society for Vascular Medicine, and Society for Vascular Surgery, *Circulation* 124:e54–e130, 2011.
22. North American Symptomatic Carotid Endarterectomy Trial Collaborators: Beneficial effect of carotid endarterectomy in symptomatic patients with high-grade carotid stenosis, *N Engl J Med* 325:445–453, 1991.
23. Barnett HJ, Taylor DW, Eliasziw M, et al: Benefit of carotid endarterectomy in patients with symptomatic moderate or severe stenosis. North American Symptomatic Carotid Endarterectomy Trial Collaborators, *N Engl J Med* 339:1415–1425, 1998.
24. European Carotid Surgery Trialists' Collaborative Group: MRC European Carotid Surgery Trial: interim results for symptomatic patients with severe (70%-99%) or with mild (0%-29%) carotid stenosis, *Lancet* 337:1235–1243, 1991.
25. Mayberg MR, Wilson SE, Yatsu F, et al: Carotid endarterectomy and prevention of cerebral ischemia in symptomatic carotid stenosis. Veterans Affairs Cooperative Studies Program 309 Trialist Group, *JAMA* 266:3289–3294, 1991.
26. Hobson RW 2nd, Fields WS, Weiss DG, et al: Efficacy of carotid endarterectomy for asymptomatic carotid stenosis. The Veterans Affairs Cooperative Study Group, *N Engl J Med* 328:221–227, 1993.
27. Yadav JS, Wholey MH, Kuntz RE, et al: Protected carotid-artery stenting versus endarterectomy in high-risk patients, *N Engl J Med* 351:1493–1501, 2004.
28. Gurm HS, Yadav JS, Fayad P, et al: Long-term results of carotid stenting versus endarterectomy in high-risk patients, *N Engl J Med* 358:1572–1579, 2008.
29. Mas JL, Chatellier G, Beyssen B, et al: Endarterectomy versus stenting in patients with symptomatic severe carotid stenosis, *N Engl J Med* 355:1660–1671, 2006.
30. Mas JL, Trinquart L, Leys D, et al: Endarterectomy versus Angioplasty in Patients with Symptomatic Severe Carotid Stenosis (EVA-3S) trial: results up to 4 years from a randomised, multicentre trial, *Lancet Neurol* 7:885–892, 2008.
31. Ringleb PA, Allenberg J, Bruckmann H, et al: 30 day results from the SPACE trial of Stent-Protected Angioplasty versus Carotid Endarterectomy in symptomatic patients: a randomised non-inferiority trial, *Lancet* 368:1239–1247, 2006.
32. Bonati LH, Jongen LM, Haller S, et al: New ischaemic brain lesions on MRI after stenting or endarterectomy for symptomatic carotid stenosis: a substudy of the International Carotid Stenting Study (ICSS), *Lancet Neurol* 9:353–362, 2010.
33. Brott TG, Hobson RW 2nd, Howard G, et al: Stenting versus endarterectomy for treatment of carotid-artery stenosis, *N Engl J Med* 363:11–23, 2010.

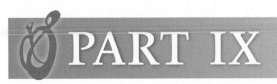
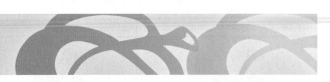
CHAPTER **34**

Pathophysiology, Clinical Evaluation, and Medical Management of Aortic Dissection

Bradley A. Maron, Patrick T. O'Gara

Acute aortic dissection is an uncommon but life-threatening emergency that requires prompt diagnosis, rapid triage, and immediate medical, endovascular, or surgical treatment. A unified effort across several international centers over the past 15 years has led to the establishment of a detailed registry that describes major aspects of presentation, management, and outcomes of patients with acute aortic dissection.[1] This longitudinal experience has given new clinical insights into an old disease and spawned additional multicenter efforts to explore its genetics and pathobiology. Although gains have been made in the delivery of life-saving care to patients with acute aortic dissection, hospital mortality rates remain distressingly high. Enhanced awareness of risk factors for aortic dissection, presentation features, diagnostic pathways, and medical, endovascular, and surgical treatment strategies is a critical first step toward improving outcomes.

Epidemiology

Published figures on the incidence of aortic dissection likely underestimate the actual occurrence rate, since misdiagnosis of this condition is common and the percentage of acute aortic dissection patients who expire before hospital presentation cannot be accurately estimated.[2] Nevertheless, acute aortic dissection is a rare event. Analysis of the Swedish National Cause of Death Register between 1987 and 2002 estimated the incidence of thoracic aortic aneurysm or dissection to be 16.3 per 100,000 men and 9.1 per 100,000 women; others have reported acute aortic dissection to affect 30 in 1 million individuals per year.[3] By comparison, acute myocardial infarction (AMI) is 140-fold more common.[1] Data from the International Registry of Aortic Dissection (IRAD) indicate that the mean age of patients at presentation with aortic dissection is 63 years, with men accounting for 63% of cases.[1]

Classification

Classifying aortic dissection according to anatomical location and time from onset of symptoms helps stratify risk and guide selection of initial treatment strategy (Fig. 34-1). The Stanford classification system designates dissections that involve the aorta proximal to the brachiocephalic artery (i.e., root and ascending aorta) as type A, and those that do not as type B.[4] This distinction is clinically important because dissection involving the ascending aorta is a key determinate of early death and major morbidity. Location of the intimal tear does not influence Stanford dissection type. In the older DeBakey classification scheme, a type I dissection *originates* within the ascending aorta and extends for a variable distance beyond the take-off the innominate artery. A DeBakey type II dissection is confined to the ascending aorta, and a type III

dissection originates in the descending thoracic aorta beyond the origin of the left subclavian artery and terminates above (type IIIA) or extends below (type IIIB) the level of the diaphragm.[5] Although there is no single universally accepted classification system, the Stanford classification scheme is most often used in practice today and will be used throughout this chapter. The terms *communicating* and *noncommunicating* refer to the presence or absence, respectively, of blood flow between the true and false lumens of the aorta.

Aortic dissection is *acute* if presentation occurs within 14 days of the onset of symptoms and *chronic* if more than 2 weeks have elapsed. Morbidity and mortality are highest within the acute phase; patients who have survived without treatment for 2 weeks are self-selected for better short- and intermediate-term outcomes.

In practice, diagnosis of aortic dissection depends on demonstration with imaging of an intimal flap with separation of true and false lumens. In type A dissection, the true lumen is usually displaced along the inner curvature of the aortic arch and continues caudally along the medial aspect of the descending thoracic aorta. Aortic branch vessel blood flow may derive from either the true or false lumen; alternatively, flow may be sluggish or absent within the false lumen, or branch vessels may be completely occluded at or near their origins.

Pathogenesis

Forces that weaken the medial layer of the aorta increase the probability of dilation, aneurysm formation, and dissection (Box 34-1). Acquired and genetic diseases that mediate this process are discussed later. In classic acute aortic dissection, the initiating event is an intimal tear through which blood rapidly surges distally into the media under systolic pressure, splitting the layers of the aortic wall and creating an intimal flap that separates the true from the false lumen.

Intimal Tear

Contemporary imaging modalities or autopsy findings identify the primary entry tear in approximately 90% of cases. It is most frequently located a few centimeters above the level of the aortic valve along the greater curvature of the aorta in cases of type A dissection and accounts for nearly 60% of all cases. Compared with other locations in the ascending aorta, the proximal few centimeters of the greater curvature are exposed to relatively greater hemodynamic, shear, and torsional force. A pivot region located in the descending thoracic aorta just beyond the insertion of the ligamentum arteriosum where the relatively mobile arch meets the fixed descending thoracic aorta is the second most common

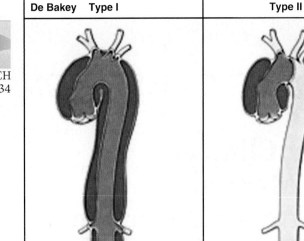

De Bakey Type I	Type II	Type III

Stanford	Type A	Type B

De Bakey

Type I	Originates in the ascending aorta, propagates at least to the aortic arch and often beyond it distally
Type II	Originates in and is confined to the ascending aorta
Type III	Originates in the descending aorta and extends distally down the aorta or, rarely, retrograde into the aortic arch and ascending aorta

Stanford

Type A	All dissections involving the ascending aorta, regardless of the site of origin
Type B	All dissections not involving the ascending aorta

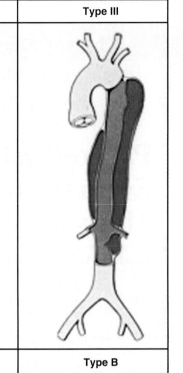

FIGURE 34-1 Aortic dissection type according to De Bakey and Stanford classification systems. *(From Nienaber C, Eagle KA: Aortic dissection: new frontiers in diagnosis and management. Part I: from etiology to diagnostic strategies. Circulation 108:628–635, 2003.)[7]*

Acute: Presentation ≤2 weeks following symptom onset

Chronic: Presentation >2 weeks following symptom onset

Box 34-1   Aortic Dissection Predisposing Factors

Genetic
Marfan's syndrome (MFS)
Ehlers-Danlos' syndrome (EDS)
Familial thoracic aortic aneurysm disease (FTAAD)
Bicuspid aortic valve (BAV) disease
Aberrant right subclavian artery
Aortic coarctation
Noonan's syndrome
Turner's syndrome
Polycystic kidney disease
Loeys-Dietz's syndrome

Acquired
Hypertension
Iatrogenic
Pregnancy
Inflammatory aortitis
Cocaine, (?)chronic amphetamine use

---

entry site for intimal tears, which will then propagate as a type B dissection (30% of cases). Arch entry occurs in 7% of cases. The abdominal aorta is the least common site for entry (3% of cases), despite the high prevalence of intima media ulcers in patients with atherosclerotic disease in this segment.[6–8]

The dissecting hematoma usually propagates in an antero-grade direction, although retrograde extension can occur. By this mechanism, as many as 20% of dissections that originate in the distal arch or descending thoracic aorta may involve the ascending aorta.[9] In rare cases, a second tear may occur, resulting in a three-channel dissection[10] (Fig. 34-2).

Blood within the false lumen may reenter the true lumen anywhere along the length of the dissection. Reentry may be protective because of spontaneous decompression of the false lumen that may reduce the risks of rupture and/or development of malperfusion syndromes.

Aortic Rupture and End-Organ Malperfusion

Aortic rupture, defined as tearing in the vessel wall that results in extravascular hemorrhage, most commonly occurs with trauma (e.g., motor vehicle collision) but may occur as a complication of the primary dissection.[11] Rupture into the pericardial space resulting in cardiac tamponade occurs in type A dissection, whereas rupture into the left pleural space is usually encountered with type B dissection. Dissection-mediated end-organ ischemia or infarction occurs from (1) mechanical compression of aortic branch vessels by false lumen hematoma, (2) extension of the dissection plane across the ostium of the branch vessel, or (3) dynamic vessel inlet obstruction caused by an oscillating intimal flap. Compromise of

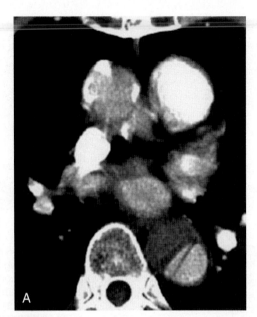
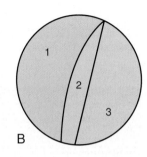

FIGURE 34-2 Three-channeled aortic dissection. A, Computed tomographic image demonstrates three-channel descending aortic dissection in Marfan syndrome patient. **B,** Schematic representation of dissection is provided: region 1 represents thrombosed false lumen, region 2 is true lumen significantly diminished in size, and region 3 designates contrast-enhanced false lumen. *(From Yoshida S, Shidoh M: Three channeled aortic dissection. Postgrad Med J 79:532, 2003.)*

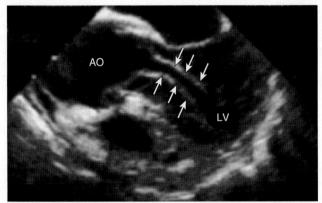

FIGURE 34-3 Aortic dissection intimal flap prolapsing into left ventricle. Horizontal plane transesophageal echocardiographic image captures prolapse of intimal flap *(arrows)* from a proximal Stanford type A aortic *(AO)* dissection into left ventricular *(LV)* cavity. *(From Rosenszweig BP, Goldstein S, Sherid M, et al: Aortic dissection with flap prolapse into the left ventricle. Am J Cardiol 77:214–216, 1996.)*

coronary, brachiocephalic, mesenteric, renal, spinal, and iliac circulations can occur and result in a myriad of clinical presentations. Occlusion of the left ventricular (LV) outflow tract by an intimal flap has been reported (Fig. 34-3).

False Lumen Thrombosis

Thrombosis of blood within the false lumen may seal the entry tear, thus eliminating communication with the true lumen and interruption of false lumen expansion. Partial thrombosis of the false lumen, however, has been identified as a risk factor for long-term death in patients with type B dissection.[12,13] Elevation of pressure with partial thrombosis within the false lumen may lead to further extrinsic compression of the true lumen and impairment of blood flow to critical organs. Alternatively, it has been proposed that partial thrombosis of the false lumen is associated with worse clinical outcomes by promoting vascular inflammation, hypoxia, and/or neovascularization with weakening of adjacent vascular structures and an increased risk for aortic rupture.[13–17]

Persistent patency of the false lumen is also associated with a higher risk of long-term complications such as late rupture or false aneurysm formation requiring operative intervention.[12,15–17] Although native aortic aneurysm disease is often a risk factor for dissection, a dissection need not result in aneurysm formation. The term "dissecting aneurysm" is an inaccurate anachronism, and

these diseases are not synonymous, a distinction that is particularly important when considering their natural histories and treatments.

Predisposing Genetic Factors

As is true for aneurysms, any process that leads to destruction or degeneration of the major supporting elements of the aortic media (elastin, collagen, smooth muscle cells [SMCs]) can predispose to development of dissection. The histopathological term *medial degeneration* refers to noninflammatory destruction or fragmentation of elastic lamellar units, dropout of SMCs, and accumulation of mucopolysaccharide ground substances (not always in distinct cystic spaces), which characterize the final common pathway for a variety of processes that affect the integrity of the aortic media (Fig. 34-4).

Marfan's syndrome (MFS) is the most common inherited connective tissue disorder, with an estimated prevalence of 1 case per 3000 to 5000 individuals irrespective of racial, ethnic, or geographic considerations.[18–21] If untreated, aortic disease in MFS is progressive and incompatible with normal longevity. Half of patients in whom aortic dissection occurs at younger than 40 years of age have a history of MFS.[22] Mutations in the gene encoding fibrillin-1 (FBN1), a critical component of the microfibrils that help form cellular adhesions in the extracellular matrix (ECM), are largely responsible for disease expression.[20] Medial degeneration is not pathognomic of MFS and may be present in numerous other conditions.[23]

Marfan's syndrome disease expression is heterogenous, but the presence of an aortic root aneurysm (aortic diameter z score ≥2) and ectopia lentis are sufficient to make the diagnosis even in the absence of a family history[24] (Box 34-2A). Conversely, in the absence of either of these two clinical features, the revised Ghent nosology for MFS outlines a scoring system based on the presence of FBN1 mutation and/or other key systemic features of MFS to make the diagnosis (Box 34-2B). Systemic features suggestive of MFS include positive wrist sign (entire distal phalanx of adducted thumb extends beyond ulnar border of the palm), positive thumb sign (tip of thumb covers entire fingernail of fifth finger when wrapped around contralateral wrist), pectus excavatum, pneumothorax, dural ectasia, hindfoot deformity, and protrusio acetabuli. Other clinical features less strongly associated with MFS include mitral valve prolapse, various abnormal facial features, and thoracolumbar kyphosis.

Using an *in vivo* murine model of MFS, Dietz et al. demonstrated that fibrillin-1 is a key target for binding of transforming growth factor (TGF)-β, a molecule involved in activation of inflammatory, fibrotic, and metalloproteinase cell signaling

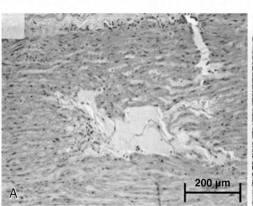
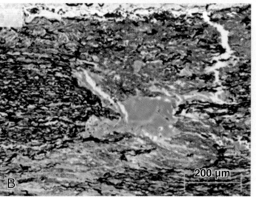

FIGURE 34-4 Cystic medial degeneration. A, Hematoxylin and eosin microscopic section of aorta reveals fragmentation and loss of elastin fibers with cyst-like structures present within media. **B,** Movat pentachrome stain emphasis medial interlamellar cystic "drop out." *(From Maleszewski JJ, Miller DV, Lu J, et al: Histopathologic findings in ascending aortas from individuals with Loeys-Dietz syndrome [LDS]. Am J Surg Pathol 33:194–201, 2009.)*

 Box 34-2A   Revised Ghent Criteria for Diagnosis of Marfan's Syndrome and Related Conditions*

In the Absence of Family History

(1) Ao ($z \geq 2$) *and* EL = MFS†
(2) Ao ($z \geq 2$) *and* FBN1 = MFS
(3) Ao ($z \geq 2$) *and* Syst (≥ 7pts) = MFS†
(4) EL *and* FBN1 with known Ao = MFS
EL with or without Syst *and* with an FBN1 not known with Ao or no FBN1 = ELS
Ao ($z <2$) *and* Syst (≥ 5 with at least one skeletal feature) without EL = MASS
MVP *and* Ao ($z <2$) *and* Syst (<5) without EL = MVPS

In the Presence of Family History

(5) EL *and* FH of MFS (as defined above) = MFS
(6) Syst (≥ 7 pts) *and* FH of MFS (as defined above) = MFS†
(7) Ao ($z \geq 2$ above 20 years old, ≥ 3 below 20 years old) + FH of MFS (as defined above) = MFS†

*In general, MFS is diagnosed in the presence of aortic root dilation/dissection and ectopia lentis; aortic root dilation/dissection plus FBN1 mutation; aortic root dilation plus sufficient systemic findings (Box 34-2B, ≥7 points); ectopia lentis plus FBN1 mutation previously associated with aortic disease; or in an individual with a positive family history of MFS, the diagnosis is made in the presence of ectopia lentis, or a systemic score ≥7 points, or aortic root dilation.
†Caveat: without discriminating features of Shprintzen-Goldberg's syndrome, Loeys-Dietz's syndrome, or vascular Ehlers-Danlos' syndrome *and* after TGFBA1/2, collagen biochemistry, COL3A1 testing if indicated. Other conditions/genes will emerge with time.
Ao, aortic diameter at the sinuses of Valsalva above indicated z-score or aortic root dissection; EL, ectopia lentis; ELS, ectopia lentis syndrome; FBN1, fibrillin-1 mutation; FBN1 not known with Ao, FBN1 mutation that has not previously been associated with aortic root aneurysm/ dissection; FBN1 with known Ao, FBN1 mutation that has been identified in an individual with aortic aneurysm; MASS, myopia, mitral valve prolapse, borderline (z <2) aortic root dilation, striae, skeletal findings phenotype; MFS, Marfan's syndrome; MVPS, mitral valve prolapse syndrome; Syst, systemic score (see Box 34-2B); z, z-score.

 Box 34-2B   Scoring of Systemic Features

Wrist and thumb sign: 3 (wrist or thumb sign: 1)
Pectus carinatum deformity: 2 (pectus excavatum or chest asymmetry: 1)
Hindfoot deformity: 2 (plain pes planus: 1)
Pneumothorax: 2
Dural ectasia: 2
Protrusio acetabuli: 2
Reduced US/LS and increased arm/height and no severe scoliosis: 1
Scoliosis or thoracolumbar kyphosis: 1
Reduced elbow extension: 1
Facial features (3/5): 1 (dolichocephaly, enophthalmos, downslanting palpebral fissures, malar hypoplasia, retrognathia)
Skin striae: 1
Myopia >3 diopters: 1
Mitral valve prolapsed (all types): 1

MAXIMUM TOTAL: 20 points; score ≥7 indicates systemic involvement.
US/LS, upper segment/lower segment ratio.
From Loeys BL, Dietz HC, Braverman AC, et al: The revised Ghent nosology for the Marfan's syndrome. J Med Genet 47:476–485, 2010.[24]

pathways.[25] To investigate the possibility that angiotensin I (AT1)-mediated TGF-β activation could represent a pharmacological target to modify development of aortic dilation in MFS, Habashi et al. studied the effects of losartan, an AT1 receptor antagonist, on aortic aneurysm formation in transgenic mice encoding a cysteine-to-glutamine substitution at position 1039 in the fibrillin-1 gene (Fbn1$^{C1039G/-}$). Mice with this fibrillin-1 mutation, the most common class of mutation associated with MFS, demonstrate significant and progressive aortic root dilation compared with wild-type mice.[26] Treatment with losartan attenuated TGF-β signaling in the aortic wall and resulted in full normalization of aortic wall thickness and a marked improvement in aortic wall architecture (i.e., a decrease in elastin fiber disruption) compared with placebo or β-adrenergic receptor antagonist therapy with propranolol.

These landmark observations have advanced understanding of the molecular basis of MFS and provided new targets for therapy. In one small clinical trial in young MFS patients, initiation of losartan resulted in a significant decrease in rate of growth of the aortic root (mean change 0.46 ± 0.62 mm/yr vs. 3.5 ± 2.8 mm/yr prior to treatment; $P < 0.001$).[27] These findings were supplemented by Ahimastos et al., who conducted a randomized placebo-controlled clinical trial testing the effect of the angiotensin-converting enzyme inhibitor (ACEI) perindopril on aortic root diameter and aortic stiffness in 17 MFS patients.[29] At 24 weeks, circulating TGF-β levels and central pulse wave velocities were lower and aortic root diameters were smaller in perindopril-treated patients. Several larger randomized clinical trials directed at modulating TGF-β signaling are ongoing (clinicaltrials.gov; NCT00683124, NCT00782327 NCT00429364, NCT00723801).

Limited forms (i.e., forme frustes) of MFS that feature cardiovascular manifestations include mitral valve prolapse syndrome (MVPS) (mitral valve prolapse, pectus excavatum, scoliosis, and mild arachnodactyly) and the MASS phenotype (myopia, mitral valve prolapse, borderline and nonprogressive aortic root dilation, skeletal findings and striae). There is increasing awareness of familial thoracic aortic aneurysm disease (FTAAD), though candidate genes affecting both matrix and SMC components have been identified in only 20% of such patients. Vascular-type Ehlers-Danlos' syndrome (EDS) is associated with arterial rupture and dissection, including the aorta.[24,28]

Ehlers-Danlos' syndrome (1:5000 births) comprises a heterogeneous group of disorders characterized clinically by hypermobile joints, hyperextensible skin, tissue fragility, and a predisposition to spontaneous vascular rupture. Aortic involvement occurs in EDS type IV, an autosomal dominant disorder attributed to structural defects in the pro-α1 (III) chain of type III collagen, encoded by the COL3A1 gene on chromosome 2q31.[30]

FTAAD has been mapped to other genetic loci, including 16p13.11 (MYH11 gene), 5q13-14, and 11q23.2-q24, which are not associated with abnormalities of fibrillin or collagen.[31,32] More than five mutations in the fibrillin-1 gene have been identified in patients with familial or spontaneous thoracic aortic aneurysm and dissection, with histopathological changes characteristic of medial degeneration, yet with no demonstrable abnormalities of collagen or fibrillin in fibroblast culture.[33,34] Polymorphisms encoding the gene vitamin K epoxide reductase complex subunit 1 (VKORC1), which results in under-carboxylation of specific matrix proteins, are associated with calcification of the arterial wall. In patients carrying the C allele (CT or CC), a relative two-fold increase in the probability of developing aortic dissection has been observed.[35] A missense mutation in the ACTA2 gene that encodes for actin filaments in SMCs is linked to 14% of patients with FTAAD.[36] As a consequence of this mutation, intracellular actin filament assembly is disrupted, promoting focal areas of SMC disarray, decreased SMC contraction, and medial degeneration of the aorta. This phenotype is felt to be associated with aortic wall weakening and increased predisposition to dissection.

Bicuspid aortic valve (BAV) disease is the most common congenital cardiac anomaly in adults (4:1000 live births) and is often accompanied by an aortopathy that is histologically similar but less severe than that observed in patients with MFS. Similar pathological changes have been described in patients with aortic coarctation (many of whom have BAV disease), Noonan's syndrome, Turner's syndrome, and polycystic kidney disease. Dilation of the root and (more commonly) the ascending aorta is present in up to 40% of patients with BAV disease and is a risk factor for dissection or rupture (Fig. 34-5).

Acquired Disorders

Systemic hypertension is the most common treatable risk factor for aortic dissection and is present in approximately 75% of patients.[2] Hypertension accelerates the normal aging process and leads to intimal thickening, SMC apoptosis, fibrosis, loss of elasticity, and compromise of nutritive blood supply. Decreased aortic compliance and vulnerability to pulsatile forces predispose to injury and create a substrate for dissection.

Iatrogenic Dissection

In the IRAD registry, iatrogenic aortic dissection after cardiac surgery or catheterization accounted for 5% of the total reported.[37] Older age, hypertension, and severe peripheral vascular disease are risk factors associated with procedure-related dissection.[38] Pain may be absent in iatrogenic dissection. Retrograde dissections created at the time of catheterization usually seal spontaneously on withdrawal of the catheter. Aortic atherosclerotic plaques may prevent longitudinal propagation of a dissection. Dissections arising from sites where the aorta has been incised or

cross-clamped may occur intraoperatively or at any time following surgery. Deceleration injury from high-speed accidents results in aortic transection with false aneurysm formation and rupture, most commonly in the region of the aortic isthmus just beyond the origin of the left subclavian artery. Transection results in a transmural tear that is different both pathologically and etiologically from aortic dissection.

Dissection in Pregnancy

Aortic dissection as a complication of pregnancy is rare, although by some estimates 50% of all dissections in women younger than 40 occur during labor, delivery, or early after childbirth.[39] Histopathological changes affecting the aortic media of pregnant women have been described, including alterations in elastic fibers and SMCs.[40] Both estrogen and relaxin are associated with alterations in matrix metalloproteinase (MMP) homeostasis and contribute to vascular remodeling and a susceptibility to injury independent of the hemodynamic stress of labor and delivery. In many cases, pregnancy unmasks primary conditions that predispose to aortic dissection (e.g., MFS). In those patients with preexisting MFS or BAV disease, aortic root size greater than 4.0 cm is a contraindication to pregnancy, owing to increased risk for spontaneous rupture or dissection.[2]

Drug Use and Other Acquired Conditions

Recent cocaine use, particularly among young men who smoke tobacco, is an additional risk factor for aortic dissection.[41] Among 38 patients with acute aortic dissection occurring over a 20-year period in an urban center, 37% reported cocaine (in particular, crack cocaine) use within the preceding 24 hours (mean 12 hours). Chronic amphetamine use and/or dependence appear to increase the probability of developing a thoracoabdominal aortic dissection in those aged 18 to 49 years.[42] Presumed mechanisms for aortic injury from cocaine and amphetamine use involve oxidant stress–mediated endothelial dysfunction and extreme catecholamine-induced shear forces, with abrupt hypertension and tachycardia that collectively lead to weakening of the aortic media and predisposition to tearing.

Inflammatory diseases of the aorta can lead to destruction of ECM proteins and SMCs, with subsequent aneurysm formation and/or dissection. Aortic dissection has been reported in patients with Takayasu's disease, giant cell aortitis, Behçet's disease, relapsing polychondritis, systemic lupus erythematosus (SLE), and the aortitis associated with inflammatory bowel disease.[2] Syphilitic aortitis, on the other hand, does not predispose to dissection, perhaps

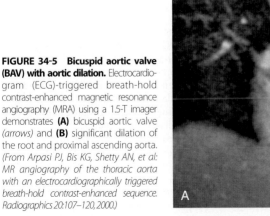
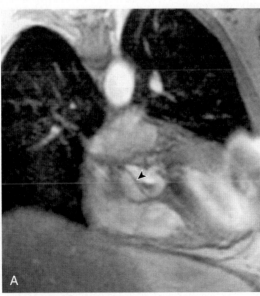
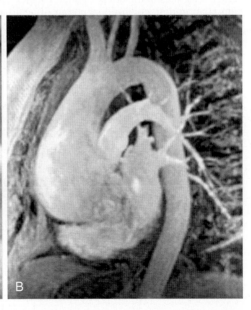

FIGURE 34-5 Bicuspid aortic valve (BAV) with aortic dilation. Electrocardiogram (ECG)-triggered breath-hold contrast-enhanced magnetic resonance angiography (MRA) using a 1.5-T imager demonstrates **(A)** bicuspid aortic valve (arrows) and **(B)** significant dilation of the root and proximal ascending aorta. (From Arpasi PJ, Bis KG, Shetty AN, et al: MR angiography of the thoracic aorta with an electrocardiographically triggered breath-hold contrast-enhanced sequence. Radiographics 20:107–120, 2000.)

CH 34

PATHOPHYSIOLOGY, CLINICAL EVALUATION, AND MEDICAL MANAGEMENT OF AORTIC DISSECTION

because of intense reactive medial scarring and fibrosis that occurs in response to the spirochetal infection. Pheochromocytoma and weight lifting (believed due to intense or repetitious Valsalva maneuvers) also predispose to aortic dissection.

Clinical Presentation

The most important element of any diagnostic algorithm for suspected acute aortic syndrome is a high clinical index of suspicion, based foremost on the presenting history and physical examination (Box 34-3). Absent an appreciation for the cardinal features of dissection, the diagnosis can be missed in a substantial number of patients. Simple clinical prediction rules have been developed to estimate probability of acute aortic dissection.[43] The IRAD investigators have recently confirmed the sensitivity of 12 clinical risk markers proposed in the 2010 American College of Cardiology Foundation/American Heart Association (ACCF/AHA) thoracic aortic disease guidelines[2] (Table 34-1). These markers, assessed at bedside, were divided into three distinct categories: predisposing factors, characteristics of the pain at time of presentation, and key physical examination findings.[44] The presence of risk factor(s) from at least one category identified 95.7% of acute aortic dissection patients in the IRAD database.

History

Diagnosis of aortic dissection may be missed on initial clinical evaluation in about a third of cases, and an equal number are detected only at autopsy.[1,44] Chest pain is the dominant feature of the clinical presentation and occurs in over 90% of patients.[2] It is qualitatively severe and may in many cases be distinguished from coronary ischemia by *abrupt* onset and maximal intensity at inception. More than 84% of aortic dissection patients described chest pain as "worst ever" in the IRAD registry.[2,45] The pain is characterized as sharp more often than tearing or ripping in nature, and may radiate or be sensed anteriorly (suggestive of type A dissection) or in the interscapular, lower back, or abdominal area (suggestive of type B dissection). Visceral discomfort or limb pain may be indicative of aortic branch vessel ischemia from malperfusion.

Syncope is a particularly ominous presenting symptom and may reflect cardiac tamponade from intrapericardial aortic rupture, cerebral malperfusion, and/or neurally mediated hypotension in response to the intense pain of the dissection. In the IRAD registry, patients with syncope were more likely to die in the hospital or suffer a stroke. Neurological complications are noted in up to 20% of aortic dissection patients. For example, paraplegia may develop when critical impairment of flow to the anterior spinal artery, thoracic intercostals, or the artery of Adamkiewicz occurs. Abdominal pain is an underrecognized symptom of acute aortic dissection; when present, it is associated with elevated in-hospital mortality and increased frequency of malperfusion syndromes.[2,43,44]

Numerous other less common clinical manifestations of aortic dissection may be evident on initial evaluation and include Horner's syndrome (compression of the superior cervical ganglion), hoarseness (pressure against the recurrent laryngeal nerve), hemoptysis (rupture into a bronchus), hematemesis (perforation into the esophagus), ischemic enterocolitis (mesenteric artery compromise), and fever of undetermined source (pyrogens released from the false lumen).

Box 34-3   Acute Aortic Syndromes

Aortic dissection
Intramural hematoma
Penetrating aortic ulcer
Rapid aneurysm expansion
Trauma

Adapted from Hiratzka LF, Bakris GL, Beckman JA, et al: 2010 ACCF/AHA/AATS/ACR/ ASA/SCA/SCAI/SIR/STS/SVM guidelines for the diagnosis and management of patients with thoracic aortic disease. J Am Coll Cardiol 55:e27, 2010.[2]

TABLE 34-1	Percentage of Patients in the International Registry of Acute Aortic Dissection (1996–2009) with Each of 12 High-Risk Clinical Markers Observed at Time of Presentation with Acute Aortic Dissection*	
AORTIC DISSECTION DETECTION RISK CATEGORY	CLINICAL CHARACTERISTICS	% OF PATIENTS (N = 2538)
1	MFS	4.3
1	Family history of aortic disease	1.9
1	Known aortic valve disease	11.9
1	Recent aortic manipulation	2.8
1	Known thoracic aortic aneurysm	14.7
2	Abrupt onset of pain	79.3
	Severe pain intensity	72.7
2	Ripping or tearing pain	21.7
3	Pulse deficit or systolic blood pressure differential	20.3
3	Focal neurological deficit (in conjunction with pain)	10.8
3	Murmur of aortic insufficiency (new or in conjunction with pain)	23.6
3	Hypotension/shock	16.0

*The aortic dissection detection (ADD) score aims to enhance early diagnosis of acute aortic dissection. The ADD score is calculated by determining the number of categories in which any of 12 high-risk clinical features are present in patients with symptoms suggestive of acute aortic dissection. For example, in a patient with a family history of aortic disease (category 1) and known thoracic aneurysm (also category 1), the ADD score would be 1. Likewise, the ADD score is 2 in a patient with Marfan's syndrome (category 1) and a blood pressure differential (category 3). A retrospective analysis of the International Registry of Acute Aortic Dissection determined that among 2538 patients with acute aortic dissection, 95.7% had an ADD score ≥1. The ADD score may therefore provide the clinician with a simple and effective bedside method to inform further diagnostic testing and/or treatment in patients with suspected aortic dissection. Importantly, the negative predictive value for acute aortic dissection in patients with an ADD score of 0 has not yet been established.
MFS, Marfan's syndrome.
From Rogers AM, Hermann LK, Booher AM, et al: Sensitivity of the aortic dissection detection risk score, a novel guideline-based tool for identification of acute aortic dissection on initial presentation. Circulation 123:2213–2218, 2011.[44]

Physical Examination

Patients with acute aortic dissection appear ill, uncomfortable, and apprehensive. Hypertension is present in more than two thirds of type B dissection patients and in approximately one third of type A patients.[1,2] A murmur of aortic regurgitation can be heard in approximately 40% of patients with type A dissection.[37] Due to rapid equilibration of aortic and LV diastolic pressure from acute aortic valve regurgitation, the murmur is usually of shorter duration, lower in pitch, and of lesser intensity than the diastolic murmur of chronic severe aortic regurgitation. Additional auscultatory findings include a soft first heart sound and a grade 1 or 2 midsystolic murmur at the base or along the left sternal border.

An inverse correlation between the presence of pulse deficits and mortality is observed in acute aortic dissection.[46] Furthermore, pulse deficits may obscure accurate blood pressure assessment, as in pseudohypotension, which arises from an inability to measure central aortic pressure when bilateral subclavian and/or femoral artery compromise is present. Thus, invasive intraarterial monitoring may be necessary in aortic dissection patients.

Elevation of jugular venous pressure, especially with pulsus paradoxus, may indicate pericardial involvement with tamponade. Superior vena cava syndrome can rarely occur with compression by an expanding false aneurysm along the greater curvature of the ascending aorta. Thoracic dullness to percussion and decreased breath sounds suggests pleural effusion, which is more common in the left chest and not necessarily indicative of rupture. In fact, pleural effusions are quite frequent with both type A and B dissections; they are usually sympathetic in nature, reflective of the intense inflammation associated with the acute tear.

Laboratory Testing

BIOMARKERS

Plasma smooth muscle myosin heavy chain protein, D-dimer, and high-sensitivity C-reactive protein (CRP) have been proposed as potentially useful biomarkers to assist with point-of-care diagnosis of aortic dissection. In one study of 95 patients with acute aortic dissection, elevated levels of circulating smooth muscle myosin heavy chain protein (>2.5 µg/L) had a sensitivity of 90% and a specificity of 98% compared with healthy controls when measured within 3 hours of presentation.[47] In this analysis, smooth muscle myosin heavy chain protein levels were elevated in all patients presenting with a proximal or type A dissection.

Soluble elastin fragment (sELAF) levels have also been proposed to be a useful biomarker for the early detection of acute aortic dissection. Despite a natural rise with age in the concentration of sELAF levels detected in plasma, a level more than 3 standard deviations above normal for age is associated with a 64% positivity rate in acute aortic dissection, compared with 2% for patients with AMI. Interestingly, patients with complete false lumen thrombosis appear to have no detectable sELAF.[48]

Suzuki et al. conducted a multicenter study of 220 patients with suspected acute aortic dissection.[49] A D-dimer level of less than 500 ng/mL when drawn within 24 hours of symptom onset was associated with a negative likelihood ratio (LR) for aortic dissection of 0.07. Consistent with these data, findings from one large meta-analysis of 734 patients demonstrated that an elevated D-dimer level had a 97% sensitivity and 96% negative predictive value for identifying acute aortic dissection. Conversely, an elevated D-dimer is less effective at "ruling-in" aortic dissection, with a specificity of 56% and positive predictive value of 60%.[50] An early rapid increase in CRP levels following acute aortic dissection has been observed, with levels falling rapidly 24 hours following symptom onset.[51] Although less well studied in aortic dissection, calponin, a counterpart protein to troponin in vascular SMCs, may provide enhanced specificity for early detection of type A aortic dissection, but requires comprehensive testing in advance of clinical application.[52]

Other Point-of-Care Tests

The chest x-ray is abnormal in 80% to 90% of patients with aortic dissection, but is an insufficient tool to rule out this condition, particularly when pathology is confined to the ascending aorta.[53] Findings suggestive of aortic dissection include mediastinal widening, disparity in the caliber of the ascending and descending thoracic aortic segments, a localized bulge or angulation along the normally smooth border of the aorta, displacement of intimal calcium (especially in the region of the aortic knob), and a double density appearance. Associated findings may include cardiomegaly (pericardial effusion) and pleural effusion (left > right). Effusions that occupy more than 50% of the chest cavity may be indicative of rupture with hemothorax.

Nonspecific electrocardiographic (ECG) repolarization abnormalities are present in approximately 40% of dissection patients.[37] Changes indicative of active ischemia may be found in 15% of patients, and findings suggestive of AMI (new Q waves, ST-segment elevation) are present in a small minority (3%) of cases.[37] A thorough assessment is critical to avoid initiation of acute reperfusion therapy in this setting.

Diagnostic Imaging

Retrograde aortography, the original diagnostic gold standard for aortic dissection, has been almost completely replaced by transesophageal echocardiography (TEE) and computed tomographic angiography (CTA). Magnetic resonance imaging/angiography (MRI/MRA) is much less frequently performed in the acute setting. Sensitivity and specificity of these three noninvasive techniques are essentially equivalent and exceed 90% in most series.[2] Choice of imaging technique depends chiefly on availability, speed, safety, and local expertise in performance and interpretation. A second test is frequently needed for clarification when the first study is abnormal but nondiagnostic. Regardless of the diagnostic sequence employed, an institutional commitment to rapid imaging of critically ill patients is critical. Essential features to be defined for both treatment and prognosis include presence or absence of ascending aortic involvement, entry and reentry sites, pericardial and aortic valve involvement, extent of the dissection, major branch vessel compromise, and the anatomical substrate for potential malperfusion syndrome(s).

TRANSESOPHAGEAL ECHOCARDIOGRAPHY

A surface transthoracic echocardiogram (TTE) alone is not sufficient for diagnosis and characterization of aortic dissection in most cases.[54] However, when combined with TEE, the sensitivity and specificity of these tests reaches 99% and 89%, respectively[54] (Fig. 34-6). Transthoracic echocardiogram should not delay performance of TEE, which can be accomplished at the bedside in the emergency department or in the operating room within 15 to 20 minutes. Oropharyngeal anesthesia and conscious sedation are required, with simultaneous monitoring of heart rate and rhythm, blood pressure, and oxygen saturation. Orthogonal and longitudinal scan planes combined with M-mode, two-dimensional (2D), and Doppler profile interrogation provide information regarding: (1) entry and reentry sites, (2) longitudinal extent and oscillation of the intimal flap, (3) flow velocity and direction within the true and false lumens, (4) spontaneous contrast or thrombus within the false lumen, (5) aortic valve competence and mechanism of regurgitation, (6) ostial coronary artery involvement, (7) pericardial effusion, and (8) global and regional LV function. In most cases, the true lumen is differentiated from the false lumen by observing systolic expansion and diastolic collapse, absence or minimal spontaneous echo contrast, and/or an antegrade Doppler signal. However, vessel diameter alone is *not* sufficient for making this determination. In ambiguous cases (e.g., with a large false lumen), a pressure gradient between true and false lumen between 10 and 25 mmHg may be observed by continuous wave Doppler interrogation.[55,56]

A series of small echo "blind spots," however, lie in the distal portion of the ascending aorta, anterior portion of the aortic arch, and anterior to the trachea and left mainstem bronchus. Signal

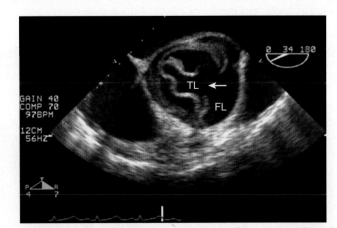

FIGURE 34-6 Proximal aortic dissection imaged by transesophageal echocardiography (TEE). Horizontal plane TEE image of Stanford type A aortic dissection reveals a true lumen *(TL)* diminished in size and false lumen *(FL)* extending circumferentially. A communication through the dissection flap that joins the TL and FL is present *(arrow). (From Meredith EL, Masani ND: Echocardiography in the emergency assessment of acute aortic syndromes. Eur J Echo 10:i31–i39, 2009.)*

dropout may occur in the presence of free fluid around the aorta or pericardium, present in some cases of traumatic aortic penetration.

COMPUTED TOMOGRAPHIC ANGIOGRAPHY

Multislice CTA using rapid acquisition protocols and postprocessing of the volumetric data (multiplanar reformatting, maximum intensity projection (MIP), shaded surface display, volumetric rendering) provides highly detailed and visually familiar anatomical images (Fig. 34-7; also see Chapter 14). The diagnostic accuracy of 64-slice CTA approaches 100% for aortic dissection.[57] The intimal flap appears as a thin, low attenuation, linear or spiral structure that separates the true and false lumens. Additional findings include displacement of intimal calcium, delayed contrast enhancement of the false lumen, and aortic widening. Branch vessel involvement anywhere along the course of the aorta to the level of the iliac arteries can be precisely displayed. In addition, CTA can visualize the proximal third of the coronary arteries. Limitations to CTA include exposure to intravenous contrast and ionizing radiation. In addition, CTA is an anatomical study; neither aortic valve nor LV function can be rapidly assessed. Motion artifact, mural thrombi, and image artifacts may negatively affect study accuracy.[57] Dedicated emergency department scanners are now widespread, and studies can be obtained, reconstructed, and interpreted within 15 to 20 minutes. Computed tomographic angiography has several advantages relative to MRA, including wider availability, quicker throughput, higher spatial resolution, absence of arterial flow-related artifacts, and the capability to visualize calcification and metallic implants.

MAGNETIC RESONANCE IMAGING/ANGIOGRAPHY

Contemporary MRI technology affords rapid scanning with the ability to cover a wide field of view and a comprehensive analysis of dissection anatomy and extraaortic involvement[57,58] (Fig. 34-8; also see Chapter 13). Magnetic resonance imaging allows for assessment of pericardial involvement, aortic regurgitation, proximal coronary artery involvement, and LV function. The 0.5-tesla (T) magnet and modern gating software allow for expedited scanning across multiple levels during a single breath hold. Despite these advances, MRI is infrequently used as the initial imaging study in patients with suspected acute aortic syndromes. Reasons for its limited use in the acute setting include lack of widespread availability, difficulties with patient transport to and monitoring within MRI scanners, and presence of implanted cardiac devices or metallic clips. Nevertheless, MRI can provide excellent imaging of false lumen thrombus, intramural hematoma, and penetrating atherosclerotic ulcers.[57,58]

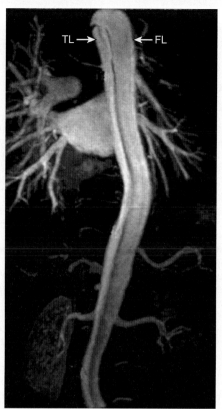

FIGURE 34-8 Contrast-enhanced magnetic resonance angiography (MRA) of aortic dissection. Maximal intensity projection (MIP) images of a thoracoabdominal aortic dissection reveal a hyperintense true lumen *(TL)* and hypointense false lumen *(FL)*. *(From Liu Q, Lu JP, Wang F, et al: Three-dimensional contrast enhanced MR angiography of aortic dissection: a pictorial essay. Radiographics 27:1311–1321, 2007.)*

INVASIVE AORTOGRAPHY

The risk for catheter-related injury, length of time required to assemble necessary personnel in an emergency situation, use of contrast and ionizing radiation, low sensitivity (77%), and availability of highly accurate noninvasive imaging techniques have significantly decreased use of invasive aortography as an initial diagnostic test for acute aortic dissection.[59] Aortography is particularly limited in diagnosing noncommunicating aortic dissections, intramural hematomas, and penetrating ulcers.[2] Inadvertent injection into the false lumen or equal and rapid opacification of true

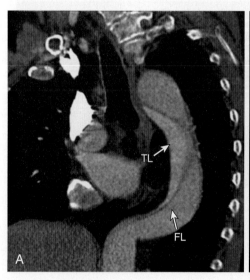

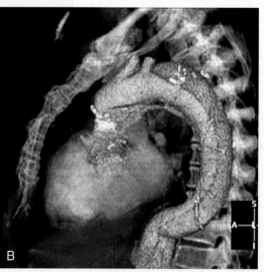

FIGURE 34-7 Planar computed tomographic angiogram (CTA) and three-dimensional (3D) reconstructed images of Stanford type A aortic dissection. A, Coronal CTA image delineates dissection plane that separates true lumen *(TL)* from false lumen *(FL).* **B,** 3D reconstruction imaging in same patient provides enhanced spatial resolution after surgical repair of aortic dissection and surrounding anatomical structures. In this case, aortic dissection extends from aortic root to innominate and left subclavian arteries, continues through aortic arch and into descending aorta, with termination near bifurcation of left common iliac artery (CIA).

and false lumens without obvious aortic dilation may make correct diagnosis of aortic dissection difficult. Invasive angiography is a feature of any catheter-based intervention.

INTRAVASCULAR ULTRASOUND

Low-frequency (<20MHz) intravascular ultrasound (IVUS) affords maximal signal penetration of the aortic wall and nearly 100% diagnostic accuracy for aortic dissection in a procedure that can be completed in less than 10 minutes.[58,60] This method provides clear delineation of several key findings, including entry points, longitudinal and circumferential extent, luminal dimensions and contour, and thrombus if present. Intravascular ultrasound is infrequently used as a second imaging technique for diagnosis in patients for whom false-negative results on invasive aortography are suspected, and femoral access has been obtained. Intravascular ultrasound may also have a role during performance of endovascular procedures.

CORONARY ANGIOGRAPHY

Selective coronary angiography is neither indicated nor advisable in anticipation of emergency surgery for type A dissection.[61] Operative mortality is generally not related to myocardial ischemia but rather to aortic rupture, so performance of angiography consumes valuable time before life-saving surgery. Systematic preoperative coronary angiography for hemodynamically stable chronic type A dissection patients is a subject of debate.[54,62] Preoperative coronary angiography is reasonable in type A dissection patients who have a history of previous coronary artery bypass graft surgery, or in type B patients with unstable angina prior to planned aortic and/or coronary intervention. Identification of high-grade atherosclerotic disease of native coronary arteries and/or coronary artery bypass graft(s) affords determination of the optimal operation for patients requiring ascending aortic surgery. However, in these instances, the potential for incorporating additional surgical procedures beyond repairing the dissection should be evaluated on a case-by-case basis.

Differential Diagnosis
Other Acute Aortic Syndromes

Aortic transection from deceleration injury and traumatic aortic valve disruption with acute severe aortic regurgitation occur in the setting of high-speed vehicular accidents or vertical falls. The nontraumatic acute aortic syndromes, however, are often *not* distinguishable from classic dissection on clinical grounds alone, but rather are delineated with cross-sectional imaging.

AORTIC INTRAMURAL HEMATOMA

Intramural hematoma (IMH) is defined as a contained collection of blood within the wall of the aorta, without evidence of an intimal flap, entry tear, or double lumen (Fig. 34-9). Mechanisms to account for IMH include primary rupture of the nutrient vasa vasorum or a limited intimal tear that cannot be detected with imaging.[62–64] Intramural hematoma is observed clinically in about 20% of cases of suspected acute aortic dissection and is discovered at autopsy in 5% to 13% of acute aortic syndrome cases.[2,64] Approximately 10% of aortic IMHs undergo spontaneous resorption. Predicting evolution to dissection, rupture, aneurysm formation, or false aneurysm development is difficult. Type A IMH thickness greater than 11 mm is an independent risk factor for death, surgery, or progression to dissection.[64,65] Likewise, an ascending aortic diameter greater than 4.8 cm is a high-risk feature.[2,62–65] Aortic IMH is managed according to the same principles that pertain to aortic dissection, including surgery for type A disease, surveillance imaging, and intervention for downstream complications.

Diagnosis of IMH by TEE requires visualization of crescentic or circumferential wall thickening of more than 0.7 cm or identification of fresh thrombus within the aortic wall. Computed tomographic angiography and MRA are more accurate than TEE for distinguishing

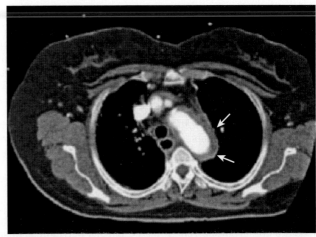

FIGURE 34-9   Aortic intramural hematoma (IMH). Axial multidetector computed tomographic angiographic (CTA) image acquired at level of aortic arch reveals circumferential rind *(arrows)* that does not enhance with contrast. *(From Takahashi K, Stanford W: Multidetector CT of the thoracic aorta. Int J Cardiovasc Imaging 21:141–153, 2005.)*

IMH from aortic aneurysm with mural thrombus, severe atherosclerosis, or aortitis with medial inflammation and edema.

PENETRATING ATHEROSCLEROTIC AORTIC ULCER

An inflamed atherosclerotic plaque that disrupts normal aortic wall architecture may result in erosion of the internal elastic membrane, allowing luminal blood to burrow into the media of the aorta and beyond. Penetrating atherosclerotic aortic ulcers (PAUs) are most commonly seen in the mid- to distal descending thoracic aorta in older persons with a heavy burden of atherosclerotic disease. They appear as irregular craters or outpouchings of contrast (Fig. 34-10) and may result in IMH formation or frank dissection. Ganaha et al. observed in a retrospective analysis of 65 symptomatic IMH patients with PAU that ulcer depth (>1.0 cm) and diameter (>2.0 cm) positively correlated with disease progression (i.e., IMH expansion, aortic rupture, propagation of dissection).[66] Others suggest that PAU location in the proximal segment of the descending thoracic aorta, and refractory symptoms rather than presence of an ulcer per se is most worrisome.[67] Medical management with vigilant clinical and radiological follow-up is advised for the initially uncomplicated descending thoracic PAU. Surgery or endovascular stent grafting when feasible can be undertaken for failed medical therapy, pseudoaneurysm, or rupture.

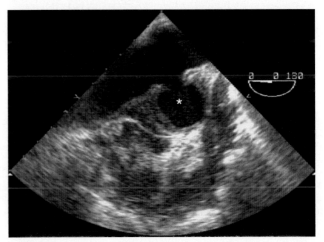

FIGURE 34-10   Penetrating atherosclerotic ulcer (PAU). Transesophageal echocardiographic (TEE) image of anterior aortic arch wall demonstrates outpouching from ulcer-like crater. *(From Firschke C, Orban M, Andrássy P, et al: Images in cardiovascular medicine. Penetrating atherosclerotic ulcer of the aortic arch. Circulation 108:e14–e15, 2003.)*

ACUTE ANEURYSM EXPANSION

Acute painful expansion of a previously established aortic aneurysm may herald impending rupture. Aortic aneurysm due to atherosclerosis (especially abdominal or descending thoracic in location) is particularly susceptible to sudden expansion, although this phenomenon occurs with aortitis and other diseases such as MFS. Imaging studies in the former disease states may reveal wall thickening and periaortic stranding or hematoma, as well as a measurable increase in aortic dimensions when compared with available past studies. Rapid expansion of the Marfan aorta occurs for reasons not related to inflammation, but when present may be even more worrisome. Urgent surgical referral is indicated.

Nonaortic Diseases

Chest or back pain may be the presenting symptom of a variety of conditions including AMI, unstable angina, pericarditis, musculoskeletal pain, pulmonary embolism (PE), pneumonia, pleuritis, and cholecystitis. Attention to the patient's description of the nature and quality of the pain, presence of predisposing factors, physical examination, and initial laboratory studies should allow early differentiation.

Initial Medical Treatment

Patients with acute aortic syndromes should be treated with intravenous medications to lower the arterial blood pressure as expeditiously as possible (Fig. 34-11). Since aortic wall strain is a function of LV contraction velocity (expressed mathematically as change in pressure divided by change in time [dP/dT]), β-adrenergic receptor antagonists, given to attenuate LV systolic

TABLE 34-2	Intravenous β-Adrenergic Receptor Antagonists for Management of Acute Aortic Dissection	
THERAPY	**DOSE**	**RECEPTOR SELECTIVITY (HALF-LIFE)**
Metoprolol	5 mg bolus every 5 min for 3 doses; additional doses of 5-10 mg every 4-6 h as needed	$\beta_1 > \beta_2$ (3-6 h)
Labetalol	10-20 mg bolus, repeat 20-40 mg bolus every 10-15 min as needed Maintenance infusion 1-2 mg/min; maximum total dose of 300 mg	α_1-, β_1-, and β_2 ($\approx$ 5.5 h)
Esmolol	0.5 mg/kg bolus, then 50 μg/kg/min infusion	β_1 (9 min)
Propranolol	0.05-0.15 mg/kg every 4-6 h as needed	$\beta_1 \approx \beta_2$ (5-7 h)

contractile force *and* decrease heart rate, are first-line therapeutic agents (Table 34-2). In patients with a contraindication or intolerance to β-adrenergic receptor antagonists, a heart rate–slowing nondihydropyridine calcium channel blocker, such as diltiazem or verapamil, may be an effective substitute.

Target systolic blood pressure and heart rate are 110 mmHg and 60 beats/min or less, respectively, but medications may require titration according to clinical evidence of impaired end-organ perfusion. β-Adrenergic receptor antagonists alone are often insufficient for achieving blood pressure control, so administration of a direct vasodilator may be necessary. Sodium nitroprusside is

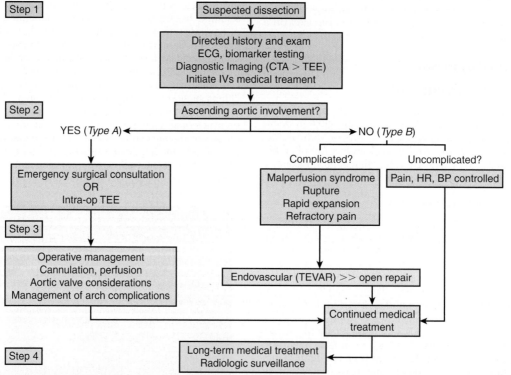

FIGURE 34-11 One proposed management pathway for acute aortic dissection. In Step 1, a low index of clinical suspicion for acute aortic dissection should prompt early diagnostic testing while medical therapy is initiated. Step 2 involves determination of ascending aortic involvement, which significantly influences importance of emergent surgical consultation. In Step 3, patients with type A aortic dissection are referred for surgery, and patients with complicated type B aortic dissection are referred for endovascular therapy or surgery. Patients with uncomplicated type B aortic dissection are continued on medical therapy and monitored for changes in clinical status. In Step 4, a care plan is established that emphasizes importance of long-term medical therapy, radiological surveillance, and lifestyle modifications to decrease risk of postdissection complications. Long-term medical therapy should include β-receptor antagonists and angiotensin receptor blockers (ARBs) or angiotensin-converting enzyme inhibitors (ACEIs) to achieve resting heart rate of 60 beats/min or less and BP of 120/80 mmHg or less, respectively. BP, blood pressure; CTA, computed tomographic angiography; ECG, electrocardiogram; HR, heart rate; IV, intravenous; TEE, transesophageal echocardiography. *(Adapted from Hiratzka LF, Bakris GL, Beckman JA, et al: 2010 ACCF/AHA/AATS/ACR/ASA/SCA/SCAI/SIR/STS/SVM guidelines for the diagnosis and management of patients with thoracic aortic disease. J Am Coll Cardiol 55:e27–e129, 2010.)[2]*

the agent of first choice in aortic dissection patients with hypertension refractory to initial β-blocker therapy, but should not be initiated without adequate heart rate control because reflex tachycardia unfavorably influences the dP/dT profile. The starting dose is 25 µg/min by continuous infusion, and adjustments are usually made in increments of 10 to 25 µg. At infusion rates above 2 µg/kg/min, the circulating concentration of the metabolite cyanide (CN^-) exceeds the rate of excretion by the kidneys. After a total nitroprusside load of 500 µg/kg, endogenous molecular CN^- buffers are depleted, increasing the probability of complications from drug toxicity, including death. In clinical practice, measuring levels of thiocyanate, a byproduct of CN^- metabolism, is critical to prevent drug-induced CN^- toxicity, particularly in patients with renal insufficiency. Alternative intravenous vasodilators available for use in the acute setting include enalaprilat, hydralazine, and nicardipine.[68] Concomitant analgesia for pain control is essential and may favorably influence blood pressure and heart rate.

For acute aortic dissection patients with *hypotension*, cardiogenic shock from hemopericardium should be considered. Volume resuscitation or pressor therapy may be necessary to maintain vital organ perfusion, but these are merely temporizing measures. Pericardiocentesis for relief of tamponade is not recommended, and surgery should be performed emergently.

Indications for Surgery

Anatomical location of disease, patient comorbidities, initial complications from the dissection, and acuity of presentation (i.e., acute vs. chronic) are key factors that influence surgical indications for treatment of aortic dissection (Box 34-4). There is evolving evidence to support a relationship between clinical outcome and operator experience in repair of aortic disease. Increasing hospital volume for open abdominal aortic aneurysm repair is associated with improved survival, particularly at centers that perform over 50 abdominal aortic aneurysm repairs annually.[69,70] Less well established are clinically useful parameters for evidence-based referral of patients with thoracic aortic disease. Ongoing public health initiatives have proposed examining the following variables to define centers of excellence for surgical repair of thoracic aortic disease: procedural volumes (operator and facility), outcome, time to

diagnosis and intervention, and logistical measures including distance to nearest referral center and services available.[2,71]

Type A Aortic Dissection

Recommendations pertaining to patient selection for surgical, endovascular, or medical treatment of acute aortic dissection are derived from consensus expert opinion because randomized trials are lacking.[2] Emergency surgery is indicated for all acute type A dissections, regardless of the site of entry.[2,72] Surgery is performed to prevent rupture with exsanguination or tamponade and to relieve aortic regurgitation when present. The extent and complexity of surgery (resection/grafting of the ascending aorta, valve resuspension or replacement, coronary artery reimplantation) is determined on a case-by-case basis. Incorporation of the aortic arch in the primary repair is indicated when the tear traverses this segment of the aorta or when it has become acutely aneurysmal.[73] Indications for and timing of surgical repair for the unusual case of chronic stable type A aortic dissection are unresolved. In this situation, surgeon preference and patient comorbidities weigh heavily in decision making, as does any information related to aortic enlargement over time. Outcomes with conservative management may not be inferior to surgical repair in the chronic phase, as suggested by limited single center experiences and retrospective data.[12,75] Endovascular stent grafts are not approved by the U.S. Food and Drug Administration (FDA) for use in the ascending aorta or arch.

Type B Aortic Dissection

Uncomplicated type B dissection is treated medically, with emphasis on tight heart rate and blood pressure control. Serial imaging is performed to monitor disease evolution. Lifestyle modifications, including the possibility of career change, may be necessary to avoid strenuous lifting, pushing, or straining that requires intense or repetitive Valsalva maneuvers.[2]

Surgery for acute type B dissection is generally reserved for those patients who have failed initial conservative therapy and have a complicated course, as indicated by refractory or recurrent pain, continued extension, early aneurysmal expansion, rupture, malperfusion syndrome, dissection location within a previously known aneurysmal aortic segment, and for patients with MFS. The importance of refractory pain in otherwise *uncomplicated* type B dissection is increasingly appreciated. In one recently published prospective analysis of 365 type B dissection patients without conventional high-risk features, the presence of pain or persistent hypertension despite medical therapy was associated with a 35-fold increase in mortality, compared with the absence of these clinical features.[74]

Presently there are insufficient data to provide comprehensive guidelines for appropriateness of endovascular stent grafting, percutaneous fenestration, and branch vessel stenting as alternatives to surgery for type B aortic dissection (Table 34-3; also see Chapter 36). Several nonrandomized small prospective trials and registries have shown that endovascular stent grafting for acute, subacute, or chronic type B dissection can be an effective lower-risk alternative to surgery.[75-77] Recent years have seen increasing adoption of endovascular stent graft treatment for complicated type B dissection, although randomized trial data are lacking. Most high-volume centers have moved in this direction, and it is unlikely that a pivotal trial versus surgery will be conducted in patients with traditional indications for surgery in type B dissection.

The Investigation of Stent Grafts in Aortic Dissection (INSTEAD) trial randomized 140 *stable* type B patients 2 weeks following dissection to optimal medical therapy or optimal medical therapy plus endovascular stent grafting.[78] Although this trial was underpowered for the primary endpoint of aorta-related death at 2 years following randomization, a substantially greater number of patients who underwent stent grafting demonstrated recovery of true lumen size and contour and false lumen thrombosis (91%) compared with those who received optimal medical therapy

---

Box 34-4 Indications for Surgery

Acute Dissection

Type A
All patients

Type B
With complications:
 Rupture
 Extension
 Rapid aneurysm expansion
 Malperfusion syndrome
 Marfan's syndrome (MFS)

Chronic Dissection

Type A
Maximal dimension ≥5.5 cm
MFS with maximum dimension ≥4.5-5 cm
Increase in dimension ≥1 cm/yr
Severe aortic regurgitation
Symptoms suggestive of expansion or compression

Type B
Maximal dimension ≥5.5-6 cm
Increase in dimension ≥1 cm/yr
Symptoms suggestive of expansion or compression

Adapted from Hiratzka LF, Bakris GL, Beckman JA, et al: 2010 ACCF/AHA/AATS/ACR/ASA/SCA/SCAI/SIR/STS/SVM guidelines for the diagnosis and management of patients with thoracic aortic disease. J Am Coll Cardiol 55:e27, 2010.[2]

TABLE 34-3 Society of Thoracic Surgeons Class I and II Recommendations for Thoracic Stent Graft Insertion

PATIENT SUBGROUP	CLASSIFICATION	LEVEL OF EVIDENCE
Acute traumatic dissection	I	C
Acute type B dissection with ischemia	I	A
Symptomatic PUA/AIH	IIa	C
Chronic dissection from trauma	IIa	B
Acute type B dissection without ischemia	IIb	C
Subacute dissection	IIb	B
Chronic dissection	IIb	B
Degenerative descending aortic dissection >5.5 cm	IIa with comorbidities IIb without comorbidities	B/C
Aortic arch dissection with morbidity prohibitive for surgery	IIb	C

AIH, aortic intramural hematoma; PUA, penetrating atherosclerotic aortic ulcer.
Adapted from Svensson LG, et al: Expert consensus document on the treatment of descending thoracic aortic disease using endovascular stent-grafts. Ann Thorac Surg 82:S1, 2008.

alone (19%; P <0.001). These data are concordant with others suggesting positive aortic remodeling in type B dissection patients following endovascular stent graft placement. It is unclear whether positive aortic remodeling will impact clinical outcomes longer term. Endoleak, stroke, and other device complications including migration and thrombosis have been reported.[76]

Indications for percutaneous balloon fenestration include false lumen compression of the true lumen with end-organ hypoperfusion. In this procedure, a balloon catheter is used to create a transverse tear across the dissection flap to attenuate compressive forces on the true lumen and improve flow to compromised organs. Placement of a bare metal stent (BMS) into side branch vessels to restore blood flow may be performed to enhance regional perfusion.[7]

Surgery for chronic type A aortic dissection is indicated for treatment of symptomatic aortic regurgitation with LV dysfunction or for management of aneurysmal disease according to conventional size criteria (≥5.5 cm for ascending aortic aneurysm, ≥5.5-6.0 cm for descending thoracic aneurysm, ≥5.5 cm for thoracoabdominal aortic aneurysm, or ≥1.0 cm/yr increase in maximal dimension).[2] Of note, in high-risk patients, such as those with MFS, elective aneurysm repair may be recommended at smaller aortic diameters.

Aneurysmal enlargement and recurrent dissection are more likely with long-term patency or partial thrombosis of the false lumen.[2] It has been proposed that partial thrombosis of the false lumen confers a worse outcome on patients with type B aortic dissection due to associated increases in pressure within the false lumen that may compromise true lumen-mediated blood flow to critical organs.[15–17]

Prognosis

The European Cooperative study group reported 1- and 2-year mortality rates for patients with type A dissection of 60% and 50%, respectively.[54] Approximately one third of aortic dissection survivors will experience rupture, extension, or require surgery for aneurysm formation within 5 years of recovery from the initial event.[7] Outcome in acute type A dissection is heavily influenced by treatment strategy; in-hospital mortality rates following presentation are 65% and 6% with medical therapy and surgical repair, respectively.[79] Nevertheless, surgical outcomes are poor in patients demonstrating signs of ischemia in renal, mesenteric, or peripheral arterial circulatory beds prior to dissection repair.[7] A bedside risk prediction tool for in-hospital mortality incorporating these variables offers clinicians, patients, and families a useful method by which to understand the complexities and hazards of the acute dissection process[72] (Fig. 34-12).

For type B dissection, overall in-hospital mortality rates approach 15%.[37] For patients with uncomplicated type B dissection managed medically, 1-month survival is 90%, whereas for patients who require surgical intervention for the indications listed previously, 1-month survival is only 75%. Independent predictors of early mortality include advanced age, rupture, and malperfusion syndromes. The excess mortality risk imposed by early complications necessitating surgical treatment, and thus operation on acutely sicker patients, has prompted investigation of endovascular stent grafting for selected patients. Nearly 2 decades of experience with thoracic endovascular aortic repair have yielded encouraging results regarding short- and long-term efficacy rates for this treatment strategy. One retrospective analysis of 87 patients undergoing endovascular stent placement to treat acute type B dissection demonstrated a 30-day survival rate of 81%, despite the presence of hemodynamic instability or shock in 62% of the study population.[80] In a type B dissection patient cohort for whom the prevalence of hemodynamic collapse was only 16%, endovascular graft placement was associated with short- and long-term survival rates of 90% and 87%, respectively.[81]

The most feared complications of type B aortic dissection are rupture, redissection, or development of malperfusion syndromes. Complete or partial false lumen patency or maximal descending thoracic aortic diameter of 4.0 cm or greater are risk factors for development of subsequent descending thoracic aortic aneurysms.[78]

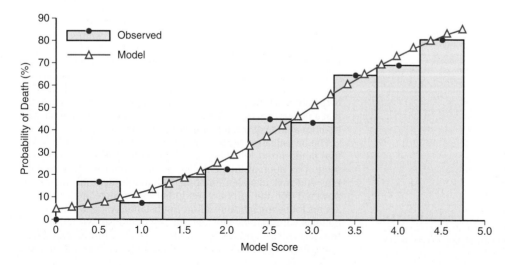

FIGURE 34-12 Observed versus predicted mortality rate for patients with acute type A dissection in the International Registry of Aortic Dissection. Variables used in the risk model include age, female gender, abrupt onset of pain, abnormal electrocardiogram (ECG), pulse deficit, renal failure, and hypotension/shock/tamponade. *(From Mehta RH, Suzuki T, Hagan PG, et al: Predicting death in patients with acute type A aortic dissection. Circulation 105:200–206, 2002.)*

Long-Term Surveillance

Because of the lifelong risk of subsequent aortic and cardiovascular complications, vigilant clinical and radiographic follow-up is mandatory for all hospital survivors. Medical management remains targeted to strict blood pressure (≤130/80 mmHg) and heart rate (≤60 beats/min) goals.[2] Statin therapy is indicated for treatment of atherosclerosis. Strenuous exercise is discouraged, and patients need be educated regarding the chronic nature of this disease, self-awareness of dissection-associated symptoms, and the importance of medication adherence. Imaging of the entire aorta is recommended pre-discharge and at 1, 3, 6, and 12 months, then annually thereafter.[82]

The continued high rates of death and disability from acute aortic dissection reinforce the urgent need for improvements in aggressive treatment of identifiable risk factors (notably hypertension), genetic and biomarker screening, clinical awareness, regional referral networks, consistent care protocols both during and after hospitalization, and possibly, surgical centers of excellence in aortic repair.

REFERENCES

1. Hagan PG, Nienaber CA, Isselbacher EM, et al: The International Registry of Acute Aortic Dissection (IRAD), JAMA 283:897, 2000.
2. Hiratzka LF, Bakris GL, Beckman JA, et al: 2010 ACCF/AHA/AATS/ACR/ASA/SCA/SCAI/SIR/STS/SVM guidelines for the diagnosis and management of patients with thoracic aortic disease, J Am Coll Cardiol 55:e27, 2010.
3. Olson C, Thelin S, Ståhle E, et al: Thoracic aortic aneurysm and dissection. Increasing prevalence and improved outcomes reported in a nationwide population-based study of more than 14,000 cases from 1987 to 2002, Circulation 114:2611, 2006.
4. Karthikesalingam A, Holt PJ, Hinchliffe RJ, et al: The diagnosis and management of aortic dissection, Vasc Endovascular Surg 44:165, 2010.
5. DeBakey ME, Beall AC Jr, Cooley DA, et al: Dissecting aneurysms of the aorta, Surg Clin North Am 46:1045, 1966.
6. Eggebrecht H, Baumgart D, Schmermund A, et al: Penetrating atherosclerotic ulcer of the aorta: treatment by endovascular stent-graft placement, Curr Opin Cardiol 18:431, 2003.
7. Nienaber C, Eagle KA: Aortic dissection: new frontiers in diagnosis and management: part I: from etiology to diagnostic strategies, Circulation 108:628, 2003.
8. Hirst AE Jr, Johns VJ Jr, Kime SW Jr: Dissecting aneurysm of the aorta: a review of 505 cases, Medicine (Baltimore) 37:217–279, 1958.
9. Lansman SL, McCullough JN, Nguyen KH, et al: Subtypes of acute aortic dissection, Ann Thorac Surg 67:1975, 1999.
10. Ando M, Okita Y, Tangusari O, et al: Surgery in three-channeled aortic dissection. A 31-patient review, Jpn J Thorac Cardiovasc Surg 48:339, 2000.
11. Richen D, Kotidis K, Neale M, et al: Rupture of the aorta following road traffic accidents in the United Kingdom 1992-199. The results of the co-operative crash injury study, Eur J Cardiothorac Surg 23:143, 2003.
12. Trimarchi S, Nienaber CA, Rampoldi V, et al: Results of surgery in acute type B aortic dissection: insights from the International Registry of Acute Aortic Dissection (IRAD), Circulation 114:I357, 2006.
13. Tsai TT, Evangelista A, Nienaber CA, et al: Partial thrombosis of the false lumen in patients with acute type B aortic dissection, N Engl J Med 357:349, 2007.
14. Li ZY, U-King-Im J, Tang TY, et al: Impact of calcification and intraluminal thrombus on the computed wall stresses of abdominal aortic aneurysm, J Vasc Surg 23:47, 2008.
15. Fillinger MF, Racusin J, Baker RK, et al: Anatomic characteristics of ruptured abdominal aortic aneurysm of conventional CT scans: implications for rupture risk, J Vasc Surg 39:1243, 2004.
16. Kazi M, Thyberg J, Religa P, et al: Influence of intraluminal thrombus on structural and cellular composition of abdominal aortic aneurysm wall, J Vasc Surg 38:1283, 2003.
17. Vorp DA, Lee PC, Wang DH, et al: Association of intraluminal thrombus in abdominal aortic aneurysm with local hypoxia and wall weakening, J Vasc Surg 34:291, 2001.
18. Nataatmadja M, West M, West J, et al: Abnormal extracellular matrix protein transport associated with increased apoptosis of vascular smooth muscle cells in Marfan syndrome and bicuspid aortic valve thoracic aortic aneurysm, Circulation 108(Suppl 1): II329, 2003.
19. LeMaire SA, Russell: Epidemiology of thoracic aortic dissection, Nat Rev Cardiol 8:103, 2011.
20. Judge DP, Dietz HC: Marfan's syndrome, Lancet 366:1965, 2005.
21. Keane MG, Pyeritz RE: Medical management of Marfan syndrome, Circulation 117:2802, 2008.
22. Januzzi JL, Isselbacher EM, Fattori R, et al: Characterizing the young patient with aortic dissection: results from the International Registry of Aortic Dissection (IRAD), J Am Coll Cardiol 43:665, 2004.
23. Gary T, Seinost G, Hafner F, et al: Cystic medial necrosis Erdheim Gsell as a rare reason for spontaneous rupture of the ascending aorta, Vasa 40:147, 2011.
24. Loeys BL, Dietz HC, Braverman AC, et al: The revised Ghent nosology for the Marfan syndrome, J Med Genet 47:476, 2010.
25. Dietz HC, Cutting GR, Pyeritz RE, et al: Marfan syndrome caused by a recurrent de novo missense mutation in the fibrillin gene, Nature 352:337, 1991.
26. Habashi JP, Judge DP, Holm TM, et al: Losartan, an AT1 antagonist, prevents aortic aneurysm in a mouse model of Marfan syndrome, Science 312:117, 2006.
27. Brooke BS, Habashi JP, Judge DP, et al: Angiotensin II blockade and aortic-root dilation in Marfan's syndrome, N Engl J Med 358:2787, 2008.
28. Malfait F, Wenstrup RJ, De Paepe A: Clinical and genetic aspects of Ehlers-Danlos syndrome, classic type, Genet Med 12:597, 2010.
29. Ahimastos AA, Dart AM, Kingwell BA: Angiotensin II blockade in Marfan's syndrome, N Engl J Med 359:1732, 2008.
30. Smith LB, Hadoke PW, Dyer E, et al: Haploinsufficiency of the murine Col3a1 locus causes aortic dissection: a novel model of the vascular type of Ehlers-Danlos syndrome, Cardiovasc Res 90:182, 2011.
31. Guo D, Hasham S, Kuang SQ, et al: Familial thoracic aortic aneurysms and dissections: genetic heterogeneity with a major locus mapping to 5q13-14, Circulation 103:2461, 2001.
32. Vaughan CJ, Casey M, He J, et al: Identification of a chromosome 11q23.2-q24 locus for familial aortic aneurysm disease, a genetically heterogeneous disorder, Circulation 103:2469, 2001.
33. Robinson PN, Godfrey M: The molecular genetics of Marfan syndrome and related microfibrillopathies, J Med Genet 37:9, 2000.
34. Pereira L, Lee SY, Gayraud B, et al: Pathogenetic sequence for aneurysm revealed in mice underexpressing fibrillin-1, Proc Natl Acad Sci U S A 96:3819, 1999.
35. Wang Y, Zhang W, Zhang Y, et al: VKORC1 haplotypes are associated with arterial vascular diseases (stroke, coronary heart disease, and aortic disease), Circulation 113:1615, 2006.
36. Guo D-C, Pannu H, Tran-Fadulu V, et al: Mutations in smooth muscle α-actin (ACTA2) lead to thoracic aortic aneurysms and dissections, Nat Genet 39:1488, 2007.
37. Januzzi JL, Sabatine MS, Eagle KA, et al: Iatrogenic aortic dissection, Am J Cardiol 89:623, 2002.
38. Ketenci B, Enc Y, Ozay B, et al: Perioperative type I aortic dissection during conventional coronary artery bypass surgery: risk factors and management, Heart Surg Forum 11:E231, 2008.
39. Braverman AC: Acute aortic dissection, Circulation 122:184, 2010.
40. Manalo-Estrella P, Barker AE: Histopathologic findings in human aortic media associated with pregnancy, Arch Pathol 83:336, 1967.
41. Hsue PY, Salinas CL, Bolger AF, et al: Acute aortic dissection related to crack cocaine, Circulation 105:1592, 2002.
42. Westover AN, Nakonezny PA: Aortic dissection in young adults who abuse amphetamines, Am Heart J 160:315, 2010.
43. von Kodolitsch Y, Schwartz AG, Nienaber CA: Clinical prediction of acute aortic dissection, Arch Intern Med 160:2977, 2000.
44. Rogers AM, Hermann LK, Booher AM, et al: Sensitivity of the aortic dissection detection risk score, a novel guideline-based tool for identification of acute aortic dissection on initial presentation, Circulation 123:2213–2218, 2011.
45. Tsai TT, Trimarchi S, Nienaber CA: Acute aortic dissection: perspectives from the International Registry of Acute Aortic Dissection (IRAD), Eur J Vasc Endovasc Surg 37:149, 2009.
46. Bossone E, Rampoldi V, Nienaber CA, et al: Usefulness of pulse deficit to predict in-hospital complications and mortality in patients with acute type A aortic dissection, Am J Cardiol 89:851, 2002.
47. Suzuki T, Katoh H, Tsuchio Y, et al: Diagnostic implications of elevated levels of smooth-muscle myosin heavy-chain protein in acute aortic dissection. The smooth muscle myosin heavy chain study, Ann Intern Med 133:537, 2000.
48. Shinohara T, Suzuki K, Okada M, et al: Soluble elastin fragments in serum are elevated in acute aortic dissection, Atheroscler Thromb Vasc Biol 23:1839, 2003.
49. Suzuki T, Distante A, Zizza A, et al: Diagnosis of acute aortic dissection by D-dimer: the International Registry of Acute Aortic Dissection Substudy on biomarkers (IRAD-Bio) experience, Circulation 119:2702, 2009.
50. Shimony A, Fillon KB, Mottillo S, et al: Meta-analysis of usefulness of D-dimer to diagnose acute aortic dissection, Am J Cardiol 107:1227–1234, 2011.
51. Schillinger M, Domanovits H, Bayegan K, et al: C-reactive protein and mortality in patients with acute aortic disease, Intensive Care Med 28:740, 2002.
52. Ranasinghe AM, Bonser RS: Biomarkers in acute aortic dissection and other aortic syndromes, J Am Coll Cardiol 56:1535, 2010.
53. von Kodolitsch Y, Nienaber CA, Dieckmann C, et al: Chest radiography for the diagnosis of acute aortic syndrome, Am J Med 116:73, 2004.
54. Erbel R, Alfonso F, Boileau C, et al: Diagnosis and management of aortic dissection: recommendations of the task force on aortic dissection, European Society of Cardiology, Eur Heart J 22:1642, 2001.
55. Bossone E, Evangelista A, Isselbacher E, et al: Prognostic role of transesophageal echocardiography in acute type A aortic dissection, Am Heart J 253:1013, 2007.
56. Flachskampf FA: Assessment of aortic dissection and hematoma, Semin Cardiothorac Vasc Anesth 10:83, 2006.
57. Macura KJ, Szarf G, Fishman EK, et al: Role of computed tomography and magnetic resonance imaging in assessment of acute aortic syndromes, Semin Ultrasound CT MR 24:232, 2003.
58. Clough RE, Schaeffter T, Taylor PR: Magnetic resonance imaging for aortic dissection, Eur J Endovasc Surg 39:514, 2010.
59. Shiga T, Wajima Z, Apfel CC, et al: Diagnostic accuracy of transesophageal echocardiography, helical computed tomography, and magnetic resonance imaging for suspected thoracic aortic dissection: systematic review and meta-analysis, Arch Intern Med 166:1350, 2006.
60. Hayashi H, Matsuoka Y, Sakamoto I, et al: Penetrating atherosclerotic ulcer of the aorta: imaging features and disease concept, Radiographics 20:995, 2000.
61. Motallebzadeh R, Batas D, Valencia O, et al: The role of coronary angiography in acute type A dissection, Eur J Cardiothorac Surg 25:231, 2004.
62. Motoyoshi N, Moizumi Y, Komatsu T, et al: Intramural hematoma and dissection involving ascending aorta: the clinical features and prognosis, Eur J Cardiothorac Surg 24:237, 2003.
63. Nienaber CA, von Kodolitsch Y, Petersen B, et al: Intramural hemorrhage of the thoracic aorta. Diagnostic and therapeutic implications, Circulation 92:1465, 1995.
64. Song JK, Kim HS, Kang DH, et al: Different clinical features of aortic intramural hematoma versus dissection involving the ascending aorta, J Am Coll Cardiol 47:1604, 2001.
65. Song JK, Yim JH, Ahn JM, et al: Outcomes of patients with acute type a aortic intramural hematoma, Circulation 120:2046, 2009.
66. Ganaha F, Miller C, Sugimoto K, et al: Prognosis of aortic intramural hematoma with and without penetrating atherosclerotic ulcer, Circulation 106:342, 2002.

67. Singhai P, Lin Z: Penetrating atheromatous ulcer of ascending aorta: a case report and review of the literature, *Heart Lung Circ* 17:380, 2008.

68. Kim KH, Moon IS, Park JS, et al: Nicardipine hydrochloride injectable phase IV open-label clinical trial: study on the anti-hypertensive effect and safety of nicardipine for acute aortic dissection, *J Int Med Res* 30:337, 2002.

69. The Leap Frog Group: *Factsheet: evidence-based hospital referral.* Available at: http://www.leapfroggroup.org/media/file/FactSheet_EBHR.pdf. Accessed. April 23, 2009.

70. Landon BE, O'Malley JA, Giles K, et al: Volume-outcome relationships and abdominal aortic aneurysm repair, *Circulation* 122:1290, 2010.

71. Luft HS, Bunker JP, Enthoven AC: Should operations be regionalized? The empirical relation between surgical volume and mortality, *Clin Orthop Relat Res* 457:3, 2007.

72. Mehta RH, Suzuki T, Hagan PG, et al: Predicting death in patients with acute type A aortic dissection, *Circulation* 105:200, 2002.

73. Sun L, Qi R, Zhu J, et al: Total arch replacement combined with stented elephant trunk implantation: a new "standard" therapy for type A dissection involving repair of the aortic arch, *Circulation* 123:971, 2011.

74. Trimarchi S, Eagle KA, Nienaber CA, et al: Importance of refractory pain and hypertension in acute type B aortic dissection: insights from the International Registry of Acute Aortic Dissection (IRAD), *Circulation* 122:1283, 2010.

75. Nienaber CA, Fattori R, Lud G, et al: Nonsurgical reconstruction of thoracic aortic dissection by stent-graft placement, *N Engl J Med* 340:1539, 1999.

76. Cambria RP, Crawford RS, Cho JS, et al: A multicenter clinical trial of endovascular stent graft repair of acute catastrophes of the descending thoracic aorta, *J Vasc Surg* 50:1255, 2009.

77. Dake M, Kato N, Mitchell RS: Endovascular stent-graft placement for the treatment of acute aortic dissection, *N Engl J Med* 340:1524, 1999.

78. Nienaber CA, Rousseau H, Eggebrecht H, et al: Randomized comparison of strategies for type B aortic dissection. The INSTEAD trial, *Circulation* 120:2519, 2009.

79. Yanagisawa S, Yuasa T, Suzuki N, et al: Comparison of medically versus surgically treated acute type A aortic dissection in patients <80 years old versus >80 years old, *Am J Cardiol* 108:453, 2011.

80. Jonker FH, Verhagen HJ, Lin PH, et al: Outcomes of endovascular repair of ruptured descending thoracic aortic aneurysms, *Circulation* 121:2718, 2010.

81. Steuer J, Eriksson MO, Nyman R, et al: Early and long-term outcome after thoracic endovascular aortic repair (TEVAR) for acute complicated type B aortic dissection, *Eur J Vasc Endovasc Surg* 41:318, 2011.

82. Yeh CH, Chen MC, Wu YC, et al: Risk factors for descending aortic aneurysm formation in medium-term follow-up of patients with type A aortic dissection, *Chest* 124:989, 2003.

CHAPTER 35

Surgical Therapy for Aortic Dissection

Joseph Huh, Joseph S. Coselli, Scott A. LeMaire

The treatment of aortic dissections remains technically challenging to surgeons. Patients can present with a wide range of anatomical and physiological derangements. Surgical decisions are made on the basis of three primary considerations: anatomical location of the dissection, time since the onset of dissection, and resulting complications of dissection. The DeBakey and Stanford classifications define dissections according to their anatomical location; both systems place great importance on the involvement of the ascending aorta[1] (Fig. 35-1). DeBakey type I dissection initiates in the ascending aorta and extends varying distances into the thoracoabdominal aorta, often reaching the aortic bifurcation. Type II dissection is confined to the ascending aorta. Type III dissection initiates in the descending thoracic aorta and extends variable distances into the thoracoabdominal aorta. Timing of the operation is important because surgical repair becomes safer as the dissection becomes older and the aorta less fragile. Risks posed by tissue fragility must be weighed against the competing risk of acute complications, which include rupture, heart failure, and malperfusion. Although arbitrary, dissection is considered *acute* within the first 14 days after the initial tear in the aortic wall. After 14 days, the dissection is described as *chronic*.

Additionally, aortic dissections can produce a wide variety of life-threatening complications that may mandate emergent surgical repair or correction. Aortic rupture can occur anywhere along the dissected aorta. Lethal proximal aortic complications include pericardial tamponade, acute aortic valve regurgitation, and myocardial infarction (MI) from coronary artery malperfusion. In subsequent aortic segments, malperfusion of branch vessels can cause stroke, paraplegia, mesenteric ischemia, renal failure, and limb-threatening ischemia (Fig. 35-2). The potential for these acute complications, combined with severe physiological derangement and extreme tissue fragility, make aortic dissection one of the most challenging conditions faced by cardiovascular surgeons. These considerations are the foundations of operative indications and strategies for aortic dissection. Surgical strategies for treating proximal aortic dissections involving the ascending aorta and transverse aortic arch differ distinctly from strategies for treating distal aortic dissections involving the descending thoracic and thoracoabdominal aorta; therefore, the proximal and distal aortic segments will be discussed independently.

Acute Proximal Dissection

Without treatment, nearly half of patients with acute proximal aortic dissection die within 48 hours.[2] Once the diagnosis is suspected, aggressive pharmacological treatment is initiated immediately, and the focus can then shift to confirming the diagnosis and assessing treatment options (see Chapter 34).

Indications for Operation

Proximal aortic repairs performed in the chronic phase uniformly have better outcomes than those performed in the acute phase. Unfortunately, the high risk associated with early operation is outweighed by the even higher risk of a fatal complication (e.g., aortic rupture) during medical management. Therefore, the presence of an acute proximal aortic dissection has traditionally been considered an absolute indication for emergency surgical repair. Many authors continue to advocate this approach.[3,4] Although controversial, delayed operative management of acute proximal aortic dissection has been proposed in specific clinical scenarios: in elderly patients; in patients with severe malperfusion; when dissection occurs after previous cardiac operation; and to enable transport to a specialized center.

ELDERLY PATIENTS

Emergent repair of proximal aortic dissection in patients with advanced age remains controversial. In recent literature, operative mortalities of nearly 50% have been reported for octogenarian patients.[5,6] Neri et al. concluded that surgical treatment is not warranted in the elderly because "it does not reverse the unfavorable prognosis of the disease."[7] A demographic study that used a Taiwanese national registry identified a significant trend toward nonoperative management of acute aortic dissections (AAD) with increasing age.[8] However, elderly patients who survived operative treatment had better long-term survival than patients who were treated medically.

Clearly, acute proximal aortic dissection in the elderly is a high-risk situation. Surgical results of institutions and communities have to be considered to optimize best outcomes.[9,10] Aggressive intraoperative strategies, such as total arch replacement and root replacement, should be weighed against the mortality risk associated with prolonged operations. In patients whose limited physiological reserve makes them poor candidates for emergency aortic repair, delayed management with initial medical optimization followed by elective surgery may be a reasonable alternative.

SEVERE MALPERFUSION

Branch-vessel obstruction due to dissection creates a spectrum of malperfusion that ranges from mild (e.g., diminished pulse in an extremity) to severe (e.g., bowel infarction). In most cases of mild to moderate malperfusion, surgical repair of the proximal aorta redirects flow into the true lumen and restores adequate peripheral blood flow; however, patients in whom ischemia has caused severe end-organ dysfunction are unlikely to benefit from immediate ascending aortic repair.[11] Stroke with resulting coma and bowel infarction with peritonitis remain ominous conditions after type I aortic dissection. Deeb et al. reported that eight of nine patients who underwent early proximal aortic repair in the setting of severe malperfusion (as defined in Box 35-1) died before discharge from the hospital. All deaths were attributed to irreversible ischemic organ damage and severe reperfusion injury after cardiopulmonary bypass (CPB). On the basis of these results, these surgeons initiated a policy of delayed surgical treatment in patients with severe malperfusion. This strategy consisted of aggressive pharmacological treatment to reduce dP/dt (rate of rise of left ventricular [LV] pressure), confirmatory arteriography, percutaneous fenestration or stenting (if needed) to restore flow to compromised branch vessels, and elective operation after complete recovery from malperfusion. Of the 20 patients treated with this strategy, 17 underwent delayed operation an average of 20 days after presentation.[12] To reduce selection bias, the authors' analysis also included the three patients who died without operation (one from rupture, two from reperfusion injury) and the two patients who died after delayed surgery. The overall survival for these patients treated without immediate operation (15/20, 75%) was significantly better than the dismal survival obtained with a strategy of immediate surgery. Fabre et al. have also advocated percutaneous intervention before operation in patients with severe ischemic sequelae.[13]

DISSECTION AFTER PRIOR CARDIAC OPERATIONS

Delayed management with elective operation has been proposed for patients who have had cardiac surgery in the remote past. Presence of prosthetic aortic valves, aortic suture lines, coronary

CH 35

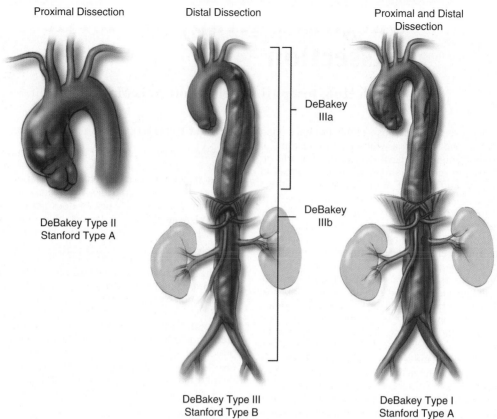

Proximal Dissection Distal Dissection Proximal and Distal Dissection

DeBakey IIIa

DeBakey IIIb

DeBakey Type II
Stanford Type A

DeBakey Type III
Stanford Type B

DeBakey Type I
Stanford Type A

FIGURE 35-1 **This simplified, descriptive classification scheme categorizes aortic dissection based on involvement of proximal aorta, distal aorta, or both segments.** Corresponding traditional classifications are included for comparison. The primary limitation of the Stanford classification is that it is based solely on presence (type A) or absence (type B) of ascending aortic involvement; it does not provide information about distal aortic involvement, a factor that has important management and prognostic implications.

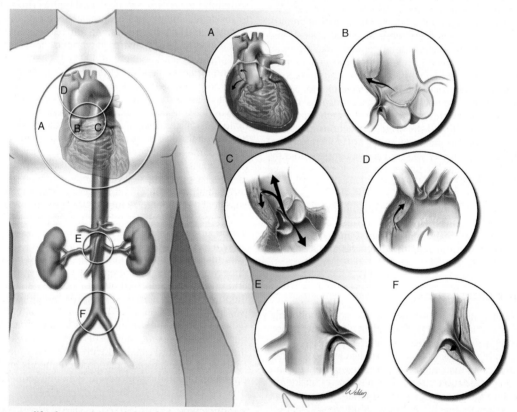

FIGURE 35-2 **Common life-threatening sequelae of aortic dissection.** Weakened aortic wall can rupture at any location and often results in fatal exsanguination. Rupture of ascending aorta into pericardial space **(A)** causes cardiac tamponade. Aortic dissection can lead to acute cardiac failure via **(B)** extension into coronary ostia, causing myocardial ischemia, and **(C)** disruption of aortic valve commissures, causing valvular insufficiency. Complications of branch vessel malperfusion include **(D)** stroke or upper-extremity ischemia when brachiocephalic branches are involved, paraplegia when segmental intercostal and lumbar arteries are compromised, **(E)** renal failure or mesenteric ischemia when visceral vessels are disrupted, and **(F)** lower-limb ischemia when iliac arteries are occluded.

Box 35-1 Definitions of Severe Malperfusion

Severe Myocardial Malperfusion
Acute infarction diagnosed by electrocardiographic changes or elevated myocardial-specific enzyme levels associated with new-onset ventricular dysfunction

Severe Cerebral Malperfusion
Generalized nonresponsiveness or severe localized neurological deficit lasting >48 hours

Severe Visceral Malperfusion
Abdominal pain, physical findings consistent with an acute abdomen, and associated abnormal laboratory findings

Severe Extremity Malperfusion
New-onset absence of pulse for more than 4 hours associated with pain, neurological symptoms, and physical findings consistent with threatened limb function

Adapted from Deeb GM, Williams DM, Bolling SF, et al: Surgical delay for acute type A dissection with malperfusion. Ann Thorac Surg 64:1669–1675, 1997.

grafts, and adhesions due to scarring and fibrosis around the aortic wall are considered protective. They can potentially prevent rupture, protect from valvular dehiscence, and prevent coronary malperfusion, the lethal complications of proximal aortic dissection. In one study by the International Registry of Acute Aortic Dissection (IRAD) investigators, patients with acute proximal dissection and a history of previous cardiac operations were less likely to present with chest pain and cardiac tamponade than those without a history of previous cardiac operations.[14] Hassan et al. explored the strategy of initial medical management in ten patients with ascending aortic dissection in the setting of prior cardiac surgery. Duration from prior cardiac surgery to dissection ranged from 2 months to 20 years. Medical therapy was successful in eight patients (80%), and all patients were discharged after the initial hospitalization. The two deaths in the series occurred at 4 months and 2 years after the dissection.[15]

It must be emphasized that the reduced risk of rupture does not apply to dissections that occur during the initial 3 weeks after cardiac surgery.[16] In fact, acute dissection during the early postoperative period carries a high risk of rupture and tamponade; these patients should undergo early operation.[17] Estrera et al. noted higher operative mortality (31% vs. 14%) and higher stroke rates (10% vs. 3%) in patients undergoing early operative repair for acute proximal dissection with prior cardiac surgery than in patients without prior cardiac surgery.[18] In their series, patients with prior cardiac surgery presented with similar incidences of tamponade and malperfusion symptoms as patients without prior cardiac surgery, although the series included patients with acute dissections occurring as early as 3 days after cardiac surgery.

TRANSPORT TO SPECIALIZED CENTERS

Patients with proximal aortic dissections frequently require transport to centers where cardiac surgery can be performed. Even in centers where cardiac surgery is available, transfer to high-volume centers can be justified in hemodynamically stable patients, and there is evidence of improved outcomes in patients transferred to specialized centers.[19–21] Before proceeding with transport, the patient's condition must be optimized. Aggressive pharmacological management should be initiated and metabolic disturbances corrected. Reliable delivery and titration of vasoactive medications during transport can be facilitated by central venous and arterial catheters, respectively. Inotropes and diuretics can be administered to patients with low cardiac output and acute ventricular distention due to aortic valvular insufficiency and volume overload. If patients with pericardial tamponade must be transferred, a pericardial drain should be placed to allow intermittent drainage during transport.[22] Whenever possible, patients with limb-threatening

ischemia should undergo revascularization—usually via femoral-to-femoral artery bypass—before transport to minimize the severe metabolic derangements that result from prolonged limb ischemia and improve chances of survival after aortic repair.[12]

Standardized treatment protocols have been developed to optimize the hemodynamic management of patients with AAD during transport. Implementation of the protocol developed by the Stanford Health Care Life Flight program decreased the number of patients who arrived at the receiving center with inadequate blood pressure control.[23] Results from a German study show that transporting patients with proximal aortic dissections by helicopter is no better than emergency ground transport with regard to survival benefit. Air transport did allow coverage of areas more than twice the distance, but at eight times the cost.[24]

Surgical Repair

PREOPERATIVE CONSIDERATIONS

With the noted considerations just discussed, most institutions repair proximal aortic dissections on an urgent or emergent basis. Important considerations that may change operative planning include the presence of connective tissue disorder and preexisting aneurysms in the aortic root or aortic arch. Dissections originating from preexisting aneurysms will likely require replacement of that segment. Preoperative computed tomography (CT) scans can provide valuable information about true lumen compression and existing malperfusion. Knowledge of which leg will access the true lumen may have implications in hemodynamic monitoring, cannulation for CPB, or subsequent requirement for adjunctive procedures such as femoral-femoral bypass. Degree of aortic valve regurgitation on preoperative echocardiography and any existing contraindications to anticoagulation will also have implications with regard to the need for aortic valve replacement and valve choice.

CARDIOPULMONARY BYPASS

Anterior exposure by median sternotomy provides standard access to the heart and proximal aorta. Most surgeons perform proximal aortic dissection repairs during a period of hypothermic circulatory arrest.[3,11,25–27] This strategy allows an "open distal anastomosis" with direct inspection of the entire arch and avoids creating additional tears that can result from placing a clamp across the fragile aorta. Peripheral options in cannulation for arterial inflow during mechanical circulation include the femoral artery and axillary artery. Many groups currently advocate axillary access by either direct cannulation or graft conduit. The axillary site usually allows perfusion of true lumen and simplifies antegrade cerebral perfusion.[28] Previously, femoral cannulation was the most common site of arterial inflow in acute dissections. One advantage is rapid access in emergent situations, although malperfusion and retrograde atheroembolization can occur. Central aortic perfusion, either by direct ascending aortic cannulation[29] or advancement of the cannula into the ascending aorta via the LV apex, is a feasible alternative. Venous drainage is typically achieved with the use of a dual-staged cannula placed in the inferior vena cava (IVC) via the right atrium.

Two methods of cerebral protection are hypothermia and cerebral perfusion. Hypothermia alone decreases metabolic activity to allow circulatory arrest, but surgeons must be aware of time limitations to ensure good neurological outcomes.[30,31] Although use of retrograde cerebral perfusion has declined over the past decade, the technique is still used in some centers. Retrograde cerebral perfusion delivers cold oxygenated blood from the pump into a cannula placed in the superior vena cava.[26,32] The initial hope was that the retrograde delivery of blood would provide oxygen to the brain. Unfortunately, accumulating evidence suggests that this technique does not provide cerebral oxygenation.[33–35] The benefits of this technique include maintenance of cerebral hypothermia and retrograde flushing of air and debris.

We and others currently use selective antegrade cerebral perfusion as a standard adjunct in proximal dissection repairs.[36,37] Direct cannulation of the innominate and left carotid arteries can be performed using flexible balloon catheters. However, right axillary cannulation for CPB can provide direct flow into the right carotid[28,38,39] (Fig. 35-3). Traditionally, circulatory arrest was initiated with deep hypothermia at 18°C, but this level of hypothermia has negative implications in CPB duration and degree of coagulopathy. Recent experience supports the safe use of moderate hypothermia during circulatory arrest.[40] Our current target temperature on CPB is 24°C. Once the target temperature is reached, CPB flows are decreased to 1 to 1.5L/min. A snare is used to occlude the innominate artery, thereby initiating circulatory arrest to the body and antegrade right cerebral perfusion. With the aorta open, we selectively use left carotid perfusion by a separate balloon catheter on the basis of the anticipated length of circulatory arrest and near-infrared spectroscopy (NIRS) cerebral monitoring. Electroencephalography (EEG) is useful during deep hypothermia when cerebral electrical silence is desired. However, with moderate hypothermia, EEG silence is usually not achieved.

DISTAL AORTIC CONSIDERATIONS

With the ascending aorta opened, the transverse aortic arch can be carefully inspected, and a decision can be made regarding the extent of aortic arch resection (Box 35-2). At the least,

most patients require graft replacement of the segment of the ascending aorta between the sinotubular junction and the origin of the innominate artery. In the setting of emergent operation for acute dissection, increasingly aggressive repairs of the aortic arch are associated with increasing early morbidity and mortality.[41] Therefore, the repair is generally only extended into the arch if the arch is aneurysmal or if the primary tear is located within the arch. When only the proximal portion of the arch is involved in the disease process, a beveled graft replacement of the lesser curvature is performed (see Fig. 35-3). This open distal hemi-arch replacement remains the most common scenario. Total arch replacement (Fig. 35-4) is performed only if the primary tear is located in the arch or if the entire arch is aneurysmal. If malperfusion was an issue preoperatively owing to true lumen compression in the descending thoracic aorta, patency of the true lumen can be assisted by open placement of an endovascular stent-graft in the descending thoracic aorta.

ASCENDING AND HEMI-ARCH REPLACEMENT

The dissecting membrane that separates the true and false lumens is excised to the distal aortic cuff (see Fig. 35-3B). The distal aortic cuff is prepared by tacking the inner and outer walls together and using surgical adhesive to obliterate the false lumen and strengthen the tissue[11,25] (see Fig. 35-3C). A Foley

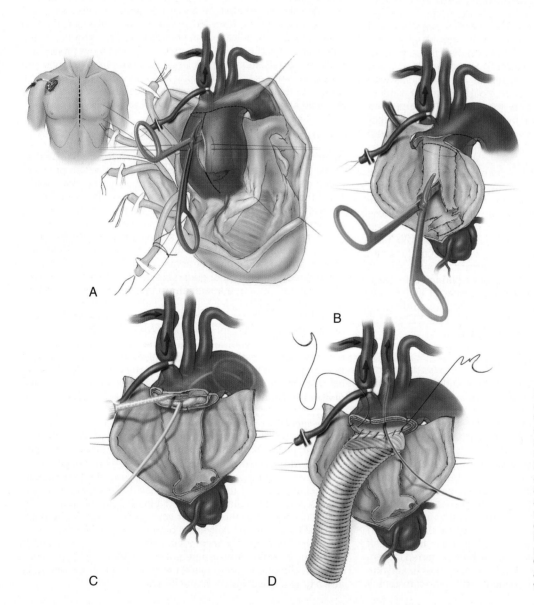

A

B

C

D

FIGURE 35-3 Graft repair of ascending aorta and proximal transverse aortic hemi-arch with concomitant aortic valve resuspension. A, Operation is performed via median sternotomy. Cardiopulmonary bypass inflow is established via the right axillary artery. **B,** After initiating circulatory arrest and antegrade cerebral perfusion, ascending aorta is opened, and dissecting membrane is excised. **C,** Distal aortic cuff is prepared using surgical adhesive; balloon catheter in descending aorta prevents distal migration of adhesive. **D,** Open distal anastomosis between graft and aorta is completed and reinforced with additional adhesive.

Continued

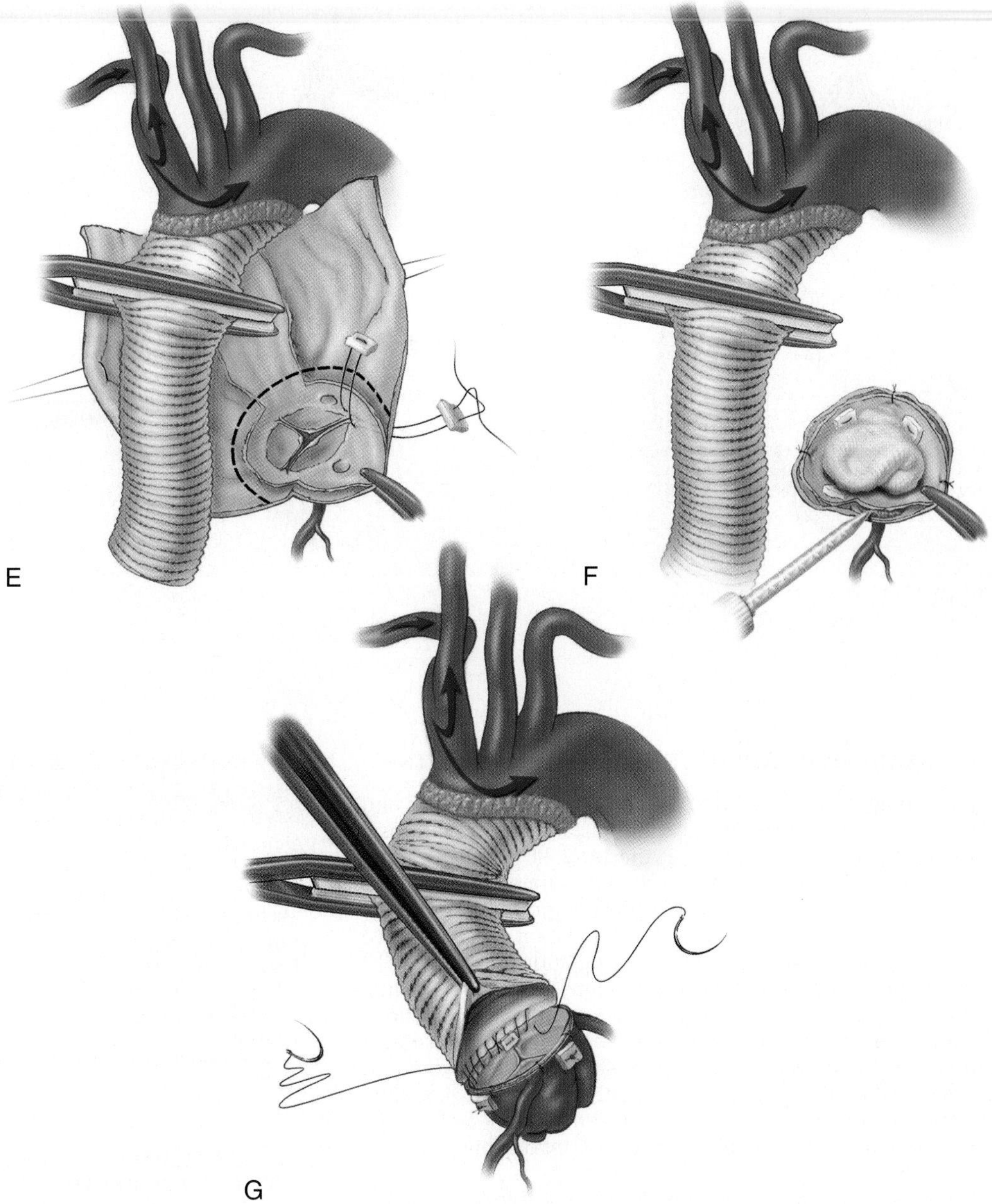

FIGURE 35-3—Cont'd E, After resuming full cardiopulmonary bypass, aortic valve is resuspended. F, Proximal aortic cuff is repaired with adhesive. G, Proximal anastomosis is performed.

Box 35-2 Options for Managing Aortic Arch During Proximal Aortic Dissection Repair

Ascending replacement only
Beveled hemi-arch replacement
Total arch replacement with island reattachment of brachiocephalic branches
Total arch replacement with bypass grafts to brachiocephalic branches
Elephant trunk technique

catheter balloon carefully inflated at the distal aortic arch can be helpful in preventing surgical adhesive from migrating distally in the false lumen. A polyester tube graft is sutured to the distal aortic cuff (see Fig. 35-3D). With the false lumen obliterated at the distal aortic cuff, the anastomosis between the graft and the aorta is constructed to a single true lumen; this often alleviates mild distal malperfusion problems that were present preoperatively. We routinely reinforce the distal anastomosis with a second suture line or interrupted pledgets. The graft is de-aired and clamped, and full CPB is resumed with the release

of the innominate snare. Rewarming is initiated, and the proximal portion of the repair is started (see Fig. 35-3E).

TOTAL AORTIC ARCH REPLACEMENT

Extensive aneurysms involving the entire arch usually require total arch replacement. Primary tears affecting the greater curvature or any of the brachiocephalic branch vessels should be resected. Distal anastomosis is created beyond the primary tear at the transverse arch or at the proximal descending thoracic aorta, using a tube graft. Our preference currently is for reattachment of the brachiocephalic vessels individually, using a trifurcated or bifurcated graft[42] (see Fig. 35-4). The single outflow to the brachiocephalic branches is anastomosed to the ascending aortic graft. In the most extreme cases, the aneurysm extends past the arch and into the descending thoracic aorta. This can be managed using Borst's elephant trunk technique for total arch replacement.[43,44] The distal anastomosis is constructed so that a portion of the graft is left suspended within the true lumen of the proximal descending thoracic aorta. In addition to directing flow into the true lumen, this "trunk" can be used to assist repair of the descending thoracic aorta during a subsequent operation.

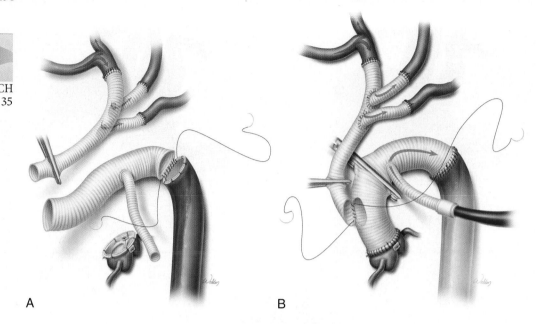

A   B

FIGURE 35-4 Graft replacement of entire transverse aortic arch involves a distal anastomosis to descending thoracic aorta and separate reattachment of brachiocephalic branches. This approach is generally reserved for patients with primary tears within the arch or large aortic arch aneurysms. *(Used with permission of Baylor College of Medicine.)*

ANTEGRADE DESCENDING THORACIC STENT-GRAFTS

Even with aggressive resection of the primary intimal tear and elimination of the false lumen at the distal aortic anatomosis, the false lumen often persists at the level of the descending thoracic aorta and beyond. The distal false lumen presents two considerations. First, presence of a false lumen after proximal aortic dissection continues to be a significant risk factor for late aneurysm formation, need for reoperation, and death.[45–47] Second, and more important in the acute setting, true lumen compression in the descending thoracic aorta can cause malperfusion in the mesenteric vessels, renal vessels, and lower extremities. Concurrent endovascular stent-graft deployment in the descending thoracic aorta with either standard ascending or hemi-arch reconstruction or in an extended total arch reconstruction in a "frozen elephant trunk" are options other investigators are exploring.[48–50]

We use an endovascular stent-graft in the descending thoracic aorta if clinically significant malperfusion (e.g., ischemia in the lower extremities, paraplegia, renal compromise) existed preoperatively with evidence of true lumen compression on imaging. The stent-graft is sized to the true lumen with care not to oversize within the friable dissected aorta. A guidewire is advanced into the true lumen of the open descending aorta under direct vision during circulatory arrest. The stent-graft is deployed in an antegrade fashion, with the proximal landing zone just distal to the left subclavian artery. One or two tacking sutures can be placed to fix the stent-graft to the distal arch to prevent migration. We do not dilate the stent-graft under hypothermic conditions. The goal of the distal stent-graft is to direct flow into the true lumen, eliminate malperfusion, and potentially help in remodeling the descending thoracic aorta by thrombosis of the false lumen. Addition of a descending stent-graft is well tolerated, although long-term outcomes remain unknown.

PROXIMAL AORTIC CONSIDERATIONS

Presence of preexisting annuloaortic ectasia/aortic root aneurysm or connective tissue disorder, the degree to which the dissection flap extends into the root, and the degree of aortic valve distortion are some of the factors for consideration when evaluating a proximal dissection for repair. Potential repairs addressing the aortic valve are listed in Box 35-3.

Box 35-3 Options for Managing Aortic Valve During Proximal Aortic Dissection Repair

Aortic valve repair:
  Commissural resuspension
  Commissural plication annuloplasty
  Resuspension and annuloplasty
Aortic valve replacement with mechanical or biological prosthesis
Aortic root replacement:
  Composite valve graft
  Aortic homograft
  Stentless porcine root
  Valve-sparing techniques (controversial)

SUPRACOMMISSURAL ANASTOMOSIS WITH AORTIC VALVE REPAIR

In the absence of intrinsic aortic root pathology and significant aortic valve distortion, the root can be repaired. The majority of these patients have separation of one or more commissures from the outer aortic wall; the resulting valve regurgitation can be corrected by resuspending the commissures into their normal position[51] (Fig. 35-5). Many surgeons use surgical adhesive within the false channel to strengthen this aortic root reconstruction.[12,25,52] The proximal aortic cuff is prepared with tacking sutures and surgical adhesive (see Fig. 35-3F) before performing the proximal aortic anastomosis (see Fig. 35-3G). If there is mild to moderate annular dilation, a commissural plication annuloplasty helps restore and maintain effective leaflet coaptation. Once the root and valve repairs are complete, the proximal aortic anastomosis is completed at the supracommissural position.

By preserving the aortic valve, long-term anticoagulation is often avoided; this is believed to favor thrombosis of the false lumen and thereby prevent subsequent dilation of the thoracoabdominal aorta. Another advantage of these valve-sparing techniques is that they only require a few stitches (usually between one and six) and can be performed quickly. Limiting the extent of repair reduces cardiac ischemia, CPB, and overall operative times and translates into lower postoperative morbidity and mortality. Therefore, although more extensive procedures can reduce risk of reoperation, limited repairs are performed whenever possible to increase the chance of

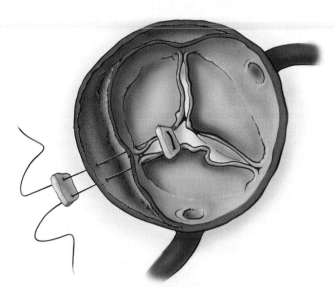

FIGURE 35-5 Cross-sectional drawing of aortic root illustrates dehiscence of two aortic valve commissures, which causes acute valvular regurgitation. Resuspending commissures onto outer aortic wall restores valve competency.

survival after the initial operation.[53] In a recent report of 200 patients who were discharged from the hospital after aortic valve repair for type A dissection, freedom from reoperation for aortic valve insufficiency was 97%, 92%, and 84% at 5, 10, and 15 years, respectively.[54]

AORTIC VALVE REPLACEMENT

Many patients undergoing proximal aortic dissection repair require concomitant correction of aortic valve pathology. Occasionally the valvular damage caused by the dissection is too severe to repair. In this case, separate replacement of the valve and graft replacement of the tubular segment of the ascending aorta are performed. This is also an option for patients who have significant preexisting aortic valvular disease (unrelated to the dissection). Separate aortic valve replacement with supracommissural graft anastomosis is generally not an option for patients with annuloaortic ectasia or Marfan's syndrome (MFS) because progressive dilation of the remaining sinus segment eventually leads to complications requiring reoperation.

AORTIC ROOT REPLACEMENT

Full aortic root replacement employs a mechanical or biological graft that has both valve and aortic conduit components. Three commercially available graft options are (1) composite valve grafts, which comprise a mechanical valve attached to a polyester tube graft, (2) aortic root homografts, which are harvested from cadavers and cryopreserved, and (3) stentless porcine aortic root grafts. Valve-sparing aortic root reimplantation is an alternative to full root replacement and involves excision of the aortic sinuses, attachment of a prosthetic graft to the native annulus, and resuspension of the native aortic valve inside the graft. Superior hemodynamics of the native valve and avoidance of anticoagulation are major advantages to this approach. Experienced centers have performed

valve-sparing root replacements in patients with acute dissection and have obtained mixed results.[55-58] Because of the substantial technical demands and lack of long-term outcome data, the role of valve-sparing root replacement in patients with AAD remains controversial, especially in patients with MFS.[59]

OUTCOMES

For operations performed from 1994 to 2007 in series including more than 100 patients with proximal aortic dissection, the reported early mortality has ranged from 14% to 24% (Table 35-1).

As operative techniques and critical care have improved, so has mortality at most centers. At one center, mortality improved in a stepwise fashion from 21% during their first quartile (1979-1980) to just 4% during their last quartile (2000-2003).[60] Reported risk factors for operative mortality include increasing patient age, cardiac tamponade, preoperative shock, preoperative neurological deficits, delay in diagnosis, repair of the aortic arch, coronary artery disease (CAD), acute myocardial infarction (AMI), concomitant coronary artery bypass, and malperfusion. Despite the substantial risks involved with surgical treatment, contemporary results are excellent compared with the lethality of unrepaired acute proximal aortic dissection.[61] In the ongoing experience of IRAD, 155 patients (17%) were managed nonoperatively, resulting in an in-hospital mortality of 59% compared with 24% in those treated surgically.[62] One-year survival after surgical repair of proximal aortic dissection ranges from 60% to 97%; survival drops to 37% to 71% at 10 years.[27,41,45,47,60,63,64] Late deaths have been multifactorial, with the majority of deaths reported being due to nonaortic etiologies such as stroke, heart failure, and malignancy.[47,65] The most common aorta-related late deaths resulted from rupture of the distal aortic segment. In recent studies focusing on long-term survival after proximal aortic dissection repair, persistent false lumen patency has been noted as a risk factor for late aorta-related mortality and need for intervention.[46,65] The incidence of patent false lumen varies significantly in the literature, from 20% to 90%. Instances of partial thrombosis have been noted, with, it appears, a higher incidence of persistent false lumen patency in the abdomen. Long-term implications of persistent false lumen patency have been the impetus for concurrent intervention at the distal segment of the initial proximal repair; however, outcomes for this strategy remain to be seen. What is certain is that patients with residual dissection in the distal aortic segments will require aggressive management and surveillance for long-term complications, including aneurysm formation.

Chronic Proximal Dissection

Occasionally, patients with proximal aortic dissection present for repair in the chronic phase. With rare exceptions, the mere presence of proximal aortic dissection continues to warrant surgical repair to prevent aortic rupture. In most regards, the operation is conducted in a manner similar to that of acute dissection repair, but the improved tissue strength in the chronic setting makes it easier to obtain secure hemostatic suture lines. Additionally, instead of obliterating the false lumen at the distal anastomosis, the dissecting membrane is fenestrated or resected into the arch to assure blood flow in both lumens and to prevent postoperative

TABLE 35-1	**In-Hospital or 30-Day Mortality for Patients with Type A Dissection**			
STUDY	YEAR PUBLISHED	NO. OF PATIENTS	SERIES RANGE (YRS)	MORTALITY
Girdauskas[99]	2009	276	1994-2008	18.8%
Fattouch[45]	2009	189	1996-2006	15.1%
Trimarchi (IRAD)[62]	2010	750	1996-2004	23.8%
Goda[100]	2010	301	1997-2007	13.6%
Song[47]	2010	118	1997-2007	17.8%

peripheral ischemia. The absence of both acute inflammation and malperfusion simplifies perioperative management considerably. These factors partially account for substantial differences in outcomes between patients who undergo surgery in the acute setting and those who undergo repair in the chronic phase. Compared with patients who undergo repairs in the acute phase, those who undergo repair of chronic dissection have lower incidences of death and stroke. Contemporary series report both early mortality and stroke rates below 8%.[37,66,67]

Acute Distal Dissection

In most centers, nonoperative management of acute distal aortic dissection results in significantly lower morbidity and mortality than open surgical treatment.[68,69] The initial strategy for medical therapy includes pharmacological treatment for blood pressure and heart rate control ("anti-impulse therapy") and close monitoring for complications of an AAD (see Chapter 34). Monitoring entails frequent clinical assessments in an intensive care unit (ICU) setting, continuous arterial line blood pressure measurement, and repeated imaging to assess for acute changes in the dissected aorta. Operative therapy is reserved for aneurysmal changes, impending rupture, or malperfusion in the acute period.[70,71]

Indications for Operation

Aortic rupture and end-organ ischemia are the most common causes of death during the acute phase, so operative indications are aimed at these complications. Specific indications for operative treatment include aortic rupture, rapid aortic expansion, uncontrolled hypertension, malperfusion, and persistent pain despite aggressive pharmacological therapy. Acute dissection superimposed on a preexisting aneurysm is considered a life-threatening condition and is also an indication for operation. Most patients with acute distal dissections have a serosanguineous left pleural effusion; this does not indicate impending rupture and is not a sole indication for surgery. However, increasing periaortic or pleural fluid associated with other worrisome findings, such as aortic expansion, warrants consideration of aortic repair. Finally, surgical treatment should be considered in patients who are noncompliant with medical therapy, provided they are otherwise satisfactory operative candidates.

Surgical Repair

OPERATIVE TECHNIQUES

A wide range of surgical techniques are potentially applicable for treating complications of acute distal aortic dissection. Therapy should be tailored to the goals of treatment, condition of the patient, anatomical considerations, and capabilities of the institution. Malperfusion of the extremities can be managed by peripheral extra-anatomical bypass. A femoral-femoral bypass or carotid-subclavian bypass may restore blood flow to an ischemic extremity and allow continued nonoperative management of the dissected aorta.

Endovascular surgical options, discussed separately in Chapter 36, have recently expanded surgical alternatives. Visceral and renal malperfusion can ideally be addressed by endovascular techniques.[25,71-73] Endovascular fenestration of the dissecting membrane or placement of stents into obstructed branch vessels can restore organ perfusion. In compromised patients with mesenteric ischemia or renal failure, endovascular reperfusion may allow clinical stabilization for other subsequent therapies or decision making. Aortic endovascular stent-grafting has also been used recently, with the goals of treating distal aortic malperfusion, excluding the dilated thoracic aorta, or promoting long-term remodeling to prevent the late sequella of aneurysm formation.[74] Aortic stent-grafting may perhaps be ideal to treat acute dilations of limited thoracic dissections. Results from the IRAD investigators show a mortality of 11% for endovascular operations, compared with 34% after open operations for acute type B dissections.[68] Long-term data are currently lacking regarding the fate

of the false lumen and the implications of late aneurysm formation after endovascular treatment of long thoracoabdominal dissections and uncomplicated dissections. Results from the only randomized prospective trial of uncomplicated chronic type B dissections for which aortic stent-grafting was performed between 2 and 52 weeks after dissection show no significant differences in mortality or adverse event rates at 2 years.[75]

When the endovascular approach is unavailable or unsuccessful in treating complications of the acute distal dissection, open surgical options—including graft replacement of the aorta, open aortic fenestration, and branch artery bypass—should be considered.[70,76] In the acute setting, the primary goals of surgery are to prevent fatal rupture and restore branch artery blood flow. A limited graft repair of the life-threatening segment can achieve these objectives while minimizing risks.[63] Because the most common site of rupture is in the upper third of the descending thoracic aorta, replacement usually extends from the level of the left subclavian artery to the mid-descending level. The distal portion of the descending thoracic aorta is also replaced if it is aneurysmal. Graft replacement of the entire thoracoabdominal aorta is only considered if there is a large coexisting aneurysm. Similarly, the repair is not extended proximally into the arch, even if the primary tear is located there, unless the arch is substantially enlarged.

Because surgery for acute distal aortic dissection carries an increased risk of postoperative paraplegia, adjuncts that provide spinal cord protection (discussed later in detail) are used liberally. Cerebrospinal fluid drainage and left heart bypass are often used, even when the planned repair is limited to the upper descending thoracic aorta. Proximal control is usually obtained by placing a clamp between the left common carotid and left subclavian arteries. Manipulation of mediastinal hematoma around the proximal descending thoracic aorta is avoided until proximal control is established. The aorta is opened, and the dissecting membrane is removed from the segment being replaced. The proximal and distal anastomoses incorporate all layers of the aortic wall, thereby obliterating the false lumen with the suture lines and directing all blood flow into the true lumen. Although there are usually multiple patent intercostal arteries, the extreme tissue fragility often precludes their reattachment.

OUTCOMES

Aggressive pharmacological management has led to a substantial decrease in mortality for patients with acute distal aortic dissection. Still, some 10% to 20% of medically treated patients die during the initial treatment phase.[69,71,77] Primary causes of death during nonoperative management include rupture, malperfusion, and cardiac failure. Risk factors associated with medical treatment failure—defined as death or need for surgery—include an enlarged aorta, persistent hypertension despite maximal treatment, oliguria, and peripheral ischemia.

Patients undergoing surgery for acute distal aortic dissection are a high-risk group that includes patients with rupture, neurological dysfunction, renal failure, and peripheral ischemia. Therefore, it is not surprising that results after surgery for AADs are often worse than those of medical therapy. Contemporary reports on acute distal dissection repairs document mortality and paraplegia rates of up to 34%.[67,69,71,74,77-81]

Despite the early survival advantage with nonoperative management compared to surgical treatment, long-term results are similar in patients in both groups. The reported actuarial survival rates with nonoperative management are 58% to 76% at 5 years and 25% to 56% at 10 years.[61,70,71] Five- and 10-year survival rates after repair range from 63% to 80% and 39% to 55%, respectively.[71,80]

Chronic Distal Dissection

Chronic aortic dissection is a progressive disease that requires lifelong management. The rationale for careful surveillance lies in the clinical history of the disease. Surgical intervention is eventually required in 25% to 35% of patients. Rupture and ischemic events related to the dissection are responsible for 15% to 30% of late deaths.[71,82]

Indications for Operation

Operative repair for a chronic distal aortic dissection is required in the setting of a type III dissection for which successful medical management initially was achieved or in the setting of residual distal disease after a previous successful proximal repair of a type I dissection. Although subsequent dissection, malperfusion, and ischemic events can occur in a chronically dissected aorta, the majority of patients will require operative intervention for the aneurysmal sequella of chronic dissections. Interval surveillance is critical in monitoring the growth of the aneurysm. Although the entire thoracoabdominal aorta may be dissected, dissection in and of itself is not an indication for graft replacement. In asymptomatic patients, an elective operation is considered when the aneurysmal segment has reached 5 to 6 cm or when it has enlarged more than 1 cm during a 1-year period. A lower threshold is often used for patients with connective tissue disorders, including Marfan, Loeys-Dietz, and other familial aortic syndromes.

Urgent operation is considered if the aneurysm becomes symptomatic. Patients with symptomatic aneurysms are at increased risk of rupture and deserve expeditious evaluation and treatment. The onset of new pain in a patient with a known aneurysm is particularly concerning and may herald significant expansion, leakage, or impending rupture. Emergent surgery is reserved for patients with clinical signs or imaging findings of rupture. Operative strategies are considerably different in emergent versus elective procedures. Patients with chronic dissection who require emergency repair because of acute pain or rupture undergo limited graft replacement of the symptomatic segment. Although the entire thoracoabdominal aorta may be dissected and aneurysmal, typically a relatively localized segment is the cause of the symptoms. Limited repair minimizes early postoperative morbidity. In appropriate surgical candidates, elective repairs replace the entire descending thoracic aorta and often extend to include the thoracoabdominal aorta (Figs. 35-6 and 35-7).

Preoperative Assessment

Given the influence of preexisting comorbidity on surgical outcomes, a careful preoperative assessment of physiological reserve is critical. Most patients undergo a thorough evaluation before undergoing elective operation. Preoperative assessment focuses on cardiovascular, pulmonary, and renal status.

CARDIOVASCULAR STATUS

Coronary artery occlusive disease is common in patients with thoracic aortic aneurysms (TAA) and contributes to a substantial proportion of early and late postoperative deaths. Additionally, valvular pathology and myocardial dysfunction have important implications when planning anesthetic management and strategies for aortic repair. Transthoracic echocardiography (TEE) is routinely obtained to evaluate both valvular and ventricular functions. Nuclear stress tests or comparable imaging studies are used selectively to identify reversible myocardial ischemia. Cardiac catheterization with coronary arteriography should be considered in patients who have evidence of coronary disease (on the basis of history or noninvasive studies) or an ejection fraction of 30% or less. Patients who have asymptomatic distal aortic aneurysms and severe coronary artery occlusive disease may undergo percutaneous angioplasty or surgical revascularization before aneurysm repair.

The hemodynamic changes that occur during thoracic aortic repair can precipitate stroke in patients with significant cerebrovascular disease. Therefore, carotid duplex ultrasound studies are also routinely obtained to detect occult carotid artery stenosis. It is recommended that significant carotid artery stenosis be corrected with an endarterectomy before proceeding with the aortic operation.

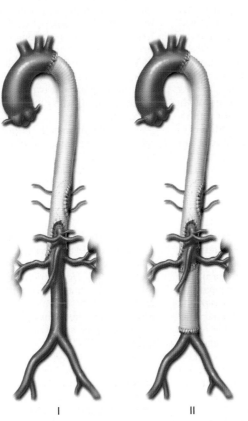
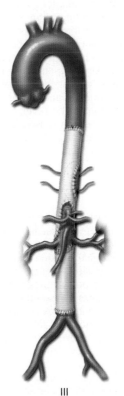
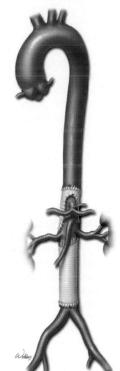

FIGURE 35-6 Crawford's classification categorizes thoracoabdominal aortic aneurysms (TAAA) based on extent of aortic repair. Extent I repairs begin in upper descending thoracic aorta, often near left subclavian artery, and extend to region of visceral and renal arteries. Extent II repairs also involve upper descending thoracic aorta but extend distally beyond renal arteries, often to aortic bifurcation. Extent III repairs begin in lower descending thoracic aorta (below sixth rib) and extend into abdominal segment. Extent IV repairs begin at diaphragmatic crura and extend distally, often involving entire abdominal aorta. *(Reproduced with permission of Coselli JS, Bozinovski J, LeMaire SA: Open surgical repair of 2286 thoracoabdominal aortic aneurysms. Ann Thorac Surg 83:S862–S864, 2007 [Fig. 1, p. S863].)*

I   II   III   IV

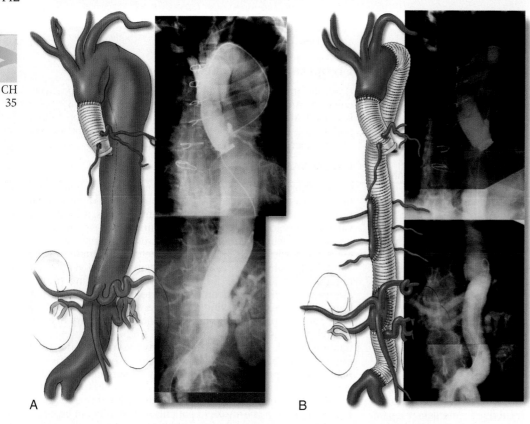

A   B

FIGURE 35-7 These drawings and aortograms illustrate presentation (A) and repair (B) of an extent II thoracoabdominal aortic aneurysm (TAAA) aneurysm that developed secondary to chronic distal aortic dissection. Patient had previously undergone repair of a proximal aortic dissection.

PULMONARY STATUS

The most common complication after descending thoracic and thoracoabdominal aortic repairs is pulmonary dysfunction.[83] Therefore, pulmonary function testing, including arterial blood gases and spirometry, is also routinely obtained before surgery to assess risk and allow optimization of the patient's pulmonary status. Patients with an forced expiratory volume in the first second of expiration (FEV_1) exceeding 1 liter and a partial pressure of carbon dioxide (Pco_2) below 45 mmHg are considered reasonable candidates for elective surgery. In selected patients, borderline pulmonary function can be improved with a 1- to 3-month regimen that includes smoking cessation, exercise, weight loss, and treatment of bronchitis. In most cases, operation is not withheld in patients with symptomatic aneurysms and poor pulmonary reserve. Surgical techniques, however, can be modified to improve the chance of recovery in these high-risk patients. For example, precautions can be taken to ensure preservation of the left recurrent laryngeal and phrenic nerves. Diaphragm-sparing techniques may also be helpful in such patients.[84]

RENAL STATUS

Preoperative renal status is evaluated on the basis of serum electrolytes, blood urea nitrogen (BUN), and creatinine (Cr) measurements. The computed tomography (CT) or magnetic resonance imaging (MRI) studies obtained to evaluate the aorta also provide information regarding kidney size and perfusion. Accurate information regarding baseline renal function has important prognostic and therapeutic implications. For example, patients with severely impaired renal function frequently require at least temporary hemodialysis after operation; these patients are also at increased risk of death.[85] Additionally, perfusion strategies and perioperative medications are adjusted on the basis of renal function. Finally, patients with poor renal function due to renal malperfusion from a dissection flap or from occlusive disease can undergo renal endarterectomy, stenting, or bypass grafting during thoracoabdominal aortic aneurysm (TAAA) repair.

Surgical Repair

OPERATIVE TECHNIQUES

Surgical strategies are determined on the basis of the extent of the aneurysm being repaired.[86,87] Descending TAAs are confined to the chest and are therefore repaired through a left thoracotomy. In patients with TAAAs, this incision is extended across the costal margin and into the abdomen (Fig. 35-8A). Extent of the thoracoabdominal replacement is defined by the Crawford classification of TAAAs (see Fig. 35-6). A double-lumen endobronchial tube is used to allow selective right lung ventilation and left lung deflation. Transperitoneal exposure of the thoracoabdominal aorta is achieved by dividing the diaphragm and performing medial visceral rotation.

Aortic repair usually is performed during a period of aortic clamping. The clamp is ideally applied distal to the left subclavian artery but is often required between the left common carotid artery (CCA) and left subclavian artery because of the anatomy of the aneurysm. In patients who have undergone previous coronary artery bypass surgery using the left internal thoracic artery, clamping proximal to the left subclavian artery can precipitate severe myocardial ischemia and cardiac arrest. When clamping at this location is anticipated in these patients, a left common carotid-to-subclavian bypass is performed to avoid cardiac complications. In certain situations, hypothermic circulatory arrest is required; the primary indication for this approach is the inability to clamp the aorta because of rupture, an extremely large aneurysm, or extension of the aneurysm into the distal transverse aortic arch.[79] Regardless of the technique, once proximal control is established, the aneurysmal segment of aorta is replaced with a polyester tube graft (Fig. 35-8B-J).

Because of the periaortic inflammation caused by the dissection, the vagus and left recurrent laryngeal nerves are often adherent to the aortic wall and susceptible to injury during repair of the proximal descending segment. Careful separation of the proximal descending thoracic aorta from the underlying esophagus before performing the proximal anastomosis minimizes the risk of a secondary aortoesophageal fistula. Important branch vessels—including the intercostal, celiac, superior mesenteric, renal, and lumbar arteries—are reattached to openings made in the graft.

When the dissection extends into the visceral or renal arteries, the membrane can be fenestrated or the false lumen can be obliterated using sutures or intraluminal stents.[88] Asymmetrical expansion of the false lumen often displaces the left renal artery laterally enough to require separate reattachment or use of a side branch graft. If the dissection stops at the level of the visceral vessels, the distal anastomosis can be beveled to include the abdominal branches. Although it is tempting to resect as much of the dissected aorta as possible, risks of the operation are incrementally increased with the greater extent of aortic replacement. Adjacent dissected aorta that is not aneurysmal is fenestrated by resecting wedges of the dissecting membrane proximally and distally from within the aortic cuffs, allowing blood to flow through both true and false channels after the reconstruction is completed. The distal anastomosis is accomplished in an open fashion with rapid direct reinfusion of the filtered whole blood via a cell saver system.

ORGAN PROTECTION

Clamping the descending thoracic aorta creates ischemia of the spinal cord and abdominal viscera. Clinically significant postoperative manifestations of hepatic, pancreatic, and bowel ischemia are relatively uncommon. Acute renal failure and spinal cord injury, however, are the main causes of morbidity and mortality after these operations. Therefore, several aspects of the operation are devoted to minimizing spinal and renal ischemia[86] (Box 35-4). A multimodality approach to spinal cord protection includes cerebrospinal fluid drainage, mild permissive hypothermia (32°C-34°C, nasopharyngeal), moderate systemic heparinization to prevent small-vessel thrombosis, distal aortic perfusion with left heart bypass during proximal anastomosis, sequential clamping of the lower aortic segments to reestablish flow to proximal organs as the proximal anastomoses are completed, and reattachment of the segmental intercostal and lumbar arteries. Cerebrospinal fluid drainage is used in extensive thoracoabdominal repairs (i.e., extents I and II) and in selected redo surgeries or other complicated situations. Benefits of cerebrospinal fluid drainage, which improves spinal perfusion by reducing cerebrospinal fluid pressure, have been confirmed by a randomized clinical trial.[89] Left heart bypass, which provides perfusion of the distal aorta and its branches during the proximal clamp period, is also used during extensive thoracoabdominal aortic repairs.[90] Because it unloads the heart, left heart bypass is also useful in patients with poor cardiac reserve. The visceral and distal aortic anastomoses are completed in an open fashion with the distal clamp off. During this time, balloon perfusion cannulas connected to the left heart bypass circuit can be used to deliver blood directly to the celiac axis and superior mesenteric artery (SMA) during their reattachment. Potential benefits of reducing hepatic and bowel ischemia include reduced risks of postoperative coagulopathy and bacterial translocation, respectively. Whenever possible, renal protection is enhanced by perfusing the kidneys with cold (4°C) crystalloid.[91,92]

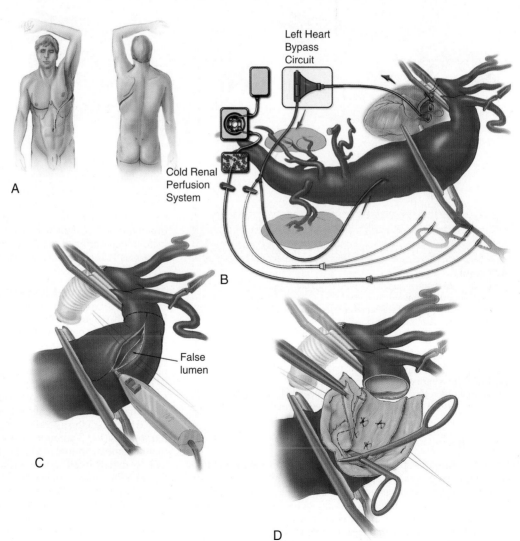

FIGURE 35-8 Surgical techniques involved in repairing an extent II thoracoabdominal aortic aneurysm (TAAA) related to chronic aortic dissection. **A,** Repair is performed through left thoracoabdominal incision. **B,** Aortic clamps are applied after establishing distal aortic perfusion via a left heart bypass circuit. **C,** The segment of aorta isolated between clamps is opened. **D,** Dissecting membrane is excised, and intercostal arteries are ligated.

Continued

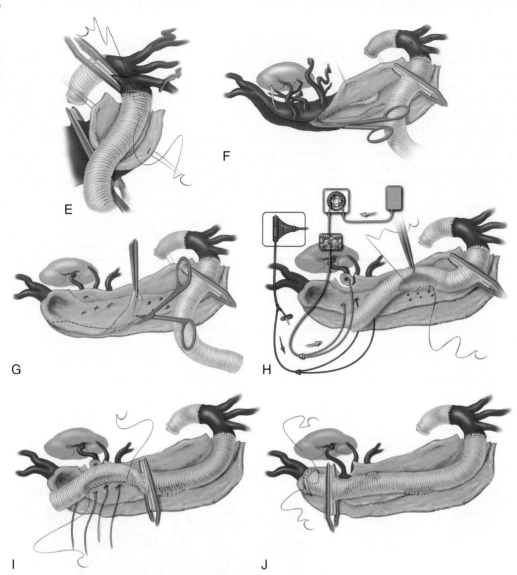

FIGURE 35-8—Cont'd E, Graft is sutured to proximal descending thoracic aorta. **F,** Clamps are repositioned to restore perfusion of left subclavian artery, left heart bypass is stopped, and remainder of aneurysm is opened. **G,** Dissecting membrane is removed to allow identification of patent segmental arteries and origins of visceral and renal arteries. **H,** Blood from left heart bypass circuit is delivered to celiac axis and superior mesenteric artery (SMA) via balloon perfusion catheters. Cold crystalloid is delivered to kidneys through catheters placed in renal arterial ostia. Critical intercostal arteries are attached to an opening in graft. **I,** Reattachment of visceral branches and **(J)** the distal aortic anastomosis complete the repair.

results in patients who require replacement of the entire thoracoabdominal aorta (extent II repairs) in chronic versus acute settings include early mortality in 5% versus 10%, paraplegia/paraparesis in 5% versus 11%, and renal failure in 13% versus 20%, respectively.[93]

Postoperative Considerations

Postoperative management remains critical in optimizing organ outcomes and preventing morbidity. Maintaining organ perfusion while preventing hypertension requires close monitoring. Aortic anastomoses are often extremely fragile during the early postoperative period, especially after acute dissection repair. Even brief episodes of postoperative hypertension can disrupt suture lines and precipitate severe bleeding or pseudoaneurysm formation. Therefore, during the initial 24 to 48 hours, aggressive blood pressure control is maintained to protect the integrity of the anastomoses. Nitroprusside and intravenous (IV) β-adrenoreceptor antagonists are routinely used to maintain mean arterial blood pressure at 80 to 90 mmHg. In patients with extremely friable aortic tissue, such as those with acute dissection or MFS, a lower target (70-80 mmHg) is used.

While preventing hypertensive episodes, maintaining adequate blood pressure, preload, and cardiac inotropic state are important in preventing delayed paraplegia and postoperative renal failure. In the absence of postoperative bleeding, blood pressure should be kept near its preoperative baseline level. Delayed paraplegia can arise hours to days after aortic surgery. In the postoperative period,

Box 35-4 Strategies for Spinal Cord, Visceral, and Renal Protection During Repair of Distal Thoracic Aortic Dissection

All Extents
Permissive mild hypothermia (32°C-34°C, nasopharyngeal)
Moderate heparinization
Aggressive reattachment of segmental arteries (especially T8-L1)
Sequential aortic clamping when possible
Perfusion of renal arteries with 4°C crystalloid solution when possible

Extent I and II Thoracoabdominal Repairs
Cerebrospinal fluid drainage
Left heart bypass during proximal anastomosis
Selective perfusion of celiac axis and superior mesenteric artery (SMA) during intercostal and visceral/renal anastomoses

OUTCOMES

When performed in specialized centers, these operations achieve excellent survival with acceptable morbidity.[67,77,78,81,93-95] Early mortality for chronic distal dissection repair ranges from 6% to 10%. Predictors of operative mortality include increasing age, congestive heart failure (CHF), aortic rupture (contained or free), and preoperative renal failure. Risk of paraplegia or paraparesis is 3% to 9%. These outcomes are significantly better than those obtained in patients who undergo surgery during the acute phase. For example, comparative strategies to reverse paraplegia include inducing systemic hypertension, decreasing cerebrospinal pressure by cerebrospinal fluid drainage, correcting anemia, preventing fever, and administering cardiac inotropes, mannitol, and steroids.[96] Recovery from paraplegia is possible, but if cord function does not return promptly after these measures are taken, such a recovery is not likely.

Aortic graft infections are a threat to anastomotic integrity and are associated with extremely high morbidity and mortality.[97] Definitive treatment often requires complete removal of the graft and complex vascular reconstruction. In an attempt to prevent this complication, administration of IV antibiotics is recommended until all drains, chest tubes, and central venous lines are removed. Similarly, all postoperative infections are treated aggressively with parenteral antibiotics to minimize the risk of secondary graft infection.

Vocal cord paresis is not uncommon after dissection at the distal arch. Resulting hoarseness is a concern that affects both voice and postoperative pulmonary toilet (owing to ineffective cough). Thyroplasty can improve functional status and is performed early before discharge.[98] An exception would be in the event of anticipated reintubation for a planned subsequent operation, such as completion of an elephant trunk. Reintubation can potentially disturb the thyroplasty; in these cases, initial vocal fold medialization can be achieved via collagen injection, and definitive thyroplasty can be performed at a later time.

The View Ahead

The landscape of thoracic aortic surgery is changing rapidly. As patient age and disease complexity continue to increase, new challenges are being met with innovative treatment strategies and technological advances. As we gain experience with endovascular aortic stent-grafts, new indications are being explored (see Chapter 36). The role of stent-grafts continues to expand in both the hybrid setting and stand-alone situations. Improvements in our understanding of the molecular mechanisms of dissection may lead to novel forms of medical treatment aimed at reducing the rate of aortic expansion and risk of fatal rupture.

ACKNOWLEDGMENTS

The authors express gratitude to Chrissie Chambers, MA, ELS, and Stephen N. Palmer, PhD, ELS, of the Texas Heart Institute, and Susan Y. Green, MPH, for editorial assistance; and Scott A. Weldon, MA, CMI, and Carol Lawson, CMI, for creating illustrations and assisting with image selection.

REFERENCES

1. Hiratzka LF, Bakris GL, Beckman JA, et al: 2010 ACCF/AHA/AATS/ACR/ASA/SCA/SCAI/SIR/STS/SVM guidelines for the diagnosis and management of patients with thoracic aortic disease: a report of the American College of Cardiology Foundation/American Heart Association Task Force on Practice Guidelines, American Association for Thoracic Surgery, American College of Radiology, American Stroke Association, Society of Cardiovascular Anesthesiologists, Society for Cardiovascular Angiography and Interventions, Society of Interventional Radiology, Society of Thoracic Surgeons, and Society for Vascular Medicine, Circulation 121(13):e266–e369, 2010.
2. Fann JI, Miller DC: Aortic dissection, Ann Vasc Surg 9(3):311–323, 1995.
3. Ehrlich MP, Ergin MA, McCullough JN, et al: Results of immediate surgical treatment of all acute type A dissections, Circulation 102(19 Suppl 3):III248–III252, 2000.
4. Estrera AL, Huynh TT, Porat EE, et al: Is acute type A aortic dissection a true surgical emergency? Semin Vasc Surg 15(2):75–82, 2002.
5. Piccardo A, Regesta T, Pansini S, et al: Should octogenarians be denied access to surgery for acute type A aortic dissection? J Cardiovasc Surg (Torino) 50(2):205–212, 2009.
6. Piccardo A, Regesta T, Zannis K, et al: Outcomes after surgical treatment for type A acute aortic dissection in octogenarians: a multicenter study, Ann Thorac Surg 88(2):491–497, 2009.
7. Neri E, Toscano T, Massetti M, et al: Operation for acute type A aortic dissection in octogenarians: is it justified? J Thorac Cardiovasc Surg 121(2):259–267, 2001.
8. Wu IH, Yu HY, Liu CH, et al: Is old age a contraindication for surgical treatment in acute aortic dissection? A demographic study of national database registry in Taiwan, J Card Surg 23(2):133–139, 2008.
9. Fehrenbacher J, Halbrook H, Siderys H: Operation for acute type A aortic dissection in octogenarians: is it justified? J Thorac Cardiovasc Surg 123(2):393–394, 2002.
10. McKneally MF: "We don't do that here": reflections on the Siena experience with dissecting aneurysms of the thoracic aorta in octogenarians, J Thorac Cardiovasc Surg 121(2):202–203, 2001.
11. Westaby S, Saito S, Katsumata T: Acute type A dissection: conservative methods provide consistently low mortality, Ann Thorac Surg 73(3):707–713, 2002.
12. Deeb GM, Williams DM, Bolling SF, et al: Surgical delay for acute type A dissection with malperfusion, Ann Thorac Surg 64(6):1669–1675, 1997.
13. Fabre O, Vincentelli A, Willoteaux S, et al: Preoperative fenestration for type A acute aortic dissection with mesenteric malperfusion, Ann Thorac Surg 73(3):950–951, 2002.
14. Collins JS, Evangelista A, Nienaber CA, et al: Differences in clinical presentation, management, and outcomes of acute type a aortic dissection in patients with and without previous cardiac surgery, Circulation 110(11 Suppl 1):II237–II242, 2004.
15. Hassan M, Carvalho EM, Macedo FI, et al: Paradigm change in the management of patients with acute type A aortic dissection who had prior cardiac surgery, J Card Surg 25(4):387–389, 2010.
16. Gillinov AM, Lytle BW, Kaplon RJ, et al: Dissection of the ascending aorta after previous cardiac surgery: differences in presentation and management, J Thorac Cardiovasc Surg 117(2):252–260, 1999.
17. Murphy DA, Craver JM, Jones EL, et al: Recognition and management of ascending aortic dissection complicating cardiac surgical operations, J Thorac Cardiovasc Surg 85(2):247–256, 1983.
18. Estrera AL, Miller CC, Kaneko T, et al: Outcomes of acute type a aortic dissection after previous cardiac surgery, Ann Thorac Surg 89(5):1467–1474, 2010.
19. Birkmeyer JD, Stukel TA, Siewers AE, et al: Surgeon volume and operative mortality in the United States, N Engl J Med 349(22):2117–2127, 2003.
20. Cowan JA Jr, Dimick JB, Henke PK, et al: Surgical treatment of intact thoracoabdominal aortic aneurysms in the United States: hospital and surgeon volume-related outcomes, J Vasc Surg 37(6):1169–1174, 2003.
21. Miyata H, Motomura N, Ueda Y, et al: Toward quality improvement of thoracic aortic surgery: estimating volume-outcome effect from nationwide survey, Eur J Cardiothorac Surg 36(3):517–521, 2009.
22. Garcia-Jimenez A, Peraza Torres A, Martinez Lopez G, et al: Cardiac tamponade by aortic dissection in a hospital without cardiothoracic surgery, Chest 104(1):290–291, 1993.
23. Perez L, Wise L: A standardized treatment protocol for blood pressure management in transport patients with a reported diagnosis of acute aortic dissection or symptomatic aortic aneurysm, Air Med J 18(3):111–113, 1999.
24. Knobloch K, Dehn I, Khaladj N, et al: HEMS vs. EMS transfer for acute aortic dissection type A, Air Med J 28(3):146–153, 2009.
25. Bavaria JE, Brinster DR, Gorman RC, et al: Advances in the treatment of acute type A dissection: an integrated approach, Ann Thorac Surg 74(5):S1848–S1852, 2002.
26. Deeb GM, Williams DM, Quint LE, et al: Risk analysis for aortic surgery using hypothermic circulatory arrest with retrograde cerebral perfusion, Ann Thorac Surg 67(6):1883–1886, 1999; discussion 91–4.
27. Kazui T, Washiyama N, Bashar AH, et al: Surgical outcome of acute type A aortic dissection: analysis of risk factors, Ann Thorac Surg 74(1):75–81, 2002.
28. Wong DR, Coselli JS, Palmero L, et al: Axillary artery cannulation in surgery for acute or subacute ascending aortic dissections, Ann Thorac Surg 90(3):731–737, 2010.
29. Kamiya H, Kallenbach K, Halmer D, et al: Comparison of ascending aorta versus femoral artery cannulation for acute aortic dissection type A, Circulation 120(11 Suppl):S282–S286, 2009.
30. Coselli JS, Crawford ES, Beall AC Jr, et al: Determination of brain temperatures for safe circulatory arrest during cardiovascular operation, Ann Thorac Surg 45(6):638–642, 1988.
31. Svensson LG, Crawford ES, Hess KR, et al: Deep hypothermia with circulatory arrest: determinants of stroke and early mortality in 656 patients, J Thorac Cardiovasc Surg 106(1):19–28, 1993.
32. Coselli JS, LeMaire SA: Experience with retrograde cerebral perfusion during proximal aortic surgery in 290 patients, J Card Surg 12(2 Suppl):322–325, 1997.
33. Hagl C, Khaladj N, Karck M, et al: Hypothermic circulatory arrest during ascending and aortic arch surgery: the theoretical impact of different cerebral perfusion techniques and other methods of cerebral protection, Eur J Cardiothorac Surg 24(3):371–378, 2003.
34. Moon MR, Sundt TM III: Influence of retrograde cerebral perfusion during aortic arch procedures, Ann Thorac Surg 74(2):426–431, 2002.
35. Wong CH, Bonser RS: Retrograde cerebral perfusion: clinical and experimental aspects, Perfusion 14(4):247–256, 1999.
36. Kazui T, Yamashita K, Washiyama N, et al: Usefulness of antegrade selective cerebral perfusion during aortic arch operations, Ann Thorac Surg 74(5):S1806–S1809, 2002.
37. Matalanis G, Hata M, Buxton BF: A retrospective comparative study of deep hypothermic circulatory arrest, retrograde, and antegrade cerebral perfusion in aortic arch surgery, Ann Thorac Cardiovasc Surg 9(3):174–179, 2003.
38. Pasic M, Schubel J, Bauer M, et al: Cannulation of the right axillary artery for surgery of acute type A aortic dissection, Eur J Cardiothorac Surg 24(2):231–235, 2003; discussion 5–6.
39. Sabik JF, Lytle BW, McCarthy PM, et al: Axillary artery: an alternative site of arterial cannulation for patients with extensive aortic and peripheral vascular disease, J Thorac Cardiovasc Surg 109(5):885–890, 1995; discussion 90–1.
40. Leshnower BG, Myung RJ, Kilgo PD, et al: Moderate hypothermia and unilateral selective antegrade cerebral perfusion: a contemporary cerebral protection strategy for aortic arch surgery, Ann Thorac Surg 90(2):547–554, 2010.
41. Crawford ES, Kirklin JW, Naftel DC, et al: Surgery for acute dissection of ascending aorta: should the arch be included? J Thorac Cardiovasc Surg 104(1):46–59, 1992.
42. LeMaire SA, Price MD, Parenti JL, et al: Early outcomes after aortic arch replacement by using the Y-graft technique, Ann Thorac Surg 91(3):700–708, 2011.
43. Borst HG, Frank G, Schaps D: Treatment of extensive aortic aneurysms by a new multiple-stage approach, J Thorac Cardiovasc Surg 95(1):11–13, 1988.
44. Schepens MA, Dossche KM, Morshuis WJ, et al: The elephant trunk technique: operative results in 100 consecutive patients, Eur J Cardiothorac Surg 21(2):276–281, 2002.
45. Fattouch K, Sampognaro R, Navarra E, et al: Long-term results after repair of type a acute aortic dissection according to false lumen patency, Ann Thorac Surg 88(4):1244–1250, 2009.
46. Song JM, Kim SD, Kim JH, et al: Long-term predictors of descending aorta aneurysmal change in patients with aortic dissection, J Am Coll Cardiol 50(8):799–804, 2007.

446

47. Song SW, Chang BC, Cho BK, et al: Effects of partial thrombosis on distal aorta after repair of acute DeBakey type I aortic dissection, *J Thorac Cardiovasc Surg* 139(4):841–847 e1, 2010; discussion 7.

48. Gorlitzer M, Weiss G, Meinhart J, et al: Fate of the false lumen after combined surgical and endovascular repair treating Stanford type A aortic dissections, *Ann Thorac Surg* 89(3):794–799, 2010.

49. Jazayeri S, Tatou E, Gomez MC, et al: Combined treatment of aortic type A dissection: ascending aorta repair and placement of a stent in the descending aorta, *Heart Surg Forum* 6(5):387–389, 2003.

50. Pochettino A, Brinkman WT, Moeller P, et al: Antegrade thoracic stent grafting during repair of acute DeBakey I dissection prevents development of thoracoabdominal aortic aneurysms, *Ann Thorac Surg* 88(2):482–489, 2009; discussion 9–90.

51. Fann JI, Glower DD, Miller DC, et al: Preservation of aortic valve in type A aortic dissection complicated by aortic regurgitation, *J Thorac Cardiovasc Surg* 102(1):62–73, 1991; discussion -5.

52. Murashita T, Kunihara T, Shiiya N, et al: Is preservation of the aortic valve different between acute and chronic type A aortic dissections? *Eur J Cardiothorac Surg* 20(5):967–972, 2001.

53. Kirsch M, Soustelle C, Houel R, et al: Risk factor analysis for proximal and distal reoperations after surgery for acute type A aortic dissection, *J Thorac Cardiovasc Surg* 123(2):318–325, 2002.

54. Piccardo A, Regesta T, Pansini S, et al: Fate of the aortic valve after root reconstruction in type A aortic dissection: a 20-year follow up, *J Heart Valve Dis* 18(5):507–513, 2009.

55. Erasmi AW, Stierle U, Bechtel JF, et al: Up to 7 years' experience with valve-sparing aortic root remodeling/reimplantation for acute type A dissection, *Ann Thorac Surg* 76(1):99–104, 2003.

56. Kallenbach K, Pethig K, Leyh RG, et al: Acute dissection of the ascending aorta: first results of emergency valve sparing aortic root reconstruction, *Eur J Cardiothorac Surg* 22(2):218–222, 2002.

57. Kerendi F, Guyton RA, Vega JD, et al: Early results of valve-sparing aortic root replacement in high-risk clinical scenarios, *Ann Thorac Surg* 89(2):471–476, 2010; discussion 7–8.

58. von Segesser LK, Lorenzetti E, Lachat M, et al: Aortic valve preservation in acute type A dissection: is it sound? *J Thorac Cardiovasc Surg* 111(2):381–390, 1996; discussion 90–1.

59. Bachet J: Acute type A aortic dissection: can we dramatically reduce the surgical mortality? *Ann Thorac Surg* 73(3):701–703, 2002.

60. Stevens LM, Madsen JC, Isselbacher EM, et al: Surgical management and long-term outcomes for acute ascending aortic dissection, *J Thorac Cardiovasc Surg* 138(6):1349–1357 e1, 2009.

61. Masuda Y, Yamada Z, Morooka N, et al: Prognosis of patients with medically treated aortic dissections, *Circulation* 84(5 Suppl):III7–III13, 1991.

62. Trimarchi S, Eagle KA, Nienaber CA, et al: Role of age in acute type A aortic dissection outcome: report from the International Registry of Acute Aortic Dissection (IRAD), *J Thorac Cardiovasc Surg* 140(4):784–789, 2010.

63. Fann JI, Smith JA, Miller DC, et al: Surgical management of aortic dissection during a 30-year period, *Circulation* 92(9 Suppl):II113–II121, 1995.

64. Pansini S, Gagliardotto PV, Pompei E, et al: Early and late risk factors in surgical treatment of acute type A aortic dissection, *Ann Thorac Surg* 66(3):779–784, 1998.

65. Kimura N, Tanaka M, Kawahito K, et al: Influence of patent false lumen on long-term outcome after surgery for acute type A aortic dissection, *J Thorac Cardiovasc Surg* 136(5):1160–1166, 6 e1–6 e3, 2008.

66. Kazui T, Yamashita K, Washiyama N, et al: Impact of an aggressive surgical approach on surgical outcome in type A aortic dissection, *Ann Thorac Surg* 74(5):S1844–S1847, 2002; discussion S57–63.

67. Safi HJ, Miller CC III, Reardon MJ, et al: Operation for acute and chronic aortic dissection: recent outcome with regard to neurologic deficit and early death, *Ann Thorac Surg* 66(2):402–411, 1998.

68. Fattori R, Tsai TT, Myrmel T, et al: Complicated acute type B dissection: is surgery still the best option? A report from the International Registry of Acute Aortic Dissection, *JACC Cardiovasc Interv* 1(4):395–402, 2008.

69. Hagan PG, Nienaber CA, Isselbacher EM, et al: The International Registry of Acute Aortic Dissection (IRAD): new insights into an old disease, *JAMA* 283(7):897–903, 2000.

70. Elefteriades JA, Hartleroad J, Gusberg RJ, et al: Long-term experience with descending aortic dissection: the complication-specific approach, *Ann Thorac Surg* 53(1):11–20, 1992.

71. Umana JP, Lai DT, Mitchell RS, et al: Is medical therapy still the optimal treatment strategy for patients with acute type B aortic dissections? *J Thorac Cardiovasc Surg* 124(5):896–910, 2002.

72. Chavan A, Lotz J, Oelert F, et al: Endoluminal treatment of aortic dissection, *Eur Radiol* 13(11):2521–2534, 2003.

73. Vedantham S, Picus D, Sanchez LA, et al: Percutaneous management of ischemic complications in patients with type-B aortic dissection, *J Vasc Interv Radiol* 14(2 Pt 1):181–194, 2003.

74. Kische S, Ehrlich MP, Nienaber CA, et al: Endovascular treatment of acute and chronic aortic dissection: midterm results from the Talent Thoracic Retrospective Registry, *J Thorac Cardiovasc Surg* 138(1):115–124, 2009.

75. Nienaber CA, Rousseau H, Eggebrecht H, et al: Randomized comparison of strategies for type B aortic dissection: the INvestigation of STEnt Grafts in Aortic Dissection (INSTEAD) trial, *Circulation* 120(25):2519–2528, 2009.

76. Panneton JM, Teh SH, Cherry KJ Jr, et al: Aortic fenestration for acute or chronic aortic dissection: an uncommon but effective procedure, *J Vasc Surg* 32(4):711–721, 2000.

77. Gysi J, Schaffner T, Mohacsi P, et al: Early and late outcome of operated and non-operated acute dissection of the descending aorta, *Eur J Cardiothorac Surg* 11(6):1163–1169, 1997.

78. Coselli JS, LeMaire SA, de Figueiredo LP, et al: Paraplegia after thoracoabdominal aortic aneurysm repair: is dissection a risk factor? *Ann Thorac Surg* 63(1):28–35, 1997.

79. Kouchoukos NT, Masetti P, Rokkas CK, et al: Hypothermic cardiopulmonary bypass and circulatory arrest for operations on the descending thoracic and thoracoabdominal aorta, *Ann Thorac Surg* 74(5):S1885–S1887, 2002.

80. Lansman SL, Hagl C, Fink D, et al: Acute type B aortic dissection: surgical therapy, *Ann Thorac Surg* 74(5):S1833–S1835, 2002; discussion S57–63.

81. Svensson LG, Crawford ES, Hess KR, et al: Dissection of the aorta and dissecting aortic aneurysms: improving early and long-term surgical results, *Circulation* 82(5 Suppl):IV24–IV38, 1990.

82. Glower DD, Speier RH, White WD, et al: Management and long-term outcome of aortic dissection, *Ann Surg* 214(1):31–41, 1991.

83. Svensson LG, Hess KR, Coselli JS, et al: A prospective study of respiratory failure after high-risk surgery on the thoracoabdominal aorta, *J Vasc Surg* 14(3):271–282, 1991.

84. Engle J, Safi HJ, Miller CC III, et al: The impact of diaphragm management on prolonged ventilator support after thoracoabdominal aortic repair, *J Vasc Surg* 29(1):150–156, 1999.

85. LeMaire SA, Miller CC III, Conklin LD, et al: A new predictive model for adverse outcomes after elective thoracoabdominal aortic aneurysm repair, *Ann Thorac Surg* 71(4):1233–1238, 2001.

86. Coselli JS, Conklin LD, LeMaire SA: Thoracoabdominal aortic aneurysm repair: review and update of current strategies, *Ann Thorac Surg* 74(5):S1881–S1884, 2002; discussion S92–8.

87. Coselli JS, LeMaire SA: Surgical techniques: thoracoabdominal aorta, *Cardiol Clin* 17(4):751–765, 1999.

88. LeMaire SA, Jamison AL, Carter SA, et al: Deployment of balloon expandable stents during open repair of thoracoabdominal aortic aneurysms: a new strategy for managing renal and mesenteric artery lesions, *Eur J Cardiothorac Surg* 26(3):599–607, 2004.

89. Coselli JS, LeMaire SA, Köksoy C, et al: Cerebrospinal fluid drainage reduces paraplegia after thoracoabdominal aortic aneurysm repair: results of a randomized clinical trial, *J Vasc Surg* 35(4):631–639, 2002.

90. Coselli JS, LeMaire SA: Left heart bypass reduces paraplegia rates after thoracoabdominal aortic aneurysm repair, *Ann Thorac Surg* 67(6):1931–1934, 1999.

91. Köksoy C, LeMaire SA, Curling PE, et al: Renal perfusion during thoracoabdominal aortic operations: cold crystalloid is superior to normothermic blood, *Ann Thorac Surg* 73(3):730–738, 2002.

92. LeMaire SA, Jone MM, Conklin LD, et al: Randomized comparison of cold blood and cold crystalloid renal perfusion for renal protection during thoracoabdominal aortic aneurysm repair, *J Vasc Surg* 49:11–19, 2009.

93. Coselli JS, LeMaire SA, Conklin LD, et al: Morbidity and mortality after extent II thoracoabdominal aortic aneurysm repair, *Ann Thorac Surg* 73(4):1107–1116, 2002.

94. Coselli JS, Bozinovski J, LeMaire SA: Open surgical repair of 2286 thoracoabdominal aortic aneurysms, *Ann Thorac Surg* 83:S862–S864, 2007.

95. Estrera AL, Miller CC III, Huynh TT, et al: Preoperative and operative predictors of delayed neurologic deficit following repair of thoracoabdominal aortic aneurysm, *J Thorac Cardiovasc Surg* 126(5):1288–1294, 2003.

96. Wong DR, Coselli JS, Amerman K, et al: Delayed spinal cord deficits after thoracoabdominal aortic aneurysm repair, *Ann Thorac Surg* 83(4):1345–1355, 2007.

97. Coselli JS, Köksoy C, LeMaire SA: Management of thoracic aortic graft infections, *Ann Thorac Surg* 67(6):1990–1993, 1999.

98. Rosingh HJ, Dikkers FG: Thyroplasty to improve the voice in patients with a unilateral vocal fold paralysis, *Clin Otolaryngol Allied Sci* 20(2):124–126, 1995.

99. Girdauskas E, Kuntze T, Borger MA, et al: Surgical risk of preoperative malperfusion in acute type A aortic dissection, *J Thorac Cardiovasc Surg* 138(6):1363–1369, 2009.

100. Goda M, Imoto K, Suzuki S, et al: Risk analysis for hospital mortality in patients with acute type a aortic dissection, *Ann Thorac Surg* 90(4):1246–1250, 2010.

CHAPTER 36 Endovascular Therapy for Aortic Dissection

Michael D. Dake

Acute aortic dissection (AAD) is a precipitous event associated with a wide range of outcomes from uncomplicated to catastrophic. Current endovascular strategies are based on identifying features that portend increased risk of death or other poor outcome and applying interventional techniques to prevent the life-threatening complications of the dissection.[1-3]

During the last 2 decades, there has been increasing interest in exploring endovascular procedures for management of aortic dissection.[4-13] Initially, endovascular approaches focused on addressing branch vessel involvement and ischemic complications associated with the dissection process[8,9] (Fig. 36-1). Subsequently, endovascular aortic stent grafts (initially developed to repair aortic aneurysms) were applied in type B aortic dissection to cover the primary entry tear of the dissection and promote thrombosis of the thoracic aortic false lumen[4,5] (Fig. 36-2). These basic endovascular tactics are now routine in the contemporary armamentarium for treatment of aortic dissection and its myriad manifestations.

Endovascular approaches are complementary to the two traditional therapeutic paradigms of open surgical repair for type A dissection and medical treatment for uncomplicated type B disease. Invasive interventional procedures fit between the existing operative and noninvasive alternatives to provide effective options for type A dissection with severe branch vessel compromise (before or after ascending aortic repair), complicated type B dissection (branch vessel involvement, descending aortic rupture, extension of disease or early aortic dilation, etc.), arch involvement, and ascending aortic intramural hematoma associated with an intimal tear distal to the left subclavian artery.

This chapter will review the specific endovascular procedures currently in use to manage aortic dissection, the patient subgroups in which these techniques are commonly employed, and the outcomes of these interventions.

Branch Vessel Interventions

Branch vessel involvement accompanying aortic dissection is a well-recognized complication occurring in over 30% of cases.[7,8,14] For appropriate intervention selection, the pathoanatomical concepts of static and dynamic branch involvement are crucial to selection of the endovascular option for reperfusion of an affected vascular bed.[15-17] As the dissection process extends distally from the primary entry tear, the dissection septum may engage the ostia of branch vessels. If the aortic flap, which consists of the intima and portion of the media shorn away from the wall, engages a branch orifice as it extends, two pathophysiological situations referred to respectively as *static* and *dynamic branch involvement* may occur (Fig. 36-3).

Static Branch Involvement

One manifestation that may arise when the advancing dissection septum intersects an aortic branch is static branch vessel involvement (Fig. 36-4). In static involvement, the aortic dissection flap extends directly into the branch for a variable distance. In contrast to the geometry described earlier, orientation of the septal trajectory is such that the branch ostium is incompletely engaged by the edge of the dissection plane. Rather than being circumferentially shorn by the septum, there is only partial circumferential involvement of the branch by the dissection. The aortic flap extends into the branch, creating a false lumen within the artery. As a result, the individual branch has both a true and false lumen like the aorta.

Similar to the aorta, a branch affected by static involvement may have multiple fates. At the end of the dissection where the flap terminates in the branch, a *reentry tear* in the false lumen may or may not occur. If a reentry tear occurs at the end of the false lumen, branch perfusion results from blood flow in both the true and false lumens. In many such cases, dual lumen perfusion is not associated with ischemic branch vessel symptoms. If reentry does not occur in cases of static branch vessel involvement, however, the false lumen within the branch has no outflow. The absence of a distal tear to allow communication with the vascular bed beyond the dissection may impair blood flow significantly. This *no reentry* state within the branch's false lumen renders perfusion limited to that contributed by the true lumen. Unfortunately, the true lumen may be compromised by the engorged false lumen. The blind pouch of the false lumen, without outflow, swells to a maximum dimension at its distal end. The pressure exerted by the false lumen severely distorts and compresses the true lumen to markedly reduce branch vessel flow. Commonly, the degree of ischemia experienced by the involved vascular bed may be significant and can lead to irreversible tissue necrosis if not relieved quickly.

In no-reentry situations, a local solution directed at improving flow within the affected artery is required because the problem is localized within the specific branch. Two options for endovascular treatment are possible. Resistance to outflow within the false lumen may be decreased by creating a distal tear or fenestration within the blind channel. This can be accomplished with the end of a guidewire or other endovascular probe placed within the false lumen through the aortic false lumen. This approach is associated with practical challenges, including the avoidance of distal extension of the dissection process, safe penetration of the false lumen wall to create an effective outflow tear, and determination of the presence of thrombus within the blind sac of stagnant false lumen blood to avoid its distal embolization.

In most cases, the preferred strategy involves increasing branch flow by decreasing the resistance to true lumen blood flow. This is performed by placing a stent in the true lumen of the branch through catheterization from the aortic true lumen. The stent is typically placed from beyond the end of the false lumen in the branch back to the aortic true lumen. A self-expanding nitinol stent is commonly employed because this distance is frequently greater than 2 cm and because there is a risk of squeezing any existing clot out of the false lumen with a balloon-expandable stent. These stents are sized to the total transarterial diameter of the branch and allowed to progressively expand on their own (post deployment) without supplemental balloon dilation. There are many successful reports of this approach in mesenteric, renal, and iliac arteries affected by no-reentry or static involvement.[8,9,18,19]

Occasionally, static branch vessel involvement with reentry anatomy and double-barrel flow may require endovascular intervention. The most common indication for stent placement in this setting occurs with involvement of a renal artery (Fig. 36-5). The kidney supplied by a dissected renal artery may be affected by the physical presence of a flap within the branch. The variable flow reduction caused by the flap, and resultant disrupted pattern of true and false lumen perfusion, may contribute to an exacerbation of hypertension. In cases where high blood pressure is sustained and recalcitrant to numerous intravenous (IV) medications, endovascular intervention may be warranted to restore a single lumen without flap. The approach to treatment involves placement of a balloon-expandable renal stent within the true lumen of the renal artery through the aortic true lumen. In most cases, this type of

448

CH
36

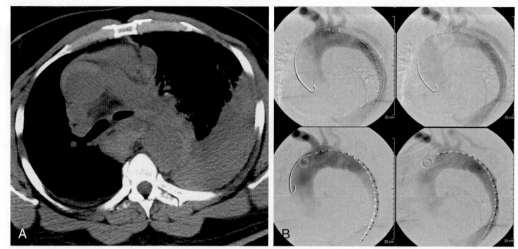

FIGURE 36-1 **Type B aortic dissection with proximal entry tear distal to left subclavian artery, retrograde extension, ascending intramural hematoma, and rupture into left chest. A,** Non–contrast-enhanced axial computed tomography (CT) image through the aorta demonstrates an ascending aortic mural-based ring with increased density, indicative of intramural hematoma. Also apparent is abnormal extravascular tissue surrounding aorta, with characteristic appearance of a rupture with clot. **B,** Series of images from a thoracic aortogram demonstrate entry tear just beyond left subclavian artery, with contrast media opacifying both the true and false lumens. Precise point of rupture is not identified.

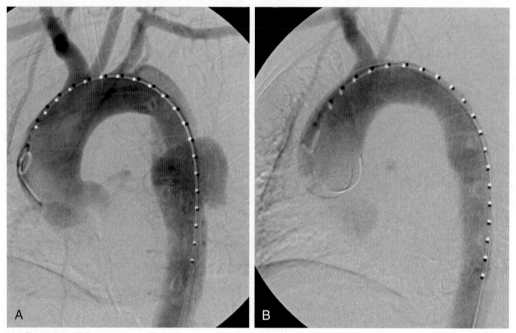

FIGURE 36-2 **Aortic dissection with rupture. A,** Thoracic aortogram demonstrates type B aortic dissection with mid-descending aortic rupture. **B,** Repeat aortogram following placement of thoracic endograft over proximal entry tear just above the site of rupture, without evidence of residual contrast extravasation.

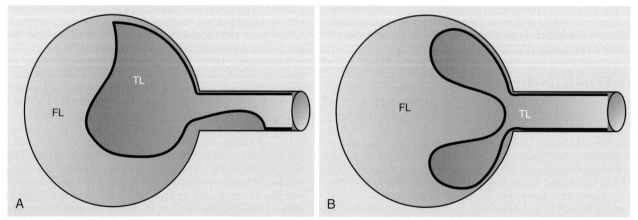

FIGURE 36-3 **A,** Static obstruction. Dissection has extended into a branch vessel. **B,** Dynamic obstruction. Membrane is lying across and obstructing origin of branch vessel. TL, true lumen; FL, false lumen.

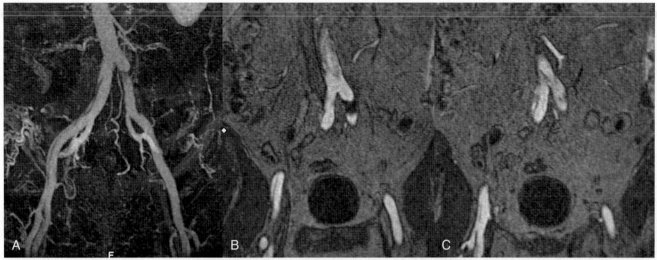

FIGURE 36-4   Magnetic resonance imaging (MRI) of static branch vessel involvement of iliac arteries. A, Coronal image of pelvis identifies a flap extending into right common iliac artery (CIA) and down to distal external iliac artery (EIA). Flow is evident in both true and false lumens within the right iliac artery. This is an example of static involvement with direct flap extension from the aorta into a branch. At the end of the dissection within the EIA, there is a distal reentry tear. This terminal tear establishes double-barrel flow within the iliac artery, which is rarely associated with ischemic symptoms. **B-C,** Similar coronal views show flap extension into left iliac system, but a segmental flow void *(black segment)* within false lumen of left CIA. This is associated with a no-reentry situation at distal extent of false lumen. No reentry within a branch is typically associated with obstruction of true lumen by a dilated false lumen cul-de-sac. The flow void noted may represent thrombosis in a blind channel or simply no blood flow. The usual consequence of this phenomenon of no reentry is branch vessel ischemia due to a lack of false lumen perfusion and compromised true lumen branch flow.

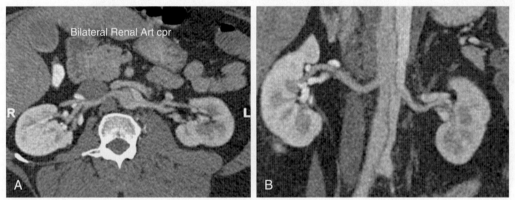

FIGURE 36-5   Computed tomography (CT) images of true and false lumen relationships to renal arteries. Axial **(A)** and coronal **(B)** CT images at level of left renal artery show that left renal artery is supplied by the false lumen (left aortic lumen). True lumen is located along right wall of aorta, and flap shows a characteristic natural fenestration or defect corresponding to left renal ostium. Flap around fenestration has small tail-like extensions pointing to the left that represent the initial few millimeters of left renal intimal lining that were torn away with the retracted aortic septum.

reentry involvement does not extend into the branch as far as the no-reentry extension. Thus, stents less than 2-cm long are typically implanted. This technique is well established at most centers that manage cases of aortic dissection frequently.

Dynamic Branch Involvement

In addition to primary branch pathology that occurs as a complication of aortic dissection, another mechanism, dynamic branch vessel involvement, may be responsible for organ ischemia. Dynamic branch involvement is a phenomenon associated with obstruction to branch vessel flow by an aortic septum that has prolapsed over the branch ostia like a curtain. In contrast to static involvement, where the aortic flap extends directly into a branch, dynamic obstruction occurs as an aortic process exclusively without an associated branch lesion. Propagation of the aortic flap may create a circumferential cleavage of the aortic wall surrounding the branch ostium (Fig. 36-6). Factors associated with this event include the flap trajectory, the resultant orientation of the septal plane proximal to the branch, and the inclusion of the ostium by the cleaved flap as it extends past. In this situation, the dissection septum surrounds the branch ostium as it tears

distally. The cleavage plane extends 1 to 2 mm into the branch, and then circumferentially reenters, creating a cylindrical tear, coring out a short segment of the intimal/medial lining of the most proximal aspect of the branch. The septum retracts into the aortic lumen with a fenestration corresponding to the branch orifice. This gives the flap a stencil-like appearance when viewed en face, with the number of holes related to the number of branch vessels involved by this phenomenon. When imaged in an axial plane, the affected artery appears to originate exclusively from the aortic false lumen. Closer inspection usually allows identification of a tear in the flap at the level or adjacent to the level of the branch. The flap often displays small projections angled from the edge of the tear, giving its outline on axial imaging an appearance similar to the contour of a metal rivet, the short-legged extensions corresponding to the amputated proximal lining of the branch.

In dynamic branch obstruction, hemodynamic flow patterns result in a large aortic false lumen with a diminutive or collapsed true lumen. There is variability, however, in the degree of true lumen obliteration related to the dynamic compromise.

In the majority of aortic dissection cases with true and false lumen aortic flow (often called *double-barrel flow*), the process described does *not* cause critical branch perfusion abnormalities.

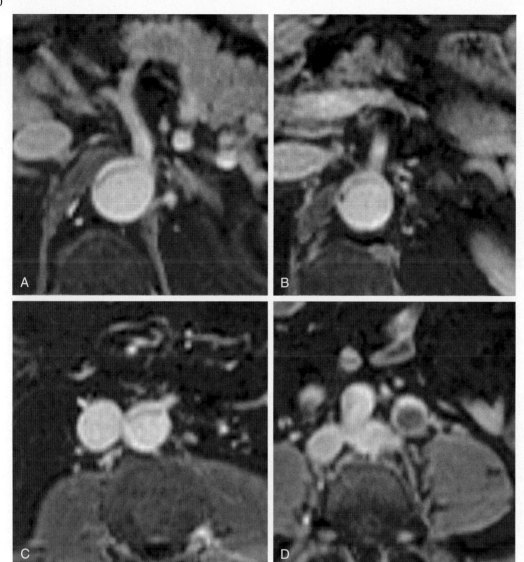

FIGURE 36-6 Magnetic resonance imaging (MRI) demonstrates dynamic branch vessel involvement, with aortic true lumen collapse and accompanying static no-reentry obstruction of left common iliac artery (CIA). A-C, Axial MRI shows wafer-thin crescent-shaped true lumen collapsed against anterior aortic wall at level of visceral arteries. Aortic septum prolapses like a curtain across the origins of branches originating from true lumen, with resultant malperfusion and multiorgan ischemia. **D,** At the level just below aortic bifurcation, there is marked asymmetry in appearance of CIAs. Lumen of left CIA has a flow void *(black circle)* due to static involvement without reentry that coexists with the dynamic process observed more proximally.

Flow to the branch originates primarily from the false lumen, with a small contribution from the true lumen through the corresponding fenestration in the aortic septum. Most of the false lumen flow usually occurs in diastole. During systole, the small contribution from the true lumen arrives through the septal window into the false lumen and branch. If the proximal primary tear is very large or the entry tear is in close proximity to the branch, the dominant flow pattern supplying branch perfusion may be in systole. In general, a branch that originates exclusively from the aortic false lumen is rarely affected by an ischemic complication.

Consistently, the aortic septum prolapses with a convex contour toward a compromised crescent-shaped true lumen. Consequently, all branches originating from the true lumen are at risk of obstruction. In this regard, the aortic septum in a dynamic obstructive process often assumes a coronal position, oriented across the aorta from left to right, in the distal descending thoracic proximal abdominal aortic segments. Consequently, the anteriorly oriented mesenteric vessels are in peril of ischemia because they frequently originate exclusively from a miniscule aortic true lumen. The likelihood of developing clinically relevant dynamic branch vessel compromise appears related in part to the area of the proximal entry tear. Although the process of dynamic involvement is dependent on multiple factors, as a general rule, the more severe the true lumen collapse, the larger or more circumferential the size of the proximal primary entry tear. Management of more than one ischemic vascular bed related to dynamic branch involvement and

an obliterated aortic true lumen that supplies the compromised branches is most expeditiously and effectively approached by an endovascular aortic procedure rather than a strategy directed at the individual branches.

More than one mechanism of branch involvement can coexist in any given patient. The clinical manifestations and the analysis of imaging for any patient requires an individualized approach that must synthesize information and aortic and branch vessel involvement to customize an optimal treatment strategy that will safely, successfully, and durably address the most compelling effects of the dissection.

Aortic Interventions

Endovascular aortic stent grafting is a less invasive alternative to open surgery for selected patients with both thoracic and abdominal aneurysms. Recently, the application of similar technology for management of acute aortic syndromes, including aortic dissection, has emerged as a focus of interest and study.[7,10–13,20,21] As with any new procedure, the key question is the determination of specific patient populations who may benefit from the new technique. In this regard, the use of traditional classification parameters for risk stratification of aortic dissection patients has advanced evaluation of the possible benefits and risks of endograft management.

Nearly all experience in endograft management of aortic dissection has been with type B disease when there is exclusive involvement of the descending thoracic aorta. Experience with endograft applications in type A dissection is limited to isolated case reports. In the United States, type B aortic dissections constitute approximately 30% to 35% of all dissections. The initial risk stratification of the type B dissection is made with the determination of the presence or absence of complications.

Medical management is the traditional treatment strategy for uncomplicated acute aortic dissection. Current reports cite a 30-day mortality rate of approximately 10%.[22,23] Use of stent grafting for stable uncomplicated patients with type B aortic dissection has yet to realize any improvement in survival compared to traditional medical therapy. Indeed, current conservative noninterventional management of uncomplicated cases is associated with 1-year survival rates of around 80%. Such results may be hard to improve upon with endograft therapy.[23,33]

Stent Grafts for Uncomplicated Type B Dissection

The Investigation of Stent Grafts in Patients with Type B Aortic Dissection (INSTEAD) trial observed that elective stent graft placement in survivors of uncomplicated chronic type B dissection does not improve 1-year survival and adverse event rates compared with medical therapy. Among the 140 patients randomized in this prospective trial, 1-year survival was 91% compared with 97% in patients randomized to medical therapy.[34,35] Moreover, aorta-related mortality was not different, and the risk for the combined endpoint of aorta-related death (rupture) and progression (including conversion or additional endovascular or open surgical intervention) was similar.

In the setting of complicated aortic dissection, medical management is associated with a high mortality rate, such that most patients will undergo surgery to address life-threatening complications.[2,4] Depending on the patient's underlying medical conditions and the nature of the complication(s), surgical mortality rates range from between 30% and 60% or higher.[24,25] It is in these high-risk scenarios that an opportunity exists to establish a role for interventional management. Thus the question becomes, *What constitutes complicated type B aortic dissection?* There is no strict definition for this category of disease, but traditionally it is relegated to two unambiguous disease manifestations: *aortic rupture* (Fig. 36-7) and *symptomatic branch vessel involvement.* These conditions are clear and their diagnosis unequivocal. Other adverse effects of the dissection process, such as uncontrollable hypertension, unrelenting pain,

and increasing pleural fluid, defy easy classification and do not have uniform criteria for comparative assessment. These so-called softer indications for intervention are commonly included as a surgical indication in most published series of acute complicated dissection.[8,26]

Endograft Treatment of Complicated Type B Dissection

The procedural goal for endovascular stent grafting in patients with complicated acute type B aortic dissection is endograft elimination of blood flow entry into the proximal entry tear. Obliterating the primary communication between the true lumen and the false redirects pulsatile flow into the true lumen, promotes false lumen thrombosis, and ultimately improves remodeling of the aorta by increasing the dimensions of the true lumen while shrinking the false lumen (Fig. 36-8).

Specific procedural techniques vary depending on the precise complication. Faced with dynamic branch vessel involvement and clinically relevant obstruction compromising flow to one or multiple branches, the procedural strategy focuses on unloading the aortic false lumen by increasing resistance to false lumen inflow or decreasing resistance to its outflow. The former is attempted by deploying an endograft over the proximal primary entry tear and rechanneling all flow into the true lumen. Logistically, this typically involves placement of a 15-cm-long (range 12-20 cm) stent graft from the nondissected segment of aorta proximal to the primary intimal tear, commonly between the origins of the left carotid and left subclavian arteries. This may require intentional partial or complete coverage of the left subclavian origin. The distal extent of the device usually remains above the diaphragm. The diameter of the implant selected is based on the transaortic dimension of the nondissected aorta just proximal to the dissection, rather than the size of the true lumen or transaortic diameter of the dissected segment.

Endovascular Treatment of Branch Vessel Involvement

The outcomes of stent graft therapy for reversal of dynamic branch vessel involvement are excellent, with procedural success in up to 95% of cases and complete false lumen thrombosis in 85% of patients.[7-9] These procedures are associated with 67.7% 5-year freedom from aortic rupture and open repair.[9] Additionally, static

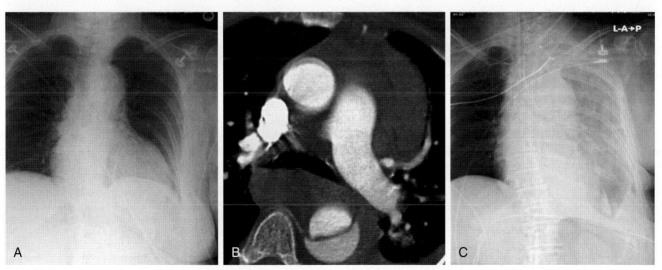

FIGURE 36-7   Acute type B aortic dissection with rupture in a 68-year-old woman. A, Frontal chest radiograph upon presentation to emergency room with severe back pain and hypertension that occurred while gardening. **B,** Axial computed tomography (CT) scan after contrast media administration shows typical appearance of aortic dissection in mid-descending aorta. **C,** Repeat chest radiograph performed after transfer to referral facility 4 hours after initial study, with marked interval change including opacification of left hemithorax from leaking blood.

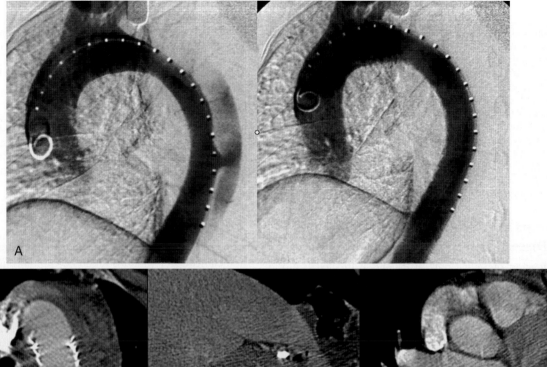

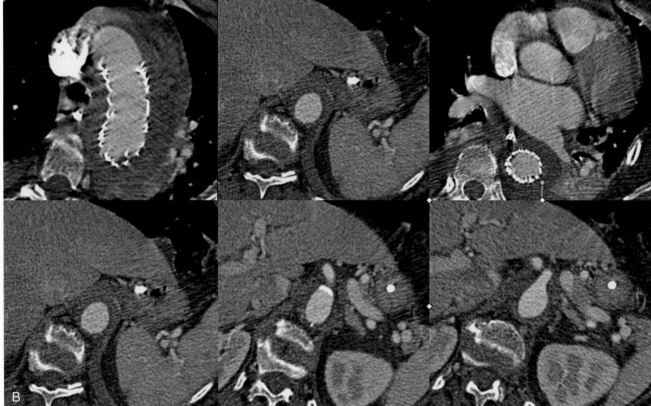

FIGURE 36-8 **Treatment and follow-up imaging of type B aortic dissection with rupture. A,** Aortograms pre- and post placement of a thoracic endograft across mid-descending aorta entry tear of a type B dissection in the 68-year-old woman described in Figure 36-7. **B,** Series of axial computed tomography (CT) images obtained 1 week postendograft management of a type B dissection with rupture. Stent graft is in good position, and false lumen is thrombosed. Residual extravascular blood and hematoma are evident.

branch involvement remote from the covered proximal aortic entry tear may require separate targeted intervention to manage residual ischemic compromise. This is especially important in cases with no-reentry anatomy complicating static branch involvement. In these situations, endovascular branch intervention should be provided emergently.

An alternative to endograft placement in dynamic branch compromise is distal flap fenestration.[9,27] Percutaneous balloon fenestration of the aortic septum has replaced the operative procedure. Balloon fenestration of the septum is designed to unload the aortic false lumen by decreasing the resistance to outflow. Technically, initial transgression of the aortic flap with a small cardiac transseptal TIPS needle and cannula usually is

performed from the small true lumen into the larger target of the false channel. The site of the needle puncture commonly lies within the infrarenal aorta at the level of the aortic bifurcation. Once successful transgression of the septum is confirmed, a wire is advanced across the flap and well into the targeted lumen. Sequentially larger balloon dilation of the flap is performed until a final size of between 20 and 25 mm is obtained.

Balloon fenestration causes a linear transverse tear in the flap that allows greater mixture of blood between the two aortic channels and decompresses the true lumen. These effects must be confirmed by aortography or intravascular ultrasound (IVUS) to ensure relief of the dynamic pattern of branch obstruction. After these two endovascular (endograft or fenestration) procedures, imaging comparisons of the anatomical effects (with computed tomography [CT], magnetic resonance imaging [MRI] or IVUS), including changes in the size of the aortic lumens, typically demonstrate a more dramatic result following endograft management. Specifically, the magnitude of true lumen expansion with stent grafting is greater than that observed after distal flap fenestration. Because false lumen fenestration promotes flow in the false lumen, whereas endograft placement promotes false lumen thrombosis, the latter is thought to be a superior method to minimize late aneurysm formation. Consequently, the opportunities for percutaneous balloon fenestration are decreasing now that thoracic endograft availability has improved. Fenestration is typically limited to situations when stent grafts are unavailable or when the specific aortic anatomy is unsuitable for endograft placement.

Aortic Rupture

Rupture that complicates aortic dissection is an interventional imperative.[28,29] The procedural considerations for aortic rupture focus on preventing exsanguination. Both open surgical and endovascular therapies are associated with high mortality and morbidity rates in the presence of aortic rupture. Recent reports suggest that endovascular approaches permit treatment of more patients, including older and less fit individuals whose operative risk in this setting is prohibitive.[21,28,29]

Localizing the precise site of rupture noninvasively is not always possible. The point of rupture through the false lumen wall may be evident by the presence of contrast enhancement beyond the anticipated aortic border, though this occurs typically in the setting of severe hemodynamic instability or shock (Fig. 36-9). More commonly, a periaortic, mediastinal, and/or pleural collection is evident on CT imaging, which has an appearance and attenuation value consistent with hematoma or complex fluid. This abnormality may be most prominent around a focal aortic segment or extend diffusely over a wider zone.

The goal of endograft management for aortic rupture is coverage of the proximal entry tear, with isolation of the false lumen, to ensure false lumen obliteration and expeditious thrombosis. It is thrombosis of the false lumen that prevents aortic leakage of blood. To facilitate rapid false lumen thrombosis, the overall endograft coverage of the aorta is often longer than that used for other thoracic pathologies. By extending the length of coverage (20-30 cm) to at least the level of the diaphragm or celiac trunk, the aortic septum is braced by the stent in the true lumen, and the

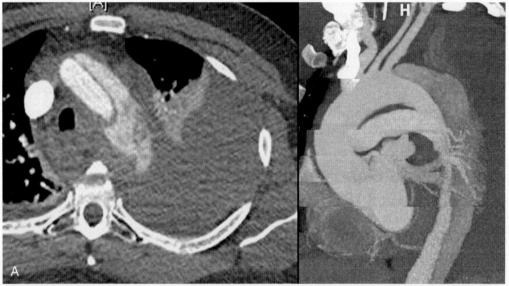

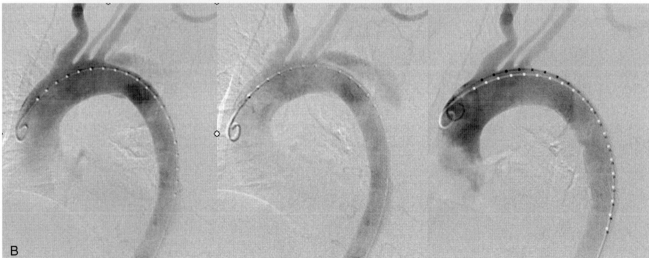

FIGURE 36-9 Endograft management of aortic dissection with rupture. A, Axial and sagittal computed tomography (CT) images of 59-year-old man with acute type B dissection with primary tear distal to left subclavian artery and retrograde extension into the proximal arch (DeBakey class IIID) complicated by rupture. Axial projection shows a large quantity of extravascular fluid, and sagittal image shows a faint wisp of contrast extravasation above aorta, just distal to subclavian artery. **B,** Three views from the stent graft procedure, with the left and middle panels before device placement, and the right panel after deployment. A good result is evident, with contrast opacification of the true lumen only.

thoracic false lumen is converted to a long, inverted cul-de-sac, or blind pouch. Then with flap pulsation limited by the buttressing stent, blood in the false lumen becomes stagnant and prone to thrombosis.[30-32]

False lumen thrombosis is critical because the precise rupture point in any individual patient is frequently unknown, and the breech may exist well below the entry tear. Simple coverage of the proximal entry may then eliminate direct flow into the false lumen, but if distal retrograde flow from abdominal sources persists, the risk of a continued leak exists and morbidity remains. Although this strategy is associated with considerable mortality and procedural complications, it represents an addition to the existing treatment armamentarium.

Other Indications for Aortic Endografts

The question of unidentified patient subgroup(s) who present with uncomplicated acute type B aortic dissection who may benefit from endograft placement remains. Some investigators have identified certain high-risk features in patients with acute uncomplicated type B dissection that may portend an increased risk of early aneurysm formation and increased mortality. These features include measurements of various aortic dimensions at the time of initial diagnosis. Initial attempts to propose high-risk criteria from CT imaging considered descriptive features associated with a poor prognosis and disease progression, such as a patent false lumen, a gaping and circumferential entry tear with resultant small true lumen, and a dominant false lumen with early fusiform expansion of the proximal descending aorta within 3 months of initial symptoms.

Marui et al. proposed that patients with uncomplicated aortic dissection and transaortic diameter greater than 40 mm were at high risk of rapid aortic expansion.[36] When applied to larger groups of patients with dissection, this benchmark provided modest prognostic value. The poor results encouraged others to focus on the issues and pursue more in-depth imaging analysis. Thereafter, Marui et al. offered an improved prognostic factor that was based on the extent of proximal descending aorta dilation at the time of initial diagnosis[37]: the *fusiform index*. This index is defined as the maximum transaortic diameter of the distal aortic arch divided by the sum of the minimum diameter of the proximal aortic arch plus the aortic diameter at the level of the pulmonary artery. A value greater than 0.64 anticipates late aortic events in patients with uncomplicated type B aortic dissection. The investigators recommended that patients with these predictors should undergo early intervention with open surgery or stent graft implantation.

Immer et al. analyzed imaging studies (CT or MRI) over the initial 18 months after diagnosis in 84 patients with acute type A aortic dissection.[38] They concluded that a large false lumen at the time of the initial diagnostic scan is the strongest predictor of subsequent downstream aortic enlargement. This was especially true if the true lumen was less than 30% of the overall transaortic area 6 months after aortic surgery for repair of type A dissection.

This concept of the initial false lumen diameter as a determinant of late clinical deterioration was evaluated for type B disease in 2007 by Song et al.[39] These authors studied 100 consecutive patients with acute aortic dissection, including 51 with type A dissection and 49 with type B dissection. Over half of the patients underwent CT imaging follow-up through 24 months. Of these, an aneurysm (diameter > 60 mm) was diagnosed in 28%, with the maximal aortic diameter located in the proximal descending segment. A greater than 22-mm initial false lumen diameter of the upper thoracic segment of the descending aorta predicted late aneurysm formation with a sensitivity of 100% and a sensitivity of 76%. The 42 patients with an initial false lumen diameter greater than 22 mm had a higher event rate than the 58 with smaller false lumen aortic diameters (aneurysm, 42% vs. 5%; or death, 12% vs. 5%).

More recently, another predictive feature for early complication and clinical deterioration was described by Tsai et al. after reviewing data from the International Registry of Aortic Dissection (IRAD).[40] They reviewed 201 cases of type B acute aortic dissection. During the index hospitalization, 114 patients (56.7%) had a patent false lumen, 68 patients (33.8%) had partial thrombosis of the false lumen, and 19 (9.5%) had complete thrombosis of the false lumen. The mean 3-year mortality rate for patients with a patent false lumen was 13.7%, for those with partial thrombosis was 31.6%, and for those with complete thrombosis was 22.6%. Although postdischarge mortality was high among patients with acute type B aortic dissection, partial thrombosis, as compared with complete patency, is a significant independent predictor of postdischarge mortality (relative risk, 2.69; 95% confidence interval [CI], 1.45-4.98; $P = 0.002$).

In the future, it is likely that more sophisticated analysis will identify additional factors beyond simple dimensional aortic measurements to better predict patients with acute type B aortic dissection who are at increased risk of disease progression, rapid deterioration, or acute rupture. As prognostic evaluation of aortic dissection improves, the use of endovascular approaches will better target and improve outcomes of this disease.

REFERENCES

1. Erbel R, Alfonso F, Boileau C, et al: Diagnosis and management of aortic dissection, *Eur Heart J* 22:1642–1681, 2001.
2. Glower DD, Speier RH, White WD, et al: Management and long-term outcome of aortic dissection, *Ann Surg* 214:21–41, 1991.
3. Wong DR, Lemaire SA, Coselli JS: Managing dissections of the thoracic aorta, *Am Surg* 74:364–380, 2008.
4. Dake MD, Kato N, Mitchell RS, et al: Endovascular stent graft placement for the treatment of acute aortic dissection, *N Engl J Med* 340:1546–1552, 1999.
5. Neinaber CA, Fattori R, Lund G, et al: Nonsurgical reconstruction of thoracic aortic dissection by stent-graft placement, *N Engl J Med* 340:1539–1545, 1999.
6. Mukherjee D, Eafle KA: Aortic dissection–an update, *Curr Probl Cardiol* 30:287–325, 2005.
7. Parker JD, Golledge J: Outcome of endovascular treatment of acute type B aortic dissection, *Ann Thorac Surg* 86:1707–1712, 2008.
8. Fattori R, Botta L, Lovato L, et al: Malperfusion syndrome in type B aortic dissection: role of the endovascular procedures, *Acta Chir Belg* 108:192–197, 2008.
9. Patel HJ, Williams DM, Meekov M, et al: Long-term results of percutaneous management of malperfusion in acute type B aortic dissection: implications for thoracic aortic endovascular repair, *J Thorac Cardiovasc Surg* 138:300–308, 2009.
10. Czermak BV, Waldenberger P, Fraedrich G, et al: Treatment of Stanford type B aortic dissection with stent grafts: preliminary results, *Radiology* 217:544–550, 2000.
11. Feezor RJ, Martin TD, Hess PJ, et al: Early outcomes after endovascular management of acute, complicated type B aortic dissection, *J Vasc Surg* 49:561–566, 2009.
12. Pearce BJ, Passman MA, Patterson MA, et al: Early outcomes of thoracic endovascular stent-graft repair for acute complicated type B dissections using the gore TAG endoprosthesis, *Ann Vasc Surg* 22:742–749, 2008.
13. Parsa CJ, Schroder JN, Daneshmand MA, et al: Midterm results for endovascular repair of complicated acute and chronic type B aortic dissection, *Ann Thorac Surg* 89:97–104, 2010.
14. Oderich GS, Panneton JM, Bower TC, et al: Aortic dissection with aortic side branch compromise: impact of malperfusion on patient outcome, *Perspect Vasc Surg Endovasc Ther* 20:190–200, 2008.
15. Apostolakis E, Baikoussis NG, Georgiopoulos M: Acute type-B aortic dissection: the treatment strategy, *Hellenic J Cardiol* 51:338–347, 2010.
16. Williams DM, Lee DY, Hamilton BH, et al: The dissected aorta: part III. Anatomy and radiological diagnosis of branch-vessel compromise, *Radiology* 203:37–44, 1997.
17. Williams DM, Lee DY, Hamilton BH, et al: The dissected aorta: percutaneous treatment of ischemic complications-principles and results, *J Vasc Interv Radiol* 8:605–625, 1997.
18. Shiiya N, Matsuzaki K, Kunihara T, et al: Management of vital organ malperfusion in acute aortic dissection: proposal of a mechanism-specific approach, *Gen Thorac Cardiovasc Surg* 55:85–90, 2007.
19. Deeb GM, Patel HJ, Williams DM: Treatment for malperfusion syndrome in acute type A and B aortic dissection: a long-term analysis, *J Thorac Cardiovasc Surg* 140:98–100, 2010.
20. Kische S, Ehrlich MP, Nienaber CA, et al: Endovascular treatment of acute and chronic aortic dissection: midterm results from the talent thoracic retrospective registry, *J Thorac Cardiovasc Surg* 138:115–124, 2009.
21. Fattori R, Tsai TT, Myrmel T, et al: Complicated acute type B dissection: is surgery still the best option?: a report from the international registry of acute aortic dissection, *JACC Cardiovasc Interv* 1:395–402, 2008.
22. Tefera G, Acher CW, Hoch JR, et al: Effectiveness of intensive medical therapy in type B aortic dissection: a single-center experience, *J Vasc Surg* 45:1114–1118, 2007.
23. Estrera AL, Miller CC, Safi HJ, et al: Outcomes of medical management of acute type B aortic dissection, *Circulation* 114:384–389, 2006.
24. Giersson A, Szeto WY, Pochettino A, et al: *Eur J Cardiothorac Surg* 32:255–262, 2007.
25. Hagan PG, Nienaber CA, Isselbacher EM, et al: The international registry of acute aortic dissection (IRAD): new insight into an old disease, *JAMA* 283:897–903, 2000.
26. Trimarchi S, Eagle KA, Neinaber CA, et al: Importance of refractory pain and hypertension in acute type B aortic dissection: insights from the international registry of acute aortic dissection (IRAD), *Circulation* 122:1283–1289, 2010.
27. Slonim SM, Miller DC, Mitchell RS, et al: Percutaneous balloon fenestration and stenting for life-threatening ischemic complications in patients with acute aortic dissections, *J Thorac Cardiovasc Surg* 117:1118–1127, 1999.

28. Xenos ES, Minion DJ, Davenport DL, et al: Endovascular versus open repair for descending thoracic aortic rupture: institutional experience and meta-analysis, *Eur J Cardiothorac Surg* 35:282–286, 2009.
29. Patel HJ, Williams DM, Upchurch GR, et al: A comparative analysis of open and endovascular repair for the ruptured descending thoracic aorta, *J Vasc Surg* 50:1265–1270, 2009.
30. Resch TA, Delle M, Falkenberg M, et al: Remodeling of the thoracic aorta after stent grafting of type B dissection: a Swedish multicenter study, *J Cardiovasc Surg (Torino)* 47:503–508, 2006.
31. Kusagawa H, Shimono T, Ishida M, et al: Changes in false lumen after transluminal stent-graft placement in aortic dissections: six years' experience, *Circulation* 111:2951–2957, 2005.
32. Sayer D, Bratby M, Brooks M, et al: Aortic morphology following endovascular repair of acute and chronic type B aortic dissection: implications for management, *Eur J Vasc Endovasc Surg* 36:522–529, 2008.
33. Tsai TT, Fattori R, Trimarchi S, et al: Long-term survival in patients presenting with type B acute aortic dissection: insights from the international registry of acute aortic dissections, *Circulation* 114:2226–2231, 2006.
34. Nienaber CA, Rousseau H, Eggebrecht H, et al: Randomized comparison of strategies for type B aortic dissection. The Investigation of Stent Grafts in Aortic Dissection (INSTEAD) trial, *Circulation* 120:2519–2528, 2009.
35. Nienaber CA, Kische S, Akin I, et al: Strategies for subacute/chronic type B aortic dissection: the Investigation of Stent Grafts in Patients with Type B Aortic Dissection (INSTEAD) trial 1-year outcome, *J Thorac Cardiovasc Surg* 140:101–108, 2010.
36. Marui A, Mochizuki T, Mitsui N, et al: Toward the best treatment for uncomplicated patients with type B acute aortic dissection: a consideration for sound surgical indication, *Circulation* 100(Suppl II):II-275–II-280, 1999.
37. Marui A, Mochizuki T, Koyama T, et al: Degree of fusiform dilation of the proximal descending aorta in type B acute aortic dissection can predict late events, *J Thorac Cardiovasc Surg* 134:1163–1170, 2007.
38. Immer F, Krahenbuhl E, Hagan U, et al: Large area of false lumen favors secondary dilation of the aorta after acute type A aortic dissection, *Circulation* 112(Suppl I):I-249–I-252, 2005.
39. Song JM, Kim JH, Kang DH, et al: Long-term predictors of descending aorta aneurismal change in patients with aortic dissection, *J Am Coll Cardiol* 50:799–804, 2007.
40. Tsai TT, Evangelista A, Nienaber CA, et al: Partial thrombosis of the false lumen in patients with acute type B aortic dissection, *N Engl J Med* 357:349–359, 2007.

CH
36

ENDOVASCULAR THERAPY FOR AORTIC DISSECTION

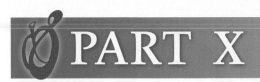

PART X

AORTIC ANEURYSM

CHAPTER 37   **Pathophysiology, Epidemiology, and Prognosis of Aortic Aneurysms**

Reena L. Pande, Joshua A. Beckman

Aortic aneurysms result in significant morbidity and mortality, accounting for nearly 13,000 deaths and 55,000 hospital discharges per year in the United States.[1] Although aneurysms may affect any part of the aorta from the aortic root down to the abdominal aorta, the prognosis and outcome in patients with aortic aneurysms vary based on location and underlying etiology. Timely and appropriate intervention may improve the natural history of the disease process. This chapter reviews the pathophysiology, epidemiology, and prognosis of aortic aneurysms.

The Normal Aorta

The aorta is the large conduit vessel through which the heart delivers blood to the entire body. It courses from the heart through the thorax and abdomen, and ultimately bifurcates into the common iliac arteries (CIAs) in the abdomen. In the thorax, the aorta can be subdivided into three segments: ascending aorta (from the base of the heart to the innominate artery), transverse aorta or aortic arch (including the great vessels and extending to the left subclavian artery), and descending aorta (from the distal edge of the subclavian artery to the level of the diaphragm) (Fig. 37-1).

Like other arterial structures, the aorta is composed of three layers: *tunica intima*, *tunica media*, and *adventitia*. The innermost surface of the tunica intima is lined by a single-cell-thick layer of endothelial cells (ECs). The intima is bound by the internal elastic lamina. The tunica media is composed of smooth muscle cells (SMCs), collagen, fibroblasts, elastin fibers, and ground substance, which together control the degree of vessel constriction and vasodilation. The presence of elastin fibers in the media defines the aorta as an elastic artery and provides the tensile strength that permits the aorta to withstand pulsatile delivery of blood from the heart. Elastin content gradually decreases with distance from the heart.[2] The outermost layer, the adventitia, is a thin layer that contains connective tissue, fibroblasts, and the nutritive vasa vasorum.

Definition of Aortic Aneurysm

In adults, the normal diameter of the aorta is approximately 3 cm at the origin, 2.5 cm in the descending thoracic aorta, and 1.8 to 2 cm in the abdominal aorta. *Aortic aneurysm* is defined as a maximal aortic dimension greater than 3.0 cm, or a 50% increase in size compared with the normal segment proximal to the aneurysm. Mild expansion that does not meet these criteria may be referred to as *aortic ectasia*. True aneurysms are classified into two major groups on the basis of morphology: (1) *fusiform* (Figs. 37-2 and 37-3), defined as a circumferential expansion of the aorta, and (2) *saccular*, representing a focal outpouching of a segment of the aorta (Fig. 37-4). Fusiform aneurysms are the most common manifestation. In contrast to true aneurysms, which involve expansion of all three layers of the aortic wall, a *pseudoaneurysm*, also known

as a *false aneurysm*, results from a disruption of the aortic wall and essentially represents a contained rupture of the aorta.

Pathophysiology of Aortic Aneurysms

A wide variety of pathological states are associated with aortic aneurysms (Box 37-1). These include degenerative diseases, inherited disorders, infections, inflammatory conditions (i.e., vasculitis), and trauma. Specific disorders associated with aortic aneurysms are discussed later in this chapter. Important determinants of aortic aneurysm formation include inflammation, proteolysis of the structural components of the aortic wall, and abnormal biomechanical forces[3] (see Fig. 37-2). Understanding the underlying pathophysiology of aneurysm formation is critical not only for prevention of initial aneurysm formation but also for limiting aneurysm growth and expansion.

Traditionally, pathological aortic aneurysm formation was ascribed to a process akin to atherogenesis. Although advances in basic and clinical investigation in both lesion types have revealed some common themes, newer studies suggest that aneurysm formation is fundamentally different from atherosclerosis. Preferential weakening of the adventitia and media—rather than an intimal proliferative process, as in atherosclerosis—results in diminished aortic resilience and tensile strength, culminating in aortic wall thinning, dilation, and increased wall stress, all of which may result in rupture. Although atherosclerotic changes may be seen in the wall of aneurysms, these changes may be a consequence of local turbulent flow as opposed to a cause of aneurysm formation.[4,5] Moreover, the degree of systemic atherosclerosis does not correlate well with the degree of aneurysm formation.[6]

Development of aneurysms is associated with loss of two critical structural elements in the aortic wall: elastin and collagen. Elastin provides radial and longitudinal support, enabling the aorta to respond to pulsatile flow while maintaining normal arterial dimensions. The importance of elastin in maintaining aortic structure is highlighted by animal models where elastase infusion results in elastin breakdown and experimental aortic aneurysm formation.[7] However, breakdown of elastin alone appears insufficient to cause aneurysmal expansion and rupture. Loss of collagen, another important structural element, is an additional contributor, and the relative balance of elastin and collagen deposition, among other factors, may be critical for determining aneurysm formation.[8] Early in aneurysm formation, the aorta compensates for loss of elastin by increasing production of collagen,[8] but as elastin content decreases, collagen (as the major source of tensile strength) is overwhelmed, and aortic expansion occurs. This is exacerbated by up-regulation of collagenases, resulting in further collagen degradation as described later.[9] Structural changes in each layer of the aortic wall develop that together promote aortic stiffness. As a consequence, decrease in the vessel's ability to distend normally with left ventricular (LV) contraction, weakening of the

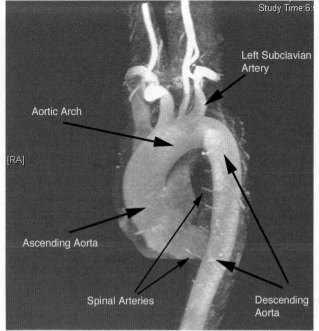

FIGURE 37-1 **Magnetic resonance angiography (MRA) of the thoracic aorta.** Note the different aortic segments: ascending aorta, aortic arch, and descending aorta. Left subclavian artery separates the aortic arch from the descending aorta.

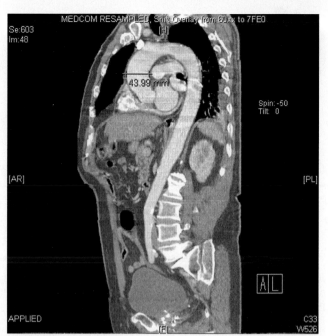

FIGURE 37-3 **Computed tomographic angiogram (CTA) of ascending aortic aneurysm.** Notice that proximal descending portion of aorta is ectatic as well. Aneurysm involves entire circumference of aorta and is thus fusiform. Normal ascending aorta size is less than 3 cm.

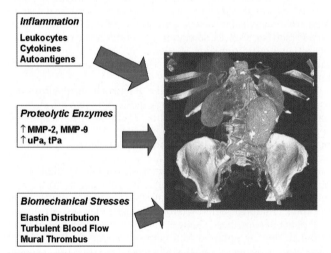

Inflammation

Leukocytes
Cytokines
Autoantigens

Proteolytic Enzymes

↑ **MMP-2, MMP-9**
↑ **uPa, tPa**

Biomechanical Stresses

Elastin Distribution
Turbulent Blood Flow
Mural Thrombus

FIGURE 37-2 **Three pathophysiological mechanisms that best characterize the process of aneurysm formation.** Aortic aneurysm specimens reveal increases in leukocyte infiltration, cytokine concentration, and leukocyte adhesion molecules. Both elastin-related and collagen-related autoantigens have been identified and may participate in initiation of process. Once process has begun, proteolytic enzymes, particularly matrix metalloproteinase (MMP)-2 and -9, increase in concentration and break down elastin and collagen. Increases in enzyme coactivators (e.g., urokinase plasminogen activator [uPA], tissue plasminogen activator [tPA]) further augment matrix breakdown. Increase in proteolysis is not accompanied by change in inhibitors of process, yielding a degenerative environment. Abdominal aorta is predisposed to aneurysm formation because of adverse blood flow patterns and its relative lack of elastin and vascular smooth muscle compared with thoracic aorta. *(Volume-rendered computed tomography image of abdominal aortic aneurysm used with permission of Joseph Schoepf, MD.)*

vessel wall, and increase in the tendency for dilation and ectasia follow.[10] Some of the changes in aortic structure that promote aneurysm formation may arise as a result of the normal aging process. With normal aging, aortic stiffness due to fragmentation of elastin fibers, deposition of glycosaminoglycans, fibronectin (FN), and collagen, and reduced bioavailability of endothelium-derived nitric oxide (NO) occurs.[11–14]

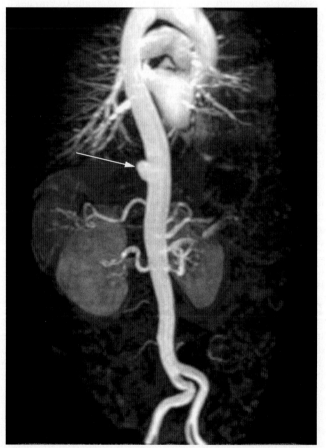

FIGURE 37-4 **Maximal intensity projection (MIP) of magnetic resonance (MR) image of saccular aneurysm.** Note outpouching of an otherwise normal descending aorta (arrow). This pattern of aneurysm is more common in infectious aneurysms.

Box 37-1 Disorders Associated with Aortic Aneurysms

Degenerative
Cystic medial necrosis
Aortic dissection

Developmental
Marfan's syndrome (MFS)
Loeys-Dietz's syndrome
Ehlers-Danlos' syndrome (EDS)
Bicuspid aortic valve (BAV)
Turner's syndrome
Aortic coarctation

Infectious
Tuberculosis
Syphilis
Staphylococcus
Salmonella

Vasculitis
Takayasu's arteritis (TA)
Giant cell arteritis (GCA)
Behçet's disease
Rheumatoid arthritis
Systemic lupus erythematosus (SLE)
Sarcoidosis
Ankylosing spondylitis
Reiter's syndrome
Relapsing polychondritis
Cogan's syndrome

Trauma

Pathophysiologically, the major determinants of aortic aneurysm formation include proteolysis of the structural components of the aortic wall, inflammation, and abnormal biomechanical forces[3] (see Fig. 37-2). Pathology of aortic aneurysms varies in different segments of the aorta and in different predisposing diseases. Frequently observed histological features include cystic medial necrosis, mucoid infiltration, and cyst formation in the setting of elastin necrosis and vascular smooth muscle apoptosis. In patients with Marfan's syndrome (MFS), bicuspid aortic valve (BAV), or Turner's syndrome, cystic medial necrosis is a common feature, but in contrast, inflammation is less prominent than in abdominal aortic aneurysms (AAAs).[15,16] On the other hand, cystic medial necrosis is less likely to be observed in AAAs. Instead, AAAs typically have disrupted elastin fibers, inflammation, greater vascular smooth muscle cell (VSMC) apoptosis, and deficient glycosaminoglycan production.[17] Elastin fragmentation occurs adjacent to the inflammatory cells. Despite differences in pathophysiology due to location and underlying etiology, formation of all aortic aneurysms involves to some degree the processes described in the following discussions (i.e., proteolytic degradation, inflammation, changes in biomechanical forces) that together facilitate aneurysm formation.

Proteolytic Degradation

Several proteolytic enzymes contribute to degradation of structural components of the arterial wall, ultimately increasing risk of aneurysm formation. Matrix metalloproteinases (MMPs) are endopeptidases that degrade one or more components of the extracellular matrix (ECM). Thus far, several classes of MMPs, comprising nearly 30 individual proteinases, have been characterized. They include collagenases, gelatinases, stromelysins, matrilysins, membrane-type (MT)-MMPs, and other MMPs.[18] Typically produced as proenzymes, MMPs may be activated both intracellularly and extracellularly, and may be secreted by endothelial cells, vascular smooth muscle cells, or adventitial fibroblasts. Extracellular regulation of activation may occur as a result of an MMP–MT-MMP interaction or via interaction with plasmin or reactive oxygen species (ROS).[19–21] The inhibitors of MMPs are the tissue inhibitors of matrix metalloproteinases (TIMPs) and plasminogen activator inhibitors (PAI) 1 and 2.[18]

Increased local production of MMPs in aortic aneurysms was first reported nearly 20 years ago.[22–24] Although elevations of several MMPs have been noted, MMP-1 (collagenase) and MMP-3 (stromelysin), MMP-2 (gelatinase A), and MMP-9 (gelatinase B) represent the principal proteinases in aortic aneurysms that result in elastin and collagen degradation.[25,26] MMP-2 and MMP-9 gelatinases specifically break down collagen. They are synthesized by local cells in the aortic wall, including infiltrating macrophages and resident aortic VSMCs.[27,28] MMP-9 is typically found in the adventitia near the vasa vasorum, localizing to infiltrating macrophages.[29] MMP-2 is synthesized constitutively by VSMCs[30] but can also be synthesized by infiltrating leukocytes.[31] Interestingly, MMP-2 production is increased in the vasculature remote from the aorta, suggesting a systemic underlying disease process that manifests with aortic aneurysmal disease.[32]

The centrality of these enzymes in aneurysm formation is supported by several lines of evidence. Studies have demonstrated that MMP-2 and MMP-9 levels are higher in tissue obtained from aortic aneurysms than in atherosclerotic plaque or normal arterial tissue.[30,31] Furthermore, MMP-9 and MMP-2 knockout mice do not form aortic aneurysms in experimental models.[33] Reinfusion of competent macrophages from wild-type mice into MMP-9 knockout mice enables aneurysm formation.[33] In addition, elevated levels of MMP-1, MMP-8 (a neutrophil collagenase), and MMP-9 have been associated with aneurysm rupture, and levels of these MMPs may vary with aneurysm size.[34–36] Relationship to aneurysm size is less clear for MMP-2.[37–40]

Elevated levels of other proteolytic enzymes such as human macrophage metalloelastase (MMP-12) and membrane type-1 metalloproteinase (MT1-MMP) have also been demonstrated in aortic aneurysms.[41] Expression of MMP-12 is increased in aortic aneurysms as a result of macrophage infiltration. However, the relevance of MMP-12 to aneurysm formation is less clear, based on the finding that MMP-12 knockout mice are not completely protected from aneurysm formation.[42] MT1-MMP, a collagenase produced by macrophages and increased in aortic aneurysms, likely has its greatest effect as an activator of the proenzyme form of MMP-2.[43,44]

In addition to increased expression of MMPs, aneurysm formation is associated with abnormal regulation of MMP levels in tissues. Matrix metalloproteinase levels are increased in states of inflammation and oxidant stress, both known to play a role in aneurysm formation. Compared with nonaneurysmal sections of aorta, superoxide anion and markers of oxidative stress are increased in aneurysmal segments, and ROS can convert proenzymes of MMPs to their active form.[45–47] In addition, MMP levels can be augmented by plasminogen activators, such as urokinase-type plasminogen activator (uPA) and tissue-type plasminogen activator (tPA), which are specific physiological regulators of MMP-2 and MMP-9 activation and overexpressed in aortic aneurysms but not in healthy aortic specimens.[48]

Matrix metalloproteinase levels are also normally regulated by TIMPs. Although early work reported decreased concentrations of TIMPs in aneurysmal tissue,[49] more recent data have been less clear, showing no difference in certain TIMP levels between aneurysmal and healthy aortic tissue.[36,43,50,51] However, the relative imbalance in MMPs to TIMPs may be the more relevant factor.[41] Nonetheless, experimental data have clearly demonstrated the significance of TIMPs to aneurysm formation. Local overexpression of TIMP-1 prevented aneurysm formation in a rat model of aortic aneurysm,[52] but TIMP knockout mice have increased MMP activity and greater aneurysm formation.[53] Similarly, lower expression of PAI-1, a regulator of plasminogen activator activity, has been reported in aneurysmal disease.[49,54] Increased expression of plasminogen activators without reciprocal changes in their inhibitors alters the balance toward fibrinolysis, MMP activation, and tissue degradation. Experimental overexpression of PAI-1 prevents aneurysm formation in a rat model of aortic aneurysm,[55] confirming the importance of relative rather than absolute concentrations.

The contribution of MMPs to the pathophysiology of aortic aneurysms is highlighted by the beneficial effect of medications known to reduce MMP levels on aneurysm expansion. For example, tetracyclines (e.g., doxycycline) have long been recognized as generalized inhibitors of metalloproteinases.[56] Their potential value in aortic aneurysmal disease has been demonstrated in both organ culture and rodent models of aneurysm formation.[36,57–59] In humans, doxycycline limits the activity of both MMP-2 and MMP-9 in aortic wall specimens, both by reducing macrophage MMP-9 messenger ribonucleic acid (mRNA) expression and diminishing activation of the proenzyme form of MMP-2.[60–62] In a few small randomized phase 2 trials, doxycycline has been shown to decrease aneurysm expansion rate.[63,64] Although these data await confirmation in larger trials, they do support the conceptual framework of the importance of proteolytic enzymes in aortic aneurysm formation and expansion.

By reducing levels of proteolytic enzymes, several other therapies may potentially be of therapeutic benefit in aneurysmal disease. HMG-CoA reductase inhibitors, or statins, have antianeurysm properties in experimental models by virtue of reducing oxidant stress and macrophage production of MMPs.[65–67] However, data in humans have been inconsistent. A meta-analysis of five studies including 697 patients with small aortic aneurysms (<55 mm) treated with or without statins suggested that statin therapy was associated with lower rates of expansion.[68] On the other hand, other human studies have not shown a benefit of preoperative statin treatment on MMP or TIMP levels in aneurysm specimens, and no difference in aneurysm expansion rate.[69–71] Indomethacin also appears to prevent aortic aneurysm formation in a rat model,[72] and the mechanism may be related to inhibition of cyclooxygenase (COX) 2, prostaglandin E_2 (PGE2), and reductions in MMP-9.[73–75] Indeed, PGE2 expression is up-regulated more than 30-fold in aortic aneurysms.[76] Prostaglandin E_2 localizes to infiltrating macrophages, and its expression is dependent on COX activity.[77] Prostaglandin E_2, through activation of interleukin (IL)-6, may increase VSMC apoptosis, further weakening the structural elements of the aorta.[75,76,78]

Inflammation

The contribution of inflammation to many pathological arterial processes has been well established.[79] In 1981, Rose and Dent[80] reported mild chronic inflammation in 72.5% and moderate inflammation in 15.7% in 51 consecutively resected AAAs. Subsequently it was discovered that lymphocytes and macrophages are found in greater quantity in the adventitia and media of AAAs than of atherosclerotic or normal aortas.[81] In addition, surgical explant specimens from patients with aortic aneurysms demonstrated higher levels of adhesion molecules, including intracellular adhesion molecule (ICAM)-1 and vascular cell adhesion molecule (VCAM)-1, than seen in atherosclerotic and normal aortas. Similarly, tissue levels of proinflammatory cytokines, such as tumor necrosis factor (TNF)-α, interleukin (IL)-1β, IL-8, monocyte chemoattractant protein (MCP)-1, interferon (IFN)-γ, and IL-6, have all been noted to be elevated in patients with aneurysms compared with control subjects.[82] Some studies have even suggested cytokine levels are higher in ruptured aortic aneurysms than in asymptomatic aortic aneurysms,[83] although the data have been inconsistent.[84] Finally, other acute-phase proteins, including C-reactive protein (CRP), D-dimer, and ceruloplasmin, are also present at increased levels in plasma and in the vessel wall.[82,85–87]

These inflammatory mediators largely derive from infiltrating macrophages, but lymphocytes and aortic ECs and SMCs also contribute to the inflammatory milieu. The presence of inflammation in aortic aneurysms is supported by positron emission tomographic imaging with[18] fluorodeoxyglucose (FDG-PET) showing greater FDG uptake in aneurysmal compared to nonaneurysmal aortic segments from matched control subjects, and by advanced magnetic resonance imaging (MRI) techniques.[88,89] Thus, immune cells

invade the aortic wall, become activated, and create an inflammatory environment that engages the activity of local stabilizing cells, initiating the process of elastin and collagen breakdown and aneurysm formation. However, the initial signals that drive inflammatory cell recruitment remain unclear. Animal studies with experimental aneurysm models have confirmed the human studies and demonstrated that increased inflammation promotes aneurysm formation.[90]

Given the contribution of inflammation to aortic aneurysms, it follows that strategies to reduce inflammation might reduce aneurysm formation or limit aneurysm growth. Indeed, as mentioned previously, some data suggest that statins, known to have beneficial antiinflammatory properties beyond their effect on cholesterol lowering, may limit aneurysm growth and expansion.[67,91,92] Recent studies have also shown that limiting inflammation can reduce aneurysm formation in animal models.[93–97] Future studies will be required to clarify whether strategies to target inflammation can prevent formation of aortic aneurysms or limit expansion in humans.

Increases in Biomechanical Wall Stress

The frequency of aneurysm formation in the abdominal aorta compared to other vascular locations suggests a predisposition in this area. Variations in biomechanical factors have been noted in the differing regions of the aorta. Relative deficiencies in structural elements combined with adverse blood flow patterns predispose the abdominal aorta to aneurysm formation. Compensatory mechanisms occur after aneurysm formation have developed, but they do not stop the process. Thus, aneurysm expansion is promoted by an imbalance of biomechanical forces and compensatory mechanisms.

Several specific structural changes may predispose the abdominal aorta to aneurysm formation. For example, elastin within the aortic wall is organized into circumferential plates, or lamellae, that respond to the pulsatile load created by the heart. Each lamellar unit consists predominantly of two elastin bundles and vascular smooth muscle. However, deposition of elastin is not uniform along the aorta, with the thoracic aorta incorporating 35 to 56 lamellar units compared to only 28 in the abdominal aorta.[98] The abdominal aorta may therefore be more susceptible to elastin breakdown due to a relative increase in pressure withstood per lamellar unit, compared with the rest of the vessel. In addition, the abdominal aorta has a decreased concentration of nutritive vasa vasorum compared to more proximal aortic segments.[99] Reductions in aortic tissue perfusion stiffen the vessel, reducing compliance and ability to withstand pulsatile stress.[100]

Vascular cells in the aorta attempt to restore elastin content in the setting of elastin degradation to compensate for reductions in tensile and radial strength. Human AAA samples show a four- to sixfold increase in tropoelastin protein compared with control arteries.[101,126] Elastin is produced by SMCs and macrophages. In areas of macrophage infiltration, elastin deposition is not organized into mature effective bundles. Indeed, compared with normal specimens, aneurysm specimens have a ninefold reduction in desmosine, a marker for mature elastin cross-linking.[101] Thus, compensatory elastin replacement is disordered and does not improve aortic compliance.

Another factor that may make the abdominal segment of the aorta more prone to aneurysm formation is blood flow patterns specific to that segment. In experimental models, the infrarenal segment of the aorta is subject to much higher levels of oscillating flow and reflected pressure waves compared with the suprarenal segment,[102] resulting in higher levels of aortic wall tension. Turbulence and pressure are exacerbated by the aneurysm's morphology, which promotes development of local vortices and turbulent flow patterns.[103] Excluding these flow patterns from the aneurysm by placing an aortic endograft rapidly reduces plasma MMP-9 levels in patients.[104,105] In a rodent elastase infusion model of aortic aneurysm, flow conditions were examined by creating a left femoral arteriovenous fistula (AVF) or left iliac artery ligation. Increases in shear stress due to fistula formation resulted in a more stable aortic phenotype with decreased oxidative stress, decreased macrophage density in the media, increased aortic ECs and vascular smooth muscle cells, and reduced apoptosis compared to the lower shear stress introduced by femoral artery ligation.[4,106,107] Improved flow decreased aortic expansion by 26%.[106]

In addition to adverse biomechanical forces creating an environment permissive for aneurysm formation, the role of intraluminal thrombus on wall stress and aneurysm expansion has recently been a focus of much study. Using finite element analysis in a three-dimensional (3D) model of the aorta derived from computed tomography (CT) scans, intraluminal thrombus was found to lower peak wall stress by up to 38%[108] relatively independent of thrombus constituents.[109] Thrombus decreases transmission of luminal pressure to the aneurysm wall and may prevent aneurysm rupture by reducing wall strain.[110-115] On the other hand, intraluminal thrombus may also contribute to further aneurysm formation,[111] given that thrombus has been demonstrated to have higher levels of proteolytic enzymes and enzyme activators than the aneurysm itself.[116] Intraluminal thrombus may act as a proteolytic enzyme reservoir through polymorphonuclear leukocytes, and enzyme accumulation provides a ready source of destructive elements for the adjacent aneurysm.[116]

Understanding biomechanical factors may help improve assessment of risk of aneurysm growth and rupture above and beyond the predictive value of lumen diameter alone.[117] Several studies have used novel computational models to incorporate biomechanical factors such as wall stress, wall strength, and extent of intraluminal thrombus for assessment of abdominal aneurysms.[112,118-123] Some studies have suggested that assessment of wall stress, wall strength, and the ratio of wall stress to wall strength may be better predictors of rupture risk than diameter.[124,125]

Epidemiology and Prognosis of Aortic Aneurysms

Abdominal Aortic Aneurysms

Aortic aneurysms are typically defined as an increase in diameter of 50% compared to the adjacent normal segment of the aorta; the upper limit of normal for the abdominal aorta is 3 cm. The absolute size definition for AAA is preferable, given that body size and baseline diameter may vary on the basis of height, sex, weight, and presence of a thoracoabdominal aortic aneurysm (TAAA). However, all these factors should be taken into consideration when considering risk in any given individual.

PREVALENCE

The prevalence of aneurysms of the abdominal aorta has been determined on the basis of several large screening studies and autopsy series (Table 37-1). In an early series of 24,000 consecutive autopsies performed over 23 years, 1.97% of the subjects were found to have an AAA.[126] Of the 473 aneurysms found, 58% were

larger than 4 cm in diameter, nearly three quarters of the patients were men, and one fourth of the aneurysms had ruptured. More recent large screening programs in targeted populations have further evaluated the prevalence of AAA. The largest screening program performed was the Aneurysm Detection and Management (ADAM) Study Screening Program, which studied 126,196 veterans 50 to 79 years of age.[127] In this cohort of predominantly male American veterans, 3.6% of subjects had an infrarenal aortic diameter greater than 3 cm, and an AAA 4 cm or larger was found in 1.2%. The Multicentre Aneurysm Screening Study (MASS) also screened 27,147 of 33,830 invited men aged 65 to 74 and reported a 4.9% prevalence of AAA 3 cm or larger.[128]

Several studies have demonstrated lower prevalence of AAA in women. The largest and most recent of these studies screened nearly 10,012 women (mean age, 69.6 years) and found an AAA prevalence rate of 0.7%, with only 4 of 74 detected aneurysms measuring larger than 5 cm.[129] These low prevalence rates were consistent with findings from earlier studies. Among 4237 subjects aged 65 to 80 who participated in a screening study among general practitioners in West Sussex, United Kingdom, 2290 women agreed to undergo abdominal ultrasonography.[130] Only 1.4% of the women had an AAA 3 cm or larger, and only 0.3% had an AAA 4 cm or larger. This dramatically lower prevalence in women has been confirmed in subsequent studies. In the Norwegian Tromso study, 2% of 2943 women aged 55 to 84 had an AAA 3 cm or larger, and 0.5% had an abdominal aneurysm 4 cm or larger.[131] Finally, among female American veterans, the prevalence of an AAA 3 cm or larger was just 1%.[132] However, an increasing number of cardiovascular risk factors does increase the risk of AAA in women, with a prevalence rate as high as 6.4% in this higher-risk group.[129]

RISK FACTORS

Three risk factors predict the vast majority of AAAs: age, gender, and cigarette smoking. Aneurysms usually affect the elderly, seldom occurring in those younger than 60 years of age, and there is a clear increase in incidence with increasing age, even when limiting the studies to older individuals.[133-135] In a Norwegian population-based study of 6386 men and women aged 25 to 84, the incidence of AAA in men increased from 0% in those aged 25 to 44, to 6% in those aged 55 to 64, and to 18.5% in those aged 75 to 84.[131] Large North American epidemiological studies have demonstrated an increase in AAA risk ranging from 58% to 300% with each additional decade of life.[136] Gender is also an important predictor of AAA formation; in all age groups, risk of AAA is two- to sixfold higher in men than women.[131,132,137-140] Cigarette smoking is the most potent modifiable risk factor and increases the risk of AAA by 60% to 850%.[141-147] In the ADAM study and the Edinburgh Artery Study, risk of an aneurysm increased threefold with any smoking history.[127,148] Risk of AAA development further increases with number of cigarettes smoked, duration of smoking, and lack of filtration, indicating a dose-response relationship.[149] In the Whitehall study of 18,403 male civil servants examined at age 40 to 64 years, aneurysm frequency increased from sixfold with manufactured cigarettes with filters to 25-fold with hand-rolled cigarettes.[150] Smoking cessation can

TABLE 37-1	Prevalence of Aortic Aneurysm in Large Epidemiological Studies				
AUTHOR	NO.	GENDER	AGE (YRS)	ANEURYSM FREQUENCY (%)	NATION
Pleumeekers[137]	5419	42% M	>55	4.1 M, 0.7 F	Netherlands
Lederle[127]	126,196	97% M	50-79	1.3	United States
Ashton[128]	27,147	M	65-74	4.9	United Kingdom
Singh[131]	2998	F	25-84	2.2	Norway
Lederle[132]	3450	F	50-79	1.0	United States
Scott[139]	9342	F	65-80	1.3	United Kingdom

F, female; M, male.

reduce the risk of aneurysm formation, with former smokers having a lower AAA risk than current smokers.[136,149,151]

Risk factors for cardiovascular disease in general (e.g., hypertension, hyperlipidemia) also increase the risk of AAA formation but are less potent risk factors than age, gender, and smoking.[127,136,152-154] In the REACH registry, there was a clear modest association of both hypertension and hyperlipidemia with AAA.[155] Earlier studies had suggested a less consistent relationship with hypertension,[138,156] but aneurysm formation seems to correlate best with diastolic blood pressure[157] or use of an antihypertensive medication.[140] Some data suggest that hypertension may be a greater risk factor for aneurysm rupture than for initial aneurysm formation.[158] The association between cholesterol and AAA is clear, although hyperlipidemia is a less potent risk factor than those mentioned previously.[135,137,159] Risk of AAA formation increased 30% per 40 mg/dL total cholesterol in the Chicago Heart Association Detection Project in Industry cohort.[138] For specific components of the lipid profile, higher levels of low-density lipoprotein (LDL) and lower levels of high-density lipoprotein (HDL) cholesterol are both associated with aneurysm formation.[133,159] Similarly, the presence of atherosclerosis increases risk of aneurysm formation,[133,134,137] although as mentioned previously, aneurysm formation is likely a process distinct from atherosclerosis. In the ADAM study of more than 100,000 subjects, hypertension, elevated cholesterol, and presence of other vascular disease increased risk of aneurysm formation by 15%, 44%, and 66%, respectively.[127] In contrast, diabetes and black race appear protective against formation of an aneurysm.[127,132,136,160] Diabetes decreases risk of aneurysm formation by 30% to 50%.[136,157]

A dramatic increase in frequency of AAA formation in relatives of patients with aortic aneurysm suggests a genetic component to the disease. Although cigarette smoking numerically accounts for the vast majority of AAAs in the population,[136] the most potent risk factor for aneurysm formation is a history of aneurysm in a first-degree relative. Norgaard et al.[161] identified an 18% incidence of aneurysms in first-degree relatives of patients with AAA. In the ADAM study, a family history doubled the risk of AAA, but was reported in only 5.1% of more than 100,000 participants.[162] Investigations specific to the impact of family history demonstrate a larger risk. Several studies have demonstrated that a family history of AAA increases the risk of AAA four- to fivefold.[157,163] Family history of AAA was also related to earlier AAA formation and rupture by nearly a decade.[164] Rate of rupture was nearly fourfold higher in patients with a family history than in sporadic AAA patients. Frydman et al.[165] screened the siblings of 400 AAA patients and found an AAA in 43% of male siblings and 16% of female siblings. More specifically, the risk of AAA formation consistently rises above 20% for men older than 50 who have a first-degree relative with AAA.[161,166-169] Using segregation analysis, Majumder et al.[170] reported that the relative risk of developing an AAA is 3.97 and 4.03 with paternal and maternal history, respectively. Risk increases to nearly 10-fold with an affected male sibling and 23-fold when a female sibling is affected.[170] Twin studies further support a genetic component to AAA formation, with one study reporting an odds ratio (OR) of 71 (95% confidence interval [CI], 27-183) for monozygotic twins and 7.6 (95% CI, 3.0-19) for dizygotic twins.[171]

Despite the wealth of data supporting a genetic component to AAA formation, no clear mode of inheritance and no single candidate gene has been identified. Early studies suggested evidence of both sex-linked and autosomal dominant patterns of inheritance. Associations have been made with blood types, haptoglobin variations, α_1-antitrypsin, and human leukocyte antigen class II (HLA-II) immune response genes.[172-174] More than 100 reports on genetic associations with AAA have appeared in the literature,[175] including genes related to cardiovascular disease, inflammation, and related signaling pathways. One study suggested an association between reduced AAA growth and five single-nucleotide polymorphisms (SNPs) in latent TGF-β binding protein (LTBP4), as well as an allelic variant of TGFB3.[176] However, another study showed no association between genetic polymorphisms in the main receptors for TGF-β and AAA formation.[177] Two genome-wide association studies (GWAS) have suggested an association between AAA and a SNP located on chromosome 3p12.3 in a region near the gene CNTN3 for contactin-3, a lipid-anchored cell adhesion molecule.[178] Another GWAS in a population from Iceland and the Netherlands found a SNP on 9q33 associated with AAA with an OR of 1.21. The same SNP has been associated with coronary artery disease (CAD), peripheral artery disease (PAD), and pulmonary embolism (PE).[179] The SNP resides in the gene coding for DAB2IP, a gene encoding a cell growth and survival inhibitor. In addition, the same gene variant associated with myocardial infarction (MI) at locus 9p21 has been associated with AAA.[180,181] Finally, of interest but of unclear significance is the association between telomere length and AAA in a small cohort in the United Kingdom.[182] This may represent the association of aging, telomere length, and aneurysm formation, but the direct pathophysiological link remains unclear.

PROGNOSIS

The natural history of AAA is one of silent coexistence and sudden lethal rupture. In a large autopsy study performed over a quarter of a century, one fourth of abdominal aneurysms were ruptured on postmortem examination.[126] The frequency of rupture was dependent largely on size in this study population, ranging from 9.5% in aneurysms smaller than 4 cm to 45.6% in aneurysms 7.1 to 10 cm in diameter. In a comparison of patients with aortic aneurysms divided into two groups at a cutoff point of 6 cm, survival was markedly decreased in the patients with larger aneurysms.[183] In a single-center study that included 60 AAA ruptures over a 30-year period, only 2 occurred in patients with an aneurysm diameter smaller than 5 cm.[184] Similarly, in a study in Rochester, Minnesota, no ruptures occurred in aneurysms smaller than 5 cm, whereas rupture occurred in 25% of AAAs larger than 5 cm.[185] In 198 patients with aneurysms 5.5 cm in diameter or larger, but who were deemed too risky for surgery, 23% had presumed rupture over a mean follow-up of 1.6 years.[186] Mortality rates as high as 64% are observed in patients who present with a ruptured aortic aneurysm.[187]

On the basis of these data, two large trials have been conducted to determine whether early recognition and treatment can alter the natural history of AAA. The U.K. Small Aneurysm Trial randomized 1090 patients aged 60 to 76 years with asymptomatic AAAs 4 to 5.5 cm in diameter to undergo early elective open surgery or ultrasonographic surveillance.[188] In the surveillance group, surgery was performed when the aneurysm reached 5.5 cm. Early surgery did not affect overall mortality. At 3 years, nearly 20% of both groups had died, although abdominal aneurysms accounted for only a quarter of the deaths in both groups. Cardiovascular mortality unrelated to the aneurysm accounted for 40% of total mortality, and cancer caused slightly more than 20% of the deaths. In a similar study performed by the U.S. Veterans Administration, 1136 subjects aged 50 to 79 years with asymptomatic AAA 4 to 5.5 cm in diameter were randomized to undergo either early elective open surgery or ultrasonographic surveillance[153] (Fig. 37-5). After 5 years, there was no significant difference in survival between the groups, each with a near 25% mortality rate. In this study, aneurysm-related deaths accounted for only 3% of total mortality. More recently, the PIVOTAL study demonstrated no difference between surveillance and early endovascular repair in patients with small aneurysms (measuring 4-5 cm), and no difference in aneurysm-related death in the two groups after 3 years of follow-up.[189] Together, these data suggest that early repair of small aneurysms does not alter outcomes.

Several factors can predict the likelihood of expansion and rupture of AAAs and can help identify which patients require intervention. The factor most predictive of rupture is initial size of the aneurysm. In one study of patients too ill for surgery, aneurysm rupture rates ranged from 9.4% for AAA of 5.5 to 5.9 cm to 32.5% for AAA of 7 cm or more.[186] In the U.K. Small Aneurysm Study, rate

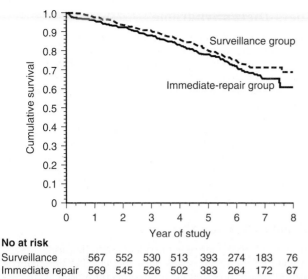

No at risk

Surveillance	567	552	530	513	393	274	183	76
Immediate repair	569	545	526	502	383	264	172	67

FIGURE 37-5 Survival curves in early surgery group compared with ultrasound surveillance group in Aneurysm Detection and Management (ADAM) Veterans Affairs Cooperative Study. No significant difference in mortality was found between the two groups. *(From Lederle FA, Wilson SE, Johnson GR, et al: Immediate repair compared with surveillance of small abdominal aortic aneurysms. N Engl J Med 346:1437, 2002.)*[153]

of rupture was 0.9% in aneurysms 3 to 3.9 cm, 2.7% in aneurysms 4 to 5.5 cm, and 27.8% in aneurysms 5.6 cm and larger.[158] Larger aneurysm size also predicted a more rapid increase in diameter.[190] Similar to factors that predispose to initial development of AAA, cigarette smoking and higher blood pressure increase the risks of rapid expansion and rupture. In contrast to the decreased risk of AAA development in women, being female actually increases risk of rupture and death after rupture in those with established AAA.[158,191,192] In the U.K. Small Aneurysm Study, women had a threefold higher risk of AAA rupture than men.[158] As mentioned previously, some have advocated use of biomechanical factors (wall stress, wall strength) to help with risk prediction. Prospective studies will be required to determine whether these factors can improve assessment of patients at high risk for aneurysm rupture and can improve selection of patients for aneurysm repair.

Thoracic and Thoracoabdominal Aortic Aneurysms

PREVALENCE

The most common location of involvement of thoracic aortic aneurysms (TAAs) is the ascending aorta and/or aortic root (noted in 60%), with the descending aorta affected in approximately 40% of cases and the aortic arch in 10%.[193] Thoracoabdominal aortic aneurysms are defined by contiguous involvement of the descending thoracic aorta and abdominal aorta and account for 5% to 10% of all aortic aneurysms.[193,194] The prevalence of isolated TAA is poorly defined but estimated at 6 persons per 100,000 per year.[195] In autopsy records reported from 63% of 70,368 deaths between 1958 and 1985 in the city of Malmo, Sweden, TAAs were diagnosed in 205 of the deceased, 53% of whom were men.[196] Of the 44,332 autopsies performed, 63 individuals (0.14%) had died of a ruptured TAA. The relative infrequency of TAA is confirmed by a retrospective analysis in Rochester, Minnesota.[197] Over 30 years, of approximately 45,000 residents, 72 (0.16%) were diagnosed with a TAA; 61% were women, and 67 patients had thoracic aortic involvement only. Most studies, however, suggest that men are twice as likely to develop a TAA as women.[197,198] Thoracoabdominal aortic aneurysms occur even more infrequently. Of the 44,332 people to undergo necropsy in Malmo, Sweden, a mere 10 had TAAA.[196]

In the Rochester, Minnesota, experience the incidence was 0.37 per 100,000 person-years of follow-up.[197] Because of the relatively small sample sizes reported in the literature, risk factors for TAAA development are less well defined. Risk factors currently associated with development of TAAA include smoking, hypertension, and atherosclerotic vascular disease.[193]

ETIOLOGY AND PATHOPHYSIOLOGY

Aneurysms involving the thoracic aorta commonly develop as a result of cystic medial necrosis, a degenerative process that histologically involves degeneration of elastic fibers and SMCs. Cystic medial degeneration can arise as an isolated abnormality or as a result of an underlying connective tissue disease, such as MFS or Ehlers-Danlos' syndrome (EDS). Degeneration of the media within the arterial wall results in impaired structural integrity of the aorta, leading to eventual aortic dilation, aneurysm formation, and risk of rupture.

As with AAA, age is a significant risk factor for development of TAA; median age for presentation varies from 64 to 69 years.[193] Cystic medial necrosis develops to some degree as a natural consequence of aging and may be accelerated by comorbid conditions such as hypertension.[199] Although a degenerative aneurysmal process is found in the majority of patients with TAAA, several other etiologies should be considered, including inherited collagen vascular disorders (e.g., MFS), BAV disease, aortic dissection, infection, and vasculitis (e.g., giant cell or Takayasu's arteritis). Rarer causes of TAA include coarctation of the aorta and trauma. Finally, some aneurysms develop because of a familial predisposition termed *familial thoracic aortic syndrome*.

NATURAL HISTORY AND PROGNOSIS

The natural history and prognosis for TAAs and TAAAs remain poor but not completely defined, in part because modern imaging techniques now allow for early detection and intervention of aneurysm before rupture, and because the natural history is dependent in large part on underlying etiology. However, in a study accumulated over 25 years that followed 94 patients with TAAAs who did not undergo operative repair, 76% died within 2 years of follow-up, with half of the deaths resulting from aneurysm rupture.[200] A more recent experience with 57 TAAA patients managed without operation revealed a 69% 2-year survival, with aneurysm rupture as the cause of death in 19%.[201] Features associated with aneurysm expansion and rupture include smoking, chronic obstructive pulmonary disease (COPD), and renal insufficiency.[202] Dissection as an underlying cause of aneurysm formation is also associated with a greater risk of rupture compared with degenerative causes.[203] Extension of a TAA into the abdomen is associated with a 50% relative increase in risk of rupture, compared with those limited to the thoracic aorta alone.[204]

The natural history of TAA depends in large part on rate of expansion. Initial aneurysm size at the time of diagnosis is the most important predictor of thoracic aneurysm growth.[193] Longitudinal data have suggested that the mean rate of growth of thoracic aneurysms averages 0.1 cm/yr.[205] Several factors also contribute to the rate of growth. Growth rate is increased in the setting of an aortic dissection. In one study, presence of a chronic aortic dissection was associated with a 0.37 cm/yr rate of growth.[205] Descending TAAs tend to increase in size more rapidly than ascending TAAs.[205,206] Those who smoke have a twofold increased rate of growth over nonsmokers.[207]

Survival rates for TAA range from 39% to 87% at 1 year and from 13% to 46% at 5 years.[201,207,208] In a study of 67 patients with TAA (mean age, 65 years), those with an aortic diameter less than 5 cm had a 90% 3-year survival rate, compared to 60% for patients with a TAA larger than 5 cm.[207] Similarly, in two other studies, patients with TAAs 6 cm or larger had a higher mortality rate than those with smaller aneurysms.[206] Based on these data, referral for surgery is recommended when the aneurysm reaches 5.5 cm or greater in the ascending aorta.[209]

However, several factors increase risk of aneurysm rupture and may prompt earlier referral for intervention. Guidelines recommend that patients with MFS or other genetic disorders (e.g., vascular Ehlers-Danlos', Loeys-Dietz's, and Turner's syndromes, BAV disease, or familial aortic aneurysm) may require intervention at smaller diameters, such as 4.0 cm to 5.0 cm, depending on clinical circumstances.[206,209-214] In addition, those with a more rapid rate of growth than expected (i.e., ≥0.5 cm/yr) may be at increased risk of rupture and require repair at diameters less than 5.5 cm.[209] Finally, repair should be considered in patients with ascending aortic diameter greater than 4.5 cm if undergoing aortic valve surgery.[209]

For aneurysms involving the aortic arch, surgery should be considered when the diameter reaches 5.5 cm or greater.[209] For degenerative descending TAAs, repair is recommended when the diameter exceeds 5.5 cm, although in individuals with TAAAs or those with high surgical risk, elective surgery is recommended when the diameter exceeds 6.0 cm.[209] Other factors reported to significantly increase rate of rupture or need for surgery include older age, history of COPD, pain possibly related to the aneurysm, higher blood pressure, and extension of the aneurysm into the abdomen.[202,204]

Inherited and Developmental Disorders

Marfan's Syndrome

Marfan's syndrome is an autosomal dominant inherited disorder of connective tissue arising from mutations in *FBN1*, a gene on chromosome 15 encoding the ECM protein fibrillin-1 (FBN1). Abnormalities in fibrillin synthesis may affect multiple tissues in patients with Marfan syndrome, including the cardiovascular, skeletal, and ocular systems. Excessive signaling through the TGF-β cascade has been suggested as a contributing factor. This is supported by experiments showing that TGF-β-neutralizing antibodies reverse aortic disease in a mouse model of Marfan syndrome, and by the demonstration that losartan, an angiotensin receptor blocker (ARB) with anti-TGF-β properties, can partially reverse aortic wall defects in these mice.[215] Clinical manifestations of MFS include ectopia lentis, hyperelasticity and ligamentous redundancy, valvular heart disease, and abnormalities in skin, fascia, skeletal muscle, and adipose tissue.

However, potentially the most lethal complication in MFS is disease of the ascending aorta resulting in aneurysm, dissection, and rupture. Dilation of the aortic root has been demonstrated early in childhood in patients with Marfan syndrome. Histologically, changes in the media seen in patients with MFS include cystic medial necrosis with fragmentation and disarray of elastic fibers, a paucity of smooth muscle cells, and separation of muscle fibers by collagen and glycosaminoglycans.[216]

Ehlers-Danlos' Syndrome

Ehlers-Danlos' syndrome type 4 (vascular type) is a rare congenital defect in the synthesis of type 3 collagen resulting from a mutation in the COL3A1 gene.[217] Patients with EDS typically present with acrogeria (distinctive facial appearance), bruising, thin skin, and vascular or visceral rupture. Histological examination reveals a thinned, fragmented internal elastic lamina.[218] Moreover, deposition of glycosaminoglycans in the media of major arteries and intima of smaller arteries, with intimal thickening, has been noted.[219] Abnormalities in type 3 collagen fiber formation reduce stability or prevent formation of collagen, decreasing vascular wall stability.[218] In a study of 199 patients with confirmed Ehlers-Danlos syndrome, 25% of patients suffered a ruptured vessel or viscus by age 20 and 80% by age 40.[220] Mean survival was 48 years. There were 131 deaths, 103 of which were due to vascular rupture. Complications of pregnancy caused the death of 15% of the women who became pregnant.

Loeys-Dietz's Syndrome

Loeys-Dietz's syndrome is an autosomal dominant condition arising from mutations in either the type I or type II receptor for TGF-β (TGFBR1 or TGFBR2). Individuals with Loeys-Dietz's syndrome have several characteristic features, including abnormal uvula, hypertelorism (increased space between the eyes), and arterial aneurysms, among other abnormalities, some of which are similar to Marfan syndrome.[214] The syndrome is characterized by particularly aggressive arterial disease manifested as aortic aneurysm with high risk of aortic dissection and rupture. As such, the average age of death of 26 years. Because of the high morbidity and mortality and the high rate of aortic dissection, even with aneurysms of less than 5.0 cm in size, early repair at smaller diameters is recommended.[209,214]

Bicuspid Aortic Valve

Presence of a BAV increases the risk of ascending aortic aneurysm formation.[193] Although it was once thought that the aneurysmal dilation was a "post-stenotic" phenomenon arising secondary to abnormal flow through a diseased aortic valve, more recent data support the notion that aortic expansion occurs independently of valvular dysfunction, severity, age, and body size.[221] Further evidence that aortic dilation is not dependent on valve dysfunction is found in a study of 118 consecutive patients with BAV in whom the diameter of the ascending aorta was not correlated with severity of aortic stenosis.[222] Moreover, abnormalities in the aortic wall can arise even when there is no hemodynamically significant aortic valve disease, and replacement of a diseased valve does not change the rate of aortic expansion.[223]

In one study comparing aorta and pulmonary artery specimens in patients with BAV and tricuspid aortic valve disease, those with BAV had decreased FBN1 concentrations in both the aortic and pulmonary specimens, suggesting a systemic disorder.[224] Vascular smooth muscle cells from patients with BAV show intracellular accumulation and reduction of extracellular distribution of several structural elements including fibrillin, fibronectin, and tenascin.[16] Surgical specimens demonstrate greater amounts of inflammation and increased expression of MMP-2 and MMP-9 in patients with BAV compared to those with tricuspid aortic valve disease.[225,226] Patients with Turner's syndrome, who are at increased risk of developing BAV, also exhibit an increased rate of aneurysm formation.[227]

Aortic Coarctation

Coarctation of the aorta represents 5% of congenital heart disease. The clinical consequences of aortic coarctation are varied, ranging from being life-threatening in infancy to remaining unappreciated until adulthood.[228] Coarctation has long been recognized as associated with *de novo* aortic aneurysm development, and aneurysms can also develop at the site of coarctation repair—specifically patch angioplasty repair—in up to 20% of patients.[229,230] Some reports indicate aneurysm formation can even occur several decades after initial repair. Intermediate follow-up studies suggest that percutaneous balloon angioplasty repair results in a 2% to 5% rate of repair-site aortic aneurysm formation.[231,232] A potential explanation for the relationship between coarctation and aortic aneurysm is the common link with the presence of BAV in approximately 15% of patients with aortic coarctation.[212]

Other Conditions Associated with Aortic Aneurysm

Although most aortic aneurysms occur as a result of degenerative processes in the aortic wall as described earlier, certain disease states including vasculitis, infection, and inherited abnormalities of structural proteins predispose patients to aortic aneurysm formation (see Box 37-1).

Vasculitides

GIANT CELL ARTERITIS

Giant cell (temporal) arteritis (GCA; see Chapter 43) is a medium-vessel chronic inflammatory vasculitis that affects the aorta and its branch vessels. It most commonly occurs in patients older than 55 years of age and is twice as common in women as men.[233] Between 1% and 20% of GCA patients develop aneurysms, most commonly in the thoracic aorta.[234] In a series of 41 patients with GCA-related TAAs, 16 developed aortic dissection, 15 had valvular annular expansion causing symptomatic aortic valve insufficiency, and 18 required surgery.[235] In a series of 168 patients with GCA, 18% developed aortic aneurysm or dissection, and these occurrences were inversely associated with development of intracranial disease manifestations.[234] Presence of an aortic aneurysm itself was not associated with increased mortality; however, the nine individuals who developed aortic dissection had significantly increased mortality.[236] The mechanism of aneurysm formation seems to be similar to patients without GCA, with increases in MMP-2- and MMP-9-associated destruction of the vessel wall.[237,238]

TAKAYASU'S ARTERITIS

Named for a Japanese professor of ophthalmology, Takayasu's arteritis (TA; see Chapter 42) is a large-vessel vasculitis that typically has its onset between the age of 10 and 30 years. The most common vascular presentation is occlusive disease, found in 80% to 94% of patients; however, aortic aneurysms may be found in up to one fourth of patients with TA.[239,240] Development of aneurysmal disease has been associated with worse outcome in a series of 120 Japanese patients followed for 13 years.[241] Blood levels of MMP-2 and MMP-9 are elevated in TA, but the mechanism of aneurysm formation remains unknown.[242]

BEHÇET'S DISEASE

Behçet's disease (see Chapter 41) is a small-vessel vasculitis originally characterized by a set of three symptoms: aphthous stomatitis, genital ulcers, and uveitis.[243] Involvement of medium-sized and large arteries, as well as veins, arises not from direct vascular inflammation but rather due to vasculitis of the small arteries of the vasa vasorum that supply the vessel wall.[244] Vascular involvement, including aneurysms, can be found in 7% to 38% of patients.[243,245] Management of aneurysmal disease in Behçet's disease depends in large part on the location of the abnormality and clinical circumstances. First-line therapy includes an antiinflammatory regimen with corticosteroids. As with other vasculitides, risk of intervention is greatest during the state of active inflammation, and there is an increased risk of rupture, dissection, and/or future aneurysmal dilation at the site of revascularization.

SERONEGATIVE SPONDYLOARTHROPATHIES

The spondyloarthropathies (see Chapter 41) are characterized by inflammation of the spine and sacroiliac joints, association with HLA-B27, and absence of rheumatoid factor (RF). These disorders are known to be associated with an increased risk of aortic aneurysm formation. Specific spondyloarthropathies include ankylosing spondylitis, Reiter's syndrome, and relapsing polychondritis.

Ankylosing spondylitis is an HLA-B27 disease that requires the presence of four of the five following features: onset younger than 40 years of age, back pain for more than 3 months, insidious onset of symptoms, morning stiffness, and improvement with exercise. Aortic root and valve disease is present in up to 80% of patients.[242] In a series of 44 outpatients, aortic root disease and valve disease were found in 82%; thickening of the aortic valve was noted in 41% of patients, and aortic dilation in 25%.[246] Aortic valve thickening manifested as nodularities of the aortic cusps, forming a characteristic subaortic bump.[242] Valve regurgitation was seen in almost half of patients, and 40% had moderate lesions.

Reiter's syndrome is a reactive arthritis that affects the lower limbs, causing an asymmetrical oligoarthritis. To make the diagnosis, patients must have evidence of a preceding infection, diarrhea, or urethritis 4 weeks preceding the syndrome.[247] Less than 1% of Reiter's syndrome patients develop cardiovascular complications. Among this group, aortic insufficiency is a late finding.

Relapsing polychondritis is a paroxysmal and progressive inflammatory disease of the cartilaginous structures, affecting the ear, nose, and hyaline cartilage of the tracheobronchial tree. Cardiovascular disease, including aortic aneurysms, is found in 25% to 50% of patients.[248]

Infectious Aortic Aneurysms

MYCOTIC ANEURYSMS

Also known as *infective endarteritis* (see Chapter 59), mycotic aneurysms are rare phenomena. Two large necropsy studies including 22,000 and 20,000 patients, respectively, revealed a combined incidence of 0.03% in the United States.[249,250] The average age of patients with mycotic aneurysms is 65, and men are threefold more likely to develop mycotic aneurysms than women.[251,252] Hematogenous seeding, such as occurs in patients with endocarditis, affects a vessel that may be "at risk" because of preexisting atherosclerosis or previous damage and represents the most common cause of mycotic aneurysms.[253] Indeed, as many as 15% of patients with endocarditis developed mycotic aneurysm before the antibiotic era.[254] Other etiologies include septic microemboli, contiguous extension, and trauma with direct contamination. In contrast to the typical degenerative or vasculitic fusiform expansion, mycotic aneurysms are more likely to be saccular (see Fig. 37-4). The outpouching may range in size from 1 mm to 10 cm and include components of acute and chronic inflammation, hemorrhage, abscess formation, and necrosis.

Clinical manifestations of mycotic aneurysm most commonly include pain and fever and, if related to a new aneurysm, should prompt directed investigation. The organisms that most commonly cause mycotic aneurysms include *Staphylococcus* and *Salmonella* species, which cause 40% and 20% of mycotic aneurysms, respectively.[255,256] Surgery should be prompt, since rupture occurs in up to 80%.[257,258] Prognosis for cerebral vascular infection is dire, with 1-year mortality for patients who have cerebrovascular mycotic aneurysms reaching as high as 90%.[258]

TUBERCULOUS ANEURYSMS

Aortic aneurysm due to tuberculosis is quite rare. In a series of more than 22,000 autopsies performed at one urban medical center in the first half of the 20th century, only 1 of 308 aortic aneurysms had tuberculous aneurysms,[249] whereas there were no tuberculous aneurysms among 20,000 autopsies performed in a rural setting.[250] Three mechanisms have been postulated to facilitate tuberculous adhesion and endarteritis. It is thought that direct extension from a contiguous source, such as the spine or lung, may cause 75% of tuberculous aneurysms.[259] Other possibilities include adhesion to a vessel damaged by atherosclerosis or infiltration of the inner layers of the aorta via the vasa vasorum.[259] The abdominal and thoracic portions of the aorta are affected similarly. The presentation of the patient with a tuberculous aneurysm varies significantly. The patient may be asymptomatic, have a palpable or radiologically visible paraaortic mass, complain of chest or abdominal pain, or present with aortic rupture and hypovolemic shock. Tuberculous aneurysms that are symptomatic or rapidly expanding and pseudoaneurysms typically require surgical repair.

SYPHILITIC ANEURYSMS

Although syphilis may once have been a common cause of aortic disease, antibiotics have greatly diminished the incidence of syphilitic aortic aneurysm (luetic aneurysm), such that fewer than 50 cases have been reported in the antibiotic era.[260] Central nervous system (CNS) and cardiovascular complications denote the tertiary stage of syphilis. Classically, this arises after a latent phase of roughly 10 to 30 years from initial spirochete infection. Syphilitic aortitis may occur in up to 10% of patients with tertiary syphilis (Fig. 37-6). Destruction of the elastic lamina occurs as a consequence of lymphoplasmacytic infiltrate around the vasa vasorum, owing to direct spirochete infection of the aortic media. This ultimately leads to expansion but also fibrosis and calcification, producing the classic "tree bark" radiographic pattern. Luetic aortic aneurysms commonly involve the ascending aorta and are saccular. Involvement of the coronary ostia may result in coronary stenosis and resultant anginal symptoms. Survival with syphilitic aortic aneurysm is worse than the general population.

Trauma

Aneurysms related to trauma are discussed in Chapter 61.

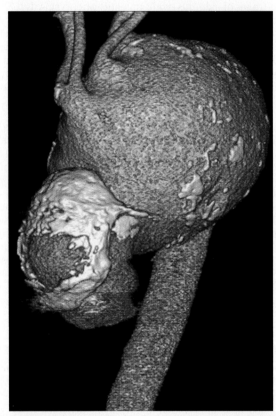

FIGURE 37-6 **Volume-rendered (VR) maximum intensity projections (MIPs) from computed tomographic angiography (CTA) of chest of patient with tertiary syphilis, showing extensively calcified thoracic aortic aneurysm (TAA) measuring 11.5 cm × 11.4 cm in short axis and 18 cm in length.** *(From Tomey MI, Murthy VL, Beckman JA: Giant syphilitic aortic aneurysm: a case report and review of the literature. Vasc Med 16:360–364, 2011.)*

REFERENCES

1. Roger VL, Go AS, Lloyd-Jones DM, et al: Heart disease and stroke statistics–2011 update: a report from the American Heart Association, *Circulation* 123(4):e18–e209, 2011.
2. Wolinsky H, Glagov S: A lamellar unit of aortic medial structure and function in mammals, *Circ Res* 20(1):99–111, 1967.
3. Wassef M, Baxter BT, Chisholm RL, et al: Pathogenesis of abdominal aortic aneurysms: a multidisciplinary research program supported by the National Heart, Lung, and Blood Institute, *J Vasc Surg* 34(4):730–738, 2001.
4. Hoshina K, Sho E, Sho M, et al: Wall shear stress and strain modulate experimental aneurysm cellularity, *J Vasc Surg* 37(5):1067–1074, 2003.
5. Golledge J, Norman PE: Atherosclerosis and abdominal aortic aneurysm: cause, response, or common risk factors? *Arterioscler Thromb Vasc Biol* 30(6):1075–1077, 2010.
6. Johnsen SH, Forsdahl SH, Singh K, et al: Atherosclerosis in abdominal aortic aneurysms: a causal event or a process running in parallel? The Tromso study, *Arterioscler Thromb Vasc Biol* 30(6):1263–1268, 2010.
7. Halpern VJ, Nackman GB, Gandhi RH, et al: The elastase infusion model of experimental aortic aneurysms: synchrony of induction of endogenous proteinases with matrix destruction and inflammatory cell response, *J Vasc Surg* 20(1):51–60, 1994.
8. Baxter BT, Davis VA, Minion DJ, et al: Abdominal aortic aneurysms are associated with altered matrix proteins of the nonaneurysmal aortic segments, *J Vasc Surg* 19(5):797–802, 1994 discussion 803.
9. Dobrin PB, Mrkvicka R: Failure of elastin or collagen as possible critical connective tissue alterations underlying aneurysmal dilatation, *Cardiovasc Surg* 2(4):484–488, 1994.
10. Groenink M, Langerak SE, Vanbavel E, et al: The influence of aging and aortic stiffness on permanent dilation and breaking stress of the thoracic descending aorta, *Cardiovasc Res* 43(2):471–480, 1999.
11. Movat HZ, More RH, Haust MD: The diffuse intimal thickening of the human aorta with aging, *Am J Pathol* 34(6):1023–1031, 1958.
12. Kawasaki T, Sasayama S, Yagi S, et al: Non-invasive assessment of the age related changes in stiffness of major branches of the human arteries, *Cardiovasc Res* 21(9):678–687, 1987.
13. Breithaupt-Grogler K, Belz GG: Epidemiology of the arterial stiffness, *Pathol Biol (Paris)* 47(6):604–613, 1999.
14. Lakatta EG: Arterial and cardiac aging: major shareholders in cardiovascular disease enterprises: part III: cellular and molecular clues to heart and arterial aging, *Circulation* 107(3):490–497, 2003.
15. Lin AE, Lippe BM, Geffner ME, et al: Aortic dilation, dissection, and rupture in patients with Turner syndrome, *J Pediatr* 109(5):820–826, 1986.
16. Nataatmadja M, West M, West J, et al: Abnormal extracellular matrix protein transport associated with increased apoptosis of vascular smooth muscle cells in Marfan syndrome and bicuspid aortic valve thoracic aortic aneurysm, *Circulation* 108(Suppl 1):II329–II334, 2003.
17. Zhang J, Schmidt J, Ryschich E, et al: Increased apoptosis and decreased density of medial smooth muscle cells in human abdominal aortic aneurysms, *Chin Med J (Engl)* 116(10):1549–1552, 2003.
18. Visse R, Nagase H: Matrix metalloproteinases and tissue inhibitors of metalloproteinases: structure, function, and biochemistry, *Circ Res* 92(8):827–839, 2003.
19. Louwrens HD, Kwaan HC, Pearce WH, et al: Plasminogen activator and plasminogen activator inhibitor expression by normal and aneurysmal human aortic smooth muscle cells in culture, *Eur J Vasc Endovasc Surg* 10(3):289–293, 1995.
20. Allaire E, Hasenstab D, Kenagy RD, et al: Prevention of aneurysm development and rupture by local overexpression of plasminogen activator inhibitor-1, *Circulation* 98(3):249–255, 1998.
21. Reilly JM, Sicard GA, Lucore CL: Abnormal expression of plasminogen activators in aortic aneurysmal and occlusive disease, *J Vasc Surg* 19(5):865–872, 1994.
22. Vine N, Powell JT: Metalloproteinases in degenerative aortic disease, *Clin Sci (Lond)* 81(2):233–239, 1991.
23. Brophy CM, Marks WH, Reilly JM, et al: Decreased tissue inhibitor of metalloproteinases (TIMP) in abdominal aortic aneurysm tissue: a preliminary report, *J Surg Res* 50(6):653–657, 1991.
24. Herron GS, Unemori E, Wong M, et al: Connective tissue proteinases and inhibitors in abdominal aortic aneurysms. Involvement of the vasa vasorum in the pathogenesis of aortic aneurysms, *Arterioscler Thromb* 11(6):1667–1677, 1991.
25. Newman KM, Malon AM, Shin RD, et al: Matrix metalloproteinases in abdominal aortic aneurysm: characterization, purification, and their possible sources, *Connect Tissue Res* 30(4):265–276, 1994.
26. Newman KM, Ogata Y, Malon AM, et al: Identification of matrix metalloproteinases 3 (stromelysin-1) and 9 (gelatinase B) in abdominal aortic aneurysm, *Arterioscler Thromb* 14(8):1315–1320, 1994.
27. Newman KM, Jean-Claude J, Li H, et al: Cellular localization of matrix metalloproteinases in the abdominal aortic aneurysm wall, *J Vasc Surg* 20(5):814–820, 1994.
28. Patel MI, Melrose J, Ghosh P, et al: Increased synthesis of matrix metalloproteinases by aortic smooth muscle cells is implicated in the etiopathogenesis of abdominal aortic aneurysms, *J Vasc Surg* 24(1):82–92, 1996.
29. Thompson RW, Holmes DR, Mertens RA, et al: Production and localization of 92-kilodalton gelatinase in abdominal aortic aneurysms. An elastolytic metalloproteinase expressed by aneurysm-infiltrating macrophages, *J Clin Invest* 96(1):318–326, 1995.
30. Davis V, Persidskaia R, Baca-Regen L, et al: Matrix metalloproteinase-2 production and its binding to the matrix are increased in abdominal aortic aneurysms, *Arterioscler Thromb Vasc Biol* 18(10):1625–1633, 1998.
31. McMillan WD, Patterson BK, Keen RR, et al: *In situ* localization and quantification of seventy-two-kilodalton type IV collagenase in aneurysmal, occlusive, and normal aorta, *J Vasc Surg* 22(3):295–305, 1995.
32. Goodall S, Crowther M, Hemingway DM, et al: Ubiquitous elevation of matrix metalloproteinase-2 expression in the vasculature of patients with abdominal aneurysms, *Circulation* 104(3):304–309, 2001.
33. Longo GM, Xiong W, Greiner TC, et al: Matrix metalloproteinases 2 and 9 work in concert to produce aortic aneurysms, *J Clin Invest* 110(5):625–632, 2002.
34. Wilson WR, Anderton M, Choke EC, et al: Elevated plasma MMP1 and MMP9 are associated with abdominal aortic aneurysm rupture, *Eur J Vasc Endovasc Surg* 35(5):580–584, 2008.
35. Wilson WR, Anderton M, Schwalbe EC, et al: Matrix metalloproteinase-8 and -9 are increased at the site of abdominal aortic aneurysm rupture, *Circulation* 113(3):438–445, 2006.
36. Petersen E, Wagberg F, Angquist KA: Proteolysis of the abdominal aortic aneurysm wall and the association with rupture, *Eur J Vasc Endovasc Surg* 23(2):153–157, 2002.
37. Nishimura K, Ikebuchi M, Kanaoka Y, et al: Relationships between matrix metalloproteinases and tissue inhibitor of metalloproteinases in the wall of abdominal aortic aneurysms, *Int Angiol* 22(3):229–238, 2003.

38. Papalambros E, Sigala F, Georgopoulos S, et al: Immunohistochemical expression of metalloproteinases MMP-2 and MMP-9 in abdominal aortic aneurysms: correlation with symptoms and aortic diameter, *Int J Mol Med* 12(6):965–968, 2003.
39. Petersen E, Gineitis A, Wagberg F, et al: Activity of matrix metalloproteinase-2 and -9 in abdominal aortic aneurysms. Relation to size and rupture, *Eur J Vasc Endovasc Surg* 20(5):457–461, 2000.
40. Petersen E, Wagberg F, Angquist KA: Serum concentrations of elastin-derived peptides in patients with specific manifestations of atherosclerotic disease, *Eur J Vasc Endovasc Surg* 24(5):440–444, 2002.
41. Tamarina NA, McMillan WD, Shively VP, et al: Expression of matrix metalloproteinases and their inhibitors in aneurysms and normal aorta, *Surgery* 122(2):264–271, 1997; discussion 271–262.
42. Pyo R, Lee JK, Shipley JM, et al: Targeted gene disruption of matrix metalloproteinase-9 (gelatinase B) suppresses development of experimental abdominal aortic aneurysms, *J Clin Invest* 105(11):1641–1649, 2000.
43. Annabi B, Shedid D, Ghosn P, et al: Differential regulation of matrix metalloproteinase activities in abdominal aortic aneurysms, *J Vasc Surg* 35(3):539–546, 2002.
44. Crowther M, Goodall S, Jones JL, et al: Localization of matrix metalloproteinase 2 within the aneurysmal and normal aortic wall, *Br J Surg* 87(10):1391–1400, 2000.
45. Henrotin YE, Bruckner P, Pujol JP: The role of reactive oxygen species in homeostasis and degradation of cartilage, *Osteoarthritis Cartilage* 11(10):747–755, 2003.
46. Miller FJ Jr, Sharp WJ, Fang X, et al: Oxidative stress in human abdominal aortic aneurysms: a potential mediator of aneurysmal remodeling, *Arterioscler Thromb Vasc Biol* 22(4): 560–565, 2002.
47. Siwik DA, Colucci WS: Regulation of matrix metalloproteinases by cytokines and reactive oxygen/nitrogen species in the myocardium, *Heart Fail Rev* 9(1):43–51, 2004.
48. Carmeliet P, Moons L, Lijnen R, et al: Urokinase-generated plasmin activates matrix metalloproteinases during aneurysm formation, *Nat Genet* 17(4):439–444, 1997.
49. Defawe OD, Colige A, Lambert CA, et al: TIMP-2 and PAI-1 mRNA levels are lower in aneurysmal as compared to athero-occlusive abdominal aortas, *Cardiovasc Res* 60(1): 205–213, 2003.
50. Saito S, Zempo N, Yamashita A, et al: Matrix metalloproteinase expressions in arteriosclerotic aneurysmal disease, *Vasc Endovasc Surg* 36(1):1–7, 2002.
51. Ailawadi G, Knipp BS, Lu G, et al: A nonintrinsic regional basis for increased infrarenal aortic MMP-9 expression and activity, *J Vasc Surg* 37(5):1059–1066, 2003.
52. Allaire E, Forough R, Clowes M, et al: Local overexpression of TIMP-1 prevents aortic aneurysm degeneration and rupture in a rat model, *J Clin Invest* 102(7):1413–1420, 1998.
53. Silence J, Collen D, Lijnen HR: Reduced atherosclerotic plaque but enhanced aneurysm formation in mice with inactivation of the tissue inhibitor of metalloproteinase-1 (TIMP-1) gene, *Circ Res* 90(8):897–903, 2002.
54. Falkenberg M, Holmdahl L, Tjarnstrom J, et al: Abnormal levels of urokinase plasminogen activator protein and tissue plasminogen activator activity in human aortic aneurysms, *Eur J Surg* 167(1):10–14, 2001.
55. Qian HS, Gu JM, Liu P, et al: Overexpression of PAI-1 prevents the development of abdominal aortic aneurysm in mice, *Gene Ther* 15(3):224–232, 2008.
56. Thompson RW, Liao S, Curci JA: Therapeutic potential of tetracycline derivatives to suppress the growth of abdominal aortic aneurysms, *Adv Dent Res* 12(2):159–165, 1998.
57. Manning MW, Cassis LA, Daugherty A: Differential effects of doxycycline, a broad-spectrum matrix metalloproteinase inhibitor, on angiotensin II-induced atherosclerosis and abdominal aortic aneurysms, *Arterioscler Thromb Vasc Biol* 23(3):483–488, 2003.
58. Bartoli MA, Parodi FE, Chu J, et al: Localized administration of doxycycline suppresses aortic dilatation in an experimental mouse model of abdominal aortic aneurysm, *Ann Vasc Surg* 20(2):228–236, 2006.
59. Chung AW, Yang HH, Radomski MW, et al: Long-term doxycycline is more effective than atenolol to prevent thoracic aortic aneurysm in Marfan syndrome through the inhibition of matrix metalloproteinase-2 and -9, *Circ Res* 102(8):e73–e85, 2008.
60. Curci JA, Mao D, Bohner DG, et al: Preoperative treatment with doxycycline reduces aortic wall expression and activation of matrix metalloproteinases in patients with abdominal aortic aneurysms, *J Vasc Surg* 31(2):325–342, 2000.
61. Baxter BT, Pearce WH, Waltke EA, et al: Prolonged administration of doxycycline in patients with small asymptomatic abdominal aortic aneurysms: report of a prospective (phase II) multicenter study, *J Vasc Surg* 36(1):1–12, 2002.
62. Lindeman JH, Abdul-Hussien H, van Bockel JH, et al: Clinical trial of doxycycline for matrix metalloproteinase-9 inhibition in patients with an abdominal aneurysm: doxycycline selectively depletes aortic wall neutrophils and cytotoxic T cells, *Circulation* 119(16): 2209–2216, 2009.
63. Mosorin M, Juvonen J, Biancari F, et al: Use of doxycycline to decrease the growth rate of abdominal aortic aneurysms: a randomized, double-blind, placebo-controlled pilot study, *J Vasc Surg* 34(4):606–610, 2001.
64. Dodd BR, Spence RA: Doxycycline inhibition of abdominal aortic aneurysm growth–a systematic review of the literature, *Curr Vasc Pharmacol* 9:471–478, 2011.
65. Nagashima H, Aoka Y, Sakomura Y, et al: A 3-hydroxy-3-methylglutaryl coenzyme A reductase inhibitor, cerivastatin, suppresses production of matrix metalloproteinase-9 in human abdominal aortic aneurysm wall, *J Vasc Surg* 36(1):158–163, 2002.
66. Ejiri J, Inoue N, Tsukube T, et al: Oxidative stress in the pathogenesis of thoracic aortic aneurysm: protective role of statin and angiotensin II type 1 receptor blocker, *Cardiovasc Res* 59(4):988–996, 2003.
67. Schouten O, van Laanen JH, Boersma E, et al: Statins are associated with a reduced infrarenal abdominal aortic aneurysm growth, *Eur J Vasc Endovasc Surg* 32(1):21–26, 2006.
68. Takagi H, Matsui M, Umemoto T: A meta-analysis of clinical studies of statins for prevention of abdominal aortic aneurysm expansion, *J Vasc Surg* 52(6):1675–1681, 2010.
69. Rahman MN, Khan JA, Mazari FA, et al: A randomized placebo controlled trial of the effect of preoperative statin use on matrix metalloproteinases and tissue inhibitors of matrix metalloproteinases in areas of low and peak wall stress in patients undergoing elective open repair of abdominal aortic aneurysm, *Ann Vasc Surg* 25(1):32–38, 2011.
70. Hurks R, Hoefer IE, Vink A, et al: Different effects of commonly prescribed statins on abdominal aortic aneurysm wall biology, *Eur J Vasc Endovasc Surg* 39(5):569–576, 2010.
71. Ferguson CD, Clancy P, Bourke B, et al: Association of statin prescription with small abdominal aortic aneurysm progression, *Am Heart J* 159(2):307–313, 2010.
72. Holmes DR, Petrinec D, Wester W, et al: Indomethacin prevents elastase-induced abdominal aortic aneurysms in the rat, *J Surg Res* 63(1):305–309, 1996.
73. Franklin IJ, Walton LJ, Greenhalgh RM, et al: The influence of indomethacin on the metabolism and cytokine secretion of human aneurysmal aorta, *Eur J Vasc Endovasc Surg* 18(1):35–42, 1999.
74. Miralles M, Wester W, Sicard GA, et al: Indomethacin inhibits expansion of experimental aortic aneurysms via inhibition of the COX2 isoform of cyclooxygenase, *J Vasc Surg* 29(5):884–892, 1999; discussion 892–883.
75. Walton LJ, Franklin IJ, Bayston T, et al: Inhibition of prostaglandin E2 synthesis in abdominal aortic aneurysms: implications for smooth muscle cell viability, inflammatory processes, and the expansion of abdominal aortic aneurysms, *Circulation* 100(1):48–54, 1999.
76. Reilly JM, Miralles M, Wester WN, et al: Differential expression of prostaglandin E2 and interleukin-6 in occlusive and aneurysmal aortic disease, *Surgery* 126(4):624–627, 1999; discussion 627–628.
77. Holmes DR, Wester W, Thompson RW, et al: Prostaglandin E2 synthesis and cyclooxygenase expression in abdominal aortic aneurysms, *J Vasc Surg* 25(5):810–815, 1997.
78. Bayston T, Ramessur S, Reise J, et al: Prostaglandin E2 receptors in abdominal aortic aneurysm and human aortic smooth muscle cells, *J Vasc Surg* 38(2):354–359, 2003.
79. Libby P: Inflammation in atherosclerosis, *Nature* 420(6917):868–874, 2002.
80. Rose AG, Dent DM: Inflammatory variant of abdominal atherosclerotic aneurysm, *Arch Pathol Lab Med* 105(8):409–413, 1981.
81. Satta J, Laurila A, Paakko P, et al: Chronic inflammation and elastin degradation in abdominal aortic aneurysm disease: an immunohistochemical and electron microscopic study, *Eur J Vasc Endovasc Surg* 15(4):313–319, 1998.
82. Golledge AL, Walker P, Norman PE, et al: A systematic review of studies examining inflammation associated cytokines in human abdominal aortic aneurysm samples, *Dis Markers* 26(4):181–188, 2009.
83. Treska V, Kocova J, Boudova L, et al: Inflammation in the wall of abdominal aortic aneurysm and its role in the symptomatology of aneurysm, *Cytokines Cell Mol Ther* 7(3):91–97, 2002.
84. Wilson WR, Wills J, Furness PN, et al: Abdominal aortic aneurysm rupture is not associated with an up-regulation of inflammation within the aneurysm wall, *Eur J Vasc Endovasc Surg* 40(2):191–195, 2010.
85. Parry DJ, Al-Barjas HS, Chappell L, et al: Markers of inflammation in men with small abdominal aortic aneurysm, *J Vasc Surg* 52(1):145–151, 2010.
86. Hellenthal FA, Buurman WA, Wodzig WK, et al: Biomarkers of abdominal aortic aneurysm progression. Part 2: inflammation, *Nat Rev Cardiol* 6(8):543–552, 2009.
87. Vainas T, Lubbers T, Stassen FR, et al: Serum C-reactive protein level is associated with abdominal aortic aneurysm size and may be produced by aneurysmal tissue, *Circulation* 107(8):1103–1105, 2003.
88. Truijers M, Kurvers HA, Bredie SJ, et al: *In vivo* imaging of abdominal aortic aneurysms: increased FDG uptake suggests inflammation in the aneurysm wall, *J Endovasc Ther* 15(4):462–467, 2008.
89. Howarth SP, Tang TY, Graves MJ, et al: Non-invasive MR imaging of inflammation in a patient with both asymptomatic carotid atheroma and an abdominal aortic aneurysm: a case report, *Ann Surg Innov Res* 1:4, 2007.
90. Tang EH, Shvartz E, Shimizu K, et al: Deletion of EP4 on bone marrow-derived cells enhances inflammation and angiotensin II-induced abdominal aortic aneurysm formation, *Arterioscler Thromb Vasc Biol* 31(2):261–269, 2011.
91. Shiraya S, Miyake T, Aoki M, et al: Inhibition of development of experimental aortic abdominal aneurysm in rat model by atorvastatin through inhibition of macrophage migration, *Atherosclerosis* 202(1):34–40, 2009.
92. Kalyanasundaram A, Elmore JR, Manazer JR, et al: Simvastatin suppresses experimental aortic aneurysm expansion, *J Vasc Surg* 43(1):117–124, 2006.
93. Schultz G, Tedesco MM, Sho E, et al: Enhanced abdominal aortic aneurysm formation in thrombin-activatable procarboxypeptidase B-deficient mice, *Arterioscler Thromb Vasc Biol* 30(7):1363–1370, 2010.
94. Leeper NJ, Tedesco MM, Kojima Y, et al: Apelin prevents aortic aneurysm formation by inhibiting macrophage inflammation, *Am J Physiol Heart Circ Physiol* 296(5):H1329–H1335, 2009.
95. Onoda M, Yoshimura K, Aoki H, et al: Lysyl oxidase resolves inflammation by reducing monocyte chemoattractant protein-1 in abdominal aortic aneurysm, *Atherosclerosis* 208(2):366–369, 2010.
96. Kaneko H, Anzai T, Morisawa M, et al: Resveratrol prevents the development of abdominal aortic aneurysm through attenuation of inflammation, oxidative stress, and neovascularization, *Atherosclerosis* 217:350–357, 2011.
97. Hannawa KK, Cho BS, Sinha I, et al: Attenuation of experimental aortic aneurysm formation in P-selectin knockout mice, *Ann N Y Acad Sci* 108:353–359, 2006.
98. Wolinsky H, Glagov S: Comparison of abdominal and thoracic aortic medial structure in mammals. Deviation of man from the usual pattern, *Circ Res* 25(6):677–686, 1969.
99. Benjamin HB, Becker AB: Etiologic incidence of thoracic and abdominal aneurysms, *Surg Gynecol Obstet* 125(6):1307–1310, 1967.
100. Stefanadis C, Vlachopoulos C, Karayannacos P, et al: Effect of vasa vasorum flow on structure and function of the aorta in experimental animals, *Circulation* 91(10): 2669–2678, 1995.
101. Krettek A, Sukhova GK, Libby P: Elastogenesis in human arterial disease: a role for macrophages in disordered elastin synthesis, *Arterioscler Thromb Vasc Biol* 23(4): 582–587, 2003.
102. Moore JE Jr, Ku DN, Zarins CK, et al: Pulsatile flow visualization in the abdominal aorta under differing physiologic conditions: implications for increased susceptibility to atherosclerosis, *J Biomech Eng* 114(3):391–397, 1992.
103. Egelhoff CJ, Budwig RS, Elger DF, et al: Model studies of the flow in abdominal aortic aneurysms during resting and exercise conditions, *J Biomech* 32(12):1319–1329, 1999.
104. Sangiorgi G, D'Averio R, Mauriello A, et al: Plasma levels of metalloproteinases-3 and -9 as markers of successful abdominal aortic aneurysm exclusion after endovascular graft treatment, *Circulation* 104(12 Suppl 1):I288–I295, 2001.

105. Lorelli DR, Jean-Claude JM, Fox CJ, et al: Response of plasma matrix metalloproteinase-9 to conventional abdominal aortic aneurysm repair or endovascular exclusion: implications for endoleak, *J Vasc Surg* 35(5):916–922, 2002.
106. Nakahashi TK, Hoshina K, Tsao PS, et al: Flow loading induces macrophage antioxidative gene expression in experimental aneurysms, *Arterioscler Thromb Vasc Biol* 22(12): 2017–2022, 2002.
107. Sho E, Sho M, Hoshina K, et al: Hemodynamic forces regulate mural macrophage infiltration in experimental aortic aneurysms, *Exp Mol Pathol* 76(2):108–116, 2004.
108. Wang DH, Makaroun MS, Webster MW, et al: Effect of intraluminal thrombus on wall stress in patient-specific models of abdominal aortic aneurysm, *J Vasc Surg* 36(3):598–604, 2002.
109. Di Martino ES, Vorp DA: Effect of variation in intraluminal thrombus constitutive properties on abdominal aortic aneurysm wall stress, *Ann Biomed Eng* 31(7):804–809, 2003.
110. Thubrikar MJ, Robicsek F, Labrosse M, et al: Effect of thrombus on abdominal aortic aneurysm wall dilation and stress, *J Cardiovasc Surg (Torino)* 44(1):67–77, 2003.
111. Speelman L, Schurink GW, Bosboom EM, et al: The mechanical role of thrombus on the growth rate of an abdominal aortic aneurysm, *J Vasc Surg* 51(1):19–26, 2010.
112. Bluestein D, Dumont K, De Beule M, et al: Intraluminal thrombus and risk of rupture in patient specific abdominal aortic aneurysm--FSI modelling, *Comput Methods Biomech Biomed Engin* 12(1):73–81, 2009.
113. Georgakarakos E, Ioannou C, Kostas T, et al: Inflammatory response to aortic aneurysm intraluminal thrombus may cause increased 18F-FDG uptake at sites not associated with high wall stress: comment on "high levels of 18F-FDG uptake in aortic aneurysm wall are associated with high wall stress", *Eur J Vasc Endovasc Surg* 39(6):795, 2010; author reply 795–796.
114. Li ZY, U-King-Im J, Tang TY, et al: Impact of calcification and intraluminal thrombus on the computed wall stresses of abdominal aortic aneurysm, *J Vasc Surg* 47(5):928–935, 2008.
115. Wiernicki I, Cnotliwy M, Baranowska-Bosiacka I, et al: Elastin degradation within the abdominal aortic aneurysm wall–relationship between intramural pH and adjacent thrombus formation, *Eur J Clin Invest* 38(12):883–887, 2008.
116. Fontaine V, Jacob MP, Houard X, et al: Involvement of the mural thrombus as a site of protease release and activation in human aortic aneurysms, *Am J Pathol* 161(5): 1701–1710, 2002.
117. Breeuwer M, de Putter S, Kose U, et al: Towards patient-specific risk assessment of abdominal aortic aneurysm, *Med Biol Eng Comput* 46(11):1085–1095, 2008.
118. Sheidaei A, Hunley SC, Zeinali-Davarani S, et al: Simulation of abdominal aortic aneurysm growth with updating hemodynamic loads using a realistic geometry, *Med Eng Phys* 33(1):80–88, 2011.
119. Georgakarakos E, Ioannou CV, Papaharilaou Y, et al: Computational evaluation of aortic aneurysm rupture risk: what have we learned so far? *J Endovasc Ther* 18(2):214–225, 2011.
120. Reeps C, Gee M, Maier A, et al: The impact of model assumptions on results of computational mechanics in abdominal aortic aneurysm, *J Vasc Surg* 51(3):679–688, 2010.
121. Malkawi AH, Hinchliffe RJ, Xu Y, et al: Patient-specific biomechanical profiling in abdominal aortic aneurysm development and rupture, *J Vasc Surg* 52(2):480–488, 2010.
122. Maier A, Gee MW, Reeps C, et al: A comparison of diameter, wall stress, and rupture potential index for abdominal aortic aneurysm rupture risk prediction, *Ann Biomed Eng* 38(10):3124–3134, 2010.
123. Georgakarakos E, Ioannou CV, Kamarianakis Y, et al: The role of geometric parameters in the prediction of abdominal aortic aneurysm wall stress, *Eur J Vasc Endovasc Surg* 39(1):42–48, 2010.
124. Vande Geest JP, Di Martino ES, Bohra A, et al: A biomechanics-based rupture potential index for abdominal aortic aneurysm risk assessment: demonstrative application, *Ann N Y Acad Sci* 1085:1–21, 2006.
125. Vande Geest JP, Dillavou ED, Di Martino ES, et al: Gender-related differences in the tensile strength of abdominal aortic aneurysm, *Ann N Y Acad Sci* 1085:400–402, 2006.
126. Darling RC, Messina CR, Brewster DC, et al: Autopsy study of unoperated abdominal aortic aneurysms. The case for early resection, *Circulation* 56(3 Suppl):II161–II164, 1977.
127. Lederle FA, Johnson GR, Wilson SE, et al: The aneurysm detection and management study screening program: validation cohort and final results. Aneurysm Detection and Management Veterans Affairs Cooperative Study Investigators, *Arch Intern Med* 160(10):1425–1430, 2000.
128. Ashton HA, Buxton MJ, Day NE, et al: The Multicentre Aneurysm Screening Study (MASS) into the effect of abdominal aortic aneurysm screening on mortality in men: a randomised controlled trial, *Lancet* 360(9345):1531–1539, 2002.
129. Derubertis BG, Trocciola SM, Ryer EJ, et al: Abdominal aortic aneurysm in women: prevalence, risk factors, and implications for screening, *J Vasc Surg* 46(4):630–635, 2007.
130. Scott RA, Ashton HA, Kay DN: Abdominal aortic aneurysm in 4237 screened patients: prevalence, development and management over 6 years [see comments], *Br J Surg* 78(9):1122–1125, 1991.
131. Singh K, Bonaa KH, Jacobsen BK, et al: Prevalence of and risk factors for abdominal aortic aneurysms in a population-based study: the Tromso Study, *Am J Epidemiol* 154(3): 236–244, 2001.
132. Lederle FA, Johnson GR, Wilson SE: Abdominal aortic aneurysm in women, *J Vasc Surg* 34(1):122–126, 2001.
133. Alcorn HG, Wolfson SK Jr, Sutton-Tyrrell K, et al: Risk factors for abdominal aortic aneurysms in older adults enrolled in the Cardiovascular Health Study, *Arterioscler Thromb Vasc Biol* 16(8):963–970, 1996.
134. Kurvers HA, van der Graaf Y, Blankensteijn JD, et al: Screening for asymptomatic internal carotid artery stenosis and aneurysm of the abdominal aorta: comparing the yield between patients with manifest atherosclerosis and patients with risk factors for atherosclerosis only, *J Vasc Surg* 37(6):1226–1233, 2003.
135. Tornwall ME, Virtamo J, Haukka JK, et al: Life-style factors and risk for abdominal aortic aneurysm in a cohort of Finnish male smokers, *Epidemiology* 12(1):94–100, 2001.
136. Lederle FA, Johnson GR, Wilson SE, et al: Prevalence and associations of abdominal aortic aneurysm detected through screening. Aneurysm Detection and Management (ADAM) Veterans Affairs Cooperative Study Group, *Ann Intern Med* 126(6):441–449, 1997.
137. Pleumeekers HJ, Hoes AW, van der Does E, et al: Aneurysms of the abdominal aorta in older adults. The Rotterdam Study, *Am J Epidemiol* 142(12):1291–1299, 1995.
138. Rodin MB, Daviglus ML, Wong GC, et al: Middle age cardiovascular risk factors and abdominal aortic aneurysm in older age, *Hypertension* 42(1):61–68, 2003.
139. Scott RA, Bridgewater SG, Ashton HA: Randomized clinical trial of screening for abdominal aortic aneurysm in women, *Br J Surg* 89(3):283–285, 2002.
140. Vardulaki KA, Walker NM, Day NE, et al: Quantifying the risks of hypertension, age, sex and smoking in patients with abdominal aortic aneurysm, *Br J Surg* 87(2):195–200, 2000.
141. Doll R, Peto R, Wheatley K, et al: Mortality in relation to smoking: 40 years' observations on male British doctors, *BMJ* 309(6959):901–911, 1994.
142. Goldberg RJ, Burchfiel CM, Benfante R, et al: Lifestyle and biologic factors associated with atherosclerotic disease in middle-aged men. 20-year findings from the Honolulu Heart Program, *Arch Intern Med* 155(7):686–694, 1995.
143. Hammond EC: Smoking in relation to the death rates of one million men and women, *Natl Cancer Inst Monogr* 19:127–204, 1966.
144. Nilsson S, Carstensen JM, Pershagen G: Mortality among male and female smokers in Sweden: a 33-year follow-up, *J Epidemiol Community Health* 55(11):825–830, 2001.
145. Rogot E, Murray JL: Smoking and causes of death among U.S. veterans: 16 years of observation, *Public Health Rep* 95(3):213–222, 1980.
146. Tang JL, Morris JK, Wald NJ, et al: Mortality in relation to tar yield of cigarettes: a prospective study of four cohorts, *BMJ* 311(7019):1530–1533, 1995.
147. Weir JM, Dunn JE Jr: Smoking and mortality: a prospective study, *Cancer* 25(1):105–112, 1970.
148. Lee AJ, Fowkes FG, Carson MN, et al: Smoking, atherosclerosis and risk of abdominal aortic aneurysm, *Eur Heart J* 18(4):671–676, 1997.
149. Wilmink TB, Quick CR, Day NE: The association between cigarette smoking and abdominal aortic aneurysms, *J Vasc Surg* 30(6):1099–1105, 1999.
150. Strachan DP: Predictors of death from aortic aneurysm among middle-aged men: the Whitehall study, *Br J Surg* 78(4):401–404, 1991.
151. Lederle FA, Nelson DB, Joseph AM: Smokers' relative risk for aortic aneurysm compared with other smoking-related diseases: a systematic review, *J Vasc Surg* 38(2):329–334, 2003.
152. Powell JT, Greenhalgh RM: Clinical practice. Small abdominal aortic aneurysms, *N Engl J Med* 348(19):1895–1901, 2003.
153. Lederle FA, Wilson SE, Johnson GR, et al: Immediate repair compared with surveillance of small abdominal aortic aneurysms, *N Engl J Med* 346(19):1437–1444, 2002.
154. Brady AR, Thompson SG, Fowkes FG, et al: Abdominal aortic aneurysm expansion: risk factors and time intervals for surveillance, *Circulation* 110(1):16–21, 2004.
155. Baumgartner I, Hirsch AT, Abola MT, et al: Cardiovascular risk profile and outcome of patients with abdominal aortic aneurysm in out-patients with atherothrombosis: data from the Reduction of Atherothrombosis for Continued Health (REACH) Registry, *J Vasc Surg* 48(4):808–814, 2008.
156. Franks PJ, Edwards RJ, Greenhalgh RM, et al: Risk factors for abdominal aortic aneurysms in smokers, *Eur J Vasc Endovasc Surg* 11(4):487–492, 1996.
157. Blanchard JF, Armenian HK, Friesen PP: Risk factors for abdominal aortic aneurysm: results of a case-control study, *Am J Epidemiol* 151(6):575–583, 2000.
158. Brown LC, Powell JT: Risk factors for aneurysm rupture in patients kept under ultrasound surveillance. UK Small Aneurysm Trial Participants, *Ann Surg* 230(3):289–296, 1999; discussion 296–287.
159. Hobbs SD, Claridge MW, Quick CR, et al: LDL cholesterol is associated with small abdominal aortic aneurysms, *Eur J Vasc Endovasc Surg* 26(6):618–622, 2003.
160. Gillum RF: Epidemiology of aortic aneurysm in the United States, *J Clin Epidemiol* 48(11):1289–1298, 1995.
161. Norrgard O, Rais O, Angquist KA: Familial occurrence of abdominal aortic aneurysms, *Surgery* 95(6):650–656, 1984.
162. Lederle FA: Ultrasonographic screening for abdominal aortic aneurysms, *Ann Intern Med* 139(6):516–522, 2003.
163. Baird PA, Sadovnick AD, Yee IM, et al: Sibling risks of abdominal aortic aneurysm, *Lancet* 346(8975):601–604, 1995.
164. Verloes A, Sakalihasan N, Koulischer L, et al: Aneurysms of the abdominal aorta: familial and genetic aspects in three hundred thirteen pedigrees, *J Vasc Surg* 21(4):646–655, 1995.
165. Frydman G, Walker PJ, Summers K, et al: The value of screening in siblings of patients with abdominal aortic aneurysm, *Eur J Vasc Endovasc Surg* 26(4):396–400, 2003.
166. Adams DC, Tulloh BR, Galloway SW, et al: Familial abdominal aortic aneurysm: prevalence and implications for screening, *Eur J Vasc Surg* 7(6):709–712, 1993.
167. Cole CW, Barber GG, Bouchard AG, et al: Abdominal aortic aneurysm: consequences of a positive family history, *Can J Surg* 32(2):117–120, 1989.
168. Webster MW, Ferrell RE, St. Jean PL, et al: Ultrasound screening of first-degree relatives of patients with an abdominal aortic aneurysm, *J Vasc Surg* 13(1):9–13, 1991 discussion 13–14.
169. Webster MW, St. Jean PL, Steed DL, et al: Abdominal aortic aneurysm: results of a family study, *J Vasc Surg* 13(3):366–372, 1991.
170. Majumder PP, St Jean PL, Ferrell RE, et al: On the inheritance of abdominal aortic aneurysm, *Am J Hum Genet* 48(1):164–170, 1991.
171. Wahlgren CM, Larsson E, Magnusson PK, et al: Genetic and environmental contributions to abdominal aortic aneurysm development in a twin population, *J Vasc Surg* 51(1):3–7, 2010; discussion 7.
172. Wiernicki I, Gutowski P, Ciechanowski K, et al: Abdominal aortic aneurysm: association between haptoglobin phenotypes, elastase activity, and neutrophil count in the peripheral blood, *Vasc Surg* 35(5):345–350, 2001; discussion 351.
173. St Jean P, Hart B, Webster M, et al: Alpha-1-antitrypsin deficiency in aneurysmal disease, *Hum Hered* 46(2):92–97, 1996.
174. Schardey HM, Hernandez-Richter T, Klueppelberg U, et al: Alleles of the alpha-1-antitrypsin phenotype in patients with aortic aneurysms, *J Cardiovasc Surg (Torino)* 39(5):535–539, 1998.
175. Hinterseher I, Tromp G, Kuivaniemi H: Genes and abdominal aortic aneurysm, *Ann Vasc Surg* 25(3):388–412, 2011.
176. Thompson AR, Cooper JA, Jones GT, et al: Assessment of the association between genetic polymorphisms in transforming growth factor beta, and its binding protein (LTBP), and the presence, and expansion, of abdominal aortic aneurysm, *Atherosclerosis* 209(2):367–373, 2010.

177. Golledge J, Clancy P, Jones GT, et al: Possible association between genetic polymorphisms in transforming growth factor beta receptors, serum transforming growth factor beta1 concentration and abdominal aortic aneurysm, *Br J Surg* 96(6):628–632, 2009.
178. Elmore JR, Obmann MA, Kuivaniemi H, et al: Identification of a genetic variant associated with abdominal aortic aneurysms on chromosome 3p12.3 by genome wide association. *J Vasc Surg* 49(6):1525–1531, 2009.
179. Gretarsdottir S, Baas AF, Thorleifsson G, et al: Genome-wide association study identifies a sequence variant within the DAB2IP gene conferring susceptibility to abdominal aortic aneurysm, *Nat Genet* 42(8):692–697, 2010.
180. Helgadottir A, Thorleifsson G, Magnusson KP, et al: The same sequence variant on 9p21 associates with myocardial infarction, abdominal aortic aneurysm and intracranial aneurysm, *Nat Genet* 40(2):217–224, 2008.
181. Thompson AR, Golledge J, Cooper JA, et al: Sequence variant on 9p21 is associated with the presence of abdominal aortic aneurysm disease but does not have an impact on aneurysmal expansion, *Eur J Hum Genet* 17(3):391–394, 2009.
182. Atturu G, Brouilette S, Samani NJ, et al: Short leukocyte telomere length is associated with abdominal aortic aneurysm (AAA), *Eur J Vasc Endovasc Surg* 39(5):559–564, 2010.
183. Szilagyi DE, Elliott JP, Smith RF: Clinical fate of the patient with asymptomatic abdominal aortic aneurysm and unfit for surgical treatment, *Arch Surg* 104(4):600–606, 1972.
184. Bickerstaff LK, Hollier LH, Van Peenen HJ, et al: Abdominal aortic aneurysms: the changing natural history, *J Vasc Surg* 1(1):6–12, 1984.
185. Nevitt MP, Ballard DJ, Hallett JW Jr: Prognosis of abdominal aortic aneurysms. A population-based study, *N Engl J Med* 321(15):1009–1014, 1989.
186. Lederle FA, Johnson GR, Wilson SE, et al: Rupture rate of large abdominal aortic aneurysms in patients refusing or unfit for elective repair, *JAMA* 287(22):2968–2972, 2002.
187. Harris LM, Faggioli GL, Fiedler R, et al: Ruptured abdominal aortic aneurysms: factors affecting mortality rates, *J Vasc Surg* 14(6):812–818, 1991 discussion 819–820.
188. Mortality results for randomised controlled trial of early elective surgery or ultrasonographic surveillance for small abdominal aortic aneurysms. The UK Small Aneurysm Trial Participants, *Lancet* 352(9141):1649–1655, 1998.
189. Ouriel K, Clair DG, Kent KC, et al: Endovascular repair compared with surveillance for patients with small abdominal aortic aneurysms, *J Vasc Surg* 51(5):1081–1087, 2010.
190. Brown PM, Sobolev B, Zelt DT: Selective management of abdominal aortic aneurysms smaller than 5.0 cm in a prospective sizing program with gender-specific analysis, *J Vasc Surg* 38(4):762–765, 2003.
191. Powell JT, Brown LC: The natural history of abdominal aortic aneurysms and their risk of rupture, *Acta Chir Belg* 101(1):11–16, 2001.
192. Evans SM, Adam DJ, Bradbury AW: The influence of gender on outcome after ruptured abdominal aortic aneurysm, *J Vasc Surg* 32(2):258–262, 2000.
193. Isselbacher EM: Thoracic and abdominal aortic aneurysms, *Circulation* 111(6):816–828, 2005.
194. Svensson LG: Natural history of aneurysms of the descending and thoracoabdominal aorta, *J Card Surg* 12(2 Suppl):279–284, 1997.
195. Ince H, Nienaber CA: Etiology, pathogenesis and management of thoracic aortic aneurysm, *Nat Clin Pract Cardiovasc Med* 4(8):418–427, 2007.
196. Svensjo S, Bengtsson H, Bergqvist D: Thoracic and thoracoabdominal aortic aneurysm and dissection: an investigation based on autopsy, *Br J Surg* 83(1):68–71, 1996.
197. Bickerstaff L, Pairolero P, Hollier L, et al: Thoracic aortic aneurysms: a population-based study, *Surgery* 92(6):1103–1108, 1982.
198. Svensson LG, Crawford ES, Hess KR, et al: Experience with 1509 patients undergoing thoracoabdominal aortic operations, *J Vasc Surg* 17(2):357–368, 1993; discussion 368–370.
199. Guo D, Hasham S, Kuang SQ, et al: Familial thoracic aortic aneurysms and dissections: genetic heterogeneity with a major locus mapping to 5q13–14, *Circulation* 103(20):2461–2468, 2001.
200. Crawford ES, DeNatale RW: Thoracoabdominal aortic aneurysm: observations regarding the natural course of the disease, *J Vasc Surg* 3(4):578–582, 1986.
201. Cambria RA, Gloviczki P, Stanson AW, et al: Outcome and expansion rate of 57 thoracoabdominal aortic aneurysms managed nonoperatively, *Am J Surg* 170(2):213–217, 1995.
202. Griepp RB, Ergin MA, Galla JD, et al: Natural history of descending thoracic and thoracoabdominal aneurysms, *Ann Thorac Surg* 67(6):1927–1930, 1999; discussion 1953–1928.
203. Pitt MP, Bonser RS: The natural history of thoracic aortic aneurysm disease: an overview, *J Card Surg* 12(2 Suppl):270–278, 1997.
204. Juvonen T, Ergin MA, Galla JD, et al: Prospective study of the natural history of thoracic aortic aneurysms, *Ann Thorac Surg* 63(6):1533–1545, 1997.
205. Davies RR, Goldstein LJ, Coady MA, et al: Yearly rupture or dissection rates for thoracic aortic aneurysms: simple prediction based on size, *Ann Thorac Surg* 73(1):17–27, discussion 27–18, 2002.
206. Elefteriades JA: Natural history of thoracic aortic aneurysms: indications for surgery, and surgical versus nonsurgical risks, *Ann Thorac Surg* 74(5):S1877–S1880, 2002; discussion S1892–1878.
207. Dapunt OE, Galla JD, Sadeghi AM, et al: The natural history of thoracic aortic aneurysms, *J Thorac Cardiovasc Surg* 107(5):1323–1332, 1994; discussion 1332–1323.
208. Pressler V, McNamara JJ: Aneurysm of the thoracic aorta. Review of 260 cases, *J Thorac Cardiovasc Surg* 89(1):50–54, 1985.
209. Hiratzka LF, Bakris GL, Beckman JA, et al: 2010 ACCF/AHA/AATS/ACR/ASA/SCA/SCAI/SIR/STS/SVM guidelines for the diagnosis and management of patients with thoracic aortic disease: a report of the American College of Cardiology Foundation/American Heart Association Task Force on Practice Guidelines, American Association for Thoracic Surgery, American College of Radiology, American Stroke Association, Society of Cardiovascular Anesthesiologists, Society for Cardiovascular Angiography and Interventions, Society of Interventional Radiology, Society of Thoracic Surgeons, and Society for Vascular Medicine, *Circulation* 121(13):e266–e369, 2010.
210. Gott VL, Greene PS, Alejo DE, et al: Replacement of the aortic root in patients with Marfan's syndrome, *N Engl J Med* 340(17):1307–1313, 1999.
211. Svensson LG, Kouchoukos NT, Miller DC, et al: Expert consensus document on the treatment of descending thoracic aortic disease using endovascular stent-grafts, *Ann Thorac Surg* 85(1 Suppl):S1–S41, 2008.
212. Tzemos N, Therrien J, Yip J, et al: Outcomes in adults with bicuspid aortic valves, *JAMA* 300(11):1317–1325, 2008.
213. Vallely MP, Semsarian C, Bannon PG: Management of the ascending aorta in patients with bicuspid aortic valve disease, *Heart Lung Circ* 17(5):357–363, 2008.
214. Loeys BL, Schwarze U, Holm T, et al: Aneurysm syndromes caused by mutations in the TGF-beta receptor, *N Engl J Med* 355(8):788–798, 2006.
215. Habashi JP, Judge DP, Holm TM, et al: Losartan, an AT1 antagonist, prevents aortic aneurysm in a mouse model of Marfan syndrome, *Science* 312(5770):117–121, 2006.
216. El-Hamamsy I, Yacoub MH: Cellular and molecular mechanisms of thoracic aortic aneurysms, *Nature Reviews Cardiology* 6(12):771–786, 2009.
217. Germain DP: Clinical and genetic features of vascular Ehlers-Danlos syndrome, *Ann Vasc Surg* 16(3):391–397, 2002.
218. Arteaga-Solis E, Gayraud B, Ramirez F: Elastic and collagenous networks in vascular diseases, *Cell Struct Funct* 25(2):69–72, 2000.
219. Nishiyama Y, Manabe N, Ooshima A, et al: A sporadic case of Ehlers-Danlos syndrome type IV: diagnosed by a morphometric study of collagen content, *Pathol Int* 45(7):524–529, 1995.
220. Pepin M, Schwarze U, Superti-Furga A, et al: Clinical and genetic features of Ehlers-Danlos syndrome type IV, the vascular type, *N Engl J Med* 342(10):673–680, 2000.
221. Nistri S, Sorbo MD, Marin M, et al: Aortic root dilatation in young men with normally functioning bicuspid aortic valves, *Heart* 82(1):19–22, 1999.
222. Keane MG, Wiegers SE, Plappert T, et al: Bicuspid aortic valves are associated with aortic dilatation out of proportion to coexistent valvular lesions, *Circulation* 102(19 Suppl 3):III35–III39, 2000.
223. Yasuda H, Nakatani S, Stugaard M, et al: Failure to prevent progressive dilation of ascending aorta by aortic valve replacement in patients with bicuspid aortic valve: comparison with tricuspid aortic valve, *Circulation* 108(Suppl 1):II291–II294, 2003.
224. Fedak PW, de Sa MP, Verma S, et al: Vascular matrix remodeling in patients with bicuspid aortic valve malformations: implications for aortic dilatation, *J Thorac Cardiovasc Surg* 126(3):797–806, 2003.
225. Schmid FX, Bielenberg K, Holmer S, et al: Structural and biomolecular changes in aorta and pulmonary trunk of patients with aortic aneurysm and valve disease: implications for the Ross procedure, *Eur J Cardiothorac Surg* 25(5):748–753, 2004.
226. Boyum J, Fellinger EK, Schmoker JD, et al: Matrix metalloproteinase activity in thoracic aortic aneurysms associated with bicuspid and tricuspid aortic valves, *J Thorac Cardiovasc Surg* 127(3):686–691, 2004.
227. Sybert VP: Cardiovascular malformations and complications in Turner syndrome, *Pediatrics* 101(1):E11, 1998.
228. Jenkins NP, Ward C: Coarctation of the aorta: natural history and outcome after surgical treatment, *QJM* 92(7):365–371, 1999.
229. Knyshov GV, Sitar LL, Glagola MD, et al: Aortic aneurysms at the site of the repair of coarctation of the aorta: a review of 48 patients, *Ann Thorac Surg* 61(3):935–939, 1996.
230. Benzaquen BS, Therrien J: Thoracic aortic aneurysm occurring at a coarctation repair site, *Can J Cardiol* 19(5):561–562, 2003.
231. Rao PS, Galal O, Smith PA, et al: Five- to nine-year follow-up results of balloon angioplasty of native aortic coarctation in infants and children, *J Am Coll Cardiol* 27(2):462–470, 1996.
232. Fletcher SE, Nihill MR, Grifka RG, et al: Balloon angioplasty of native coarctation of the aorta: midterm follow-up and prognostic factors, *J Am Coll Cardiol* 25(3):730–734, 1995.
233. Beckman JA: Giant cell arteritis, *Curr Treat Options Cardiovasc Med* 2(3):213–218, 2000.
234. Nuenninghoff DM, Hunder GG, Christianson TJ, et al: Incidence and predictors of large-artery complication (aortic aneurysm, aortic dissection, and/or large-artery stenosis) in patients with giant cell arteritis: a population-based study over 50 years, *Arthritis Rheum* 48(12):3522–3531, 2003.
235. Evans JM, Bowles CA, Bjornsson J, et al: Thoracic aortic aneurysm and rupture in giant cell arteritis. A descriptive study of 41 cases, [published erratum appears in Arthritis Rheum 38(2):290, 1995], *Arthritis Rheum* 37(10):1539–1547, 1994.
236. Nuenninghoff DM, Hunder GG, Christianson TJ, et al: Mortality of large-artery complication (aortic aneurysm, aortic dissection, and/or large-artery stenosis) in patients with giant cell arteritis: a population-based study over 50 years, *Arthritis Rheum* 48(12):3532–3537, 2003.
237. Nikkari ST, Hoyhtya M, Isola J, et al: Macrophages contain 92-kd gelatinase (MMP-9) at the site of degenerated internal elastic lamina in temporal arteritis, *Am J Pathol* 149(5): 1427–1433, 1996.
238. Tomita T, Imakawa K: Matrix metalloproteinases and tissue inhibitors of metalloproteinases in giant cell arteritis: an immunocytochemical study, *Pathology* 30(1):40–50, 1998.
239. Subramanyan R, Joy J, Balakrishnan KG: Natural history of aortoarteritis (Takayasu's disease), *Circulation* 80(3):429–437, 1989.
240. Kerr GS, Hallahan CW, Giordano J, et al: Takayasu arteritis, *Ann Intern Med* 120(11):919–929, 1994.
241. Ishikawa K, Maetani S: Long-term outcome for 120 Japanese patients with Takayasu's disease. Clinical and statistical analyses of related prognostic factors, *Circulation* 90(4):1855–1860, 1994.
242. Roldan CA, Chavez J, Wiest PW, et al: Aortic root disease and valve disease associated with ankylosing spondylitis, *J Am Coll Cardiol* 32(5):1397–1404, 1998.
243. Sakane T, Takeno M, Suzuki N, et al: Behcet's disease, *N Engl J Med* 341(17):1284–1291, 1999.
244. Yazici H, Yurdakul S, Hamuryudan V: Behcet disease, *Curr Opin Rheumatol* 13(1):18–22, 2001.
245. Ehrlich GE: Vasculitis in Behcet's disease, *Int Rev Immunol* 14(1):81–88, 1997.
246. Roldan CA, Chavez J, Wiest PW, et al: Aortic root disease and valve disease associated with ankylosing spondylitis, *J Am Coll Cardiol* 32(5):1397–1404, 1998.
247. Amor B: Reiter's syndrome. Diagnosis and clinical features, *Rheum Dis Clin North Am* 24(4):677–695, vii, 1998.
248. Letko E, Zafirakis P, Baltatzis S, et al: Relapsing polychondritis: a clinical review, *Semin Arthritis Rheum* 31(6):384–395, 2002.
249. Parkhurst GF, Dekcer JP: Bacterial aortitis and mycotic aneurysm of the aorta; a report of twelve cases, *Am J Pathol* 31(5):821–835, 1955.
250. Sommerville RL, Allen EV, Edwards JE: Bland and infected arteriosclerotic abdominal aortic aneurysms: a clinicopathologic study, *Medicine (Baltimore)* 38:207–221, 1959.
251. Bennett DE, Cherry JK: Bacterial infection of aortic aneurysms. A clinicopathologic study, *Am J Surg* 113(3):321–326, 1967.

252. Sedwitz MM, Hye RJ, Stabile BE: The changing epidemiology of pseudoaneurysm. Therapeutic implications, *Arch Surg* 123(4):473–476, 1988.

253. Mansur AJ, Grinberg M, Leao PP, et al: Extracranial mycotic aneurysms in infective endocarditis, *Clin Cardiol* 9(2):65–72, 1986.

254. Anderson CB, Butcher HR Jr, Ballinger WF: Mycotic aneurysms, *Arch Surg* 109(5):712–717, 1974.

255. Jarrett F, Darling RC, Mundth ED, et al: The management of infected arterial aneurysms, *J Cardiovasc Surg (Torino)* 18(4):361–366, 1977.

256. Vogelzang RL, Sohaey R: Infected aortic aneurysms: CT appearance, *J Comput Assist Tomogr* 12(1):109–112, 1988.

257. Taylor LM Jr, Deitz DM, McConnell DB, et al: Treatment of infected abdominal aneurysms by extraanatomic bypass, aneurysm excision, and drainage, *Am J Surg* 155(5):655–658, 1988.

258. Johansen K, Devin J: Mycotic aortic aneurysms. A reappraisal, *Arch Surg* 118(5):583–588, 1983.

259. Long R, Guzman R, Greenberg H, et al: Tuberculous mycotic aneurysm of the aorta: review of published medical and surgical experience, *Chest* 115(2):522–531, 1999.

260. Pugh PJ, Grech ED: Syphilitic aortitis, *N Engl J Med* 346(9):676, 2002.

CHAPTER 38 Clinical Evaluation of Aortic Aneurysms

Joshua A. Beckman, Mark A. Creager

The vast majority of aortic aneurysms are asymptomatic, accounting for a much higher disease prevalence than hospitalization and mortality statistics would suggest (see Chapter 37). These data underscore the central challenge in aortic aneurysmal disease: a common clinical problem that is silent until rupture and death. Aortic aneurysms typically increase in size slowly over years or decades, with few warning signs. The management of aortic aneurysmal disease, therefore, requires suspicion and diligence to avoid adverse outcomes. This chapter will focus on the history, physical examination, and diagnostic tests important to clinical evaluation of aortic aneurysms.

Clinical History

Thoracic Aortic Aneurysms

Aneurysms of the thoracic aorta typically produce no symptoms, but a variety of symptom complexes may arise related to aneurysm size and location within the thorax.

Patients with aneurysmal dilation of the ascending thoracic aorta may develop clinical manifestations of congestive heart failure (CHF) as a consequence of aortic valvular regurgitation. Enlargement of the sinuses of Valsalva may cause myocardial ischemia or infarction due to direct compression of the coronary arteries or coronary arterial thromboembolism. Right ventricular (RV) outflow tract obstruction and tricuspid regurgitation may result from aneurysmal deformation of the noncoronary sinus. Aneurysms of the sinuses of Valsalva may rupture directly into the RV cavity, right atrium, or pulmonary artery, causing heart failure associated with a continuous murmur. Chest pain may occur when the aneurysm compresses surrounding structures or erodes into adjacent bone such as the ribs or sternum. Compression of the superior vena cava may produce venous congestion of the head, neck, and upper extremities. Symptoms are frequently a harbinger of rupture or death. Rupture may occur into the left pleural space, pericardium, pulmonary artery, or superior vena cava.

Aneurysms of the aortic arch may produce symptoms by compression of contiguous structures, but most are asymptomatic. Dyspnea or cough may be caused by compression of the trachea or mainstem bronchi, dysphagia by compression of the esophagus, or hoarseness secondary to left vocal cord paralysis related to compression of the left recurrent laryngeal nerve. The superior vena cava syndrome and pulmonary artery stenosis result when these vessels are compressed.[1,2] Chest pain, related either to compression of adjacent structures or to erosion of ribs or vertebrae, is typically positional. Aneurysms of the aortic arch may rupture into the mediastinum, pleural space, tracheobronchial tree (causing hemoptysis), or esophagus (causing hematemesis). Arteriovenous fistulas (AVFs) may result from rupture into the superior vena cava or pulmonary artery. Tuberculous aneurysms, akin to other causes of thoracic aortic aneurysms (TAAs), may present with pain but are commonly asymptomatic or may present with hypovolemic shock as a consequence of rupture.

Symptoms of descending TAAs include chest pain from compression of surrounding soft tissues or erosion of vertebrae. Irritation of the recurrent laryngeal nerve may produce hoarseness. Dyspnea may result from bronchial compression, and hemoptysis from direct erosion into the lung parenchyma. Dysphagia and hematemesis are features of esophageal compression or erosion. Rupture may occur into the mediastinum or left pleural space.

Thoracoabdominal Aortic Aneurysms

Although most patients with thoracoabdominal aortic aneurysms (TAAA) are asymptomatic, discomfort occasionally develops in the epigastrium or left upper quadrant of the abdomen. Back or flank pain may occur when the patient lies in left lateral decubitus position. Erosion of the anterior surfaces of the vertebral bodies may occur, leading to radiculopathy. Visceral artery occlusion may occur, but frank ischemia and infarction are infrequent. Patients who complain of claudication also may have occlusive atherosclerotic disease of the aorta, iliac, or more distal arteries. Because mural thrombosis is so common in atherosclerotic aneurysms, they may be the source of peripheral atheroembolism, causing occlusion of distal vessels. Rupture of the thoracic component of these aneurysms generally occurs into the left pleural space, producing a hemothorax; the abdominal component may rupture into the retroperitoneum, inferior vena cava, or duodenum.

Abdominal Aortic Aneurysms

Most patients with abdominal aortic aneurysms (AAAs) are asymptomatic, yet symptoms may take the form of abdominal discomfort or back pain; some patients become aware of abdominal pulsation. Less frequently, pain may occur in the legs, chest, or groin; anorexia, nausea, vomiting, constipation, or dyspnea may develop. Compression of the left iliac vein may cause left leg swelling, just as compression of the left ureter may cause hydronephrosis, or compression of testicular veins may cause varicocele. As the aneurysm expands and compresses vertebrae and lumbar nerve roots, pain may develop in the lower back and radiate to the posterior aspects of the legs. Flank pain radiating to the anterior left thigh or scrotum may reflect compression of the left genitofemoral nerve. Nausea and vomiting may occur as the aneurysm compresses the duodenum. Bladder compression may cause urinary frequency or urgency.

Occasionally, nascent or frank rupture occurs and causes symptoms indicating a life-threatening emergency. The mortality of patients with AAA rupture is 60%; patients with symptoms suggestive of rupture require emergent surgical referral. The classical triad associated with AAA rupture includes hypotension, back pain, and a pulsatile abdominal mass; however, fewer than 50% of patients have all components of this triad. Diverticulitis, renal colic, and gastrointestinal hemorrhage represent common disorders in the differential diagnosis in these patients.

In the absence of patient complaints, physicians must intuit the presence of aneurysm based on the clinical characteristics of the patient. Risk factors for aortic aneurysm disease (see Chapter 37) can be used to guide directed physical examination and, if necessary, diagnostic testing.

Physical Examination

Physical examination is usually unhelpful in diagnosing TAAs because the rib cage precludes palpation of the aorta. Physical examination may demonstrate right sternoclavicular lift or tracheal deviation. Dilation of the aortic root may cause aortic valve regurgitation.

The key physical finding for an AAA is a pulsatile abdominal mass. The patient should be positioned supine with the knees flexed. A pulsatile epigastric or periumbilical mass may be visible as well as palpable. To distinguish an AAA from paraaortic masses

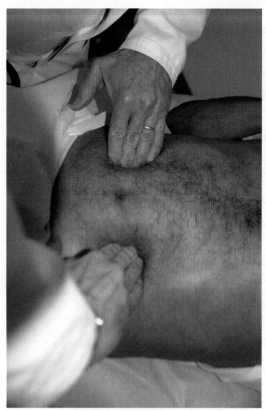

FIGURE 38-1 Examination to detect lateral borders of an aortic aneurysm should be performed with fingertips of both hands. Aneurysm should expand laterally with each heart beat. Aortic aneurysm transverse diameter may be estimated as distance between closest fingers.

only about 40% of such aneurysms are associated with bruits. Proper physical examination of the abdomen may detect the presence of an AAA in 30% to 48% of patients with AAA.[3,4] In a review of 15 studies, sensitivity of abdominal examination for aneurysm detection was 49%[4] (Table 38-1).

Several factors limit the potential for AAA diagnosis. First, palpation for an aneurysm requires consideration of the diagnosis prior to examination. Routine physical examination decreases the sensitivity of the exam. Second, size matters; as the size of an aneurysm increases, so does the likelihood of making the diagnosis. Sensitivity of palpation increases to 75% in patients with aneurysms greater than 5 cm in diameter.[4] Third, increasing abdominal girth decreases the likelihood of discovery. In one study of 201 patients, all six aneurysms present were diagnosed in patients with an abdominal girth less than 100 cm, but only 3 of 12 were detected when the abdominal girth exceeded 100 cm.[5] So although the directed physical examination has moderate sensitivity and specificity for AAA diagnosis, routine examination misses the diagnosis more commonly than making it.

The finding of a pulsatile mass in the groin, suggesting an iliac artery aneurysm, or in the popliteal fossa, suggesting a popliteal artery aneurysm, should raise the index of suspicion that an AAA may be present, since multiple aneurysms often coexist. Physical signs such as carotid bruits or diminished arterial pulses in the lower extremities may reflect atherosclerosis of other vessels.

Rupture of an AAA usually produces the clinical picture of extreme distress as a result of abdominal catastrophe. Despite surgical advances, mortality is still the rule because of the abrupt nature of circulatory collapse, which prevents timely intervention in most cases. Patients frequently have severe abdominal or back pain, but the pattern of pain varies considerably and may be either persistent or intermittent, sharp or dull, constricting or burning. The aneurysm may rupture into the retroperitoneum or into the peritoneal or pleural cavities. Patients may develop hypotension, tachycardia, pallor, diaphoresis, or shock, depending on the extent of rupture and associated blood loss into the extravascular space. On occasion, rupture occurs directly into the duodenum, causing an aortoduodenal fistula and acute gastrointestinal bleeding. This possibility should be considered when gastrointestinal bleeding is evident along with signs of an aneurysm on physical examination.

requires that the examiner's hands address the lateral borders (Fig. 38-1). *An aneurysm expands laterally with each systole.* This technique also permits estimation of the transverse diameter of the aneurysm. Auscultation may reveal a bruit over the mass, but abdominal bruits are not specific for aneurysm formation, and

TABLE 38-1	Sensitivity and Specificity of Physical Examination for Abdominal Aortic Aneurysm							
SOURCE	AGE RANGE	NO. SCREENED	ALL AAA	SENSITIVITY	4-4.9 CM AAA	SENSITIVITY	≥5 CM AAA	SENSITIVITY
Cabellon[55]	43-79	73	9	22%	NA	NA	NA	NA
Ohman[56]	50-88	50	3	0%	1	0%	0	NA
Twomey[57]	>50	200	14	64%	3	100%	4	75%
Allen[58]	>65	168	3	0%	0	NA	1	0%
Allardice[59]	39-90	100	15	33%	3	100%	2	100%
Lederle[5]	60-75	201	20	45%	5	20%	5	80%
Collin[60]	65-74	426	23	35%	NA	NA	NA	NA
Shapira[61]	31-83	101	4	0%	0	NA	2	0%
Andersson[62]	38-86	288	14	29%	NA	NA	NA	NA
Spiridonov[63]	17-67	163	10	70%	4	100%	3	100%
MacSweeney[64]	NA	200	55	24%	16	44%	6	100%
Karanjia[65]	55-82	89	9	100%	5	100%	2	100%
Molnar[66]	65-83	411	7	43%	3	33%	2	50%
al-Zahrani[67]	60-80	392	7	57%	4	50%	2	100%
Arnell[68]	55-81	96	1	100%	0	NA	0	NA
Fink[69]	51-88	200	99	68%	44	69%	14	82%
SUMMARY		3155	293	49%				

AAA, abdominal aortic aneurysm; NA, not available.
Adapted from Lederle FA, Simel DL: The rational clinical examination. Does this patient have abdominal aortic aneurysm? JAMA 281:77–82, 1999.

Rupture may also occur into the inferior vena cava or iliac veins, producing an arteriovenous fistula; this is suggested by rapid development of leg swelling or so-called high-output CHF in the presence of an AAA.

Screening and Surveillance of Aortic Aneurysms

Several trials have evaluated the possibility of reducing AAA event rates as a result of screening. In a study from Chichester, United Kingdom, 15,775 men and women aged 65 to 80 years were divided in two, and half were invited for an abdominal ultrasound screening.[6] Nearly 70% of those offered screening accepted the invitation, and aneurysm was detected in 4%. A 55% reduction in rate of aneurysm rupture (2.8 per 1000 vs. 6.2 per 1000 subjects) and a 42% reduction in AAA-related mortality in men only (3 per 1000 vs. 5.3 per 1000 male subjects) were noted in the screening group compared to controls. A similar study in Denmark offered 12,658 65- to 73-year-old males a screening invitation, of whom 9620 accepted and 3038 declined.[7] There was a tenfold reduction in AAA-related death in the group that accepted the invitation compared with those who did not (.006% vs. .06%). Only one trial has assessed the impact of screening on total mortality. The Multicentre Aneurysm Screening Study (MASS) assessed the impact of AAA screening in 67,800 men aged 65 to 74 years.[8] Half were invited for AAA screening, and the others were not. Long-term mortality was monitored in both groups. In the screened group, there was a 42% relative risk reduction in aneurysm-related mortality from 0.33% to 0.19%, representing 48 fewer deaths. Reduction in absolute mortality, however, was a statistically insignificant 0.27%.

Some clinical features exist to suggest which patients should definitely undergo screening for aortic aneurysm, and AAA in particular. These include patients with a family history for aneurysm and inherited disorders of connective tissue (e.g., Marfan's syndrome [MFS]) and those with arteritis (e.g., Takayasu and giant cell arteritis [GCA]). Siblings of patients with an AAA have a 25% chance of having an aneurysm.[9]

On the basis of these data, the American College of Cardiology/American Heart Association (ACC/AHA) Practice Guidelines for the Management of Peripheral Arterial Disease recommends that "Men 60 years of age or older who are either the siblings or offspring of patients with AAAs" and "men who are 65 to 75 years of age who have ever smoked should undergo a physical examination and one-time ultrasound screening for detection of AAAs."[10] The U.S. Preventive Services Task Force recommends one-time screening for AAA by ultrasonography in men aged 65 to 75 who have ever smoked, but does not recommend routine screening in women.[11] Medicare will pay for a one-time ultrasound screen during the "Welcome to Medicare" preventive visit if the patient has a family history of AAA or is a man aged 65 to 75 who has smoked at least 100 cigarettes in his lifetime.

Screening for TAAs is less well established. Recent data have shown that bicuspid aortic valve (BAV) disease is an autosomal dominant condition that may be associated with TAA formation. Interestingly, patients with this condition may manifest the valvular or aneurysmal findings alone or in tandem.[12] Thus, the ACC/AHA thoracic aortic disease guidelines recommend that all patients with a BAV should have both the aortic root and ascending thoracic aorta evaluated for evidence of aortic dilatation. In pedigree analysis of more than 500 patients with TAA, Albornoz et al. have shown that one in five non-MFS patients have an inherited pattern of disease.[13]

Because of the frequency of both known and unknown genetic conditions associated with TAA, the ACC/AHA thoracic aortic disease guidelines recommend that first-degree relatives of patients with a bicuspid aortic valve, premature onset of thoracic aortic disease with minimal risk factors, and/or a familial form of TAA and dissection should be evaluated for the presence of a BAV and asymptomatic thoracic aortic disease.[14]

Diagnostic Testing

Major objectives of imaging studies include identifying the aorta and its branches, diagnosing and characterizing the type of aneurysm (fusiform or saccular), determining the transverse and longitudinal dimensions of the aneurysm, and detecting associated pathology that may affect treatment. Imaging studies are also indicated for longitudinal surveillance of known aneurysms, or for anatomical definition before endovascular or surgical repairs. An understanding of the benefits and limitations of the several imaging modalities will enable appropriate test selection (Table 38-2).

Chest roentgenography may provide the first indication of a TAA (Fig. 38-2). Aneurysms of the ascending thoracic aorta are usually evident on the right side of the mediastinum. Aneurysms of the aortic arch widen the mediastinal shadow and may project more toward the left. These aneurysms may displace or compress the trachea or left mainstem bronchus. Descending TAAs typically appear as mediastinal masses extending into the left hemithorax. Assessment of the aorta by chest roentgenography requires both posteroanterior and lateral projections. Failure to detect TAA roentgenographically, however, does not exclude the diagnosis, since aneurysms may not become apparent until considerable dilation has occurred.

Similarly, plain abdominal roentgenography frequently discloses an unsuspected AAA.[3] Anteroposterior and lateral views of the abdomen may disclose a curvilinear rim of calcification in the wall of the aneurysm, and the diameter of the aneurysm may be estimated when such calcification is visible in two opposing walls. In 25% to 50% of suspected cases, however, the walls of the aneurysm are not sufficiently calcified to permit radiographic identification. Furthermore, it may underestimate anteroposterior aneurysm size by 15%.

TABLE 38-2 Abdominal Aortic Aneurysm Imaging Modalities: Strengths and Weaknesses

MODALITY	ADVANTAGES	DISADVANTAGES	OPTIMAL USE
Ultrasound	Highly accurate sizing Inexpensive	Unable to discern longitudinal extent Cannot define branch artery anatomy	Initial diagnosis Follow-up until repair
CT	Highly accurate sizing Defines branch artery involvement well	Ionizing radiation Contrast required	Pre-repair assessment Stent graft follow-up
MRA	Highly accurate sizing No ionizing radiation Defines branch artery involvement well	Cannot image some stent grafts	Pre-repair assessment
Contrast angiography	Defines branch artery involvement well	Cannot size aneurysm Invasive Ionizing radiation Contrast required	Stent graft implantation

NOTE: Sensitivity and specificity of each examination exceed 95% for diagnosis of abdominal aortic aneurysm (AAA). CT, computed tomography; MRA, magnetic resonance angiography.

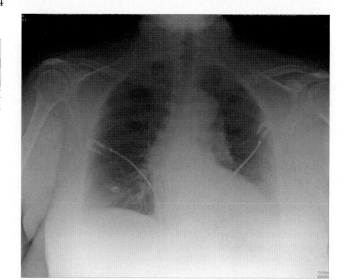

FIGURE 38-2 Posterior-anterior chest radiograph demonstrating widened mediastinum in patient with a 5-cm ascending thoracic aortic aneurysm (TAA).

Ultrasound

Ultrasonography is the most commonly used method for identification and characterization of AAA. It is the least expensive modality, does not expose the patient to ionizing radiation, and can accurately determine the anteroposterior, transverse, and longitudinal dimensions of an AAA (Fig. 38-3). Sensitivity for diagnosis of an AAA 3 cm or larger approaches 100%.[10] The examination is rapid and easily performed. The abdominal aorta is subject to anteroposterior, transverse, and longitudinal evaluation. Sonographic classification of AAA begins when the maximum diameter exceeds 3 cm in either anteroposterior or transverse dimensions. Care must be taken to image the aorta perpendicular to its longitudinal axis to avoid eccentricity, which may lead to overestimating its true diameter. Thrombus is frequently identified within the lumen, and echodense calcification may be present in or adjacent to the aortic wall. Beyond determining the size of an aneurysm, ultrasound imaging may help define the relation of major arterial branches and adjacent organs. Certain ultrasound characteristics have potential value in predicting rupture. Intramural hematoma, appearing as a hypoechoic soft-tissue mass surrounding the aorta that may silhouette the psoas muscle, appears to represent such a sign.[15] This may be indistinguishable from periaortic fibrosis, which appears on ultrasound examination as a hypoechoic mantle surrounding the aortic wall in patients with inflammatory aortic aneurysms.

Several groups have recently demonstrated the reliability of a "quick screen" in emergency departments.[16,17] In a prospective study of 125 emergency department patients, quick evaluations did not miss an AAA. Emergency department testing had 100% sensitivity and 98% specificity.[18] Indeed, accuracy is maintained at 100% when the "quick screen" and classical examination approaches are compared within a noninvasive vascular laboratory.[19]

Accuracy of ultrasonography should be considered in respect to other imaging modalities (see later discussion). In the Abdominal Aortic Aneurysm Detection and Management (ADAM) Veterans Administration Cooperative Study Group study, computed tomography (CT) and ultrasound were compared. Although both techniques demonstrated sizing variability between local and central reading sites,[20] in a third of subjects, the variation between ultrasound and CT was 0.5 cm or more. Ultrasonographic evaluation undersized the aneurysm by a mean of 0.27 cm compared with CT measurements. Similarly, in 334 patients participating in an aneurysm endograft study, CT reported a greater aneurysm diameter than ultrasound 95% of the time.[21] The correlation between the two measurements was strong at 0.7, but in nearly half the patients, aortic diameter varied by a centimeter or more between the ultrasound and CT studies. Smaller studies confirm both the high sensitivity yet consistent undersizing by ultrasound.

Despite these observations, two large surgical trials have shown that ultrasonography is an appropriate method to evaluate and follow AAA. The U.K. Small Aneurysm Trial[22] and the Aneurysm Detection and Management Trial[23] used ultrasonographic monitoring to determine the time of surgical repair in the group of patients randomized to surveillance. More recently, in the Comparison of Surveillance versus Aortic Endografting for Small Aneurysm Repair (CAESAR) trial, which compared early endovascular repair to watchful waiting, ultrasonographic monitoring was used similarly for monitoring.[24] In the absence of any clinical data suggesting the inadequacy of ultrasound, it remains the primary tool for diagnosis and follow-up.

Postoperatively, ultrasound can evaluate important ongoing clinical issues including perianeurysm aortic size and anastomotic aneurysm and pseudoaneurysm formation. Currently, duplex ultrasonography is not the ideal imaging test following endovascular aneurysm repair (EVAR). Its sensitivity and specificity are less than computed tomographic angiography (CTA) for a variety of problems encountered after endovascular aortic stent grafting (e.g., endoleaks, device migration, thrombosis), so it should not be used as the primary method of follow-up.[25] Improvements in technique, including contrast agents and three-dimensional (3D) imaging, are currently in development and likely will improve ultrasound's accuracy to diagnose complications of endografts.[26–28] Indeed, recent data suggest that ultrasonography may be approaching acceptability for EVAR follow-up.[29] In a prospective study, 108 patients underwent color Doppler ultrasound, contrast-enhanced ultrasonography, CTA, and magnetic resonance angiography (MRA) for follow-up after EVAR. Contrast-enhanced ultrasonography demonstrated accuracy similar to CTA and MRA, while all three were superior to color Doppler ultrasonography.[30]

Ultrasound can also be employed to diagnose and monitor TAA. Transthoracic echocardiography (TTA) visualizes the aortic root and a portion of the ascending aorta. Transesophageal echocardiography (TEE) images much of the thoracic aorta well,

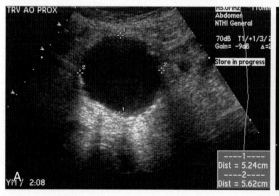
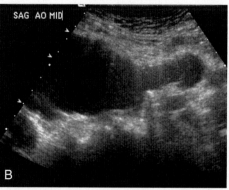

FIGURE 38-3 **A,** Transverse B-mode ultrasound image of widest portion of abdominal aorta. Electronic calipers have been applied and demonstrate a 5.6-cm transverse diameter and 5.2-cm anteroposterior diameter. **B,** Sagittal view of same vessel demonstrating transition from normal to aneurysmal aorta.

with sensitivity and specificity both above 95%[31] except where obscured by the trachea. The limitation of TEE for routine diagnostic purposes is that it requires sedation and is relatively invasive compared to other techniques to evaluate TAA, such as CT and magnetic resonance imaging (MRI) examinations (see later discussion).

Computed Tomography

Rapid advances in technology have put CTA in the forefront of aortic imaging (see Chapter 14). Contemporary multidetector-row CTA can acquire 320 simultaneous helices, creating high-resolution images and providing better sensitivity and specificity than could be obtained previously[32] (Figs. 38-4 and 38-5). Yet even with single-detector scanners, CT was able to determine aortic aneurysm size to within 0.2 mm.[33]

Computed tomographic angiography is now a preferred imaging modality for preoperative definition of aortic aneurysms because of its accuracy. Computed tomography can define the proximal and distal extension of AAAs[34] and determine the relationship of the aneurysm to branch arteries.[35] In a study of 30 patients undergoing AAA repair, both spiral CT and conventional contrast angiography were performed. Spiral CT had 100% sensitivity for determining aneurysm extent and better sized the aneurysm than angiography, but it revealed only 2 of 9 accessory renal arteries.[36] In one study comparing CTA to conventional angiography, CTA had 93% sensitivity and 96% specificity in determining clinically significant branch vessel stenoses (≥85%) and the presence of aneurysm.[37] Computed tomographic angiography has replaced angiography as the primary presurgical examination because it is noninvasive and provides detailed information about the vessel walls, such as inflammation, mural thrombus, and vascular calcification. Moreover, CTA creates better anatomical definition with various 3D visualization techniques[38] (Fig. 38-6). Also, it can diagnose abnormalities in adjacent structures. Recent data suggest that multidetector CTA has similar image quality and diagnostic accuracy as MRA, with 91% sensitivity and 98% specificity.[39]

Computed tomographic angiography also can demonstrate mural calcification and, with 3D reconstruction, show aortic angulation.[40] Placement of aortic stent grafts for AAA requires acquisition of specific anatomical information prior to the procedure. The most important parameter measured prior to placement of an endograft is the diameter of the neck. Modalities that create a cross-sectional image, including CT, can accurately determine vessel diameter.[41,42] Helical CT, MRA, and digital subtraction angiography (DSA) were compared in a prospective study of 61 patients planned for aortic stent graft placement.[43] Magnetic resonance angiography and helical CT were similar in their ability to determine proximal aneurysm extent and aortic diameter, but CT performed better in imaging accessory renal arteries and detecting

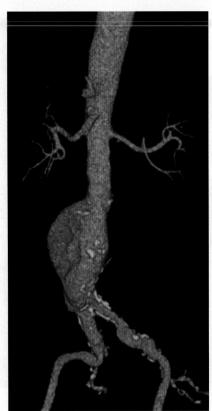

FIGURE 38-5 Three-dimensional (3D) reconstruction of abdominal aortic aneurysm (AAA) from a multidetector computer tomography angiographic (CTA) scan. Note infrarenal location of aneurysm, vascular calcification in white, and tortuosity of iliac arteries.

renal artery stenosis. Currently, 3D CTA reconstruction is becoming routine and may provide even better results than 2D images.[44]

Postoperatively, CT imaging is directed at the primary complications of stent grafts: endoleaks, device failure, aneurysm expansion, and aneurysm rupture. Determining the type of endoleak has important prognostic implications. In a study of 40 aortic stent graft patients, CTA was superior to DSA in determining the presence of endoleak, with a sensitivity of 92% for CTA and only 63% for DSA. Computed tomographic angiography also is effective in detecting stent graft migration, distortion, and destruction. Thus, CT imaging is indicated for preprocedural planning and post-endograft surveillance. After the implantation, imaging typically is performed at 3, 6, and 12 months and yearly thereafter.[42]

Computed tomographic angiography also is useful to image the thoracic aorta for diagnosis, follow-up, and perioperative management of TAA (Fig. 38-7). Computed tomographic can be used to follow aneurysm growth,[45] detecting changes as small as a millimeter. Use of contrast permits evaluation of aneurysms from any angle and the creation of 3D images. In one study of 49 patients, CT accurately assessed spinal cord circulation and predicted the requirement for hypothermic circulatory arrest 94% of the time.[46] Computed tomographic may also play an important role in follow-up of thoracic endovascular grafts by demonstrating volumetric changes in the aneurysm and thrombus suggestive of a successful repair.[47] Computed tomographic angiography accurately assess the thoracic aorta prior to operation, assists in operative planning, and is the standard imaging modality for follow-up.

Magnetic Resonance Imaging

Magnetic resonance imaging and angiography are also used to image and characterize aortic aneurysms (see Chapter 13). The technique has been used for diagnosis of AAA for more than 20 years[48] and is quite acceptable for preoperative evaluation (Fig. 38-8). Magnetic resonance angiography can determine aneurysm diameter, longitudinal extent, involvement of branch vessels,

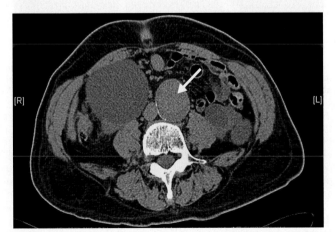

FIGURE 38-4 Coronal section of an x-ray multidetector computed tomographic (CT) scan of abdomen. Large white arrow indicates the abdominal aortic aneurysm.

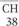

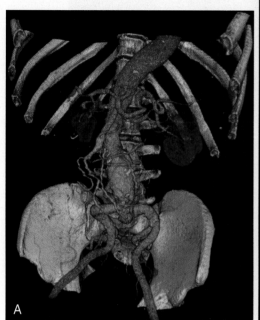

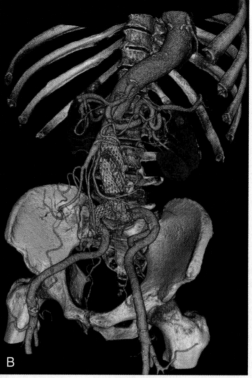

FIGURE 38-6 A 62-year-old man with abdominal aortic aneurysm (AAA) before (A) and after (B) placement of aortic stent. A, Patient underwent contrast-enhanced computed tomography (CT) for preinterventional evaluation of abdominal aorta and aneurysm, and for planning. **B,** After successful placement of stent, CT scan demonstrates effective exclusion of aneurysm and restitution of aortic lumen.

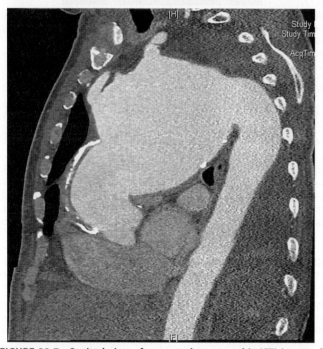

FIGURE 38-7   Sagittal view of computed tomographic (CT) image of thorax, demonstrating aneurysm involving ascending aorta and aortic arch, measuring more than 10 cm in diameter. *(From Tomey MI, Murthy VL, Beckman JA: Giant syphilitic aortic aneurysm: A case report and review of the literature. Vasc Med 16:360–364, 2011.)*

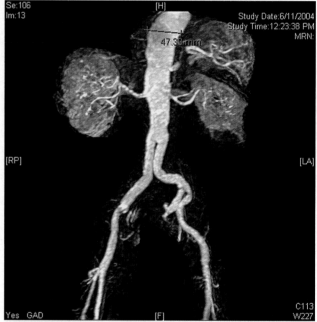

FIGURE 38-8 Maximal intensity projection (MIP) of magnetic resonance angiogram (MRA) demonstrating a 4.7-cm suprarenal abdominal aortic aneurysm (AAA).

and proximity to renal arteries. Both MRI and gadolinium-enhanced MRA have better than 90% sensitivity and specificity for determination of TAA.[49] Moreover, MRA has better than 90% sensitivity and specificity for detecting concordant stenoses in splanchnic, renal, or iliac branches.[50]

Magnetic resonance angiography is an accurate method for defining aortic anatomy, required prior to aortic endograft, and is superior to duplex ultrasonography.[41,51] Magnetic resonance angi-

ography is at least as good as CTA for postprocedural surveillance of stent grafts. In a study of 108 patients, MRA diagnosed endoleaks with sensitivity and specificity of 96% and 100%, respectively, compared with 83% and 100% for CTA.[30] Cine-MRA can show the pulsatility of the aneurysm and quantify AAA wall motion before and after endovascular graft placement to help identify endoleaks.

One of the more important issues associated with repair of the thoracic aorta is identifying the artery of Adamkiewicz. This artery arises most commonly from the left side of the aorta between T8 and L4 and supplies perfusion to the lower two thirds of the spinal cord. Both CT and MR, with their high spatial resolution, visualize

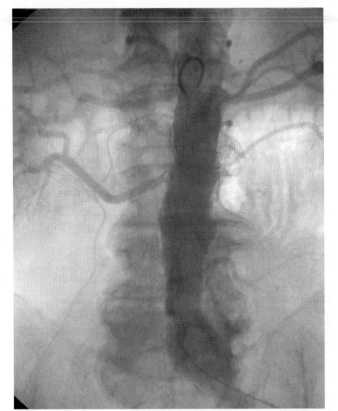

FIGURE 38-9 Contrast abdominal aortography revealing infrarenal abdominal aortic aneurysm (AAA). Note that angiogram cannot determine aneurysm size, but can show that renal arteries are not involved.

the artery well.[52,53] In a series of 30 patients with TAA, both MRA and CTA visualized the artery of Adamkiewicz via a clear identification of the vascular anatomy.[54]

Contrast Angiography

Contrast angiography is useful to define branch vessel anatomy and the longitudinal extent of aortic aneurysms (Fig. 38-9). Angiography, which provides information about the aortic lumen, cannot accurately size an aneurysm because it does not visualize the vessel wall or aneurysm thrombus. Digital subtraction angiography has similar accuracy to MRA and CTA in defining aneurysm length and aortic anatomy prior to endograft placement. In a study of 20 patients prior to endograft placement, length and diameter measurements were similar between MRA and CT, but superior to DSA.[51] Contrast angiography is less commonly performed than noninvasive imaging studies because of its invasive nature, the nephrotoxicity of contrast, and the lack of diagnostic superiority.

Once an aortic aneurysm is diagnosed, serial imaging studies should be performed every 3 to 12 months until the rate of expansion is 1 cm or more per year, or the diameter increases to a point that merits surgical or endovascular repair (see Chapters 39 and 40).

REFERENCES

1. Tomey MI, Murthy VL, Beckman JA: Giant syphilitic aortic aneurysm: a case report and review of the literature, *Vasc Med* 16:360–364, 2011.
2. Boulia SP, Metaxas E, Augoulea M, et al: Superior vena cava syndrome due to giant aortic aneurysm, *Asian Cardiovasc Thorac Ann* 18:396–397, 2010.
3. Karkos CD, Mukhopadhyay U, Papapostas I, et al: Abdominal aortic aneurysm: the role of clinical examination and opportunistic detection, *Eur J Vasc Endovasc Surg* 19:299–303, 2000.
4. Lederle FA, Simel DL: The rational clinical examination. Does this patient have abdominal aortic aneurysm? *JAMA* 281:77–82, 1999.
5. Lederle FA, Walker JM, Reinke DB: Selective screening for abdominal aortic aneurysms with physical examination and ultrasound, *Arch Intern Med* 148:1753–1756, 1988.
6. Scott RA, Wilson NM, Ashton HA, et al: Influence of screening on the incidence of ruptured abdominal aortic aneurysm: 5-year results of a randomized controlled study, *Br J Surg* 82:1066–1070, 1995.
7. Lindholt JS, Juul S, Fasting H, et al: Hospital costs and benefits of screening for abdominal aortic aneurysms. Results from a randomised population screening trial, *Eur J Vasc Endovasc Surg* 23:55–60, 2002.
8. Ashton HA, Buxton MJ, Day NE, et al: The Multicentre Aneurysm Screening Study (MASS) into the effect of abdominal aortic aneurysm screening on mortality in men: a randomised controlled trial, *Lancet* 360:1531–1539, 2002.
9. Frydman G, Walker PJ, Summers K, et al: The value of screening in siblings of patients with abdominal aortic aneurysm, *Eur J Vasc Endovasc Surg* 26:396–400, 2003.
10. Hirsch AT, Haskal ZJ, Hertzer NR, et al: ACC/AHA 2005 practice guidelines for the management of patients with peripheral arterial disease (lower extremity, renal, mesenteric, and abdominal aortic): a collaborative report from the American Association for Vascular Surgery/Society for Vascular Surgery, Society for Cardiovascular Angiography and Interventions, Society for Vascular Medicine and Biology, Society of Interventional Radiology, and the ACC/AHA Task Force on Practice Guidelines (Writing Committee to Develop Guidelines for the Management of Patients With Peripheral Arterial Disease): endorsed by the American Association of Cardiovascular and Pulmonary Rehabilitation; National Heart, Lung, and Blood Institute; Society for Vascular Nursing; TransAtlantic Inter-Society Consensus; and Vascular Disease Foundation, *Circulation* 113:e463–e654, 2006.
11. Screening for abdominal aortic aneurysm: recommendation statement, *Ann Intern Med* 142:198–202, 2005.
12. Loscalzo ML, Goh DL, Loeys B, et al: Familial thoracic aortic dilation and bicommissural aortic valve: a prospective analysis of natural history and inheritance, *Am J Med Genet A* 143A:1960–1967, 2007.
13. Albornoz G, Coady MA, Roberts M, et al: Familial thoracic aortic aneurysms and dissections–incidence, modes of inheritance, and phenotypic patterns, *Ann Thorac Surg* 82:1400–1405, 2006.
14. Hiratzka LF, Bakris GL, Beckman JA, et al: 2010 ACCF/AHA/AATS/ACR/ASA/SCA/SCAI/SIR/STS/SVM guidelines for the diagnosis and management of patients with thoracic aortic disease: a report of the American College of Cardiology Foundation/American Heart Association Task Force on Practice Guidelines, American Association for Thoracic Surgery, American College of Radiology, American Stroke Association, Society of Cardiovascular Anesthesiologists, Society for Cardiovascular Angiography and Interventions, Society of Interventional Radiology, Society of Thoracic Surgeons, and Society for Vascular Medicine, *Circulation* 121:e266–e369, 2010.
15. Cumming MJ, Hall AJ, Burbridge BE: Psoas muscle hematoma secondary to a ruptured abdominal aortic aneurysm: case report, *Can Assoc Radiol J* 51:279–280, 2000.
16. Kuhn M, Bonnin RL, Davey MJ, et al: Emergency department ultrasound scanning for abdominal aortic aneurysm: accessible, accurate, and advantageous, *Ann Emerg Med* 36:219–223, 2000.
17. Salen P, Melanson S, Buro D: ED screening to identify abdominal aortic aneurysms in asymptomatic geriatric patients, *Am J Emerg Med* 21:133–135, 2003.
18. Tayal VS, Graf CD, Gibbs MA: Prospective study of accuracy and outcome of emergency ultrasound for abdominal aortic aneurysm over two years, *Acad Emerg Med* 10:867–871, 2003.
19. Lee TY, Korn P, Heller JA, et al: The cost-effectiveness of a "quick-screen" program for abdominal aortic aneurysms, *Surgery* 132:399–407, 2002.
20. Lederle FA, Wilson SE, Johnson GR, et al: Variability in measurement of abdominal aortic aneurysms. Abdominal Aortic Aneurysm Detection and Management Veterans Administration Cooperative Study Group, *J Vasc Surg* 21:945–952, 1995.
21. Sprouse LR 2nd, Meier GH 3rd, Lesar CJ, et al: Comparison of abdominal aortic aneurysm diameter measurements obtained with ultrasound and computed tomography: is there a difference? *J Vasc Surg* 38:466–471, 2003 discussion 471–462.
22. Mortality results for randomised controlled trial of early elective surgery or ultrasonographic surveillance for small abdominal aortic aneurysms. The UK Small Aneurysm Trial Participants, *Lancet* 352:1649–1655, 1998.
23. Lederle FA, Wilson SE, Johnson GR, et al: Immediate repair compared with surveillance of small abdominal aortic aneurysms, *N Engl J Med* 346:1437–1444, 2002.
24. Cao P, De Rango P, Verzini F, et al: Comparison of surveillance versus aortic endografting for small aneurysm repair (CAESAR): results from a randomised trial, *Eur J Vasc Endovasc Surg* 41:13–25, 2011.
25. Teodorescu VJ, Morrissey NJ, Olin JW: Duplex ultrasonography and its impact on providing endograft surveillance, *Mt Sinai J Med* 70:364–366, 2003.
26. van Essen JA, Gussenhoven EJ, Blankensteijn JD, et al: Three-dimensional intravascular ultrasound assessment of abdominal aortic aneurysm necks, *J Endovasc Ther* 7:380–388, 2000.
27. Leotta DF, Paun M, Beach KW, et al: Measurement of abdominal aortic aneurysms with three-dimensional ultrasound imaging: preliminary report, *J Vasc Surg* 33:700–707, 2001.
28. Bendick PJ, Bove PG, Long GW, et al: Efficacy of ultrasound scan contrast agents in the noninvasive follow-up of aortic stent grafts, *J Vasc Surg* 37:381–385, 2003.
29. Nagre SB, Taylor SM, Passman MA, et al: Evaluating outcomes of endoleak discrepancies between computed tomography scan and ultrasound imaging after endovascular abdominal aneurysm repair, *Ann Vasc Surg* 25:94–100, 2011.
30. Cantisani V, Ricci P, Grazhdani H, et al: Prospective comparative analysis of colour-Doppler ultrasound, contrast-enhanced ultrasound, computed tomography and magnetic resonance in detecting endoleak after endovascular abdominal aortic aneurysm repair, *Eur J Vasc Endovasc Surg* 41:186–192, 2011.
31. Chirillo F, Cavallini C, Longhini C, et al: Comparative diagnostic value of transesophageal echocardiography and retrograde aortography in the evaluation of thoracic aortic dissection, *Am J Cardiol* 74:590–595, 1994.
32. Hein PA, Romano VC, Lembcke A, et al: Initial experience with a chest pain protocol using 320-slice volume MDCT, *Eur Radiol* 19:1148–1155, 2009.
33. Todd GJ, Nowygrod R, Benvenisty A, et al: The accuracy of CT scanning in the diagnosis of abdominal and thoracoabdominal aortic aneurysms, *J Vasc Surg* 13:302–310, 1991.
34. Simoni G, Perrone R, Cittadini G Jr, et al: Helical CT for the study of abdominal aortic aneurysms in patients undergoing conventional surgical repair, *Eur J Vasc Endovasc Surg* 12:354–358, 1996.

35. Posacioglu H, Islamoglu F, Apaydin AZ, et al: Predictive value of conventional computed tomography in determining proximal extent of abdominal aortic aneurysms and possibility of infrarenal clamping, *Tex Heart Inst J* 29:172–175, 2002.

36. Errington ML, Ferguson JM, Gillespie IN, et al: Complete pre-operative imaging assessment of abdominal aortic aneurysm with spiral CT angiography, *Clin Radiol* 52:369–377, 1997.

37. Raptopoulos V, Rosen MP, Kent KC, et al: Sequential helical CT angiography of aortoiliac disease, *AJR Am J Roentgenol* 166:1347–1354, 1996.

38. Filis KA, Arko FR, Rubin GD, et al: Three-dimensional CT evaluation for endovascular abdominal aortic aneurysm repair. Quantitative assessment of the infrarenal aortic neck, *Acta Chir Belg* 103:81–86, 2003.

39. Willmann JK, Wildermuth S, Pfammatter T, et al: Aortoiliac and renal arteries: prospective intraindividual comparison of contrast-enhanced three-dimensional MR angiography and multi-detector row CT angiography, *Radiology* 226:798–811, 2003.

40. Broeders IA, Blankensteijn JD: Preoperative imaging of the aortoiliac anatomy in endovascular aneurysm surgery, *Semin Vasc Surg* 12:306–314, 1999.

41. Lutz AM, Willmann JK, Pfammatter T, et al: Evaluation of aortoiliac aneurysm before endovascular repair: comparison of contrast-enhanced magnetic resonance angiography with multidetector row computed tomographic angiography with an automated analysis software tool, *J Vasc Surg* 37:619–627, 2003.

42. Whitaker SC: Imaging of abdominal aortic aneurysm before and after endoluminal stent-graft repair, *Eur J Radiol* 39:3–15, 2001.

43. Thurnher SA, Dorffner R, Thurnher MM, et al: Evaluation of abdominal aortic aneurysm for stent-graft placement: comparison of gadolinium-enhanced MR angiography versus helical CT angiography and digital subtraction angiography, *Radiology* 205:341–352, 1997.

44. Pitoulias GA, Donas KP, Schulte S, et al: Two-dimensional versus three-dimensional CT angiography in analysis of anatomical suitability for stentgraft repair of abdominal aortic aneurysms, *Acta Radiol* 52:317–323, 2011.

45. Masuda Y, Takanashi K, Takasu J, et al: Expansion rate of thoracic aortic aneurysms and influencing factors, *Chest* 102:461–466, 1992.

46. Quint LE, Francis IR, Williams DM, et al: Evaluation of thoracic aortic disease with the use of helical CT and multiplanar reconstructions: comparison with surgical findings, *Radiology* 201:37–41, 1996.

47. Czermak BV, Fraedrich G, Schocke MF, et al: Serial CT volume measurements after endovascular aortic aneurysm repair, *J Endovasc Ther* 8:380–389, 2001.

48. Amparo EG, Hoddick WK, Hricak H, et al: Comparison of magnetic resonance imaging and ultrasonography in the evaluation of abdominal aortic aneurysms, *Radiology* 154:451–456, 1985.

49. Krinsky GA, Rofsky NM, DeCorato DR, et al: Thoracic aorta: comparison of gadolinium-enhanced three-dimensional MR angiography with conventional MR imaging, *Radiology* 202:183–193, 1997.

50. Prince MR, Narasimham DL, Stanley JC, et al: Gadolinium-enhanced magnetic resonance angiography of abdominal aortic aneurysms, *J Vasc Surg* 21:656–669, 1995.

51. Engellau L, Albrechtsson U, Dahlstrom N, et al: Measurements before endovascular repair of abdominal aortic aneurysms. MR imaging with MRA vs. angiography and CT, *Acta Radiol* 44:177–184, 2003.

52. Yamada N, Okita Y, Minatoya K, et al: Preoperative demonstration of the Adamkiewicz artery by magnetic resonance angiography in patients with descending or thoracoabdominal aortic aneurysms, *Eur J Cardiothorac Surg* 18:104–111, 2000.

53. Kudo K, Terae S, Asano T, et al: Anterior spinal artery and artery of Adamkiewicz detected by using multi-detector row CT, *AJNR Am J Neuroradiol* 24:13–17, 2003.

54. Yoshioka K, Niinuma H, Ohira A, et al: MR angiography and CT angiography of the artery of Adamkiewicz: noninvasive preoperative assessment of thoracoabdominal aortic aneurysm, *Radiographics* 23:1215–1225, 2003.

55. Cabellon S Jr, Moncrief CL, Pierre DR, et al: Incidence of abdominal aortic aneurysms in patients with atheromatous arterial disease, *Am J Surg* 146:575–576, 1983.

56. Ohman EM, Fitzsimons P, Butler F, et al: The value of ultrasonography in the screening for asymptomatic abdominal aortic aneurysm, *Ir Med J* 78:127–129, 1985.

57. Twomey A, Twomey E, Wilkins RA, et al: Unrecognised aneurysmal disease in male hypertensive patients, *Int Angiol* 5:269–273, 1986.

58. Allen PI, Gourevitch D, McKinley J, et al: Population screening for aortic aneurysms, *Lancet* 2:736, 1987.

59. Allardice JT, Allwright GJ, Wafula JM, et al: High prevalence of abdominal aortic aneurysm in men with peripheral vascular disease: screening by ultrasonography, *Br J Surg* 75:240–242, 1988.

60. Collin J, Araujo L, Walton J, et al: Oxford screening programme for abdominal aortic aneurysm in men aged 65 to 74 years, *Lancet* 2:613–615, 1988.

61. Shapira OM, Pasik S, Wassermann JP, et al: Ultrasound screening for abdominal aortic aneurysms in patients with atherosclerotic peripheral vascular disease, *J Cardiovasc Surg (Torino)* 31:170–172, 1990.

62. Andersson AP, Ellitsgaard N, Jorgensen B, et al: Screening for abdominal aortic aneurysm in 295 outpatients with intermittent claudication, *Vasc Surg* 25:516–520, 1991.

63. Spiridonov AA, Omirov ShR: Selective screening for abdominal aortic aneurysms by using the clinical examination and ultrasonic scanning, *Grud Serdechnososudistaia Khir* 33–36, 1992.

64. MacSweeney ST, O'Meara M, Alexander C, et al: High prevalence of unsuspected abdominal aortic aneurysm in patients with confirmed symptomatic peripheral or cerebral arterial disease, *Br J Surg* 80:582–584, 1993.

65. Karanjia PN, Madden KP, Lobner S: Coexistence of abdominal aortic aneurysm in patients with carotid stenosis, *Stroke* 25:627–630, 1994.

66. Molnar LJ, Langer B, Serro-Azul J, et al: Prevalence of intraabdominal aneurysm in elderly patients, *Rev Assoc Med Bras* 41:43–46, 1995.

67. al-Zahrani HA, Rawas M, Maimani A, et al: Screening for abdominal aortic aneurysm in the Jeddah area, western Saudi Arabia, *Cardiovasc Surg* 4:87–92, 1996.

68. Arnell TD, de Virgilio C, Donayre C, et al: Abdominal aortic aneurysm screening in elderly males with atherosclerosis: the value of physical exam, *Am Surg* 62:861–864, 1996.

69. Fink HA, Lederle FA, Roth CS, et al: The accuracy of physical examination to detect abdominal aortic aneurysm, *Arch Intern Med* 160:833–836, 2000.

CHAPTER 39

Surgical Treatment of Abdominal Aortic Aneurysms

David H. Stone, Jack L. Cronenwett

Abdominal aortic aneurysms (AAAs) remain a leading cause of death in the elderly. In the United States, ruptured AAAs are the 15th leading cause of death overall and the 10th leading cause of death in men older than age 55.[1] In addition, 30% to 40% of patients with ruptured AAAs die after reaching a hospital, but without operation.[2] When combined with an operative mortality rate of 40% to 50%,[3-7] this results in an overall mortality rate of 80% to 90% for AAA rupture.[8-10] Unfortunately, this high mortality rate has not changed over the past 20 years despite improvements in operative technique and perioperative critical care management that have reduced the elective surgical mortality rate to less than 5% in most series.[3] Ruptured aneurysms also impose a substantial financial burden on overall healthcare costs. One report estimated that as much as $50 million and 2000 lives could have been saved in 1 year if AAAs had been repaired prior to rupture.[11] Another study showed that emergency operations for AAAs resulted in a mean financial loss to the hospital of $24,655 per patient.[12] These data have significant implications in an era of healthcare cost containment. For all these reasons, AAAs remain a central focus for vascular surgeons and an important healthcare problem for all physicians.

Definition

Most aortic aneurysms are true aneurysms involving all layers of the aortic wall and are infrarenal in location. As shown by Pierce et al.,[13] normal aortic diameter gradually decreases from the thorax (28 mm in men) to the infrarenal location (20 mm in men). At all anatomical levels, normal aortic diameter is approximately 2 mm larger in men than in women and increases with age and increased body surface area.[13] Because the average infrarenal aortic diameter is 2 cm, using a 3-cm definition for an infrarenal AAA has been recommended, without the need to consider a more complicated definition based on factors such as gender or body surface area. Although such definitions are useful for large patient groups, in clinical practice with individual patients, defining an aneurysm based on a 50% or greater diameter enlargement compared with the adjacent nonaneurysmal aorta has been recommended.[14] This is particularly true for patients with unusually small arteries, in whom even a 2.5-cm local dilation of the infrarenal aorta might be aneurysmal if the adjacent aorta were only 1.5 cm in diameter.

Decision Making for Elective Abdominal Aortic Aneurysm Repair

The choice between observation and elective surgical repair of an AAA for an individual patient at any given point should take into account the (1) rupture risk under observation, (2) operative risk of repair, (3) patient's life expectancy, and (4) personal preferences of the patient.[15,16] Two randomized trials have provided substantial information to assist with this decision-making process. The U.K. Small Aneurysm Trial was the first randomized trial to compare early surgery with surveillance of 4- to 5.5-cm diameter AAAs in 1090 patients aged 60 to 76.[17] Those undergoing surveillance underwent repeat ultrasound every 6 months for AAAs 4 to 4.9 in diameter cm, and every 3 months for those 5 to 5.5 cm. If AAA diameter exceeded 5.5 cm, the expansion rate was more than 1 cm/yr, the AAA became tender, or repair of an iliac or thoracic aneurysm was necessary, elective surgical repair was recommended. At the initial report in 1998, after a mean 4.6 years' follow-up, there was no difference in survival between the two groups. After 3 years, patients who had undergone early surgery had better

late survival, but the difference was not significant. It was notable that more than 60% of patients randomized to surveillance eventually underwent surgery at a median time of 2.9 years. Rupture risk among those undergoing careful surveillance was 1% per year.

In 2002, the U.K. trial participants published results of long-term follow-up.[18] At 8 years, there was a small survival advantage in the early surgery group (7.2% improved survival). However, the proportion of deaths due to rupture of an unrepaired AAA was low (6%). The early surgery group had a higher rate of smoking cessation, which may have contributed to a reduction in overall mortality. An additional 12% of surveillance patients underwent surgical repair during extended follow-up to bring the total to 74%. Fatal rupture occurred in only 5% of men but 14% of women in the surveillance group. Risk of rupture was more than four times higher for women than men. This prompted participants to recommend a lower-diameter threshold for elective AAA repair in women.

The Aneurysm Detection and Management (ADAM) study conducted at the U.S. Department of Veterans Affairs (VA) hospitals was published in 2002.[19] In this trial, 1163 veterans (99% male) aged 50 to 79 with AAAs 4 to 5.4 cm in diameter were randomized to either surveillance or early surgery. Surveillance entailed ultrasound or computed tomography (CT) scan every 6 months, with elective surgery for expansion to 5.5 cm, expansion of greater than 0.7 cm in 6 months or greater than 1 cm in 1 year, or development of symptoms attributable to the AAA. Computed tomography was used for initial evaluation, with AAA diameter defined as the maximal cross-sectional measurement in any plane that was perpendicular to the aorta. Ultrasound was used for the majority of surveillance visits, but CT was used when the diameter reached 5.3 cm. Patients with severe heart or lung disease were excluded, as were those who were not likely to comply with surveillance. As in the U.K. trial, there was no survival difference between the two strategies after a mean follow-up of 4.9 years. Similarly, more than 60% of patients in the surveillance arm underwent repair. Initial AAA diameter predicted subsequent surgical repair in the surveillance group; 27% of those with AAAs initially 4 to 4.4 cm underwent repair during follow-up, compared with 53% of those with 4.5 to 4.9 cm, and 81% of those with 5- to 5.4-cm diameter AAAs. Operative mortality was 2.7% in the early surgery group and 2.1% in the surveillance group. Rupture risk in those undergoing surveillance was 0.6% per year. This trial confirmed the results of the U.K. trial, demonstrating lack of benefit of early surgery for AAAs 4 to 5.5 cm, even if operative mortality is low. Compliance with surveillance was high in both trials. More recently, Ouriel et al. reported results of 728 patients who were randomized to either ultrasound surveillance or early endovascular AAA repair (EVAR). Mean follow-up of 20 ± 12 months demonstrated no difference in AAA rupture, aneurysm-related death, or overall mortality between groups.[20]

Taken together, these two large randomized studies indicate that it is generally safe to wait for AAA diameter to reach 5.5 cm before performing surgery in selected men who are compliant with surveillance, even if their operative mortality is predicted to be low even in the endovascular era. However, compliance in these carefully monitored trials of selected patients was high. In another VA population, Valentine et al.[21] reported that 32 of 101 patients undergoing AAA surveillance were noncompliant despite several appointment reminders, and 3 or 4 of these 32 patients experienced rupture. Additionally, the increased rupture risk for women seen in the U.K. trial highlights the need to individualize treatment on the basis of a careful assessment of individual patient characteristics (rupture risk, operative risk, life expectancy, and patient preferences).

Elective Operative Risk

As expected, considerable variation in operative risk occurs among individual patients and depends on specific risk factors. A meta-analysis by Steyerberg et al.[22] identified seven prognostic factors that were independently predictive of operative mortality with elective AAA repair and calculated the relative risk for these factors (Table 39-1). The most important risk factors for increased operative mortality were renal dysfunction (creatinine (Cr) >1.8 mg/dL), congestive heart failure (CHF) (cardiogenic pulmonary edema, jugular vein distension, or the presence of a gallop rhythm), and ischemic changes on resting electrocardiogram (ECG; ST depression >2 mm). Age had a limited effect on mortality when corrected for the highly associated comorbidities of cardiac, renal, and pulmonary dysfunction (mortality increased only 1.5-fold per decade). This explains the excellent results reported in multiple series in which selected octogenarians have undergone elective AAA repair, with mortality comparable to younger patients.[23]

On the basis of their analysis, Steyerberg et al.[22] developed a clinical prediction rule to estimate the operative mortality for individual patients undergoing elective AAA repair (Table 39-2). This scoring system takes into account the seven independent risk factors plus the average overall elective mortality for a specific center. To demonstrate the impact of the risk factors on a hypothetical patient, it can be seen that the predicted operative mortality for a 70-year-old man in a center with an average operative mortality of 5% could range from 2% if no risk factors were present to more than 40% if cardiac, renal, and pulmonary comorbidities were all present. Obviously this would have a substantial impact on the decision to perform elective AAA repair. A similar Bayesian model for perioperative cardiac risk assessment in vascular patients has been reported by L'Italien et al.,[24] which demonstrated the added predictive value of dipyridamole-thallium studies in patients with intermediate risk for cardiac death. This study also demonstrated the protective effect of coronary artery bypass surgery within the previous 5 years, which reduced the risk of myocardial infarction (MI) or death following AAA repair by 2.2-fold. Although this type of statistical modeling cannot substitute for experienced clinical judgment, it helps identify high-risk patients who might benefit from further evaluation, risk factor reduction, or medical management instead of surgery if AAA rupture risk is not high.

The review of Hallin et al.[5] supports the findings of Steyerberg's group that renal failure is the strongest predictor of mortality, with a four- to ninefold increased mortality risk. Cardiac disease (a history of either coronary artery disease [CAD], CHF, or prior MI) was associated with a 2.6- to 5.3-fold greater operative mortality risk. Older age and female gender appeared to be associated with increased risk, but the evidence was not as strong. Valuable data regarding predictors of operative risk have been generated by prospective trials. In the Canadian Aneurysm Study, overall operative mortality

TABLE 39-1	Independent Risk Factors for Operative Mortality After Elective Abdominal Aortic Aneurysm Repair		
RISK FACTOR	**ODDS RATIO***	**95% CONFIDENCE INTERVAL**	
Cr >1.8 mg/dL	3.3	1.5-7.5	
CHF	2.3	1.1-5.2	
ECG ischemia	2.2	1-5.1	
Pulmonary dysfunction	1.9	1-3.8	
Older age (per decade)	1.5	1.2-1.8	
Female gender	1.5	0.7-3	

*Indicates relative risk compared with patients without that risk factor.
CHF, congestive heart failure; Cr, creatinine; ECG, electrocardiogram.
From Steyerberg EW, Kievit J, de Mol Van Otterloo JC, et al: Perioperative mortality of elective abdominal aortic aneurysm surgery. A clinical prediction rule based on literature and individual patient data. Arch Intern Med 155:1998–2004, 1995.[22]

TABLE 39-2	Predicting Operative Mortality After Elective Abdominal Aortic Aneurysm Repair					
1. Surgeon-specific average operative mortality:						
Mortality (%):	3	4	5	6	8	12
Score:	−5	−2	0	+2	+5	+10 ___

2. Individual patient risk factors:

Age (yrs):	60	70	80
Score:	−4	0	+4
Gender:	Female	Male	
Score:	+4	0	
Cardiac comorbidity:	MI	CHF	ECG Ischemia
Score:	+3	+8	+8
Renal comorbidity:	Cr >1.8 mg/dL		
Score:	+12		
Pulmonary comorbidity:	COPD, dyspnea		
Score:	+7		

3. Estimated individual		**surgical mortality**				**TOTAL SCORE:** ___				
TOTAL SCORE:	−5	0	5	10	15	20	25	30	35	40
MORTALITY (%):	1	2	3	5	8	12	19	28	39	51

Based on total score from sum of scores for each risk factor (line 2), including surgeon-specific average mortality for elective AAA repair (line 1), estimate patient-specific mortality from the table (line 3).
AAA, abdominal aortic aneurysm; CHF, congestive heart failure; COPD, chronic obstructive pulmonary disease; Cr, creatinine; ECG, electrocardiogram; MI, myocardial infarction.
From Steyerberg EW, Kievit J, de Mol Van Otterloo JC, et al. Perioperative mortality of elective abdominal aortic aneurysm surgery. A clinical prediction rule based on literature and individual patient data. Arch Intern Med 155:1998–2004, 1995.[22]

was 4.8%.[25] Preoperative predictors of death were ECG evidence of ischemia, chronic pulmonary disease, and renal insufficiency. The randomized U.K. Small Aneurysm Trial found older age, lower forced expiratory volume in 1 second (FEV$_1$), and higher Cr to be associated with mortality on univariate analysis.[26] With multivariate analysis, the effect of age was diminished, whereas renal disease and pulmonary disease remained strong predictors of operative mortality. The predicted mortality ranged from 2.7% for younger patients with below average Cr and above average FEV$_1$ to 7.8% in older patients with above average Cr and below average FEV$_1$. The U.K. trialists noted that the Steyerberg prediction rule did not work well for the U.K. trial patients. However, they did not gather information on a history of CHF (one of the strongest predictors in Steyerberg's analysis) in the randomized trial. Female gender has also been found to be associated with higher operative risk in several population-based studies using administrative data.[3,22,27,28] However, these databases may suffer from inaccurate coding of comorbidities and thereby lack of ability to fully adjust for comorbid conditions.[29] Gender has not been found to be associated with operative mortality in prospective trials.[26,30]

More recently, a study by Beck et al. from the Vascular Study Group of New England assessed risk factors associated with 1-year mortality following open AAA repair and EVAR. In this study, 1387 consecutive patients between 2003 and 2007 underwent elective AAA repair, including 748 who underwent open repair and 639 who underwent EVAR. Consistent with other studies, factors associated independently with 1-year mortality following open AAA repair included age (>70 years), chronic obstructive pulmonary disease (COPD), chronic renal insufficiency (Cr >1.8 mg/dL) and suprarenal aortic clamp site. Likewise, factors associated with 1-year mortality following EVAR included CHF and AAA diameter. One-year mortality correlated linearly with the number of risk factors present, and accordingly should be factored into decision making when considering elective AAA repair.[31]

Life Expectancy

Assessment of life expectancy is crucial to determine whether an individual patient will benefit from prophylactic repair of an AAA. Many patients with AAAs have been long-term smokers. Most AAA patients also have extensive comorbid disease, particularly CAD, COPD, hypertension, hyperlipidemia, cerebrovascular disease, and cancer.[32–37] Many of these chronic conditions increase operative risk, as noted earlier. In addition, these factors impact life expectancy. Patients who survive elective AAA repair have a reduced life expectancy compared to age- and gender-matched populations.[38–40] In 2001, Norman et al.[41] reviewed 32 publications over 20 years that described long-term survival after AAA repair. They found that the mean 5-year survival after AAA repair was 70%, compared with 80% in the age- and gender-matched population without AAA. Predictors of late death after successful AAA repair include age, cardiac disease, chronic pulmonary disease, renal insufficiency, and continued smoking.[38,42,43] The U.K. trialists found (after adjustment for age, gender, and AAA diameter but not cardiac disease) that both FEV_1 and current smoking status (plasma cotinine) predicted late death.[43]

Surgical Decision Making

In patients with symptomatic AAAs, operative repair is nearly always appropriate because of the high mortality associated with rupture or thrombosis and the high likelihood of limb loss associated with peripheral embolism. Occasionally, high-risk patients or those with short life expectancies may choose to forego emergency repair of symptomatic AAAs, but in general, surgical decision making for symptomatic AAAs is straightforward. A contemporary analysis of outcomes of symptomatic AAAs by De Martino et al. from the Vascular Study Group of New England recently assessed 2386 AAA repairs in whom 1959 were elective, 156 were symptomatic, and 271 were ruptured. EVAR was successfully performed in 945 elective patients, 60 symptomatic patients, and 33 ruptured AAA patients, respectively. Hospital mortality was 1.7% for elective AAA, compared to 1.3% for the symptomatic cohort. One- and 4-year survival was determined to be 83% and 68%, respectively, among the symptomatic group, which compared favorably to the elective group with 89% and 73% 1- and 4-year survival.[44]

For those with asymptomatic AAAs, randomized trials have provided assurance that the typical male patient can generally be safely monitored with careful ultrasound surveillance until the AAA reaches 5.5 cm, at which time elective repair can be performed. However, decision analyses and cost-effectiveness modeling have previously demonstrated that individual patient rupture risk, operative risk, and life expectancy have to be considered to determine the optimal threshold for intervention.[15,16,45,46] Both the U.K. and ADAM trials excluded patients who were considered "unfit" for repair, highlighting the fact that those with high operative risk and short life expectancy should have a threshold diameter greater than 5.5 cm. In the U.K. trial, the rupture risk for women was 4.5-fold higher than for men, prompting the authors to recommend a lower threshold for women than men, so it seems logical to consider other factors that may make rupture more likely during surveillance as well. In both randomized trials, 60% to 75% of patients undergoing surveillance eventually underwent AAA repair.[19,47] In the U.K. trial, 81% of those with initial diameters 5 to 5.4 cm eventually underwent repair. Clearly, for many patients with this size AAA, the question is not *whether* to perform AAA repair but *when*. Therefore, in patients with AAA diameters approaching 5.5 cm whose life expectancy is expected to be more than 5 years and whose operative risk is estimated to be low, the patient should be informed that AAA repair would likely be required within the next few years. This subgroup of patients could be offered surgery at a time when it is convenient for them, with the understanding that waiting for expansion to 5.5 cm has little risk. In these cases, patient preference should weigh heavily in the decision-making process. For those with multiple risk factors for rupture, long life expectancy, and low operative risk, it would seem prudent to recommend AAA repair at less than 5.5 cm. Additionally, the ability of the patient to comply with careful surveillance should be considered. Although the recent randomized trials have provided a great deal of information to guide decision making, clinicians should

not adopt a one-size-fits-all policy for treating patients with AAA. Moreover, with a progressively aging population in mind, quality-of-life assessments should likely be factored into decision-making analyses as well.

Preoperative Assessment

Patient Evaluation

A careful history, physical examination, and basic laboratory data are the most important factors for estimating perioperative risk and subsequent life expectancy. These factors may not only influence the decision to perform elective AAA repair, but they may focus preoperative management to reduce modifiable risk. Assessments of activity level, stamina, and stability of health are important and can be translated into metabolic equivalents to help assess both cardiac and pulmonary risks.[48] Because COPD is an independent predictor of operative mortality,[26,30] it should be assessed by pulmonary function studies as well as room air arterial blood gas measurement in patients who have apparent pulmonary disease. In some cases, preoperative treatment with bronchodilators and pulmonary toilet can reduce operative risk.[49] In more extreme cases, pulmonary risk may substantially reduce life expectancy, and in these patients, formal pulmonary consultation may be helpful to estimate survival. Serum Cr is one of the most important predictors of operative mortality[25] and must be assessed. The impact of other diseases such as malignancy on expected survival should also be carefully considered.

It is well established that patients with AAAs have a high prevalence of CAD. By performing routine preoperative coronary arteriography at the Cleveland Clinic in 1979, Hertzer et al.[50] reported that only 6% of patients with AAAs had normal arteries; 29% had mild to moderate CAD, 29% had advanced compensated CAD, 31% had severe correctable CAD, and 5% had severe uncorrectable CAD. Furthermore, this study established that clinical prediction of the severity of CAD was imperfect because 18% of patients without clinically apparent CAD had severe correctable CAD on arteriography, compared with 44% of patients whose CAD was clinically apparent. This pivotal study has led to intense efforts to identify risk factors and algorithms that more accurately predict the presence of severe CAD that would justify its correction before AAA repair, or would lead to avoiding AAA repair. A number of clinical parameters such as angina, history of MI, Q-wave on ECG, ventricular arrhythmia, CHF, diabetes, and increasing age have been reported to increase the risk of postoperative cardiac events.[51] Various combinations of these risk factors have been used to generate prediction algorithms for perioperative cardiac morbidity.[48] In general, these algorithms identify low-risk, high-risk, or intermediate-risk patients. For high-risk patients, such as those with unstable angina, more sophisticated cardiac evaluation is required, whereas low-risk patients may undergo elective AAA repair without further testing. For intermediate-risk patients, who comprise the vast majority with AAAs, decision making is more difficult and may be assisted by additional cardiac testing.[51]

Aneurysm Evaluation

Most surgeons recommend a preoperative imaging study using CT scanning, magnetic resonance imaging or angiography (MRI/MRA), or arteriography. Contrast-enhanced CT appears to be the most useful study for preoperative AAA evaluation when considering information obtained, invasiveness, and cost (also see Chapter 14). This is particularly true for spiral CT scanning, with thin "slices" in the region of interest. This allows not only accurate size measurements but also accurate definition of the relationship of an AAA to visceral and renal arteries. Furthermore, CT scanning aids in identifying venous anatomical anomalies (e.g., retroaortic left renal vein, duplicated vena cava) or renal abnormalities (e.g., horseshoe or pelvic kidney) that would influence operative techniques and approach. Computed tomography is the technique of choice to identify suspected inflammatory aneurysms and may reveal unsuspected abdominal pathology such as associated malignancy or gallbladder disease. In centers with experience with these techniques, CT angiography has made percutaneous intraarterial angiography unnecessary in the vast majority of AAA patients. Moreover, in the EVAR era, CT is vital for case planning and accurate detailed anatomical assessment of aortic neck anatomy, iliac artery anatomy and tortuosity, and perirenal mural thrombus burden among other factors. In addition, three-dimensional (ED) modeling of contemporary CT scanning is useful prior to EVAR as well as open AAA repair and has largely supplanted the role of conventional angiography.

Magnetic resonance imaging is comparable with CT in terms of AAA measurement accuracy and other preoperative planning issues (also see Chapter 13). It avoids intravenous contrast, which may represent an advantage over CT for some patients. Because it is more expensive and time consuming, it also is not as widely used as CT. When MRA is included with this technique, however, it can significantly increase the value in patients where additional imaging would otherwise be required.

Surgical Treatment

For the past 40 years, AAAs have been repaired using the technique of endoaneurysmorrhaphy with intraluminal graft placement, as described by Creech.[52] This procedure is described later in the section on transperitoneal approach. Development of this technique was based in part on the failure of previous "nonresective" operations now of only historical interest, including aneurysm ligation, wrapping, and attempts at inducing aneurysm thrombosis that yielded uniformly dismal results. Abdominal aortic aneurysm thrombosis by iliac ligation combined with axillobifemoral bypass enjoyed a brief resurgence in popularity for high-risk patients but demonstrated a high complication rate, including late aneurysm rupture, and an operative mortality rate comparable with conventional repair in similar patients.[53-57] Thus this technique was similarly abandoned. As an alternative to standard open AAA repair, Shah and Leather et al.[58] proposed exclusion of an AAA with bypass to reduce operative blood loss. However, this group has recently published long-term follow-up and no longer recommends this procedure owing to persistent flow in the excluded AAA sac and rupture in rare cases.[59] In another attempt to reduce the invasiveness of open AAA repair, the use of laparoscopy as an adjunct has been suggested to assist AAA repair. This approach uses laparoscopic techniques to dissect the aneurysm neck and iliac arteries, followed by a standard endoaneurysmorrhaphy through a mini-laparotomy. Cohen et al.[60] have reported their results in 20 patients to demonstrate the feasibility of this approach, but a clear benefit has not been shown; intraoperative, intensive care unit (ICU), and total hospital duration were comparable with conventional AAA repair. Further experience with this technique may identify a subgroup of patients for whom a laparoscopic-assisted AAA repair is advantageous.

EVAR (see Chapter 40) repair was introduced by Parodi in 1991 and has rapidly gained in popularity in the United States after reports of clinical trials and subsequent U.S. Food and Drug Administration (FDA) approval.[61] Endovascular AAA repair has been shown to reduce operative morbidity, mortality, length of stay, and disability compared with open repair.[62-65] Recovery time is shorter after endovascular repair than open repair,[63,66] but endovascular repair may not be as durable.[67-74] Frequent and lifelong surveillance is required after endovascular repair, along with reintervention or conversion to open repair in some. There appears to be a small ongoing risk of rupture after endografting as well. Decision analysis suggests that there is little difference in outcome between open and endovascular repair for most patients.[72] However, endovascular AAA repair is usually recommended for those with good anatomy for EVAR or those with marginal anatomy but high operative risk for open surgery. Open surgery may be preferred for younger, healthier patients in whom there is little difference in operative risk between the two strategies, and for whom long-term

durability is a concern, although contemporary stent grafts appear to have improved durability from their initial constructs and are now recommended for most patients with acceptable anatomy (see Chapter 40).

To date, there are several important randomized trials comparing open AAA repair with endovascular repair. Specifically, in the EVAR I and DREAM trials, patients were randomized to either open repair or EVAR. The EVAR I study demonstrated a 3% lower initial mortality associated with endovascular treatment, with a persistent associated reduction in AAA-related death at 4 years. However, there was no overall improvement in all-cause mortality between groups. Likewise, the DREAM trial demonstrated an operative mortality advantage associated with EVAR compared to open surgical repair, but 1-year survival was similar between groups. The EVAR II study randomized patients unfit for open AAA repair to either EVAR or no surgical therapy. This trial failed to demonstrate a survival advantage for the EVAR treatment group compared to the no treatment group. It should be noted, however, that most ruptures in the EVAR group occurred during a prolonged delay before surgery, making the results in this group appear worse. In addition, 27% of patients in EVAR II crossed over from the no treatment group to the EVAR group, potentially limiting the study's findings.[71,75-77] Likewise, the VA Open vs. Endovascular AAA repair (OVER) study randomized patients to either open AAA repair or EVAR. Results demonstrated diminished perioperative mortality in the EVAR group compared to the open repair group (0.5% vs. 3.0%). However, there was no observed difference in mortality at 2 years between groups. This study also demonstrated diminished median procedure times, blood loss, transfusion requirement, duration of mechanical ventilation, hospital length of stay, and ICU length of stay in the EVAR group.[78]

These trials illustrate many of the advantages of EVAR therapy or open surgery. However, the ultimate treatment must be individually tailored to specific patients, especially those with high associated surgical risk. Ongoing rapid advances in stent graft technology will have to be considered in the future as device applicability and accompanying morbidity change.

Perioperative Management

Preoperative intravenous antibiotics are administered to reduce the risk of prosthetic graft infection.[79] Ample intravenous access, intraarterial pressure recording, and Foley catheter monitoring of urine output are routine. For patients with significant cardiac disease, pulmonary artery catheters are frequently used to guide volume replacement and vasodilator or inotropic drug therapy, both intraoperatively and in the early postoperative period. Mixed venous oxygen tension measurement, available with these catheters, can provide an additional estimate of global circulatory function. Transesophageal echocardiography (TEE) can be useful in certain patients to monitor ventricular volume and cardiac wall motion abnormalities and to guide fluid administration and use of vasoactive drugs. Despite the frequent use of pulmonary artery catheters, studies examining their use during AAA surgery have not demonstrated added value.[80,81] However, these studies have usually excluded high-risk patients who are most likely to benefit from such monitoring. These techniques are not without risk, so selective use is probably more appropriate than routine application.

The volume of blood lost during AAA repair often requires blood replacement. Therefore, intraoperative autotransfusion as well as preoperative autologous blood donation has become popular, primarily to avoid the infection risk associated with allogeneic transfusion. Studies of the cost-effectiveness of such procedures, however, question their routine use.[82-84] Autologous blood donation is less important for elderly patients in whom life expectancy is shorter than the usual time for development of transfusion-associated viral illness. Autologous blood donation does not appear to be cost-effective in elderly cardiovascular patients, because the allogenic blood pool has become safer and the transfusion requirement for elective AAA repairs lower.[82]

Intraoperative autotransfusion during AAA repair is widely used because of the documented safety of this technique.[85] Because it is usually difficult to predict the volume of blood loss during AAA repair, most surgeons employ autotransfusion in case blood loss becomes extensive. Optimizing oxygen delivery to patients with reduced cardiac output by maintaining an adequate hematocrit appears beneficial in patients undergoing AAA repair. One study has shown that a postoperative hematocrit of less than 28% was associated with significant cardiac morbidity in vascular surgery patients.[86]

Maintenance of normal body temperature during aortic surgery is important to prevent coagulopathy, allow extubation, and maintain normal metabolic function. In a review of patients undergoing elective AAA repair, Bush et al.[87] noted significantly more organ dysfunction (53% vs. 29%) and higher mortality (12% vs. 1.5%) in hypothermic patients (temperature <34.5°C) compared with normothermic patients. The only predictor of intraoperative hypothermia was female gender, whereas prolonged hypothermia was related to initial hypothermia, indicating the difficulty in rewarming cold patients. A recent randomized trial found significantly reduced cardiac morbidity (1.4% vs. 6.3%) in patients who were normothermic (36.7°C) rather than hypothermic (35.4°C) intraoperatively.[88] To prevent hypothermia, a recirculating warm forced-air blanket should be placed in contact with the patient, and intravenous fluids, including any blood returned from an autotransfusion device, should be warmed before administration.

The role of ischemic preconditioning in lowering the incidence of perioperative MI during open AAA repair remains undefined, although there are data to support its potential benefit. In the largest study to date, Ali et al. randomized 82 patients undergoing elective open AAA repair to receive remote ischemic preconditioning or not. The technique involves sequential clamping of each common iliac artery (CIA) for 10 minutes, followed by 10 minutes of respective reperfusion. The authors demonstrated that patients undergoing remote ischemic preconditioning had both diminished rates of postoperative MI and diminished critical care length of stay compared with the control groups.[89]

Anesthesia

Nearly all patients undergo general anesthesia for AAA repair. Supplemental use of continuous epidural anesthesia, begun immediately preoperatively and continued for postoperative pain control, is increasing in popularity.[90] This technique allows a lighter level of general anesthesia to be maintained while controlling pain through the epidural blockade. Additional benefits may include a reduction in the sympathetic catecholamine stress response, which might decrease cardiac complications. One randomized trial comparing general anesthesia with combined general and epidural anesthesia demonstrated decreased deaths, cardiac events, infection, and overall complications.[91] These benefits, however, were not observed in another randomized trial,[92] suggesting that the details of perioperative management and patient selection may determine the impact of epidural anesthesia. Furthermore, it is possible that the major benefit of epidural anesthesia accrues in the postoperative period rather than intraoperatively.[93]

Perioperative β-adrenergic blockade remains somewhat more controversial, given recent findings of randomized controlled trials.[94] Earlier studies by Pasternack et al.[95] demonstrated that patients who underwent vascular surgery and received metoprolol immediately before operation had significantly lower heart rates and less intraoperative myocardial ischemia than untreated controls. Mangano et al.[96] performed the first randomized placebo-controlled trial to assess the effect of atenolol (given intravenously immediately before and after surgery and orally during that hospitalization) in patients at risk for CAD who underwent noncardiac surgery. A significant reduction in mortality extending 2 years after discharge was observed in the atenolol-treated patients (3% vs. 14% 1-year mortality) because of reduction in death from cardiac causes. In a separate analysis, they noted that

atenolol-treated patients had a 50% lower incidence of myocardial ischemia during the first 48 hours after surgery and a 40% lower incidence during postoperative days 0 to 7.[97] Patients with perioperative myocardial ischemia were significantly more likely to die within 2 years after surgery. Poldermans et al.[98] performed a randomized trial of perioperative β-blockade with bisoprolol in patients with abnormal dobutamine echocardiograms undergoing aortic or lower-extremity arterial reconstruction. They found that perioperative cardiac death was significantly reduced from 17% (placebo) to 3% (bisoprolol). Additionally, nonfatal MI occurred in 17% of those given placebo but in none of those given bisoprolol. A subsequent publication from the same authors demonstrated that during a mean follow-up of 22 months, cardiac events were significantly lower in those who had received perioperative β-blockade (12% vs. 32%).[99]

More recently, however, results from the POISE trial, a randomized controlled trial reflecting 190 hospitals, 23 countries, and an enrollment of 8351 patients, provided different results. This study compared the effects of perioperative extended release metoprolol succinate with a limited titration scheme to placebo among patients undergoing noncardiac surgery. Results demonstrated that there was a significant reduction in the composite endpoint of cardiovascular death, nonfatal MI, and nonfatal cardiac arrest among patients receiving perioperative β-blocker therapy. However, the study also revealed that there were more deaths and strokes among the treated group compared to placebo.[94] Although these findings seemingly conflict, perioperative β-blocker use is valuable when titrated to heart rate, but not when applied at initial high dose or without respect to the patient's hemodynamics.[100]

Given this knowledge, it has been suggested that β-blockers are underused, likely because of fears about use in patients with COPD or prior heart failure. However, chronic β-blocker usage is now known to improve outcomes in patients with heart failure.[101,102] Additionally, Gottlieb et al.[101] demonstrated that COPD should not be considered a contraindication for β-blockade. They found a 40% reduction in risk of death after MI in patients with COPD who were taking β-blockers compared with those who were not. In Mangano's trial, the only exclusion criteria were preexisting ECG abnormalities that would preclude detection of new ischemic events. β-Blockers were withheld during the trial only for a heart rate of less than 55 beats/min, systolic blood pressure less than 100 mmHg, acute bronchospasm, current evidence of CHF, or third-degree heart block. The weight of evidence supports routine use of β-blockers for nearly all patients undergoing AAA repair.

Antiplatelet use remains common in this patient cohort, concordant with American College of Cardiology/American Heart Association (ACC/AHA) guidelines for noncardiac surgery. Associated bleeding risk with such agents, including aspirin and clopidogrel, remains controversial. In a recent study by the Vascular Study Group of New England, however, preoperative antiplatelet use (aspirin alone, clopidogrel alone, combined dual therapy) was not significantly associated with increased serious bleeding complications, measured as reoperation for bleeding across a spectrum of commonly performed vascular procedures including EVAR, open AAA repair, carotid endarterectomy, and lower-extremity bypass.[103]

Choice of Incision

Abdominal aortic aneurysm repair can be accomplished through an anterior transperitoneal incision (midline or transverse; Fig. 39-1) or through a retroperitoneal approach (Fig. 39-2). Midline transperitoneal incisions can be performed rapidly and provide wide access to the abdomen, but they may be associated with more pulmonary complications due to postoperative splinting from upper abdominal pain. Transverse abdominal incisions just above or below the umbilicus require more time to open and close, but may be associated with fewer pulmonary complications and late incisional hernias, although this has not yet been proven. Retroperitoneal incisions, from the lateral rectus margin extending

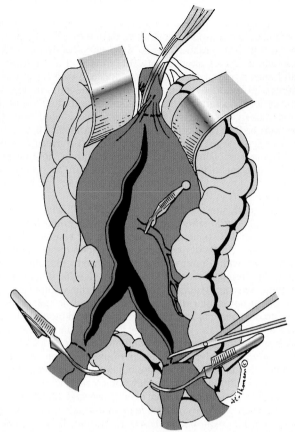

FIGURE 39-1 Transperitoneal abdominal aortic aneurysm (AAA) exposure, vascular clamps in place, incising the aneurysm.

into the 10th or 11th intercostal space, afford good exposure of both the infrarenal and suprarenal aorta, but limit exposure of the contralateral renal and iliac arteries. In addition, this exposure does not allow access to intraabdominal organs unless the peritoneum is purposely opened. The left retroperitoneal approach is usually favored over the right for exposure of the upper abdominal aorta because the spleen is easier to mobilize and retract than the liver. The right retroperitoneal approach is used when specific abdominal problems, such as a stoma, preclude the left-sided approach.[104]

In recent years, the left retroperitoneal approach has enjoyed a resurgence in popularity owing to suggestions that pulmonary morbidity, ileus, and intravenous fluid requirements are decreased postoperatively. Randomized trials have reached different conclusions about the potential advantages of retroperitoneal over transabdominal incisions, however. Sicard et al.[105] reported more prolonged ileus, small-bowel obstruction, and overall complications after transabdominal compared with retroperitoneal aortic surgery, although pulmonary complications were similar. Cambria et al.[106] found no differences in these incisions in terms of pulmonary complications, fluid or blood requirements, or other postoperative complications, except for slightly prolonged return to oral intake after the transperitoneal approach.

In the most recent randomized trial, Sieunarine et al.[107] found no differences in operating time, cross-clamp time, blood loss, fluid requirement, analgesia requirement, gastrointestinal function, ICU stay, or hospital stay for transperitoneal versus retroperitoneal approaches for aortic surgery. In long-term follow-up, however, there were significantly more wound problems (hernias, bulging, and pain) in the retroperitoneal group. These results suggest that in most cases, the choice of incision for AAA repair is a matter of personal preference. However, both the transperitoneal and retroperitoneal approaches have advantages in certain patients. Relative indications for retroperitoneal exposure include a "hostile" abdomen due to multiple previous transperitoneal

operations, an abdominal wall stoma, a horseshoe kidney, an inflammatory aneurysm, or anticipated need for suprarenal endarterectomy or anastomosis, mindful that the retroperitoneal approach provides facilitated access to the visceral aorta or even supraceliac aortic segments. Relative indications for a transperitoneal approach include a ruptured AAA, coexistent intraabdominal pathology, uncertain diagnosis, left-sided vena cava, large bilateral iliac artery aneurysms, or need for access to both renal arteries. Advantages of each approach make it advisable for surgeons to become proficient with both techniques.

TRANSPERITONEAL APPROACH

After entering the abdomen through a transperitoneal incision, the abdomen is thoroughly explored to exclude other pathology and assess extent of the aneurysm. The transverse colon is then retracted superiorly, and the ligament of Treitz is divided to allow retraction of the small bowel to the right. Exposure is greatly assisted using a fixed self-retaining retractor. A longitudinal incision is made in the peritoneum just to the left of the base of the small-bowel mesentery to expose the aneurysm. This incision extends from the inferior border of the pancreas proximally to the level of normal iliac arteries distally. Care must be taken to avoid the ureters, especially if exposure includes the iliac bifurcation where the ureters normally cross. Autonomic nerves to the pelvis course anterior to the proximal segment of the left CIA and should be retracted with associated retroperitoneal tissue rather than incised, to prevent sexual dysfunction in men. The left renal vein should be identified and retracted superiorly if necessary to fully expose the neck of the aneurysm. Care must be taken not to avulse renal vein tributaries, particularly a descending lumbar vein, frequently encountered to the left of the aorta, which must be divided before the left renal vein is mobile enough to allow upward retraction. Rarely, proximal exposure cannot be obtained without division of the left renal vein. In such cases, this should be done at its junction with the vena cava to maintain patency of collateral drainage via adrenal and gonadal branches. In a recent study by Sampson et al., 56 patients underwent left renal vein division and ligation during open aortic surgery; none developed directly related complications.[108] If necessary, reanastomosis can be performed if renal vein engorgement suggests inadequate collateral drainage.

After obtaining adequate aortoiliac exposure, the normal aorta and iliac arteries are dissected sufficiently to place a vascular clamp proximal and distal to the aneurysm. Regardless of the proximal extent of an infrarenal AAA, it is desirable to construct the proximal aortic anastomosis near the renal arteries to avoid subsequent aneurysmal degeneration of residual infrarenal aorta. When an AAA approaches or involves the renal arteries, it can be safer to apply the cross-clamp proximal to the celiac artery, rather than between the renal arteries and the superior mesenteric artery (SMA). Green et al.[109] demonstrated much higher operative mortality (32% vs. 3%) and renal failure requiring dialysis (23% vs. 3%) after infrarenal AAA repair when clamping was performed between the SMA and renal arteries rather than proximal to the celiac artery. They attributed this to the greater likelihood of dislodging atherosclerotic debris in the pararenal aorta as opposed to the supraceliac aorta, which is usually less diseased. Complications resulted from atheroembolization to the kidneys, legs, and intestine or injury to the aorta or renal arteries.

Others have also noted the relative safety of clamping the supraceliac aorta, which can easily be accessed by dividing the gastrohepatic ligament and the diaphragmatic crus.[110] However, aortic clamping between the renal arteries and the SMA is also safe when performed in properly selected patients without extensive plaque in this region.[111] Occasionally it is possible to obtain distal control of an AAA on the aorta, but usually aneurysmal changes or calcification in this location make iliac artery clamping preferred. A disease-free area of proximal aorta and iliac arteries should be identified for clamping to minimize the possibility of clamp injury or embolization of arterial debris. Some iliac arteries may be so

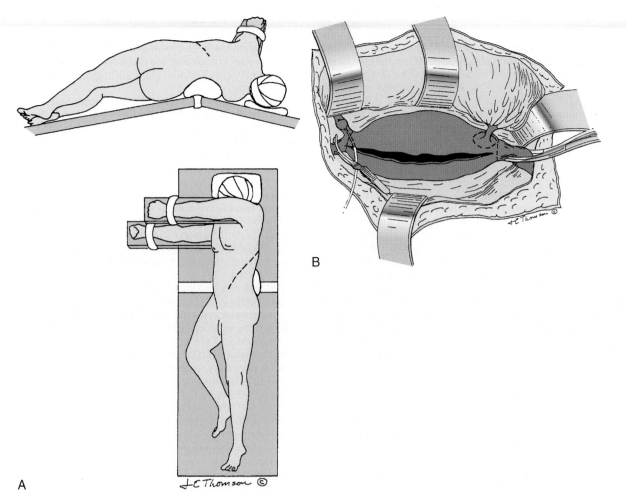

FIGURE 39-2   A, Positioning and skin incision for retroperitoneal approach for abdominal aortic aneurysm (AAA) repair. **B,** Retroperitoneal aortic exposure with left kidney retracted anteriorly for repair of suprarenal AAA. Left renal artery will be reimplanted as a Carrel patch. Right iliac artery is controlled with a balloon catheter.

diffusely calcified that clamping without injury is impossible. In such cases, internal occlusion with a balloon catheter or extension of the graft to the femoral arteries is required. In most cases, it is unnecessary to completely encircle the aorta and iliac arteries because vascular clamps can be placed in the anteroposterior direction, leaving the back wall undissected. This minimizes the likelihood of injury to both lumbar and iliac veins. Sometimes posterior arterial plaque necessitates placement of a vascular clamp transversely on either the aorta or iliac arteries, which then require careful posterior dissection precisely on the plane of the artery to avoid venous injury.

Abdominal aortic aneurysm repair can be accomplished with a straight ("tube") graft in 40% to 50% of patients, without extension onto the iliac arteries.[30,112] Although concern has been raised about the potential for future aneurysm development in the iliac arteries after tube graft repair of AAAs, late follow-up has shown that this is not clinically significant if the iliac arteries were not aneurysmal at the time of AAA repair.[113] Extension to the iliac arteries with a bifurcated graft for AAA repair is necessary in the remaining 50% to 60% of patients because of aneurysmal involvement of the iliac arteries or severe calcification of the aortic bifurcation. Extension of the graft to the femoral artery level is indicated for severe concomitant iliac occlusive disease or rarely because of technical difficulties associated with a deep pelvic anastomosis. Iliac artery anastomoses are preferred, however, owing to decreased infection and pseudoaneurysm complications compared with femoral artery anastomoses.

Prosthetic grafts available for AAA repair include knitted Dacron, knitted Dacron impregnated with collagen or gelatin to decrease porosity, woven Dacron, and polytetrafluoroethylene (PTFE). There is no clear evidence that any of these graft types provides superior outcome. In a prospective randomized comparison of PTFE and Dacron, long-term patency was equivalent, but PTFE had a higher incidence of early graft failure and graft sepsis.[114] In contrast, in a smaller trial with shorter follow-up, PTFE was found to be superior.[115] Most surgeons prefer an impervious graft to avoid the need for preclotting and thus select impregnated knitted Dacron, PTFE, or woven Dacron.[116] This not only saves time and more reliably prevents bleeding through the graft but also allows graft selection to be delayed until the aneurysm is opened so that a graft diameter corresponding to the inner diameter of the normal proximal aorta can be selected. It also allows delayed selection of a straight versus bifurcated graft that may not always be obvious before the aneurysm is open and the distal aorta can be carefully inspected.

Most surgeons use heparin anticoagulation during aortic cross-clamping to reduce lower-extremity thrombotic complications. Heparin dosage varies from 50 to 150 units/kg, based on personal preference. Activated clotting time (ACT) measurement is useful to determine the need for supplemental heparin in prolonged cases and the appropriate dose of protamine sulfate to reverse anticoagulation after declamping.[117] The sequence for applying proximal and distal vascular clamps is selected to apply the initial clamp in the area of least atherosclerotic disease to reduce the risk of distal embolization. The aneurysm is opened longitudinally along its anterior surface, away from the inferior mesenteric artery (IMA) in case this requires later reimplantation. The proximal aorta is then incised horizontally at the level selected for proximal anastomosis (see Fig. 39-1). To avoid potential injury to posterior veins, this incision does not have to extend through the back wall of the aorta, although some surgeons prefer complete transection for better exposure. Intraluminal thrombotic material and atherosclerotic debris are extracted from the aneurysm sac, which usually discloses several backbleeding lumbar artery orifices that require suture ligation. If the IMA is patent, it should be controlled temporarily with a small vascular clamp (see Fig. 39-1) so its need for reimplantation can be assessed after the revascularization is completed. Inferior mesenteric artery revascularization may be advised if the hypogastric arteries are diseased or if one requires ligation for technical reasons.

Once hemostasis within the opened aneurysm sac has been achieved, the proximal anastomosis is performed. There is often a distinct ring at the aneurysm neck that defines the appropriate level for this anastomosis. Usually polypropylene suture is used, taking large aortic "bites" and incorporating a double thickness of posterior aortic wall for added strength. If the aortic wall is friable, pledgets of Teflon or Dacron can be incorporated into the suture line. After completing the proximal anastomosis, the graft is clamped and the proximal aortic clamp released briefly to check for and correct any suture-line bleeding. If the distal anastomosis is to the aorta, a similar technique is used just above its bifurcation, suturing from within the lumen and encompassing both iliac artery orifices within the suture line. If iliac artery aneurysms exist, these are incised anteriorly so the limbs of a bifurcated graft can be sutured to the normal iliac artery beyond these aneurysms (Fig. 39-3). Often this requires graft extension to the CIA bifurcation, including the orifices of both the internal and external iliac arteries within the distal anastomosis. In rare instances, aneurysmal involvement of the distal CIA may preclude anastomosis to both the internal and external iliac artery orifices because these are widely separated. In such cases, an external iliac artery (EIA) anastomosis can be constructed, but care must be taken to preserve adequate pelvic blood flow, which may mean direct revascularization of at least one internal iliac artery (IIA). The need for internal iliac revascularization is usually assessed by the extent of back-bleeding, as discussed later in this chapter (isolated iliac aneurysms). For large aneurysms of the left iliac artery, medial

reflection of the sigmoid mesocolon assists a retroperitoneal approach to the distal CIA and prevents unnecessary dissection of autonomic nerves crossing the proximal left common iliac artery. Before completing the distal anastomoses, arterial clamps are carefully removed, and vigorous irrigation is used to flush out any thrombus or debris.

When the first iliac artery (or distal aortic) anastomosis is completed, flow into that extremity should be restored, releasing the clamp slowly to minimize "declamping" hypotension. Declamping shock is rare if adequate IV fluid replacement has been administered. However, sudden restoration of blood flow into a dilated distal vascular bed and the associated venous return of vasoactive substances that have accumulated in the ischemic limbs usually causes some hypotension. Declamping should therefore be gradual and carefully coordinated with the anesthesia team because additional volume administration can be required. In some cases, the clamp must be intermittently reapplied to allow adequate volume resuscitation and prevent hypotension. After restoration of lower-extremity and pelvic blood flow, the IMA and sigmoid colon are inspected.

The IMA can be ligated with a transfixing suture applied to its internal orifice if it is small and not associated with known SMA occlusive disease, if it has good backflow on release of its vascular clamp, if the sigmoid colon and arterial pulsations are good, and if at least one IIA is patent. In questionable cases, Doppler signals from the sigmoid colon or an assessment of IMA stump pressure[118] may be necessary to determine the need for IMA reimplantation. In the rare circumstances when sigmoid colon perfusion appears marginal, a circular cuff of the aortic wall around the IMA orifice is excised (Carrel patch) and anastomosed to the left side of the graft (Fig. 39-4). Next, the adequacy of lower-extremity blood flow is determined by visual inspection of the feet, palpation of distal pulses, or more sophisticated Doppler or pulse volume recording. If reduced blood flow is detected, intraoperative arteriography can differentiate thrombosis or embolism from peripheral vasoconstriction, which is relatively common if the procedure is prolonged and the patient is cold. Embolism or thrombosis requires prompt surgical correction, whereas vasoconstriction requires correction of any volume deficit and rewarming.

After assuring adequate intestinal and lower-extremity circulation, heparin is reversed with protamine sulfate if sufficient heparin

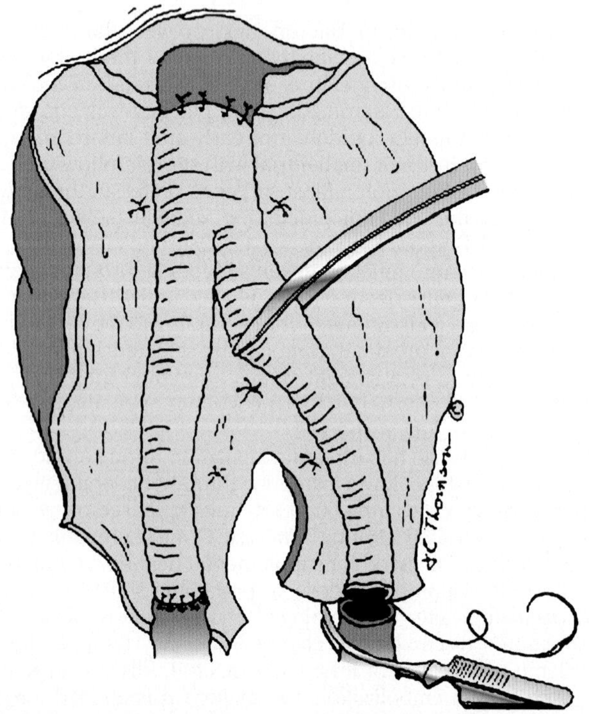

FIGURE 39-3 Completing the iliac anastomosis of an abdominal aortic aneurysm (AAA) repair. Lumbar artery orifices have been suture ligated. Flow has already been established through the right graft limb.

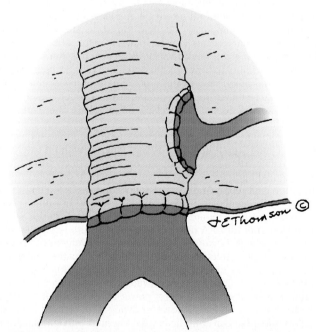

FIGURE 39-4 Reimplanting inferior mesenteric artery (IMA) with a Carrel patch technique after abdominal aortic aneurysm (AAA) repair with tube graft.

For infrarenal aneurysm exposure, it is often sufficient to proceed anteriorly and leave the left kidney in its normal position. For juxtarenal or suprarenal aneurysms that require more cephalad exposure, the kidney is mobilized anteriorly to approach the aorta from behind the left renal artery (see Fig. 39-2B). If the need for higher exposure is anticipated, the incision should be directed more cephalad over the 9th or 10th rib and the shoulders positioned as perpendicularly as possible to the table. In this case, more table flexion is required to open the space between the pelvis and ribs, and the trunk is twisted so that the angle between the pelvis and the table is about 30 degrees. When approaching the aorta from behind the left renal artery, it is necessary to divide a large lumbar branch of the left renal vein to mobilize the kidney and renal vein anteriorly. The ureter must be identified and retracted medially with the kidney, taking care to separate it from the iliac bifurcation distally.

Medial mobilization of the peritoneal contents exposes the IMA, which usually is divided for more complete exposure of the aortic bifurcation and right renal artery, depending on the size of the AAA. Exposure is greatly assisted by using a fixed self-retaining retractor. If necessary, exposure of the right iliac artery and right renal artery is easier after opening and decompressing the AAA. Right iliac artery control is often best accomplished by using a balloon occlusion catheter after entering the aneurysm (see Fig. 39-2B). After achieving adequate exposure, repair of the AAAs is usually carried out as described earlier for the transperitoneal approach. The retroperitoneal technique does not normally afford an opportunity to inspect colonic and intestinal viability, but the peritoneum can be opened to accomplish this if any concern exists.

Associated Arterial Disease

Indications for concomitant mesenteric or renal artery revascularization during elective AAA repair are comparable with those used for isolated disease in these arteries. Occasionally, patients with asymptomatic high-grade stenoses of these arteries warrant "prophylactic" concomitant reconstruction if the patient is at low operative risk and the AAA repair proceeds uneventfully. Although the natural history of asymptomatic mesenteric artery stenosis is not well characterized, it appears that patients with critical disease of all three mesenteric arteries are at sufficiently high risk for future complications of mesenteric ischemia that concomitant revascularization is justified.[119] Progression of renal artery stenosis has been better documented,[120,121] but the ultimate clinical impact of such progression appears minimal in nonhypertensive patients with normal renal function.[122] The adjacency of the renal arteries to the operative field for AAA repair has led some to recommend prophylactic repair of critical but asymptomatic renal artery stenoses.[123] Although this may be appropriate in younger good-risk patients, it adds morbidity and mortality to the AAA repair, leading others to recommend the combined procedure only for standard indications of hypertension or ischemic nephropathy.[124,125]

Complications of Abdominal Aortic Aneurysm Repair

Despite improvements in the outcome of elective AAA repair, major complications occur and must be correctly managed or avoided to maintain the low mortality necessary to justify prophylactic AAA repair. Myocardial infarction is the leading single-organ cause of both early and late mortality in patients undergoing AAA repair[25] and must be carefully assessed and managed to reduce mortality. In a recent review of patients undergoing elective AAA repair, however, Huber et al.[84] found that multisystem organ failure (MSOF) caused more deaths (57%) than cardiac events (25%). Visceral organ dysfunction was the most common cause of MSOF, followed by postoperative

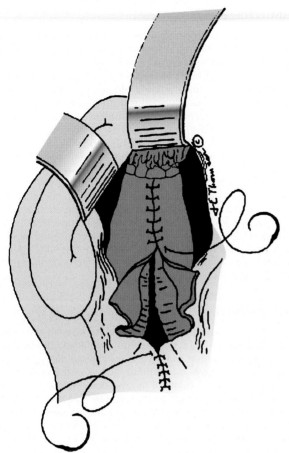

FIGURE 39-5 Closing aneurysm sac and retroperitoneum between graft and duodenum.

has been given to justify reversal, and hemostasis is achieved. The aneurysm wall and retroperitoneum are then closed over the graft to provide a tissue barrier between the prosthesis and the adjacent intestine (Fig. 39-5). The aortic prosthesis and upper anastomosis must be isolated from the overlying duodenum during closure; if necessary, a pedicle of greater omentum can be interposed to achieve this purpose. The small bowel should be inspected carefully and replaced in its normal position before abdominal closure.

RETROPERITONEAL APPROACH

Proper patient positioning is essential to achieve optimal exposure using the retroperitoneal approach. For most infrarenal AAAs, a left retroperitoneal incision centered on the 11th or 12th rib is employed. The patient's left shoulder is elevated at a 45- to 60-degree angle relative to the table, and the pelvis is positioned relatively flat. The table is flexed with the break positioned at a level midway between the iliac crest and the costal margin (see Fig. 39-2A). An air-evacuating "beanbag" is helpful to maintain proper positioning. Beginning at the lateral border of the left rectus muscle midway between the pubis and umbilicus, the skin incision is carried superiorly and then curved laterally up to the tip of the 11th or 12th rib. If extensive exposure of the right iliac artery is required, the incision can be extended inferolaterally into the right lower quadrant, or a separate right lower quadrant retroperitoneal incision can be used. The underlying lateral abdominal wall muscles are divided, exposing the underlying peritoneum and the anterior edge of the properitoneal fat layer at the lateral aspect of this exposure. Dissection in the retroperitoneal plane is then developed, either anterior or posterior to the left kidney, until the aorta is encountered.

pneumonia. However, most patients with MSOF had associated cardiac dysfunction that may have aggravated visceral ischemic injury. Several factors may be responsible for the emergence of MSOF as a more prominent cause of death following elective AAA repair. First, with modern techniques of intensive care, it is uncommon for patients to die with single-system failure (even cardiac) following AAA repair. Second, strict attention to cardiac risk in these patients may have reduced the relative impact of cardiac complications. Finally, older patients with more associated visceral and renal artery disease underwent AAA repair in this series and had the highest likelihood of MSOF postoperatively. The relative frequency of single-system complications following elective AAA repair is listed in Table 39-3.

Cardiac Complications

The majority of cardiac ischemic events occur within the first 7 days following surgery, during which time intensive care monitoring is appropriate for high-risk patients. Maximizing myocardial function with adequate preload, controlling oxygen consumption by the reduced heart rate and blood pressure product, ensuring adequate oxygenation, β-blockade, and establishing effective analgesia are important techniques for preventing myocardial ischemia postoperatively. Patients with cardiac dysfunction have a greater risk of MI when the postoperative hematocrit is below 28%, even though this is well tolerated by normal individuals.[126] Postoperative epidural analgesia, in addition to providing excellent pain control, may reduce myocardial complications by decreasing the catecholamine stress response.[91]

TABLE 39-3	Early (30-Day) Complications After Elective Abdominal Aortic Aneurysm Repair*
COMPLICATION	FREQUENCY
Death	<5%
All cardiac	15%
MI	2%-8%
All pulmonary	8%-12%
Pneumonia	5%
Renal insufficiency	5%-12%
Dialysis dependent	1%-6%
DVT	8%
Bleeding	2%-5%
Ureteral injury	<1%
Stroke	1%
Leg ischemia	1%-4%
Colon ischemia	1%
Spinal cord ischemia	<1%
Wound infection	<5%
Graft infection	<1%
Graft thrombosis	<1%

*Estimated from the following surgical series: Johnston KW: Multicenter prospective study of nonruptured abdominal aortic aneurysm. Part II. Variables predicting morbidity and mortality. J Vasc Surg 9:437–447, 1989; Johnston KW, Scobie TK: Multicenter prospective study of nonruptured abdominal aortic aneurysms. I. Population and operative management. J Vasc Surg 7:69–81, 1988; Olsen PS, Schroeder T, Agerskov K, et al: Surgery for abdominal aortic aneurysms. A survey of 656 patients. J Cardiovasc Surg 32:636–642, 1991; AbuRahma AF, Robinson PA, Boland JP, et al: Elective resection of 332 abdominal aortic aneurysms in a southern West Virginia community during a recent five-year period. Surgery 109:244–251, 1991; Diehl JT, Cali RF, Hertzer NR, Beven EG: Complications of abdominal aortic reconstruction. An analysis of perioperative risk factors in 557 patients. Ann Surg 197: 49–56, 1983; and Richardson JD, Main KA: Repair of abdominal aortic aneurysms. A statewide experience. Arch Surg 126:614–616, 1991. DVT, deep vein thrombosis; MI, myocardial infarction.[25,30,112,152–154]

Hemorrhage

Intraoperative or postoperative hemorrhage usually results from difficulties with the proximal aortic anastomosis or from iatrogenic venous injury. Proximal suture line bleeding, particularly when posterior, can be difficult to control, especially if the proximal anastomosis is juxtarenal. Venous bleeding usually results from injury to the iliac or left renal veins during initial exposure. Often the distal aortic aneurysm or common iliac aneurysm is densely adherent to the associated iliac vein, making circumferential arterial dissection hazardous. In such cases, vascular clamps can usually be applied successfully without complete dissection of the posterior wall of the iliac artery or vascular control obtained with balloon occlusion catheters. A posterior left renal vein or a large lumbar vein may pose similar hazards during the proximal dissection. If undetected by preoperative CT scanning, such anomalies pose a high risk for venous injury. Diffuse bleeding after substantial intraoperative blood loss is usually due to exhausted coagulation factors and platelets, combined with hypothermia. Aggressive rewarming with platelet and coagulation factor replacement is required to overcome this complication.

Renal Failure

Although once common after infrarenal AAA repair, renal failure is now rare because of adequate volume replacement and maintenance of normal cardiac output and renal blood flow. Precautions are still required, however, to reduce the risk of this complication. Because of the renal toxicity of intravenous contrast, it is prudent to delay AAA repair following arteriography or contrast-enhanced CT to be certain that renal dysfunction has not been induced. A more likely cause of renal failure following infrarenal AAA repair is embolization of aortic atheromatous debris into the renal arteries during proximal aortic cross-clamping. Preoperative CT scanning may reveal pararenal atheromatous debris or thrombus, which should prompt temporary supraceliac cross-clamping until the infrarenal aorta is open. Preoperative renal insufficiency is the best predictor of postoperative renal failure,[25,127] so special precautions are appropriate in such patients. Some evidence supports a beneficial effect of intravenous mannitol when given before aortic cross-clamping ($\approx 25\,g$).[127] Although some have advocated maintenance of higher urine volume using furosemide, the efficacy of this approach has not been proven and may hinder assessment of fluid balance by artificially increasing urine output.

Gastrointestinal Complications

Some degree of bowel dysfunction occurs after any major abdominal procedure. However, the paralytic ileus that follows evisceration and dissection of the base of the mesentery during transperitoneal AAA repair often lasts longer than that occurring after other procedures. Consequently, one must use caution in reinstituting oral feeding postoperatively. Anorexia, periodic constipation, or diarrhea is commonly seen in the first few weeks following aneurysm surgery.

Sigmoid colon ischemia following AAA repair is a rare but devastating complication that occurs after approximately 1% of elective AAA repairs.[128,129] This may result from embolization into, or ligation of, the IMA or IIAs. Although the IMA is often chronically occluded, ligation too far from the aneurysm wall can obliterate important SMA collaterals. Fortunately, the abundance of collateral flow to the sigmoid colon usually prevents ischemia. Sigmoid ischemia is three to four times more likely following ruptured AAA repair, presumably due to the associated hypotension and shock added to the usual risk of this complication.[128–130] Careful inspection of the sigmoid colon following graft placement is important and may be facilitated by Doppler insonation of the bowel wall and mesentery. Preoperatively, patent IMAs should be carefully inspected for back-bleeding following the aortic reconstruction, and ligated only when back-bleeding is pulsatile and colon viability is assured. In questionable circumstances, IMA reimplantation or direct internal iliac revascularization is indicated.[131]

Postoperatively, colon ischemia should be suspected in the presence of early diarrhea (usually containing blood), left lower quadrant abdominal pain, unexplained fever or leukocytosis, or excessive intravenous fluid or pressor requirement. This should prompt immediate flexible sigmoidoscopy or colonoscopy. In most cases, patchy partial-thickness mucosal necrosis and sloughing are detected and often resolve with antibiotic therapy and bowel rest. In more severe cases of transmural infarction, however, early reexploration is indicated to avoid the high mortality rate associated with delayed treatment of this complication. Treatment requires sigmoid resection and colostomy, rarely combined with aortic graft excision followed by extra-anatomical bypass if substantial graft contamination has occurred.

Distal Embolization

Lower-extremity ischemia may occur after AAA repair, usually from embolization of aneurysmal debris that occurs during aneurysm mobilization or aortoiliac clamping. Usually such emboli are small (termed *microemboli*) and not amenable to surgical removal, and they result in transient patchy areas of dusky skin or "blue toes" (also see Chapter 47). This can result in persistent pain or skin loss, occasionally necessitating amputation. Management is largely expectant. Occasionally, larger emboli or distal intimal flaps, particularly in diseased iliac arteries, may require operative intervention. For this reason, the legs should be carefully inspected intraoperatively for ischemia after AAA repair, while the incision is still open and arterial access can be easily obtained if necessary.

Paraplegia

Paraplegia due to spinal cord ischemia is rare following infrarenal AAA repair. It can result when important spinal artery collateral flow via the IIAs or an abnormally low origin of the accessory spinal artery (arterial magna radicularis or artery of Adamkiewicz) is obliterated or embolized during AAA repair.[132] Because the accessory spinal artery normally originates from the descending thoracic or upper abdominal aorta, this complication is much more common following thoracoabdominal aneurysm repair.

Impaired Sexual Function

Impotence or retrograde ejaculation due to injury of autonomic nerves during paraaortic dissection may result after AAA repair.[133] The incidence of this complication is difficult to determine because of the multiple causes of impotence in this age group and frequent underreporting. In the recent ADAM trial in U.S. VA hospitals, 40% of men had impotence before AAA repair.[134] Contrary to most other reports that asked patients retrospectively if they had impotence before AAA repair, in the ADAM trial, less than 10% developed new impotence in the first year after repair. However, the proportion reporting new impotence increased over time such that by 4 years after AAA repair, more than 60% reported having impotence, which underscores the multifactorial etiology of impotence in this age group. Careful preservation of nerves, particularly as they course along the left side of the infrarenal aorta, around the IMA, and cross the proximal left CIA has been shown to substantially reduce this complication, which has reportedly occurred in up to 25% of patients.[135,136] Other possible causes of postoperative impotence include reduction in pelvic blood flow due to internal iliac occlusion or embolization. Sexual dysfunction is not confined to open AAA repair patients. A recent study by Pettersson et al. demonstrated that a group of patients, when asked about their respective sexual function following EVAR, reported increased postoperative impotence and ejaculatory function 1 year following AAA repair.[137]

Venous Thromboembolism

Pulmonary embolism (PE) and deep vein thrombosis (DVT) are less common after AAA repair than after other abdominal operations, perhaps because of intraoperative anticoagulation. Unrecognized DVT, however, can occur in up to 18% of untreated patients.[138] Therefore, perioperative prophylaxis with intermittent pneumatic compression stockings or subcutaneous heparin or low-molecular-weight heparin (LMWH) is appropriate.

Functional Outcome

Williamson et al.[139] recently reviewed their experience with open AAA repair with regard to functional outcome. They found that two thirds of patients experienced complete recovery at an average time of 4 months, whereas one third had not fully recovered at an average time of nearly 3 years. Additionally, 18% said they would not undergo AAA repair again after knowing the recovery process, despite appearing to understand the implications of AAA rupture. Eleven percent were initially discharged to a skilled nursing facility, with an average stay of 3.7 months. This is similar to a 9% rate of discharge to a facility other than home, as reported in a review of national administrative data by Huber et al.[140] All patients in Williamson's review were ambulatory preoperatively, but at a mean of 25 months' follow-up, only 64% were fully ambulatory, whereas 22% required assistance, and 14% were nonambulatory. Although it is difficult to determine the extent of the disability that is due to the AAA repair, this report highlights the high rate of disability after open AAA repair. More research into long-term functional outcomes and quality-of-life assessment is clearly necessary.

Long-Term Survival

As noted previously, early (30-day) mortality after elective AAA repair in properly selected patients is 5% or less, whereas early mortality after ruptured AAA repair averages 54% (not including patients who died from rupture before repair).[5,15] Five-year survival after successful AAA repair in modern series is approximately 70%, compared with approximately 80% in the age- and gender-matched general population.[41,42,112,141–145] Ten-year survival after AAA repair is approximately 40%. Although survival is similar in men and women, women without AAA have longer survival than men. Therefore, survival relative to gender-specific norms is lower in women after AAA repair than in men.[146] Survival after successful ruptured AAA repair versus successful elective repair was similar in one report[147] but reduced in others.[148,149] In a population-based analysis from Western Australia, survival after ruptured or elective AAA repair was similar for men but significantly reduced for women with ruptured AAA.[146] Overall, survival after AAA repair is reduced compared with an age- and sex-matched population because of greater associated comorbidity in patients with aneurysms.[33,142] Not surprisingly, systemic complications of atherosclerosis cause most late deaths after AAA repair in this predominately elderly male population. The cause of late deaths after AAA repair are cardiac disease (44%), cancer (15%), rupture of another aneurysm (11%), stroke (9%), and pulmonary disease (6%).[141,142,150] Combining cardiac causes, aneurysmal disease, and stroke indicates that vascular complications account for two thirds of late deaths following AAA repair.

When outcome is stratified according to these risk factors, the 5-year survival rate improves to 84% in patients without heart disease, which is substantially better than the 54% survival rate observed in patients with known heart disease.[141] Hypertension also reduces 5-year survival after AAA repair from 84% to 59%.[141] In patients without hypertension or heart disease, late survival after AAA repair is identical to normal age-matched controls.[142] Multivariate analysis indicates that uncorrected CAD is the most significant variable associated with late mortality after AAA repair, but that age, renal dysfunction, COPD, and peripheral occlusive disease also contribute.[41,42,112,151] One analysis of coronary artery bypass grafting performed in preparation for AAA repair indicates that it may improve long-term survival in patients younger than age 70 but that older patients do not benefit from this aggressive approach.[151] A recent prospective multicentered study identified not only age, cardiac, carotid, and renal disease as independent predictors of late mortality following elective AAA repair but also aneurysm extent, as judged by size, suprarenal extension, and external iliac involvement.[143]

REFERENCES

1. Upchurch GR Jr, Schaub TA: Abdominal aortic aneurysm, *Am Fam Physician* 73(7):1198–1204, 2006.
2. Bengtsson H, Nilsson P, Bergqvist D: Natural history of abdominal aortic aneurysm detected by screening, *Br J Surg* 80(6):718–720, 1993.
3. Heller JA, Weinberg A, Arons R, et al: Two decades of abdominal aortic aneurysm repair: have we made any progress? *J Vasc Surg* 32(6):1091–1100, 2000.
4. Adam DJ, Mohan IV, Stuart WP, et al: Community and hospital outcome from ruptured abdominal aortic aneurysm within the catchment area of a regional vascular surgical service, *J Vasc Surg* 30(5):922–928, 1999.
5. Hallin A, Bergqvist D, Holmberg L: Literature review of surgical management of abdominal aortic aneurysm, *Eur J Vasc Endovasc Surg* 22(3):197–204, 2001.
6. Bown MJ, Sutton AJ, Bell PR, et al: A meta-analysis of 50 years of ruptured abdominal aortic aneurysm repair, *Br J Surg* 89(6):714–730, 2002.
7. Ernst CB: Abdominal aortic aneurysm, *N Engl J Med* 328(16):1167–1172, 1993.
8. Heikkinen M, Salenius JP, Auvinen O: Ruptured abdominal aortic aneurysm in a well-defined geographic area, *J Vasc Surg* 36(2):291–296, 2002.
9. Kantonen I, Lepantalo M, Brommels M, et al: Mortality in ruptured abdominal aortic aneurysms. The Finnvasc Study Group, *Eur J Vasc Endovasc Surg* 17(3):208–212, 1999.
10. Bengtsson H, Bergqvist D: Ruptured abdominal aortic aneurysm: a population-based study, *J Vasc Surg* 18(1):74–80, 1993.
11. Pasch AR, Ricotta JJ, May AG, et al: Abdominal aortic aneurysm: the case for elective resection, *Circulation* 70(3 Pt 2):I1–I4, 1984.
12. Breckwoldt WL, Mackey WC, O'Donnell TF Jr: The economic implications of high-risk abdominal aortic aneurysms, *J Vasc Surg* 13(6):798–803, 1991 discussion 803–794.
13. Pearce WH, Slaughter MS, LeMaire S, et al: Aortic diameter as a function of age, gender, and body surface area, *Surgery* 114(4):691–697, 1993.
14. Johnston KW, Rutherford RB, Tilson MD, et al: Suggested standards for reporting on arterial aneurysms. Subcommittee on Reporting Standards for Arterial Aneurysms, Ad Hoc Committee on Reporting Standards, Society for Vascular Surgery and North American Chapter, International Society for Cardiovascular Surgery, *J Vasc Surg* 13(3):452–458, 1991.
15. Katz DA, Littenberg B, Cronenwett JL: Management of small abdominal aortic aneurysms. Early surgery vs. watchful waiting, *JAMA* 268(19):2678–2686, 1992.
16. Brewster DC, Cronenwett JL, Hallett JW Jr, et al: Guidelines for the treatment of abdominal aortic aneurysms. Report of a subcommittee of the Joint Council of the American Association for Vascular Surgery and Society for Vascular Surgery, *J Vasc Surg* 37(5):1106–1117, 2003.
17. Brown LC, Powell JT: Risk factors for aneurysm rupture in patients kept under ultrasound surveillance. UK Small Aneurysm Trial Participants, *Ann Surg* 230(3):289–296, 1999. discussion 296–287.
18. Mortality results for randomised controlled trial of early elective surgery or ultrasonographic surveillance for small abdominal aortic aneurysms. The UK Small Aneurysm Trial Participants, *Lancet* 352(9141):1649–1655, 1998.
19. Lederle FA, Wilson SE, Johnson GR, et al: Immediate repair compared with surveillance of small abdominal aortic aneurysms, *N Engl J Med* 346(19):1437–1444, 2002.
20. Ouriel K, Clair DG, Kent KC, et al: Endovascular repair compared with surveillance for patients with small abdominal aortic aneurysms, *J Vasc Surg* 51(5):1081–1087, 2010.
21. Valentine RJ, Decaprio JD, Castillo JM, et al: Watchful waiting in cases of small abdominal aortic aneurysms–appropriate for all patients? *J Vasc Surg* 32(3):441–448, 2000. discussion 448–450.
22. Steyerberg EW, Kievit J, de Mol Van Otterloo JC, et al: Perioperative mortality of elective abdominal aortic aneurysm surgery. A clinical prediction rule based on literature and individual patient data, *Arch Intern Med* 155(18):1998–2004, 1995.
23. Kazmers A, Perkins AJ, Jacobs LA: Outcomes after abdominal aortic aneurysm repair in those > or = 80 years of age: recent Veterans Affairs experience, *Ann Vasc Surg* 12(2):106–112, 1998.
24. L'Italien GJ, Paul SD, Hendel RC, et al: Development and validation of a Bayesian model for perioperative cardiac risk assessment in a cohort of 1,081 vascular surgical candidates, *J Am Coll Cardiol* 27(4):779–786, 1996.
25. Johnston KW: Multicenter prospective study of nonruptured abdominal aortic aneurysm. Part II. Variables predicting morbidity and mortality, *J Vasc Surg* 9(3):437–447, 1989.
26. Brady AR, Fowkes FG, Greenhalgh RM, et al: Risk factors for postoperative death following elective surgical repair of abdominal aortic aneurysm: results from the UK Small Aneurysm Trial. On behalf of the UK Small Aneurysm Trial participants, *Br J Surg* 87(6):742–749, 2000.
27. Katz DJ, Stanley JC, Zelenock GB: Gender differences in abdominal aortic aneurysm prevalence, treatment, and outcome, *J Vasc Surg* 25(3):561–568, 1997.
28. Katz DA, Cronenwett JL: The cost-effectiveness of early surgery versus watchful waiting in the management of small abdominal aortic aneurysms, *J Vasc Surg* 19(6):980–990, 1994. discussion 990–981.
29. Iezzoni LI: Assessing quality using administrative data, *Ann Intern Med* 127(8 Pt 2):666–674, 1997.
30. Johnston KW, Scobie TK: Multicenter prospective study of nonruptured abdominal aortic aneurysms. I. Population and operative management, *J Vasc Surg* 7(1):69–81, 1988.
31. Beck AW, Goodney PP, Nolan BW, et al: Predicting 1-year mortality after elective abdominal aortic aneurysm repair, *J Vasc Surg* 49(4):838–843, 2009. discussion 843–834.
32. Lederle FA, Johnson GR, Wilson SE, et al: The aneurysm detection and management study screening program: validation cohort and final results. Aneurysm Detection and Management Veterans Affairs Cooperative Study Investigators, *Arch Intern Med* 160(10):1425–1430, 2000.
33. Newman AB, Arnold AM, Burke GL, et al: Cardiovascular disease and mortality in older adults with small abdominal aortic aneurysms detected by ultrasonography: the cardiovascular health study, *Ann Intern Med* 134(3):182–190, 2001.
34. Rodin MB, Daviglus ML, Wong GC, et al: Middle age cardiovascular risk factors and abdominal aortic aneurysm in older age, *Hypertension* 42(1):61–68, 2003.
35. Singh K, Bonaa KH, Jacobsen BK, et al: Prevalence of and risk factors for abdominal aortic aneurysms in a population-based study: the Tromso Study, *Am J Epidemiol* 154(3):236–244, 2001.
36. Tornwall ME, Virtamo J, Haukka JK, et al: Life-style factors and risk for abdominal aortic aneurysm in a cohort of Finnish male smokers, *Epidemiology* 12(1):94–100, 2001.
37. Wilmink AB, Quick CR: Epidemiology and potential for prevention of abdominal aortic aneurysm, *Br J Surg* 85(2):155–162, 1998.
38. Johnston KW: Nonruptured abdominal aortic aneurysm: six-year follow-up results from the multicenter prospective Canadian aneurysm study. Canadian Society for Vascular Surgery Aneurysm Study Group, *J Vasc Surg* 20(2):163–170, 1994.
39. Batt M, Staccini P, Pittaluga P, et al: Late survival after abdominal aortic aneurysm repair, *Eur J Vasc Endovasc Surg* 17(4):338–342, 1999.
40. Aune S, Amundsen SR, Evjensvold J, et al: Operative mortality and long-term relative survival of patients operated on for asymptomatic abdominal aortic aneurysm, *Eur J Vasc Endovasc Surg* 9(3):293–298, 1995.
41. Norman PE, Semmens JB, Lawrence-Brown MM: Long-term relative survival following surgery for abdominal aortic aneurysm: a review, *Cardiovasc Surg* 9(3):219–224, 2001.
42. Hertzer NR, Mascha EJ, Karafa MT, et al: Open infrarenal abdominal aortic aneurysm repair: the Cleveland Clinic experience from 1989 to 1998, *J Vasc Surg* 35(6):1145–1154, 2002.
43. Smoking, lung function and the prognosis of abdominal aortic aneurysm. The UK Small Aneurysm Trial Participants, *Eur J Vasc Endovasc Surg* 19(6):636–642, 2000.
44. De Martino RR, Nolan BW, Goodney PP, et al: Outcomes of symptomatic abdominal aortic aneurysm repair, *J Vasc Surg* 52(1):5–12 e11, 2010.
45. Michaels JA: The management of small abdominal aortic aneurysms: a computer simulation using Monte Carlo methods, *Eur J Vasc Surg* 6(5):551–557, 1992.
46. Schermerhorn ML, Birkmeyer JD, Gould DA, et al: Cost-effectiveness of surgery for small abdominal aortic aneurysms on the basis of data from the United Kingdom small aneurysm trial, *J Vasc Surg* 31(2):217–226, 2000.
47. Long-term outcomes of immediate repair compared with surveillance of small abdominal aortic aneurysms, *N Engl J Med* 346(19):1445–1452, 2002.
48. Eagle KA, Berger PB, Calkins H, et al: ACC/AHA guideline update for perioperative cardiovascular evaluation for noncardiac surgery–executive summary. A report of the American College of Cardiology/American Heart Association Task Force on Practice Guidelines (Committee to Update the 1996 Guidelines on Perioperative Cardiovascular Evaluation for Noncardiac Surgery), *Anesth Analg* 94(5):1052–1064, 2002.
49. Fagevik Olsen M, Hahn I, Nordgren S, et al: Randomized controlled trial of prophylactic chest physiotherapy in major abdominal surgery, *Br J Surg* 84(11):1535–1538, 1997.
50. Hertzer NR, Young JR, Kramer JR, et al: Routine coronary angiography prior to elective aortic reconstruction: results of selective myocardial revascularization in patients with peripheral vascular disease, *Arch Surg* 114(11):1336–1344, 1979.
51. Eagle KA, Coley CM, Newell JB, et al: Combining clinical and thallium data optimizes preoperative assessment of cardiac risk before major vascular surgery, *Ann Intern Med* 110(11):859–866, 1989.
52. Creech O Jr: Endo-aneurysmorrhaphy and treatment of aortic aneurysm, *Ann Surg* 164(6):935–946, 1966.
53. Hollier LH, Reigel MM, Kazmier FJ, et al: Conventional repair of abdominal aortic aneurysm in the high-risk patient: a plea for abandonment of nonresective treatment, *J Vasc Surg* 3(5):712–717, 1986.
54. Inahara T, Geary GL, Mukherjee D, et al: The contrary position to the nonresective treatment for abdominal aortic aneurysm, *J Vasc Surg* 2(1):42–48, 1985.
55. Karmody AM, Leather RP, Goldman M, et al: The current position of nonresective treatment for abdominal aortic aneurysm, *Surgery* 94(4):591–597, 1983.
56. Lynch K, Kohler T, Johansen K: Nonresective therapy for aortic aneurysm: results of a survey, *J Vasc Surg* 4(5):469–472, 1986.
57. Schwartz RA, Nichols WK, Silver D: Is thrombosis of the infrarenal abdominal aortic aneurysm an acceptable alternative? *J Vasc Surg* 3(3):448–455, 1986.
58. Shah DM, Chang BB, Paty PS, et al: Treatment of abdominal aortic aneurysm by exclusion and bypass: an analysis of outcome, *J Vasc Surg* 13(1):15–20, 1991. discussion 20–12.
59. Darling RC 3rd, Ozsvath K, Chang BB, et al: The incidence, natural history, and outcome of secondary intervention for persistent collateral flow in the excluded abdominal aortic aneurysm, *J Vasc Surg* 30(6):968–976, 1999.
60. Kline RG, D'Angelo AJ, Chen MH, et al: Laparoscopically assisted abdominal aortic aneurysm repair: first 20 cases, *J Vasc Surg* 27(1):81–87, 1998. discussion 88.
61. Parodi JC, Palmaz JC, Barone HD: Transfemoral intraluminal graft implantation for abdominal aortic aneurysms, *Ann Vasc Surg* 5(6):491–499, 1991.
62. Moore WS, Brewster DC, Bernhard VM: Aorto-uni-iliac endograft for complex aortoiliac aneurysms compared with tube/bifurcation endografts: results of the EVT/Guidant trials, *J Vasc Surg* 33(Suppl 2):S11–S20, 2001.
63. Matsumura JS, Brewster DC, Makaroun MS, et al: A multicenter controlled clinical trial of open versus endovascular treatment of abdominal aortic aneurysm, *J Vasc Surg* 37(2):262–271, 2003.
64. Zarins CK, White RA, Schwarten D, et al: AneuRx stent graft versus open surgical repair of abdominal aortic aneurysms: multicenter prospective clinical trial, *J Vasc Surg* 29(2):292–305, 1999. discussion 306–298.
65. Lee WA, Carter JW, Upchurch G, et al: Perioperative outcomes after open and endovascular repair of intact abdominal aortic aneurysms in the United States during 2001, *J Vasc Surg* 39(3):491–496, 2004.
66. Aquino RV, Jones MA, Zullo TG, et al: Quality of life assessment in patients undergoing endovascular or conventional AAA repair, *J Endovasc Ther* 8(5):521–528, 2001.

67. Bernhard VM, Mitchell RS, Matsumura JS, et al: Ruptured abdominal aortic aneurysm after endovascular repair, J Vasc Surg 35(6):1155–1162, 2002.

68. Harris PL, Vallabhaneni SR, Desgranges P, et al: Incidence and risk factors of late rupture, conversion, and death after endovascular repair of infrarenal aortic aneurysms: the EUROSTAR experience. European Collaborators on Stent/graft techniques for aortic aneurysm repair, J Vasc Surg 32(4):739–749, 2000.

69. Holzenbein TJ, Kretschmer G, Thurnher S, et al: Midterm durability of abdominal aortic aneurysm endograft repair: a word of caution, J Vasc Surg 33(2 Suppl):S46–S54, 2001.

70. Schermerhorn ML, Finlayson SR, Fillinger MF, et al: Life expectancy after endovascular versus open abdominal aortic aneurysm repair: results of a decision analysis model on the basis of data from EUROSTAR, J Vasc Surg 36(6):1112–1120, 2002.

71. Prinssen M, Verhoeven EL, Buth J, et al: A randomized trial comparing conventional and endovascular repair of abdominal aortic aneurysms, N Engl J Med 351(16):1607–1618, 2004.

72. Blankensteijn JD, de Jong SE, Prinssen M, et al: Two-year outcomes after conventional or endovascular repair of abdominal aortic aneurysms, N Engl J Med 352(23):2398–2405, 2005.

73. Zarins CK, White RA, Fogarty TJ: Aneurysm rupture after endovascular repair using the AneuRx stent graft, J Vasc Surg 31(5):960–970, 2000.

74. Ohki T, Veith FJ, Shaw P, et al: Increasing incidence of midterm and long-term complications after endovascular graft repair of abdominal aortic aneurysms: a note of caution based on a 9-year experience, Ann Surg 234(3):323–334, 2001. discussion 334–325.

75. Endovascular aneurysm repair versus open repair in patients with abdominal aortic aneurysm (EVAR trial 1): randomised controlled trial, Lancet 365(9478):2179–2186, 2005.

76. Endovascular aneurysm repair and outcome in patients unfit for open repair of abdominal aortic aneurysm (EVAR trial 2): randomised controlled trial, Lancet 365(9478):2187–2192, 2005.

77. Rutherford RB: Randomized EVAR trials and advent of level I evidence: a paradigm shift in management of large abdominal aortic aneurysms? Semin Vasc Surg 19(2):69–74, 2006.

78. Lederle FA, Freischlag JA, Kyriakides TC, et al: Outcomes following endovascular vs. open repair of abdominal aortic aneurysm: a randomized trial, JAMA 302(14):1535–1542, 2009.

79. Kaiser AB, Clayson KR, Mulherin JL Jr, et al: Antibiotic prophylaxis in vascular surgery, Ann Surg 188(3):283–289, 1978.

80. Bender JS, Smith-Meek MA, Jones CE: Routine pulmonary artery catheterization does not reduce morbidity and mortality of elective vascular surgery: results of a prospective, randomized trial, Ann Surg 226(3):229–236, 1997. discussion 236–227.

81. Ziegler DW, Wright JG, Choban PS, et al: A prospective randomized trial of preoperative "optimization" of cardiac function in patients undergoing elective peripheral vascular surgery, Surgery 122(3):584–592, 1997.

82. Birkmeyer JD, AuBuchon JP, Littenberg B, et al: Cost-effectiveness of preoperative autologous donation in coronary artery bypass grafting, Ann Thorac Surg 57(1):161–168, 1994. discussion 168–169.

83. Goodnough LT, Monk TG, Sicard G, et al: Intraoperative salvage in patients undergoing elective abdominal aortic aneurysm repair: an analysis of cost and benefit, J Vasc Surg 24(2):213–218, 1996.

84. Huber TS, Carlton LC, Irwin PB, et al: Intraoperative autologous transfusion during elective infrarenal aortic reconstruction, J Surg Res 67(1):14–20, 1997.

85. Ouriel K, Shortell CK, Green RM, et al: Intraoperative autotransfusion in aortic surgery, J Vasc Surg 18(1):16–22, 1993.

86. Nelson AH, Fleisher LA, Rosenbaum SH: Relationship between postoperative anemia and cardiac morbidity in high-risk vascular patients in the intensive care unit, Crit Care Med 21(6):860–866, 1993.

87. Bush HL Jr, Hydo LJ, Fischer E, et al: Hypothermia during elective abdominal aortic aneurysm repair: the high price of avoidable morbidity, J Vasc Surg 21(3):392–400, 1995. discussion 400–392.

88. Frank SM, Fleisher LA, Breslow MJ, et al: Perioperative maintenance of normothermia reduces the incidence of morbid cardiac events. A randomized clinical trial, JAMA 277(14):1127–1134, 1997.

89. Ali ZA, Callaghan CJ, Lim E, et al: Remote ischemic preconditioning reduces myocardial and renal injury after elective abdominal aortic aneurysm repair: a randomized controlled trial, Circulation 116(11 Suppl):I98–I105, 2007.

90. Mason RA, Newton GB, Cassel W, et al: Combined epidural and general anesthesia in aortic surgery, J Cardiovasc Surg (Torino) 31(4):442–447, 1990.

91. Yeager MP, Glass DD, Neff RK, et al: Epidural anesthesia and analgesia in high-risk surgical patients, Anesthesiology 66(6):729–736, 1987.

92. Baron JF, Bertrand M, Barre E, et al: Combined epidural and general anesthesia versus general anesthesia for abdominal aortic surgery, Anesthesiology 75(4):611–618, 1991.

93. Raggi R, Dardik H, Mauro AL: Continuous epidural anesthesia and postoperative epidural narcotics in vascular surgery, Am J Surg 154(2):192–197, 1987.

94. Devereaux PJ, Yang H, Yusuf S, et al: Effects of extended-release metoprolol succinate in patients undergoing non-cardiac surgery (POISE trial): a randomised controlled trial, Lancet 371(9627):1839–1847, 2008.

95. Pasternack PF, Grossi EA, Baumann FG, et al: Beta blockade to decrease silent myocardial ischemia during peripheral vascular surgery, Am J Surg 158(2):113–116, 1989.

96. Mangano DT, Layug EL, Wallace A, et al: Effect of atenolol on mortality and cardiovascular morbidity after noncardiac surgery. Multicenter Study of Perioperative Ischemia Research Group, N Engl J Med 335(23):1713–1720, 1996.

97. Wallace A, Layug B, Tateo I, et al: Prophylactic atenolol reduces postoperative myocardial ischemia. McSPI Research Group, Anesthesiology 88(1):7–17, 1998.

98. Poldermans D, Boersma E, Bax JJ, et al: The effect of bisoprolol on perioperative mortality and myocardial infarction in high-risk patients undergoing vascular surgery. Dutch Echocardiographic Cardiac Risk Evaluation Applying Stress Echocardiography Study Group, N Engl J Med 341(24):1789–1794, 1999.

99. Poldermans D, Boersma E, Bax JJ, et al: Bisoprolol reduces cardiac death and myocardial infarction in high-risk patients as long as 2 years after successful major vascular surgery, Eur Heart J 22(15):1353–1358, 2001.

100. Fleisher LA, Beckman JA, Brown KA, et al: 2009 ACCF/AHA focused update on perioperative beta blockade incorporated into the ACC/AHA 2007 guidelines on perioperative cardiovascular evaluation and care for noncardiac surgery: a report of the American College of Cardiology Foundation/American Heart Association Task Force on Practice Guidelines, Circulation 120(21):e169–e276, 2009.

101. Gottlieb SS, McCarter RJ, Vogel RA: Effect of beta-blockade on mortality among high-risk and low-risk patients after myocardial infarction, N Engl J Med 339(8):489–497, 1998.

102. Cleland JG, McGowan J, Clark A, et al: The evidence for beta blockers in heart failure, BMJ 318(7187):824–825, 1999.

103. Stone DH, Goodney PP, Schanzer A, et al: Clopidogrel is not associated with major bleeding complications during peripheral arterial surgery, J Vasc Surg 54(3):779–784, 2011.

104. Chang BB, Paty PS, Shah DM, et al: The right retroperitoneal approach for abdominal aortic surgery, Am J Surg 158(2):156–158, 1989.

105. Sicard GA, Reilly JM, Rubin BG, et al: Transabdominal versus retroperitoneal incision for abdominal aortic surgery: report of a prospective randomized trial, J Vasc Surg 21(2):174–181, 1995. discussion 181–173.

106. Cambria RP, Brewster DC, Abbott WM, et al: Transperitoneal versus retroperitoneal approach for aortic reconstruction: a randomized prospective study, J Vasc Surg 11(2):314–324, 1990. discussion 324–315.

107. Sieunarine K, Lawrence-Brown MM, Goodman MA: Comparison of transperitoneal and retroperitoneal approaches for infrarenal aortic surgery: early and late results, Cardiovasc Surg 5(1):71–76, 1997.

108. Samson RH, Lepore MR Jr, Showalter DP, et al: Long-term safety of left renal vein division and ligation to expedite complex abdominal aortic surgery, J Vasc Surg 50(3):500–504, 2009. discussion 504.

109. Green RM, Ricotta JJ, Ouriel K, et al: Results of supraceliac aortic clamping in the difficult elective resection of infrarenal abdominal aortic aneurysm, J Vasc Surg 9(1):124–134, 1989.

110. Breckwoldt WL, Mackey WC, Belkin M, et al: The effect of suprarenal cross-clamping on abdominal aortic aneurysm repair, Arch Surg 127(5):520–524, 1992.

111. Nypaver TJ, Shepard AD, Reddy DJ, et al: Repair of pararenal abdominal aortic aneurysms. An analysis of operative management, Arch Surg 128(7):803–811, 1993. discussion 811–803.

112. Olsen PS, Schroeder T, Agerskov K, et al: Surgery for abdominal aortic aneurysms. A survey of 656 patients, J Cardiovasc Surg (Torino) 32(5):636–642, 1991.

113. Provan JL, Fialkov J, Ameli FM, et al: Is tube repair of aortic aneurysm followed by aneurysmal change in the common iliac arteries? Can J Surg 33(5):394–397, 1990.

114. Polterauer P, Prager M, Holzenbein T, et al: Dacron versus polytetrafluoroethylene for Y-aortic bifurcation grafts: a six-year prospective, randomized trial, Surgery 111(6):626–633, 1992.

115. Lord RS, Nash PA, Raj BT, et al: Prospective randomized trial of polytetrafluoroethylene and Dacron aortic prosthesis. I. Perioperative results, Ann Vasc Surg 2(3):248–254, 1988.

116. Piotrowski JJ, McCroskey BL, Rutherford RB: Selection of grafts currently available for repair of abdominal aortic aneurysms, Surg Clin North Am 69(4):827–836, 1989.

117. Mabry CD, Thompson BW, Read RC: Activated clotting time (ACT) monitoring of intraoperative heparinization in peripheral vascular surgery, Am J Surg 138(6):894–900, 1979.

118. Ernst CB, Hagihara PF, Daugherty ME, et al: Inferior mesenteric artery stump pressure: a reliable index for safe IMA ligation during abdominal aortic aneurysmectomy, Ann Surg 187(6):641–646, 1978.

119. Thomas JH, Blake K, Pierce GE, et al: The clinical course of asymptomatic mesenteric arterial stenosis, J Vasc Surg 27(5):840–844, 1998.

120. Tollefson DF, Ernst CB: Natural history of atherosclerotic renal artery stenosis associated with aortic disease, J Vasc Surg 14(3):327–331, 1991.

121. Zierler RE, Bergelin RO, Davidson RC, et al: A prospective study of disease progression in patients with atherosclerotic renal artery stenosis, Am J Hypertens 9(11):1055–1061, 1996.

122. Dean RH, Benjamin ME, Hansen KJ: Surgical management of renovascular hypertension, Curr Probl Surg 34(3):209–308, 1997.

123. Cambria RP, Brewster DC, L'Italien G, et al: Simultaneous aortic and renal artery reconstruction: evolution of an eighteen-year experience, J Vasc Surg 21(6):916–924, 1995. discussion 925.

124. Benjamin ME, Hansen KJ, Craven TE, et al: Combined aortic and renal artery surgery. A contemporary experience, Ann Surg 223(5):555–565, 1996. discussion 565–557.

125. Williamson WK, Abou-Zamzam AM Jr, Moneta GL, et al: Prophylactic repair of renal artery stenosis is not justified in patients who require infrarenal aortic reconstruction, J Vasc Surg 28(1):14–20, 1998. discussion 20–12.

126. Nennhaus HP, Javid H: The distinct syndrome of spontaneous abdominal aortocaval fistula, Am J Med 44(3):464–473, 1968.

127. Miller DC, Myers BD: Pathophysiology and prevention of acute renal failure associated with thoracoabdominal or abdominal aortic surgery, J Vasc Surg 5(3):518–523, 1987.

128. Jarvinen O, Laurikka J, Salenius JP, et al: Mesenteric infarction after aortoiliac surgery on the basis of 1752 operations from the National Vascular Registry, World J Surg 23(3):243–247, 1999.

129. Bast TJ, van der Biezen JJ, Scherpenisse J, et al: Ischaemic disease of the colon and rectum after surgery for abdominal aortic aneurysm: a prospective study of the incidence and risk factors, Eur J Vasc Surg 4(3):253–257, 1990.

130. Welling RE, Roedersheimer LR, Arbaugh JJ, et al: Ischemic colitis following repair of ruptured abdominal aortic aneurysm, Arch Surg 120(12):1368–1370, 1985.

131. Ernst CB: Prevention of intestinal ischemia following abdominal aortic reconstruction, Surgery 93(1 Pt 1):102–106, 1983.

132. Szilagyi DE, Hageman JH, Smith RF, et al: Spinal cord damage in surgery of the abdominal aorta, Surgery 83(1):38–56, 1978.

133. DePalma RG, Levine SB, Feldman S: Preservation of erectile function after aortoiliac reconstruction, Arch Surg 113(8):958–962, 1978.

134. Lederle FA, Johnson GR, Wilson SE, et al: Quality of life, impotence, and activity level in a randomized trial of immediate repair versus surveillance of small abdominal aortic aneurysm, J Vasc Surg 38(4):745–752, 2003.

135. Flanigan DP, Schuler JJ, Keifer T, et al: Elimination of iatrogenic impotence and improvement of sexual function after aortoiliac revascularization, Arch Surg 117(5):544–550, 1982.

136. Weinstein MH, Machleder HI: Sexual function after aorto-iliac surgery, Ann Surg 181(6):787–790, 1975.

137. Pettersson M, Mattsson E, Bergbom I: Prospective follow-up of sexual function after elective repair of abdominal aortic aneurysms using open and endovascular techniques, *J Vasc Surg* 50(3):492–499, 2009.

138. Olin JW, Graor RA, O'Hara P, et al: The incidence of deep venous thrombosis in patients undergoing abdominal aortic aneurysm resection, *J Vasc Surg* 18(6):1037–1041, 1993.

139. Williamson WK, Nicoloff AD, Taylor LM Jr, et al: Functional outcome after open repair of abdominal aortic aneurysm, *J Vasc Surg* 33(5):913–920, 2001.

140. Huber TS, Wang JG, Derrow AE, et al: Experience in the United States with intact abdominal aortic aneurysm repair, *J Vasc Surg* 33(2):304–310, 2001. discussion 310–301.

141. Crawford ES, Saleh SA, Babb JW 3rd, et al: Infrarenal abdominal aortic aneurysm: factors influencing survival after operation performed over a 25-year period, *Ann Surg* 193(6):699–709, 1981.

142. Hollier LH, Plate G, O'Brien PC, et al: Late survival after abdominal aortic aneurysm repair: influence of coronary artery disease, *J Vasc Surg* 1(2):290–299, 1984.

143. Koskas F, Kieffer E: Long-term survival after elective repair of infrarenal abdominal aortic aneurysm: results of a prospective multicentric study. Association for Academic Research in Vascular Surgery (AURC), *Ann Vasc Surg* 11(5):473–481, 1997.

144. Soreide O, Lillestol J, Christensen O, et al: Abdominal aortic aneurysms: survival analysis of four hundred thirty-four patients, *Surgery* 91(2):188–193, 1982.

145. Vohra R, Reid D, Groome J, et al: Long-term survival in patients undergoing resection of abdominal aortic aneurysm, *Ann Vasc Surg* 4(5):460–465, 1990.

146. Norman PE, Semmens JB, Lawrence-Brown MM, et al: Long-term relative survival after surgery for abdominal aortic aneurysm in western Australia: population based study, *BMJ* 317(7162):852–856, 1998.

147. Stonebridge PA, Callam MJ, Bradbury AW, et al: Comparison of long-term survival after successful repair of ruptured and non-ruptured abdominal aortic aneurysm, *Br J Surg* 80(5):585–586, 1993.

148. Kazmers A, Perkins AJ, Jacobs LA: Aneurysm rupture is independently associated with increased late mortality in those surviving abdominal aortic aneurysm repair, *J Surg Res* 95(1):50–53, 2001.

149. Cho JS, Gloviczki P, Martelli E, et al: Long-term survival and late complications after repair of ruptured abdominal aortic aneurysms, *J Vasc Surg* 27(5):813–819, 1998. discussion 819–820.

150. Hertzer NR: Fatal myocardial infarction following abdominal aortic aneurysm resection. Three hundred forty-three patients followed 6–11 years postoperatively, *Ann Surg* 192(5):667–673, 1980.

151. Reigel MM, Hollier LH, Kazmier FJ, et al: Late survival in abdominal aortic aneurysm patients: The role of selective myocardial revascularization on the basis of clinical symptoms, *J Vasc Surg* 5(2):222–227, 1987.

152. AbuRahma AF, Robinson PA, Boland JP, et al: Elective resection of 332 abdominal aortic aneurysms in a southern West Virginia community during a recent five-year period, *Surgery* 109(3 Pt 1):244–251, 1991.

153. Diehl JT, Cali RF, Hertzer NR, et al: Complications of abdominal aortic reconstruction. An analysis of perioperative risk factors in 557 patients, *Ann Surg* 197(1):49–56, 1983.

154. Richardson JD, Main KA: Repair of abdominal aortic aneurysms. A statewide experience, *Arch Surg* 126(5):614–616, 1991.

CHAPTER 40

Endovascular Therapy for Abdominal Aortic Aneurysms

Matthew J. Eagleton, Gilbert R. Upchurch, Jr.

Surgical treatment of abdominal aortic aneurysms (AAAs) dates back centuries. Some of the initial approaches involved techniques similar in some fashion to modern endovascular techniques. In 1684, Moore reported on the use of large quantities of wire placed intraluminally into the aneurysm sac to induce thrombosis of an AAA.[1] Later, electric currents were passed through the wire to further promote thrombosis. A self-expanding endoluminally placed umbrella device was reported by Colt in the early 1900s to treat AAA.[2] In the mid-1900s, the use of endoluminally placed wire with the passage of electricity through it was revived and remained the procedure of choice until conventional operative therapy of AAA was introduced.[3] Operative repair of AAA evolved during the second half of the 20th century. Early techniques ranged from simple aortic ligation to aortic wrapping with cellophane.[4,5] Neither was successful. In 1951, the first replacement of an aortic aneurysm with an aortic homograft was described by Dubost et al.[6] Homografts, however, became aneurysmal over time, and the procedure evolved to the use of prosthetic material to reconstruct the aorta.[7,8] This technique was later modified by Creech, who reported on endoaneurysmorrhaphy with intraluminal graft placement, leaving the aneurysm sac *in situ*[9]; this has become the mainstay of treatment.

Although excellent results have been obtained with conventional aneurysm repair, it remains a complex, challenging operation that initiates great physiological stress for patients. The pursuit of a less invasive approach to AAA repair has subsequently evolved. Parodi et al.[10] reported the first use of endovascular AAA repair (EVAR). This approach allowed for intraluminal exclusion of an aneurysm with placement, through the femoral arteries, of an endograft. The hope was that this would decrease the morbidity and mortality of aneurysm repair and allow repairs to be performed in patients with significant comorbidities. The original endograft was constructed of a Dacron tube sutured to a Palmaz stent. Several generations of endografts have since been developed, tested, and put into general clinical use. With the evolution of aortic endografting, our knowledge about the pathophysiology of AAA has changed. Our understanding of the complexities of this mode of treatment is only just being realized and examined. This chapter reviews what is currently understood about endograft repairs of abdominal aortic aneurysms.

Indications

The indications for endovascular repair of an AAA remain the same as conventional repair with regard to the size of the aneurysm and its rate of growth. The classic teaching is that rupture rates for aneurysms depend on the size of the aneurysm. Rupture rates of 5% to 7% per year are estimated for aneurysms between 5 and 7 cm in diameter, and a greater than 20% rupture rate per year is estimated for larger aneurysms.[11] Compared with observation, surgical treatment for patients with these larger aneurysms significantly improves mortality.[12] Although it is known that small aneurysms do have the potential to rupture, the U.K. Small Aneurysm Trial, which randomized patients with AAAs between 4.5 and 5.5 cm to either surgery or observation, suggested that early repair did not improve survival.[13] The operative arm of this study, however, had a mortality rate of 5.8%, which is high compared with other large series of elective open AAA repair.[14] Perhaps with lower mortality rates in the operative arm, the conclusions of the study would have been reversed.[15]

Endovascular AAA repair is a less invasive technique than open surgery and offers several potential benefits over conventional AAA repair. It requires small femoral incisions instead of a large abdominal incision, which may decrease the incidence of postoperative pulmonary complications. Avoidance of extensive retroperitoneal dissection decreases the risk for perioperative bleeding. The period of aortic occlusion is minimal and accounts for the lower incidence of intraoperative hemodynamic and metabolic stress compared with patients undergoing open surgery.[16] Given these differences, endovascular aneurysm repair may be reasonable in patients who are "unfit" for conventional AAA surgery.[17] Proving its durability as a replacement for conventional surgery in relatively healthy patients is the aim of many clinical trials, the results of which will be discussed in more detail later.

Anatomical Requirements

The exact anatomical requirements for placing an aortic endograft vary with device design. There are key aspects of each device and aortic anatomy to be aware of when assessing a patient as a potential candidate for endograft repair. Preprocedural imaging is paramount for proper assessment of proximal and distal sites of fixation, as well as the path the endograft will traverse before taking its postdeployment position.

Imaging

Successful endograft placement is completely dependent on adequate and accurate preoperative planning. One of the major elements distinguishing preoperative planning in open aneurysm repair from endovascular repair is the latter's increased dependency on imaging to provide information necessary for clinical decisions. Preprocedural imaging allows the surgeon to determine whether a patient is an acceptable candidate for endovascular aortic grafting and which device is best suited for a particular patient; this ultimately allows for determining the proper size of the endograft.

Historically, contrast aortography was used as a routine adjunct to axial imaging because it was felt to allow for a more accurate determination of vessel length and angulation before computed tomography (CT) reformatting was widely available. Preoperative angiography is now rarely employed and reserved for cases where an adjunctive therapeutic intervention (i.e., coil embolization) is necessary.[18] Recently the advent of flat panel technology has allowed for development of rotational angiography techniques that facilitate construction of three-dimensional (3D) images found to be comparable to standard multidetector computed tomographic angiography (CTA). This technique has been termed *C-arm cone-beam CT* or *fluoro-CT*. Fluoro-CT uses a modified C-arm with specialized software and allows for precise measurements to be performed without using standard CT imaging.[19] Its routine use in preoperative planning prior to EVAR is currently under investigation.[20]

Spiral CT of the abdomen and pelvis is the mainstay of aortoiliac imaging. The imaging protocol is different from the standard protocol for most abdominal CT scans. Acquisition should use a 1:1.5 helical pitch and 3- to 5-mm collimation.[21] Two- to 3-mm slices are ideal for providing adequate information for stent graft planning. The two-dimensional (2D) images, however, can often be misinterpreted. The axial images may "cut" vessels at an angle, particularly iliac arteries that have some degree of tortuosity, thus creating an ellipse as opposed to visualization of the true lumen diameter. Due to this problem, some physicians recommend 3D image processing as a better method to evaluate aortoiliac anatomy for endograft therapy.[22] Although it was common initially to perform an angiogram in addition to a CT scan, recent evaluations suggest that high-quality 3D CT scans alone may provide sufficient data for endovascular graft planning.[18,23] Currently, proprietary products for CT postprocessing provide the ability to evaluate the 3D reconstruction of the aortoiliac system rapidly, rotate the images on the screen to obtain better vessel diameter measurements, and provide "virtual endograft" simulation.

Magnetic resonance angiography (MRA) can provide information similar to that of a CT scan. It too can provide thin-slice reconstructions and 3D postprocessing. Its usefulness, however, is often limited by availability and physician expertise. Magnetic resonance imaging may provide a useful modality to avoid use of iodinated contrast agents in patients.

Intravascular ultrasound (IVUS) is not routinely used in the preoperative evaluation of an endograft candidate. It is an invasive procedure, often performed at the time of angiography. Images produced by IVUS have a similar problem as viewing axial images on a 2D CT scan. Unless the catheter remains centerline within the aorta, the images produced will be elliptical, which may also provide shorter-than-required length measurements. Its primary use is at the time of stent graft placement to assess graft position relative to the renal artery ostia; this can help diminish the amount of contrast agent required.

Aortic Neck

The *aortic neck* is defined as the area of the aorta cephalad to the aneurysm in which the aortic endograft is placed (Fig. 40-1). This zone of the aorta is important for two reasons during aortic endografting. First, it is the site of proximal fixation that will prevent the device from migrating distally. Second, a circumferential seal must be obtained between the graft and the aorta in this area to prevent leakage of blood into the aneurysm sac. The exact length of aortic neck required is somewhat device dependent, but most commercially available devices require a 10- to 15-mm length of aortic neck

below the level of the most caudal renal artery. Some investigational devices may allow for shorter necks. Several devices employ the use of a suprarenal uncovered (or bare) stent to provide additional protection against graft migration. Suprarenal stent fixation may be useful, particularly in patients who have a shorter aortic neck, because it transfers protection against migration to a more normal segment of aorta. The suprarenal stent, however, does not provide any function with regard to creating a circumferential seal.

In addition to the length of the neck, other anatomical characteristics are important when determining whether patients are suitable candidates for endovascular aneurysm repair. These include aortic neck angulation, the shape of the neck, and the quality of the neck. *Neck angulation* refers to an alteration in the direction the aorta takes with regard to the centerline pathway. Acute angulation of the aortic neck can greatly affect the endograft's ability to obtain a proximal seal. Aortic neck angulation of greater than 60 degrees compared to the centerline is often considered prohibitive for endovascular aneurysm repair. The shape of the aortic neck also affects the ability of the graft to obtain a seal as well as fixation. A conical-shaped neck (Fig. 40-2) is generally felt to be unstable and predisposes to distal migration.[24] An increase in diameter from the top of the neck to the bottom of greater than 10% is often believed to be a contraindication to routine aortic endografting. Presence of circumferential thrombus or aortic calcification can also negatively affect an endograft's ability to obtain a proximal seal.

Iliac Arteries

The iliofemoral arterial system is important in endograft placement for two reasons. First, most endografts are placed through the common femoral artery (CFA) and must traverse the iliofemoral system to reach the aorta. Iliac artery diameter and tortuosity can adversely affect the ease with which the endograft traverses this course. This topic is covered in more detail below. Certainly the presence of significant atherosclerotic disease can cause arterial narrowing that inhibits placement of the device. In addition, tortuosity of the iliac arteries can hinder placement of the grafts (Fig. 40-3). Second, the iliofemoral system is important because it is the site of the distal seal between the endograft and the iliac artery, preventing retrograde flow of blood into the aneurysm sac.

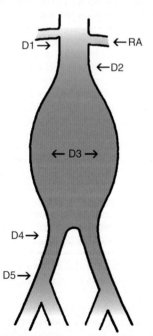

FIGURE 40-1 Diagram of abdominal aortic aneurysm (AAA). D1 represents diameter at proximal aspect of aortic neck, and D2 represents diameter at distal aspect of aortic neck. Distance between D1 and D2, in general, must be 10-15 mm to adequately place an endograft. Difference between diameter at D1 and D2 should not exceed 10%. D3 represents aortic diameter. D4 and D5 represent diameter within common iliac artery (CIA) where the distal fixation point of the aortic endograft occurs. Distance between D4 and D5 should exceed 15 mm. RA is the left and, in this case, most caudal renal artery.

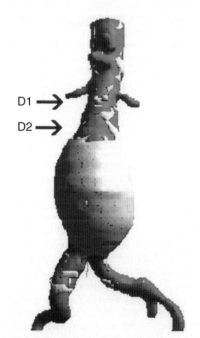

FIGURE 40-2 Three-dimensional (3D) reconstruction from spiral computed tomography (CT) scan of abdominal aortic aneurysm (AAA). This is representative of a conical neck. Distance between D1 and D2 is 15 mm. Diameter at D1 is 23 mm and at D2 is 28 mm, representing a >10% increase. Patient was not a suitable endograft candidate.

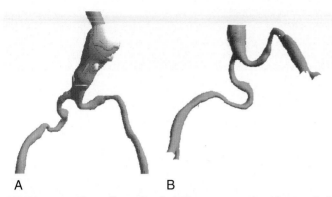

FIGURE 40-3 Three-dimensional (3D) reconstruction from spiral computed tomography (CT) scan of abdominal aortic aneurysm (AAA). Note tortuous iliac arteries **(A)**. Degree of tortuosity may be underestimated in direct anterior-posterior view, but on a more oblique angle **(B)**, a more significant degree of tortuosity is visible.

Many of the features necessary for an adequate aortic neck are also necessary for the distal landing zone. Presence of thrombus, calcification, and tortuosity can significantly hinder the iliac limb seal. Ectatic or aneurysmal iliac arteries obviously affect the ability of the graft to seal against the iliac limb. Most available endograft systems require at least a 15-mm segment of iliac artery to be of adequate caliber and free of significant disease to obtain a distal seal. If this is not present, adjunct interventions can be performed to assist in placing the device (i.e., iliac artery conduit placement, coil embolization of the internal iliac artery [IIA]). Management of these complicated situations is discussed in more detail later.

Endograft Design

Endograft design can greatly affect the ability of the device to be placed in patients, particularly in those with complex anatomy. Alterations in graft characteristics are what distinguish one manufacturer's device from another. Some key elements in endograft design are outlined in the following discussions.

Delivery System

Standard endograft insertion involves placement of the device through an arteriotomy in the common femoral artery, from where the graft traverses the external iliac and common iliac arteries (CIAs). The ability to deliver the endograft safely and effectively in this fashion is a prerequisite for effective repair. Three factors are important determinants of device delivery.[25]

DELIVERY SYSTEM SIZE

With the placement of most endografts through the iliofemoral arterial system, any site along this pathway can represent a size limitation, the most common of which is the external iliac artery (EIA). Inadequate diameter or presence of extensive calcifications can exclude standard endograft placement. It is intuitive that the size of the delivery system cannot be larger than the size of the iliac arteries it traverses. Most sheaths are sized based on inner diameter, so knowledge of the outer diameter of the sheaths is necessary for safe graft placement. Different manufacturers' devices have different size measurements for the delivery systems, so one device may be suitable for placement, whereas another is not. Most delivery systems easily traverse an iliofemoral segment of 7 to 8 mm in diameter (or a sheath that does not exceed 21 F), although several designs that provide a lower-profile system are currently in clinical trials in the United States.

FLEXIBILITY

Tortuosity, another anatomical variant, affects the ability to adequately deliver the endograft system. Tortuous iliac vessels can be "straightened" with the use of stiff guidewires, but this is not always possible or desirable. The ideal delivery system easily traverses these arteries on the basis of an intrinsic degree of flexibility. Again, different delivery systems have different abilities to track through tortuous iliac arteries, and some may be more successfully placed than others in this anatomical variant. Delivery systems composed of long, flexible, tapered tips pass more easily than those with short, stiff, blunt tips. In addition, other aspects of device construction, such as metallic struts that provide columnar strength, increase device rigidity and limit use in tortuous vessels.[25]

DELIVERABILITY

A number of features have been noted to affect the deliverability of endograft devices. As stated previously, long, flexible, tapered tips pass more easily than short, blunt, stiff ones. This allows for easier maneuverability through tortuous vessels, as well as past sites of narrowing. Larger-caliber devices are also more difficult to deliver, particularly in patients with smaller-diameter arteries.[25] Some delivery systems allow for placement of the endograft system through alternate sheaths, whereas other systems necessitate use of the manufacturer's own delivery system. This can greatly affect placement of specific endografts in specific anatomical variants. A thorough understanding of the patient's arterial anatomy and the limitations of different endograft systems are important. The complexity of the delivery system also affects the ease with which it is placed. Some devices generally provide a simple maneuver to deploy the graft, whereas others have several complicated steps.

Endograft Features

The ideal endograft should be flexible enough to maneuver through tortuous and angulated vessels but also rigid enough to prevent kinking. It should have a low profile (having a small external diameter) that would allow it to be placed through as small an arteriotomy as possible. Two general classifications of endografts exist: unibody and modular. A unibody device is a single-piece graft—including the main body and both limbs. Although this decreases the risk of endoleaks at the graft-graft interface, the unibody design often requires a larger delivery system, and sizing can be more difficult. The modular system includes endografts that are composed of two to three pieces. Generally there is a main body that may have one attached limb and one or two docking limbs. These devices can be introduced through smaller delivery systems and offer a greater degree of flexibility with regard to placement. With multiple sites of graft-graft interface, however, there is an increased risk of endoleak, as explained later.

Graft material is variable and can range from thin-walled polytetrafluoroethylene (PTFE) to polyester. The graft material is typically supported by a metal framework that is commonly stainless steel, its modified version Elgiloy, or nitinol. The graft support can be placed inside the graft material (endoskeleton) or outside the graft (exoskeleton). Grafts can be fully supported, having stent material throughout, or only partially supported, with aspects of the device composed only of graft material and no metal. The graft skeleton provides several key elements to endograft make-up. First, it assists in graft fixation and in obtaining a seal. These stents provide some degree of radial force that helps provide a seal, as well as providing a point of fixation. Some devices have hooks or barbs in the proximal aspect of the skeleton that help anchor the graft onto the aortic wall and prevent migration. In addition, some devices employ a metal framework that extends above the fabric and is used to engage the aorta in the pararenal or suprarenal location. The second function of the skeleton is to provide columnar strength, which may prevent graft migration. The skeleton can also prevent kinking and occlusion of limbs as they traverse the aortoiliac anatomy. Lack of stents, however, may allow a graft to adapt more readily to morphological changes without dislocation of attachment sites. The interplay of the stent and fabric materials can lead to eventual erosion of the fabric.

TABLE 40-1	**Description of a Variety of Commercially Available Endografts**							
COMPANY	DEVICE	INITIAL FDA APPROVAL DATE	DEPLOYMENT TYPE	GRAFT MATERIAL	STENT MATERIAL	BIFURCATED DEVICE DESIGN	MAIN BODY SHEATH SIZE (OD)	FIXATION
Cook (Bloomington, Ind.)	Zenith	May 2003	Self-expanding	Dacron	Stainless steel	Modular	21F-26F	Suprarenal
Gore (Flagstaff, Ariz.)	Excluder	November 2002	Self-expanding	ePTFE	Nitinol	Modular	20F-23F	Infrarenal
Endologix (Irvine, Calif.)	Powerlink	October 2004	Self-expanding	High-density ePTFE	Cobalt chromium alloy	Unibody	21F	Anatomical (with either suprarenal or infrarenal proximal orientation)
Medtronic (Minneapolis, Minn.)	AneuRx	September 1999	Self-expanding	Dacron	Nitinol	Modular	21F	Infrarenal
Medtronic (Minneapolis, Minn.)	Talent	June 2008	Self-expanding	Dacron	Nitinol	Modular	22F-24F	Suprarenal

ePTFE, expanded polytetrafluoroethylene; FDA, U.S. Food and Drug Administration; OD, outer diameter.

Specific Grafts

Various endografts are currently commercially available or in clinical trials in the United States. A brief description of the currently commercially available endograft systems (in the United States) is outlined in Table 40-1 and depicted in Figure 40-4.

Graft Placement and Postoperative Management

Once the patient is deemed an endograft candidate, the best graft has been chosen, and the device properly sized, the patient can undergo implantation. The majority of endografts are placed through the femoral arteries that have been operatively exposed. The majority of surgeons prefer the use of the transverse incision as it associated with a lower rate of wound complications (12.7% in transverse incision vs. 47.5% in vertical incisions).[26] Percutaneous access for EVAR is growing in popularity, and its use will become even more widespread with the further development of low-profile devices. Suture-mediated closure devices facilitate this process, and using a "preclose" technique has been described to allow closure of sheaths as large as 24 F.[27] Use of this procedure has been associated with 70% to 100% technical success, and immediate failures mandate surgical exploration of the femoral artery. Prospective analysis has demonstrated that use of a percutaneous approach may shorten operating times and reduce the rate of wound-related complications, without a significant increase in overall procedural cost.[27–29] The aorta is then cannulated with a guidewire and catheter. Small boluses of contrast agent are delivered to further define the anatomy and localize the renal arteries. With an angulated aorta, it is important to remember that the best view of the renal arteries and visualization of the fixation zone may not be in a direct anterior-posterior plane but at a more cranial-caudal angle. The device is then generally advanced over a stiff guidewire and correctly positioned to allow the most extensive coverage within the aortic neck without intruding on the orifice of the renal arteries. Each device has its own unique instruction for actual deployment. Once the main body and ipsilateral limb have been placed, the contralateral limb has to be placed. The sequence of events for this varies depending on graft design—whether unibody or modular.

Recovery following EVAR is generally rapid and uncomplicated, and most patients are discharged home on the first or second postoperative day. Return to activities of daily living has been shown to be quicker following endovascular repair than open surgery. In addition, most patients report less postoperative pain. Aortic remodeling following EVAR, however, is a slow process that continues for several years. Anatomical changes in the native vessel, particularly at the proximal neck, can cause conformational changes in the implanted device that mandate close follow-up. In addition, late failures have been identified that have required reintervention.[30] Given these facts, routine surveillance following EVAR is universally recommended, although there are no standard regimens, and the requirements of a standard intensive regimen are debated. Nordon et al. performed a meta-analysis evaluating secondary intervention rates based on contemporary graft implants.[31] Their findings demonstrated that surveillance imaging alone initiated the secondary intervention in 1.4% to 9% of cases. Over 90% of EVAR cases, however, received no benefit from surveillance scans. Based on these findings, the group recommended that surveillance should be directed toward those patients identified as having a high risk for postoperative complications. Identification of this group, however, is not obvious but may be necessary in patients with complicated aortic neck anatomy or in patients in whom the device was used outside of the indications for use (IFU).

Contrast-enhanced CT is the most widely used modality for follow-up after EVAR. It is widely available, has rapid data acquisition, reproducibility, and is uniform across institutions. The major concerns associated with this modality are use of a contrast agent and the potential associated nephrotoxicity, radiation exposure, and cost. It is considered the gold standard for assessing aortic diameter, with nearly 100% sensitivity and specificity. Sensitivity and specificity rates for endoleak detection with CT are better than those with conventional angiography: 92% and 90% for CT vs. 63% and 77% for angiography, respectively.[32–34] Triphasic CT (noncontrasted phase, arterial phase, and delayed phase) results in the greatest amount of information but at the cost of increased radiation exposure. Unenhanced CT imaging is useful for differentiation of endoleaks from calcifications from the metallic portion of a stent graft, and can help detect small perigraft leaks better than arterial-phase images. Use of arterial phase alone has a lower diagnostic value than combined arterial and delayed-phase scanning.[35]

Repeated CT scanning subjects the patient to potential carcinogenic risks associated with ionizing radiation exposure. The estimated lifetime attributable risk of death from cancer following an abdominal CT scan in a patient older than 50 years of age is 0.02%.[31,36] Although this effect in itself is small, the cumulative effects over time with repeat imaging can be significant. Repetitive use of iodinated contrast can have a cumulative deleterious effect on renal function, especially in the elderly and those patients with preexisting renal impairment.[37] Given this, as well as the expense, the use of alternate modes of surveillance has been evaluated.

Magnetic resonance imaging (MRI) and MRA provide much of the same imaging information that can be acquired by CT scanning.

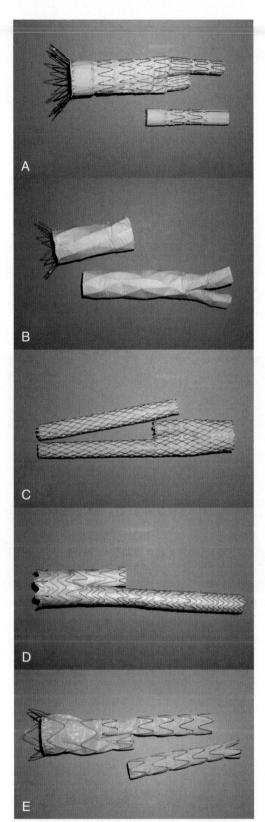

FIGURE 40-4 Several endograft systems illustrating different features.
A, Zenith endograft (Cook Inc., Bloomington, Ind.) represents a three-piece modular system with a main body and separate bilateral limbs. This graft design uses a bare suprarenal stent and internal stents at the sealing zones and is otherwise supported by a stainless steel Z-stent exoskeleton. **B,** Powerlink graft (Endologix, Irvine, Calif.) constructed of expanded polytetrafluoroethylene (ePTFE) and a cobalt alloy skeleton. **C,** AneuRx stent graft system (Medtronic AVE, Santa Rosa, Calif.) composed of nitinol exoskeleton. **D,** Excluder endograft (WL Gore and Associates, Flagstaff, Ariz.), which represents a two-piece modular system. Graft is constructed from ePTFE and is fully supported by a nitinol exoskeleton. **E,** Talent endograft system (Medtronic AVE, Santa Rosa, Calif.) represents a two-piece modular system composed of a suprarenal bare stent and then a nitinol endoskeleton.

Multiple format MR images (T1, T2, gadolinium-enhanced) can be viewed in 2D and be reformatted into 3D volumes, allowing dimensional measurements, assessment of luminal patency, device positioning, and detecting the presence of an endoleak. Limitations of MRA/MRI include potential magnet-induced *in vivo* metallic heating or motion, which may prevent imaging in the immediate postimplant time period. In addition, postimplant artifacts, in particular with ferromagnetic metallic stents, will limit morphological assessments. Furthermore, there is a risk of nephrogenic systemic fibrosis associated with gadolinium contrast use in patients with renal insufficiency.[38] Benefits of MRI are related to the lack of exposure to ionizing radiation and low nephrotoxicity of MR contrast medium. Disadvantages of MRI are its lack of wide availability, longer procedure time than CT, patient claustrophobia, and contraindications for patients with cardiac pacemakers.

Color duplex ultrasonography (US) is a convenient, noninvasive, inexpensive portable means of postimplant surveillance. Its reliability as a useful surveillance tool, however, is still debated. Grayscale US is accurate for measurement of aortic aneurysm diameter. Endoleak detection by US requires color duplex. The reported specificity rates of color duplex US for endoleak detection are high (89%-97%), but the sensitivity and diagnostic power of color duplex US for endoleak detection compared with CT is still debated.[39] The use of duplex US to detect an endoleak has a sensitivity of approximately 77%, with a specificity approaching 94%.[40] The addition of US contrast agents increases sensitivity to 98%, with no significant change in specificity.[40] Contrast agents are useful in identifying slow leaks that are not readily discernible on CT.[41,42] Detection of flow direction of the endoleak is also an advantage of US that is not easily discernable with CT.[43] Presence of a "to-and-fro" flow pattern is associated with spontaneous closure of the endoleak, whereas a monophasic or biphasic waveform is consistent with endoleak persistence.[43] Limitations of color duplex US include its operator dependence, variation based on patient physical size, and the need for optimal patient preparation. The substitution of duplex US imaging for CT, however, may result in long-term cost savings.[44]

Problems with Endografting and Management

Various problems can arise in the planning and placement of abdominal aortic endografts. Once the grafts are in place, several complications can arise over time that may require intervention to prevent subsequent expansion and possible rupture of the previously excluded aneurysm. In the following section, several of the more common problems that occur following endograft placement are outlined.

Iliac Artery Disease

When iliac artery disease is present, whether it be aneurysmal disease, atherosclerotic disease, or severe tortuosity, the use of an iliac conduit can provide a safe route to deliver the endograft.[45] In cases of iliac artery lumen narrowing resulting from atherosclerotic disease or increased vessel tortuosity, advancement of the device, despite the presence of resistance, can result in rupture of the iliac artery. Iliac artery rupture has been reported in 1% to 2% of cases.[46,47] To circumvent prohibitive iliac artery anatomy, an iliac conduit can be used. An iliac conduit involves suturing a prosthetic graft (generally 8-10 mm in diameter) to the mid–CIA even if it is aneurysmal. This can be done in an end-to-end or end-to-side fashion, although the latter often provides a greater lumen for passage of the device. The device is placed through the prosthetic graft, and the iliac limb of the endovascular graft traverses the CIA and anastomosis and seals within the conduit. The distal end of the graft is tunneled along the natural course of the iliac artery and anastomosed to the femoral artery. The distal end of the CIA is oversewn to allow retrograde flow through the EIA to supply the ipsilateral hypogastric artery. Alternatively, the hypogastric artery can be anastomosed directly to the conduit.

Iliac artery ectasia or aneurysms can present a problem in obtaining a distal seal. Enlarged CIAs are present in up to 30% of patients presenting for endovascular aneurysm repair.[48–51] Many available endografts do not allow for ectatic or aneurysmal common iliac arteries, so the distal seal may have to be obtained within the external iliac artery, which is often of normal caliber. If the distal seal occurs in the external iliac artery, the hypogastric artery is generally sacrificed using coil embolization. Presence of a hypogastric artery aneurysm would necessitate the same approach. Rarely, bilateral hypogastric artery embolization is required. Hypogastric artery embolization can occur before aneurysm repair or concurrently. If bilateral embolization is planned, it is generally performed in a staged fashion, although its occlusion is not always planned. Hypogastric artery embolization is not without risk, and side effects can occur in up to 50% of patients.[49] Buttock claudication is the predominant complaint after hypogastric artery occlusion. This occurs in 12% to 50% of patients, but in most it generally resolves after several months.[48–53] Some 5% to 25% of men complain of new-onset erectile dysfunction (ED).[51,52] Buttock ischemia and bowel ischemia requiring resection are of theoretical concern, but they have not been described in any of the larger series. Patients requiring embolization in the more distal branches of the hypogastric artery (as might be done with the presence of an IIA aneurysm) and those in whom coil placement was not adequately controlled are at higher risk of developing pelvic symptoms.[53] Bilateral hypogastric artery embolization has not been associated with increased symptoms when compared with unilateral occlusion.[49,50,52] Coil embolization of the IIA is not necessary if it is not aneurysmal. In the face of CIA aneurysms, Wyers et al.[54] have shown that if there is a 5-mm neck of iliac artery proximal to the hypogastric artery in addition to a 15-mm neck in the external iliac artery, coil embolization of the hypogastric artery is not necessary to obtain a distal seal. This may be possible in up to two thirds of patients requiring coverage of the hypogastric artery.

Endoleaks

An *endoleak* is the persistence of blood flow outside the endograft, but in the aneurysm sac. Endoleaks are classified according to their etiology, and currently five types have been described[47,48] (Table 40-2). A type 1 endoleak (Fig. 40-5) arises from inadequate sealing at either the proximal aortic (allowing antegrade flow) or distal iliac (allowing retrograde flow) attachment sites. Type 2 endoleaks (Fig. 40-6) arise from patent branch vessels off of the aortic sac that allow for retrograde flow into the aneurysm. Such branches may include a patent lumbar or inferior mesenteric artery (IMA). Type 3 endoleaks develop from defects in the fabric of the graft or at the junction zone between modular components. Type 4 endoleaks develop secondary to diffuse "leaking" of blood between the interstices of the fabric or where the graft is sutured to a stent. Type 5 endoleaks describe a scenario in which the aneurysm sac remains pressurized and the aneurysm enlarges, but no demonstrable flow of blood into the sac can be visualized on current imaging modalities. These may be due to imaging that is not sophisticated enough to discern these leaks

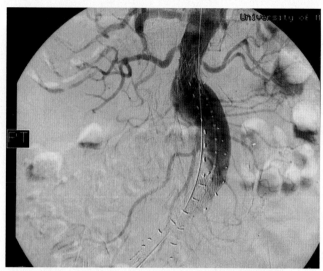

FIGURE 40-5 **Angiogram demonstrating a type 1 endoleak.** Contrast can be seen leaking around proximal part of graft and filling aneurysm sac. Patient subsequently had a giant Palmaz stent placed in the aortic neck, and this ameliorated the endoleak.

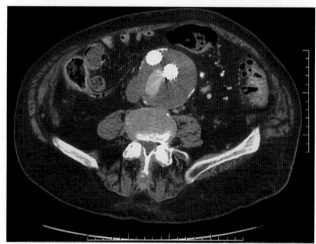

FIGURE 40-6 **Computed tomography (CT) scan representative of a type 2 endoleak.** There is contrast within aneurysm sac but outside limbs of endograft. This aneurysm had continued expansion until patient underwent embolization of inferior mesenteric artery (IMA).

or due to intermittent episodes of leakage.[49] The pressure applied to the aneurysm sac causing it to continue to expand in this situation, has been termed *endotension*.[50,51] Controversy with regard to this concept exists, in particular with the ability of the thrombus to transmit pressure to the aneurysm wall. It is argued that these merely represent a type 1, 2, or 3 endoleak in which the defect is large enough to allow blood to flow into the sac and transmit pressure to the sac, but the exit site is not present or too small to be detected.

Type 1 and type 3 endoleaks are associated with significant risks of aneurysm enlargement and possible rupture, and these should be treated.[55,56] This may be accomplished with placement of an extension cuff limb over the site of the leak. If the leak is a type 1 and the graft is juxtaposed to the inferior border of the renal arteries, a large balloon-expandable stent can be placed in the proximal aspect of the endograft. This provides increased radial force, causing better juxtaposition of the graft and aortic wall, thus ameliorating the leakage. If this is unsuccessful, open repair and graft explantation are generally indicated. Fabric tears are easily managed if the site of the leak is localized. In these situations, the tear can be covered with a cuff or extension. When it is more

TABLE 40-2	Endoleak Classification	
ENDOLEAK	**CAUSE**	**BLOOD FLOW INTO SAC**
Type 1	Inadequate seal at aortic or iliac attachment sites	Antegrade or retrograde
Type 2	Patent branches off aneurysm sac	Retrograde
Type 3	Fabric defects or component junctions	Antegrade
Type 4	Leak at fabric interstices	Antegrade
Type 5	Endotension	No clear leak

diffuse, the entire endograft can be relined with a second endograft, or the device can be removed and the aneurysm repaired in an open fashion.

Type 2 endoleaks are rarely associated with aneurysm rupture.[57] At least 10% to 15% of patients are identified with a type 2 endoleak during follow-up.[58–61] Warfarin treatment is not associated with an increased incidence of early or delayed postoperative endoleak, but type 2 endoleaks are less likely to undergo spontaneous resolution in these patients.[62] Type 2 endoleaks are generally observed unless they are associated with an increase in aneurysm size or aortic pulsatility on physical examination. In these situations, arteriography is the next step to identify the source of the endoleak. Superior mesenteric artery injection reveals retrograde IMA flow as the source, whereas selective hypogastric artery injection demonstrates a lumbar artery filling the aneurysm. Super-selective arterial canalization can then be performed with embolization of the feeding vessels. Another approach is through direct aneurysm sac puncture.[63] With direct sac puncture, one can measure sac pressure and inject the sac directly with contrast agent to precisely identify the leak. The systolic sac pressure is related to the size of the leak, and the pulse amplitude is related to the resistance of the outflow vessels and sac compliance.[64] After localization of the leak, feeding vessels can be directly accessed and embolized.[65] In addition, the sac can be filled with substances such as coils, glue, or gel foam to further prevent flow. Differences in outcomes between these two different approaches has not been realized.[66]

Measurement of intrasac pressures may help determine whether an endoleak is present at the time of the original surgery or if an endoleak has been adequately treated if it has been approached through direct sac puncture. In an *ex vivo* model of endoleaks, Parodi et al.[67] evaluated pressure changes in the aortic sac with various types and sizes of endoleaks. In this model, sac pressures were significantly higher than systemic pressures in the presence of all endoleaks. This obviously places the aneurysm at significant risk for rupture. Presence of patent side branches significantly reduced the pressure within the sac, particularly the mean pressure and diastolic pressure. Clinically, persistent side branches augment the development of type 2 endoleaks and influence early sac behavior.[68,69] Gawenda et al.[70] evaluated the use of sac pressure monitoring and found it helpful in the detection and treatment of endoleaks. They noted, however, that intrasac pressure measurements did not correlate with AAA size change over ensuing follow-up. This may be an effective modality for monitoring aneurysms after endograft exclusion once less invasive methods of pressure measurement are developed.

Structural Failure

Material failure represents one of the most concerning problems for potential failure of endograft placement. This is a difficult event to identify because patients are often asymptomatic and may not present with any acute changes in their endograft evaluation. Three modes of structural failure have been described in aortic endografting and involve fabric erosion, suture disruption, and metal fracture.[71]

Development of endoleaks secondary to graft erosion has been documented with some first-generation endograft devices[72,73] (Fig. 40-7). It has been speculated that the areas of graft erosion are secondary to friction between the stent material and the fabric, which can be confounded by pulsation of the aorta. Predicting the incidence of fabric fatigue is difficult, and although this does occur in grafts placed by conventional open aneurysm repair, it occurs much more rapidly and more commonly in the endograft systems.[74,75] In several device designs, the graft fabric is attached to the metal skeleton through the use of sutures. Disruption of these sutures is believed to explain graft failure in some instances.[76–78] The mechanism for suture failure is believed to be the same as for fabric erosion—namely, motion of the stents with aortic pulsations causes friction and wear of the sutures, with subsequent suture fracture.

The most common structural problem identified in aortic endograft systems has been metallic stent fractures.[75] Stent and hook

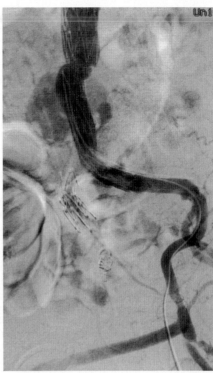

FIGURE 40-7 **Angiogram revealing a type 3 endoleak that developed at site of a tear in graft fabric.** This was a "homemade" aorto-uniiliac graft that had been in place for approximately 5 years. Patient presented with new-onset abdominal pain and had a computed tomography (CT) scan that revealed an aneurysm sac that had significantly expanded in diameter. Tear was sealed by placement of a new endograft.

fractures in the phase 1 trial of the Endovascular Technologie's graft resulted in suspension of the program and redesign of the metallic attachment system.[79] In a review of 686 patients who underwent endovascular aneurysm repair, Jacobs et al. identified 60 patients who had material failure.[75] Forty-three (72%) of these failures were due to metallic stent fractures and occurred in various different endografts with different stent composition. The cause of metal failure has been attributed to stress fatigue and metal corrosion, particularly in nitinol stents.[80] Corrosion has not been seen in next-generation endografts and may reflect improved nitinol processing.[81–83] Tortuosity of the arterial system can also stress the stent graft system and lead to metal fracture. This has been reported in the longitudinal bar of the Talent and Gore stent graft devices.[75]

Limb Thrombosis

Endograft limb thrombosis after endovascular repair of infrarenal AAA is a recognized complication occurring in up to 11% of patients.[84–90] Various underlying factors have been purported to place patients at increased risk for limb thrombosis. One reported risk factor is the lack of device support. Although Carroccio et al.[85] reported on the results of 351 bifurcated grafts with no significant association between use of unsupported devices and graft thrombosis, others have suggested there is a significant relationship. Baum et al.[91] specifically evaluated the rates of graft limb kinking and thrombosis between supported and unsupported abdominal aortic stent grafts. In total, 12% of the limbs in their series required an intervention for kinking. In the supported limbs, 5% required subsequent placement of arterial stents; 2% required these for evidence of kinking at the time of the initial operation, and 3% required stenting in the postoperative period after the patients presented with limb thrombosis. In the unsupported grafts, there was an intervention rate of 44%. About half of these had an additional stent placed at the time of the initial procedure, and the remainder had a subsequent stent placed in the postoperative follow-up period, owing to limb thrombosis or severe stenosis.

Another factor increasing the risk of limb thrombosis is oversizing of the iliac limb. Oversizing causes the graft material to have a significant amount of infolding, reducing the intraluminal diameter.[87] Along these lines, significant intraluminal vessel narrowing from underlying atherosclerotic disease or tortuosity can result in flow abnormalities and eventually cause graft limb thrombosis.[91] Extension of the graft limb into the EIA has also been described as a risk factor for developing limb thrombosis.[85] It was believed that transition into the EIA caused both a significant reduction in arterial diameter and a kink in the graft due to acute angulation of the limb as it passed through the pelvis. Damage to the distal iliac or femoral artery, such as dissection during graft placement, can subsequently cause outflow obstruction and graft limb thrombosis.[84]

Management of patients presenting with limb thrombosis depends on the severity of the patient's symptoms. In the series by Carroccio et al.,[85] nearly a third of the patients presenting with symptoms had such mild symptoms that no intervention was required. Most patients, however, underwent a femoral-femoral bypass to restore flow to the affected extremity. Few patients are successfully treated with thrombolysis or graft thrombectomy followed by endovascular repair of the underlying problem. In most series, patients with limb problems generally present early, within the first 6 months following endograft repair.[84,91–95] In fact, Sampram et al.[93] reported that no limb occlusions presented after 30 months of follow-up.

Migration

Distal stent graft migration after abdominal aortic endografting has been reported to occur in 9% to 45% of patients.[61,96–99] Migration certainly has been identified as a risk for development of a type 1 endoleak and delayed aneurysm rupture or late conversion to open repair. The pathophysiology behind aortic endograft migration is complex, and various factors contribute to its occurrence.[100] A number of forces are at play within the aortic endograft, but blood flow acts as the main displacing force. As the tube of the aortic graft curves, there is a change in the velocity of the blood, resulting in an increased displacement force. For many endografts, the forces providing protection against migration are friction forces of the graft against the aortic wall and the columnar strength of the graft. The friction forces depend on the apposition of the graft fabric and the aortic wall and obviously can be affected by aortic wall composition (thrombus, calcifications), size of the aorta, radial force of the stent, and the nature of the graft fabric. It has been suggested that the presence of barbs or hooks in the proximal portion of the stent graft may provide additional protection.[101]

The infrarenal aortic neck length and its maximum diameter, shape, and angulation have all been implicated as causes of stent graft migration.[96,102,103] All of these work to decrease the friction between the stent graft and aortic wall. Albertini et al.[102] evaluated the development of proximal perigraft endograft leak and device migration following endovascular aneurysm repair. Fifteen patients had graft migration, and 31 of 184 repairs developed a proximal endoleak. Neck angulation was the only factor found to be significant in the development of device migration, whereas neck angulation and neck diameter were the two factors important in developing a proximal perigraft endoleak.[102] Lee et al.,[104] however, were unable to identify any specific anatomical correlate and device migration. They did observe that any device that migrated distally by more than 1 cm subsequently required an intervention.

Other hypotheses as to the cause of device migration have focused on morphological changes in the aneurysm and aortic neck after endovascular AAA repair. Specifically, aortic neck dilation, longitudinal sac shrinkage, and graft shortening have been described.[96,97,105,106] One of the more widely accepted hypotheses is aortic neck dilation following aortic endografting. After endovascular aneurysm repair, the aneurysm neck has been documented to dilate significantly, mostly in the first 2 years after graft placement.[107] In a review by Cao et al.,[99] 17 (15%) of 148 patients had

an episode of device migration. The only two independent risk factors for device migration were neck dilation postoperatively and an AAA diameter of greater than 55 mm. Others have argued that neck dilation is not a significant event, provided adequate graft oversizing was performed at initial endograft placement.[104] The amount the aortic neck dilated did not exceed the size of the original aortic endograft placed. Larger aneurysms have also been noted to have increased risks of developing type 1 endoleak, graft migration, and the subsequent need for open surgical conversion compared with larger aneurysms.[108]

Outcomes

Results of Aortic Endografting

Endovascular AAA repair generally has a low mortality rate (1%-3%) compared to open repair, and subsequent rates of aneurysm rupture after endovascular repair are reduced to 1% per year.[56,61,93,109] Endograft placement is not free of adverse events, however, and there is frequent need for secondary interventions. Naslund et al.[110] reported technical complications in 26% of 34 endografts placed. Fairman et al. evaluated the occurrence of critical events during deployment of their initial 75 endografts, and patients were divided into three groups corresponding to the time period in which the graft was placed.[94] Critical events were defined as unanticipated technical difficulties that occurred during the course of operation that threatened the success of the procedure. Difficulty in obtaining access occurred in nearly one quarter of all patients. Although it would be expected that the latter 25 patients should not have experienced as great a difficulty in obtaining access, these patients had increased complexity of their aortoiliac anatomy compared with endograft patients earlier in their experience. This group had a greater frequency of iliac artery balloon angioplasty, as well as the use of iliac artery conduits. Deployment difficulties existed and were composed mostly of graft foreshortening, necessitating the placement of additional distal covered extensions. Other deployment issues encountered included suprarenal graft displacement, infrarenal graft displacement, and device-related issues such as iliac limb kinking or twisting. Malplacement of the graft did not correlate with anatomical complexity.

The need for subsequent secondary procedures has been evaluated by several large series of patients who had an abdominal aortic endograft placed.[88,93,111,112] The Eurostar registry reported the results of 1023 patients with a follow-up of 12 months or longer.[111] Overall, 186 (18%) patients required a secondary intervention. The majority of these interventions (76%) involved a transfemoral procedure, whereas the remaining patients required transabdominal (12%) or extra-anatomical (11%) surgery. The rates of freedom from intervention at 1, 3, and 4 years were 89%, 67%, and 62%, respectively. The transfemoral procedures performed most frequently were aortic or iliac limb extension for graft migration or endoleak. Late death was more frequent in those patients requiring a secondary intervention resulting in a 3-year cumulative survival of 85%, which is lower than the 90% rate ($P < 0.05$) observed in those that did not require reintervention. In addition, death was more frequently associated with those requiring a transabdominal procedure.

The Montefiore Medical Center and the Cleveland Clinic Foundation have published their single-institution results on the durability of aortic endografting. Montefiore reported on 239 endografts placed over 9 years, with a technical success rate of 88.7%.[88] The 5-year survival rate in this group was only 37%. Secondary interventions were required in 10% of the patients, with more than half of the secondary procedures being performed for presence of an endoleak. Sampram et al.[93] reported the results from the Cleveland Clinic Foundation on 703 patients undergoing endovascular aortic endografting, with follow-up averaging 1 year. Survival in this group was 90% at 1 year and declined to 70% at 3 years. Overall, 128 secondary interventions were performed in 105 patients (15%). Freedom from intervention mirrored that of the Eurostar registry, with freedom from intervention rates of 88%, 76%, and 65% at 1, 2, and

3 years, respectively. Mortality related to the secondary procedure was 8% but rose to 18% in those requiring a transabdominal procedure. Univariate analysis revealed that secondary procedures were more common in patients with larger major and minor sac axes, in patients who received a large aortic stent because of a proximal endoleak present at initial aneurysm repair, and in patients who received treatment later in the course of the review. This last finding is felt to be secondary to the increased complexity of cases approached in an endovascular fashion.

The Cleveland Clinic Foundation review included the use of six different devices, which included two Zenith grafts—one that was part of the multicenter national trial and one group that was part of a sponsor-investigator investigational device exemption trial.[25] The overall freedom from risk of rupture was 98.7% at 2 years. Results of this review reveal that there are significant differences in outcomes between groups with different endovascular devices, in particular with regard to limb occlusion and rate of endoleak. Limb occlusion occurred most frequently with the Ancure device, at a rate of 11% at 2 years. Endoleak of any kind was most common with the Excluder device, at a rate of 64% at 1 year. Modular separations were the most frequent with the Zenith graft at 3.5%. Aneurysm sac shrinkage correlated inversely with the frequency of endoleaks, and aneurysm sac shrinkage was most common in the Zenith and Talent groups but least common in the Excluder group. There were no differences with regard to rate of secondary procedures, conversion to open repair, or migration. Sternbergh et al.[113] have reported similar findings. Outcomes were compared between the Zenith device and the AneuRx device, and it was determined that the Zenith graft was associated with fewer endoleaks and a higher rate and amount of aneurysm sac shrinkage. Bertges et al.[114] also reported similar findings in their evaluation. Regression of AAA size after endograft placement was more significant after placement of the Talent and Ancure endografts than with the AneuRx or Excluder devices. During the first 2 years of follow-up, the initial size of the AAA, presence of an endoleak, and type of graft used were significant predictors of sac shrinkage. After 2 years, however, only graft type was significant. Ouriel et al.[108] have additionally concluded that the outcome after endovascular AAA repair depends on the initial size of the aneurysm.

Comparison with Open Surgery

Endovascular AAA repair has been shown to be associated with lower postoperative morbidity, shorter length of hospital stay, and quicker return to normal function.[115] Direct comparison to open surgery utilizing randomized prospective trials, however, has only recently been available for evaluation. There have been three randomized prospective trials evaluating the use of EVAR compared with open surgery. The EVAR-1 trial enrolled 1082 patients with AAA who were healthy enough to be suitable candidates for surgery.[115] They were randomized to either EVAR or open repair. Results from this trial demonstrated that the 30-day mortality rate was lower after EVAR (1.7%) than open surgery (4.7%, P <0.0001). At 4-years follow-up, the aneurysm-related mortality rate in the EVAR group was half that in the open group (P = 0.04), but there was no difference in all-cause mortality (26% for the EVAR group and 29% for the open group). The Dutch Randomized Endovascular Aneurysm Management (DREAM) trial was a prospective randomized trial that enrolled 351 patients. As in EVAR-1, the 30-day mortality rate was lower in patients who underwent endovascular repair than in those who underwent open surgical reconstruction, but the 2-year outcomes were similar between the two groups. In addition, the results of the Open versus Endovascular Repair (OVER) Veterans Affairs Cooperative Study Group results have been reported.[116] In this trial, 881 patients suitable for open or EVAR were randomized to one of the two surgical techniques. As with the other two trials, 30-day mortality was lower in the EVAR arm (0.5%) than the open surgery arm (3.0%, P = 0.004). This difference, however, resolved by 2-year follow-up time points (7.0% vs. 9.8%, respectively). Patients undergoing EVAR had shorter hospital stays, shorter operative

durations, and required fewer blood transfusions, but they had increased exposure to fluoroscopy and contrast. Given its promising initial results, it is not surprising EVAR has become increasingly popular with both patients and providers over the past decade.

One of the most controversial aspects of AAA repair, however, is when to perform EVAR and when to perform conventional open surgery. Open surgical repair of AAA has long been considered the gold standard, and there is evidence this option provides good long-term durability.[117,118] Endovascular AAA repair however, given its young age, does not have similar time-tested outcomes data. Recently, longer-term outcomes from both EVAR-1 and DREAM have been reported.[30,119] For EVAR-1,[30] the median follow-up was 6 years (range, 5-10 years), and at follow-up, the overall aneurysm-related mortality was 1.0 deaths per 100 person-years in the EVAR group and 1.2 deaths per 100 person-years in the open repair group (P = 0.73). All-cause mortality was 7.2 deaths per 100 person-years (EVAR) and 7.1 deaths per 100 person-years (open surgery). Graft-related complication rates were higher in the EVAR group (12.6 per 100 person-years) compared to the open surgical arm (2.5 per 100 person-years; P < 0.001), and significantly more patients in the EVAR group required reintervention (5.1 per 100 person-years vs. 1.7 per 100 person-years; P <0.001). In fact, new graft-related complications and reinterventions were reported for as long as 8 years following EVAR. For DREAM,[119] at a median follow-up of 6.4 years (5.1-8.2 years), cumulative survival rates were 69.9% for open repair and 68.9% for EVAR. The cumulative rates of freedom from secondary interventions were 81.9% for the open repair group and 70.4% for EVAR (P = 0.03). Based on these data, it is clear that EVAR is not without its drawbacks. These factors may change as the technology improves and we gain a better understanding of the long-term implications of placing an endovascular graft in the aorta.

Initial applications of EVAR were geared toward patients considered high risk for conventional surgery, but this concept has come under some scrutiny after the results of the EVAR-2 trial.[120] In this trial, the outcomes of 404 patients with large AAAs (≥5.5 cm in diameter) who were considered to be physically ineligible for open repair were evaluated. Of this cohort, 197 patients were assigned to undergo endovascular repair, while 207 were assigned to have no intervention. The 30-day operative mortality rate for the EVAR group was 7.3%, and the overall rate of aneurysm rupture in the observation group was 12.4 per 100 person years. Aneurysm-related mortality was lower in the endovascular repair group, but this did not provide an advantage when evaluating all-cause mortality, and during follow-up, EVAR required a considerable increase in expense. These results called into question the appropriateness of using EVAR in high-risk patients. The results, however, have been refuted by others demonstrating lower rates of perioperative mortality and better long-term survivals in these high-risk patients.[121] These improved outcomes are likely due to an aggressive multidisciplinary approach to managing these patients' comorbidities.

Other Considerations

EVAR for Small Abdominal Aortic Aneurysms

Randomized prospective trials have demonstrated that there is no benefit to open repair of AAA for aneurysms that are less than 5.5 cm in diameter.[122,123] Operative mortality rates of 2.7% and 5.8% in these two trials raised the question of whether a procedure with lower operative mortality might provide benefit compared with observation in patients with smaller AAA. The Positive Impact of Endovascular Options for Treating Aneurysms Early (PIVOTAL) trial sought to evaluate whether endovascular repair of small AAA (4-5 cm) might provide a survival advantage compared with surveillance.[124] In this trial, 728 patients were randomly assigned to either EVAR (n = 366) or ultrasound surveillance (n = 362). Of the patients randomized to EVAR, 89% underwent repair, and of those assigned to surveillance, 31% subsequently underwent repair during the course of the study (mean follow-up 20 ± 12 months, range

0-41 months). The unadjusted hazard ratio (95% confidence interval [CI]) for mortality after EVAR was 1.01 (0.49-2.07; $P = 0.98$), with 15 deaths (4.1%) occurring in each group. No survival advantage was demonstrated with EVAR.

Endovascular Treatment of Ruptured Abdominal Aortic Aneurysms

With the widespread application of EVAR for repair of AAA, its use in the repair of ruptured AAA has similarly expanded. Initially there were several limitations to the application of this technology to treat the devastating problem of ruptured AAA: (1) unavailability of preoperative CT in patients with ruptured AAA, (2) unavailability of a dedicated operating room and ancillary staff equipped to perform emergent EVAR at all times, (3) unavailability of off-the-shelf stent grafts; and (4) lack of data from multicenter randomized trials.[125] Many large-volume centers, however, have developed protocols that allow treatment teams to overcome these hurdles and provide emergent care for ruptured AAA with endovascular devices.[125-128] Gerassimidis et al.[126] reported on the treatment of 69 patients with a ruptured AAA. Of these, 42 patients (63%) were suitable for EVAR. The in-hospital and 30-day mortality rates were 36% and 41%, respectively. Veith et al.[128] reported the worldwide experience with treating ruptured AAA with endovascular grafts. Data were collected from 49 centers at which 1037 patients were treated with EVAR for ruptured AAA. Overall 30-day mortality was 21%, which was significantly lower than the 30-day mortality rate for the 763 patients undergoing open repair (36%, $P < 0.001$) for ruptured AAA at these same institutions during the same time period. Given these experiences, there is a trend toward even more centers instituting a program of EVAR for ruptured AAA. Certainly, longer-term follow-up and larger series will be required to assess whether EVAR has ultimately affected outcomes from ruptured AAA.

Fenestrated and Branched Aortic Endografts

The most common reason for excluding patients from EVAR is lack of a suitable proximal implantation site between the renal arteries and the aneurysm. Although commercially available devices provide a mechanism for supplementing fixation within the suprarenal aorta without detrimentally affecting renal function,[129] such a practice has not been advocated to treat juxtarenal aneurysms. Despite evidence of short-term success with treatment of short necks with devices intended to treat infrarenal aneurysms,[130] the risk of later failure remains high.[131] To overcome this, fenestrated stent graft technology was developed. The devices used currently are hybrids of original abdominal devices. The primary goal of treating an aneurysm with a fenestrated graft is to move the sealing and fixation region of the repair into healthy aorta with a parallel neck and without wall defects. A fenestration (hole in the graft) allows the stent graft to occupy this more proximal location while providing for transgraft flow to the renal arteries (or other significant branches) (Fig. 40-8). It is designed to incorporate the minimum number of visceral vessels required to achieve fixation

and seal within healthy aorta. The fenestrations are constructed to match the ostial diameter of the visceral vessels and maximize the sealing zone. Several large series of fenestrated endograft deployments have been reported, demonstrating the midterm safety and efficacy of fenestrated stent grafting.[132-134] One of the largest series is reported by O'Neill et al.[132] They outline a series of 119 patients with mean follow-up of 19 months. There was only one perioperative death, and survival at 12, 24, and 36 months was 92%, 83%, and 79%, respectively. The 30-day endoleak rate was 10%, and all endoleaks were type II in nature. Regression of the aneurysm sac was noted in 79% of the patients by 12 months. Complications related to the renal arteries was noted in 10 of the 231 stented renal arteries, and only one patient who did not have significant renal dysfunction preoperatively went on to require dialysis. Incorporation of the renal arteries raises questions about the effect of fenestrated stent graft repair on long-term renal function.

Application of fenestrated technology has advanced to allow for the treatment of thoracoabdominal aortic aneurysms (TAAA) in which the aneurysm involves the renal and visceral vessels. When treating TAAA with an endograft, however, use of a simple fenestration is inadequate. Unlike fenestrated grafts where a hole in the graft suffices, in more complex aneurysms such as TAAA, the branch arteries arise from the aneurysm. In this scenario, blood flow has to be carried from the endograft, across the aneurysm, and to the target vessel, without extravasation into the aneurysm (Fig. 40-9). There are two modes by which this can be assured. The first is the fenestrated branched stent graft[135] or reinforced fenestrated graft[136] (see Fig. 40-8). In this style, the addition of a covered bridging stents converts a fenestrated stent graft into a form of branched stent graft.[137] Sealing between the covered stent and the fenestration is tenuous because there is very limited overlap of material. A nitinol ring is added to the fenestration to reinforce the site of interaction between the covered stent and the fenestration. These are termed reinforced fenestrations. The second mode of branched graft design is the cuffed branched stent graft[138] or directional branched stent graft[136] (see Fig. 40-8). The cuff or branch creates an overlap zone between the stent graft and the branch artery. It provides a segment of overlap that can be used to provide better sealing and fixation than the thin joint between a reinforced fenestration and mating visceral stent graft. A longer overlap affords one the ability to use a self-expanding stent graft rather than a balloon-expandable stent graft. This may provide a means to better accommodate tortuosity and diameter discrepancies and may limit type 1 endoleaks and component separation from this region.

Investigators tend to pool results of fenestrated branch grafts and cuffed branched grafts, with few series containing significant numbers of patients.[139-145] The largest single-center experience has been reported by the Cleveland Clinic. Greenberg et al.[143] performed a retrospective analysis on patients who underwent elective open surgical repair (N = 372) or endovascular repair (N = 352) of descending thoracic or thoracoabdominal aortic aneurysms. The group of patients treated with endovascular repair was older and had more comorbid conditions than those undergoing open repair. Open repair, however, was more frequently applied

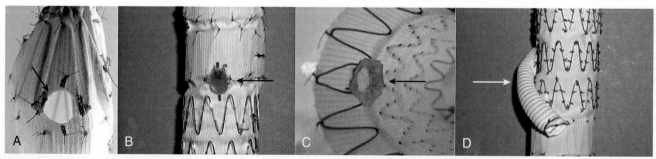

FIGURE 40-8 A, Example of endograft with fenestration *(arrow)* within endograft body to accommodate a renal artery. **B,** Reinforced fenestration *(arrow)* that allows for placement of **(C)** covered stent graft, creating a form of a branched endograft for treatment of a thoracoabdominal aortic aneurysm (TAAA). **D,** True directional branch *(arrow)* used to allow for continued flow to a visceral vessel when treating thoracoabdominal aortic aneurysm.

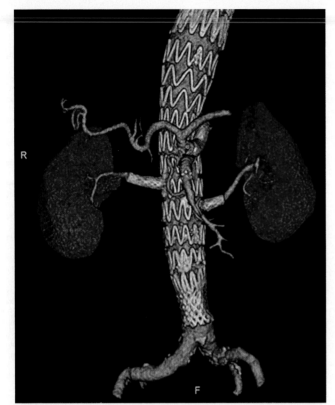

FIGURE 40-9   Example of thoracoabdominal aortic aneurysm (TAAA) that has been treated with a branched endograft that incorporates all of the visceral vessels.

to patients with type II or type III aneurysms and those that were associated with a chronic dissection. Despite the differences in patient age and comorbid conditions, mortality rates at 30 days (5.7% vs. 8.3%) and 12 months (15.6% vs. 15.9%) were not different between endovascular repair and surgical repair, nor was there a difference in the development of spinal cord ischemia (4% vs. 8%, respectively; $P = 0.08$). Bakoyiannis et al. performed a meta-analysis of all English language literature published between 2000 and 2009 on endovascular procedures using fenestrated and/or branched technology.[145] The results of this analysis demonstrated that complex endografting can be performed with a technical success rate of 94%, with a 30-day mortality of 7%. Typically these procedures were performed in patients who were deemed high risk for conventional surgery. The 1-year mortality was 1.3%. The application of fenestrated and branched technology is very much in its infancy. As the technology progresses, we will be able to better discern who will best benefit from these procedures, and ultimately replace open surgery with this less invasive option.

Summary

Abdominal aortic endografting provides a less invasive method of treating AAA. It provides a beneficial way of treating aneurysms in patients who are at high risk for conventional open surgical repair, and results of randomized trials suggest, at least in the short-term, it provides clinical equipoise with conventional surgery. The durability of this procedure is still under evaluation. It is likely, however, that the application of endovascular technology will replace current open surgical options, and ultimately the entire aortic tree will be treated with endovascular options.

REFERENCES

1. Criado FJ, Barnatan MF, Lingelbach JM, et al: Abdominal aortic aneurysm: overview of stent-graft devices, *J Am Coll Surg* 194(1 Suppl):S88, 2002.
2. Power D: Palliative treatment of aneurysms by wiring with Colt's apparatus, *Br J Surg* 9:27, 1927.
3. Blakemore A, King B: Electrothermic coagulation of aortic aneurysms, *JAMA* 111:1821, 1938.
4. Matas R: Ligation of the abdominal aorta: report of the ultimate result. 1 year, 5 months and 9 days after the ligation of the abdominal aorta for aneurysm of the bifurcation, *Ann Surg* 81:457, 1925.
5. Rea C: Surgical treatment of aneurysm of the abdominal aorta, *Minn Med* 31:153, 1948.
6. Dubost C, Allary M, Oeconomos N: Resection of an aneurysm of the abdominal aorta: resection of the continuity by a preserved arterial graft, with result after five months, *Arch Surg* 64:405, 1952.
7. Voorhees A, Jaretski A, Blakemore A: Use of tubes constructed from Vinyon "N" cloth in bridging arterial defects: a preliminary report, *Ann Surg* 135:322, 1952.
8. Edwards W, Tapp J: Chemically treated nylon tubes as arterial grafts, *Surgery* 38:61, 1955.
9. Creech O: Endo-aneurysmorrhaphy and treatment of aortic aneurysm, *Ann Surg* 164:935, 1966.
10. Parodi J, Palmaz J, Barone H: Transfemoral intraluminal graft implantation for abdominal aortic aneurysms, *Ann Vasc Surg* 5:491, 1991.
11. Ernst C: Abdominal aortic aneurysm, *N Engl J Med* 1993:1167, 1993.
12. Szilagyi D, Smith R, DeRusso F, et al: Contributions of abdominal aortic aneurysmectomy to prolongation of life, *Ann Surg* 164:678, 1966.
13. United Kingdom Small Aneurysm Trial Participants: Long-term outcomes of immediate repair compared with surveillance of small abdominal aortic aneurysms, *N Engl J Med* 346:1445, 2002.
14. Hertzer NR, Mascha EJ, Karafa MT, et al: Open infrarenal abdominal aortic aneurysm repair: the Cleveland Clinic experience from 1989 to 1998, *J Vasc Surg* 35:1145, 2002.
15. Cronenwett J, Johnston K: The United Kingdom Small Aneurysm Trial: implications for surgical treatment of abdominal aortic aneurysms, *J Vasc Surg* 29:191, 1999.
16. Baxendale B, Baker D, Hutchinson A, et al: Haemodynamic and metabolic response to endovascular repair of infra-renal aortic aneurysms, *Br J Anaesth* 77:581, 1996.
17. Laheij RJ, Van Marrewijk CJ: Endovascular stenting of abdominal aortic aneurysm in patients unfit for elective open surgery. Eurostar group. EUROpean collaborators registry on Stent-graft Techniques for abdominal aortic Aneurysm Repair, *Lancet* 356:832, 2000.
18. Beebe H, Kritpracha B, Serres S, et al: Endograft planning without preoperative arteriography: a clinical feasibility study, *J Endovasc Ther* 7:8, 2000.
19. Eide K, Odegard A, Myhre H, et al: DynaCT during EVAR - a comparison with multidetector CT, *Eur J Endovasc Surg* 37:23, 2009.
20. Nordon I, Hinchcliffe R, Malkawi A, et al: Validation of DynaCT in the morphological assessment of abdominal aortic aneurysm for endovascular repair, *J Endovasc Ther* 17:183, 2010.
21. Beebe H, Kritpracha B: Imaging of abdominal aortic aneurysm: current status, *Ann Vasc Surg* 17:111, 2003.
22. Beebe H, Jackson T, Pigott J: Aortic aneurysm morphology for planning endovascular aortic grafts: limitations of conventional imaging methods, *J Endovasc Surg* 2:139, 1995.
23. Truijers M, Resch T, Van Den Berg JC, et al: Endovascular aneurysm repair: state-of-art imaging techniques for preoperative planning and surveillance, *J Cardiovasc Surg (Torino)* 50:423, 2009.
24. Resch T, Ivancev K, Brunkwall J, et al: Distal migration of stent-grafts after endovascular repair of abdominal aortic aneurysms, *J Vasc Interv Radiol* 10:257–264, 1999.
25. Ouriel K: Endovascular repair of abdominal aortic aneurysms: the Cleveland Clinic experience with five different devices, *Semin Vasc Surg* 16(2):88–94, 2003.
26. Swinnen J, Chao A, Tiwari A, et al: Vertical or transverse incisions for access to the femoral artery: a randomized control study, *Ann Vasc Surg* 24:336–341, 2010.
27. Lee W, Brown M, Nelson P, et al: Total percutaneous access for endovascular aortic aneurysm repair ("preclose" technique), *J Vasc Surg* 45:1095–1101, 2007.
28. McDonnell C, Forlee M, Dowdall J, et al: Percutaneous endovascular abdominal aortic aneurysm repair leads to a reduction in wound complications, *Ir J Med Sci* 177:49–52, 2008.
29. Smith S, Timaran C, Valentine R, et al: Percutaneous access for endovascular abdominal aortic aneurysm repair: can selection criteria be expanded? *Ann Vasc Surg* 23:621–626, 2009.
30. The United Kingdom EVAR Trial Investigators: Endovascular versus open repair of abdominal aortic aneurysm, *N Engl J Med* 362:1863–1871, 2010.
31. Nordon I, Karthikesalingam R, Hinchliffe R, et al: Secondary interventions following endovascular aneurysm repair (EVAR) and the enduring value of graft surveillance, *Eur J Endovasc Surg* 39:547–554, 2010.
32. Armerding M, Rubin G, Beaulieu C, et al: Aortic aneurysmal disease: assessment of stent-graft treatment - CT versus conventional angiography, *Radiology* 215:138–146, 2000.
33. Rozenblit A, Marin M, Veith F, et al: Endovascular repair of abdominal aortic aneurysm: value of postoperative follow-up with helical CT, *Am J Roentgenol* 165:1473–1479, 1995.
34. Gorich J, Rlinger N, Sokirnaski R, et al: Leakages after endovascular repair of aortic aneurysms: classification based on findings at CT, angiography, and radiography, *Radiology* 213:767–772, 1999.
35. Buth J, Harris P, Marrewijk C: Causes and outcomes of open conversion and aneurysm rupture after endovascular abdominal aortic aneurysm repair: can type II endoleaks be dangerous? *J Am Coll Surg* 194:S98–S102, 2002.
36. Brenner D, Hall E: Computed tomography - an increasing source of radiation exposure, *N Engl J Med* 357:2277–2284, 2007.
37. Solomon R, DuMouchel W: Contrast media and nephropathy: findings from systematic analysis and food and drug administration reports of adverse effects, *Invest Radiol* 41:651–660, 2006.
38. Broome D, Giguis M, Baron P, et al: Gadodiamide-associated nephrogenic systemic fibrosis: why radiologists should be concerned, *Am J Roentgenol* 189:586–592, 2007.
39. Sun Z: Diagnostic value of color duplex ultrasonography in the follow-up of endovascular repair of abdominal aortic aneurysm, *J Vasc Interv Radiol* 17:759–764, 2006.
40. Mirza T, Karthikesalingam A, Jackson D, et al: Duplex ultrasound and contrast-enhanced ultrasound versus computed tomography for the detection of endoleak after EVAR: systematic review and bivariate meta-analysis, *Eur J Vasc Endovasc Surg* 39:418–428, 2010.

41. Napoli V, Bargellini I, Sardella S, et al: Abdominal aortic aneurysm: contrast-enhanced US for missed endoleaks after endoluminal repair, *Radiology* 233:217–225, 2004.

42. Henao E, Hodge M, Felkai D, et al: Contrast-enhanced duplex surveillance after endovascular abdominal aortic aneurysm repair: improved efficacy using a continuous infusion technique, *J Vasc Surg* 43:259–264, 2006.

43. Parent F, Meier G, Godziachvili V, et al: The incidence and natural history of type I and II endoleak: a 5-year follow-up assessment with 1 color duplex ultrasound scan, *J Vasc Surg* 35:474–481, 2002.

44. Beeman B, Doctor L, Doerr K, et al: Duplex ultrasound imaging alone is sufficient for midterm endovascular aneurysm repair surveillance: a cost analysis study and prospective comparison with computed tomography scan, *J Vasc Surg* 50:1019–1024, 2009.

45. Yao O, Faries P, Morrissey N, et al: Ancillary techniques to facilitate endovascular repair of aortic aneurysms, *J Vasc Surg* 34:69, 2001.

46. Zarins CK: The US AneuRx Clinical Trial: 6-year clinical update 2002, *J Vasc Surg* 37:904–908, 2003.

47. May J, White G, Waugh R, et al: Improved survival after endoluminal repair with second-generation prostheses compared with open repair in the treatment of abdominal aortic aneurysms: a 5-year concurrent comparison using life table method, *J Vasc Surg* 33:S21–S26, 2001.

48. Lee WA, O'Dorisio J, Wolf YG, et al: Outcome after unilateral hypogastric artery occlusion during endovascular aneurysm repair, *J Vasc Surg* 33:921–926, 2001.

49. Wolpert LM, Dittrich KP, Hallisey MJ, et al: Hypogastric artery embolization in endovascular abdominal aortic aneurysm repair, *J Vasc Surg* 33:1193–1198, 2001.

50. Criado FJ, Wilson EP, Velazquez OC, et al: Safety of coil embolization of the internal iliac artery in endovascular grafting of abdominal aortic aneurysms, *J Vasc Surg* 32:684–688, 2000.

51. Schoder M, Zaunbauer L, Holzenbein T, et al: Internal iliac artery embolization before endovascular repair of abdominal aortic aneurysms: frequency, efficacy, and clinical results, *AJR Am J Roentgenol* 177:599–605, 2001.

52. Mehta M, Veith F, Ohki T, et al: Unilateral and bilateral hypogastric artery interruption during aortoiliac aneurysm repair in 154 patients: a relatively innocuous procedure, *J Vasc Surg* 33:S27–S32, 2001.

53. Kritpracha B, Pigott JP, Price CI, et al: Distal internal iliac artery embolization: a procedure to avoid, *J Vasc Surg* 37:943–948, 2003.

54. Wyers MC, Schermerhorn ML, Fillinger MF, et al: Internal iliac occlusion without coil embolization during endovascular abdominal aortic aneurysm repair, *J Vasc Surg* 36:1138–1145, 2002.

55. Zarins CK, White RA, Hodgson KJ, et al: Endoleak as a predictor of outcome after endovascular aneurysm repair: AneuRx multicenter clinical trial, *J Vasc Surg* 32:90–107, 2000.

56. Holzenbein T, Kretschmer G, Thurnher S, et al: Midterm durability of abdominal aortic aneurysm endograft repair: a word of caution, *J Vasc Surg* 33:S46–S54, 2001.

57. Buth J, Harris PL, Van MC, et al: The significance and management of different types of endoleaks, *Semin Vasc Surg* 16:95–102, 2003.

58. Chuter TA, Faruqi RM, Sawhney R, et al: Endoleak after endovascular repair of abdominal aortic aneurysm, *J Vasc Surg* 34:98–105, 2001.

59. Buth J, Laheji R: Early complications and endoleaks after endovascular abdominal aortic aneurysm repair: report of a multicenter study, *J Vasc Surg* 31:134–146, 2000.

60. Dattilo JB, Brewster DC, Fan CM, et al: Clinical failures of endovascular abdominal aortic aneurysm repair: incidence, causes, and management, *J Vasc Surg* 35:1137–1144, 2002.

61. Zarins C: The US AneuRx clinical trial: 6-year clinical update 2002, *J Vasc Surg* 37:904–908, 2003.

62. Fairman R, Carpenter J, Baum R, et al: Potential impact of therapeutic warfarin treatment on type II endoleaks and sac shrinkage rates on midterm follow-up examination, *J Vasc Surg* 35:679, 2002.

63. Baum RA, Carpenter JP, Cope C, et al: Aneurysm sac pressure measurements after endovascular repair of abdominal aortic aneurysms, *J Vasc Surg* 33:32–41, 2001.

64. Marty B, Sanchez LA, Ohki T, et al: Endoleak after endovascular graft repair of experimental aortic aneurysms: does coil embolization with angiographic "seal" lower intraaneurysmal pressure? *J Vasc Surg* 27:454–461, 1998.

65. Baum R, Cope C, Fairman R, et al: Translumbar embolization of type 2 endoleaks after endovascular repair of abdominal aortic aneurysms, *J Vasc Interv Radiol* 12:111–116, 2001.

66. Stavropoulos S, Park J, Fairman R, et al: Type 2 endoleak embolization comparison: translumbar embolization versus modified transarterial embolization, *J Vasc Interv Radiol* 20:1299–1302, 2009.

67. Parodi J, Berguer R, Ferreira L, et al: Intra-aneurysmal pressure after incomplete endovascular exclusion, *J Vasc Surg* 33:909, 2001.

68. Back MR, Bowser AN, Johnson BL, et al: Patency of infrarenal aortic side branches determines early aneurysm sac behavior after endovascular repair, *Ann Vasc Surg* 17:27–34, 2003.

69. Fan CM, Rafferty EA, Geller SC, et al: Endovascular stent-graft in abdominal aortic aneurysms: the relationship between patent vessels that arise from the aneurysmal sac and early endoleak, *Radiology* 218:176–182, 2001.

70. Gawenda M, Heckenkamp J, Zaehringer M, et al: Intra-aneurysm sac pressure--the holy grail of endoluminal grafting of AAA, *Eur J Vasc Endovasc Surg* 24:139–145, 2002.

71. Jacobs T, Teodorescu V, Morrissey N, et al: The endovascular repair of abdominal aortic aneurysm: an update analysis of structural failure modes of endovascular stent grafts, *Semin Vasc Surg* 16:103–112, 2003.

72. Stelter W, Umscheid T, Ziegler P: Three-year experience with modular stent-graft devices for endovascular AAA treatment, *J Endovasc Surg* 4:362–369, 1997.

73. Beebe HG: Lessons learned from aortic aneurysm stent graft failure; observations from several perspectives, *Semin Vasc Surg* 16:129–138, 2003.

74. Riepe G, Loos J, Imig H, et al: Long-term *in vivo* alterations of polyester vascular grafts in humans, *Endovasc Surg* 13:540, 1997.

75. Jacobs TS, Won J, Gravereaux EC, et al: Mechanical failure of prosthetic human implants: a 10-year experience with aortic stent graft devices, *J Vasc Surg* 37:16–26, 2003.

76. Alimi YS, Chakfe N, Rivoal E, et al: Rupture of an abdominal aortic aneurysm after endovascular graft placement and aneurysm size reduction, *J Vasc Surg* 28:178–183, 1998.

77. Riepe G, Heilberger P, Umscheid T, et al: Frame dislocation of body middle rings in endovascular stent tube grafts, *Eur J Vasc Endovasc Surg* 17:28–34, 1999.

78. Krajcer Z, Howell M, Dougherty K: Unusual case of AneuRx stent-graft failure two years after AAA exclusion, *J Endovasc Ther* 8:465–471, 2001.

79. Moore W, Rutherford R: Transfemoral endovascular repair of abdominal aortic aneurysm: results of the North American EVT phase I trial, *J Vasc Surg* 34:353, 1996.

80. Heintz C, Riepe G, Birken L, et al: Corroded nitinol wires in explanted aortic endografts: an important mechanism of failure? *J Endovasc Ther* 8:248–253, 2001.

81. Trepanier C, Tabrizian M, Yahia L, et al: Effect of modification of oxide layer on NiTi stent corrosion resistance, *J Biomed Mater Res B Appl Biomater* 43:433, 1998.

82. Duerig T, Pelton A, Stockel D: An overview of nitinol medical applications, *Mater Sci Eng* A273–275:149, 1999.

83. Starosvetsky E, Gotman I: Corrosion behavior of titanium nitride coated Ni-Ti shape memory surgical alloy, *Biomaterials* 22:1853, 2001.

84. Fairman R, Baum R, Carpenter J, et al: Limb intervention in patients undergoing treatment with an unsupported bifurcated aortic endograft system: a review of the phase II EVT trial, *J Vasc Surg* 36:118–126, 2002.

85. Carroccio A, Faries P, Morrissey N, et al: Predicting iliac limb occlusion after bifurcated aortic stent grafting: anatomic and device-related causes, *J Vasc Surg* 36:679–684, 2002.

86. Baum R, Shetty S, Carpenter J, et al: Limb kinking in supported and unsupported abdominal aortic stent-grafts, *J Vasc Interv Radiol* 11:1165–1171, 2000.

87. Amesur NB, Zajko AB, Orons PD, et al: Endovascular treatment of iliac limb stenoses or occlusions in 31 patients treated with the Ancure endograft, *J Vasc Interv Radiol* 11:421–428, 2000.

88. Ohki T, Veith FJ, Shaw P, et al: Increasing incidence of midterm and long-term complications after endovascular graft repair of abdominal aortic aneurysms: a note of caution based on a 9-year experience, *Ann Surg* 234:323–334, 2001.

89. Carpenter JP, Neschis DG, Fairman RM, et al: Failure of endovascular abdominal aortic aneurysm graft limbs, *J Vasc Surg* 33:296–302, 2001.

90. Cao P, De RP, Verzini F, et al: Endoleak after endovascular aortic repair: classification, diagnosis and management following endovascular thoracic and abdominal aortic repair, *J Cardiovasc Surg (Torino)* 51:53–69, 2010.

91. Baum RA, Shetty SK, Carpenter JP, et al: Limb kinking in supported and unsupported abdominal aortic stent-grafts, *J Vasc Interv Radiol* 11:1165–1171, 2000.

92. Carroccio A, Faries PL, Morrissey NJ, et al: Predicting iliac limb occlusions after bifurcated aortic stent grafting: anatomic and device-related causes, *J Vasc Surg* 36:679–684, 2002.

93. Sampram ES, Karafa MT, Mascha EJ, et al: Nature, frequency, and predictors of secondary procedures after endovascular repair of abdominal aortic aneurysm, *J Vasc Surg* 37:930–937, 2003.

94. Fairman RM, Velazquez O, Baum R, et al: Endovascular repair of aortic aneurysms: critical events and adjunctive procedures, *J Vasc Surg* 33:1226–1232, 2001.

95. Conners M III, Sternbergh W III, Carter G, et al: Secondary procedures after endovascular aortic aneurysm repair, *J Vasc Surg* 36:992, 2002.

96. Resch T, Ivancev K, Brunkwall J, et al: Distal migration of stent-grafts after endovascular repair of abdominal aortic aneurysms, *J Vasc Interv Radiol* 10:257–264, 1997.

97. Harris P, Vallavhaneni S, Desgranges P, et al: Incidence and risk factors of late rupture, conversion, and death after endovascular repair of infrarenal aortic aneurysms: the EUROSTAR experience, *J Vasc Surg* 32:739–749, 2000.

98. Albertini N, Kalliafas S, Travis S, et al: Anatomical risk factors for proximal perigraft endoleak and graft migration following endovascular repair of abdominal aortic aneurysms, *Eur J Endovasc Surg* 19:308–312, 2000.

99. Cao P, Verzini F, Zannetti S, et al: Device migration after endoluminal abdominal aortic aneurysm repair: analysis of 113 cases with a minimum follow-up period of 2 years, *J Vasc Surg* 35:229–235, 2002.

100. Lawrence-Brown M, Semmens J, Hartley D, et al: How is durability related to patient selection and graft design with endoluminal grafting for abdominal aortic aneurysm? In Greenhalgh R, editor: *Durability of vascular and endovascular surgery*, London, 1999, WB Saunders, pp 375–385.

101. Resch T, Malina M, Lindblad B, et al: The impact of stent-graft development on outcome of AAA repair–a 7-year experience, *Eur J Vasc Endovasc Surg* 22:57–61, 2001.

102. Albertini J, Kalliafas S, Travis S, et al: Anatomical risk factors for proximal perigraft endoleak and graft migration following endovascular repair of abdominal aortic aneurysms, *Eur J Vasc Endovasc Surg* 19:308–312, 2000.

103. Malina M, Lindblad B, Ivancev K, et al: Endovascular AAA exclusion: will stents with hooks and barbs prevent stent-graft migration? *J Endovasc Surg* 5:310–317, 1998.

104. Lee J, Lee J, Aziz I, et al: Stent-graft migration following endovascular repair of aneurysms with large proximal necks: anatomical risk factors and long-term sequelae, *J Endovasc Ther* 9:652–664, 2002.

105. White G, May J, Waugh R, et al: Shortening of endografts during deployment in endovascular AAA repair, *J Endovasc Ther* 6:4, 1999.

106. Prinssen M, Wever J, Mali W, et al: Concerns for the durability of the proximal abdominal aortic aneurysm endograft fixation from a 2-year and 3-year longitudinal tomography angiography study, *J Vasc Surg* 33:S64–S69, 2001.

107. Badran MF, Gould DA, Raza I, et al: Aneurysm neck diameter after endovascular repair of abdominal aortic aneurysms, *J Vasc Interv Radiol* 13(9 Pt 1):887–892, 2002.

108. Ouriel K, Srivastava SD, Sarac TP, et al: Disparate outcome after endovascular treatment of small versus large abdominal aortic aneurysm, *J Vasc Surg* 37:1206–1212, 2003.

109. Becker G, Kovacs M, Mathison M, et al: Risk stratification and outcomes of transluminal endografting for abdominal aortic aneurysm: 7-year experience and long-term follow-up, *J Vasc Interv Radiol* 12:1033–1046, 2003.

110. Naslund TC, Edwards WH Jr, Neuzil DF, et al: Technical complications of endovascular abdominal aortic aneurysm repair, *J Vasc Surg* 26:502–509, 1997.

111. Laheji R, Buth J, Harris P, et al: Need for secondary interventions after endovascular repair of abdominal aortic aneurysms. Intermediate-term follow-up results of a European collaborative registry (EUROSTAR), *Br J Surg* 87:1666, 2000.

112. May J, White G, Waugh R, et al: Life-table analysis and assisted success following endoluminal repair of abdominal aortic aneurysms: the role of supplementary endovascular intervention in improving outcome, *Eur J Vasc Endovasc Surg* 19:648, 2000.

113. Sternbergh W III, Conners M, Tonnessen B, et al: Aortic aneurysm sac shrinkage after endovascular repair is device-dependent: a comparison of Zenith and AneuRx endografts, *Ann Vasc Surg* 17:49, 2003.

114. Bertges D, Chow K, Wyers M, et al: Abdominal aortic aneurysm size regression after endovascular repair is endograft dependent, *J Vasc Surg* 37:716, 2003.

115. EVAR Trial Participants: Endovascular aneurysm repair versus open repair in patients with abdominal aortic aneurysm (EVAR trial 1): randomised controlled trial, *Lancet* 365:2179, 2005.

116. Lederle F, Freischlag J, Kyriakides T, et al: Outcomes following endovascular vs. open repair of abdominal aortic aneurysm. A randomized trial, *J Am Med Assoc* 302:1535–1542, 2009.

117. Hallet J Jr, Marshall D, Petterson T, et al: Graft-related complications after abdominal aortic aneurysm repair: reassurance from a 36-year population-based experience, *J Vasc Surg* 25:277–284, 1997.

118. Conrad M, Crawford R, Pedraza J, et al: Long-term durability of open abdominal aortic aneurysm repair, *J Vasc Surg* 46:669–675, 2007.

119. De Bruin J, Baas A, Buth J, et al: Long-term outcome of open or endovascular repair of abdominal aortic aneurysm, *N Engl J Med* 362:1881–1889, 2010.

120. The United Kingdom EVAR Trial Investigators: Endovascular repair of aortic aneurysm in patients physically ineligible for open repair, *N Engl J Med* 362:1872–1880, 2010.

121. Sobocinski J, Maurel B, Delsart P, et al: Should we modify our indications after the EVAR-2 trial conclusions? *Ann Vasc Surg* 25:590–597, 2011.

122. Lederle F, Wilson S, Johnson G, et al: Immediate repair compared with surveillance of small abdominal aneurysms, *N Engl J Med* 346:1437–1444, 2002.

123. Powell J, Brown L, Forbes J, et al: Final 12-year follow-up of surgery versus surveillance in the UK small aneurysm trial, *Br J Surg* 94:702–708, 2007.

124. Ouriel K, Clair D, Kent C, et al: Endovascular repair compared with surveillance for patients with small abdominal aortic aneurysms, *J Vasc Surg* 51:1081–1087, 2010.

125. Mehta M, Taggert J, Darling RC III, et al: Establishing a protocol for endovascular treatment of ruptured abdominal aortic aneurysms: outcomes of a prospective analysis, *J Vasc Surg* 44:1–8, 2006.

126. Gerassimidis TS, Karkos CD, Karamanos DG, et al: Endovascular management of ruptured abdominal aortic aneurysms: an 8-year single-centre experience, *Cardiovasc Intervent Radiol* 32:241–249, 2009.

127. Starnes B, Quiroga E, Hutter C, et al: Management of ruptured abdominal aortic aneurysm in the endovascular era, *J Vasc Surg* 51:9–18, 2010.

128. Veith F, Lachat M, Mayer D, et al: Collected world and single center experience with endovascular treatment of ruptured abdominal aortic aneurysms, *Ann Vasc Surg* 250:818–824, 2009.

129. Greenberg RK, Chuter TA, Sternbergh WC III, et al: Zenith AAA endovascular graft: intermediate-term results of the US multicenter trial, *J Vasc Surg* 39:1209–1218, 2004.

130. Greenberg R, Fairman R, Srivastava S, et al: Endovascular grafting in patients with short proximal necks: an analysis of short-term results, *Cardiovasc Surg* 8:350–354, 2000.

131. Waasdorp EJ, de Vries JP, Hobo R, et al: Aneurysm diameter and proximal aortic neck diameter influence clinical outcome of endovascular abdominal aortic repair: a 4-year EUROSTAR experience, *Ann Vasc Surg* 19:755–761, 2005.

132. O'Neill S, Greenberg RK, Haddad F, et al: A prospective analysis of fenestrated endovascular grafting: intermediate-term outcomes, *Eur J Vasc Endovasc Surg* 32:115–123, 2006.

133. Greenberg RK, Sternbergh WC III, et al: Intermediate results of a United States multicenter trial of fenestrated endograft repair for juxtarenal abdominal aortic aneurysms, *J Vasc Surg* 50:730–737, 2009.

134. Greenberg RK, Haulon S, O'Neill S, et al: Primary endovascular repair of juxtarenal aneurysms with fenestrated endovascular grafting, *Eur J Vasc Endovasc Surg* 27:484–491, 2004.

135. Chuter TA: Fenestrated and branched stent-grafts for thoracoabdominal, pararenal and juxtarenal aortic aneurysm repair, *Semin Vasc Surg* 20:90–96, 2007.

136. Greenberg R: Aortic aneurysm, thoracoabdominal aneurysm, juxtarenal aneurysm, fenestrated endografts, branched endografts, and endovascular aneurysm repair, *Ann N Y Acad Sci* 1085:187–196, 2006.

137. Anderson J, Adam D, Berce M, et al: Repair of thoracoabdominal aortic aneurysms with fenestrated and branched endovascular stent grafts, *J Vasc Surg* 42:600–607, 2005.

138. Chuter TA: Fenestrated and branched stent-grafts for thoracoabdominal, pararenal and juxtarenal aortic aneurysm repair, *Semin Vasc Surg* 20:90–96, 2007.

139. Anderson JL, Adam DJ, Berce M, et al: Repair of thoracoabdominal aortic aneurysms with fenestrated and branched endovascular stent grafts, *J Vasc Surg* 42:600–607, 2005t.

140. Chuter TA: Fenestrated and branched stent-grafts for thoracoabdominal, pararenal and juxtarenal aortic aneurysm repair, *Semin Vasc Surg* 20:90–96, 2007.

141. Chuter TA, Rapp JH, Hiramoto JS, et al: Endovascular treatment of thoracoabdominal aortic aneurysms, *J Vasc Surg* 47:6–16, 2008.

142. Roselli EE, Greenberg RK, Pfaff K, et al: Endovascular treatment of thoracoabdominal aortic aneurysms, *J Thorac Cardiovasc Surg* 133:1474–1482, 2007.

143. Greenberg R, Lu Q, Roselli E, et al: Contemporary analysis of descending thoracic and thoracoabdominal aneurysm repair. A comparison of endovascular and open techniques, *Circulation* 118:808–817, 2008.

144. Vourliotakis G, Bos WT, Beck AW, et al: Fenestrated stent-grafting after previous endovascular abdominal aortic aneurysm repair, *J Cardiovasc Surg (Torino)* 51:383–389, 2010.

145. Bakoyiannis CN, Economopoulos KP, Georgopoulos S, et al: Fenestrated and branched endografts for the treatment of thoracoabdominal aortic aneurysms: a systematic review, *J Endovasc Ther* 17:201–209, 2010.

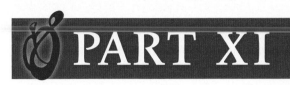

CHAPTER **41**   **Overview of Vasculitis**

Peter A. Merkel

The vasculitides are a group of rare diseases linked by the pathological consequences of vascular inflammation, including bleeding, ischemia, and infarction of downstream organs (Box 41-1). However, the clinical spectrum of these diseases is wide ranging and includes a myriad of clinical and pathological findings. Not all disease phenotypes that occur in the vasculitides are due to true "vasculitis" (i.e., inflammation of vascular structures). Some damage in vasculitis is due to nonvascular inflammation. For example, arthritis, uveitis, and pulmonary nodules are parts of different vasculitides but are not due to interruption of vascular flow. The pathophysiology of vasculitis is covered in Chapter 9 and in individual chapters on Takayasu's arteritis (TA) (Chapter 42), giant cell arteritis (GCA; Chapter 43), and Kawasaki disease (Chapter 45).

The diseases outlined in this chapter are rare, and all are considered "orphan" diseases, with fewer than 200,000 cases in the United States at any time. As with most rare diseases, few well-controlled clinical treatment trials have been performed for this group of disorders. Much of the clinical investigation stems from studies of patient cohorts at large referral centers. In the past 2 decades, however, increasing international cooperation among vasculitis centers has resulted in several important randomized controlled treatment trials that have had significant impacts on the care and management of patients with vasculitis. Similarly, advances in diagnostic imaging and laboratory testing have improved clinicians' ability to diagnose and evaluate patients with vasculitis.

This chapter reviews the major types of vasculitis, discusses evaluation of suspected cases of vasculitis, and outlines approaches to treatment and management of these disorders. There is a focus on differentiating *inflammatory* from *noninflammatory* disease as it relates to the types of patients physicians specializing in vascular medicine are likely to encounter in a consultative practice (Table 41-1). The newest advances in diagnosis and treatment are also reviewed briefly.

Classification of Vasculitis

The classification and nomenclature of vasculitis can be unnecessarily confusing. The most important first step in approaching these disorders is for clinicians to consider the possibility of "some sort of vasculitis" and, once clinical proof is found, to narrow down the specific type. Nevertheless, knowledge of the classification criteria is quite useful when considering treatment and clinical follow-up. Establishing a treatment plan for a case of vasculitis relies on both an understanding of the prognosis of a specific type and applying results of clinical trials that always include patients who meet specific classification criteria. For example, a patient with arthritis, purpura, and abdominal pain might well be treated with glucocorticoids alone if believed to have Henoch-Schönlein Purpura HSP, but would also receive an additional immunosuppressive drug (e.g., methotrexate, cyclophosphamide) if determined to have granulomatosis with polyangiitis (GPA [Wegener's]). Similarly, the nature of follow-up visits, examinations, and subsequent evaluations are also heavily influenced by the specific type of vasculitis. For example, new-onset hemoptysis in a patient believed to be in remission after treatment for GCA would be concerning for infection or malignancy, whereas the same finding in a patient with GPA would usually prompt immediate reinstitution of high-dose glucocorticoids to treat potential alveolar hemorrhage while further evaluations, including for infection, are put in place.

Two major classification systems for vasculitis exist: the American College of Rheumatology (ACR) system[1] and the Chapel Hill Consensus Conference definitions.[2] These systems were not meant to be strictly diagnostic systems, but rather classification systems. These are definitions to apply to established vasculitis and differentiate one vasculitis from another. The main use of these systems has been for clinical trials and other types of clinical research. Nevertheless, these systems have been adapted for use by clinicians as helpful guides to practice. Not all types of vasculitis are included in the ACR or Chapel Hill systems; both are currently undergoing reevaluation and revision.[3]

The practice of differentiating among the inflammatory vasculitides by associated diagnostic antibodies is at this time limited to use of antineutrophil cytoplasmic antibodies (ANCAs). Specifically, many authors refer to *ANCA-associated vasculitis*, which includes GPA, microscopic polyangiitis (MPA), renal-limited pauci-immune glomerulonephritis, and the Churg-Strauss' syndrome (CSS). Although it is convenient to refer to these related diseases as "ANCA-associated" vasculitis, it is important to realize that patients may have any of these diseases and still test negative for the presence of ANCA.

Perhaps the simplest method of sorting out the vasculitides, albeit also incomplete and not fully accurate, is to list them according to the size of artery (predominantly but not necessarily exclusively) involved (see Box 41-1). This results in considering *small-vessel*, *medium-vessel*, and *large-vessel vasculitides*. This system, although not applied for clinical trials or even clinically for treatment purposes, is an easy one to use as a first approach to describing the diseases and their major manifestations, and is used to outline the descriptions of the vasculitides in this chapter. However, when specific diseases and results of treatment trials are mentioned, the ACR and Chapel Hill Consensus systems are applied.

Large-Vessel Vasculitis

The large-vessel vasculitides are disorders in which the aorta and its main branches are affected, including the subclavian, carotid, vertebral, renal, mesenteric, and iliac arteries[4] (Fig. 41-1). Because such vessels are so frequently involved in noninflammatory vascular diseases, and patients with these diseases are frequently encountered by specialists in vascular medicine, these disorders are particularly highlighted in this textbook. Also included are individual chapters on TA (Chapter 42), giant cell (temporal) arteritis (Chapter 43), and Kawasaki disease (Chapter 45). The vasculitides involving large arteries are briefly described in this section, but it is important to realize that many of them also involve smaller-sized vessels.

> ### Box 41-1 Classification of Vasculitis* by Predominant Size of Vessel Involvement
>
> **Large Vessel**
> GCA
> TA
> Behçet's disease
> Relapsing polychondritis
> Cogan's syndrome
> Aortitis associated with spondyloarthropathies
> Retroperitoneal fibrosis
> Idiopathic aortitis
>
> **Medium Vessel**
> PAN
> GPA (Wegener's)
> MPA
> CSS
> Kawasaki disease
>
> **Small Vessel**
> HSP
> CV
> Primary angiitis of the CNS
> Anti-GBM Disease
> Goodpasture's syndrome
> Rheumatoid arthritis (rheumatoid vasculitis)
> Sjögren's syndrome
> SLE
> Systemic sclerosis (scleroderma)
> Drug-induced vasculitis
>
> *Most of these diseases can involve vessels of varying sizes but are listed here by the size of the most commonly affected arteries for convenience purposes. This is not an exhaustive list of vasculitides.
> CNS, central nervous system; CSS, Churg-Strauss' syndrome; CV; cryoglobulinemic vasculitis; GBM, glomerular basement membrane; GCA, giant-cell arteritis; GPA, granulomatosis with polyangiitis; HSP, Henoch-Schönlein purpura; MPA, microscopic polyangiitis; PAN, polyarteritis nodosa; SLE, systemic lupus erythematosus; TA, Takayasu's arteritis.

Giant Cell Arteritis

Giant-cell arteritis, also commonly known as *temporal arteritis* and described in detail in Chapter 43, is the most common of the idiopathic vasculitides.[4,5] Giant-cell arteritis affects men and women aged 50 and older but is especially prevalent after age 70. Many vascular and systemic manifestations are seen in this disease. Vascular disease occurs in the aorta and its branches, with predilection for the branches of the carotid arteries, especially the ophthalmic artery, with resulting headaches, jaw claudication, and visual impairment. Rapid-onset irreversible monocular blindness is the most feared complication, but stroke, limb ischemia, and aortic disease can occur, the latter more common than generally appreciated, especially several years after the initial presentation. Common systemic manifestations include fever, anemia, proximal arthralgias (polymyalgia rheumatica), and fatigue. Diagnosis is often established on finding arteritis on temporal artery biopsy, but this is not required for a diagnosis. Elevated acute phase reactants are seen in 90% of cases. Treatment with high-dose glucocorticoids is highly effective but often results in significant drug-related morbidity.

Takayasu's Arteritis

Takayasu's arteritis, described in detail in Chapter 42, is a vasculitis that involves the aorta and all its major branches and the pulmonary arteries, including but not limited to the brachiocephalic, carotid, vertebral, subclavian, renal, femoral, and coronary arteries. This disease often results in stenoses, occlusions, and ischemic damage to end organs and limbs.[4,6] Stroke, myocardial infarction (MI), limb claudication, and severe renovascular hypertension are all complications well known to occur in this disease. It is mostly seen in women and usually first presents clinically in the second or third decade, but it can occur at older ages. Many patients have associated systemic symptoms of fever, arthralgias, and malaise. The disease has a waxing and waning course, and delay in diagnosis is common. Treatment involves glucocorticoids in almost all patients and often the addition of immunosuppressive medications. Surgical bypass procedures may be necessary in some cases.

Behçet's Disease

Behçet's disease is a systemic inflammatory disease with multiple mucocutaneous manifestations, especially including genital and oral ulcers and often severe sight-threatening inflammatory eye disease.[7] Arthritis, gastrointestinal disease (including mucosal lesions), epididymitis, and secondary amyloidosis can also occur. Although its prevalence is markedly increased in countries in the Eastern Mediterranean, Middle East, and East Asia and descendents of people from these regions, Behçet's disease is found in populations worldwide.

Vasculitis occurs in up to one third of patients with Behçet's disease and is unique among the inflammatory vasculitides for the relatively common clinical involvement of venous disease. Both arterial and venous manifestations may occur in the same patients. Venous involvement includes superficial phlebitis, varices, and thromboses of deep veins, vena cava, cerebral sinuses, and other major veins.

The arterial lesions in Behçet's disease are often in large vessels and frequently result in aneurysms, stenoses, or rupture. The most common sites of arteritis are the aorta and its branches and the pulmonary arteries; however, Behçet's disease may also involve medium and small vessels.

Behçet's disease can involve a huge range of different types of histopathologies, consistent with the protean disease manifestations. The oral and genital ulcers do not have specific pathognomonic features. Similarly, biopsy specimens of the gastrointestinal lesions cannot differentiate Behçet's disease from inflammatory bowel disease. Although the vascular lesions can include large and small arteries as well as veins, these lesions are similar to those of other vasculitides.

Treatment of Behçet's disease varies with the manifestation being addressed and may range from colchicine and topical glucocorticoids for aphthous ulcers to large doses of glucocorticoids for many problems including mucocutaneous, vascular, and eye lesions. The uveitis is treated with long-term immunosuppressive agents, including cyclosporine, azathioprine, chlorambucil, and cyclophosphamide. Inhibitors of tumor necrosis factor (TNF)-α are now also used to treat this disorder. Many treatment protocols are based on expert opinion, but in recent years an increasing number of controlled clinical trials have been performed, especially involving eye disease. Behçet's disease can be a highly aggressive form of vasculitis that frequently results in significant morbidity and mortality.

Relapsing Polychondritis

Relapsing polychondritis is a rare connective tissue disease that predominantly affects the cartilaginous structures of the eyes, ears, nose, and subglottis/trachea, but may also affect a wide variety of other organ systems and is associated with vasculitis, especially of large vessels.[8] The cardinal feature of polychondritis is auriculitis, inflammation of the outer ear, usually sparing the noncartilaginous lobe. Auriculitis, which is also a feature of GPA and CSS but virtually of no other diseases, is readily treated with glucocorticoids and can result in disfigurement if allowed to go untreated. Other common manifestations include inflammatory eye disease that can lead to blindness, destruction of nasal cartilage leading to internal derangement and external disfigurement, sensorineural hearing loss and vertigo, arthritis, and subglottic inflammation with resulting stenosis, a life-threatening condition. Each of these features can also be seen in GPA, although auriculitis is rare in this disease, and relapsing polychondritis is not associated with parenchymal pulmonary manifestations.

The vasculitis seen in relapsing polychondritis can affect vessels of any size, but large-vessel vasculitis is the most common. Aortitis

TABLE 41-1 Manifestations of Vasculitis That Mimic Noninflammatory Cardiovascular Disease

TYPE OF VASCULITIS	THORACIC AORTIC DISEASE	ABDOMINAL AORTIC DISEASE	CAROTID/ VERTEBRAL ARTERIAL DISEASE	STROKE DUE TO SMALL- OR MEDIUM-ARTERY DISEASE	UPPER- AND LOWER-EXTREMITY ARTERIAL STENOSIS	RENAL ARTERIAL DISEASE	CORONARY ARTERY DISEASE	MESENTERIC ARTERITIS	MYOCARDITIS	PERICARDITIS
GCA	++*	+†			+	+	Rare‡	Rare		
TA	+++§	++			+++	++	+	+	Rare	Rare
Behçet's disease	+	++	Rare	Rare	+	Rare	Rare		+	Rare
Other large-vessel diseases (RPC, CS, RPF, IA)	++	+	+	Rare	+	+	Rare	+	Rare	Rare
PAN				+	+	+	Rare	+++	+	+
GPA (Wegener's)	Rare			Rare	+	Rare	Rare	+	Rare	+
MPA				Rare		Rare	Rare	+	Rare	+
CSS				Rare			Rare	+	++	++
Kawasaki disease			Rare	Rare			+++		++	+
HSP								+++		
CV				Rare			Rare	Rare	+++	
Primary angiitis of CNS			++	++						
Small-vessel vasculitis of RA, SS, SLE, or SSc			Rare	+	Rare	+	+	++	+	+++

*Moderately common manifestation.
†Well described but relatively uncommonly seen.
‡Reported but quite rare.
§Common manifestation.

CNS, central nervous system; CS, Cogan's syndrome; CSS, Churg-Strauss' syndrome; CV, cryoglobulinemic vasculitis; GCA, giant-cell arteritis; GPA, granulomatosis with polyangiitis; HSP, Henoch Schönlein purpura; IA, idiopathic aortitis; MPA, microscopic polyangiitis; PAN, polyarteritis nodosa; RPC, relapsing polychondritis; RA, rheumatoid arthritis; RPF, retroperitoneal fibrosis; SLE, systemic lupus erythematosus; SS, Sjögren syndrome; SSc, systemic sclerosis (scleroderma); TA, Takayasu's arteritis.

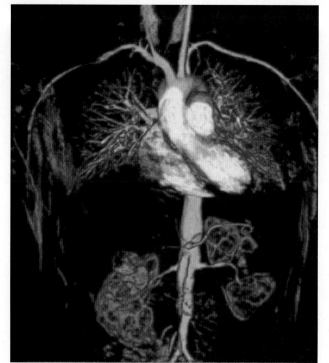

FIGURE 41-1 (See also Color Plate 41-1.) **Large-vessel vasculitis with stenotic lesions of abdominal aorta and left subclavian, left carotid, and bilateral renal arteries as imaged using three-dimensional (3D) dynamic gadolinium-enhanced magnetic resonance angiography (MRA)**.

with associated aortic valvular dysfunction and accompanied by thoracic or abdominal aortic aneurysms is fairly common and can lead to heart failure, aneurysmal rupture or dissection, and involvement of branch arteries. Small-vessel disease can affect nerves, eyes, kidneys, and other systems.

The histopathology of relapsing polychondritis includes destructive inflammation of various types of cartilage, necrotizing aortitis, vasculitis in small vessels (e.g., skin, glomeruli), and direct inflammatory infiltration of eye structures, heart valves, pericardium, skin, and other tissues.

Relapsing polychondritis has been associated with various other primary autoimmune diseases, such as inflammatory bowel disease, lupus, and others. The rarity of this syndrome has precluded comprehensive research that might help both better differentiate cases from other conditions and learn more about the pathophysiology. Treatment almost always involves systemic glucocorticoids, and immunosuppressive agents are frequently prescribed for this often rapidly progressive disease.

Cogan's Syndrome

Cogan's syndrome is a rare disorder characterized by inflammatory eye and inner ear/vestibular disease that can also involve inflammatory vasculitis.[9] It is a disease of young adults, usually first affecting patients before age 40, although both children and older patients have also been affected.

The characteristic clinical manifestations of Cogan's syndrome are interstitial keratitis, sensorineural hearing loss, and vestibulatory dysfunction. Although interstitial keratitis is the most common eye problem in Cogan's syndrome, uveitis, scleritis, and many other types of ophthalmological inflammation can occur. The eye and ear damage is often permanent and can be quite debilitating. The combination of inflammatory eye disease and inner ear problems is required for a diagnosis of Cogan's syndrome, but these findings can occur in other diseases as well, such as infections, malignancies, sarcoidosis, and various autoimmune diseases, including other vasculitides (e.g., GPA, relapsing polychondritis, Behçet's disease). Other organ systems are less commonly involved.

Vasculitis occurs in up to 15% of patients with Cogan's syndrome and is mostly large-vessel disease, with some medium-vessel manifestations reported. The large-vessel disease in Cogan's syndrome is similar to that of TA and includes aortitis with aortic insufficiency, stenoses of the carotid and subclavian and other aortic branch arteries, and even coronary artery disease (CAD). Treatment of Cogan's syndrome includes both glucocorticoids and immunosuppressive drugs, appropriate rehabilitation (e.g., vestibular retraining), surgical correction of eye damage, and use of hearing aides or surgical correction of hearing loss.

Idiopathic Aortitis

Aortitis may be found in the absence of any other manifestations of a systemic inflammatory disease.[10-12] These cases often come to the attention of vascular medicine specialists when patients undergoing surgical repair of aortic aneurysms and dissections are found to have inflammation consistent with aortitis on pathological specimens. Autopsies and studies of large numbers of surgical specimens have demonstrated that noninfectious aortitis occurs in 4% to 15% of cases. Although on detailed investigation, many of these patients are retrospectively found to have had evidence of GCA, TA, relapsing polychondritis, GPA, or another definable vasculitis, it is common among these cases to find *no* evidence of more systemic inflammatory disease. The majority of cases of so-called idiopathic aortitis involve thoracic lesions, in contrast to the overall predominance of abdominal aortic lesions for noninflammatory disease.

It is possible that cases of isolated inflammatory aortic aneurysms will be increasingly identified earlier as magnetic resonance imaging (MRI) technology continues to improve and helps demonstrate inflammation in the arterial wall. It can, however, be difficult to differentiate inflammation due to true idiopathic aortitis and vasculitis from the vascular and periaortic inflammations seen in association with atherosclerotic disease. Currently, in the absence of pathological specimens or other evidence of a vasculitis, MRI alone is not diagnostic for inflammation. The emergence of positron emission tomography (PET) scanning for large-vessel disease may also help in the evaluation of such patients.

The approach to treatment of idiopathic aortitis is unclear; many patients never develop other findings of vasculitis. However, new aneurysms and significant vascular disease do occur in some cases.[11] Comprehensive evaluation of evidence of systemic disease is necessary and should include a detailed physical examination, diagnostic imaging, laboratory studies, and other approaches outlined later in this chapter. Appropriate treatment should be given if inflammatory disease other than that seen in the surgical specimen is found, but not all patients require glucocorticoids, especially in the postoperative period. Furthermore, regular follow-up of such patients by a specialist knowledgeable about vasculitis is imperative because lesions may develop subtly and only years after the initial pathological diagnosis is made.

Miscellaneous Forms of Large-Vessel Vasculitis

Although large-vessel vasculitis is only rarely seen with other systemic inflammatory conditions, it is important to recognize these potential associations. Aortitis is rarely associated with long-standing seronegative spondyloarthropathies (ankylosing spondylitis, reactive arthritis, psoriatic arthritis, and inflammatory bowel disease) and can result in aortic insufficiency. Retroperitoneal fibrosis, a rare disease of proliferating fibroblasts usually causing ureteral obstruction and at times aortic stenosis and periaortitis, is also associated with true inflammatory aortitis. There have been a few case reports of large-vessel vasculitis in patients with rheumatoid arthritis, systemic lupus erythematosus (SLE), and GPA.

Medium-Vessel Vasculitis

Among the inflammatory vasculitides, the medium-vessel diseases have the greatest variety of clinical manifestations, which result from the broad range of vessel sizes actually involved in the process. As stated earlier, classifying the vasculitides by affected vessel size can be problematic, but particularly with the medium-vessel disorders.

Specialists in vascular medicine need to be aware of protean presentations of active medium-vessel disease and the lasting damage they can cause. As with large-vessel disease, these disorders can mimic noninflammatory cardiac, renal, cerebral, and other vascular problems. This fascinating set of diseases comprises the vasculitides for which the highest quality and quantity of clinical trial data are available to help guide therapy.

Polyarteritis Nodosa

Polyarteritis nodosa (PAN) is among the "purer" vasculitides in that most of its manifestations are due to true vascular inflammation.[13] With the identification of other types of vasculitis, the spectrum of what is now diagnosed as PAN has narrowed over the past 50 years. Although characterized as a medium-vessel disease, PAN may also involve small vessels such as those in the skin. Polyarteritis nodosa frequently involves inflammation leading to multiple small aneurysms that often appear angiographically as a "string of beads." Ischemia and infarction of kidneys, intestines, and skin are common in PAN, with arthralgias, myalgias, and fevers also frequently seen. Diagnosis is based on angiographic appearance (Fig. 41-2) or tissue pathology, often from surgical specimens such as a resected ischemic bowel segment. Interestingly, PAN in one subset of patients is associated with either hepatitis B or hepatitis C infections.[13,14] Importantly, there is a difference between hepatitis C–associated PAN and hepatitis C–associated cryoglobulinemic vasculitis (CV, see later section). Cardiac manifestations of PAN are due to coronary arteritis or malignant hypertension (secondary to renal artery disease) and include myocardial ischemia, heart failure, and arrhythmias.

Treatment of PAN almost always involves high-dose glucocorticoids followed by a slow tapering of the dose. In more severe cases, an immunosuppressive agent is added. Hepatitis-associated PAN is now often treated with short courses of glucocorticoids and prolonged courses of antiviral agents. The rate of disease relapse in PAN is lower than that for many other types of vasculitis, and this relatively good prognosis is another important factor to take into consideration when deciding on a therapeutic regimen. Due to the rarity of the disease, controlled clinical trials for PAN are unlikely to occur; treatment is based on case series and expert opinion.

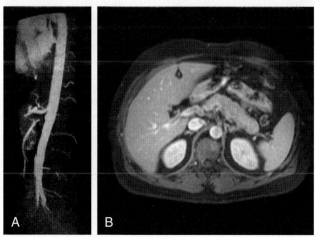

FIGURE 41-2 Polyarteritis nodosa (PAN) with stenotic lesions (A) and wall thickening and enhancement (B) of celiac and superior mesenteric arteries imaged using three-dimensional (3D) dynamic gadolinium-enhanced magnetic resonance angiography (MRA).

Granulomatosis with Polyangiitis (Wegener's)

Granulomatosis with polyangiitis is characterized by the triad of inflammation and destruction of tissue in the upper airway and sinuses (Fig. 41-3), lower airway (Fig. 41-4), and kidneys (Fig. 41-5), as well as the development of ANCAs.[15,16] Approximately 70% of patients with GPA are positive for ANCA at diagnosis, although some will develop the antibodies later in the course of their illness. Among patients with GPA and glomerulonephritis, more than 90% are positive for ANCA. Although the combination of these features is common in GPA, many patients present with only a subset of these findings. Granulomatosis with polyangiitis also frequently involves many other organ systems. The upper airway lesions include destructive rhinitis, often leading to nasal bridge collapse and the "saddle nose" deformity, sinusitis, and subglottic inflammation that can lead to life-threatening tracheal stenosis. The most severe form of pulmonary disease in GPA is alveolar hemorrhage, and this is a common cause of early death. Other common pulmonary lesions

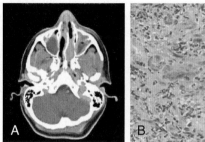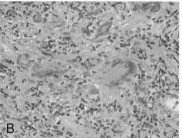

FIGURE 41-3 (See also Color Plate 41-3.) **Severe sinusitis in a patient with granulomatosis with polyangiitis (GPA; Wegener's). A,** Computed tomography (CT) scan during an acute flare of disease. **B,** H&E stain of a sinus biopsy from this patient demonstrates characteristic inflammation, including a giant cell.

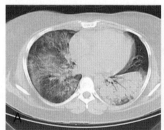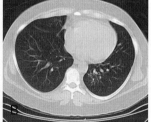

FIGURE 41-4 **Pulmonary hemorrhage in a patient with granulomatosis with polyangiitis (GPA; Wegener's) as seen on chest computed tomography (CT) scans. A,** During acute flare of disease. **B,** Same patient after treatment with glucocorticoids and cyclophosphamide. Patient's dyspnea and plain radiographic changes mostly resolved within 2 weeks of starting glucocorticoids.

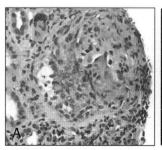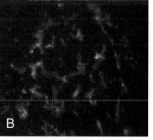

FIGURE 41-5 (See also Color Plate 41-5.) **Renal biopsy in a patient with granulomatosis with polyangiitis (GPA; Wegener's same patient as in Fig. 41-4) with rapidly progressive glomerulonephritis. A,** H&E stain demonstrates marked glomerular destruction as well as a multinucleated giant cell *(upper left).* **B,** Characteristic "pauci-immune" immunofluorescent staining seen in GPA and microscopic polyangiitis (MPA).

include nodules, with or without cavitation, and tracheobronchitis. Other common features of GPA are retroorbital pseudotumor with resulting proptosis, conductive and sensorineural hearing loss, mononeuritis multiplex, arthritis, and purpura. Peripheral vascular involvement with gangrene is seen in GPA and may be the presenting feature (Fig. 41-6).

Inflammatory cardiac disease is rare in GPA but can include myocarditis and pericarditis. Aortic or large-vessel involvement in GPA is extremely uncommon.

Venous thromboses, including both deep vein thromboses (DVTs) and pulmonary emboli (PEs), occur frequently in GPA and may be associated with active disease.[17,18] Although some of the pathology in GPA is indeed granulomatous with histiocytes, piecemeal necrosis, and occasional giant cells and eosinophils, other manifestations of inflammation are also seen in the disease. True vasculitis occurs and includes capillaritis. The renal disease of GPA is identical to other ANCA-positive diseases, and the pathology is that of rapidly progressive glomerulonephritis.

Untreated, GPA most often leads to death or serious damage.[19] Glucocorticoids are always used for treatment, but the prognosis of GPA changed considerably when a protocol using cyclophosphamide was introduced in the 1970s at the National Institutes of Health (NIH). The morbidity and mortality of GPA was markedly improved by cytotoxic therapy: 1-year mortality changed from more than 80% to less than 20%.[16,19,20] However, serious side effects are common with the use of cyclophosphamide, and the rate of recurrent disease in GPA after therapy is above 50%. In recent years, new treatment protocols have been tested in open and controlled trials that incorporate less toxic immunosuppressive drugs, including methotrexate and azathioprine.[21-23] Two multicentered randomized controlled trials (RCTs) have demonstrated that treatment with rituximab, a monoclonal antibody directed against the CD20 receptor on B cells, was equivalent to cyclophosphamide for induction of remission in ANCA-associated vasculitis (GPA and MPA).[24,25] In 2011, the U.S. Food and Drug Administration (FDA) approved rituximab for the treatment of GPA and MPA, and it has quickly become an established alternative to cyclophosphamide.

Microscopic Polyangiitis

With the publication of the Chapel Hill Consensus Conference classification system, recognition of MPA as a separate entity gained acceptance.[2,13] Microscopic polyangiitis is a mostly small- to medium-vessel ANCA-associated vasculitis with manifestations that strongly overlap with GPA. Its key features include glomerulonephritis, alveolar hemorrhage, skin lesions, and mononeuritis multiplex, but many other organ systems may be involved as well. Unlike GPA, the pathology of MPA is nongranulomatous and does not involve the type of nonvascular disease seen in GPA or CSS. The glomerulonephritis of MPA is identical to that seen in GPA. Most patients with MPA are positive for ANCA, and the predominant ANCA antigen specificity is myeloperoxidase. Cardiac manifestations of MPA are uncommon, but peripheral artery disease (PAD) and gangrene are seen and may be confused with noninflammatory vascular disease. Microscopic polyangiitis should be differentiated from classic PAN. Polyarteritis nodosa is more of a medium-vessel disease and does not include glomerulonephritis or pulmonary capillaritis. Microscopic polyangiitis does not produce the microaneurysms seen in PAN. Treatment of MPA is essentially identical to that for GPA.

Churg-Strauss' Syndrome

Churg-Strauss' syndrome, also known as *allergic granulomatous angiitis*, is a rare disease characterized by the triad of asthma, pulmonary infiltrates, and hypereosinophilia.[26,27] Churg-Strauss' syndrome can, however, involve almost all the clinical features seen in GPA, including the presence of ANCA in some cases (30%-40%).

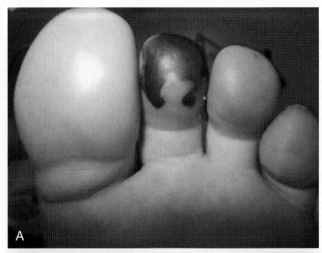

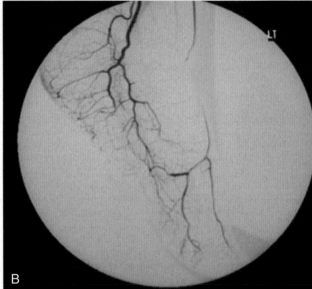

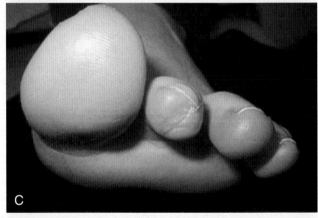

FIGURE 41-6 (See also Color Plate 41-6.) **Gangrenous toe in a patient with granulomatosis with polyangiitis (GPA; Wegener's). A,** Gangrenous left second toe pretreatment. **B,** Conventional angiogram of left foot at time of gangrene seen in **A,** demonstrating marked stenosis/occlusion of dorsal pedal artery and runoff. **C,** Same toe months after initiation of glucocorticoids and cyclophosphamide. Only minimal tissue loss resulted, and toe is now well perfused.

As with GPA, much of the pathology seen in CSS is due to inflammation that is not "vasculitis" per se but is every bit as damaging as vascular inflammation. Tissue eosinophilia, although seen in other types of vasculitis, is particularly common in CSS and often striking. More than 90% of patients have asthma, often severe; the hypereosinophilia may be a marker of disease activity for some patients but is not always present. Pulmonary manifestations include dense infiltrates that rapidly clear with glucocorticoid therapy. Additionally, neuropathies—especially mononeuritis multiplex and gastrointestinal ischemia—are common features and quite damaging. Diagnosis is based on the combination of clinical findings, hypereosinophilia, and pathology specimens that often show granulomatous and eosinophilic inflammation.

Cardiovascular manifestations of CSS are fairly common and include myocarditis with resultant congestive heart failure (CHF) and pericarditis. Angina is rare in CSS. Cardiac involvement in CSS may be rapid in onset and fatal.

Glucocorticoids are the mainstay of treatment for CSS, but immunosuppressive agents are increasingly being used for more severe cases and to help wean patients from glucocorticoids. It is important to avoid overtreating the asthma component of the syndrome; asthma is not in itself a reason to start cytotoxic medications.

Kawasaki Disease

Kawasaki disease, a vasculitis of young children involving medium and small arteries, is a leading cause of acquired CAD in children.[28] The disease manifests as a systemic illness with high fevers, conjunctival injection, erythematous oropharyngeal lesions, erythematous rashes and skin desquamation, lymphadenopathy, and other signs and symptoms. Cardiac involvement is frequent in Kawasaki disease and can result in long-term morbidity. Myocarditis and pericarditis are common and can be serious, but coronary artery aneurysms are the most feared aspect of the disease. Both panarteritis and granulomas can be seen in the vessels, with subsequent scarring and aneurysm formation. Treatment includes aspirin and intravenous immunoglobulin (IVIG); such regimens have been shown to markedly reduce the incidence of coronary complications. Kawasaki disease is described in detail in Chapter 45.

Small-Vessel Vasculitis

Henoch-Schönlein Purpura

Henoch-Schönlein purpura is a small-vessel vasculitis that classically involves the clinical triad of inflammatory arthritis, ischemic abdominal pain, and purpura, although not all cases exhibit all three manifestations.[29] The most feared manifestation of HSP is glomerulonephritis, which can lead to renal failure. Cardiac disease is not a feature of HSP, but hypertension from renal insufficiency can be severe. The lesions in HSP often involve leukocytoclasia and immunoglobulin (Ig)A deposition. An elevated serum IgA level is commonly seen in patients with HSP.

Henoch-Schönlein purpura is much more common among young children and is probably the most common type of vasculitis in this age group. Nevertheless, HSP is also seen in adults. The disease is more often self-limited among children and more likely to lead to chronic renal insufficiency in adults. Relapse is common in all age groups. Treatment of HSP varies from watchful waiting in some cases of pediatric HSP, to high-dose glucocorticoids, to the addition of immunosuppressive agents. However, it is not clear whether immunosuppressive therapy substantially alters long-term outcomes for HSP.

Cryoglobulinemic Vasculitis

Cryoglobulinemic vasculitis occurs when cryoglobulins, any of various types of Igs that precipitate from serum at temperatures below body temperature, induce an immune complex–mediated inflammatory process in any organ.[30] Several types of cryoglobulins can occur, and cryoglobulinemia is subclassified based on the mix of IgG and IgM antibodies that make up the cryoglobulin portion of serum (the "cryocrit"), and whether the excess cryoproteins are polyclonal or monoclonal.

Cryoglobulinemic vasculitis was previously considered to be a quite rare phenomenon sometimes seen in chronic inflammatory diseases such as lupus or rheumatoid arthritis or associated with lymphoproliferative disorders. Once the association between hepatitis C infection and type 2 mixed CV was established, however, it became apparent that coincident with the worldwide rise in hepatitis C infection, CV has been increasingly identified as a cause of vasculitis. The vast majority of cases of CV now seen are associated with hepatitis C infection.

Major clinical manifestations of CV include cutaneous vasculitis (purpura), arthralgias, peripheral neuropathy, and nephropathy with associated renal insufficiency or nephrotic syndrome (or both). Cardiovascular manifestations of CV include Raynaud's phenomenon, hypertension, and congestive heart failure. The hypertension in CV, which is often associated with renal disease, can be severe and lead to cardiac failure.

The histopathology of CV includes necrotizing vasculitis but may also involve Ig and complement deposition detected by immunofluorescence staining.

Treatment of CV is somewhat controversial. However, there is consensus that for patients with CV who are infected with hepatitis C virus, treatment with antiviral agents, even in the absence of significant liver disease, is important. For acute disease exacerbations or when antiviral therapy is not efficacious or possible, treatment may include glucocorticoids, cytotoxic agents, and plasmapheresis. There is increasing evidence that rituximab (ant-CD20 B cell depleting agent) is effective in treating CV.

Primary Angiitis of the Central Nervous System

Primary angiitis of the central nervous system (PACNS) is a quite rare necrotizing angiitis limited to the central nervous system (CNS).[31,32] PACNS is frequently associated with subacute nonfocal neurological deficits and chronic meningitis, although strokes and hemorrhage can also be seen.

Diagnosis of PACNS necessitates first suspecting this rare disease. Conventional angiography may be helpful in identifying other entities, such as aneurysms and emboli, but is often not diagnostic for vasculitis for several reasons (Fig. 41-7). First, in older patients the endothelial changes of atherosclerosis may mimic those of vasculitis. Second, vasospasm can be confused with stenosis from either atherosclerosis or inflammation. Finally, the resolution of conventional angiography is such that small arteries are not well visualized, and thus many cases of vasculitis may be missed by this technique. Leptomeningeal biopsies or larger tissue samples from affected brain areas are often necessary to demonstrate PACNS and provide the level of evidence required to institute therapy. The histopathology is that of vasculitis, but granulomas and giant cells are not always seen; there may be no inflammation in the vasospastic variant. Tests of cerebrospinal fluid are often normal in patients with PACNS, but are important in evaluating patients for other conditions, especially infection or malignancy.

Experts in vascular medicine need to be aware of PACNS because it can easily be mistaken for atherosclerotic disease with multiple infarcts. PACNS is extremely rare, but the approach to treatment is quite different from atherosclerotic disease.

Treatment recommendations are based solely on case series and an incomplete understanding of the pathophysiology. PACNS is treated with glucocorticoids, with immunosuppressive agents often added.

It is imperative to differentiate PACNS from the increasingly recognized set of reversible cerebral vasoconstrictive syndromes (RCVS) previously referred to as *benign PACNS*[33]; RCVS is *not* a vasculitis. It is characterized by acute onset of severe headache ("thunderclap headaches") and a focal neurological event. RCVS is treated with aggressive vasodilators, including calcium channel blockers, and strict avoidance of smoking and vasoconstricting drugs and substances, such as caffeine, cocaine, sympathomimetics, and serotonin receptor agonists (e.g., sumatriptan).

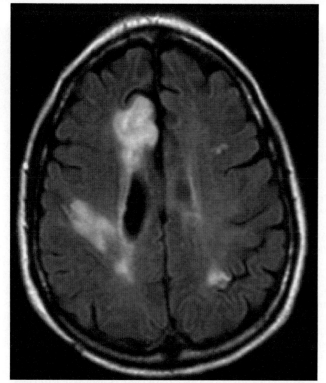

FIGURE 41-7 Multiple areas of brain infarction secondary to primary angiitis of the central nervous system (PACNS) as seen on gadolinium-enhanced magnetic resonance angiography (MRA). The cerebral angiogram on this patient was unremarkable, but brain biopsy demonstrated small-vessel vasculitis.

Vasculitis Secondary to Autoimmune/Connective Tissue Diseases

Vasculitis, especially of small arteries, can be seen in various systemic autoimmune diseases, including SLE, rheumatoid arthritis, Sjögren's syndrome, and systemic sclerosis (scleroderma). In these diseases, vasculitis usually accompanies evidence of severe disease in other organs or long-standing disease (e.g., rheumatoid arthritis). Skin vasculitis is common, but mesenteric and CNS vasculitis are the most feared and dangerous vascular manifestations seen in these diseases.

Although coronary arteritis is rarely seen in these systemic autoimmune disorders, there is an increased recognition of early accelerated atherosclerotic CAD among patients with SLE, rheumatoid arthritis, and other chronic inflammatory diseases. The pathophysiology of this problem is under active investigation and parallels the increased attention vascular biologists are paying to the contribution of inflammation to atherosclerosis. When vasculitis occurs in SLE or rheumatoid arthritis, it is frequently severe and often necessitates treatment with high-dose glucocorticoids and cyclophosphamide.

Drug-Induced Vasculitis

Many drugs or other toxins have been implicated as causing inflammatory vasculitis involving vessels of all sizes, especially small arteries. A full list of drugs considered to be causative for vasculitis and details regarding the clinical syndromes of drug-induced vasculitis are available in recent reviews.[34,35] There is an interesting subset of patients with ANCA-associated vasculitis whose disease is caused by exposure to certain medications.[36]

The clinical manifestations of drug-induced vasculitis range from skin-only disease to widespread life-threatening multisystemic disease. No clinical, laboratory, or pathological findings differentiate drug-induced from other types of vasculitis. Given that agents from most classes of drugs have been implicated in vasculitis, it is important that clinicians consider the possible contribution of not only every medication the patient was taking at the time of clinical presentation but also medications, supplements, and illegal drugs used in the previous year. The temporal association between drug exposure and disease, combined with the pattern of illness and evidence for or against a different vasculitic process, are helpful in establishing a diagnosis of drug-induced vasculitis.

Management of drug-induced vasculitis always includes discontinuation of the putative causative agent when possible, but may also involve treatment with clinical observation alone, glucocorticoids, or immunosuppressive agents. Patients should be followed for an extended period, even after apparent disease resolution, to ensure the diagnosis of drug-induced vasculitis rather than waxing and waning idiopathic vasculitis.

Evaluation and Diagnosis of Possible Vasculitis

When evaluating cases of potential vasculitis, the clinician's first challenge is to consider that one of these rare diseases is a possibility. Rather than quickly focusing on a specific type of vasculitis, it is best to consider first whether "some sort of" vasculitis is present and determine the specific type once more information becomes available. It is common that when clinicians are evaluating patients for vasculitis, they are also conducting parallel evaluations for non-vasculitic diseases, an appropriate approach given the rarity of vasculitis and the urgency to diagnose and treat conditions that mimic vasculitis, such as infection.

Due to the protean potential manifestations of the vasculitides, clinicians must be comprehensive in their evaluation of patients for possible inflammatory vascular disease. By "looking everywhere" at all organ systems with complete history-taking, physical examinations, and selective laboratory and radiographic diagnostic tests, evidence is sought for both the presence of vasculitis and the size of vessel involved. Finding the "worst" manifestation of any new diagnosis or flare of disease is important, but the goal is to determine the diagnosis of a vasculitis and ensure all manifestations are documented. Treatment protocols will differ based on extent of disease, and later assessment of response depends on accurate baseline evaluation of all features of disease.

With the exception of tissue pathology, no single test is fully diagnostic for vasculitis. A comprehensive initial medical evaluation including medical history, physical examination, and routine laboratory studies can provide most of the information clinicians need to either dismiss the diagnosis of vasculitis or focus on more specific diagnostic testing. Finally, clinicians must reconsider a diagnosis of vasculitis or consider a coexisting problem when either the clinical course changes or treatment response is not characteristic for vasculitis.

Medical History

Medical history and physical examination remain key elements of evaluation for vasculitis. A comprehensive review of systems is essential, and the potential queries related to vasculitis are numerous. Examples of symptoms to inquire about include any visual changes or eye symptoms, changes in hearing, nasal discharge or epistaxis, sinusitis, headaches, any mental status change, any neurological symptom, stridor, wheezing, cough, hemoptysis, pleuritic chest pain, jaw or limb claudication, abdominal pain, any skin lesion, arthralgias, arthritis, myalgias, weakness, fevers, weight loss, and many other symptoms.

A full and accurate medication and drug use history is mandatory and should include any prescription drugs, over-the-counter products, illegal drugs, and alternative/herbal products taken within the *prior 6 to 12 months*, as well as accurate stop and start dates. If patients have been prescribed medications to address specific symptoms that may be vasculitic, documenting the response to these treatments may be important.

Physical Examination

A full physical examination is required whenever a patient is evaluated for potential vasculitis, and several examination findings should always prompt consideration of vasculitis in any patient. Blood pressure should be measured in both arms for discrepancies. Obtaining pressures in the legs may be appropriate if lower-extremity stenoses are suspected. Hypertension may result from renal artery stenoses (RAS) from vasculitis, and similar physiology occurs with some tight suprarenal aortic stenoses. A full examination of bilateral pulses should include radial, ulnar, brachial, carotid, femoral, popliteal, posterior tibial, and dorsalis pedis pulses. Bruits should be listened for over the aorta and the carotid, femoral, axillary, subclavian, and renal arteries. Presence of blood pressure discrepancies, absent pulses, or arterial bruits are each highly specific for major arterial disease but are not highly sensitive for major arterial lesions in large-vessel vasculitis.[37]

Careful examination of skin and mucosal surfaces can reveal many clues to vasculitis. Although palpable purpura is the classic vasculitis skin lesion, not all purpura is vasculitis, and not all skin vasculitis manifests as purpura. Macular lesions, both flat and raised, as well as bullae and nonerythematous lesions, can all occur in vasculitis. Livedo reticularis may be a clue to vasculitis or vasospasm. One should examine the patient for oral or genital aphthous ulcers. Extremity cyanosis and pallor may be seen and may be variable depending on the ambient temperature and limb positioning. Ulcerations and crusting should be sought in the nasopharynx. Nailfold capillary changes can be seen on bedside microscopic examination with an ophthalmoscope. Signs of capillary fragility, especially over sites of blood pressure cuff or tourniquet application, may be seen.

The rest of a full physical examination is also essential in evaluating for vasculitis. Lung examination may reveal any of the many abnormalities commonly seen in vasculitis, including rhonchi, pleural rubs, dullness due to effusions, and wheezing. Careful cardiac auscultation might reveal evidence of aortic regurgitation, as seen in aortitis or pericardial rubs. Gross inspection of the eyes may reveal signs of inflammation, and funduscopic examinations may show retinal pallor or other signs of ischemia. A full ophthalmological examination including slit lamp is necessary for any patient suspected of vasculitis with eye symptoms. A full joint examination may reveal even asymptomatic effusions. Detailed neurological examination is essential; subtle cranial and peripheral neuropathies often go unnoticed by both patients and physicians, but are clues to severe disease.

Laboratory Studies

ACUTE PHASE REACTANTS

Acute phase reactants, including the Westergren erythrocyte sedimentation rate (ESR), C-reactive protein (CRP), and others, are perhaps the most misunderstood and misused tests in the evaluation of vasculitis. Erythrocyte sedimentation rate should never be considered a screening test for vasculitis because acute phase reactants are neither highly sensitive nor specific diagnostically for any type of vasculitis. There is good evidence that a normal ESR can be found in active TA, GCA, GPA, PACNS, drug-induced vasculitis, and other vasculitides. Although ESR is most helpful in evaluating patients for possible GCA, even in that disease, up to 10% of patients with documented GCA have normal sedimentation rates at the time of diagnosis. Furthermore, an elevated ESR can be seen in most of the disorders usually considered in the differential diagnosis of patients with possible vasculitis, notably infections and malignancies, thus emphasizing the lack of diagnostic usefulness of this test. Acute phase reactants are somewhat useful for monitoring disease activity and therefore in some cases may be supportive of a disease flare.

RENAL FUNCTION TESTS

Laboratory tests of renal function are an essential part of evaluating patients for possible vasculitis. A properly performed urinalysis is mandatory. Glomerulonephritis is a major feature of many small- and medium-vessel vasculitides and may manifest first as subtle findings on urinalysis, including proteinuria and hematuria. If the urine dipstick is abnormal, clinicians need to examine the urinary sediment. Clinicians must not count on hospital or reference laboratories to perform a manual urine sediment analysis because urinary casts are often dissolved by the time laboratory personnel run the test. If clinicians are not comfortable examining the sediment themselves, they should consult a nephrologist or another provider expert in this key test. Creatinine (Cr) elevations may reflect both acute renal disease and long-standing damage and scarring from prior flares of disease, and knowing a patient's baseline value is always important. Furthermore, the doses of many drugs used for patients with vasculitis are modified based on renal function; these include cyclophosphamide, methotrexate, cyclosporine, and nonsteroidal antiinflammatory drugs (NSAIDs). Hematuria may also be a clue to bladder toxicity from cyclophosphamide, including hemorrhagic cystitis and transitional cell carcinoma.

COMPLETE BLOOD CELL COUNTS AND WHITE BLOOD CELL DIFFERENTIAL COUNTS

No findings from a blood count and review of a blood smear are diagnostic for vasculitis, but the tests may provide clues to other diagnoses. Many, but certainly not all, patients with systemic vasculitis are anemic at initial presentation. Although eosinophilia is frequently present in CSS, GPA, drug-induced disease, and other vasculitides, this finding is also neither sensitive nor specific enough for diagnosis. Significant eosinophilia does, however, help narrow the potential diagnoses and may help in classifying patients with established vasculitis. Additionally, it is not uncommon for patients with CSS to have an increase in total eosinophil count before or during a flare of disease.

ANTINEUTROPHIL CYTOPLASMIC AUTOANTIBODIES TESTING

The discovery of ANCAs and their association with GPA, microscopic polyangiitis, CSS, and renal-only pauci-immune glomerulonephritis was extremely important in the evolution of diagnostic testing for vasculitis.[38] ANCA testing, when performed properly, is highly specific for these syndromes, and in the correct clinical setting may be the last piece of data necessary to establish a diagnosis, even in the absence of a tissue biopsy. Additionally, the finding of a positive test for ANCA in a patient with already established vasculitis essentially narrows the diagnosis to one of four ANCA-associated diseases.

Currently, the methodology for conducting ANCA testing is not standardized, which leads to problems with reliability and interpretation of test results. At a minimum, a laboratory should perform both immunofluorescence testing to identify the cytoplasmic ("C") ANCA pattern or perinuclear ("P") pattern, as well as conduct enzyme-linked immunosorbent assay (ELISA) testing for antibodies to proteinase 3 (anti-PR3) and antibodies to myeloperoxidase (anti-MPO). Antigen-specific ELISA tests are less prone to false-positive results (for the diagnosis of vasculitis) than the somewhat subjective immunofluorescence tests. Positive ANCA testing by the combined presence of C-pattern/anti-PR3 or P-pattern/anti-MPO is extremely specific for vasculitis, with other types of ANCA not helpful diagnostically.

Specificity of properly performed ANCA testing is better than 90% and may be closer to 99% in certain laboratories.[38,39] Sensitivity of ANCA testing varies with the type of disease and clinical manifestations. Although more than 90% of patients with GPA who have renal involvement are ANCA positive, this rate drops to about 70% for patients without renal disease. Most patients with MPA and renal-limited pauci-immune glomerulonephritis are ANCA positive, but the rate of ANCA positivity among patients with CSS varies in the literature from 40% to 80%. Thus, although ANCA is highly specific for vasculitis when present, a negative test by no means excludes the diagnosis.

OTHER IMMUNOLOGY TESTS

Antinuclear antibodies (ANAs) and rheumatoid factor (RF) should be tested only in selected cases. Antinuclear antibody is a useful screening test for SLE because 99% of patients with SLE have a positive ANA test, especially if they have vasculitis. However, a positive ANA is by no means specific for any autoimmune disease. In the absence of arthritis, a test for RF is rarely useful diagnostically because it can be seen in various infections and in type 2 cryoglobulinemia. Also, the test often has false-positive results. Furthermore, it is not diagnostic in itself for rheumatoid arthritis but is almost always positive in patients with rheumatoid vasculitis.

Testing for the presence of cryoglobulins is important. Their presence may not only help make the diagnosis, but treatment may be different and include plasmapheresis or antiviral agents (or both) in cases of hepatitis C–associated disease. Testing for cryoglobulins is not simple and is frequently done incorrectly. The blood specimen must be kept at body temperature (37°C) from the moment it is drawn through transport to the laboratory, where it must be allowed to clot in a warm water bath or heated box. Once the clot forms at 37°C, further special processing is required. From a Bayesian perspective, it is not unreasonable to repeat testing for cryoglobulins when the likelihood of their presence is medium to high, especially if the patient is infected with hepatitis C virus.

MICROBIOLOGICAL TESTING

Cultures of blood, urine, and other specimens are often appropriate when evaluating patients with vasculitis. Furthermore, patients with established vasculitis are at considerably increased risk of infection when undergoing immunosuppressive therapy, necessitating a low threshold to test for infection in this population. Finally, it is important that some biopsy specimens, especially lung tissue, be sent for culture for both typical and atypical/opportunistic pathogens.

Diagnostic Vascular Imaging

Radiographic assessment of vascular structures has long been an important tool for diagnosing patients with vasculitis. This is especially true when medium and large vessels are involved because they are much more likely to be visualized by the techniques available.[40] Although small- and even medium-sized arteries can often be seen on diagnostic biopsies or surgical specimens, large vessels are not usually amenable to tissue biopsy. Thus diagnostic imaging is crucial to assessment and management of patients with large-vessel vasculitis. The two great challenges inherent in interpretation of imaging of large vessels are (1) differentiating inflammatory disease from atherosclerotic disease and (2) trying to determine whether vascular lesions represent "active" disease. In recent years, interest in large-vessel vascular imaging has greatly increased as investigators and clinicians working in vasculitis strive to properly incorporate advances in various radiological modalities into practice. Imaging of organs and tissues other than arteries themselves is of obvious benefit for specific syndromes to help understand the extent of disease, facilitate choice of tissue biopsy, and rule out other pathology.

Specialists in vascular medicine need to be aware of the capabilities and limitations of various modalities for imaging the vascular system and differentiating atherosclerotic from inflammatory disease. Vascular imaging is much more commonly obtained to evaluate suspected atherosclerotic or structural disease, and thus it is vital that inflammatory disease is recognized, even when it is not expected. The increased recognition that atherosclerosis may have an inflammatory component and that vasculitis can result in some changes seen in atherosclerosis makes this differentiation even more challenging. Marked differences in treatment and prognosis for these different disorders make continued cooperative work by experts in cardiology, rheumatology, radiology, vascular surgery, and other specialties essential in evaluating patients and interpreting imaging data. The following sections summarize the progress to date in using various imaging modalities for evaluating vascular disease in the inflammatory vasculitides.

CONVENTIONAL ANGIOGRAPHY

Conventional angiography with intravascular injection of radiocontrast dye remains the gold standard for detecting stenoses and aneurysms in medium and large arteries and in diagnosing patients with vasculitis, especially TA and PAN. It is important to ask radiologists to view the distal runoffs of arteries beyond the trunk; diagnostic and critical lesions more distally (e.g., axillary artery) may be missed by undue concentration on the proximal vessels. Additional advantages to conventional angiography include the ability to measure intraarterial blood pressure directly. Such pressure readings are especially important when caring for patients with subclavian or proximal aortic stenoses, where peripheral pressure readings may be inaccurate. Finally, conventional angiography is the only current imaging modality that assists catheter-based intervention, including angioplasty and stent placement.

There are several problems with and limitations to conventional angiography for evaluation of potential vasculitis. The direct toxicities of the contrast dye have the potential for hypersensitivity reactions, renal insufficiency, and volume overload. Catheters can potentially cause vascular injury. The resolution of conventional angiography is limited, and most small-vessel disease, such as in the brain or mesentery, is not well imaged by this technique. Additionally, serial studies by conventional angiography, although sometimes necessary, are impractical, incur additive toxicity, and are thus not routinely performed to monitor patients. Finally, conventional angiography does not provide any information about the biological state of the arterial wall and therefore, except with serial images, cannot determine disease activity.

MAGNETIC RESONANCE IMAGING

The use of MRI to help in the diagnosis and management of vasculitis continues to gain acceptance rapidly, although there are few properly done studies on the reliability of MRI for these purposes. Magnetic resonance imaging and magnetic resonance angiography (MRA) provide detailed information on luminal structures, arterial wall thickness and edema, tissue enhancement (by gadolinium contrast), and blood flow for large and some medium vessels. These structural measures have been proposed as useful in determining vasculitis disease activity. Magnetic resonance imaging and MRA can be performed repeatedly with little risk to the patient and can thus provide important serial data. The technology for magnetic resonance (MR) continues to improve, and it is anticipated that the reliability and breadth of information it provides in evaluating patients with vasculitis will continue to increase substantially in the next few years, especially for large-vessel pathology.

Several problems remain in the use of MR for diagnosing and following patients with vasculitis. First, not all vascular structures are easily imaged, and false-positive scans due to problems with imaging artifact (and possibly other reasons) do occur. Second, neither the protocols for data acquisition nor the methods of image interpretation are standardized, making comparison of research data and studies from different institutions or even different machines problematic. The specificity of MR as a disease activity measure remains controversial. Unlike conventional angiography, MR does not allow for pressure readings or catheter-based interventions. Finally, MR is currently not helpful for small- or even most medium-vessel disease, although resolution is improving.

COMPUTED TOMOGRAPHY

Computed tomography (CT) is another promising imaging technique for large-vessel vasculitis. Computed tomography can demonstrate arterial calcification well and, with the newer machines and software, quite precise images are possible. Major drawbacks to CT include the associated toxicities of ionizing radiation and iodinated contrast dye. The best future use of CT may be in combination with other modalities, especially PET (see later discussion).

ULTRASOUND

Ultrasound has been used to evaluate vascular disease for many years, and well-developed literature is available on this technique. The noninvasive nature, widespread availability, and relatively low cost of ultrasound make it an attractive technique for vascular imaging. However, the work in ultrasound has mostly been on atherosclerotic disease and has focused on specific anatomical areas including the carotid, vertebral, and ophthalmic arterial systems and the abdominal aorta. Recently, investigators have become more interested in using ultrasound for inflammatory disease, but experience and research in this area are still quite limited.

Ultrasound is often the first vascular imaging test obtained for patients with suspected carotid or vertebral arterial disease or aortic aneurysms. Recognition by the examiner that the disease process may be something *other* than atherosclerosis is vital for proper early diagnosis. Greater awareness of the differences in foci of disease and in the size and appearances of lesions between atherosclerosis and vasculitis are important to emphasize.

Future use of ultrasound in evaluating inflammatory vascular disease depends on both (1) improved technology that better evaluates arterial wall structures and allows for examination of smaller-caliber vessels and (2) demonstration that ultrasound provides insight beyond that obtained from other modalities such as MR.

POSITRON EMISSION TOMOGRAPHY

Positron emission tomography is an intriguing imaging modality for vascular disease. Because it relies on uptake of an isotope, it may be able to provide a biological link to disease activity. Cases series on the use of PET in evaluating aortitis provide evidence that it may help detect and diagnose aortitis that is not otherwise apparent. However, the rate of so-called false-positive tests is not clear, and data from PET studies must be carefully considered within the clinical context. It has not been demonstrated that serial PET studies are helpful in either evaluating disease activity or guiding treatment for large-vessel vasculitis. The work on PET for large-vessel vasculitis is still in the early stages, and lack of standardization, paucity of direct comparisons with MRI, and high cost are all important issues to consider.

Tissue Biopsy

Given the need to often exclude infection, malignancy, or other processes, as well as the need for immunosuppressive medications for vasculitis, biopsy evidence is often crucial, and empirical therapy is strongly discouraged. With the exception of some cases of large-vessel vasculitis and some situations in patients with ANCA-positive disease, tissue biopsy is usually necessary to establish a firm diagnosis of vasculitis.

A temporal artery biopsy is almost always appropriate when GCA is a consideration, even if there are no cranial symptoms. A positive biopsy is such strong evidence for GCA that although a negative temporal artery biopsy does not exclude the diagnosis, a second contralateral biopsy is sometimes advised if the initial specimen is nondiagnostic.

For large-vessel diseases other than GCA, a vessel biopsy is almost never obtained because a medium- to full-thickness biopsy of the aorta or its main branches has obvious morbidity. Obtaining surgical specimens during bypass procedures or biopsies under highly controlled situations such as during aortic valve or graft surgery should, however, be considered when a diagnosis of large-vessel disease has not yet been established or when disease activity status is unclear.

For the other vasculitides, it is usually preferred to obtain a biopsy from the most accessible tissue. Skin biopsies are simple, have low risk of morbidity, and can be instrumental in diagnosis. Too often, purpuric lesions are assumed to be vasculitis, and biopsies not performed. Additionally, skin biopsies can be examined for evidence of embolic, thrombotic, or infectious diseases.

In the proper setting, biopsies of kidneys or lungs involve moderate risks but can be of high yield, whereas biopsies of other tissues (e.g., sinus mucosa, nerve, myocardium) are lower risk but also have lower diagnostic yields. Biopsies of other organs, such as intestine and liver, offer low yields and higher risks but may be appropriate, especially during a surgical procedure, in certain circumstances.

Treatment of Vasculitis

The goals of treatment for inflammatory vasculitis are to stop the active inflammation and prevent permanent damage. Unlike many other systemic inflammatory diseases, true clinical remission is not only possible in many cases of vasculitis but should be the goal of treatment. Thus, protocols are increasingly being referred to as involving either "remission induction" or "remission maintenance" treatments. The mainstays of therapy for vasculitis remain glucocorticoids and various immunosuppressive drugs. Treatment protocols are tailored to the specific type of vasculitis and the extent of disease. Clinical trial data are increasingly available to guide treatment for GPA, microscopic polyangiitis, Kawasaki disease, and GCA, whereas other diseases rely on either case series for guidance or extrapolated data from studies in related, but not identical, vasculitides. Box 41-2 outlines the treatments used for patients with inflammatory vasculitis.

Ensuring long-term follow-up of patients with inflammatory vasculitis is extremely important. Relapse of vasculitis, even after complete remission, is quite common in many forms, including both large- and small-vessel diseases. Relapse may occur weeks to years from the time of clinical remission and manifest with different clinical findings than those seen on initial presentation. For example, aortic aneurysms may be seen in patients with GCA years after

---

Box 41-2 Treatments for Inflammatory Vasculitis

Commonly Used Medications/Treatments
Aspirin
Glucocorticoids
Cyclophosphamide
Azathioprine
Methotrexate
Mycophenolate mofetil
Cyclosporine and tacrolimus (FK506)
Antiviral agents
Plasmapheresis
IVIG

Newer and/or Experimental Agents
Rituximab (anti-CD20)
Leflunomide
Inhibitors of TNF-α
Abatacept
Inhibitors of IL-6
Other experimental "biologics"

Surgical/Invasive Treatments
Balloon angioplasty
Intravascular stents (±drug-eluting coating)
Vascular bypass or replacement grafts
Reconstructive surgery

IL, interleukin; IVIG, intravenous immunoglobulin; TNF, tumor necrosis factor.

the patient was believed to be in "remission." Other manifestations may also occur, even in the absence of clinical symptoms, and are more likely missed when patients are believed to be "cured" of their vasculitis. For example, inadequate surveillance may allow renal insufficiency in patients with ANCA-associated vasculitis to go undetected until end-stage renal failure has occurred.

Medical Therapies for Vasculitis

Medical management of patients with vasculitis should only be directed by physicians familiar with both the use of chronic immunosuppressive agents and the clinical presentation and management of vasculitis. The acute and chronic toxicities of these drugs should not be underestimated and can result in significant morbidity. Treatment protocols are beyond the scope of this chapter, but the most commonly used medications for vasculitis are briefly outlined. Many different agents have been used for vasculitis (see Box 41-2).

Glucocorticoids are used for almost all patients with almost all types of vasculitis during the acute presentation or during flares. They have a rapid onset of action, and high doses often stabilize patients even with severe manifestations such as alveolar hemorrhage or glomerulonephritis. The toxicities of glucocorticoids, especially with prolonged use, are serious and common and include weight gain, osteoporosis, osteonecrosis, glucose intolerance, Cushingoid habitus, adrenal suppression, hypertension, mood disturbances, frank psychosis, cataracts, glaucoma, and many others (IV).

Immunosuppressive drugs are often used in conjunction with glucocorticoids, either to provide more effective therapy and induce a remission or to act as "steroid-sparing" drugs, allowing for safe tapering of the glucocorticoids.

Cyclophosphamide is widely considered the most effective agent for inducing and maintaining remission in various types of vasculitis.[16] The introduction of cyclophosphamide-based therapy changed the prognosis of many of these diseases. Although cyclophosphamide is extremely effective, its multiple toxicities are severe and include cytopenias, especially neutropenia with associated infections, gonadal failure, teratogenicity, hemorrhagic cystitis, transitional cell carcinoma of the bladder, myelodysplasia, mucositis, hair loss, and others. Controversy exists about the best route of administration for cyclophosphamide, orally or intravenously (IV).

Multiple alternative agents have been tested and proposed to limit use of cyclophosphamide. Methotrexate, taken orally or intramuscularly (IM) weekly, has demonstrated efficacy as both a remission-induction agent and remission-maintenance agent for GPA and is used for both purposes for multiple vasculitides.[41] The toxicities of methotrexate include cytopenias, gastrointestinal upset, oral ulcers, teratogenicity, and hepatic disease. Azathioprine is another commonly used agent for remission maintenance in vasculitis.[21] Azathioprine can cause cytopenias, infections, nausea, mucositis, hair loss, pancreatitis, and other problems, but like methotrexate, is usually well tolerated even for extended periods. Mycophenolate mofetil is also used for vasculitis. Cyclosporine has long been used in Behçet's disease and occasionally in other vasculitides.

Rituximab has been demonstrated in two RCTs to have similar efficacy to cyclophosphamide for induction of remission in ANCA-associated vasculitis (GPA and MPA). The risks of rituximab include allergic reactions and potential for infections.

Plasmapheresis (plasma exchange) has a central role in treating anti–glomerular basement membrane antibody-associated disease (Goodpasture's syndrome) and is used at some centers to treat both alveolar hemorrhage and severe glomerulonephritis in ANCA-associated vasculitis. The role of plasmapheresis in GPA and MPA is the focus of a currently enrolling international clinical trial. Pheresis is frequently used to treat acute manifestations of CV and occasionally other vasculitides. Intravenous IG is a mainstay of therapy for Kawasaki disease and has been advocated for several other types of vasculitis, often as a second- or third-line regimen, and based mostly on small case series.

Many biological agents ("biologics") have been and continue to be studied as treatment for vasculitides[23] (see Box 41-2). This rapidly expanding group of agents that inhibit specific targets within the immune system are having a remarkable impact on the care of patients with a wide variety of autoimmune and systemic inflammatory diseases. The studies of rituximab for GPA and MPA demonstrated efficacy of the new agent.[24,25] However, despite initial enthusiasm from open-label studies, randomized trials studying the use of inhibitors of TNF-α did not demonstrate efficacy of this class of drug for treatment of either GPA[42] or GCA.[43] This experience highlights the need for properly conducted randomized clinical trials in vasculitis. Studies testing the efficacy of several other biologics for various forms of vasculitis are either currently in process or in the planning stages.

Surgical or Procedural Interventions for Vasculitis

In addition to medical therapies, interventional and surgical treatments for vasculitis remain options for certain types of problems, especially in larger vessels after damage has become permanent. Angioplasty and stent placement have been performed for patients with TA and other diseases when severe arterial stenoses occur in large vessels. Results of these interventions are mixed, with restenosis a commonly reported problem. Whether or not drug-eluting stents (DESs) will offer advantages for the vasculitides remains to be demonstrated.

Surgical bypass or grafts of stenotic vessels, including the aorta and coronary, subclavian, carotid, and renal arteries, are an option for patients with large-vessel vasculitides. Several questions are unanswered regarding the proper timing of such surgery in the presence of "active" disease or when patients are on chronic glucocorticoids. Reconstructive surgery also plays a role in the care of patients with vasculitis, especially in patients with GPA who suffer deforming damage from nasal collapse or other upper airway and retroorbital disease.

Miscellaneous Issues in the Treatment of Vasculitis

PNEUMOCYSTIS JIROVECI PNEUMONIA PROPHYLAXIS

It is now standard practice to prescribe trimethoprim-sulfamethoxazole or another agent for prophylaxis against *Pneumocystis jiroveci* (formerly *carinii*) pneumonia for patients on medium to high doses of glucocorticoids in combination with an immunosuppressive agent.

GONADAL FUNCTION AND PREGNANCY-RELATED PROBLEMS

Treatment of vasculitis often involves drugs that adversely affect patients' gonadal function or are problematic during pregnancy, or both.[44] Cyclophosphamide can cause both male and female sterility and is a highly teratogenic agent. Methotrexate is teratogenic and an abortifacient drug. Glucocorticoids cause significant maternal and some fetal problems. Several of the other treatments in Box 41-2 are either directly contraindicated during pregnancy, or their safety during pregnancy has not been established.

It is imperative that patients in their reproductive years be counseled at the time of diagnosis and regularly thereafter regarding issues of fertility, pregnancy, and contraception. Full discussion of these issues often leads to careful planning that may involve freezing sperm, empirical ovarian-preserving medication protocols, and reevaluation of contraceptive choices.

OSTEOPOROSIS PREVENTION

Because patients with inflammatory vasculitis are often treated with repeated courses of high-dose glucocorticoids, it is essential that treating physicians give consideration to preservation of bone mass and assessments of osteoporosis. Most patients need to be given calcium and vitamin D supplementation, and many patients

OVERVIEW OF VASCULITIS

may be candidates for bisphosphonates or other treatments for prophylaxis or treatment of glucocorticoid-induced osteoporosis. A baseline bone density scan is often useful for risk stratification.

ACCELERATED ATHEROSCLEROSIS

Although there is little firm evidence yet, concern is growing that patients with inflammatory vasculitis are at increased risk of accelerated atherosclerosis and coronary artery disease, as is seen in patients with other chronic inflammatory diseases such as rheumatoid arthritis and SLE.[45] The etiology of the atherosclerosis is likely multifactorial but includes glucocorticoid usage, lipid disorders associated with disease and treatment regimens, and other treatment-related problems, such as nephrotic syndrome and diabetes mellitus. The impact of chronic inflammation itself, however, may be the most important factor in the development of atherosclerosis. Ongoing research is directed at the interaction between inflammation and atherogenesis. Whether or not chronic therapy with statins or other agents that act via lipid or inflammatory pathways is appropriate has yet to be proved in clinical studies.

REFERENCES

1. Bloch DA, Michel BA, Hunder GG, et al: The American College of Rheumatology 1990 criteria for the classification of vasculitis. Patients and methods, *Arthritis Rheum* 33: 1068–1073, 1990.
2. Jennette JC, Falk RJ, Andrassy K, et al: Nomenclature of systemic vasculitides. Proposal of an international consensus conference, *Arthritis Rheum* 37:187–192, 1994.
3. Watts RA, Suppiah R, Merkel PA, et al: Systemic vasculitis--is it time to reclassify? *Rheumatology (Oxford)* 50:643–645, 2011.
4. Kissin GY, Merkel PA: Large-vessel vasculitis. In Coffman JD, Eberhardt RT, editors: *Peripheral arterial disease: diagnosis and treatment*, Totawa, NJ, 2002, Humana Press, pp 319.
5. Weyand CM, Goronzy JJ: Giant-cell arteritis and polymyalgia rheumatica, *Ann Intern Med* 139:505–515, 2003.
6. Kerr GS, Hallahan CW, Giordano J, et al: Takayasu arteritis, *Ann Intern Med* 120:919–929, 1994.
7. Sakane T, Takeno M, Suzuki N, et al: Behcet's disease, *N Engl J Med* 341:1284–1291, 1999.
8. Sridharan ST: Relapsing polychondritis. In Hoffman GS, Weyand CM, editors: *Inflammatory diseases of blood vessels*, New York, 2001, Marcel Dekker, pp 675.
9. St Clair EW, McCallum RM: Cogan's syndrome, *Curr Opin Rheumatol* 11:47–52, 1999.
10. Liang KP, Chowdhary VR, Michet CJ, et al: Noninfectious ascending aortitis: a case series of 64 patients, *J Rheumatol* 36:2290–2297, 2009.
11. Merkel PA: Noninfectious ascending aortitis: staying ahead of the curve, *J Rheumatol* 36:2137–2140, 2009.
12. Rojo-Leyva F, Ratliff NB, Cosgrove DM 3rd, et al: Study of 52 patients with idiopathic aortitis from a cohort of 1,204 surgical cases, *Arthritis Rheum* 43:901–907, 2000.
13. Guillevin L: Polyarteritis nodosa and microscopic polyangiitis. In Ball GV, Bridges L, editors: *Vasculitis*, New York, 2002, Oxford University Press, pp 300.
14. Guillevin L, Lhote F, Cohen P, et al: Polyarteritis nodosa related to hepatitis B virus. A prospective study with long-term observation of 41 patients, *Medicine (Baltimore)* 74: 238–253, 1995.
15. Hoffman GS, Gross WL: Wegener's granulomatosis: clinical aspects. In Hoffman GS, Weyand CM, editors: *Inflammatory diseases of blood vessels*, New York, 2001, Marcel Dekker, pp 381.
16. Hoffman GS, Kerr GS, Leavitt RY, et al: Wegener's granulomatosis: an analysis of 158 patients, *Ann Intern Med* 116:488–498, 1992.
17. Allenbach Y, Seror R, Pagnoux C, et al: High frequency of venous thromboembolic events in Churg-Strauss syndrome, Wegener's granulomatosis and microscopic polyangiitis but not polyarteritis nodosa: a systematic retrospective study on 1130 patients, *Ann Rheum Dis* 68:564–567, 2009.
18. Merkel PA, Lo GH, Holbrook JT, et al: Brief communication: high incidence of venous thrombotic events among patients with Wegener granulomatosis: the Wegener's Clinical Occurrence of Thrombosis (WeCLOT) Study, *Ann Intern Med* 142:620–626, 2005.
19. Walton EW: Giant-cell granuloma of the respiratory tract (Wegener's granulomatosis), *BMJ* 2:265–270, 1958.
20. Reinhold-Keller E, Beuge N, Latza U, et al: An interdisciplinary approach to the care of patients with Wegener's granulomatosis: long-term outcome in 155 patients, *Arthritis Rheum* 43:1021–1032, 2000.
21. Jayne D, Rasmussen N, Andrassy K, et al: A randomized trial of maintenance therapy for vasculitis associated with antineutrophil cytoplasmic autoantibodies, *N Engl J Med* 349: 36–44, 2003.
22. Langford CA: Treatment of ANCA-associated vasculitis, *N Engl J Med* 349:3–4, 2003.
23. Langford CA, Sneller MC: Biologic therapies in the vasculitides, *Curr Opin Rheumatol* 15:3–10, 2003.
24. Jones RB, Tervaert JW, Hauser T, et al: Rituximab versus cyclophosphamide in ANCA-associated renal vasculitis, *N Engl J Med* 363:211–220, 2010.
25. Stone JH, Merkel PA, Spiera R, et al: Rituximab versus cyclophosphamide for ANCA-associated vasculitis, *N Engl J Med* 363:221–232, 2010.
26. Guillevin L, Lhote F, Cohen P: Churg-Strauss syndrome: clinical aspects. In Hoffman GS, Weyand CM, editors: *Inflammatory diseases of blood vessels*, New York, 2001, Marcel Dekker, pp 399.
27. Guillevin L, Cohen P, Gayraud M, et al: Churg-Strauss syndrome. Clinical study and long-term follow-up of 96 patients, *Medicine (Baltimore)* 78:26–37, 1999.
28. Barron KS: Kawasaki disease: etiology, pathogenesis, and treatment, *Cleve Clin J Med* 69(Suppl 2):SII69–SII78, 2002.
29. Saulsbury FT: Henoch-Schonlein purpura, *Curr Opin Rheumatol* 13:35–40, 2001.
30. Cacoub P, Costedoat-Chalumeau N, Lidove O, et al: Cryoglobulinemia vasculitis, *Curr Opin Rheumatol* 14:29–35, 2002.
31. Calabrese LH, Duna GF, Lie JT: Vasculitis in the central nervous system, *Arthritis Rheum* 40:1189–1201, 1997.
32. Hajj-Ali RA, Singhal AB, Benseler S, et al: Primary angiitis of the CNS, *Lancet Neurol* 10: 561–572, 2011.
33. Calabrese LH, Dodick DW, Schwedt TJ, et al: Narrative review: reversible cerebral vasoconstriction syndromes, *Ann Intern Med* 146:34–44, 2007.
34. Merkel PA: Drug-induced vasculitis, *Rheum Dis Clin North Am* 27:849–862, 2001.
35. Merkel PA: Drug-induced vasculitis. In Hoffman GS, Weyand CM, editors: *Inflammatory diseases of blood vessels*, New York, 2001, Marcel Dekker, pp 727.
36. Choi HK, Merkel PA, Walker AM, et al: Drug-associated antineutrophil cytoplasmic antibody-positive vasculitis: prevalence among patients with high titers of antimyeloperoxidase antibodies, *Arthritis Rheum* 43:405–413, 2000.
37. Grayson PC, Tomasson G, Cuthbertson D, et al: Association of vascular physical examination findings and arteriographic lesions in large vessel vasculitis, *J Rheumatol* 39:303–309, 2012.
38. Niles JL: Antineutrophil cytoplasmic antibodies in the classification of vasculitis, *Annu Rev Med* 47:303–313, 1996.
39. Merkel PA, Polisson RP, Chang Y, et al: Prevalence of antineutrophil cytoplasmic antibodies in a large inception cohort of patients with connective tissue disease, *Ann Intern Med* 126:866–873, 1997.
40. Kissin EY, Merkel PA: Diagnostic imaging in Takayasu arteritis, *Curr Opin Rheumatol* 16: 31–37, 2004.
41. Langford CA, Sneller MC, Hoffman GS: Methotrexate use in systemic vasculitis, *Rheum Dis Clin North Am* 23:841–853, 1997.
42. WGET Research Group: Etanercept plus standard therapy for Wegener's granulomatosis, *N Engl J Med* 352:351–361, 2005.
43. Hoffman GS, Cid MC, Rendt-Zagar KE, et al: Infliximab for maintenance of glucocorticosteroid-induced remission of giant cell arteritis: a randomized trial, *Ann Intern Med* 146:621–630, 2007.
44. Langford CA, Kerr GS: Pregnancy in vasculitis, *Curr Opin Rheumatol* 14:36–41, 2002.
45. Hahn BH: Systemic lupus erythematosus and accelerated atherosclerosis, *N Engl J Med* 349:2379–2380, 2003.

CHAPTER 42 Takayasu's Arteritis

Kathleen Maksimowicz-McKinnon, Gary S. Hoffman

Takayasu's arteritis is a rare chronic inflammatory large-vessel disease with a female bias. It affects the aorta and its primary branches. Initially thought to be an illness of young Asian women, it is now recognized worldwide. Chronic vascular inflammation leads to vessel stenosis and, less commonly, aneurysm formation.

Epidemiology

Takayasu's arteritis is a rare disorder that has variable incidence and prevalence depending on the country where it has been studied. In the United States, incidence estimates from Olmstead County, Minnesota, are 2.6 cases/million/yr, whereas in Sweden they are 1.2 cases/million/yr.[1,2] Autopsy studies in Japan document a high prevalence, with evidence of Takayasu's arteritis found in 1 of every 3000 individuals.[3] Similar postmortem studies have not been performed elsewhere to provide comparative data.

The peak incidence of Takayasu's arteritis is in the third decade of life, but not all investigators adhere to guidelines that exclude women beyond reproductive age. Consequently, some series may include women beyond their seventh decade of life.

Pathogenesis

Differences in disease prevalence and characteristics among different racial and ethnic cohorts suggest a genetic predisposition; however, no definite allelic associations have been found consistently across all groups of patients with Takayasu's arteritis. The well-established association between certain infections and secondary vasculitis has propelled a search for an infectious etiology. Special attention has been directed toward mycobacterial pathogens because of the increased prevalence of *Mycobacterium tuberculosis* (TB) infection in countries (e.g., India, Korea, Mexico) with a high prevalence of Takayasu's arteritis, associations of Takayasu's arteritis with previous mycobacterial infection, and TB skin test positivity in patients with Takayasu's arteritis. In several small studies, patients with Takayasu's arteritis were demonstrated to have increased immunological responses to mycobacterial proteins when compared to healthy controls, but these inflammatory responses can be nonspecific and do not prove causality.[4,5]

Vessel injury results from the influx and actions of macrophages, cytotoxic T cells, γδT cells, natural killer cells,[6] and B cells. Access of leukocytes to the vessel wall is through the vasa vasorum, with subsequent migration toward the large lumen intima. Various cytokines, including perforin, interleukin (IL)-6, RANTES (regulated, upon activation, normal T-cell expressed, and secreted), tumor necrosis factor (TNF)-α,[7,8] and B-cell activating factor (BAFF),[9] enhance vascular inflammation. Although the most common response to this process is myointimal proliferation that leads to wall thickening and luminal stenosis, destruction of smooth muscle cells (SMCs), elastic fibers, and other matrix proteins may lead to aneurysm formation, especially in the aortic root and arch (Fig. 42-1). Disease progression leads to secondary vessel stiffening associated with atherosclerosis.[10]

Clinical Manifestations

Systemic symptoms and signs occur in less than half of all patients and include fever, weight loss, malaise, and generalized arthralgias and myalgias. Patients more often present with signs and/or symptoms of tissue ischemia, never having had an associated systemic illness. The most common symptom of Takayasu's arteritis is upper-extremity claudication, occurring in more than 60% of patients and reflecting disease predilection for aortic arch vessels (≈90% of cases)[11] (Figs. 42-2 through 42-4). The most frequent clinical findings include blood pressure asymmetry in paired extremities, and bruits found most often over the carotid, subclavian, and aortic vessels.[12] Aneurysms most often affect the aortic root, stretching the atrioventricular annulus and producing valvular regurgitation (≈20% of patients); valve leaflets are not a site of inflammation. Many within this subset require surgical intervention.

Hypertension occurs in at least 40% of patients in U.S. cohorts and is even more common in Japanese and Indian cohorts (80%). Hypertension is most frequently due to renal artery stenosis (RAS), but it may also result from suprarenal aortic stenosis or loss of aortic compliance[11,13] (Figs. 42-5 through 42-7). The diagnosis of hypertension can easily be missed in patients with disease involving both upper extremities, where peripheral cuff measurements in either arm will be an inaccurate reflection of central aortic pressure. Hypertension with vascular bruits or claudication, especially in younger patients, should lead to a suspicion of Takayasu's arteritis and to further evaluation of all four extremity pulses and blood pressures for asymmetry. Vascular imaging of the entire aorta and primary branch vessels should then confirm anatomical abnormalities compatible with the diagnosis and delineate the extent of disease and types of lesions.

Coronary arteritis may produce obstructive coronary artery disease (CAD) or coronary artery aneurysms. Patients may develop myocardial ischemia, dysrhythmias, congestive heart failure (CHF), or myocarditis.

Classification of Takayasu's arteritis is based on sites of arterial involvement. One of the most widely accepted schemes separates patients into the following types (Fig. 42-8):
- Type I: branches of the aortic arch.
- Type IIa: ascending aorta, aortic arch, and its branches.
- Type IIb: type IIa plus thoracic descending aorta.
- Type III: thoracic descending aorta, abdominal aorta, or renal arteries, or a combination.
- Type IV: only abdominal aorta or renal arteries, or both.
- Type V: segments of the entire aorta and its branches.

Type V is the most common.

Morbidity results primarily from extremity claudication, less often from cardiac, renal, and central nervous system (CNS) vascular disease. Undetected and/or untreated hypertension is a significant cofactor in these disease sequelae. Mortality estimates range from just 3% at 8 years to 35% at 5 years' follow-up. Causes of death include stroke, congestive heart failure, sudden death of uncertain cause, and unrecognized or inadequately treated hypertension.[14,15]

Differential Diagnosis

A thorough and careful investigation is necessary to distinguish Takayasu's arteritis from its mimics (Box 42-1). Congenital and acquired disorders of tissue matrix may present with aortic root diltation, valvular insufficiency, and aneurysms in other sites; however, they are not generally associated with large-vessel stenoses, the hallmark of Takayasu's arteritis. In many cases, there are also genetic studies and extravascular features that help identify the syndromic disorders (e.g., Marfan, Loeys-Dietz, Ehlers-Danlos syndromes). Exceptions better known for matrix abnormalities usually leading to stenoses are fibromuscular dysplasia and Grange's syndrome.[16]

Although other autoimmune disorders can be associated with large-vessel vasculitis, they are most often distinguished by their other associated disease manifestations and age preferences. Aortitis restricted to the aortic arch has emerged as one of

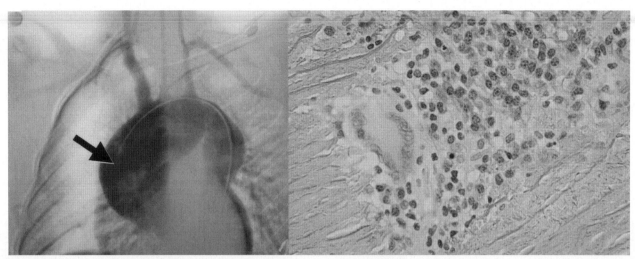

FIGURE 42-1   Destruction of muscle and elastic fibers of the thoracic aorta, with aneurysm formation *(arrow)*.

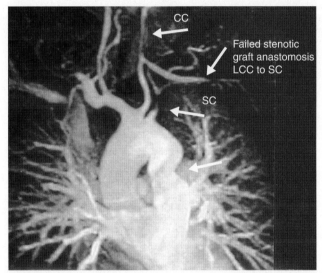

CC

Failed stenotic
graft anastomosis
LCC to SC

SC

FIGURE 42-2 Magnetic resonance angiography (MRA) illustrating stenotic lesions involving aorta, left common carotid *(CC)*, and left subclavian *(SC)* arteries.

numerous examples of single-organ vasculitis. Distinguishing it from Takayasu's arteritis requires complete evaluation of the large-vessel anatomy and careful follow-up over years to be certain that it is not the first sign of Takayasu's arteritis. It is important to distinguish isolated aortitis from Takayasu's arteritis because after surgical intervention, further therapy is usually not required.[10,17,18]

A significant and often underappreciated overlap exists between Takayasu's arteritis and giant cell arteritis[GCA], a disease of the elderly (mean age at diagnosis ≈70). A recent comparative cohort study of Takayasu's arteritis and GCA identified numerous shared features of disease, much of this coming to light with the advent and increased use of noninvasive vascular imaging studies.[19] Takayasu's arteritis and GCA may be indistinguishable in patients who present in middle age (45-55 years of age) with large-artery stenoses and less often aneurysms, especially of the aortic root.

Infectious causes of large-vessel aneurysms should always be considered irrespective of age or gender. Stenosis of large vessels is unusual in the setting of infection, where aneurysms dominate.

Diagnosis

Serological tests do not exist to identify Takayasu's arteritis. Rarely, the diagnosis is first considered after a surgical procedure provides biopsy findings that are compatible with the diagnosis. Most often

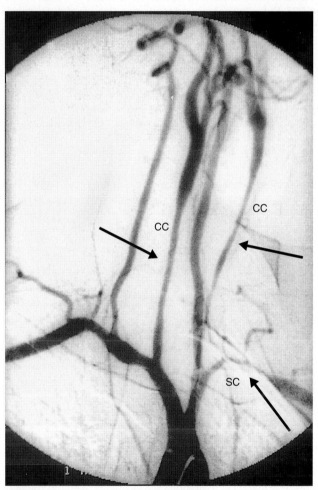

CC

CC

CC

SC

FIGURE 42-3   Angiography demonstrating stenoses of left subclavian *(SC)* and bilateral common carotid *(CC)* arteries.

the diagnosis is based on clinical findings in the presence of compatible vascular imaging abnormalities.[20,21]

Catheter-directed angiography allows for luminal imaging and pressure measurements and provides opportunities for intervention (e.g., angioplasty), but it provides little direct information about the vessel wall. Computed tomography (CT) or magnetic resonance imaging and angiography (MRI/MRA) provide more information regarding vessel wall thickening and edema, but the clinical implications of these findings, although suggestive of

522

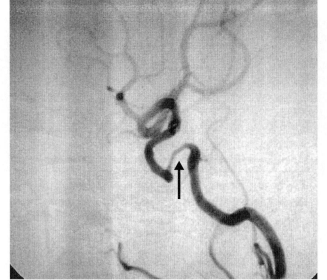

FIGURE 42-4 Angiography demonstrating stenosis of distal internal carotid artery (ICA).

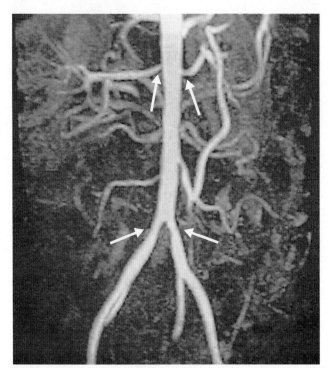

FIGURE 42-5 Magnetic resonance angiography (MRA) showing bilateral common iliac and renal arterial stenoses.

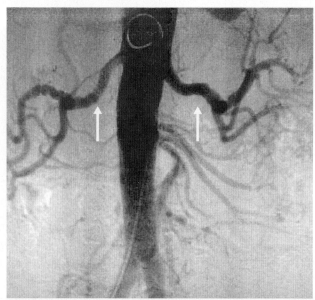

FIGURE 42-6 Angiography demonstrating bilateral renal artery lesions mimicking fibromuscular dysplasia (FMD).

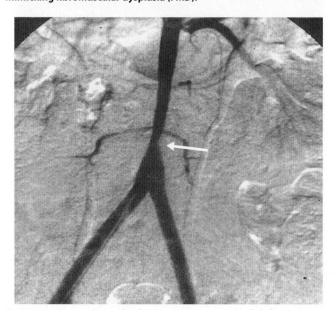

FIGURE 42-7 Angiography demonstrating stenosis of abdominal aorta.

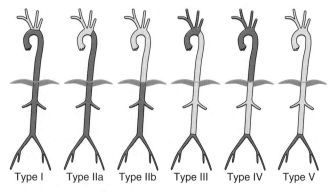

Angiographic Classification of Takayasu's Arteritis

Type I   Type IIa   Type IIb   Type III   Type IV   Type V

Types can be further modified by:
C: involved coronary artery
P: involved pulmonary artery

FIGURE 42-8 Classification of Takayasu's arteritis based on vessel involvement according to the International Conference on Takayasu Arteritis (1994).

active vascular disease, do not always correlate with disease activity or progression.[22] Studies examining the use of combined CT and positron emission tomography (PET) imaging are underway to determine whether more useful information may be derived about the vessel lumen and wall. The presence or absence of increased tagged glucose uptake within large vessels may have improved sensitivity and specificity for identifying active disease in Takayasu's arteritis.[23,24]

Although systemic signs and symptoms or elevated acute-phase reactants may be suggestive of active disease, they are inadequately sensitive in patients who only have vascular symptoms or findings. Sequential angiographic evaluations have revealed progression of disease, based on the presence of new vascular abnormalities,

Box 42-1 Differential Diagnosis of Takayasu's Arteritis

Autoimmune Disease
Behçet disease
Cogan's syndrome
Relapsing polychondritis
Ankylosing spondylitis
Sarcoidosis
Kawasaki disease
Sjögren's syndrome*
Systemic lupus erythematosus (SLE)*
Wegener's granulomatosis*
Rheumatoid arthritis*
Juvenile idiopathic arthritis*
Immunoglobulin (Ig)G4 systemic disease with aortitis
Idiopathic single-organ vasculitis restricted to the aortic arch

Collagen Vascular Disease (Congenital or Acquired)
Fibromuscular dysplasia (FMD)
Marfan's syndrome (MFS)
Loeys-Dietz's syndrome
Ehlers-Danlos' syndrome (EDS)
Grange's syndrome
Idiopathic aortic dissection/aneurysm

Infectious
Tuberculosis
Syphilis
Staphylococcus aureus
Salmonella typhimurium
Coxiella burnetii

Other
Atherosclerotic vascular disease
Aortic aneurysm associated with congenital bicuspid aortic valve (BAV)

*When vasculitis is a complication of these diseases, it most often takes the form of small-vessel disease.

in more than 50% of patients with normal erythrocyte sedimentation rates.[13] In addition, histopathological proof of vascular inflammation has been documented in 44% of bypass specimens from patients with Takayasu's arteritis who underwent surgery at a time when their disease was believed to be quiescent.

Treatment

Essential to effective treatment is accurate determination of disease activity, a goal that may not always be possible. Kerr et al.[13] define *active disease* as any two or more of the following. New or worsening:

- Signs or symptoms of vascular ischemia or inflammation.
- Increase in sedimentation rate.
- Angiographic features.
- Systemic symptoms not attributable to another disease.

Although these features are helpful when present, their absence does not guarantee disease remission. These criteria combined with sequential imaging are currently the best, albeit imperfect, means of monitoring disease activity.

Glucocorticoid therapy induces improvement in nearly all patients and initial disease remission in about 50%, but in 96% of patients, relapses occur during the course of tapering medication (with a mean of 2.8 relapses per patient in one study).[13,19] Therapy with other immunosuppressive agents may aid in achieving lower glucocorticoid requirements in such individuals or those with glucocorticoid-responsive and relapsing disease. Low-dose methotrexate was determined to be efficacious in diminishing glucocorticoid requirements in 13 of 16 patients in a National Institutes of Health (NIH) study.[25] Shelhamer et al.[26] demonstrated that cyclophosphamide administered with glucocorticoid induced remission in four of six patients with relapsing disease on glucocorticoid treatment alone. The authors recommend cyclophosphamide only

for patients with severe active disease. Patients generally achieve remission within 3 to 6 months, at which point cyclophosphamide should be changed to maintenance therapy with another immunosuppressive agent, such as methotrexate or azathioprine, to minimize the risk of cyclophosphamide toxicity. More recently, Molloy et al.[27] treated 25 Takayasu's arteritis patients who had refractory disease with anti–tumor necrosis factor therapy (principally infliximab) and found that 60% of them were able to achieve glucocorticoid-free disease remission, and an additional 28% achieved remission requiring less than 10 mg/day of prednisone. Randomized controlled trials are needed to assess the impact of such therapy in a larger cohort, with particular attention paid to the risk of reactivation of tuberculosis.

About 80% of patients require chronic immunosuppressive therapy over extended periods. Only over the past 15 years have investigators recognized the chronic and relapsing nature of Takayasu's arteritis. Studies that have incorporated sequential angiography have demonstrated that the majority of patients continue to develop new lesions in new vascular territories, even if they appear clinically to be in remission.[11,13,15,19] Because clinical symptoms and serological tests are often unreliable in monitoring disease activity, serial imaging studies are routinely used for assessment of disease progression.

Hypertension is a major source of morbidity and mortality in Takayasu's arteritis. Delay in the diagnosis of hypertension is common because of the high frequency of subclavian and innominate artery involvement, which may result in underestimation of central aortic pressure. Stenotic lesions also may be present in lower-extremity vessels, leaving some patients without any extremity capable of providing cuff blood pressure measurements that reliably represent those within the aortic root (Figs. 42-9 and 42-10). This emphasizes the need for complete vascular imaging at the time of diagnosis and during extended follow-up. Imaging should include the entire aorta and its primary branches. If stenoses of extremity vessels and/or the abdominal aorta preclude accurate determination of cen-

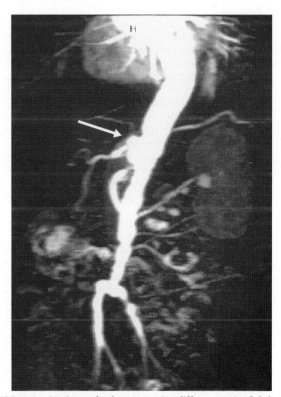

FIGURE 42-9 Angiography demonstrating diffuse ectasia of abdominal aorta and bilateral common iliac arteries, significant stenosis of left iliac artery, and dilation of origin of celiac artery *(arrow).*

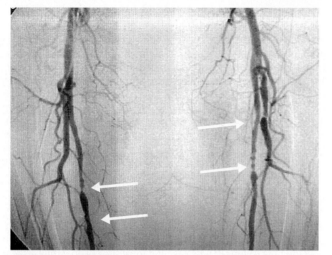

FIGURE 42-10   Angiography demonstrating multiple stenoses of deep femoral arteries (DFAs).

tral aortic pressure by using an extremity blood pressure cuff, invasive angiography should be considered to obtain direct central aortic pressure measurements and gradient determinations. Effective blood pressure management is crucial and can be complex in Takayasu's arteritis. Even with reliable peripheral recordings, determining and attaining a target pressure range without causing compromised perfusion in the setting of arterial stenotic lesions affecting major organs (e.g., cerebral or coronary stenoses) can be challenging. For this reason, careful monitoring is essential when intervention for blood pressure control is necessary. In addition, angiotensin-converting enzyme inhibitors (ACEIs) should be used with caution in the setting of renal artery stenosis, because this therapy blunts the renal autoregulatory response to decreased glomerular pressure. Decrease in glomerular filtration rate (GFR) results with lowering of blood pressure and may lead to a clinically significant decline in renal function.

Arterial stenoses may affect any organ system. Intervention to correct lesions should be considered in the setting of severely impaired daily function or evidence of significant organ ischemia. Multiple studies demonstrate impressive initial patency rates of 80% to 100% with percutaneous angioplasty.[28–30] However, vascular restenosis occurs in 20% to 71% of cases followed up to 45 months post procedure. Case reports of drug-eluting stents (DES) in Takayasu's arteritis are encouraging and may increase patency duration. However, long-term studies in large numbers of patients will have to be performed before their use can be endorsed.

Bypass procedures also may be complicated by vessel restenosis, but rates of sustained patency are higher than with angioplasty (65%-88%; mean follow-up period 44-60 months).[30,31] One postoperative observational study of 29 patients demonstrated that disease activity at the time of surgery is a significant factor in bypass outcomes. In this study, patients with active disease at the time of operative intervention had 53% bypass graft patency rate at 5 years, whereas patients who were operated on when disease was quiescent had an 88% patency rate over the same period.[32] Thus, when interventions are planned, it is preferred that they occur in the setting of disease remission. Tissue should be obtained from the origin or insertion of grafts, since histopathological examination can provide critical information in assessing disease activity and later assist in medical management.

Patients with Takayasu's arteritis are generally young, but disease-related complications may increase their surgical risk. A retrospective review of 106 consecutive patients with the disease noted 12 perioperative deaths (11.3%) following operative intervention.[33] Most deaths were due to cardiovascular complications,

but other series document perioperative mortality as low as 0% to 3%.[13,34] Surgical outcomes can be significantly affected by the experience of the surgical team and medical center in caring for patients with Takayasu's arteritis.

A multidisciplinary approach to the care of Takayasu's arteritis patients is essential for optimizing patient outcomes. The team should include a rheumatologist, cardiovascular physician, imaging specialist, and in the setting of critical stenoses or aneurysms, vascular and cardiothoracic surgeons.

REFERENCES

1. Hall S, Barr W, Lie JT, et al: Takayasu arteritis: a study of 32 North American patients, *Medicine* 64:89, 1985.
2. Waern AU, Anderson P, Hemmingsson A: Takayasu's arteritis: a hospital-region based study on occurrence, treatment, and prognosis, *Angiology* 34:311, 1983.
3. Nasu T: Takayasu's truncoarteritis in Japan: a statistical observation of 76 autopsy cases, *Pathol Microbiol (Basel)* 43:140, 1975.
4. Chauhan SK, Tripathy NK, Sinha N, et al: Cellular and humoral immune responses to mycobacterial heat shock protein-65 and its human homologue in Takayasu's arteritis, *Clin Exp Immunol* 138:547, 2004.
5. Chauhan SK, Tripathy NK, Nityanand S: Antigenic targets and pathogenicity of anti-aortic endothelial cell antibodies in Takayasu's arteritis, *Arthritis Rheum* 54:2326, 2006.
6. Seko Y, Minota S, Kawasaki A, et al: Perforin-secreting killer cell infiltration and expression of a 65 kD heat shock protein in aortic tissue of patients with Takayasu's arteritis, *J Clin Invest* 93:750, 1994.
7. Inder SJ, Bobryshev YV, Cherian SM, et al: Immunophenotypic analysis of the aortic wall in Takayasu's arteritis: involvement of lymphocytes, dendritic cells, and granulocytes in immuno-inflammatory reactions, *Cardiovasc Surg* 8:141, 2000.
8. Noris M, Daina E, Gamba S, et al: Interleukin-6 and RANTES in Takayasu arteritis: a guide for therapeutic decisions? *Circulation* 100:55, 1999.
9. Nishino Y, Tamai M, Kawakami A, et al: Serum levels of BAFF for assessing the disease activity of Takayasu arteritis, *Clin Exp Rheumatol* 28(1 Suppl 57):14, 2010.
10. Hoffman GS: Large-vessel vasculitis: unresolved issues, *Arthritis Rheum* 48:2406, 2003.
11. Numano F: Takayasu's arteritis: clinical aspects. In Hoffman GS, Weyand CM, editors: *Inflammatory diseases of blood vessels*, New York, 2002, Marcel Dekker, p 455.
12. Hotchi M: Pathologic studies on Takayasu arteritis, *Heart Vessels Suppl* 7:11, 1992.
13. Kerr G, Hallahan C, Giordano J, et al: Takayasu arteritis, *Ann Intern Med* 120:919, 1994.
14. Lupi-Herrara E, Sanchez-Torrez G, Marchushamer J, et al: Takayasu arteritis: clinical study of 107 cases, *Am Heart J* 93:94, 1977.
15. Numano F, Kobayashi Y: Takayasu arteritis—beyond pulselessness, *Intern Med* 38:226, 1999.
16. Grange DK, Balfour IC, Chen SC, et al: Familial syndrome of progressive arterial occlusive disease consistent with fibromuscular dysplasia, hypertension, congenital cardiac defects, bone fragility, brachysyndactyly, and learning disabilities, *Am J Med Genet* 75:469, 1998.
17. Rojo-Leyva F, Ratliff N, Cosgrove DM, et al: Study of 52 patients with idiopathic aortitis from a cohort of 1,204 surgical cases, *Arthritis Rheum* 43:901, 2000.
18. Hernandez-Rodriguez J, Molloy ES, Hoffman GS: Single organ vasculitis, *Curr Opin Rheumatol* 20:40, 2008.
19. Maksimowicz-McKinnon, Clark TM, Hoffman GS: Takayasu arteritis and giant cell arteritis: a spectrum within the same disease? *Medicine (Baltimore)* 88:221, 2009.
20. Arnaud L, Haroche J, Limal N, et al: Takayasu arteritis in France: a single-center, retrospective study of 82 cases comparing white, North African, and black patients, *Medicine* 89:1, 2010.
21. Bicakcigil M, Aksu K, Ozbalkan Z, et al: Takayasu's arteritis in Turkey-clinical and angiographic features of 248 patients, *Clin Exp Rheumatol* 27(Suppl 52):S59, 2009.
22. Tso E, Flamm SD, White RD, et al: Takayasu arteritis. Utility and limitations of magnetic resonance imaging in diagnosis and treatment, *Arthritis Rheum* 46:1634, 2002.
23. Webb M, Chambers A, Al-Nahhas A, et al: The role of 18-FDG PET in characterizing disease activity in Takayasu arteritis, *Eur J Nucl Med* 31:627, 2004.
24. Walter MA, Melzer RA, Schindler C, et al: The value of F-18 FDG-PET in the diagnosis of large-vessel vasculitis and the assessment of activity and extent of disease, *Eur J Nucl Med Mol Imaging* 32:674, 2005.
25. Hoffman GS, Leavitt RY, Kerr GS, et al: Treatment of glucocorticoid-resistant or relapsing Takayasu arteritis with methotrexate, *Arthritis Rheum* 37:578, 1994.
26. Shelhamer JH, Volkman DJ, Parrillo JE, et al: Takayasu's arteritis and its therapy, *Ann Intern Med* 103:121, 1985.
27. Molloy ES, Langford CA, Clark TM, et al: Anti-tumour necrosis factor therapy in patients with refractory Takayasu arteritis: long-term follow-up, *Ann Rheum Dis* 67:1567, 2008.
28. Sharma BK, Jain S, Bali HK, et al: A follow-up study of balloon angioplasty and de-novo stenting in Takayasu arteritis, *Int J Cardiol* 75:S147, 2000.
29. Tyagi S, Gambhir DS, Kaul UA, et al: A decade of subclavian angioplasty: aortoarteritis versus atherosclerosis, *Indian Heart J* 48:667, 1996.
30. Bali HK, Bhargava M, Jain AK, et al: De novo stenting of descending thoracic aorta in Takayasu arteritis: intermediate-term follow-up results, *J Invasive Cardiol* 12:612, 2000.
31. Liang P, Tan-Ong M, Hoffman GS: Takayasu's arteritis: vascular interventions and outcomes, *J Rheumatol* 31:102, 2004.
32. Pajari R, Hekali P, Harjola PT: Treatment of Takayasu's arteritis: an analysis of 29 operated patients, *Thorac Cardiovasc Surg* 34:176, 1986.
33. Miyata T, Sato O, Koyama H, et al: Long-term survival after surgical treatment of patients with Takayasu's arteritis, *Circulation* 108:1474, 2003.
34. Lagneau P, Michel JB, Vuong PN: Surgical treatment of Takayasu's disease, *Ann Surg* 205:157, 1987.

CHAPTER 43 Giant Cell Arteritis

Maria C. Cid, Peter A. Merkel

Giant-cell (temporal) arteritis (GCA) is a chronic inflammatory arteritis that preferentially involves large and medium-sized arteries and affects persons older than 50 years of age. Although autopsy studies have shown that the aorta and its major tributaries are almost invariably involved, most of the major clinical manifestations and complications of the disease arise from involvement of the carotid artery branches and include headaches, visual loss, and stroke.[1–3] Aneurysms due to aortitis, as well as extremity arterial occlusions and claudication, can also be seen in GCA, especially in late disease.[4,5] Histopathological diagnosis is usually determined from examination of a biopsy of the superficial temporal artery (Figs. 43-1 and 43-2).

Some 50% of patients with GCA develop *polymyalgia rheumatica* (PMR), a clinically defined syndrome consisting of aching and stiffness in the neck, shoulders, or pelvic girdle. Polymyalgia rheumatica can also exist as a distinct entity with no evidence of vascular involvement.[6]

This chapter presents the epidemiology, pathophysiology, clinical manifestations, and treatment options for GCA, with particular reference to manifestations likely encountered by vascular medicine specialists.

Epidemiology

Giant-cell arteritis characteristically occurs in people older than 50 years of age, and its frequency increases with age. Maximal incidence of GCA occurs in persons between 75 and 85, and it is twice as frequent in women as men. Although there is a markedly increased incidence of GCA among Caucasians in northern Europe and in populations with similar ethnic background,[7] the disease can occur in all populations. Giant-cell arteritis is not an uncommon disease. Studies conducted in northern Europe and North America disclose an annual incidence of 19 to 32 cases per 100,000 people older than 50[8,9] and a rate of 49 per 100,000 for individuals in their 80s.[7,9] In Mediterranean countries, the annual incidence is lower, about 6 to 10 cases per 100,000.[10,11] Isolated PMR is even more frequent, with an average annual incidence of 52 per 100,000 among people older than age 50.[6,7]

Pathology

In the large and medium-sized arteries involved in GCA, the vessel wall is infiltrated by T lymphocytes and macrophages, frequently forming a granulomatous reaction with the presence of multinucleated giant cells[12] (see Fig. 43-2). Scattered polymorphonuclear leukocytes can be occasionally identified. B lymphocytes are scarce and natural killer (NK) cells are virtually absent.[13]

Inflammatory infiltrates usually reach the artery through the adventitial layer and subsequently expand to involve the entire vessel thickness. Extent of inflammatory infiltrates is highly variable among patients and even varies in different sections of the same specimen. The internal elastic lamina is usually disrupted, and giant cells often accumulate in its vicinity but are not required for the diagnosis. In well-developed lesions, the lumen is occluded by intimal hyperplasia. In some specimens, inflammation of the vasa vasorum and small vessels surrounding the temporal artery is the only apparent abnormality.[14] When inflammation of small branches is the only abnormality, other forms of systemic small- and medium-vessel vasculitis must be excluded.

Inflammatory lesions are typically segmental and preferentially distributed along the carotid and vertebral arteries. Intracranial vessels are usually spared. Small arteries and arterioles in the vicinity of the superficial temporal artery are almost invariably involved.[14] Autopsy studies have demonstrated that inflammatory infiltrates are often detected in the aorta and its major tributaries.[15]

Histopathological findings in PMR include chronic synovitis and bursitis of proximal joints.[16,17] Synovitis is usually mild, and inflammatory infiltrates contain CD4 T lymphocytes and macrophages, with scarce granulocytes. Muscle biopsies do not disclose specific abnormalities.

Pathogenesis

Genetic Predisposition

The predominance of GCA and PMR among Caucasians, especially those of northern European origin, strongly suggests a genetic component in the pathogenesis of GCA and PMR. A higher prevalence of HLA class II alleles DRB1*04 has been reported among patients with GCA and PMR compared to the general population.[18] Certain polymorphisms of genes involved in immune and inflammatory responses, such as tumor necrosis factor (TNF)-α, vascular endothelial growth factor (VEGF),[19,20] endothelial nitric oxide synthase (eNOS),[21] intercellular adhesion molecule (ICAM)-1,[22] interleukin (IL)-6, and mannose-binding lectin[23] among others,[24] appear to be more frequent in patients with GCA than in the general population. The influence of these polymorphisms in the development of GCA remains undefined but is under active investigation.

Possible Triggering Agents

Several observations suggest that GCA may be caused by an environmental triggering agent yet to be defined. Cyclic fluctuations in the incidence of GCA occurring every 6 or 7 years have been reported.[9] Additionally, the characteristic granulomatous reaction with multinucleated giant cells has also prompted a search for an infectious agent that may cause a delayed-type hypersensitivity reaction. However, attempts to identify specific pathogens, including *Chlamydia pneumoniae* and parvovirus B19, have led to conflicting results,[25,26] and the search for an infectious etiology of GCA continues.[27]

Immunopathogenic Mechanisms

It has been postulated that inflammatory lesions in GCA develop as a consequence of an antigen-specific immune response against antigens present in the vessel wall. Activated dendritic cells have been detected in inflammatory lesions of GCA,[13,28] where they are thought to serve as antigen-presenting cells and provide co-stimulatory signals for CD4 T-cell activation. Innate immune system activation through Toll-like receptors (TLRs) seems to be relevant in the activation of dendritic cells.[29] Immunopathological studies have demonstrated that inflammatory infiltrates in GCA mainly consist of activated macrophages and T lymphocytes, particularly of the CD4 subset.[13] Expansion of CD4 T-lymphocyte clones derived from different areas of temporal artery biopsy specimens has shown that some of them share identical sequences at the third complementary determining region of the T-cell receptor,[30] suggesting a specific immune recognition of a disease-relevant antigen. CD4 T lymphocytes undergo T helper 1 (T$_H$1) differentiation, with vigorous production of interferon (IFN)-γ, a key cytokine in macrophage activation and granuloma formation.[31] Interleukin-17 is also produced in GCA lesions, providing evidence for the participation of T$_H$17-mediated responses in the pathophysiology of GCA.[32]

Mechanisms of Vascular Injury

Multiple processes have been implicated in the vascular injury seen in GCA. Activated macrophages produce oxygen radicals and proteolytic enzymes that participate in disruption of the vessel wall

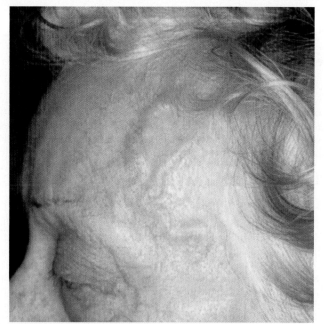

FIGURE 43-1 Enlarged, hardened, and pulseless temporal and frontal arteries in a patient with giant cell arteritis (GCA).

and tissue destruction.[33,34] Increased levels of lipid peroxidation products, aldose reductase, inducible nitric oxide synthase (iNOS), and functionally active matrix metalloproteases MMP-2 and MMP-9 have been demonstrated in GCA.[33,35]

Systemic Inflammatory Response

Activated macrophages produce proinflammatory cytokines IL-1, TNF-α, and IL-6, which are major inducers of the systemic inflammatory response (fever, weight loss, anemia, and hepatic synthesis of acute-phase proteins) often prominent in patients with GCA. Expression of these cytokines in the arterial tissue of patients, as well as circulating levels of TNF-α and IL-6, correlate with the intensity of the systemic inflammatory reaction.[36] As discussed later, these cytokines are able to activate proinflammatory cascades such as chemokine release, adhesion molecule expression, and angiogenesis. Although each of these cascades may amplify and maintain the inflammatory process,[37] some of their effects on vessel wall components might be protective against vascular occlusion.

Vascular Response to Inflammation

Vessel wall components, particularly endothelial cells (ECs) and smooth muscle cells (SMCs), actively react to cytokines and growth factors released by infiltrating leukocytes. Vascular response to inflammation leads to amplification and perpetuation of the inflammatory process and vessel occlusion.[37] Inflammation-induced angiogenesis is remarkable in GCA lesions and preferentially occurs at the adventitial layer and within inflammatory infiltrates, particularly in granulomatous areas at the intima media junction.[38,39]

Neovessels may have a protective role at distal sites where providing new blood supply may prevent organ ischemia.[39] Additionally, neovessels provide a population of ECs that may exert a variety of proinflammatory activities.[38] Vascular response to inflammation may eventually lead to vessel occlusion, with subsequent ischemia of the tissues supplied by involved vessels. In GCA, vessel occlusion results mostly from intimal hyperplasia driven by proliferation and matrix production by myointimal cells; platelet-derived growth factor (PDGF) and transforming growth factor (TGF)-β appear to be crucial cytokines in this process.[37]

Clinical Manifestations

Patients with GCA may present with a wide variety of clinical features, summarized in Table 43-1. Disease-related manifestations may appear rapidly or develop insidiously. A delay of weeks or even months between the onset of clinical symptoms and diagnosis is common, particularly in patients with predominantly systemic complaints in whom more prevalent diseases (e.g., infections, malignancies) are usually suspected. Ischemic complications tend to accumulate in some patients and are frequently early events during the course of the disease.[40,41]

Some data suggest that an initial presentation of GCA that includes signs and symptoms of systemic inflammation (elevated acute phase reactants, fever, anemia, weight loss) is associated with a specific pattern of clinical illness. For unclear reasons, patients with a strong systemic inflammatory response are at lower risk of ischemic events but are more refractory to therapy[40,42] than patients with a seemingly weaker initial inflammatory response. Similarly, as with cranial ischemic complications, symptomatic stenosis of large vessels has been shown to be negatively associated with prominent inflammatory markers at the time of diagnosis.[43]

Systemic Manifestations

Patients with GCA or PMR frequently experience malaise, anorexia, weight loss, and depression.[1,3,44] Nearly 50% of patients with GCA have fever, and in some patients, fever or constitutional symptoms are the most prominent findings. Approximately 10% of patients present with fever of unknown origin with subtle or no cranial manifestations.[6]

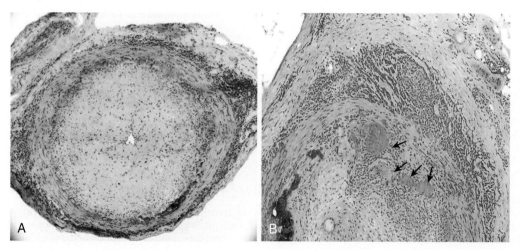

FIGURE 43-2 Classic fully developed lesions in temporal artery biopsy specimens from patients with giant cell arteritis (GCA). A, Inflammatory infiltrates involving entire arterial wall and predominating at adventitial layer and intima media junction, where a granulomatous reaction around internal elastic lamina can be appreciated. Note prominent intimal hyperplasia virtually occluding lumen. **B,** Enlargement of another specimen. Thin arrows indicate multinucleated giant cells.

TABLE 43-1	Clinical Findings in a Series of 250 Patients with Giant Cell Arteritis
General Features	
Age (mean, range)	75 (50-94)
Sex (female/male)	178/72
Weight loss	61%
Fever	47%
Cranial Symptoms	**86%**
Headache	77%
Temporal artery abnormality (swollen, tender, weak/absent pulse)	74%
Jaw claudication	44%
Scalp tenderness	39%
Facial pain	18%
Earache	18%
Odynophagia	12%
Ocular pain	8%
Tongue pain	5%
Carotodynia	5%
Toothache	5%
Trismus	1%
Ophthalmic Events	**22%**
Blindness (permanent)	14%
Amaurosis fugax	10%
Transient diplopia	4%
Cerebrovascular Accident	**2%**
Symptomatic Large Vessel Involvement (Claudication and/or Bruit)	**5%**
Polymyalgia Rheumatica (PMR)	**48%**

Modified and reprinted from Cid MC, Hernandez-Rodriquez J, Grau JM: Vascular manifestations in giant-cell arteritis. In Asherson RA, Cervera R, editors: Vascular manifestations of systemic autoimmune diseases, London, 2001, CRC Press.

Clinical Manifestations of Cranial Arterial Involvement

Headache is one of the most common and classic symptoms and occurs in 60% to 98% of cases of GCA.[6] Intensity and location of headache are highly variable, but it frequently predominates at the temporal areas. Scalp tenderness is also common. About 40% of patients experience jaw claudication when eating, a symptom highly specific for GCA but occasionally seen in other vascular diseases (e.g., necrotizing vasculitis, systemic amyloidosis). Other manifestations, such as facial swelling, tongue ischemia, or edema,

are less frequently seen[6,45] (see Table 43-1). Patients may also present with a variety of unusual pains in the craniofacial area, including ocular pain, earache, toothache, odynophagia, odontalgia, and carotidynia. When certain of these symptoms predominate, a substantial delay in diagnosis is common.

Visual impairment is the most feared complication of GCA and occurs in approximately 15% of cases. Blindness is most commonly due to anterior ischemic optic neuropathy derived from inflammatory involvement of posterior ciliary arteries supplying the optic nerve. Less frequently, central retinal artery occlusion, retrobulbar neuritis, or cortical blindness can occur. Visual loss can be bilateral or unilateral, complete or partial. It usually appears suddenly but is often preceded by transient visual loss (*amaurosis fugax*), diplopia, or occasionally, blue vision.

Less common ischemic complications include stroke due to involvement of carotid or vertebral tributaries, and scalp or tongue necrosis. Strokes, when they do occur, are more frequent in territories supplied by the vertebral arteries (Fig. 43-3). Additional ischemic manifestations include hearing loss and vestibular dysfunction.[46]

Cardiac, Aortic, and Peripheral Vascular Manifestations

Aortitis and inflammatory involvement of the main branches of the aorta are more common in GCA than generally appreciated (Fig. 43-4). In a small autopsy series, aortic inflammation was observed in 12 out of 13 patients with GCA. Imaging techniques are now used to indirectly measure aortic inflammation in living individuals. Evidence of probable aortic involvement can be detected by positron emission tomography (PET) or computed tomographic angiography (CTA) in 50% to 65% of patients at the time of diagnosis[47,48] (see Fig. 43-4). Aortic involvement is asymptomatic unless aortic dissection or dilation occurs (Fig. 43-5). Systematic screening of 54 patients revealed that aortic dilatation occurs in 22.5% of patients after a median follow-up of 5.6 years. Interestingly, unlike noninflammatory aortic disease, there is a markedly increased ratio of thoracic to abdominal aortic aneurysms in patients with GCA, and the risk of thoracic disease may be 17-fold higher among patients with a history of GCA.[49]

Giant cell arteritis may also involve aortic branches (see Fig. 43-4). Positron emission tomography scan studies show that subclavian arteries may be involved in 70% of patients, axillary arteries in 40%, iliac arteries in 37%, and femoral arteries in 37%. Studies using color duplex ultrasonography (US) have disclosed abnormalities in these territories in about one third of patients.[50] Distal lower-limb arteries (e.g., femoropopliteal, tibial, peroneal) may also be affected.[5] Although in most instances, extremity involvement is asymptomatic, some

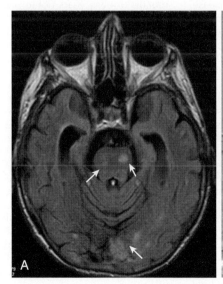
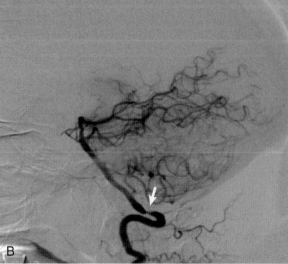

FIGURE 43-3 Neurological complications in giant cell arteritis (GCA). **A,** Magnetic resonance imaging (MRI) discloses multiple ishemic lesions in vertebral territory in patient with GCA presenting with subacute dementia and ataxia. **B,** Stenosis in left vertebral artery in patient with GCA presenting with recurrent transient ischemic attacks (TIAs).

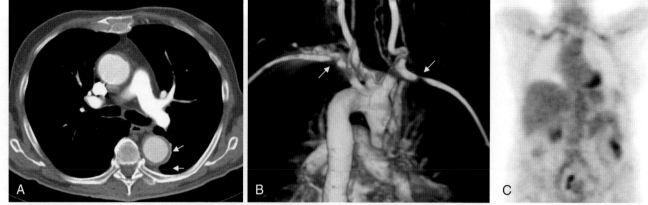

FIGURE 43-4 **Large-artery involvement in giant cell arteritis (GCA). A,** Concentric thickening with contrast enhancement of thoracic descending aorta in patient with newly diagnosed GCA (computed tomographic angiography [CTA]). **B,** Bilateral subclavian stenosis in patient with newly diagnosed GCA and subclavian bruits (magnetic resonance angiogram [MRA]). **C,** Subclavian, axillary, aortic, and iliac arteries fluorodeoxyglucose-18 (^{18}F-FDG) uptake in patient with active GCA (positron emission tomography [PET] scan).

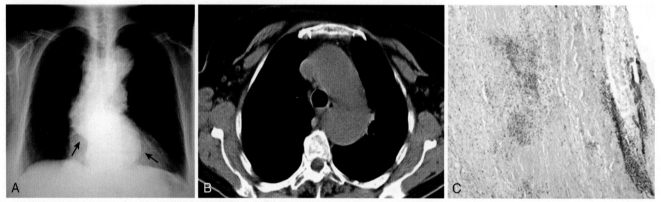

FIGURE 43-5 **Aortic aneurysm in patient with giant cell arteritis (GCA) discovered 5 years after diagnosis. A,** Plain chest radiography. **B,** Computed tomography (CT). **C,** Histology from surgical specimen showing remaining scattered inflammatory infiltrates.

patients develop claudication and even critical ischemia when significant vascular stenoses occur. Large-vessel occlusions are usually late manifestations of GCA, often occurring years after initial diagnosis. When they become clinically significant, they often are misdiagnosed as secondary to atherosclerotic disease. For this reason, the frequency of clinically relevant peripheral artery disease in GCA is not well known.

Patients with GCA should be followed indefinitely for complications of large-vessel disease, even when there is no evidence of other active disease. In patients with GCA, aortic valvular disease, aortic aneurysms or dissections, and peripheral vascular occlusions should all be considered possibly related to vasculitis. New vascular bruits or cardiac murmurs, asymmetry in blood pressure readings, weak or absent peripheral pulses, and limb claudication or ischemia are all warning signs easily inquired about and examined for in physicians' offices.

Myocardial or mesenteric infarction due to GCA is seen infrequently.[51] Because GCA occurs in older people, some cases of inflammatory coronary or mesenteric arteritis may be misdiagnosed as due to atherosclerotic disease. Even among patients with GCA, however, atherosclerosis is a much more common cause of cardiac or mesenteric ischemia than vasculitis. With increased interest in the role of inflammation in coronary artery disease (CAD) and new tools to study the disease process, investigators are now better able to study the contributions, if any, of inflammatory arteritis to CAD among patients with GCA and other vasculitides.

Polymyalgia Rheumatica

Approximately 50% of patients with GCA present with symptoms of PMR, a syndrome clinically defined by the presence of aching and stiffness in the neck, shoulders, or pelvic girdle. Pain is exacerbated with movement. Morning stiffness is a prominent finding and may last for many hours. Proximal muscles are usually tender, but true weakness or myopathy is not seen. Ultrasonography, magnetic resonance imaging (MRI), and PET studies indicate that the underlying abnormalities are synovitis and bursitis of proximal joints.[44,52]

Polymyalgia rheumatica can appear simultaneously with cranial symptoms or may precede development of GCA symptoms by months or even years. Some patients without PMR develop PMR symptoms during GCA relapses, and PMR may sometimes be the only clinical manifestation of GCA.[53]

Polymyalgia rheumatica can exist as an isolated entity without any evidence of vascular inflammation. The epidemiology and immunogenetic backgrounds of patients with isolated PMR are similar to those reported for GCA. Temporal artery biopsies disclosing GCA can be demonstrated in about 10% to 20% of patients with apparently isolated PMR. This frequency is much lower when cranial symptoms are ruled out by a detailed inquiry, and abnormalities at careful physical examination of the temporal arteries are excluded. It is important that patients with PMR be followed with the same rigor as patients with GCA.

Patients with GCA may develop peripheral synovitis; knees, wrists, and metacarpophalangeal joints are most frequently involved. Peripheral manifestations usually occur in patients with PMR but may also occasionally appear in patients without proximal symptoms of PMR. Other associated manifestations include tenosynovitis, carpal tunnel syndrome, and distal swelling with pitting edema.[44,54] Some patients develop a clinical picture indistinguishable from seronegative rheumatoid arthritis.[44]

Incidentally Discovered Giant Cell Arteritis

Occasionally, GCA may be unexpectedly diagnosed when vascular surgical specimens reveal arteritis with or without giant cells. In these patients, retrospective investigation may reveal prior signs or symptoms attributable to GCA. Several retrospective surgical or autopsy series of aortic specimens have demonstrated rates of nonsyphilitic aortitis ranging from 1% to 15%.[55,56] In most instances, aortitis involved the thoracic aorta, and the majority of cases were in women. Fewer than 50% of these cases were associated with an identifiable clinical syndrome such as GCA. In a series of 1204 aortic surgical specimens from one institution, 52 (4.3%) demonstrated idiopathic aortitis, and only 12 of the 52 were found to have a non-GCA inflammatory disease.[55] Because a subset of patients with idiopathic aortitis may go on to develop additional clinically important manifestations of GCA, it seems prudent to evaluate and follow such patients as one would cases of more clearly diagnosed GCA.[57]

Physical Examination

Physical examination is extremely important, not only for initial evaluation of patients with possible GCA but also for following patients after the diagnosis has been established. Blood pressure measurements should be taken in both arms at each visit (and periodically in both legs). Asymmetry of pressures may indicate aortic, subclavian, or other peripheral artery involvement. A careful comprehensive examination of all pulses is key to evaluating GCA. The temporal arteries may be swollen, hard, or pulseless in GCA, although they may appear fully normal even in arteries later found to have active arteritis. At times, just a slight asymmetry, decrease, or irregularity in the pulse can be detected in temporal or other cranial arteries. Auscultation for bruits should be performed over carotid, subclavian, axillary, renal, iliac, and other arteries and the aorta. The scalp should be examined for tenderness. Ophthalmological examination, including funduscopy, visual field assessment, and acuity testing, should be performed for evidence of optic ischemia or other abnormalities of GCA. Evidence of synovitis or enthesitis should be sought. A comprehensive examination is important to help evaluate patients for disorders with overlapping features of GCA.

Laboratory Findings

With few exceptions, both GCA and PMR are characterized by a strong acute-phase reaction. The erythrocyte sedimentation rate (ESR) is usually markedly elevated, frequently around 100 mm/h (Westergren method). Plasma concentrations of acute-phase proteins such as C-reactive protein (CRP), haptoglobin, and fibrinogen are also elevated. Protein electrophoresis shows an increase in α_2 globulins. Thrombocytosis and chronic disease–type anemia are common, and some patients have abnormal liver function tests, particularly increased levels of alkaline phosphatase.[6] Hyperbilirubinemia with visible jaundice is rare but may also occur. Symptomatic anemia may occasionally be the first clinical manifestation of GCA. Nonspecific immunological abnormalities, such as decreased numbers of circulating CD8 lymphocytes and elevated levels of soluble IL-2 receptors, are common in GCA and PMR.[6]

Several monocyte and EC activation products can be detected at increased concentrations in plasma from patients with GCA and PMR. These include cytokines such as IL-6 and TNF-α, soluble adhesion molecules such as ICAM-1, and von Willebrand factor (vWF) antigen.[6,37,58,59] The role these or other cytokines or cellular markers may play in the diagnosis and management of GCA is an area of active investigation.

Diagnosis

Diagnosis of GCA is arrived at by a combination of clinical history, physical examination findings, laboratory studies, and arterial biopsy results. No one feature or finding is fully diagnostic on its own, since even "positive" temporal artery biopsies can occasionally be seen in other types of arteritis, and other disorders can also result in similar systemic features, headaches, or visual changes. Nonetheless, a positive temporal artery biopsy is an extremely strong finding and is almost always diagnostic. Similarly, no feature or finding is absolutely required to make the diagnosis. For example, the ESR may be normal in up to 10% of patients with GCA at presentation, but certain symptoms and findings should prompt a high suspicion of GCA. It is the initial consideration of GCA that is crucial for initiating the diagnostic process that often leads to empirical treatment even before a diagnosis is fully established.

In parallel with an evaluation of GCA itself, physicians will usually need to consider alternative diagnoses such as brain lesions, infections, or malignancies and conduct appropriate evaluations for these disorders. Even if GCA is established by history and biopsy, other inflammatory vasculitides, such as granulomatosis with polyangiitis (GPA; Wegner's) or polyarteritis nodosa (PAN), must at least be considered and screened for, since they can rarely present with temporal artery involvement. Finally, although there are differences between patients with GCA and Takayasu's arteritis (TA) in terms of the frequency of specific clinical manifestations, responses to therapy, use of non-glucocorticoid immunosuppressive agents, and outcomes, there are many similar features. Thus all patients with either diagnosis should be screened for manifestations of the other.

In evaluating and treating patients with GCA, the best management often includes collaboration among rheumatologists, ophthalmologists, neurologists, and vascular medicine specialists.

Temporal Artery Biopsy

Histopathological examination of a temporal artery biopsy often provides the definitive diagnosis of GCA.[12] The area to be excised is carefully selected, guided by symptoms and physical examination findings. At least a 2- to 3-cm fragment should be removed, and multiple sections examined histologically. When the initial biopsy is negative for evidence of GCA, excision of the contralateral artery is not routinely recommended but may increase diagnostic sensitivity in selected cases. Temporal artery biopsy is highly sensitive for the diagnosis of GCA.[60] Occasionally, the temporal artery may be involved in the context of other systemic vasculitides or other disorders such as systemic amyloidosis.[12,61,62] When systemic necrotizing vasculitis involves the temporal artery or its tributaries, it may present with cranial symptoms and complications similar to GCA.

Although the diagnostic yield of a temporal artery biopsy (if performed appropriately) is high, a normal temporal artery biopsy does not necessarily exclude GCA, owing to the segmental distribution of inflammatory infiltrates or involvement of other arteries. In only 10% of patients with negative temporal artery biopsy results obtained from biopsy performed and processed under optimal conditions is clinical suspicion strong enough to recommend long-term glucocorticoid therapy.[60] Given the frequent existence of overlapping features among vasculitides, criteria sets have been established to classify patients with vasculitis into specific categories. The most commonly used classification criteria are those of the American College of Rheumatology[63]; the criteria for GCA are outlined in Box 43-1. Although not intended for use diagnostically, these criteria are useful when evaluating patients. Also, they are adopted for use as inclusion criteria for most research studies of GCA. However, to ensure that patients with nonvasculitic conditions are not mistakenly labeled as having GCA, caution must be exercised when applying these criteria. Classification criteria for this and other vasculitides are currently under reconsideration.[64]

Diagnostic Imaging

A variety of imaging modalities are under investigation for use in the diagnosis and long-term management of GCA.[65] These modalities include ultrasound, MRI, PET or PET-computed tomography

Box 43-1   American College of Rheumatology Criteria for Classification of Giant Cell (Temporal) Arteritis

1. Age at disease onset ≥50 years
2. New onset of headache or new type of localized pain in the head
3. Temporal artery tenderness or decreased pulsation
4. ESR ≥50 mm/h (Westergren)
5. Temporal artery biopsy showing vasculitis with a predominance of mononuclear cells or granulomatous inflammation, usually with multinucleated giant cells

A patient is considered to have giant cell arteritis (GCA) if at least three of the above criteria are present. Presence of any three or more criteria yields a sensitivity of 93.5% and a specificity of 91.2%.
ESR, erythrocyte sedimentation rate.
From Hunder GG, Bloch DA, Michel BA, et al: The American College of Rheumatology 1990 criteria for the classification of giant cell arteritis. Arthritis Rheum 33:1122–1128, 1990.

(CT), and conventional contrast angiography (see Fig. 43-4). Lack of standardization for these modalities, wide variations in available equipment, absence of proper validation studies or long-term data, necessity of differentiating GCA findings from those of atherosclerotic disease, and the high cost of some studies are all limiting factors to more widespread adoption, but are all areas where progress is anticipated in the next decade. Furthermore, as these imaging techniques continue to be used extensively for evaluation of patients with fever of unknown origin, presumed cancer, or atherosclerotic disease, additional patients who actually have inflammatory vascular disease are likely to be encountered and diagnosed. Thus, vascular medicine specialists, vascular surgeons, and vascular radiologists will need to consider GCA more when reviewing such imaging studies.

Color duplex US and high-resolution MRI of the cranial arteries may be particularly useful in diagnosing GCA. The ultrasonographic finding of a dark hypoechoic halo surrounding the lumen, or MRI evidence of thickening and contrast enhancement of the artery wall, have remarkable specificity.[66] Although temporal artery biopsy is the gold standard for diagnosis, these other techniques may be useful for biopsy site selection. They are increasingly considered as potential surrogates when biopsy is not feasible or when other arteries such as the occipital or axillary arteries are involved.[50] Imaging techniques also may have a complementary role in evaluating other vascular territories; this is an area of active investigation.

Conventional invasive contrast angiography may confirm involvement of large vessels in patients with bruits or limb claudication. Additional advantages of angiography include the ability to measure blood pressure at various locations to evaluate the functional effect of stenoses and as a prelude for intervention with angioplasty or stent placement. The invasive nature and risks of conventional angiography preclude its routine use for screening purposes or for serial examinations.

MRI/MRA and CT/CTA are increasingly used imaging modalities for screening and evaluating large-vessel disease in GCA.[65,67,68] Although MR or CT can detect luminal narrowing, arterial wall thickness, and wall enhancement, corresponding to inflammation, specificity of these findings as indicators of active vasculitis is unclear, and the tests are not sufficiently reliable to be the sole basis of treatment decisions. Nevertheless, MR is a relatively low risk method to screen and monitor patients for large-vessel disease in GCA and is increasingly part of the standard management for such patients.

Fluorodeoxyglucose-18 (^{18}F-FDG) PET is another promising modality for evaluating patients with suspected GCA. Positron emission tomography scans may demonstrate FDG uptake in the aorta and its branches in patients with GCA, and also in some patients thought to have just PMR.[69] As with MRI/MRA testing, the prognostic importance of detecting large arterial changes by ^{18}F-FDG PET in asymptomatic patients with GCA is unclear. Furthermore, FDG uptake in the abdominal aorta and arteries of the lower limbs also can be seen in severe atherosclerosis, so specificity is lower in these locations.[70] Its diagnostic sensitivity and specificity have to be tested in larger studies, but ^{18}F-FDG PET may have a role in evaluation of vascular inflammation in patients with atypical symptoms, patients with fever of unknown origin, and when assessing vascular involvement in patients with apparently isolated PMR. The combination of PET with CT imaging may also have a role in evaluating these patients because it takes advantage of the properties of both techniques.

Diagnosis of Polymyalgia Rheumatica

Diagnosis of PMR relies at present on clinical criteria; imaging modalities may provide supportive evidence.[71] Magnetic resonance imaging, PET, and ultrasound are able to detect subdeltoid or trochanteric bursitis, biceps tenosynovitis, or glenohumeral or hip synovitis, the sources of many polymyalgic symptoms.[44,52,71,72] Recently an American College of Rheumatology/European League Against Rheumatic Disease classification algorithm[71] has been proposed (Table 43-2). Polymyalgia rheumatica diagnosis requires evaluation to exclude other disorders, particularly rheumatoid arthritis, but also inflammatory myopathies, other vasculitides, and infections that occasionally present with similar symptoms.

TABLE 43-2   Polymyalgia Rheumatica Classification Criteria Scoring Algorithm*

CRITERIA	POINTS WITHOUT ULTRASOUND (0-6)	POINTS WITH ULTRASOUND (0-8)†
Morning stiffness >45 minutes	2	2
Hip pain or limited range of motion	1	1
Normal RF or ACPA	2	2
Absence of other joint movement	1	1
At least one shoulder with subdeltoid bursitis and/or biceps tenosynovitis and/or glenohumeral synovitis (either posterior or axillary) *and* At least one hip with synovitis and/or trochanteric bursitis	NA	1
Both shoulders with subdeltoid bursitis, biceps tenosynovitis, or glenohumeral synovitis	NA	1

*Required criteria: age ≥50 years, bilateral shoulder aching, and abnormal CRP and/or ESR. A score of 4 or more is categorized as polymyalgia rheumatica (PMR) in the algorithm without ultrasound and a score of 5 or more is categorized as PMR in the algorithm with ultrasound.
†Optional ultrasound criteria.
ACPA, anticitrullinated protein antibody; CRP, C-reactive protein; ESR, erythrocyte sedimentation rate; NA, not applicable; RF, rheumatoid factor.
From Dasgupta B, Cimmino MA, Maradit-Kremers H, et al: International Polymyalgia Rheumatica Classification Criteria Work Group. European League Against Rheumatism/American College of Rheumatology classification criteria for polymyalgia rheumatica. Ann Rheum Dis 71: 484–492, 2012.

Treatment and Management

Glucocorticoid therapy is the treatment of choice for GCA and in most cases induces a dramatic amelioration of disease manifestations within a few days. The most widely recommended initial dose is 40 to 60 mg/day of prednisone (or equivalent glucocorticoid). Presence of transient ocular manifestations (e.g., amaurosis fugax, diplopia, blurred vision) should be considered a medical emergency. Treatment should be started immediately, even before histological confirmation of GCA is obtained. Glucocorticoid treatment for several days, and even weeks, does not clear the inflammatory infiltrates and therefore should not hinder histopathological diagnosis.[73–75] When visual loss is established, glucocorticoid pulses of 1 g/day of methylprednisolone (or equivalent glucocorticoid) for 3 days is frequently recommended, although it has not been clearly demonstrated that this dose regimen is more effective than the standard oral treatment. Treatment within the first 12 to 24 hours appears to be the major determinant of visual recovery, which can be expected in only 4% to 12% of cases.[74–76] It is reasonable to recommend antiplatelet drugs, but their efficacy is not proven. Some patients with visual symptoms experience further visual loss during the first 1 to 2 weeks of glucocorticoid treatment. Visual loss beyond this point or during controlled relapses is rare.

The starting dose of prednisone (or equivalent) is maintained for 2 to 4 weeks. The daily dose is then tapered progressively by approximately 5 mg/wk. Although most patients do well with a daily maintenance dose of 7.5 to 10 mg, some patients require higher doses. Tapering is guided primarily by clinical evaluation. The ESR is a useful parameter for following patients with GCA, but therapeutic decisions must not rely solely on ESR values.[6] The usual initial dose of prednisone for patients with isolated PMR is 10 to 20 mg/day. Guidelines for reduction are similar to those recommended for GCA. Some patients with PMR with mild symptoms may respond to nonsteroidal antiinflammatory drugs.[54]

Total duration of therapy may vary, but most patients require treatment for about 2 to 3 years. Reduction in dose below the maintenance doses must be made gradually to avoid relapses, which are common during the first 2 years after diagnosis. Approximately 40% to 60% of patients require low-dose glucocorticoid therapy for longer periods of time, some perhaps indefinitely.[77]

In the majority of patients, the ESR normalizes quickly after initiation of glucocorticoid therapy. Other inflammatory markers, however (e.g., IL-6, C-reactive protein, haptoglobin, vWF antigen) are elevated persistently in many patients who appear to be in clinical remission, possibly indicating persistent low-level inflammatory activity.[37,78] Long-term consequences of persistent subclinical activity are unknown. Subclinical inflammatory activity does not appear to be associated with a higher incidence of delayed complications of GCA, such as aneurysm or vascular occlusion.[4] Persistent modest elevation of inflammatory markers should not lead to an increase in glucocorticosteroid dose in the setting of clinical remission.

Complications of glucocorticoid therapy are quite common among patients with GCA and PMR. These include osteoporosis, weight gain, mood and sleep disturbances, glucose intolerance, congestive heart failure (CHF), cataracts, glaucoma, hypertension, and other problems. Giant-cell arteritis affects elderly patients, a population particularly susceptible to serious complications of glucocorticoid therapy. Physicians treating GCA should anticipate such complications, screen for them, and when feasible, prescribe prophylactic treatments such as calcium, vitamin D, and bisphosphonate therapy to prevent osteoporosis.

Other immunosuppressive drugs may be considered as "steroid sparing agents" to reduce the cumulative toxicity of glucocorticoid therapy. The most carefully investigated of these agents is methotrexate, which was evaluated in three randomized placebo-controlled double-blind studies.[79–81] An individual patient–level meta-analysis of these trials demonstrated modest but significant benefits of methotrexate, including prevention of relapses and reduction of glucocorticoid use.[82] Although small case series

reported beneficial effects of TNF blockers for GCA, TNF-α blockade with infliximab was not superior to placebo in maintaining glucocorticoid-induced remission in an international randomized double-masked placebo-controlled trial.[83] The efficacy in GCA of interfering with CD28-mediated T-cell activation with abatacept is currently being tested in a clinical trial. Although the potential for treatment of GCA through B-cell depletion (rituximab) or by neutralizing IL-6 (tocilizumab) are intriguing, case reports alone are not adequate evidence of efficacy, and randomized trials are needed to establish the roles, if any, of these or other agents.

Patients with both GCA and PMR require long-term follow-up care, often for many years if not for their lifetime, following apparent disease remission. Disease relapse is common, and the long-term problems of large-vessel disease are now being fully appreciated. Finally, it is imperative that patients and their family members be educated and reminded about the warning symptoms of GCA, which necessitate urgent medical evaluation.

REFERENCES

1. Hunder G: Giant cell arteritis and polymyalgia rheumatica, *Med Clin North Am* 81:195–219, 1997.
2. Cid MC, Coll-Vinent B, Grau JM: Large vessel vasculitides, *Curr Opin Rheumatol* 10:18–28, 1998.
3. Salvarani C, Cantini F, Boiardi L: Polymyalgia rheumatica and giant-cell arteritis, *N Engl J Med* 347:261–271, 2002.
4. Garcia-Martinez A, Hernandez-Rodriguez J, Arguis P, et al: Development of aortic aneurysm/dilatation during the followup of patients with giant cell arteritis: a cross-sectional screening of fifty-four prospectively followed patients, *Arthritis Rheum* 59:422–430, 2008.
5. Assie C, Janvresse A, Plissonnier D: Long-term follow-up of upper and lower extremity vasculitis related to giant cell arteritis: a series of 36 patients, *Medicine (Baltimore)* 90:40–51, 2011.
6. Salvarani C, Cantini F, Hunder GG: Polymyalgia rheumatica and giant-cell arteritis, *Lancet* 372:234–245, 2008.
7. Hunder GG: Epidemiology of giant-cell arteritis, *Cleve Clin J Med* 69(Suppl 2):SII79–SII82, 2002.
8. Baldursson O, Steinsson K, Bjornsson J: Giant cell arteritis in Iceland. An epidemiologic and histopathologic analysis, *Arthritis Rheum* 37:1007–1012, 1994.
9. Salvarani C, Gabriel SE, O'Fallon WM: The incidence of giant cell arteritis in Olmsted County, Minnesota: apparent fluctuations in a cyclic pattern, *Ann Intern Med* 123:192–194, 1995.
10. Gonzalez-Gay MA, Vazquez-Rodriguez TR, Lopez-Diaz MJ, et al: Epidemiology of giant cell arteritis and polymyalgia rheumatica, *Arthritis Rheum* 61:1454–1461, 2009.
11. Sonnenblick M, Nesher G, Friedlander Y: Giant cell arteritis in Jerusalem: a 12-year epidemiological study, *Br J Rheumatol* 33:938–941, 1994.
12. Lie J: Histopathologic specificity of systemic vasculitis, *Rheum Dis Clin North Am* 21:883–909, 1995.
13. Cid MC, Campo E, Ercilla G, et al: Immunohistochemical analysis of lymphoid and macrophage cell subsets and their immunologic activation markers in temporal arteritis. Influence of corticosteroid treatment, *Arthritis Rheum* 32:884–893, 1989.
14. Esteban MJ, Font C, Hernandez-Rodriguez J, et al: Small-vessel vasculitis surrounding a spared temporal artery: clinical and pathological findings in a series of twenty-eight patients, *Arthritis Rheum* 44:1387–1395, 2001.
15. Ostberg G: Temporal arteritis in a large necropsy series, *Ann Rheum Dis* 30:224–235, 1971.
16. Meliconi R, Pulsatelli L, Uguccioni M, et al: Leukocyte infiltration in synovial tissue from the shoulder of patients with polymyalgia rheumatica. Quantitative analysis and influence of corticosteroid treatment, *Arthritis Rheum* 39:1199–1207, 1996.
17. Meliconi R, Pulsatelli L, Melchiorri C, et al: Synovial expression of cell adhesion molecules in polymyalgia rheumatica, *Clin Exp Immunol* 107:494–500, 1997.
18. Weyand CM, Hicok KC, Hunder GG: The HLA-DRB1 locus as a genetic component in giant cell arteritis. Mapping of a disease-linked sequence motif to the antigen binding site of the HLA-DR molecule, *J Clin Invest* 90:2355–2361, 1992.
19. Mattey DL, Hajeer AH, Dababneh A, et al: Association of giant cell arteritis and polymyalgia rheumatica with different tumor necrosis factor microsatellite polymorphisms, *Arthritis Rheum* 43:1749–1755, 2000.
20. Boiardi L, Casali B, Nicoli D, et al: Vascular endothelial growth factor gene polymorphisms in giant cell arteritis, *J Rheumatol* 30:2160–2164, 2003.
21. Salvarani C, Casali B, Nicoli D, et al: Endothelial nitric oxide synthase gene polymorphisms in giant cell arteritis, *Arthritis Rheum* 48:3219–3223, 2003.
22. Salvarani CC, Boiardi B, Ranzi L, et al: Intercellular adhesion molecule 1 gene polymorphisms in polymyalgia rheumatica/giant cell arteritis: association with disease risk and severity, *J Rheumatol* 27:1215–1221, 2000.
23. Jacobsen S, Baslund B, Madsen HO, et al: Mannose-binding lectin variant alleles and HLA-DR4 alleles are associated with giant cell arteritis, *J Rheumatol* 29:2148–2153, 2002.
24. Martinez-Taboada VM, Alvarez L, RuizSoto M, et al: Giant cell arteritis and polymyalgia rheumatica: role of cytokines in the pathogenesis and implications for treatment, *Cytokine* 44:207–220, 2008.
25. Regan MJ, Wood BJ, Hsieh YH, et al: Temporal arteritis and *Chlamydia pneumoniae*: failure to detect the organism by polymerase chain reaction in ninety cases and ninety controls, *Arthritis Rheum* 46:1056–1060, 2002.
26. Salvarani C, Farnetti E, Casali B, et al: Detection of parvovirus B19 DNA by polymerase chain reaction in giant cell arteritis: a case-control study, *Arthritis Rheum* 46:3099–3101, 2002.
27. Weck KE, Dal Canto AJ, Gould JD, et al: Murine gamma-herpesvirus 68 causes severe large-vessel arteritis in mice lacking interferon-gamma responsiveness: a new model for virus- induced vascular disease, *Nat Med* 3:1346–1353, 1997.

28. Krupa WM, Dewan M, Jeon MS, et al: Trapping of misdirected dendritic cells in the granulomatous lesions of giant cell arteritis, *Am J Pathol* 161:1815–1823, 2002.

29. Palomino-Morales R, Torres O, Vazquez-Rodriguez TR, et al: Association between toll-like receptor 4 gene polymorphism and biopsy-proven giant cell arteritis, *J Rheumatol* 36:1501–1506, 2009.

30. Weyand CM, Schonberger J, Oppitz U, et al: Distinct vascular lesions in giant cell arteritis share identical T cell clonotypes, *J Exp Med* 179:951–960, 1994.

31. Weyand CM, Tetzlaff N, Bjornsson J, et al: Disease patterns and tissue cytokine profiles in giant cell arteritis, *Arthritis Rheum* 40:19–26, 1997.

32. Deng J, Younge BR, Olshen RA, et al: Th17 and Th1 T-cell responses in giant cell arteritis, *Circulation* 121:906–915, 2010.

33. Rittner HL, Kaiser M, Brack A, et al: Tissue-destructive macrophages in giant cell arteritis, *Circ Res* 84:1050–1058, 1999.

34. Weyand CM, Goronzy JJ: Medium- and large-vessel vasculitis, *N Engl J Med* 349:160–169, 2003.

35. Segarra M, Garcia-Martinez A, Sanchez M, et al: Gelatinase expression and proteolytic activity in giant-cell arteritis, *Ann Rheum Dis* 66:1429–1435, 2007.

36. Hernandez-Rodriguez J, Segarra M, Vilardell C, et al: Tissue production of pro-inflammatory cytokines (IL-1beta, TNF-alpha and IL-6) correlates with the intensity of the systemic inflammatory response and with corticosteroid requirements in giant-cell arteritis, *Rheumatology (Oxford)* 43:294–301, 2004.

37. Lozano E, Segarra M, Garcia-Martinez A, et al: New therapeutic targets in giant-cell arteritis. Considerations based on the current pathogenic model and the availability of new therapeutic agents, *Clin Exp Rheumatol* 26:S141–S150, 2008.

38. Cid MC, Cebrian M, Font C, et al: Cell adhesion molecules in the development of inflammatory infiltrates in giant cell arteritis: inflammation-induced angiogenesis as the preferential site of leukocyte-endothelial cell interactions, *Arthritis Rheum* 43:184–194, 2000.

39. Cid MC, Hernandez-Rodriguez J, Esteban MJ, et al: Tissue and serum angiogenic activity is associated with low prevalence of ischemic complications in patients with giant-cell arteritis, *Circulation* 106:1664–1671, 2002.

40. Cid MC, Ercilla G, Vilaseca J, et al: Polymyalgia rheumatica: a syndrome associated with HLA-DR4 antigen, *Arthritis Rheum* 31:678–682, 1988.

41. Font CC, Cid MC, Coll-Vinent B, et al: Clinical features in patients with permanent visual loss due to biopsy–Proven giant cell arteritis, *Br J Rheumatol* 36:251–254, 1997.

42. Hernandez-Rodriguez J, Segarra M, Vilardell C, et al: Elevated production of interleukin-6 is associated with a lower incidence of disease-related ischemic events in patients with giant-cell arteritis: angiogenic activity of interleukin-6 as a potential protective mechanism, *Circulation* 107:2428–2434, 2003.

43. Nuenninghoff DM, Hunder GG, Christianson TJ, et al: Incidence and predictors of large-artery complication (aortic aneurysm, aortic dissection, and/or large-artery stenosis) in patients with giant cell arteritis: a population-based study over 50 years, *Arthritis Rheum* 48:3522–3531, 2003.

44. Salvarani C, Macchioni P, Boiardi L: Polymyalgia rheumatica, *Lancet* 350:43–47, 1997.

45. Huston KA, Hunder GG, Lie JT, et al: Temporal arteritis: a 25-year epidemiologic, clinical, and pathologic study, *Ann Intern Med* 88:162–167, 1978.

46. Amor-Dorado JC, Llorca J, Garcia-Porrua C, et al: Audiovestibular manifestations in giant cell arteritis: a prospective study, *Medicine (Baltimore)* 82:13–26, 2003.

47. Blockmans D, de Ceuninck L, Vanderschueren S, et al: Repetitive 18F-fluorodeoxyglucose positron emission tomography in giant cell arteritis: a prospective study of 35 patients, *Arthritis Rheum* 55:131–137, 2006.

48. Cid MC, Prieto-Gonzalez S, Arguis P, et al: The spectrum of vascular involvement in giant-cell arteritis: clinical consequences of detrimental vascular remodelling at different sites, *APMIS Suppl* 10–20, 2009.

49. Evans JM, O'Fallon WM, Hunder GG: Increased incidence of aortic aneurysm and dissection in giant cell (temporal) arteritis. A population-based study, *Ann Intern Med* 122:502–507, 1995.

50. Schmidt WA, Seifert A, Gromnica-Ihle E, et al: Ultrasound of proximal upper extremity arteries to increase the diagnostic yield in large-vessel giant cell arteritis, *Rheumatology (Oxford)* 47:96–101, 2008.

51. Scola CJ, Li C, Upchurch KS: Mesenteric involvement in giant cell arteritis. An underrecognized complication? Analysis of a case series with clinicoanatomic correlation, *Medicine (Baltimore)* 87:45–51, 2008.

52. Camellino D, Cimmino MA: Imaging of polymyalgia rheumatica: indications on its pathogenesis, diagnosis and prognosis, *Rheumatology (Oxford)* 2011 May 12 [Epub ahead of print].

53. Hernandez-Rodriguez J, Font C, Garcia-Martinez A, et al: Development of ischemic complications in patients with giant cell arteritis presenting with apparently isolated polymyalgia rheumatica: study of a series of 100 patients, *Medicine (Baltimore)* 86:233–241, 2007.

54. Chuang TY, Hunder GG, Ilstrup DM, et al: Polymyalgia rheumatica: a 10-year epidemiologic and clinical study, *Ann Intern Med* 97:672–680, 1982.

55. Rojo-Leyva F, Ratliff NB, Cosgrove DM 3rd, et al: Study of 52 patients with idiopathic aortitis from a cohort of 1,204 surgical cases, *Arthritis Rheum* 43:901–907, 2000.

56. Liang KP, Chowdhary VR, Michet CJ, et al: Noninfectious ascending aortitis: a case series of 64 patients, *J Rheumatol* 36:2290–2297, 2009.

57. Merkel PA: Noninfectious ascending aortitis: staying ahead of the curve, *J Rheumatol* 36:2137–2140, 2009.

58. Roche NE, Fulbright JW, Wagner AD, et al: Correlation of interleukin-6 production and disease activity in polymyalgia rheumatica and giant cell arteritis, *Arthritis Rheum* 36:1286–1294, 1993.

59. Coll-Vinent B, Vilardell C, Font C, et al: Circulating soluble adhesion molecules in patients with giant cell arteritis. Correlation between soluble intercellular adhesion molecule-1 (sICAM-1) concentrations and disease activity, *Ann Rheum Dis* 58:189–192, 1999.

60. Vilaseca J, Gonzalez A, Cid MC, et al: Clinical usefulness of temporal artery biopsy, *Ann Rheum Dis* 46:282–285, 1987.

61. Genereau T, Lortholary O, Pottier MA, et al: Temporal artery biopsy: a diagnostic tool for systemic necrotizing vasculitis. French Vasculitis Study Group, *Arthritis Rheum* 42:2674–2681, 1999.

62. Duran E, Merkel PA, Sweet S, et al: ANCA-associated small vessel vasculitis presenting with ischemic optic neuropathy, *Neurology* 62:152–153, 2004.

63. Hunder GG, Bloch DA, Michel BA, et al: The American College of Rheumatology 1990 criteria for the classification of giant cell arteritis, *Arthritis Rheum* 33:1122–1128, 1990.

64. Basu N, Watts R, Bajema I, et al: EULAR points to consider in the development of classification and diagnostic criteria in systemic vasculitis, *Ann Rheum Dis* 69:1744–1750, 2010.

65. Kissin EY, Merkel PA: Diagnostic imaging in Takayasu arteritis, *Curr Opin Rheumatol* 16:31–37, 2004.

66. Arida A, Kyprianou M, Kanakis M, et al: The diagnostic value of ultrasonography-derived edema of the temporal artery wall in giant cell arteritis: a second meta-analysis, *BMC Musculoskelet Disord* 11:44, 2010.

67. Blockmans D: Utility of imaging studies in assessment of vascular inflammation, *Cleve Clin J Med* 69(Suppl 2):SII95–SII99, 2002.

68. Tso E, Flamm SD, White RD, et al: Takayasu arteritis: utility and limitations of magnetic resonance imaging in diagnosis and treatment, *Arthritis Rheum* 46:1634–1642, 2002.

69. Blockmans D, Stroobants S, Maes A, et al: Positron emission tomography in giant cell arteritis and polymyalgia rheumatica: evidence for inflammation of the aortic arch, *Am J Med* 108:246–249, 2000.

70. Yun M, Jang S, Cucchiara A, et al: 18F FDG uptake in the large arteries: a correlation study with the atherogenic risk factors, *Semin Nucl Med* 32:70–76, 2002.

71. Dasgupta B, Cimmino MA, Maradit-Kremers H, et al: European League Against Rheumatism/American College of Rheumatology classification criteria for polymyalgia rheumatica, *Ann Rheum Dis* 71:484–492, 2012.

72. Cantini F, Salvarani C, Olivieri I, et al: Shoulder ultrasonography in the diagnosis of polymyalgia rheumatica: a case-control study, *J Rheumatol* 28:1049–1055, 2001.

73. Achkar AA, Lie JT, Hunder GG, et al: How does previous corticosteroid treatment affect the biopsy findings in giant cell (temporal) arteritis? *Ann Intern Med* 120:987–992, 1994.

74. Hayreh SP PA, Zimmerman B: Occult giant cell arteritis: ocular manifestations, *Am J Ophthalmol* 125:521–526, 1998.

75. Foroozan R, Deramo VA, Buono LM, et al: Recovery of visual function in patients with biopsy-proven giant cell arteritis, *Ophthalmology* 110:539–542, 2003.

76. Gonzalez-Gay MA, Blanco R, Rodriguez-Valverde V, et al: Permanent visual loss and cerebrovascular accidents in giant cell arteritis: predictors and response to treatment, *Arthritis Rheum* 41:1497–1504, 1998.

77. Proven A, Gabriel SE, Orces C, et al: Glucocorticoid therapy in giant cell arteritis: duration and adverse outcomes, *Arthritis Rheum* 49:703–708, 2003.

78. Weyand CM, Fulbright JW, Hunder GG, et al: Treatment of giant cell arteritis: interleukin-6 as a biologic marker of disease activity, *Arthritis Rheum* 43:1041–1048, 2000.

79. Jover JA, Hernandez-Garcia C, Morado IC, et al: Combined treatment of giant-cell arteritis with methotrexate and prednisone. a randomized, double-blind, placebo-controlled trial, *Ann Intern Med* 134:106–114, 2001.

80. Spiera RF, Mitnick HJ, Kupersmith M, et al: A prospective, double-blind, randomized, placebo controlled trial of methotrexate in the treatment of giant cell arteritis (GCA), *Clin Exp Rheumatol* 19:495–501, 2001.

81. Hoffman G, Cid M, Hellmann D, et al: A multicenter placebo-controlled study of methotrexate (MTX) in giant cell arteritis (GCA) [abstract], *Arthritis Rheum* 43, 2002.

82. Mahr AD, Jover JA, Spiera RF, et al: Adjunctive methotrexate for treatment of giant cell arteritis: an individual patient data meta-analysis, *Arthritis Rheum* 56:2789–2797, 2007.

83. Hoffman GS, Cid MC, Rendt-Zagar KE, et al: Infliximab for maintenance of glucocorticosteroid-induced remission of giant cell arteritis: a randomized trial, *Ann Intern Med* 146:621–630, 2007.

CHAPTER 44

Thromboangiitis Obliterans (Buerger's Disease)

Gregory Piazza, Jeffrey W. Olin

Thromboangiitis obliterans (TAO) describes a segmental non-atherosclerotic inflammatory disorder that primarily involves the small and medium arteries, veins, and nerves of the extremities.[1-3] Although TAO was initially thought to be a disease confined exclusively to men, recent epidemiological studies demonstrate a growing population of women with the disorder. Also known as *Buerger's disease*, TAO has an extremely strong pathophysiological relationship with tobacco use, usually in the form of heavy cigarette smoking.

In 1879, von Winiwarter provided the first description of a patient with TAO. He presented the case of a 57-year-old man who had reported pain in his feet for 12 years. Histopathological examination of an amputation specimen from this patient demonstrated intimal proliferation, luminal thrombosis, and fibrosis; von Winiwarter hypothesized that the endarteritis and endophlebitis observed were distinct from atherosclerosis.[4] In his landmark paper 29 years later,[5] Leo Buerger published a detailed report of the pathological findings of 11 amputated limbs from patients with the disease and coined the term *thromboangiitis obliterans* to describe the characteristic observations of endarteritis and endophlebitis. Similar to von Winiwarter, Buerger made a point to distinguish the clinical and pathological findings of TAO from those of atherosclerosis.

In 1928, Allen and Brown described the clinical and pathological characteristics of 200 cases of TAO seen at the Mayo Clinic from 1922 to 1926.[6] The majority of cases occurred among Jewish men, and all patients were heavy smokers. The pathological findings in this report were virtually identical to those described in Buerger's original paper.

Epidemiology

Although it is observed worldwide, TAO is more prevalent in the Middle East and Far East than North America and Western Europe.[7,8] Prior to the late 1960s, overdiagnosis of TAO was frequent. Of 205 cases originally diagnosed as TAO at Mount Sinai Hospital from 1933 to 1963, only 33 were later believed to be compatible with the diagnosis, 28 were considered questionable, and 144 were determined incorrect.[9]

Adoption of stricter diagnostic criteria and a reduction in tobacco use have caused the reported number of new patients diagnosed with TAO in the United States and Europe to decline. Overall incidence of TAO is higher in regions of the world where consumption of tobacco is greater. At the Mayo Clinic over a 40-year period, the prevalence rate of patients with the diagnosis of TAO has decreased from 104 per 100,000 patient registrations in 1947 to 13 per 100,000 patient registrations in 1986.[7] The prevalence rate of TAO in patients with peripheral artery disease (PAD) varies across Europe and Asia: 1% to 3% in Switzerland, 0.5% to 5% in West Germany, 1.2% to 5.6% in France, 4% in Belgium, 0.5% in Italy, 0.25% in the United Kingdom, 3.3% in Poland, 6.7% in East Germany, 11.5% in Czechoslovakia, 39% in Yugoslavia, 80% in Israel (among Ashkenazi Jews), 45% to 53% in India, and 16% to 66% in Japan and Korea.[10] In Asia, a greater proportion of patients with limb ischemia has been attributed to TAO than in the United States and Europe.

Overall incidence of TAO also appears to be declining in South Asia and Japan.[11,12] During the 1990s, the ratio of new patients with TAO to new patients with atherosclerotic PAD was reported to be 1:3 in a vascular outpatient clinic in Japan.[13] Since 2000, the ratio has declined to 1:10.[13]

Thromboangiitis obliterans has been associated with manual labor and lower socioeconomic status in some series. In particular areas of Southeast Asia, including India, TAO has been associated with lower socioeconomic class and smoking unrefined homemade tobacco cigarettes called *bidi*. In a study of 28 cases of TAO from Korea, 23 patients were farmers or manual laborers and belonged to the lowest socioeconomic class.[14] In another analysis of 106 patients with TAO in Java, Indonesia, the majority of patients were from the lowest socioeconomic class.[15] However, in a study of 8858 Japanese patients with the disease, there was no significantly greater prevalence among manual laborers.[16]

Although it has been considered a disease of young men, TAO also occurs in women. Reported incidence was less than 2% in the majority of published case series before 1970. More recent studies have demonstrated a much higher prevalence, ranging from 11% to 23%.[17-20] The increasing prevalence of TAO among women has been attributed to rising consumption of tobacco products.

Etiology and Pathogenesis

Thromboangiitis obliterans is a vasculitis characterized by a highly cellular inflammatory thrombus with relative sparing of the vessel wall; its precise etiology remains unknown. Thromboangiitis obliterans is distinct from other vasculitides because levels of acute-phase reactants such as erythrocyte sedimentation rate and C-reactive protein (CRP). Commonly measured autoantibodies are typically normal, but it has been suggested that abnormalities in immunoreactivity and other factors may contribute to the inflammatory process.

Tobacco

Exposure to tobacco is critical to initiation, maintenance, and progression of TAO. Although smoking tobacco is by far the most frequent precipitating factor, chewing tobacco and using snuff[21] or marijuana have also been implicated in its development.[22,23] The association between heavy tobacco use and TAO is so strong, it is typically considered a sine qua non for the diagnosis.[17,24] Patients with TAO have higher tobacco consumption and carboxyhemoglobin levels than those with atherosclerotic vascular disease or healthy controls.[25] It has been hypothesized that some patients develop an immunological reaction to a constituent of tobacco that triggers small-vessel occlusive disease.[26,27] Because only a small proportion of smokers worldwide eventually develop TAO, other factors are believed to play a contributory role in disease pathogenesis.

As noted earlier, in South Asia, a large proportion of patients diagnosed with TAO belong to the lowest socioeconomic class and smoke bidi. Bidi smoking is believed to account for the higher incidence of TAO in the Indian population. A case-control study from Bangladesh reported that 35% of patients with TAO were cigarette smokers and 65% were bidi smokers, compared with 69.9% and 30.1%, respectively, of controls.[28] After adjusting for confounding factors and using 10-per-day smoking frequency as a reference, the study found that smoking 11 to 20 bidi per day was associated with a seven fold increased risk of developing TAO, and smoking over 20 bidi per day led to a 35-fold increased risk. The authors concluded that bidi smoking carried greater risk than cigarette smoking for consequent TAO.[28]

In addition to its role in disease initiation, tobacco use is a critical factor in disease progression and continued symptoms associated with TAO.[2] Although second-hand or passive smoking has not been associated with TAO onset, it may play an important role in continuation of the disease process. In a study of 40 patients with TAO, cotinine, the major metabolite of nicotine, was used as a measure of exposure to tobacco smoke. Urinary cotinine levels were measured to classify them as smokers (cotinine levels >50 ng/mg creatinine), passive smokers (cotinine levels 10-50 ng/mg creatinine), and nonsmokers who did not experience noticeable passive smoking (cotinine levels <10 ng/mg creatinine).[29] Using these criteria, 10 patients were classified as smokers, 9 as passive smokers, and 21 as nonsmokers. Seven of the 10 smokers, none of the 9 passive smokers, and 4 of the 21 nonsmokers experienced disease exacerbation. Of the four nonsmokers who experienced disease exacerbation, three had continued to smoke and one had been exposed to second-hand tobacco smoke in the workplace at the time of relapse. Among active smokers, the seven whose conditions had worsened showed significantly higher urinary cotinine levels than the three remaining patients who remained in remission.

Genetic Predisposition

Several studies have suggested there may be a genetic predisposition to developing TAO. Although there appears to be an association between certain human lymphocyte antigen (HLA) haplotypes and development of TAO, no consistent pattern has been identified across patient populations. In the United Kingdom, HLA-A9 and HLA-B5 are particularly prevalent in patients with TAO.[30] In a U.S. study, HLA testing was performed in 11 patients with TAO, and no specific pattern could be identified.[18] Lack of consistency in HLA haplotype predominance among various populations with TAO is likely due to genetic diversity and methodological differences in each of the studies.[31]

Polymorphisms of CD14, a main receptor for bacterial lipopolysaccharide, (37.4% vs. 24.2%; $P = 0.008$; odds ratio [OR] = 1.87; 95% confidence interval [CI], 1.18-2.97), HLA-DRB1 (34.4% vs. 13.2%; $P < 0.001$; OR = 3.44; 95% CI, 2.06-5.73), and HLA-DPB1 (79.4% vs. 55.1%; $P < 0.001$; OR = 3.14; 95% CI, 1.93-5.11) have been observed to have a significantly higher frequency in patients with TAO than in controls.[32] Stratification analyses of these polymorphisms suggested synergistic roles with ORs that ranged from 4.72 to 12.57 in individuals carrying any two of these three markers. These data suggest that susceptibility to TAO may be controlled in part by genes involved in innate and adaptive immunity.

In a study comparing 21 TAO patients with healthy age-, gender-, and race-matched controls, frequency of mutations associated with arterial vasospasm (stromelysin-1 5A/6A, endothelial nitric oxide synthase [eNOS] T-786 C) was evaluated.[33] Homozygosity for 5A/6A stromelysin-1 was present in 7 of 21 (33%) TAO cases, compared with 5 of 21 (24%) controls (risk ratio 1.4; 95% CI, 0.5-3.7). Homozygosity for eNOS T-786 C was present in 3 of 21 (14%) TAO cases, compared with 1 of 21 (5%) controls (risk ratio 3.0; 95% CI, 0.3-26.6).

In another recent study, eNOS 894 G→T and endothelin-1 (ET-1) 8000 T→C polymorphisms were assessed to determine whether either played a role in development of TAO.[34] Investigators found that the T allele of the eNOS 894 G→T polymorphism was protective against TAO.

Hypercoagulable States

The role of hypercoagulable states in TAO pathogenesis remains unclear; studies have failed to demonstrate a consistent pattern of association. In a comparison of patients with TAO and healthy controls, levels of urokinase-plasminogen activator (uPA) were twofold higher, and free plasminogen activator inhibitor-1 (PAI-1) were 40% lower, in patients with the disease.[35] During venous occlusion, tissue plasminogen activator (tPA) antigen concentrations increased to a greater extent in controls while PAI-1 levels were lower in patients with TAO. Patients with TAO also appear to have an enhanced platelet response to serotonin[36] and higher platelet contractile force.[37]

In one case-control study, the frequencies of factor V Leiden and prothrombin gene 20210A mutations were similar in patients with TAO and healthy subjects.[38] However, in another case-control study, OR for the prothrombin 20210 A allele compared with the G allele was 7.98 (95% CI, 2.45-25.93) in patients with TAO.[39] Elevated plasma homocysteine levels have been reported in patients with TAO and may be associated with a higher amputation rate.[40]

Increased levels of anticardiolipin antibodies have been reported in patients with TAO.[40–42] In one study, anticardiolipin antibodies were measured in 47 patients with TAO, 48 patients with premature atherosclerosis, and 48 otherwise healthy individuals.[42] Prevalence of anticardiolipin antibodies was significantly higher in patients with TAO (36%) compared with those with premature atherosclerosis (8%; $P = 0.01$) and healthy controls (2%; $P < 0.001$). Compared with those without detectable autoantibodies, patients with TAO and elevated anticardiolipin antibody titers were younger at age of onset and had increased rates of major amputation. A smaller study, however, did not demonstrate increased amputation rates in TAO patients with elevated anticardiolipin antibodies.[40]

Immunological Mechanisms

Abnormalities in immunoreactivity are believed to play a critical role in the inflammatory process that characterizes TAO. In a study of 39 patients with TAO, cellular and humoral immune responses to native human collagen type I and type III were evaluated.[43] Cell-mediated sensitivity to these collagens as measured by an antigen-sensitive thymidine incorporation assay was significantly higher in patients with TAO than in patients with atherosclerosis or in healthy male controls. Lymphocytes from 77% of the patients with TAO demonstrated cellular sensitivity to type I or type III collagens or both. In 17 of 39 serum samples (44%) from the patients with TAO, a low but significant level of anticollagen antibody activity was detected, whereas no antibody activity was observed in serum samples from controls. Circulating immune complexes found in peripheral arteries of patients with TAO provide further evidence for an immunological basis for this disease.[44,45]

In a study of nine patients with TAO, immunohistochemical analysis was performed on 33 specimens.[46] Architecture of blood vessel walls was well preserved regardless of the stage of disease, but cell infiltration involving the thrombus and intima was observed. Among infiltrating cells, CD3+ T cells greatly outnumbered CD20+ B cells, and CD68+ macrophages or S-100+ dendritic cells were detected in the intima during acute and subacute phases. Deposits of immunoglobulins (Ig)G, IgA, and IgM and complement factors 3d and 4c were noted along the internal elastic lamina. These data indicate that TAO represents an endarteritis characterized by both T cell– (cellular) and B cell–mediated (humoral) immunity in association with activation of antigen-presenting cells in the intima.

Immunohistochemical and TUNEL (terminal dUTP nick end labeling) studies were conducted on arterial walls obtained from eight patients with TAO to phenotype infiltrating cells with CD4+ (helper T cell), CD8+ (cytotoxic T cell), CD56 (natural killer cell), and CD68 (macrophage) to (1) identify cell activation with vascular cell adhesion molecule-1 (VCAM-1) and inducible nitric oxide synthase (iNOS), (2) determine the presence of cell death with TUNEL analysis, and (3) detect inflammatory cytokines with reverse transcriptase-polymerase chain reaction (RT-PCR).[47] T cells were identified mainly in the thrombus, intima, and adventitia. Among infiltrating cells, CD4+ T cells greatly outnumbered CD8+ cells. VCAM-1 and iNOS were expressed in endothelial cells (ECs) around the intima in patent segments or in vaso vasorum in occluded segments. These findings suggest that a T cell–mediated immune response may play an important role in development of TAO.

An immunohistochemistry study compared 58 amputated lower extremities from patients with TAO to 5 autopsy controls.[48] In patients with a definite diagnosis of TAO, as determined by clinical criteria, linear arrangement of macrophages, B lymphocytes, and T lymphocytes along vascular elastic fibers was found to be a predictable and specific inflammatory response to the internal elastic lamina of affected vessels. This finding indicates that elastic fibers are important immunogens in TAO pathogenesis.

Endothelial Dysfunction

Abnormalities of endothelial function also appear to contribute to TAO pathogenesis. Although various autoantibodies commonly observed in vasculitides are typically absent, elevations in antiendothelial cell antibody titers have been documented in patients with active TAO.[49] In one study, seven patients with active TAO had antiendothelial cell antibody titers of 1857 ± 450 arbitrary units (AU), compared with 461 ± 41 AU in 21 patients in remission ($P < 0.01$) and 126 ± 15 AU in 30 control subjects ($P < 0.001$).[49] If these findings can be confirmed, measurement of antiendothelial cell antibody titers may serve as a useful tool in following disease activity.

Patients with TAO also demonstrate impairment of endothelium-dependent vasodilation in the peripheral vasculature. Changes in forearm blood flow induced by the endothelium-dependent vasodilator acetylcholine, the endothelium-independent vasodilator sodium nitroprusside, and occlusion-induced reactive hyperemia were measured plethysmographically in the nondiseased limb in eight patients with TAO and in eight healthy controls matched for age and smoking status.[50] The increase in forearm blood flow response to intraarterial acetylcholine infusion was diminished in patients with TAO compared with healthy controls (22.9 ± 2.9 vs. 14.1 ± 2.8 mL/min per dL of tissue volume; $P < 0.01$). In contrast, there was no significant difference in the increase in forearm blood flow response to sodium nitroprusside infusion and reactive hyperemia between the two study groups. These data suggest that peripheral endothelium-dependent vasodilation is impaired even in the nondiseased limbs of patients with TAO.

In a study designed to evaluate the role of circulating progenitor cells in endothelial function in patients with TAO and atherosclerosis obliterans, investigators measured flow-mediated vasodilation, nitroglycerin-induced vasodilation, and circulating progenitor cells in 30 patients with TAO, 30 age- and sex-matched healthy subjects, and 40 patients with atherosclerosis obliterans.[51] Flow-mediated vasodilation was decreased in both the TAO group and atherosclerosis obliterans group compared with controls (6.6% ± 2.7%, 5.7% ± 3.3% vs. 9.5% ± 3.1%, $P < 0.0001$, respectively). However, there was no significant difference in flow-mediated vasodilation between the TAO group and atherosclerosis obliterans group. Nitroglycerin-induced vasodilation was similar in the three groups. The number and migration of circulating progenitor cells were similar in the TAO group and control group, but were significantly decreased in the atherosclerosis obliterans group. There was a significant relationship between the number and migration of circulating progenitor cells and flow-mediated vasodilation ($r = 0.43$ and $r = 0.40$, $P < 0.0001$, respectively). Flow-mediated vasodilation was impaired in patients with TAO and patients with atherosclerosis obliterans compared with control subjects, but the number and function of circulating progenitor cells were not decreased in patients with TAO.

In a study of surgical biopsies obtained from femoral and iliac arteries of patients with TAO, expression of intercellular adhesion molecule-1 (ICAM-1), VCAM-1, and E-selectin was increased on endothelial and inflammatory cells in the thickened intima.[52] Immunohistochemistry demonstrated contacts between mononuclear cells and morphologically activated ECs expressing ICAM-1 and E-selectin. These findings provide evidence for EC activation, tumor necrosis factor (TNF)-α secretion by tissue-infiltrating inflammatory cells, ICAM-1, VCAM-1 and E-selectin expression on ECs, and leukocyte adhesion in TAO.

Infection

Chronic anaerobic periodontal infection may represent an additional risk factor for development of TAO.[53] Nearly two thirds of patients with TAO have severe periodontal disease. Polymerase chain reaction (PCR) analysis demonstrated deoxyribonucleic acid (DNA) fragments from anaerobic bacteria, in particular *Treponema denticola*, in both arterial lesions and oral cavities of patients with TAO, but not in arterial samples from healthy control subjects. However, the higher prevalence of periodontal infection in TAO may simply be a marker of lower socioeconomic status in patients who develop the disease, rather than a pathogenic correlate.

Pathology

Pathologically, TAO is distinguished by inflammatory thrombus that affects small- and medium-sized arteries and veins. Histopathology of involved blood vessels varies according to the stage at which the tissue sample is obtained. Thromboangiitis obliterans involves three phases: acute, subacute, and chronic (Fig. 44-1). Histopathology is most likely to be diagnostic of TAO

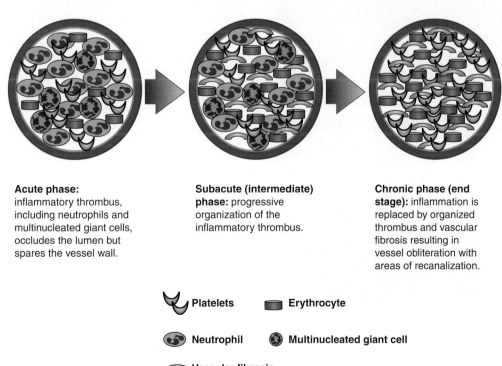

Acute phase: inflammatory thrombus, including neutrophils and multinucleated giant cells, occludes the lumen but spares the vessel wall.

Subacute (intermediate) phase: progressive organization of the inflammatory thrombus.

Chronic phase (end stage): inflammation is replaced by organized thrombus and vascular fibrosis resulting in vessel obliteration with areas of recanalization.

⤹ Platelets   ▬ Erythrocyte

◉ Neutrophil   ✸ Multinucleated giant cell

〰 Vascular fibrosis

FIGURE 44-1   Histopathological stages of thromboangiitis obliterans (TAO).

in samples obtained during the acute phase of the disease. As the disease progresses from the subacute to chronic phases, the histopathology of TAO becomes virtually indistinguishable from other obstructive vascular diseases that result in fibrosis of the blood vessels in their end stage. Because the histological appearance can vary from patient to patient and depends upon the stage of the disease, a pathological diagnosis of TAO may be challenging in some cases.[54] Furthermore, pathological diagnosis may be inconclusive if only amputated specimens or occluded arteries and veins are examined. Subacute and chronic phase lesions have far fewer characteristic features and therefore are rarely diagnostic for TAO.

Acute Phase

The acute phase of TAO consists of an occlusive, highly cellular, inflammatory thrombus. Polymorphonuclear neutrophils, microabscesses, and multinucleated giant cells are often present around the periphery of the thrombus (Fig. 44-2). Presence of multinucleated giant cells is characteristic of but not specific for TAO.[55]

Inflammatory thrombus is observed with greatest frequency in biopsies of areas demonstrating acute superficial thrombophlebitis taken from patients with TAO. It is unclear whether the vascular lesions of TAO are primarily thrombotic or inflammatory, but the pattern of intense inflammatory cell infiltration and cellular proliferation observed in the acute phase of the disease is particularly distinctive. Acute phlebitis without thrombosis, acute phlebitis with thrombosis, and acute phlebitis with thrombus containing microabscesses and giant cells may coexist in different segments of the same affected vein if it is biopsied at an early stage. These lesions correspond with the clinical finding of thrombophlebitis migrans.[56]

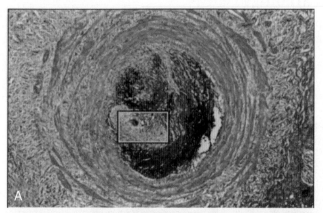

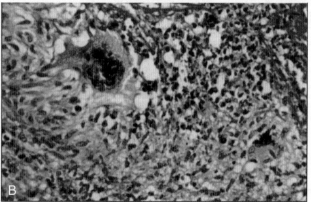

FIGURE 44-2 **A,** Typical acute histological lesion in vein obtained from patient with thromboangiitis obliterans (TAO). **B,** Close-up of boxed area in **A,** demonstrating a microabscess in the thrombus and two multinucleated giant cells (hematoxylin and eosin, ×64 [**A**] and ×400 [**B**]). *(Reproduced with permission from Lie JT: Thromboangiitis obliterans (Buerger's disease) revisited. Pathol Annu 23:257–291, 1988.)*

Subacute (Intermediate) Phase

During the subacute or intermediate phase, progressive organization of the inflammatory thrombus takes place in affected arteries and veins. Although some degree of inflammatory infiltrate remains within the thrombus, the vessel wall is generally spared. Partial recanalization of the vessel and disappearance of microabscesses may also be observed in the subacute phase.[46]

Chronic (End-Stage) Phase

The chronic phase is characterized by organized thrombus with areas of extensive recanalization, prominent vascularization of the media, and adventitial and perivascular fibrosis. Because they represent the end products of vascular injury and occlusive thrombosis, chronic-phase arterial lesions are the least distinctive of the three morphological stages of TAO. However, focal residual inflammation within the organized thrombus may suggest TAO in an end-stage lesion. Chronic-phase lesions in TAO frequently mimic atherosclerotic vascular disease. In some patients, especially those older than 40 years of age, both TAO and atherosclerotic vascular disease may coexist and thereby create further diagnostic uncertainty.

Additional Histopathological Features

In all three phases of TAO, normal architecture of the vessel wall adjacent to the occlusive thrombus, including the internal elastic lamina, remains intact. This observation distinguishes TAO from atherosclerotic vascular disease and from other systemic vasculitides in which there is typically disruption of the internal elastic lamina and the media. "Skip" areas in which normal vessel segments are observed between diseased ones are common in TAO. In addition, the intensity of the periadventitial inflammatory reaction can be quite variable in different segments of the same vessel.

Immunohistochemical Features

Studies focusing on immunohistochemistry have provided limited understanding of the role of the cytoskeleton and other cellular elements in TAO.[44–48,52,57] Soon after the inflammatory thrombus has occluded the vessel lumen, spindle cells migrate from the media through fenestrations in the internal elastic lamina into the intima to populate the periphery of the thrombus. These spindle cells express vimentin and α_1-actin and originate from smooth muscle cells (SMCs) of the media. Capillaries appear along thrombus margins. Endothelial cells express factor VIII–related antigen and *Ulex europaeus* agglutinin.

As the thrombus organizes during later disease stages, spindle cells differentiate into fibroblasts and lose their positive staining for α_1-actin. Demonstration of the internal elastic lamina by collagen type IV markers confirms that the lamina remains intact in TAO, and that SMCs migrate from the media to the intima via fenestrations. Newly formed capillaries within the thrombus are noted.

Immunohistochemically, the process of thrombus organization in TAO is virtually identical to that of ordinary thrombus, with the exception of the characteristic inflammatory component. However, infiltration of SMCs from the media results in a more hypercellular thrombus and rapid organization.

Clinical Presentation

The typical patient with TAO is a young man with a history of heavy tobacco smoking who presents with onset of ischemic symptoms of the extremities before age 45 years. However, patients should be questioned about chewing tobacco as well as snuff and marijuana use, especially if they deny smoking and present with a history compatible with TAO. Ischemic symptoms result from stenosis or occlusion of the distal small arteries and veins. Thromboangiitis obliterans frequently progresses proximally and involves multiple limbs. Large-artery involvement is atypical and rarely occurs in the absence of small-vessel occlusive disease.[58] The most common

TABLE 44-1	Presenting Symptoms and Signs in 112 patients with Thromboangiitis Obliterans Evaluated at Cleveland Clinic Between 1970 and 1987*	
CLINICAL FINDING	**N (%)**	
Intermittent claudication	70 (63)	
Rest pain	91 (81)	
Ischemic ulcerations:	85 (76)	
Upper extremity	24 (28)	
Lower extremity	39 (46)	
Both	22 (26)	
Thrombophlebitis	43 (38)	
Raynaud phenomenon	49 (44)	
Sensory findings	77 (69)	
Abnormal Allen test	71 (63)	

*Data from Olin JW, Young JR, Graor RA, et al: The changing clinical spectrum of thromboangiitis obliterans (Buerger's disease). Circulation 82:3–8, 1990.

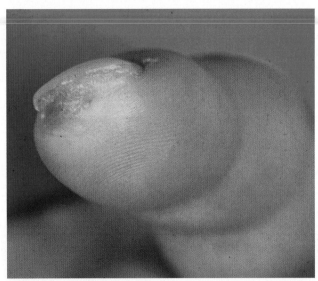

FIGURE 44-4 Ischemic ulceration of index finger in patient with thromboangiitis obliterans (TAO).

symptoms result from arterial occlusive disease, secondary vasospasm, and superficial thrombophlebitis (Table 44-1).

Arterial Occlusive Disease

Arterial occlusive disease due to TAO most often presents as intermittent claudication of the feet, legs, hands, or arms. In a study of 112 patients with TAO evaluated at the Cleveland Clinic from 1970 to 1987, intermittent claudication occurred in 70 patients (63%).[17] In a retrospective study of 344 patients treated surgically for TAO in Turkey, major complaints included foot coldness in 312 (90.6%) patients, color changes in 290 (84.3%), rest pain in 160 (46.5%), claudication in 166 (48.2%), and necrotic ulcers in 185 (53.1%).[59] Foot or arch claudication may be a presenting symptom and is frequently attributed to an orthopedic problem, resulting in diagnostic delay. As lower-extremity disease progresses proximally, patients with TAO may report classic calf claudication.

Symptoms and signs of critical limb ischemia, including rest pain, ulcerations, and digital gangrene, occur with advanced arterial occlusive disease. At the time of presentation, 76% of patients have ischemic ulcerations (Fig. 44-3A and Fig. 44-4).[17] With early recognition of symptoms and signs of TAO, many patients can be identified and treated before critical limb ischemia develops.

Although only one limb may be affected clinically, arterial occlusive disease always involves two or more extremities on angiographic evaluation. In one series of patients with TAO, two limbs were affected in 16% of patients, three limbs in 41%, and all four limbs in 43%.[60] The Intractable Vasculitis Syndromes Research Group of Japan reported isolated lower limb involvement in 75%, isolated upper limb involvement in 5%, and both upper and lower limb involvement in 20% of patients with TAO.[61]

Raynaud Phenomenon

A common complaint in TAO, cold sensitivity may represent one of the earliest manifestations of the disease. Indeed, presentations of TAO appear to be more common in the winter.[62] Cold sensitivity likely results from ischemia or markedly increased muscle sympathetic nerve activity, which has been demonstrated in TAO patients compared with controls.[63] Raynaud phenomenon is present in over 40% of patients with TAO and may be asymmetrical.[2] The extremities, particularly the digits, may be characterized by either rubor or cyanosis. This discoloration has been termed *Buerger's color.*[64]

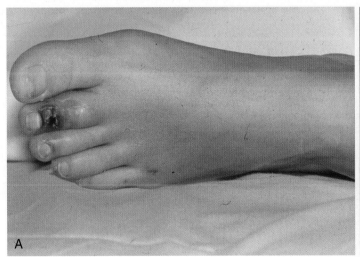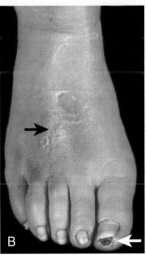

FIGURE 44-3 A, Ischemic ulceration on second toe in young woman with thromboangiitis obliterans. **B,** Superficial thrombophlebitis on dorsum of the right foot *(black arrow)* in patient with TAO. Note ischemic ulceration on distal right great toe. *(Reproduced with permission from Olin JW, Lie JT: Current management of hypertension and vascular disease. In Cooke JP, Frohlich ED, editors: Thromboangiitis obliterans (Buerger's disease), St. Louis, 1992, Mosby-Yearbook, p 65.)*

Superficial Thrombophlebitis

Although it may also be observed in Behçet disease, superficial thrombophlebitis differentiates TAO from other vasculitides and atherosclerotic vascular disease (see Fig. 44-3B). Superficial thrombophlebitis occurs in approximately 40% of patients with TAO.[17] Superficial thrombophlebitis may predate the onset of ischemic symptoms caused by arterial occlusive disease[56] and may parallel disease activity.[65] Some patients may describe a migratory pattern of tender nodules that follow a venous distribution (thrombophlebitis migrans).[56]

Neurological Findings

Sensory abnormalities are common in TAO and were observed in up to 70% of cases in a series from the Cleveland Clinic.[17] Sensory findings are most likely due to ischemic neuropathy, a late finding in the course of TAO. Sensory findings may also be due to primary involvement of the nerves themselves, since earlier studies have suggested that inflammatory cell infiltrate may surround the nerves.[5]

Unusual Presentations

TAO is typically a disease affecting vessels in distal parts of the extremities, but it has also been reported to involve unusual vascular beds: the great vessels and pulmonary, proximal extremity, mesenteric, cerebral, coronary, renal, pelvic, and ophthalmic arteries. Thromboangiitis obliterans in atypical vascular beds is characterized by similar pathological findings as found in the extremities. Of note, reports of TAO in unusual locations should be interpreted with caution because the diagnosis of TAO in such cases may not meet criteria suggested in this chapter.

Thromboangiitis obliterans of large elastic arteries such as the pulmonary[66] and iliac arteries[58] has been rarely documented. Visceral involvement may present as abdominal pain, nausea, vomiting, diarrhea, melena, hematochezia, weight loss, and anorexia and result in mesenteric ischemia or infarction.[67–72] Cerebrovascular involvement may manifest as transient ischemic attack (TIA), ischemic stroke, and psychotic disorders.[73–77]

Coronary artery involvement may present as myocardial ischemia or infarction.[78–82] Thromboangiitis obliterans affecting the intrarenal arterial branches has been reported.[83] Rarely, TAO may involve the pelvic vessels, including the pudendal arteries and veins, resulting in erectile dysfunction.[84] Thromboangiitis obliterans involving the temporal and ophthalmic arteries may mimic giant cell arteritis (GCA).[85,86]

Involvement of saphenous vein bypass grafts in patients with TAO is a truly rare occurrence.[87]

Differential Diagnosis

A clinical diagnosis of TAO requires exclusion of disorders that may mimic the disease (Box 44-1). The most important disorders to exclude are atherosclerotic vascular disease, thromboembolic disease, and autoimmune diseases such as scleroderma or CREST (calcinosis, Raynaud phenomenon, esophageal dysmotility, sclerodactyly, telangiectasia) syndrome. In most cases, the combination of serological testing, echocardiography, and arteriography can exclude these disorders and help establish the diagnosis of TAO.

A scleroderma or CREST syndrome diagnosis is typically suggested by clinical presentation, including skin findings. Nailfold capillaroscopy may be performed and is usually quite distinctive in patients with these disorders. However, characteristic findings of capillary loop dropout in scleroderma or CREST syndrome may also be observed in some patients with TAO. Detection of serological markers such as anti-ACL-70 or anticentromere antibodies provides further evidence for scleroderma or CREST syndrome.

Clinicians should evaluate patients for features of other autoimmune diseases such as systemic lupus erythematosus, rheumatoid arthritis, and other vasculitides. Serological markers are often

Box 44-1 Disorders That May Mimic Thromboangiitis Obliterans

- Atherosclerotic vascular disease
- Thromboembolic disease
- Rheumatological disorders:
  - Scleroderma
  - CREST syndrome
  - Systemic lupus erythematosus
  - Rheumatoid arthritis
  - Mixed connective tissue diseases
  - Other vasculitides
- Hypercoagulable states:
  - Antiphospholipid antibody syndrome
- Syndromes of repetitive mechanical trauma:
  - Hypothenar hammer syndrome
  - Vibration-related vascular injury
- Thoracic outlet syndrome
- Popliteal entrapment syndrome
- Cystic adventitial disease
- Drugs:
  - Ergotamine abuse
  - Cocaine abuse
  - Amphetamine abuse

CREST, calcinosis, Raynaud phenomenon, esophageal dysmotility, sclerodactyly, telangiectasia.

helpful in excluding such disorders. Patients with antiphospholipid antibody syndrome pose a particular diagnostic challenge because they may present with both arterial and venous thrombotic events. Antiphospholipid antibody syndrome is suggested by detection of lupus-type anticoagulants or presence of elevated titers of anticardiolipin antibodies. Of note, lupus anticoagulant and anticardiolipin antibodies may be detected in some patients with TAO, but may also indicate an unrelated thrombophilia.[1] Pathological examination can clearly differentiate between the two disorders because antiphospholipid antibody syndrome is characterized by the presence of bland thrombosis, whereas TAO results in an inflammatory thrombus.

Thromboangiitis obliterans is differentiated from other vasculitides in that it results in distal extremity ischemia, whereas patients with Takayasu's arteritis or GCA present with more proximal arterial involvement. Arteriographic features of TAO are also quite distinctive from those observed in Takayasu's arteritis or giant cell arteritis. In addition, vasculitides such as Takayasu's arteritis and GCA are typically associated with elevations in inflammatory markers, including erythrocyte sedimentation rate and C-reactive protein.

Clinicians evaluating patients with suspected TAO should inquire about possible ergotamine or cocaine abuse, in addition to disorders of repetitive mechanical trauma such as vibration-induced vascular injury and hypothenar hammer syndrome. Serum ergotamine levels can be obtained to exclude vascular injury caused by this drug. Because it can mimic TAO, all patients should be questioned about cocaine abuse. A complete toxicology screen is recommended in patients who present with a history and physical compatible with TAO, especially if they deny tobacco use.

Diagnosis

Thromboangiitis obliterans is a clinical diagnosis that requires a compatible history in combination with supportive physical examination findings and vascular abnormalities on imaging studies (Fig. 44-5).

Physical Examination

Physical examination of a patient with suspected TAO should include a detailed vascular evaluation with palpation of peripheral pulses, auscultation for arterial bruits, and measurement of ankle:brachial indices. Extremities should be carefully inspected

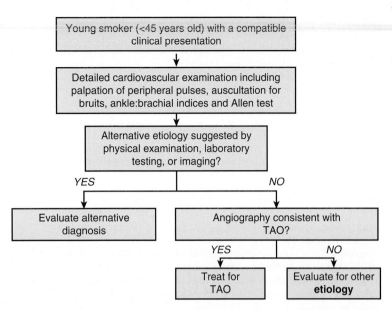

FIGURE 44-5   Diagnostic algorithm for patients with suspected thromboangiitis obliterans (TAO).

for superficial thrombophlebitis, which may present as tender superficial venous nodules and cords. Hands and feet should be examined for findings of digital ischemia. Neurological examination may document peripheral nerve involvement in the form of sensory deficits.

Although nonspecific, an abnormal Allen test in a young smoker with digital ischemia is strongly suggestive of TAO because it provides evidence for small-vessel disease (Fig. 44-6). In a series from the Cleveland Clinic, 63% of patients with TAO had an abnormal Allen test.[17] Documentation of an abnormal Allen test is helpful because the distal nature of TAO and involvement of both upper and lower extremities distinguishes it from atherosclerotic vascular disease. With the exception of chronic kidney disease patients with diabetes or those who have undergone renal transplantation, atherosclerosis does not involve the hands and rarely occurs distal to the subclavian artery.

Diagnostic Criteria

Several diagnostic criteria have been proposed for evaluating patients with suspected TAO. The Shionoya criteria require all five of the following to establish the diagnosis of TAO: history of smoking, onset before 50 years of age, infrapopliteal arterial occlusive disease, either upper extremity involvement or superficial thrombophlebitis, and absence of risk factors for atherosclerosis other than smoking.[88]

Papa and Adar proposed criteria that incorporated various clinical, angiographic, histopathological, and exclusionary elements, and then subsequently devised a point-scoring system for the diagnosis of TAO.[89,90]

Mills and Porter use a set of major and minor criteria for the diagnosis.[91] Commonly used clinical criteria include age younger than 45, current or recent history of tobacco use,

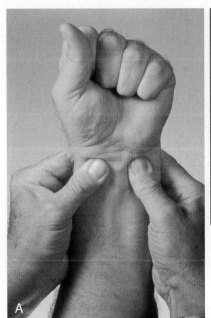

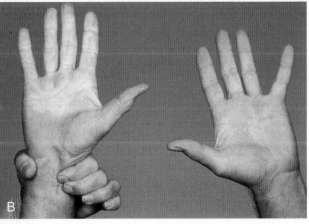

FIGURE 44-6   **A,** Allen test with occlusion of radial and ulnar pulses by manual compression. **B,** When compression of ulnar pulse is released while continuing to compress radial artery, hand does not fill with blood. Pallor of right hand compared with left is consistent with distal arterial occlusive disease of the ulnar artery *(right portion of image). (Reproduced with permission from Olin JW, Lie JT: Current management of hypertension and vascular disease. In Cooke JP, Frohlich ED, editors: Thromboangiitis obliterans (Buerger's disease), St. Louis, 1992, Mosby-Yearbook, p 65.)*

BOX 44-2 Common Criteria for the Diagnosis of Thromboangiitis Obliterans

- Age younger than 45 years at disease onset
- Current or recent history of tobacco use
- Symptoms and signs of distal extremity ischemia with confirmation by noninvasive testing
- Consistent angiographic findings
- Exclusion of thrombophilia, autoimmune disease, diabetes mellitus, and a proximal source of emboli
- Supportive tissue biopsy in patients with unusual presentations such as large-artery involvement or age older than 45-50 years at symptom onset

distal extremity ischemia confirmed by noninvasive testing, consistent angiographic findings, and exclusion of thrombophilia, autoimmune disease, diabetes mellitus, and a proximal source of emboli[2] (Box 44-2).

An increasing number of individuals who fulfill clinical criteria for TAO have risk factors for atherosclerotic vascular disease (e.g., hypertension, hyperlipidemia). A subset of these patients may subsequently develop concomitant atherosclerotic vascular disease after the original diagnosis of TAO. Accordingly, if patients meet criteria of distal extremity involvement, tobacco use, and exclusion of a proximal source of emboli, atherosclerosis, and thrombophilia, hyperlipidemia, or hypertension should not exclude the diagnosis of TAO.

Laboratory Evaluation

Although there are no specific blood tests to aid in the diagnosis, laboratory evaluation in patients with suspected TAO is useful for excluding alternative diagnoses. Initial laboratory studies should include a complete blood cell count (CBC), chemistry panel, liver function tests, fasting blood glucose, urinalysis, inflammatory markers such as erythrocyte sedimentation rate and C-reactive protein, cold agglutinins, and cryoglobulins. In addition, serological markers of autoimmune disease, including antinuclear antibody, rheumatoid factor, anticentromere antibody, and anti-SCL-70 antibody, should be obtained and are typically negative in patients with TAO. Evaluation for hypercoagulable states is frequently performed. Of note, antiphospholipid and anticardiolipin antibodies are detected in some patients with TAO but may also indicate an isolated thrombophilia.

Imaging

Imaging in patients with suspected TAO is not only used to establish the diagnosis but also to exclude alternative etiologies for the presentation that may require a radically different therapeutic approach. For example, echocardiography is frequently indicated to exclude a cardiac source of embolism that results in acute arterial occlusion. Likewise, catheter-based angiography provides evidence for TAO, but also excludes proximal sources of artery-to-artery embolism.

Noninvasive vascular laboratory studies such as segmental arterial pressure measurements with pulse volume recordings demonstrating distal abnormalities in the absence of proximal disease suggest a diagnosis of TAO. Digital plethysmography, finger and toe pressures, and transcutaneous oxygen measurement may be useful in documenting distal small-vessel disease in the absence of more proximal upper- or lower-extremity abnormalities in patients with TAO. Arterial duplex scanning can also be used to exclude proximal atherosclerotic lesions and identify distal arterial occlusive disease. "Corkscrew collaterals," a finding frequently observed in patients with TAO, may also be visualized on arterial duplex scanning.[32] Abdominal aortic ultrasonography may be used to exclude abdominal aortic aneurysm or atherosclerosis as a source of distal embolization to the lower extremities.

Computed tomography angiography (CTA), magnetic resonance angiography (MRA), or catheter-based angiography may be performed to exclude a proximal arterial source of embolism and define the anatomy and severity of distal arterial occlusive disease. Although advances in CTA and MRA have shown promise for imaging distal vessels, the majority of patients will require catheter-based angiography to provide the spatial resolution necessary to detect small-artery pathology, especially of the hands and feet. In patients with ischemic ulcerations and in whom secondary infection is a concern, magnetic resonance (MR) may be useful in determining the presence of osteomyelitis.[93]

Catheter-based angiography plays a critical role in establishing the diagnosis of TAO and excluding proximal arterial pathology that may result in distal arterial occlusive disease.[94,95] Although there are no pathognomonic angiographic findings in TAO, angiography helps establish the diagnosis when taken in the context of a compatible clinical presentation. The classic angiographic picture of TAO consists of arterial occlusive disease confined to the distal circulation, most often infrapopliteal and infrabrachial, with proximal arteries free of atheroma, aneurysms, and other sources of emboli (Fig. 44-7). There are often areas of disease interspersed with normal-appearing vessels (skip areas). In the absence of diabetes, isolated arterial occlusive disease distal to the popliteal artery virtually never occurs in atherosclerosis. Commonly, angiographic abnormalities are observed in the digital arteries of the fingers and toes, the palmar and plantar arteries of the hands and feet, and the radial, ulnar, anterior tibial, posterior tibial, and peroneal arteries.[96,97]

Distal small- to medium-artery involvement, segmental occlusions, and corkscrew-shaped collaterals around areas of occlusions are characteristic angiographic findings in TAO (Fig. 44-8). Corkscrew collaterals are not specific for TAO, however, and may be observed with any disease process that results in small-vessel occlusive disease. In particular, arterial occlusive disease due to scleroderma or CREST syndrome can closely mimic the angiographic appearance of TAO. Findings of arterial wall irregularity, vascular calcification, and proximal artery involvement should call a diagnosis of TAO into question.

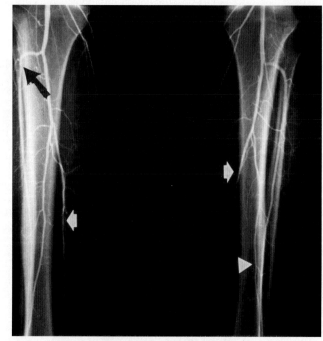

FIGURE 44-7 Catheter-based angiogram demonstrating severe infrapopliteal arterial occlusive disease in patient with thromboangiitis obliterans (TAO). In right leg, anterior tibial artery *(black arrow)* occludes just distal to its origin. Posterior tibial artery tapers and then occludes in the mid- to distal calf *(white arrow)*. In left leg, anterior tibial artery is patent, but posterior tibial *(white arrow)* occludes several centimeters after its origin. Peroneal artery *(arrowhead)* tapers in mid-calf.

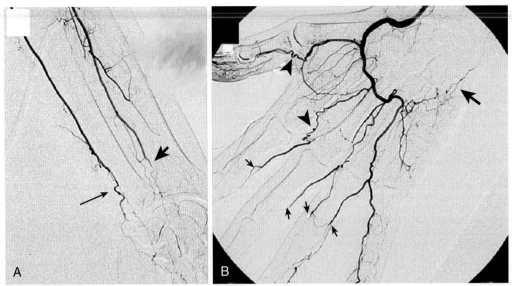

FIGURE 44-8 **A,** Catheter-based angiogram of left forearm and hand, demonstrating tapering occlusion of left radial artery *(arrowhead)* and ulnar artery *(arrow)* at the wrist. All proximal arteries were normal. **B,** Right hand of same patient demonstrated an occluded ulnar artery at the wrist *(large arrow)*. A patent radial artery fills the deep palmar arch. Multiple segmental digital artery occlusions are present *(small arrows)*. Numerous "corkscrew collaterals" *(arrowheads)*, which represent collateralization around occluded segments, are visualized. *(Reproduced with permission from Olin JW, Shih A: Thromboangiitis obliterans (Buerger's disease). Curr Opin Rheumatol 18:18–24, 2006.)*

Role for Biopsy

Tissue biopsy is rarely required for the diagnosis of TAO unless the clinical presentation involves an unusual vascular territory or a patient older than 45 or 50 years of age at the onset of symptoms. Biopsy is most likely to be diagnostic when obtained from a vein with superficial thrombophlebitis during the acute phase of the disease. A highly inflammatory thrombus, relative sparing of the blood vessel wall, and preservation of the internal elastic lamina in arterial biopsies are characteristic histological findings in TAO.

Prognosis

Prognosis for patients with TAO greatly depends on their ability to discontinue tobacco use. In a retrospective series of 110 patients with TAO (106 men, 4 women; mean age, 40 years), the natural history of the disease was compared in those who quit smoking and those who did not.[98] Seven of 110 study patients (6%) died during a mean follow-up of 10.6 years. Forty-seven patients (43%) underwent 108 amputation procedures, including either major amputation (13 patients) or minor amputation (34 patients) of an upper or lower extremity. Of 69 patients who continued smoking, 13 patients (19%) underwent major amputation. None of those who stopped smoking underwent amputation. Continued smoking correlated with the risk of limb amputation ($P = 0.007$).

Quality of life is substantially diminished in patients with TAO.[98,99] In the retrospective analysis referenced above, 11 of 13 patients (85%) who underwent major lower-limb amputation lost their jobs, compared to only 9 of 97 patients (9%) without major amputation.[98] Limb amputation strongly correlated with job loss ($P < 0.0001$).

Management

Although various options exist for TAO management, discontinuation of tobacco use is the definitive and most effective therapy for the disease (Box 44-3). Efficacy of alternative therapies in TAO is profoundly limited in the setting of ongoing tobacco use.

BOX 44-3 Therapeutic Options for the Management of Thromboangiitis Obliterans

- Tobacco cessation
- Vasodilators:
  - Prostacyclin analogs
  - α-Adrenergic receptor antagonists
  - Calcium channel antagonists
  - Phosphodiesterase (PDE) inhibitors (cilostazol, sildenafil)
  - Transdermal nitrates
- Peripheral periarterial sympathectomy
- Regional sympathetic blockade
- Spinal cord stimulation
- Intermittent pneumatic compression
- Therapeutic angiogenesis
- Endovascular therapy
- Surgical revascularization:
  - Arterial bypass surgery
  - Omental transfer
  - Amputation
- Local wound care:
  - Debridement
  - Vacuum-assisted wound closure

Tobacco Cessation

Again, the cornerstone of therapy for TAO is *total discontinuation* of any tobacco use (Box 44-4). Even a few cigarettes a day may drive disease progression and culminate in amputation.[1,17,100,101] Patients should be counseled to abstain from using smokeless tobacco as well as smoking marijuana; both have been associated with TAO.[21–23] Patient education on the role of tobacco exposure in initiation, maintenance, and progression of TAO is of paramount importance. Adjunctive measures to assist in discontinuing tobacco use (e.g., pharmacotherapy, smoking-cessation groups) should be made available to all patients with TAO. However, nicotine replacement therapy should be avoided in these patients because it may contribute to disease activity. Agents such as bupropion and varenicline may be preferred as smoking-cessation aids in patients with TAO. Although it remains unclear whether passive smoke exposure can cause TAO, patients with active disease should be advised to avoid second-hand smoke as much as possible.

Box 44-4 Pearls for Tobacco Cessation in Patients with Thromboangiitis Obliterans

- Educate patients on the critical role of tobacco in the initiation, maintenance, and progression of thromboangiitis obliterans (TAO).
- Counsel patients and members of their households about the role of secondhand smoke exposure in perpetuating the disease process.
- Ask the patient at every office visit if they have been successful in tobacco cessation. This approach lets the patient know that tobacco cessation is the single most important aspect in treating this disease.
- Explain to patients the limited efficacy of alternative therapies for TAO in the absence of complete and continued tobacco cessation.
- Measure urinary nicotine, cotinine, and cannabis in patients who continue to have signs and symptoms consistent with active disease, despite claims of tobacco cessation.
- Offer adjunctive therapies such as pharmacotherapy and smoking-cessation groups to assist with discontinuation of tobacco use.
- Prescribe bupropion and varenicline as the preferred pharmacological adjuncts to assist in tobacco cessation because nicotine replacement therapy may contribute to continued disease activity.

It has been stated in the past that patients with TAO have a greater degree of tobacco dependence than those with atherosclerotic cardiovascular disease, but this is not an accurate assumption. Patients with TAO may have a higher frequency of tobacco cessation than those with atherosclerotic vascular disease. In a study of 112 patients with TAO followed over a mean of 92 months, 43 (48%) patients stopped smoking for a mean of 80 months.[17] A case-control study compared 103 patients with TAO confirmed on angiography, biopsy, or noninvasive testing with 273 patients with coronary artery disease (CAD) confirmed by angiography to determine patterns of tobacco dependence.[102] Degree of tobacco dependence in each group was ascertained by questionnaire. Kaplan-Meier curves demonstrated no significant difference in time to tobacco cessation after initial diagnosis. Patients with TAO smoked fewer cigarettes per day than those with CAD (22.3 ± 10.7 vs. 27.7 ± 15.3 cigarettes/day, $P = 0.003$). Among 170 current smokers in the analysis, patients with TAO smoked fewer cigarettes/day (20.2 ± 8.2 vs. 24.6 ± 12.7, $P = 0.03$) and were more likely to have made a serious attempt to quit smoking (97% vs. 90%, $P = 0.03$). Based on these data, the study investigators concluded that patients with TAO did not appear to have greater tobacco dependence than CAD patients.

Patients with TAO should be reassured that if they are able to discontinue tobacco use, the disease will become quiescent and the risk of amputation will greatly diminish, provided critical limb ischemia is not present. If significant arterial occlusive disease has developed, symptoms of intermittent claudication and secondary vasospasm (Raynaud phenomenon) may continue but should not progress. Alternative therapies such as vasodilators may help reduce symptoms in such patients.

Vasodilators

The use of vasodilators in patients with TAO is largely palliative. The most extensive clinical experience with vasodilators in TAO comes from trials evaluating the prostacyclin analog iloprost. In a prospective randomized double-blind trial, 133 patients with TAO and critical limb ischemia were randomly allocated to receive iloprost or low-dose aspirin for 28 days.[103] Lower-extremity ischemic ulcerations were present in 98 patients. At 1-month follow-up, 58 (85%) of 68 iloprost-treated patients showed ulcer healing or relief of rest pain, compared with 11 (17%) of 65 in the aspirin-treated group. Compared with 18 (28%) on aspirin, 43 (63%) treated with iloprost had complete relief of pain. Ulcers healed completely in 18 of 52 (35%) treated with iloprost, compared with 6 of 46 (13%) who received aspirin. At 6-month follow-up, the response rate was 45 of 51 (88%) patients treated with iloprost, compared with 12 of 44 (21%) patients treated with aspirin.

A pharmacokinetic study demonstrated that an oral extended-release preparation of iloprost had pharmacological equivalence to the intravenous formulation in patients with TAO.[104] Based on these findings, a double-blind randomized trial comparing oral iloprost with placebo was conducted in 319 TAO patients with rest pain, trophic lesions, or both.[105] The primary study end point was total healing of the most important lesion; a secondary end point was relief of rest pain without need of analgesic medications. A combined end point included amputation-free survival, absence of trophic lesions and rest pain, and need for analgesic medications. Total healing of trophic lesions was not significantly different between study groups at any time point. Low-dose oral iloprost was significantly more effective than placebo at end of follow-up in relieving rest pain, without the need for analgesic medications, and improving the benefit over placebo. Based on these studies, iloprost may be considered for patients with TAO who have critical limb ischemia and require symptomatic relief early in the treatment period while they discontinue tobacco use.

Phosphodiesterase (PDE) inhibitors with vasodilator properties have the potential to play a role in the management of TAO, but require evaluation in prospective trials. Although not specifically described in patients with TAO, cilostazol has been reported to aid in healing ischemic ulcerations in patients who were ineligible for revascularization.[106,107] Although it is helpful in treating claudication due to atherosclerotic peripheral vascular disease, clinical experience with cilostazol for this indication in patients with TAO is limited. Sildenafil may represent another option in this drug class for patients with TAO, but requires investigation.

Other vasodilators such as α-adrenergic receptor antagonists, calcium channel antagonists, and transdermal nitrates may be helpful in patients who experience vasospasm, but these agents have not been studied in prospective clinical trials.

Periarterial Sympathectomy and Sympathetic Blockade

Peripheral periarterial sympathectomy may be considered for patients with refractory pain and digital ischemia due to TAO but remains controversial. Sympathectomy has anecdotally been reported to occasionally assist the healing of ischemic ulcerations, but a series from the Cleveland Clinic demonstrated no difference in amputation rate in patients undergoing the procedure compared to those who did not.[17] In a single case report, intravenous regional sympathetic blockade (Bier block) with guanethidine and lidocaine increased finger blood flow and resulted in complete disappearance of fingertip ischemic ulcerations and rest pain in a patient with advanced TAO.[108]

Spinal Cord Stimulation

Epidural spinal cord stimulation has been evaluated in a limited number of patients to decrease ischemic pain and avoid amputation when revascularization is not feasible and other therapeutic interventions have not been effective.[109-112] In a retrospective study, 29 patients were evaluated to determine the effect of epidural spinal cord stimulation in the treatment of TAO.[113] The regional perfusion index (ratio between foot and chest transcutaneous oxygen pressure) at baseline was 0.27 ± 0.25. Three months after spinal cord stimulation implantation, the regional perfusion index increased to 0.41 ± 0.22. During the 1- and 3-year follow-up period, sustained improvement in microcirculation was recorded. The most pronounced improvement in regional perfusion index values was observed in the subgroup of 13 patients with trophic lesions. In this group, the regional perfusion index increased significantly from 0.17 ± 0.21 to 0.4 ± 0.18 ($P < 0.02$) after a mean follow-up of 5.7 years. Limb survival rate was 93.1%.

Intermittent Pneumatic Compression

Intermittent pneumatic compression of the foot and calves has been used to augment perfusion to the lower extremities in patients with severe claudication or critical limb ischemia who are not candidates for revascularization because of advanced distal arterial occlusive disease, including those with TAO. In a retrospective study at the Mayo Clinic, the effect of intermittent pneumatic compression on nonhealing wounds was evaluated in 101 patients with critical limb ischemia and lower-extremity ulcerations.[114] Of all ulcerations, 64% were multifactorial in etiology, and 60% had associated transcutaneous oxygen tension levels below 20 mmHg. Patients were instructed to use the intermittent compression device on the affected limbs for 6 hours daily. Complete wound healing with limb preservation was achieved in 40% of patients with transcutaneous oxygen tension levels below 20 mmHg, 48% with osteomyelitis or active wound infection, 46% with insulin-requiring diabetes mellitus, and 28% with a previous amputation. Intermittent pneumatic compression appears to be most beneficial for patients with distal arterial occlusive disease and in whom revascularization is not feasible.

Therapeutic Angiogenesis and Cell-Based Therapy

A limited number of options for patients with severe distal arterial occlusive disease and critical limb ischemia due to TAO has driven a growing interest in therapeutic angiogenesis. In a study of seven limbs in six patients with TAO and critical limb ischemia, direct intramuscular injection of naked plasmid DNA-encoding vascular endothelial growth factor (VEGF) resulted in complete healing of ischemic ulcerations that were nonhealing for more than 1 month in three of five limbs.[115] Nocturnal rest pain was relieved in the remaining two patients with ulcerations. Evidence of improved perfusion to the distal ischemic limb included an increase of more than 0.1 in the ankle:brachial index in three limbs, improved flow shown by MR imaging in all seven limbs studied, and newly formed collateral vessels demonstrated on serial catheter-based angiography in all seven limbs studied. Two patients with advanced distal-extremity gangrene ultimately required below-knee amputation despite evidence of improved perfusion. The efficacy of therapeutic angiogenesis with VEGF gene transfer for patients with TAO requires confirmation in a prospective controlled trial.

Several studies have evaluated autologous bone marrow mononuclear cell implantation for patients with critical limb ischemia due to TAO.[116–119] Although short-term results with autologous bone marrow mononuclear cell implantation have been promising, long-term safety and efficacy remain to be demonstrated.[120] Autologous whole bone marrow stem cell transplantation may represent another promising avenue for therapeutic angiogenesis in patients with TAO.[121,122]

Revascularization Strategies

ENDOVASCULAR THERAPY

Endovascular therapy for arterial revascularization in patients with TAO remains controversial. Selective intraarterial infusion of fibrinolytic therapy has been reported as an adjunctive treatment in these patients.[123–126] In one series, selective low-dose intraarterial streptokinase (10,000 unit bolus followed by 5000 units/h infusion) was administered to 11 patients with TAO of the lower limbs that caused variable degrees of gangrene or pregangrene of the toes or feet, and who had no other possible therapeutic options except major amputation.[125] The investigators noted the overall success rate (defined as an altered or avoided amputation) to be 58.3%. Notably, bleeding complications were observed in 16.6% of the total at-risk limbs included in the study.

The efficacy of intraarterial fibrinolysis for TAO may not be as high as initially reported. From a pathological standpoint, the highly inflammatory thrombus observed in TAO is quickly invaded by fibroblasts and subsequently organized, making it quite resistant to fibrinolysis. In patients facing amputation and in whom no other alternatives for revascularization exist, a short trial of intraarterial fibrinolysis may be reasonable to avoid amputation in the absence of contraindications.

Other percutaneous techniques, including angioplasty and stent placement, have a very limited role in TAO treatment because of the distal and small-vessel nature of the disease.

SURGICAL REVASCULARIZATION

Surgical revascularization is usually not possible in patients with TAO because of the distal and diffuse nature of the disease, with extremely poor runoff. In addition, there is rarely a suitable distal target vessel for bypass. Short- and long-term patency rates are poor. Superficial thrombophlebitis of the lower extremities frequently limits the number and quality of venous conduits available for bypass surgery. However, surgical bypass using autologous vein may be considered in selected patients with severe ischemia, suitable distal target vessels, and good-quality venous conduits. In a series of 236 patients with TAO, only 11 (4.6%) had occlusive lesions that were amenable to surgery.[127] In a retrospective study of 101 patients with TAO who were followed for a mean of 10.6 years, outcomes after surgical bypass were often suboptimal, with primary patency rates of 41%, 32%, and 30% and secondary patency rates of 54%, 47%, and 39% at 1, 5, and 10 years, respectively.[98] Graft patency rates are nearly 50% lower in TAO patients who continue to smoke after surgical revascularization.[128] For reasons already mentioned, lower-extremity bypass surgery in patients with TAO is rarely carried out in the United States.[1–3,17–19]

Long-term patency of surgical bypass grafts is limited, but short-term patency may be sufficient to allow healing of ischemic ulcerations due to TAO and preservation of the at-risk limb. In a study of 94 patients with TAO, 27 of 36 (81%) patients who were eligible for surgery underwent revascularization.[129] During 36-month follow-up, patency rates at 12, 24, and 36 months were 59.2%, 48%, and 33.3%, respectively. Despite these low patency rates, limb salvage rate was 92.5%.

Another surgical option for patients with TAO consists of omental transfer.[130–134] In a study of 50 patients with TAO who underwent omental transfer, all had intermittent claudication, and 40 had evidence of critical limb ischemia such as rest pain, nonhealing ulcers, or gangrene.[134] All patients demonstrated improved skin temperature, 36 reported improved rest pain, and 48 noted increased claudication-free walking distance. Ischemic ulcerations healed in 32 of 36 patients. Despite these data, omental transfer has not been adopted by most major centers. The reason for this remains unclear but may be due to the lack of published data from centers outside of India where the technique was pioneered.

Unfortunately for a subset of patients with TAO, amputation is necessary to treat refractory rest pain or prevent progression of local infection, including osteomyelitis. In a registry of 111 patients with TAO followed for a mean of 15.6 years at the Mayo Clinic, risk of any amputation was reported to be 25% at 5 years, 38% at 10 years, and 46% at 20 years.[99] Risk of major amputation was observed to be 11% at 5 years, 21% at 10 years, and 23% at 20 years. Amputation rate was substantially reduced among patients who discontinued tobacco use compared with those who did not. The authors noted that the increased risk of amputation in former smokers was eliminated by 8 years after tobacco cessation.

Local Wound Care

For patients with areas of frank or threatened ischemic ulceration due to TAO, local wound care is of paramount importance. Consultation with wound care specialists can provide recommendations for dressings and other local interventions to aid wound

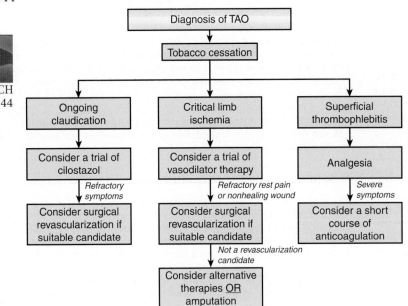

FIGURE 44-9 Overall therapeutic algorithm for patients with thromboangiitis obliterans (TAO).

healing. In addition, wound care specialists can educate patients about daily care and warning signs of progression or infection. In patients with more advanced ischemic ulcerations or gangrene, local débridement and appropriate antibiotic therapy may be required. Vacuum-assisted wound closure may be promising in patients with TAO and ischemic ulcerations, but requires further investigation.[135]

Supportive Care

Supportive care in patients with TAO and ischemic rest pain or ulcerations is identical to that for patients with critical limb ischemia due to any other arterial occlusive disease. A reverse Trendelenburg position should be used in patients who have severe ischemic rest pain. Adequate analgesia, with narcotics if required, should be used to manage periods of severe ischemic pain. Maintenance of central and peripheral warmth is crucial to reduce cold-induced vasospasm. Meticulous skin care of the hands and feet is important to prevent new ulcerations.

Unproven Therapies

Other alternative therapies that remain unproven in the treatment of patients with TAO include antiplatelet agents, anticoagulants, and hyperbaric oxygen therapy. Although they may be prescribed on an individual basis, the role of antiplatelet agents such as aspirin and clopidogrel has not been established in TAO. Likewise, therapeutic anticoagulation has never been shown to be effective in TAO treatment. Despite this, some clinicians have used anticoagulation in an effort to delay amputation and improve collateral flow in severe critical limb ischemia. A short 30- to 45-day course of anticoagulation may also be used in patients with severe symptoms due to superficial thrombophlebitis.[136,137] Pentoxifylline increases red blood cell membrane flexibility and has been used with limited benefit in patients with claudication due to atherosclerotic peripheral vascular disease of the lower extremities. Its role, if any, in TAO remains to be defined. Hyperbaric oxygen therapy has shown promise in the healing of cutaneous wounds due to a variety of disorders but has not been evaluated in treating TAO patients. Although they have pleomorphic effects that include modulation of inflammatory pathways, which may benefit patients with TAO, the role of statins in managing this disorder is unclear.

Overall Therapeutic Algorithm

An overall therapeutic algorithm for patients with TAO emphasizes tobacco cessation and then addresses symptoms based on extent of arterial and venous occlusive disease (Fig. 44-9).

Future Perspectives

Although the pathophysiology of TAO is not completely understood, the role of tobacco use in disease initiation and activity is indisputable. Continued population- and individual-based efforts to decrease the frequency of tobacco use will not only prevent TAO but also other smoking-related illnesses such as lung cancer, chronic obstructive pulmonary disease, and atherosclerotic cardiovascular disease.

For patients who are unable to discontinue tobacco use or for those who require palliative therapy to help them get through an episode of critical limb ischemia, more effective therapeutic alternatives would be beneficial. Gene therapy or cell-based therapy holds the greatest promise in this regard. Prospective randomized trials will have to be conducted to determine whether therapeutic angiogenesis is in fact a useful treatment strategy for patients with TAO. Since TAO is a vasculitis characterized by inflammatory thrombus, improved understanding of the mechanisms of inflammation in this disease as well as medications that modulate vascular inflammation may result in more effective therapy for this disorder.

REFERENCES

1. Piazza G, Creager MA: Thromboangiitis obliterans, *Circulation* 121:1858–1861, 2010.
2. Olin JW: Thromboangiitis obliterans (Buerger's disease), *N Engl J Med* 343:864–869, 2000.
3. Mills JL Sr: Buerger's disease in the 21st century: diagnosis, clinical features, and therapy, *Semin Vasc Surg* 16:179–189, 2003.
4. von Winiwarter F: Ueber eine eigenthumliche form von endarteritis und endophlebitis mit gangran des fusses, *Arch Klin Chir* 23:202–225, 1879.
5. Buerger L: Thrombo-angiitis obliterans: a study of the vascular lesions leading to presenile spontaneous gangrene, *Am J Med Sci* 136:567–580, 1908.
6. Allen EV, Brown GE: Thrombo-angiitis obliterans: a clinical study of 200 cases, *Ann Intern Med* 1:535–549, 1928.
7. Lie JT: The rise and fall and resurgence of thromboangiitis obliterans (Buerger's disease), *Acta Pathol Jpn* 39:153–158, 1989.
8. Lie JT: Thromboangiitis obliterans (Buerger's disease) revisited, *Pathol Annu* 23(Pt 2):257–291, 1988.
9. Herman BE: Buerger's syndrome, *Angiology* 26:713–716, 1975.
10. Cachovan M: Epidemiologie und geographisches verteilungsmuster der thromboangiitis obliterans. In Heidrich J, editor: *Thromboangiitis obliterans morbus Winiwarter-Buerger*, Stuttgart, New York, 1988, George Thieme, pp 31–36.

11. Matsushita M, Nishikimi N, Sakurai T, et al: Decrease in prevalence of Buerger's disease in Japan, *Surgery* 124:498–502, 1998.
12. Laohapensang K, Rerkasem K, Kattipattanapong V: Decrease in the incidence of Buerger's disease recurrence in northern Thailand, *Surg Today* 35:1060–1065, 2005.
13. Kobayashi M, Nishikimi N, Komori K: Current pathological and clinical aspects of Buerger's disease in Japan, *Ann Vasc Surg* 20:148–156, 2006.
14. McKusick VA, Harris WS: The Buerger syndrome in the Orient, 1961 *Bull Johns Hopkins Hosp*.
15. Hill GL, Moeliono J, Tumewu F, et al: The Buerger syndrome in Java A description of the clinical syndrome and some aspects of its aetiology, *Br J Surg* 60:606–613, 1973.
16. Nishikimi N, Shionoya S, Mizuno S: Result of national epidemiological study of Buerger's disease, *J Jpn Coll Angiol* 27:1125–1130, 1987.
17. Olin JW, Young JR, Graor RA, et al: The changing clinical spectrum of thromboangiitis obliterans (Buerger's disease), *Circulation* 82:IV3–IV8, 1990.
18. Mills JL, Taylor LM Jr, Porter JM: Buerger's disease in the modern era, *Am J Surg* 154: 123–129, 1987.
19. Lie JT: Thromboangiitis obliterans (Buerger's disease) in women, *Medicine (Baltimore)* 66:65–72, 1987.
20. Leu HJ: Buerger's thromboangiitis obliterans. Pathologico-anatomical analysis of 53 cases, *Schweiz Med Wochenschr* 115:1080–1086, 1985.
21. Lie JT: Thromboangiitis obliterans (Buerger's disease) and smokeless tobacco, *Arthritis Rheum* 31:812–813, 1988.
22. Disdier P, Granel B, Serratrice J, et al: Cannabis arteritis revisited–ten new case reports, *Angiology* 52:1–5, 2001.
23. Combemale P, Consort T, Denis-Thelis L, et al: Cannabis arteritis, *Br J Dermatol* 152: 166–169, 2005.
24. Olin JW, Shih A: Thromboangiitis obliterans (Buerger's disease), *Curr Opin Rheumatol* 18:18–24, 2006.
25. Kjeldsen K, Mozes M: Buerger's disease in Israel. Investigations on carboxyhemoglobin and serum cholesterol levels after smoking, *Acta Chir Scand* 135:495–498, 1969.
26. Westcott FN, Wright IS: Tobacco allergy and thromboangiitis obliterans, *J Allergy* 9:555–564, 1938.
27. Harkavy J: Tobacco sensitivities in thromboangiitis obliterans, migratory phlebitis, and coronary artery disease, *Bull N Y Acad Med* 9:318–322, 1933.
28. Rahman M, Chowdhury AS, Fukui T, et al: Association of thromboangiitis obliterans with cigarette and bidi smoking in Bangladesh: a case-control study, *Int J Epidemiol* 29: 266–270, 2000.
29. Matsushita M, Shionoya S, Matsumoto T: Urinary cotinine measurement in patients with Buerger's disease–effects of active and passive smoking on the disease process, *J Vasc Surg* 14:53–58, 1991.
30. McLoughlin GA, Helsby CR, Evans CC, et al: Association of HLA-A9 and HLA-B5 with Buerger's disease, *BMJ* 2:1165–1166, 1976.
31. Papa M, Bass A, Adar R, et al: Autoimmune mechanisms in thromboangiitis obliterans (Buerger's disease): the role of tobacco antigen and the major histocompatibility complex, *Surgery* 111:527–531, 1992.
32. Chen Z, Takahashi M, Naruse T, et al: Synergistic contribution of CD14 and HLA loci in the susceptibility to Buerger disease, *Hum Genet* 122:367–372, 2007.
33. Glueck CJ, Haque M, Winarska M, et al: Stromelysin-1 5A/6A and eNOS T-786C polymorphisms, MTHFR C677T and A1298C mutations, and cigarette-cannabis smoking: a pilot, hypothesis-generating study of gene-environment pathophysiological associations with Buerger's disease, *Clin Appl Thromb Hemost* 12:427–439, 2006.
34. Adiguzel Y, Yilmaz E, Akar N: Effect of eNOS and ET-1 polymorphisms in thromboangiitis obliterans, *Clin Appl Thromb Hemost* 16:103–106, 2010.
35. Choudhury NA, Pietraszek MH, Hachiya T, et al: Plasminogen activators and plasminogen activator inhibitor 1 before and after venous occlusion of the upper limb in thromboangiitis obliterans (Buerger's disease), *Thromb Res* 66:321–329, 1992.
36. Pietraszek MH, Choudhury NA, Koyano K, et al: Enhanced platelet response to serotonin in Buerger's disease, *Thromb Res* 60:241–246, 1990.
37. Carr ME Jr, Hackney MH, Hines SJ, et al: Enhanced platelet force development despite drug-induced inhibition of platelet aggregation in patients with thromboangiitis obliterans–two case reports, *Vasc Endovascular Surg* 36:473–480, 2002.
38. Brodmann M, Renner W, Stark G, et al: Prothrombotic risk factors in patients with thrombangitis obliterans, *Thromb Res* 99:483–486, 2000.
39. Avcu F, Akar E, Demirkilic U, et al: The role of prothrombotic mutations in patients with Buerger's disease, *Thromb Res* 100:143–147, 2000.
40. Olin JW, Childs MB, Bartholomew JR, et al: Anticardiolipin antibodies and homocysteine levels in patients with thromboangiitis obliterans, *Arthritis Rheum* 39:S-47, 1996.
41. Olin JW: Are anticardiolipin antibodies really important in thromboangiitis obliterans (Buerger's disease)? *Vasc Med* 7:257–258, 2002.
42. Maslowski L, McBane R, Alexewicz P, et al: Antiphospholipid antibodies in thromboangiitis obliterans, *Vasc Med* 7:259–264, 2002.
43. Adar R, Papa MZ, Halpern Z, et al: Cellular sensitivity to collagen in thromboangiitis obliterans, *N Engl J Med* 308:1113–1116, 1983.
44. Roncon de Albuquerque R, Delgado L, Correia P, et al: Circulating immune complexes in Buerger's disease. Endarteritis obliterans in young men, *J Cardiovasc Surg (Torino)* 30:821–825, 1989.
45. Gulati SM, Saha K, Kant L, et al: Significance of circulatory immune complexes in thromboangiitis obliterans (Buerger's disease), *Angiology* 35:276–281, 1984.
46. Kobayashi M, Ito M, Nakagawa A, et al: Immunohistochemical analysis of arterial wall cellular infiltration in Buerger's disease (endarteritis obliterans), *J Vasc Surg* 29:451–458, 1999.
47. Lee T, Seo JW, Sumpio BE, et al: Immunobiologic analysis of arterial tissue in Buerger's disease, *Eur J Vasc Endovasc Surg* 25:451–457, 2003.
48. Kurata A, Machinami R, Schulz A, et al: Different immunophenotypes in Buerger's disease, *Pathol Int* 53:608–615, 2003.
49. Eichhorn J, Sima D, Lindschau C, et al: Antiendothelial cell antibodies in thromboangiitis obliterans, *Am J Med Sci* 315:17–23, 1998.
50. Makita S, Nakamura M, Murakami H, et al: Impaired endothelium-dependent vasorelaxation in peripheral vasculature of patients with thromboangiitis obliterans (Buerger's disease), *Circulation* 94:II211–II215, 1996.
51. Idei N, Nishioka K, Soga J, et al: Vascular function and circulating progenitor cells in thromboangiitis obliterans (Buerger's disease) and atherosclerosis obliterans, *Hypertension* 57:70–78, 2011.
52. Halacheva K, Gulubova MV, Manolova I, et al: Expression of ICAM-1, VCAM-1, E-selectin and TNF-alpha on the endothelium of femoral and iliac arteries in thromboangiitis obliterans, *Acta Histochem* 104:177–184, 2002.
53. Iwai T, Inoue Y, Umeda M, et al: Oral bacteria in the occluded arteries of patients with Buerger disease, *J Vasc Surg* 42:107–115, 2005.
54. Dible JH: *The pathology of limb ischemia*, Edinburgh, 1966, Oliver & Boyd.
55. Leu HJ, Bollinger A: Migrating phlebitis, *Vasa* 7:440–442, 1978.
56. Fazeli B, Modaghegh H, Ravrai H, et al: Thrombophlebitis migrans as a footprint of Buerger's disease: a prospective-descriptive study in north-east of Iran, *Clin Rheumatol* 27:55–57, 2008.
57. Wang MH, Jin X, Wu XJ, et al: Phosphatidylcholine-specific phospholipase C activity and level increase evidently in thromboangiitis obliterans, *Biofactors* 36:196–200, 2010.
58. Shionoya S, Ban I, Nakata Y, et al: Involvement of the iliac artery in Buerger's disease (pathogenesis and arterial reconstruction), *J Cardiovasc Surg (Torino)* 19:69–76, 1978.
59. Ates A, Yekeler I, Ceviz M, et al: One of the most frequent vascular diseases in northeastern of Turkey: thromboangiitis obliterans or Buerger's disease (experience with 344 cases), *Int J Cardiol* 111:147–153, 2006.
60. Shionoya S: Buerger's disease (thromboangiitis obliterans). In Rutherford RB, editor: *Vascular surgery*, ed 3, Philadelphia, 1989, WB Saunders, pp 207–217.
61. Sasaki S, Sakuma M, Kunihara T, et al: Distribution of arterial involvement in thromboangiitis obliterans (Buerger's disease): results of a study conducted by the Intractable Vasculitis Syndromes Research Group in Japan, *Surg Today* 30:600–605, 2000.
62. Tavakoli H, Rezaii J, Esfandiari K, et al: Buerger's disease: a 10-year experience in Tehran, Iran, *Clin Rheumatol* 27:369–371, 2008.
63. Yamamoto K, Iwase S, Mano T, et al: Muscle sympathetic outflow in Buerger's disease, *J Auton Nerv Syst* 44:67–75, 1993.
64. Kimura T, Yoshizaki S, Tsushima N, et al: Buerger's colour, *Br J Surg* 77:1299–1301, 1990.
65. Papa MZ, Adar R: A critical look at thromboangiitis obliterans (Buerger's disease), *Vasc Surg* 5:1–21, 1992.
66. Alpaslan M, Akgun G, Doven O, et al: Thrombus in the main pulmonary artery of a patient with thromboangiitis obliterans: observation by transthoracic echocardiography, *Eur J Echocardiogr* 2:139–140, 2001.
67. Siddiqui MZ, Reis ED, Soundararajan K, et al: Buerger's disease affecting mesenteric arteries: a rare cause of intestinal ischemia–a case report, *Vasc Surg* 35:235–238, 2001.
68. Leung DK, Haskal ZJ: SIR 2006 film panel case: mesenteric involvement and bowel infarction due to Buerger disease, *J Vasc Interv Radiol* 17:1087–1089, 2006.
69. Kobayashi M, Kurose K, Kobata T, et al: Ischemic intestinal involvement in a patient with Buerger disease: case report and literature review, *J Vasc Surg* 38:170–174, 2003.
70. Hassoun Z, Lacrosse M, De Ronde T: Intestinal involvement in Buerger's disease, *J Clin Gastroenterol* 32:85–89, 2001.
71. Cho YP, Kwon YM, Kwon TW, et al: Mesenteric Buerger's disease, *Ann Vasc Surg* 17:221–223, 2003.
72. Cho YP, Kang GH, Han MS, et al: Mesenteric involvement of acute-stage Buerger's disease as the initial clinical manifestation: report of a case, *Surg Today* 35:499–501, 2005.
73. Zulch KJ: The cerebral form of von Winiwarter-Buerger's disease: does it exist? *Angiology* 20:61–69, 1969.
74. No YJ, Lee EM, Lee DH, et al: Cerebral angiographic findings in thromboangiitis obliterans, *Neuroradiology* 47:912–915, 2005.
75. Lippmann HI: Cerebrovascular thrombosis in patients with Buerger's disease, *Circulation* 5:680–692, 1952.
76. Bozikas VP, Vlaikidis N, Petrikis P, et al: Schizophrenic-like symptoms in a patient with thrombo-angiitis obliterans (Winiwarter-Buerger's disease), *Int J Psychiatry Med* 31:341–346, 2001.
77. Berlit P, Kessler C, Reuther R, et al: New aspects of thromboangiitis obliterans (von Winiwarter-Buerger's disease), *Eur Neurol* 23:394–399, 1984.
78. Tamura A, Aso N, Kadota J: Corkscrew appearance in the right coronary artery in a patient with Buerger's disease, *Heart* 92:944, 2006.
79. Hsu PC, Lin TH, Su HM, et al: Frequent accelerated idioventricular rhythm in a young male of Buerger's disease with acute myocardial infarction, *Int J Cardiol* 127:e64–e66, 2008.
80. Hoppe B, Lu JT, Thistlewaite P, et al: Beyond peripheral arteries in Buerger's disease: angiographic considerations in thromboangiitis obliterans, *Catheter Cardiovasc Interv* 57:363–366, 2002.
81. Hong TE, Faxon DP: Coronary artery disease in patients with Buerger's disease, *Rev Cardiovasc Med* 6:222–226, 2005.
82. Abe M, Kimura T, Furukawa Y, et al: Coronary Buerger's disease with a peripheral arterial aneurysm, *Eur Heart J* 28:928, 2007.
83. Goktas S, Bedir S, Bozlar U, et al: Intrarenal arterial stenosis in a patient with thromboangiitis obliterans, *Int J Urol* 13:1243–1244, 2006.
84. Yavas US, Calisir C, Kaya T: Vasculogenic impotence as a symptom in late-onset Buerger's disease, *J Clin Ultrasound* 35:469–472, 2007.
85. Lie JT, Michet CJ Jr: Thromboangiitis obliterans with eosinophilia (Buerger's disease) of the temporal arteries, *Hum Pathol* 19:598–602, 1988.
86. Flammer J, Pache M, Resink T: Vasospasm, its role in the pathogenesis of diseases with particular reference to the eye, *Prog Retin Eye Res* 20:319–349, 2001.
87. Lie JT: Thromboangiitis obliterans (Buerger's disease) in a saphenous vein arterial graft, *Hum Pathol* 18:402–404, 1987.
88. Shionoya S: What is Buerger's disease? *World J Surg* 7:544–551, 1983.
89. Papa MZ, Rabi I, Adar R: A point scoring system for the clinical diagnosis of Buerger's disease, *Eur J Vasc Endovasc Surg* 11:335–339, 1996.
90. Adar R, Papa MZ, Schneiderman J: Thromboangiitis obliterans: an old disease in need of a new look, *Int J Cardiol* 75(Suppl 1):S167–S170, 2000; discussion S171–S163.
91. Mills JL, Porter JM: Buerger's disease: a review and update, *Semin Vasc Surg* 6:14–23, 1993.
92. Fujii Y, Nishioka K, Yoshizumi M, et al: Images in cardiovascular medicine. Corkscrew collaterals in thromboangiitis obliterans (Buerger's disease), *Circulation* 116:e539–e540, 2007.

93. Jaccard Y, Walther S, Anderson S, et al: Influence of secondary infection on amputation in chronic critical limb ischemia, *Eur J Vasc Endovasc Surg* 33:605–609, 2007.

94. Olin JW, Lie JT: Thromboangiitis obliterans (Buerger's disease). In Cooke JP, Frohlich ED, editors: *Current management of hypertension and vascular disease*, St. Louis, 1992, Mosby-Yearbook, pp 265–271.

95. Lambeth JT, Yong NK: Arteriographic findings in thromboangiitis obliterans with emphasis on femoropopliteal involvement, *Am J Roentgenol Radium Ther Nucl Med* 109:553–562, 1970.

96. McKusick VA, Harris WS, Ottsen OE: Buerger's disease: a distinct clinical and pathologic entity, *JAMA* 181:93–100, 1962.

97. McKusick VA, Harris WS, Ottsen OE: The Buerger's syndrome in the United States: arteriographic observations with special reference to involvement of the upper extremities and the differentiation from atherosclerosis and embolism, *Bull Johns Hopkins Hosp* 110:145–176, 1962.

98. Ohta T, Ishioashi H, Hosaka M, et al: Clinical and social consequences of Buerger disease, *J Vasc Surg* 39:176–180, 2004.

99. Cooper LT, Tse TS, Mikhail MA, et al: Long-term survival and amputation risk in thromboangiitis obliterans (Buerger's disease), *J Am Coll Cardiol* 44:2410–2411, 2004.

100. Gifford RW Jr, EA Hines Jr: Complete clinical remission in thromboangiitis obliterans during abstinence from tobacco: report of case, *Proc Staff Meet Mayo Clin* 26:241–245, 1951.

101. Corelli F: Buerger's disease: cigarette smoker disease may always be cured by medical therapy alone. Uselessness of operative treatment, *J Cardiovasc Surg (Torino)* 14:28–36, 1973.

102. Cooper LT, Henderson SS, Ballman KV, et al: A prospective, case-control study of tobacco dependence in thromboangiitis obliterans (Buerger's disease), *Angiology* 57:73–78, 2006.

103. Fiessinger JN, Schafer M: Trial of iloprost versus aspirin treatment for critical limb ischaemia of thromboangiitis obliterans. The TAO Study, *Lancet* 335:555–557, 1990.

104. Hildebrand M: Pharmacokinetics and tolerability of oral iloprost in thromboangiitis obliterans patients, *Eur J Clin Pharmacol* 53:51–56, 1997.

105. The European TAO Study Group: Oral iloprost in the treatment of thromboangiitis obliterans (Buerger's disease): a double-blind, randomised, placebo-controlled trial, *Eur J Vasc Endovasc Surg* 15:300–307, 1998.

106. Dean SM, Vaccaro PS: Successful pharmacologic treatment of lower extremity ulcerations in 5 patients with chronic critical limb ischemia, *J Am Board Fam Pract* 15:55–62, 2002.

107. Dean SM, Satiani B: Three cases of digital ischemia successfully treated with cilostazol, *Vasc Med* 6:245–248, 2001.

108. Paraskevas KI, Trigka AA, Samara M: Successful intravenous regional sympathetic blockade (Bier's Block) with guanethidine and lidocaine in a patient with advanced Buerger's disease (thromboangiitis obliterans)–a case report, *Angiology* 56:493–496, 2005.

109. Swigris JJ, Olin JW, Mekhail NA: Implantable spinal cord stimulator to treat the ischemic manifestations of thromboangiitis obliterans (Buerger's disease), *J Vasc Surg* 29:928–935, 1999.

110. Pace AV, Saratzis N, Karokis D, et al: Spinal cord stimulation in Buerger's disease, *Ann Rheum Dis* 61:1114, 2002.

111. Chierichetti F, Mambrini S, Bagliani A, et al: Treatment of Buerger's disease with electrical spinal cord stimulation–review of three cases, *Angiology* 53:341–347, 2002.

112. Boari B, Salmi R, Manfredini R: Buerger's disease: spinal cord stimulation may represent a useful tool for delaying amputation in young patients, *Eur J Intern Med* 18:259, 2007.

113. Donas KP, Schulte S, Ktenidis K, et al: The role of epidural spinal cord stimulation in the treatment of Buerger's disease, *J Vasc Surg* 41:830–836, 2005.

114. Montori VM, Kavros SJ, Walsh EE, et al: Intermittent compression pump for nonhealing wounds in patients with limb ischemia. The Mayo Clinic experience (1998-2000), *Int Angiol* 21:360–366, 2002.

115. Isner JM, Baumgartner I, Rauh G, et al: Treatment of thromboangiitis obliterans (Buerger's disease) by intramuscular gene transfer of vascular endothelial growth factor: preliminary clinical results, *J Vasc Surg* 28:964–973, 1998; discussion 973–965.

116. Saito Y, Sasaki K, Katsuda Y, et al: Effect of autologous bone-marrow cell transplantation on ischemic ulcer in patients with Buerger's disease, *Circ J* 71:1187–1192, 2007.

117. Saito S, Nishikawa K, Obata H, et al: Autologous bone marrow transplantation and hyperbaric oxygen therapy for patients with thromboangiitis obliterans, *Angiology* 58:429–434, 2007.

118. Matoba S, Tatsumi T, Murohara T, et al: Long-term clinical outcome after intramuscular implantation of bone marrow mononuclear cells (Therapeutic Angiogenesis by Cell Transplantation [TACT] trial) in patients with chronic limb ischemia, *Am Heart J* 156:1010–1018, 2008.

119. Durdu S, Akar AR, Arat M, et al: Autologous bone-marrow mononuclear cell implantation for patients with Rutherford grade II-III thromboangiitis obliterans, *J Vasc Surg* 44:732–739, 2006.

120. Miyamoto K, Nishigami K, Nagaya N, et al: Unblinded pilot study of autologous transplantation of bone marrow mononuclear cells in patients with thromboangiitis obliterans, *Circulation* 114:2679–2684, 2006.

121. Kim SW, Han H, Chae GT, et al: Successful stem cell therapy using umbilical cord blood-derived multipotent stem cells for Buerger's disease and ischemic limb disease animal model, *Stem Cells* 24:1620–1626, 2006.

122. Kim DI, Kim MJ, Joh JH, et al: Angiogenesis facilitated by autologous whole bone marrow stem cell transplantation for Buerger's disease, *Stem Cells* 24:1194–1200, 2006.

123. Lang EV, Bookstein JJ: Accelerated thrombolysis and angioplasty for hand ischemia in Buerger's disease, *Cardiovasc Intervent Radiol* 12:95–97, 1989.

124. Kubota Y, Kichikawa K, Uchida H, et al: Superselective urokinase infusion therapy for dorsalis pedis artery occlusion in Buerger's disease, *Cardiovasc Intervent Radiol* 20:380–382, 1997.

125. Hussein EA, A el Dorri: Intra-arterial streptokinase as adjuvant therapy for complicated Buerger's disease: early trials, *Int Surg* 78:54–58, 1993.

126. Hodgson TJ, Gaines PA, Beard JD: Thrombolysis and angioplasty for acute lower limb ischemia in Buerger's disease, *Cardiovasc Intervent Radiol* 17:333–335, 1994.

127. Inada K, Iwashima Y, Okada A, et al: Nonatherosclerotic segmental arterial occlusion of the extremity, *Arch Surg* 108:663–667, 1974.

128. Sasajima T, Kubo Y, Inaba M, et al: Role of infrainguinal bypass in Buerger's disease: an eighteen-year experience, *Eur J Vasc Endovasc Surg* 13:186–192, 1997.

129. Dilege S, Aksoy M, Kayabali M, et al: Vascular reconstruction in Buerger's disease: is it feasible? *Surg Today* 32:1042–1047, 2002.

130. Talwar S, Prasad P: Single-stage lumbar sympathectomy and omentopexy: a new surgical approach towards patients with Buerger's disease, *Trop Doct* 31:73–75, 2001.

131. Talwar S, Jain S, Porwal R, et al: Free versus pedicled omental grafts for limb salvage in Buerger's disease, *Aust N Z J Surg* 68:38–40, 1998.

132. Talwar S, Jain S, Porwal R, et al: Pedicled omental transfer for limb salvage in Buerger's disease, *Int J Cardiol* 72:127–132, 2000.

133. Talwar S, Choudhary SK: Omentopexy for limb salvage in Buerger's disease: indications, technique and results, *J Postgrad Med* 47:137–142, 2001.

134. Singh I, Ramteke VK: The role of omental transfer in Buerger's disease: New Delhi's experience, *Aust N Z J Surg* 66:372–376, 1996.

135. Canter HI, Isci E, Erk Y: Vacuum-assisted wound closure for the management of a foot ulcer due to Buerger's disease, *J Plast Reconstr Aesthet Surg* 62:250–253, 2009.

136. Geerts WH, Bergqvist D, Pineo GF, et al: Prevention of venous thromboembolism: American College of Chest Physicians evidence-based clinical practice guidelines (8th edition), *Chest* 133:381S–453S, 2008.

137. Decousus H, Prandoni P, Mismetti P, et al: Fondaparinux for the treatment of superficial-vein thrombosis in the legs, *N Engl J Med* 363:1222–1232, 2010.

CHAPTER 45 Kawasaki Disease

David R. Fulton, Jane W. Newburger

Kawasaki disease, initially described by Dr. Tomisaku Kawasaki in 1967,[1] is an acute systemic vasculitis of uncertain etiology that predominantly affects infants and young children. The disease has been described worldwide and occurs in all populations. The classic presentation of the illness is marked by at least 4 days of fever, oral mucositis, nonexudative conjunctivitis, erythematous nonvesicular rash, changes in the hands and feet including edema or erythema, and cervical lymphadenopathy[2] (Box 45-1). Coronary artery dilation or aneurysms affect up to 25% of those who are not treated with intravenous gamma globulin (IVIG) early in the course of the disease. In patients who develop aneurysms, angina, myocardial infarction (MI), and death may ensue during the acute phase[3] or months to years later.[4]

Epidemiology

Despite its description in diverse areas of the world, by far the greatest number of cases have been reported in Japan. Indeed, in the most recent Japanese nationwide survey performed in calendar years 2007 and 2008, the incidence rate was over 200 per 100,000 children younger than 5 years of age.[5] In Japan, 1.4% of cases occur in children with a previously affected sibling. The disease can recur (≈3.5% in Japan), but person-to-person transmission is unusual. Lack of a mandatory national reporting system in the United States hinders epidemiological analysis, but administrative data from hospital discharge abstracts suggested that more than 4000 U.S. hospitalizations were associated with Kawasaki disease in the year 2000.[6] Among children younger than age 5, occurrence was greatest in Asians (33.3/100,000), somewhat less in African Americans (23.4/100,000), and lowest in Caucasians (12.7/100,000).[6] Outbreaks are more likely in the late winter and early spring, suggesting an infectious etiology, but a steady background activity of cases is noted throughout the remainder of the year. Males outnumber females, generally in a ratio of 1.4:1. Although Kawasaki disease is most common in children younger than age 5, the illness is being more commonly recognized in older children and adolescents.[7]

Etiology and Pathogenesis

The search for an etiological agent has been wide-ranging over the course of the past 3 decades, but to date the cause of Kawasaki disease is unknown. Although Kawasaki disease is not spread by person-to-person transmission, features suggesting an infectious etiology include its peak incidence in young children; clinical features including fever, rash, and conjunctivitis; the increase in incidence in winter and early spring; and the past occurrence of nationwide epidemics in Japan. Prior exposure of index cases to freshly cleaned carpets has been reported to be a risk factor by some investigators,[8] although other studies have not confirmed this association,[9] and no specific organism or toxin has been identified in the rugs. Some researchers hold that Kawasaki disease is caused by a single agent,[10] but others believe the marked immune response typical in Kawasaki disease can be triggered by a variety of different agents.[11] Reports of selective expansion of $V_\beta 2$ and $V_\beta 8$ T-cell receptor families have implicated specific superantigens, including TSST-1-secreting strains of *Staphylococcus aureus* and streptococcal pyrogenic exotoxin B- and C-producing streptococci.[12] The only animal model of Kawasaki disease, which uses *Lactobacillus casei* to induce coronary arteritis in mice, implicates a toxin-mediated etiology.[13] By contrast, Rowley has found support for a typical antigen-driven response by demonstrating oligoclonal immunoglobulin (Ig)A plasma cells and IgA heavy chain genes, as

well as macrophages and CD8 T lymphocytes in inflamed arterial tissue of individuals with fatal Kawasaki disease.[14] With a synthetic IgA antibody, these investigators have demonstrated intracytoplasmic inclusion bodies with aggregates of nucleic acids and viral proteins in the proximal bronchial epithelium and coronary arteries in most postmortem specimens from Kawasaki disease.[15] These ribonucleic acid (RNA)-containing cytoplasmic inclusion bodies were demonstrated in 85% of postmortem specimens from Kawasaki disease patients but few young age-matched children. The finding that 25% of older children but adult controls have such inclusion bodies postmortem is consistent with the hypothesis that Kawasaki disease could be caused by a ubiquitous RNA virus that persists and causes the clinical features of Kawasaki disease in susceptible children.[16,17]

Kawasaki disease is accompanied by significant derangements in the immunoregulatory system that lead to coronary inflammation and coronary artery abnormalities (dilation, aneurysm formation, and giant aneurysms) in some patients. Profound immune activation is evidenced by release of proinflammatory cytokines and growth factors, endothelial cell (EC) activation, and infiltration of the coronary arterial wall first by neutrophils, and then by CD68+ monocyte/macrophages, CD8+, CD3+, and CD20+ lymphocytes, and IgA plasma cells.[18-26]

Release of matrix metalloproteinases (MMPs) may further disrupt arterial wall integrity, leading to aneurysms of the coronary arteries and occasionally of other extraparenchymal medium-sized muscular arteries.[27] Kawasaki disease patients with coronary artery lesions have higher levels of MMPs and higher ratios of MMPs to tissue inhibitors of metalloproteinases (TIMPs) than those without coronary abnormalities,[28] suggesting these circulating proteins may play an active role in coronary arterial remodeling. Data to suggest an important role for MMPs in the pathogenesis of aneurysms also comes from recent research on genetic risk factors, showing that MMP-3 rs3025058 (–/T) and haplotypes containing MMP-3 rs3025058 (–/T) and MMP-12 rs2276109 (A/G) were associated with a higher risk of aneurysm formation.[29]

Genetic factors have long been recognized to play an important role in susceptibility to Kawasaki disease. Children of Japanese ancestry have a relative risk 10 to 15 times higher than that of Caucasian children, whether they live in Japan or the United States. Furthermore, siblings have a relative risk 6 to 10 times greater than that of children without a family history. The parents of Japanese children with Kawasaki disease are twice as likely to have had the disease themselves in childhood than expected in the general population.[30] In addition to MMP haplotypes, increased susceptibility to Kawasaki disease has been related to genetic variations in the transforming growth factor (TGF)-β pathway,[31] CC chemokine receptor 5 (CCR5) and/or its ligand CCL3L1,[32] and ITPKC (a negative regulator of T cell activation)[33] among others. In a genome-wide association study, investigators recently identified a single functional network containing LNX1, CAMK2D, ZFHX3, CSMD1, and TCP1, believed to be relevant to inflammation and apoptosis.[34] Functional genomics may eventually allow development of new diagnostic tests and therapies for Kawasaki disease.

Pathology

Because mortality in this disease is uncommon (ranging from 0%-0.17% in the United States), published studies on the histopathology of early Kawasaki disease are limited.[35,36] The original pathological description of Kawasaki disease by Fujiwara and Hamashima was based on autopsy findings of children dying in the acute and subacute phases of Kawasaki disease

Box 45-1   Principal Clinical Findings in Kawasaki Disease*

Fever persisting at least 4 days or more without other source in association with at least 4 principal features:
1. Oral changes that may include erythema or cracking of the lips, strawberry tongue, erythema of the oral mucosa
2. Bilateral nonexudative conjunctival injection
3. Polymorphous rash, generally truncal involvement, nonvesicular
4. Changes of extremities that may include erythema and edema of the hands or feet; desquamation of fingers and toes 1 to 3 weeks after onset of illness
5. Cervical lymphadenopathy, often unilateral, with at least 1 node ≥1.5 cm

*Patients with fever and fewer than four criteria can be diagnosed with the presence of coronary artery disease (CAD) by two-dimensional (2D) echocardiography or coronary angiography. Adapted from American Heart Association Scientific Statement: Diagnosis, treatment, and long-term management of Kawasaki disease. Circulation 110:2751, 2004.

before available treatment with IVIG.[35] In this early study, they established four categories of illness on the basis of time from onset of the disease: stage 1 (0-9 days), stage 2 (12-25 days), stage 3 (28-31 days), and stage 4 (40 days-4 years). Stage 1 was characterized by vasculitis of small vessels and microvessels, perivasculitis and endarteritis of the coronary vessels, and pancarditis. Pancarditis was seen also in stage 2, with coronary artery vasculitis, sometimes with aneurysm formation and coronary thrombosis. By stage 3, the acute inflammation had subsided, but myointimal proliferation of the coronary arteries was evident. In stage 4, coronary artery stenosis was noted for the first time. In stage 1, death resulted from arrhythmia and myocarditis, with evolution to ischemia and infarction with greater time from onset of disease to postmortem examination. Indeed, patients who die late after Kawasaki disease often have coronary artery stenoses resulting from neointimal proliferation and fibrosis.[35,36] Within aneurysms, the internal elastic lamina is disrupted, and medial smooth muscle is replaced by fibroblasts and extracellular matrix (ECM).[37] Finally, growth factors are expressed in the areas subjected to the greatest shear stress, particularly at the proximal and distal ends of an aneurysm.[38] Peripheral artery aneurysms (e.g., occurring in axillary or iliac arteries) are found only among patients with giant coronary artery aneurysms.

Clinical Presentation

Because no laboratory test or pathognomonic feature is available for Kawasaki disease, the diagnosis must be made on clinical grounds. First described by Kawasaki on the basis of his observations in Japanese children,[39] the classic criteria have continued to serve as the standard adopted by the American Heart Association (AHA; see Box 45-1) for arriving at the diagnosis.[2] They include fever for 4 days or more and at least 4 of the 5 following findings: (1) a nonexudative bilateral conjunctivitis, (2) oral changes with erythematous or dry cracked lips, strawberry tongue, or pharyngitis, (3) a nonvesicular rash, often involving the trunk, perineum, and extremities, (4) erythema of the palmar and plantar surfaces, edema of the hands or feet, or periungual desquamation 2 weeks after illness onset, and (5) anterior cervical lymphadenopathy of 1.5 cm or greater, usually unilateral. Alternatively, the diagnosis can be made with fewer than 4 of 5 criteria in the presence of coronary artery abnormalities. Not all criteria have to be present simultaneously to make the diagnosis; indeed, it is common for some findings to resolve as others appear, making serial evaluation of the child essential.

The epidemiological case definition is not fulfilled in almost a third of children who develop coronary artery aneurysms.[40] To capture incomplete cases, the 2004 AHA recommendations include an algorithm for evaluation and treatment of suspected Kawasaki disease in children with at least 5 days of fever and only two or three clinical criteria.[2] Furthermore, infants younger than 6 months of age present a particular challenge because they often have incomplete criteria, yet are at greater risk for development of coronary artery abnormalities. The diagnosis should be considered and echocardiography performed in young infants who have fever for

Box 45-2   Other Significant Clinical and Laboratory Findings in Kawasaki Disease

Cardiovascular
On auscultation, gallop rhythm or distant heart sounds; ECG changes (arrhythmias, abnormal Q waves, prolonged PR or QT intervals or both; occasionally low-voltage or ST-T wave changes); chest x-ray abnormalities (cardiomegaly); echocardiographic changes (pericardial effusion, coronary aneurysms, or decreased contractility); mitral or aortic valvular insufficiency or both; and (rarely) aneurysms of peripheral arteries (e.g., axillary), angina pectoris, or MI

Gastrointestinal
Diarrhea, vomiting, abdominal pain, hydrops of gallbladder, paralytic ileus, mild jaundice, and mild increase of serum transaminase levels

Blood
Increased ESR, leukocytosis with left shift, positive CRP, hypoalbuminemia, and mild anemia in acute phase of illness (thrombocytosis in subacute phase)

Urine
Sterile pyuria of urethral origin and occasional proteinuria

Skin
Perineal rash and desquamation in subacute phase and transverse furrows of fingernails (Beau's lines) during convalescence

Respiratory
Cough, rhinorrhea, and pulmonary infiltrate

Joints
Arthralgia and arthritis

Neurological
Mononuclear pleocytosis in cerebrospinal fluid, striking irritability, and (rarely) facial palsy

CRP, C-reactive protein; ECG, electrocardiogram; ESR, erythrocyte sedimentation rate; MI, myocardial infarction. Adapted from American Heart Association Scientific Statement: Diagnosis, treatment, and long-term management of Kawasaki disease. Circulation 110:2751, 2004.

at least 7 days without documented source and whose laboratory tests indicate substantial systemic inflammation.[2]

Other supportive signs are present in many children with Kawasaki disease (Box 45-2). The rash, when perineal in location, often desquamates by the end of the first week of illness. Anterior uveitis can be identified by slit-lamp examination in 83% of patients early in the course.[41] Arthralgia and arthritis of large and small joints may be severe enough that children refuse to walk or perform tasks with their hands, but the arthritis is virtually never chronic. Abdominal signs including vomiting, diarrhea, or hydrops of the gallbladder are common.

Laboratory values in the acute phase are consistent with systemic inflammation. Acute-phase reactants, including erythrocyte sedimentation rate (ESR) and C-reactive protein (CRP), are markedly increased. White blood cell (WBC) count is elevated with a leftward shift, and a normochromic, normocytic anemia is noted within the first week of illness. Thrombocytosis is usually present by the second week of the disease, often peaking at counts greater than 1,000,000 mm[3] in association with hypercoagulability. These parameters often persist over the first month of the illness and gradually decline. Hepatocellular inflammation is accompanied by increases in γ-glutamyl transferase. Sterile pyuria and pleocytosis of cerebrospinal fluid,[42] both with mononuclear cells, are found frequently. Laboratory measures of systemic inflammation usually return to normal by 6 to 8 weeks after illness onset.

Cardiac Manifestations

Coronary Artery Abnormalities

Kawasaki disease causes coronary artery abnormalities in 15% to 25% of patients who are not treated in the acute phase of the disease with high-dose IVIG. Lesions may be observed by echocardiography as early as 1 week from the onset of fever, with further progression of aneurysms ensuing in the next 3 to 4 weeks. Given the difficulty in reaching diagnostic confirmation of the illness using the classic criteria, identification of those at higher risk for coronary disease and for whom early treatment could reduce extent of involvement has led investigators to focus on predictive factors for coronary artery abnormalities. Many studies have explored predictors of coronary artery aneurysms. Late diagnosis and treatment with IVIG is the most important modifiable risk factor.[43] Infants younger than age 6 months are at the highest risk for developing aneurysms, even when they are treated within the first 10 days of illness. The youngest infants frequently present with incomplete or atypical features, further increasing their risk of aneurysms by delaying diagnosis and IVIG treatment. Older children are also at higher risk for coronary aneurysms, in part because care providers do not consider Kawasaki disease as high in the differential diagnosis of the older child with fever.[44] Many studies have highlighted the association of coronary aneurysms with persistent and recrudescent fever, as well as with IVIG resistance.[45,46] Greater derangement of laboratory measures of the acute-phase response, reflecting more severe vasculitis, is also predictive and include lower hematocrit or hemoglobin (Hb), lower serum albumin, lower serum sodium, higher alanine aminotransferase, higher CRP and ESR, lower baseline serum IgG, and elevations in interleukin (IL)-6, IL-8, and other biomarkers.[47–49] In addition, genetic polymorphisms (e.g., MMP haplotypes,[29] polymorphisms of vascular endothelial growth factor [VEGF] and its receptors[50]) affect host susceptibility to aneurysms.

Myocarditis

In acute Kawasaki disease, myocarditis is a frequent finding at autopsy and by biopsy.[51,52] Gallium-67 citrate scans[53] and technetium-99 m-labeled WBC scans[54] have also identified inflammatory myocardial changes in 50% to 70% of patients. Congestive heart failure (CHF) in the acute phase of the illness is generally the result of myocarditis and improves rapidly with IVIG treatment, in many cases within 24 hours from initiation of treatment.[55] Later implications of these early changes is speculative, but several investigators have evaluated pathology and clinical function late after Kawasaki disease. Myocardial biopsies in patients with long-term follow-up have shown fibrosis, abnormal branching, and hypertrophy of myocytes unrelated to duration from illness onset.[56] Although late noninvasive studies of myocardial function are encouraging, data on long-term myocardial function should accrue as the earliest Japanese cohorts reach middle age.[57]

Valve Regurgitation

Mitral and aortic regurgitation have been associated with Kawasaki disease in both early and chronic phases of the disease. In the acute stage, one in four children has mitral regurgitation of mild to moderate severity detected by two-dimensional (2D) echocardiography, which resolves in most children by the convalescent phase.[58] The frequency of aortic regurgitation has been reported to be as high as 5% in Japanese children[59] but only 1% in a recent North American population with Kawasaki disease,[58] and there are rare reports of late-onset aortic regurgitation necessitating valve replacement.[60,61] The cause for aortic insufficiency is not known; however, it has been reported that the aortic root enlarges from baseline and remains dilated during the first year after illness onset,[58,62] raising the possibility that coaptation of the leaflets is disturbed.

Other Cardiac Findings

Rarely, patients in the acute or subacute phase of Kawasaki disease can develop tamponade due to a pericardial effusion, although effusions greater than 1 mm occur in fewer than 5%

of patients.[58,63] Rupture of a giant aneurysm into the pericardial space is an even rarer cause of pericardial tamponade.[64–66]

Cardiac Testing

Electrocardiographic (ECG) findings are nonspecific and include sinus tachycardia, prolonged PR interval, and diffuse ST-T wave changes. In children with coronary artery aneurysms, ECG abnormalities are useful in detecting myocardial ischemia and infarction.

Using 2D echocardiography, visualization of the proximal coronary arteries in young children is almost always possible, and measurements correlate closely with those identified by angiography. In addition to measurements of the proximal left main, anterior descending, circumflex, proximal, and middle right and posterior descending branches, assessment of ventricular function, pericardial fluid, and mitral and aortic regurgitation should be obtained. Coronary artery dilation may be present as early as the end of the first week of illness. In addition, findings on echocardiography are used to determine the need for IVIG treatment of children with suspected Kawasaki disease on the basis of fever and incomplete criteria.[2] As a result, echocardiography should be undertaken when the diagnosis is entertained, particularly as an incomplete clinical picture, with coronary artery abnormalities sufficient to make the diagnosis and initiate therapy.[2,67] Serial studies are obtained at 10 to 14 days from onset of illness to assess for the presence of aneurysm development and at the end of the subacute phase, 6 to 8 weeks from onset. Echocardiography should be performed more frequently in the child with coronary dilation at baseline, persistent fever, or other factors raising the likelihood of development of coronary aneurysms. Finally, children with giant aneurysms are at highest risk for development of coronary thrombosis in the first months after illness onset. For this reason, echocardiography may be performed once or twice a week until 8 weeks after illness onset or until coronary arteries stop enlarging and systemic inflammation has subsided.

The definition of normal coronary artery dimensions has been the subject of some controversy. Criteria established by the Japanese Ministry of Health in 1984 defined as abnormal those coronary arteries with lumen diameter greater than 3 mm in children younger than 5 years, or greater than 4 mm in those older than age 5; lumen diameter 1.5 times the size of an adjacent segment; or irregular lumen.[68] Others have shown that coronary artery size in normal children correlates linearly with increasing body size. In patients with Kawasaki disease whose coronary arteries are classified as normal by Japanese Ministry of Health criteria, the dimensions are larger than expected when adjusted for body surface area (BSA) in all phases of the disease.[69] Indeed, the median coronary z score at presentation in a multicenter trial was 1.43, significantly larger than the expected population norm in afebrile children of 0.[49] Of note, normative data for febrile children are not available.

Echocardiography in the acute phase of Kawasaki disease is also useful for assessing left ventricular (LV) dysfunction.[55] Among patients without coronary aneurysms, systolic function rapidly improves following IVIG administration.[58] Diastolic function, specifically relaxation, is impaired in acute Kawasaki disease; patients with coronary aneurysms may continue to have long-term diastolic dysfunction, even when systolic function is preserved.[70]

Although echocardiography has high sensitivity and specificity for detection of dilation in the proximal coronary arteries, it is less useful for detection of coronary stenoses and aneurysms in the distal coronary vasculature. The quality of coronary imaging by echocardiography also diminishes as children grow larger, limiting its utility in long-term follow-up of the patient with Kawasaki disease. Therefore, imaging of the coronary arteries by ultrafast computed tomographic angiography (CTA) and magnetic resonance angiography (MRA) are used to obtain high-resolution images.[71–75] Because the long-term effects of ionizing radiation are of special concern in children, CTA is used sparingly.

Although the quality of coronary artery images may be superior with CTA, MRA does not require ionizing radiation and, in the child who is too young to exercise on a treadmill or bicycle, can be used with dobutamine or adenosine stress to delineate reversible ischemia.

Stress testing for inducible ischemia is an important component of periodic testing for patients with Kawasaki disease, but literature is limited to case series.[76-79] As in so many other domains of care of the child with this disease, choice of stress test type is based upon literature related to adults with atherosclerotic coronary disease. As already noted, additional considerations include risks of repeated exposure to ionizing radiation and inability of the youngest children to exercise on a treadmill or bicycle, in whom pharmacological stress is required. To avoid false-positive test results, stress testing should only be performed in children with a history of coronary artery aneurysms.

Coronary angiography has been used extensively for diagnostic assessment of coronary abnormalities. With rapid technical improvement in noninvasive imaging modalities and concerns about the use of ionizing radiation in children, invasive studies are generally reserved for children with aneurysms in whom noninvasive testing is insufficient to guide treatment or in whom revascularization is needed. Aneurysms are described as *localized* or *extensive*, the former being further subclassified as *fusiform* or *saccular* (Fig. 45-1). Extensive aneurysms, those that involve more than one segment, are *ectatic* (dilated uniformly; Fig. 45-2) or *segmented* (multiple dilated segments joined by normal or stenotic segments). Aneurysms may also involve other medium- to large-sized extraparenchymal arteries, particularly the subclavian, axillary, femoral, iliac, renal, and mesenteric arteries. Occasionally, aneurysms of the aorta may occur.

Clinical Course

Persistent Coronary Aneurysms

After expansion in diameter over the first 4 to 6 weeks after illness onset, coronary aneurysms in Kawasaki disease tend to regress over time. In a study of 594 patients, regression occurred over a 13.6-year period in 54% of those with aneurysms, with 90% regressing within 2 years from the onset of illness.[80] Substantial regression in aneurysm diameter after 2 years is unlikely. The potential for aneu-

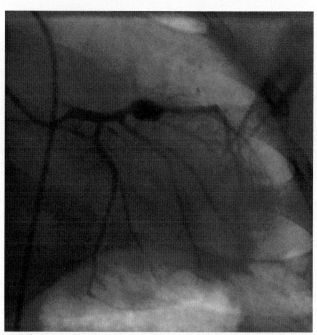

FIGURE 45-2 Ectatic giant aneurysm of right coronary artery (maximum diameter 11 mm) from same patient as in Figure 45-1.

rysm regression to normal internal lumen diameter is determined by the initial size of the aneurysm, with smaller abnormalities more likely to improve.[81] Giant aneurysms (i.e., diameter ≥8 mm) are least likely to regress.[82] In regressed aneurysms, intravascular ultrasound examination reveals myointimal thickening,[83,84] worst in patients whose coronary diameters were initially the largest.[83] Furthermore, coronary and peripheral vascular reactivity may be impaired in patients with either persistent or regressed aneurysms.[84]

Among patients with persistent coronary aneurysms, prevalence of arterial stenosis increases linearly with time, owing to myointimal proliferation at the entrance or exit of the aneurysm. Giant aneurysms (diameter >8 mm) are at highest risk; stenoses commonly occur at the distal end of these lesions (Fig. 45-3) and, together with

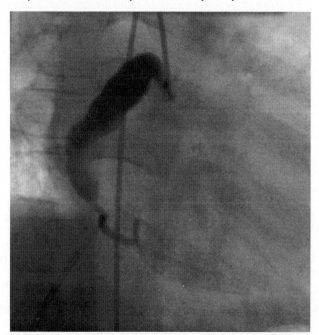

FIGURE 45-1 Isolated giant aneurysm of left anterior descending (LAD) coronary artery in a 7-year-old boy who received multiple doses of intravenous gamma globulin (IVIG) and plasmapheresis for persistent fever.

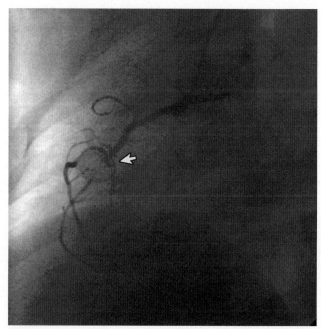

FIGURE 45-3 Calcified thrombotic right coronary artery giant aneurysm in a 10-year-old boy diagnosed with Kawasaki disease at 1 year of age. Lesion is stenotic proximally (arrow), with recanalized distal vessels.

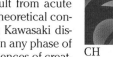

sluggish blood flow in the grossly dilated arterial segment, predispose to thrombosis and infarction. Relative to smaller aneurysms, giant aneurysms are more frequently associated with late sudden death from infarction. In a recent review, coronary artery stenoses had developed at 15-year follow-up in half of aneurysms with maximum diameter of at least 6 mm.[85] In the largest reported series of patients with giant aneurysms (median observation 19 years), survival rates at 10, 20, and 30 years after disease onset were 95%, 88%, and 88%, and cumulative rates of coronary intervention at 5, 15, and 25 years were 28%, 43%, and 59%, respectively.[82]

In addition to stenoses, coronary arteries that have been affected by aneurysm formation may become increasingly tortuous and calcified, and they are prone to thrombotic occlusion. Rupture of an aneurysm is a rare event that occurs in the first months after illness onset in children whose aneurysms are expanding rapidly.

Myocardial infarction due to Kawasaki disease, although infrequent, is a feared complication. In the largest series of cases from Japan, many patients were asymptomatic before their event.[86] Most (73%) had infarction in the initial year following onset of illness, and approximately 50% of infarctions occurred within the first 3 months after illness onset. Symptoms were more common in those older than 4 years (83%) compared with younger children (17%) and included crying, chest pain, shock, abdominal pain, vomiting, dyspnea, and arrhythmia. Often, infarction occurred during rest or sleep rather than during exercise or play. First MI was associated with a mortality rate of 22%, most often the result of obstruction of the left main coronary artery or of both the right and left anterior descending (LAD) coronary arteries. Survivors tended to have involvement of a single artery other than the left main. Mortality rose to 62.5% after a second infarct and to nearly 100% in those with a third infarct. At later follow-up, a sizable proportion (41%) reported no symptoms. Not surprisingly, ejection fraction is a significant predictor of long-term survival after MI, with poor 30-year survival when ejection fraction is 45% or less.[87]

Regressed Coronary Aneurysms

Regression of aneurysms occurs as a result of myointimal proliferation, identified at postmortem examination with use of transluminal ultrasound.[88] Histological examination of regressed aneurysms shows pathological findings similar to those seen in atherosclerosis,[89] raising concern that individuals with Kawasaki disease might be predisposed to early onset of coronary disease. In a study of patients with Kawasaki disease receiving isosorbide dinitrate at catheterization, those segments with regressed aneurysms, as well as regions with persistent aneurysms, had diminished reactivity relative to coronary arteries that had never been dilated or to coronary arteries of control patients.[84] Furthermore, the decreased reactivity in abnormal areas progressed as duration from illness increased.

No Detectable Lesions

In the absence of a history of coronary aneurysms, Kawasaki disease has not been associated with an increase in standardized mortality ratio in adulthood. Concerns that have been raised about the health of the coronary vasculature thus are based solely on studies searching for preclinical disease. Autopsy studies of incidental deaths are limited. In one series, five children who died of incidental causes following Kawasaki disease underwent postmortem examination.[56] Microscopic examination of the coronary arteries revealed intimal thickening and fibrosis indistinguishable from that of atherosclerosis, but correlation with clinical status was not possible. On positron emission tomography (PET), Kawasaki patients who never had aneurysms, compared to controls, had lower myocardial reserve and higher total coronary resistance without regional perfusion abnormalities, suggesting an abnormal coronary microcirculation.[90] Testing coronary endothelial function by infusing acetylcholine in the epicardial coronary arteries of Kawasaki patients and comparison patients has

yielded conflicting results,[91,92] as have studies on peripheral arterial stiffness and brachial reactivity.[93–96] Finally, some investigators have speculated that long-term sequelae may result from acute myocarditis that occurs during the acute illness.[57] Theoretical concerns about coronary and myocardial sequelae in Kawasaki disease patients without detectable coronary dilation in any phase of illness should be tempered by the adverse consequences of creating "cardiac non-disease."[97]

Treatment

Therapy in the acute phase of the illness is aimed at reducing the systemic inflammatory response, minimizing the occurrence of coronary artery aneurysms, and preventing acute coronary thrombosis among those in whom such aneurysms develop. Late management focuses on prevention of myocardial ischemia and infarction among patients with persistent aneurysms, and reduction in risk factors for later atherosclerotic coronary artery disease (CAD) in all patients.

Antiinflammatory Therapy During Acute Kawasaki Disease

ASPIRIN

Aspirin has been a mainstay of therapy for Kawasaki disease, for both its antiinflammatory and antithrombotic effects. Most clinicians use high-dose aspirin, 80 to 100 mg/kg/day divided into four daily doses until defervescence, and then reduce the dosage to 3 to 5 mg/kg/day, administered once daily until the end of the subacute phase (6-8 weeks; Box 45-3) to reduce the likelihood for Reye's syndrome or gastrointestinal bleeding. Meta-analysis has shown that low-dose or high-dose aspirin regimens in conjunction with IVIG have a similar incidence of coronary abnormalities at 30 and 60 days from onset of illness.[98] In patients with aneurysms, low-dose aspirin therapy is continued, sometimes in combination with anticoagulants or other antiplatelet agents.

INTRAVENOUS GAMMA GLOBULIN

Intravenous Ig was first administered to children with Kawasaki disease in 1984[99] and shown to have beneficial effects in reducing the likelihood of coronary aneurysms and the inflammatory response in the acute phase. Many subsequent studies have confirmed the efficacy of high-dose IVIG; the lowest incidence of coronary artery lesions occurs in those patients treated with IVIG 2 g/kg, administered as a single dose over 8 to 12 hours[98,100] (see Box 45-3). The mechanism of action of IVIG remains unknown. Children who are acutely ill with Kawasaki disease should be administered IVIG 2 g/kg as a single dose no later than the 10th day of illness and ideally within the first 7 days.[101] Patients with fever beyond 10 days of illness should also receive IVIG,[102] as should those with aneurysm formation and evidence for persistent inflammation. Approximately 15% of children have persistent or recrudescent fever after IVIG treatment (so-called IVIG resistance).[103] Although not tested in a randomized trial, retreatment with IVIG 2 g/kg is generally administered if recurrent or

Box 45-3   Accepted Therapy for Acute Kawasaki Disease

Intravenous gamma globulin (IVIG) 2 g/kg single infusion over 8 to 12 hours
and:
Aspirin 80 to 100 mg/kg divided equally 4 times daily until afebrile at least 48 hours
followed by:
Aspirin 3 to 5 mg/kg as a single daily dose until patient is afebrile for 48 hours, discontinued if echo is normal at 6 to 8 weeks

recrudescent fever is present more than 36 hours after completion of an initial course of IVIG.[2] If a second dose of IVIG is ineffective in diminishing fever, particularly in the presence of worsening coronary dilation, alternative antiinflammatory therapies are often administered (see later) discussion.

CORTICOSTEROIDS

Corticosteroids are widely used in the treatment of other vasculitides, but data on the efficacy of primary and secondary (rescue) steroid therapy in Kawasaki disease are mixed. Although uncontrolled studies and one open multicenter trial previously suggested benefit for primary steroid therapy,[104–109] a randomized multicenter placebo-blind study showed that primary therapy with pulsed-dose intravenous (IV) methylprednisolone did not improve coronary outcomes when added to conventional treatment with IVIG and aspirin.[103] However, efficacy of other corticosteroid dosage regimens for primary treatment are currently being studied.

Corticosteroids are often used as rescue therapy in the patient with IVIG-resistant Kawasaki disease, with most reports comprising case series.[110–112] Similar to findings in primary steroid treatment, rescue treatment with pulsed steroids was reported to shorten fever duration and length of hospital stay, but did not improve coronary outcomes in a randomized trial of pulsed steroid therapy.[112] Based on the differing dosage regimens that have been used in studying the effect of steroids on coronary outcomes, and the limited power for randomized trials of rescue therapy, data are insufficient to conclude whether steroids have a place in the armamentarium of IVIG-resistant Kawasaki disease. Most experts consider use of steroids, either as a pulsed dose or chronic oral regimen in children who have persistent or recrudescent fever despite at least two courses of IVIG 2 g/kg.

Additional Therapies

Limited data are available concerning efficacy of other therapies that can be used in the IVIG-resistant patient. Plasmapheresis has been reported to lower the incidence of coronary disease,[113] but it is technically complex, requiring placement of large-bore catheters and the commitment of the local blood bank to assist in the exchange. Abciximab, a platelet glycoprotein (GP) IIb/IIIa receptor inhibitor that prevents platelet aggregation, has been used as an antithrombotic agent in acute Kawasaki disease. A retrospective study reported that patients treated with abciximab, compared to those who were not, had smaller aneurysm size and a greater percentage decrease in aneurysm diameter.[114] Infliximab, a chimeric monoclonal antibody to tumor necrosis factor (TNF)-α, has been used as rescue therapy in IVIG-resistant patients.[115,116] A two-center retrospective study suggested that infliximab as rescue therapy shortens fever duration but does not reduce prevalence or size of aneurysms.[117] Finally, in the most refractory cases of Kawasaki disease where coronary aneurysms are progressively enlarging despite all other medical therapies, treatment with cytotoxic agents has been reported.[111,118]

ANTITHROMBOTIC THERAPY

The combination of active vasculitis with endothelial damage, thrombocytosis, and hypercoagulable state create the clinical setting for thrombosis of coronary arteries. Peak occurrence for such events is 15 to 45 days from onset of illness. The current recommendation for therapy is aspirin 3 to 5 mg/kg/day for 6 to 8 weeks. If the echocardiogram is normal at that time, aspirin is discontinued, but in the presence of dilation or aneurysms, aspirin is continued until regression to normal vessel lumen size. For patients with moderate to large aneurysms, some clinicians use combination antiplatelet therapy consisting of aspirin together with an inhibitor of adenosine diphosphate (ADP)-induced platelet aggregation (e.g., thienopyridine).[2]

Finally, patients with *giant aneurysms*, defined as those with an internal lumen diameter of 8 mm or greater or a *z* score of 10 or more,[119] have the greatest risk for coronary thrombosis and are conventionally treated with a combination of anticoagulation and aspirin. One series has shown that patients with giant aneurysms have a lower risk of MI if treated with aspirin and warfarin than with aspirin alone.[120] Low-molecular-weight heparin (LMWH) may be used in those for whom warfarin management is difficult. Newer oral direct thrombin inhibitors and factor Xa inhibitors have not yet been approved for use in the pediatric population but hold promise for future treatment of Kawasaki disease patients requiring anticoagulation. Women of childbearing age who have giant coronary aneurysms and are contemplating pregnancy should be counseled about the effects of warfarin and, once pregnant, should be treated in accordance with a protocol similar to that used for the pregnant woman with a mechanical prosthetic valve.[121]

THROMBOLYTIC THERAPY

On the basis of experience in adult patients with acute coronary thrombosis, thrombolytic therapy has been used in those with acute ischemic events or evolving MI following Kawasaki disease. No prospective randomized study has been undertaken to assess the preferred thrombolytic medication in Kawasaki disease because adequate power is precluded by the limited number of affected patients. Therapy should be instituted as soon as possible. After reperfusion of the affected vessel, anticoagulation is started with the combination of IV heparin and aspirin. This regimen is converted to warfarin or LMWH in place of IV (unfractionated) heparin (UFH) for chronic therapy.

Coronary Revascularization

The criteria for coronary revascularization in Kawasaki disease are based upon consensus of experts, experience in adult patients with atherosclerotic CAD, and small retrospective reviews of experience in Kawasaki disease.[122–125]

Coronary Artery Bypass Surgery

The decision to undertake coronary artery bypass graft (CABG) surgery is generally based on a combination of factors, including evidence of reversible ischemia on stress-imaging tests, viable myocardium in the region of distribution of the affected vessel, and absence of evidence for severe disease distal to the site of the planned graft.[126] Initial reports of bypass grafting in Kawasaki disease involved use of saphenous veins, but early failures, particularly among younger children, led to introduction of internal mammary artery grafts. In the current era, systemic arterial grafts (e.g., internal mammary, radial) are preferred because they increase in length and diameter with somatic growth.[122–124] Even young children have undergone successful surgical revascularization, but freedom from reintervention is longer when bypass is performed at an older age. Kitamura et al. recently reported his single-center experience; at 25 years, freedom from reintervention was only 60%, but patient survival was 95%.[124]

Percutaneous Coronary Intervention

Experience with percutaneous coronary intervention (PCI) in children affected by Kawasaki disease is even more limited than CABG, but techniques for interventional catheterization procedures used in these patients are similar to those in adults. Based on recommendations of the Research Committee of the Japanese Ministry of Health, Labor, and Welfare, patients with the following criteria should be considered for PCI: ischemic symptoms, presence of reversible ischemia on stress testing, or at least 75% stenosis of the LAD coronary artery.[127] These recommendations suggest that CABG is superior to PCI in the setting of severe LV dysfunction or presence of multiple ostial or long-segment coronary artery stenoses. Although early success rates for percutaneous transluminal coronary angioplasty, rotational ablation, and stent placement are all high, restenosis is common.[128]

Furthermore, neoaneurysm formation is a risk of percutaneous dilation related to use of high inflation pressures necessary to dilate the heavily calcified arteries found in Kawasaki disease patients.[128] For this reason, rotational ablation and stent placement are generally preferred to percutaneous transluminal coronary angioplasty, after a few years have passed since disease onset. Because pediatric cardiologists have limited experience with interventional coronary artery techniques, percutaneous intervention should be performed by adult invasive cardiologists, with support from pediatric teams when children are small.

Randomized clinical trials of CABG versus PCI have not been conducted; sample size and power would be limited by the infrequency with which revascularization is required, even in Japanese children. Using survey data comparing outcomes in patients whose first intervention was either PCI or CABG, rates of mortality and MI were similar. However, repeat revascularization therapies were administered more often to children whose first intervention was percutaneous.[129]

Cardiac transplantation is reserved for patients with end-stage ischemic cardiomyopathy who can no longer be helped by coronary revascularization.

Preventive Cardiology

Patients who have regressed or persistent aneurysms are likely to be at increased risk for premature atherosclerotic cardiovascular disease. Histopathological findings have noted atherosclerosis on autopsies performed in children who die years after illness onset.[130] Those with a history of aneurysms have increased myointimal thickness in the coronary arteries on intravascular ultrasound,[83] and evidence of premature atherosclerosis is seen on carotid artery ultrasound 6 to 20 years after illness onset.[131] Late after Kawasaki disease, peripheral arteries with coronary aneurysms have been noted to be stiffer with diminished vascular reactivity, compared to normal controls.[84] High-sensitivity CRP levels are greater in Kawasaki disease patients with a history of aneurysms than among those who never developed aneurysms or in normal children.[132,133] Data about future risk in children who never had coronary aneurysms continue to be controversial.

All patients with a history of Kawasaki disease should be counseled about risk factors for atherosclerotic cardiovascular disease, including the importance of a heart-healthy diet, exercise, avoidance of smoking, and for parents, the importance of maintaining a smoke-free home. In the AHA recommendations, the threshold for pharmacological treatment of hypertension and hyperlipidemia is lower for children with current and regressed coronary aneurysms.[134] Exercise recommendations for participation in competitive sports depend upon severity of coronary disease, but all patients with a history of Kawasaki disease should avoid a sedentary life style.[135]

Summary

Kawasaki disease is an acute vasculitis of uncertain etiology in children. Coronary artery aneurysms occur in 2% to 4% of individuals treated in the acute phase of the disease if they are treated within 10 days, and ideally 7 days, of illness onset with IVIG 2 g/kg and aspirin. Many coronary aneurysms regress to normal lumen diameter by myointimal proliferation, but larger aneurysms may persist and can be associated with progressive stenoses leading to ischemia and MI. Patients with coronary aneurysms are followed with regular stress testing to guide the need for invasive testing and catheter or surgical interventions. The question of whether individuals with Kawasaki disease without detected coronary aneurysms have increased relative risk for atherosclerotic cardiovascular disease will not be answered until the earliest Japanese cohorts reach middle age. Until then, patients with a history of Kawasaki disease should be followed at regular intervals appropriate to the severity of their heart disease. With such surveillance, the long-term natural history of Kawasaki disease, including its effects on vascular health and myocardial function, will continue to be delineated.

REFERENCES

1. Kawasaki T: Acute febrile mucocutaneous syndrome with lymphoid involvement with specific desquamation of the fingers and toes in children (Japanese), Jpn J Allergy 116(3):178–222, 1967.
2. Newburger JW, Takahashi M, Gerber MA, et al: Diagnosis, treatment, and long-term management of Kawasaki disease. A statement for health professionals from the Committee on Rheumatic Fever, Endocarditis and Kawasaki Disease, Council on Cardiovascular Disease in the Young, American Heart Association, Circulation 110(17):2747–2771, 2004.
3. Hayasaka S, Nakamura Y, Yashiro M, et al: Analyses of fatal cases of Kawasaki disease in Japan using vital statistical data over 27 years, J Epidemiol 13(5):246–250, 2003.
4. Tsuda E, Matsuo M, Naito H, et al: Clinical features in adults with coronary arterial lesions caused by presumed Kawasaki disease, Cardiol Young 17(1):84–89, 2007.
5. Nakamura Y, Yashiro M, Uehara R, et al: Epidemiologic features of Kawasaki disease in Japan: results of the 2007-2008 nationwide survey, J Epidemiol 20(4):302–307, 2010.
6. Holman RC, Curns AT, Belay ED, et al: Kawasaki syndrome hospitalizations in the United States, 1997 and 2000, Pediatrics 112(3 Pt 1):495–501, 2003.
7. Stockheim JA, Innocentini N, Shulman ST: Kawasaki disease in older children and adolescents, J Pediatr 137(2):250–252, 2000.
8. Rauch AM, Glode MP, Wiggins JW Jr, et al: Outbreak of Kawasaki syndrome in Denver, Colorado: association with rug and carpet cleaning, Pediatrics 87(5):663–669, 1991.
9. Burns JC, Mason WH, Glode MP, et al: Clinical and epidemiologic characteristics of patients referred for evaluation of possible Kawasaki disease, J Pediatr 118(5):680–686, 1991.
10. Rowley AH, Shulman ST: Recent advances in the understanding and management of Kawasaki disease, Curr Infect Dis Rep 12(2):96–102, 2010.
11. Burns JC, Glode MP: Kawasaki syndrome, Lancet 364(9433):533–544, 2004.
12. Leung DYM: Superantigens related to Kawasaki syndrome, Springer Semin Immunopathol 17(4):385–396, 1996.
13. Yeung RS: Lessons learned from an animal model of Kawasaki disease, Clin Exp Rheumatol 25(1 Suppl 44):S69–S71, 2007.
14. Rowley AH: Kawasaki disease: novel insights into etiology and genetic susceptibility, Annu Rev Med 62:69–77, 2011.
15. Rowley AH, Baker SC, Shulman ST, et al: Cytoplasmic inclusion bodies are detected by synthetic antibody in ciliated bronchial epithelium during acute Kawasaki disease, J Infect Dis 192(10):1757–1766, 2005.
16. Rowley AH, Baker SC, Shulman ST, et al: RNA-containing cytoplasmic inclusion bodies in ciliated bronchial epithelium months to years after acute Kawasaki disease, PLoS ONE 3(2):e1582, 2008.
17. Rowley AH, Baker SC, Shulman ST, et al: Ultrastructural, immunofluorescence, and RNA evidence support the hypothesis of a "new" virus associated with Kawasaki disease, J Infect Dis 203(7):1021–1030, 2011.
18. Rowley AH, Shulman ST, Spike BT, et al: Oligoclonal IgA response in the vascular wall in acute Kawasaki disease, J Immunol 166(2):1334–1343, 2001.
19. Brown TJ, Crawford SE, Cornwall ML, et al: CD8 T lymphocytes and macrophages infiltrate coronary artery aneurysms in acute Kawasaki disease, J Infect Dis 184(7):940–943, 2001.
20. Yasukawa K, Terai M, Shulman ST, et al: Systemic production of vascular endothelial growth factor and FMS-like tyrosine kinase-1 receptor in acute Kawasaki disease, Circulation 105(6):766–769, 2002.
21. Asano T, Ogawa S: Expression of monocyte chemoattractant protein-1 in Kawasaki disease: the anti-inflammatory effect of gamma globulin therapy, Scand J Immunol 51(1):98–103, 2000.
22. Freeman AF, Crawford SE, Finn LS, et al: Inflammatory pulmonary nodules in Kawasaki disease, Pediatr Pulmonol 36(2):102–106, 2003.
23. Ohno T, Yuge T, Kariyazono H, et al: Serum hepatocyte growth factor combined with vascular endothelial growth factor as a predictive indicator for the occurrence of coronary artery lesions in Kawasaki disease, Eur J Pediatr 161(2):105–111, 2002.
24. Nomura Y, Masuda K, Maeno N, et al: Serum levels of interleukin-18 are elevated in the subacute phase of Kawasaki syndrome, Int Arch Allergy Immunol 135(2):161–165, 2004.
25. Terai M, Honda T, Yasukawa K, et al: Prognostic impact of vascular leakage in acute Kawasaki disease, Circulation 108(3):325–330, 2003.
26. Takahashi K, Oharaseki T, Naoe S, et al: Neutrophilic involvement in the damage to coronary arteries in acute stage of Kawasaki disease, Pediatr Int 47(3):305–310, 2005.
27. Takeshita S, Tokutomi T, Kawase H, et al: Elevated serum levels of matrix metalloproteinase-9 (MMP-9) in Kawasaki disease, Clin Exp Immunol 125(2):340–344, 2001.
28. Gavin PJ, Crawford SE, Shulman ST, et al: Systemic arterial expression of matrix metalloproteinases 2 and 9 in acute Kawasaki disease, Arterioscler Thromb Vasc Biol 23(4):576–581, 2003.
29. Shimizu C, Matsubara T, Onouchi Y, et al: Matrix metalloproteinase haplotypes associated with coronary artery aneurysm formation in patients with Kawasaki disease, J Hum Genet 55(12):779–784, 2010.
30. Uehara R, Yashiro M, Nakamura Y, et al: Kawasaki disease in parents and children, Acta Paediatr 92(6):694–697, 2003.
31. Shimizu C, Jain S, Davila S, et al: Transforming growth factor-beta signaling pathway in patients with Kawasaki disease, Circ Cardiovasc Genet 4(1):16–25, 2011.
32. Mamtani M, Matsubara T, Shimizu C, et al: Association of CCR2-CCR5 haplotypes and CCL3L1 copy number with Kawasaki disease, coronary artery lesions, and IVIG responses in Japanese children, PLoS ONE 5(7):e11458, 2010.
33. Onouchi Y, Gunji T, Burns JC, et al: ITPKC functional polymorphism associated with Kawasaki disease susceptibility and formation of coronary artery aneurysms, Nat Genet 40(1):35–42, 2008.
34. Burgner D, Davila S, Breunis WB, et al: A genome-wide association study identifies novel and functionally related susceptibility Loci for Kawasaki disease, PLoS Genet 5(1):e1000319, 2009.

35. Fujiwara H, Hamashima Y: Pathology of the heart in Kawasaki disease, *Pediatrics* 61(1):100–107, 1978.
36. Naoe S, Takahasha M, Masuda H, et al: Kawasaki disease with particular emphasis on arterial lesions, *Acta Pathol Jpn* 41(1):785–797, 1991.
37. Burns JC: Kawasaki disease update, *Indian J Pediatr* 76(1):71–76, 2009.
38. Suzuki A, Miyagawa-Tomita S, Komatsu K, et al: Active remodeling of the coronary arterial lesions in the late phase of Kawasaki disease: immunohistochemical study, *Circulation* 101(25):2935–2941, 2000.
39. Kawasaki T, Kosaki F, Okawa S, et al: A new infantile acute febrile mucocutaneous lymph node syndrome (MLNS) prevailing in Japan, *Pediatrics* 54(3):271–276, 1974.
40. Yellen ES, Gauvreau K, Takahashi M, et al: Performance of 2004 American Heart Association recommendations for treatment of Kawasaki disease, *Pediatrics* 125(2):e234–e241, 2010.
41. Burns JC, Joffe L, Sargent RA, et al: Anterior uveitis associated with Kawasaki syndrome, *Pediatr Infect Dis* 4(3):258–261, 1985.
42. Dengler LD, Capparelli EV, Bastian JF, et al: Cerebrospinal fluid profile in patients with acute Kawasaki disease, *J Ped Inf Dis* 17(6):478–481, 1998.
43. Minich LL, Sleeper LA, Atz AM, et al: Delayed diagnosis of Kawasaki disease: what are the risk factors? *Pediatrics* 120(6):e1434–e1440, 2007.
44. Muta H, Ishii M, Sakaue T, et al: Older age is a risk factor for the development of cardiovascular sequelae in Kawasaki disease, *Pediatrics* 114(3):751–754, 2004.
45. Song D, Yeo Y, Ha K, et al: Risk factors for Kawasaki disease-associated coronary abnormalities differ depending on age, *Eur J Pediatr* 168(11):1315–1321, 2009.
46. Kim T, Choi W, Woo CW, et al: Predictive risk factors for coronary artery abnormalities in Kawasaki disease, *Eur J Pediatr* 166(5):421–425, 2007.
47. Beiser AS, Takahashi M, Baker AL, et al: A predictive instrument for coronary artery aneurysms in Kawasaki disease, *Am J Cardiol* 81(9):1116–1120, 1998.
48. Sabharwal T, Manlhiot C, Benseler SM, et al: Comparison of factors associated with coronary artery dilation only versus coronary artery aneurysms in patients with Kawasaki disease, *Am J Cardiol* 104(12):1743–1747, 2009.
49. McCrindle BW, Li JS, Minich LL, et al: Coronary artery involvement in children with Kawasaki disease: risk factors from analysis of serial normalized measurements, *Circulation* 116(2):174–179, 2007.
50. Kariyazono H, Ohno T, Khajoee V, et al: Association of vascular endothelial growth factor (VEGF) and VEGF receptor gene polymorphisms with coronary artery lesions of Kawasaki disease, *Pediatr Res* 56(6):953–959, 2004.
51. Fujiwara H, Hamashima Y: Pathology of the heart in Kawasaki disease, *Pediatrics* 61(1):100–107, 1978.
52. Yutani C, Okano K, Kamiya T, et al: Histopathological study on right endomyocardial biopsy of Kawasaki disease, *Br Heart J* 43(5):589–592, 1980.
53. Matsuura H, Ishikita T, Yamamoto S, et al: Gallium-67 myocardial imaging for the detection of myocarditis, *Br Heart J* 58(4):385–392, 1987.
54. Kao CH, Hsieh KS, Wang YL, et al: Tc-99m HMPAO labeled WBC scan for the detection of myocarditis in different phases of Kawasaki disease, *Clin Nucl Med* 17(3):185–190, 1992.
55. Moran AM, Newburger JW, Sanders SP, et al: Abnormal myocardial mechanics in Kawasaki disease: rapid response to gamma-globulin, *Am Heart J* 139(2 Pt 1):217–223, 2000.
56. Tanaka N, Naoe S, Masuda H, et al: Pathological study of sequelae of Kawasaki disease (MCLS). With special reference to the heart and coronary arterial lesions, *Acta Pathol Jpn* 36(10):1513–1527, 1986.
57. Gordon JB, Kahn AM, Burns JC: When children with Kawasaki disease grow up: myocardial and vascular complications in adulthood, *J Am Coll Cardiol* 54(21):1911–1920, 2009.
58. Printz BF, Sleeper LA, Newburger JW, et al: Noncoronary cardiac abnormalities are associated with coronary artery dilation and with laboratory inflammatory markers in acute Kawasaki disease, *J Am Coll Cardiol* 57(1):86–92, 2010.
59. Nakano H, Nojima K, Saito A, et al: High incidence of aortic regurgitation following Kawasaki disease, *J Pediatr* 107(1):59–63, 1985.
60. Gidding SS: Late onset valvular dysfunction in Kawasaki disease, *Prog Clin Biol Res* 250:305–309, 1987.
61. Gidding SS, Shulman ST, Ilbawi M, et al: Mucocutaneous lymph node syndrome (Kawasaki disease): delayed aortic and mitral insufficiency secondary to active valvulitis, *J Am Coll Cardiol* 7(4):894–897, 1986.
62. Ravekes WJ, Colan SD, Gauvreau K, et al: Aortic root dilation in Kawasaki disease, *Am J Cardiol* 87(7):919–922, 2001.
63. Ozdogu H, Boga C: Fatal cardiac tamponade in a patient with Kawasaki disease, *Heart Lung* 34(4):257–259, 2005.
64. Kuppuswamy M, Gukop P, Sutherland G, et al: Kawasaki disease presenting as cardiac tamponade with ruptured giant aneurysm of the right coronary artery, *Interact Cardiovasc Thorac Surg* 10(2):317–318, 2010.
65. Imai Y, Sunagawa K, Ayusawa M, et al: A fatal case of ruptured giant coronary artery aneurysm, *Eur J Pediatr* 165(2):1–4, 2005.
66. Maresi E, Passantino R, Midulla R, et al: Sudden infant death caused by a ruptured coronary aneurysm during acute phase of atypical Kawasaki disease, *Hum Pathol* 32(12):1407–1409, 2001.
67. Council on Cardiovascular Disease in the Young Committee on Rheumatic Fever Endocarditis and Kawasaki Disease American Heart Association: Diagnostic guidelines for Kawasaki disease, *Circulation* 103(2):335–336, 2001.
68. Research Committee on Kawasaki Disease: *Report of subcommittee on standardization of diagnostic criteria and reporting of coronary artery lesions in Kawasaki disease*, Tokyo, Japan, 1984, Ministry of Health and Welfare.
69. de Zorzi A, Colan SD, Gauvreau K, et al: Coronary artery dimensions may be misclassified as normal in Kawasaki disease, *J Pediatr* 133(2):254–258, 1998.
70. Tierney ES, Newburger JW, Graham D, et al: Diastolic function in children with Kawasaki Disease, *Int J Cardiol* 148(3):309–312, 2009.
71. Greil GF, Stuber M, Botnar RM, et al: Coronary magnetic resonance angiography in adolescents and young adults with Kawasaki disease, *Circulation* 105(8):908–911, 2002.
72. Danias PG, Stuber M, Botnar RM, et al: Coronary MR angiography: clinical applications and potential for imaging coronary artery disease, *Magn Reson Imaging Clin N Am* 11(1): 81–99, 2003.
73. Mavrogeni S, Papadopoulos G, Douskou M, et al: Magnetic resonance angiography is equivalent to x-ray coronary angiography for the evaluation of coronary arteries in Kawasaki disease, *J Am Coll Cardiol* 43(4):649–652, 2004.
74. Sohn S, Kim HS, Lee SW: Multidetector row computed tomography for follow-up of patients with coronary artery aneurysms due to Kawasaki disease, *Pediatr Cardiol* 25(1):35–39, 2004.
75. Schmidt WA: Use of imaging studies in the diagnosis of vasculitis, *Curr Rheumatol Rep* 6(3):203–211, 2004.
76. Muhling O, Jerosch-Herold M, Nabauer M, et al: Assessment of ischemic heart disease using magnetic resonance first-pass perfusion imaging, *Herz* 28(2):82–89, 2003.
77. Kaul S, Ito H: Microvasculature in acute myocardial ischemia: part I: evolving concepts in pathophysiology, diagnosis, and treatment, *Circulation* 109(2):146–149, 2004.
78. Zilberman MV, Witt SA, Kimball TR: Is there a role for intravenous transpulmonary contrast imaging in pediatric stress echocardiography? *J Am Soc Echocardiogr* 16(1):9–14, 2003.
79. Ishii M, Himeno W, Sawa M, et al: Assessment of the ability of myocardial contrast echocardiography with harmonic power Doppler imaging to identify perfusion abnormalities in patients with Kawasaki disease at rest and during dipyridamole stress, *Pediatr Cardiol* 23(2):192–199, 2002.
80. Kato H, Sugimura T, Akagi T, et al: Long-term consequences of Kawasaki disease. A 10- to 21-year follow-up study of 594 patients, *Circulation* 94(6):1379–1385, 1996.
81. Kamiya T, Suzuki A, Ono Y, et al: Angiographic follow-up study of coronary artery lesion in the cases with a history of Kawasaki disease - with a focus on the follow-up more than ten years after the onset of the disease. In Kato H, editor: *Kawasaki disease. Proceedings of the 5th International Kawasaki Disease Symposium, Fukuoka, Japan, May 22-25, 1995*, The Netherlands, 1995, Elsevier Science B.V, pp 569–573.
82. Suda K, Iemura M, Nishiono H, et al: Long-term prognosis of patients with Kawasaki disease complicated by giant coronary aneurysms: a single-institution experience, *Circulation* 123(17):1836–1842, 2011.
83. Tsuda E, Kamiya T, Kimura K, et al: Coronary artery dilatation exceeding 4.0 mm during acute Kawasaki disease predicts a high probability of subsequent late intima-medial thickening, *Pediatr Cardiol* 23(1):9–14, 2002.
84. Iemura M, Ishii M, Sugimura T, et al: Long term consequences of regressed coronary aneurysms after Kawasaki disease: vascular wall morphology and function, *Heart* 83(3):307–311, 2000.
85. Tsuda E, Kamiya T, Ono Y, et al: Incidence of stenotic lesions predicted by acute phase changes in coronary arterial diameter during Kawasaki disease, *Pediatr Cardiol* 26(1):73–79, 2005.
86. Kato H, Ichinose E, Kawasaki T: Myocardial infarction in Kawasaki disease: clinical analyses in 195 cases, *J Pediatr* (6);108:923–927, 1986.
87. Tsuda E, Hirata T, Matsuo O, et al: The 30-year outcome for patients after myocardial infarction due to coronary artery lesions caused by Kawasaki disease, *Pediatr Cardiol* 32(2):176–182, 2010.
88. Sugimura T, Kato H, Inoue O, et al: Intravascular ultrasound of coronary arteries in children. Assessment of the wall morphology and the lumen after Kawasaki disease, *Circulation* 89(1):258–265, 1994.
89. Sasaguri Y, Kato H: Regression of aneurysms in Kawasaki disease: a pathological study? *J Pediatr* 100(2):225–231, 1982.
90. Muzik O, Paridon SM, Singh TP, et al: Quantification of myocardial blood flow and flow reserve in children with a history of Kawasaki disease and normal coronary arteries using positron emission tomography, *J Am Coll Cardiol* 28(3):757–762, 1996.
91. Mitani Y, Okuda Y, Shimpo H, et al: Impaired endothelial function in epicardial coronary arteries after Kawasaki disease, *Circulation* 96:454–461, 1997.
92. Yamakawa R, Ishii M, Sugimura T, et al: Coronary endothelial dysfunction after Kawasaki disease: evaluation by intracoronary injection of acetylcholine, *J Am Coll Cardiol* 31(5):1074–1080, 1998.
93. Cheung YF, Wong SJ, Ho MH: Relationship between carotid intima-media thickness and arterial stiffness in children after Kawasaki disease, *Arch Dis Child* 92(1):43–47, 2007.
94. McCrindle BW, McIntyre S, Kim C, et al: Are patients after Kawasaki disease at increased risk for accelerated atherosclerosis? *J Pediatr* 151(3):244–248, 2007.
95. Deng YB, Li TL, Xiang HJ, et al: Impaired endothelial function in the brachial artery after Kawasaki disease and the effects of intravenous administration of vitamin C, *Pediatr Infect Dis J* 22(1):34–39, 2003.
96. Gupta-Malhotra M, Gruber D, Abraham SS, et al: Atherosclerosis in survivors of Kawasaki disease, *J Pediatr* 155(4):572–577, 2009.
97. Gersony WM: The adult after Kawasaki disease: the risks for late coronary events, *J Am Coll Cardiol* 54(21):1921–1923, 2009.
98. Durongpisitkul K, Gururaj VJ, Park JM, et al: The prevention of coronary artery aneurysm in Kawasaki disease: a meta-analysis on the efficacy of aspirin and immunoglobulin treatment, *Pediatrics* 96(6):1057–1061, 1995.
99. Furusho K, Kamiya T, Nakano H, et al: High-dose intravenous gammaglobulin for Kawasaki disease, *Lancet* 2(8411):1055–1058, 1984.
100. Red Book: Report of the Committee on Infectious Disease. Kawasaki Disease. In Pickering LK, editor: ed 26, Elk Grove Village, IL, 2003, American Academy of Pediatrics, p 394.
101. Tse SM, Silverman ED, McCrindle BW, et al: Early treatment with intravenous immunoglobulin in patients with Kawasaki disease, *J Pediatr* 140(4):450–455, 2002.
102. Marasini M, Pongiglione G, Gazzolo D, et al: Late intravenous gamma globulin treatment in infants and children with Kawasaki disease and coronary artery abnormalities, *Am J Cardiol* 68(8):796–797, 1991.
103. Newburger JW, Sleeper LA, McCrindle BW, et al: Randomized trial of pulsed corticosteroid therapy for primary treatment of Kawasaki disease, *N Engl J Med* 356(7):663–675, 2007.
104. Sundel RP, Baker AL, Fulton DR, et al: Corticosteroids in the initial treatment of Kawasaki disease: report of a randomized trial, *J Pediatr* 142(6):611–616, 2003.
105. Okada Y, Shinohara M, Kobayashi T, et al: Effect of corticosteroids in addition to intravenous gamma globulin therapy on serum cytokine levels in the acute phase of Kawasaki disease in children, *J Pediatr* 143(3):363–367, 2003.
106. Shinohara M, Sone K, Tomomasa T, et al: Corticosteroids in the treatment of the acute phase of Kawasaki disease, *J Pediatr* 135(4):465–469, 1999.

107. Nonaka Z, Maekawa K, Okabe T, et al: Randomized controlled study of intravenous prednisolone and gamma globulin treatment in 100 cases with Kawasaki disease. In *Proceedings of the Fifth International Symposium on Kawasaki Disease*, 1995, pp 328–331.

108. Asano T, Sudoh M, Watanabe M, et al: Transient thrombocytopenia with large platelets in Kawasaki disease, *Pediatr Hematol Oncol* 24(7):551–554, 2007.

109. Wooditch AC, Aronoff SC: Effect of initial corticosteroid therapy on coronary artery aneurysm formation in Kawasaki disease: a meta-analysis of 862 children, *Pediatrics* 116(4):989–995, 2005.

110. Dale RC, Saleem MA, Daw S, et al: Treatment of severe complicated Kawasaki disease with oral prednisolone and aspirin, *J Pediatr* 137(5):723–726, 2000.

111. Wallace CA, French JW, Kahn SJ, et al: Initial intravenous gammaglobulin treatment failure in Kawasaki disease, *Pediatrics* 105(6):E78, 2000.

112. Hashino K, Ishii M, Iemura M, et al: Re-treatment for immune globulin-resistant Kawasaki disease: a comparative study of additional immune globulin and steroid pulse therapy, *Pediatr Int* 43(3):211–217, 2001.

113. Imagawa T, Mori M, Miyamae T, et al: Plasma exchange for refractory Kawasaki disease, *Eur J Pediatr* 163(4–5):263–264, 2004.

114. Williams RV, Wilke VM, Tani LY, et al: Does abciximab enhance regression of coronary aneurysms resulting from Kawasaki disease? *Pediatrics* 109(1):E4, 2002.

115. Weiss JE, Eberhard BA, Chowdhury D, et al: Infliximab as a novel therapy for refractory Kawasaki disease, *J Rheumatol* 31(4):808–810, 2004.

116. Burns JC, Best BM, Mejias A, et al: Infliximab treatment of intravenous immunoglobulin-resistant Kawasaki disease, *J Pediatr* 153(6):833–838, 2008.

117. Son MB, Gauvreau K, Burns JC, et al: Infliximab for intravenous immunoglobulin resistance in Kawasaki disease: a retrospective study, *J Pediatr* 158(4):644–649, 2011.

118. Kuijpers TW, Biezeveld M, Achterhuis A, et al: Longstanding obliterative panarteritis in Kawasaki disease: lack of cyclosporin A effect, *Pediatrics* 112(4):986–992, 2003.

119. Manlhiot C, Brandao LR, Somji Z, et al: Long-term anticoagulation in Kawasaki disease: initial use of low molecular weight heparin is a viable option for patients with severe coronary artery abnormalities, *Pediatr Cardiol* 31(6):834–842, 2010.

120. Sugahara Y, Ishii M, Muta H, et al: Warfarin therapy for giant aneurysm prevents myocardial infarction in Kawasaki disease, *Pediatr Cardiol* 29(2):398–401, 2008.

121. Tsuda E, Ishihara Y, Kawamata K, et al: Pregnancy and delivery in patients with coronary artery lesions caused by Kawasaki disease, *Heart* 91(11):1481–1482, 2005.

122. Tsuda E, Kitamura S, Kimura K, et al: Long-term patency of internal thoracic artery grafts for coronary artery stenosis due to Kawasaki disease: comparison of early with recent results in small children, *Am Heart J* 153(6):995–1000, 2007.

123. Tsuda E, Kitamura S: National survey of coronary artery bypass grafting for coronary stenosis caused by Kawasaki disease in Japan, *Circulation* 110(11 Suppl 1):II61–II66, 2004.

124. Kitamura S, Tsuda E, Kobayashi J, et al: Twenty-five-year outcome of pediatric coronary artery bypass surgery for Kawasaki disease, *Circulation* 120(1):60–68, 2009.

125. Akagi T: Interventions in Kawasaki disease, *Pediatr Cardiol* 26(2):206–212, 2005.

126. Subcommittee of Cardiovascular Sequelae, Subcommittee of Surgical Treatment, Kawasaki Disease Research Committee: Guidelines for treatment and management of cardiovascular in Kawasaki disease, *Heart Vessels* 3(1):50–54, 1987.

127. Ishii M, Ueno T, Akagi T, et al: Guidelines for catheter intervention in coronary artery lesion in Kawasaki disease, *Pediatr Int* 43(5):558–562, 2001.

128. Ishii M, Ueno T, Ikeda H, et al: Sequential follow-up results of catheter intervention for coronary artery lesions after Kawasaki disease: quantitative coronary artery angiography and intravascular ultrasound imaging study, *Circulation* 105(25):3004–3010, 2002.

129. Muta H, Ishii M: Percutaneous coronary intervention versus coronary artery bypass grafting for stenotic lesions after Kawasaki disease, *J Pediatr* 157(1):120–126, 2010.

130. Takahashi K, Ohharaseki T, Naoe S: Pathological study of postcoronary arteritis in adolescents and young adults: with reference to the relationship between sequelae of Kawasaki disease and atherosclerosis, *Pediatr Cardiol* 22(2):138–142, 2001.

131. Noto N, Okada T, Yamasuge M, et al: Noninvasive assessment of the early progression of atherosclerosis in adolescents with Kawasaki disease and coronary artery lesions, *Pediatrics* 107(5):1095–1099, 2001.

132. Cheung YF, Ho MH, Tam SC, et al: Increased high sensitivity C reactive protein concentrations and increased arterial stiffness in children with a history of Kawasaki disease, *Heart* 90(11):1281–1285, 2004.

133. Mitani Y, Sawada H, Hayakawa H, et al: Elevated levels of high-sensitivity c-reactive protein and serum amyloid-A late after Kawasaki disease. Association between inflammation and late coronary sequelae in Kawasaki disease, *Circulation* 111(1):38–43, 2005.

134. Kavey RE, Allada V, Daniels SR, et al: Cardiovascular risk reduction in high-risk pediatric patients: a scientific statement from the American Heart Association Expert Panel on Population and Prevention Science; the Councils on Cardiovascular Disease in the Young, Epidemiology and Prevention, Nutrition, Physical Activity and Metabolism, High Blood Pressure Research, Cardiovascular Nursing, and the Kidney in Heart Disease; and the Interdisciplinary Working Group on Quality of Care and Outcomes Research, *Circulation* 114(24):2710–2738, 2006.

135. Graham TP Jr, Driscoll DJ, Gersony WM, et al: Task Force 2: congenital heart disease, *J Am Coll Cardiol* 45(8):1326–1333, 2005.

KAWASAKI DISEASE

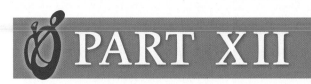

PART XII

ACUTE LIMB ISCHEMIA

CHAPTER **46** **Acute Arterial Occlusion**

Piotr S. Sobieszczyk

Nontraumatic acute occlusion of arterial supply to a limb or organ presents with a constellation of symptoms specific to the tissue suddenly deprived of arterial perfusion. Irrespective of the arterial segment involved, this syndrome represents a vascular emergency. Irreversible organ injury may occur within seconds in the case of acute embolic occlusion of a middle cerebral artery (MCA) or take hours when arterial supply of a lower limb is involved. In everyday clinical practice, *acute arterial occlusion* is synonymous with *acute limb ischemia*. Rapid recognition and treatment are required to prevent limb loss and life-threatening morbidity. *Acute limb ischemia* is thus defined as sudden limb-threatening decrease in arterial perfusion of less than 14 days' duration. It can occur as a result of embolic occlusion or *in situ* arterial thrombosis. Over the last several decades, the etiology of acute limb ischemia has varied with changing prevalence of causative conditions. Management of the syndrome has evolved, but the diagnostic skills required to recognize this clinical entity remain unchanged.

Epidemiology of Acute Limb Ischemia

Acute limb ischemia is a rare vascular event, and its incidence eludes exact quantification. It has been influenced by the ever-changing medical landscape. Increasing numbers of patients treated with antiplatelet and antithrombotic therapies, effective therapy for atrial fibrillation, and advances in treatment of valvular and ischemic heart disease have had an impact on the incidence of acute limb ischemia by decreasing the number of embolic events. This may be counterbalanced by increasing numbers of patients undergoing elective surgical and endovascular revascularization therapies, which carry a low but measurable risk of graft or stent thrombosis. An estimate in the 1990s proposed that a vascular center serving a community of 500,000 may expect an annual incidence of 75 patients with acute limb ischemia of the lower extremity.[1] Other studies report similar data, estimating the incidence of acute lower-limb ischemia between 13 and 17 cases per 100,000 people per year, with mortality as high as 18% even in the modern era.[2,3] Contemporary studies report amputation rates as high as 13% in patients presenting with acute limb ischemia of the lower extremity.[4]

Acute limb ischemia affects men and women equally. It is infrequent in patients with established peripheral artery disease (PAD), except in those who underwent surgical or endovascular revascularization and developed acute thrombosis of the conduit, graft, or stent. Acute limb ischemia is typically a disease of the middle-aged and older population but can affect younger patients when unusual clinical events such as paradoxical embolism, intracardiac masses and endocarditis, or hypercoagulable syndromes affect the arterial circulation.

Acute nontraumatic ischemia of the upper extremity is even more uncommon. It is less likely to result in limb loss, and thus its importance has been overshadowed by lower-extremity ischemic syndromes. Few published series have been reported, and there are no randomized trials evaluating this clinical syndrome and its treatment. However, the consequences of functional impairment in the upper extremity can be equally devastating to the patient.[5] On average, acute arm ischemia accounts for 16.6% of cases of acute ischemia of the extremities and, by extrapolation, occurs with an incidence of 1.2 to 3.5 cases per 100,000 per year.[6] However, these estimates are based primarily on surgical series, which usually include only patients who underwent surgical treatment. Surveys of all patients presenting with acute arm ischemia estimate an incidence of 1.13 per 100,000 per year.[7] In the absence of more meticulous population studies, the true incidence can only be estimated. Patients with upper-extremity ischemia tend to be older than those with lower-extremity ischemia, with mean ages of 74 and 70 respectively.[8]

Amputation-free survival is influenced by many modifiable and nonmodifiable factors.[9] Among the former, delay in diagnosis stands out as a major factor. Non-Caucasian race, older age, malignancy, congestive heart failure (CHF), and low body weight decrease, whereas systemic atherosclerosis increases the likelihood of amputation-free survival.[9,10] Among patients older than 75 years of age, overall 30-day mortality rates approach 42%.[11] Survival and functional recovery among patients with acute limb ischemia are directly related to underlying comorbidities and delay in diagnosis and treatment.

Etiology of Acute Limb Ischemia
Acute Upper-Extremity Ischemia

The most common sites of arterial occlusion in the upper extremity are the brachial and axillary arteries, representing 85% of cases of embolic occlusion.[6] The subclavian artery is thought to be the most frequent site of occlusion in uncommon cases of *in situ* thrombosis (Fig. 46-1).

IATROGENIC CAUSES

In the past, acute ischemia of the arm was primarily caused by cardiac catheterization performed via brachial artery access (Fig. 46-2). In a series from the 1980s reporting on 37 cases of acute arm ischemia treated surgically over a period of 5 years, 56% of cases were caused by this iatrogenic complication, 24% were related to embolic events, and the remainder were due to stab wounds.[12] Since brachial artery catheterization fell out of favor, causes of upper-extremity ischemia have changed. In a later series of 65 patients with acute arm ischemia treated surgically over a span of 8 years, a cardioembolic source was identified in 41% of patients, 17% of events were attributed to an arterial source of embolism, and 28% of cases were related to iatrogenic occlusion, mainly a result of cardiac catheterization.[13] The resurgence of interest in radial artery access for coronary procedures is unlikely to result in a rise in frequency of upper-extremity ischemia. Occlusion of the radial artery, seen in up to 5% of procedures, is unlikely to compromise perfusion of the hand in a patient with proper preprocedural assessment of a patent palmar arch.

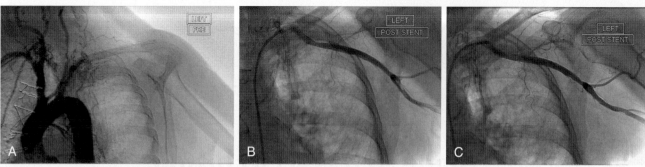

FIGURE 46-1 *In situ* thrombosis of subclavian artery in a patient presenting with an inferior ST-segment elevation myocardial infarction (MI) and symptoms of acute left arm and hand ischemia. **A,** Occlusion of subclavian artery, with angiographic changes suggestive of *in situ* thrombosis. **B,** After balloon angioplasty and stenting of subclavian artery, thrombotic component of lesion is seen trapped in filter embolic protection device positioned in axillary artery. **C,** Patent vessel after filter retrieval.

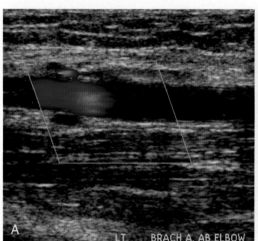

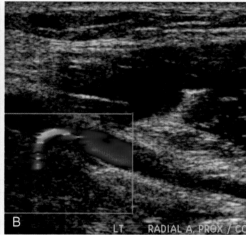

FIGURE 46-2 Acute hand ischemia after coronary angiography via left brachial artery access. **A,** Occlusion of left brachial artery. **B,** Radial artery reconstitutes via collaterals.

EMBOLISM

Embolic occlusion is the most frequent cause of acute arm ischemia, accounting for 74% to 100% of cases in several reported series.[6,7,13–15] Of these, 72% are thought to be cardioembolic in origin, 12% originate from the proximal vessel, and the remainder are of unknown origin.[6] Atrial fibrillation and left ventricular (LV) thrombus in patients with ventricular dysfunction are the most frequent causes of cardiac emboli. Common causes of embolization include atrial myxoma[16,17] and paradoxical embolism.[18] Proximal arteries of the arm can be a source of arterial embolism. Artery-to-artery embolization may cause occlusion of a large- or medium-caliber artery but more commonly presents with digital embolization. Atherosclerotic stenosis of the subclavian artery is a rare cause of embolism but can result in acute hand or arm ischemia.[19–21] The rare primary subclavian artery aneurysm or one caused by external compression in a thoracic outlet syndrome (TOS) can result in thromboembolic occlusion of upper-extremity arteries.[20,22–24] Aortic arch atheroma has also been implicated as the source of acute arm ischemia.[15,25] Other rare arterial sources of embolic events are malignant emboli or paradoxical embolism through intracardiac shunting[26,27] (Fig. 46-3).

THROMBOSIS

Atherosclerotic disease is much less frequent in the upper extremity than the lower limb. Consequently, *in situ* thrombosis is uncommon and has been estimated to account for 5% of ischemic cases in population studies and 5% to 35% of cases in surgical series.[7,14,15,28] Many of the proximal arterial lesions responsible for distal embolization can cause *in situ* thrombosis. Arteritis, radiation injury, and hypercoagulable syndromes have been reported as rare causes of *in situ* arterial thrombosis of the upper extremity.[20,22,29,30]

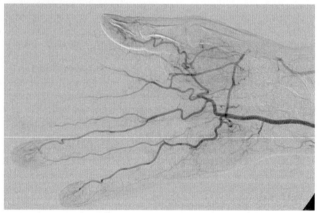

FIGURE 46-3 Embolic occlusion of right radial artery and ischemia of index and middle fingers in patient with patent foramen ovale.

Acute Lower-Extremity Ischemia

The distinction between embolism and *in situ* thrombosis should not detract from the need to establish a rapid diagnosis and institute immediate therapy. Nevertheless, embolic etiology is more commonly associated with rapid onset of symptoms, history of cardiac disease, and absence of prior history of PAD. The contralateral limb is likely to have a normal exam, without stigmata of systemic atherosclerosis. Some of the causes of acute limb ischemia are listed in Box 46-1.

IN SITU THROMBOSIS

In situ thrombosis rather than embolism was responsible for 85% of the acute limb ischemia cases enrolled in the Thrombolysis or Peripheral Arterial Surgery (TOPAS) trial. Rates of embolic cases

Box 46-1 Causes of Acute Limb Ischemia

Embolism
Cardiac Source of Embolism
Atrial fibrillation
Left ventricular (LV) thrombus
Cardiac myxoma
Valvular heart disease:
  Infectious endocarditis
  Prosthetic valve thrombosis
  Rheumatic valve disease
Paradoxical embolism via patent foramen ovale

Artery-to-Artery Source
Arterial aneurysm
Atherosclerotic plaque

Iatrogenic
Catheter-associated embolism
Vascular closure device malfunction

Other
Tumor embolism
Amniotic fluid
Fat embolism
Air

***In Situ* Thrombosis**
Atherosclerotic Peripheral Artery Disease
Iatrogenic
Catheter-associated *in situ* thrombosis

Stent and Graft Thrombosis
Restenosis
Intimal hyperplasia
Stent or stent graft underexpansion
Mechanical

Arterial Aneurysm
Popliteal aneurysm thrombosis

Hypercoagulable States
Antiphospholipid antibody syndrome
Advanced malignancy
Hyperviscosity syndromes

Low-Flow States
Cardiogenic shock and preexisting peripheral artery disease (PAD)
Vasopressor-induced vasospasm

Arterial Dissection
Access-site artery dissection
Aortic dissection

Other Causes
Trauma
Vasospasm
Ergotism
Cocaine use
Phlegmasia cerulea dolens

have been decreasing over the last few decades. In a Greek study evaluating the causes of acute limb ischemia at a referral center between 2000 and 2004, 40% of cases were caused by embolic events, *in situ* thrombosis was responsible for 50% of cases, and the remaining 10% were due to trauma, iatrogenic injury, vasculitis, or dissection.[31] As many as 78% of embolic events were due to a cardiac source; the source of 9% of embolic events could not be determined. Among cases of *in situ* thrombosis, 30% involved native arteries, and 70% involved thrombosis of vessels after an intervention (65% represented graft thrombosis and 5% iliac or infrainguinal stent thrombosis). Surgical graft thrombosis represented 30% of all cases of acute limb ischemia. Patients with surgical grafts can develop graft thrombosis and symptoms of acute limb ischemia

due to graft degeneration or mechanical problems such as anastomotic stenosis or retained valves. Graft compression or kink can also cause its thrombosis. With the advent of stent grafting for aortoiliac aneurysmal disease, acute stentgraft thrombosis has been added as a cause of acute limb ischemia (Fig. 46-4).

In situ thrombosis of a popliteal artery aneurysm usually presents with acute limb ischemia. A review of nearly 900 patients presenting with acute limb ischemia secondary to a thrombosed popliteal aneurysm reported amputation rates of 14%. In this study, catheter-directed thrombolysis prior to surgery did not lower the likelihood of amputation, but it significantly improved the long-term patency of the graft, presumably by maximizing patency of the tibial vessel.[32] The decision to perform catheter-directed thrombolysis must depend on the clinical situation and urgency of revascularization. In a Swedish vascular registry, amputation rates for acute thrombosis of the popliteal aneurysm were 17% in patients presenting with acute ischemia and only 1.8% for asymptomatic electively repaired aneurysms.[33]

EMBOLISM

Acute limb ischemia is often caused by an embolic event, commonly from a cardiac source. The embolus most frequently lodges in the aortoiliac bifurcation, femoral bifurcation, or popliteal trifurcation. Over the last several decades, the etiology of cardioembolic events has evolved. Embolic events caused by rheumatic mitral stenosis with left atrial enlargement have become a rare occurrence because the prevalence of rheumatic valve disease has decreased substantially. Age-related atrial fibrillation and LV dysfunction with apical thrombus formation are the most common causes of cardioembolic events (Fig. 46-5). Less common causes include endocarditis, intracardiac myxoma, or paradoxical embolism due to a patent foramen ovale allowing transit of venous thrombus into the arterial circulation. Acute embolic occlusion related to aortic aneurysmal disease and intramural thrombus is rare.

IATROGENIC CAUSES

Iatrogenic acute limb ischemia can be caused by arterial access in the common femoral artery (CFA) and injury of the vessel at the access site, be it by deployment of a vascular closure device or direct injury to the common femoral or iliac artery. Similarly, catheter-associated thrombosis and embolism of the popliteal artery can occur.

OTHER CAUSES

Intense vasospasm, such as can be caused by ergotism[34,35] or cocaine ingestion,[36] have been reported to cause acute limb ischemia. Aortic dissection can result in occlusion of the distal aorta and iliac vessels when the true lumen is compressed by a pressurized false lumen. Iliofemoral deep vein thrombosis (DVT) with massive swelling of the thigh can compromise arterial inflow to the leg. The syndrome of phlegmasia cerulea dolens requires urgent catheter direct thrombolysis of the venous thrombus to restore venous outflow and thus arterial inflow to the limb.

Pathophysiology of Acute Limb Ischemia

Most emboli lodge in points of arterial branching: aortic, iliac, femoral, or popliteal bifurcations in the leg, and brachial bifurcation in the arm. *In situ* thrombosis most commonly affects the femoral or popliteal artery, particularly in the setting of an existing arterial bypass, ruptured atherosclerotic plaque, or low-output state. Sudden cessation of arterial flow to the extremity triggers a series of complex pathophysiological processes. Malperfused tissues shift from aerobic to anaerobic metabolism. The shift in lactate-to-pyruvate ratio further increases lactate production, increases the concentration of hydrogen ions, and induces acidosis. Progressive ischemia

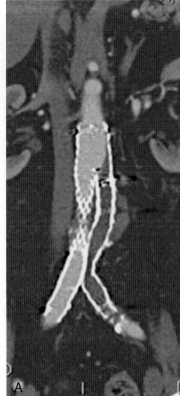

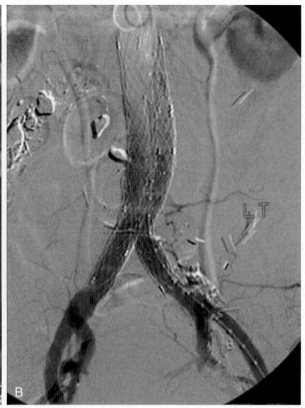

FIGURE 46-4 A, Acute limb ischemia due to collapse of right iliac endograft limb. **B,** Treated with ultrasound-accelerated thrombolysis.

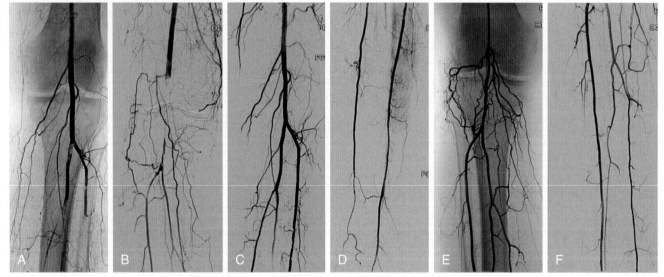

FIGURE 46-5   Bilateral acute limb ischemia in patient with atrial fibrillation and interrupted anticoagulation. Left anterior tibial artery and tibioperoneal trunk are occluded **(A)**, as is right popliteal artery **(B)**. Mechanical thrombectomy and catheter suction embolectomy restored flow in left **(C-D)** and right calf **(E-F)**.

results in cell dysfunction and eventual cell death. Muscle hypoxia depletes intracellular adenosine triphosphate (ATP) stores, and the consequent dysfunction of the sodium/potassium-ATPase and calcium/sodium pumps causes leakage of intracellular calcium into myocytes.[37] Intracellular free calcium levels rise and interact with actin, myosin, and proteases, leading to necrosis of muscle fibers. As the cellular membranes and microvascular integrity fail, intracellular potassium, phosphate, creatinine (Cr) kinase, and myoglobin leak into the systemic circulation. Reperfusion further amplifies these cellular changes.

Nerve and muscle tissue are quite susceptible to ischemic injury, so presence or absence of neuromotor deficit is of paramount importance in assessing the severity of acute limb ischemia.

Irreversible muscle damage begins after 3 hours of ischemia and is nearly complete after 6 hours.[38] In addition to myocyte injury, progressive microvascular damage follows skeletal muscle injury. The more severe the cellular damage, the greater the microvascular changes. In the setting of muscle necrosis, microvascular flow stops within a few hours. Traditionally, a window of 6 hours has been assumed before irreversible functional injury occurs. This time window may be longer in a "preconditioned" limb with collateral pathways.

Ischemic insult sets the stage for reperfusion injury, a process triggered by restoration of perfusion and mediated by a complex cascade of cytokines, reactive oxygen species (ROS), and neutrophils. Reactive oxygen species (e.g., superoxide anion, hydrogen peroxide, hydroxyl radicals, peroxynitrite) are produced by activated neutrophils and xanthine oxidase, an enzyme located on microvascular endothelial cells (ECs) of skeletal muscle and activated during ischemic conditions.[39] Under normal conditions, xanthine dehydrogenase uses nicotinamide adenine dinucleotide to oxidize hypoxanthine to xanthine. Xanthine dehydrogenase is converted to xanthine oxidase after 2 hours of ischemia.[40] During ischemia, ATP is degraded to hypoxanthine, but xanthine oxidase requires oxygen to convert hypoxanthine to xanthine. Thus, hypoxanthine accumulates during ischemia. When oxygen is reintroduced during reperfusion, xanthine dehydrogenase isoform becomes active again. Conversion of massive amounts of hypoxanthine generates reactive oxygen species.[41]

The essential substrate for production of these radicals, molecular oxygen, is provided by reperfusion. Xanthine oxidase–derived oxidants mediate the increased vascular permeability in postischemic muscle. The importance of elemental oxygen and the role of oxygen radicals in reperfusion injury is underscored by studies showing that reperfusion initially with deoxygenated autologous blood prevents increase in permeability after ischemia. Changing the perfusate to oxygenated blood during reperfusion mimicked the microvascular injury response seen after normoxic reperfusion.[42] Similarly, gradual reintroduction of oxygen early in reperfusion decreases postischemic injury.[42] Additional supplementation with free radical scavengers and reduced oxygen delivery further reduces injury of postischemic necrosis.[43]

Activated neutrophils are the principal agents responsible for local and systemic damage caused by reperfusion. Leukocytes play an equally important role in reperfusion injury. Activated neutrophils accumulate in the reperfusing muscle and produce reactive oxygen metabolites, release cytotoxic enzymes, and occlude microcirculation pathways.[44] Leukocyte depletion has been shown to reduce the ischemia-reperfusion injury. Reperfusion with oxygenated blood depleted of leukocytes by the use of filters completely prevents development of vascular permeability in canine skeletal muscle.[45,46] Interestingly, inducing neutropenia before ischemia in rats restores transmembrane potential and contractile function in postischemic rat muscle.[47,48]

Skeletal muscle ischemia and reperfusion triggers a number of additional inflammatory cascades that include complement activation, increased expression of adhesion molecules, cytokine release, eicosanoid synthesis, free radical formation, cytoskeletal alterations, adenine nucleotide depletion, alterations in calcium and phospholipid metabolism, leukocyte activation, and endothelial dysfunction.[40] Interleukin (IL)-1β and tumor necrosis factor (TNF)-α are detected soon after reperfusion and induce adhesion molecules on the surface of endothelial cells, increase capillary leak, and stimulate production of IL-6 and IL-8, which further increase endothelial permeability, destroy endothelial integrity, and activate leukocytes.[49–53]

The clinical impact of these cellular responses to reperfusion results in tissue swelling, a catastrophic event in the closed spaces of the forearm, thigh, calf, and buttock. Elevated compartment pressures within fascial boundaries cause a *compartment syndrome*: elevated compartment pressures that reduce the perfusion gradient and capillary blood flow below the metabolic requirement, resulting in further ischemia and necrosis. Release of myoglobin can result in renal injury. Increased endothelial permeability can lead to acute lung injury, a process attenuated in animal models by chemically induced neutropenia, suggesting that activation and transmigration of neutrophils and loss of endothelial integrity are critical in acute lung injury in reperfusion injury.[54] Thus, noncardiogenic pulmonary edema can develop after reperfusion of lower limbs, a process that can be prevented by granulocyte depletion.[54,55]

The reperfusion syndrome consists of two components. The local response to reperfusion triggers tissue swelling, while the systemic response can result in multiorgan failure and death. It is the latter that mitigates intervention in advanced and irreversible limb ischemia. The degree of inflammatory response following reperfusion is variable. There is little inflammatory response when muscle necrosis is uniform. The degree of ischemic damage, however,

will vary depending on proximity of the tissue to the occlusion and efficiency of the collateral supply. The magnitude of the inflammatory response will be determined by the extent of the ischemic, but not completely necrotic, zone. Thus, reperfusion of large muscle groups with advanced ischemic injury and tissue necrosis will result in release of large amounts of toxic inflammatory mediators into the systemic circulation. This detrimental effect of reperfusion favors amputation in patients with irreversible ischemic injury.

Diagnosis of Acute Limb Ischemia

The diagnosis of acute limb ischemia may be elusive, especially in patients who present with sensory and motor deficits that direct attention toward neurological evaluation. Clinical signs and symptoms of acute limb ischemia manifest as a spectrum of findings directly related to the severity of ischemia and duration of arterial malperfusion. Diagnosis of acute limb ischemia is made on the basis of physical examination. Confirmatory imaging with computed tomographic angiography (CTA) or magnetic resonance angiography (MRA) introduces a potentially costly delay in therapeutic intervention. Bedside duplex ultrasonography can be performed rapidly and can add information about the level of occlusion and the arterial access strategy for an endovascular procedure. A careful physical examination, including Doppler evaluation of arterial and venous signals, is usually sufficient for obtaining this information. A good physical examination can determine the level of arterial occlusion and obviate the need for additional imaging.

The classic symptoms and physical examination findings of an acutely ischemic limb are commonly known as the *six Ps: pulselessness, pallor, pain, poikilothermia, paralysis, and paresthesia*. Pain is the most common symptom and progresses with ischemia. Pallor is an early finding in an ischemic extremity and is caused by complete emptying and vasospasm of the arteries (Fig. 46-6). Subsequent stagnation of microvascular circulation will cause mottling of the skin, which initially blanches with pressure. As ischemia continues, paresthesia develops, and numbness replaces pain, often falsely reassuring both patient and physician. In the final stages of ischemic injury, paralysis sets in, and skin mottling is fixed and nonblanching. Loss of motor function and marble-like appearance of the skin herald irreversible ischemic injury.

A careful physical examination can determine the level of occlusion by detecting a temperature gradient along the limb and a deficit in pulses either on palpation or by arterial Doppler exam. The cutaneous changes of pallor and temperature are detected one level below the occluded arterial segment. Physical examination must also include a search for potential sources of acute limb ischemia. Recognition of atrial fibrillation, a cardiac murmur of valvular disease, or symptoms of CHF may implicate a cardioembolic cause of the event. Systemic symptoms of fevers, night sweats, and chills may hint at endocarditis as the etiology of cardiac embolism. Stigmata of PAD in the contralateral limb or signs of prior surgical revascularization point to an *in situ* arterial thrombosis, whereas chest pain, hypertension, and asymmetry in arterial pulses of the upper extremity may require additional imaging to exclude an aortic dissection.

More importantly, it is the physical examination that allows classification of the severity of ischemia, urgency of revascularization, and prognosis after revascularization[56] (Table 46-1). These clinical classes are also useful for determining the best intervention strategies. In general, Rutherford class I represents a viable and nonthreatened limb, akin to patients with chronic and noncritical ischemia. Rutherford class II symptoms describe a directly threatened limb. A class IIa limb is characterized by intact sensory and motor examination despite absent arterial Doppler signals in the foot. This limb is marginally threatened. Class IIb includes patients with an immediately threatened limb, characterized by sensory loss, mild motor function impairment, and absent Doppler arterial signals. This limb can be salvaged if treated immediately. Irreversible limb ischemia falls into Rutherford class III, with permanent nerve damage, profound sensory loss and motor paralysis,

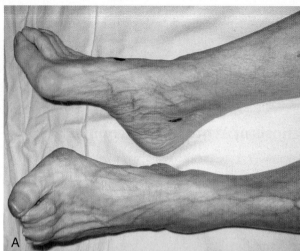

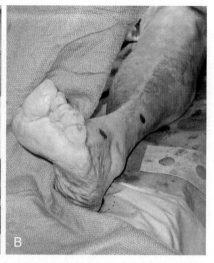

FIGURE 46-6 **Acute limb ischemia due to left common femoral artery (CFA) embolism.** Marked pallor of left foot **(A)** resolves after surgical embolectomy **(B)**. *(Image courtesy Dr. Edwin Gravereaux.)*

TABLE 46-1 **Rutherford Classification of Acute Limb Ischemia**						
RUTHERFORD CLASS	**PROGNOSIS**	**SENSORY EXAM**	**MOTOR EXAM**	**ARTERIAL DOPPLER SIGNAL**	**VENOUS DOPPLER SIGNAL**	**SKIN EXAM**
Class I: viable, not threatened	Threatened	Normal sensory exam	Normal	Audible	Audible	Normal capillary return
Class IIa: marginally threatened	Salvageable with prompt therapy	Minimal sensory loss	Normal	Often audible	Audible	Decreased capillary return
Class IIb: immediately threatened	Salvageable if treated immediately	Mild sensory loss and rest pain	Mildly to moderately abnormal	Usually inaudible	Audible	Pallor
Class III: irreversible	Irreversible tissue and nerve damage	Profound sensory loss	Paralysis and rigor	Inaudible	Inaudible	No capillary return, skin marbling

Adapted from Rutherford RB, Baker JD, Ernst C, et al: Recommended standards for reports dealing with lower extremity ischemia: revised version. J Vasc Surg 26:517–538, 1997.[56]

and absent arterial and venous Doppler signals. Revascularization of such a limb is harmful; amputation is required.

The presence of preexisting arterial occlusive disease may "precondition" the limb by fostering development of collaterals that lessen the severity of tissue malperfusion when acute occlusion occurs. Thus, patients with thrombosis *in situ* in an atherosclerotic vessel and those with graft failure may tolerate acute ischemia better than patients with no underlying arterial disease who develop acute limb ischemia due to a cardioembolic or an iatrogenic event. Several clinical characteristics may allow differentiation between an embolic event and *in situ* thrombosis. Patients with the former report a more abrupt onset of pain with clearer demarcation of ischemic temperature change and skin mottling. These patients usually present with symptoms and signs in Rutherford class IIb and III. Patients with *in situ* arterial thrombosis usually have signs of established PAD and report a more vague onset of symptoms. Physical examination findings are less striking, with a less distinct demarcation of ischemic changes and more cyanosis than pallor. These patients often fall into Rutherford class I and IIa categories.

Treatment of Acute Limb Ischemia

Prompt recognition of acute limb ischemia and rapid restoration of arterial perfusion are cornerstones of therapy. The decision whether revascularization or primary amputation should be undertaken depends largely on the viability of the affected limb. In patients with a salvageable limb, selection of the type of revascularization therapy is equally important. The two major factors affecting morbidity and mortality among patients with acute limb ischemia are the burden of medical comorbidities and the delay in recognition and treatment of the ischemic limb. Other factors associated

with lower amputation-free survival are increased age, race, diabetes, and absence of prompt initiation of anticoagulation.[57]

Surgical intervention has been traditionally associated with high perioperative mortality rates. In a compilation of 3000 patients treated surgically for acute limb ischemia in 30 centers between 1963 and 1978, 30-day mortality rates were as high as 25%.[58] Despite rapid advances in surgical and anesthesia techniques, Jivegard reported a 20% mortality rate a decade later.[10] Even in the 1990s, 30-day mortality after surgical intervention among selected patients enrolled in the TOPAS, Surgery versus Thrombolysis for Ischemia of the Lower Extremity (STILE), and Rochester randomized trials ranged from 5% to 18%.[9,59,60]

The high burden of cardiopulmonary disease and high surgical mortality in the population affected by acute limb ischemia provided an impetus for development of less invasive endovascular strategies. Evidence from randomized trials suggests equipoise between endovascular and surgical therapies in selected patients, particularly those with class I and IIa symptoms. The cause of limb ischemia, location of the occlusion, Rutherford class, as well as patient characteristics play a crucial role in selection of appropriate revascularization strategy. The Rochester, STILE, and TOPAS trials form a framework for selection of patients for endovascular therapies.[9,59,60] These trials demonstrated that patients with underlying PAD or graft thrombosis and Rutherford class I and IIa thrombolytic-based endovascular therapies do indeed have better outcomes. Patients with cardioembolic events usually present with Rutherford class IIb symptoms and are best treated with prompt surgical embolectomy.[4]

In modern practice, a rigid division between open surgical and endovascular treatment is artificial. Although many patients can be treated with an entirely endovascular approach, and others require traditional surgical embolectomy, large numbers of patients are treated with hybrid approaches. Indeed, routine use of perioperative angiography suggests a high rate of residual thrombus, necessitating additional combined surgical and endovascular intervention in up to 90% of complex cases.[61]

In addition to revascularization therapies, the sequelae of acute limb ischemia include ischemia-reperfusion injury, which may range from mild injury without functional or systemic consequences to systemic inflammatory response and multiorgan failure. Treatment of these metabolic consequences of acute limb ischemia is essential to patients' survival.

Initial Medical Management

Regardless of the revascularization strategy selected, the basic principles of initial therapy are the same: fluid resuscitation, analgesia, and administration of antithrombin and antiplatelet therapy. After decades of clinical experience, heparin therapy has been shown to decrease ischemic injury, reduce thrombus propagation, and improve survival.[4,62-64] Some studies dispute the benefit of perioperative anticoagulation, even in patients with a cardiac source of emboli, but the overwhelming amount of data support perioperative anticoagulation with heparin.[65] Unfractionated heparin (UFH) should be administered at high doses (100-150 units/ kg), with a goal of rapidly achieving a therapeutic level of anticoagulation and a rise in partial thromboplastin time (PTT) by a factor of 2 to 2.5 above baseline. Patients with heparin-induced thrombocytopenia (HIT) should be treated with intravenous (IV) direct thrombin inhibitors (DTI) such as lepirudin or argatroban. Bivalirudin, another DTI commonly used in coronary and endovascular interventions, has a relatively short half-life and is more familiar to most vascular specialists. The decision regarding long-term anticoagulation must be made based on the etiology of the ischemic event, outcome of revascularization, and the balance between bleeding and thrombotic risk.

Correction of laboratory abnormalities and stabilization of the underlying acute medical condition are imperative to achieve best clinical outcomes. Certain laboratory characteristics predict ultimate therapeutic success. Patients presenting with elevated Cr kinase and neutrophil count have a 50% risk of amputation as compared to a 5% risk among those with normal enzyme and neutrophil levels.[66] This finding underscores the poor clinical outcomes in patients with advanced ischemic injury of skeletal muscle. In patients who present with irreversible tissue loss, alkalinization of urine may be required to prevent renal injury from myoglobinuria. In some cases, the cause of acute limb ischemia is itself immediately life threatening, such as myocardial infarction (MI) complicated by LV thrombus and cardiogenic shock, or aortic dissection or infective endocarditis

with hemodynamic compromise due to valvular incompetence. In such cases, the principle of "life over limb" should guide best therapeutic strategy.

Endovascular Therapy of Acute Limb Ischemia

The basic principle behind endovascular therapy is to restore arterial flow, either by thrombus lysis or unmasking and treating an underlying lesion, thus eliminating the need for surgery or reducing the extent of surgical procedure.

Endovascular therapy for acute limb ischemia became possible when Tillet and Garner discovered the fibrinolytic properties of hemolytic streptococcus in 1933.[67] It was not long after the first use of IV streptokinase in healthy volunteers by Tillet et al. in 1955 that Cliffton reported on the therapeutic use of streptokinase to dissolve pathological thrombi in arteries and veins in 1957.[68,69] Catheter-based delivery of intraarterial (IA) streptokinase was pioneered by Charles Dotter et al. in 1974.[70] Berridge et al. subsequently confirmed that catheter delivery of fibrinolytic agents directly into the affected artery was superior to an IV administered thrombolytic, and improved limb salvage rates (80% vs. 45%) and lowered hemorrhagic complications.[71]

Modern thrombolytic agents work by enhancing the intrinsic fibrinolytic process through activation of plasminogen and its conversion into plasmin, which degrades fibrin (Table 46-2). The conversion of plasminogen into plasmin requires hydrolysis of a lysine-arginine bond, a step catalyzed by tissue-type plasminogen activator (tPA), the model for today's recombinant plasminogen activators. Technical success of catheter-directed thrombolysis is defined as restoration of antegrade flow and complete or near-complete resolution of thrombus. Clinical success is defined as relief of acute ischemic symptoms or reduction of the level of the subsequent surgical intervention or amputation.[72] Enzymatic dissolution of thrombus may be more complete compared to surgical embolectomy, particularly in the distal arterial beds and in cases of distal embolization. Endovascular therapies evolved and became more effective as cumulative experience grew in the 1980s and 1990s. Development of multihole infusion catheters and recognition of the importance of traversing the thrombotic occlusion with the infusion catheter and infusing the drug into the clot rather than above the occlusion have markedly increased the efficacy of these procedures.

Three randomized trials performed in the 1990s compared endovascular therapy to surgical intervention in patients with acute limb ischemia. The Rochester trial randomized 114 patients with limb-threatening ischemia from embolic and thrombotic occlusion of native vessels or grafts to treatment with IA delivery of urokinase or surgery.[60] Catheter-directed thrombolysis resulted in resolution of thrombus in 70% of patients. After 1 year, amputation rates were identical in both arms at 18%, but

ACUTE ARTERIAL OCCLUSION

CH 46

TABLE 46-2	Properties of Thrombolytic Agents Used in Treatment of Acute Limb Ischemia						
THROMBOLYTIC AGENT	PROPERTIES	HALF-LIFE	DOSAGE	MAJOR BLEEDING COMPLICATIONS	FIBRIN AFFINITY	FIBRIN SPECIFICITY
Urokinase	Direct plasminogen activator; cleavage of plasminogen converts it into active plasmin	7-20 min	240,000 IU/h for 4 h, then 120,000 IU/h	5.6%-12.5%	Low	Low
Alteplase (rtPA)	Recombinant tissue plasminogen activator; fibrin-mediated conversion of plasminogen to active plasmin	3-6 min	0.5-1 mg/h; maximum dose 40 mg	6.1%-6.8%	High	High
Reteplase (rPA)	Superior thrombus penetration	14-18 min	0.25-2 units/h; maximum dose 20 units in 24 h	6.1%-6.8%	Low	Moderate
Tenecteplase (TNK-rtPA)	Increased fibrin affinity and longer half-life	20-24 min	0.25-1 mg/h Low-dose regimen: 0.125 mg/h	5.4%-13.3% 2.9%	Low	Very high

IU, international units.

mortality was significantly higher in the surgical arm: 16% vs. 42%, with the majority of deaths in the surgical arm related to cardiopulmonary complications. Thrombolytic therapy was also associated with lower cost.

The larger STILE trial enrolled 393 patients with native vessel or graft thrombosis of less than 6 months duration who were randomized to surgical intervention or thrombolytic therapy.[59] The trial was handicapped by inclusion of patients with chronic ischemic symptoms unlikely to respond to thrombolysis. Indeed, 70% of patients in the thrombolytic arm had symptoms of a chronic nature. Technical failure accounted for a large fraction of clinical failures in the fibrinolytic arms. Failure to traverse the occlusive lesion was noted in 28% of patients. In patients who underwent successful catheter placement, patency was restored in 81% of bypass grafts and 69% of native arteries (P = NS). The ability to cross the lesion with a wire was predictive of therapeutic success, a key finding that has guided endovascular therapy for acute limb ischemia ever since.

In the fibrinolytic arm, patients received either recombinant tPA (rtPA) at a dose of 0.05 mg/kg/h for up to 12 hours or urokinase for up to 36 hours. The dose of tPA used in this trial was much larger than usual doses of 1 mg/h used in clinical practice today. The trial was terminated early after the combined endpoint of death, major amputation, and recurrent ischemia occurred in 61.7% and 36.1% of patients, respectively, in the lytic and surgical arms (P <0.001). The 30-day mortality rates were 4.0% in the thrombolysis arm and 4.9% in the surgical arm (P = NS), with amputation rates of 5.2% and 6.3%, respectively (P = NS). The difference in major morbidity of 21% in the thrombolysis arm and 16% in the surgical group stemmed primarily from the hemorrhagic and vascular access complications and recurrent ischemia observed in the former group. Patients in the thrombolysis arm had a reduction in the extent of surgical revascularization.

A post hoc analysis stratified patients according to the duration of symptoms: among patients with symptoms less than 14 days in duration, thrombolytic therapy was associated with a trend toward a lower rate of major amputation compared to surgical intervention (5.7% vs. 17.9%; P = 0.06). Among patients with longer duration of symptoms, 5.3% of those in the thrombolytic arm and 2.1% in the surgical arm underwent amputation (P = NS). Among patients with symptoms for 14 days, the rates of death and amputation at 6 months were 15.3% in the fibrinolytic arm and 37.5% in the surgical arm (P = 0.01). This study firmly established that thrombolytic therapy was not effective in most cases of chronic limb ischemia.

The TOPAS trial, the third trial comparing surgical intervention to catheter-directed thrombolysis, enrolled only patients with symptoms of less than 14 days' duration.[9] Thrombotic events were the predominant etiology of acute limb ischemia, responsible for 85% of cases, and occurred more frequently in arterial grafts than native arteries. In addition, only 19% of the grafts consisted of autologous vein conduits, a departure from modern practice. The first dose-finding phase of the trial randomized 213 patients to initial infusion of variable doses of urokinase, followed by prolonged low-dose infusion. Complete thrombolysis was achieved in 71% of patients, without statistically significant difference in 12-month limb salvage or mortality rates in the surgical and urokinase arms. Patients treated with urokinase had a prohibitively high rate of intracranial hemorrhage (2.1%), particularly associated with use of a higher urokinase dose. In the second phase of the trial, 542 patients were randomized to surgical intervention or treatment with the safest dose of urokinase infusion. Recanalization occurred in 79.7% of patients and complete thrombolysis in 67.9% of patients. After 1 year, amputation-free survival in the thrombolytic and surgical arms was nearly identical (65% vs. 69.9%; P = NS) but came at a cost of higher rates of intracranial hemorrhage of 1.6% in the thrombolytic arm. Intracranial hemorrhage was associated with concomitant infusion of therapeutic doses of UFH and occurred in as many as 4.8% of patients receiving doses aimed at full systemic anticoagulation, compared to 0.5% of patients who received subtherapeutic doses of heparin.

Major bleeding complications were higher in the thrombolytic arm than in the surgical group (12.5% vs. 5.5%; P = 0.005). At the time of discharge, death occurred in 5.9% of surgical patients and 8.8% of urokinase-treated patients (P = NS). Thrombolytic therapy with urokinase was associated with higher rate of bleeding complications, but effectively reduced the need for surgical interventions without compromising amputation-free survival in patients with primarily thrombotic rather than embolic etiology of acute limb ischemia.

A Cochrane review of five trials of catheter-directed thrombolysis included 1283 patients and reported that there was no significant difference between the two strategies when limb salvage or mortality are compared at 30 days or 1 year. Patients undergoing catheter-directed thrombolysis were more likely to suffer bleeding complications (8.8% vs. 3.3%; 95% confidence interval [CI]: 1.7-4.6) and stroke (1.3% vs. 0%; 95% CI: 1.57, 26.22).[73] A "real-world" experience with catheter-directed thrombolysis was reported in the National Audit of Thrombolysis for Acute Leg Ischemia (NATALI) registry of 1133 patients treated with thrombolytic drugs between 1990 and 1999. This study showed amputation-free survival of 75%, with amputation and death rates each at 12% in the first 30 days, and a 7.8% rate of major hemorrhage. It is not clear whether registries of such type included patients in whom thrombolytic therapy was selected because of high perioperative mortality risk.[74]

Multivariable analysis identified several factors predicting success of thrombolytic therapy.[75] Ability to traverse the thrombus and position the thrombolytic infusing catheter directly into the thrombus favored successful fibrinolysis. Similarly, native artery or a prosthetic graft were more responsive to thrombolysis, whereas patients with diabetes were less likely to have successful treatment.

The success of thrombolytic therapy has led to an intense search for the optimal agent and dosing regimen in an ongoing effort to provide maximal thrombolysis effect with minimal bleeding complications. The largest experience in arterial thrombolysis comes from streptokinase, urokinase, and rtPA. Urokinase has been shown to achieve more rapid thrombolysis and fewer bleeding complications than streptokinase.[76] Streptokinase use has therefore been abandoned owing to its immunogenic effects, platelet-activating effects, and higher bleeding rates compared to later-generation agents. Urokinase was withdrawn from production in 1999 after concerns about contamination in the production process. Since that time, rtPA agents have become the dominant fibrinolytics used in clinical practice. Three agents are available in this class: alteplase, reteplase, and tenecteplase.

Alteplase and tenecteplase have higher affinity for activation of fibrin-bound plasminogen than urokinase and reteplase, which are less fibrin specific. Reduced fibrin binding of reteplase could allow greater availability of unbound drug for thrombus penetration and faster lysis compared to tPA. Alteplase is commonly used for catheter-directed thrombolysis. Catheter-directed thrombolysis using rtPA has been shown to be superior to streptokinase, achieving better angiographic results and superior 30-day limb salvage rates.[71] When compared with urokinase, alteplase was found to have superior efficacy in thrombus resolution but a price of higher incidence of access-site hematoma.[77] In the STILE trial, however, there were no differences between urokinase and alteplase. A review of multiple studies evaluating alteplase concluded that the risk of bleeding was directly related to the duration of infusion and overall dose, but did not differ from complications encountered with urokinase.[78] Reteplase, a third-generation tPA derivative has a longer half-life of 13 to 16 minutes and has been successfully tested in a small number of patients with acute limb ischemia.[79,80] Proliferation of adjunctive endovascular treatments has made direct comparisons between various lytic agents increasingly difficult, but there is no convincing evidence that one rtPA thrombolytic is superior to another in terms of efficacy and safety.

Adjuvant therapy with the glycoprotein (GP) IIb/IIIa inhibitor abciximab was piloted in a small trial of thrombolysis with reteplase. Study results suggested that combined therapy allowed shorter thrombolytic infusion without an increase in bleeding complications.[81] Efficacy of combining infusion of fibrinolytics and GP IIb/IIIa inhibitors was further evaluated in the randomized RELAX trial (official title: Phosphodiesterase-5 Inhibition to Improve Clinical Status and Exercise Capacity in Diastolic Heart Failure [RELAX]). In this study, 74 patients with acute occlusion received variable does of reteplase alone or reteplase and abciximab infusion.[82] At 90 days, the composite endpoint in patients treated with a tPA dose of 1 mg/h did not differ, whether they received concomitant placebo or abciximab. Interestingly, no instances of intracranial hemorrhage were observed in either arm. Use of these adjuvant agents has not been accepted as standard therapy. Unfractionated heparin, on the other hand, is routinely infused through the catheter's side arm to achieve a PTT of 40 to 50. Subgroup analysis of the STILE trial suggested that heparin administration during alteplase infusion was associated with reduction in the composite endpoint of death, amputation, major morbidity, and recurrent ischemia. More importantly, adjunctive infusion of heparin in either urokinase or alteplase arms was not associated with increased bleeding.[56] Infusion of heparin through the sidearm also lowers the risk of catheter thrombosis.[83] Thus, low-dose heparin 400 to 600 units/h should be administered; some authors recommend a lower dose of 100 units/h.

Risk of hemorrhagic complications increases with duration of therapy. It has been estimated that the risk of major complications associated with thrombolytic therapy increases with duration of infusion, from 4% at 8 hours to 34% at 40 hours.[84] The optimal duration of thrombolytic infusion is not well defined. There has been a gradual decrease in therapy duration from 48-hour infusions in early trials to 6- to 18-hour infusions used currently in the era of adjunctive techniques. Monitoring of fibrinogen levels during thrombolytic infusion has long been advocated. Fibrinogen levels are checked serially during infusion, and a level below 100 to 150 mg/dL indicates significant dysfibrinogenemia and requires lowering the drug dose or stopping the infusion altogether. Lower fibrinogen levels correlated with bleeding in the STILE trial, but it is not clear whether the fibrinogen level is a reliable predictor of bleeding complications.

One of the drawbacks of catheter-directed thrombolysis are the prolonged infusion times, high costs of fibrinolytic agents, need for repeat angiographic imaging, and monitoring of patients in intensive care units (ICUs). Delays in restoring vessel patency made this therapy unsuitable for patients who require immediate revascularization, so surgical intervention has been recommended for patients with Rutherford class IIb symptoms. The drive to overcome these shortcomings, reduce the dose of thrombolytics required to achieve clinical success, and lower hemorrhagic complications has led to development of several adjunctive techniques and devices designed to achieve more rapid reperfusion of the threatened limb.[85-87] Mechanical thrombectomy, pulse-spray thrombectomy, and ultrasound-accelerated thrombolysis are examples of these techniques. In modern practice, endovascular procedures for acute limb ischemia combine catheter-directed thrombolysis with mechanical thrombectomy, pulse-spray thrombectomy, catheter suction embolectomy, ultrasound-assisted thrombolysis, distal embolic protection devices, and angioplasty and stenting. Despite a variety of adjunctive therapies, certain basic principles apply to endovascular thrombolysis: the entire occluded segment must be crossed, and an infusion with multiple side holes positioned across the thrombus to directly infuse the thrombolytic drug into the thrombus must be given. Recombinant tissue plasminogen activator is the most commonly used thrombolytic agent, infused at a rate of 0.5 to 1 mg/h for a minimum of 12 hours.

Mechanical Thrombectomy Devices

The AngioJet Xpeedior rheolytic thrombectomy catheter (Medrad Interventional/Possis, Warrendale, Pa.) is the most commonly used mechanical thrombectomy catheter. This small-caliber catheter uses a system of forced saline jets at its tip to fragment the thrombus, while the vacuum created proximal to the jets by the Venturi effect aids in aspiration of the fragmented debris. A simple modification allows substitution of saline for thrombolytic agents, which can be sprayed into the thrombus without concomitant aspiration. Some 20 to 30 minutes after such pulse-spray treatment, the thrombus laced with fibrinolytic is fragmented and aspirated in standard thrombectomy mode, reducing the thrombotic burden and restoring arterial flow.[88] Mechanical thrombectomy can be performed without the pulse spray technique to restore flow in patients intolerant of thrombolytic drugs. In early trials, thrombectomy with the AngioJet catheter in acute limb ischemia of native arteries and bypass grafts reestablished arterial flow in 90% of patients. Clinical improvement was seen in 82% of patients, with distal embolization of thrombus occurring in only 2%.[89] Catheter-directed thrombolysis is routinely used with this adjuvant therapy, but the dose and duration of fibrinolytic therapy is reduced.[90]

Rheolytic thrombectomy was evaluated in a small multicenter registry of patients with mostly class IIa and IIb symptoms who were treated with catheter-directed infusion before or after rheolytic thrombectomy. After adjunctive angioplasty and stenting or elective surgery was performed in 80% of these patients, amputation rates were 7.1% and mortality 4.0% at 30 days.[91] Experience with rheolytic thrombectomy suggests that it is particularly effective in cases of *in situ* thrombosis, irrespective of the conduit type[90] (Fig. 46-7). The thrombectomy devices fail to remove organized

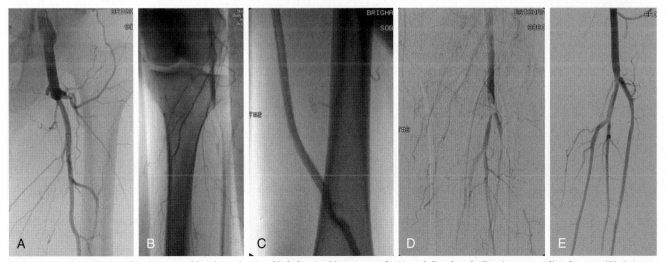

FIGURE 46-7 Acute limb ischemia caused by thrombosis of left femoral bypass graft (A) and distal embolization to popliteal artery (B). Pulse-spray thrombectomy restored patency of graft **(C)** and reduced thrombotic burden in popliteal artery **(D)**, allowing catheter-directed thrombolysis to restore patency **(E)**.

and adherent thrombus and are best used to treat acute thrombus. Overall technical success rates with the AngioJet range from 56% to 95%, with distal embolization rates of 9.5% and amputation-free survival rates reaching 75% at 2 years. The device can be also used without concomitant thrombolytics, with limb salvage rates reported to be as high as 95%.[90,92-94]

Several other devices are used for percutaneous mechanical thrombectomy. The Trellis device consists of a catheter with multiple infusion holes bordered by proximal and distal balloons that when inflated, localize the thrombolytic to the thrombosed segment and potentially limit the systemic effect of these agents. A battery-powered sinusoidal wire rotates around the catheter, effectively mixing the thrombus and thrombolytic agents. Before the balloons are deflated, the debris contained between the balloons is aspirated. The use of this device, more common in venous thrombosis, has been described in a handful of patients with arterial occlusions, but its use was associated with a 11.5% rate of distal embolization.[95] The Rotarex device (Straub Medical AG, Wangs, Switzerland) is available in Europe and has been tested to be safe and effective in peripheral arterial thromboembolic disease.[96] This over-the-wire catheter is designed for thrombus removal in peripheral vessels. A spiral at the catheter's tip rotates at 40,000 rpm, and fragments and aspirates particles at 180 mL/min. The catheter is advanced into the thrombus and gently withdrawn during aspiration. The strength of suction can be adjusted to avoid collapse and injury of the vessel around the catheter. The Hydrolyser catheter (Cordis, Warren, N.J.) was originally designed for management of dialysis access thrombosis. This 6 F 0.018-inch guidewire-compatible catheter uses the Venturi effect to create a vacuum when powered by a standard contrast injector filled with saline. It has been reported effective in treatment of graft thrombosis, and *in vitro* evaluations have found a lower distal embolization rate compared to the AngioJet.[97] Technical success rates of 88% in grafts and 73% in native arteries, with amputation rates of 11%, have been reported.[98]

All thrombectomy devices require frequent use of thrombolysis. None of these devices have been studied rigorously, but they firmly belong in the arsenal of adjunctive devices accelerating reperfusion and decreasing the amount of thrombolytic drug used. Reduction in procedural time and thrombolytic dose is likely counterbalanced by more traumatic effect compared to pharmacotherapy alone. The thrombolytic drug also affects patency of side branches and collateral vessels that are too small to be treated with these devices.

Suction Embolectomy

Percutaneous aspiration thrombectomy may be particularly effective for popliteal and tibial vessels (Figs. 46-8 and 46-9). A large-lumen catheter (6F-8F) connected to a 60-mL syringe is advanced into the proximal aspect of the occlusion, vacuum is attached by aspirating the syringe, and the thrombus is aspirated into the catheter and removed from the artery.[99,100] Combination catheter suction embolectomy and thrombolysis can result in success rates of up to 90%, with a limb salvage rate of 86% at 4-year follow-up.[101]

Ultrasound-Assisted Thrombolysis

Ultrasound-emitting catheters have been used to assist and accelerate thrombolysis. Administration of high-energy ultrasound can mechanically fragment thrombus,[102,103] whereas low-energy ultrasound accelerates enzymatic thrombus lysis by dissociating fibrin strands, exposing more fibrin binding sites, and increasing thrombus permeability and penetration by thrombolytics.[104,105] These effects have the potential for accelerating reperfusion and reducing hemorrhagic complications of thrombolytic therapy.

Four small studies investigated ultrasound-assisted thrombolysis for acute limb ischemia. The EKOS EndoWave low-energy system (EKOS Corp., Bothell, Wash.) was tested in 25 patients with acute lower-extremity arterial occlusion. Complete thrombus resolution was noted in 88% of patients after mean therapy time of only 16.9 ± 10.9 hours.[106] Another study compared ultrasound accelerated thrombolysis with mechanical thrombectomy using the Rotarex device in 20 patients with acute femoropopliteal graft occlusion.[107] Motarjeme used ultrasound-accelerated thrombolysis

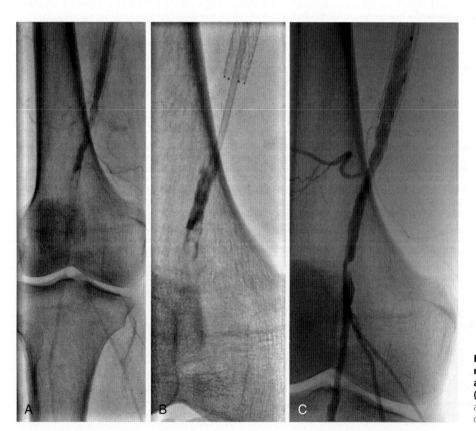

FIGURE 46-8 Acute limb ischemia due to restenosis and thrombosis of superficial femoral artery (SFA). Embolic occlusion noted distal to stent **(A)** is engaged with a catheter under suction **(B)** and retrieved, unmasking additional atherosclerotic disease **(C)**.

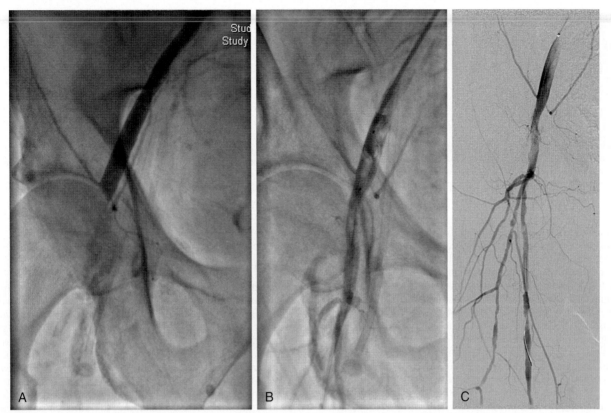

FIGURE 46-9   Acute limb ischemia after manual compression of right common femoral artery (CFA) access site. A, Thrombotic occlusion of right common femoral artery. **B,** Thrombus is trapped in a filter embolic protection device and withdrawn from artery toward a sheath. Arterial flow is restored immediately after percutaneous thrombus removal, with evidence of calcified atherosclerotic disease in CFA **(C)**.

to treat 24 subacute arterial occlusions, with a technical success rate of 100% and complete thrombus lysis in 96% of cases after a mean treatment period of 16.4 hours (range, 3-25 hours).[108] The mean duration of thrombolytic infusion in the ultrasound arm was 15 hours, with a technical success rate of 90%. Another prospective study of 21 patients treated with ultrasound-accelerated thrombolysis showed that complete lysis was achieved in 20 patients, without hemorrhagic complications and 30-day vessel or graft patency of 81%.[109] The Dutch DUET study will compare the efficacy of standard catheter-directed thrombolysis and ultrasound-assisted thrombolysis in a randomized trial of acute and chronic thrombosis of native and bypassed infrainguinal vessels with class I and IIa symptoms.[94]

Gradual dissolution of thrombus may provoke distal embolization of smaller fragments into the distal circulation. This complication can occur in 5% of procedures and is manifested by sudden worsening of pain or loss of distal pulses.[2] This complication requires temporary increase in the thrombolytic dose and, if symptoms do not improve in the course of the next 1 to 2 hours, repeat angiography may be warranted.

In modern practice, the distinction between surgical and endovascular techniques is often blurred, and patients with acute ischemic symptoms are often treated with catheter-directed thrombolysis followed by either endovascular, combined, or open procedures.[110] In a recent series of 119 patients with acute limb ischemia, 54% of cases involved solely endovascular techniques, 13% open techniques, and 25% combined techniques.[110] Femoropopliteal and tibial thrombosis was associated with less favorable outcomes compared to patients who had occlusion of the aortoiliac segment. After 30 days, 82% of patients in this series were alive without limb loss. Complications included access-site hematoma in 11% of patients, transfusion-requiring bleeding in 8%, and compartment syndrome in 4% of patients. Thirty-day mortality was observed in

6% of patients, most of them associated with surgical amputation, while limb salvage and survival at 1 year were 74.6% and 85.7%, respectively.

Surgical Therapy of Acute Limb Ischemia

Modern surgical therapy for acute limb ischemia was introduced in 1963 in a landmark study by Fogarty et al.[111] Prior to development of the Fogarty catheter, emboli were retrieved by direct exposure of the occluded artery and its exploration with rigid instruments and suction devices. These methods were not only largely ineffective but also damaging to the artery.[112,113] Fogarty's technique allowed arterial exposure away from the occluded segment, with much lower risk of arterial injury. Physical examination guides the site of surgical exposure; absence of a palpable popliteal pulse requires femoral artery exposure regardless of the presence of a femoral pulse. This approach allows embolectomy of the iliac, superficial femoral, profunda, and popliteal arteries. Physical examination supporting infrapopliteal occlusion will guide popliteal artery exposure and allow cannulation of individual tibial vessels. In cases of upper-extremity acute limb ischemia, the brachial artery is the preferred exposure site. Appropriately sized balloon-tipped embolectomy catheters are advanced into the occluded artery, inflated distally, and pulled back, removing the thrombus (Fig. 46-10). Appropriate technique is essential to avoid arterial dissection and excessive endothelial injury.

When embolectomy does not reconstitute pedal perfusion, intraoperative angiography is performed to determine whether adjunctive surgical or endovascular intervention is required to treat residual distal thrombus. Direct exploration of the tibial vessels at the ankle is associated with high rates of rethrombosis, so intraoperative fibrinolytic therapy may be a more effective therapy. Intraoperative angiography should be performed to confirm

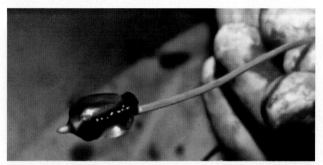

FIGURE 46-10 Fogarty embolectomy balloon with thrombus removed from popliteal artery. *(Image courtesy Dr. Edwin Gravereaux.)*

complete embolectomy. Residual thrombus can be seen in as many as 30% of embolectomy procedures.[114,115] Similarly, Doppler examination should accompany completion angiography to document restoration of arterial perfusion, although arterial spasm may attenuate the detected signals. Arterial rupture, perforation, intimal injury, and distal embolization can complicate embolectomy and underscore the importance of performing completion angiography.

In cases of acute limb ischemia caused by embolism, embolectomy is usually sufficient. Removal of the intravascular debris from a healthy vessel restores perfusion without the need for additional intervention. In patients with acute ischemia due to thrombosis, the underlying atherosclerotic disease must be addressed, either by a surgical bypass or hybrid endovascular approach with angioplasty or stent placement. Indeed, as the population presenting with acute limb ischemia has shifted toward elderly patients with preexisting PAD and *in situ* thrombosis, Fogarty embolectomy has ceased to be a standalone technique. Instead, modern surgical therapy for acute limb ischemia incorporates complex vascular reconstruction, embolectomy, angiography, and hybrid endovascular techniques.[114]

Treatment of Upper-Extremity Ischemia

Most reported series regarding management of ischemia of the upper extremities come from surgical experience, and therefore carry an inherent bias by underreporting the outcomes of conservative management. The development of simple and well-tolerated embolectomy techniques has increased the frequency of surgical interventions for upper-extremity ischemia.

Before surgical embolectomy techniques gained popularity, conservative management included warming, pharmacological vasodilation, and anticoagulation, with sympathectomy reserved for intractable pain. Baird reported a series of 95 patients treated before the advent of the Fogarty balloon. Among the 78 patients treated conservatively, 68% did not suffer any residual effect, 24% suffered from residual weakness or claudication, and 8% required amputation or had complete loss of function in the extremity. These results and the superior collateral circulation of the upper extremity led to recommendations for conservative treatment, a practice largely abandoned today in favor of surgical embolectomy. Subsequent reports indicated that as many as 50% of patients treated conservatively were left with significant functional impairment, strengthening the argument for more aggressive intervention.[116]

Prior to the development of balloon embolectomy, surgical interventions involved arteriotomies at multiple sites and removal of the clot by "milking out" the arm or use of corkscrew wires and forceps. Introduction of the Fogarty balloon catheter enabled removal of thrombus under local anesthesia through a single brachial arteriotomy in the antecubital fossa. Modern surgical techniques result in amputation and symptom-free outcomes in 80% to 90% of patients.[117,118] A more recent series of 251 patients treated with surgical embolectomy over a period of 2 decades reported amputation rates of 2% and a mortality rate of 5.6% from cardiac and cerebrovascular complications, despite the fact that general anesthesia was used in only 3% of procedures.[119] The high perioperative mortality and 40% subsequent mortality underscores the severity of coexisting medical conditions in patients with acute arterial occlusions.

Catheter-directed thrombolysis has not been widely used in the treatment of acute arm ischemia. Upper-limb salvage rates are much higher than in lower-limb arterial occlusion, and the risk of bleeding associated with thrombolytic therapy may thus be more justified in lower-extremity interventions. Nevertheless, initial reports of catheter-directed thrombolysis have been successful. Coulon et al. described a series of 13 patients with acute occlusion of the axillary and brachial arteries largely due to atrial fibrillation. Catheter-directed thrombolysis resulted in complete thrombus resolution in 8 patients, full recovery in 11, and no limb loss.[120] Others have reported similar results in small groups of patients.[121,122] Thrombolytic therapy may be particularly useful in cases of digital vessel thrombosis.

Compartment Syndrome

Compartment syndrome follows intracranial hemorrhage as the most feared complication of revascularization procedures in patients with acute limb ischemia. Post-reperfusion compartment syndrome most frequently occurs in patients with surgically treated class IIb and III symptoms, but can also occur in patients with less severe ischemia undergoing endovascular therapies. Ischemic reperfusion injury can occur even after only an hour of ischemia.[123] Mortality from this syndrome ranged from 7.5% to 41% in the 1960s and 1970s and remains high today.[124] The likelihood of developing compartment syndrome is directly related to the duration of ischemia; the longer the ischemic period, the higher the likelihood of reperfusion syndrome and worse clinical outcome. Reperfusion within 12 hours of ischemia onset has been associated with mortality and limb salvage rates of 12% and 93%, respectively. Reperfusion after more than 12 hours of ischemia carries a much worse prognosis: mortality rates can be as high as 31%, with limb salvage rates of 78%.[125]

Compartment syndrome is caused by tissue swelling following restoration of blood flow and reperfusion injury.[126] The tissue injury initiated during the ischemic period is continued by reperfusion with oxygenated blood, with introduction of oxygen free radicals and inflammatory cells. Free radicals peroxidate the lipid component of cell membranes, thus enhancing capillary permeability and muscle edema.[123,127] Compartment syndrome occurs when high pressure in a confined fascial space reduces capillary perfusion below a level needed to maintain tissue viability.[128] The resulting pressure decreases venous drainage from swollen muscle groups encased in firm fascial layers. Pressure in the limb compartment increases to further decrease venous and capillary flow, and eventually overcomes arterial pressure and stops arterial perfusion. Unless rapidly decompressed, the compartment pressures will result in irreversible neuromuscular damage.

Clinical signs and symptoms of the syndrome include rapidly progressive pain out of proportion to the clinical situation. Clinical examination is characterized by pain on passive stretch of the muscle in the affected compartment, paresthesias of the muscles in the compartment, and hypoesthesia in the distribution of the nerve traversing the affected compartment. Limb examination is notable for a pale and painful swollen calf, thigh, or forearm. Distal pulses may become undetectable if the pressure becomes severe enough, but their presence does not exclude the syndrome.[129] Timely recognition of this complication is crucial because compartment pressure exceeding 30 mmHg for 6 to 8 hours leads to irreversible limb injury and limb loss. Some reports indicate that untreated compartment syndrome results in muscle necrosis within 3 hours.[130] Diagnosis of the syndrome is established by physical examination, but compartment pressure measurement can help confirm the diagnosis in some cases. The compartment pressure criteria used to guide the decision for urgent fasciotomy vary from 30 mmHg, 45 mmHg, or any pressure exceeding the diastolic arterial pressure by 10 to 30 mmHg.[131–135]

Once recognized, urgent fasciotomy of the three compartments in the thigh or four compartments in the calf (anterior, lateral, deep posterior, and superficial posterior) is recommended. Delay in therapy results in limb loss, rhabdomyolysis, tissue necrosis, renal failure, and death.[136,137] Even after successful fasciotomy, amputation rates can be as high as 11% to 21%.[138,139] Among patients undergoing fasciotomy for reperfusion injury, even successful limb salvage leaves 36% of the limbs with some degree of dysfunction.[139]

The frequency of fasciotomies after revascularization has been reported to be as high as 16% to 22%, although many of these procedures are performed prophylactically to prevent compartment syndrome.[140,141] Patients undergoing thrombolysis usually have less severe ischemia, and reperfusion is more gradual. Consequently, compartment syndrome rates in patients treated with endovascular therapies occurs in 2% of procedures. Some increase in compartment pressure is routinely seen after revascularization of an ischemic limb, but the pressure rarely reaches levels high enough to cause a clinical syndrome.[142,143] Experimental evidence suggests that prophylactic fasciotomies performed at the time of reperfusion reduce the amount of muscle injury, compared to fasciotomies performed several hours later. Some authors recommend prophylactic fasciotomies in cases when ischemia exceeds 6 hours, the patients are young, reperfusion is incomplete, and tissue swelling develops immediately upon or even before reperfusion.[129,140,144]

Adjunctive Medical Therapy

In addition to the underlying medical comorbidities, reperfusion injury is the principal cause of mortality and morbidity after revascularization. To reduce ischemic reperfusion injury, gradual reperfusion with modified reperfusate has been evaluated in experimental animal models. Hypothermia and low initial flow rates have been shown to decrease the severity of reperfusion injury in animal skeletal muscle.[145] Controlled reperfusion consists of a 30-minute infusion of crystalloid reperfusion solution mixed with oxygenated blood directly into the revascularized artery and muscle bed.[146] Controlled reperfusion does not eliminate reperfusion injury, but may significantly attenuate it with a decrease in tissue edema and preservation of muscle viability and contraction force.[147,148] Other strategies have been proposed over the years, but none have penetrated into clinical practice. Administration of free radical scavengers and antiinflammatory agents has been shown to mitigate the deleterious effects of reperfusion.[43] Controlled reperfusion with blood mixed with crystalloid to obtain an alkalotic, hypocalcemic, and substrate-rich perfusate has been shown to successfully reduce the degree of reperfusion injury.[146,149-151] Patients undergoing controlled reperfusion have superior functional recovery and a lower rate of amputation.[152]

Iloprost, a synthetic analog of prostacyclin, has been investigated as adjunctive therapy to reduce limb-related complications by improving microcirculation. In a randomized study of 300 patients with acute limb ischemia, patients treated with IA and IV infusion of iloprost had a statistically significant lower 90-day mortality rate compared to patients in the placebo arm.[153] There was, however, no difference in the rate of amputation. None of these investigational therapies have reached the mainstream of modern clinical practice.

REFERENCES

1. Earnshaw JJ: Demography and etiology of acute leg ischemia, *Semin Vasc Surg* 14:86–92, 2001.
2. Davies B, Braithwaite BD, Birch PA, et al: Acute leg ischaemia in Gloucestershire, *Br J Surg* 84:504–508, 1997.
3. Bergqvist D, Troeng T, Elfstrom J, et al: Auditing surgical outcome: ten years with the Swedish Vascular Registry--Swedvasc. The Steering Committee of Swedvasc, *Eur J Surg Suppl* 3–8, 1998.
4. Eliason JL, Wainess RM, Proctor MC, et al: A national and single institutional experience in the contemporary treatment of acute lower extremity ischemia, *Ann Surg* 238:382–389, 2003 discussion 9–90.
5. Williams N, Bell PR: Acute ischaemia of the upper limb, *Br J Hosp Med* 50:579–582, 1993.
6. Eyers P, Earnshaw JJ: Acute non-traumatic arm ischaemia, *Br J Surg* 85:1340–1346, 1998.
7. Dryjski M, Swedenborg J: Acute ischemia of the extremities in a metropolitan area during one year, *J Cardiovasc Surg (Torino)* 25:518–522, 1984.
8. Stonebridge PA, Clason AE, Duncan AJ, et al: Acute ischaemia of the upper limb compared with acute lower limb ischaemia; a 5-year review, *Br J Surg* 76:515–516, 1989.
9. Ouriel K, Veith FJ, Sasahara AA: A comparison of recombinant urokinase with vascular surgery as initial treatment for acute arterial occlusion of the legs. Thrombolysis or Peripheral Arterial Surgery (TOPAS) Investigators, *N Engl J Med* 338:1105–1111, 1998.
10. Jivegard L, Holm J, Schersten T: Acute limb ischemia due to arterial embolism or thrombosis: influence of limb ischemia versus pre-existing cardiac disease on postoperative mortality rate, *J Cardiovasc Surg (Torino)* 29:32–36, 1988.
11. Braithwaite BD, Davies B, Birch PA, et al: Management of acute leg ischaemia in the elderly, *Br J Surg* 85:217–220, 1998.
12. Lambert M, Ball C, Hancock B: Management of acute brachial artery occlusion due to trauma or emboli, *Br J Surg* 70:639–640, 1983.
13. Katz SG, Kohl RD: Direct revascularization for the treatment of forearm and hand ischemia, *Am J Surg* 165:312–316, 1993.
14. Wirsing P, Andriopoulos A, Botticher R: Arterial embolectomies in the upper extremity after acute occlusion. Report on 79 cases, *J Cardiovasc Surg (Torino)* 24:40–42, 1983.
15. James EC, Khuri NT, Fedde CW, et al: Upper limb ischemia resulting from arterial thromboembolism, *Am J Surg* 137:739–744, 1979.
16. Darling RC, Austen WG, Linton RR: Arterial embolism, *Surg Gynecol Obstet* 124:106–114, 1967.
17. Kaar G, Broe PJ, Bouchier-Hayes DJ: Upper limb emboli. A review of 55 patients managed surgically, *J Cardiovasc Surg (Torino)* 30:165–168, 1989.
18. Gazzaniga AB, Dalen JE: Paradoxical embolism: its pathophysiology and clinical recognition, *Ann Surg* 171:137–142, 1970.
19. Bryan AJ, Hicks E, Lewis MH: Unilateral digital ischaemia secondary to embolisation from subclavian atheroma, *Ann R Coll Surg Engl* 71:140–142, 1989.
20. Rapp JH, Reilly LM, Goldstone J, et al: Ischemia of the upper extremity: significance of proximal arterial disease, *Am J Surg* 152:122–126, 1986.
21. Keen RR, McCarthy WJ, Shireman PK, et al: Surgical management of atheroembolization, *J Vasc Surg* 21:773–780, 1995 discussion 80–1.
22. Ricotta JJ, Scudder PA, McAndrew JA, et al: Management of acute ischemia of the upper extremity, *Am J Surg* 145:661–666, 1983.
23. Banis JC Jr, Rich N, Whelan TJ Jr: Ischemia of the upper extremity due to noncardiac emboli, *Am J Surg* 134:131–139, 1977.
24. Nehler MR, Taylor LM Jr, Moneta GL, et al: Upper extremity ischemia from subclavian artery aneurysm caused by bony abnormalities of the thoracic outlet, *Arch Surg* 132:527–532, 1997.
25. Sachatello CR, Ernst CB, Griffen WO Jr: The acutely ischemic upper extremity: selective management, *Surgery* 76:1002–1009, 1974.
26. Prioleau PG, Katzenstein AL: Major peripheral arterial occlusion due to malignant tumor embolism: histologic recognition and surgical management, *Cancer* 42:2009–2014, 1978.
27. Lorentzen JE, Roder OC, Hansen HJ: Peripheral arterial embolism. A follow-up of 130 consecutive patients submitted to embolectomy, *Acta Chir Scand Suppl* 502:111–116, 1980.
28. Jivegard LE, Arfvidsson B, Holm J, et al: Selective conservative and routine early operative treatment in acute limb ischaemia, *Br J Surg* 74:798–801, 1987.
29. Vohra R, Lieberman DP: Arterial emboli to the arm, *J R Coll Surg Edinb* 36:83–85, 1991.
30. Quraishy MS, Cawthorn SJ, Giddings AE: Critical ischaemia of the upper limb, *J R Soc Med* 85:269–273, 1992.
31. Klonaris C, Georgopoulos S, Katsargyris A, et al: Changing patterns in the etiology of acute lower limb ischemia, *Int Angiol* 26:49–52, 2007.
32. Kropman RH, Schrijver AM, Kelder JC, et al: Clinical outcome of acute leg ischaemia due to thrombosed popliteal artery aneurysm: systematic review of 895 cases, *Eur J Vasc Endovasc Surg* 39:452–457, 2010.
33. Ravn H, Bergqvist D, Bjorck M: Nationwide study of the outcome of popliteal artery aneurysms treated surgically, *Br J Surg* 94:970–977, 2007.
34. Marine L, Castro P, Enriquez A, et al: Four-limb acute ischemia induced by ergotamine in an AIDS patient treated with protease inhibitors, *Circulation* 124:1395–1397, 2011.
35. Zavaleta EG, Fernandez BB, Grove MK, et al: St. Anthony's fire (ergotamine induced leg ischemia)--a case report and review of the literature, *Angiology* 52:349–356, 2001.
36. Mirzayan R, Hanks SE, Weaver FA: Cocaine-induced thrombosis of common iliac and popliteal arteries, *Ann Vasc Surg* 12:476–481, 1998.
37. Knochel JP: Mechanisms of rhabdomyolysis, *Curr Opin Rheumatol* 5:725–731, 1993.
38. Blaisdell FW: The pathophysiology of skeletal muscle ischemia and the reperfusion syndrome: a review, *Cardiovasc Surg* 10:620–630, 2002.
39. Gillani S, Cao J, Suzuki T, et al: The effect of ischemia reperfusion injury on skeletal muscle, *Injury* 2011, epub ahead of print; http://dx.doi.org/10.1016/j.injury.2011.03.008.
40. Rubin BB, Romaschin A, Walker PM, et al: Mechanisms of postischemic injury in skeletal muscle: intervention strategies, *J Appl Physiol* 80:369–387, 1996.
41. Collard CD, Gelman S: Pathophysiology, clinical manifestations, and prevention of ischemia-reperfusion injury, *Anesthesiology* 94:1133–1138, 2001.
42. Korthuis RJ, Smith JK, Carden DL: Hypoxic reperfusion attenuates postischemic microvascular injury, *Am J Physiol* 256:H315–H319, 1989.
43. Walker PM, Lindsay TF, Labbe R, et al: Salvage of skeletal muscle with free radical scavengers, *J Vasc Surg* 5:68–75, 1987.
44. Jerome SN, Akimitsu T, Korthuis RJ: Leukocyte adhesion, edema, and development of postischemic capillary no-reflow, *Am J Physiol* 267:H1329–H1336, 1994.
45. Korthuis RJ, Grisham MB, Granger DN: Leukocyte depletion attenuates vascular injury in postischemic skeletal muscle, *Am J Physiol* 254:H823–H827, 1988.
46. Carden DL, Smith JK, Korthuis RJ: Neutrophil-mediated microvascular dysfunction in postischemic canine skeletal muscle. Role of granulocyte adherence, *Circ Res* 66:1436–1444, 1990.
47. Walden DL, McCutchan HJ, Enquist EG, et al: Neutrophils accumulate and contribute to skeletal muscle dysfunction after ischemia-reperfusion, *Am J Physiol* 259:H1809–H1812, 1990.
48. Yokota J, Minei JP, Fantini GA, et al: Role of leukocytes in reperfusion injury of skeletal muscle after partial ischemia, *Am J Physiol* 257:H1068–H1075, 1989.

49. Welbourn R, Goldman G, O'Riordain M, et al: Role for tumor necrosis factor as mediator of lung injury following lower torso ischemia, *J Appl Physiol* 70:2645–2649, 1991.

50. Yassin MM, Harkin DW, Barros D'Sa AA, et al: Lower limb ischemia-reperfusion injury triggers a systemic inflammatory response and multiple organ dysfunction, *World J Surg* 26:115–121, 2002.

51. Ascer E, Mohan C, Gennaro M, et al: Interleukin-1 and thromboxane release after skeletal muscle ischemia and reperfusion, *Ann Vasc Surg* 6:69–73, 1992.

52. Hashimoto M, Shingu M, Ezaki I, et al: Production of soluble ICAM-1 from human endothelial cells induced by IL-1 beta and TNF-alpha, *Inflammation* 18:163–173, 1994.

53. Sato N, Goto T, Haranaka K, et al: Actions of tumor necrosis factor on cultured vascular endothelial cells: morphologic modulation, growth inhibition, and cytotoxicity, *J Natl Cancer Inst* 76:1113–1121, 1986.

54. Klausner JM, Anner H, Paterson IS, et al: Lower torso ischemia-induced lung injury is leukocyte dependent, *Ann Surg* 208:761–767, 1988.

55. Welbourn CR, Goldman G, Paterson IS, et al: Pathophysiology of ischaemia reperfusion injury: central role of the neutrophil, *Br J Surg* 78:651–655, 1991.

56. Rutherford RB, Baker JD, Ernst C, et al: Recommended standards for reports dealing with lower extremity ischemia: revised version, *J Vasc Surg* 26:517–538, 1997.

57. Henke PK: Contemporary management of acute limb ischemia: factors associated with amputation and in-hospital mortality, *Semin Vasc Surg* 22:34–40, 2009.

58. Blaisdell FW, Steele M, Allen RE: Management of acute lower extremity arterial ischemia due to embolism and thrombosis, *Surgery* 84:822–834, 1978.

59. Results of a prospective randomized trial evaluating surgery versus thrombolysis for ischemia of the lower extremity. The STILE trial, *Ann Surg* 220:251–266, 1994 discussion 66–8.

60. Ouriel K, Shortell CK, DeWeese JA, et al: A comparison of thrombolytic therapy with operative revascularization in the initial treatment of acute peripheral arterial ischemia, *J Vasc Surg* 19:1021–1030, 1994.

61. Zaraca F, Stringari C, Ebner JA, et al: Routine versus selective use of intraoperative angiography during thromboembolectomy for acute lower limb ischemia: analysis of outcomes, *Ann Vasc Surg* 24:621–627, 2010.

62. Tawes RL Jr, Harris EJ, Brown WH, et al: Arterial thromboembolism. A 20-year perspective, *Arch Surg* 120:595–599, 1985.

63. Hobson RW 2nd, Neville R, Watanabe B, et al: Role of heparin in reducing skeletal muscle infarction in ischemia-reperfusion, *Microcirc Endothelium Lymphatics* 5:259–276, 1989.

64. Wright JG, Kerr JC, Valeri CR, et al: Heparin decreases ischemia-reperfusion injury in isolated canine gracilis model, *Arch Surg* 123:470–472, 1988.

65. Jivegard L, Holm J, Bergqvist D, et al: Acute lower limb ischemia: failure of anticoagulant treatment to improve one-month results of arterial thromboembolectomy. A prospective randomized multi-center study, *Surgery* 109:610–616, 1991.

66. Currie IS, Wakelin SJ, Lee AJ, et al: Plasma creatine kinase indicates major amputation or limb preservation in acute lower limb ischemia, *J Vasc Surg* 45:733–739, 2007.

67. Tillet WS: The fibrinolytic activity of hemolytic streptococci, *J Exp Med* 58:485–502, 1933.

68. Tillett WS, Johnson AJ, McCarty WR: The intravenous infusion of the streptococcal fibrinolytic principle (streptokinase) into patients, *J Clin Invest* 34:169–185, 1955.

69. Clifton EE: The use of plasmin in humans, *Ann N Y Acad Sci* 68:209–229, 1957.

70. Dotter CT, Rosch J, Seaman AJ: Selective clot lysis with low-dose streptokinase, *Radiology* 111:31–37, 1974.

71. Berridge DC, Gregson RH, Hopkinson BR, et al: Randomized trial of intra-arterial recombinant tissue plasminogen activator, intravenous recombinant tissue plasminogen activator and intra-arterial streptokinase in peripheral arterial thrombolysis, *Br J Surg* 78:988–995, 1991.

72. Karnabatidis D, Spiliopoulos S, Tsetis D, et al: Quality improvement guidelines for percutaneous catheter-directed intra-arterial thrombolysis and mechanical thrombectomy for acute lower-limb ischemia, *Cardiovasc Intervent Radiol* 34:1123–1136, 2011.

73. Berridge DC, Kessel D, Robertson I: Surgery versus thrombolysis for acute limb ischaemia: initial management, *Cochrane Database Syst Rev* 2002 CD002784.

74. Earnshaw JJ, Whitman B, Foy C: National Audit of Thrombolysis for Acute Leg Ischemia (NATALI): clinical factors associated with early outcome, *J Vasc Surg* 39:1018–1025, 2004.

75. Ouriel K, Shortell CK, Azodo MV, et al: Acute peripheral arterial occlusion: predictors of success in catheter-directed thrombolytic therapy, *Radiology* 193:561–566, 1994.

76. Olin JW, Graor RA: Thrombolytic therapy in the treatment of peripheral arterial occlusions, *Ann Emerg Med* 17:1210–1215, 1988.

77. Schweizer J, Altmann E, Stosslein F, et al: Comparison of tissue plasminogen activator and urokinase in the local infiltration thrombolysis of peripheral arterial occlusions, *Eur J Radiol* 22:129–132, 1996.

78. Semba CP, Murphy TP, Bakal CW, et al: Thrombolytic therapy with use of alteplase (rt-PA) in peripheral arterial occlusive disease: review of the clinical literature. The Advisory Panel, *J Vasc Interv Radiol* 11:149–161, 2000.

79. Hanover TM, Kalbaugh CA, Gray BH, et al: Safety and efficacy of reteplase for the treatment of acute arterial occlusion: complexity of underlying lesion predicts outcome, *Ann Vasc Surg* 19:817–822, 2005.

80. Laird JR, Dangas G, Jaff M, et al: Intra-arterial reteplase for the treatment of acute limb ischemia, *J Invasive Cardiol* 11:757–762, 1999.

81. Drescher P, Crain MR, Rilling WS: Initial experience with the combination of reteplase and abciximab for thrombolytic therapy in peripheral arterial occlusive disease: a pilot study, *J Vasc Interv Radiol* 13:37–43, 2002.

82. Ouriel K, Castaneda F, McNamara T, et al: Reteplase monotherapy and reteplase/abciximab combination therapy in peripheral arterial occlusive disease: results from the RELAX trial, *J Vasc Interv Radiol* 15:229–238, 2004.

83. McNamara TO, Fischer JR: Thrombolysis of peripheral arterial and graft occlusions: improved results using high-dose urokinase, *AJR Am J Roentgenol* 144:769–775, 1985.

84. Sullivan KL, Gardiner GA Jr, Shapiro MJ, et al: Acceleration of thrombolysis with a high-dose transthrombus bolus technique, *Radiology* 173:805–808, 1989.

85. Ritchie JL, Hansen DD, Vracko R, et al: Mechanical thrombolysis: a new rotational catheter approach for acute thrombi, *Circulation* 73:1006–1012, 1986.

86. Drasler WJ, Jenson ML, Wilson GJ, et al: Rheolytic catheter for percutaneous removal of thrombus, *Radiology* 182:263–267, 1992.

87. Schmitz-Rode T, Gunther RW, Muller-Leisse C: US-assisted aspiration thrombectomy: *in vitro* investigations, *Radiology* 178:677–679, 1991.

88. Allie DE, Hebert CJ, Lirtzman MD, et al: Novel simultaneous combination chemical thrombolysis/rheolytic thrombectomy therapy for acute critical limb ischemia: the power-pulse spray technique, *Catheter Cardiovasc Interv* 63:512–522, 2004.

89. Mathie AG, Bell SD, Saibil EA: Mechanical thromboembolectomy in acute embolic peripheral arterial occlusions with use of the AngioJet Rapid Thrombectomy System, *J Vasc Interv Radiol* 10:583–590, 1999.

90. Kasirajan K, Gray B, Beavers FP, et al: Rheolytic thrombectomy in the management of acute and subacute limb-threatening ischemia, *J Vasc Interv Radiol* 12:413–421, 2001.

91. Ansel GM, George BS, Botti CF, et al: Rheolytic thrombectomy in the management of limb ischemia: 30-day results from a multicenter registry, *J Endovasc Ther* 9:395–402, 2002.

92. Wagner HJ, Muller-Hulsbeck S, Pitton MB, et al: Rapid thrombectomy with a hydrodynamic catheter: results from a prospective, multicenter trial, *Radiology* 205:675–681, 1997.

93. Silva JA, Ramee SR, Collins TJ, et al: Rheolytic thrombectomy in the treatment of acute limb-threatening ischemia: immediate results and six-month follow-up of the multicenter AngioJet registry. Possis Peripheral AngioJet Study AngioJet Investigators, *Cathet Cardiovasc Diagn* 45:386–393, 1998.

94. Muller-Hulsbeck S, Kalinowski M, Heller M, et al: Rheolytic hydrodynamic thrombectomy for percutaneous treatment of acutely occluded infra-aortic native arteries and bypass grafts: midterm follow-up results, *Invest Radiol* 35:131–140, 2000.

95. Sarac TP, Hilleman D, Arko FR, et al: Clinical and economic evaluation of the trellis thrombectomy device for arterial occlusions: preliminary analysis, *J Vasc Surg* 39:556–559, 2004.

96. Stanek F, Ouhrabkova R, Prochazka D: Mechanical thrombectomy using the Rotarex catheter--safe and effective method in the treatment of peripheral arterial thromboembolic occlusions, *Vasa* 39:334–340, 2010.

97. Bucker A, Schmitz-Rode T, Vorwerk D, et al: Comparative *in vitro* study of two percutaneous hydrodynamic thrombectomy systems, *J Vasc Interv Radiol* 7:445–449, 1996.

98. Reekers JA, Kromhout JG, Spithoven HG, et al: Arterial thrombosis below the inguinal ligament: percutaneous treatment with a thrombosuction catheter, *Radiology* 198:49–53, 1996.

99. Wagner HJ, Starck EE: Acute embolic occlusions of the infrainguinal arteries: percutaneous aspiration embolectomy in 102 patients, *Radiology* 182:403–407, 1992.

100. Zehnder T, Birrer M, Do DD, et al: Percutaneous catheter thrombus aspiration for acute or subacute arterial occlusion of the legs: how much thrombolysis is needed? *Eur J Vasc Endovasc Surg* 20:41–46, 2000.

101. Wagner HJ, Starck EE, Reuter P: Long-term results of percutaneous aspiration embolectomy, *Cardiovasc Intervent Radiol* 17:241–246, 1994.

102. Siegel RJ, Fishbein MC, Forrester J, et al: Ultrasonic plaque ablation. A new method for recanalization of partially or totally occluded arteries, *Circulation* 78:1443–1448, 1988.

103. Steffen W, Fishbein MC, Luo H, et al: High intensity, low frequency catheter-delivered ultrasound dissolution of occlusive coronary artery thrombi: an *in vitro* and *in vivo* study, *J Am Coll Cardiol* 24:1571–1579, 1994.

104. Braaten JV, Goss RA, Francis CW: Ultrasound reversibly disaggregates fibrin fibers, *Thromb Haemost* 78:1063–1068, 1997.

105. Francis CW, Blinc A, Lee S, et al: Ultrasound accelerates transport of recombinant tissue plasminogen activator into clots, *Ultrasound Med Biol* 21:419–424, 1995.

106. Wissgott C, Richter A, Kamusella P, et al: Treatment of critical limb ischemia using ultrasound-enhanced thrombolysis (PARES Trial): final results, *J Endovasc Ther* 14:438–443, 2007.

107. Wissgott C, Kamusella P, Richter A, et al: Treatment of acute femoropopliteal bypass graft occlusion: comparison of mechanical rotational thrombectomy with ultrasound-enhanced lysis, *Rofo* 180:547–552, 2008.

108. Motarjeme A: Ultrasound-enhanced thrombolysis, *J Endovasc Ther* 14:251–256, 2007.

109. Schrijver AM, Reijnen MM, van Oostayen JA, et al: Initial results of catheter-directed ultrasound-accelerated thrombolysis for thromboembolic obstructions of the aortofemoral arteries: a feasibility study, *Cardiovasc Intervent Radiol* 35:279–285, 2012.

110. Kashyap VS, Gilani R, Bena JF, et al: Endovascular therapy for acute limb ischemia, *J Vasc Surg* 53:340–346, 2011.

111. Fogarty TJ, Cranley JJ, Krause RJ, et al: A method for extraction of arterial emboli and thrombi, *Surg Gynecol Obstet* 116:241–244, 1963.

112. Dale WA: Endovascular suction catheters for thrombectomy and embolectomy, *J Thorac Cardiovasc Surg* 44:557–558, 1962.

113. Green RM, DeWeese JA, Rob CG: Arterial embolectomy before and after the Fogarty catheter, *Surgery* 77:24–33, 1975.

114. Hill SL, Donato AT: The simple Fogarty embolectomy: an operation of the past? *Am Surg* 60:907–911, 1994.

115. Plecha FR, Pories WJ: Intraoperative angiography in the immediate assessment of arterial reconstruction, *Arch Surg* 105:902–907, 1972.

116. Galbraith K, Collin J, Morris PJ, et al: Recent experience with arterial embolism of the limbs in a vascular unit, *Ann R Coll Surg Engl* 67:30–33, 1985.

117. Davies MG, O'Malley K, Feeley M, et al: Upper limb embolus: a timely diagnosis, *Ann Vasc Surg* 5:85–87, 1991.

118. Pentti J, Salenius JP, Kuukasjarvi P, et al: Outcome of surgical treatment in acute upper limb ischaemia, *Ann Chir Gynaecol* 84:25–28, 1995.

119. Hernandez-Richter T, Angele MK, Helmberger T, et al: Acute ischemia of the upper extremity: long-term results following thrombembolectomy with the Fogarty catheter, *Langenbecks Arch Surg* 386:261–266, 2001.

120. Coulon M, Goffette P, Dondelinger RF: Local thrombolytic infusion in arterial ischemia of the upper limb: mid-term results, *Cardiovasc Intervent Radiol* 17:81–86, 1994.

121. Michaels JA, Torrie EP, Galland RB: The treatment of upper limb vascular occlusions using intraarterial thrombolysis, *Eur J Vasc Surg* 7:744–746, 1993.

122. Widlus DM, Venbrux AC, Benenati JF, et al: Fibrinolytic therapy for upper-extremity arterial occlusions, *Radiology* 175:393–399, 1990.

123. Beyersdorf F: Protection of the ischemic skeletal muscle, *Thorac Cardiovasc Surg* 39:19–28, 1991.

124. Dormandy J, Heeck L, Vig S: Acute limb ischemia, *Semin Vasc Surg* 12:148–153, 1999.

125. Abbott WM, Maloney RD, McCabe CC, et al: Arterial embolism: a 44 year perspective, *Am J Surg* 143:460–464, 1982.
126. Perry MO: Compartment syndromes and reperfusion injury, *Surg Clin North Am* 68: 853–864, 1988.
127. McCord JM: Oxygen-derived free radicals in postischemic tissue injury, *N Engl J Med* 312:159–163, 1985.
128. Mubarak SJ, Hargens AR: Acute compartment syndromes, *Surg Clin North Am* 63: 539–565, 1983.
129. Hyde GL, Peck D, Powell DC: Compartment syndromes. Early diagnosis and a bedside operation, *Am Surg* 49:563–568, 1983.
130. Vaillancourt C, Shrier I, Vandal A, et al: Acute compartment syndrome: how long before muscle necrosis occurs? *CJEM* 6:147–154, 2004.
131. Mubarak SJ, Owen CA, Hargens AR, et al: Acute compartment syndromes: diagnosis and treatment with the aid of the wick catheter, *J Bone Joint Surg Am* 60:1091–1095, 1978.
132. Rorabeck CH: The treatment of compartment syndromes of the leg, *J Bone Joint Surg Br* 66:93–97, 1984.
133. Matsen FA 3rd, Winquist RA, Krugmire RB Jr: Diagnosis and management of compartmental syndromes, *J Bone Joint Surg Am* 62:286–291, 1980.
134. Whitesides TE, Haney TC, Morimoto K, et al: Tissue pressure measurements as a determinant for the need of fasciotomy, *Clin Orthop Relat Res* 43–51, 1975.
135. Frink M, Hildebrand F, Krettek C, et al: Compartment syndrome of the lower leg and foot, *Clin Orthop Relat Res* 468:940–950, 2010.
136. Rush DS, Frame SB, Bell RM, et al: Does open fasciotomy contribute to morbidity and mortality after acute lower extremity ischemia and revascularization? *J Vasc Surg* 10: 343–350, 1989.
137. Jensen SL, Sandermann J: Compartment syndrome and fasciotomy in vascular surgery. A review of 57 cases, *Eur J Vasc Endovasc Surg* 13:48–53, 1997.
138. Finkelstein JA, Hunter GA, Hu RW: Lower limb compartment syndrome: course after delayed fasciotomy, *J Trauma* 40:342–344, 1996.
139. Heemskerk J, Kitslaar P: Acute compartment syndrome of the lower leg: retrospective study on prevalence, technique, and outcome of fasciotomies, *World J Surg* 27:744–747, 2003.
140. Papalambros EL, Panayiotopoulos YP, Bastounis E, et al: Prophylactic fasciotomy of the legs following acute arterial occlusion procedures, *Int Angiol* 8:120–124, 1989.
141. Allenberg JR, Meybier H: The compartment syndrome from the vascular surgery viewpoint, *Chirurg* 59:722–727, 1988.
142. Qvarfordt P, Christenson JT, Eklof B, et al: Intramuscular pressure after revascularization of the popliteal artery in severe ischaemia, *Br J Surg* 70:539–541, 1983.
143. Melberg PE, Styf J, Biber B, et al: Muscular compartment pressure following reconstructive arterial surgery of the lower limbs, *Acta Chir Scand* 150:129–133, 1984.
144. Patman RD: Compartmental syndromes in peripheral vascular surgery, *Clin Orthop Relat Res* 103–110, 1975.
145. Wright JG, Belkin M, Hobson RW 2nd: Hypothermia and controlled reperfusion: two non-pharmacologic methods which diminish ischemia-reperfusion injury in skeletal muscle, *Microcirc Endothelium Lymphatics* 5:315–334, 1989.
146. Beyersdorf F, Schlensak C: Controlled reperfusion after acute and persistent limb ischemia, *Semin Vasc Surg* 22:52–57, 2009.
147. Dick F, Li J, Giraud MN, et al: Basic control of reperfusion effectively protects against reperfusion injury in a realistic rodent model of acute limb ischemia, *Circulation* 118:1920–1928, 2008.
148. Anderson RJ, Cambria R, Kerr J, et al: Sustained benefit of temporary limited reperfusion in skeletal muscle following ischemia, *J Surg Res* 49:271–275, 1990.
149. Defraigne JO, Pincemail J, Laroche C, et al: Successful controlled limb reperfusion after severe prolonged ischemia, *J Vasc Surg* 26:346–350, 1997.
150. Walker PM, Romaschin AD, Davis S, et al: Lower limb ischemia: phase 1 results of salvage perfusion, *J Surg Res* 84:193–198, 1999.
151. Mowlavi A, Neumeister MW, Wilhelmi BJ, et al: Local hypothermia during early reperfusion protects skeletal muscle from ischemia-reperfusion injury, *Plast Reconstr Surg* 111: 242–250, 2003.
152. Wilhelm MP, Schlensak C, Hoh A, et al: Controlled reperfusion using a simplified perfusion system preserves function after acute and persistent limb ischemia: a preliminary study, *J Vasc Surg* 42:690–694, 2005.
153. de Donato G, Gussoni G, de Donato G, et al: The ILAILL study: iloprost as adjuvant to surgery for acute ischemia of lower limbs: a randomized, placebo-controlled, double-blind study by the Italian Society for Vascular and Endovascular Surgery, *Ann Surg* 244:185–193, 2006.

CHAPTER 47

Atheroembolism

Roger F.J. Shepherd

Atheroembolism is a rare but serious disorder with significant morbidity from stroke, renal failure, and limb loss. This systemic disorder affects multiple organs and carries a high mortality rate. Atheroembolism can be a single event or recurrent. It can occur spontaneously or following an invasive vascular procedure. It can originate from atherosclerotic or aneurysmal disease and involve single or multiple sites. There is no specific laboratory test that can reliably distinguish cholesterol embolization from other disorders. A definitive diagnosis can only be made with biopsy of involved tissue and histological examination. A high index of clinical suspicion is necessary because atheroembolism may mimic a number of other disorders, leading to potential misdiagnosis. The focus of this chapter will be review of pathophysiology, precipitating factors, clinical syndromes, and management of atheroembolic disease. Prognosis is determined by the extent of systemic involvement and risk of recurrent episodes. As in many vascular disorders, prevention is the best treatment.

Atheroembolism occurs when tiny fragments of an atherosclerotic plaque (in particular, cholesterol crystals) break off from a proximal artery and travel distally in the circulation, ending up in small arteries downstream from its origin. The consequence of this event is microvascular obstruction with tissue ischemia. The abdominal aorta is the most common origin for atheroembolism to the abdominal organs and lower extremities, but any artery with atheromatous disease may be a potential embolic source. End-organ targets include the brain, eye, heart, kidney, gastrointestinal tract, fingers, toes, and skin. The kidneys and skin are the two most common targets in many cases.[1] In the setting of an elderly patient who develops sudden onset of pain and ischemia of the distal extremities and unexplained renal failure after an invasive angiographic procedure, atheroembolism should be high on the list of likely diagnoses.[2]

Atheroembolism can present in a number of distinct clinical syndromes (Box 47-1). The *blue toe syndrome* occurs when arteries to the distal parts of the feet and toes become obstructed by atheromatous embolization causing toe ischemia (Fig. 47-1). *Livedo reticularis* (localized mottling of the skin) occurs when the atheroembolism involves small cutaneous vessels (Figs. 47-2 and 47-3). When present, this can be an important diagnostic indicator of atheroembolism. *Acute and chronic kidney failure* can result from aortic or renal artery atheroembolism. Atheroemboli can also travel to the mesenteric arteries, causing *intestinal necrosis*, or to the splenic, hepatic, or pancreatic arteries, causing *localized infarction*. *Transient ischemic episodes and stroke* may result from atheromatous disease of the aortic arch, internal carotid, or vertebral arteries. Atheroembolism to the retinal arteries may present with temporary horizontal monocular visual loss called *amaurosis fugax*. Funduscopic examination may identify a bright reflection from a cholesterol crystal in a retinal artery known as a *Hollenhorst plaque*.[3] The unifying cause of all atheroembolic syndromes is the presence of atheromatous disease in a proximal artery and ischemic damage to a distal organ or extremity when these fragments embolize and lodge in distal vessels.

A number of terms for this syndrome are used interchangeably in the literature, including *cholesterol crystal embolization*, *atheromatous embolization*, and *atheroembolism*. Vascular medicine covers a great deal of internal medicine, and atheroembolism should be in the differential diagnosis of many diseases including vasculitis, infective endocarditis, malignancy, hematological diseases, atypical infections, Raynaud's syndrome, and acute and chronic renal failure. Atheroembolism has been called "the great masquerader" because it may resemble many other conditions.[4] Diagnosis of atheroembolism is usually made on the basis of clinical suspicion, by history and examination, but most importantly by an astute clinician who considers this entity when presented with unusual vascular diseases.

Pathobiology

Atheroembolism originates from atherosclerotic plaque. The pathobiology of atherosclerosis is reviewed in detail in Chapter 8.

Etiology

Atheroembolism may occur spontaneously or be precipitated by angiographic or surgical procedures (iatrogenic). Earlier reports indicated spontaneous episodes of atheroembolism were more common.[5,6] Today with increased numbers of vascular procedures, iatrogenic catheter-induced atheroembolism outnumbers spontaneous cases. Currently, over three fourths of atheroembolic renal disease is procedure-related, occurring during or after an angiographic or endovascular procedure[7,8] (Figs. 47-4 through 47-6).

Spontaneous Atheroembolism

WHO IS AT RISK?

Spontaneous atheroembolism occurs in older patients with advanced atherosclerosis. In Fine's review of 221 cases of atheroembolism in the English literature, he noted a predominance of patients with underlying atherosclerotic disease including cardiac, carotid, and kidney disease. In particular, many had significant preexisting chronic kidney disease (CKD) evidenced by elevated serum creatinine (Cr) (CKD stage 3 or 4). There was also a high incidence of aortic aneurysms, present in 25% of these patients.[5] Many patients with atheroembolic events present with multisystem manifestations. Common presentations of spontaneous atheroembolism included blue toe syndrome, livedo, and progressive renal failure. Stroke/transient ischemic events due to carotid atherosclerosis is one of the best examples of a spontaneous atheroembolic episode. The mechanism of blue toe syndrome has been likened to a brain transient ischemic attack (TIA), but affecting a lower extremity.[9] Today, many cases of unexplained progressive renal failure may be due to unsuspected atheroembolism.

In most series, males outnumber females, with mean ages ranging from 63 to 69 years.[1,5,10] Skin lesions and renal failure are often the two most common manifestations.[1,5] Skin lesions may be the initial clinical sign of atheroembolization (see Fig. 47-3), of which blue toes and livedo reticularis make up 88% of cutaneous findings.[1] African Americans are less likely to be diagnosed with atheroembolism, perhaps because the faint cutaneous pattern of livedo is more difficult to see in skin that is more deeply pigmented[11] (Fig. 47-7).

HOW COMMON IS SPONTANEOUS ATHEROEMBOLISM?

Autopsies studies from the 1940s found an atheroembolic incidence of 3.4% (9 of 267 patients with aortic atherosclerosis).[12] A larger and more recent autopsy study involving 2126 elderly patients over a period of 7 years found only 16 cases of spontaneous atheroembolism (incidence <0.1%) despite the high prevalence of severe aortoiliac atheromatous disease and aortic aneurysms.[13] Another autopsy study of 372 patients found spontaneous cholesterol embolization occurred in only seven individuals; all were over age 60, and all but one were male, for an incidence of 1.9%. Lesions of different ages were noted, suggesting recurrent episodes to the kidneys and spleen.[10] A review of autopsy data at Johns Hopkins from 1973 to 1995 found 0.7% had histological features of atheroembolism.[14]

Box 47-1 Clinical Syndromes and Manifestations of Atheroembolism

Skin
Livedo reticularis
Petechiae
Purpura
Splinter hemorrhages
Fissures and nodules
Ulceration and skin necrosis

Extremities
Blue toe syndrome
Digital gangrene
Trash foot

Renal
Acute and chronic renal failure
Progressive renal failure
Proteinuria
Renal infarction
Worsening or uncontrolled hypertension

Gastrointestinal
Abdominal pain
Nausea/vomiting
Gastrointestinal hemorrhage
Bowel perforation/infarction
Pancreatitis
Cholecystitis
Splenic infarcts
Abnormal liver transaminases

Central Nervous System
Amaurosis fugax
Hollenhorst plaque
Transient ischemic attack (TIA)/stroke
Spinal cord infarction

Cardiac
Myocardial infarction (MI)

General Symptoms
Myalgias
Fever
Malaise
Weight loss
Anorexia

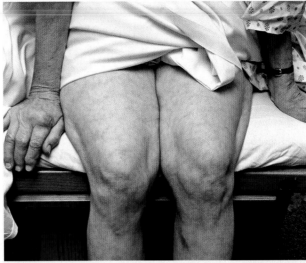

FIGURE 47-2 Patient with previously undiagnosed abdominal aortic aneurysm (AAA) presenting with atheroembolism to lower extremities. Note typical lacy reticular skin pattern of both thighs.

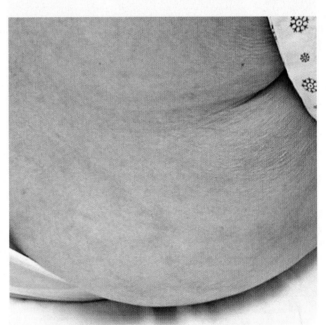

FIGURE 47-3 Atheroembolism to buttock and flank. Same patient as in Figure 47-2, with renal failure and livedo reticularis as presenting symptoms of previously unknown abdominal aortic aneurysm (AAA).

The actual incidence of spontaneous atheroembolism is difficult to determine; symptoms may be vague, and clinical features can be subtle or not recognized.[15]

Procedure-Related Atheroembolism

CARDIOVASCULAR SURGERY

Atheroembolism can occur as a complication of any invasive cardiac or vascular procedure or operation. Atheroembolism has been reported following abdominal aortic aneurysm (AAA) repair, aortoiliac bypass, and aortic and renal arteriography. Atheromatous debris can be dislodged during left heart catheterization, external cardiac message, blunt abdominal trauma, coronary artery bypass surgery, and many endovascular procedures.[2,16]

The advent of aortography in the 1930s transformed our ability to make accurate vascular diagnosis and expanded treatment options, but brought with it the risk of atheroembolism, especially

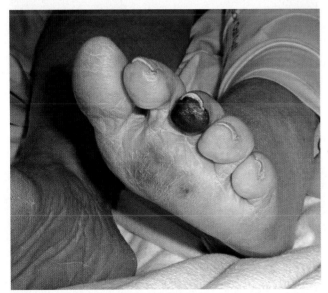

FIGURE 47-1 Classic blue toe syndrome. Note impending infarction of affected third toe, with livedo of the plantar surface.

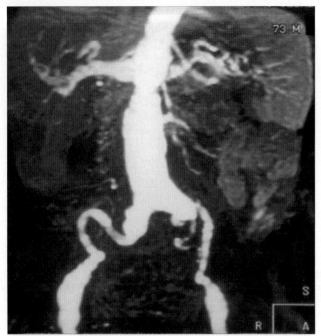

FIGURE 47-4 Abdominal magnetic resonance imaging (MRI) showing diffuse atherosclerosis of aorta, with "arteriomegaly." This disease has a high risk of atheroembolism.

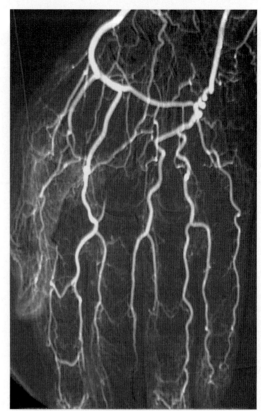

FIGURE 47-6   Upper-extremity angiogram in patient with hypothenar hammer syndrome, multiple digital artery occlusions resulting in critical ischemia of fingers. Note abnormal ulnar artery tortuosity secondary to local trauma to hand.

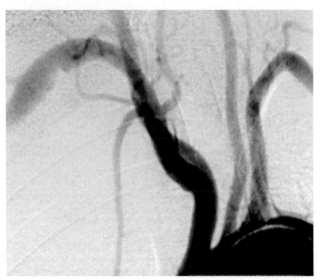

FIGURE 47-5   Arch aortogram showing right subclavian aneurysm with ulcerated atheromatous disease in nonsmoking young woman with thoracic outlet syndrome, presenting with atheroemboli to fingers.

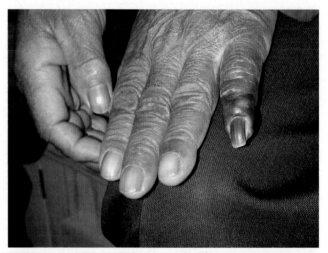

FIGURE 47-7   Atheroembolism to left fifth finger. Origin is from subclavian atheromatous plaque.

in patients with atheromatous or aneurysmal disease. A 30% incidence of atheroembolism after abdominal aortography was reported in patients who subsequently died within 6 months of the procedure. The organs most commonly affected were the kidneys and spleen.[17]

In the 1950s, Thurlbeck and Castleman first reported atheroembolism associated with vascular surgery and attributed this to operative manipulations that included arterial incisions, cannulation, and clamping of major arteries. Postmortem examination of those who died following AAA repair found cholesterol embolization to the kidneys in as many as 77% of patients.[18] In a more recent large retrospective series of 1011 patients undergoing angiographic procedures prior to aortic or infrainguinal vascular surgery, 2.9% (29 patients) were identified with atheroembolism. The majority of iatrogenic cases were attributed to aortography as opposed to surgery. The primary sources of embolism in these

patients were the abdominal aorta, iliac arteries, and femoropopliteal arteries.[19]

Massive atheroembolism following aortoiliac stent placement for treatment of aortic aneurysmal disease has been reported but is uncommon.[20,21] A study using Doppler ultrasound to identify microembolism found a significantly higher degree of peripheral embolization during endovascular aneurysm repair, compared to conventional surgical aneurysm repair.[22]

Atheroembolism can also occur after coronary artery bypass grafting (CABG) and valve surgery. Fatal myocardial infarction (MI) due to atheroembolism has been reported during coronary artery bypass operations.[23] Procedures that provoke atheroembolism include aortic cannulation, initiation of cardiopulmonary bypass (CPB), and transecting and anastomosis of bypass grafts to the ascending aorta during cardiac surgery. Atheroemboli may originate from the aortic root at the origin of vein grafts or from ruptured plaque in a coronary artery. In one series of 29 patients who died after cardiac surgery, atheroembolism was the causative factor in 22% of all deaths. In this series, atheroembolism to the coronary circulation caused cardiac failure; to the brain caused massive stroke; and to the gastrointestinal tract caused abdominal pain and bleeding.[14] Fortunately this is rare. Of 4095 CABG procedures, atheroembolism was found in only nine patients, for an incidence of 0.22%.[23] Those undergoing reoperation were found to have a higher incidence of 2.3%.[23]

Atherosclerosis involving the ascending aorta is a major risk factor for stroke during cardiac surgery. A large autopsy study of 221 patients found severe atherosclerosis of the ascending aorta in patients who died from atheroembolism after cardiac procedures. Atheroembolism occurred in 46 of 123 patients with severe ascending aortic disease, but only 2 of 98 (2%) without ascending aortic disease.[24] The incidence of atheroembolism was three times as high after CABG than valve surgery (26.1% vs. 8.9%).[24] Older patients with more advanced atheromatous disease of the ascending aorta were at the highest risk. Atheroemboli traveled to the brain in 16%, the spleen in 11%, kidney in 10%, and pancreas in 7%. Two thirds of patients had multiple sites of atheroembolism.[24] A 12% stroke risk during CPB was noted in a more recent study if aortic arch atheromas are seen with intraoperative transesophageal echocardiography (TEE).[25]

Transcranial Doppler (TCD) has documented that the greatest number of microembolic events was found during aortic clamping and initiation of bypass.[26] A study where an intraaortic filter was deployed and left in place until the patient was weaned from bypass found that 62% of filters contained atheroma in addition to platelet and fibrin strands.[27]

Off-pump CABG may reduce cerebral damage due to microembolism.[28] A study comparing effects of CABG with and without CPB assessed retinal microembolization by fluorescein angiography and fundus photography. Doppler high-intensity transient signals (HITS) was used to assess emboli to the brain. Five of nine pump patients had retinal microvascular damage, but none was evident in the off-pump patients. Doppler HITS were 20 times more frequent in the CPB patients.[28] Off-pump coronary artery bypass may have less risk of atheroembolism by avoiding arterial cannulation and the abrasive effect of CPB on the arterial wall.[24,28]

CARDIAC CATHETERIZATION

Cholesterol embolization after left heart catheterization is rare but can be devastating when it occurs. Coronary angiography is the most common invasive procedure associated with atheroembolism.[8] Clinically detectable cholesterol embolization occurring after cardiac catheterization has resulted in stroke, renal failure, mesenteric ischemia, and lower-extremity tissue loss with gangrene. In some situations it has a high fatality rate.[29–33]

A retrospective British study by Drost et al. reported 7 cases out of a total of 4587 cardiac catheterization procedures. Most had extensive atherosclerosis and suffered multisystem atheroembolization, with a retinal embolism in one patient, renal failure in five patients, and three requiring toe amputations. Six of the seven had extensive atherosclerosis. Four of these patients died within 4.5 months of this procedure.[29]

In a large prospective Japanese study, Fukumoto et al. prospectively reviewed 1786 consecutive patients undergoing left heart catheterization in a multicenter study. Diagnostic criteria for atheroembolism included livedo reticularis, blue toe syndrome, digital gangrene, or renal dysfunction. They found an incidence of 1.4% (25 patients), of which cutaneous findings and renal failure were the two most common clinical findings. If only definite cases were counted, the incidence was lower at 0.75%. Prognosis is poor in some patients, with an in-hospital mortality rate of 16%.[34]

Saklayen et al. prospectively evaluated 267 patients undergoing coronary angiography at a Veterans Administration (VA) medical center. A rise in Cr of 0.5 mg/dL or more at 3 weeks after the procedure was the main indicator of atheroembolism. They found an incidence of atheroembolic renal dysfunction of 1.9% (5/263 of patients undergoing coronary angiography).[31] Frock identified 17 patients with atheroembolic renal disease out of 14,998 angiographic procedures, an incidence of 0.1%.[35] In a prospective study of 1579 patients, Johnson et al. also found the incidence of cholesterol embolization to be very low: a single patient in 1579 coronary angiograms (0.06%).[36]

Passage of a catheter into the aorta for any endovascular procedure may not only loosen atheromatous plaque but can also scrape off aortic debris into the coronary guiding catheters. During contrast injection, this debris could be injected into the coronary or cerebral artery. In a study of 1000 consecutive coronary interventions, the amount of atheromatous material entering a guiding catheter from passage up the aorta was assessed by allowing blood to passively exit the back of the catheter into a sterile towel. Depending on the catheter shape, aortic debris was recovered in 24% to 65% of interventional cases. Surprisingly, the finding of aortic debris did not correlate with clinically apparent neurological, coronary, or renal ischemic events. Allowing adequate back-bleeding of guiding catheters before injecting contrast was suggested to decrease the risk of atheroembolism found in the guiding catheter from scraping the wall of the aorta during placement.[37]

Today with more advanced surgical techniques and greater awareness of atheroembolic risk, the incidence of atheroembolism during vascular and cardiac procedures is less common. The promise of distal protection devices to decrease the risk of atheroembolism during a procedure is still being assessed. Atheromatous debris can be recovered from the majority of angioplasty procedures. Development of more flexible catheters and lower-profile devices, along with improved operator technique, should allow for lower incidence of atheroembolic events in the future.[38]

Intraaortic Balloon Pumps

Karalis et al. addressed the risk of atheroembolism in patients undergoing catheterization when they have a so-called shaggy aorta. In this study, 70 patients were identified with aortic debris found on echocardiography, and 10 had a procedure-related embolic episode. A brachial approach may be a better option in these patients.[39]

Intraaortic balloon pumps have especially high potential for embolization when placed in an aorta with atherosclerotic debris. In one study, 5 of 10 patients (50%) had an embolic event related to placement of an intraaortic balloon pump.[39] If aortic debris is mobile, risk of embolization is especially high.

Spinal cord atheroembolism is a very rare complication of angiography.[13,40,41] Spinal cord infarction likely occurs secondary to embolic occlusion of small spinal cord arteries.

Anticoagulation/Thrombolysis Issues

The concern that warfarin could precipitate atheroembolism was first raised in 1961 by Fedar and Auerbach, who reported six patients who had developed painful purple toes after initiation of an oral anticoagulant.[42] Since then, anecdotal reports have linked warfarin with spontaneous atheroembolism. Clinical improvement of atheroembolism manifestations, including livedo reticularis, abdominal pain, and even renal function, has been reported after oral anticoagulants were discontinued.[43,44] Other anecdotal reports have indicated improvement in skin necrosis and livedo when low-molecular-weight heparin (LMWH) was discontinued.[43,45] It is hypothesized that anticoagulation could dissolve or prevent formation of a protective thrombus over an atherosclerotic plaque, leaving it vulnerable to rupture and embolization.

To the contrary, a number of large studies have shown no increased risk of atheroembolism in patients treated with warfarin. Blackshear et al. addressed concerns of warfarin anticoagulation in patients with atrial fibrillation and documented aortic plaque.

The SPAF III (Stroke Prevention in Atrial Fibrillation) trial looked at patients with atrial fibrillation and aortic plaque documented by TEE and found that patients assigned to warfarin therapy had an annual cholesterol embolization rate of 0.7 per patient-year, which was lower than those randomized to warfarin plus aspirin. The authors conclude that "elderly patients with AF and aortic plaque can receive adjusted-dose warfarin with a relatively low risk of cholesterol embolism."[46] The French Study of Aortic Plaques in Stroke found no difference in recurrent brain infarction in patients receiving warfarin compared to those on aspirin.[47]

Many cardiovascular patients are on anticoagulation, and in most case reports, causation is difficult to prove. Elderly patients are most likely to have advanced atherosclerosis and yet have chronic disorders such as atrial fibrillation requiring long-term anticoagulation. Often these patients had undergone other procedures including angiography, which is more likely an explanation for atheroembolic events. Delayed recognition of an acute event or recurrent showers in patients with shaggy aortas may account for the temporal association of atheroembolism with an oral anticoagulant.[48]

A sensible conclusion is to continue anticoagulation when compelling conditions exist, such as atrial fibrillation and thromboembolism, but consider stopping it if there is a lesser indication.[38]

Atheroembolism has also been reported to occur after thrombolytic therapy for myocardial infarction.[49–52] In some of these case reports, atheroembolism occurred in the absence of any invasive procedure, therefore implicating thrombolysis as a possible culprit. The mechanism of atheroembolism is thought to be dissolution of thrombus overlying atheromatous plaque, exposing ulcerated plaque to the arterial circulation that can embolize distally. Large trials of thrombolysis for acute myocardial infarction (AMI), including GISSI 2 and GUSTO, did not cite atheroembolism as a complication of thrombolytic therapy, so concern of atheroembolization should not be a reason to withhold thrombolysis.[53]

Blankenship et al. prospectively followed 60 patients with AMI who later underwent CABG. Half of these patients received thrombolytic therapy and half did not. It was concluded the prevalence of cholesterol embolization was not higher in those who received thrombolytic therapy.[54]

Atheroembolic Syndromes

Livedo and Skin Atheroembolism

Skin findings are the earliest and at times the only clinical finding of atheroembolism. Livedo reticularis is the most common manifestation of skin involvement, noted in 49% of patients.[55,56] The incidence of cutaneous manifestations of atheroembolism ranges from 35% to 96%.[1,57,58] Livedo has been labeled an underutilized clue to the diagnosis of atheroembolism because it should be considered an important and common indicator of atheroembolism elsewhere—in particular, to the kidneys or mesenteric organs.[55,59] For example, the suspicion of renal atheroembolism is markedly strengthened by the finding of livedo reticularis affecting the trunk or abdomen.

Livedo reticularis has a classic appearance as a reddish-blue lacy or netlike color pattern of the skin (Fig. 47-8). It is noted when the cutaneous venous plexus becomes visible owing to desaturated venous blood. In the presence of atheroembolism, small arteries are obstructed, reducing flow into the venous plexus and resulting in stasis of deoxygenated blood.[60] Characteristics of livedo reticularis include blanching with local pressure. It is more prominent when the patient is upright and may not be apparent if the patient is examined in the supine position.[55] Atheroembolism is less frequently diagnosed in nonwhite individuals because darker skin may disguise visible manifestations.[11] Livedo is most commonly seen on the feet and legs, but thighs, buttocks, lower back, abdomen, and upper-extremities can also be affected, depending on the source of the atheroembolism.[1]

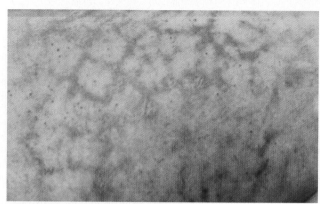

FIGURE 47-8 Unusual nonblanching livedo reticularis of thigh in patient with suspected livedo vasculitis.

Less common cutaneous findings in atheroembolism include splinter hemorrhages, petechiae, purpura, and erythematous nodules. Cholesterol embolism to the skin has been called a *pseudovasculitic syndrome*.[61] Livedo due to atheroembolism has been mistaken for small-vessel vasculitis in 16% of patients.[62] The diagnosis of atheroembolism can be confirmed by skin biopsy, and is positive in 92% of cases.[57,62]

In young women, livedo reticularis may be a common normal finding due to cold-induced vasospasm of skin vessels, and classically disappears with warming. It can also be seen in a number of diseases including collagen vascular disorders, antiphospholipid antibody syndrome, disseminated intravascular coagulation (DIC), vasculitides such as systemic lupus erythematosus (SLE) and polyarteritis nodosa, infective endocarditis, cryoglobulinemia, and hyperviscosity disorders.[38]

Atheroembolic Renal Disease

About half of all reported cases of atheroembolism involve the kidney.[7] The kidney receives a major percentage of the cardiac output and is the most common site for atheroembolism, followed by skin and gastrointestinal tract.[1,63] In clinical practice, it has been estimated that up to 10% of all cases of acute renal failure may be due to atheroembolism.[64]

Atheroembolic renal disease is defined as a syndrome of renal failure secondary to obstruction of small kidney arteries, arterioles, and glomerular capillaries by cholesterol crystal atheroembolism dislodged from the aorta or proximal renal arteries.[65] Renal atheroembolism may occur spontaneously in patients who have advanced atheromatous disease of the abdominal aorta, but more frequently it occurs as a complication of an angiographic or endovascular procedure. As noted earlier, passage of a catheter or guidewire through the aorta or renal arteries may dislodge atheromatous plaque fragments that travel to the kidneys, where they remain in small vessels. Today, approximately three fourths of renal atheroembolization cases are iatrogenic secondary to invasive procedures, in particular angiography. Coronary angiography is the most common angiographic procedure.[7,8]

The exact incidence of spontaneous atheroembolic renal disease is difficult to determine because most studies are retrospective. However, approximately 20% of atheroembolic episodes to the kidneys are thought to be unprovoked spontaneous episodes.[65] In addition, many atheroembolic episodes are subclinical, difficult to diagnose, and may be missed unless specifically looked for.

In renal biopsy studies, the prevalence of renal atheroembolism in all patients and age groups is quite low, ranging from 0.31% to 2.4%.[8,10] Moolenaar and Lamers reviewed the Netherlands experience of 842 cases of cholesterol crystal embolization in the Dutch National Pathology Information System and found an incidence of 6.0 cases per million population. Among autopsy reports, they also found a low incidence of 0.31%.[63] In other renal biopsy series, Greenberg et al. found 24/500 had atheroembolic findings.[66]

In another large series of 755 renal biopsies, atheroemboli were discovered in 8 patients (1.1%).[67] Selection bias may account for the low prevalence; these patients were selected for biopsy because of unexplained recent worsening of renal function.

Atheroembolism to the kidneys can also occur during any vascular surgical procedure, in particular AAA resection, renal revascularization, and aortoiliac or aortofemoral bypass. In those who died after aortic surgery or an angiographic procedure, the finding of atheroembolism at autopsy ranged from 12% to 77%.[8] Atheromatous emboli to the kidney was documented in 77% of patients following surgical repair of abdominal aortic aneurysms.[2]

Atheroembolism to the kidneys also occurs as complication of endovascular procedures (Box 47-2). Modi and Rao reports 85% of patients presenting with atheroembolic renal disease underwent an invasive vascular procedure within the prior 3 months (abdominal aorta, coronary, or carotid angiography).[65] Olin has stated that atheroembolism likely occurs in every patient undergoing an endovascular procedure (renal artery angioplasty and stent) for atherosclerotic renal disease.[68] A study by Kawarada et al. used intrarenal duplex ultrasound to detect microembolic signals and found that emboli occurred in all 13 patients undergoing renal artery stent implantation, in particular post dilation of the stent.[69] Underappreciation of this frequent occurrence is because clinicians attribute acute renal failure after a procedure to another cause such as contrast-induced nephropathy.

A prospective study at a VA medical center looked at renal failure after cardiac catheterization. Atheroembolism was suspected on the basis of a 0.5 mg/dL or more rise in Cr 3 weeks after a coronary angiogram. Although the incidence of renal impairment was low in this group, two of the five died of renal failure. Of note, none of the five had skin signs of livedo, and the diagnosis of atheroembolism would have been missed on examination.[31]

Atheroembolism to the kidneys is underrecognized as a cause of acute and chronic renal disease. In one review of 259 patients who underwent renal biopsy for acute renal failure, cholesterol emboli were found in 6.9% of cases. Of note, 15 of 18 of these patients were clinically unsuspected to have atheroembolism as a cause of renal failure. Another study found 7.5% of patients with acute renal failure had documented atheroembolism on renal biopsy.[70]

In one review, Mayo and Swartz estimated that 4% of all inpatient nephrology consults were due to atheroembolism.[64] This may be a conservative estimate because older patients with multiple risk factors accounted for a higher proportion of in-hospital nephrology consults. Of those consults seen with acute renal failure, 5% to 10% were felt to be due to atheroembolic renal disease.[64]

Atheromatous emboli and cholesterol crystals tend to lodge in arcuate and interlobar arteries which are 150 to 200 microns in diameter.[8,65] Cholesterol crystal emboli not only cause mechanical vessel obstruction but also set up an endothelial inflammatory reaction that some have labeled *microcrystalline angiitis*.[8] This is characterized by polymorphonuclear leukocyte and eosinophil infiltration around the vessel, and subsequently mononuclear cells with giant cell formation in the perivascular tissues. Endothelial distortion, intimal proliferation, perivascular fibrosis, and sometimes extraluminalization of crystals can be seen.[67] With thrombus formation, there is further microvascular occlusion of renal vessels. Over 2 to 4 weeks, there is a progressive gradual decline in renal function following an acute atheroembolic episode. Renal infarction or necrosis is rare because the process is patchy and does not obstruct the larger feeding arteries to the kidney.

Atheroembolic renal disease presents as acute or subacute renal dysfunction in older patients, rarely younger than age 50, usually affecting those with preexisting renal insufficiency.[5,35,65,71] Patients with atheroembolism have multiple risk factors including smoking, diabetes, hypertension, and hyperlipidemia. A review of 52 cases of atheroembolic renal failure at the Massachusetts General Hospital from 1981 to 1990 found these patients were more likely to have significant hypertension and coronary and peripheral artery disease (PAD).[72]

The clinical course may be variable. In contrast-induced nephropathy, renal failure occurs immediately after dye infusion, with a peak in Cr within several days and resolving in less than 2 weeks.[8] Unlike contrast-induced nephropathy, atheroembolic renal failure may slowly worsen over a period of weeks to months, likely because of recurrent spontaneous showers of emboli. The kidney responds to ischemic damage with inflammatory changes that lead to glomerular sclerosis, tubular atrophy, and interstitial fibrosis.[38,65] Sometimes, features of focal segmental necrotizing glomerulonephritis and crescentic glomerulonephritis are seen in renal biopsy specimens.[65,66,73]

Atheroembolism to kidneys may be subclinical. Subacute presentation is more common with progressive renal failure over several weeks. In one report, the average time interval between an angiographic procedure and diagnosis of atheroembolic renal disease was 5 weeks.[35] Renal function declined over 3 to 8 weeks.[72]

A chronic form of renal failure may be mild and can be clinically silent. Atheroembolism may present acutely, with onset within 1 week, or be subacute with delayed onset of renal impairment 2 to 6 weeks after an inciting procedure. A step-and-plateau drop in renal function has been described, perhaps owing to intermittent recurrent showers of cholesterol crystals over a period of time. One to two thirds of patients with atheroembolic renal disease will need dialysis. Lye et al. reviewed the English literature in 1993, noting that 40% of patients required dialysis.[6] Only 20% to 30% will recover sufficient renal function to stop dialysis.[6,8,74]

Clinical features are often absent but may include flank pain and gross hematuria due to renal infarction. Abdominal pain, nausea, vomiting, and blood loss can result from embolization to the gastrointestinal tract. In approximately half of these patients, there may be livedo reticularis or purple toe discoloration due to cholesterol embolization to the skin. Fever, malaise, and weight loss may be accompanying systemic symptoms.[65]

Severe or resistant hypertension has been noted in up to half of patients with atheroembolic renal disease.[6,15] Hypertension may result from activation of renin angiotensin system, or be volume mediated secondary to inability of the kidney to excrete excess fluid. Malignant hypertension can occur with atheromatous embolization to the kidneys.[75]

LABORATORY TESTING

Laboratory testing generally shows nonspecific findings. Although elevated creatinine, proteinuria, and eosinophilia have been reported in up to 80% of patients in the acute stage, these findings are inconsistently found.[15,76] Anemia, leukocytosis, thrombocytopenia,

Box 47-2 Differential Diagnosis of Renal Failure After Procedure

Contrast-Induced Nephropathy
ATN: rapid rise in Cr, peaks in 3 days and back to baseline in 2 weeks

Ischemic Renal Failure
Renal artery stenosis, often severe hypertension

Small-Vessel Vasculitis
Active urine sediment, autoimmune markers (ANA or ANCA)

Drug-Induced Interstitial Nephritis
Drug fever, rash, eosinophilia

Thrombotic Thrombocytopenic Purpura
Smear for schistocytes

Bacterial Endocarditis
TEE

ANA, antinuclear antibody; ANCA, antineutrophil cytoplasmic autoantibody; ATN, acute tubular necrosis; Cr, creatinine; TEE, transesophageal echocardiogram.

and elevated inflammatory markers including sedimentation rate and C-reactive protein (CRP) are occasionally noted.[1]

The finding of eosinophils in the urine has been considered to be a very important diagnostic feature of renal atheroembolism. In a report by Wilson et al., urine eosinophils were found in 8 of 24 patients who had biopsy-proven atheroembolic disease. Six of the eight patients had more than 5% of urinary white cells as eosinophils.[77] Hansel's stain may increase the identification of urinary eosinophils. Urinary eosinophils, however, can be seen in other kidney disorders such as acute interstitial nephritis and other allergic disorders. Urinalysis may show hyaline or granular casts. Proteinuria may be present but is rarely severe enough to cause nephrotic syndrome.[78] Urine sediment is usually inactive and unremarkable.[78,79]

Blood tests may show eosinophilia ranging from 14% to 80%, but again this is not a consistent finding.[8,72] Eosinophilia is thought to be due to inflammatory changes in the kidney with immune activation. Kasinath et al. reviewed the literature and observed that 29 of 36 reports noted eosinophilia in association with renal atheroembolism. In this patient series, they found eosinophil counts ranging from 540 to 2000 cells/mm^3.[76] Modi and Rao found that 60% of patients had eosinophilia,[65] and Lye et al. reported an incidence of 71%.[6] Eosinophilia may be transient and seen only in the acute phase. Despite not always being present, if the eosinophil count is greater than 500 cells per μL, many clinicians feel this is a contributing finding, helpful in establishing a possible diagnosis of atheroembolism.[7]

The definitive diagnosis of atheroembolic kidney disease is confirmed histologically by the demonstration of cholesterol crystals in arcuate and interlobular arteries of the kidney. The sensitivity of a single renal biopsy may be only 75% owing to the patchy distribution of atheroembolism; however, with two biopsies, 94% are positive.[65]

Renal biopsies are not done in every patient with renal insufficiency, but a high degree of suspicion of atheroembolism in the appropriate setting (e.g., after an invasive vascular procedure) is necessary to make the correct diagnosis. It is important to be aware of many potential causes of renal failure in vascular patients, including contrast nephropathy, volume depletion from diuretics, renal artery or vein thrombosis, renal artery stenosis, nephrotoxic agents (e.g., antiinflammatory agents, angiotensin inhibitors), drug-induced interstitial nephritis, and glomerulonephritis. Atheroembolic renal disease can also mimic vasculitis. In many cases, renal failure after an angiographic procedure is incorrectly attributed to contrast-induced acute tubular necrosis. Clinical differentiation between the two is important.

PROGNOSIS AND TREATMENT

The prognosis for atheroembolic renal disease is generally poor.[1] Some 30% to 40% of patients with recurrent atheroembolic events have irreversible end-stage kidney failure requiring long-term hemodialysis.[6,80,81] Dialysis dependency is also an indicator of poor prognosis. In one study, those who progressed to end-stage renal failure had a mortality rate of 75%, compared to 17% in those who recovered renal function.[35] Scolari et al. reported poor outcomes for 354 subjects followed for 2 years, of whom 116 required dialysis and 102 died. These patients were elderly with advanced cardiovascular disease and comorbidities including heart failure and renal disease.[7,82] Another series also reported an overall mortality rate of 58% over 15 months. Most of these patients died of cardiac failure.[1] The overall outcome and prognosis is influenced by severity of atheroembolism and presence of preexisting kidney and cardiovascular comorbidities.

Treatment of renal atheroembolism is preventive (to avoid further episodes of atheroembolism) and supportive.[8] General measures include avoidance of nephrotoxic agents, including angiographic contrast and antiinflammatory drugs. Hypertension and congestive heart failure (CHF) should be managed with appropriate medications such as vasodilators and diuretics. Aggressive management of hypertension may decrease proteinuria.[79] Dialysis may be needed for uremia, volume excess, and electrolyte imbalances.

Belenfant et al. showed positive outcomes with aggressive supportive care in 67 patients admitted to a renal intensive care unit (ICU) for management of acute renal failure in the setting of multisystem cholesterol embolization. Clinical features included pulmonary edema, gastrointestinal ischemia, cutaneous ischemia, and retinal embolism. Treatment consisted of anticoagulation withdrawal, avoidance of invasive procedures, management of CHF with angiotensin-converting enzyme (ACE) inhibitors, and loop diuretics. Ultrafiltration or hemodialysis was used when needed for renal support. Enteral or parenteral nutrition supplementation was provided when needed. Some patients were treated empirically with steroids. Improved outcomes in multiorgan cholesterol embolism were reported, although the in-hospital mortality rate was 16%. Of the 56 patients who survived initial hospitalization and were ultimately discharged, there was a 77% 1-year and 52% 4-year survival; 32% remained on maintenance hemodialysis for irreversible renal failure.[80]

Pharmacological treatment for renal atheroembolism is empirical because there are no prospective clinical trials, and no definitive treatment has been established. Anecdotal reports suggest the use of steroids to reduce the inflammatory response associated with atheroembolism to the kidney.[83,84] Cholesterol crystals act like foreign bodies setting up an inflammatory reaction with a cascade of systemic mediators of inflammation. Steroids reduce the inflammatory reaction and may have a favorable response.[85,86] Belenfant et al. treated those with new cholesterol embolization, as well as those with declining clinical status, with corticosteroids and noted improved constitutional symptoms and nutrition.[80] Scolari et al. found the risk of dialysis and death was lower in those patients on steroids.[7]

In an anecdotal report, simvastatin (40 mg daily) was associated with improved renal function in some patients with renal biopsy–documented atheroembolism.[87] Corticosteroids and plasma exchange for treatment of atheroembolic renal disease has been tried for management.[88] Treatment of cyanotic toes with lovastatin was noted in a case report of a man with diffuse atheromatous disease and gangrenous toes.[89]

Prevention is the best management, in particular avoiding additional invasive angiographic procedures in high-risk patients with extensive atheromatous disease of the aorta. If procedures are necessary, distal embolic protection devices may improve outcomes for arterial interventions.[90]

Gastrointestinal Tract Atheroembolism

The gastrointestinal tract is one of the common sites for aortic atheroembolism and ranks as the third most frequently affected organ system after skin and renal involvement.[63] Cholesterol embolization should be in the differential diagnosis of all patients with atherosclerosis presenting with gastrointestinal symptoms after a vascular interventional procedure. Symptoms may be nonspecific and difficult to diagnose but include abdominal pain, fever, and diarrhea. Gastrointestinal bleeding due to mucosal infarcts and ulceration caused by bowel ischemia may occur.[57,91,92] In severe cases, intestinal infarction may require urgent surgery for necrotic bowel or bowel perforation. The colon is most commonly involved. Multiple emboli over time may result in stricture formation, bowel obstruction, or polypoid lesions.[93–95] Rarely, atheroembolism to the gut can mimic colon cancer.[96] Sometimes symptoms may be misdiagnosed for months until a catastrophic event such as small-bowel perforation with peritonitis or bleeding occurs.[97] The liver, gallbladder, and pancreas are also uncommon sites for atheroembolism, but there are case reports of acute pancreatitis and acute acalculous cholecystitis from aortic atheroembolism.[98–103] Cholesterol embolization has been reported after protracted vomiting.[104] The stomach is rarely involved. An endoscopic biopsy should include submucosa to detect cholesterol clefts in small arterioles.[91] Most patients with atheroembolism to the gastrointestinal tract have advanced atherosclerosis, and atheroembolism affects multiple organs.[92] When atheroembolism involves the gastrointestinal tract, cholesterol embolization can also be seen as livedo reticularis or associated blue toe syndrome.[97] At least half of these cases are precipitated by an angiographic procedure and have a high mortality rate.[91]

Lower Extremities and Blue Toe Syndrome

In 1961, Feder and Auerbach described six patients who presented with painful purple toes and noted findings of dark-tinged discoloration of the plantar surfaces and sides of the first and second toes bilaterally. He noted the toes were painful and tender to touch, and that the blue discoloration of the skin blanched with local pressure, which he felt differentiated this entity from localized hematoma or purpura. These patients were older, with ages ranging from 53 to 69, and had atherosclerotic cardiovascular diseases including diabetes, stroke, or congestive heart failure. Most of these patients had intact peripheral pulses.[42] Feder and Auerbach associated these skin changes with initiation of warfarin anticoagulation but recognized these features were not due to warfarin-induced skin necrosis.

Fifteen years later in 1976, Karmody et al. established the term *blue toe syndrome*, recognizing that the sudden onset of pain and cyanosis was the result of a microembolic event to the digital arteries. Angiography in a number of these patients localized the source of embolism to the femoral, popliteal, or aortoiliac arteries.[9]

The typical patient with blue toe syndrome presents with sudden onset of painful cyanotic skin lesions that may involve one or many toes. Cyanosis results from decreased arterial inflow along with impaired venous outflow, leading to stasis of desaturated blood. Initially, the cyanosis blanches with pressure, but with worsening ischemia and tissue damage, the blue discoloration may become nonblanchable. The affected toe is dark blue in color, painful due to ischemia, and exquisitely tender to touch. Digital ischemia can progress to cause skin necrosis, ulceration, and black gangrene. Livedo reticularis of the foot may also be present involving the base of the affected toe, forefoot, plantar surface, or heel (Figs. 47-9 through 47-13). Myalgias due to muscle atheroembolism may occur, with clinical features of local muscle tenderness, sometimes with actual myonecrosis.[105]

Clinical examination should be the initial step to determine the source of atheroembolism. In 78% of patients, peripheral pulses including pedal pulses are intact.[1] Although distal pulses are palpable in the classic case of blue toe syndrome, occlusive arterial disease is present in up to half of patients, based on ankle-brachial indices (ABIs) less than 0.9.[106] Careful pulse examination with auscultation for bruits may suggest proximal arterial disease. A widened expansile common femoral or popliteal pulse may

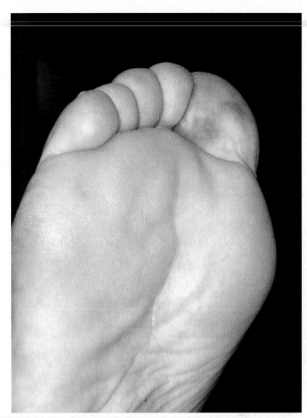

FIGURE 47-10 Atheroembolic mottling of the big toe.

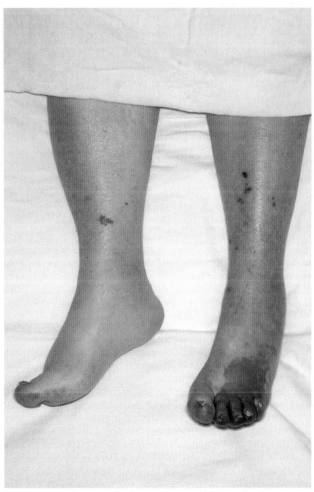

FIGURE 47-11 Severe episode of atheroembolism to forefoot.

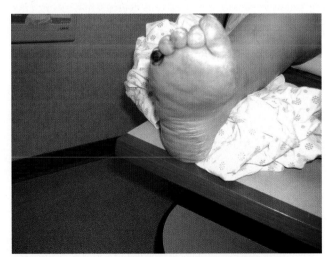

FIGURE 47-9 Blue toe syndrome with infarction of fifth toe.

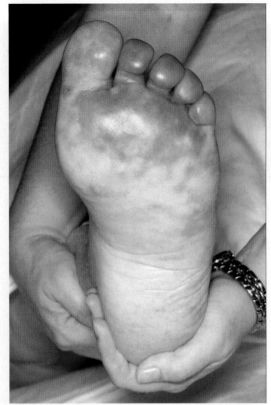

FIGURE 47-12 Plantar surface of same patient as in Figure 47-11, showing purple toes and severe atheroembolism to forefoot.

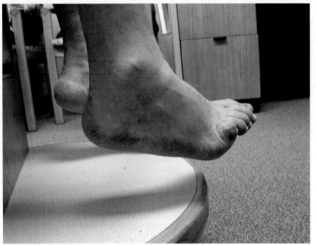

FIGURE 47-13 Livedo reticularis from atheroembolism involving lateral aspect of foot and heel.

When no embolic source is readily identifiable, imaging of the thoracic aorta is important and may reveal a coral reef (see later discussion) or mobile plaque as the source of distal atheroemboli. Sometimes a solitary embolic source cannot be isolated, owing to the diffuse nature of atherosclerosis. For example, in one study, arteriograms showed diffuse disease at both aortoiliac and femoropopliteal levels in 40% of patients, making it difficult to discern the likely source of atheroembolism.

Only a few years ago, angiography was the gold standard to search for a culprit lesion, but now with advances in noninvasive imaging, computed tomographic angiography (CTA), magnetic resonance angiography (MRA), duplex ultrasound, and TEE are all first-line well-established methods to image the aorta.[110,111]

Blue toes due to atheroembolism should be differentiated from other skin and systemic disorders (Fig. 47-14). Blue toes can also be caused by benign cold-induced reversible vasospasm, similar to Raynaud's phenomenon of the fingers. Other vascular diseases that can present with a blue toe include pernio, thromboangiitis obliterans (TAO) (Buerger's disease), and digital artery thrombosis. Paraproteinemia (e.g., myeloma) or myeloproliferative disorders (e.g., polycythemia vera, essential thrombocytosis) may cause small-vessel thrombosis. Cryofibrinogenemia results from complexes of fibrinogen, fibrin, and proteins that precipitate with cold. Secondary forms are associated with cancers, rheumatological diseases, and infections. Cryoglobulinemia results from immunoglobulins (Igs) that precipitate in the cold. There are three types: type 1 cryoglobulinemia occurs in association with lymphoproliferative disease (e.g., chronic lymphocytic lymphoma); types 2 and 3 may be associated with viral hepatitis infections. Hirschmann and Raugi defines the blue toe syndrome as a "blue or violaceous discoloration of one or more toes in the absence of trauma (fracture or strain), cold-induced injury (pernio or frostbite), or disorders that produce systemic cyanosis (methemoglobinemia or hypoxia)".[60]

The short- and long-term outcome after an atheroembolic episode is variable depending on the extent of atheroembolism and resulting tissue damage. For many patients, the prognosis for atheroembolism is poor, sometimes requiring limb amputation. Improvement may occur but may take several weeks for pain to slowly subside, and longer for skin color changes to improve. In more severe cases, the affected toe(s) may progress to necrosis with black gangrene. If carefully managed, the gangrene may stay dry and demarcate from healthy tissue, allowing future autoamputation of the distal or entire toe. Wet gangrene may lead to infection and may require surgical amputation. A toe amputation may heal satisfactorily at a demarcation line if large-vessel arterial perfusion is intact.

Although some individuals recover after a single episode of atheroembolism, a recurrent episode can cause further irreparable damage resulting in extensive tissue damage and necrosis. Spontaneous embolic episodes tend to be recurrent. With very extensive atheroembolism, skin necrosis may occur, affecting much of the foot; this has been referred to as *trash foot*[19] (Fig. 47-15). This is potentially limb threatening and is associated

suggest an aneurysm. Palpation of the abdomen may reveal an aortic aneurysm. The location of livedo, such as the foot, thigh, or abdomen, suggests a more proximal site.

Lower-extremity atheromatous emboli can originate from focal or diffuse atherosclerosis, from stenotic or aneurysmal disease, and from disease above or below the inguinal ligament.[106] If both lower extremities are involved, this suggests the origin of the atheroembolism is proximal to the aortic bifurcation. In unilateral blue toe syndrome, the culprit site is likely at or distal to the iliac artery. Common sites of atherosclerosis are the common or external iliac artery (EIA), the superficial femoral artery (SFA) at the adductor hiatus (due to stenotic disease), and the popliteal artery (arising from a local aneurysm). The aortoiliac segment is the most common origin for atheroembolism, accounting for two thirds of cases.[106–109] One third of cases are found to arise from the femoropopliteal arteries.[106]

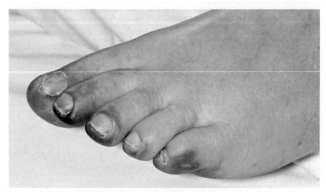

FIGURE 47-14 Blue toes from unknown cause.

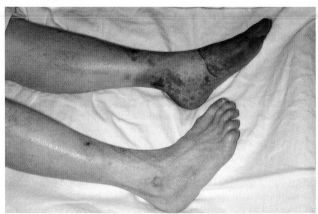

FIGURE 47-15 Postangiographic atheroembolism to foot, resulting in critical irreversible foot ischemia requiring below-knee amputation.

with a high mortality rate, owing to coexistent multisystem disease. In one study where trash foot occurred in 19 of 29 patients (7 bilateral) following abdominal aorta or lower-extremity revascularization, 8 patients underwent major amputations, and 5 minor amputations.[19] The risk of major amputation after extensive atheroembolism varies from 10% to 27% depending on the reported series.[9,106,112] Mortality is also significant in multisystem atheroembolism, as in one recent study where 31% of patients died during a follow-up period of 15 months.[113]

OPERATIVE MANAGEMENT

Once lower-extremity atheroembolism occurs, management principles are to prevent recurrent embolic episodes and provide local care for the affected extremity. General treatment measures are discussed later under the section on treatment.

Surgical or endovascular intervention has been advocated because of the high likelihood of recurrent atheroembolic events leading to worsening irreversible tissue ischemia with risk of limb amputation.[9,112] Embolic recurrence may be as high as 50% to 80%, with a 40% to 60% risk of tissue loss.[106,107] The goal of surgical intervention is to remove or exclude the source of embolization and prevent recurrent episodes leading to organ and extremity loss. Treatment choice is determined by location and severity of disease. The optimal surgical intervention depends on the individual patient. Arterial bypass, endarterectomy, and angioplasty with stent placement have been reported to be effective in selected patients by preventing recurrent embolization.[107,114]

A retrospective study at Washington University Medical Center found 62 patients with renal or cutaneous manifestations of atheroembolism. Angiography was done in almost all patients. The aorta and iliac arteries (80%) were felt to be the most common source of atheroembolism, followed by femoral (13%), popliteal (3%), and subclavian (3%) arteries.[108] Bypass grafting procedures were performed on 42 patients to exclude the native diseased artery. Other patients underwent a combination of endarterectomy and bypass grafts. Limb salvage was accomplished in 98%, although 31% had minor amputations. No further episodes of atheroembolism occurred over a mean follow-up period of 20 months.[108]

Keen et al. reviewed his experience of surgical management of atheroembolism in 100 patients with lower-extremity, visceral, and upper-extremity atheroembolism who were followed for 12 years.[109] Aortoiliac occlusive disease was present in 47 patients, and aortic aneurysm was present in 20 patients (average size, 3.5 cm). Operations to exclude the embolic source included aortic bypass or aortoiliac endarterectomy, femoral and popliteal endarterectomy, or bypass graft. Several patients underwent extra-anatomical reconstruction.[109] Despite surgery, 6 of 97 had recurrent events, and 9 required major leg amputations with 10 toe amputations.

Friedman and Krishnasastry reviewed a small group of high-risk surgical patients presenting with rest pain, ulceration, or gangrene due to atheroemboli to both lower extremities. These patients, who were not candidates for direct aortic reconstruction because of preexisting medical comorbidities, underwent ligation of the EIA with axillary-bifemoral bypass. Initial limb salvage was accomplished in all, with no limb loss over the next 52 months.[115] Kaufman et al. also reported a small group of high-risk patients in whom limb salvage and healing of foot ulcers was accomplished in the majority with an axillobifemoral bypass with exclusion of the external iliacs.[116]

Hollier et al. reviewed 88 patients with shaggy aorta syndrome who suffered atheromatous embolization (Fig. 47-16). Surgical correction was performed in 27 patients, including endarterectomy, external iliac ligation, and graft replacement. The best outcome (lowest morbidity and mortality) for those with lower-extremity atheroembolism was with ligation of the distal EIA and extra-anatomical bypass.[117] The author noted that surgery was not always successful in preventing visceral infarction or renal failure.[117]

Primary angioplasty for iliac or superficial femoral lesions can also be successful for focal high-grade stenotic lesions of the iliac or superficial femoral artery.[114,118] Although there may be concern of provoking further embolization, some studies show good results. In one series of 10 patients treated with primary angioplasty, none had embolization at the time of the procedure, and 8 of the 10 had no recurrent atheroembolic episodes. The patients in this series were more likely to have single focal high-grade stenotic lesions of an iliac or SFA amenable to angioplasty, as opposed to more diffuse proximal atherosclerotic plaque.[112,114]

A self-expanding stent has been used to treat atheroembolism arising from an isolated segment of the iliac artery.[107] For more complex plaques, a covered stent has been successfully deployed and offers the advantage of excluding the diseased segment by trapping the atheroma and thrombus under the covered stent.[107,119] In one case report of three patients with iliac artery disease treated with a self-expanding stent covered with Dacron, no recurrences

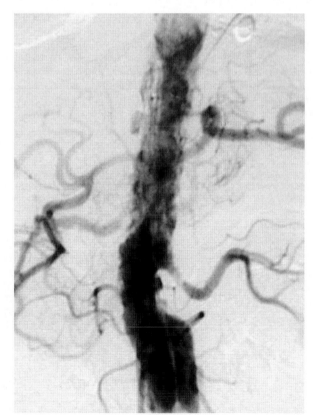

FIGURE 47-16 Aortogram demonstrating diffuse atheromatous disease, so-called shaggy aorta, with high atheroembolic potential.

of microembolism were noted after 16 months, and the toe lesions healed.[107]

Aortic stent grafting is now commonly used in the management of abdominal aortic aneurysms. In a retrospective study of 19 patients with symptomatic lower-extremity atheroembolism presenting with ischemic ulcers or toe gangrene and an abdominal aneurysm, an aortic stent graft was deployed to exclude an abdominal aortic aneurysm. At 1-year follow-up, eight of nine patients had resolution of ischemic toe symptoms.[113] The authors note that although stent graft repair of AAA may prevent future embolization, it is important to not miss coexisting thoracic aortic disease.

Arterial filters have also been employed in the superficial femoral artery, carotid, renal, and many other vessels. As filter development continues to advance, this may become an adjunctive procedure in the future.[120]

Upper-Extremity Atheroembolism

In the upper extremity, atheroembolism is said to be uncommon.[108] Atherosclerosis may involve the aortic arch and branch vessels. Two sites in particular are important. The subclavian artery is a common site for atherosclerosis. Unequal upper-extremity blood pressures should raise suspicion of disease at or proximal to the subclavian artery level. Most individuals with subclavian atherosclerotic disease are asymptomatic, but this can be a source of atheroembolism to the arm and the fingers (Fig. 47-17). Thoracic outlet syndrome causes extrinsic compression of the subclavian artery as it passes under the clavicle and over the first rib. This is a site for aneurysm formation and subsequent atheroembolism to the hand and fingers. Finally, at the wrist level, repetitive pounding injury to the hypothenar side of the palm, as occurs in carpenters and car mechanics, can result in ulnar artery aneurysm with atheroembolism to the hand and fingers.

Coral Reef Plaque

A coral reef plaque is an exophytic calcified discrete mass that is prone to distal embolization.[121] These are more commonly located in the posterior wall of the suprarenal aorta.[122] Although unusual, they occur in patients with generalized atherosclerosis. They can be treated by surgical thromboendarterectomy or bypass.[123,124] Endovascular stent placement has also been successful in patients symptomatic with claudication from aortic lumen compromise by a coral reef.[125]

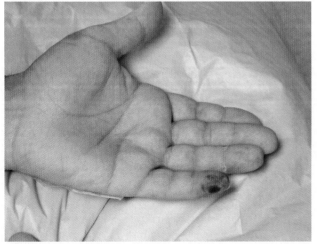

FIGURE 47-17 Cutaneous infarction of fifth finger due to atheroembolism. Note subtle ischemic mottling of other fingers.

Ascending Aorta/Arch Atheroma and Stroke

Sixty years ago, cerebral vasospasm was speculated to cause stroke. Today, carotid artery disease and atrial fibrillation are known to be major causes of nonhemorrhagic stroke. With the advent of TEE, aortic arch plaque has been identified as an important potential source of cerebral embolic stroke.[126,127] Case-controlled prospective studies have shown a clear association between atherosclerotic disease of the ascending aorta/aortic arch and risk of ischemic stroke.[128] Autopsy studies found ulcerated plaque in the aortic arch to be present in 26% of 239 patients with cerebrovascular disease (both stroke and brain hemorrhage) but only 5% of patients with another neurological diagnosis.[128,129] Another large study using TEE to detect aortic atheroma compared 215 consecutive patients with first stroke or TIA to 202 control subjects and confirmed that atheroma in the ascending aorta and arch are a significant risk factor for stroke.[130]

Characterization of aortic plaque morphology (hypoechoic plaque, ulceration, calcification, sessile or mobile thrombus) is important in prediction of stroke.[131] In particular, the thickness of plaque in the ascending aorta and arch correlates with risk of stroke. When patients with acute stroke were compared to consecutive controls, 28% had plaques of 4 mm or more in thickness in those with unexplained stroke, compared to 8% of 172 patients who had a known or suspected cause of brain infarct.[128] In the French Study of Aortic Plaques in Stroke, TEE was done to quantify aortic arch atheromatous disease in 331 patients aged 60 or older admitted to hospital with an acute stroke. The incidence of recurrent brain infarction was 11.9% per 100 person-years in those with aortic plaque thickness greater than 4 mm, compared to 2.8% for those with minimal plaque (<1 mm). The presence of atherosclerotic arch plaque thickness of 4 mm or greater was found to be an independent predictor of recurrent brain infarction and cardiovascular events.[132] Even moderate atheromatous disease (defined as intimal thickness of the ascending aorta and arch of > 2 mm) is a significant risk factor for stroke after cardiac surgery.[133]

Mobile Atheroma

Atheromatous plaque that is protruding and pedunculated has been correlated with an increased risk of stroke. The presence of mobile components, however, denotes the highest risk for stroke.[109,132,134–141] In a study of 118 elderly patients studied with intraoperative TEE, 3 of 12 patients (25%) with a mobile aortic arch atheroma had suffered a perioperative stroke, compared to 2 of 118 (2%) patients without a mobile atheroma.[134] A mobile mass overlying an atheromatous plaque is likely adherent thrombus and therefore is more likely to respond to anticoagulation than the underlying plaque itself. Whether to use anticoagulation for mobile thrombus in the aorta, however, remains controversial.

Warfarin anticoagulation has been advocated for the management of mobile aortic atheroma. A study by Dressler et al. documented effectiveness of warfarin in preventing recurrent embolic events in those with symptomatic thoracic aorta mobile atheroma compared to those not receiving anticoagulation.[142] He reviewed 31 patients with mobile aortic atheroma who presented with a systemic embolic event. At follow-up, those patients not receiving warfarin had a much higher incidence of vascular events (45% vs. 5%). Recurrent strokes occurred in 38% of patients. There were no strokes in those on warfarin.[142] Of note, those with small mobile atheroma were not treated with warfarin, and recurrent strokes occurred in 37% of these patients.[142]

Warfarin was noted to be more effective than antiplatelet medications in another study of patients with severe ascending aortic atheromatous disease.[140] Further randomized controlled trials would be needed to address anticoagulation vs. antiplatelet therapy for this important issue.

In case examples, peripheral embolization from plaque-related mobile thrombus in the thoracic aorta has been successfully treated with warfarin. In one case report, a 71-year-old man had atheroembolism to the toes after vomiting. A large mobile mass in the descending thoracic aorta was identified by TEE. After 3 months of warfarin anticoagulation, there was virtual resolution of the aortic mass, suggesting it was thrombus covering atheromatous plaque. The toe pain and discoloration from atheroembolism also resolved completely.[104]

Stroke due to atheroembolism can occur during carotid surgery. Microemboli occurs during carotid endarterectomy and can be detected by TCD ultrasound. Ackerstaff et al. found a positive correlation with the occurrence of microembolism during carotid endarterectomy and perioperative TIA and stroke. Magnetic resonance imaging also documented new ischemic brain lesions in these patients.[143]

Carotid sinus massage may reproduce syncope in patients with carotid sinus hypersensitivity but also cause inadvertent atheroembolic stroke in patients with carotid atherosclerosis.[144]

Embolic stroke should be suspected in the proper clinical setting. In young patients with unexplained embolism, TEE has identified unsuspected mobile aortic arch thrombus on atherosclerotic plaque.[127] Brain imaging characteristically shows multiple small ischemic lesions. Brain pathology has also documented multiple cholesterol emboli.[145] Lacunar infarcts are generally thought to be due to small brain infarcts from hypertension. It is possible some lacunar infarcts may be due to cholesterol emboli.[146]

General Treatment Measures for Atheroembolic Disease

Preventive

It has been said many times that the best treatment for many diseases is prevention.[147] Angiography is the most common iatrogenic cause of atheroembolism, responsible for up to 80% of cases, so safer angiographic techniques and newer technologies may decrease the incidence of catheter-induced atheroembolism.[8] For example a "no touch technique" has been advocated to reduce potential for intimal disruption during renal artery stenting. A second guide is placed within the guide catheter to minimize contact between the guide catheter and aorta.[148] Arterial filters have also been successfully employed in the superficial artery.[120] Distal protection devices are available for renal and cerebral angioplasty.[149–151] Cerebral protection devices may reduce stroke during carotid artery stenting, but device-related complications can occur.[147,152]

Reduction of atherosclerotic burden and plaque stabilization has been a major focus for preventing coronary events and should also be a focus for preventing atheroembolism. Reducing lipid content in the plaque core, decreasing inflammation and inflammatory cells, and reducing vasa vasorum neovascularization are future strategies.

Control of lifestyle-related risk factors includes cessation of cigarette smoking and avoidance of all tobacco products, avoiding obesity, adult-onset diabetes, and elevated triglycerides, with recognition and management of the metabolic syndrome and decreasing salt in the diet. Avoiding physical inactivity by pursuing an aerobic exercise program is an important step to preventing progression of atheromatous disease and therefore lessening the risk of atheroembolism.[153]

Pharmacological therapy consists of statin medications, antiplatelet agents, ACE inhibitors, often in combination, as well as medications to control hyperglycemia and hypertension.

HMG-CoA reductase inhibitors, or statins, are well-established medications for lowering cholesterol and reducing cardiovascular mortality. Statin medications likely have multiple effects that include antiinflammatory properties, improvement in endothelial function, and reducing blood thrombogenicity. They may also have immunomodulatory effects, decreasing recruitment of monocytes and T cells into the arterial wall and stabilizing arterial plaque, thus decreasing the risk of plaque rupture.[154]

Many large trials have confirmed the benefits of statin agents in secondary prevention of cardiovascular events.[153,155] Slowing atherosclerosis progression is a laudable goal. Recently, regression of atheroma volume (of almost 7%) has been documented in the ASTEROID trial, which achieved an average low-density lipoprotein (LDL) decline from 130.4 to 60.8 mg/dL and increase in high-density lipoprotein (HDL) by 14.7%.[156] Cholesterol education program guidelines for lipid management suggest an initial treatment goal of LDL less than 100 mg/dL, except in those at highest risk with established atheromatous disease, who should have an LDL goal of less than 70 mg/dL.[153]

There are no large randomized trials of statin medications in atheroembolism, but there are a number of observational case reports. Tunick et al. looked at the rate of cholesterol embolism in 519 patients with complex aortic plaque seen during TEE in a retrospective study in which atheroembolism occurred in 21%. Although treatment was not randomized, multivariate analysis showed a benefit of statin medication, with absolute risk reduction of 17%. No protective effect was found for warfarin or antiplatelet drugs.[157]

Antiplatelet agents prevent platelet activation and thrombosis. Commonly used oral antiplatelet agents include aspirin (75-365 mg/day), dipyridamole plus aspirin, and clopidogrel 75 mg daily. Many clinical trials have documented the effectiveness of combined antiplatelet therapy in coronary disease. Aspirin blocks the enzyme cyclooxygenase (COX)-1 to prevent synthesis of thromboxane A_2 (TxA_2), thus inhibiting platelet aggregation. Thienopyridines act by blocking adenosine diphosphate (ADP)-mediated platelet aggregation via the glycoprotein (GP)-IIb/IIIa receptor. Dipyridamole is a phosphodiesterase (PDE) inhibitor that reduces the breakdown of cyclic adenosine and guanine monophosphate (cAMP and cGMP) and increases activity of prostacyclin (PGI_2), which inhibits platelet aggregation.[158] It is not known whether antiplatelet agents prevent recurrent atheroembolism.

Cilostazol has antiplatelet and vasodilatory effects. One small study of five patients reported healing of distal limb ulcers and improved large- and small-vessel perfusion, but there was no control group and therefore no compelling evidence that ulcer healing was related to this drug.[159] Iloprost therapy has been used for cholesterol emboli syndrome.[160] Anecdotal treatment of blue toe syndrome has included nifedipine and pentoxifylline.[161] With fixed microvascular disease, there is no clear benefit of vasodilator therapy in the majority of patients with atheroembolism.

Although anticoagulation may be of benefit for mobile thrombus overlying atheromatous plaque, it is not routinely used in asymptomatic patients with nonmobile atheroma.[162]

Supportive

Organ failure has to be treated. Kidney disease has to be monitored, with correction of electrolyte abnormalities, volume excess, and uremia. Renal replacement therapy with dialysis may be temporary or permanent. Heart failure and hypertension should be managed with diuretics, renin-angiotensin-aldosterone system (RAAS) antagonists, β-blockers, and vasodilators. The HOPE trial showed benefit for ACE inhibitors in patients with vascular disease or diabetes, with reduced rates of stroke, myocardial infarction, and overall death.[163] The efficacy of renin-angiotensin system inhibition in preventing recurrent atheroembolism is not known.

Wound care may be needed for management of lower-extremity skin necrosis, using surgical wound débridement and application of topical agents and dressings. Limited amputation of toes or forefoot is necessary in some patients, and limb amputations may be necessary for patients with irreversible ischemia with gangrene. Antibiotics may be necessary for infection. A fluffy, soft vascular boot can protect the ischemic foot from trauma. Pneumatic arterial pumps can improve arterial perfusion in some patients.

Effective pain control is very important; ischemic pain can be severe and persist for weeks after lower-extremity atheroembolism.[164] The degree of pain from blue toe syndrome may seem to be out of proportion to the extent of tissue involvement but reflects microvascular necrosis. Besides narcotic and neurotransmitter pharmaceutical agents, several other modalities have been used for pain associated with lower-extremity ischemia.

Lumbar sympathectomy was popular 50 years ago when surgical options for PAD were more limited. There has always been controversy regarding actual benefit in patients with atherosclerotic disease.[165-168] Lumbar sympathectomy historically has been done for critical leg ischemia with gangrene, ischemic ulcerations, and rest pain. A 60% improvement rate has been reported, although not all respond. In one retrospective review of 45 patients (50 limbs) with toe gangrene treated with lumbar sympathectomy, amputation rate remained high at 40%.[169,170] More recently, some surgeons continue to advocate lumbar sympathectomy for selected patients in situations of threatened tissue loss.[162] The hope is that this may improve collateral blood flow and open arteriovenous connections by relieving smooth muscle constriction.[162] Some studies do show improved tissue perfusion and enhanced healing in addition to surgical reconstruction.

Today, a lumbar sympathetic block may be done by local injection, with the goal of improving skin warmth and pain. A spinal cord stimulator has been of benefit in a few selected patients.[164]

Other treatment options may include hyperbaric oxygen or pneumatic leg compression to improve distal perfusion in selected cases of extremity atheroembolism.[171]

Conclusions

Atheroembolism is a rare but serious disorder that can occur spontaneously or be a complication of invasive cardiac and vascular procedures. Angiography is the most common iatrogenic cause, responsible for up to 80% of cases.[8] Be aware that atheroembolic skin changes may mimic other disorders.

A presumptive diagnosis is often based on clinical features. The diagnosis requires a high index of suspicion in an appropriate clinical setting, such as exposure to a precipitating factor, unexplained renal failure, and cutaneous signs of atheroembolization.[2]

A definitive diagnosis requires histological confirmation of cholesterol crystals in a biopsy of muscle, skin, or affected organ. There is no single definitive laboratory test except biopsy of involved tissue to confirm the diagnosis of atheroembolic disease.

It is important to determine the most likely embolic source. When atheroembolism involves the lower extremities, atherosclerotic or aneurysmal disease of the aortoiliac segment accounts for two thirds of cases.[107,108]

Atheroembolism can be recurrent, and in those patients there is a 40% to 60% risk of tissue loss.[106,107] The goal of surgical and endovascular treatment is to exclude the embolic source and prevent recurrent episodes. A covered stent or extra-anatomical bypass may be an option in high-risk patients.

Management of mobile atheroma is controversial, but warfarin seems to be effective in preventing symptomatic thromboembolism in some patients.[142] Anticoagulation is not routine therapy in patients with diffuse atherosclerosis.

The best treatment of atheroembolism is prevention. Ultimately, prevention of atherosclerosis will prevent atheroembolism.

REFERENCES

1. Jucgla A, Moreso F, Muniesa C, et al: Cholesterol embolism: still an unrecognized entity with a high mortality rate, J Am Acad Dermatol 55:786–793, 2006.
2. Kiechle FL, McLaughlin JH, Yang SS, et al: Atheromatous embolization, Am J Emerg Med 1:299–301, 1983.
3. Hollenhorst RW: Significance of bright plaques in the retinal arterioles, Trans Am Ophthalmol Soc 59:252–273, 1961.
4. Lie JT: Cholesterol atheromatous embolism. The great masquerader revisited, Pathol Annu 27(Pt 2):17–50, 1992.
5. Fine MJ, Kapoor W, Falanga V: Cholesterol crystal embolization: a review of 221 cases in the English literature, Angiology 38:769–784, 1987.
6. Lye WC, Cheah JS, Sinniah R: Renal cholesterol embolic disease. Case report and review of the literature, Am J Nephrol 13:489–493, 1993.
7. Scolari F, Ravani P, Gaggi R, et al: The challenge of diagnosing atheroembolic renal disease: clinical features and prognostic factors, Circulation 116:298–304, 2007.
8. Scolari F, Ravani P: Atheroembolic renal disease, Lancet 375:1650–1660, 2010.
9. Karmody AM, Powers SR, Monaco VJ, et al: "Blue toe" syndrome. An indication for limb salvage surgery, Arch Surg 111:1263–1268, 1976.
10. Cross SS: How common is cholesterol embolism? J Clin Pathol 44:859–861, 1991.
11. Saklayen MG: Atheroembolic renal disease: preferential occurrence in whites only, Am J Nephrol 9:87–88, 1989.
12. Flory C: Arterial occlusions produced by emboli from eroded aortic atheromatous plaques, Am J Pathol 21:549–565, 1945.
13. Kealy WF: Atheroembolism, J Clin Pathol 31:984–989, 1978.
14. Doty JR, Wilentz RE, Salazar JD, et al: Atheroembolism in cardiac surgery, Ann Thorac Surg 75:1221–1226, 2003.
15. Rosman HS, Davis TP, Reddy D, et al: Cholesterol embolization: clinical findings and implications, J Am Coll Cardiol 15:1296–1299, 1990.
16. Hertzer NR: Peripheral atheromatous embolization following blunt abdominal trauma, Surgery 82:244–247, 1977.
17. Ramirez G, O'Neill WM Jr, Lambert R, et al: Cholesterol embolization: a complication of angiography, Arch Internal Med 138:1430–1432, 1978.
18. Thurlbeck WM, Castleman B: Atheromatous emboli to the kidneys after aortic surgery, N Engl J Med 257:442–447, 1957.
19. Sharma PV, Babu SC, Shah PM, et al: Changing patterns of atheroembolism, Cardiovasc Surg 4:573–579, 1996.
20. Lindholt JS, Sandermann J, Bruun-Petersen J, et al: Fatal late multiple emboli after endovascular treatment of abdominal aortic aneurysm. Case report, Int Angiol 17:241–243, 1998.
21. Zempo N, Sakano H, Ikenaga S, et al: Fatal diffuse atheromatous embolization following endovascular grafting for an abdominal aortic aneurysm: report of a case, Surg Today 31:269–273, 2001.
22. Thompson MM, Smith J, Naylor AR, et al: Microembolization during endovascular and conventional aneurysm repair, J Vasc Surg 25:179–186, 1997.
23. Keon WJ, Heggtveit HA, Leduc J: Perioperative myocardial infarction caused by atheroembolism, J Thorac Cardiovasc Surg 84:849–855, 1982.
24. Blauth CI, Cosgrove DM, Webb BW, et al: Atheroembolism from the ascending aorta. An emerging problem in cardiac surgery, J Thorac Cardiovasc Surg 103:1104–1111, 1992; discussion 1111–1102.
25. Tunick PA, Krinsky GA, Lee VS, et al: Diagnostic imaging of thoracic aortic atherosclerosis, AJR Am J Roentgenol 174:1119–1125, 2000.
26. Baker AJ, Naser B, Benaroia M, et al: Cerebral microemboli during coronary artery bypass using different cardioplegia techniques, Ann Thorac Surg 59:1187–1191, 1995.
27. Harringer W: Capture of particulate emboli during cardiac procedures in which aortic cross-clamp is used. International Council of Emboli Management Study Group, Ann Thorac Surg 70:1119–1123, 2000.
28. Ascione R, Ghosh A, Reeves BC, et al: Retinal and cerebral microembolization during coronary artery bypass surgery: a randomized, controlled trial, Circulation 112:3833–3838, 2005.
29. Drost H, Buis B, Haan D, et al: Cholesterol embolism as a complication of left heart catheterisation. Report of seven cases, Br Heart J 52:339–342, 1984.
30. Colt HG, Begg RJ, Saporito JJ, et al: Cholesterol emboli after cardiac catheterization. Eight cases and a review of the literature, Medicine 67:389–400, 1988.
31. Saklayen MG, Gupta S, Suryaprasad A, et al: Incidence of atheroembolic renal failure after coronary angiography. A prospective study, Angiology 48:609–613, 1997.
32. Gaines PA, Cumberland DC, Kennedy A, et al: Cholesterol embolisation: a lethal complication of vascular catheterisation, Lancet 1:168–170, 1988.
33. Gjesdal K, Orning OM, Smith E: Fatal atheromatous emboli to the kidneys after left-heart catheterisation, Lancet 2:405, 1977.
34. Fukumoto Y, Tsutsui H, Tsuchihashi M, et al: Cholesterol Embolism Study I. The incidence and risk factors of cholesterol embolization syndrome, a complication of cardiac catheterization: a prospective study, J Am Coll Cardiol 42:211–216, 2003.
35. Frock J, Bierman M, Hammeke M, et al: Atheroembolic renal disease: experience with 22 patients, Nebr Med J 79:317–321, 1994.
36. Johnson LW, Esente P, Giambartolomei A, et al: Peripheral vascular complications of coronary angioplasty by the femoral and brachial techniques, Cathet Cardiovasc Diagn 31:165–172, 1994.
37. Keeley EC, Grines CL: Scraping of aortic debris by coronary guiding catheters: a prospective evaluation of 1,000 cases, J Am Coll Cardiol 32:1861–1865, 1998.
38. Liew YP, Bartholomew JR: Atheromatous embolization, Vasc Med 10:309–326, 2005.
39. Karalis DG, Quinn V, Victor MF, et al: Risk of catheter-related emboli in patients with atherosclerotic debris in the thoracic aorta, Am Heart J 131:1149–1155, 1996.
40. Blankenship JC, Mickel S: Spinal cord infarction resulting from cardiac catheterization, Am J Med 87:239–240, 1989.
41. Harrington D, Amplatz K: Cholesterol embolization and spinal infarction following aortic catheterization, Am J Roentgenol Radium Ther Nucl Med 115:171–174, 1972.
42. Feder W, Auerbach R: "Purple toes": an uncommon sequela of oral coumarin drug therapy, Ann Intern Med 55:911–917, 1961.
43. Bruns FJ, Segel DP, Adler S: Control of cholesterol embolization by discontinuation of anticoagulant therapy, Am J Med Sci 275:105–108, 1978.
44. Hyman BT, Landas SK, Ashman RF, et al: Warfarin-related purple toes syndrome and cholesterol microembolization, Am J Med 82:1233–1237, 1987.
45. Carron PL, Florea A, Ducloux D, et al: Atheroembolic disease associated with the use of low-molecular-weight heparin during haemodialysis, Nephrol Dial Transplant 14:520–521, 1999.
46. Blackshear JL, Zabalgoitia M, Pennock G, et al: Warfarin safety and efficacy in patients with thoracic aortic plaque and atrial fibrillation. SPAF TEE Investigators. Stroke Prevention and Atrial Fibrillation. Transesophageal echocardiography, Am J Cardiol 83:453–455.
47. Atherosclerotic disease of the aortic arch as a risk factor for recurrent ischemic stroke. The French Study of Aortic Plaques in Stroke Group, N Engl J Med 334:1216–1221, 1996.
48. Bols A, Nevelsteen A, Verhaeghe R: Atheromatous embolization precipitated by oral anticoagulants, Int Angiol 13:271–274, 1994.

49. Boudes P: Cholesterol emboli and streptokinase therapy, *JAMA* 259:1180, 1988.

50. Gupta BK, Spinowitz BS, Charytan C, et al: Cholesterol crystal embolization-associated renal failure after therapy with recombinant tissue-type plasminogen activator, *Am J Kidney Dis* 21:659–662, 1993.

51. Wong FK, Chan SK, Ing TS, et al: Acute renal failure after streptokinase therapy in a patient with acute myocardial infarction, *Am J Kidney Dis* 26:508–510, 1995.

52. Arora RR, Magun AM, Grossman M, et al: Cholesterol embolization syndrome after intravenous tissue plasminogen activator for acute myocardial infarction, *Am Heart J* 126:225–228, 1993.

53. GUSTO: An international randomized trial comparing four thrombolytic strategies for acute myocardial infarction. The GUSTO investigators, *N Engl J Med* 329:673–682, 1993.

54. Blankenship JC, Butler M, Garbes A: Prospective assessment of cholesterol embolization in patients with acute myocardial infarction treated with thrombolytic vs. conservative therapy, *Chest* 107:662–668, 1995.

55. Chaudhary K, Wall BM, Rasberry RD: Livedo reticularis: an underutilized diagnostic clue in cholesterol embolization syndrome, *Am J Med Sci* 321:348–351, 2001.

56. Faraggiana T, Muda AO: Atheromatous embolism, *Contrib Nephrol* 119:67–73, 1996.

57. Ben-Horin S, Bardan E, Barshack I, et al: Cholesterol crystal embolization to the digestive system: characterization of a common, yet overlooked presentation of atheroembolism, *Am J Gastroenterol* 98:1471–1479, 2003.

58. Scolari F, Tardanico R, Zani R, et al: Cholesterol crystal embolism: a recognizable cause of renal disease, *Am J Kidney Dis* 36:1089–1109, 2000.

59. Chesney TM: Atheromatous embolization to the skin, *Am J Dermatopathol* 4:271–273, 1982.

60. Hirschmann JV, Raugi GJ: Blue (or purple) toe syndrome, *J Am Acad Dermatol* 60:1–20, 2009 quiz 21–22.

61. Cappiello RA, Espinoza LR, Adelman H, et al: Cholesterol embolism: a pseudovasculitic syndrome, *Semin Arthritis Rheum* 18:240–246, 1989.

62. Falanga V, Fine MJ, Kapoor WN: The cutaneous manifestations of cholesterol crystal embolization, *Arch Dermatol* 122:1194–1198, 1986.

63. Moolenaar W, Lamers CB: Cholesterol crystal embolization in the Netherlands, *Arch Internal Med* 156:653–657, 1996.

64. Mayo RR, Swartz RD: Redefining the incidence of clinically detectable atheroembolism, *Am J Med* 100:524–529, 1996.

65. Modi KS, Rao VK: Atheroembolic renal disease, *J Am Soc Nephrol* 12:1781–1787, 2001.

66. Greenberg A, Bastacky SI, Iqbal A, et al: Focal segmental glomerulosclerosis associated with nephrotic syndrome in cholesterol atheroembolism: clinicopathological correlations, *Am J Kidney Dis* 29:334–344, 1997.

67. Jones DB, Iannaccone PM: Atheromatous emboli in renal biopsies. An ultrastructural study, *Am J Pathol* 78:261–276, 1975.

68. Olin JW: Atheroembolic renal disease: underdiagnosed and misunderstood, *Catheter Cardiovasc Interv* 70:789–790, 2007.

69. Kawarada O, Yokoi Y, Takemoto K: The characteristics of dissemination of embolic materials during renal artery stenting, *Catheter Cardiovasc Interv* 70:784–788, 2007.

70. Haas M, Spargo BH, Wit EJ, et al: Etiologies and outcome of acute renal insufficiency in older adults: a renal biopsy study of 259 cases, *Am J Kidney Dis* 35:433–447, 2000.

71. Hara S, Asada Y, Fujimoto S, et al: Atheroembolic renal disease: clinical findings of 11 cases, *J Atheroscler Thromb* 9:288–291, 2002.

72. Thadhani RI, Camargo CA Jr, Xavier RJ, et al: Atheroembolic renal failure after invasive procedures. Natural history based on 52 histologically proven cases, *Medicine* 74:350–358, 1995.

73. Goldman M, Thoua Y, Dhaene M, et al: Necrotising glomerulonephritis associated with cholesterol microemboli, *Br Med J (Clin Res Ed)* 290:205–206, 1985.

74. Theriault J, Agharazzi M, Dumont M, et al: Atheroembolic renal failure requiring dialysis: potential for renal recovery? A review of 43 cases, *Nephron* 94:c11–c18, 2003.

75. Dalakos TG, Streeten DH, Jones D, et al: "Malignant" hypertension resulting from atheromatous embolization predominantly of one kidney, *Am J Med* 57:135–138, 1974.

76. Kasinath BS, Corwin HL, Bidani AK, et al: Eosinophilia in the diagnosis of atheroembolic renal disease, *Am J Nephrol* 7:173–177, 1987.

77. Wilson DM, Salazer TL, Farkouh ME: Eosinophiluria in atheroembolic renal disease, *Am J Med* 91:186–189, 1991.

78. Haqqie SS, Urizar RE, Singh J: Nephrotic-range proteinuria in renal atheroembolic disease: report of four cases, *Am J Kidney Dis* 28:493–501, 1996.

79. Williams HH, Wall BM, Cooke CR: Reversible nephrotic range proteinuria and renal failure in atheroembolic renal disease, *Am J Med Sci* 299:58–61, 1990.

80. Belenfant X, Meyrier A, Jacquot C: Supportive treatment improves survival in multivisceral cholesterol crystal embolism, *Am J Kidney Dis* 33:840–850, 1999.

81. Herzog AL, Wanner C: Case report: atheroembolic renal disease in a 72-year-old patient through coronary intervention after myocardial infarction, *Hemodial Int* 12:406–411, 2008.

82. Scolari F, Ravani P, Pola A, et al: Predictors of renal and patient outcomes in atheroembolic renal disease: a prospective study, *J Am Soc Nephrol* 14:1584–1590, 2003.

83. Fabbian F, Catalano C, Lambertini D, et al: A possible role of corticosteroids in cholesterol crystal embolization, *Nephron* 83:189–190, 1999.

84. Nakayama M, Nagata M, Hirano T, et al: Low-dose prednisolone ameliorates acute renal failure caused by cholesterol crystal embolism, *Clin Nephrol* 66:232–239, 2006.

85. Graziani G, Santostasi S, Angelini C, et al: Corticosteroids in cholesterol emboli syndrome, *Nephron* 87:371–373, 2001.

86. Hasegawa M, Sugiyama S: Apheresis in the treatment of cholesterol embolic disease, *Ther Apher Dial* 7:435–438, 2003.

87. Woolfson RG, Lachmann H: Improvement in renal cholesterol emboli syndrome after simvastatin, *Lancet* 351:1331–1332, 1998.

88. Hasegawa M, Kawashima S, Shikano M, et al: The evaluation of corticosteroid therapy in conjunction with plasma exchange in the treatment of renal cholesterol embolic disease. A report of 5 cases, *Am J Nephrol* 20:263–267, 2000.

89. Cabili S, Hochman I, Goor Y: Reversal of gangrenous lesions in the blue toe syndrome with lovastatin–a case report, *Angiology* 44:821–825, 1993.

90. Dubel GJ, Murphy TP: Distal embolic protection for renal arterial interventions, *Cardiovasc Intervent Radiol* 31:14–22, 2008.

91. Moolenaar W, Lamers CB: Gastrointestinal blood loss due to cholesterol crystal embolization, *J Clin Gastroenterol* 21:220–223, 1995.

92. Paraf F, Jacquot C, Bloch F, et al: Cholesterol crystal embolization demonstrated on GI biopsy, *Am J Gastroenterol* 96:3301–3304, 2001.

93. Blundell JW: Small bowel stricture secondary to multiple cholesterol emboli, *Histopathology* 13:459–462, 1988.

94. Mulliken JB, Bartlett MK: Small bowel obstruction secondary to atheromatous embolism. A case report and review of the literature, *Ann Surg* 174:145–150, 1971.

95. Gramlich TL, Hunter SB: Focal polypoid ischemia of the colon: atheroemboli presenting as a colonic polyp, *Arch Pathol Lab Med* 118:308–309, 1994.

96. Chan T, Levine MS, Park Y: Cholesterol embolization as a cause of cecal infarct mimicking carcinoma, *AJR Am J Roentgenol* 150:1315–1316, 1988.

97. Fujiyama A, Mori Y, Yamamoto S, et al: Multiple spontaneous small bowel perforations due to systemic cholesterol atheromatous embolism, *Intern Med* 38:580–584, 1999.

98. Funabiki K, Masuoka H, Shimizu H, et al: Cholesterol crystal embolization (CCE) after cardiac catheterization: a case report and a review of 36 cases in the Japanese literature, *Japan Heart J* 44:767–774, 2003.

99. Orvar K, Johlin FC: Atheromatous embolization resulting in acute pancreatitis after cardiac catheterization and angiographic studies, *Arch Intern Med* 154:1755–1761, 1994.

100. Moolenaar W, Kreuning J, Eulderink F, et al: Ischemic colitis and acalculous necrotizing cholecystitis as rare manifestations of cholesterol emboli in the same patient, *Am J Gastroenterol* 84:1421–1422, 1989.

101. Moolenaar W, Lamers CB: Cholesterol crystal embolization and the digestive system, *Scand J Gastroenterol* 188:69–72, 1991.

102. Harvey RL, Doberneck RC, Black WC 3rd: Infarction of the stomach following atheromatous embolization. Report of a case and literature review, *Gastroenterology* 62:469–472, 1972.

103. Bourdages R, Prentice RS, Beck IT, et al: Atheromatous embolization to the stomach: an unusual cause of gastrointestinal bleeding, *Am J Dig Dis* 21:889–894, 1976.

104. Blackshear JL, Jahangir A, Oldenburg WA, et al: Digital embolization from plaque-related thrombus in the thoracic aorta: identification with transesophageal echocardiography and resolution with warfarin therapy, *Mayo Clin Proc* 68:268–272, 1993.

105. Donohue KG, Saap L, Falanga V: Cholesterol crystal embolization: an atherosclerotic disease with frequent and varied cutaneous manifestations, *J Eur Acad Dermatol Venereol* 17:504–511, 2003.

106. Wingo JP, Nix ML, Greenfield LJ, et al: The blue toe syndrome: hemodynamics and therapeutic correlates of outcome, *J Vasc Surg* 3:475–480, 1986.

107. Kumins NH, Owens EL, Oglevie SB, et al: Early experience using the wall graft in the management of distal microembolism from common iliac artery pathology, *Ann Vasc Surg* 16:181–186, 2002.

108. Baumann DS, McGraw D, Rubin BG, et al: An institutional experience with arterial atheroembolism, *Ann Vasc Surg* 8:258–265, 1994.

109. Keen RR, McCarthy WJ, Shireman PK, et al: Surgical management of atheroembolization, *J Vasc Surg* 21:773–780, 1995; discussion 780–771.

110. Applebaum RM, Kronzon I: Evaluation and management of cholesterol embolization and the blue toe syndrome, *Curr Opin Cardiol* 11:533–542, 1996.

111. Spittell PC, Seward JB, Hallett JW Jr: Mobile thrombi in the abdominal aorta in cases of lower extremity embolic arterial occlusion: value of extended transthoracic echocardiography, *Am Heart J* 139:241–244, 2000.

112. Matchett WJ, McFarland DR, Eidt JF, et al: Blue toe syndrome: treatment with intra-arterial stents and review of therapies, *J Vasc Interv Radiol* 11:585–592, 2000.

113. Carroccio A, Olin JW, Ellozy SH, et al: The role of aortic stent grafting in the treatment of atheromatous embolization syndrome: results after a mean of 15 months follow-up, *J Vasc Surg* 40:424–429, 2004.

114. Kumpe DA, Zwerdlinger S, Griffin DJ: Blue digit syndrome: treatment with percutaneous transluminal angioplasty, *Radiology* 166:37–44, 1988.

115. Friedman SG, Krishnasastry KV: External iliac ligation and axillary-bifemoral bypass for blue toe syndrome, *Surgery* 115:27–30, 1994.

116. Kaufman JL, Saifi J, Chang BB, et al: The role of extraanatomic exclusion bypass in the treatment of disseminated atheroembolism syndrome, *Ann Vasc Surg* 4:260–263, 1990.

117. Hollier LH, Kazmier FJ, Ochsner J, et al: "Shaggy" aorta syndrome with atheromatous embolization to visceral vessels, *Ann Vasc Surg* 5:439–444, 1991.

118. Brewer ML, Kinnison ML, Perler BA, et al: Blue toe syndrome: treatment with anticoagulants and delayed percutaneous transluminal angioplasty, *Radiology* 166:31–36, 1988.

119. Dougherty MJ, Calligaro KD: Endovascular treatment of embolization of aortic plaque with covered stents, *J Vasc Surg* 36:727–731, 2002.

120. Van Thielen J, Hendriks JMH, Hertoghs M, et al: Filters placed in the superficial femoral arteries for limb salvage in a high-surgical-risk patient with atheroembolism: results at 2 years, *J Endovasc Ther* 17:399–401.

121. Rosenberg GD, Killewich LA: Blue toe syndrome from a "coral reef" aorta, *Ann Vasc Surg* 9:561–564, 1995.

122. Schlieper G, Grotemeyer D, Aretz A, et al: Analysis of calcifications in patients with coral reef aorta, *Ann Vasc Surg* 24:408–414, 2010.

123. Schulte KM, Reiher L, Grabitz L, et al: Coral reef aorta: a long-term study of 21 patients, *Ann Vasc Surg* 14:626–633, 2000.

124. Teebken OE, Pichlmaier MA, Kuhn C, et al: Severe obstructive calcifications affecting the descending and suprarenal abdominal aorta without coexisting peripheral atherosclerotic disease–coral reef aorta, *Vasa* 35:206–208, 2006.

125. Holfeld J, Gottardi R, Zimpfer D, et al: Treatment of symptomatic coral reef aorta by endovascular stent-graft placement, *Ann Thorac Surg* 85:1817–1819, 2008.

126. Bernard Y: Value of transoesophageal echocardiography for the diagnosis of embolic lesions from the thoracic aorta, *J Neuroradiol* 32:266–272, 2005.

127. Laperche T, Laurian C, Roudaut R, et al: Mobile thromboses of the aortic arch without aortic debris. A transesophageal echocardiographic finding associated with unexplained arterial embolism. The Filiale Echocardiographie de la Société Française de Cardiologie, *Circulation* 96:288–294, 1997.

128. Amarenco P, Cohen A, Tzourio C, et al: Atherosclerotic disease of the aortic arch and the risk of ischemic stroke, *N Engl J Med* 331:1474–1479, 1994.

129. Amarenco P, Duyckaerts C, Tzourio C, et al: The prevalence of ulcerated plaques in the aortic arch in patients with stroke, *N Engl J Med* 326:221–225, 1992.

130. Jones EF, Kalman JM, Calafiore P, et al: Proximal aortic atheroma. An independent risk factor for cerebral ischemia, *Stroke* 26:218–224, 1995.

131. Cohen A, Tzourio C, Bertrand B, et al: Aortic plaque morphology and vascular events: a follow-up study in patients with ischemic stroke. FAPS Investigators. French Study of Aortic Plaques in Stroke, *Circulation* 96:3838–3841, 1997.

132. Di Tullio MR, Homma S, Jin Z, et al: Aortic atherosclerosis, hypercoagulability, and stroke the APRIS (Aortic Plaque and Risk of Ischemic Stroke) study, *J Am Coll Cardiol* 52:855–861, 2008.

133. Djaiani G, Fedorko L, Borger M, et al: Mild to moderate atheromatous disease of the thoracic aorta and new ischemic brain lesions after conventional coronary artery bypass graft surgery, *Stroke* 35:e356–e358, 2004.

134. Katz ES, Tunick PA, Rusinek H, et al: Protruding aortic atheromas predict stroke in elderly patients undergoing cardiopulmonary bypass: experience with intraoperative transesophageal echocardiography, *J Am Coll Cardiol* 20:70–77, 1992.

135. Karalis DG, Chandrasekaran K, Victor MF, et al: Recognition and embolic potential of intraaortic atherosclerotic debris, *J Am Coll Cardiol* 17:73–78, 1991.

136. Tunick PA, Kronzon I: Protruding atherosclerotic plaque in the aortic arch of patients with systemic embolization: a new finding seen by transesophageal echocardiography, *Am Heart J* 120:658–660, 1990.

137. Tunick PA, Perez JL, Kronzon I: Protruding atheromas in the thoracic aorta and systemic embolization, *Ann Intern Med* 115:423–427, 1991.

138. Tunick PA, Rosenzweig BP, Katz ES, et al: High risk for vascular events in patients with protruding aortic atheromas: a prospective study, *J Am Coll Cardiol* 23:1085–1090, 1994.

139. Tunick PA, Kronzon I: Atheromas of the thoracic aorta: clinical and therapeutic update, *J Am Coll Cardiol* 35:545–554, 2000.

140. Ferrari E, Vidal R, Chevallier T, et al: Atherosclerosis of the thoracic aorta and aortic debris as a marker of poor prognosis: benefit of oral anticoagulants, *J Am Coll Cardiol* 33:1317–1322, 1999.

141. Naghavi M, Libby P, Falk E, et al: From vulnerable plaque to vulnerable patient: a call for new definitions and risk assessment strategies: Part I, *Circulation* 108:1664–1672, 2003.

142. Dressler FA, Craig WR, Castello R, et al: Mobile aortic atheroma and systemic emboli: efficacy of anticoagulation and influence of plaque morphology on recurrent stroke, *J Am Coll Cardiol* 31:134–138, 1998.

143. Ackerstaff RG, Jansen C, Moll FL, et al: The significance of microemboli detection by means of transcranial Doppler ultrasonography monitoring in carotid endarterectomy, *J Vasc Surg* 21:963–969, 1995.

144. Beal MF, Park TS, Fisher CM: Cerebral atheromatous embolism following carotid sinus pressure, *Arch Neurol* 38:310–312, 1981.

145. Ezzeddine MA, Primavera JM, Rosand J, et al: Clinical characteristics of pathologically proved cholesterol emboli to the brain, *Neurology* 54:1681–1683, 2000.

146. Laloux P, Brucher JM: Lacunar infarctions due to cholesterol emboli, *Stroke* 22:1440–1444, 1991.

147. Cremonesi A, Manetti R, Setacci F, et al: Protected carotid stenting: clinical advantages and complications of embolic protection devices in 442 consecutive patients, *Stroke* 34:1936–1941, 2003.

148. Feldman RL, Wargovich TJ, Bittl JA: No-touch technique for reducing aortic wall trauma during renal artery stenting, *Catheter Cardiovasc Interv* 46:245–248, 1999.

149. Henry M, Henry I, Klonaris C, Polydorou, et al: Renal angioplasty and stenting under protection: the way for the future? *Catheter Cardiovasc Interv* 60:299–312, 2003.

150. Henry M, Henry I, Klonaris C, et al: Benefits of cerebral protection during carotid stenting with the PercuSurge GuardWire system: midterm results, *J Endovasc Ther* 9:1–13, 2002.

151. Kawarada O, Yokoi Y, Takemoto K, et al: Double-wire technique in balloon-protected carotid artery stenting, *J Interv Cardiol* 20:55–62, 2007.

152. Kastrup A, Groschel K, Krapf H, et al: Early outcome of carotid angioplasty and stenting with and without cerebral protection devices: a systematic review of the literature, *Stroke* 34:813–819, 2003.

153. Grundy SM, Cleeman JI, Merz CNB, et al: Coordinating Committee of the National Cholesterol Education Program. Implications of recent clinical trials for the National Cholesterol Education Program Adult Treatment Panel III Guidelines, *J Am Coll Cardiol* 44:720–732, 2004.

154. Blanco-Colio LM, Tunon J, Martin-Ventura JL, et al: Anti-inflammatory and immuno-modulatory effects of statins, *Kidney Int* 63:12–23, 2003.

155. Cannon CP, Steinberg BA, Murphy SA, et al: Meta-analysis of cardiovascular outcomes trials comparing intensive versus moderate statin therapy, *J Am Coll Cardiol* 48:438–445, 2006.

156. Nissen SE, Nicholls SJ, Sipahi I, et al: Effect of very high-intensity statin therapy on regression of coronary atherosclerosis: the ASTEROID trial, *JAMA* 295:1556–1565, 2006.

157. Tunick PA, Nayar AC, Goodkin GM, et al: Effect of treatment on the incidence of stroke and other emboli in 519 patients with severe thoracic aortic plaque, *Am J Cardiol* 90:1320–1325, 2002.

158. Ling G, Ovbiagele B: Oral antiplatelet therapy in the secondary prevention of atherothrombotic events, *Am J Cardiovasc Drugs* 9:197–209, 2009.

159. Dean SM, Vaccaro PS: Successful pharmacologic treatment of lower-extremity ulcerations in 5 patients with chronic critical limb ischemia, *J Am Board Fam Pract* 15:55–62, 2002.

160. Elinav E, Chajek-Shaul T, Stern M: Improvement in cholesterol emboli syndrome after iloprost therapy, *BMJ* 324:268–269, 2002.

161. Carr ME Jr, Sanders K, Todd WM: Pain relief and clinical improvement temporally related to the use of pentoxifylline in a patient with documented cholesterol emboli–a case report, *Angiology* 45:65–69, 1994.

162. Jennings WC, Corder CN, Jarolim DR, et al: Atheromatous embolism: varied clinical presentation and prognosis, *South Med J* 82:849–852, 1989.

163. Yusuf S, Sleight P, Pogue J, et al: Effects of an angiotensin-converting-enzyme inhibitor, ramipril, on cardiovascular events in high-risk patients. The Heart Outcomes Prevention Evaluation Study Investigators, [Erratum appears in *N Engl J Med* 2000 Mar 9;342(10):748.] [Erratum appears in 2000 May 4;342(18):1376.] *N Engl J Med* 342:145–153, 2000.

164. Ghilardi G, Massaro F, Gobatti D, et al: Temporary spinal cord stimulation for peripheral cholesterol embolism, *J Cardiovasc Surg (Torino)* 43:255–258, 2002.

165. Haimovici H, Steinman C, Karson IH: Evaluation of lumbar sympathectomy. Advanced occlusive arterial disease, *Arch Surg* 89:1089–1095, 1964.

166. Fulton RL, Blakeley WR: Lumbar sympathectomy: a procedure of questionable value in the treatment of arteriosclerosis obliterans of the legs, *Am J Surg* 116:735–744, 1968.

167. Berardi RS, Siroospour D: Lumbar sympathectomy in the treatment of peripheral vascular occlusive disease. Ten-year study, *Am J Surg* 130:309–314, 1975.

168. Berry RE, Flotte CT, Coller FA: A critical evaluation of lumbar sympathectomy for peripheral arteriosclerotic vascular disease, *Surgery* 37:115–129, 1955.

169. Kim GE, Ibrahim IM, Imparato AM: Lumbar sympathectomy in end stage arterial occlusive disease, *Ann Surg* 183:157–160, 1976.

170. Lee BY, Madden JL, Thoden WR, et al: Lumbar sympathectomy for toe gangrene. Long-term follow-up, *Am J Surg* 145:398–401, 1983.

171. Vella A, Carlson LA, Blier B, et al: Circulator boot therapy alters the natural history of ischemic limb ulceration, [Erratum appears in *Vasc Med* 2000;5(2):128.] *Vasc Med* 5:21–25, 2000.

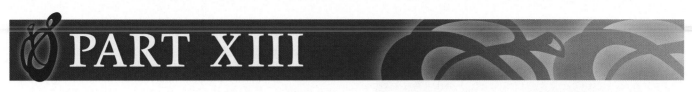

PART XIII

VASOSPASM AND OTHER RELATED VASCULAR DISEASES

CHAPTER **48** **Raynaud's Phenomenon**

Mark A. Creager, Todd S. Perlstein, Jonathan L. Halperin

In its simplest form, local syncope is a condition perfectly compatible with health. Persons who are attacked with it are ordinarily females. Under the least stimulus, sometimes without appreciable cause, one or many fingers become pale and cold all at once; in many cases, it is the same finger that is always first attacked; the others become dead successively and in the same order. It is the phenomenon known as "dead finger." The attack is indolent, the duration varies from a few minutes to many hours. The determining cause is often the impression of cold; but that which is only commonly produced under the influence of the most severe cold, appears in the subjects of whom I speak on the occasion of the least lowering of temperatures; sometimes even a simple mental emotion is enough ... the skin of the affected parts assumes a dead white or sometimes a yellow colour; it appears completely exsanguine. The cutaneous sensibility becomes blunted, then annihilated; the fingers become like foreign bodies to the subject ... the slight importance of this local abolition of the circulation is probably due to the fact that it is so transient ... the attack is followed by a period of reaction, which is often very painful, and which gives place to a sensation quite analogous to that of being numbed by cold ... and in the more pronounced cases, which the patients compared to tingling from cold, or to the stinging of nettles... Finally, a patch of deep red is formed on the extremities of the fingers. This patch gives place to the normal pink colour, and then the skin is found to have entirely returned to the primitive condition.

— Maurice Raynaud[1]

Episodic vasospastic ischemia of the digits was first described by Maurice Raynaud in the quotation above[1] (Fig. 48-1). Raynaud's phenomenon comprises sequential development of digital blanching, cyanosis, and rubor following cold exposure and subsequent rewarming[2] (Fig. 48-2). Emotional stress also precipitates Raynaud's phenomenon. The color changes are usually well demarcated and primarily confined to fingers or toes. Blanching, or pallor, occurs during the ischemic phase of the phenomenon and is secondary to digital vasospasm. During ischemia, arterioles, capillaries, and venules dilate. Cyanosis results from the deoxygenated blood in these vessels. Cold, numbness, or paresthesias of the digits often accompany the phases of pallor and cyanosis. With rewarming, digital vasospasm resolves, and blood flow dramatically increases into the dilated arterioles and capillaries. This "reactive hyperemia" imparts a bright red color to the digits. In addition to rubor and warmth, patients often experience a throbbing sensation during the hyperemic phase. Thereafter, the color of the digits gradually returns to normal. Although the triphasic color response is typical of Raynaud's phenomenon, some patients may develop only pallor and cyanosis. Others may experience only cyanosis.

The classification of Raynaud's phenomenon is broadly separated into two categories: (1) the idiopathic variety, termed *primary Raynaud's phenomenon*, and (2) the secondary variety, associated with other disease states or known causes of vasospasm (Box 48-1). Secondary causes of Raynaud's phenomenon include collagen vascular diseases, arterial occlusive disease, thoracic outlet syndrome, several neurological disorders, blood dyscrasias, trauma, and several drugs.

Overview of Primary Raynaud's Phenomenon

Primary Raynaud's phenomenon, or idiopathic episodic digital vasospasm, is the most common diagnosis of patients who present with Raynaud's phenomenon.[2] The diagnosis is based on criteria originally established by Allen and Brown,[3] including (1) intermittent attacks of ischemic discoloration of the extremities, (2) absence of organic arterial occlusions, (3) bilateral distribution, (4) trophic changes—when present, limited to the skin and never consisting of gross gangrene, (5) absence of any symptoms or signs of systemic disease that might account for the occurrence of Raynaud's phenomenon, and (6) symptom duration for 2 years or longer. If a normal erythrocyte sedimentation rate (ESR), normal nailfold capillary examination, and negative test for antinuclear antibodies (ANAs) are added to these criteria, the diagnosis is more secure.

Women are affected approximately five times more frequently than men. In one large study, the average age of onset of Raynaud's phenomenon was 31 years; 78% of the patients were younger than 40 when symptoms began.[4] Onset of symptoms in women may occur between menarche and menopause. Raynaud's phenomenon is also known to occur in young children.[5,6] Prevalence of primary Raynaud's phenomenon varies with climate, with 4.6% of the population affected in warm climates, compared with 17% in cooler climates.[6] There is a significant familial aggregation of primary Raynaud's phenomenon. Approximately 26% of patients may know of one or more relatives who have the phenomenon, suggesting a genetic predisposition.[7]

In the vast majority of patients, the fingers are the initial sites of involvement.[2] At first, blanching or cyanosis may involve only one or two fingers (Fig. 48-3). Later, color changes may develop in additional fingers, and symptoms occur bilaterally. In about 40% of patients, Raynaud's phenomenon involves the toes as well as the fingers. Isolated Raynaud's phenomenon of the toes occurs in only 1% to 2% of patients. Rarely, the ear lobes, tip of the nose, or tongue are affected.

Episodes of Raynaud's phenomenon are usually precipitated by exposure to a cool environment or by direct exposure of the extremities to low temperatures. Some patients may experience Raynaud's phenomenon during either cold exposure or emotional stress; infrequently, emotional stress may be the only precipitating factor. Duration, frequency, and severity of Raynaud's phenomenon increase during cold months.

Several studies have correlated Raynaud's phenomenon with migraine headaches and variant angina, suggesting a common mechanism for vasospasm.[8-10] An association with vasospasm in the kidney,[11] retina,[12] and pulmonary[13] vessels has also been described. Further evidence is the report of a family with three generations of systemic arterial vasospastic disease involving Raynaud's phenomenon, variant angina, and migraine headaches.[14] Differences in the responses of pharmacological intervention make the hypothesis of a common mechanism less appealing.[15] Propranolol has been successfully used to prevent migraine headaches.[16] In contrast, β-adrenoceptor blockers are not beneficial in variant angina and may cause Raynaud's phenomenon.[17,18] Similarly, nitrates are used for variant angina but are not beneficial in Raynaud's phenomenon and often cause headaches. Ergot alkaloids are effective for treating migraine headaches but can cause coronary and digital vasospasm.[19,20]

Physical examination of patients with primary Raynaud's phenomenon is often entirely normal. Sometimes the fingers and toes are cool and may perspire excessively. The pulse examination is normal; radial, ulnar, and pedal pulses should be easily palpable. Trophic changes such as sclerodactyly (thickening and tightening of the digital subcutaneous tissue) have been reported in up to 10% of patients, but these studies preceded nailfold capillaroscopy and ANA tests. The physical examination is most important to exclude secondary causes of Raynaud's phenomenon.

Of all the forms of Raynaud's phenomenon, primary Raynaud's phenomenon has the most benign prognosis. In the group of patients identified by Gifford and Hines[4] followed for a period of 1 to 32 years (average 12 years), 16% reported worsening of their symptoms, and 38%, 36%, and 10%, respectively, reported no change, improvement, or disappearance of symptoms. Sclerodactyly or trophic changes of the digits occurred in approximately 3% of patients during follow-up, and less than 1% of patients lost part of a digit. In some patients, scleroderma may develop after Raynaud's phenomenon has been present as the only symptom for more than 20 years. Wollersheim et al.[21] reported that measuring ANAs by immunofluorescence and immunoblotting in patients with Raynaud's phenomenon had a positive predictive value of 65%

FIGURE 48-1 A patient with Raynaud's phenomenon. *(From Raynaud M: Local asphyxia and symmetrical gangrene of the extremities, London, 1862, New Sydenham Society. Courtesy Boston Medical Library in the Francis A. Countway Library of Medicine.)*

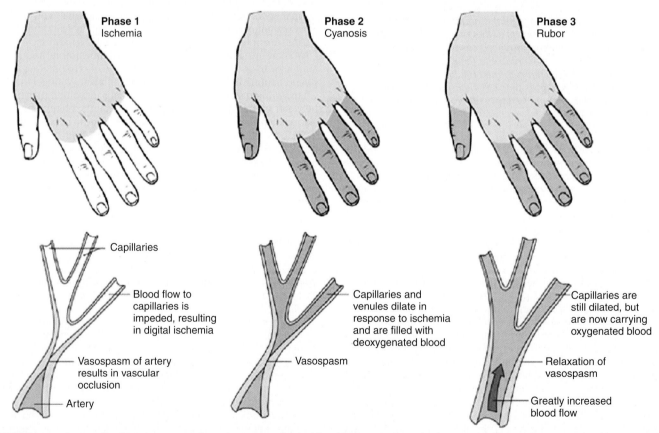

FIGURE 48-2   Raynaud's phenomenon may have three color phases: blanching, cyanosis, and rubor. *(From Creager MA: Raynaud's phenomenon. Med Illus 2:84, 1983.)*

Box 48-1   Secondary Causes of Raynaud's Phenomenon

Collagen Vascular Diseases
Systemic sclerosis (scleroderma)
Systemic lupus erythematosus (SLE)
Rheumatoid arthritis
Dermatomyositis and polymyositis
Mixed connective tissue disease (MCTD)
Sjögren's syndrome
Necrotizing vasculitis

Arterial Occlusive Disease
Atherosclerosis of the extremities
Thromboangiitis obliterans (TAO) (Buerger's disease)
Thromboembolism

Neurological Disorders
Carpal tunnel syndrome
Reflex sympathetic dystrophy
Stroke
Intervertebral disk disease
Syringomyelia
Poliomyelitis

Thoracic Outlet Syndrome

Trauma
Exposure to vibrating tools ("vibration white finger")
Electric shock injury

Thermal injury
Percussive injury
Hypothenar hammer syndrome

Drugs and Toxins
Ergot alkaloids
Methysergide
Vinblastine
Bleomycin
Gemcitabine
β-Adrenoceptor antagonists
Vinyl chloride

Blood Dyscrasias
Hyperviscosity syndrome
Cold agglutinin disease
Cryoglobulinemia
Cryofibrinogenemia

Myeloproliferative Disease

Miscellaneous Causes
Hypothyroidism
Arteriovenous fistula (AVF)
Pulmonary hypertension

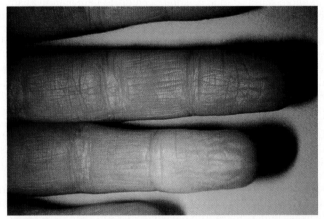

FIGURE 48-3   Raynaud's phenomenon presenting as blanching of one finger.

Box 48-2   Possible Pathophysiological Mechanisms of Raynaud's Phenomenon

Vasoconstrictive Stimuli
Digital vascular hyperreactivity ("local fault")
Increased sympathetic nervous system activity
β-Adrenoceptor blockade
Circulating vasoactive hormones
Angiotensin II (Ang II)
Serotonin
Thromboxane
Endothelin-1 (ET-1)
Exogenous administration of vasoconstrictor agents
Ergot alkaloids
Sympathomimetic drugs

Decreased Intravascular Pressure
Low systemic blood pressure
Arterial occlusive disorder (e.g., atherosclerosis, thromboangiitis obliterans [TAO])
Digital arterial occlusions (e.g., scleroderma)
Hyperviscosity

and 71%, and a negative predictive value of 93% and 83%, respectively, for development of a connective tissue disease.

Pathophysiology

The precise cause of Raynaud's phenomenon has not been clearly identified. It is quite likely that a variety of physiological and pathological conditions may contribute to or cause digital vasospasm[2] (Box 48-2 and Fig. 48-4).

Normally, regulation of peripheral blood flow depends on several factors that include intrinsic vascular tone, sympathetic nervous system activity, hemorrheological properties such as blood viscosity, and various circulating hormonal substances. In contrast to other regional circulations that are supplied by both vasoconstrictor and vasodilator sympathetic fibers, the cutaneous vessels of the hands and feet are innervated only by sympathetic adrenergic vasoconstrictor fibers. In these vascular beds, neurogenic vasodilation occurs by *withdrawal* of a sympathetic stimulus. Cooling evokes reflex sympathetic-mediated vasoconstriction in the hands and feet via neurons originating in cutaneous receptors. Environmental cooling or cooling of specific body parts, such as

the head, neck, or trunk, normally causes a reduction in digital blood flow. Local digital cooling also induces vasoconstriction, but digital vasoconstriction caused by local cooling is not mediated by the sympathetic nervous system. Thus digital vasoconstriction may be a physiological response to local cooling or to reflex activation of the sympathetic nervous system by environmental cold exposure or emotional stress.

Raynaud's phenomenon is not a normal physiological response but rather an episode of digital artery vasospasm causing cessation of blood flow to the digits. The term *vasospasm* must be distinguished from *vasoconstriction*. *Vasoconstriction* may be defined as the expected reduction in vessel lumen size as a result of endogenous neural, hormonal, or metabolic factors that cause smooth muscle contraction. *Vasospasm* implies an excessive vasoconstrictor response to stimuli that would normally cause modest smooth muscle contraction, but that instead has resulted in obliteration of the vascular lumen. Patency of the digital artery depends on a

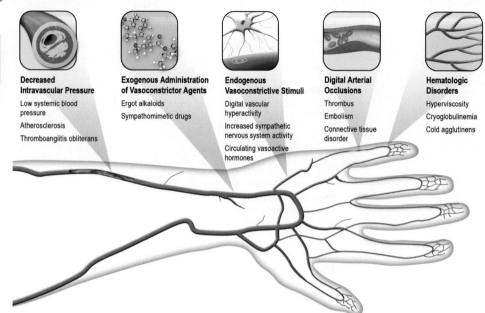

Decreased Intravascular Pressure
Low systemic blood pressure
Atherosclerosis
Thromboangiitis obliterans

Exogenous Administration of Vasoconstrictor Agents
Ergot alkaloids
Sympathomimetic drugs

Endogenous Vasoconstrictive Stimuli
Digital vascular hyperactivity
Increased sympathetic nervous system activity
Circulating vasoactive hormones

Digital Arterial Occlusions
Thrombus
Embolism
Connective tissue disorder

Hematologic Disorders
Hyperviscosity
Cryoglobulinemia
Cold agglutinens

FIGURE 48-4   Pathophysiology of digital vasospasm. Digital vasospasm may be due to vasoconstrictive stimuli, decreased intravascular pressure, or both. Mechanisms that contribute to exercise vasoconstriction include local vascular hypersensitivity to vasoactive stimuli (e.g., increased α-adrenoceptor sensitivity), sympathetic efferent activity, and local or circulating vasoactive hormones such as angiotensin II (Ang II), endothelin-1 (ET-1), serotonin, or thromboxane A_2 (TxA$_2$). Low blood pressure, even in a healthy young person, may predispose to Raynaud's phenomenon when the person encounters vasoconstrictive stimuli. Pathological conditions that may decrease intravascular pressure include arterial occlusion in proximal arteries (e.g., atherosclerosis), digital vascular occlusion (e.g., scleroderma), or hyperviscosity. TAO, thromboangiitis obliterans.

favorable balance between the contractile forces of the muscular wall of the digital artery and its intraluminal pressure. Thus a situation in which there is excessive vasoconstrictive force or decreased intravascular pressure upsets this balance and results in vasospasm. It is with these rather simple concepts that several theories have been proposed to explain the episodic digital vasospasm that defines Raynaud's phenomenon.

Increased Vasoconstrictive Stimuli

Several theories implicate excessive vasoconstrictive stimuli as a cause of Raynaud's phenomenon. Postulated causes include local vascular hyperreactivity, increased sympathetic nervous system activity, elevated levels of vasoconstrictor hormones (e.g., angiotensin II (Ang II), serotonin, thromboxane A_2 (TxA$_2$)), and exogenously administered agents such as ergot alkaloids and sympathomimetic drugs.

Local Vascular Hyperreactivity

The observation that episodic digital vasospasm occurs during cold exposure has led several investigators to consider the possibility that Raynaud's phenomenon occurs as a result of a local vascular hyperreactivity. In 1929, Sir Thomas Lewis observed that following exposure of the finger to cold, vasospasm could be produced even after nerve blockade or sympathectomy.[22] These experiments were repeated and confirmed 60 years later.[23] Therefore, the vasospastic response of the Raynaud's phenomenon may occur in the absence of efferent digital nerves. The possibility of local vascular hyperreactivity was examined by Jamieson et al.[24] They compared the magnitude of reflex vasoconstriction in each hand following application of ice to the neck while one hand was kept at 26°C and the other at 36°C.[9] At 36°C, the reflex vasoconstrictor response was comparable in normal subjects and patients with primary Raynaud's phenomenon. In the hand cooled to 26°C, however, reflex vasoconstriction was exaggerated in patients with Raynaud's phenomenon. This response led these investigators to hypothesize that digital α_1 adrenoceptors were sensitized by cold exposure.

A series of studies by Vanhoutte et al.[25] have supported the hypothesis that cooling potentiates the vascular response to sympathetic nerve activation. Vasoconstriction, in response to exogenous norepinephrine, also is increased by cooling. Augmentation of adrenergic-mediated vasoconstriction by cooling occurs despite generalized depression of contractile machinery and diminished release of norepinephrine from sympathetic nerve endings in the

vessel wall. The most likely hypothesis is that cold causes changes at the level of the adrenoceptor, such as an increase in the affinity for norepinephrine or greater efficacy of the agonist/receptor complex. Vanhoutte et al.[25] have reported that α_2 adrenoceptors are more sensitive than α_1 adrenoceptors to temperature change. Whereas cooling slightly depresses α_1 adrenergic–mediated vasoconstriction, it markedly augments α_2 adrenergic–mediated responses. Conversely, warming augments α_1-adrenergic vasoconstriction and depresses α_2-adrenergic vasoconstriction.[26]

These experimental observations may have important implications regarding the pathophysiology of Raynaud's phenomenon. Flavahan et al.[27] examined the distribution of α_1 and α_2 adrenoceptors in arterial tissue from amputated limbs of patients who did not have vascular disease. They reported that α_2 adrenoceptors were more prominent in digital arteries. Chotani et al.[28] found that human dermal arterioles selectively expressed α_{2C} adrenoceptors. Jeyaraj et al.[29] observed that cooling redistributed α_{2C} adrenoceptors from the Golgi to the plasma membrane in human embryonic kidney cells. It is therefore an intriguing observation by Keenan and Porter that the density of α_2 adrenoreceptors is increased in platelets from patients with Raynaud's disease.[30]

In support of these findings, Coffman and Cohen reported that α_2 adrenoceptors were more important than α_1 adrenoceptors in mediating sympathetic nerve–induced vasoconstriction in the fingers.[31] They administered the α_1-antagonist prazosin and the α_2-antagonist yohimbine to patients with Raynaud's phenomenon during reflex sympathetic vasoconstriction caused by body cooling. Whereas prazosin caused no significant change in finger blood flow or finger vascular resistance, yohimbine significantly increased finger blood flow and decreased finger vascular resistance. This study confirmed that postjunctional α_2 adrenoceptors are present in human digits and strongly suggested that these receptors contribute to digital vasoconstriction during environmental cooling in patients with Raynaud's phenomenon.

Thereafter, Coffman and Cohen demonstrated that compared to normal subjects, patients with Raynaud's phenomenon were hypersensitive to the vasoconstrictor effects of clonidine, an α_2-adrenoceptor agonist, but not to phenylephrine, an α_1-adrenoceptor agonist.[31] Cooke et al.[32] found that both α_1- and α_2-adrenoceptor antagonists induced digital vasodilation in patients with acute Raynaud's phenomenon, yet did not inhibit digital vasoconstriction caused by local digital cooling. Although still speculative, these studies suggest that episodic digital vasospasm may be secondary to a predominance of postjunctional α_2 adrenoceptors in digits of patients with primary Raynaud's phenomenon.

Increased Sympathetic Nervous System Activity

Although appealing as a potential mechanism for digital vaso-spasm, the concept of exaggerated reflex sympathetic vasoconstrictor responses to cold environment has not been convincingly demonstrated. Increased concentrations of epinephrine and nor-epinephrine in peripheral venous blood at the wrist were found to be higher in patients with primary Raynaud's phenomenon than in normal subjects by one investigator,[33] but others found normal local levels of norepinephrine in brachial arterial and venous blood samples.[34] The latter group of investigators reported that the reflex vasoconstrictor response of the hand to a cold stimulus in affected patients is similar to that in a control group, and there were comparable vasoconstrictor responses to the intraarterial infusion of tyramine, a drug that causes vasoconstriction by releasing norepinephrine from sympathetic nerve terminals. Central thermoregulatory control of skin temperature has also been reported to be comparable in normal individuals and patients with primary Raynaud's phenomenon.[35] Finally, microelectrode recordings of skin sympathetic nerve activity do not demonstrate an abnormality in patients with primary Raynaud's phenomenon.[36] There was no hypersensitivity of the vessels to strong sympathetic stimuli or abnormal increase in sympathetic outflow.

β-Adrenergic Blockade

Raynaud's phenomenon is observed frequently in individuals treated with β-adrenoceptor antagonists.[37–39] It may be inferred from this observation that β-adrenergic vasodilation normally attenuates digital vasoconstrictor tone. Cohen and Coffman[40] examined the effect of isoproterenol and propranolol on fingertip blood flow after vasoconstriction had been induced by a brachial artery infusion of norepinephrine or angiotensin, or reflexly by environmental cooling. Intraarterial isoproterenol administration increased fingertip blood flow during infusions of norepinephrine and angiotensin, but not during reflex sympathetic vasoconstriction. Conversely, propranolol served to potentiate vasoconstriction caused by intraarterial norepinephrine, but not that caused by reflex sympathetic vasoconstriction. These investigators concluded that a β-adrenergic vasodilator mechanism may be active in human digits, but does not modulate sympathetic vasoconstriction. There is no evidence to support the contention that decreased sensitivity or number of β adrenoceptors contributes to the pathophysiology of Raynaud's phenomenon in the absence of pharmacological blockade of β adrenoceptors.

Vasoconstriction Caused by Circulating Vascular Smooth Muscle Agonists

Various neurotransmitters, hormones, and platelet release byproducts are capable of constricting vascular smooth muscle and causing digital vasoconstriction. These include Ang II, serotonin, TxA_2, and endothelin-1 (ET-1). It would be difficult to attribute all causes of Raynaud's phenomenon to excessive levels of these vasoconstrictor agents, but in some secondary causes of Raynaud's phenomenon, any one of them might contribute to vasoconstriction.

Serotonin (5-hydroxytryptamine [5-HT]) is a neurotransmitter that is synthesized and released by selective neurons and enterochromaffin cells. Serotonin can cause vasoconstriction by directly activating serotoninergic receptors on the smooth muscle cells (SMCs). Vasoconstriction may also be caused by direct activation of α adrenoceptors on SMCs or indirectly by facilitating release of norepinephrine from adrenergic nerve terminals. Although some evidence implicates a role for serotonin in the pathophysiology of Raynaud's phenomenon, the contribution of serotonin to digital vasospasm remains speculative.

The possibility that vasoconstrictors released during platelet aggregation may be pertinent to the pathophysiology of Raynaud's phenomenon has been further evaluated by studies that have either measured levels of TxA_2 or administered a thromboxane synthetase inhibitor.[41,42] Coffman and Rasmussen compared the thromboxane synthetase inhibitor dazoxiben to placebo in patients with either primary or secondary Raynaud's phenomenon.[41] Dazoxiben did not affect total fingertip blood flow or fingertip capillary blood flow, whether measured in a warm (28.3 °C) or cool (20 °C) environment. With chronic treatment, there was a small decrease in frequency of vasospastic episodes in patients with primary Raynaud's phenomenon. To date, however, there is insufficient evidence to support a role for TxA_2 in digital vasospasm.

Plasma concentration of the potent vasoconstrictor Ang II is rarely elevated in patients with Raynaud's phenomenon. This hormone is therefore unlikely to contribute to the pathophysiology of digital vasospasm in most patients.

Endothelin-1 is an endothelium-derived, powerful, and prolonged-acting vasoconstrictor agent suggested to play a part in the pathogenesis of Raynaud's phenomenon. It rises in response to a cold pressor test and constricts cutaneous blood vessels.[43] Studies measuring ET-1 in primary or secondary Raynaud's phenomenon have been conflicting.[44] Controlled clinical trials of ET-1 receptor antagonism in the treatment of Raynaud's disease have achieved little success.[45,46] It is therefore doubtful that it plays a role in Raynaud's phenomenon.

Decreased Intravascular Pressure

Patency of a blood vessel requires balance between arterial wall tension (favoring closure of the vessel) and intravascular distending pressure. Landis measured intravascular pressure in patients with Raynaud's phenomenon by introducing a micropipette into a large digital capillary.[47] During cyanosis, capillary pressure fell to approximately 5 mmHg, and flow ceased. These findings suggested that the site of closure was proximal to the capillaries at the arterial level. Interestingly, Thulesius reported that brachial artery blood pressure in patients with primary Raynaud's phenomenon was significantly lower than that in a normal control population.[48] Cohen and Coffman also found that blood pressure was lower in patients with primary Raynaud's phenomenon compared with normal subjects.[49] In addition to lower brachial blood pressure, systolic blood pressure (SBP) measured at the proximal and distal digital arteries averaged 18 mmHg less than that in normal digits.

A low digital artery pressure may occur in various disorders associated with Raynaud's phenomenon, such as large-vessel arterial occlusive disease secondary to atherosclerosis, embolism, or thoracic outlet syndrome. When extrinsic vasoconstrictor force is applied, these vessels may collapse and cause digital ischemia. Distal vascular occlusions secondary to thromboangiitis obliterans (TAO), vasculitis, or vibration injury may also reduce digital arterial pressure distal to the diseased vascular segment.

Hyperviscosity may reduce blood flow velocity in digital vessels, leading to a decrease in intravascular pressure. Indeed, Raynaud's phenomenon occurs in patients with hyperviscosity due to polycythemia vera or Waldenström macroglobulinemia.[50,51] In patients with Raynaud's phenomenon secondary to disorders such as cryoglobulinemia and cold agglutinin disease, hyperviscosity caused by cooling may contribute to digital vasospasm.[52–54] Indeed, cooling has been shown to abolish hand blood flow in patients with cold agglutinins, possibly because the vessels become occluded by agglutinated red cells.[54] Data invoking hyperviscosity as a cause of Raynaud's phenomenon in patients who do not have an established blood dyscrasia, however, are less compelling.

Secondary Causes of Raynaud's Phenomenon

The secondary causes of Raynaud's phenomenon include collagen vascular diseases, arterial occlusive disorders, thoracic outlet syndrome, several neurological disorders, blood dyscrasias, trauma, and several drugs (see Box 48-1).

Collagen Vascular Diseases

SYSTEMIC SCLEROSIS (SCLERODERMA)

Raynaud's phenomenon occurs in 80% to 90% of patients with systemic sclerosis; it may be the presenting symptom in approximately 33% of patients. In some patients, scleroderma may develop after Raynaud's phenomenon has been present as the only symptom for many years. Frequency and severity of Raynaud's phenomenon in patients with systemic sclerosis is often worse than that observed in patients with primary Raynaud's phenomenon. The incidence of digital ulceration and gangrene is increased, possibly leading to amputation. Diagnosis of systemic sclerosis is suggested by the appearance of typical sclerotic skin changes. These include tightness, thickening, and nonpitting induration involving the extremities, face, neck, or trunk. When present in the digits, these abnormalities produce changes in the contour of the fingers and toes, referred to as *sclerodactyly*. Other manifestations of systemic sclerosis include pitting scars of the tips of the digits, normal skin pigmentation, and telangiectasia. Visceral manifestations include pulmonary fibrosis, esophageal dysmotility, and colonic sacculation. The kidney and heart may also be involved. As the disease progresses, skin and subcutaneous tissue of the fingers become stiffer, joints become immobile, and contractures develop. A variant of systemic sclerosis is the CREST syndrome, a form of limited scleroderma that includes calcinosis, Raynaud's phenomenon, esophageal dysmotility, sclerodactyly, and telangiectasia in the absence of internal organ involvement.

Several serological studies are consistent with the diagnosis of scleroderma. Erythrocyte sedimentation rate may be elevated, and ANAs are present in the majority of individuals with this disorder. Patients may have antibodies to nucleolar antigens, nuclear ribonucleoprotein, and to the centromeric region of metaphase chromosomes. In patients with systemic sclerosis and Raynaud's phenomenon, capillary microscopy often demonstrates enlarged and deformed capillary loops surrounded by relatively avascular areas, particularly in the nailfolds.[55] Angiography frequently demonstrates digital vascular obstruction.

SYSTEMIC LUPUS ERYTHEMATOSUS

Raynaud's phenomenon occurs in approximately 10% to 35% of patients with systemic lupus erythematosus (SLE). Persistent digital vasospasm, often due to proliferative endarteritis of the small digital vessels, also occurs and may result in gangrene. Diagnosis of SLE is based on the presence of at least 4 of the following 11 criteria:

1. Malar rash.
2. Discoid rash.
3. Photosensitivity.
4. Oral ulcers.
5. Arthritis.
6. Serositis, including pleuritis or pericarditis.
7. Renal disorders, including persistent proteinuria or cellular casts.
8. Neurological disorders, such as seizures and psychosis.
9. Hematological disorders, including hemolytic anemia, leukopenia, lymphopenia, or thrombocytopenia.
10. Immunological disorders.
11. Abnormal titers of antinuclear antibody, especially antideoxyribonucleic acid (DNA)[56]

RHEUMATOID ARTHRITIS

Raynaud's phenomenon also occurs in patients with rheumatoid arthritis. These patients may have vasculitis of medium-sized vessels, as well as proliferative endarteritis of small vessels. Crops of small brown spots may be observed in the nail beds and digital pulp. Digital blood flow is often reduced in patients with rheumatoid arthritis, and angiography frequently reveals occlusions of one or more digital arteries.[57] The diagnosis is suggested in patients who have at least one joint with synovitis, with the synovitis not explained by another disease, and who score 6/10 points or more on the following consensus diagnostic criteria[58]:

1. Involvement of 2 to 10 large joints (1 point).
2. 1 to 3 small joints (2 points).
3. 4 to 10 small joints (3 points).
4. More than 10 joints (5 points).
5. Low-positive rheumatoid factor (RF) or low-positive anticitrullinated protein/peptide (ACPA) (2 points).
6. High-positive RF or high-positive ACPA (3 points).
7. Abnormal C-reactive protein (CRP) or abnormal ESR (1 point).
8. Duration of symptoms 6 weeks or more (1 point).

DERMATOMYOSITIS AND POLYMYOSITIS

Thirty percent of patients with dermatomyositis and polymyositis have associated Raynaud's phenomenon. Muscular manifestations include weakness of the proximal girdle muscles, particularly those involving the lower extremities. Patients may also experience aching in the buttocks, thighs, and calves. Some patients complain of dysphagia or dyspnea. Myocarditis develops in approximately one third of these individuals. The dermatological abnormalities in dermatomyositis include localized or diffuse erythema, a maculopapular rash, and eczematoid dermatitis. A purplish (heliotrope) rash may develop on the upper eyelids, face, chest, limbs, or around the nail beds. Laboratory diagnosis of dermatomyositis and polymyositis is based on elevated serum levels of the skeletal muscle enzymes, including creatine kinase, aldolase, serum glutamic oxaloacetic transaminase, and lactic acid dehydrogenase. There may be myoglobinuria, and ESR is often elevated. Electromyogram reveals evidence of a myopathy.

PRIMARY SJÖGREN'S SYNDROME

Sjögren's syndrome is an autoimmune disease that mainly affects exocrine glands and leads to dryness of the eyes and mouth, but it can have extraglandular manifestations. Raynaud's phenomenon has been reported in 13% to 33% of patients and may precede the sicca symptomatology in many.[59] Presence of anticentromere antibody increases the likelihood of associated Raynaud's phenomenon, possibly because of an association with an increase in fibrous tissues.[60] The clinical course is usually milder than in patients with systemic sclerosis. Antinuclear antibody tests are often positive, but the diagnosis is usually made by the clinical picture.

MIXED CONNECTIVE TISSUE DISEASE

Mixed connective tissue disease (MCTD) is a disorder with overlapping clinical features of SLE, scleroderma, and myosomitis, and presence of a distinctive antibody against U1-ribonucleoprotein (RNP). Raynaud's phenomenon is the main symptom in mixed connective tissue disease, and trophic abnormalities of the fingers are frequently observed. Elevated anti-U1-RNP antibody titers and an abnormal capillaroscopic pattern are specific for the condition.[61]

Arterial Occlusive Disease

Occlusive disease of arteries proximal to the digital vessels is often associated with Raynaud's phenomenon. Proximal arterial occlusive disease may decrease intravascular pressure and upset the balance between tension in the arterial wall and intravascular distending pressure. This may make the vessel more prone to vasospasm when subjected to sympathetic nervous system stimuli.

Atherosclerosis of the extremities tends to occur most frequently in males older than 50 years of age and females older than 60. When Raynaud's phenomenon occurs in these individuals, it tends to be unilateral and related to the affected extremity. Usually only one or two digits are involved. The diagnosis is suggested by clinical history and physical examination. Symptoms of claudication or findings that would suggest atherosclerosis elsewhere, such as in the coronary or cerebral vasculature, often indicate the underlying disorder. Physical findings are noteworthy for decreased or absent pulses in the involved extremity. These abnormalities can be confirmed by noninvasive vascular testing. Severe ischemia may manifest as persistent digital pallor or cyanosis and must be distinguished from the episodic digital vasospasm of Raynaud's phenomenon.

Thromboangiitis obliterans (or Buerger's disease) is an inflammatory occlusive vascular disorder involving small- and medium-sized arteries and veins, often accompanied by Raynaud's phenomenon (see Chapter 44). In addition to Raynaud's phenomenon, clinical features of TAO include claudication of the affected extremity and migratory superficial vein thrombosis in a young male.

Thoracic Outlet Syndrome

Compression of the neurovascular bundle as it courses through the neck and shoulder can result in a symptom complex that includes Raynaud's phenomenon as well as shoulder and arm pain, weakness, paresthesias, and claudication of the affected upper extremity (see Chapter 62). Raynaud's phenomenon may result from the decreased intravascular pressure caused by extrinsic compression of the subclavian artery. Whether compression of the brachial plexus alters sympathetic nervous system activity is unknown.

Neurological Disorders

Various neurological conditions, particularly those causing disuse of the limb, may be associated with disorders of circulatory vasomotion. These include stroke, syringomyelia, intervertebral disk disease, spinal cord tumors, and poliomyelitis. The affected limb, including the hand or foot in addition to the digits, may be cool and cyanotic. In contrast to the episodic nature of Raynaud's phenomenon, these changes tend to be persistent.

Raynaud's phenomenon has been reported in approximately 10% of patients with carpal tunnel syndrome.[62] This entrapment neuropathy is due to compression of the median nerve as it passes through the carpal tunnel. It may result from pregnancy, localized tenosynovitis, trauma, hypothyroidism, amyloidosis, or activities associated with repeated motion of the wrist. Patients usually experience paresthesias or weakness in the distribution of the median nerve. The diagnosis is suggested when symptoms are reproduced by tapping the volar surface of the wrist (Tinel sign) or by maintaining flexion of the wrist (Phalen maneuver). Nerve conduction tests usually demonstrate abnormalities of the median nerve at the wrist. Supportive treatment includes splints and antiinflammatory drugs. With severe persistent symptoms, surgical release of the carpal ligament may be beneficial.

Complex regional pain syndrome, previously known as *reflex sympathetic dystrophy* or *causalgia*, is another neurological disorder associated with cyanotic extremities and involves pain and tenderness of a distal extremity, with accompanying vasomotor instability (see Chapter 52).

Blood Dyscrasias

Hyperviscosity syndromes, cold-precipitable plasma proteins, abnormalities of red cell agglutination, and certain myeloproliferative disorders are associated with Raynaud's phenomenon, as well as with persistent digital ischemia.

Patients with cold agglutinins occasionally develop Raynaud's phenomenon. It is generally thought that Raynaud's phenomenon develops when proteins precipitate on red blood cells and agglutinate within the digital vessel during exposure to cold. Prolonged exposure may cause thrombosis and subsequent digital gangrene. Cold agglutinin disease usually involves immunoglobulin (Ig) M antibodies that are reactive with I antigen.[63] The antibody titer is high at 4°C and low at 37°C. These antibodies also may cause cold-induced hemolysis. Agglutination usually does not occur in temperatures above 32°C. Cold agglutinins may arise spontaneously or occur in patients with mycoplasma pneumonia, infectious mononucleosis, or lymphoproliferative disorders. Cold agglutinin disease may be short lived in patients with infectious causes but is often persistent in patients with lymphoproliferative disease.

Cryoglobulins are a group of proteins that precipitate in cold serum and may cause Raynaud's phenomenon.[64] Cryoglobulins are associated with monoclonal and polyclonal gammopathies in disorders such as Waldenström macroglobulinemia, SLE, and rheumatoid arthritis. Cryoglobulinemia has been categorized into three subtypes. Type I cryoglobulins include monoclonal immunoglobulins of a single class, usually associated with lymphoproliferative disorders such as multiple myeloma. Type II encompasses mixed cryoglobulins containing monoclonal IgM or rheumatoid factor and polyclonal IgG. This may occur in patients with Waldenström macroglobulinemia or chronic active hepatitis. In patients with Waldenström macroglobulinemia, about 10% of macroglobulins are cryoglobulins. Type III cryoglobulinemia includes polyclonal IgM and IgG immunoglobulins, as may occur in SLE. Indeed, approximately 80% of patients with lupus have cold-insoluble precipitates. In these patients, there is a significantly higher level of cryoprecipitating IgM class rheumatoid factors than in other patients. Most patients with mixed cryoglobulinemia have a chronic hepatitis C infection.

Cryofibrinogenemia is a rare condition that may be associated with digital vasospasm.[65] The plasma, but not the serum, of patients with cryofibrinogenemia forms a gelatinous precipitate at 4°C. Disorders associated with cryofibrinogenemia include disseminated intravascular coagulation, collagen vascular diseases, thromboembolism, and diabetes mellitus.

Trauma

Various traumatic injuries are associated with Raynaud's phenomenon and have been designated *traumatic vasospastic diseases*. Causes of traumatic vasospastic disease include electric shock injury, thermal injuries such as frostbite, and mechanical percussive injury associated with piano playing and typing. The most common traumatic cause of Raynaud's phenomenon is repeated exposure to vibrating tools. This has occasionally been referred to as *vibration white finger syndrome*. It has been reported in lumberjacks and other users of chainsaws, stonecutters who use air hammers, operators of pneumatic hand grinders and impact wrenches in the engine manufacturing industry, and road drillers. Prevalence of Raynaud's phenomenon induced by vibration ranges from 33% to 71% among members of populations at risk and increases with exposure time.[66,67] It has been suggested that the combination of vibration and cold exposure in many of these workers is responsible for development of Raynaud's phenomenon.[68] Pathophysiological changes may involve both the vascular and neurological systems in these individuals and may contribute to digital vasospasm. Intimal thickening of peripheral arteries has been reported in animals exposed to repeated vibration, but pathological changes of the blood vessels have not consistently been demonstrated.[69] Medial muscular hypertrophy and subintimal fibrosis have been found in biopsy specimens of digital arteries of patients in one study, but not in others. Nailbed capillaroscopy has shown a reduction in the number of capillaries. Arteriograms of these patients have shown arterial occlusion of the distal radial and ulnar arteries and frequently of the palmar arch.

Neurophysiological abnormalities have not been consistently demonstrated in patients with Raynaud's phenomenon secondary to vibration. Although some have found a high instance of abnormal electromyograms, others have found that episodes of Raynaud phenomena occur independently of electromyographic abnormalities.[70] Peripheral nerve conduction velocities are often abnormal in vibrating tool operators, and pathological changes have also been reported in the nerves of patients with vibration white finger, including axonal degeneration, demyelination, and collagenization of perineurium and endoperineurium. Thus the precise pathophysiology of Raynaud's phenomenon in patients repeatedly exposed to vibratory stimuli is unclear. Some have suggested that overexcitation of the Pacinian corpuscles causes reflex efferent sympathetic nerve activity. Others have suggested that following vibration, cutaneous vessels become more reactive to sympathetic stimuli.

Another trauma-induced cause of Raynaud's phenomenon is the hypothenar hammer syndrome. Patients develop an ulnar artery thrombosis after hammering with the palms of their hands or practicing karate.

Drugs and Toxins

Various drugs have been implicated in producing Raynaud's phenomenon or digital vasospasm (see Box 48-1). Although some of these drugs act by directly causing vasoconstriction, the mechanism whereby others cause Raynaud's phenomenon is not known.

Ergot derivatives cause vasospasm, primarily by stimulating α adrenoceptors. Ergotamine may stimulate serotonergic receptors as well. Vasospasm usually occurs when excessive doses of these drugs have been administered. Spasm may affect digital vessels as well as the coronary, carotid, and femoral vessels and the coronary, carotid, femoral, and splanchnic arteries. Bromocriptine mesylate, an ergot derivative with dopamine agonist activity used to treat Parkinson's disease, hyperprolactinemia, and acromegaly, has been associated with Raynaud's phenomenon. Methysergide, used to treat migraine headaches, is another ergot derivative that has been associated with digital ischemia. The tricyclic antidepressant imipramine and the amphetamines also have been reported to cause arterial spasm.

Raynaud's phenomenon has also been associated with use of at least three chemotherapeutic agents: vinblastine, gemcitabine, and bleomycin. Although it is unknown how these compounds cause Raynaud's phenomenon, it has been reported that bleomycin causes pathological changes in small blood vessels. Vinblastine can induce peripheral neuropathy and perhaps interfere with the autonomic reflexes. Gemcitabine therapy has been associated with Raynaud's phenomenon and digital ischemia due to endothelial damage secondary to inflammatory changes, and from thrombotic microangiopathy.[71]

Industrial exposure to vinyl chloride polymerization processes may cause acro-osteolysis of the distal phalanges of the fingers, changes that are occasionally associated with Raynaud's phenomenon, but one recent study found the phenomenon less frequent among workers than in the population.[72]

β-Adrenoceptor blocking drugs may cause Raynaud's phenomenon. Although the mechanism of action is unknown, possibilities include unopposed stimulation of vascular α adrenoceptors or reflex sympathetic vasoconstriction initiated by the central cardiovascular depressant effect of β-adrenergic blockade. It remains controversial whether cardioselective β-adrenoceptor blocking drugs cause Raynaud's phenomenon less frequently than nonselective drugs, and whether there is less digital vasospasm with drugs that also have α-adrenoceptor blocking properties or intrinsic sympathomimetic activity. One placebo-controlled study examined both cardioselective and nonselective β-adrenoceptor blockers in patients who already had Raynaud's phenomenon.[73] Compared with placebo, neither metoprolol nor propranolol decreased fingertip blood flow, despite exposure to a cool environment. Furthermore, chronic treatment did not increase the number of vasospastic attacks in patients receiving either drug compared with placebo. One might conclude from these observations that β-adrenoceptor blocking drugs may cause Raynaud's phenomenon in some individuals, but these drugs do not seem to adversely affect frequency of vasospastic attacks, nor do they decrease finger blood flow in patients with Raynaud's phenomenon.

Miscellaneous Causes

Hypothyroidism may be associated with Raynaud's phenomenon.[74] In these cases, thyroid replacement alleviates the episodes of digital vasospasm. Although the mechanism is unknown, peripheral vasoconstriction may occur in hypothyroid patients to conserve heat. Alternatively, edematous thickening of the vascular wall could predispose to vessel closure during normal sympathetic stimuli.

Patients with arteriovenous fistula (AVF) may develop Raynaud's phenomenon; it is particularly prevalent in patients undergoing hemodialysis.[75] This may be secondary to decreased blood flow and blood pressure in the digits of the limb with the fistula.

Pulmonary hypertension and Raynaud's phenomenon may occur in the same patients. Some of these may have a connective tissue disorder such as scleroderma.[76] Approximately 30% of patients with pulmonary arterial hypertension (PAH) have elevated titers of antinuclear antibody.[77,78] Ten percent of women with PAH have Raynaud's phenomenon.[78] This frequency is not different from that occurring in the general population, so it is not clear whether the association of primary pulmonary hypertension and Raynaud's phenomenon is coincidence or related to a common neurohumoral or immunological mechanism.

Paraneoplastic Raynaud's phenomenon is a rare complication of a number of different malignancies (e.g., carcinomas, sarcomas, lymphomas, leukemias), at times accompanied by paraneoplastic dermatomyositis and characterized by capillaroscopic findings similar to scleroderma.[79,80]

Diagnostic Tests

Noninvasive vascular tests may be employed to evaluate patients with Raynaud's phenomenon (see Chapter 12). The effect on finger systolic pressure of local cooling with ischemia is an objective test for Raynaud's phenomenon,[81] but this is too cumbersome a test for routine use because it involves measuring digital systolic pressure with cooling plus 5 minutes of ischemia at four different temperatures (Fig. 48-5). Patients with Raynaud's phenomenon have a greater reduction or loss of finger systolic pressure with cooling compared with normal subjects, who show a gradual decrease.

The pulse volume waveform may distinguish patients with Raynaud's phenomenon who have digital ischemia secondary to vascular occlusive lesions (Fig. 48-6). During local digital warming, the vessels dilate. The pulse waveform is usually normal during warming in patients with Raynaud's phenomenon if obstructive lesions are not present, and may be abnormal if atherosclerosis, TAO, or other fixed obstructive digital vascular pathology impairs digital blood flow.

Various serological studies such as for collagen vascular disorders or blood dyscrasias are useful to screen for secondary causes of Raynaud's phenomenon. These tests include ESR,

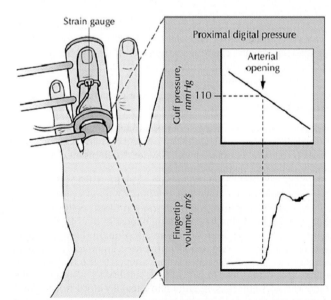

FIGURE 48-5 **Measurement of proximal finger systolic blood pressure (SBP) using strain gauge to detect increase in fingertip volume as proximal cuff is slowly deflated from suprasystolic pressure.** Fingertip pulsations and volume increase are not detected until cuff pressure deflates to 110 mmHg, the point of digital artery opening.

RAYNAUD'S PHENOMENON

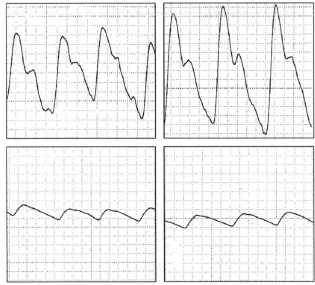

FIGURE 48-6 Digital pulse volume recordings (PVRs). Digital pulse volume waveforms were recorded during cooling (*left; 24°C*) and rewarming (*right; 44°C*). In healthy subject (*top*), pulse volume amplitude increased during warming. In patient with digital ischemia secondary to vascular occlusion, pulse volume amplitude is diminished during both cooling and rewarming (*bottom*).

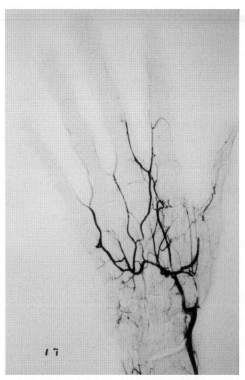

FIGURE 48-8   Angiogram from young woman with persistent digital ischemia. Multiple areas demonstrate digital vascular occlusion. Blood vessel biopsy was performed to make the diagnosis of necrotizing vasculitis.

serum protein electrophoresis, and assays for antinuclear antibody, rheumatoid factor, cryoglobulins, and cold agglutinins. Indications for these and other serological studies are usually suggested by the history and physical examination. Nailfold capillary microscopy may be used to detect the deformed capillary loops and avascular areas typical of collagen vascular disorders[55] (Fig. 48-7). Roentgenography of the cervical spine is used to detect cervical ribs.

Angiography is rarely indicated, since Raynaud's phenomenon is a diagnosis based primarily on history. Angiography may be indicated, however, in patients with persistent digital ischemia secondary to atherosclerosis, TAO, or emboli from a subclavian artery aneurysm, in order to plan revascularization procedures (Fig. 48-8).

Treatment

Treatment programs must be individualized and designed according to the underlying cause of Raynaud's phenomenon and severity of symptoms. Therapy directed specifically at the symptoms of Raynaud's phenomenon can be categorized as (1) conservative measures, (2) pharmacological intervention, and (3) surgical sympathectomy (Box 48-3). In individuals with well-defined secondary causes of Raynaud's phenomenon, treatment should also be directed specifically at the underlying cause. For example, if a patient has been taking a vasoactive medication, such as an ergot alkaloid, or has been treated with a β-adrenergic blocking drug for hypertension, removal of the offending agent may reduce or eliminate the Raynaud's phenomenon. Similarly, specific treatment may be directed at other secondary causes such as arterial occlusive disorders, connective tissue diseases, and blood dyscrasias. The following discussion focuses on treatment designed to palliate Raynaud's phenomenon.

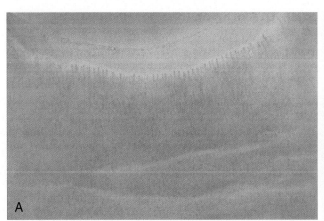
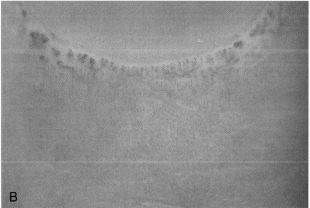

FIGURE 48-7   Nailfold capillary microscopy is performed using magnifying glass, ophthalmoscope, or compound microscope (magnification, × 10) to view clean nailfold covered with immersion oil. A, Normally, superficial capillaries are regularly spaced hairpin loops. **B,** Results of this test are abnormal in patients with connective tissue disorders. Avascular areas and enlarged and deformed capillary loops are present in nailfold of this patient with scleroderma. Disorganized nailfold capillaries associated with avascular areas and hemorrhage are present in patients with dermatomyositis and polymyositis (magnification, × 10). *(Courtesy H. Maricq, MD.)*

Box 48-3   Treatment of Raynaud's Phenomenon

Conservative Measures
Warm clothing
Avoidance of cold exposure
Abstinence from nicotine
Remove offending drug (if present)
Behavioral therapy

Pharmacological Interventions
Calcium channel blockers
Nifedipine
Diltiazem
Felodipine
Isradipine
Amlodipine

Sympathetic Nervous System Inhibitors
Prazosin
Reserpine
Guanethidine
Phenoxybenzamine

Phosphodiesterase Type-5 Inhibitors
Sildenafil
Tadalafil

Classes of Drugs with Unproven Efficacy
Serotonin antagonists
Ketanserin
Fluoxetine
Vasodilator prostaglandins (PGs)
Iloprost
Thromboxane inhibitors
Angiotensin-converting enzyme inhibitors (ACEIs)
Angiotensin receptor antagonists
Endothelin receptor antagonists
Organic nitrates

Sympathectomy
Stellate ganglionectomy
Lumbar sympathectomy
Digital sympathectomy

Botulinum Toxin Injection

Conservative Measures

Patients with primary Raynaud's phenomenon often benefit from reassurance. An explanation describing the frequency of the disease in the general population, its precipitating factors, and its benign prognosis is reassuring and allays fears of amputation. Patients should avoid unnecessary cold exposure and should wear loose, warm clothing. In addition to gloves and adequate foot protection, the trunk and head should be kept warm to avoid reflex vasoconstriction. Moving to a warmer climate is rarely feasible; furthermore, vasospasm may be induced after a move by even small changes in environmental temperature. Patients should use a moisturizing cream on their digits to prevent drying and cracking. Cigarette smoking should be avoided, since nicotine causes cutaneous vasoconstriction. Because the sympathetic nervous system mediates the vasoconstrictor response to cold and emotional distress, behavioral therapy has been proposed as a means of ameliorating the symptoms of Raynaud's phenomenon. Studies have been reported both supporting and refuting the efficacy of biofeedback training in this disorder.[78,82–87] The techniques used for biofeedback training in most of these studies were different. Furthermore, objective means of assessing responses varied from determination of digital temperature during cold exposure to queries regarding symptomatic improvement. Several uncontrolled studies indicated that following biofeedback training, patients were able to increase digital temperature and possibly decrease the frequency of vasospastic attacks.[78,82–85] Patients usually trained to increase their digital

temperature during either local or environmental cold exposure. In one controlled study that compared temperature biofeedback with nifedipine for treatment of primary Raynaud's phenomenon, biofeedback was not better than control treatment, and inferior to the drug.[88] Another form of behavioral therapy, Pavlovian conditioning, has been shown to increase digital temperature during cold exposure.[89] Although behavioral therapy may be effective in some individuals, there are insufficient data to support its routine use for patients with Raynaud's phenomenon.

Pharmacological Intervention

Two classes of drugs are effective for treatment of Raynaud's phenomenon: calcium channel blockers and sympathetic nervous system inhibitors.[2,90,91] Other classes of drugs for which efficacy has not been firmly established include serotonin antagonists, angiotensin-converting enzyme inhibitors (ACEIs), and direct-acting smooth muscle relaxants such as nitrates, endothelin antagonists, phosphodiesterase type 5 (PDE5) inhibitors, and vasodilator prostaglandins (PGs).

CALCIUM CHANNEL BLOCKERS

Calcium entry blockers are the most effective drugs for treating Raynaud's phenomenon. Most of the evidence accumulated to date involves nifedipine, which interferes with vascular smooth muscle contraction by antagonizing calcium influx. This drug decreases digital vascular resistance in patients with Raynaud's phenomenon during environmental cold exposure and increases digital SBP and digital skin temperature during local cold exposure.[92,93] In multiple placebo-controlled trials, nifedipine decreased frequency and severity of Raynaud's phenomenon.[2,90] It has also been reported to be effective treatment in children.[94] Although nifedipine is not of benefit in all patients, symptoms improve in about two thirds of individuals. Patients with both primary and secondary Raynaud's phenomenon have shown improvement. Extended-action preparations should be used, starting with 30 mg daily and increasing to 60 mg, 90 mg, and 120 mg if necessary.[2,95] Side effects include hypotension, lightheadedness, indigestion, and peripheral edema.

Less information is available about the other calcium channel blocking drugs. Diltiazem, however, has been reported in several studies to improve symptoms of Raynaud's phenomenon.[96,97] One preliminary report also indicated that it was effective in patients with Raynaud's phenomenon secondary to vibration injury.[98] Felodipine, at a dose of 2.5 or 5 mg, may be as effective as nifedipine but has not been as extensively studied.[99,100] Isradipine and amlodipine have been reported beneficial in small studies. In contrast, verapamil has not been shown to be effective in patients with Raynaud's phenomenon.[101]

SYMPATHETIC NERVOUS SYSTEM INHIBITORS

The vasoconstrictor response to cold exposure or emotional stress is mediated via the sympathetic nervous system. Sympathetic nervous system inhibitors that have been used to treat Raynaud's phenomenon include prazosin, reserpine, guanethidine, phenoxybenzamine, and methyldopa.

Prazosin hydrochloride is an α_1-adrenoceptor blocker. Since postsynaptic α_1 adrenoceptors are found on digital vessels, clinical improvement following administration of this drug might be anticipated.[2,91] However, one study reported only modest increases in digital blood flow during intraarterial infusion of prazosin. Uncontrolled observations have suggested that prazosin is effective in roughly 50% of patients with Raynaud's phenomenon. A few small placebo-controlled double-blind studies suggest that prazosin in doses ranging from 1 to 4 mg twice daily reduce the frequency of Raynaud's phenomenon.[102–104] Tachyphylaxis may occur with prazosin, often necessitating dosage increments up to 10 mg three times daily. Side effects of prazosin include hypotension, particularly after the first few doses, leading to lightheadedness or syncope. In addition, patients may develop headache, drowsiness, or fatigue. Long acting α_1-adrenoceptor blockers, such as doxazosin and terazosin, have not been studied in patients with Raynaud's phenomenon, but would probably have effects similar to prazosin.

SELECTIVE SEROTONIN REUPTAKE INHIBITORS

One small study found that fluoxetine, a selective serotonin reuptake inhibitor (SSRI), reduced the number and severity of vasospastic attacks in 53 patients with primary or secondary Raynaud's phenomenon compared with nifedipine; more clinical trial data are needed.[105] Erythromelalgia has been reported as a complication of SSRI therapy for Raynaud's phenomenon.[106]

RENIN-ANGIOTENSIN SYSTEM INHIBITORS

Angiotensin II is unlikely to mediate digital vasospasm in most patients with Raynaud's phenomenon.[107] If elevation of this hormone is due to other pathological conditions, it could conceivably contribute to digital vasospasm in patients already predisposed to Raynaud's phenomenon. One such population is patients with systemic sclerosis and malignant hypertension. One report described two patients with systemic sclerosis, malignant hypertension, renal failure, and digital ischemia who were treated with the ACEI captopril. Hypertension, renal insufficiency, and digital ischemia all improved following drug administration.[108] However, another study reported that captopril decreased vasospastic attacks in patients with primary Raynaud's phenomenon, but not in patients with Raynaud's phenomenon secondary to scleroderma.[109] Other uncontrolled studies have suggested that captopril reduces symptoms in Raynaud's disease. The angiotensin receptor antagonist losartan has been reported to decrease the frequency and severity of vasospastic attacks in 15 patients with primary Raynaud's phenomenon.[110] More studies of this class of drug are necessary.

ENDOTHELIN RECEPTOR ANTAGONISTS

Case reports and case series have described success in the use of endothelin receptor antagonists in the treatment of refractory Raynaud's phenomenon.[111-113] In a small placebo-controlled trial of patients with Raynaud's phenomenon secondary to systemic sclerosis, bosentan, a dual endothelin receptor antagonist, did not lessen frequency, duration, pain or severity of attacks.[45] In a large multicenter double-blind, placebo-controlled trial of 24 weeks of therapy in 188 patients with systemic sclerosis, bosentan reduced occurrence of new digital ulcers but had no effect on ulcer healing; other secondary endpoints such as pain and disability were negative.[46]

PHOSPHODIESTERASE TYPE 5 INHIBITORS

The PDE5 inhibitors prevent breakdown of cyclic guanosine monophosphate (cGMP), causing relaxation of vascular smooth muscle cells (VSMCs) and vasodilation. Accumulating evidence supports use of these agents in patients with Raynaud's phenomenon.[114] In a placebo-controlled crossover trial in patients with secondary Raynaud's phenomenon resistant to vasodilator therapy, the PDE5 inhibitor sildenafil reduced frequency of vasospasm and shortened attack duration while improving mean capillary flow velocity.[115] In a trial of similar design, the PDE5 inhibitor tadalafil reduced frequency and severity of vasospastic attacks and caused resolution of digital ulcers.[116] Sildenafil also reduced frequency of vasospastic attacks in a placebo-controlled study of 57 patients with Raynaud's phenomenon secondary to limited cutaneous systemic sclerosis.[117]

DIRECT VASCULAR SMOOTH MUSCLE RELAXANTS

The problem with most vasodilators is that they cause a general reduction in vascular resistance and may actually divert blood flow from the affected digits. As a result, patients often experience adverse side effects, including hypotension, without deriving any benefit for Raynaud's phenomenon.

Organic nitrate preparations including nitropaste are often used in patients with Raynaud's phenomenon. One study reported that topical glyceryl trinitrate was an effective therapy for patients with Raynaud's phenomenon, but limited in utility because of headache.[118] A novel formulation of topical nitroglycerin, MQX-503 gel, may offer relief in Raynaud's phenomenon and be better tolerated than nitropaste.[119] Nitroprusside has been used to treat severe ergotism-caused vasospasm. No other convincing evidence exists that chronic treatment with nitrate preparations ameliorates Raynaud's phenomenon.[90]

PROSTAGLANDINS

Prostaglandins inhibit platelet aggregation and are vasodilators. Several uncontrolled studies have suggested that intravenous (IV) infusions of prostaglandin E_1 (PGE_1) promote healing of digital ulcers in patients with scleroderma.[2,90] In a placebo-controlled multicenter study, however, IV PGE_1 was no more effective than placebo in reducing symptoms of Raynaud's phenomenon or healing digital ulcers. Several placebo-controlled studies, however, have reported long-term benefit in the treatment of severe Raynaud's phenomenon with IV iloprost, a prostacyclin (PGI_2) analog, for 3 to 5 days, or with prostacyclin for 3 weeks.[2,90] There were significant decreases in frequency, duration, and severity of vasospastic attacks, or increases in indices of finger blood flow for up to 9 weeks. In one study that compared IV iloprost with oral nifedipine, both drugs were of benefit subjectively, but parameters of finger blood flow were only increased with iloprost. Side effects of iloprost depend on dosage and include headaches, flushing, nausea, vomiting, and jaw pain. Oral prostacyclin preparations, unfortunately, have not proven of value in the treatment of Raynaud's phenomenon.

STATINS

HMG-CoA reductase inhibitors ("statins") exhibit pleiotropic effects on endothelial function and therefore might be anticipated to retard the vascular pathology of Raynaud's phenomenon. One prospective placebo-controlled clinical trial of atorvastatin 40 mg daily demonstrated improvement in digital ulcers in patients with Raynaud's phenomenon secondary to systemic sclerosis.[120]

N-ACETYLCYSTEINE

N-acetylcysteine, a powerful antioxidant, is postulated to decrease free radical injury of the endothelium. A pilot study of IV N-acetylcysteine for 5 days in 22 patients with Raynaud's phenomenon due to systemic sclerosis decreased vasospastic attack frequency and severity, compared with pretreatment values.[121] Controlled studies are needed with this interesting compound, which is used safely in other disorders.

OTHER AGENTS

Agents no longer commonly used in the treatment of Raynaud's phenomenon include reserpine and guanethidine (which decrease norepinpehrine release from nerve terminals), the adrenergic blocking drugs α-methyldopa and phenoxybenzamine, the serotonin antagonist ketanserin, and the thromboxane synthetase inhibitor dazoxiben.

Sympathectomy

The success rate of sympathectomy for episodic digital vasospasm of the upper extremity is not as good as might be anticipated. Raynaud's phenomenon recurs in the majority of patients.[2,122,123] Successful relief of digital ischemia is less in patients with secondary forms of Raynaud's phenomenon than in patients with primary Raynaud's phenomenon. In contrast, the majority of patients experience improvement in symptoms in their lower extremities following lumbar sympathectomy. Possibly, lumbar sympathectomy is more complete than thoracodorsal sympathectomy, in which residual sympathetic pathways may develop following surgery.

Digital sympathectomy, also referred to as *adventitial stripping*, has been advocated by some surgeons for treatment of digital ischemia, particularly that secondary to severe Raynaud's phenomenon.[124] This technique may improve digital blood flow and allow healing of digital ulcerations.[2,88,90]

Botulinum Injection

Botulinum toxin type A is a neurotoxin that results in flaccid muscle paralysis. Injection of botulinum toxin into the perineurovascular tissue of the wrist or the distal palm, or along the digits, has been reported to relieve recalcitrant Raynaud's phenomenon in several case series, but no controlled clinical trial has been reported.[125,126]

REFERENCES

1. Raynaud M: *L'Asphyxie Locale et de la Gangrene Symmetrique des Extremities*, London, 1862, New Sydenham Society.
2. Wigley FM: Clinical practice. Raynaud's Phenomenon, *N Engl J Med* 347:1001–1008, 2002.
3. Allen EV, Brown GE: Raynaud's disease: a critical review of minimal requisites for diagnosis, *Am J Med Sci* 183, 1932.
4. Gifford RW Jr, Hines EA Jr: Raynaud's disease among women and girls, *Circulation* 16:1012–1021, 1957.
5. Guntheroth WG, Morgan BC, Harbinson JA, et al: Raynaud's disease in children, *Circulation* 36:724–729, 1967.
6. Maricq HR, Carpentier PH, Weinrich MC, et al: Geographic variation in the prevalence of Raynaud's phenomenon: Charleston, SC, USA, vs Tarentaise, Savoie, France, *J Rheumatol* 20:70–76, 1993.
7. Freedman RR, Mayes MD: Familial aggregation of primary Raynaud's disease, *Arthritis Rheum* 39:1189–1191, 1996.
8. O'Keeffe ST, Tsapatsaris NP, Beetham WP Jr: Increased prevalence of migraine and chest pain in patients with primary Raynaud disease, *Ann Intern Med* 116:985-989, 1992.
9. Miller D, Waters DD, Warnica W, et al: Is variant angina the coronary manifestation of a generalized vasospastic disorder? *N Engl J Med* 304:763–766, 1981.
10. Zahavi I, Chagnac A, Hering R, et al: Prevalence of Raynaud's phenomenon in patients with migraine, *Arch Intern Med* 144:742–744, 1984.
11. Cannon PJ, Hassar M, Case DB, et al: The relationship of hypertension and renal failure in scleroderma (progressive systemic sclerosis) to structural and functional abnormalities of the renal cortical circulation, *Medicine (Baltimore)* 53:1–46, 1974.
12. Salmenson BD, Reisman J, Sinclair SH, et al: Macular capillary hemodynamic changes associated with Raynaud's phenomenon, *Ophthalmology* 99:914–919, 1992.
13. Vergnon JM, Barthelemy JC, Riffat J, et al: Raynaud's phenomenon of the lung. A reality both in primary and secondary Raynaud syndrome, *Chest* 101:1312–1317, 1992.
14. Krumholz HM, Goldberger AL: Systemic arterial vasospastic syndrome: familial occurrence with variant angina, *Am J Med* 92:334–335, 1992.
15. Coffman JD, Cohen RA: Vasospasm–ubiquitous? *N Engl J Med* 304:780–782, 1981.
16. Tokola R, Hokkanen E: Propranolol for acute migraine, *Br Med J* 2:1089, 1978.
17. Marshall AJ, Roberts CJ, Barritt DW: Raynaud's phenomenon as side effect of beta-blockers in hypertension, *BMJ* 1:1498–1499, 1976.
18. Yasue H, Touyama M, Shimamoto M, et al: Role of autonomic nervous system in the pathogenesis of Prinzmetal's variant form of angina, *Circulation* 50:534–539, 1974.
19. Curry RC Jr, Pepine CJ, Sabom MB, et al: Effects of ergonovine in patients with and without coronary artery disease, *Circulation* 56:803–809, 1977.
20. Schroeder JS, Bolen JL, Quint RA, et al: Provocation of coronary spasm with ergonovine maleate. New test with results in 57 patients undergoing coronary arteriography, *Am J Cardiol* 40:487–491, 1977.
21. Wollersheim H, Thien T, Hoet MH, et al: The diagnostic value of several immunological tests for anti-nuclear antibody in predicting the development of connective tissue disease in patients presenting with Raynaud's phenomenon, *Eur J Clin Invest* 19:535–541, 1989.
22. Lewis T: Experiments relating to the peripheral mechanism involved in spasmodic arrest of the circulation in the fingers, a variety of Raynaud's disease, *Heart* 15:7-101, 1929.
23. Freedman RR, Mayes MD, Sabharwal SC: Induction of vasospastic attacks despite digital nerve block in Raynaud's disease and phenomenon, *Circulation* 80:859–862, 1989.
24. Jamieson GG, Ludbrook J, Wilson A: Cold hypersensitivity in Raynaud's phenomenon, *Circulation* 44:254–264, 1971.
25. Vanhoutte PM, Cooke JP, Lindblad LE, et al: Modulation of postjunctional alpha-adrenergic responsiveness by local changes in temperature, *Clin Sci (Lond)* 68(Suppl 10):121s–123s, 1985.
26. Cooke JP, Shepherd JT, Vanhoutte PM: The effect of warming on adrenergic neurotransmission in canine cutaneous vein, *Circ Res* 54:547–553, 1984.
27. Flavahan NA, Cooke JP, Shepherd JT, et al: Human postjunctional alpha-1 and alpha-2 adrenoceptors: differential distribution in arteries of the limbs, *J Pharmacol Exp Ther* 241:361–365, 1987.
28. Chotani MA, Mitra S, Su BY, et al: Regulation of alpha(2)-adrenoceptors in human vascular smooth muscle cells, *Am J Physiol Heart Circ Physiol* 286:H59–H67, 2004.
29. Jeyaraj SC, Chotani MA, Mitra S, et al: Cooling evokes redistribution of alpha2C-adrenoceptors from Golgi to plasma membrane in transfected human embryonic kidney 293 cells, *Mol Pharmacol* 60:1195–1200, 2001.
30. Keenan EJ, Porter JM: Alpha-adrenergic receptors in platelets from patients with Raynaud's syndrome, *Surgery* 94:204–209, 1983.
31. Coffman JD, Cohen RA: Role of alpha-adrenoceptor subtypes mediating sympathetic vasoconstriction in human digits, *Eur J Clin Invest* 18:309–313, 1988.
32. Cooke JP, Creager SJ, Scales KM, et al: Role of digital artery adrenoceptors in Raynaud's disease, *Vasc Med* 2:1–7, 1997.
33. Peacock JH: Peripheral venous blood concentrations of epinephrine and norepinephrine in primary Raynaud's disease, *Circ Res* 7:821–827, 1959.
34. Kontos HA, Wasserman AJ: Effect of reserpine in Raynaud's phenomenon, *Circulation* 39:259–266, 1969.
35. Downey JA, LeRoy EC, Miller JM 3rd, et al: Thermoregulation and Raynaud's phenomenon, *Clin Sci* 40:211–219, 1971.
36. Fagius J, Blumberg H: Sympathetic outflow to the hand in patients with Raynaud's phenomenon, *Cardiovasc Res* 19:249–253, 1985.
37. Greenblatt DJ, Koch-Weser J: Adverse reactions to beta-adrenergic receptor blocking drugs: a report from the Boston collaborative drug surveillance program, *Drugs* 7:118–129, 1974.
38. Marshall A, Barritt DW, Roberts CJ: Letter: Raynaud's phenomenon as side effect of beta-blockers, *Br Med J* 2:301, 1976.
39. Eliasson K, Lins LE, Sundqvist K: Peripheral vasospasm during beta-receptor blockade - a comparison between metoprolol and pindolol, *Acta Med Scand Suppl* 665:109–112, 1982.
40. Cohen RA, Coffman JD: Beta-adrenergic vasodilator mechanism in the finger, *Circ Res* 49:1196–1201, 1981.
41. Coffman JD, Rasmussen HM: Effect of thromboxane synthetase inhibition in Raynaud's phenomenon, *Clin Pharmacol Ther* 36:369–373, 1984.
42. Luderer JR, Nicholas GG, Neumyer MM, et al: Dazoxiben, a thromboxane synthetase inhibitor, in Raynaud's phenomenon, *Clin Pharmacol Ther* 36:105–115, 1984.
43. Zamora MR, O'Brien RF, Rutherford RB, et al: Serum endothelin-1 concentrations and cold provocation in primary Raynaud's phenomenon, *Lancet* 336:1144–1147, 1990.
44. Smyth AE, Bell AL, Bruce IN, et al: Digital vascular responses and serum endothelin-1 concentrations in primary and secondary Raynaud's phenomenon, *Ann Rheum Dis* 59:870–874, 2000.
45. Nguyen VA, Eisendle K, Gruber I, et al: Effect of the dual endothelin receptor antagonist bosentan on Raynaud's phenomenon secondary to systemic sclerosis: a double-blind prospective, randomized, placebo-controlled pilot study, *Rheumatology (Oxford)* 49:583–587, 2010.
46. Matucci-Cerinic M, Denton CP, Furst DE, et al: Bosentan treatment of digital ulcers related to systemic sclerosis: results from the RAPIDS-2 randomised, double-blind, placebo-controlled trial, *Ann Rheum Dis* 70:32–38, 2011.
47. Landis EM: Micro-injection studies of capillary blood pressure in Raynaud's disease, *Heart* 15:247, 1930.
48. Thulesius O: Methods for the evaluation of peripheral vascular function in the upper extremities, *Acta Chir Scand Suppl* 465:53–54, 1976.
49. Cohen RA, Coffman JD: Reduced fingertip arterial pressure in Raynaud's disease, *J Vasc Med Biol* 1:21, 1989.
50. Imhof JW, Baars H, Verloop MC: Clinical and haematological aspects of macroglobulinaemia Waldenstrom, *Acta Med Scand* 163:349–366, 1959.
51. Jahnsen T, Nielsen SL, Skovborg F: Blood viscosity and local response to cold in primary Raynaud's phenomenon, *Lancet* 2:1001–1002, 1977.
52. Marshall RJ, Shepherd JT, Thompson ID: Vascular responses in patients with high serum titres of cold agglutinins, *Clin Sci (Lond)* 12:255–264, 1953.
53. McGrath MA, Penny R: Blood hyperviscosity in cryoglobulinaemia: temperature sensitivity and correlation with reduced skin blood flow, *Aust J Exp Biol Med Sci* 56:127–137, 1978.
54. Hillestad LK: The peripheral circulation during exposure to cold in normals and in patients with the syndrome of high-titre cold haemagglutination. I. The vascular response to cold exposure in normal subjects, *Acta Med Scand* 164:203–229, 1959.
55. Maricq HR, LeRoy EC, D'Angelo WA, et al: Diagnostic potential of *in vivo* capillary microscopy in scleroderma and related disorders, *Arthritis Rheum* 23:183–189, 1980.
56. Tan EM, Cohen AS, Fries JF, et al: The 1982 revised criteria for the classification of systemic lupus erythematosus, *Arthritis Rheum* 25:1271–1277, 1982.
57. Fischer M, Mielke H, Glaefke S, et al: Generalized vasculopathy and finger blood flow abnormalities in rheumatoid arthritis, *J Rheumatol* 11:33–37, 1984.
58. Aletaha D, Neogi T, Silman AJ, et al: 2010 Rheumatoid arthritis classification criteria: an American College of Rheumatology/European League Against Rheumatism collaborative initiative, *Arthritis Rheum* 62:2569–2581, 2010.
59. Garcia-Carrasco M, Siso A, Ramos-Casals M, et al: Raynaud's phenomenon in primary Sjogren's syndrome. Prevalence and clinical characteristics in a series of 320 patients, *J Rheumatol* 29:726–730, 2002.
60. Nakamura H, Kawakami A, Hayashi T, et al: Anti-centromere antibody-seropositive Sjogren's syndrome differs from conventional subgroup in clinical and pathological study, *BMC Musculoskelet Disord* 11:140, 2010.
61. Lambova SN, Kuzmanova SI: Raynaud's phenomenon in common rheumatic diseases, *Folia Med (Plovdiv)* 48:22–28, 2006.
62. Waller DG, Dathan JR: Raynaud's syndrome and carpal tunnel syndrome, *Postgrad Med J* 61:161–162, 1985.
63. Cooper RA, Bunn HF: Hemolytic anemia. In Braunwald E, et al, editors: *Harrison's Principles of Internal Medicine*, New York, 1987, McGraw-Hill.
64. Trejo O, Ramos-Casals M, Garcia-Carrasco M, et al: Cryoglobulinemia: study of etiologic factors and clinical and immunologic features in 443 patients from a single center, *Medicine (Baltimore)* 80:252–262, 2001.
65. Jager BV: Cryofibrinogenemia, *N Engl J Med* 266:579–583, 1962.
66. Letz R, Cherniack MG, Gerr F, et al: A cross sectional epidemiological survey of shipyard workers exposed to hand-arm vibration, *Br J Ind Med* 49:53–62, 1992.
67. Mirbod SM, Yoshida H, Nagata C, et al: Hand-arm vibration syndrome and its prevalence in the present status of private forestry enterprises in Japan, *Int Arch Occup Environ Health* 64:93–99, 1992.
68. Davies TA, Glaser EM, Collins CP: Absence of Raynaud's phenomenon in workers using vibratory tools in a warm climate, *Lancet* 272:1014–1016, 1957.
69. Okada A, Inaba R, Furuno T: Occurrence of intimal thickening of the peripheral arteries in response to local vibration, *Br J Ind Med* 44:470–475, 1987.
70. Hisanaga H: Studies of peripheral nerve conduction velocities in vibrating tool operators, *Sangyo Igaku* 24:284–293, 1982.

71. Kuhar CG, Mesti T, Zakotnik B: Digital ischemic events related to gemcitabine: report of two cases and a systematic review, *Radiol Oncol* 44:257–261, 2010.

72. Laplanche A, Clavel-Chapelon F, Contassot JC, et al: Exposure to vinyl chloride monomer: results of a cohort study after a seven-year follow up. The French VCM Group, *Br J Ind Med* 49:134–137, 1992.

73. Coffman JD, Rasmussen HM: Effects of beta-adrenoreceptor-blocking drugs in patients with Raynaud's phenomenon, *Circulation* 72:466–470, 1985.

74. Nielsen SL, Parving HH, Hansen JE: Myxoedema and Raynaud's phenomenon, *Acta Endocrinol (Copenh)* 101:32–34, 1982.

75. Nielsen SL, Lokkegaard H: Cold hypersensitivity and finger systolic blood pressure in hemodialysis patients, *Scand J Urol Nephrol* 15:319–322, 1981.

76. Preston IR, Hill NS: Evaluation and management of pulmonary hypertension in systemic sclerosis, *Curr Opin Rheumatol* 15:761–765, 2003.

77. Fuster V, Steele PM, Edwards WD, et al: Primary pulmonary hypertension: natural history and the importance of thrombosis, *Circulation* 70:580–587, 1984.

78. Rich S, Dantzker DR, Ayres SM, et al: Primary pulmonary hypertension. A national prospective study, *Ann Intern Med* 107:216–223, 1987.

79. Schildmann EK, Davies AN: Paraneoplastic Raynaud's phenomenon–good palliation after a multidisciplinary approach, *J Pain Symptom Manage* 39:779–783, 2010.

80. Lambova S, Muller-Ladner U: Capillaroscopic pattern in paraneoplastic Raynaud's phenomenon, *Rheumatol Int* published online 21 Jan 2011 (DOI: 10.1007/s00296-010-1715-8).

81. Nielsen SL: Raynaud phenomena and finger systolic pressure during cooling, *Scand J Clin Lab Invest* 38:765–770, 1978.

82. Keefe FJ, Surwit RS, Pilon RN: A 1-year follow-up of Raynaud's patients treated with behavioral therapy techniques, *J Behav Med* 2:385–391, 1979.

83. Keefe FJ, Surwit RS, Pilon RN: Biofeedback, autogenic training, and progressive relaxation in the treatment of Raynaud's disease: a comparative study, *J Appl Behav Anal* 13:3–11, 1980.

84. Yocum DE, Hodes R, Sundstrom WR, et al: Use of biofeedback training in treatment of Raynaud's disease and phenomenon, *J Rheumatol* 12:90–93, 1985.

85. Stambrook M, Hamel ER, Carter SA: Training to vasodilate in a cooling environment: a valid treatment for Raynaud's phenomenon? *Biofeedback Self Regul* 13:9–23, 1988.

86. Guglielmi RS, Roberts AH, Patterson R: Skin temperature biofeedback for Raynaud's disease: a double-blind study, *Biofeedback Self Regul* 7:99–120, 1982.

87. Freedman RR, Ianni P, Wenig P: Behavioral treatment of Raynaud's phenomenon in scleroderma, *J Behav Med* 7:343–353, 1984.

88. Comparison of sustained-release nifedipine and temperature biofeedback for treatment of primary Raynaud phenomenon. Results from a randomized clinical trial with 1-year follow-up, *Arch Intern Med* 160:1101–1108, 2000.

89. Jobe JB, Sampson JB, Roberts DE, et al: Induced vasodilation as treatment for Raynaud's disease, *Ann Intern Med* 97:706–709, 1982.

90. Coffman JD: Raynaud's phenomenon, *Curr Treat Options Cardiovasc Med* 2:219–226, 2000.

91. Belch JJ, Ho M: Pharmacotherapy of Raynaud's phenomenon, *Drugs* 52:682–695, 1996.

92. Creager MA, Pariser KM, Winston EM, et al: Nifedipine-induced fingertip vasodilation in patients with Raynaud's phenomenon, *Am Heart J* 108:370–373, 1984.

93. Nilsson H, Jonason T, Leppert J, et al: The effect of the calcium-entry blocker nifedipine on cold-induced digital vasospasm. A double-blind crossover study versus placebo, *Acta Med Scand* 221:53–60, 1987.

94. Matucci Cerinic M, Falcini F, Bartolozzi G, et al: Nifedipine treatment of Raynaud's phenomenon in a paediatric age, *Int J Clin Pharmacol Res* 5:67–69, 1985.

95. Jobe JB, Beetham WP Jr, Roberts DE, et al: Induced vasodilation as a home treatment for Raynaud's disease, *J Rheumatol* 12:953–956, 1985.

96. Kahan A, Amor B, Menkes CJ: A randomised double-blind trial of diltiazem in the treatment of Raynaud's phenomenon, *Ann Rheum Dis* 44:30–33, 1985.

97. Rhedda A, McCans J, Willan AR, et al: A double blind placebo controlled crossover randomized trial of diltiazem in Raynaud's phenomenon, *J Rheumatol* 12:724–727, 1985.

98. Matoba T, Chiba M: Effects of diltiazem on occupational Raynaud's syndrome (vibration disease), *Angiology* 36:850–856, 1985.

99. Schmidt JF, Valentin N, Nielsen SL: The clinical effect of felodipine and nifedipine in Raynaud's phenomenon, *Eur J Clin Pharmacol* 37:191–192, 1989.

100. Kallenberg CG, Wouda AA, Meems L, et al: Once daily felodipine in patients with primary Raynaud's phenomenon, *Eur J Clin Pharmacol* 40:313–315, 1991.

101. Kinney EL, Nicholas GG, Gallo J, et al: The treatment of severe Raynaud's phenomenon with verapamil, *J Clin Pharmacol* 22:74–76, 1982.

102. Nielsen SL, Vitting K, Rasmussen K: Prazosin treatment of primary Raynaud's phenomenon, *Eur J Clin Pharmacol* 24:421–423, 1983.

103. Wollersheim H, Thien T, Fennis J, et al: Double-blind, placebo-controlled study of prazosin in Raynaud's phenomenon, *Clin Pharmacol Ther* 40:219–225, 1986.

104. Russell IJ, Lessard JA: Prazosin treatment of Raynaud's phenomenon: a double blind single crossover study, *J Rheumatol* 12:94–98, 1985.

105. Coleiro B, Marshall SE, Denton CP, et al: Treatment of Raynaud's phenomenon with the selective serotonin reuptake inhibitor fluoxetine, *Rheumatology (Oxford)* 40:1038–1043, 2001.

106. Rey J, Cretel E, Jean R, et al: Serotonin reuptake inhibitors, Raynaud's phenomenon and erythromelalgia, *Rheumatology (Oxford)* 42:601–602, 2003.

107. Challenor VF: Angiotensin converting enzyme inhibitors in Raynaud's phenomenon, *Drugs* 48:864–867, 1994.

108. Lopez-Ovejero JA, Saal SD, D'Angelo WA, et al: Reversal of vascular and renal crises of scleroderma by oral angiotensin-converting-enzyme blockade, *N Engl J Med* 300:1417–1419, 1979.

109. Tosi S, Marchesoni A, Messina K, et al: Treatment of Raynaud's phenomenon with captopril, *Drugs Exp Clin Res* 13:37–42, 1987.

110. Dziadzio M, Denton CP, Smith R, et al: Losartan therapy for Raynaud's phenomenon and scleroderma: clinical and biochemical findings in a fifteen-week, randomized, parallel-group, controlled trial, *Arthritis Rheum* 42:2646–2655, 1999.

111. Selenko-Gebauer N, Duschek N, Minimair G, et al: Successful treatment of patients with severe secondary Raynaud's phenomenon with the endothelin receptor antagonist bosentan, *Rheumatology (Oxford)* 45(Suppl 3):iii45–iii48, 2006.

112. Ramos-Casals M, Brito-Zeron P, Nardi N, et al: Successful treatment of severe Raynaud's phenomenon with bosentan in four patients with systemic sclerosis, *Rheumatology (Oxford)* 43:1454–1456, 2004.

113. Tsifetaki N, Botzoris V, Alamanos Y, et al: Bosentan for digital ulcers in patients with systemic sclerosis: a prospective 3-year followup study, *J Rheumatol* 36:1550–1552, 2009.

114. Levien TL: Phosphodiesterase inhibitors in Raynaud's phenomenon, *Ann Pharmacother* 40:1388–1393, 2006.

115. Fries R, Shariat K, von Wilmowsky H, et al: Sildenafil in the treatment of Raynaud's phenomenon resistant to vasodilatory therapy, *Circulation* 112:2980–2985, 2005.

116. Shenoy PD, Kumar S, Jha LK, et al: Efficacy of tadalafil in secondary Raynaud's phenomenon resistant to vasodilator therapy: a double-blind randomized cross-over trial, *Rheumatology (Oxford)* 49:2420–2428, 2010.

117. Herrick AL, van den Hoogen F, Gabrielli A, et al: Modified-release sildenafil reduces Raynaud's phenomenon attack frequency in limited cutaneous systemic sclerosis, *Arthritis Rheum* 63:775–782, 2011.

118. Teh LS, Manning J, Moore T, et al: Sustained-release transdermal glyceryl trinitrate patches as a treatment for primary and secondary Raynaud's phenomenon, *Br J Rheumatol* 34:636–641, 1995.

119. Chung L, Shapiro L, Fiorentino D, et al: MQX-503, a novel formulation of nitroglycerin, improves the severity of Raynaud's phenomenon: a randomized, controlled trial, *Arthritis Rheum* 60:870–877, 2009.

120. Abou-Raya A, Abou-Raya S, Helmii M: Statins: potentially useful in therapy of systemic sclerosis-related Raynaud's phenomenon and digital ulcers, *J Rheumatol* 35:1801–1808, 2008.

121. Sambo P, Amico D, Giacomelli R, et al: Intravenous N-acetylcysteine for treatment of Raynaud's phenomenon secondary to systemic sclerosis: a pilot study, *J Rheumatol* 28:2257–2262, 2001.

122. Coffman JD: *Raynaud phenomenon*, New York, 1989, Oxford University Press.

123. de Trafford JC, Lafferty K, Potter CE, et al: An epidemiological survey of Raynaud's phenomenon, *Eur J Vasc Surg* 2:167–170, 1988.

124. Yee AM, Hotchkiss RN, Paget SA: Adventitial stripping: a digit saving procedure in refractory Raynaud's phenomenon, *J Rheumatol* 25:269–276, 1998.

125. Fregene A, Ditmars D, Siddiqui A: Botulinum toxin type A: a treatment option for digital ischemia in patients with Raynaud's phenomenon, *J Hand Surg Am* 34:446–452, 2009.

126. Neumeister MW: Botulinum toxin type A in the treatment of Raynaud's phenomenon, *J Hand Surg Am* 35:2085–2092, 2010.

CHAPTER 49

Acrocyanosis

Veerendra Chadachan, Robert T. Eberhardt

The term *acrocyanosis* is derived from the Greek words *akron* (meaning "extremity") and *kyanos* (meaning "blue"). As a medical condition, acrocyanosis is an uncommon functional vasospastic disorder characterized by persistent bluish discoloration, primarily of the hands and feet. The original description of acrocyanosis is credited to Crocq in 1896, thus the eponym *Crocq's disease*. Classically, acrocyanosis affects young asthenic females in regions with cooler climates. In contrast to Raynaud's syndrome, the bluish discoloration of acrocyanosis is persistent rather than episodic and is not associated with discomfort.[1] *Primary acrocyanosis* is not associated with an identifiable cause and is usually a benign disorder with a good prognosis; skin ulceration and tissue loss are extremely rare. Patients with primary disease usually do well with behavioral measures such as avoidance of exposure to cold; pharmacological therapy is rarely necessary. *Secondary acrocyanosis* occurs in association with another underlying disorder. An acrocyanotic appearance may be seen in conjunction with any disease that causes central cyanosis or markedly decreases blood flow to the extremity. Treatment and prognosis of secondary acrocyanosis depends on the underlying condition.[1]

Epidemiology

Limited information is available on many of the epidemiological aspects of primary acrocyanosis, including its precise incidence and prevalence. Acrocyanosis is believed to occur more frequently with a low body mass index (BMI), outdoor occupations, and in areas with cooler climates.[2] Despite early reports suggesting similar gender predilection, acrocyanosis seems to affect women more frequently than men, with a female-to-male ratio of 6:1.[3] It is more common in younger individuals, the typical age range being 20 to 45 years.[4] In addition, occurrence of acrocyanosis seems to decrease with increasing age, regardless of the regional climate.[5] It is seen frequently in patients with anorexia nervosa, affecting up to 20% of women with this disorder.[6] It has been suggested that as many as 10% of patients have a family history of acrocyanosis in one of the first-degree relatives, suggesting a genetic basis.[4]

Etiology

As already noted, acrocyanosis is commonly a primary or idiopathic disorder that is not associated with an identifiable cause. It also occurs as a secondary condition in association with connective tissue disorders, some hematological conditions, anorexia nervosa, neurovascular disorders, drugs, toxins, infections, heritable metabolic diseases, and some malignancies.[7] An acrocyanotic appearance also occurs in conjunction with any disease that causes central cyanosis or markedly decreases blood flow to the extremities (Box 49-1).

Pathophysiology

Acrocyanosis is due to a decrease in the amount of oxygen delivered to the tissues of the extremities. Several mechanisms for primary acrocyanosis have been proposed, but the precise mechanism remains elusive. Potential pathophysiological disturbances include abnormal arteriolar tone, alteration of microvascular responsiveness with capillary and venular dilation and stasis, and abnormal sympathetic nervous system activity (Box 49-2).

The essential abnormality in primary acrocyanosis seems to be peripheral cutaneous vasoconstriction due to increased tone of the arterioles, associated with secondary vasodilation of capillaries and subpapillary venous plexi.[8] Arteriolar vasoconstriction produces the cyanotic discoloration, and compensatory venular dilation in the postcapillary sphincter leads to excessive sweating. Persistent vasoconstriction at the precapillary sphincter creates a local hypoxic environment that may cause increased release of vasodilatory mediators such as adenosine in the capillary beds.[9] This in turn leads to dilation of postcapillary venules. The difference in the vessel tone may create a countercurrent exchange system in an attempt to retain heat, and this leads to sweating. Potential mediators that may contribute to the pathogenesis of acrocyanosis include serotonin, adrenaline, noradrenaline, and endothelin (ET)-1. Levels of these mediators have been shown to be increased in acrocyanosis.[3,10]

The exact cause of the disordered arteriolar tone in acrocyanosis is unknown. Most evidence points to local sensitivity of the arterioles to cold and an exaggerated sympathetic nervous system response. Earlier studies suggested an exaggerated digital arteriolar vasoconstrictive response to cold stimuli,[11] whereas subsequent studies have implicated the sympathetic nervous system.[1] An interesting case described normalization of cutaneous thermal-induced vasoreactivity in the hands of a young girl with acrocyanosis during phenobarbital-induced sleep. In this state, her hands responded in the same manner as the rest of body to heat and cold exposure. This finding supports the hypothesis that the abnormal vascular tone in acrocyanosis may be of central origin.[12] Other mechanisms hypothesized include increased blood viscosity,[13] decreased distal blood flow at low temperatures, and persistently elevated vasoconstrictive mediators such as endothelin-1 levels,[14] but convincing supporting evidence for these is not readily available.

Clinical Presentation

Primary acrocyanosis typically occurs in thin young women who are not physically active. They commonly present with persistent bluish discoloration of the hands and feet. The distribution of the discoloration is symmetrical.[5] It less frequently involves forearms, ears, lips, nose, or nipples. It is the discoloration that usually prompts patients to seek medical care. Patients may also describe a sensation of coolness of the affected areas, but generally will not have pain. There may be slight swelling of the digits and increased perspiration. Although the discoloration is persistent, emotion and cold temperature can intensify the acrocyanotic appearance, and warmth can diminish it.[1] Discoloration and coolness are worse in cold weather, but typically persist even during the summer months.

Examination reveals bluish discoloration of the hands and feet, which are cool and often sweaty (Fig. 49-1). The color has also been described as bluish-pink or orange-like tinged with red, and differing hues may be seen at various times. A brownish-yellow color on the dorsum of hands and feet has been described and attributed to exposure to the warmth of the sun because it is most obvious in summer. Pressure on the discolored skin causes pallor, and color returns slowly and irregularly. Fingers may be puffy, but trophic changes do not occur.

In patients with primary disease, there are no other abnormal physical findings. Arterial pulses are normal, suggesting there is no large-vessel arterial obstruction.[8] Elevation of a cyanotic limb above heart level produces pallor, suggesting venous obstruction is not present. Patients with secondary acrocyanosis may have clinical features of the underlying condition. Episodes of digital pallor or rubor do not occur, although patients may have both acrocyanosis and Raynaud's phenomenon. This is especially true in patients with scleroderma or systemic lupus erythematosus (SLE) as an underlying cause.

Box 49-1 Differential Diagnosis for Acrocyanosis

Primary or Idiopathic Acrocyanosis

Secondary Acrocyanosis
Connective Tissue Disorders
Scleroderma
Systemic lupus erythematosus (SLE)
Rheumatoid arthritis
Mixed connective tissue disease
Antiphospholipid antibody syndrome

Hematological
Cryoglobulins
Cold agglutinins
Lymphoproliferative disorders

Infections
Mycoplasma pneumonia
Mononucleosis
Hepatitis C

Medications and Toxins
Tricyclic antidepressants, interferon alpha (IFN-α), amphotericin B deoxycholate, Blasticidin S
Arsenic, butyl nitrate

Anorexia Nervosa

Heritable Disorders
Ethylmalonic aciduria
Mitochondrial disease
Fucosidosis
Fabry's disease

Neurovascular Disorders
Spinal cord injury
Complex regional pain syndrome
Postural orthostatic tachycardia syndrome

Malignancy
Lymphoma

Cardiopulmonary Disease
Pulmonary hypertension (PH)
Cyanotic heart disease
Respiratory failure

Arterial Occlusive Disease
Atheromatous embolism
Disseminated intravascular coagulation (DIC)
Heparin-induced thrombocytopenia (HIT)
Septic embolism

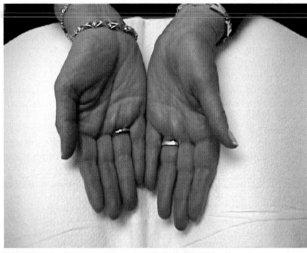

FIGURE 49-1   Primary acrocyanosis involving the hands.

pulse examination is normal, excluding significant peripheral artery occlusive disease. Pulse oximetry reveals normal oxygen saturation.

Secondary acrocyanosis is suggested by asymmetrical distribution of the discoloration, presence of pain, or trophic changes of the fingers or toes. Hypoxemia or absent pulses suggest central cyanosis or arterial obstructive disease, respectively. Selected laboratory tests are necessary to confirm the diagnosis of secondary acrocyanosis. Arterial blood gas is appropriate to evaluate for hypoxemia. Antinuclear antibodies (ANAs) are typically absent, but if present suggest an underlying connective tissue disorder. If the history and physical examination are suggestive, directed testing for cryoglobulins, antiphospholipid antibodies, cold agglutinins, or antibodies to Epstein-Barr virus should be performed.

Nailfold capillaroscopy is often abnormal in acrocyanosis. Features include abnormal capillary morphology, pericapillary edema, and even hemorrhage. Findings on capillaroscopy are often nondiagnostic and may be associated with secondary disease. It has been shown that mean capillary density is decreased in patients with acrocyanosis compared with normal subjects, but not to the extent seen in patients with Raynaud's phenomenon due to scleroderma.[16] Other capillary abnormalities include capillary loops of diameter larger than normal. The presence of megacapillaries and areas of sparse or absent capillaries suggest underlying scleroderma or mixed connective tissue, whereas bushy capillaries suggest underlying systemic lupus erythematosus. Other findings such as decreased oscillations over the radial artery and decreased digital vessel sounds when assessed by Doppler have been described but are nonspecific.[17]

Histopathology

Cutaneous biopsy is usually unnecessary for the diagnosis of acrocyanosis. Findings described on biopsy are thickening of the medial coat of arterioles and dilation of papillary and subpapillary capillaries. Other features include mild perivascular infiltration, mild dermal edema, and skin fibrosis with formation of new blood vessels.[4]

Differential Diagnosis

Primary acrocyanosis should be distinguished from other cold-related vasospastic conditions such as Raynaud's syndrome, pernio, and livedo reticularis.[15] This determination is based upon general appearance, distribution, and persistence of the cyanosis. Then the finding of acrocyanosis requires consideration of other local or systemic features that would suggest an underlying secondary disorder.[18]

Box 49-2   Proposed Pathophysiological Mechanisms of Primary Acrocyanosis

Abnormal arteriolar tone
Alteration in microvascular reactivity
Abnormal sympathetic nervous system activity
Increased blood viscosity
Persistently elevated vasoconstrictive mediators

Diagnosis

Primary acrocyanosis is diagnosed clinically based on a careful history and physical examination. Laboratory or imaging studies typically are not necessary.[15] Cyanosis is symmetrical in distribution and will be present at the time of examination, since it is persistent. In addition, there are usually no associated trophic skin changes, localized pain, or ulcerations. Peripheral

602

CH
49

Systemic hypoxemia with increased deoxyhemoglobin is a common etiology of an acrocyanotic appearance. Presence of central cyanosis with arterial hypoxemia should prompt a search for underlying cardiopulmonary disease.[19] Peripheral cyanosis may result from an alteration in hemoglobin (Hb), with accumulation of the oxidized form, methemoglobin.[20] This may be seen with exposure to oxidizing agents such as aniline, benzocaine, dapsone, phenazopyridine, nitrates, and naphthalene. Cold agglutinins and cryoglobulinemia may cause acrocyanosis.[21,22] Cold agglutinins may be associated with infectious mononucleosis and *Mycoplasma* pneumonia and also occur in lymphoproliferative disorders. Acrocyanosis has been reported as a presenting feature of Hodgkin lymphoma.[23] Acrocyanosis is also caused by cryoglobulinemia associated with hepatitis C infection and several other diseases.[24]

Acrocyanosis is well described in anorexia nervosa.[25] It tends to occur in the more severely ill and malnourished patients. Typically these patients have pallor of the face and trunk, slower pulse rates, and high fasting plasma glucose levels. These patients also have decreased distal blood flow and impaired vasodilation to a heat stimulus.[6]

Numerous connective tissue disorders may manifest acrocyanosis, but other signs of these diseases are usually present. Patients with scleroderma and SLE may have both acrocyanosis and episodic attacks of Raynaud's phenomenon.[16,26] Antinuclear antibodies may be detected in patients with connective tissue disorders. Acrocyanosis is also present in up to one third of patients with antiphospholipid antibodies, and may be seen in conjunction with other cutaneous manifestations such as dermatographism, urticaria, livedo reticularis, cutaneous nodules, ulceration, and purpura.[27,28]

Several medications and toxins are associated with acrocyanosis, including tricyclic antidepressants, interferon alpha (IFN-α)-2a, amphotericin B, arsenic, and butyl nitrite.[29-33] Therefore, it is important to consider medications or toxic substances as a potential cause.

Acrocyanosis has been observed in several neurological disorders with suspected neurovascular instability. An acrocyanotic appearance may be seen following spinal cord injuries or with complex regional pain syndrome.[34] This later disorder often occurs following trauma and is typified by pain and autonomic dysregulation. Acrocyanosis and lower-extremity edema has also been described in postural orthostatic tachycardia syndrome and is ascribed to venous pooling.[35]

Acrocyanosis secondary to inherited metabolic disorders is more likely to present during childhood or adolescence. These disorders are suspected when other characteristic associated manifestations are present. Infants with ethylmalonic aciduria have petechiae, diarrhea, pyramidal signs, and mental retardation.[36] Children with mitochondrial disease may have hair abnormalities, pigmentation disorders, and hypertrichosis.[37]

Acrocyanosis may also be present in patients with microemboli, microthrombi, or atheromatous embolism. Patients with atheromatous emboli are typically older with other signs of atherosclerosis, and they have other cutaneous signs such as petechiae, livedo reticularis, and painful skin lesions on the toes (so-called blue toe syndrome).[38] Microthrombi and/or microemboli may occur in acutely ill patients with disseminated intravascular coagulation (DIC), heparin-induced thrombocytopenia (HIT), or septic embolism due to endocarditis.[39]

Treatment

Primary acrocyanosis is a benign condition that usually requires only conservative measures; there is no effective curative medical or surgical treatment (Box 49-3). Treatments typically focus on symptom relief or more often cosmetic appearance. Some patients are so affected they avoid social contact.[15] Reassurance and behavioral measures, such as avoidance of exposure to cold and use of protective clothing, often improve the discoloration.[40] In addition, psychophysiological measures such as biofeedback

Box 49-3 Treatment of Primary Acrocyanosis

Reassurance
Behavioral measures:
    Avoidance of exposure to cold
    Use of protective clothing
Psychophysiological measures:
    Biofeedback training
    Conditioning of reflexes
    Hypnosis
Pharmacological interventions:
    Calcium channel blockers
    Nicotinic acid derivatives
    Adrenergic blocking agents
    Cyclandelate
    Topical minoxidil
    Bromocriptine
Sympathectomy

training, conditioning of reflexes, and hypnosis may give partial relief.

Pharmacological intervention is rarely necessary. Various drugs have been advocated, although no controlled studies have been performed. Calcium channel blockers, nicotinic acid derivatives, adrenergic blocking agents (rauwolfia, guanethidine, reserpine, and α-blockers), cyclandelate, topical minoxidil, and rutin compounds have been claimed to provide symptomatic improvement.[18] Bromocriptine has been reported to relieve acrocyanosis in a few days, but may induce Raynaud's phenomenon in about one third of patients.[41] Sympathectomy or disrupting the fibers of the sympathetic nervous system to the area usually will alleviate acrocyanosis. However, such a drastic procedure is rarely appropriate for a benign disease.[42]

Treatment of secondary acrocyanosis depends on the underlying cause.

Prognosis

Although there is no cure, the prognosis of primary acrocyanosis is very good. It is not associated with increased risk of death, amputation, or other complications. Apart from the discoloration, patients with primary acrocyanosis usually have no other signs or symptoms such as pain, skin ulcerations, or tissue loss. Patients can expect to lead normal lives. In contrast, the prognosis of secondary acrocyanosis seems to vary widely depending upon the underlying condition.

REFERENCES

1. Coffman JD: Acrocyanosis and livedo reticularis, *Raynaud's phenomenon*, New York, 1989, Oxford University Press, pp 167–170.
2. Carpentier PH: Definition and epidemiology of vascular acrosyndromes, *Rev Prat* 48: 1641–1646, 1998.
3. Davis E: Clinical aspects of acrocyanosis, *Adv Microcirc* 10:101–106, 1982.
4. Stern ES: The aetiology and pathology of acrocyanosis, *Br J Derm* 49:100–108, 1937.
5. Creager MA, Dzau VJ: Vascular disease of the extremity. In Kasper DL, Fauci AS, Lango DL, editors: *Harrison's principles of internal medicine*, ed 16, New York, 2005, McGraw-Hill, pp 1490–1495.
6. Hediger C, Rost B, Itin P: Cutaneous manifestations in anorexia nervosa, *Schweiz Med Wochenschr* 130:565–575, 2000.
7. Brown PJ, Zirwas MJ, English JC: The purple digit an algorithmic approach to diagnosis, *Am J Clin Dermatol* 11:103–116, 2010.
8. Mansilha A, Sampaio S: Vasospastic disorders of the upper extremities. In Liapis CD, Balzer K, Benedetti-Valentini F, Fernandes J, editors: *European manual of medicine: vascular surgery*, Berlin, 2007, Springer-Verlag, Part 3, pp 237–246.
9. Bollinger A: Function of the precapillary vessels in peripheral vascular disease, *J Cardiovasc Pharmacol* 7:S147–S151, 1985.
10. Kurklinsky AK, Miller VM, Rooke TW: Acrocyanosis: the Flying Dutchman, *Vasc Med* 16: 288–301, 2011.
11. Lottenbach K: Vascular response to cold in acrocyanosis, *Helvetia Medica Acta* 33:437–444, 1967.
12. Day R, Klingman WO: The effect of sleep on the skin temperature reactions in a case of acrocyanosis, *J Clin Invest* 8:271–276, 1939.
13. Coperman PW: Acrocyanosis: a blood disease? *Proc R Soc Med* 66:741–742, 1973.
14. Mangiafico RA, Malatino LS, Santonocito M, et al: Plasma endothelin-1 concentrations during cold exposure in essential acrocyanosis, *Angiology* 47:1033–1038, 1996.

15. Heidrich H: Functional vascular diseases: Raynaud's syndrome, acrocyanosis and erythromelalgia, *Vasa* 39:33–41, 2010.
16. Monticone G, Colonna L, Palmeri G, et al: Quantitative nailfold capillary microscopy findings in patients with acrocyanosis compared with patients having systemic sclerosis and normal subjects, *J Am Acad Dermatol* 42:787–790, 2000.
17. Davis E: Oscillometry of radial artery in acrocyanosis and cold sensitivity, *J Mal Vasc* 17: 214–217, 1992.
18. Nousari HC, Kimyai-Asadi A, Anhalt GJ: Chronic idiopathic acrocyanosis, *J Am Acad Dermatol* 45:S207–S208, 2001.
19. Golombek SG, Ally S, Woolf PK: A newborn with cardiac failure secondary to a large vein of Galen malformation, *South Med J* 97:516–518, 2004.
20. Jiminez MA, Polena S, Coplan NL, et al: Methemoglobinemia and transesophageal echo, *Proc West Pharmacol Soc* 50:134–135, 2007.
21. Cholongitas E, Ioannidou D: Acrocyanosis due to cold agglutinins in a patient with rheumatoid arthritis, *J Clin Rheumatol* 15:375, 2009.
22. Sinha A, Richardson G, Patel RT: Cold agglutinin related acrocyanosis and paroxysmal haemolysis, *Eur J Vasc Endovasc Surg* 30:563–565, 2005.
23. Solak Y, Aksoy S, Kilickap S, et al: Acrocyanosis as a presenting symptom of Hodgkin lymphoma, *Am J Hematol* 81:151–152, 2006.
24. Trejo O, Ramos-Casals M, Garcia-Carrasco M, et al: Cryoglobulinemia: study of etiological factors and clinical and immunologic features in 443 patients from a single center, *Medicine* 80:252–262, 2001.
25. Strumia R: Skin signs in anorexia nervosa, *Dermatoendocrinol* 1:268–270, 2009.
26. Richter JG, Sander O, Schneider M, et al: Diagnostic algorithm for Raynaud's phenomenon and vascular skin lesions in systemic lupus erythematosus, *Lupus* 19:1087–1095, 2010.
27. Vayssairat M, Abauf N, Baudot N, et al: Abnormal IgG cardiolipin antibody titers in patients with Raynaud's phenomenon and/or related disorders: prevalence and clinical significance, *J Am Acad Dermatol* 38:555–558, 1998.
28. Diógenes MJ, Diógenes PC, de Morais Carneiro RM, et al: Cutaneous manifestations associated with antiphospholipid antibodies, *Int J Dermatol* 43:632–637, 2004.
29. Anderson RP, Morris BA: Acrocyanosis to imipramine, *Arch Dis Child* 63:204–205, 1988.
30. Ozaras R, Yemisen M, Mete B, et al: Acrocyancosis developed with amphotericin B deoxycholate but not amphotericin B lipid complex, *Mycoses* 50:242, 2007.
31. Campo-Voegeli A, Estrach T, Marti RM, et al: Acrocyanosis induced by interferon alpha (2a), *Dermatology* 196:361–363, 1998.
32. Hall AH: Chronic arsenic poisoning, *Toxicol Lett* 128:69–72, 2002.
33. Hoegl L, Thoma-Greber E, Poppinger J, et al: Butyl nitrite-induced acrocyanosis in an HIV infected patient, *Arch Dermatol* 135:90–92, 1999.
34. Glazer E, Pacanowski JP, Leon LR: Asymptomatic lower extremity acrocyanosis: report of two cases and review of the literature, *Vascular* 19:105–110, 2011.
35. Steward JM, Gewitz MH, Weldon A, et al: Patterns of orthostatic intolerance: the orthostatic tachycardia syndrome and adolescent chronic fatigue, *J Pediatr* 135:218–221, 1999.
36. Burlina AB, Dionisi-Vici C, Bennett MJ, et al: A new syndrome with ethylmalonic aciduria and normal fatty acid oxidation in fibroblasts, *J Pediatr* 124:79–86, 1994.
37. Boderman C, Rötig A, Rustin P, et al: Hair and skin disorders as signs of mitochondrial diseases, *Paediatrics* 103:428–433, 1999.
38. Yücel AE, Kart-Köseoglu H, Demirhan B, et al: Cholesterol crystal embolization mimicking vasculitis: success with corticosteroid and cyclophosphamide therapy in two cases, *Rheumatol Int* 26:454–460, 2006.
39. Sharma BD, Kabra SR, Gupta B: Symmetrical peripheral gangrene, *Trop Doct* 34:2–4, 2004.
40. Planchon B, Becker E, Carpentier PH, et al: Acrocyanosis: changing concepts and nosological limitations, *J Mal Vasc* 26:5–15, 2001.
41. Morrish DW, Crockford PM: Acrocyanosis treated with bromocriptine, *Lancet* 2:851, 1976.
42. Grima MR: Nursing case study: bilateral cervical sympathectomy for acrocyanosis, *Nurs Times* 71:1850–1852, 1975.

CHAPTER 50

Erythromelalgia

Mark D.P. Davis, Thom W. Rooke

Definition and Historical Perspective

Erythromelalgia is a rare condition of the extremities characterized by the triad of redness, warmth, and pain. The symptom complex of intermittent acral warmth, pain, and erythema that defines erythromelalgia has been well documented in the medical literature for more than 150 years. Graves[1] described cases of "hot and painful legs" in 1834. The term *erythromelalgia* was coined in 1878 by Mitchell[2] from *erythros* (red), *melos* (extremity), and *algos* (pain); some have since referred to it as *Mitchell's disease*. As we discover more about the link between a vasculopathy and neuropathy in this syndrome, it seems that Mitchell was prophetically accurate when he entitled the original manuscript "On a Rare Vasomotor Neurosis of the Extremities." Smith and Allen[3] emphasized another essential component of this syndrome when they renamed it *erythermalgia* in 1938 to denote the heat (*thermé*) in the affected extremity during periods of redness. Although many authors agree that *erythermalgia* is perhaps more accurate, *erythromelalgia* is the term most commonly used, and it is the term used in this chapter.

Although poorly characterized inititally,[4-6] there have been considerable advances in the characterization of this clinical syndrome, with large case series[7-10] published. Although the condition is mysterious, it is not as mysterious as was once believed.[9,10] It has been argued that William Harvey could have had erythromelalgia, not gout.[11] Much of our current understanding of erythromelalgia derives from the larger case series reported.[7,8,10,12,13]

Nomenclature

Considerable confusion exists regarding the nomenclature of erythromelalgia.[14] Many terms have been used, and some authors have proposed that these terms should refer to different forms of erythromelalgia, as detailed later. However, these synonyms are not widely used, and most authors now use the term *erythromelalgia* as originally used by Silas Weir Mitchell (1829-1914). Related names used by some include *Weir-Mitchell's disease*, *Mitchell's disease*, and *acromelalgia*. Michiels et al.[15] proposed that the term *erythromelalgia* be restricted to cases due to myeloproliferative disorders responsive to aspirin therapy. They used the term *erythermalgia* to describe idiopathic conditions or conditions due to other diseases that are unresponsive to aspirin therapy. An unwieldy term, *erythermomelalgia*, accounts for the four cardinal symptoms and signs of the condition, but it is not in general use.[16] *Erythralgia* has been used.[5,17] *Erythroprosopalgia*, derived from *prosopon* (face), is used in the German literature to describe facial erythromelalgia.[5,14,17]

Criteria for Diagnosis

No objective criteria exist for the diagnosis of erythromelalgia, making it difficult to interpret some of the cases reported in the literature.[14] The diagnosis is most often clinically based, dependent on the medical history and physical findings, because no objective diagnostic or laboratory tests are available,[14] and because the physical findings of erythromelalgia may be absent owing to the frequently intermittent nature of the condition.[8]

Different diagnostic criteria have been suggested by different authors. Weir Mitchell[2,8] applied the three inclusion criteria used in the original description of the syndrome: red, hot, and painful extremities. Brown[18] added three additional criteria in 1932: induction and exacerbation of symptoms by warming, relief by cooling, and unresponsiveness to therapy. The criteria were described as follows: (1) during attacks (bilateral or symmetrical burning pain in hands and feet), affected parts are flushed, congested, and warm; (2) attacks are initiated or aggravated by standing, exercising, or exposing the extremity to temperatures warmer than 34 °C; (3) symptoms are relieved by elevation of the extremity or exposure of the extremity to cold; and (4) the condition is refractory to treatment. Thompson et al.[19] suggested the following five criteria: (1) burning extremity pain, (2) pain aggravated by warming, (3) pain relieved by cooling, (4) erythema of the affected skin, and (5) increased temperature of the affected skin. These five criteria have been used in several publications.[10,14,20-23]

Lazareth et al.[24] used three major and two of four minor criteria to satisfy the diagnosis. Major criteria were paroxysmal pain, burning pain, and redness of affected skin. Minor criteria were typical precipitating factors (heat exposure, effort), typical relieving factors (cold, rest), elevated skin temperature in affected skin, and response of symptoms to acetylsalicylic acid. Drenth et al.[25-28] distinguished three types of red, congested, and painful conditions of the extremities that must be distinguished for effective treatment according to their cause: (1) erythromelalgia in thrombocythemia, (2) primary erythermalgia, and (3) secondary erythermalgia. Kurzrock and Cohen[29] used a classification of early-onset erythromelalgia and late-onset erythromelalgia, irrespective of the cause.

Littleford et al.[30] used a classification of type 1 erythromelalgia (the typical form) and type 2 erythromelalgia (the abortive form), in which the burning nature of the pain is absent and symptomatic relief is not always provided by cooling or elevation of the limb. Mørk and Kvernebo[14] made the following distinctions: (1) *Syndrome* is used when initial and gradual symptoms localized to the feet and legs appear in childhood or adolescence, and when there is a family history of erythromelalgia; *phenomenon* is used for all other cases. (2) Erythromelalgia is *primary* when it is idiopathic. It is *secondary* when symptoms are caused by a primary disease such as a hemorrheological, metabolic, connective tissue, musculoskeletal, or infective disease; are induced by drugs; or are part of a paraneoplastic phenomenon. (3) *Acute* is used when symptoms reach maximal strength within 1 month after onset of symptoms. (4) *Borderline erythromelalgia*, *erythromelalgia*, and *severe erythromelalgia* may be useful.[14]

Clinical Controversies

Several controversies persist concerning erythromelalgia: nomenclature, diagnostic criteria, scoring systems for clinical severity, and pathogenesis. Classification of erythromelalgia into primary and secondary types may be controversial when comorbid conditions are mislabeled as underlying diseases that cause erythromelalgia. Classification of incomplete forms of erythromelalgia is also controversial; for example, some patients report that their feet are blue when symptoms are present. The problem with all definitions is that each criterion depends on clinical subjective judgment. The diagnosis of erythromelalgia is based on history because there are no objective physical findings. This may lead to an erroneous diagnosis.

Clinical Presentation

The essential elements of this clinical syndrome, as described by its name, are intermittent (occasionally continuous) redness of an acral area (i.e., extremities, head and neck area) associated with heat and pain. Common terms used to describe the pain include "piercing," "burning," and "discomfort."[8] The pain and

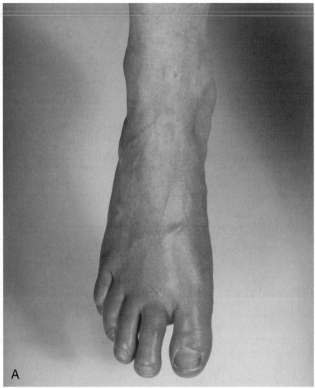

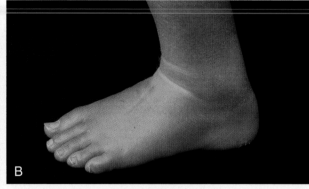

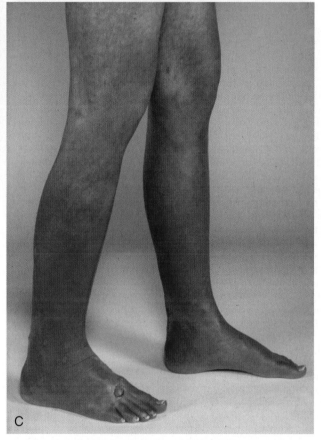

FIGURE 50-1 Erythromelalgia (red, hot, acral areas) involving lower extremities may affect toes only, distal forefoot (A), entire foot (B), or may extend up the leg, even beyond the knee (C). It is usually bilateral **(C)**.

burning sensation can be extremely severe. Patients report that they make major adjustments to their lifestyles to avoid precipitating an event. During an episode, they try to cool their feet in many ways, sometimes resorting to extraordinary measures to alleviate the pain, such as putting their feet in ice or walking barefoot in snow.

Erythromelalgia involves the feet in most circumstances (Fig. 50-1A-B); a minority of these patients have similar symptoms involving the hands.[8] Occasionally, only the hands are involved. Erythromelalgia may extend proximally to the knees in the lower extremities (Fig. 50-1C) and to the elbows in the upper extremities. Involvement of the extremities is generally symmetrical. Rarely, erythromelalgia involves the ears and face. In the largest reported series (168 patients), symptoms predominantly involved feet (148 patients, 88.1%) and hands (43 patients, 25.6%).[8]

In the majority of patients, symptoms are intermittent; episodes, precipitated by specific triggers, can last from minutes to hours. In a minority of patients, erythromelalgia symptoms are continuous, although they may wax and wane. Patients with continuous symptoms usually report that their symptoms started intermittently and then became more frequent and prolonged until they were continuous. In the series of 168 patients,[8] symptoms were intermittent in 163 patients (97%) and continuous in 5 (3%).

The specific precipitant for erythromelalgia varies from person to person, but the most frequent precipitant is an increase in temperature of the affected acral area. This may be caused by an increase in ambient temperature, and patients may experience increases in severity and frequency of attacks during the summer. Erythromelalgia affecting the feet is often precipitated by an increase in local temperature from aerobic exercise. Symptoms can also be precipitated or intensified by lowering the affected part. Common aggravating factors include warm rooms, floors, or water; placing the extremity near heating appliances; sleeping under bedcovers; and wearing shoes and gloves. Walking, exercise, sitting, dependency of the extremities, and application of skin pressure may intensify symptoms. Some patients relate that episodes of erythromelalgia occur spontaneously without clear precipitating factors.

Aspirin may dramatically relieve symptoms in a subset of patients with underlying myeloproliferative disease, but otherwise aspirin is rarely effective. Other agents that have been reported to relieve symptoms are presented later in the section on treatment. Many patients report that plunging their feet into ice water during an episode relieves their symptoms. Patients frequently report that the affected extremities must be exposed to cold surfaces or air-conditioned rooms or be immersed in buckets of cool or ice water to relieve their symptoms. A decrease in local temperature may decrease the severity of erythromelalgia or even abort an episode. Some patients sleep with their extremities outside the bedcovers, and some engage in unusual behaviors such as sleeping with their feet out a window, putting their feet in a refrigerator, walking barefoot in the snow, or storing shoes in a freezer. Kvernebo[10] described a patient who, for almost 25 years day and night, lived with a bucket of ice water at her side, immersing her feet intermittently for 15 to 30 minutes an hour. Thus, in what superficially appears to be the antithesis of Raynaud's phenomenon, patients seek relief by cooling the affected extremity.

Symptoms of erythromelalgia are intermittent, and the clinical examination is often normal. If the patient is examined during an episode of erythromelalgia, the affected extremity is tender, erythematous, and objectively hot. In up to two thirds of patients, affected extremities are discolored (blue/cyanotic, red, or mottled) and cool or cold to the touch, with varying degrees of discomfort between episodes. Raynaud's phenomenon is not uncommon between episodes, occurring in 15% of one series.[31]

The syndrome of erythromelalgia is frequently worsened when patients try to relieve their symptoms. For example, patients soak their feet in water and ice, which can lead to immersion irritant contact dermatitis or even frostbite. Allergic contact dermatitis due to substances that have been applied to the affected feet can occur. Other common vascular problems in the lower extremities such as edema, venous insufficiency, and lymphedema can be worsened by erythromelalgia. Patients may have high requirements for pain medications and become addicted to or dependent on narcotic analgesics. Psychiatric problems such as depression and obsessive-compulsive behaviors to avoid episodes of erythromelalgia can occur. The syndrome can be socially disabling if patients avoid exercising, walking, participating in sports, or leaving their homes, which leads to a sense of disablement, isolation, and loneliness. The syndrome frequently affects performance in the workplace (especially with manual work or jobs that entail standing) and at home.

Erythromelalgia predominantly affects individuals who are white and of any age. In the largest published series,[8] all 168 patients were white, the female-to-male ratio was approximately 3:1, and the mean age was 55.8 years (range, 5-91 years). Symptoms had been present since childhood in seven patients (4.2%), and six patients (3.6%) had a first-degree relative with erythromelalgia.

Erythromelalgia can also occur in the pediatric age group. In the largest pediatric series reported—32 patients (girls, 22 [69%]) seen at the Mayo Clinic[32]—mean age was 14.1 years (range, 5-18 years), and the diagnosis was delayed; mean time to diagnosis was 5.2 years. Seven patients (22%) had a first-degree relative with erythromelalgia; four were from the same family. Physical activity was limited in 21 patients (66%), and school attendance was affected in 11 patients (34%). Hypertension was not a feature of these patients. In contrast, Drenth et al.[33] described nine children in whom erythromelalgia was transient (seven girls and two boys, mean age 11.6 years); in seven, hypertension was directly related to the symptoms, and treatment of the hypertension with intravenous (IV) sodium nitroprusside relieved symptoms.

Diagnosis

Making the diagnosis is often a problem because objective findings may not be present during the physical examination, so the diagnosis may rest on history alone. However, because the differential diagnosis includes many possibilities, it is best to have evidence to support the diagnosis. The following may help:

1. Examine and assess the patient both during an episode and between episodes. Ask the patient to engage in an activity, such as climbing stairs, that will precipitate an episode.
2. If it is not possible to examine a patient during an episode, ask the patient to obtain a photograph of the affected areas during an episode.

Classification

Most authors agree on the fundamentals of the diagnosis of erythromelalgia, but there are many described criteria for diagnosis and many subclassifications of erythromelalgia. Use of these subclassifications may depend on whether one is a "lumper" or "splitter."[28,29,34] The most popular classification of erythromelalgia is into primary and secondary forms.

Primary Erythromelalgia

Primary erythromelalgia is defined by patients in whom no identifiable cause is found. This group includes the hereditary forms.

Secondary Erythromelalgia

Potential causes of secondary erythromelalgia are presented in Box 50-1. Erythromelalgia has been reported in association with myeloproliferative diseases, blood disorders, drugs, infectious diseases, food ingestion (mushrooms), neoplasms, connective tissue disease, physiological conditions (pregnancy), and neuropathies. An epidemic in China has been described.[66] The relationship of many underlying disorders to erythromelalgia is sometimes unclear, and the disorder may be a coincidental comorbidity rather than an underlying disease.

Among the reported series, the association with myeloproliferative disease seems most constant.[8,35–37] Evidence of underlying myeloproliferative disease should be sought at diagnosis and subsequently. Erythromelalgia can herald the onset of underlying myeloproliferative disease. In one series, erythromelalgia was the presenting symptom of essential thrombocythemia in 26 of 40 patients (65%)[36]; in another series, erythromelalgia was the presenting symptom in 11 of 268 patients with thrombocythemia (4%).[37]

Incidence

In a population-based study from Olmsted County, Minnesota, the overall age- and sex-adjusted incidence rate (95% confidence interval [95% CI]) was calculated to be 1.3 (0.8-1.7) per 100,000 persons per year. The incidence of primary and secondary erythromelalgia was 1.1 (0.7-1.5) and 0.2 (0.02-0.4) per 100,000 persons per year, respectively.[89] The incidence was noted to have increased over the past 3 decades. This incidence was approximately five times higher than that reported from Norway, where the incidence was calculated to be 2.5 to 3.3 per 1 million inhabitants per year in the Norwegian population, with a corresponding annual prevalence of 18 to 20 per 1 million.[10] Cases of borderline erythromelalgia were not included in these figures.[9,10]

Pathophysiology

The pathophysiology of erythromelalgia is not clearly understood. Part of the difficulty in understanding this disorder has been the heterogeneity of the affected population.[90] The underlying pathological mechanisms most likely involve a complex dysregulation of cutaneous blood flow that ultimately results in microvascular ischemia. Determining the nature of this dysfunction has also been challenging because control of cutaneous blood flow depends on an intricate interplay of systemic and local signals and is not completely understood.[90] A small-fiber neuropathy likely contributes to this dysregulation.[91,92]

Box 50-1 Reported Causes of Secondary Erythromelalgia

Condition or Agent

Myeloproliferative Diseases and Blood Disorders
Myeloproliferative disorders[8,35]
Essential thrombocythemia[36–41]
Polycythemia rubra vera[42,43]
Myelodysplastic syndrome[44]
Pernicious anemia[45]
Thrombotic thrombocytopenic purpura[46]
Idiopathic thrombocytopenic purpura[47]

Drugs
Cyclosporin[48]
Norephedrine[49]
Verapamil[50]
Nicardipine[51,52]
Nifedipine[53–55]
Pergolide mesylate[56]
Bromocriptine[57–59]

Infectious Diseases
Human immunodeficiency virus (HIV)[60,61]
Hepatitis B vaccine[62]
Influenza vaccine[63]
Infectious mononucleosis[64]
Pox virus[65]
Unknown agent[66]

Ingestion
Mushrooms[22,60]

Neoplastic
Abdominal cancer[67]
Paraneoplastic[68]
Astrocytoma[69]
Malignant thymoma[70]

Connective Tissue Disease
Systemic lupus erythematosus (SLE)[71–74]
Vasculitis[75]

Physiologic
Pregnancy[76]

Neuropathic
Hereditary sensory neuropathy[77]
Neuropathy[78]
Polyneuropathy[79]
Riley-Day's syndrome[80]
Multiple sclerosis[81]
Acute diabetic neuropathy[82]
Neurofibromatosis[83]

Inherited
X-linked dominant?[84]
Autosomal dominant[85]
Unknown[86]
Familial[87,88]

Erythromelalgia: a Vasculopathy?

Thermoregulatory control of human skin blood flow is vital to maintenance of normal body temperatures during challenges to thermal homeostasis. Sympathetic neural control of skin blood flow includes the noradrenergic vasoconstrictor system and a sympathetic active vasodilator system, the latter being responsible for 80% to 90% of the substantial cutaneous vasodilation that occurs with whole-body heat stress. With body heating, the magnitude of skin vasodilation is striking; skin blood flow can reach 6 to 8 L/min during hyperthermia.[93]

Erythromelalgia is a cutaneous microvascular disorder. Pathophysiology appears to relate to disorders of local or reflex thermoregulatory control of skin circulation.[93] Two paradoxical observations concerning blood flow during an episode of erythromelalgia have been made. During symptoms, there is increased blood flow. Sandroni et al.,[92] Mørk et al.,[9] and Kvernebo[10] confirmed that the observed erythema and warmth are associated with increased blood flow. Using laser Doppler, Sandroni et al. measured blood flow during symptoms and demonstrated increased perfusion during attacks. Paradoxically, however, this increased blood flow is accompanied by local hypoxia. Although there is increased perfusion during attacks, the values for transcutaneous oxygen tension are critically low, low, or unchanged—in other words, during symptoms, transcutaneous oximetry values decrease or do not change.[9,10,91,92] To explain this paradox, Mørk et al.[23] theorized and demonstrated that the increased blood flow is probably due to shunting through arteriovenous anastomoses, which results in hypoperfusion of the more superficial nutritive capillaries. If available blood is shunted away from normal skin capillaries, the skin will be hypoxic. Mørk et al. demonstrated that despite increased overall blood flow to the skin, the induction of erythromelalgia symptoms is accompanied by decreased perfusion of the superficial vascular plexus, as evidenced by a decreased density of skin capillaries. Thus their hypothesis is that dilation of arteriovenous anastomoses is directly responsible for shunting nutritive blood flow away from the superficial vascular plexus. Furthermore, Mørk et al.[21] postulated that erythromelalgia is not a disease, but rather a physiological response to stimuli such as infection, trauma, or tumor, and symptoms are caused by tissue hypoxia induced by maldistribution of microvascular blood flow in the skin, with increased thermoregulatory flow and inadequate perfusion.

Sandroni et al.[92] theorized that the effects of diminished perfusion could be exacerbated by increased metabolic demands in response to hyperthermia, ultimately resulting in hypoxic tissue damage and pain. Pain relief by cooling could be explained by a resultant decrease in the metabolic rate and a corresponding decrease in the need for oxygen.

Littleford et al.[30] described an underlying vasoconstrictor tendency in patients with erythromelalgia that may be related to functional or structural changes in skin microvessels, and noted that basal skin erythrocyte flux and skin temperature were lower in patients with a history of erythromelalgia than in controls. As noted earlier, Raynaud's phenomenon has been described in patients with erythromelalgia.[94,95] Acrocyanosis has also been described.[94] Davis et al.[91] have also noted that at baseline, the skin is cool and occasionally cyanotic between episodes in two thirds of patients.[31]

Erythromelalgia: a Neuropathy?

Several lines of evidence suggest that a neuropathy is associated with erythromelalgia, since the disorder has been described in association with many types of neuropathy. Both large- and small-fiber neuropathies are observed in a large proportion of patients with erythromelalgia (see Box 50-1).[91,92,96]

Among 57 patients with erythromelalgia who were evaluated with use of an autonomic reflex screen, results for 49 (86%) were abnormal, indicating a small-fiber neuropathy. The most common abnormalities were sudomotor abnormalities (i.e., absent or reduced sweat production).[91] In an earlier series, findings were similar for 17 of 27 patients (63%); whether the observed neuropathy led to erythromelalgia, or vice versa, is unclear.[92,98] In support of this, thermoregulatory sweat testing results were abnormal in 28 (88%) of 32 patients, and quantitative sudomotor axon reflex test results were abnormal in 22 patients (69%); abnormalities noted on thermoregulatory sweat testing varied from local hypohidrosis or anhidrosis to global anhidrosis.[96]

Conversely, in a series of 321 cases of disorders of autonomic neuropathy, the majority had erythromelalgia.[99] Orstavik et al.[100] used erythromelalgia as a model to study chronic pain and found changes in the conductive properties of C fibers in patients with erythromelalgia that were indicative of a small-fiber neuropathy. Additionally, an active contribution of mechanoinsensitive fibers to chronic pain was postulated. Uno and Parker[101] reported that the density of both acetylcholinesterase-positive and catecholamine-containing nerve terminals in the periarterial and sweat gland plexuses was much less in the skin of the erythermalgic foot than in the unaffected skin of the same patient, and much less than in the foot skin of a healthy person.

Layzer[102] wrote that it seems plausible to regard erythromelalgia as a problem of polymodal C-fiber receptors in sensitized skin. The threshold of C fibers to activation by heat would decrease to between 32 °C and 36 °C; activated C fibers would cause vasodilation by axon reflexes, resulting in redness, heat, and swelling. With cooling, the threshold for the nociceptors would increase.

Kazemi et al.[97] reported that 72.7% of the patients studied had abnormal sympathetic reflexes, which may result from an abnormality of the sympathetic nerves. Normal sympathetic nerve activity in skin without an associated vasoconstriction response has been found in a patient.[103] Littleford et al.[104] also noted findings suggesting that patients with erythromelalgia have diminished sympathetic vasoconstrictor responses to both cold challenge of the contralateral arm and inspiratory gasp; an interplay between neural and vasoactive agents was postulated.

Inherited Erythromelalgia

There is a subset of erythromelalgia that is inherited. In the largest reported series, the proportion of cases that are inherited was approximately 5%.[8] Inheritance in familial autosomal dominant (29 persons were affected in five generations) and X-linked dominant fashions have been reported. Clinical onset in familial cases usually occurs in childhood, most frequently prior to the age of 5 or 6, but occasionally is seen up to 10 or 12 years of age and, in rare families, at even older ages.

GAIN-OF-FUNCTION MUTATIONS IN SENSORY NERVES AND CONSEQUENT NERVE HYPEREXCITABILITY

In the inherited forms of erythromelalgia, there have been new developments in understanding the disease. It now appears that mutations in particular sodium channels in the nociceptors of sensory nerves lead to firing of nerves with little provocation; in other words, sensory nerves are hyperexcitable. In 2001, Drenth et al. investigated DNA from five families with hereditary erythromelalgia using linkage analysis and located the gene responsible to chromosome 2q31-32.[105] Based on this work, Yang et al. subsequently reported that mutations in the gene SCN9A on this chromosome caused primary erythromelalgia.[106] Cummins et al. showed that functionally this gene encoded the Nav 1.7 sodium channel; mutations in this gene leads to altered channel function in nerves.[107] These mutations are preferentially expressed by the dorsal root ganglion and sympathetic ganglion neuron. In 2005, Michiels et al. reported that a mutation in this gene occurred in all five affected members of a Flemish family and in none of five unaffected members.[108] Han et al. described a patient with onset of erythromelalgia in the second decade and suggested that mutations that lead to lesser changes in sodium channel activation are associated with lesser neuron excitability and later onset of clinical signs.[109]

The implications of these findings are significant, since these mutated sodium channels could be a therapeutic target, and more widely, other pain syndromes also involve altered sodium channel function.[110] In an editorial in 2005, Waxman and Dib-Hajj stated, "Erythromelalgia is the first human disorder in which it has been possible to associate an ion channel mutation with chronic neuropathic pain … erythromelalgia may emerge as a model disease that holds more general lessons about the molecular neurobiology of chronic pain."[111]

It is important to bear in mind that these findings have been described in the inherited form of erythromelalgia thus far and not the more common noninherited forms. Additionally, SCN9A mutation is not always present in inherited erythromelalgia. Drenth et al. identified this mutation in only 1 of 15 patients with a family history of the disease.[112]

ERYTHROMELALGIA ASSOCIATED WITH A MYELOPROLIFERATIVE DISEASE

Erythromelalgia in the setting of thrombocythemia or myeloproliferative diseases seems to be a separate entity, although it presents similarly to other forms of erythromelalgia. Recognition of the associated myeloproliferative disease is vital because in these specific types of erythromelalgia, aspirin provides immediate and long-lived relief from symptoms. Thrombin, platelet function, and genetics have been considered in studies of erythromelalgia. Van Genderen et al.[113] noted that thrombocythemia-associated erythromelalgia may develop despite treatment with oral anticoagulants or heparin, suggesting that generation of thrombin is not a prerequisite for development of erythromelalgia. Disordered platelet function affecting the microvasculature has been implicated in thrombocythemia-related erythromelalgia.[114]

Pathophysiological Controversies

Several questions about erythromelalgia remain. Does a neuropathy cause the vasculopathy, or does the vasculopathy cause a neuropathy?[91] What causes the neuropathy if it is not caused by the vasculopathy? In the inherited form, mutations in the sodium channel lead to hyperexcitability of sensory nerves. Similar mutations have not been described in the sporadic form, which accounts for 95% of cases. What is the pathophysiology in these forms? How does dysfunction of the precapillary sphincter affect this disease? Schechner[90] pointed out that it is unknown whether shunting of blood through arteriovenous anastomoses alone can induce hypoxia severe enough to induce pain, particularly in areas that contain few arteriovenous anastomoses. Potentially inadequate compensatory dilation, or even inappropriate constriction of the precapillary sphincter, may compound the effects of the relative hypoperfusion. What factors are responsible for vascular dysfunction? Both autonomic neuropathy[21,92] and endothelial injury[115] have been observed in patients with erythromelalgia, but it is not known whether this damage to critical vasoregulatory components is primary or secondary to chronic hypoxia.

Differential Diagnosis

Any condition causing extremity pain could be mistaken for erythromelalgia. In particular, unwarranted diagnosis of erythromelalgia can result from any clinical situation that includes burning sensations in the limbs.[116] However, the syndrome of erythromelalgia is specific for red, hot extremities. The following conditions are included in the differential diagnosis:

- Neuropathies: peripheral neuropathy, small-fiber neuropathy, reflex sympathetic dystrophy.
- Vascular: large vessel disease, small-vessel disease, Raynaud's phenomenon, Raynaud's disease, arterial insufficiency, venous insufficiency (which can produce sensations of warm feet, often at bedtime, with edema and an increase in local heat).
- Metabolic: painful crises associated with Fabry's disease (a hereditary sphingolipidosis transmitted on chromosome X that occurs predominantly in men, often starting early in childhood with a burning sensation in the limbs).
- Skin: dermatitis, immersion foot.
- Infectious: erysipelas.
- Bone: osteomyelitis.
- Exogenous: acrodynia (a rare disease caused by excessive mercury intake and confirmed by high mercury levels in the urine, in which the main sign is vasomotor impairment in the limbs, and the red hands and feet have an intense, paroxysmal, burn-type pain).

Investigations

To investigate the possibility of erythromelalgia, the clinician should take the following steps:

1. Get a detailed history, and perform a physical examination with respect to each element of the history outlined earlier.
2. If signs of erythromelalgia are not present during the examination, ask the patient to photograph the affected area when symptoms are apparent.
3. Evaluate the results of a complete blood cell (CBC) count, including total and differential leukocyte counts.
4. Investigate the possibility of underlying disease, as indicated by the patient's age, history, and physical examination.
5. Consider further investigations as outlined in Box 50-2, especially for small-fiber neuropathy and large-fiber neuropathy, and for noninvasive vascular studies during symptoms and between symptoms (as detailed by Davis et al.[91]) to better define the pathophysiology. Results of these tests are useful to confirm the diagnosis and help guide therapy.
6. In the inherited form, molecular genetic testing for mutations in SCN9A is available on a clinical basis.

Biopsy Findings

Reports of skin biopsies for erythromelalgia are scant. In the series reported by Davis et al.,[8] only 12 of the 168 patients with primary erythromelalgia had a biopsy, and the biopsy specimens showed no specific abnormalities. Three cases of primary erythromelalgia were reported by Drenth et al.,[115] and similarly, the biopsy specimens showed nonspecific changes.

The histopathological changes in cases of erythromelalgia related to thrombocythemia have been characterized by Michiels and associates.[36] Arteriolar inflammation, fibromuscular intimal proliferation, and thrombotic occlusions were noted.[117] Croue et al.[118] noted similar changes in a case of erythromelalgia related to essential thrombocythemia. Biopsies from a few patients with drug-induced erythromelalgia have been described. Biopsies from a patient with verapamil-induced erythromelalgia showed mild perivascular mononuclear infiltrate and moderate perivascular edema.[50] Among three patients with erythromelalgia due to bromocriptine, biopsies showed a prominent perivascular lymphocytic infiltration and perivascular edema of the dermis without frank vasculitis.[58]

Natural History and Prognosis

Information concerning the prognosis of this condition is limited.[8,12] In a study of the natural history of erythromelalgia in which 168 patients were studied, with a mean follow-up of 8.7 years (range, 1.3-20 years), Kaplan-Meier survival curves showed a significant decrease in survival compared with expected survival among people matched for age and sex from the U.S. general population ($P<.001$).[8] Of 94 patients questioned about their symptoms, 30 (31.9%) reported that their symptoms had worsened, 25 (26.6%) had not changed, 29 (30.9%) had improved, and 10 (10.6%) had completely resolved.

At the time of the most recent follow-up, 45 of the 168 patients (26.8%) had died. Causes of death included myeloproliferative disease, cardiovascular disease, and cancer. Importantly, three patients with severe symptoms had committed suicide. In a series of patients with pediatric erythromelalgia, one patient had committed suicide.[32]

Kalgaard et al.[12] reported that about two thirds of 87 patients studied had primary cases, and about three quarters had some form of chronic condition. Over time in the patients with erythromelalgia, the condition gradually became worse. In patients with primary or secondary acute erythromelalgia, the condition improved, and in patients with primary or secondary chronic erythromelalgia, the condition remained stable.

Thus overall, it can be concluded from these studies that some patients become worse, some have a stable course, and some get better or even have full resolution of erythromelalgia with time. It is notable that some patients experienced cure.[8]

Quality of Life

Erythromelalgia has a markedly negative effect on quality of life. One study has directly measured quality-of-life parameters.[8] The Medical Outcomes Study 36-Item Short Form Health Survey was used, and the results of this questionnaire were compared with scores obtained from a cohort from the U.S. general population. The questionnaire is a standard survey that measures health-related quality-of-life outcomes and measures each of eight health concepts (or domains) on a five-point Likert scale: physical functioning, role limitations due to physical disease, bodily pain, general health, vitality (energy and fatigue), social functioning, role limitations due to emotional problems, and mental health (psychological stress and psychological well-being). Scores for all but one of the health domains were significantly less in the study population than in the U.S. general population. The lowest scores were in the physical functioning domain.

Management

Management of erythromelalgia is difficult. There are no randomized controlled studies of treatments for erythromelalgia, and no single treatment is effective in all cases. The literature is replete with case reports and small case series describing a response to one treatment or another. When a larger group of erythromelalgia patients was surveyed, the majority reported that no treatment was very effective. Various treatments used in the management of erythromelalgia have been reviewed.[119]

One algorithmic approach to the management of erythromelalgia is as follows:

1. General measures:
   a. Patient education regarding the condition.
   b. Avoidance of factors that precipitate events.
   c. Judicious use of factors to relieve pain during symptoms.
   d. Patient support groups such as the Erythromelalgia Association.

> ### Box 50-2　Investigation Protocol for Patients Presenting with Erythromelalgia
>
> **Clinical**
> History
> Physical examination
>
> **Peripheral Vascular Laboratory**
> Studies of the following parameters in affected extremities, with and without symptoms:
> Color change
> Skin temperature and core temperature
> Blood flow (laser Doppler flowmetry)
> Oxygen saturation (transcutaneous oximetry)
> Ankle-brachial indices (ABIs)
>
> **Neurological Evaluation**
> Electromyography
> Autonomic nerve studies:
> 　Quantitative sudomotor axon reflex test (QSART)
> 　Heart rate response to deep breathing and Valsalva ratio (cardiovagal functioning)
> 　Adrenergic function testing
> Thermoregulatory sweat testing
> Consultation with neurologist specializing in autonomic nerve studies if results of the above tests are abnormal

Modified from Davis MDP, Sandroni P, Rooke TW, et al: Erythromelalgia: vasculopathy, neuropathy, or both? A prospective study of vascular and neurophysiologic studies in erythromelalgia. Arch Dermatol 139:1337, 2003.[91]

2. Topical medications:
    a. Lidocaine patches.[120,121]
    b. Amitriptyline/ketamine.[122]
3. Systemic medications (see later discussion).
4. Pain rehabilitation program.[123]

Aspirin[3,36,42] has been reported to abolish erythromelalgia, especially in initial reports of the syndrome. It has become increasingly evident that aspirin may be effective in erythromelalgia due to myeloproliferative disease, but it is rarely effective in other forms of erythromelalgia.[8,124]

Increasingly, drugs acting on the nervous system are reported to be useful in inducing remission of disease or in controlling symptoms. These include selective serotonin reuptake inhibitors (SSRIs) such as venlafaxine and sertraline,[125,126] tricyclic antidepressants such as amitriptyline,[77] and anticonvulsants such as gabapentin.[127] Intravenous lidocaine followed by oral mexiletine[128] induced remission in a patient with long-standing erythromelalgia. Topical capsaicin was helpful in one report[129] but not in others.[8] Benzodiazepines such as clonazepam are effective occasionally.[72] Sympathectomy and sympathetic nerve blocks have been reported to both relieve and exacerbate erythromelalgia.[16,130-133] Stereotactic thalamotomy,[134] ankle nerve crushing and neurectomy,[135] and spinal cord stimulation[136] have been reported to be helpful. Drugs acting on the vascular system (vasoactive drugs) may be effective. β-Blockers such as propranolol[137] and labetalol[33] have been reported to be successful in single cases. Calcium antagonists have been reported to both relieve and exacerbate erythromelalgia.[8,124] Various doses of magnesium have been reported to relieve symptoms.[138] Sodium nitroprusside infusions may be helpful in children with erythromelalgia,[139-142] but one adult experienced worsening of the disease with this medication.[124] Prostaglandin E$_1$ (PGE$_1$), a potent vasodilator and platelet inhibitor administered intravenously, has successfully induced remission.[10,30,139] Iloprost, a synthetic prostacyclin analog, improved patients' symptoms more than placebo did.[143] Use of ergot alkaloids, such as methysergide maleate, has been described in isolated case reports.[82,144] Low-molecular-weight heparin (LMWH) has been reported to exacerbate erythromelalgia.[140]

Control of pain is an extremely important factor in erythromelalgia. Anesthetics have been used, including topical lidocaine (lidocaine patch),[145] a combination of topical amitriptyline and ketamine,[122] and epidural infusion of narcotic analgesic medications such as bupivacaine, sometimes in combination with other narcotic drugs.[146-149] Narcotic analgesic drugs may be administered by various routes—oral, intravenous, intramuscular (IM),[150] epidural,[149] or intrathecal,[151] alone or in combination with other drugs. Nonsteroidal antiinflammatory drugs (NSAIDs) such as piroxicam[152] may be helpful occasionally.

Pizotyline, a benzocycloheptathiophene derivative used primarily for migraine prophylaxis, has been used for erythromelalgia.[33,153,154] Systemic corticosteroids, including prednisone[155] and prednisolone,[156] and growth hormone[157] have been useful in single cases. Antihistamines such as cyproheptadine[158] have been reported to help, but many patients find them unhelpful.

A combination of pharmacological interventions may be of benefit.[63,159] Nonmedicinal therapies such as acupuncture, biofeedback, hypnosis, and magnets have been variably effective.[124,160]

Pain rehabilitation is a useful method for managing pain-related impairment in physical and emotional functioning in patients with severe forms of erythromelalgia.[123]

REFERENCES

1. Graves RJ: *Clinical lectures on the practice of medicine*, Dublin, 1834, Fannin.
2. Mitchell SW: On a rare vaso-motor neurosis of the extremities and on the maladies with which it may be confounded, *Am J Med Sci* 76:17, 1878.
3. Smith LA, Allen EV: Erythermalgia (erythromelalgia) of the extremities: a syndrome characterized by redness, heat, and pain, *Am Heart J* 16:175, 1938.
4. Housley E: What is erythromelalgia and how should it be treated? *BMJ* 293:117, 1986.
5. Lewis T: Clinical observations and experiments relating to burning pain in extremities and to so-called "erythromelalgia" in particular, *Clin Sci* 1:175, 1933.
6. Snapper I, Kahn AI: *Bedside medicine*, ed 2, London, 1967, William Heinemann Medical Books p 106.
7. Babb RR, Alarcon-Segovia D, Fairbairn JF II: Erythermalgia: review of 51 cases, *Circulation* 29:136, 1964.
8. Davis MD, O'Fallon WM, Rogers RS III, et al: Natural history of erythromelalgia: presentation and outcome in 168 patients, *Arch Dermatol* 136:330, 2000.
9. Mørk C, Kalgaard OM, Kvernebo K: Erythromelalgia: a clinical study of 102 cases (abstract), *Australas J Dermatol* 38(Suppl 2):50, 1997.
10. Kvernebo K: Erythromelalgia: a condition caused by microvascular arteriovenous shunting, *VASA J Vasc Dis Suppl* 51:1, 1998.
11. Hart FD: William Harvey and his gout, *Ann Rheum Dis* 43:125, 1984.
12. Kalgaard OM, Seem E, Kvernebo K: Erythromelalgia: a clinical study of 87 cases, *J Intern Med* 242:191, 1997.
13. Levesque H: Classification of erythermalgia [French], *J Mal Vasc* 21:80, 1996.
14. Mørk C, Kvernebo K: Erythromelalgia: a mysterious condition? *Arch Dermatol* 136:406, 2000.
15. Michiels JJ, Drenth JP, Van Genderen PJ: Classification and diagnosis of erythromelalgia and erythermalgia, *Int J Dermatol* 34:97, 1995.
16. Zoppi M, Zamponi A, Pagni E, et al: A way to understand erythromelalgia, *J Auton Nerv Syst* 13:85, 1985.
17. Regli F: Facial neuralgia and vascular facial pain [German], *Praxis* 58:210, 1969.
18. Brown GE: Erythromelalgia and other disturbances of the extremities accompanied by vasodilatation and burning, *Am J Med Sci* 183:468, 1932.
19. Thompson GH, Hahn G, Rang M: Erythromelalgia, *Clin Orthop* 144:249, 1979.
20. Mørk C, Asker CL, Salerud EG, et al: Microvascular arteriovenous shunting is a probable pathogenetic mechanism in erythromelalgia, *J Invest Dermatol* 114:643, 2000.
21. Mørk C, Kalgaard OM, Kvernebo K: Impaired neurogenic control of skin perfusion in erythromelalgia, *J Invest Dermatol* 118:699, 2002.
22. Mørk C, Kalgaard OM, Myrvang B, et al: Erythromelalgia in a patient with AIDS, *J Eur Acad Dermatol Venereol* 14:498, 2000.
23. Mørk C, Kvernebo K, Asker CL, et al: Reduced skin capillary density during attacks of erythromelalgia implies arteriovenous shunting as pathogenetic mechanism, *J Invest Dermatol* 119:949, 2002.
24. Lazareth I, Fiessinger JN, Priollet P: Erythermalgia, rare acrosyndrome: 13 cases [French], *Presse Med* 17:2235, 1988.
25. Drenth JP, Michiels JJ, van Joost T: Primary and secondary erythermalgia [Dutch], *Ned Tijdschr Geneeskd* 138:2231, 1994.
26. Drenth JP, Michiels JJ: Erythromelalgia and erythermalgia: diagnostic differentiation, *Int J Dermatol* 33:393, 1994.
27. Drenth JP, Michiels JJ: Erythromelalgia versus primary and secondary erythermalgia, *Angiology* 45:329, 1994.
28. Drenth JP, van Genderen PJ, Michiels JJ: Thrombocythemic erythromelalgia, primary erythermalgia, and secondary erythermalgia: three distinct clinicopathologic entities, *Angiology* 45:451, 1994.
29. Kurzrock R, Cohen PR: Classification and diagnosis of erythromelalgia, *Int J Dermatol* 34:146, 1995.
30. Littleford RC, Khan F, Belch JJ: Skin perfusion in patients with erythromelalgia, *Eur J Clin Invest* 29:588, 1999.
31. Davis MD, Wilkins F, Rooke TW: Between episodes of erythromelalgia: a spectrum of colors, *Arch Dermatol* 142:1085, 2006.
32. Cook-Norris RH, Tollefson MM, Cruz-Inigo AE, et al: Pediatric erythromelalgia: a retrospective review of 32 cases evaluated at Mayo Clinic over a 37-year period, *J Am Acad Dermatol* 66:416, 2012.
33. Drenth JPH, Michiels JJ, Özsoylu S: Erythermlgia Multidisciplinary Study Group: acute secondary erythermalgia and hypertension in children, *Eur J Pediatr* 154:882, 1995.
34. Michiels JJ, Drenth JP: Erythromelalgia and erythermalgia: lumpers and splitters, *Int J Dermatol* 33:412, 1994.
35. Kurzrock R, Cohen PR: Erythromelalgia and myeloproliferative disorders, *Arch Intern Med* 149:105, 1989.
36. Michiels JJ, Abels J, Steketee J, et al: Erythromelalgia caused by platelet-mediated arteriolar inflammation and thrombosis in thrombocythemia, *Ann Intern Med* 102:466, 1985.
37. Itin PH, Winkelmann RK: Cutaneous manifestations in patients with essential thrombocythemia, *J Am Acad Dermatol* 24:59, 1991.
38. Michiels JJ, ten Kate FJ: Erythromelalgia in thrombocythemia of various myeloproliferative disorders, *Am J Hematol* 39:131, 1992.
39. McCarthy L, Eichelberger L, Skipworth E, et al: Erythromelalgia due to essential thrombocythemia, *Transfusion* 42:1245, 2002.
40. Michiels JJ, van Genderen PJ, Lindemans J, et al: Erythromelalgic, thrombotic and hemorrhagic manifestations in 50 cases of thrombocythemia, *Leuk Lymphoma* 22(Suppl 1): 47, 1996.
41. Naldi L, Brevi A, Cavalieri d'Oro L, et al: Painful distal erythema and thrombocytosis: erythromelalgia secondary to thrombocytosis, *Arch Dermatol* 129:105, 1993.
42. Ongenae K, Janssens A, Noens L, et al: Erythromelalgia: a clue to the diagnosis of polycythemia vera, *Dermatology* 192:408, 1996.
43. Kudo I, Soejima K, Morimoto S, et al: Polycythemia vera associated with erythromelalgia [Japanese], *Rinsho Ketsueki* 29:1055, 1988.
44. Coppa LM, Nehal KS, Young JW, et al: Erythromelalgia precipitated by acral erythema in the setting of thrombocytopenia, *J Am Acad Dermatol* 48:973, 2003.
45. Mehle AL, Nedorost S, Camisa C: Erythromelalgia, *Int J Dermatol* 29:567, 1990.
46. Yosipovitch G, Krause I, Blickstein D: Erythromelalgia in a patient with thrombotic thrombocytopenic purpura, *J Am Acad Dermatol* 26:825, 1992.
47. Rey J, Cretel E, Jean R, et al: Erythromelalgia in a patient with idiopathic thrombocytopenic purpura (letter), *Br J Dermatol* 148:177, 2003.
48. Thami GP, Bhalla M: Erythromelalgia induced by possible calcium channel blockade by ciclosporin, *BMJ* 326:910, 2003.
49. Wagner DR, Spengel F, Middeke M: Erythromelalgia unmasked during norephedrine therapy: a case report, *Angiology* 44:244, 1993.
50. Drenth JP, Michiels JJ, Van Joost T, et al: Verapamil-induced secondary erythermalgia, *Br J Dermatol* 127:292, 1992.

51. Levesque H, Moore N, Wolfe LM, et al: Erythromelalgia induced by nicardipine (inverse Raynaud's phenomenon?), *BMJ* 298:1252, 1989.

52. Drenth JP: Erythromelalgia induced by nicardipine (letter), *BMJ* 298:1582, 1989.

53. Albers GW, Simon LT, Hamik A, et al: Nifedipine versus propranolol for the initial prophylaxis of migraine, *Headache* 29:215, 1989.

54. Brodmerkel GJ Jr: Nifedipine and erythromelalgia (letter), *Ann Intern Med* 99:415, 1983.

55. Fisher JR, Padnick MB, Olstein S: Nifedipine and erythromelalgia, *Ann Intern Med* 98:671, 1983.

56. Monk BE, Parkes JD, Du Vivier A: Erythromelalgia following pergolide administration, *Br J Dermatol* 111:97, 1984.

57. Dupont E, Illum F, Olivarius BF: Bromocriptine and erythromelalgia-like eruptions (letter), *Neurology* 33:670, 1983.

58. Eisler T, Hall RP, Kalavar KA, et al: Erythromelalgia-like eruption in parkinsonian patients treated with bromocriptine, *Neurology* 31:1368, 1981.

59. Calne DB, Plotkin C, Williams AC, et al: Long-term treatment of parkinsonism with bromocriptine, *Lancet* 1:735, 1978.

60. Dolan CK, Hall MA, Turlansky GW: Secondary erythermalgia in an HIV-1-positive patient, *AIDS Read* 113:91, 2003.

61. Itin PH, Courvoisier S, Stoll A, et al: Secondary erythermalgia in an HIV-infected patient: is there a pathogenic relationship? *Acta Derm Venereol* 76:332, 1996.

62. Rabaud C, Barbaud A, Trechot P: First case of erythermalgia related to hepatitis B vaccination, *J Rheumatol* 26:233, 1999.

63. Confino I, Passwell JH, Padeh S: Erythromelalgia following influenza vaccine in a child, *Clin Exp Rheumatol* 15:111, 1997.

64. Clayton C, Faden H: Erythromelalgia in a twenty-year-old with infectious mononucleosis, *Pediatr Infect Dis J* 12:101, 1993.

65. Zheng ZM, Specter S, Zhang JH, et al: Further characterization of the biological and pathogenic properties of erythromelalgia-related poxviruses, *J Gen Virol* 73:2011, 1992.

66. Mo YM: An epidemiological study on erythromelalgia [Chinese], *Zhonghua Liu Xing Bing Xue Za Zhi* 10:291, 1989.

67. Mørk C, Kalgaard OM, Kvernebo K: Erythromelalgia as a paraneoplastic syndrome in a patient with abdominal cancer (letter), *Acta Derm Venereol* 79:394, 1999.

68. Kurzrock R, Cohen PR: Paraneoplastic erythromelalgia, *Clin Dermatol* 11:73, 1993.

69. Levine AM, Gustafson PR: Erythromelalgia: case report and literature review, *Arch Phys Med Rehabil* 68:119, 1987.

70. Lantrade P, Didier A, Ille H, et al: Thymome malin et acrosyndromes vasculaires paroxystiques: une observation, *Ann Med Interne (Paris)* 131:228, 1980.

71. Cailleux N, Levesque H, Courtois H: Erythermalgia and systemic lupus erythematosus [French], *J Mal Vasc* 21:88, 1996.

72. Kraus A: Erythromelalgia in a patient with systemic lupus erythematosus treated with clonazepam, *J Rheumatol* 17:120, 1990.

73. Michiels JJ: Erythermalgia in SLE, *J Rheumatol* 18:481, 1991.

74. Alarcon-Segovia D, Diaz-Jouanen E: Case report: erythermalgia in systemic lupus erythematosus, *Am J Med Sci* 266:149, 1973.

75. Drenth JP, Michiels JJ, Van Joost T, et al: Erythermalgia secondary to vasculitis, *Am J Med* 94:549, 1993.

76. Garrett SJ, Robinson JK: Erythromelalgia and pregnancy, *Arch Dermatol* 126:157, 1990.

77. Herskovitz S, Loh F, Berger AR, et al: Erythromelalgia: association with hereditary sensory neuropathy and response to amitriptyline, *Neurology* 43:621, 1993.

78. Staub DB, Munger BL, Uno H, et al: Erythromelalgia as a form of neuropathy, *Arch Dermatol* 128:1654, 1992.

79. Nagamatsu M, Ueno S, Teramoto J, et al: A case of erythromelalgia with polyneuropathy [Japanese], *Nippon Naika Gakkai Zasshi* 78:418, 1989.

80. Tridon P, Vidailhet C, Schweitzer F: The acrodynic form of the Riley-Day syndrome [French], *Pediatrie* 44:455, 1989.

81. Cendrowski W: Secondary erythromelalgia in multiple sclerosis [Polish], *Wiad Lek* 41:1477, 1988.

82. Vendrell J, Nubiola A, Goday A, et al: Erythromelalgia associated with acute diabetic neuropathy: an unusual condition, *Diabetes Res* 7:149, 1988.

83. Kikuchi I, Inoue S, Tada S: A unique erythermalgia in a patient with von Recklinghausen neurofibromatosis, *J Dermatol* 12:436, 1985.

84. van Genderen PJ, Michiels JJ, Drenth JP: Hereditary erythermalgia and acquired erythromelalgia, *Am J Med Genet* 45:530, 1993.

85. Finley WH, Lindsey JR Jr, Fine JD, et al: Autosomal dominant erythromelalgia, *Am J Med Genet* 42:310, 1992.

86. Michiels JJ, van Joost T, Vuzevski VD: Idiopathic erythermalgia: a congenital disorder, *J Am Acad Dermatol* 21:1128, 1989.

87. Cohen IJ, Samorodin CS: Familial erythromelalgia, *Arch Dermatol* 118:953, 1982.

88. Krebs A, Andres HU: On the clinical features of erythromelalgia: familial incidence of an idiopathic form in mother and daughter [German], *Schweiz Med Wochenschr* 99:344, 1969.

89. Reed KB, Davis MD: Incidence of erythromelalgia: a population-based study in Olmsted County, Minnesota, *J Eur Acad Dermatol Venereol* 23:13, 2009.

90. Schechner J: Red skin re-read, *J Invest Dermatol* 119:781, 2002.

91. Davis MDP, Sandroni P, Rooke TW, et al: Erythromelalgia: vasculopathy, neuropathy, or both? A prospective study of vascular and neurophysiologic studies in erythromelalgia, *Arch Dermatol* 139:1337, 2003.

92. Sandroni P, Davis MDP, Harper CM Jr, et al: Neurophysiologic and vascular studies in erythromelalgia: a retrospective analysis, *J Clin Neuromuscul Dis* 1:57, 1999.

93. Charkoudian N: Skin blood flow in adult human thermoregulation: how it works, when it does not, and why, *Mayo Clin Proc* 78:603, 2003.

94. Lazareth I, Priollet P: Coexistence of Raynaud's syndrome and erythromelalgia (letter), *Lancet* 335:1286, 1990.

95. Slutsker GE: Coexistence of Raynaud's syndrome and erythromelalgia (letter), *Lancet* 335:853, 1990.

96. Davis MD, Genebriera J, Sandroni P, et al: Thermoregulatory sweat testing in patients with erythromelalgia, *Arch Dermatol* 142:1583–1588, 2006.

97. Kazemi B, Shooshtari SM, Nasab MR, et al: Sympathetic skin response (SSR) in erythromelalgia, *Electromyogr Clin Neurophysiol* 43:165, 2003.

98. Davis MD, Rooke TW, Sandroni P: Mechanisms other than shunting are likely contributing to the pathophysiology of erythromelalgia, *J Invest Dermatol* 115:1166, 2000.

99. Liu Y: A study of erythromelalgia in relation to the autonomic nervous system: report of 321 cases of functional disorders of the autonomic nervous system [Chinese], *Zhonghua Shen Jing Jing Shen Ke Za Zhi* 23:47, 1990.

100. Orstavik K, Weidner C, Schmidt R, et al: Pathological C-fibres in patients with a chronic painful condition, *Brain* 126:567, 2003.

101. Uno H, Parker F: Autonomic innervation of the skin in primary erythermalgia, *Arch Dermatol* 119:65, 1983.

102. Layzer RB: Hot feet: erythromelalgia and related disorders, *J Child Neurol* 16:199, 2001.

103. Sugiyama Y, Hakusui S, Takahashi A, et al: Primary erythromelalgia: the role of skin sympathetic nerve activity, *Jpn J Med* 30:564, 1991.

104. Littleford RC, Khan F, Belch JJ: Impaired skin vasomotor reflexes in patients with erythromelalgia, *Clin Sci (Lond)* 96:507, 1999.

105. Drenth JP, Finley WH, Breedveld GJ, et al: The primary erythromelalgia-susceptibility gene is located on chromosome 32, *Am J Hum Genet* 68:1277, 2001.

106. Yang Y, Wang Y, Li S, et al: Mutations in SCN9A, encoding a sodium channel alpha subunit, in patients with primary erythromelalgia, *J Med Genet* 41:171, 2004.

107. Cummins TR, Dib-Hajj SD, Waxman SG: Electrophysiological properties of mutant Nav1.7 sodium channels in a painful inherited neuropathy, *J Neurosci* 24:8232, 2004.

108. Michiels JJ, te Morsche RH, Jansen JB, et al: Autosomal dominant erythermalgia associated with a novel mutation in the voltage-gated sodium channel alpha subunit Nav1.7, *Arch Neurol* 62:1587, 2005.

109. Han C, Dib-Hajj SD, Lin Z, et al: Early- and late-onset inherited erythromelalgia: genotype-phenotype correlation, *Brain* 132:1711, 2009.

110. Estacion M, Waxman SG, Dib-Hajj SD: Effects of ranolazine on wild-type and mutant hNav1.7 channels and on DRG neuron excitability, *Mol Pain* 6:35, 2010.

111. Waxman SG, Dib-Hajj S: Erythromelalgia: molecular basis for an inherited pain syndrome, *Trends Mol Med* 11:555, 2005.

112. Drenth JP, Te Morsche RH, Mansour S, et al: Primary erythermalgia as a sodium channelopathy: screening for SCN9A mutations: exclusion of a causal role of SCN10A and SCN11A, *Arch Dermatol* 144:320, 2008.

113. van Genderen PJ, Lucas IS, van Strik R, et al: Erythromelalgia in essential thrombocythemia is characterized by platelet activation and endothelial cell damage but not by thrombin generation, *Thromb Haemost* 76:333, 1996.

114. Kurzrock R, Cohen PR: Erythromelalgia: review of clinical characteristics and pathophysiology, *Am J Med* 91:416, 1991.

115. Drenth JP, Vuzevski V, Van Joost T, et al: Cutaneous pathology in primary erythromelalgia, *Am J Dermatopathol* 18:30, 1996.

116. Lazareth I: False erythromelalgia [French], *J Mal Vasc* 21:84, 1996.

117. Michiels JJ, ten Kate FW, Vuzevski VD, et al: Histopathology of erythromelalgia in thrombocythaemia, *Histopathology* 8:669, 1984.

118. Croue A, Gardembas-Pain M, Verret JL, et al: Histopathologic lesions in erythromelalgia during essential thrombocythemia [French], *Ann Pathol* 13:128, 1993.

119. Davis MD, Rooke T: Erythromelalgia, *Curr Treat Options Cardiovasc Med* 4:207, 2002.

120. Davis MD, Sandroni P: Lidocaine patch for pain of erythromelalgia: follow-up of 34 patients, *Arch Dermatol* 141:1320, 2005.

121. Davis MD, Sandroni P: Lidocaine patch for pain of erythromelalgia, *Arch Dermatol* 138:17–19, 2002.

122. Sandroni P, Davis MD: Combination gel of 1% amitriptyline and 0.5% ketamine to treat refractory erythromelalgia pain: a new treatment option? *Arch Dermatol* 142:283, 2006.

123. Durosaro O, Davis MD, Hooten WM, et al: Intervention for erythromelalgia, a chronic pain syndrome: comprehensive pain rehabilitation center, Mayo Clinic, *Arch Dermatol* 144:1578, 2008.

124. Cohen JS: Erythromelalgia: new theories and new therapies, *J Am Acad Dermatol* 43:841, 2000.

125. Rudikoff D, Jaffe IA: Erythromelalgia: response to serotonin reuptake inhibitors, *J Am Acad Dermatol* 37:281, 1997.

126. Moiin A, Yashar SS, Sanchez JE, et al: Treatment of erythromelalgia with a serotonin/noradrenaline reuptake inhibitor, *Br J Dermatol* 146:336, 2002.

127. McGraw T, Kosek P: Erythromelalgia pain managed with gabapentin, *Anesthesiology* 86:988, 1997.

128. Kuhnert SM, Phillips WJ, Davis MD: Lidocaine and mexiletine therapy for erythromelalgia, *Arch Dermatol* 135:1447, 1999.

129. Muhiddin KA, Gallen IW, Harries S, et al: The use of capsaicin cream in a case of erythromelalgia, *Postgrad Med J* 70:841, 1994.

130. Postlethwaite JC: Lumbar sympathectomy: a retrospective study of 142 operations on 100 patients, *Br J Surg* 60:878, 1973.

131. Shiga T, Sakamoto A, Koizumi K, et al: Endoscopic thoracic sympathectomy for primary erythromelalgia in the upper extremities, *Anesth Analg* 88:865, 1999.

132. Takeda S, Tomaru T, Higuchi M: A case of primary erythromelalgia (erythermalgia) treated with neural blockade [Japanese], *Masui* 38:383, 1989.

133. Seishima M, Kanoh H, Izumi T, et al: A refractory case of secondary erythermalgia successfully treated with lumbar sympathetic ganglion block, *Br J Dermatol* 143:868, 2000.

134. Kandel EI: Stereotactic surgery of erythromelalgia, *Stereotact Funct Neurosurg* 54–55:96, 1990.

135. Sadighi PJ, Arbid EJ: Neurectomy for palliation of primary erythermalgia, *Ann Vasc Surg* 9:197, 1995.

136. Graziotti PJ, Goucke CR: Control of intractable pain in erythromelalgia by using spinal cord stimulation, *J Pain Symptom Manage* 8:502, 1993.

137. Bada JL: Treatment of erythromelalgia with propranolol, *Lancet* 2:412, 1977.

138. Cohen JS: High-dose oral magnesium treatment of chronic, intractable erythromelalgia, *Ann Pharmacother* 36:255, 2002.

139. Kvernebo K, Seem E: Erythromelalgia—pathophysiological and therapeutic aspects: a preliminary report, *J Oslo City Hosp* 37:9, 1987.

140. Conri CL, Azoulai P, Constans J, et al: Erythromelalgia and low molecular weight heparin [French], *Therapie* 49:518, 1994.

141. Ozsoylu S, Coskun T: Sodium nitroprusside treatment in erythromelalgia, *Eur J Pediatr* 141:185, 1984.

142. Stone JD, Rivey MP, Allington DR: Nitroprusside treatment of erythromelalgia in an adolescent female, *Ann Pharmacother* 31:590, 1997.

143. Kalgaard OM, Mørk C, Kvernebo K: Prostacyclin reduces symptoms and sympathetic dysfunction in erythromelalgia in a double-blind randomized pilot study, *Acta Derm Venereol* 83:442, 2003.

144. Pepper H: Primary erythermalgia: report of a patient treated with methysergide maleate, *JAMA* 203:1066, 1968.

145. Davis MD, Sandroni P: Lidocaine patch for pain of erythromelalgia, *Arch Dermatol* 138:17, 2002.

146. Stricker LJ, Green CR: Resolution of refractory symptoms of secondary erythermalgia with intermittent epidural bupivacaine, *Reg Anesth Pain Med* 26:488, 2001.

147. D'Angelo R, Cohen IT, Brandom BW: Continuous epidural infusion of bupivacaine and fentanyl for erythromelalgia in an adolescent, *Anesth Analg* 74:142, 1992.

148. Rauck RL, Naveira F, Speight KL, et al: Refractory idiopathic erythromelalgia, *Anesth Analg* 82:1097, 1996.

149. Mohr M, Schneider K, Grosche M, et al: Cervical epidural infusion of morphine and bupivacaine in severe erythromelalgia [German], *Anasthesiol Intensivmed Notfallmed Schmerzther* 29:371, 1994.

150. Trapiella Martinez L, Quiros JF, Caminal Montero L, et al: Treatment of erythromelalgia with buprenorphine (letter) [Spanish], *Rev Clin Esp* 197:792, 1997.

151. Macres S, Richeimer S: Successful treatment of erythromelalgia with intrathecal hydromorphone and clonidine, *Clin J Pain* 16:310, 2000.

152. Calderone DC, Finzi E: Treatment of primary erythromelalgia with piroxicam, *J Am Acad Dermatol* 24:145, 1991.

153. H'Mila R, Samoud A, Souid M, et al: Erythermalgia: a rare vascular acrosyndrome [French], *Arch Fr Pediatr* 48:555, 1991.

154. Guillet MH, Le Noach E, Milochau P, et al: Familial erythermalgia treated with pizotifen [French], *Ann Dermatol Venereol* 122:777, 1995.

155. Drenth JP, Michiels JJ: Treatment options in primary erythermalgia? (letter), *Am J Hematol* 43:154, 1993.

156. Kasapcopur O, Akkus S, Erdem A, et al: Erythromelalgia associated with hypertension and leukocytoclastic vasculitis in a child, *Clin Exp Rheumatol* 16:184, 1998.

157. Cimaz R, Rusconi R, Fossali E, et al: Unexpected healing of cutaneous ulcers in a short child, *Lancet* 358:211, 2001.

158. Sakakibara R, Fukutake T, Kita K, et al: Treatment of primary erythromelalgia with cyproheptadine, *J Auton Nerv Syst* 58:121, 1996.

159. Suh DH, Kim SD, Ahn JS, et al: A case of erythromelalgia successfully controlled by systemic steroids and pentazocine: is it related to a unique subtype of neutrophilic dermatosis? *J Dermatol* 27:204, 2000.

160. Chakravarty K, Pharoah PD, Scott DG, et al: Erythromelalgia: the role of hypnotherapy, *Postgrad Med J* 68:44, 1992.

CHAPTER 51 Pernio (Chilblains)

Jeffrey W. Olin, Amjad Al Mahameed

Pernio, commonly known as *chilblains*, is a cold-induced localized inflammatory condition presenting as skin lesions predominantly on unprotected acral areas. Typically there is swelling of the dorsa of the proximal phalanges of fingers and toes (Fig. 51-1). *Pernio* is a Latin term meaning "frostbite." *Chilblains* is an Anglo-Saxon term used in older literature and means "cold sore." The tissue and vascular damage is less severe in pernio than in frostbite, in which the skin is actually frozen. The numerous names that were used to describe this syndrome created much confusion and misunderstanding of this entity[1] (Box 51-1). In the mid-1800s, there were attempts to better classify the disease[2] and in 1894, Corlett was the first to describe the clinical characteristics of pernio, which he called *dermatitis hiemalis*.[3]

Epidemiology

The first epidemiological study to explicate the prevalence of chilblains and its impact on productivity in servicewomen was carried out in 1942 by the U.S. Medical Department of the War Office.[4] The study concluded that at least 50% of questionnaire participants had chilblains by age 40 during World War II (1939-1943). Although pernio is most common in young women, it has also been reported in all ages and both sexes.[5–8] The number of reported cases of pernio is higher during times of wet near-freezing weather, and less common in dry freezing weather or in a bitterly cold climate.[9] Pernio is most commonly encountered in the northern and western parts of the United States; isolated cases have been reported in warmer climates in times of cooler damp weather.[5,6,10–12]

As shown by a recently reported cross-sectional study conducted by the U.S. Army, the yearly rate of cold weather injuries declined from 38.2/100,000 in 1985 to 0.2/100,000 in 1999.[13] This and other observations from clinical practice suggest that the disease is becoming less common with higher standards of home and workplace heating and greater use of appropriate clothing during the cold winter months. Also, the study confirmed previous investigations that cold weather injuries in African American men and women occurred approximately 4 and 2.2 times as often, respectively, as in their Caucasian counterparts.

Pathophysiology

The first response to cold exposure is vasoconstriction in the dermis and subcutaneous tissue. Heat loss is minimized by shutting down distal capillary beds and diminishing blood supply to the acral portions of the extremities to maintain central body temperature. Stasis and shunting of blood flow away from the superficial vessels occurs secondary to arteriolar constriction, venular relaxation, and cold-associated increased blood viscosity. The result of these changes is superficial tissue anoxia and ischemia.[7,9,14–16] The arteriolar vasoconstriction described in pernio has been demonstrated in pathological and radiographic studies.[6,7] Female predominance may be related to increased responsiveness of their cutaneous circulation to cold. Indeed, there is a higher frequency of vasomotor instability, cold hands and feet, and Raynaud's phenomenon in women.[8,17–19]

Humidity has an important role in the pathophysiology of pernio because it enhances air conductivity, promoting heat loss from the skin.[5,8] Most individuals tolerate exposure to nonfreezing damp cold, but others may experience pernio, Raynaud's phenomenon, acrocyanosis, or cold urticaria.[8,18] The clinical manifestations of cold injuries are related to duration, severity, and dampness of cold exposure as well as the individual's underlying predisposition to cold injury and the stage at which medical attention was

sought.[7] The exposed skin of affected subjects remains cool longer and warms slower than that of controls, further highlighting the importance of individual susceptibility for development of pernio after cold exposure.[6–8,20] The increased incidence of pernio among relatives of affected patients suggests the possibility of genetic predisposition.[4] Several other conditions have been proposed to promote vulnerability to the disease (Box 51-2).

Why one patient exposed to cold develops Raynaud's phenomenon and another pernio is unclear. Raynaud's phenomenon and pernio frequently coexist in the same patient, so these diseases may be part of a continuum, with Raynaud's phenomenon representing acute and readily reversible vasospasm, and pernio representing more prolonged vasospasm with more chronic changes.[8,21]

A number of conditions have been associated with pernio. Weston and Morelli reported the presence of cryoproteins in four of eight children presenting with pernio.[11,22] Since cryoproteins and cold agglutinins may be detected transiently after viral infections, they hypothesized that exposure to cold wet weather during the brief cryoproteinemia may lead to exaggerated tissue injury manifesting as pernio. Pernio has been described both in women with large amounts of leg fat and in women with inadequate fat pads, as seen in anorexia nervosa.[5–7]

The possibility that pernio may be a manifestation of a pre-leukemic state, namely the chronic myelomonocytic type, has been suggested in several case reports in which skin lesions and a clinical course similar to that of pernio were observed.[5,23–25] In some of these cases, leukemia was diagnosed 6 to 36 months after the pernio-like illness.

Viguier et al. reported observations over 38 months on a cohort of 33 patients with severe chilblains, defined as duration of lesions greater than 1 month.[21] Two thirds of the patients had clinical and/or laboratory features supporting a diagnosis of connective tissue disorders: 12 patients had systemic lupus erythematosus (SLE) and 10 patients presented with at least one of the American College of Rheumatology revised criteria for SLE at the time of the diagnosis of pernio. In the latter group, all patients except one had positive antinuclear antibody (ANA) titers. These observations led the authors to conclude that when the lesions persist beyond the cold season, perniotic lesions may be a clue to underlying SLE. Therefore, targeted laboratory investigations to search for conditions listed in Box 51-2, as well as long-term follow-up, are recommended for patients who present with pernio.[26]

Histopathology

Although not routinely required to establish the diagnosis, biopsies are occasionally sought by healthcare providers unfamiliar with the disease.[27] The histopathological features of perniotic lesions may vary depending upon the chronological stage of the disease and presence or absence of superimposed secondary pathology such as infection or ulceration.[7,28,29]

The characteristic histopathological features of pernio are usually seen in the dermis and subcutaneous tissue, but are not pathognomonic. These consist of edema of the papillodermis, vasculitis characterized by perivascular infiltration of the arterioles and venules of the dermis and subcutaneous fat by mononuclear and lymphocytic cells, thickening and edema of blood vessel walls, fat necrosis, and chronic inflammatory reaction with giant cell formation.[8] Not all these changes are necessarily present, and fat necrosis and giant cell formation are frequently absent. The most consistent feature is perivascular lymphocytic or mononuclear infiltrates.[28]

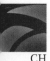

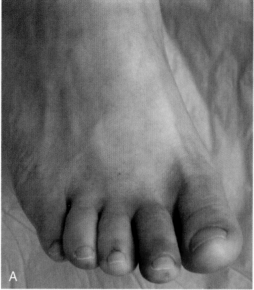

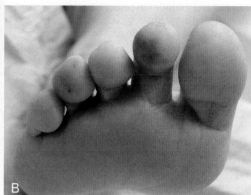

FIGURE 51-1 Typical changes of pernio on dorsal portion of toes (A) and on pads of toes (B). Distribution around nail beds **(A)** and swollen toes with brownish yellow lesions **(B)** are characteristic of pernio. At this stage, affected extremities often itch and burn.

Box 51-1 Different Names Used in the Literature to Describe Pernio or Pernio-like Conditions

Pernio
Chilblains
Nodular vasculitis
Erythrocyanosis
Erythrocyanose sur malléolair
Erythema induratum
Lupus pernio
Kibes
Perniosis
Dermatitis hiemalis
Frostschaeden
Erythrocyanosis frigida
Erythrocyanosis crurum puellaris
Bazin's disease
L'engelune
Cold panniculitis

Box 51-2 Categories of Diseases Associated with Pernio

Defective Cutaneous Vasomotor Reactivity
Raynaud's phenomenon
Acrocyanosis
Complex regional pain syndrome (reflex sympathetic dystrophy [RSD])
Anterior poliomyelitis
Syringomyelia
Livedo reticularis

Underlying Chronic Limb Ischemia
Peripheral artery disease (PAD)
Erythromelalgia (advanced stage)

Hyperviscosity Syndrome
Leukemia
Systemic lupus erythematosus (SLE)
Dysproteinemia (cryoproteins)

Abnormal Fat Distribution
Obesity with excess leg fat
Inadequate fat pads (anorexia nervosa)

Repeated episodes of vasospasm or prolonged vasospasm may cause tissue anoxia, thus causing the identical histopathological picture that occurs in pernio.[1] The histological pattern of pernio lesions may mimic cutaneous vasculitis but typically lacks fibrinoid deposition, inflammatory cells in the vessel wall, and thrombosis, typical of true vasculitis.[5–7,11,27,29–33] Blood vessels in long-standing pernio resemble those of any chronic occlusive vascular disease. The occlusion and fibrosis present are due to long-standing injury; this histopathological appearance may be seen in many other types of vascular disease.

Review of published case series and case reports support the notion that pernio may display different and loosely related histological features.[33] Cribier et al. retrospectively compared the biopsies of hand lesions from 17 patients with chilblains to those of 10 patients with proven SLE and associated pernio-like hand lesions.[27] The study included only acute lesions (<1 month duration) occurring during the cold period of the year. The most characteristic finding in chilblains (47% of cases) was the association of edema and reticular dermis infiltrate that showed a perieccrine reinforcement: dermal edema (70% of chilblains lesions vs. 20% of SLE lesions), superficial (papillary) and deep (reticular) infiltrate (82% vs. 80%), and deep perieccrine reinforcement (76% vs. 0%). The infiltrate was composed primarily of T cells, which were predominantly CD3+. Remarkably, 29% of the chilblain lesions in this group showed evidence of microthrombi (compared to 10% in the lupus group), usually a feature seen in vasculitis, and 6% had conspicuous vacuolation (compared to 60% in the lupus group).

In another study, Viguier et al. prospectively studied 33 patients with severe prolonged chilblains (i.e., lesions persisted >1 month) and attempted to differentiate the histopathological characteristics of lesions of "idiopathic" pernio from those of pernio-like lesions in patients with connective tissue diseases or lupus pernio.[21] Skin punch biopsies were performed on 5 of 11 patients of the "idiopathic" pernio group, and these showed deep dermal, perisudoral lymphocytic infiltrate (100%), dermal edema (75%), keratinocyte necrosis (62.5%), and keratinocyte vacuolization (50%). In comparison, biopsies from 7 of the 12 patients with the diagnosis of SLE (LE chilblain), demonstrated perisudoral cellular infiltrate in only two patients (vs. 8/8 in the "idiopathic" chilblains group; $P = .007$). Biopsy is rarely needed to make the diagnosis of pernio, but a biopsy may be helpful in differentiating atheromatous embolization from pernio in an ischemic-looking lesion (Fig. 51-2).

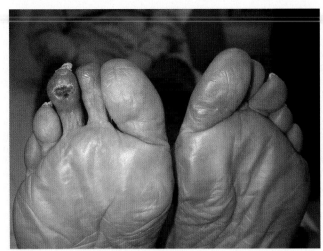

FIGURE 51-2 Advanced stage of pernio. Toes are cyanotic, and there is a shallow ulcer on right third toe. This stage of pernio is often quite painful and may be mistaken for atheromatous embolization in the elderly patient.

Clinical Features

Pernio most commonly affects females in adolescence and early adulthood, but may occur at any age and in either gender. The lesions typically affect the acral areas of the toes and the dorsa of the proximal phalanges but may involve the nose, ears, and thighs[1-4,7,21,34-38] (Fig. 51-3). The location of the lesions seems to depend on occupation, lifestyle, and clothing habits. Hands and

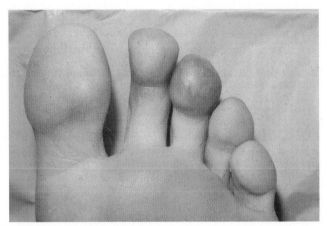

FIGURE 51-3 Typical appearance of pernio. Note characteristic bulbous swelling and brownish yellow appearance of left third toe. Flaking, itching, burning, and pain are common.

fingers appear more commonly affected in milkers and gardeners, the buttocks have been involved in women driving tractors in winter, and involvement of the lateral thighs have been described in women who wear thin pants and ride horses or motorcycles in winter.[3,18,39-44] There was a recent report of perniotic lesions on the hips of young girls wearing tight-fitting jeans with a low waistband.[45] The distal shins and calves are common sites of involvement in young women who wear short skirts.[46] Facial lesions have been described in infants and rarely in adults.[21,47]

Typically the initial presentation is one of *acute pernio*, where the lesions appear during the cold months and disappear when the weather warms up. This may recur for several years and follows a similar seasonal pattern.[7,8] Lesions vary in shape, number, and size and usually are associated with functional symptoms such as itching, burning, or pain. They can be described as brownish, yellow, or cyanotic on a base of doughy subcutaneous swelling or erythema (see Figs. 51-1 and 51-3). They may be cool to the touch or cooler than surrounding skin. Acute lesions may be self-limited and resolve within a few days to few weeks (especially in children) unless cold exposure persists, the lesions become infected, or the skin is broken by iatrogenic causes such as self-treatment with severe heat or vigorous massage.[38,48] Otherwise, ulceration is not common in acute pernio, and when it happens, the lesions are usually shallow with a hemorrhagic base[7,8] (see Fig. 51-2).

Chronic pernio ensues if repeated and prolonged exposure to cold persists throughout the acute phase and/or the patient goes through several seasons of acute pernio. The lesions of chronic pernio are similar to those seen in acute pernio but, if they occur over many seasons, may be associated with scarring, atrophy, permanent discoloration, and possibly ulceration (see Fig. 51-2). Initially, pernio may start late in the fall or early winter and resolve in early spring. If left untreated, the lesions of pernio may start earlier in the cold season and resolve later, until eventually all seasonal variation is lost.

Pernio tends to be more severe in adults and may, if left untreated, eventually cause macrovascular occlusive disease.[6,8] Children, on the other hand, tend to have recurrent acute pernio over several seasons.[38] Although most children outgrow the disease, middle-aged individuals presenting with pernio may occasionally recall a history of acute pernio during childhood. Several different forms of pernio have been described.

Milker's pernio usually affects the hands and could be debilitating and force the affected individual to quit milking[42] (Fig. 51-4). *Kibe* is defined as a chapped or inflamed area on the skin, especially on the heel, resulting from exposure to cold or an ulcerated chilblain.[49] This has been described in overweight women who ride horses and wear tight pants, in women who ride motorcycles and wear thin pants, and in men who cross cold rivers with their thighs inadequately clothed.[18,39] Lesions tend to localize on the outer thighs and often cause severe pain and disability. The pain may last up to a week and usually resolves once the lesions heal.[18] A similar form has been described in women who drive tractors in winter, who tend to have lesions on the buttocks.[44]

FIGURE 51-4 This woman was exposed to a cold wet climate, resulting in pernio. Note brown and yellow flaking lesion on thumb **(A)** and healing lesions on index and ring fingers **(B)**.

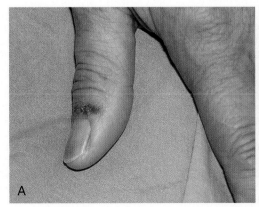

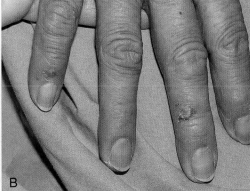

Lupus pernio applies to papular lesions involving the extremities and is associated with SLE.[50] Whether this is a subtype of pernio or a pernio-like lupus manifestation remains controversial. Some authors suggested that most lupus pernio patients have lesions on the hands, but this anatomical localization was not a differentiating factor between idiopathic pernio and lupus pernio according to others.[8,21,26] Features that suggest pernio secondary to SLE include onset of pernio during the third decade, female sex, African origin, and presence of pernio long after the cold weather has abated.

Erythrocyanosis affects adolescent girls and young women and typically involves the lower extremities. Some have classified this as the "nodular chronic form" of pernio; lesions take on a swollen, dusky red appearance.[8]

Diagnosis

Pernio usually is not difficult to diagnose. A comprehensive history and complete physical exam are the primary means by which the diagnosis of pernio can be correctly established. Chronological correlation between nonfreezing cold and onset of typical lesions that improve with onset of warm weather should strongly suggest the diagnosis.

Within hours of exposure to damp cold, and commonly at the onset of winter, the patient develops violet or yellow blisters, brown plaques, or shallow ulcers on the toes, which often burn, itch, or become painful. These lesions typically disappear when the weather warms up at the beginning of spring. However, in some chronic cases in which the lesions do not disappear in warm weather, or in which the lesions cause severe pigmentation and disfiguration of the lower part of the leg, the diagnosis may be more difficult.

The main obstacle to establishing the diagnosis of pernio is unfamiliarity of the healthcare provider with the disease. Since many of the dermatological manifestations associated with pernio overlap with other serious diseases, it is not uncommon for pernio patients to be subjected to unnecessary investigations and suffer needless delay in proper treatment.[5,47,51] Characteristically, peripheral pulses and peripheral blood pressure measurements are normal unless the patient has underlying peripheral artery disease (PAD) or the pernio has been of such long duration that chronic occlusive vascular disease has developed.[6] Pulse volume recordings (PVR) and segmental blood pressures may be abnormal in patients with pernio. This may be due to either vasospasm (the study will normalize with warming of the extremity) or fixed vascular disease due to long-standing pernio.[52]

Because the diagnosis of pernio is a clinical diagnosis, sophisticated laboratory tests are often not needed, but it is important to rule out other entities that can mimic pernio. The following tests may be obtained: complete blood cell count (CBC) with differential, ANA titer, rheumatoid factor (RF), comprehensive metabolic panel, cryoglobulin, cryofibrinogen, cold agglutinin, and serum viscosity measurements. Arteriography and skin biopsy are not warranted to establish the diagnosis of pernio, except in the occasional case where a clear history could not be obtained or a concomitant vascular pathology (e.g., atheromatous embolization) is suspected.

The differential diagnosis of pernio includes a variety of diseases. Atheromatous emboli (blue toe syndrome) is the most challenging diagnostic entity to differentiate from pernio because similar lesions may be present in each disorder (see Chapter 47).[53] When the history of cold exposure is uncertain and in patients with established or suspected atherosclerosis, imaging studies often are warranted to demonstrate atheroma in the aorta or iliac vessels. A biopsy of these lesions showing characteristic cholesterol clefts establishes the diagnosis of atheromatous emboli.[53]

The next group of diseases that may be confused with pernio include those with chronic recurrent erythematous, nodular, and ulcerative lesions: erythema induratum, nodular vasculitis, erythema nodosum, and cold panniculitis. Erythema induratum (Bazin's disease) is often but not always a cutaneous form of tuberculosis that affects adolescent girls and is manifested by nodular ulcerating lesions of the calves.[7,54] Nontuberculous forms of recurrent painful nodules are called *nodular vasculitis*.[54] Women over the age of 30 years are usually affected, and no apparent cause is known. Although the nodules of nodular vasculitis are extremely painful, they rarely ulcerate. Erythema nodosum may be differentiated from pernio in that it may be associated with fever, arthralgias, malaise, and an underlying disease. The lesions are painful and generally do not ulcerate. Cold panniculitis is another important entity characterized by painful nodules that appear on the skin after cold exposure and can be reproduced by application of an ice cube. The histology of these lesions reveals fat necrosis.[55] The palpable purpuric lesion sometimes present in pernio must be differentiated from other types of vasculitis, especially leukocytoclastic vasculitis. Lack of the systemic manifestations and laboratory abnormalities that occur in leukocytoclastic vasculitis and the relation of the lesions to cold exposure in pernio serve to separate these two conditions. Rarely, a skin biopsy may be needed to make a definitive diagnosis.

Treatment

Since the primary trigger for development of pernio is cold exposure, prevention is the mainstay of management. Working in a damp cold basement or living in a poorly heated apartment may necessitate change of profession or moving to a properly heated residence. Patients do not always volunteer information about the climate of their residence and workplace, so the physician may need to ask specifically about the quality of heating systems and the degree of humidity present. The patient should be instructed on methods of proper dress. Adequate body insulation with gloves, stockings, footwear, and headwear may be needed. As is the case in the treatment of Raynaud's phenomenon, the entire body must be kept warm.

A dihydropyridine calcium channel blocker, such as nifedipine, is quite effective in patients with pernio. In a double-blind placebo-controlled randomized crossover pilot study, Dowd et al. reported that treatment with 20 mg of nifedipine three times daily, when given shortly after the appearance of lesions, led to resolution of the lesions within 7 to 10 days, compared to 20 to 28 days with placebo. In addition, the pain disappeared within 5 days in the treated group, compared to 20 to 25 days in the group receiving placebo.[56] In a double-blind placebo-controlled randomized trial, Rustin et al. have shown that nifedipine given at a daily dose of 20 to 60 mg was shown to reduce severity of symptoms, shorten their duration, enhance resolution of existing lesions, and prevent development of new lesions.[57] Based upon these studies and the authors' experience, all patients are prescribed either nifedipine or amlodipine to facilitate healing of the lesions and prevent their recurrence. Others have had success with α-blocking agents such as prazocin.[52] When spring and summer approach, the medications can be discontinued and then restarted the following fall. These pharmacological therapies should be used in conjunction with other preventive strategies already discussed.

A recent study reported improvement in symptoms in four of five patients treated with hydroxychloraquin.[58] However, it should be noted that all four of the patients showing improvement had an underlying connective tissue disease (Sjögren's syndrome [1], SLE [2], or a family history of connective tissue disease [1]).

Despite speculation that it may enhance resolution of active lesions and provide subjective improvement, sympathectomy does not prevent recurrence of new lesions and has little effect if any on pigmentation and thickness at the sites of perniotic lesions. Conflicting reports exist about use of other treatment modalities such as topical vasodilators, topical or systemic corticosteroids, calcium, vitamin D, and intramuscular (IM) vitamin K. Given the controversy and lack of prospective studies, routine use of these agents is not recommended.[8,19]

REFERENCES

1. McGovern T, Wright IS, Kruger E: Pernio: a vascular disease, *Am Heart J* 22:583, 1941.
2. Bazin E: *Lecons theoriques et cliniques sur la scrofule* Paris 1861.
3. Corlett WT: *Cold as an etiological factor in diseases of the skin* 1894.
4. Winner A, Cooper-Willis E: Chilblains in service women, *Lancet* 1:663, 1946.
5. Goette DK: Chilblains (perniosis), *J Am Acad Dermatol* 23:257–262, 1990.
6. Jacob JR, Weisman MH, Rosenblatt SI, et al: Chronic pernio. A historical perspective of cold-induced vascular disease, *Arch Intern Med* 146:1589–1592, 1986.
7. Lynn RB: Chilblains, *Surg Gynecol Obstet* 99:720, 1954.
8. Olin JW, Arrabi W: Vascular diseases related to extremes in environmental temperature. In Young JR, Olin JW, Bartholomew JR, editors: *Peripheral vascular disease*, ed 2 , St. Louis, 1996, Mosby-Year Book, Inc, pp 611–613.
9. Purdue GF, Hunt JL: Cold injury: a collective review, *J Burn Care Rehabil* 7:417–421, 1986.
10. Wessagowit P, Asawanonda P, Noppakun N: Papular perniosis mimicking erythema multiforme: the first case report in Thailand, *Int J Dermatol* 39:527–529, 2000.
11. Weston WL, Morelli JG: Childhood pernio and cryoproteins, *Pediatr Dermatol* 17:97–99, 2000.
12. Chan Y, Tang WY, Lam WY, et al: A cluster of chilblains in Hong Kong, *Hong Kong Med J* 14:185–191, 2008.
13. DeGroot DW, Castellani JW, Williams JO, et al: Epidemiology of U.S. Army cold weather injuries, 1980-1999, *Aviat Space Environ Med* 74:564–570, 2003.
14. Eubanks RG: Heat and cold injuries, *J Ark Med Soc* 71:53–58, 1974.
15. Kulka JP: Vasomotor microcirculatory insufficiency: observations on nonfreezing cold injury of the mouse ear, *Angiology* 12:491–506, 1961.
16. Lewis T: Observations upon the reactions of the vessels of the human skin to cold, *Heart* 15:177–208, 1930.
17. Goodfield M: Cold-induced skin disorders, *Practitioner* 233:1616–1620, 1989.
18. Price RD, Murdoch DR: Perniosis (chilblains) of the thigh: report of five cases, including four following river crossings, *High Alt Med Biol* 2:535–538, 2001.
19. Almahameed A, Pinto DS: Pernio (chilblains), *Curr Treat Options Cardiovasc Med* 10: 128–135, 2008.
20. Lewis ST: Observations on some normal and injurious effects of cold upon the skin and underlying tissues: chilblains and allied conditions, *BMJ* 2:837, 1941.
21. Viguier M, Pinquier L, Cavelier-Balloy B, et al: Clinical and histopathologic features and immunologic variables in patients with severe chilblains. A study of the relationship to lupus erythematosus, *Medicine (Baltimore)* 80:180–188, 2001.
22. Yang X, Perez OA, English JC III: Adult perniosis and cryoglobulinemia: a retrospective study and review of the literature, *J Am Acad Dermatol* 62:e21–e22, 2010.
23. Baker H: Chronic monocytic leukemia with necrosis of pinnae, *Br J Dermatol* 76:480–481, 1946.
24. Kelly JW, Dowling JP: Pernio. A possible association with chronic myelomonocytic leukemia, *Arch Dermatol* 121:1048–1052, 1985.
25. Marks R, Lim CC, Borrie PF: A perniotic syndrome with monocytosis and neutropenia; a possible association with a preleukaemic state, *Br J Dermatol* 81:327–332, 1969.
26. Stagaki E, Mountford WK, Lackland DT, et al: The treatment of lupus pernio: results of 116 treatment courses in 54 patients, *Chest* 135:468–476, 2009.
27. Cribier B, Djeridi N, Peltre B, et al: A histologic and immunohistochemical study of chilblains, *J Am Acad Dermatol* 45:924–929, 2001.
28. Herman EW, Kezis JS, Silvers DN: A distinctive variant of pernio. Clinical and histopathologic study of nine cases, *Arch Dermatol* 117:26–28, 1981.
29. Wall LM, Smith NP: Perniosis: a histopathological review, *Clin Exp Dermatol* 6:263–271, 1981.
30. Corbett D, Benson P: Military dermatology. In Zajtchuk R, Bellamy RF, editors: *Textbook of military medicine. Part III. Diseases of the environment*, Washington, DC, 1994, Office of the Surgeon General.
31. Inoue G, Miura T: Microgeodic disease affecting the hands and feet of children, *J Pediatr Orthop* 11:59–63, 1991.
32. Page EH, Shear NH: Temperature-dependent skin disorders, *J Am Acad Dermatol* 18:1003–1019, 1988.
33. Boada A, Bielsa I, Fernandez-Figueras MT, et al: Perniosis: clinical and histopathological analysis, *Am J Dermatopathol* 32:19–23, 2010.
34. Gourlay RJ: The problem of chilblains: with a note of their treatment with nicotinic acid, *BMJ* 1:336–339, 1948.
35. Parra SL, Wisco OJ: What is your diagnosis? Perniosis (chilblain), *Cutis* 84:15, 27–15, 29, 2009.
36. Prakash S, Weisman MH: Idiopathic chilblains, *Am J Med* 122:1152–1155, 2009.
37. McCleskey PE, Winter KJ, Devillez RL: Tender papules on the hands. Idiopathic chilblains (perniosis), *Arch Dermatol* 142:1501–1506, 2006.
38. Simon TD, Soep JB, Hollister JR: Pernio in pediatrics, *Pediatrics* 116:e472–e475, 2005.
39. Winter kibes in horsey women, *Lancet* 2:1345, 1980.
40. Beacham BE, Cooper PH, Buchanan CS, et al: Equestrian cold panniculitis in women, *Arch Dermatol* 116:1025–1027, 1980.
41. De Silva BD, McLaren K, Doherty VR: Equestrian perniosis associated with cold agglutinins: a novel finding, *Clin Exp Dermatol* 25:285–288, 2000.
42. Duffill MB: Milkers' chilblains, *N Z Med J* 106:101–103, 1993.
43. Fisher DA, Everett MA: Violaceous rash of dorsal fingers in a woman. Diagnosis: chilblain lupus erythematosus (perniosis), *Arch Dermatol* 132:459, 462, 1996.
44. Thomas EW: Chapping and chilblains, *Practitioner* 193:755–760, 1964.
45. Weismann K, Larsen FG: Pernio of the hips in young girls wearing tight-fitting jeans with a low waistband, *Acta Derm Venereol* 86:558–559, 2006.
46. Walsh S: More red toes, *J Pediatr Health Care* 14:193, 205–193, 206, 2000.
47. Giusti R, Tunnessen WW Jr: Picture of the month. Chilblains (pernio), *Arch Pediatr Adolesc Med* 151:1055–1056, 1997.
48. Gardinal-Galera I, Pajot C, Paul C, et al: Childhood chilblains is an uncommon and invalidant disease, *Arch Dis Child* 95:567–568, 2010.
49. *The American Heritage® Dictionary for the English Language*, 2000.
50. Millard LG, Rowell NR: Chilblain lupus erythematosus (Hutchinson). A clinical and laboratory study of 17 patients, *Br J Dermatol* 98:497–506, 1978.
51. Parlette EC, Parlette HL III: Erythrocyanotic discoloration of the toes, *Cutis* 65:223–224, 226, 2000.
52. Spittell JA Jr, Spittell PC: Chronic pernio: another cause of blue toes, *Int Angiol* 11:46–50, 1992.
53. Olin JW, Bartholomew JR: Atheromatous embolization syndrome. In Cronenwett JL, Johnston KW, editors: *Rutherford's vascular surgery*, ed 7, Philadelphia, 2010, W.B. Saunders Co, pp 2422–2434.
54. Montgomery H, O'Leary PA, Barker NW: Nodular vascular disease of the legs, *JAMA* 128:335, 1945.
55. Solomon LM, Beerman H: Cold panniculitis, *Arch Dermatol* 88:897, 1961.
56. Dowd PM, Rustin MH, Lanigan S: Nifedipine in the treatment of chilblains, *BMJ (Clin Res Ed)* 293:923–924, 1986.
57. Rustin MH, Newton JA, Smith NP, et al: The treatment of chilblains with nifedipine: the results of a pilot study, a double-blind placebo-controlled randomized study and a long-term open trial, *Br J Dermatol* 120:267–275, 1989.
58. Yang X, Perez OA, English JC III: Successful treatment of perniosis with hydroxychloroquine, *J Drugs Dermatol* 9:1242–1246, 2010.

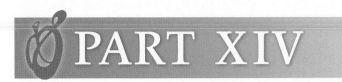

PART XIV

VENOUS THROMBOEMBOLIC DISEASE

CHAPTER **52** **Venous Thrombosis**

Jeffrey I. Weitz, John W. Eikelboom

Definitions

Deep vein thrombosis (DVT) refers to an obstruction of a deep vein by thrombus, usually in the legs or pelvis but occasionally in the arms. Thrombus from these sites can travel to the lungs to produce pulmonary embolism (PE), which occurs when the thrombus obstructs a pulmonary artery. This process is known as *venous thromboembolism* (VTE). Blockage of blood flow through the lungs and the resultant increased pressure in the right ventricle are responsible for the symptoms and signs of PE,[1] whereas obstructed outflow of blood from occluded veins in the legs or arms produces symptoms and signs of DVT.

Epidemiology

Venous thromboembolism, which includes DVT and PE, represents the third most common cause of cardiovascular death after myocardial infarction (MI) and strokes. A first episode of VTE occurs in about 1 person per 1000 each year in the United States.[2] The incidence rises exponentially with age, with 5 cases per 1000 persons per year by the age of 80 years. Although men and women are affected equally, the incidence is higher in Caucasians and African Americans than in Hispanic persons and Asian Pacific Islanders.[3]

Approximately one third of patients with symptomatic VTE present with PE; the remainder present with DVT alone.[4] Up to half of patients with a first episode of VTE have no identifiable risk factors and are described as having unprovoked or idiopathic VTE. The remainder develop VTE secondary to well-recognized transient risk factors such as surgery or immobilization. Pulmonary embolism accounts for an estimated 15% of deaths in hospitalized patients, with at least 100,000 deaths from PE each year in the United States.

Pathobiology

Pulmonary embolism and DVT are part of the spectrum of VTE and share the same genetic and acquired risk factors that determine the intrinsic risk of VTE for each individual[5] (Fig. 52-1). Genetic risk factors include abnormalities associated with hypercoagulability of the blood, the most common of which are factor V Leiden and the prothrombin 20210 gene mutations. Acquired risk factors include advanced age, history of previous VTE, obesity, and active cancer, all of which limit mobility and may be associated with hypercoagulability. Superimposed on this background risk, VTE often occurs in the presence of a triggering factor that increases risk above the critical threshold. Such triggering factors (e.g., surgery, pregnancy, estrogen therapy) lead to vascular damage, stasis, and/or hypercoagulability, the components of *Virchow's triad*.

In at least 90% of patients, PE originates from DVT in the lower limbs, and up to 70% of patients with proven PE still have demonstrable DVT upon presentation. Thrombi usually start in the calf veins.[4] About 20% of these calf vein thrombi then extend into the popliteal and more proximal veins of the leg, from which they are more likely to embolize. Although often asymptomatic, PE can be detected in about 50% of patients with proximal DVT. Upper-extremity DVT involving the axillary and/or subclavian veins also can give rise to PE, but only 10% to 15% of such patients develop PE. Upper-extremity DVT most often occurs in patients with cancer, particularly those with indwelling central venous catheters. Unprovoked upper-extremity DVT, usually involving the dominant arm, can occur with strenuous effort—the so-called Paget-Schroetter's syndrome.[6]

Clinical Manifestations

Recognizing VTE can be challenging because the symptoms and signs of both DVT and PE are neither sensitive nor specific for these disorders.[1] A high index of suspicion is needed because DVT is often asymptomatic, and many cases of fatal PE go unsuspected prior to death. The clinical suspicion of VTE should be prompted by a constellation of risk factors, symptoms, signs, findings on electrocardiography, chest radiography, echocardiography, and blood test results. Although clinical assessment alone is insufficient to establish or exclude the diagnosis of VTE, clinical prediction rules are useful for establishing a pretest probability in which patients can either be classified as being at low, medium, or high probability of having DVT and/or PE, or as being unlikely or likely to have DVT and/or PE based on the estimated prevalence of the disease. Therefore, clinical pretest probability assessment serves as the root of algorithms for the diagnosis of DVT and PE.[7]

Symptoms and Signs

Although most DVT originates in the calf veins, symptoms and signs are uncommon until there is extension into the more proximal veins, which obstructs outflow of blood from the leg. The symptoms and signs of DVT may be acute and progressive, or they may resolve spontaneously if the thrombus undergoes lysis or embolism. Clinical manifestations of DVT may include tenderness or pain, swelling, and warmth and erythema of the skin. Pain on forced dorsiflexion of the foot (Homans sign) is neither sensitive nor specific for DVT. The differential diagnosis of DVT should be framed in the context of clinical presentation and underlying risk factors for VTE. Trauma, cellulitis, ruptured Baker cyst, musculoskeletal pain, or asymmetrical swelling unrelated to DVT may produce signs and symptoms compatible with acute DVT.

Diagnosis of Deep Vein Thrombosis

Because the clinical features are nonspecific, diagnosis of DVT requires objective testing. Patients who need such testing can be identified by their pretest likelihood of DVT, using validated

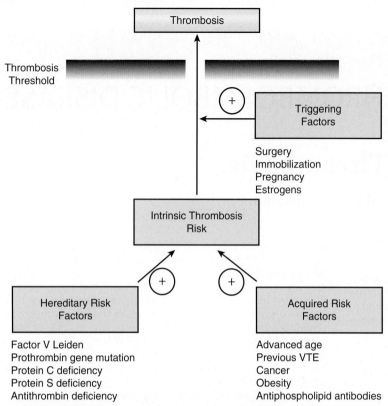

FIGURE 52-1 **Thrombosis threshold.** Hereditary and acquired risk factors combine to create an intrinsic risk of thrombosis for each individual. This risk is increased by extrinsic triggering factors. If intrinsic and extrinsic forces exceed a critical threshold where thrombin generation overwhelms protective mechanisms, thrombosis occurs. VTE, venous thrombembolism.

TABLE 52-1	Wells Clinical Prediction Model for Likelihood of Deep Vein Thrombosis	
VARIABLE		**POINTS**
Predisposing Factors		
Active cancer		1
Paralysis, paresis, or recent cast immobilization		1
Bedridden more than 3 days or recent major surgery		1
Previous VTE		1
Symptoms		
Localized tenderness along deep veins		1
Swelling of entire leg		1
Signs		
Calf swelling over 3 cm compared with asymptomatic limb		1
Pitting edema		1
Collateral superficial veins		1
Clinical Judgment		
Alternative diagnosis at least as likely		− 2

CLINICAL PROBABILITY	TOTAL POINTS
Low	<1
Intermediate	1-2
High	>2
Unlikely	<2
Likely	≥2

VTE, venous thromboembolism.
Adapted from Scarvelis D, Wells PS: Diagnosis and treatment of deep-vein thrombosis. CMAJ 175:1087–1092, 2006.

clinical prediction rules (Table 52-1) that include components of the clinical assessment, presence of risk factors for VTE, and absence of an alternative diagnosis to explain the symptoms and signs.[8] Based on the results of such an assessment, the pretest likelihood of VTE can be designated either as low, moderate, or high, or as unlikely or likely, and this assessment then guides subsequent selection of blood tests, such as the D-dimer assay, and noninvasive

or invasive tests for definitive diagnosis of DVT. Tests for diagnosis of DVT also are relevant in patients with suspected PE because a diagnosis of proximal DVT in such patients provides sufficient grounds for initiation of treatment, and the treatment of DVT and PE are usually the same. Noninvasive tests include computed tomographic (CT) pulmonary angiography or ventilation/perfusion (V/Q) lung scanning for diagnosis of PE, and venous compression ultrasound for diagnosis of DVT. These tests have largely replaced pulmonary angiography (for the diagnosis of PE) and venography (for the diagnosis of DVT).

Diagnostic Tests

D-DIMER

A plasmin-derived degradation product of cross-linked fibrin, D-dimer can be measured in whole blood or plasma to provide an indirect index of ongoing activation of the coagulation system. Sensitivity of an elevated D-dimer level for the diagnosis of VTE ranges from 85% to 98%, but all available D-dimer assays have low specificities.[9] False-positive D-dimer elevations can occur with advanced age, chronic inflammatory conditions, malignancy, and during the later stages of pregnancy and the postpartum period. In addition, hospitalized patients are more likely to have an elevated D-dimer level than outpatients, which renders the test less useful in this setting. Because of this lack of specificity, the value of the D-dimer assay resides with its high negative predictive value and the ability of a normal D-dimer to reduce the probability of VTE sufficiently to avoid further diagnostic testing in patients with a low or moderate pretest likelihood, who represent up to 30% of patients with suspected VTE.

COMPRESSION ULTRASOUND

The diagnosis of DVT (also see Chapter 12) is usually based on venous compression ultrasound (Fig. 52-2), which has a sensitivity and specificity of about 95% for the diagnosis of proximal DVT.[10] For calf DVT, the sensitivity of compression ultrasound is only about 73%. Because of the reduced sensitivity for detection of calf DVT, many centers restrict ultrasound testing to the proximal veins and only scan the region of the calf veins where they join the popliteal vein.

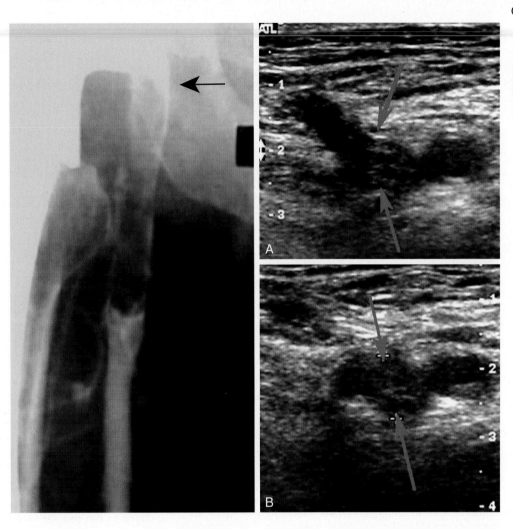

FIGURE 52-2 A venogram and venous compression ultrasound (CUS) demonstrating deep vein thrombosis (DVT). Venogram reveals intraluminal filling defect in proximal femoral vein, extending into iliac vein. CUS examination reveals noncompressibility of common femoral vein (**A** and **B**).

COMPUTED TOMOGRAPHIC VENOGRAPHY

When combined with CT pulmonary angiography, CT venography is a simple test to diagnose DVT because both tests require only one injection of contrast dye. Compared with CT pulmonary angiography alone, the combination of CT pulmonary angiography plus CT venography increases sensitivity from 83% to 90%, but specificity remains unchanged, thereby resulting in only a modest increase in negative predictive value.[8] Computed tomography venography adds significant radiation exposure and only marginally increases overall detection rate, so venous compression ultrasound is preferred because it provides the same information without exposing patients to ionizing radiation. Standard venography is not recommended in patients with suspected PE.

CONTRAST VENOGRAPHY

Although contrast venography remains the gold standard for diagnosing DVT,[11] the test is rarely performed in many centers (see Fig. 52-2). Venography is generally safe, but it can be uncomfortable and may be complicated by hypersensitivity reactions or superficial phlebitis. If the test is available, it should be considered when noninvasive testing is not diagnostic.

Diagnostic Strategies

Diagnostic strategies usually start with assessment of the pretest probability of VTE, using validated risk assessment models for either DVT (see Table 52-1) or PE (see Chapter 14), depending on the clinical presentation.[12] Patients can be classified as having a low, intermediate, or high pretest likelihood of VTE, or as being unlikely or likely to have VTE, and can then undergo further evaluation according to the appropriate algorithm.

ALGORITHM FOR DIAGNOSIS OF DEEP VEIN THROMBOSIS

Patients with a low pretest likelihood of DVT or those unlikely to have DVT should undergo D-dimer testing (Fig. 52-3). A negative D-dimer test excludes the diagnosis of DVT, whereas a positive test should prompt compression ultrasound examination.[13] A negative ultrasound excludes the diagnosis, whereas a positive test establishes it. Patients with an intermediate or high pretest likelihood of DVT or those likely to have DVT should be sent directly for compression ultrasound examination. A positive compression ultrasound establishes the diagnosis. If the ultrasound is negative, it is helpful to then perform D-dimer testing. If the D-dimer test is negative, the diagnosis of DVT can be excluded. In contrast, a positive D-dimer test should prompt a follow-up compression ultrasound in 1 week to exclude the possibility of calf DVT with interval extension. Follow-up ultrasound testing in 1 week should be done routinely if D-dimer testing is not performed. The diagnosis of DVT can be excluded if the follow-up test is negative.

Whole-leg compression ultrasound examination can prevent the need for a follow-up examination in 1 week.[14] This more time-consuming technique, which involves careful evaluation of the entire venous system, requires a high-performance scanner and an experienced operator. The advantage of this approach is that it will detect calf DVT as well as those in the more proximal veins. However, the accuracy of compression ultrasound for detection of calf DVT is lower than that for proximal DVT. Consequently,

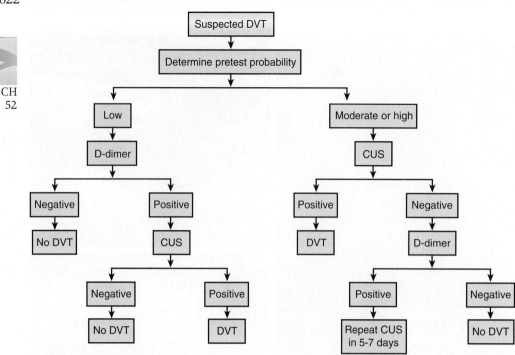

FIGURE 52-3 Clinical management of patients with suspected deep vein thrombosis (DVT). CUS; venous compression ultrasound.

whole-leg ultrasound examination should only be performed in centers where the test has been validated.

OTHER TESTS

Once a diagnosis of DVT has been established, other routinely ordered tests should include a complete blood cell count (CBC), platelet count, baseline international normalized ratio (INR), and activated partial thromboplastin time (APTT) to help guide anticoagulation. A creatinine (Cr) level and blood urea nitrogen (BUN) level also provide useful information to guide the choice of therapy, as do serum electrolytes and liver enzymes.

Thrombophilia testing has been advocated to identify patients with unprovoked (idiopathic) VTE who are at high risk of recurrence and who may therefore benefit from indefinite anticoagulation therapy. Although the common inherited thrombophilic disorders (see Fig. 52-1) are predictive of an increased risk of first-ever VTE, they do not appear to be associated with an increased risk of recurrence in patients who have already had an episode of VTE. Consequently, the results of thrombophilia testing rarely alter clinical management.[15] Exceptions may include rare patients who are homozygous for factor V Leiden or prothrombin gene mutations, those with antithrombin, protein C, or protein S deficiency, patients with more than one thrombophilic disorder, and those with antiphospholipid antibody syndrome; such patients may benefit from long-term anticoagulation treatment (see Treatment).

Treatment

Although anticoagulant therapy remains the mainstay of treatment of VTE, patients with severe PE may require urgent reperfusion therapy to increase blood flow to the pulmonary arteries, thereby reducing pulmonary artery pressure. Therefore, rapid risk stratification is crucial to help guide treatment (see Chapter 14). The role of reperfusion therapy in patients with DVT is less clear. Venous thromboembolism patients who have contraindications to anticoagulant therapy may require insertion of an inferior vena cava filter.

Reperfusion Therapy

Patients with severe PE associated with hypotension or shock may benefit from pharmacological, mechanical, or surgical reperfusion therapy. Pharmacological reperfusion therapy involves systemic administration of a fibrinolytic agent. Mechanical reperfusion includes percutaneous catheter embolectomy with thrombus fragmentation, an approach that avoids the need for fibrinolytic drugs altogether,[16] or catheter-directed fibrinolytic therapy, which requires lower doses of fibrinolytic agents than used for systemic administration. In some centers, surgical pulmonary embolectomy may be an option for patients who have severe PE and are at high risk for bleeding with systemic fibrinolytic therapy or who have failed such treatment.[17] Mechanical techniques require skilled operators but provide useful alternatives to systemic fibrinolytic therapy for patients who have severe PE and are at high risk for bleeding.

The role of reperfusion therapy for DVT is less certain.[18] Typically, such treatment is reserved for patients with extensive DVT involving the iliac and femoral veins. Systemic fibrinolytic therapy is rarely effective in this setting, so catheter-directed fibrinolysis or pharmacomechanical therapy is preferred. Pharmacomechanical therapy, which involves the use of clot maceration or extraction devices in conjunction with fibrinolytic therapy, not only produces more rapid lysis than that achieved with catheter-directed fibrinolytic therapy but is also associated with less bleeding because lower doses of fibrinolytic drugs are employed.

Although there is mounting evidence that reperfusion therapy results in higher rates of patency than are achieved with anticoagulant therapy alone, which lowers the risk of postthrombotic syndrome, definitive evidence of long-term benefit is lacking. Consequently, reperfusion therapy should only be considered for patients who are at low risk of bleeding and for those whose life expectancy is such that delayed benefits may be realized. For patients with extensive iliofemoral DVT or inferior vena cava thrombosis that is threatening the limb, reperfusion therapy may be the best option. In patients with less extensive DVT involving the iliac-femoral or femoral-popliteal veins, an ongoing clinical trial is assessing whether reperfusion therapy results in more rapid improvement in symptoms and reduces the risk of postthrombotic syndrome compared with anticoagulation therapy alone (www.clinicaltrials.gov: NCT00790335).

Anticoagulation Therapy

Anticoagulation therapy is the cornerstone of VTE treatment and should be initiated immediately with parenteral anticoagulants such as heparin, low-molecular-weight heparin (LMWH), or fondaparinux, even while patients with suspected VTE are awaiting results of confirmatory tests.[19] Heparin is generally preferred in patients with severe PE or extensive DVT because neither LMWH nor fondaparinux has been well evaluated in this setting. Heparin also should be used in patients with severe renal impairment (Cr clearance <30 mL/min) because LMWH and fondaparinux are cleared by the kidneys. If LMWH or fondaparinux is used for extended periods in patients with moderate renal impairment (Cr clearance of 30 to 50 mL/min), anti–factor Xa levels should be measured at trough to ensure there is no accumulation.

Heparin should be administered by continuous intravenous (IV) infusion and dosed using weight-based nomograms. Typically, an 80 unit/kg bolus is followed by an infusion at the rate of 18 units/kg/h, and subsequent doses are adjusted based on results of the APTT.[20] Rapid achievement and maintenance of a therapeutic APTT are important to reduce the risk of recurrent VTE. In addition to APTT monitoring, platelet count should be measured frequently because of the risk of heparin-induced thrombocytopenia (HIT).

Low-molecular-weight heparin or fondaparinux can be used for the majority of patients with DVT, using the regimens illustrated in Table 52-2.[19] Unlike heparin, these agents do not require coagulation monitoring. In addition, the risk of HIT is lower with LMWH than with heparin, and the risk is minimal with fondaparinux. Out-of-hospital management is safe for low-risk PE patients and for most patients with DVT. In PE patients at intermediate risk, outpatient management can be considered, but brief admission to hospital may be a safer approach.

After initial treatment with a parenteral anticoagulant, most patients with VTE receive extended therapy with a vitamin K antagonist (e.g., warfarin) to prevent recurrent DVT and PE. In most patients with DVT, warfarin can be started on the same day parenteral anticoagulant therapy is initiated. Parenteral anticoagulant therapy should be continued for at least 5 days and should only be stopped when the INR has been within the therapeutic range of 2 to 3, which is needed for long-term therapy, for 2 consecutive days. Initiation of warfarin therapy should be delayed in patients with extensive DVT involving the iliac-femoral veins; such patients should receive treatment with a parenteral anticoagulant until they have stabilized.

There are several emerging options to replace warfarin. These include dabigatran etexilate, an oral thrombin inhibitor,[21] and rivaroxaban, apixaban, and edoxaban, which are oral factor Xa inhibitors. With no food interactions and few drug-drug interactions, these new oral anticoagulants produce such a predictable level of anticoagulation that they can be given in fixed doses without routine coagulation monitoring.[22] In patients with VTE, rates of recurrent VTE and bleeding were similar with dabigatran (150 mg twice daily) and dose-adjusted warfarin. Dabigatran etexilate has been licensed as an alternative to warfarin for stroke prevention in patients with atrial fibrillation,[23] but the drug has not yet been approved for VTE treatment.

Rivaroxaban has been compared with conventional anticoagulation therapy (LMWH followed by warfarin) in patients with DVT[24];

a study in PE patients has been completed, but results have not yet been reported. In DVT patients, rates of recurrent VTE and bleeding with rivaroxaban (15 mg twice daily for 3 weeks, followed by 20 mg once daily thereafter) were similar to those with conventional anticoagulation therapy. Ongoing trials are investigating apixaban or edoxaban as other alternatives to warfarin.

Patients who develop VTE as a complication of a reversible risk factor such as surgery, trauma, or medical illness have a low risk of recurrence when anticoagulant therapy is stopped.[19] Consequently, a 3-month course of warfarin therapy represents adequate treatment in such patients, provided their risk factors have resolved. Women who develop VTE with estrogen therapy also can be treated for 3 months, provided hormonal treatment is withdrawn.

In contrast, patients with unprovoked VTE have a higher rate of recurrence when anticoagulant therapy stops, and often receive longer-duration treatment. Some experts recommend indefinite anticoagulant therapy, provided risk of bleeding remains low.[19] At 1 month after stopping anticoagulant therapy, an elevated D-dimer level or residual venous compression ultrasound abnormalities identify patients at higher risk for recurrence who may benefit from indefinite anticoagulation therapy.[25,26] After a minimum 3-month course of usual-intensity warfarin (target INR between 2 and 3), a lower-intensity regimen (target INR between 1.5 and 2.0) may simplify management by decreasing frequency of INR monitoring and reducing risk of bleeding, but the risk of recurrent VTE is slightly higher with this lower-intensity warfarin regimen.[27]

Caval Filters

Inferior vena cava filters, which are inserted percutaneously, are usually placed below the level of the renal veins, but can be placed higher for thrombus in the inferior vena cava. Both permanent and retrievable filters reduce the risk of recurrent PE but have not been shown to prolong survival, possibly because permanent filters can be associated with long-term complications that include inferior vena cava occlusion due to thrombus, recurrent DVT, and post-thrombotic syndrome.[28] Retrievable filters, designed to be removed within 2 to 4 weeks of implantation, can circumvent these long-term complications, but device migration or thrombosis occur in up to 10% of patients with temporary filters because the majority are not removed. Owing to these potential problems, caval filters should be restricted to patients who have high risk for recurrent PE and an absolute contraindication for anticoagulation, such as patients who develop a PE in the lead-up to or shortly after major surgery, those who experience major bleeding with anticoagulant therapy, or pregnant women who have a PE shortly before delivery. Retrievable filters should be used in these cases, and the devices should be removed as soon as anticoagulant therapy can safely be administered. Permanent filters are suitable for patients who have ongoing contraindications to anticoagulation. If a permanent filter is implanted, lifelong anticoagulation therapy should be considered once the contraindications have resolved, so as to reduce the risk of clotting of the filter.[29]

Specific Patient Subgroups

Patients with VTE in the setting of active cancer, women who suffer VTE during pregnancy, and patients with chronic thromboembolic pulmonary hypertension require special treatment. In addition, management of upper-extremity DVT and superficial thrombophlebitis also are worthy of comment.

CANCER

Active cancer and its treatment with chemotherapy, radiation therapy, and growth factors or other biological agents increase the risk of VTE.[30] Patients with advanced cancer often have limited mobility, which adds to their risk of VTE. In addition, indwelling central venous access catheters can trigger upper-extremity DVT, which can lead to PE. Therefore, the index of suspicion should be high in cancer patients who present with symptoms and signs suggestive

TABLE 52-2	Low-Molecular-Weight Heparin and Fondaparinux Regimens for Treatment of Venous Thromboembolism	
AGENT	**DOSE**	**INTERVAL**
Enoxaparin	1 mg/kg	Twice daily
	1.5 mg/kg	Once daily
Dalteparin	100 units/kg	Twice daily
	200 units/kg	Once daily
Tinzaparin	175 units/kg	Once daily
Fondaparinux	5 mg (weight <50 kg)	Once daily
	7.5 mg (weight 50-100 kg)	Once daily
	10 mg (weight >100 kg)	Once daily

of PE and/or DVT.[31] With advances in diagnostic imaging, incidental PE may be discovered on CT scans performed for staging purposes or for monitoring response to treatment. Although 20% of patients with VTE have an underlying malignancy, there is no evidence of a benefit of routine cancer screening in patients with VTE.[32]

As in patients without cancer, initial treatment of VTE in cancer patients involves administration of a rapidly acting parenteral anticoagulant. For extended treatment, however, LMWH reduces the risk of recurrent VTE to a greater extent than warfarin.[33] In addition, in the face of poor nutritional intake, severe nausea and vomiting, transient thrombocytopenia, or invasive procedures, LMWH is easier to manage than warfarin.

Cancer patients who develop VTE after curative surgery or with adjuvant chemotherapy for limited-stage disease should be treated for at least 3 months or until they have completed their chemotherapy. Those with VTE against a background of advanced cancer have a risk of recurrence of at least 20% in the first year after stopping anticoagulant therapy, so they require indefinite treatment.[21]

VENOUS THROMBOEMBOLISM IN PREGNANCY

Treatment of VTE in pregnancy centers mainly on heparin or LMWH because, unlike warfarin, these agents do not cross the placenta.[34] Although both agents can be given subcutaneously, weight-adjusted LMWH has advantages over heparin because it can be given once daily without routine monitoring, and because the risks of HIT and osteoporosis are lower with LMWH than with heparin.[35] Anti–factor Xa monitoring of LMWH should be considered in women at extremes of body weight or in those with renal impairment. Fondaparinux should be considered for pregnant women who have a history of HIT or develop injection-site reactions to heparin or LMWH.

Heparin or LMWH should be continued throughout pregnancy. Warfarin must be avoided because it crosses the placenta and can cause bone and central nervous system (CNS) abnormalities, fetal hemorrhage, or placental abruption.[36] During labor and delivery, epidural analgesia should be avoided unless prophylactic-dose LMWH has been stopped at least 12 hours and therapeutic dose LMWH has been stopped at least 24 hours before insertion of the epidural catheter; treatment can be resumed within 6 hours of catheter withdrawal.[37] After delivery, anticoagulation therapy should be continued for at least 3 months; warfarin can be used because it does not appear in breast milk.

Fibrinolytic agents have been used successfully for treatment of severe PE in pregnancy but can cause bleeding, usually from the genital tract. If PE develops late in pregnancy, a retrievable filter may prevent recurrence during delivery when anticoagulant therapy must be withheld.

UPPER-EXTREMITY DEEP VEIN THROMBOSIS

Usually involving the axillary and/or subclavian veins, upper-extremity DVT can be unprovoked, related to effort, or can be secondary to indwelling central venous catheters.[38] Unprovoked upper-extremity DVT is unusual. More common is effort-related upper-extremity DVT, known as *Paget-Schroetter's syndrome*, which usually affects the dominant arm of young, otherwise healthy individuals and occurs after strenuous exercise such as rowing or weight lifting. It is likely the unusual exertion causes injury to the vein wall, and with repeated trauma, this is sufficient to induce thrombosis, particularly if there is associated mechanical obstruction to blood flow. Such obstruction can result from compression of the subclavian vein as it exits the thoracic inlet, which can be caused by muscle hypertrophy or anomalies of the cervical ribs or spine. These abnormalities can often be detected on plain radiographs of the chest and cervical spine. However, most cases of upper-extremity DVT develop in patients with central venous catheters, particularly in patients with cancer.

Patients with upper-extremity DVT usually present with pain and swelling in the arm and may complain of associated shoulder or neck discomfort. If the DVT extends to involve the superior vena cava, there may be edema of the neck and face. Patients with thoracic outlet syndrome may have pain radiating to the fourth and fifth digits as a result of concomitant injury to the brachial plexus, and symptoms may be exacerbated by hyperabduction of the shoulder or lifting heavy objects.

The diagnosis of upper-extremity DVT is usually established by compression ultrasonography.[39] Contrast venography or magnetic resonance (MR) venography can be helpful if the ultrasound is inconclusive. D-dimer testing may be less useful for upper-extremity DVT diagnosis than it is for the diagnosis of lower-extremity DVT because of the smaller thrombus volume in the upper limbs. Therefore, a negative D-dimer test is insufficient to exclude the possibility of upper-extremity DVT.

Anticoagulation is the cornerstone of treatment for upper-extremity DVT.[19] Treatment usually starts with LMWH, and patients can then be transitioned to warfarin. Treatment should be given for at least 3 months. Patients with catheter-related upper-extremity DVT in the setting of cancer are best treated with extended LMWH, which should be continued as long as the catheter remains in place. Because of the importance of venous access in such patients, central venous catheters do not have to be removed, provided they are functional. Catheter-directed or pharmacomechanical fibrinolytic therapy can be considered for young, healthy patients with extensive upper-extremity DVT to reduce the risk of postthrombotic syndrome. This is an important consideration because recent evidence suggests that postthrombotic syndrome is a frequent and often disabling complication of upper-extremity DVT, particularly DVT involving the dominant arm.[40] Surgical decompression of thoracic outlet obstruction can be considered if symptoms fail to resolve with more conservative treatment.[41]

SUPERFICIAL THROMBOPHLEBITIS

Thrombosis in superficial veins can occur spontaneously or as a complication of IV catheter insertion.[42] Spontaneous thrombophlebitis is sterile; thrombophlebitis complicating catheter placement may be sterile or septic. Sterile thrombophlebitis is characterized by a tender cord that follows the course of superficial veins, usually on an extremity. The overlying skin may be erythematous and warm to touch. These features are magnified with septic thrombophlebitis, and a purulent discharge from a previous IV catheter puncture site is a common finding.

Superficial thrombophlebitis can extend into the deep venous system via perforating veins and can lead to PE.[43] Therefore, ultrasonography should be performed to exclude DVT in patients whose superficial thrombophlebitis is associated with limb swelling, or in those with involvement of the proximal segment of the greater saphenous vein.

Septic thrombophlebitis often requires antibiotic treatment. Localized sterile thrombophlebitis can be treated with antiinflammatory agents such as ibuprofen or naproxen. Patients with severe symptoms or with more extensive disease obtain faster relief with anticoagulation therapy with either LMWH or fondaparinux.[44,45] Therapeutic doses of these drugs can be given subcutaneously for 4 to 6 weeks or until symptoms have resolved.

Most patients with superficial thrombophlebitis have an excellent prognosis. Patients with superficial thrombophlebitis complicating varicose veins often benefit from graduated compression stockings. Recurrent or migratory superficial thrombophlebitis can occur in patients with vasculitis, such as polyarteritis nodosa or Buerger's disease, or in patients with cancer, particularly pancreatic cancer.

Venous Thromboembolism Prevention

At least half of outpatients with newly diagnosed VTE have a history of recent hospitalization, and most failed to receive thromboprophylaxis during their hospital stay. As a result, PE is the most common preventable cause of death in hospitalized patients in the United States. Guidelines for primary prophylaxis are available and should be followed.[46]

Prognosis

With the diagnosis established and adequate anticoagulant therapy initiated, most patients with VTE survive.[47,48] Case fatality rates 1 month after diagnosis of DVT or PE are 6% and 12%, respectively. Patients with severe PE who present with shock have the highest mortality, and many die within an hour of presentation. Although the case fatality rate in patients with PE is twice that in those with DVT, many deaths are the result of comorbid conditions rather than the PE itself, and are therefore unlikely to be prevented by anticoagulant therapy. Factors associated with early mortality after VTE include presentation as PE, advanced age, cancer, and underlying cardiovascular disease. The most serious long-term complication of PE is chronic thromboembolic pulmonary hypertension, a rare condition associated with significant morbidity and mortality (discussed earlier).

Postthrombotic syndrome is the major complication of lower-extremity DVT[49] (also see Chapter 55). Characterized by dependent leg swelling and discomfort, skin induration, itchiness and telangiectasias, the incidence of postthrombotic syndrome ranges from 20% to 40%. The incidence of severe postthrombotic syndrome, which can lead to venous ulcers, is about 3% at 1 year and 9% after 5 years, even with the use of graduated compression stockings.

Postthrombotic syndrome is triggered by damage to the venous valves. Venous occlusion due to residual thrombus and reflux of blood through incompetent valves leads to increased venous pressure, reduced calf muscle perfusion, increased vascular permeability, and subsequent dependent edema and discomfort. Catheter-directed or pharmacomechanical fibrinolytic therapy may improve venous patency in patients with extensive DVT and prevent valve damage, thereby reducing the risk of postthrombotic syndrome.

Inadequate anticoagulation therapy and recurrent DVT are risk factors for postthrombotic syndrome.[50] Therefore, adequate intensity and duration of anticoagulation therapy is a goal of DVT treatment. Patients with extensive proximal DVT are more likely to develop postthrombotic syndrome than those with distal DVT. Use of graduated compression stockings by DVT patients appears to reduce the risk of postthrombotic syndrome.

Despite anticoagulant therapy, about 6% of patients suffer recurrent VTE during the first 6 months. While on anticoagulation treatment, patients with unprovoked VTE and those with secondary VTE have similar risks of recurrence. In contrast, when anticoagulant therapy is stopped, patients with unprovoked VTE have a risk of recurrence of 10% at 1 year and 30% at 5 years, whereas those with secondary VTE have recurrence rates of 3% at 1 year and 10% at 5 years. Recurrent events often mirror the index events; after an initial PE, about 60% of recurrences are PE, whereas after an initial DVT, about 60% of the recurrences are DVT. Because of the high risk of recurrence in patients with unprovoked VTE, many experts recommend indefinite anticoagulant therapy for such patients.[19] In contrast, because of the lower risk of recurrence, anticoagulation therapy can be stopped after 3 months in patients with secondary VTE whose risk factors have resolved.

REFERENCES

1. Torbicki A, Perrier A, Konstantinides S, et al: Guidelines on the diagnosis and management of acute pulmonary embolism: the Task Force for the Diagnosis and Management of Acute Pulmonary Embolism of the European Society of Cardiology (ESC), Eur Heart J 29(18):2276–2315, 2008.
2. Silverstein MD, Heit JA, Mohr DN, et al: Trends in the incidence of deep vein thrombosis and pulmonary embolism: a 25-year population-based study, Arch Intern Med 158(6):585–593, 1998.
3. White RH, Zhou H, Romano RS: Incidence of idiopathic deep venous thrombosis and secondary thromboembolism among ethnic groups in California, Ann Intern Med 128(9):737–740, 1998.
4. Kearon C: Natural history of venous thromboembolism, Circulation 107(23 Suppl 1):122–130, 2003.
5. Lijfering WM, Rosendaal FR, Cannegieter SC: Risk factors for venous thrombosis – current understanding from an epidemiological point of view, Br J Haematol 149(6):824–833, 2010.
6. Bernardi E, Pesavento R, Prandoni P: Upper extremity deep venous thrombosis, Semin Thromb Hemost 32(7):729–736, 2006.
7. Agnelli G, Becattini C: Acute pulmonary embolism, N Engl J Med 363(3):266–274, 2010.
8. van Belle A, Buller HR, Huisman MV, et al: Effectiveness of managing suspected pulmonary embolism under an algorithm combining clinical probability, D-dimer testing and computed tomography, JAMA 295(2):172–179, 2006.
9. Stein PD, Hull RD, Patel KC, et al: D-dimer for the exclusion of acute venous thrombosis and pulmonary embolism: a systematic review, Ann Intern Med 140(8):589–602, 2004.
10. Lensing AWA, Prandoni P, Brandjes DPM, et al: Detection of deep-vein thrombosis by real-time B-mode ultrasonography, N Engl J Med 320(6):342–345, 1989.
11. Lensing AWA, Buller HR, Prandoni P, et al: Contrast venography, the gold standard for the diagnosis of deep-vein thrombosis: improvement in observer agreement, Thromb Haemost 67(1):8–12, 1992.
12. Goodacre S, Sutton AJ, Sampson FC: Meta-analysis: the value of clinical assessment in the diagnosis of deep venous thrombosis, Ann Intern Med 143(2):129–139, 2005.
13. Wells PS, Anderson DR, Bormanis J, et al: Value of assessment of pretest probability of deep-vein thrombosis in clinical management, Lancet 350(9094):1795–1798, 1997.
14. Elias AD, Colombier D, Victor G, et al: Diagnostic performance of complete lower limb venous ultrasound in patients with clinically suspected acute pulmonary embolism, Thromb Haemost 91(1):187–195, 2004.
15. Middeldorp S, van Hylckama Vlieg A: Does thrombophilia testing help in the clinical management of patients? Br J Haematol 143(3):321–335, 2008.
16. Brady AJ, Crake T, Oakley CM: Percutaneous catheter fragmentation and distal dispersion of proximal pulmonary embolus, Lancet 338(8776):1186–1189, 1991.
17. Leacche M, Unic D, Goldhaber SZ, et al: Modern surgical treatment of massive pulmonary embolism: results in 47 consecutive patients after rapid diagnosis and aggressive surgical approach, J Thorac Cardiovasc Surg 129(5):1018–1023, 2005.
18. Watson LI, Armon MP: Thrombolysis for acute deep vein thrombosis, Cochrane Database Syst Rev 4: CD002783, 2004.
19. Kearon C, Kahn SR, Agnelli G, et al: Antithrombotic therapy for venous thromboembolic disease: American College of Chest Physicians Evidence-Based Clinical Practice Guidelines (8th edition), Chest 133(6 Suppl):454S–545S, 2008.
20. Raschke RA, Gollihare B, Peirce JC: The effectiveness of implementing the weight-based heparin nomogram as a practice guideline, Arch Intern Med 156(15):1645–1649, 1996.
21. Schulman S, Kearon C, Kakkar AK, et al: Dabigatran versus warfarin in the treatment of acute venous thromboembolism, N Engl J Med 361(24):2342–2352, 2009.
22. Eikelboom JW, Weitz JI: New anticoagulants, Circulation 121(13):1523–1532, 2010.
23. Connolly SJ, Ezekowitz MD, Yusuf S, et al: Dabigatran versus warfarin in patients with atrial fibrillation, N Engl J Med 361(12):1139–1151, 2009.
24. Einstein Investigators, Bauersachs R, Berkowitz SD, et al: Oral rivaroxaban for symptomatic venous thromboembolism, N Engl J Med 363(26):2499–2510, 2010.
25. Bruinstroop E, Klok FA, Van De Ree MA, et al: Elevated D-dimer levels predict recurrence in patients with idiopathic venous thromboembolism: a meta-analysis, J Thromb Haemost 7(4):611–618, 2009.
26. Prandoni P, Lensing AWA, Prins MH, et al: Residual venous thrombosis as a predictive factor of recurrent venous thromboembolism, Ann Intern Med 137(12):955–960, 2002.
27. Ridker PM, Goldhaber SZ, Danielson E, et al: Long-term, low-intensity warfarin therapy for the prevention of recurrent venous thromboembolism, N Engl J Med 348(15):1425–1434, 2003.
28. PREPIC Study Group: Eight-year follow-up of patients with permanent vena cava filters in the prevention of pulmonary embolism: the PREPIC (Prevention du Risque d'Embolie Pulmonaire par Interruption Cave) randomized study, Circulation 112(3):416–422, 2005.
29. Decousus H, Leizorovicz A, Parent F, et al: A clinical trial of vena caval filters in the prevention of pulmonary embolism in patients with proximal deep-vein thrombosis, N Engl J Med 338(7):409–415, 1998.
30. Heit JA, Silverstein MD, Mohr DN, et al: Risk factors for deep vein thrombosis and pulmonary embolism: a population-based case-control study, Arch Intern Med 160(6):809–815, 2000.
31. Blom JW, Doggen CJ, Osanto S, et al: Malignancies, prothrombotic mutations, and the risk of venous thrombosis, JAMA 293(6):715–722, 2005.
32. Monreal M, Lensing AWA, Prins MH, et al: Screening for occult cancer in patients with acute deep vein thrombosis or pulmonary embolism, J Thromb Haemost 2(6):876–881, 2004.
33. Lee AYY, Levine MN, Baker RI, et al: Low-molecular-weight heparin versus a coumarin for the prevention of recurrent venous thromboembolism in patients with cancer, N Engl J Med 349(2):146–153, 2003.
34. Bates SM, Greer IA, Pabinger I, et al: Venous thromboembolism, thrombophilia, antithrombotic therapy, and pregnancy: American College of Chest Physicians: evidence-based clinical practice guidelines (8th edition), Chest 133(6 Suppl):844S–886S, 2008.
35. Bourjeily G, Paidas MJ, Khalil H, et al: Pulmonary embolism in pregnancy, Lancet 375(9713):500–512, 2010.
36. Shaul WL, Hall JG: Multiple congenital anomalies associated with oral anticoagulants, Am J Obstet Gynecol 127(2):191–198, 1977.
37. Horlocker TT, Wedel DJ, Benzon H, et al: Regional anesthesia in the anticoagulated patient: defining the risks (the second ASRA Consensus Conference on Neuraxial Anesthesia and Anticoagulation), Reg Anesth Pain Med 28(3):172–197, 2003.
38. Joffe HV, Kucher N, Tapson VF, et al: Upper-extremity deep vein thrombosis: a prospective registry of 592 patients, Circulation 110(12):1605–1611, 2004.
39. Prandoni P, Polistena P, Bernardi E, et al: Upper-extremity deep vein thrombosis. Risk factors, diagnosis and complications, Arch Intern Med 157(1):57–62, 1997.
40. Elman EE, Kahn SR: The post-thrombotic syndrome after upper extremity deep venous thrombosis in adults: a systematic review, Thromb Res 117(6):609–614, 2006.
41. Becker DM, Philbrick JT, Walker FB IV: Axillary and subclavian venous thrombosis. Prognosis and treatment, Arch Intern Med 151(10):1934–1943, 1991.
42. Leon L, Giannoukas AD, Dodd D, et al: Clinical significance of superficial vein thrombosis, Eur J Vasc Endovasc Surg 29(1):10–17, 2005.
43. Decousus H, Quere I, Presles E, et al: Superficial venous thrombosis and venous thromboembolism in a large, prospective epidemiologic study, Ann Intern Med 152(4):218–224, 2010.
44. Di Nisio M, Wichers IM, Middeldorp S: Treatment for superficial thrombophlebitis of the leg, Cochrane Database Syst Rev 2: CD004982, 2007.

45. Decousus H, Prandoni P, Mismetti P, et al: Fondaparinux for the treatment of superficial-vein thrombosis of the legs, *N Engl J Med* 363(13):1222–1232, 2010.

46. Geerts WH, Bergqvist D, Pineo GF, et al: Prevention of venous thromboembolism: American College of Chest Physicians evidence-based clinical practice guidelines (8th edition), *Chest* 133(6 Suppl):381S–453S, 2008.

47. Kasper W, Konstantinides S, Geibel A, et al: Management strategies and determinants of outcome in acute major pulmonary embolism: results of a multicenter registry, *J Am Coll Cardiol* 30(5):1165–1171, 1997.

48. Goldhaber SZ, Visani L, De Rosa M: Acute pulmonary embolism: clinical outcomes in the International Cooperative Pulmonary Embolism Registry (ICOPER), *Lancet* 353(9162):1386–1389, 1999.

49. Prandoni P, Lensing AWA, Cogo A, et al: The long-term clinical course of acute deep venous thrombosis, *Ann Intern Med* 125(1):1–7, 1996.

50. van Dongen CJ, Prandoni P, Frulla M, et al: Relation between quality of anticoagulant treatment and the development of the postthrombotic syndrome, *J Thromb Haemost* 3(5):939–942, 2005.

CHAPTER 53 Pulmonary Embolism

Samuel Z. Goldhaber, Jeffrey I. Weitz, Gregory Piazza

Pulmonary embolism (PE) and deep venous thrombosis (DVT) comprise venous thromboembolism (VTE), a complex illness that warrants primary management or consultation by vascular medicine specialists. The Surgeon General estimates that PE causes between 100,000 and 180,000 deaths in the United States alone, and singles out PE as the most preventable cause of in-hospital death.[1] Pulmonary embolism and DVT have attracted national attention among healthcare providers, policy makers, and the public. Advances in understanding PE's epidemiology, prevention, diagnosis, and treatment are evolving at a rapid pace.

Epidemiology of Venous Thromboembolism

A cardinal misperception is that PE is much more benign than arterial cardiovascular diseases such as acute myocardial infarction (AMI). In fact, the case fatality rate for PE is much higher than that for MI, probably because PE is more difficult to detect and lacks wide application of definitive therapies such as thrombolysis or mechanical coronary revascularization. In an international PE registry at 52 institutions in 7 countries, the death rate was 17% after 3 months of follow-up. This registry had no exclusion criteria.[2]

The high mortality rate after PE is only the tip of the iceberg. Pulmonary embolism is associated with a multitude of adverse events. In a Dutch registry of 866 PE patients, a group of adverse events was tracked over time: death, recurrent VTE, arterial cardiovascular events, cancer, and chronic thromboembolic pulmonary hypertension (CTEPH). Some 30% of the Dutch PE cohort suffered adverse events within 1 year; the proportion increased to more than 40% after 2 years, and to more than 50% after 4 years.[3] Chronic thromboembolic pulmonary hypertension[4] used to be considered a rare complication of PE, but contemporary epidemiological studies indicate that it evolves in 1% to 3% of patients with acute PE. This complication causes marked dyspnea and makes patients vulnerable to sudden cardiac death. About half of patients with VTE will develop chronic venous insufficiency, also known as *postthrombotic syndrome* (see Chapter 55). This problem causes chronic leg swelling and discomfort, especially with standing. Brownish skin pigmentation can develop, especially in the medial malleolus. In extreme cases, venous ulceration may occur. Postthrombotic syndrome does not cause mortality, but does reduce quality of life for those who are stricken with it.[5]

Although the frequency of PE diagnosis among hospitalized patients is increasing in the United States, the mortality rate is decreasing. There were an estimated 127,000 cases of diagnosed PE in 1998, and this case load rose to 230,000 in 2005. These data reflect marked underestimates because most PEs are misdiagnosed as cardiac conditions such as AMI or sudden cardiac death. Nevertheless, the case fatality rate from PE decreased from 12.3% in 1998 to 8.2% in 2005. During this same time period, the estimated cost per hospitalized patient with PE almost doubled from $25,000 in 1995 to $44,000 in 2005.[6]

The incidence of VTE ranges between 1 and 2 per 1000 among adults in the United States. Prevalence is similar in men and women, and frequency of PE increases with age. There are about twice as many DVT as PE cases. About half are idiopathic (called *primary PE*) and half are provoked (called *secondary PE*) and occur after surgery, trauma, immobilization, or in association with cancer, birth control pill use, pregnancy, or postmenopausal hormone replacement. Certain genetic mutations such as factor V Leiden or the prothrombin gene mutation predispose to VTE (see Chapter 10).

In about half of cases, VTE is associated with acquired (Box 53-1) or inherited (Box 53-2) risk factors. Prior VTE increases the risk of recurrence. Risk factors for VTE are often modifiable and overlap with risk factors for coronary artery disease (CAD). Abstaining from cigarettes, maintaining lean weight, limiting red meat intake, and controlling hypertension might lower the risk of PE and DVT. Hospitalized patients at especially high risk include the elderly and those with cancer, congestive heart failure (CHF),[7] or chronic obstructive pulmonary disease (COPD), as well as those undergoing surgery.[8]

Three of four PEs occur in the outpatient setting. Outpatients presenting with PE who are at high risk for adverse outcomes include those with a history of congestive heart failure, cancer, and severe infection.[9]

In the prospective DVT FREE registry of 5451 patients,[10] the most common acquired comorbidities were hypertension (50%), surgery within 3 months (38%), immobility within 30 days (34%), cancer (32%), and obesity (27%).

Cancer augments the risk of VTE[11] through numerous mechanisms that include intrinsic tumor procoagulant activity and extrinsic factors such as chemotherapeutic agents and indwelling central venous catheters. Pancreatic, lung, gastric, genitourinary tract, and breast malignancies are associated with a particularly high risk of DVT and PE. In the California Cancer Registry,[12] the highest incidence of VTE in cancer patients occurred during the first year of follow-up. The number of VTE events per 100 patient-years was 20 for pancreatic cancer, 11 for stomach cancer, 8 for bladder cancer, 6 for renal and uterine cancer, and 5 for lung cancer. Cancer chemotherapy increases levels of coagulation factors, suppresses anticoagulant and fibrinolytic activity, and directly damages the endothelium. Some patients with newly diagnosed VTE, especially idiopathic and unprovoked, harbor an occult cancer.[13]

Fatal PE associated with long-haul air travel has captivated the attention of the lay public. Although rare, the risk of massive PE increases progressively when the flight distance exceeds 5000 kilometers.[14] There appears to be a dose-response relationship, with an estimated 18% higher risk of VTE for each 2-hour incremental increase in travel duration.[15]

Venous thromboembolism can adversely affect women's health. Oral contraceptives,[16] pregnancy,[17] and postmenopausal hormone replacement therapy[18] increase the risk of PE and DVT. Most oral contraceptives are second-generation agents that double or triple VTE risk. Newer third-generation agents have desogestrel or gestodene as the progestogen component and cause less acne and hirsutism, but they appear to cause acquired resistance to activated protein C (APC), with an incremental doubling or tripling of the VTE risk compared with second-generation contraceptives.

The antiphospholipid antibody syndrome is the most ominous acquired risk factor and is associated with arterial and venous thromboembolism as well as recurrent pregnancy loss. Autoantibodies bind to endothelial receptors to promote the release of tissue factor and suppress cell surface plasminogen activation.[19]

Thrombophilia is often inherited. A family history of VTE should be sought in all patients with DVT or PE. Whether laboratory testing should routinely be undertaken for patients with PE is controversial. The factor V Leiden mutation, a single-base mutation (substitution of A for G at position 506), is a common genetic polymorphism associated with APC resistance (Fig. 53-1). This genetic mutation is also a risk factor for recurrent pregnancy loss, probably due to placental vein thrombosis. The prothrombin gene mutation is a thrombophilic mutation identified in the 3′ untranslated region of the prothrombin gene (substitution of A for G at position 20210). This mutation causes increased prothrombin

Box 53-1 Common Acquired Risk Factors for Venous Thromboembolism

Immobilization/trauma/surgery
Cancer
Prior venous thromboembolism (VTE)
Medical comorbidities, including obesity, heart failure, chronic kidney disease, chronic obstructive pulmonary disease (COPD), infection, and atherosclerosis
Increasing age
Pregnancy/postpartum
Oral contraceptives/hormonal replacement therapy
Indwelling central venous catheter
Lupus anticoagulant/antiphospholipid antibody syndrome
Long-haul air travel

Box 53-2 Inherited Hypercoagulable States Associated with Venous Thromboembolism

Factor V Leiden
Prothrombin G20210 mutation
Protein C deficiency
Protein S deficiency
Antithrombin III deficiency
Dysfibrinogenemia
Disorders of plasminogen

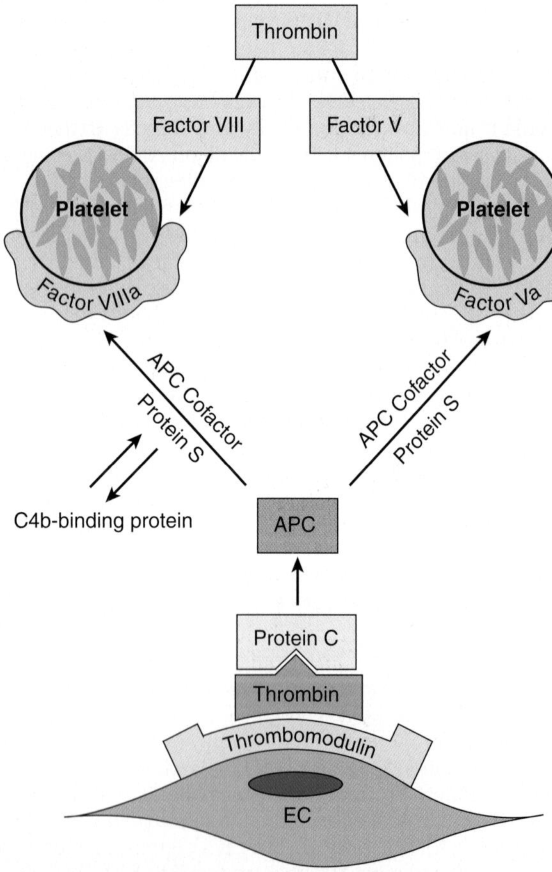

FIGURE 53-1 Thrombin converts factors VIII and V to their activated forms, factors VIIIa and Va. A complex of thrombin with the endothelial cell (EC) receptor thrombomodulin activates protein C (APC). APC inactivates factors VIIIa and Va on the platelet surface. This reaction is accelerated by APC cofactor, which is thought to be inactivated factor V, as well as by free protein S. *(From Bauer KA: Hypercoagulability—a new cofactor in the protein C anticoagulant pathway. N Engl J Med 330:566, 1994.)*

concentration and is associated with an increased risk of VTE. Use of oral contraceptives by patients with factor V Leiden or the prothrombin gene mutation is associated with a high risk of VTE.

Pathophysiology

In 1856, Rudolf Virchow postulated a triad of factors that predispose to VTE: local trauma to the vessel wall, hypercoagulability, and stasis. Venous thrombi, composed primarily of fibrin and red blood cells, often arise at sites of vessel damage. They usually form first in the veins of the calf and then extend proximally to the popliteal, femoral, and pelvic veins. The reasons why thrombi detach from the leg and pelvic veins and then embolize to the pulmonary arteries remain uncertain. About half of patients with PE do not have evidence of DVT on venous ultrasound examination, probably because the thrombus has already broken off and embolized to the lungs. With embolization, pulmonary artery pressure (PAP) usually increases right ventricular (RV) afterload, with consequent elevation of RV wall tension leading to RV dilation and dysfunction. The interventricular septum then shifts toward the left ventricle, with subsequent underfilling and decreased left ventricular (LV) diastolic distensibility. This change can decrease cardiac output, impair coronary perfusion, and produce myocardial ischemia. A downward spiral can ensue, with reduced right coronary artery blood flow, increased RV myocardial oxygen demand, RV infarction, circulatory collapse, and death.

Pulmonary embolism can manifest the following pathophysiological cardiopulmonary effects[20]: (1) increased pulmonary vascular resistance (PVR) due to vascular obstruction, neurohumoral agents, pulmonary artery baroreceptors, or increased pulmonary artery pressure; (2) impaired gas exchange due to increased alveolar dead space from vascular obstruction and hypoxemia from alveolar hypoventilation, low ventilation/perfusion (V/Q) units, and right-to-left shunting, as well as impaired carbon monoxide transfer owing to loss of gas exchange surface; (3) alveolar hyperventilation from reflex stimulation of irritant receptors; (4) increased airway resistance due to bronchoconstriction; and (5) decreased pulmonary compliance due to lung edema, lung hemorrhage, and loss of surfactant.

Arterial hypoxia and an increase in the alveolar-arterial oxygen tension gradient are the most common gas exchange abnormalities. Mismatching of ventilation and perfusion is the most common cause of impaired pulmonary oxygen transfer. Pulmonary embolism causes redistribution of blood flow so that some lung gas exchange units have low ratios of ventilation to perfusion, whereas other lung units have excessively high ratios of ventilation to perfusion. A right-to-left shunt further contributes to arterial hypoxia because venous blood enters the systemic arterial system without passing through ventilated gas exchange units of the lung. Low cardiac output due to RV dysfunction leads to increased extraction of oxygen in the tissues, thereby further decreasing the partial pressure of oxygen in venous blood. Hypercapnia suggests massive PE and results from increased anatomical and physiological dead space.

Hemodynamic alterations are common in patients with acute PE. Increased PVR and PAP cause RV shear stress and microinfarction. Increased myocardial shear stress can be quantified with brain natriuretic peptide (BNP) levels.[21] Elevated troponin levels indicate myocardial ischemia and microinfarction.[22] Myocardial ischemia and microinfarction are probably caused by two mechanisms: increased oxygen demand of the failing right ventricle and reduced coronary perfusion secondary to decreased systemic cardiac output.

Prevention

Pulmonary embolism is easier and less expensive to prevent than to diagnose or treat. A policy of routine VTE prophylaxis is cost-effective.[23] Virtually all patients hospitalized for more than a day should receive prophylactic measures against VTE. Detailed

TABLE 53-1   Possible Prophylaxis Strategies

CONDITION	PROPHYLAXIS STRATEGY
General surgery	Enoxaparin 40 mg once daily Dalteparin 2500 or 5000 units once daily UFH 5000 units bid/tid
Total hip replacement	Enoxaparin 40 mg once daily Fondaparinux 2.5 mg once daily Warfarin
Total knee replacement	Enoxaparin 40 mg once daily Fondaparinux 2.5 mg once daily
Hip fracture surgery	Enoxaparin 40 mg once daily Fondaparinux 2.5 mg once daily
Neurosurgery	GCS and IPC PLUS UFH 5000 units bid or enoxaparin 40 mg once daily, PLUS predischarge venous ultrasound in patients with brain tumor
Trauma (not brain)	Enoxaparin 40 mg once daily
Thoracic surgery	GCS, IPC, and UFH 5000 units tid
Medical patients	UFH 5000 units SC tid GCS or IPC Enoxaparin 40 mg once daily Dalteparin 5000 units once daily

bid, twice daily; GCS, graduated compression stockings; IPC, intermittent pneumatic compression; SC, subcutaneous; tid, three times daily; UFH, unfractionated heparin.

guidelines for prevention of VTE are available from various consensus conferences. The most widely influential consensus is sponsored by the American College of Chest Physicians and recommends that "every hospital develop a formal strategy that addresses the prevention of VTE."[24] The type of prophylaxis strategy selected should match the level of risk for developing venous thrombosis (Table 53-1).

Despite the availability of effective measures to prevent VTE, prophylaxis continues to be underused, even among high-risk hospitalized patients. Only half of high risk patients received prophylaxis in a survey of 15,000 acutely ill medical patients enrolled from 52 hospitals in 12 countries.[25] In the even larger ENDORSE Study of 68,000 patients, with 32 countries participating from 6 continents, only 58% of surgical service and 40% of medical service patients received prophylaxis among those at moderate or high risk for VTE.[26] However, failure to prevent in-hospital PE and DVT will no longer be tolerated by government regulators, hospital quality improvement committees, or the medicolegal system. For example, Medicare has stopped reimbursing hospitals for the incremental care needed to treat postoperative total hip or knee replacement patients who develop VTE.[27] Whether this new policy is wise or equitable is debatable,[28] but its influence in augmenting VTE prophylaxis and decreasing the rate of postoperative VTE is indisputable.

Prevention programs should be implemented to establish and enforce protocols that are streamlined and standardized.[29] Computer-generated prompting can increase utilization of prophylactic measures.[30,31] In a randomized trial of 2500 high-risk patients, a computer alert program increased physicians' use of VTE prophylaxis and reduced the rate of symptomatic DVT and PE by more than 40%.[32] At Brigham and Women's Hospital (Boston, Mass.), the computer alert was upgraded from the initial single-screen version to a multiscreen set of alerts. The advanced algorithm increased use of VTE prophylaxis among physicians who had declined to order preventive measures following an initial traditional single-screen alert reminder.[33] The multiscreen alert also provides a default option that automatically orders VTE prophylaxis unless the physician specifically "opts out."

Many hospitals do not have the necessary electronic and information technology infrastructure to support sophisticated electronic alert systems for VTE prophylaxis. An alternative strategy uses a human alert. This system consists of a direct page from a hospital staff member to the attending physician when high-risk hospitalized patients are not receiving prophylaxis. In a multicenter randomized trial, this program of direct notification of the physician by a staff member tended to increase prophylaxis use and reduce the rate of symptomatic DVT and PE by about 20%, but the improvement was not statistically significant.[34]

Venous thromboembolism related events afflict 2 of every 100 acutely ill hospitalized medical patients. Most frequently affected are patients with heart failure, respiratory failure, pneumonia, and cancer. With probability modeling, symptomatic DVT, PE, and deaths from VTE will be halved if universal prophylaxis is used.[35] Furthermore, long-term benefits will persist for at least 5 years by drastically reducing the number of cases of delayed complications such as postthrombotic syndrome and CTEPH.[36]

Mechanical prophylaxis measures use graduated compression stockings (GCS) and intermittent pneumatic compression (IPC). Graduated compression stockings increase venous blood flow and prevent perioperative venodilation of the legs. Intermittent pneumatic compression devices compress the veins more forcefully than GCS and also stimulate the endogenous fibrinolytic system. Mechanical VTE prophylaxis should be ordered for patients with active bleeding or extraordinarily high risk for major bleeding; however, pharmacological prophylaxis appears to be much more effective than IPC for preventing VTE in general surgery patients.[37] Furthermore, in a large study of patients with major debilitating strokes, thigh-high GCS that were applied without pharmacological prophylaxis did not confer any protection against the development of proximal leg DVT.[38]

Subcutaneous administration of unfractionated (UFH) or low-molecular-weight heparin (LMWH) helps prevent VTE. Low-molecular-weight heparin has several advantages over UFH. It exhibits less binding to plasma proteins and endothelial cells than UFH. Consequently, it tends to have a more predictable dose response, a more dose-independent mechanism of clearance, and a longer plasma half-life than UFH. Osteoporosis and heparin-induced thrombocytopenia (HIT) appear to be less common with LMWH than with UFH. In most VTE prevention trials, LMWH is administered as a once-daily subcutaneous injection in fixed or weight-adjusted doses, without laboratory monitoring or dose adjustment.

Fondaparinux, a pentasaccharide, is an anti–factor Xa agent and is effective in preventing VTE after orthopedic surgery in a fixed low dose of 2.5 mg daily. It also appears to markedly reduce VTE incidence among high-risk medical patients.[39]

In addition to anticoagulants, two novel pharmacological approaches appear promising for VTE prophylaxis: vitamin E supplementation and rosuvastatin. The Women's Health Study randomized 39,876 women to receive 600 units of vitamin E or placebo. After a median follow-up of 10 years, there was a 21% reduction in VTE among women assigned to vitamin E. The reduction was most marked among women with VTE prior to randomization and in women with either the factor V Leiden or prothrombin gene mutation.[40]

The JUPITER Trial studied statin therapy for VTE prophylaxis among 17,802 apparently healthy men and women with both normal low-density lipoprotein (LDL) cholesterol levels and elevated high-sensitivity C-reactive protein (CRP) levels. They were randomized to receive rosuvastatin 20 mg per day or placebo. During a median follow-up period of 1.9 years, symptomatic VTE was reduced by 43% in the rosuvastatin group.[41]

In a study of middle-aged women undergoing surgery, the risk of VTE was substantially increased during the first 12 postoperative weeks, especially for those undergoing hip or knee replacement or cancer surgery.[42] In the large RIETE Registry of VTE, the average time elapsed from surgery to VTE was 3 weeks.[43] These findings suggest the need to extend the duration of VTE prophylaxis in high-risk patients beyond hospital discharge.

A large-scale randomized controlled trial tested the concept of extended-duration VTE prophylaxis in hospitalized acutely ill medical patients with reduced mobility.[44] All patients initially received 6 to 14 days of enoxaparin 40 mg open-label VTE prophylaxis. Some patients completed this initial prophylaxis as outpatients. Those who remained at high risk were then randomized to enoxaparin 40 mg daily for 28 days or to placebo. The extended-duration enoxaparin prophylaxis group had a reduction in VTE from 4% to 2.5%, at a cost of an increase in major bleeding events from 0.3% to 0.8%. The benefits of extended duration enoxaparin appeared to be limited to women, patients older than 75 years, and those with marked immobility who did not have bathroom privileges. The trial was criticized because criteria for immobility were made stricter in a protocol amendment that was implemented about halfway through the trial.[45]

Diagnosis

Clinical Suspicion of Pulmonary Embolism

Pulmonary embolism is difficult to diagnose, despite the availability of contemporary imaging techniques such as chest computed tomography (CT) scanning. Therefore, maintaining a high degree of clinical suspicion for possible PE is of paramount importance. The most common symptoms and signs are nonspecific: dyspnea, tachypnea, chest pain, and tachycardia. Usually, patients who present with chest pain or hemoptysis have an anatomically small PE near the periphery of the lung where nerve innervation is greatest and pulmonary infarction is most likely to occur, owing to poor collateral circulation. Ironically, patients with life-threatening PEs often have a painless presentation characterized by dyspnea, syncope, or cyanosis.

Assessment of the clinical pretest probability may improve the diagnostic accuracy in patients with suspected PE. Wells and coworkers[46] have tested a bedside assessment score to estimate the clinical pretest probability for PE. The following clinical variables are required to calculate the score: signs or symptoms of DVT (3 points), no alternative diagnosis (3 points), a heart rate greater than 100 beats/min (1.5 points), immobilization or surgery within 4 weeks (1.5 points), a history of VTE (1.5 points), hemoptysis (1 point), and cancer (1 point). In this study, more than one third of the patients had a low Wells score of 2 or less. Pulmonary embolism was confirmed in only 2% of these patients. In contrast, half of the patients with a Wells score above 6 had PE diagnosed on further testing.

Pulmonary embolism should be suspected in hypotensive patients when (1) there is evidence of or predisposing factors for venous thrombosis, and (2) there is clinical evidence of acute cor pulmonale, such as distended neck veins, an S3 gallop, or an RV heave, especially if there is electrocardiographic (ECG) evidence of acute cor pulmonale manifested by a new S1Q3T3 pattern, new incomplete right bundle branch block, or T-wave inversion in V_1 through V_4 (Box 53-3).

Tests for Pulmonary Embolism

ELECTROCARDIOGRAPHY

The ECG may be normal or might show sinus tachycardia. More specific findings occur at times in the presence of RV dysfunction. These include the S1Q3T3 pattern or T-wave inversion in leads V_1 through V_4.

Box 53-3 Electrocardiographic Findings in Pulmonary Embolism

Sinus tachycardia
Incomplete or complete right bundle branch block
S1Q3T3
T-wave inversion in leads V_1-V_4

CHEST RADIOGRAPHY

A near-normal chest radiograph in the setting of severe respiratory compromise suggests massive PE. Focal oligemia (Westermark sign) indicates massive central embolic occlusion. A peripheral wedge-shaped density above the diaphragm (Hampton hump) points toward pulmonary infarction. The chest radiograph can also help exclude diseases such as lobar pneumonia or pneumothorax that may mimic PE; however, these latter patients can also have concomitant PE.

ARTERIAL BLOOD GAS ANALYSIS

Neither room air arterial blood gases nor calculation of the alveolar-arterial oxygen gradient helps differentiate patients with a confirmed PE at angiography from those with a normal pulmonary angiogram.[47] Therefore, arterial blood gases should not be obtained as a screening test in patients suspected of PE.

D-DIMER

D-dimer is a specific proteolytic degradation product released into the circulation by endogenous fibrinolysis of a cross-linked fibrin clot. An abnormally elevated level of plasma D-dimer (>500 ng/mL) performed with a quantitative enzyme-linked immunosorbent assay (ELISA; Fig. 53-2) has a greater than 90% sensitivity for angiographically proven PE.[48] Although elevated plasma concentrations of D-dimers are sensitive for the presence of PE, they are not specific. Levels are elevated for at least 1 week postoperatively and are increased in patients with pregnancy, MI, sepsis, cancer, or almost any other systemic illness. Therefore, this assay has greatest utility among outpatients or emergency department patients who have suspected PE but no coexisting acute systemic illness.

VENTILATION/PERFUSION SCAN

Ventilation/perfusion lung scanning used to be the principal noninvasive diagnostic test, but it has been supplanted by chest CT scanning. Consider lung scanning in patients with allergy to radiographic contrast agents, severe renal insufficiency, or pregnancy. Ventilation/perfusion scanning is nondiagnostic (low- or intermediate-probability scans) in the majority of patients with suspected PE. The diagnostic accuracy of lung scanning may improve when scans are interpreted in conjunction with clinical pretest probability[49] (Table 53-2).

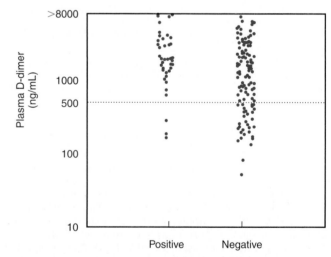

FIGURE 53-2 Distribution of plasma D-dimer enzyme-linked immunosorbent assay (ELISA) levels, sorted according to angiographic findings, among 173 patients with suspected acute pulmonary embolism (PE). *(From Goldhaber SZ, Simons GR, Elliott CG, et al: Quantitative plasma D-dimer levels among patients undergoing pulmonary angiography for suspected pulmonary embolism. JAMA 270:2819, 1993.)*

TABLE 53-2   PIOPED: Pulmonary Embolism Status

LUNG SCAN CATEGORY	Clinical Probability (%)			
	80-100 n/n (%)	20-79 n/n (%)	0-19 n/n (%)	0-100 n/n (%)
High	28/29 (96)	70/80 (88)	5/9 (56)	103/118 (87)
Intermediate	27/41 (66)	66/236 (28)	11/68 (16)	104/345 (30)
Low	6/16 (40)	30/191 (16)	4/90 (4)	40/296 (14)
Very low	0/5 (0)	4/62 (6)	1/61 (2)	5/128 (4)
Total	61/90 (68)	170/569 (30)	21/228 (9)	252/887 (28)

Modified from the PIOPED Investigators: Value of the ventilation/perfusion (V/Q) scan in acute pulmonary embolism. Results of the prospective investigation of pulmonary embolism diagnosis (PIOPED). JAMA 263:2753–2759, 1990.

CONTRAST-ENHANCED CHEST COMPUTED TOMOGRAPHY

Chest CT has become the most useful imaging test in patients with clinically suspected acute PE.[50] The clinical validity of using a CT scan to rule out PE is similar to that reported for invasive pulmonary angiography.[51] Rapid, continuous volume acquisitions obtained during a single breath enable imaging in critically ill patients. The latest generation of multidetector CT scanners (Fig. 53-3) permits image acquisition of the entire chest with 1-mm or submillimeter resolution and a breath hold of less than 10 seconds. Chest CT can also detect alternative or concomitant cardiopulmonary disease such as aortic dissection, pneumonia, or pericardial tamponade.

PULMONARY ANGIOGRAPHY

Classic invasive contrast pulmonary arteriography is the established gold-standard imaging test for diagnosis of PE. Currently, pulmonary angiography is rarely performed for diagnostic purposes because multiplanar chest CT scanning seems to be equally accurate. However, pulmonary angiography is undertaken during therapeutic interventions such as catheter embolectomy.

GADOLINIUM-ENHANCED MAGNETIC RESONANCE ANGIOGRAPHY

Magnetic resonance angiography (MRA) avoids ionizing radiation or iodinated contrast agents. Magnetic resonance angiography is superb for assessment of left and RV function and size.

Unfortunately, MRA is often technically inadequate owing to the requirement of prolonged breath holding in dyspneic and tachypneic patients, and has low sensitivity for the diagnosis of acute PE.[52]

VENOUS ULTRASONOGRAPHY

Ultrasonography of the deep veins is noninvasive, cost-effective, and accurate in diagnosing proximal leg DVT in symptomatic patients.[53] Ultrasound is considered diagnostic for PE if it confirms DVT in patients with PE symptoms. However, one third to one half of PE patients have no ultrasound or venogram evidence of leg DVT, probably because the thrombus has already embolized to the lungs. Therefore, if clinical suspicion of PE is high, patients without clinical or imaging evidence of DVT should still be worked up for PE.

ECHOCARDIOGRAPHY

Echocardiography is not useful routinely to diagnose PE because it is normal in about half of consecutive patients with suspected PE. However, echocardiography does detect RV overload among patients with large PE. Moderate or severe RV hypokinesis, persistent pulmonary hypertension (PH), a patent foramen ovale, and free-floating thrombus in the right atrium or right ventricle are ominous prognostic signs in PE patients. Echocardiography can also help identify illnesses that may mimic PE, such as MI or pericardial disease. For those patients in whom transthoracic imaging is unsatisfactory, transesophageal echocardiography (TEE) can be

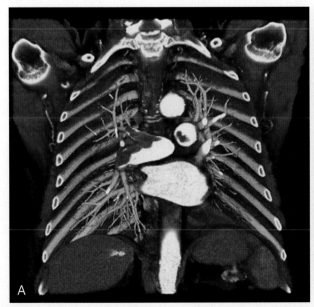
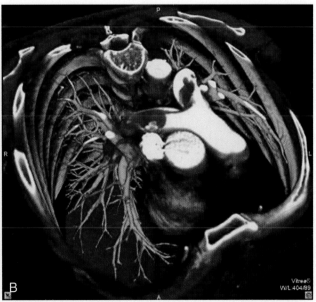

FIGURE 53-3   Contrast-enhanced multislice computed tomography (CT) in a 72-year-old man with acute central pulmonary embolism (PE) showing a "saddle embolus." Colored volume rendering technique seen from an anterior cranial **(A)** and anterior **(B)** perspective allows intuitive visualization of location and extent of embolism. *(Figures kindly provided by Joseph Schoepf, MD, Department of Radiology, Brigham and Women's Hospital, Boston, MA.)*

carried out. For critically ill patients who cannot be safely transported from the intensive care unit (ICU), TEE at the bedside may be especially useful.[54]

Overall Diagnostic Strategy

The initial assessment includes a history, physical examination, ECG, and chest radiograph. A plasma D-dimer ELISA should be obtained in all outpatient or emergency department patients. If the D-dimer is below the assay-specific cut-off level and clinical suspicion is not high, PE is essentially excluded. Chest CT scanning is indicated for diagnosis in most patients if D-dimer levels are elevated or clinical suspicion is high (Fig. 53-4). In patients with impaired renal function, pregnancy, or allergy to contrast agents, V/Q scanning may be performed as the primary imaging test. When the diagnosis remains uncertain, a venous ultrasound study is the next step. Thereafter, if high clinical suspicion for PE persists despite a negative ultrasound study, consider empirical anticoagulation or invasive diagnostic pulmonary angiography.

Management

Risk Stratification

Pulmonary embolism outcome spans a wide clinical spectrum ranging from benign to fatal. With rapidly achieved therapeutic levels of anticoagulation, the majority of patients have favorable outcomes, but some PE patients suffer rapid clinical deterioration, with manifestations of RV failure.[55] These patients often have a poor prognosis if therapy is limited to anticoagulation alone. They may require thrombolysis, embolectomy, mechanical ventilation, inotropic support, or vasopressor agents.

Rapid and accurate risk stratification is paramount in selecting the appropriate management strategy.[56] Patients used to be considered at high risk only if they had *massive PE*, defined as a systemic arterial systolic pressure less than 90 mmHg unresponsive to pressor agents. Contemporary risk stratification focuses on rapid and early detection of *submassive PE*, defined as moderate or severe RV dysfunction despite normal systemic arterial pressure. Such patients often have an ominous prognosis if managed with anticoagulation alone.[57]

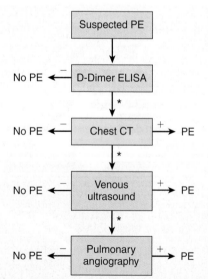

FIGURE 53-4 Suggested diagnostic strategy for patients with suspected pulmonary embolism (PE) without cardiogenic shock. In this strategy, chest computed tomography (CT) is used as the principal imaging test. *Further testing should be considered if the test is inconclusive or negative, with a persistent suspicion of PE. ELISA, enzyme-linked immunosorbent assay.

Clinical Evaluation

Severe dyspnea, cyanosis, and syncope usually indicate life-threatening PE. The clinical examination may detect signs of acute RV dysfunction, such as tachycardia, low arterial blood pressure, distended neck veins, an accentuated pulmonic component of the second heart sound, or a tricuspid regurgitation murmur. The Pulmonary Embolism Severity Index has gained traction as a semi-quantitative clinical assessment tool to assess prognosis and help triage patients with acute PE.[58] However, it is cumbersome because it requires computation of a weighted score based upon 11 different variables. This index has been simplified for greater ease of use.[59] The revised version classifies PE patients as high risk if they have even one of the following clinical variables: age older than 80 years, cancer, chronic cardiopulmonary disease, heart rate 110 beats/min or more, systolic blood pressure (SBP) less than 100 mmHg, or oxygen saturation level less than 90%.

Echocardiography

Transthoracic echocardiography (TTE) has emerged as the most important imaging tool for risk assessment because it evaluates RV size and function. Right ventricular systolic function is usually assessed qualitatively. Patients with acute PE may show a specific regional wall motion abnormality of the right ventricle known as the *McConnell sign*: hypokinesis of the RV free wall combined with preserved systolic contraction of the RV apex.[60] Right ventricular dilation is an indirect sign of RV pressure overload. An RV–to–LV diameter ratio of 1 or greater in the apical four-chamber view indicates RV dilation. Right ventricular pressure overload may cause a paradoxical (systolic) septal motion toward the left ventricle. In the parasternal short-axis view, the interventricular septum may flatten and cause a D-shaped left ventricle (Fig. 53-5). Other indirect signs of RV dysfunction include increased tricuspid regurgitant velocity greater than 2.6 m/s and reduced inspiratory collapse of a dilated inferior vena cava (IVC).

Cardiac Biomarkers

Cardiac troponins I and T, as well as N-terminal pro–brain natriuretic peptide (NT-proBNP) and BNP, have emerged as promising tools for risk stratification in PE. Cardiac troponins are the most sensitive and specific markers of myocardial cell damage. Elevations of troponin levels in PE patients are minor compared with patients with acute coronary syndromes (ACS). The stimulus for BNP synthesis and secretion in acute PE is cardiomyocyte stretch. Heart-type fatty acid–binding protein appears to be an especially useful biomarker to risk stratify normotensive patients with acute PE.[61]

Anticoagulation

When DVT or PE is diagnosed or strongly suspected, anticoagulation therapy should be initiated immediately unless a major contraindication exists.

UNFRACTIONATED HEPARIN AS A BRIDGE TO WARFARIN

A bolus of intravenous (IV) UFH (80 units/kg) followed by 18 units/kg/h is an effective and safe approach to initiate anticoagulation.[62] The activated partial thromboplastin time (aPTT) should be followed at 6-hour intervals until it remains consistently therapeutic at 1.5 to 2.5 times the upper limit of normal. The short half-life of UFH is advantageous for patients who might require thrombolysis or embolectomy. Oral anticoagulation with warfarin can be started as soon as the aPTT is within therapeutic range. Patients should receive at least 5 days of heparin overlap while an adequate level of oral anticoagulation is established.

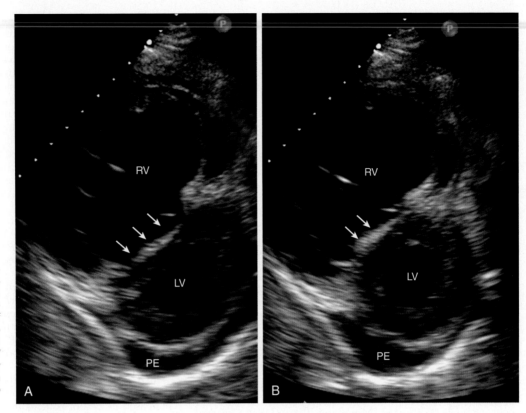

FIGURE 53-5 Parasternal short-axis views of the right ventricle (RV) and left ventricle (LV) in diastole (A) and systole (B). There is diastolic and systolic bowing of interventricular septum *(arrows)* into LV, compatible with RV volume and pressure overloads, respectively. RV is appreciably dilated and markedly hypokinetic, with little change in apparent RV area from diastole to systole. PE, small pericardial effusion.

LOW-MOLECULAR-WEIGHT HEPARIN

Chemical depolymerization of UFH yields LMWH, which improves bioavailability and lowers the risk of HIT compared with unfractionated heparin. Low-molecular-weight heparin is prescribed in a fixed dose according to weight, without the need for laboratory coagulation monitoring. The dose must be adjusted downward for patients with chronic kidney disease because LMWH is metabolized by the kidneys. In 2007, the U.S. Food and Drug Administration (FDA) approved the LMWH dalteparin as monotherapy without warfarin to treat cancer patients with acute VTE. This approval was based on a randomized trial that demonstrated that cancer patients with acute VTE have a 50% lower recurrence rate of VTE if managed with dalteparin as monotherapy rather than dalteparin as a bridge to warfarin.[63]

FONDAPARINUX

Fondaparinux is a synthetic anticoagulant composed of the five saccharide units that function as the active site where heparin binds antithrombin. The fondaparinux-antithrombin complex inhibits factor Xa. Fondaparinux has a long 17-hour half-life, does not cross-react with heparin-induced antibodies, and is often used off-label to manage HIT without thrombosis. It is FDA approved for initial treatment of acute PE and DVT as a bridge to warfarin. Fondaparinux is cleared by the kidney.

PARENTERAL DIRECT THROMBIN INHIBITORS

These agents bind directly to thrombin. Four have been FDA approved: hirudin and argatroban to treat HIT, bivalirudin as an anticoagulant during percutaneous coronary intervention (PCI), and desirudin to prevent VTE in the setting of total hip replacement.

WARFARIN

The vitamin K antagonist warfarin sodium inhibits γ-carboxylation activation of coagulation factors II, VII, IX, and X and proteins C and S. The full anticoagulant effect of warfarin requires about 5 days of therapy even if the target international normalized ratio (INR) is reached more quickly. Warfarin is a difficult drug to dose and monitor, with multiple drug-drug and drug-food interactions. Inadequate warfarin anticoagulation predisposes to recurrent VTE and stroke. Excessive warfarin anticoagulation may cause intracranial hemorrhage and massive gastrointestinal bleeding.

Major bleeding is best managed with prothrombin complex concentrate. Fresh frozen plasma can be used in patients with non–life-threatening bleeding who can tolerate large volumes of fluid. Recombinant human coagulation factor VIIa (rFVIIa) is an off-label option for catastrophic bleeding but may precipitate thrombosis. To manage minor bleeding or an excessively high INR without bleeding, oral vitamin K may be administered.

Centralized anticoagulation clinics, usually staffed by pharmacists or nurses, have improved the quality of warfarin dosing. An excellent anticoagulation clinic can maintain an overall time within therapeutic INR range of at least 60%.

Point-of-care INR testing devices use whole blood from fingertip puncture to provide the INR result within 2 minutes. Appropriately selected patients can self-test their INRs, and some can be taught to self-manage their warfarin dosing, analogous to diabetic patients who self-manage their insulin dosing.

Major genetic determinants of warfarin dose-response include (1) CYP2C9-variant alleles that impair hydroxylation of S-warfarin, resulting in extremely low warfarin dose requirements, such as 1 to 2 mg daily to achieve an INR within the 2.0 to 3.0 range; and (2) variants in the gene encoding vitamin K epoxide reductase complex 1 (VKORC1). Pharmacogenomic algorithms for initiating warfarin appear to be of greatest benefit among those patients requiring very high (>7 mg) or very low (≤3 mg) doses of warfarin.[64]

Using pharmacogenomic information may be cost-effective when initiating warfarin in atrial fibrillation patients at high risk for hemorrhage.[65] An observational study using historical controls found that rapid turnaround genetic testing for CYP2C9 alleles and VKORC1 haplotypes reduced hospitalization rates, including the risk of hospitalization for bleeding or thromboembolism.[66] To help determine the best warfarin anticoagulation dosing strategy, the National Heart, Lung, and Blood Institute (NHLBI) is sponsoring a large trial (NCT00839657) entitled Clarification of Optimal Anticoagulation through Genetics (COAG). More than 1200 patients are being randomized to a genotype-guided versus clinical-guided warfarin dosing algorithm. The primary endpoint is the percentage of time within therapeutic INR range. Results should be available in 2014.

NEW ANTICOAGULANT DRUGS

Novel oral anticoagulants provide rapid onset of action and are administered in fixed doses without routine laboratory coagulation monitoring.[67] Because their half-life is short, when they must be stopped for a diagnostic or surgical procedure, no bridging with a parenteral anticoagulant is needed. These medications have few drug-drug or drug-food interactions, making them more convenient to use than warfarin.[68] Dabigatran, a direct thrombin inhibitor (DTI), is noninferior to warfarin in a large-scale randomized double-blind double-dummy trial of acute VTE treatment.[69] Dabigatran is metabolized primarily by the kidney, whereas the anti–factor Xa agents rivaroxaban and apixaban depend less than dabigatran upon renal clearance. Rivaroxaban is noninferior to enoxaparin as a bridge to warfarin for treatment of acute VTE.[70]

Optimal Duration and Intensity of Anticoagulation

Optimal duration of anticoagulation depends mostly on whether the VTE was unprovoked and idiopathic or provoked by surgery, trauma, birth control pills, pregnancy, or postmenopausal estrogen replacement. Idiopathic VTE has a much higher rate of recurrence ($\approx$40%-50% over the ensuing 10 years) than provoked VTE ($\approx$20% over the ensuing 10 years) after cessation of anticoagulation. American College of Chest Physicians Guidelines recommend consideration of indefinite duration anticoagulation for idiopathic VTE if consistent with patient preference.[71] For provoked (secondary) VTE, these guidelines recommend 3 months of anticoagulation.[71] In the United States, however, many experts recommend anticoagulation for approximately 6 months to treat proximal leg DVT or PE.

Sometimes it is difficult to classify a patient's event as idiopathic or provoked. In this situation, a time-limited duration of therapy can be justified by favorable prognostic indicators such as whether there is vein recanalization on repeat venous ultrasound of the legs[72] or whether the D-dimer level has reverted to normal after stopping anticoagulation for about one month.[73] A hypercoagulability workup also can be useful under these circumstances. For example, patients with antiphospholipid antibody syndrome benefit from indefinite duration anticoagulation.

Cancer patients with acute VTE receive LMWH as monotherapy for 3 months and then continue either LMWH or switch to warfarin. Anticoagulation should continue until the cancer is cured.

The optimal intensity of anticoagulation in patients with idiopathic VTE is controversial. In PREVENT,[74] a double-blind randomized controlled trial of idiopathic VTE patients who had completed an average of 6 months of full-intensity warfarin, low-intensity warfarin (target INR of 1.5 to 2) for an average of 2 years reduced the recurrence rate by two thirds. Patients required INR testing only once every 8 weeks. The strategy of long-term low-intensity warfarin was highly effective in preventing recurrence in all subgroups, even in those with factor V Leiden or the prothrombin gene mutation. In the ELATE study of 739 patients with idiopathic VTE,[75] indefinite-duration full-intensity warfarin (target INR 2 to 3) was more effective and as safe as indefinite-duration low-intensity warfarin therapy (target INR 1.5 to 1.9).

Thrombolytic Therapy

Systemic thrombolysis is lifesaving and considered standard therapy in patients with massive PE and cardiogenic shock.[76] Thrombolysis rapidly reverses severe RV dysfunction by dissolution of pulmonary arterial thrombi that might otherwise lead to chronic pulmonary hypertension. Thrombolysis may also dissolve much of the source of the residual thrombus in the deep veins, thereby minimizing the likelihood of recurrent PE. In patients with acute PE, thrombolysis is effective up to 2 weeks after the onset of symptoms. The only contemporary FDA-approved thrombolytic regimen is a continuous IV infusion of alteplase 100 mg/2 h.

In the absence of PE-related cardiogenic shock, PE is classified as submassive if there is evidence of RV dysfunction. Administration of systemic thrombolysis remains controversial in these patients, because significant mortality reduction with thrombolysis has not yet been shown.[57] In the largest thrombolysis study (MAPPET-3) of patients with submassive PE, heparin plus alteplase as a continuous infusion over 2 hours was compared with heparin alone.[77] Compared with heparin alone, thrombolysis markedly reduced adverse clinical outcomes from 25% to 11%, defined as the need for cardiopulmonary resuscitation, mechanical ventilation, administration of pressors, secondary rescue thrombolysis, or surgical embolectomy. No significant increase in major bleeding occurred, and there was no intracranial bleeding with alteplase among these carefully selected PE patients.

There are only 10 randomized PE trials of thrombolysis versus heparin alone, with a total of 717 patients. In an overview, there is a trend toward a one third reduction in the combined endpoint of mortality or recurrent PE, but a doubling of major hemorrhage.[78] The American College of Chest Physicians 2008 Guidelines recommend consideration of thrombolysis for submassive PE patients who have a low bleeding risk.[71]

In a prospective study of 200 patients with submassive PE, pulmonary artery systolic pressure 6 months after diagnosis increased in 27% of patients treated with heparin alone. Almost half of these patients with increased PAP were symptomatic with dyspnea. Overall, in this cohort of submassive PE patients, the median 6-month decrease in estimated pulmonary artery systolic pressure was 2 mmHg in heparin-alone patients, compared with 22 mmHg in patients treated with alteplase. None of the alteplase-treated patients experienced an increase in PAP during the 6 months of follow-up.[79]

The Pulmonary Embolism International Thrombolysis Trial (PEITHO) is an ongoing randomized trial of submassive PE, with the primary endpoint of all-cause mortality or hemodynamic collapse within 7 days of diagnosis (NCT00639743). Patients are randomized to tenecteplase plus heparin versus heparin alone. More than half of the anticipated 1000 patients have been enrolled. The trial should be completed by 2013.

Catheter Intervention

Interventional thrombus fragmentation with or without embolectomy (Table 53-3) is an alternative to systemic thrombolysis or surgical embolectomy in patients with massive PE.[80] Catheter fragmentation, aspiration, or rheolysis can be combined with local or systemic thrombolysis.[81] This combined approach is called *pharmacomechanical therapy*.

TABLE 53-3	Interventional Devices for Treatment of Massive Pulmonary Embolism
DEVICE	**MECHANISM**
Greenfield catheter	Suction embolectomy
Pigtail catheter	Fragmentation via catheter rotation without embolectomy
Amplatz device	Clot maceration via high-speed impeller rotation that pulverizes, fragments, and recirculates small particles
AngioJet	Embolectomy via high-pressure saline injection (Venturi effect)
Aspirex catheter	Clot maceration and extraction
EKOS	Ultrasound-facilitated thrombolysis

Surgical Embolectomy

Emergency pulmonary embolectomy should be considered in patients with life-threatening PE in the setting of (1) a high bleeding risk from thrombolysis, (2) failed thrombolysis, or (3) presence of right atrial and ventricular thrombi. The operation involves a median sternotomy incision, institution of cardiopulmonary bypass, and deep hypothermia with circulatory arrest periods. Optimal results are obtained if the PE is centrally located and if surgery is undertaken prior to development of cardiogenic shock and multisystem organ failure.[82]

Vena Cava Interruption

The two principal indications for vena cava filter placement are major contraindications to anticoagulation and recurrent embolism despite adequate therapy. Filters reduce the risk of PE but increase the risk of DVT.[83] Complications of IVC filter failure include filter migration or improper filter positioning, allowing thromboemboli to bypass the filter. Occasionally, IVC obstruction due to complete filter thrombosis may occur. Temporary retrievable filters can be used in patients with a contraindication to anticoagulation that is expected to resolve over time.

Overall Management Strategy

Treatment decisions in acute PE are primarily based on the hemodynamic presentation of the patient (Fig. 53-6). Rapid institution of therapeutic levels of anticoagulation remains the foundation of therapy. Patients with massive PE and cardiogenic shock should receive a reperfusion regimen such as thrombolysis, catheter embolectomy, or surgical embolectomy. Optimal management of submassive PE patients with preserved systemic arterial pressure and RV dysfunction remains controversial. At especially high risk are normotensive PE patients (who may initially appear deceptively stable from a clinical viewpoint) with both RV enlargement and troponin elevation.[84]

Anticoagulation is usually discontinued after 3 to 6 months in patients with transient VTE risk factors such as surgery or trauma. Indefinite-duration anticoagulation with warfarin is effective and safe for most patients with idiopathic PE.

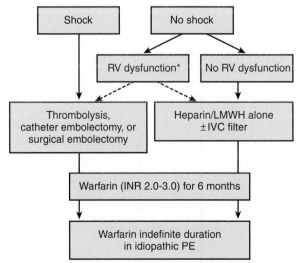

PE TREATMENT ALGORITHM

FIGURE 53-6 Suggested management strategy for pulmonary embolism (PE). Patients with right ventricular (RV) dysfunction and a preserved arterial blood pressure are candidates for thrombolysis in the absence of contraindications. INR, International Normalized Ratio; IVC, inferior vena cava; LMWH, low-molecular-weight heparin.

Emotional Support

Although PE can be as devastating emotionally as MI, the psychological burden for PE patients may be greater because the general public does not have as good an understanding of PE, particularly regarding the possibility of long-term disability and incomplete recovery. Young patients with PE repeatedly voice a common theme. Although they appear healthy, they often have difficulty expressing their fears and feelings about this potentially life-threatening illness to close family and friends.

Discussion of the implications of VTE with the patient and family may help reduce the emotional burden. One example is a PE support group led by a nurse-physician team. Although these sessions have an educational component, the major emphasis is peer support to alleviate anxieties that occur in the aftermath of PE.

Nonthrombotic Pulmonary Embolism

Nonthrombotic material that can embolize to the lungs includes fat, air, amniotic fluid, tumor cells, talc in IV drug abusers, and medical devices.

Fat Embolism Syndrome

EPIDEMIOLOGY

Fat embolism syndrome usually occurs in the setting of trauma, particularly after fracture of long bones or the pelvis.[85] The risk increases with the number of fractured bones, and the syndrome occurs more often with closed fractures than with open ones. Fat embolism also can complicate orthopedic surgery or trauma to tissues rich in fat, such as may occur with liposuction.

PATHOBIOLOGY

Characterized by a combination of respiratory, neurological, hematological, and cutaneous manifestations, fat embolism syndrome reflects a combination of vascular obstruction by fat globules, as well as the deleterious effects of free fatty acids released from these fat globules by the action of lipoprotein lipases.[86] These free fatty acids increase vascular permeability, induce a capillary leak syndrome, and can trigger platelet aggregation.

CLINICAL MANIFESTATIONS

Symptoms typically develop 24 to 72 hours after trauma or surgery.[87] Patients often complain of vague chest pain and shortness of breath. Tachypnea and fever associated with disproportionate tachycardia are common. The syndrome can rapidly progress to severe hypoxemia that requires mechanical ventilation. Neurological manifestations, which often start after the respiratory distress, include drowsiness, confusion, decreased level of consciousness, and seizures. Patients may have petechiae, particularly involving the conjunctiva, oral mucosa, and upper half of the body.

DIAGNOSIS

Fat embolism syndrome should be suspected when respiratory distress occurs a day or more after major trauma or orthopedic surgery, particularly when there are associated neurological defects and petechiae. The chest radiograph may reveal diffuse alveolar infiltrates.[88] Although fat droplets may be found in bronchoalveolar lavage fluid, this finding lacks specificity for the fat embolism syndrome.

PREVENTION, TREATMENT, AND PROGNOSIS

Early stabilization of long-bone fractures reduces the risk of fat embolization. Supportive treatment should be provided, including oxygen and mechanical ventilation. The utility of corticosteroids remains controversial. Although mortality rates as high as 10% have been reported, the prognosis is generally good.[85]

Venous Air Embolism

EPIDEMIOLOGY

Venous air embolism, which involves entrapment of environmental air or exogenous gas in the venous system, requires direct communication between the air and a vein, as well as a pressure gradient that favors entry of air into the vein.[89] Air can be introduced via indwelling central venous catheters, as a consequence of invasive surgical or medical procedures, or after barotrauma.

PATHOBIOLOGY

Large venous air emboli obstruct the RV pulmonary outflow tract, whereas mixtures of air bubbles and fibrin thrombi can obstruct pulmonary arterioles. In either case, RV failure can result. With a patent foramen ovale, venous air emboli can enter the coronary, cerebral or systemic circulation.

CLINICAL MANIFESTATIONS

Symptoms and signs depend on the volume of air and the rapidity of its entry into the circulation.[90] Large rapid boluses of air are tolerated less well than slow entry of smaller amounts. Small air emboli may be asymptomatic. With larger emboli, patients often complain of dyspnea and retrosternal chest discomfort, and they may feel lightheaded. Physical findings include tachypnea, tachycardia, and evidence of respiratory distress. Patients may have signs of right heart failure. A continuous drum-like mill-wheel murmur, which reflects air in the right ventricle, may be heard.

DIAGNOSIS

Patients may present with ECG evidence of RV dysfunction associated with elevated levels of troponin, indicative of myocardial injury. Echocardiography or chest CT may reveal air in the right ventricle. Patients may have hypoxemia and hypercapnia, and the platelet count may be low.[91]

PREVENTION AND TREATMENT

All catheters should be removed using techniques that minimize air embolism. Air should be removed from syringes prior to injection, and care should be taken during surgery to ensure that air bubbles do not form in blood vessels.[92] To avoid air embolism associated with barotrauma, divers require training in how to dive and surface safely.

The source of any air embolism should be identified so further embolism can be prevented. Left lateral decubitus positioning may benefit patients who have a large air bubble trapped in the RV outflow tract; such positioning places the outflow tract below the RV cavity, thereby allowing the air bubble to migrate into a nonobstructing position. Aspiration of air from the right ventricle via a central venous catheter may also be of benefit. Patients should receive high-flow supplemental oxygen, and hyperbaric oxygenation should be considered for patients with cardiac or neurological dysfunction.

PROGNOSIS

Outcome depends on the extent of air embolism. With good supportive care, the mortality rate can be less than 10%, even in patients with major air emboli. However, residual neurological defects often persist.

Amniotic Fluid Embolism

EPIDEMIOLOGY AND PATHOBIOLOGY

Amniotic fluid embolism is a rare but catastrophic complication of pregnancy, occurring in about 1 in 8000 to 1 in 80,000 pregnancies.[93] The syndrome develops when amniotic fluid and fetal cells enter the maternal bloodstream through small tears in the uterine veins during labor. Emboli to the heart and lungs cause cardiac dysfunction and respiratory distress. In addition, amniotic fluid and other debris activate the coagulation system, and the resultant thrombin then triggers fibrin formation and platelet activation to induce disseminated intravascular coagulation (DIC).

CLINICAL MANIFESTATIONS AND DIAGNOSIS

The syndrome often starts with the abrupt onset of dyspnea, cyanosis, and hypotension that can rapidly progress to cardiovascular collapse and death. Patients who survive this stage often develop manifestations of DIC characterized by diffuse bleeding, petechiae, and ecchymoses.[94]

The diagnosis should be suspected in women late in pregnancy, often in labor, who present with sudden onset of respiratory distress followed by cyanosis, hypotension, and shock. These findings are often associated with confusion or reduced level of consciousness, seizures, and evidence of a consumptive coagulopathy.

TREATMENT

Supportive measures include oxygen, mechanical ventilation, and hemodynamic support. Fresh frozen plasma, cryoprecipitate, and platelet transfusions can be given to replace consumed clotting factors and platelets. Heparin, often in low therapeutic doses, may be useful in some cases. If amniotic fluid embolism occurs before or during delivery, the fetus often has a poor outcome. As soon as the mother stabilizes, therefore, every attempt should be made to deliver the fetus.

PROGNOSIS

Although rare, amniotic fluid embolism remains a leading cause of maternal death during labor and the first few hours after delivery. Despite advances in critical care management, maternal and fetal mortality continue to be about 60% and 20%, respectively, with up to half of the survivors, both mother and baby, suffering from permanent hypoxia-induced neurological dysfunction.

Other Embolic Material

Many substances such as talc, starch, and cellulose are used as fillers in the manufacture of drugs. Some of these drugs are ground up by drug users, mixed in liquids, and then injected intravenously. The filler particles can then be trapped in the pulmonary vasculature where they can induce granuloma formation.[95]

Tumor emboli in the lung can mimic pneumonia, tuberculosis, or interstitial lung disease on the chest radiograph. Cancers of the prostate and breast are the most common sources of such emboli, followed by hepatoma and cancers of the stomach and pancreas. Although found in up to 26% of autopsies in patients with advanced cancer, tumor emboli are infrequently identified before death.

Various types of intravascular devices can embolize to the lungs, including vena cava filters, broken catheter tips, guidewires, stent fragments, and coils used for embolization. Many of these devices lodge in the right atrium, right ventricle, or pulmonary arteries. Intravascular retrieval can recover most of these devices; open surgery may be required for the remainder.

REFERENCES

1. www.surgeongeneral.Gov/topics/deepvein/. Accessed November 2010.
2. Goldhaber SZ, Visani L, De Rosa M: Acute pulmonary embolism: clinical outcomes in the International Cooperative Pulmonary Embolism Registry (ICOPER), *Lancet* 353:1386–1389, 1999.
3. Klok FA, Zondag W, van Kralingen KW, et al: Patient outcomes after acute pulmonary embolism. A pooled survival analysis of different adverse events, *Am J Respir Crit Care Med* 181:501–506, 2009.
4. Hoeper MM, Mayer E, Simonneau G, et al: Chronic thromboembolic pulmonary hypertension, *Circulation* 113:2011–2020, 2006.
5. Vazquez SR, Kahn SR: Postthrombotic syndrome. Cardiology patient page, *Circulation* 121:e217–e219, 2010.
6. Park B, Messina L, Dargon P, et al: Recent trends in clinical outcomes and resource utilization for pulmonary embolism in the united states: findings from the nationwide inpatient sample, *Chest* 136:983–990, 2009.

7. Ng TM, Tsai F, Khatri N, et al: Venous thromboembolism in hospitalized patients with heart failure: incidence, prognosis, and prevention, *Circ Heart Fail* 3:165–173, 2010.

8. Goldhaber SZ: Risk factors for venous thromboembolism, *J Am Coll Cardiol* 56:1–7, 2010.

9. Spencer FA, Goldberg RJ, Lessard D, et al: Factors associated with adverse outcomes in outpatients presenting with pulmonary embolism: the Worcester venous thromboembolism study, *Circ Cardiovasc Qual Outcomes* 3:390–394, 2010.

10. Goldhaber SZ, Tapson VF: A prospective registry of 5,451 patients with ultrasound-confirmed deep vein thrombosis, *Am J Cardiol* 93:259–262, 2004.

11. Undas A, Sydor WJ, Brummel K, et al: Aspirin alters the cardioprotective effects of the factor xiii val34leu polymorphism, *Circulation* 107:17–20, 2003.

12. Chew HK, Wun T, Harvey D, et al: Incidence of venous thromboembolism and its effect on survival among patients with common cancers, *Arch Intern Med* 166:458–464, 2006.

13. Carrier M, Le Gal G, Wells PS, et al: Systematic review: the Trousseau syndrome revisited: should we screen extensively for cancer in patients with venous thromboembolism? *Ann Intern Med* 149:323–333, 2008.

14. Lapostolle F, Surget V, Borron SW, et al: Severe pulmonary embolism associated with air travel, *N Engl J Med* 345:779–783, 2001.

15. Chandra D, Parisini E, Mozaffarian D: Meta-analysis: travel and risk for venous thromboembolism, *Ann Intern Med* 151:180–190, 2009.

16. Petitti DB: Clinical practice. Combination estrogen-progestin oral contraceptives, *N Engl J Med* 349:1443–1450, 2003.

17. Greer IA: Prevention and management of venous thromboembolism in pregnancy, *Clin Chest Med* 24:123–137, 2003.

18. Rossouw JE, Anderson GL, Prentice RL, et al: Risks and benefits of estrogen plus progestin in healthy postmenopausal women: principal results from the Women's Health Initiative randomized controlled trial, *JAMA* 288:321–333, 2002.

19. Joffe HV, Goldhaber SZ: Laboratory thrombophilias and venous thromboembolism, *Vasc Med* 7:93–102, 2002.

20. Goldhaber SZ, Elliott CG: Acute pulmonary embolism: part I: epidemiology, pathophysiology, and diagnosis, *Circulation* 108:2726–2729, 2003.

21. Kucher N, Printzen G, Goldhaber SZ: Prognostic role of brain natriuretic peptide in acute pulmonary embolism, *Circulation* 107:2545–2547, 2003.

22. Lankeit M, Friesen D, Aschoff J, et al: Highly sensitive troponin t assay in normotensive patients with acute pulmonary embolism, *Eur Heart J* 31:1836–1844, 2010.

23. Deitelzweig SB, Becker R, Lin J, et al: Comparison of the two-year outcomes and costs of prophylaxis in medical patients at risk of venous thromboembolism, *Thromb Haemost* 100:810–820, 2008.

24. Geerts WH, Bergqvist D, Pineo GF, et al: Prevention of venous thromboembolism: American College of Chest Physicians evidence-based clinical practice guidelines (8th edition), *Chest* 133:381S–453S, 2008.

25. Tapson VF, Decousus H, Pini M, et al: Venous thromboembolism prophylaxis in acutely ill hospitalized medical patients: findings from the International Medical Prevention Registry on venous thromboembolism, *Chest* 132:936–945, 2007.

26. Cohen AT, Tapson VF, Bergmann JF, et al: Venous thromboembolism risk and prophylaxis in the acute hospital care setting (ENDORSE Study): a multinational cross-sectional study, *Lancet* 371:387–394, 2008.

27. Streiff MB, Haut ER: The CMS ruling on venous thromboembolism after total knee or hip arthroplasty: weighing risks and benefits, *JAMA* 301:1063–1065, 2009.

28. Pronovost PJ, Goeschel CA, Wachter RM: The wisdom and justice of not paying for "preventable complications", *JAMA* 299:2197–2199, 2008.

29. Piazza G, Goldhaber SZ: Improving clinical effectiveness in thromboprophylaxis for hospitalized medical patients, *Am J Med* 122:230–232, 2009.

30. Piazza G, Goldhaber SZ: Physician alerts to prevent venous thromboembolism, *J Thromb Thrombolysis* 30:1–6, 2009.

31. Piazza G, Goldhaber SZ: Computerized decision support for the cardiovascular clinician: applications for venous thromboembolism prevention and beyond, *Circulation* 120:1133–1137, 2009.

32. Kucher N, Koo S, Quiroz R, et al: Electronic alerts to prevent venous thromboembolism among hospitalized patients, *N Engl J Med* 352:969–977, 2005.

33. Fiumara K, Piovella C, Hurwitz S, et al: Multi-screen electronic alerts to augment venous thromboembolism prophylaxis, *Thromb Haemost* 103:312–317, 2010.

34. Piazza G, Rosenbaum EJ, Pendergast W, et al: Physician alerts to prevent symptomatic venous thromboembolism in hospitalized patients, *Circulation* 119:2196–2201, 2009.

35. Piazza G, Fanikos J, Zayaruzny M, et al: Venous thromboembolic events in hospitalised medical patients, *Thromb Haemost* 102:505–510, 2009.

36. Fanikos J, Piazza G, Zayaruzny M, et al: Long-term complications of medical patients with hospital-acquired venous thromboembolism, *Thromb Haemost* 102:688–693, 2009.

37. Turpie AG, Bauer KA, Caprini JA, et al: Fondaparinux combined with intermittent pneumatic compression vs. intermittent pneumatic compression alone for prevention of venous thromboembolism after abdominal surgery: a randomized, double-blind comparison, *J Thromb Haemost* 5:1854–1861, 2007.

38. Dennis M, Sandercock PA, Reid J, et al: Effectiveness of thigh-length graduated compression stockings to reduce the risk of deep vein thrombosis after stroke (CLOTS Trial 1): a multicentre, randomised controlled trial, *Lancet* 373:1958–1965, 2009.

39. Cohen AT, Davidson BL, Gallus AS, et al: Efficacy and safety of fondaparinux for the prevention of venous thromboembolism in older acute medical patients: randomised placebo controlled trial, *BMJ* 332:325–329, 2006.

40. Glynn RJ, Ridker PM, Goldhaber SZ, et al: Effects of random allocation to vitamin e supplementation on the occurrence of venous thromboembolism: report from the Women's Health Study, *Circulation* 116:1497–1503, 2007.

41. Glynn RJ, Danielson E, Fonseca FA, et al: A randomized trial of rosuvastatin in the prevention of venous thromboembolism, *N Engl J Med* 360:1851–1861, 2009.

42. Sweetland S, Green J, Liu B, et al: Duration and magnitude of the postoperative risk of venous thromboembolism in middle aged women: prospective cohort study, *BMJ* 339:b4583, 2009.

43. Arcelus JI, Monreal M, Caprini JA, et al: Clinical presentation and time-course of postoperative venous thromboembolism: results from the RIETE Registry, *Thromb Haemost* 99:546–551, 2008.

44. Hull RD, Schellong SM, Tapson VF, et al: Extended-duration venous thromboembolism prophylaxis in acutely ill medical patients with recently reduced mobility: a randomized trial, *Ann Intern Med* 153:8–18, 2010.

45. Kent DM, Lindenauer PK: Aggregating and disaggregating patients in clinical trials and their subgroup analyses, *Ann Intern Med* 153:51–52, 2010.

46. Wells PS, Anderson DR, Rodger M, et al: Derivation of a simple clinical model to categorize patients probability of pulmonary embolism: increasing the models utility with the simplified D-dimer, *Thromb Haemost* 83:416–420, 2000.

47. Stein PD, Terrin ML, Hales CA, et al: Clinical, laboratory, roentgenographic, and electrocardiographic findings in patients with acute pulmonary embolism and no pre-existing cardiac or pulmonary disease, *Chest* 100:598–603, 1991.

48. Goldhaber SZ, Simons GR, Elliott CG, et al: Quantitative plasma d-dimer levels among patients undergoing pulmonary angiography for suspected pulmonary embolism, *JAMA* 270:2819–2822, 1993.

49. Value of the ventilation/perfusion scan in acute pulmonary embolism. Results of the Prospective Investigation of Pulmonary Embolism Diagnosis (PIOPED). The PIOPED investigators, *JAMA* 263:2753–2759, 1990.

50. Hunsaker AR, Lu MT, Goldhaber SZ, et al: Imaging in acute pulmonary embolism with special clinical scenarios, *Circ Cardiovasc Imaging* 3:491–500, 2010.

51. Quiroz R, Kucher N, Zou KH, et al: Clinical validity of a negative computed tomography scan in patients with suspected pulmonary embolism: a systematic review, *JAMA* 293: 2012–2017, 2005.

52. Stein PD, Chenevert TL, Fowler SE, et al: Gadolinium-enhanced magnetic resonance angiography for pulmonary embolism: a multicenter prospective study (PIOPED III), *Ann Intern Med* 152:434–443, W142–W433, 2010.

53. Johnson SA, Stevens SM, Woller SC, et al: Risk of deep vein thrombosis following a single negative whole-leg compression ultrasound: a systematic review and meta-analysis, *JAMA* 303:438–445, 2010.

54. Goldhaber SZ: Echocardiography in the management of pulmonary embolism, *Ann Intern Med* 136:691–700, 2002.

55. Piazza G, Goldhaber SZ: The acutely decompensated right ventricle: pathways for diagnosis and management, *Chest* 128:1836–1852, 2005.

56. Kucher N, Goldhaber SZ: Risk stratification of acute pulmonary embolism, *Semin Thromb Hemost* 32:838–847, 2006.

57. Piazza G, Goldhaber SZ: Management of submassive pulmonary embolism, *Circulation* 122:1124–1129, 2010.

58. Donze J, Le Gal G, Fine MJ, et al: Prospective validation of the pulmonary embolism severity index. A clinical prognostic model for pulmonary embolism, *Thromb Haemost* 100: 943–948, 2008.

59. Jimenez D, Aujesky D, Moores L, et al: Simplification of the pulmonary embolism severity index for prognostication in patients with acute symptomatic pulmonary embolism, *Arch Intern Med* 170:1383–1389, 2010.

60. McConnell MV, Solomon SD, Rayan ME, et al: Regional right ventricular dysfunction detected by echocardiography in acute pulmonary embolism, *Am J Cardiol* 78:469–473, 1996.

61. Dellas C, Puls M, Lankeit M, et al: Elevated heart-type fatty acid-binding protein levels on admission predict an adverse outcome in normotensive patients with acute pulmonary embolism, *J Am Coll Cardiol* 55:2150–2157, 2010.

62. Raschke RA, Reilly BM, Guidry JR, et al: The weight-based heparin dosing nomogram compared with a "standard care" nomogram. A randomized controlled trial, *Ann Intern Med* 119:874–881, 1993.

63. Lee AY, Levine MN, Baker RI, et al: Low-molecular-weight heparin versus a coumarin for the prevention of recurrent venous thromboembolism in patients with cancer, *N Engl J Med* 349:146–153, 2003.

64. Klein TE, Altman RB, Eriksson N, et al: Estimation of the warfarin dose with clinical and pharmacogenetic data, *N Engl J Med* 360:753–764, 2009.

65. Eckman MH, Rosand J, Greenberg SM, et al: Cost-effectiveness of using pharmacogenetic information in warfarin dosing for patients with nonvalvular atrial fibrillation, *Ann Intern Med* 150:73–83, 2009.

66. Epstein RS, Moyer TP, Aubert RE, et al: Warfarin genotyping reduces hospitalization rates results from the MM-WES (Medco-Mayo Warfarin Effectiveness Study), *J Am Coll Cardiol* 55:2804–2812, 2010.

67. Ahrens I, Lip GY, Peter K: New oral anticoagulant drugs in cardiovascular disease, *Thromb Haemost* 104:49–60, 2010.

68. Eikelboom JW, Weitz JI: New anticoagulants, *Circulation* 121:1523–1532, 2010.

69. Schulman S, Kearon C, Kakkar AK, et al: Dabigatran versus warfarin in the treatment of acute venous thromboembolism, *N Engl J Med* 361:2342–2352, 2009.

70. Bauersachs R, Berkowitz SD, Brenner B, et al: Oral rivaroxaban for symptomatic venous thromboembolism, *N Engl J Med* 363:2499–2510, 2010.

71. Kearon C, Kahn SR, Agnelli G, et al: Antithrombotic therapy for venous thromboembolic disease: American College of Chest Physicians evidence-based clinical practice guidelines (8th edition), *Chest* 133:454S–545S, 2008.

72. Prandoni P, Prins MH, Lensing AW, et al: Residual thrombosis on ultrasonography to guide the duration of anticoagulation in patients with deep venous thrombosis: a randomized trial, *Ann Intern Med* 150:577–585, 2009.

73. Bruinstroop E, Klok FA, Van De Ree MA, et al: Elevated D-dimer levels predict recurrence in patients with idiopathic venous thromboembolism: a meta-analysis, *J Thromb Haemost* 7:611–618, 2009.

74. Ridker PM, Goldhaber SZ, Danielson E, et al: Long-term, low-intensity warfarin therapy for the prevention of recurrent venous thromboembolism, *N Engl J Med* 348:1425–1434, 2003.

75. Kearon C, Ginsberg JS, Kovacs MJ, et al: Comparison of low-intensity warfarin therapy with conventional-intensity warfarin therapy for long-term prevention of recurrent venous thromboembolism, *N Engl J Med* 349:631–639, 2003.

76. Jaff MR, McMurtry MS, Archer SL, et al: Management of massive and submassive pulmonary embolism, iliofemoral deep vein thrombosis, and chronic thromboembolic pulmonary hypertension: a scientific statement from the American Heart Association, *Circulation* 123:1788–1830, 2011.

CH
53

77. Konstantinides S, Geibel A, Heusel G, et al: Heparin plus alteplase compared with heparin alone in patients with submassive pulmonary embolism, *N Engl J Med* 347:1143–1150, 2002.

78. Wan S, Quinlan DJ, Agnelli G, et al: Thrombolysis compared with heparin for the initial treatment of pulmonary embolism: a meta-analysis of the randomized controlled trials, *Circulation* 110:744–749, 2004.

79. Kline JA, Steuerwald MT, Marchick MR, et al: Prospective evaluation of right ventricular function and functional status 6 months after acute submassive pulmonary embolism: frequency of persistent or subsequent elevation in estimated pulmonary artery pressure, *Chest* 136:1202–1210, 2009.

80. Kucher N: Catheter embolectomy for acute pulmonary embolism, *Chest* 132:657–663, 2007.

81. Kuo WT, Gould MK, Louie JD, et al: Catheter-directed therapy for the treatment of massive pulmonary embolism: systematic review and meta-analysis of modern techniques, *J Vasc Interv Radiol* 20:1431–1440, 2009.

82. Leacche M, Unic D, Goldhaber SZ, et al: Modern surgical treatment of massive pulmonary embolism: results in 47 consecutive patients after rapid diagnosis and aggressive surgical approach, *J Thorac Cardiovasc Surg* 129:1018–1023, 2005.

83. Eight-year follow-up of patients with permanent vena cava filters in the prevention of pulmonary embolism: the PREPIC (Prevention du Risque d'Embolie Pulmonaire par Interruption Cave) randomized study, *Circulation* 112:416–422, 2005.

84. Stein PD, Matta F, Janjua M, et al: Outcome in stable patients with acute pulmonary embolism who had right ventricular enlargement and/or elevated levels of troponin i, *Am J Cardiol* 106:558–563, 2010.

85. Mellor A, Soni N: Fat embolism, *Anaesthesia* 56:145–154, 2001.

86. Sevitt S: The significance and pathology of fat embolism, *Ann Clin Res* 9:173–180, 1977.

87. Carr JB, Hansen ST: Fulminant fat embolism, *Orthopedics* 13:258–261, 1990.

88. Rossi SE, Goodman PC, Franquet T: Nonthrombotic pulmonary emboli, *AJR Am J Roentgenol* 174:1499–1508, 2000.

89. Jorens PG, Van Marck E, Snoeckx A, et al: Nonthrombotic pulmonary embolism, *Eur Respir J* 34:452–474, 2009.

90. O'Quin RJ, Lakshminarayan S: Venous air embolism, *Arch Intern Med* 142:2173–2176, 1982.

91. Mirski MA, Lele AV, Fitzsimmons L, et al: Diagnosis and treatment of vascular air embolism, *Anesthesiology* 106:164–177, 2007.

92. Orebaugh SL: Venous air embolism: clinical and experimental considerations, *Crit Care Med* 20:1169–1177, 1992.

93. O'Shea A, Eappen S: Amniotic fluid embolism, *Int Anesthesiol Clin* 45:17–28, 2007.

94. Gist RS, Stafford IP, Leibowitz AB, et al: Amniotic fluid embolism, *Anesth Analg* 108:1599–1602, 2009.

95. Torbicki A, Perrier A, Konstantinides S, et al: Guidelines on the diagnosis and management of acute pulmonary embolism: the Task Force for the Diagnosis and Management of Acute Pulmonary Embolism of the European Society of Cardiology (ESC), *Eur Heart J* 29:2276–2315, 2008.

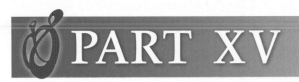

PART XV

CHRONIC VENOUS DISORDERS

CHAPTER **54** **Varicose Veins**

Alfonso J. Tafur, Suman Rathbun

Epidemiology

Varicose veins (VVs) are tortuous, dilated, bulging, superficial veins typically measuring 4 mm or larger.[1] Varicose veins are the most common manifestation of chronic venous insufficiency (CVI) and affect up to 25% of women and 15% of men.[1,2] In the Framingham Study, which includes men and women between the ages of 30 and 62 from the town of Framingham, Massachusetts, the annual incidence of VVs is 2.6% among women and 1.9% among men.[3] Risk factors include female gender, advancing age, family history, pregnancy, prolonged standing, obesity, vascular malformations, and hormone therapy.[1,4] Varicose veins are more common in patients of European ancestry compared to Blacks or Asians.[3] Approximately 4% of the women presenting with VVs have pelvic vein reflux as the underlying etiology.[5] Pregnancy and deep venous reflux are also associated with VV recurrence after treatment.[4]

Other patterns of venous pathology include reticular veins, which are smaller, 1- to 3-mm diameter, flat, blue-green colored, less tortuous veins.[1] Telangiectasias, or spider veins, are 1 mm or less, and blue, black, purple, or reddish in appearance.[1] A cross-sectional study of a random sample of 1566 subjects 18 to 64 years of age from the general population in Scotland found that telangiectasias and reticular veins were each present in approximately 80% of men and 85% of women.[6]

The chronic nature of VVs has a major impact on healthcare resources. It is estimated that venous ulcers cause the loss of approximately 2 million working days annually, generating a cost of more than $3 billion per year in the United States alone.[3] Moreover, beyond the purely economical impact of VVs, chronic venous disease is associated with reduced quality of life, with particularly negative impact on pain, physical function, and mobility measures.[3] The same is true for patients who develop venous ulcers, with effect on quality of life directly related to severity of disease.[3]

Anatomy

Broadly, the veins of the lower extremity are divided into three systems confluent in a single network, which ultimately drains into the external iliac vein. This venous network includes the superficial veins, deep venous system, and their mutual connections, as well as the perforators (Fig. 54-1). The *deep compartment* includes the deep venous system and it is bordered by the fascia muscularis. The *superficial compartment* is externally bordered by the dermis.[7] The tissue situated under the dermis is called the *tela subcutanea* (subcutaneous tissue) and contains the saphenous vein. Within the superficial compartment, a narrow anatomical space called the *saphenous compartment* can be identified by ultrasound evaluation. Externally bordered by the saphenous fascia, this compartment covers the proper venae saphenae and their beginnings. The term *perforating veins* or *perforators* is reserved only for those veins that penetrate the fascia muscularis to connect the superficial system to the deep venous system. Conversely, communicating veins connect veins of the same venous system.

The *great saphenous vein* (GSV) is the longest vein in the entire human body. It starts at the medial side of the foot and courses proximally along the medial side of the calf as the marginal medial vein together with the saphenous nerve.[7] The main tributaries are the posterior accessory GSV and the anterior accessory GSV. The vein continues alone on the medial side of the thigh and crosses through the saphenous hiatus into the common femoral vein. The normal caliber of the GSV is 3 to 4 mm, and it has 10 to 20 valves.[7] The GSV is bifid in about 20% of legs, but two venous trunks of the GSV in the same compartment, constituting a true duplication, occurs in only 1% of cases. The *small saphenous vein* (SSV) is the second largest vein of the lower limb. It begins on the lateral side of the foot dorsum and runs along the lateral margin of the foot as the lateral marginal vein. It penetrates the popliteal fascia into the popliteal vein. In one third of cases, blood flows via various communicating veins to the system of the great saphenous. In one tenth of cases, it flows via the gastrocnemii veins and perforating veins into the deep venous system. The SSV is usually 3 mm wide and contains 7 to 13 valves. It is accompanied by the small saphenous artery, which must not be confused with the vein during sclerotherapy injection.[7]

Some of the perforating veins are consistently located. The *thigh perforators* include the medial thigh (formerly Hunter's perforator), anterior thigh, lateral thigh, and posterior thigh perforating veins, and the pudendal perforating vein. The *knee perforators* include the medial knee (formerly Boyd's perforator), suprapatellar, lateral knee, infrapatellar, and popliteal fossa perforating veins. The *leg perforators* include the paratibial, posterior tibial (formerly Cockett's perforating vein), anterior leg, lateral leg, and posterior leg (medial and lateral gastrocnemius, intergemellar, para-Achillean) perforating veins. Other groups include the gluteal, ankle, and foot perforating veins. The perforator system does play a key role in calf muscle pump function (Fig. 54-2A).

A system of subcutaneous veins spreads on the lateral aspect of the thigh and leg as a developmental remnant of the embryonic lateral marginal vein, which fades out and is replaced with the system of the saphenous veins and may be abnormally developed in patients with Klippel-Trénaunay's or Parkes-Weber's syndromes. In relation to the surface, there are three levels of venous plexuses: dermal, hypodermal, and deep. The dermal veins involve the superficial subpapillary venous plexus and the deep dermal venous plexus[7] (Fig. 54-3).

Pathogenesis

Varicose veins are caused by weakness in the vein wall, and according to their underlying etiology can be divided into primary or secondary. *Primary VVs* result from idiopathic structural or functional defects in the venous system. *Secondary VVs* result from underlying venous obstruction, most commonly deep vein thrombosis (DVT) or underlying deep venous insufficiency[1] (see Fig. 54-2B-C). Primary valvular incompetence is more frequent. Approximately 8 in 10 individuals with VVs have primary valvular incompetence.

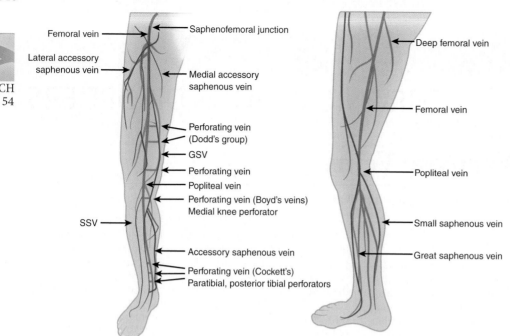

Femoral vein
Saphenofemoral junction
Lateral accessory saphenous vein
Medial accessory saphenous vein
Perforating vein (Dodd's group)
GSV
Perforating vein
Popliteal vein
Perforating vein (Boyd's veins)
Medial knee perforator
SSV
Accessory saphenous vein
Perforating vein (Cockett's)
Paratibial, posterior tibial perforators

Deep femoral vein
Femoral vein
Popliteal vein
Small saphenous vein
Great saphenous vein

FIGURE 54-1 Lower-extremity venous anatomy schematics. GSV, great saphenous vein; SSV, small saphenous vein.

Secondary valvular reflux is usually due to trauma or thrombosis. Congenital anomalies only occur in about 2% of cases.[3] Secondary chronic venous disease progresses faster than primary.

A key factor in the development of VVs is venous hypertension. Venous pressure is directly proportional to the weight of the column of blood from the right atrium to the foot and is reduced by pressures generated by muscle contractions. When standing, venous pressure is as high as 90 mmHg. It temporarily increases with muscle pumping, but then rapidly decreases as the functioning venous valves guide blood flow toward the heart. A well-functioning calf muscle pumping mechanism decreases the venous pressure to less than 30 mmHg.[3] The constant insult of increased venous pressure degenerates in stretching, splitting, tearing, thinning, and adhesion of valves, causing inflammation.[3] Adjuvant factors for development of excessive venous hypertension include failure of the calf muscle pump and obesity. Ultimately, prolonged venous hypertension leads to venous valvular incompetence or reflux and venous dilation.[1] Venous defects increase venous hypertension and cause weakened venous walls, abnormal distension of the surrounding connective tissue, and separation of valve cusps.

Elevated venous pressure may also generate edema. Prominent swelling is not a usual feature of VVs, but episodic ankle edema is common.[8] A small percentage of patients develop complications including dermatitis, superficial thrombophlebitis, or bleeding. Thrombophlebitis may occur spontaneously or result from an injury. Skin changes in chronic venous disease are proportionately related to the severity of venous hypertension. Up to 100% of patients with postexercise venous pressures of more than 90 mmHg develop venous ulcers.[3] Patients with CVI and deep vein incompetence are at greatly increased risk of developing ulcers.[9] Conversely, frequent dorsiflexion of the ankle and an effective calf muscle pump are protective factors (see Fig. 54-2A). Poor prognostic factors favoring progression include the combination of reflux and obstruction, ipsilateral recurrent DVT, and multisegmental involvement.[10]

Inflammatory changes also contribute to the genesis of VVs. Blood returning from feet that have been passively dependent for 40 to 60 minutes is depleted of leukocytes, suggesting that leukocytes accumulate and locally participate in the inflammatory cascade.[3] Circulating leukocytes and vascular endothelial cells (ECs) express several types of adhesion molecules. Integrin binding promotes firm adhesion of leukocytes, the starting point for their migration out of the vasculature and degranulation. The activated leucocytes shed L-selectin into the plasma and express members of the integrin family.[3] This is the backbone of the microvascular leukocyte-trapping hypothesis. Local inflammation associated with intercellular adhesion molecule (ICAM)-1 expression increases monocyte and macrophage adhesion. The valve damage is augmented by disturbed excessive collagen type 1 synthesis, which increases venous rigidity.[3] Finally, matrix metalloproteinases (MMPs) and serine proteinases favor the accumulation of extracellular matrix (ECM) material in VVs.[3,11]

Clinical Manifestations

Clinical manifestations of VV range from cosmetic problems to severe symptoms, including ulceration. Chronic venous insufficiency can be classified by clinical presentation, etiology, anatomy, and pathophysiology (CEAP Classification)[8,12] (see Chapter 55). Clinically, however, the patterns may be classified as *complicated* and *uncomplicated varices*. Uncomplicated VVs may need only cosmetic treatment or reassurance. Patients with complicated VVs may develop heaviness, fatigue, local pain, spontaneous bleeding, and superficial thrombophlebitis. Varicose veins may cause edema, pain, and skin changes such as stasis dermatitis and ulceration. Venous ulcerations can take more than 9 months to heal, with one study reporting that 66% of ulcers last longer than 5 years.[1] All these symptoms impair activities of daily living.[1]

Multiple questionnaires and instruments measure the effect of venous disease on quality of life. Most are subjective and completed by the patient. The Chronic Venous Insufficiency Questionnaire (CIVIQ) was validated in a sample of 2001 patients and measures the psychological, social, physical, and pain domains. A revised version of the instrument, the CIVIQ 2, equally weighted the categories across 20 questions to provide a global score. This measure is used to follow quality-of-life (QOL) improvement after therapy for chronic venous insufficiency, including VVs. The Aberdeen Varicose Vein Questionnaire (AVVQ) includes 13 questions on physical symptoms and social issues, including pain, ankle edema, ulcers, compression therapy use, and the effect of VVs on daily activities. The disease-specific index is graded from 0 to 100 (extreme venous symptoms).[13] This measure has also been validated for patient follow-up after intervention.[14] The Venous Insufficiency Epidemiological and Economic Study (VEINES) instrument consists of 35 items in two categories

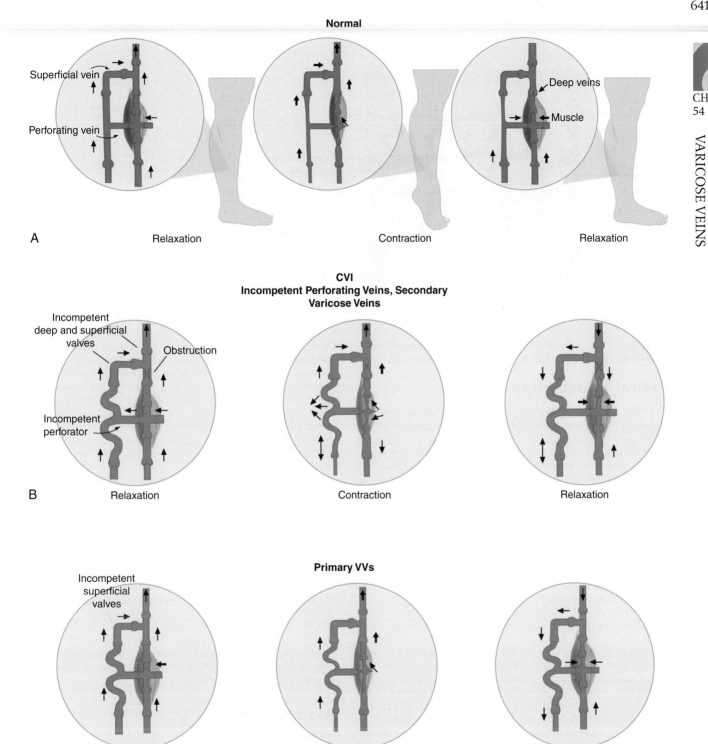

FIGURE 54-2 Calf "muscle pump" and varicose veins (V Vs). A, Normal calf muscle pump physiology during relaxation and contraction. **B,** Deep vein obstruction heralds perforator vein incompetence and associated secondary VV. **C,** Conversely, deep venous system and perforator system are independent of primary VV. CVI, chronic venous insufficiency. *(Adapted from Sumner DS: venous dynamics–varicosities. Clin Obstet Gynecol 24:743–760, 1981.)*

to generate two summary scores. It includes the VEINES-QOL, with 25 QOL questions, and the VEINES-Sym, with 10 symptom questions.[14] The focus of this measure is on physical symptoms of venous disease, in particular postthrombotic syndrome. It has been validated in patients with DVT. In 2004, Kahn et al. compared the VEINES and the 36-item Short-Form Health Survey (SF-36) with CEAP classification in 1531 patients from four countries to examine the effect of patient-related QOL reporting on interpreting outcomes in venous studies. Higher CEAP class was directly associated

with and predictive of the VEINES-QOL.[14] The Charing Cross Venous Ulceration Questionnaire (CXVUQ) was developed for patients with venous ulcers, and its performance is not impaired by the treatment option selected.[14] Finally, the Venous Severity Score (VSS) system was derived from the CEAP classification and has three elements: the venous disability score (VDS), venous segmental disease score (VSDS), and venous clinical severity score (VCSS). The VCSS has been recently revised and includes multiple parameters: pain, VVs, inflammation, edema, skin induration, pigmentation, ulcers (size,

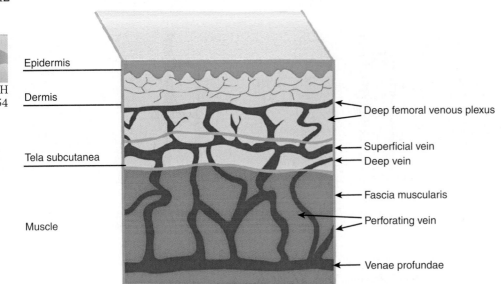

Epidermis

Dermis

Tela subcutanea

Muscle

Deep femoral venous plexus

Superficial vein
Deep vein

Fascia muscularis

Perforating vein

Venae profundae

FIGURE 54-3 Venous drainage of the lower limb. *(Adapted from Kachlik D, Pechacek V, Baca V, Musil V: The superficial venous system of the lower extremity: new nomenclature. Phlebology 25:113–123, 2010.)*

number, duration), and compression therapy.[15] The Venous Clinical Severity Score is useful for following changes with treatment.[14,15]

Physical Examination

Initial inspection of the leg may reveal edema, prominent VVs, cyanosis, plethora, hyperpigmentation, lipodermatosclerosis, or ulcerations. On inspection, VVs may be observed as tortuous, dilated, bulging, superficial veins measuring 4 mm or larger; the patient is ideally examined in the standing position to allow venous reflux.[1] *Lipodermatosclerosis* is a consequence of localized chronic inflammation and fibrosis of the skin and subcutaneous tissue of the lower part of the leg.[16] The skin changes will often occur at the "gaiter area" above the medial malleolus. *Atrophie blanche* is a localized circular, whitish, avascular, atrophic skin area surrounded by capillaries and sometimes hyperpigmentation, consistent with severe chronic venous insufficiency. Similarly, a *phlebectatic crown* (fan-shaped small intradermal veins on medial or lateral aspects of the foot) may herald severe venous insufficiency.

Trendelenburg and Perthes tests may be used during the exam to differentiate superficial from deep venous insufficiency (also see Chapter 55). In the Trendelenburg test, the leg is elevated and a tourniquet applied above the knee. This obstructs the superficial veins, which will promptly fill after standing if the patient has deep vein incompetence (secondary VVs). If after standing, the vein requires more than 20 seconds to refill, but prompt filling follows tourniquet removal, the exam is consistent with primary VVs. In the Perthes test, the leg is elevated and the tourniquet placed at the midthigh or proximal calf. When the patient stands and walks, the VVs will refill owing to incompetent perforators[16] (Figs. 54-4 and 55-5). These maneuvers may be complemented with Brodie Trendelenburg percussion: a finger is placed over the distal area of a VV while the proximal segment of the vein is percussed. A transmitted impulse at the lower end suggests incompetence.

Imaging and Physiological Testing

Duplex ultrasonography is useful in the evaluation of VVs (also see Chapter 12). The test is performed with the patient standing or in reverse Trendelenburg position, and is used to detect acute or chronic thrombosis, postthrombotic changes, obstructive flow, and incompetence in the deep veins. Reflux, demonstrated by reversal of flow, is pathological whenever longer than 0.5 seconds.[17] Duplex ultrasonography is not reliable for assessment of the iliac and caval veins, but it is sensitive for evaluation of saphenous vein reflux and useful for identification of incompetent perforator veins.

Impedance plethysmography, strain gauge plethysmography, and air plethysmography may be used to detect venous obstruction and reflux in large veins above the knee. Photoplethysmography, most commonly used with and without a tourniquet, can be employed to evaluate superficial venous insufficiency. A venous refilling time less than 20 seconds *without* a tourniquet that normalizes to over 20 seconds *with* a tourniquet is compatible with GSV incompetence.[17]

Venography may provide information regarding pelvic vein obstruction in patients with postthrombotic disease.[16] Ascending venography is performed with the patient at 45 degrees, non–weight-bearing, with legs down as contrast is infused. Contrast filling the superficial vein denotes incompetence. Ascending venography is useful to determine vein obstruction, collateralization, and recanalization. Descending venography is more useful to diagnose venous insufficiency. In this scenario, the contrast is injected into the common femoral vein above the saphenofemoral junction. The patient is initially in supine position, and after the contrast dye injection, the table is tilted feet downward. Contrast leakage to the knee or distally is abnormal.[17] Venography is usually indicated in the setting of endovenous intervention, but is difficult in the setting of a swollen leg. There is limited experience with magnetic resonance venography (MRV) or computed tomography (CT) to evaluate venous insufficiency and VVs.

Management

Treatment Suitability

Varicose veins treatment may be divided into conservative and invasive modalities. Conservative treatment for VVs and subsequent CVI include lifestyle modifications, compression therapy, and pharmacotherapy. All patients are appropriate for conservative measures. The use of more invasive techniques depends on the size of the vein and the presence of complications. Most commonly, ablation of an incompetent or varicose Great saphenous veins is performed first to decompress more distal varicosities; however, most patients require additional treatments for adequate therapeutic and cosmetic results. Thermal ablation of the GSV using endovenous laser therapy (EVLT) or radiofrequency ablation (RFA) is the most frequently employed technique. GSVs with diameters of 3 to 12 mm are candidates for RFA; EVLT is an option for those larger than 3 mm. A less invasive technique, foam sclerotherapy of the GSV, may also be performed in veins smaller than 1 cm, but has

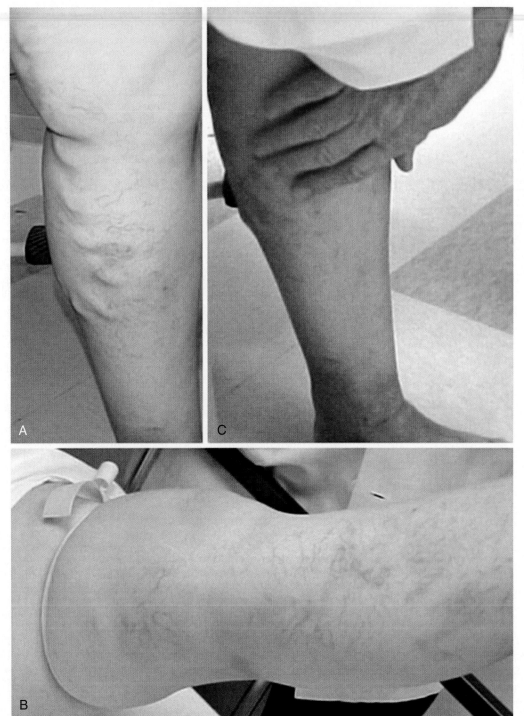

FIGURE54-4 Physical examination of varicose veins (VVs). A, Medial great saphenous vein (GSV) VVs are observed on a right leg. **B,** Limb is elevated and tourniquet positioned above knee; with tourniquet applied and patient standing, VVs are not evident. This is suggestive of primary venous incompetence.

been used to treat larger veins as well.[18] When the GSV is larger than 12 mm in diameter, surgery is an option.[19] Tortuosity of the vessel is also relevant. For RFA and EVLT, the straight segment of the GSV should extend 15 to 20 cm immediately distal to the saphenofemoral junction.[18]

In a study of 577 patients with GSV reflux, 55% were suitable for RFA or EVLT, and 57% were suitable for foam sclerotherapy. Stressing the need for careful patient selection, only 41% of the limbs were suitable for all the procedures.[18] In one study evaluating patients with recurrent VVs, less than 40% had limbs suitable for RFA or EVLT, while foam sclerotherapy was an option in 58% of the cases.[18] Owing to the risk of skin burns, superficial tributary veins are not suitable for catheter-based thermal

ablation. Optimal therapeutic results may be achieved with an approach of combined modalities.[18]

Conservative Management

DIET AND LIFESTYLE CHANGES

Prolonged standing or sitting may exacerbate signs and symptoms of VVs. The patient should elevate the legs above the level of the heart as much as possible, lose excess weight, and exercise to minimize swelling and improve calf muscle function.[20] Furthermore, moderate-intensity lower-limb exercise training improves microvascular endothelial vasodilator function in postsurgical VV patients.[21]

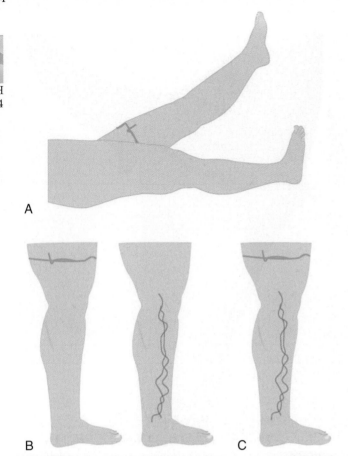

FIGURE 54-5 Physical examination of varicose veins (VVs). A, Leg is elevated so VVs are drained. **B,** Return of VVs only after tourniquet is removed. **C,** Findings suggestive of incompetent perforator veins, consistent with secondary varicosities.

COMPRESSION

External compression is the cornerstone of therapy for VVs. Compression therapy, including graduated elastic compression stockings and short-stretch bandages, is effective in reducing lower-extremity pain and swelling and preventing progression of VVs and CVI to venous ulceration.[20] Among patients with venous ulcerations, improved healing is achieved with multicomponent compression systems. Compression garments should be individualized for maximal patient compliance.[20,22]

PHARMACOTHERAPY

Low-dose diuretics are often prescribed for patients with significant edema due to VVs, but they are minimally effective in reducing the symptoms of pain and discomfort.[20] Patients with stasis dermatitis may be treated with a short course of topical corticosteroids to reduce inflammation. Antibiotics with gram-positive coverage are prescribed to treat cellulitis or infected ulcerations. Antibiotic coverage should be expanded to include gram-negative and anaerobic organisms in diabetic patients.[20] Because of the increasing problem of bacterial resistance to antibiotics, current prescribing guidelines recommend that antibacterial preparations should only be used in cases of clinical infection and not for bacterial colonization. At present, there is no evidence to support routine use of systemic antibiotics to promote healing in venous leg ulcers.[23]

HERBAL SUPPLEMENTS

Short-term studies have shown the efficacy of horse chestnut seed (*Aesculus hippocastanum*) extract in reducing edema, ankle and calf circumference, and symptoms of VVs with insufficiency.

The horse chestnut is native to southeast Europe, with aescin the active ingredient.[20,24] This extract has anti-inflammatory and vasoconstrictive properties that may exert a positive influence on venous tone and increase the flow velocity of venous blood.[24] It can be administered orally as a 20- or 50-mg dose. In a meta-analysis by Suter et al., a treated population of 219 adults with CVI stage I/II showed improvement; eight patients reported gastrointestinal upset.[24]

Micronized purified flavonoid fraction (MPFF) consists of 90% diosmin and 10% flavonoids. MPFF protects the microcirculation from raised ambulatory venous pressure. It decreases the interaction between leucocytes and ECs by inhibiting expression of endothelial ICAM-1 and vascular cell adhesion molecule (VCAM).[25] A meta-analysis of randomized prospective studies using MPFF that included 723 patients with venous ulcers suggested improved healing at 6 months among those who used MPFF compared with conventional therapy alone.[25]

French maritime pine bark extract and rutosides have demonstrated inconsistent results.[20] Although herbal products may be beneficial short term, their efficacy and safety have not been proven long term, and these preparations with varying amounts of active and inactive ingredients are not regulated by the U.S. Food and Drug Administration (FDA).

Invasive Therapy

For large VVs, invasive therapy is divided into endovenous procedures, including chemical and thermal ablation, and surgical procedures (Table 54-1).

CHEMICAL SCLEROTHERAPY

Liquid sclerosants have been a treatment for VVs for almost a century. The introduction of endovenous foam sclerotherapy (EFS) in 1944, with standardization of the method by Cabrera in the early 1990s, improved the nonsurgical obliteration of VVs. Endovenous foam sclerotherapy is especially effective when administered using ultrasound guidance.[20]

Procedure

A chemical sclerosant (e.g., polidocanol, sodium morrhuate, sodium tetradecyl sulfate) is combined with carbon dioxide/oxygen (CO_2/O_2) or room air to produce foam (concentration 1%-3%; volume 6-10 mL) using the two-syringe, or Tessari, method[26] (Fig. 54-6). Because it is more soluble in blood and water than the nitrogen in room air, CO_2/O_2 may reduce the risk of microbubble embolization. The Tessari method generates foam by pumping the contents of two disposable syringes, one containing the liquid sclerosant and the other containing air, backward and forward through a two-way stopcock.[26] Ultrasound is performed to localize the most superficially accessible segment of the varicosity or GSV proper into which a catheter can be easily inserted. The foam is prepared immediately before the procedure and injected into the GSV or its tributaries under ultrasound guidance.[26] The leg is elevated 45 degrees during injection, and the foam is massaged distally to fill the tributaries. Subsequently, a compression garment is applied to the treated leg.[26,27]

The foam displaces the blood in the vein, resulting in local inflammation, sclerosis, and obliteration of the VV over 1 to 2 weeks.[26,28] The effectiveness of foam sclerotherapy lies in the utilization of detergent sclerosants that work by denaturation of proteins. By forming a lipid bilayer, the endothelial surface is disrupted in the absence of essential proteins, which produces a delayed cell death.[27]

A systematic review of EFS by van den Bos et al.[29] that selected 64 studies and assessed 12,320 limbs followed for an average of 32 months determined an overall obliteration rate of 82.1% at 3 months (95% confidence interval [CI], 72.5-88.9), 80.9% at 1 year (95% CI, 71.8-87.6), and 73.5% at 5 years (95% CI, 62.8-82.1) (see Table 54-1). Contrary to catheter thermal-based techniques, increasing age does not impact sclerotherapy suitability.[18] Endovenous foam sclerotherapy is also effective in treating venous stasis ulcers

TABLE 54-1 Comparison of Varicose Vein Treatment Outcomes

	Percent Obliteration (95% CI)			
TREATMENT	**1 YEAR**	**3 YEARS**	**5 YEARS**	**COMPLICATIONS**
Saphenofemoral ligation and stripping	79.7% (71.8-85.8)	77.8% (70.0-84.0)	75.7% (67.9-82.1)	Hematomas (<30%) Paresthesias (4%-25%) Wound infection (2%-15%) DVT (<2%)
EVLT	93.3% (91.1-95.0)	94.5% (87.2-97.7)	95.4% (79.7-99.1)	Pain (50%) Ecchymosis (40%) Hematoma (24%) Phlebitis (12%) Paresthesias (10%) DVT (7%) Hyperpigmentation (<4%)
RFA	87.7% (83.1-91.2)	84.2% (75.5-90.4)	79.9% (59.9-91.5)	Bruising (50%) Paresthesias (3%-20%) DVT (16%) Hematoma (<7%) Burns (2%-7%) Infection (<2%)
EFS	80.9% (71.8-87.6)	77.4% (68.7-84.3)	73.5% (62.8-82.1)	Pain (common) Hyperpigmentation (common) Phlebitis (5%) DVT (<1%) TIA (<1%) Skin necrosis (rare)

CI, confidence interval; DVT, deep vein thrombosis; EFS, endovenous foam sclerotherapy; EVLT, endovenous laser therapy; RFA, radiofrequency ablation; TIA, transient ischemic attack.
Adapted from Nael R, Rathbun S: Treatment of varicose veins. Curr Treat Options Cardiovasc Med 11:91–103, 2009; and van den Bos R, Arends L, Kockaert M, et al: Endovenous therapies of lower extremity varicosities: a meta-analysis. J Vasc Surg 49:230–239, 2009.

and congenital vascular malformations.[1] In a study by Barrett et al. that analyzed a total of 100 randomly chosen legs with VVs treated with ultrasound-guided EFS, patient satisfaction was rated highly, with a 90% improvement in QOL 2 years after treatment with EFS[1] (see Table 54-1). In the van den Bos review, after adjusting for follow-up, foam therapy and RFA were as effective as surgical stripping.[29] In the absence of large comparative randomized clinical trials between multiple techniques, the minimally invasive techniques appear to be at least as effective as surgery in the treatment of lower-extremity VVs. Endovenous foam sclerotherapy is often used in conjunction with thermal ablation for sclerosis of tributary VVs.

In a study of 1931 treatment sessions that included 852 patients treated with ultrasound-guided EFS, the risk of deep venous occlusion was lower when treating veins less than 5 mm in diameter, and when restricting the volume of foam injected to less than 10 mL.[30] The most common complications include mild to moderate pain and hyperpigmentation (up to 30%).[1,13] Hyperpigmentation typically resolves within 6 to 12 months.[1] Less common adverse events include superficial thrombophlebitis, DVT and pulmonary embolism (PE), trapped coagulum, hematoma, skin necrosis, transient neurological events (migraines, visual disturbance), and pulmonary symptoms (cough). Trapped coagulum resulting in superficial thrombophlebitis occurs in less than 5% of treated veins. Deep vein thrombosis results from propagation of foam into the deep venous system and typically involves the popliteal and calf veins. The incidence of DVT/PE is less than 1%.[1,12] Transient neurological events may occur with the use of large amounts of foam in patients with a patent foramen ovale. To date, there have been three reported cases of major posttreatment neurological events (transient ischemic attack [TIA] and cerebrovascular accident) suspected to be associated with EFS. In all three cases, symptoms were associated with the presence of patent foramen ovale and resolved within 2 weeks.[1,12,31]

ClariVein, recently approved by the FDA, is a novel sclerotherapy approach for large VVs that uses a mechanical rotating dispersion wire to mix and disperse a sclerosant on the vessel wall. Potential advantages are that it does not require tumescence anesthesia,

can be used near nerve bundles, is fully disposable, and does not require a generator.[32] However, to date, no large-scale comparative studies have been published.

ENDOVENOUS LASER THERAPY

Endovenous laser therapy was introduced in 1999 for obliteration of the GSV and its tributaries. The direct action of the laser on the vein wall and heating of the venous blood result in damage to the vein wall and, over weeks to months, obliteration of the varicosity.[20] The pattern of injury is eccentrically distributed, with maximum injury occurring along the path of laser contact. Temperatures during EVLT may reach 1000 °C at the fiber tip and 300 °C in the firing zone. There is also steam generated during the photothermolytic process, but this accounts only for 2% of applied energy dose.[33] The occlusion and complication rate after EVLT are proportional to the total energy (joules) per centimeter of vein (J/cm). The laser energy can be applied in continuous or pulsed mode, the continuous mode being more effective.

Procedure

Endovenous laser therapy is performed using tumescent anesthesia. A 5-mL syringe with a 25-gauge needle may be used to subcutaneously infiltrate 2 mL of tumescent anesthetic solution (420 mL of normal saline, 60 mL of 1% lidocaine with epinephrine, and 20 mL of sodium bicarbonate) over the access site. This solution is delivered manually or with an infusion pump under ultrasound guidance, aiming to surround the vein segment to be treated.[20,34] A laser-tipped catheter is inserted into the GSV at the level of the knee and advanced just distal to the saphenofemoral junction with ultrasound guidance. The laser is continuously pulled distally in the GSV as continuous energy is applied to the vein.

The systematic review by van den Bos et al. (see Table 54-1) reported an overall obliteration rate of 92.9% at 3 months (95% CI, 90.2-94.8), 93.3% at 1 year (95% CI, 91.1-95.0), and 95.4% at 5 years (95% CI, 79.7-99.1).[29] Several studies have reported that EVLT is more effective than venous stripping and other endovenous procedures in terms of obliteration and recurrence rates.[1] Endovenous

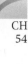

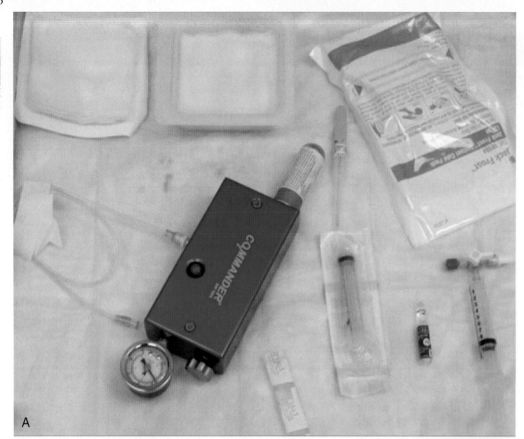

A

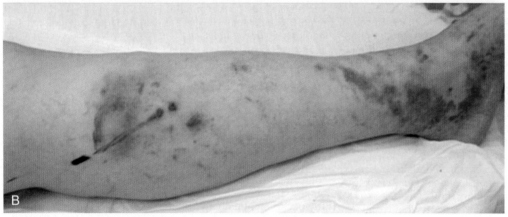

B

FIGURE 54-6 Tray prepared for sclerotherapy, and leg marked for access.

laser therapy recurrence of reflux in the treated vein occurs secondary to new incompetent perforators in the thigh and calf, and new saphenofemoral junction incompetence accounted for the progression of new vein disease.[35] In a study of 3000 treated limbs by Ravi et al., overall patient satisfaction, as assessed by symptom relief and absence of VVs after ablation, was 86%.[36] There are no absolute contraindications for EVLT.[37] Relative contraindications include uncorrectable coagulopathy, liver dysfunction limiting local anesthetic use, immobility, pregnancy, and breastfeeding.[37]

Higher energy results in increased occlusion rates but is associated with higher complication rates, including paresthesia and thermal injuries. Other complications include pain, edema, erythema, ecchymosis, hematoma, vesiculation, hypo- or hyperpigmentation, superficial thrombophlebitis, and DVT.[1,38] In a meta-analysis of 29 studies, Luebke and Brunkwall described more than a 50% incidence of ecchymosis in 12 of the studies where this complication was reported.[13] In the same meta-analysis, the incidence of paresthesias was 1.7%. Moderate pain along the treated vein and superficial thrombophlebitis occurs in up to 50% and 12% of the limbs, respectively.[39] In the same meta-analysis, seven studies with a total of 9317 patients reported only

27 cases of incident DVT (0.3%). In other studies, the incidence of DVT has been reported to be as much as 7%.[1,13] Pulmonary embolism has not been a reported complication with EVLT.[13] Because EVLT is usually performed in the outpatient setting, it may be more cost-effective than surgical treatment for VVs.[1]

RADIOFREQUENCY ABLATION

Radiofrequency ablation, introduced in the United States in 1999, results in obliteration of the GSV and its tributaries by delivering controlled heat using radiofrequency energy passed through an endovenous electrode.[1]

The theoretical advantage of segmental RFA is greater consistency in the vein treatment and increased speed of ablation; each 7-cm segment can be treated in 20 seconds.[40]

Procedure

Radiofrequency ablation is performed under general or local anesthesia. Tumescent anesthesia is required, and a dilute mixture of lidocaine in normal saline may be used (50 mL of 1% lidocaine with 1:200,000 epinephrine in 500 mL 0.9% saline for unilateral

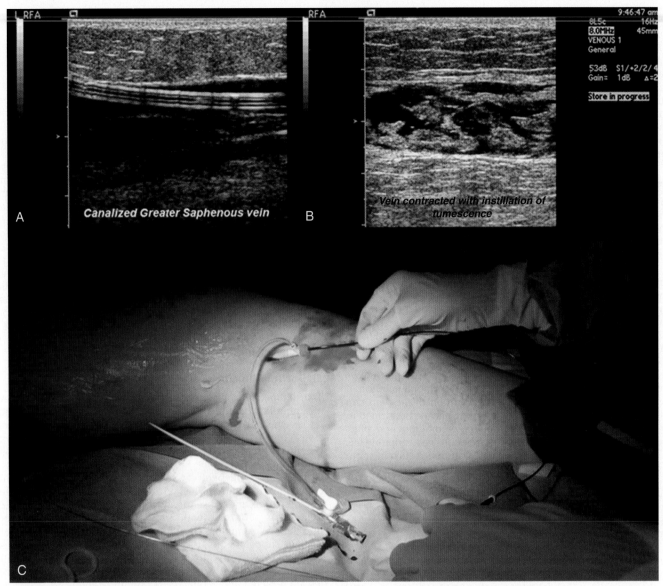

L RFA   CT   RFA   CT   9:46:47 am

                                                                          6L5c   16Hz
                                                                          8.0MHz   45mm
                                                                          VENOUS 1
                                                                          General

                                                                          53dB   S1/+2/2/4
                                                                          Gain= 1dB   Δ=2

                                                                          Store in progress

Canalized Greater Saphenous vein   Vein contracted with instillation of
                                                      tumescence

A   B

C

FIGURE 54-7 Insertion of radiofrequency catheter, with ultrasound visualization of inserted catheter and tumescence.

procedures, or in 1000 mL 0.9% saline for bilateral procedures). The volumes of tumescence are commonly between 75 and 100 mL per 10 cm of vein.[40] Ultrasound is used for catheter placement and guidance during the procedure (Fig. 54-7). The GSV is cannulated at the knee, and the catheter is advanced to the saphenofemoral junction.

Radiofrequency ablation's mechanism of action is based on resistive (or ohmic) heating caused by current. The heat generated in the vein wall (not in the catheter tip) is then dissipated and causes controlled collagen contraction or total thermocoagulation of the vein. The outcome is controlled tissue destruction that ultimately seals the lumen with minimal thrombus or coagulum.[41] The thermal effect is proportional to the temperature and treatment time. For instance, with a temperature of 85 °C to 90 °C and a pullback speed of 3 to 4 cm/min, the thermal effect is sufficient to cause collagen contraction and occlude the lumen.[41]

A compression garment is applied for several days after the procedure. Recovery time is 3 to 5 days. Complications include paresthesia, hematoma, skin burns, infection, bruising, and thrombophlebitis/thromboembolism. Transient paresthesia is reported in up to in 15%, hematoma in 5%, skin burns in 2.1%, superficial thrombophlebitis in 2.1%, DVT in 16%, and nonfatal PE in 1% of 286

treated limbs.[1] Venous size of less than 2 mm or more than 15 mm, previous superficial thrombophlebitis with residual obstruction, and GSV tortuosity are relative contraindications for RFA.[37]

In a systematic review of more than 12,000 limbs of patients who received stripping, foam sclerotherapy, or thermal ablation, the overall occlusion rate for RFA was 88.8% at 3 months (95% CI, 83.6-92.5), 87.7% at 1 year (95% CI, 83.1-91.2), and 79.9% at 5 years (95% CI, 59.5-91.5).[29] Symptomatic improvement was reported in 85% to 94% of limbs with anatomical success and 70% to 80% of limbs with anatomical failures.[1] In a meta-analysis by Luebke et al., the QOL at 72 hours and 1 week was significantly better with RFA than with surgery.[19]

Ultrasound examination is recommended within 72 hours to 1 week after the procedure to evaluate for DVT. Although no studies exist validating efficacy and safety of VTE prevention, patients with high thromboembolic risk can be considered for medical thromboprophylaxis after the procedure.[1] Radiofrequency ablation requires less hospitalization and recovery time than surgical procedures. In a study of 458 patients treated with RFA followed at 3 months and 1 year, the main predictors of long-term occlusion were pullback speed (odds ratio [OR] 3.7; 95% CI, 1.1-12.4) and CEAP classification (OR 3.1; 95% CI, 1.7-5.6).[42]

SURGICAL PROCEDURES

Surgical interventions were traditionally the alternative treatment for VVs when conservative management had been unsuccessful. These are now rarely performed. Surgical treatments of VVs include saphenous vein stripping, ligation of the saphenofemoral junction, and ambulatory phlebectomy.[1] The hemodynamic effectiveness of surgical procedures is supported by air plethysmography studies. In a study of 2120 limbs by Park et al., hemodynamic parameters including venous volume, venous filling index, residual volume function, and ejection fraction were significantly improved after surgery.[43]

Saphenous Vein Stripping

First reported in 1844, this procedure is performed in patients with incompetent GSVs or SSVs, reflux through the saphenofemoral or saphenopopliteal junctions, or superficial thrombophlebitis identified by duplex ultrasounds.[1] Additional chemical sclerotherapy is often needed for residual tributary VVs.[44]

Saphenous vein stripping is performed under general anesthesia and involves making an incision in the groin, along with ligation of the GSV and its major branches. A stiff but flexible wire is inserted into the free end of the GSV and advanced along its length and out through a second incision at the upper calf. The vein is then tied to the wire in the groin and retrieved through the second incision at the upper calf, stripping the entire GSV. The incisions are then closed and compression bandages applied.[1]

Of note, venous stripping from ankle to groin is not always necessary. Ligation of the vein at the saphenofemoral junction in conjunction with removal of the thigh portion of the vein can also reduce venous reflux. Venous stripping may be performed in conjunction with ligation of the saphenofemoral junction, phlebectomy, or chemical sclerotherapy. Saphenous vein stripping has a higher initial cost due to hospitalization and results in more time lost from work compared with endovenous procedures.[1] Recovery time varies from 2 to 3 weeks. The procedure is contraindicated in patients with a history of DVT, Klippel-Trénaunay's syndrome, or the presence of severe peripheral artery disease (PAD) or neuropathy, which may impede wound healing and increase the risk of infection.

In a large systematic review, there was persistent GSV and SSV obliteration of 80.4% (95% CI, 72.3-86.5) at 3 months, 79.7% (95% CI, 71.8-85.8) at 1 year, and 75.7% (95% CI, 67.9-82.1) at 5 years after saphenous vein stripping.[1,29] In a study of 245 extremities in 210 patients operated on for either GSV or SSV incompetence, there was a recurrence rate of 30%, as determined by ultrasound examination 14 years after the procedure, with only 6.9% having clinically significant recurrence of their VVs.[11] A multicenter study evaluated predictors of persistence or redevelopment of reflux in 1638 limbs. After adjustment for follow-up, independent predictors were found to be: groin mapping by ultrasound (OR, 0.28; 95% CI, 0.20-0.40), less than 3-cm groin incisions at or below groin crease (OR, 0.50; 95% CI, 0.32-0.78), prior parity (OR, 2.69; 95% CI, 1.45-4.97), body mass index (BMI) over 29 (OR, 1.65; 95% CI, 1.12-2.43), less than 3-cm suprainguinal incisions (OR, 3.71; 95% CI, 1.70-5.88), stripping to the ankle (OR, 2.43; 95% CI, 1.71-3.46), and interim pregnancy (OR, 4.74; 95% CI, 2.47-9.12).[45] Perforating vein incompetence and postthrombotic deep vein incompetence are also relevant considerations for postoperative VV recurrence.[46] The exact causes of VV recurrence are speculative, but may include neovascularization, presence of superficial and deep venous insufficiency, presence of incompetent perforator veins, or surgical failure.[4,8]

Although saphenous vein stripping improves the QOL for patients with symptomatic VVs, in a multicenter retrospective analysis of 376 limbs of 296 patients treated for primary VVs due to GSV insufficiency, the patient satisfaction rate decreased from 86% at 1 year to 74% at 5 years.[4] Complications of venous stripping include pain, bleeding (24%), infection (2%-15%), nerve injury (25%), superficial thrombophlebitis, and venous thromboembolism (<2%).[47]

Ligation of the Saphenofemoral Junction

Ligation of the saphenofemoral junction can be performed in patients with saphenofemoral reflux. However, owing to the high VV recurrence rate, it is typically performed in conjunction with venous stripping, phlebectomy, or EFS.[1]

Ligation is performed under local anesthesia through an incision made parallel to the inguinal ligament at the site of the saphenofemoral junction. Saphenous vein tributaries are identified and ligated until reaching the saphenofemoral junction. The GSV is then ligated at its junction with the common femoral vein. The incision is then closed, and compression garments are applied.[1] Ligation has been used with endovenous ablation techniques to improve efficacy and safety. In one study of 210 legs in 182 patients with primary saphenofemoral junction incompetence, the recurrence rate for saphenofemoral junction ligation was 5.4% at 1 year and 35.5% at 4 years. The relative risk of recurrence after ligation of the saphenofemoral junction alone is 2.4 times greater than that of venous stripping.[48] However, the percentage of patients with symptomatic recurrence of their varicosities is low.[1] In a study with long-term follow-up of 10 years of 245 extremities in 210 patients operated on for either GSV or SSV incompetence, only 7% of the limbs had recurrence (>3 mm diameter), with neovascularization as the main cause.[49] Complications of saphenofemoral ligation include pain, bleeding and hematoma (<30%), infection (2%-15%), nerve injury (4%-25%), thrombophlebitis, and DVT/PE (<2%).[47] Contraindications are similar to saphenous vein stripping.[1]

Stab or Transilluminated Phlebectomy

Transilluminated phlebectomy (TIPP) was proposed in 2000 as a more reliable and less invasive outpatient alternative to saphenous vein stripping.[1] The use of TIPP is associated with fewer incisions compared with conventional stab phlebectomy, but with a potentially higher cost, longer operating time, and greater complication rate.

For incision phlebectomy, small incisions are made along the GSV and its tributaries, which are retrieved with the use of a phlebectomy hook and subsequently avulsed.[1] Transilluminated phlebectomy is performed with a fiberoptic light channel inserted into the GSV. A mixture of saline and local anesthetic is infused into the subcutaneous tissue to produce tumescence and transilluminate the vein. With an endoscopic dissector, provided with a rotating blade and suction channel, the GSV and its tributaries are resected and aspirated.[50] Contraindications are similar to those for saphenous vein stripping.

A randomized prospective trial on 188 limbs comparing stab phlebectomy with TIPP reported a significant difference in the number of incisions for phlebectomy between the two groups (29 ± 1.28 vs. 5 ± 0.17; P <0.001). However, there was a higher recurrence rate at 52 weeks with TIPP (21.2% vs. 6.2%), with no significant difference in complication rates.[51] Complications include pain, hyperpigmentation (<2%), cellulitis (<3%), hematoma (5%-12%), and nerve injury (up to 25%).[1] The rate of calf hematoma is higher for TIPP than for stab phlebectomy (25% vs. 2.5%).[1] Phlebectomy is useful for larger truncal veins, in which higher venous flow limits the use of endovenous procedures, and in younger patients with thicker vein walls.[1] This procedure is often performed in conjunction with traditional surgical ligation of the saphenofemoral junction.[1] Both stab phlebectomy and TIPP prolong the return to work and resumption of activities of daily living. However, most patients recover fully by 6 weeks post surgery.[52]

Microphlebectomy

Dr. Robert Muller, a Swiss dermatologist from Neuchâtel, Switzerland, rediscovered this technique in 1956.[53] Ambulatory phlebectomy is a minimally invasive technique that can be performed in an office-based practice. This technique may be suitable for GSV, SSV, and pudendal veins in the groin, but more commonly is used to treat reticular varices in the popliteal fold or lateral part of the thigh.[53]

The VVs are carefully identified with a marking pen while the patient is standing. After tumescent anesthesia, with the patient in Trendelenburg position, cutaneous incisions are made with a #11 scalpel blade or 18-gauge needle, vertically oriented along the thigh and lower leg following the skin lines at the knee or the ankle.[53] The distance between the incisions is determined by experience, anatomy, and history of phlebitis. The vein is then dissected with the phlebectomy hook and mosquito forceps. Incompetent perforators can be dissected and eliminated with gentle traction or torsion, but this is more difficult. Venous ligation is not necessary, since hemostasis may be achieved with local compression during and after surgery. No skin closure is needed with small incisions of 1 to 3 mm. Postoperative bandaging is essential.[54] Dressings are removed after 24 or 48 hours. Ongoing compression therapy with elastic bandages or compression stockings is recommended for up to 3 weeks. Complementary chemical sclerotherapy may be used several weeks after the initial procedure.

Complications are minor and benign and usually resolve spontaneously. Periprocedurally, patients should avoid early sun exposure because hyperpigmentation may result at the puncture or incision sites.[53] Complications include edema, bleeding, hematoma formation, scarring, trauma-induced telangiectatic matting, neotelangiectasia, occasional nerve injury with sensory disturbances, and blisters due to wound dressings.[54] Very rarely, skin necrosis due to the high pH caused by adding excess bicarbonate to the anesthetic solution may occur. Deep venous thrombosis has not been reported.[54] Contraindications to ambulatory phlebectomy include reflux at the saphenofemoral or saphenopopliteal junctions. These junctions may be treated by thermal ablation.[53] Small studies and case series have reported a high rate of success with this procedure.

CHIVA CURE

This is a relatively new outpatient method described by Franceschi in 1988. "Cure Conservatrice et Hémodynamique de l'Insuffisance Veineuse en Ambulatoire" (CHIVA), or "Ambulatory Conservative Hemodynamic Management of Varicose Veins," aims for preservation of the superficial venous system and its cutaneous and subcutaneous drainage. The CHIVA method consists of breaking up the hydrostatic pressure column by disconnecting venous shunts. This is achieved by using venous ligatures guided by hemodynamic and duplex ultrasonography data derived from the deep and superficial venous system.[55] A variation of the CHIVA technique may be done using sclerotherapy.[56] Recurrence at 5 years of follow-up were 44.3% cured, 24.6% improved, and 31.1% failure in a study by Pares et al.[55] There were no occurrences of DVT, pulmonary thromboembolism, saphenous vein neuralgia, or deaths. Potential complications include bruises (47.5%), wound infection (2.5%), and phlebitis (1.3%).[55] Although the technique was invented in 1988, it is not yet widely available in United States. The practice guidelines of the American Venous Forum and the Society for Vascular Surgery do not currently endorse widespread use of the CHIVA technique.[37]

Management of Incompetent Perforator Veins

Poor deep venous function caused by venous reflux, obstruction, or calf muscle pump failure will ultimately lead to an increase in ambulatory venous pressure and recurrence of VV through incompetent perforators, resulting in chronic venous insufficiency. Incompetent perforator veins in patients with venous ulcerations were previously treated with ligation using the open Linton procedure, and now occasionally with subfascial endoscopic perforator surgery (SEPS).[1] More commonly, endovenous thermal ablation or sclerotherapy is the treatment of choice for patients with venous ulcers who have failed conservative compression therapy and require ablation of incompetent perforator veins. The current Society for Vascular Surgery and American Venous Forum guidelines do suggest treatment of so-called pathological perforating veins, defined as those with outward flow of 500-ms duration, diameter of 3.5 mm, and located beneath a healed or open venous ulcer.[37]

Surgical Treatments of Incompetent Perforator Veins

Patients who undergo ligation of perforator veins typically have severe resistant CVI complicated by venous ulcerations. The Linton procedure was introduced in the 1950s for treating perforator veins and has largely been replaced by SEPS. About 45% of incompetent perforator veins are located in an area 10 to 15 cm above the medial malleolus, the typical Cockett 2/3 area, but the anatomy of the subfascial compartments makes only 32% of Cockett 2, 4% of Cockett 3, and 40% of Cockett 4 perforators available in the superficial posterior compartment for interruption via a SEPS procedure.[57]

LINTON OR SUBFASCIAL ENDOSCOPIC PERFORATOR SURGERY PROCEDURE

The Linton procedure involves making a long incision across the calf including the diseased tissue, forming a skin/soft tissue/fascial flap, and ligating the perforator veins under direct visualization.[1] SEPS can be performed in the ambulatory care setting, with less time away from work required. The SEPS procedure involves making two incisions below the knee and inserting ports into the subfascial space.[1] The subfascial plane is kept open with infusion of CO_2 for visualization of the structures. The perforator veins are identified and ligated.

As noted, the Linton procedure has largely been replaced by SEPS because of higher complication rates, including wound infections (40%-50%), nerve injury (11%), and DVT (4%). Complications associated with SEPS are less frequent and include wound infection (5%-7%), nerve injury (6%), superficial thrombophlebitis (3%), and cellulitis (2.5%).[18,20,51] Presence of peripheral artery disease, which carries the risk of poor wound healing, is a relative contraindication to these procedures. Similarly, performance of these procedures in patients with deep vein occlusion is associated with poor outcomes.[58]

Lower-extremity activity is limited for 5 to 7 days.[1] SEPS may be performed in conjunction with other surgical and endovenous procedures that ablate an incompetent GSV.

SCLEROTHERAPY

Ultrasound-guided sclerotherapy uses a relatively small catheter to gain access to the incompetent perforator or its tributary. Masuda et al. treated 80 limbs in 68 patients by sclerotherapy using liquid sodium morrhuate. The initial incompetent perforator closure rate was 90%, but fell to 70% at a mean follow-up of 20 months.[57] After treatment, the VCSS was improved from a median of 8 to 2. Skin necrosis is a reported adverse effect.

ENDOVENOUS ABLATION

Percutaneous endovenous RFA of incompetent perforator veins can be carried out with a small incision or puncture site in the calf. However, because this entry site is usually made in compromised skin directly over the perforator, there may be risk of infection or exacerbation of the wound. In a meta-analysis of 1573 incompetent perforator veins treated by RFA, the occlusion rate varied from 64% to 99% during a short follow-up.[57] In a study of 37 patients who underwent Doppler ultrasound surveillance 5 years after incompetent perforator ablation, of 125 incompetent perforators analyzed, 101 were closed (81%).[59] Although this is a promising procedure, data regarding ulcer healing rates and long-term efficacy are limited.[57]

Management of Telangiectasia/Reticular Veins

Surface Transcutaneous Laser Therapy

Surface transcutaneous laser therapy has been used for treating telangiectasias and reticular veins since the 1970s. Laser obliterates the vein by heating the hemoglobin (Hb) within the vessel and injuring the endothelium. New advances in laser technology have allowed delivery of sufficient energy to achieve pan-endothelial necrosis without affecting structures in the epidermal layer. High-intensity pulsed light therapy was developed in 1990 for treating small VVs. It differs from laser by emitting a spectrum of light, rather than a wavelength, to obliterate the vein.

PROCEDURE

Patients undergo skin cooling with water-cooled chambers applied to the skin, cooling coupling gel, air-blowing cooling devices, or refrigerated cooling sprays before and after the procedure to provide comfort during the procedure and minimize postprocedure adverse effects. The amount of pre-cooling depends on the patient's skin type and size of varicosities; those with higher amounts of melanin in their skin require longer pre-cooling. The amount of postcooling depends on the size of the vessels to be treated, with smaller vessels requiring longer postcooling.

The laser is applied to the surface of the skin and targets a wavelength of light to the Hb within the vessel, resulting in heating and obliteration of the vessel. Small (<1 mm) superficial vessels with higher oxygenated Hb content are treated with shorter wavelengths (580-1064 nm), shorter pulse durations (15-30 ms), higher fluences (350-600 J/cm²), and smaller spot sizes (<2 mm).[40] Larger, deeper vessels with lower oxygenated Hb content are treated with longer wavelengths (800-1064 nm), longer pulse durations (30-50 ms), moderate fluences (100-350 J/cm²), and larger spot sizes (2-8 mm).[1] Pulsed light therapy delivers a high-intensity spectrum of light to the vessel, resulting in its obliteration. Pulsed light therapy generally is used for longer vessels. Typically, one to three laser treatments are scheduled at 6- to 12-week intervals.[1]

Reports of effectiveness are based on case series reporting small numbers of patients. In a study of 40 female patients 24 to 58 years old, the leg veins were treated with synchronized micropulses from a long-pulsed 1064-nm Nd:YAG laser, 6-mm diameter spot size, and 130 and 140 J/cm.[2] After one to three laser treatment sessions, there was a 50% to 75% disappearance of veins in approximately 60% of the limbs at 4 weeks, and in more than 80% of the limbs at 12 weeks. The patient subjective satisfaction index, measuring cosmetics, increased from 42.5% at 6 months to 75% at 12 months. Objective improvement in cosmetic appearance, measured with computer-assessed medical photography, increased from 57% at 6 months to 82.5% at 12 months.[60]

Postprocedure pain is a common side effect of laser and light therapy. Other complications include edema, erythema, bruising, vesiculation, hypo/hyperpigmentation, transient hemosiderin staining, telangiectatic matting, and scarring. This procedure is contraindicated during pregnancy and in those with tanned or dark skin, history of photosensitivity disorder, or keloidal scarring. Patients are advised to avoid tanning before the procedure to avoid absorption of shorter wavelengths from the laser by sun-induced melanin, resulting in blistering and hyperpigmentation.[3] Sunscreen is advised after treatment with laser.

Laser and light therapies are more expensive than liquid sclerotherapy, owing to the cost of equipment.

Chemical Sclerotherapy

Sclerotherapy for treating telangiectasias and reticular veins is generally performed using liquid sclerosant (glycerin, hypertonic saline, polidocanol, and sodium tetradecyl sulfate) rather than foam, although foam can also be used in lower volumes. To decrease telangiectatic matting and postsclerosis hyperpigmentation, a reduced amount of foam per injection (0.5 mL) and per treatment session is recommended for telangiectasias and reticular veins. *Telangiectatic matting* describes a network of tiny vessels less than 0.2 mm in diameter that may appear after sclerotherapy treatment.[61] In a large retrospective analysis of 2120 patients, the overall incidence of telangiectatic matting was 16%.[61]

Follow-Up and Prognosis

A relevant disclosure before treating the patient with VVs is that current methodologies continue to require long-term follow-up and retreatment. The possibility of recurrence at 5 years is 5% to 30%, depending on the treatment administered and ongoing risk factors. Obesity, multiple pregnancies, incompetent perforators, and saphenofemoral junction incompetence are some of the often-mentioned risk factors for recurrence. Regular compression stocking use will minimize the signs and symptoms associated with recurrent VVs and progression of chronic venous insufficiency. However, patients will commonly return for repeated treatments over their lifetime.[45,46]

REFERENCES

1. Nael R, Rathbun S: Treatment of varicose veins, *Curr Treat Options Cardiovasc Med* 11(2):91–103, 2009.
2. Callam MJ: Epidemiology of varicose veins, *Br J Surg* 81(2):167–173, 1994.
3. Bergan JJ, et al: Chronic venous disease, *N Engl J Med* 355(5):488–498, 2006.
4. Miyazaki K, et al: Long-term results of treatments for varicose veins due to greater saphenous vein insufficiency, *Int Angiol* 24(3):282–286, 2005.
5. Marsh P, et al: Pelvic vein reflux in female patients with varicose veins: comparison of incidence between a specialist private vein clinic and the vascular department of a National Health Service District General Hospital, *Phlebology* 24(3):108–113, 2009.
6. Evans CJ, et al: Prevalence of varicose veins and chronic venous insufficiency in men and women in the general population: Edinburgh Vein Study, *J Epidemiol Community Health* 53(3):149–153, 1999.
7. Kachlik D, Pechacek V, Baca V, et al: The superficial venous system of the lower extremity: new nomenclature, *Phlebology* 25:113–123, 2010.
8. Raju S, Neglen P: Clinical practice. Chronic venous insufficiency and varicose veins, *N Engl J Med* 360(22):2319–2327, 2009.
9. Robertson L, et al: Risk factors for chronic ulceration in patients with varicose veins: a case control study, *J Vasc Surg* 49(6):1490–1498, 2009.
10. Labropoulos N, et al: Secondary chronic venous disease progresses faster than primary, *J Vasc Surg* 49(3):704–710, 2009.
11. Raffetto JD, Khalil RA: Matrix metalloproteinases in venous tissue remodeling and varicose vein formation, *Curr Vasc Pharmacol* 6(3):158–172, 2008.
12. Rutherford RB, et al: Venous severity scoring: an adjunct to venous outcome assessment, *J Vasc Surg* 31(6):1307–1312, 2000.
13. Luebke T, Brunkwall J: Systematic review and meta-analysis of endovenous radiofrequency obliteration, endovenous laser therapy, and foam sclerotherapy for primary varicosis, *J Cardiovasc Surg (Torino)* 49(2):213–233, 2008.
14. Vasquez MA, Munschauer CE: Venous Clinical Severity Score and quality-of-life assessment tools: application to vein practice, *Phlebology* 23(6):259–275, 2008.
15. Vasquez MA, et al: Revision of the Venous Clinical Severity Score: venous outcomes consensus statement: special communication of the American Venous Forum Ad Hoc Outcomes Working Group, *J Vasc Surg.* 52:1387–1396, 2010.
16. Rathbun S: Chronic venous disease and lymphatic disease. In Rooke T, editor: *Vascular medicine and endvascular interventions*, Oxford, UK, 2009, Blackwell, pp 44–58.
17. Rumwell C, McPharlin M: *Vascular technology*, ed 4, Pasadena, CA, 2009, Davies.
18. Goode SD, et al: Suitability of varicose veins for endovenous treatments, *Cardiovasc Intervent Radiol* 32(5):988–991, 2009.
19. Luebke T, et al: Meta-analysis of endovenous radiofrequency obliteration of the great saphenous vein in primary varicosis, *J Endovasc Ther* 15(2):213–223, 2008.
20. Rathbun SW, Kirkpatrick AC: Treatment of chronic venous insufficiency, *Curr Treat Options Cardiovasc Med* 9(2):115–126, 2007.
21. Klonizakis M, et al: Exercise training improves cutaneous microvascular endothelial function in post-surgical varicose vein patients, *Microvasc Res* 78(1):67–70, 2009.
22. Milic DJ, et al: The influence of different sub-bandage pressure values on venous leg ulcers healing when treated with compression therapy, *J Vasc Surg* 51(3):655–661, 2010.
23. O'Meara S, et al: Antibiotics and antiseptics for venous leg ulcers, *Cochrane Database Syst Rev* (1): CD003557, 2010.
24. Suter A, Bommer S, Rechner J: Treatment of patients with venous insufficiency with fresh plant horse chestnut seed extract: a review of 5 clinical studies, *Adv Ther* 23(1):179–190, 2006.
25. Coleridge-Smith P, Lok C, Ramelet AA: Venous leg ulcer: a meta-analysis of adjunctive therapy with micronized purified flavonoid fraction, *Eur J Vasc Endovasc Surg* 30(2):198–208, 2005.
26. Breu FX, Guggenbichler S: European Consensus Meeting on Foam Sclerotherapy, April, 4-6, 2003, Tegernsee, Germany, *Dermatol Surg* 30(5):709–717, 2004 discussion 717.
27. Bergan J, Cheng V: Foam sclerotherapy for the treatment of varicose veins, *Vascular* 15(5):269–272, 2007.

28. Belcaro G, et al: Foam-sclerotherapy, surgery, sclerotherapy, and combined treatment for varicose veins: a 10-year, prospective, randomized, controlled, trial (VEDICO trial), *Angiology* 54(3):307–315, 2003.

29. van den Bos R, et al: Endovenous therapies of lower extremity varicosities: a meta-analysis, *J Vasc Surg* 49(1):230–239, 2009.

30. Myers KA, Jolley D: Factors affecting the risk of deep venous occlusion after ultrasound-guided sclerotherapy for varicose veins, *Eur J Vasc Endovasc Surg* 36(5):602–605, 2008.

31. Morrison N, Neuhardt DL: Foam sclerotherapy: cardiac and cerebral monitoring, *Phlebology* 24(6):252–259, 2009.

32. PRNewswire: *ClariVein®: New method for vein ablation introduced in Europe,* 2010. [cited 2010 October 3, 2010]; Available from: http://www.vasculardiseasemanagement.com/content/clarivein%C2%AE-new-method-vein-ablation-introduced-europe.

33. Fan CM, Rox-Anderson R: Endovenous laser ablation: mechanism of action, *Phlebology* 23(5):206–213, 2008.

34. Perkowski P, et al: Endovenous laser ablation of the saphenous vein for treatment of venous insufficiency and varicose veins: early results from a large single-center experience, *J Endovasc Ther* 11(2):132–138, 2004.

35. King J: Progression and recurrence of vein disease in patients treated with endovenous laser ablation: one year experience. In *The 11th Annual Scientific Meeting & Workshops,* Sydney, Australia, 2007.

36. Ravi R, et al: Endovenous thermal ablation of superficial venous insufficiency of the lower extremity: single-center experience with 3000 limbs treated in a 7-year period, *J Endovasc Ther* 16(4):500–505, 2009.

37. Gloviczki P, et al: The care of patients with varicose veins and associated chronic venous diseases: clinical practice guidelines of the Society for Vascular Surgery and the American Venous Forum, *J Vasc Surg* 53(5 Suppl):2S–48S.

38. Nwaejike N, Srodon PD, Kyriakides C: 5-years of endovenous laser ablation (EVLA) for the treatment of varicose veins - a prospective study, *Int J Surg* 7(4):347–349, 2009.

39. Pannier-Fischer F, Rabe E: Endovenous laser therapy and radiofrequency ablation of saphenous varicose veins, *J Cardiovasc Surg (Torino)* 47(1):3–8, 2006.

40. Gohel MS, Davies AH: Radiofrequency ablation for uncomplicated varicose veins, *Phlebology* 24(Suppl 1):42–49, 2009.

41. Roth SM: Endovenous radiofrequency ablation of superficial and perforator veins, *Surg Clin North Am* 87(5):1267–1284, xii, 2007.

42. Boon R, Akkersdijk GJ, Nio D: Percutaneous treatment of varicose veins with bipolar radiofrequency ablation, *Eur J Radiol* 75(1):43–47.

43. Park UJ, et al: Analysis of the postoperative hemodynamic changes in varicose vein surgery using air plethysmography, *J Vasc Surg* 51(3):634–638, 2010.

44. Nishibe T, et al: Fate of varicose veins after great saphenous vein stripping alone, *Int Angiol* 28(4):311–314, 2009.

45. Fischer R, et al: Patient characteristics and physician-determined variables affecting saphenofemoral reflux recurrence after ligation and stripping of the great saphenous vein, *J Vasc Surg* 43(1):81–87, 2006.

46. Allegra C, Antignani PL, Carlizza A: Recurrent varicose veins following surgical treatment: our experience with five years follow-up, *Eur J Vasc Endovasc Surg* 33(6):751–756, 2007.

47. Beale RJ, Gough MJ: Treatment options for primary varicose veins–a review, *Eur J Vasc Endovasc Surg* 30(1):83–95, 2005.

48. Winterborn RJ, et al: Randomised trial of flush saphenofemoral ligation for primary great saphenous varicose veins, *Eur J Vasc Endovasc Surg* 36(4):477–484, 2008.

49. Hartmann K, et al: Recurrent varicose veins: sonography-based re-examination of 210 patients 14 years after ligation and saphenous vein stripping, *Vasa J Vasc Dis* 35(1):21–26, 2006.

50. Beale RJ, Gough MJ: Treatment options for primary varicose veins - a review, *Eur J Vasc Endovasc Surg* 30(1):83–95, 2005.

51. Aremu MA, et al: Prospective randomized controlled trial: conventional versus powered phlebectomy, *J Vasc Surg* 39(1):88–94, 2004.

52. Chetter IC, et al: Randomized clinical trial comparing multiple stab incision phlebectomy and transilluminated powered phlebectomy for varicose veins, *Br J Surg* 93(2):169–174, 2006.

53. Ramelet AA: Phlebectomy. Technique, indications and complications, *Int Angiol* 21(2 Suppl 1):46–51, 2002.

54. Weiss RA, Dover JS: Leg vein management: sclerotherapy, ambulatory phlebectomy, and laser surgery, *Semin Cutan Med Surg* 21(1):76–103, 2002.

55. Pares JO, et al: Varicose vein surgery: stripping versus the CHIVA method: a randomized controlled trial, *Ann Surg* 251(4):624–631, 2010.

56. Bernardini E, et al: Echo-sclerosis hemodynamic conservative: a new technique for varicose vein treatment, *Ann Vasc Surg* 21(4):535–543, 2007.

57. Donnell TF: The role of perforators in chronic venous insufficiency, *Phlebology* 25(1):3–10, 2010.

58. Gloviczki P, et al: Mid-term results of endoscopic perforator vein interruption for chronic venous insufficiency: lessons learned from the North American subfascial endoscopic perforator surgery registry. The North American Study Group, *J Vasc Surg* 29(3):489–502, 1999.

59. Bacon JL, et al: Five-year results of incompetent perforator vein closure using trans-luminal occlusion of perforator, *Phlebology* 24(2):74–78, 2009.

60. Trelles MA, et al: Long pulse Nd:YAG laser for treatment of leg veins in 40 patients with assessments at 6 and 12 months, *Lasers Surg Med* 35(1):68–76, 2004.

61. Davis LT, Duffy DM: Determination of incidence and risk factors for postsclerotherapy telangiectatic matting of the lower extremity: a retrospective analysis, *J Dermatol Surg Oncol* 16(4):327–330, 1990.

CHAPTER 55 Chronic Venous Insufficiency

Nitin Garg, Peter Gloviczki

An estimated 25 to 40 million Americans have varicose veins, and more than 2 million have chronic venous insufficiency, including venous edema, skin changes, or venous ulcers.[1] The cost of venous ulcer care is greater than $3 billion in the United States; in the United Kingdom, estimates are greater than $1 billion annually.[2,3] Patients with advanced venous disease have decreased quality of life and occasionally, severe disease that is limb threatening.[4,5]

Definition

Chronic venous disease (CVD) includes a series of clinical conditions of varying severity, from varicose veins at one end of the spectrum to venous ulcers at the other. Chronic venous insufficiency (CVI) is the diagnosis given to patients with venous dysfunction causing edema, skin changes, or ulcerations (CEAP class 3-6; Box 55-1). The CEAP classification is used to define, categorize, and grade the severity of all chronic venous disorders.[6] This classification provides insight into the clinical presentation (C), etiology (E), anatomy (A), and pathophysiology (P) of the underlying venous disorder.

Clinical Presentation

Varicose veins (CEAP class C2) are dilated superficial veins (>3 mm in diameter in the upright position)[7] (see Chapter 54). Chronic venous insufficiency includes patients with more advanced disease, with or without varicose veins. These patients have edema, skin changes like dermatosclerosis, pigmentation, corona phlebectatica or eczema, or healed or active venous ulcer[8,9] (see Box 55-1).

Increased ambulatory venous hypertension leads to a series of changes in subcutaneous tissue and skin, mostly in the "gaiter" area of the leg, at or above the ankle (Fig. 55-1). These are caused by activation of the endothelial cells (ECs), extravasation of macromolecules and red blood cells, diapedesis of leukocytes, tissue edema, and chronic inflammatory changes.[7] These changes are all consequences of either venous valvular incompetence or venous obstruction, or a combination of both.

Etiology

Most cases of venous insufficiency have underlying primary etiology. The most frequent cause is likely intrinsic morphological or biochemical abnormality in the vein wall. The origin of venous reflux in patients with primary varicose veins can be local or multifocal structural weakness of the vein wall, and this can occur together or independently of proximal saphenous vein valvular incompetence.[10] Chronic venous insufficiency can also develop as a result of secondary causes such as previous deep venous thrombosis (DVT), deep venous obstruction, superficial thrombophlebitis, or arteriovenous fistula (AVF). May-Thurner's syndrome (occlusion or stenosis of the left iliac vein due to compression by the overriding right common iliac artery [CIA]) is a cause of CVI that is likely much more frequent than previously thought (Fig. 55-2). Varicose veins may also be congenital and present as venous malformation and eventually lead to CVI. Primary venous insufficiency accounts for approximately 70% of advanced CVI (class 4-6), with the remainder occurring in legs following DVT.[11,12]

Anatomy

Significant changes have been made to venous terminology over the last decade, and these have been uniformly adopted and promoted by international vascular societies.[13,14] Superficial veins of the lower limbs are those located between the deep fascia, covering the muscles of the limb, and the skin. The main superficial veins are the great saphenous vein (GSV) and the small saphenous vein (SSV; Fig. 55-3). All previous names used to describe these vessels (greater, long, and lesser) should be abandoned. The GSV originates from the medial superficial veins of the dorsum of the foot and ascends in front of the medial malleolus along the medial border of the tibia, behind the saphenous nerve. There are posterior and anterior accessory saphenous veins in the calf and the thigh. The saphenofemoral junction (SFJ) is the confluence of superficial inguinal veins comprising the GSV and superficial circumflex iliac, superficial epigastric, and external pudendal veins. The GSV in the thigh lies in the saphenous subcompartment of the superficial compartment between the saphenous fascia and deep fascia. The SSV is the primary superficial vein of the posterior aspect of the lower leg and originates posterior to the lateral malleolus and courses posterolaterally in the lower leg to drain into the popliteal vein, behind the knee. The intersaphenous vein (vein of Giacomini) connects the SSV in the posterior thigh with the GSV.[15]

Deep veins follow the arterial circulation in the limb and pelvis and are usually paired in the lower leg, accompanying tibial arteries by the same name. The popliteal or the femoral vein can also be paired. The femoral vein runs parallel to the superficial femoral artery (SFA) and replaces the term superficial femoral vein to avoid confusion regarding its importance as a deep vein.[14] The pelvic veins include the external, internal, and common iliac veins (CIVs), which drain into the inferior vena cava (IVC). Large gonadal veins drain into the IVC on the right and left renal vein on the left.

Perforator veins traverse the deep muscular fascia and communicate between the superficial and deep venous system at multiple levels in the lower extremity (see Fig. 55-3). These primarily function to drain the superficial system into the deep venous system. The most important leg perforating veins are the medial calf perforators.[16] The posterior tibial perforating veins ("Cockett perforators" in the old nomenclature) connect the posterior accessory GSV with the posterior tibial veins and form the lower, middle, and upper groups. They are located just behind the medial malleolus (lower), at 7 to 9 cm (middle) and 10 to 12 cm (upper) from the lower edge of the malleolus. The distance between these perforators and the medial edge of the tibia is 2 to 4 cm.[16] Paratibial perforators connect the main GSV trunk with the posterior tibial veins. In the distal thigh, perforators of the femoral canal connect, usually directly, the GSV to the femoral vein.

Bicuspid venous valves are present in all superficial and deep lower-extremity veins and are important in assisting normal unidirectional venous flow. The GSV usually has at least six valves (maximum 14-25),[17] with a constant valve present within 2 to 3 cm of the SFJ in 85% of cases (preterminal valve).[18] The SSV has a median of 7 to 10 valves (range, 4-13).[17] There are valves in the deep veins of the lower limb, but the common femoral or external iliac vein has only one valve in about 63% of cases.[17] In 37%, there is no valve in the common iliac vein. The internal iliac vein has a valve in 10%; its tributaries have valves in 9%.[19]

Although isolated severe incompetence of the superficial system may lead to development of ulcers with high ambulatory pressures, most venous ulcers have underlying multisystem (superficial, deep, perforator) incompetence involving at least two of the three venous systems.[20,21] Of 239 patients with venous ulcers evaluated with duplex scanning in three different studies, 144 (60.3%) had incompetent perforating veins, and 141 (59%) had deep vein incompetence or obstruction.[22–24]

Pathophysiology

Most patients with CVI have primary or secondary venous valvular incompetence. Venous outflow obstruction can be the result of primary venous disease (e.g., May-Thurner's syndrome),[25] or it can

Box 55-1 The CEAP Classification (Basic)

1. Clinical classification:
   - C0 No visible or palpable signs of venous disease
   - C1 Telangiectases or reticular veins
   - C2 Varicose veins
   - C3 Edema
   - C4a Pigmentation and/or eczema
   - C4b Lipodermatosclerosis and/or atrophie blanche
   - C5 Healed venous ulcer
   - C6 Active venous ulcer
   - S   Symptoms including ache, pain, tightness, skin irritation, heaviness, muscle cramps, as well as other complaints attributable to venous dysfunction
   - A   Asymptomatic
2. Etiological classification:
   - Ec Congenital
   - Ep Primary
   - Es Secondary (postthrombotic)
   - En No venous etiology identified
3. Anatomical classification:
   - As Superficial veins
   - Ap Perforator veins
   - Ad Deep veins
   - An No venous location identified
4. Pathophysiological classification:
   - Pr   Reflux
   - Po   Obstruction
   - Pr,o Reflux and obstruction
   - Pn   No venous pathophysiology identifiable

Adapted from Eklof B, Rutherford RB, Bergan JJ, et al: Revision of the CEAP classification for chronic venous disorders: consensus statement. J Vasc Surg 40:1248–1252, 2004; used with permission.

be the result of a previous DVT. Occasionally, congenital anomalies like deep vein agenesis or hypoplasia result in venous outflow obstruction.

Venous obstruction results in venous congestion, distal venous hypertension, and venous claudication. Obstruction alone may also result in skin changes and venous ulcerations. Depending on the extent of the collateral circulation, these patients will have pain, swelling, and heaviness of the limb; rarely, the most severe forms of venous obstruction may even interfere with viability of the limb.

Patients with valvular incompetence may have similar symptoms as those with obstruction: varicosity, edema, skin changes, or venous ulcers. Venous claudication or feeling fullness and edema are usually not as severe as with venous obstruction, and relief with limb elevation is immediate.

Recent evidence suggests that venous obstruction could be more important than valvular incompetence. Among 504 patients who underwent iliac vein stenting for venous obstruction, symptoms resolved after stenting, despite associated valvular incompetence.[26]

Diagnostic Evaluation

A thorough history and physical examination should be complemented by duplex scan of the superficial and deep veins to evaluate obstruction and valvular incompetence, as recommended by the recent guidelines of the Society for Vascular Surgery and the American Venous Forum (recommendation grade 1A).[27] Subsequent diagnostic testing is carried out based on clinical presentation and examination findings.

History

Symptoms related to CVI can include tingling, aching, burning, pain, muscle cramps, swelling, sensation of throbbing or heaviness, itching skin, restless legs, leg tiredness, fatigue, or ulceration in extreme cases.[28] These symptoms suggest CVI, particularly if patients notice exacerbation by heat or dependency during the course of the day and relief by resting or leg elevation or use of compression therapy.[29] Pain during and after exercise that is relieved with rest and leg elevation (venous claudication) can also be caused by venous outflow obstruction from previous DVT (postthrombotic syndrome) or obstruction of CIVs (May-Thurner's syndrome).[28] Diffuse pain is more frequently associated with axial venous reflux, whereas poor venous circulation in bulging varicose veins usually causes local pain. The Guideline Committee recommends using the revised Venous Clinical Severity Score (VCSS; Table 55-1)[30] to grade and document the presenting symptoms of patients with CVD.[27]

A detailed medical history may establish the diagnosis of primary, secondary, or congenital venous problems. Adequate history should address previous DVT or thrombophlebitis, personal or family history of thrombophilia, medication history (particularly oral contraceptive pills), smoking, obstetric history, and a family history of venous disorders (most patients with varicose veins would be able to relate their parents' or grandparents'

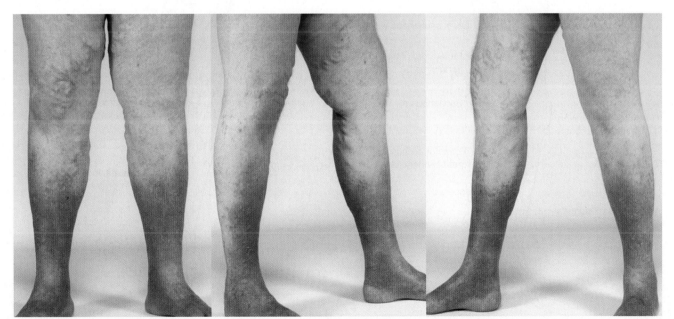

FIGURE 55-1 A 53-year-old man with chronic venous insufficiency (CVI) CEAP class C4, showing extensive skin changes of venous hypertension, with hyperpigmentation, eczema, and lipodermatosclerosis.

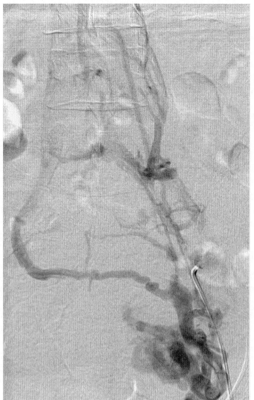

FIGURE 55-2 **Iliac venogram demonstrating chronic left iliac vein occlusion, likely as a result of compression from the iliac artery (May-Thurner's syndrome) in a 44-year-old woman with left leg swelling and suprapubic varicosities.**

disease). Premenopausal women with varicose veins should also be questioned for symptoms of pelvic congestion syndrome (pelvic pain, aching, or heaviness; dyspareunia). Advanced age is the most important risk factor for varicose veins and CVI. A positive family history and obesity are risk factors for CVI.[31]

Physical Examination

Examination should always be performed with the patient in the standing position in a warm room with good light, and should establish the size, location, and distribution of varicose veins and also focus on other signs of venous disease such as edema (partially pitting or nonpitting), skin changes (induration, pigmentation, lipodermatosclerosis, atrophie blanche, eczema, dermatitis, skin discoloration, increased skin temperature), and ulceration (healed or active). Inspection and palpation are essential parts of the examination, and auscultation (for bruits) is particularly helpful in those with vascular malformation and arteriovenous fistula.[32] Varicose dilations or venous aneurysms, palpable cord in the vein, tenderness, thrill, bruit, or pulsatility should be recorded. Ankle mobility should also be examined because patients with advanced venous disease frequently have decreased mobility in the ankle joints. Sensory and motor functions of the limb and foot are assessed to help differentiate from diabetic neuropathy or any underlying neurological problem. An abdominal mass or lymphadenopathy can provide a clue to venous compression and outflow obstruction.

Corona phlebectatica (ankle flare or malleolar flare) is a fan-shaped pattern of small intradermal veins located around the ankle or the dorsum of the foot.[27] This is considered to be an early sign of advanced venous disease. Inspection of the abdominal wall and perineal and inguinal region should be routinely performed. Perineal, vulvar, or groin varicosities can be seen in iliac vein obstruction or internal iliac vein or gonadal vein incompetence causing

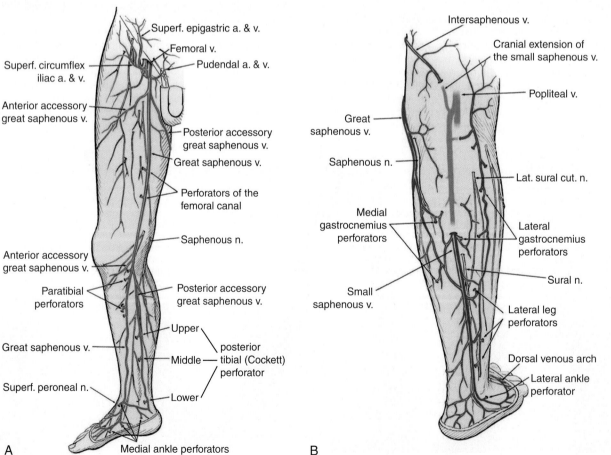

FIGURE 55-3 **A,** Medial superficial and perforating veins of the lower limb. **B,** Posterior superficial and perforating veins of the leg. *(Used with permission of Mayo Foundation for Medical Education and Research.)*

TABLE 55-1   Revised Venous Clinical Severity Score

PAIN	NONE: 0	MILD: 1	MODERATE: 2	SEVERE: 3
Or other discomfort (i.e., aching, heaviness, fatigue, soreness, burning); presumes venous origin		Occasional pain or other discomfort (i.e., not restricting regular daily activity)	Daily pain or other discomfort (i.e., interfering with but not preventing regular daily activities)	Daily pain or discomfort (i.e., limits most regular daily activities)
VARICOSE VEINS	**NONE: 0**	**MILD: 1**	**MODERATE: 2**	**SEVERE: 3**
"Varicose" veins must be ≥3 mm in diameter to qualify in the standing position		Few scattered (i.e., isolated branch varicosities or clusters); also includes corona phlebectatica (ankle flare)	Confined to calf or thigh	Involves calf and thigh
VENOUS EDEMA	**NONE: 0**	**MILD: 1**	**MODERATE: 2**	**SEVERE: 3**
Presumes venous origin		Limited to foot and ankle area	Extends above ankle but below knee	Extends to knee and above
SKIN PIGMENTATION	**NONE: 0**	**MILD: 1**	**MODERATE: 2**	**SEVERE: 3**
Presumes venous origin; does not include focal pigmentation over varicose veins or pigmentation due to other chronic diseases (e.g., vasculitis purpura)	None or focal	Limited to perimalleolar area	Diffuse over lower third of calf	Wider distribution above lower third of calf
INFLAMMATION	**NONE: 0**	**MILD: 1**	**MODERATE: 2**	**SEVERE: 3**
More than just recent pigmentation (i.e., erythema, cellulitis, venous eczema, dermatitis)		Limited to perimalleolar area	Diffuse over lower third of calf	Wider distribution above lower third of calf
INDURATION	**NONE: 0**	**MILD: 1**	**MODERATE: 2**	**SEVERE: 3**
Presumes venous origin of secondary skin and subcutaneous changes (e.g., chronic edema with fibrosis, hypodermitis); includes white atrophy and lipodermatosclerosis		Limited to perimalleolar area	Diffuse over lower third of calf	Wider distribution above lower third of calf
NO. OF ACTIVE ULCERS	**0**	**1**	**2**	**≥3**
Active ulcer duration (longest active)	N/A	<3 mo	>3 mo but <1 y	Not healed for >1 y
Active ulcer size (largest active)	N/A	Diameter <2 cm	Diameter 2-6 cm	Diameter >6 cm
USE OF COMPRESSION THERAPY	**NONE: 0**	**OCCASIONAL: 1**	**FREQUENT: 2**	**ALWAYS: 3**
	Not used	Intermittent use of stockings	Wears stockings most days	Full compliance with stockings

Adapted from Vasquez MA, Rabe E, McLafferty RB, et al: Revision of the venous clinical severity score: venous outcomes consensus statement: special communication of the American Venous Forum Ad Hoc Outcomes Working Group. J Vasc Surg 52:1387–1396, 2010; used with permission.

pelvic congestion syndrome. Scrotal varicosity may be a sign of gonadal vein incompetence, left renal vein compression between the superior mesenteric artery (SMA) and aorta (nutcracker syndrome), or occasionally even IVC lesions or renal carcinoma.

Classic tourniquet tests for saphenous or perforator incompetence or deep venous occlusion (Trendelenburg test, Ochsner-Mahorner test, Perthes test) are rarely used today. They are mostly of historical interest and should be used in rare instances when duplex scanning or Doppler studies are unavailable.[32] Distal palpation and proximal percussion of the saphenous vein, however, are useful tests to suggest valvular incompetence.

Skin lesions other than those already described (e.g., capillary malformations, tumors, onychomycosis, excoriations) should also be noted. An aneurysmal saphenous vein can be misdiagnosed as a femoral hernia or vice versa. Presence of a longer limb, lateral varicosity noted soon after birth, and associated capillary malformations are tipoffs for congenital venous malformation (Klippel-Trénaunay's syndrome).[33] Edema of the dorsum of the foot, squaring of the toes, thick skin, and nonpitting edema are signs of chronic lymphedema. A complete pulse examination should be performed to exclude underlying peripheral arterial disease. The physical examination can be complemented by a handheld Doppler examination, although the latter does not replace evaluation of the venous circulation with color duplex scanning.

The aim of the clinical evaluation is not only to determine the presenting signs and symptoms and type of venous disease

(primary, secondary, congenital) but also exclude other etiologies (peripheral artery disease, rheumatoid disease, infection, tumor, or allergies). The physician should also establish the degree of disability caused by the venous disease and its impact on the patient's quality of life.

Duplex Scanning

Duplex scanning is safe, noninvasive, cost-effective, and reliable and is recommended as the first diagnostic test for all patients with suspected CVD[27,34,35] (also see Chapter 12). B-mode imaging permits accurate placement of the pulsed Doppler sample volume, and color flow evaluation makes it easier to establish obstruction, turbulence, and direction of venous and arterial flow,[36] increasing diagnostic accuracy in comparison to continuous wave Doppler ultrasonography in the assessment of venous insufficiency.[37] Duplex scanning is excellent for evaluation of both infrainguinal venous obstruction and valvular incompetence[38] (Fig. 55-4).

The appropriate technique of venous duplex scanning has been described in detail by several authors.[39] An 8.4- to 9-MHz linear array pulsed-wave Doppler transducer is used most frequently for the deeper veins, with the higher-frequency probe (up to 18 MHz) for detailed assessment of the superficial veins. Evaluation of reflux should be performed with the patient in the upright position, with the leg rotated outward, heel on the ground, and weight taken on the opposite limb.[35] The supine position gives both false-positive

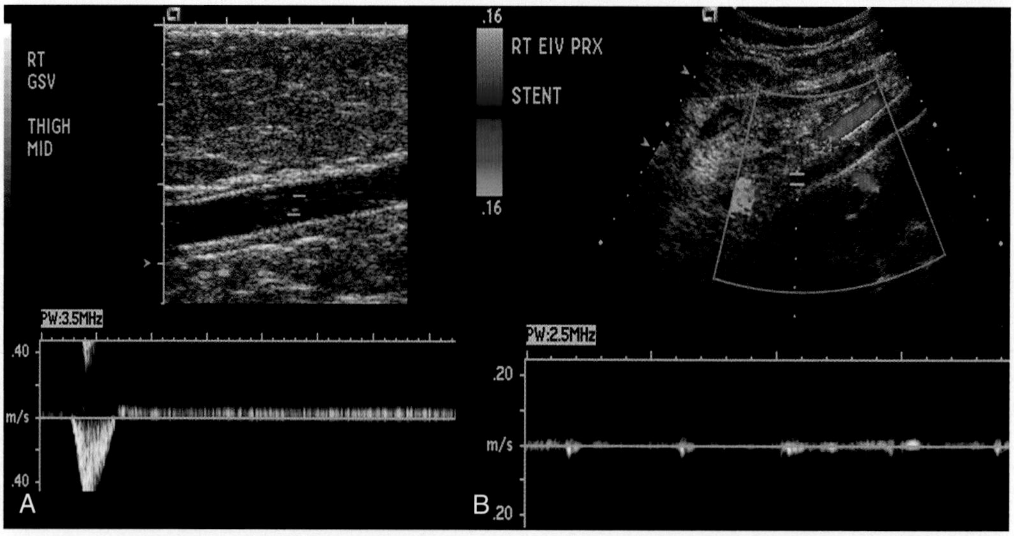

FIGURE 55-4 A, Duplex of right great saphenous vein (GSV) showing marked incompetence. **B,** Color duplex of left iliac vein showing absence of flow in stented venous segment, suggesting occlusion.

and false-negative results of reflux.[40] All deep veins of the leg are evaluated, followed by evaluation of the superficial veins, including the GSV, SSV, accessory saphenous veins, and perforating veins for a complete examination.

The four essential components of a complete duplex scanning examination for CVD are visibility, compressibility, venous flow, and augmentation. Asymmetry in flow velocity, lack of respiratory variations in venous flow, and waveform patterns at rest and during flow augmentation in the common femoral veins indicate proximal obstruction. Reflux can be elicited in two ways: (1) increased intraabdominal pressure using a Valsalva maneuver for the common femoral vein or SFJ or (2) manual/cuff compression and release of the limb distal to the point of examination. The first is more appropriate for evaluation of reflux in the common femoral vein and at the SFJ, whereas compression and release is the preferred technique more distally on the limb.[40] The guidelines recommend the cutoff value for abnormally reversed venous flow (reflux) as 1.0 second in the deep femoropopliteal veins and 500 milliseconds in the superficial and perforator veins.[27]

Perforating veins are evaluated in patients with advanced disease, usually CEAP class C5-C6, or in those with recurrent varicose veins after previous interventions. The diameter of a clinically relevant "pathological perforator" (e.g., beneath healed or open venous ulcer) can predict valve incompetence. The SVS/AVF Guideline Committee definition of "pathological" perforating veins includes those with outward flow of more than 500 milliseconds, with a diameter of greater than 3.5 mm, located beneath a healed or open venous ulcer (CEAP class C5-C6).[27]

Plethysmography

Air or strain-gauge venous plethysmography can provide noninvasive evaluation of calf muscle pump function, global venous reflux, and venous outflow obstruction[41-44] (Figs. 55-5 and 55-6). Strain-gauge plethysmography is usually performed with a modified Struckmann protocol, validated by comparison with simultaneously recorded ambulatory venous pressure measurements.[45] Strain-gauge or air plethysmography consists of exercise venous plethysmography, measurement of passive refill and drainage, and outflow plethysmography. Plethysmography quantifies venous reflux and obstruction and has been used to monitor venous functional changes and assess physiological outcome of surgical treatments.[46,47] Venous plethysmography provides information on venous function in patients with CVI and is a complementary examination to duplex scanning. These studies are especially helpful in patients with suspected outflow obstruction but normal duplex findings, or those suspected of having venous disease due to calf muscle pump dysfunction, but no reflux or obstruction

was noted on duplex scanning. Air plethysmography remains one of the few noninvasive techniques that can quantify reflux; other parameters have been reported to be variably useful.[44,47] According to the new guidelines, use of air plethysmography is encouraged as best practice in evaluation of patients with CVI (C3-6).[27]

Intravascular Ultrasound

Recent assessment of patients with iliofemoral venous occlusion suggested that intravascular ultrasound (IVUS) should be used for evaluation of all patients with suspected or confirmed iliac vein obstruction. Intravascular ultrasound can be used in veins with obstruction without occlusion to assess venous wall morphology and mural thickness and identify trabeculations and recanalization, frozen valves, and external compression. Some of these lesions, as emphasized by Raju and Neglen, are not seen with conventional planar venography and provide measurements in assessing the degree of stenosis.[48] In addition, in patients who have had an endovenous intervention, IVUS confirms position of the stent in the venous segment and resolution of the stenosis.[48]

Contrast Venography and Hemodynamic Studies

Ascending or descending (or both) contrast venography for CVI is performed selectively in patients with deep venous obstruction, postthrombotic syndrome, thrombotic or nonthrombotic pelvic vein obstruction (May-Thurner's syndrome), pelvic congestion syndrome, nutcracker syndrome, vascular malformations, venous trauma, tumors, and if endovenous or open surgical treatment is planned. Descending venography is used to study venous valve incompetence. The Valsalva maneuver is used to grade the severity of reflux (grade 1-4: 1 = to upper thigh, 2 = to distal thigh, 3 = popliteal reflux, 4 = reflux to tibials and perforators).[49,50] Since open valve repair is rarely performed today, this test has been less frequently used in recent years. Ascending venography is performed in a standing position to evaluate patency of the superficial and/or deep venous system (Fig. 55-7). It can be used together with direct venous pressure measurements to evaluate patients with varicose veins and associated iliac vein obstruction (May-Thurner's syndrome). Contrast venography is routinely used in CVD to perform endovenous procedures such as angioplasty or venous stenting or open venous reconstructions. A pressure gradient across iliofemoral obstruction at rest in the supine patient (3 mmHg) is indicative of functional venous obstruction. Arm/foot venous pressure measurements and ambulatory venous pressure (AVP) measurement in a dorsal foot vein are additional tests that can be performed. Detailed descriptions and techniques for these tests are provided in the consensus statement.[2]

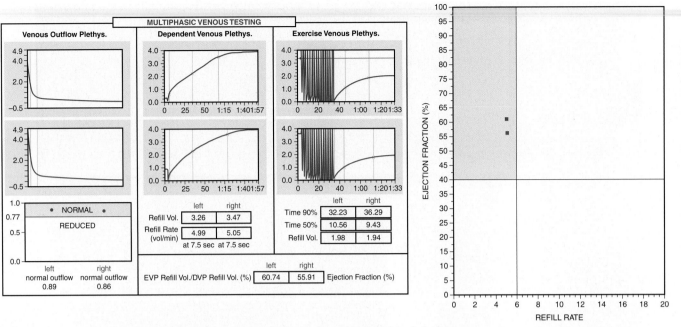

FIGURE 55-5 Multiphasic venous plethysmography showing normal venous physiology in both legs.

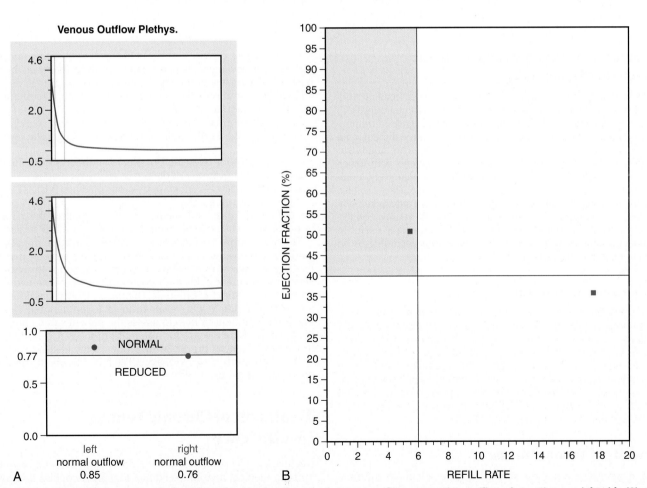

FIGURE 55-6 Multiphasic venous plethysmography showing decreased venous outflow, suggesting outflow obstruction on right side (A) and increased refill rate suggesting incompetence (B).

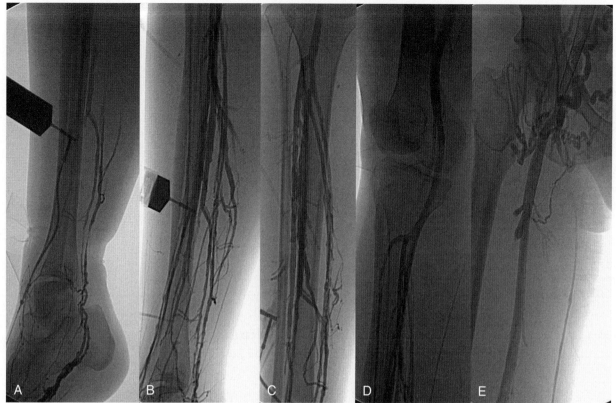

FIGURE 55-7 **A-E,** Ascending venogram performed by contrast injection in the pedal veins reveals evidence of chronic thrombotic changes and irregularity in the paired tibial veins **(C)** and normal popliteal and femoral vein segment **(D).** Large venous collaterals and absence of contrast in right iliac vein stent suggest obstruction **(E).**

Computed Tomography and Magnetic Resonance Venography

Early venous disease (C1-2) rarely requires advanced imaging studies other than duplex ultrasonography. Computed tomography (CT) and magnetic resonance imaging (MRI) have progressed tremendously in the last decade and provide excellent three-dimensional (3D) imaging of the venous system. Both modalities are suitable to identify pelvic or iliac venous obstruction in patients with lower-limb varicosity when proximal obstruction or iliac vein compression (May-Thurner's syndrome) is suspected.[48] They are also suitable to establish left renal vein compression (nutcracker syndrome),[51] gonadal vein incompetence, and pelvic venous congestion syndrome. Gadolinium-enhanced MRI is especially useful in evaluating patients with vascular malformations, including those with congenital varicose veins.[52]

Laboratory Evaluation

Based on their history, selected patients with recurrent DVT, thrombosis at a young age, or thrombosis in an unusual site should undergo screening for thrombophilia.[27] Laboratory examination is also needed in patients with long-standing recalcitrant venous ulcers, since a small percentage of these patients could have an underlying secondary etiology, including neoplasia, chronic inflammation, and other disorders.[53] Patients who undergo general anesthesia for treatment of CVI should undergo appropriate testing to assess suitability for such procedures.

Severity of Venous Disease

The diagnostic evaluation should provide adequate information to quantify and classify the severity of venous disease, using CEAP clinical class and VCSS.[6,30] The revised VCSS documents are used to establish disease severity at the first examination and will quantify improvement or deterioration during follow-up. In the basic CEAP classification, only the highest score is used to denote clinical class, and only the main anatomical groups (superficial, perforating, deep) are noted.

The revised format of the classification[6] includes two elements in addition to the CEAP findings, the date and diagnostic level of the evaluation:

- Level 1: history, physical, Doppler examination (handheld).
- Level 2: noninvasive—duplex scan, plethysmography.
- Level 3: invasive—venography, venous pressure, IVUS, CT venography, MR venography.

Recording the date and method used to confirm the clinical impression can be added in parentheses after the CEAP recording.

The main purpose of using the CEAP classification in patients with varicose veins is to distinguish primary venous disease causing simple varicose veins from secondary postthrombotic venous insufficiency.[7] Evaluation and treatment of the two conditions are distinctly different. Complete CEAP classification and quality-of-life (QOL) evaluation is recommended before and after treatment to help to assess the patient's perception of the burden of the disease for research purposes. A general QOL instrument such as the SF-36 and one of the disease-specific QOL instruments (e.g., VEINES, CIVIQ 2, Aberdeen, Charing cross) should be used.[4,54–56]

Treatment of Chronic Venous Insufficiency

Treatment of CVI requires a multimodality approach and has roles for both medical and interventional therapy. A concise flowchart for surgical/interventional treatment decision making is presented in Figure 55-8.

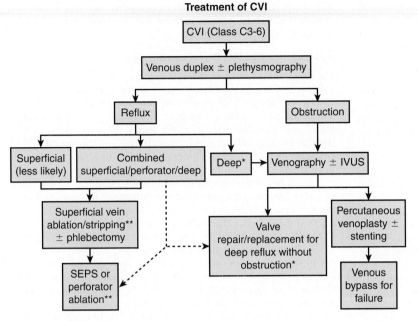

Treatment of CVI

FIGURE 55-8 Evaluation and management of chronic venous insufficiency (CVI). Good compression therapy, although not listed, is a must in any treatment protocol. *, Essential to rule out occult underlying obstruction; ** and dotted lines, in selected cases only. IVUS, intravascular ultrasound; SEPS, subfascial endoscopic perforator surgery.

Noninvasive Treatment

DRUG TREATMENT

In the United States, no phlebotonic drug is approved by the U.S. Food and Drug Administration (FDA) for treatment of CVI. Elsewhere, multiple phlebotonic drugs are available to treat symptoms of CVI; they have also been used to decrease ankle swelling and accelerate ulcer healing. Many compounds have been tried with varying success, but the most promising drugs include γ-benzopyrones (flavonoids) such as rutoside, diosmin, and hesperidin, micronized purified flavonoid fraction (MPFF), saponins like horse chestnut seed extract (aescin), pentoxifylline, and other plant extracts like French maritime pine bark extract. Synthetic products include calcium dobesilate, naftazone, aminophtone, and chromocarb.[57]

Precise mechanisms of action of most of these drugs is unknown, but they are postulated to improve venous tone and capillary permeability. Flavonoids appear to affect leukocytes and the endothelium by modifying the degree of inflammation and reducing edema.[9] Two different Cochrane reviews found that flavonoids[58] and aescin[59] appeared to have an effect on edema and restless legs syndrome, but these meta-analyses concluded there is insufficient evidence to support the global use of phlebotonics to treat CVD.

Recent randomized controlled trials (RCTs) for pentoxifylline have shown some benefit in venous ulcer healing, although all three trials failed to show any statistically significant benefit.[60–62] The venous guidelines of the American College of Chest Physicians (ACCP) suggest the use of oral pentoxifylline (400 mg three times daily) in patients with venous ulcers, in addition to local care, a compression garment, or intermittent compression pump (ICP; grade 2B).[63] A meta-analysis of five RCTs that included 723 patients with venous ulcers found that at 6 months, the chance of ulcer healing was 32% better in patients treated with adjunctive MPFF than in those managed by conventional therapy alone (relative risk reduction, 32%; 95% confidence interval [CI], 3%-70%).[64] For patients with persistent venous ulcers, flavonoids in the form of MPFF given orally or sulodexide administered intramuscularly (IM) and then orally, are suggested in the ACCP guidelines (grade 2B).[63]

COMPRESSION THERAPY

Compression therapy remains the standard of care for patients with CVI and venous ulcers (class C3-C6). Compression is recommended to decrease ambulatory venous hypertension in patients with CVI, in addition to lifestyle modifications that include

weight loss, exercise, and elevation of the legs whenever possible. Ambulatory compression techniques and devices include elastic compression stockings, paste gauze boots (Unna boot), multilayer elastic wraps, dressings, and elastic and nonelastic bandages and nonelastic garments. Pneumatic compression devices (e.g., ICP), applied primarily at night, are also used for patients with refractory edema and venous ulcers.[65] The rationale of compression treatment is to compensate for the increased ambulatory venous hypertension. Pressures to compress the superficial veins in supine patients range from 20 to 25 mmHg. In the upright position, pressures around 35 to 40 mmHg have been shown to narrow the superficial veins, and pressures higher than 60 mmHg are needed to occlude them.[66]

Compression therapy improves calf muscle pump function and decreases reflux in vein segments in patients with CVI.[67,68] Although graded compression is effective as primary treatment to aid healing of venous ulceration and as adjuvant therapy to interventions to prevent recurrence of venous ulcers, compliance is important.[69] In one study, ulcer healing was 97% in compliant patients and 55% in noncompliant patients (P <0.0001), and recurrence was 16% in compliant patients and 100% in noncompliant patients.[69]

Systematic reviews of compression treatment for venous ulcers concluded that compression treatment improves ulcer healing compared with no compression, and that high compression is more effective than low compression.[70,71] A recent meta-analysis examined data of 692 ulcer patients in eight RCTs and found that ulcer healing was faster by an average of 3 weeks with stockings than with bandages (P = 0.0002), and pain was significantly less (P <0.0001).[72] There is no evidence that hydrocolloid or other dressings beneath compression is more effective than compression alone.[73]

The ESCHAR trial randomized 500 patients with leg ulcers to either compression treatment alone or compression in combination with superficial venous surgery.[74,75] Compression consisted of multilayer compression bandaging followed by class 2 (medium compression, 18-24 mmHg) below-knee stockings. Compression treatment alone was as effective as compression with surgery for ulcer healing (65% vs. 65%; hazard ratio, 0.84 [95% CI, 0.77-1.24]), but 12-month ulcer recurrence rates were reduced in the compression with surgery group vs. those with compression alone (12% vs. 28%; hazard ratio, −2.76 [95% CI, −1.78 to −4.27]). This difference in ulcer recurrence rates persisted between the two groups at 4 years.[76] Unfortunately, this trial did not have a surgery-only arm; data suggest that saphenous vein disconnection improves venous function and may heal venous ulcers even without compression bandaging in patients with normal deep veins.[77]

Surgical Treatment

TREATMENT OF SUPERFICIAL VEIN INCOMPETENCE

Superficial reflux treatment is the primary treatment modality in patients with CVI. Treatment of superficial reflux leads to decrease in ulcer recurrence, as proved in the ESCHAR trial.[74,75] We refer readers to Chapter 54 for details on technique and results of surgical treatment of superficial venous incompetence.

High Ligation, Division, and Stripping

Surgical stripping of the GSV and/or SSV is performed selectively nowadays with the advent of endovenous ablation techniques. Patients who could benefit from open vein stripping include those with a very superficial great or accessory saphenous vein, with large tortuous or aneurysmal saphenous veins, and with partially recanalized veins after thrombophlebitis that cannot be cannulated using the ablation probe. There are limited data for preservation of the GSV using CHIVA[78] or ASVAL[79] techniques for CVI patients, and these are used selectively in few centers.

Phlebectomy

Ambulatory phlebectomy or powered phlebectomy can be used to eliminate large venous tributaries.[80,81] These are important adjuncts to treatment of superficial and/or perforator incompetence and can be safely performed even in patients with CVI.

TREATMENT OF PERFORATOR VEIN INCOMPETENCE

An association between incompetent perforating veins and venous ulcers was established more than a century ago by Gay,[82] and surgical perforator interruption was recommended by multiple authors to treat venous ulcers.[83–86] The importance of incompetent perforators in CVI is supported by the observation that most skin changes and ulcers are seen in the gaiter area, where large incompetent medial perforating veins are located. A correlation between number and size of duplex-based incompetent perforating veins and severity of CVI has been demonstrated.[20] Still, the contribution of perforator incompetence to CVI changes is debated, and further randomized studies to establish a firm connection are warranted.

Perforator interruption is reserved for patients with advanced CVI (CEAP classes 5-6) and documented perforator reflux on duplex scanning (see established criteria above). Usually superficial reflux is corrected first. In many cases, superficial reflux correction would lead to resolution of some of the perforator vein incompetence,[74,87] although one study showed conflicting results.[88] Contraindications to perforator interruption include moderate to severe arterial occlusive disease, infected ulcer, or medically unfit or nonambulatory patient. Relative contraindications include diabetes, renal/liver failure, morbid obesity, autoimmune disorders, recent DVT, and severe lymphedema. Popliteal or proximal deep venous obstruction is also a relative contraindication. A brief description of the anatomy of perforator veins is described in the preceding section and illustrated in Figure 55-1, and details can be found in the article by Mozes et al.[16] All identified incompetent perforators are marked on the skin with nonerasable marker during perioperative duplex.

Open Perforator Interruption

Linton's original open subfascial ligation[83] was abandoned because of a wound complication rate of up to 24%.[89,90] Many modifications were proposed to this technique, and currently the only potential role for open perforator ligation is in the lateral fascial compartment, owing to limited space in this compartment. Open perforator ligation using duplex guidance and small incisions may limit the extent of surgery. One RCT observed a significantly higher rate of wound complications after open perforator ligation using a modified Linton procedure than after endoscopic perforator ligation (53% vs. 0%; $P < 0.001$).[91]

Subfascial Endoscopic Perforator Surgery

Hauer's technique of subfascial endoscopic perforator surgery (SEPS), introduced in 1985,[92] uses a single port and is practiced mostly in Europe. O'Donnell was the first to use laparoscopic instrumentation with a two-port technique[93]; the Mayo Clinic team[94] and Conrad[95] improved the technique and added carbon dioxide insufflation to the procedure. Between 1992 and 2008, SEPS became the technique of choice for perforator ablation, primarily because of the reduced rate of wound complications.[91,96]

SEPS is performed under general or epidural anesthesia. Either single or double endoscopic port techniques can be used for dissection and division of medial calf perforators. Most authors use balloon dissection, carbon dioxide insufflation with a pressure of 30 mmHg, and a pneumatic thigh tourniquet inflated to 300 mmHg to avoid any bleeding in the surgical field.[97] Division of the fascia of the deep posterior compartment with a paratibial fasciotomy is required to identify all important medial perforating veins. Occlusion of the perforators can be done with endoscopic clips, although most surgeons use an ultrasonic harmonic scalpel for division and transection of the perforators. The wounds are closed, the tourniquet is deflated, and the extremity is wrapped with an elastic bandage. The operation is an outpatient procedure, and patients are encouraged to ambulate 3 hours after the operation.

The North American SEPS registry[11] reported on results of SEPS performed in 17 U.S. centers on 155 limbs, 85% with class C5 and C6 disease. Ulcer healing at 1 year was 88%, with the median time to ulcer healing of 54 days. Ulcer recurrence was 16% at 1 year and 28% at 2 years. In this registry, there were 27 patients with class C6 disease who underwent SEPS alone; 78% of the ulcers healed, and the ulcer healing rate was significantly lower (79%) at 2 years than it was in those who had SEPS and superficial ablation (95%; $P < 0.05$). The ulcer recurrence rate (35%) in the SEPS-only group at 2 years was, however, not significantly worse than that in patients who underwent SEPS and superficial ablation alone (25%).

In a systematic review, Tenbrook et al.[98] reported results of the SEPS procedure performed with or without superficial ablation on 1140 limbs in one RCT and 19 case series. Ulcers in 88% of limbs healed but recurred in 13% at a mean time of 21 months. Risk factors for nonhealing and recurrence included postoperative incompetent perforating veins, pathophysiological obstruction, previous DVT, and ulcer diameter greater than 2 cm. The authors concluded that surgical treatment including SEPS, with or without saphenous ablation, is recommended for patients with venous ulcers, but RCTs are needed to discern the contributions of compression therapy, superficial venous surgery, and SEPS in patients with advanced CVI. A recent meta-analysis of SEPS by Luebke and Brunkwall[99] reviewed data of studies published between 1985 and 2008 and concluded that SEPS used as part of a treatment regimen for severe CVI benefits most patients in the short term, regarding ulcer healing and prevention of ulcer recurrence, but further prospective RCTs are needed to define the long-term benefits of SEPS.

TREATMENT OF DEEP VEIN INCOMPETENCE

The first open venous *valve reconstruction* was reported by Kistner in 1968.[100,101] Since then, many techniques have been developed and modified to treat deep venous insufficiency. Deep valve reconstruction is reserved for advanced CVI patients who have failed other treatment strategies, including compression therapy. Preoperative assessment includes venography in all patients, primarily to rule out underlying proximal venous obstruction causing secondary valvular reflux, but also to grade severity of reflux as described earlier. No specific strategies exist to quantify reflux at a single valve station. Pathological appearance of valves would vary depending on the underlying cause for incompetence, with both primary and secondary (postthrombotic) deep vein reflux contributing to about half the cases.[102] In primary valve reflux patients, valves grossly have normal texture with a widened commissure. On the other hand, postthrombotic valves have fibrosis of the vein wall and valve cusp thickening, trabeculation, and sometimes complete destruction of the valve structure. In cases with extensive damage to valve structure, valvuloplasty is not an option; reconstruction is usually carried out using valve or vein transposition.

Exposure and preparation of valves is similar for both repair and transfer techniques. An arm is prepped out to provide access to the axillary/brachial vein in case vein transfer is needed. Usually only one valve is repaired, the first femoral vein valve, despite reflux at multiple stations in the femoral vein. The deep femoral vein (DFV) valve is also repaired in case it is incompetent. Meticulous dissection is carried out to identify the valve attachment lines, which may require subadventitial dissection in some postthrombotic cases. Intact valve lines signify preserved valve apparatus that can be repaired in most cases, in contrast to absence or disruption of valve attachment lines when repair is not possible.[102] A strip test is used to confirm valve incompetence.

Valvuloplasty can be performed from within (internal as originally described by Kistner) or from outside (external). The goal for both approaches is to appose the commissure and achieve valve tightening. An obvious advantage of internal valvuloplasty is repair under direct vision, although opening the vein increases the risk of surgical trauma to the vein and valve apparatus. To overcome this disadvantage of external valvuloplasty, we have used an angioscopic external valvuloplasty technique where an angioscope is introduced from a tributary proximal to the repaired valve and helps with visualization during suture placement.[103]

Valve transfer can be achieved using two methods: either transfer of a segment of vein with a competent valve and using it as an interposition graft (usually an axillary/brachial vein segment from the arm); or transposition of the incompetent vein onto a competent vein segment (usually femoral vein is transposed to the adjacent GSV or DFV). Vein transposition requires an adjacent patent competent vein, which is not always true in many cases where the GSV has already been ablated/stripped and the DFV is also incompetent. Also, long-term competence is a concern, owing to increased chance of reflux with dilation as a result of increased flow.[104] Axillary vein transfer is technically demanding, with 40% incidence of incompetent axillary valves *in situ*, and carries additional morbidity of a second incision.

Other less commonly used techniques include *prosthetic sleeve reconstruction, de novo valve reconstruction, cryopreserved allograft,* and *artificial venous valves*. None of these techniques have been widely adopted, and all previous attempts at artificial or cryopreserved valves were met with miserable failure. A new "neovalve" technique described by Maleti and Lugli[105] holds tremendous promise, but their excellent results, at least in the short term, have not been duplicated at other centers.

Perioperative complications are rare, with minimal or no mortality in these cases. The incidence of DVT has been reported to be between 0% and 11%, with higher rates in postthrombotic patients.[49,106] Long-term outcomes of deep vein incompetence have reported 60% to 80% ulcer healing,[102] with better outcomes in primary disease and better outcomes with valvuloplasty compared to valve transfer techniques.[49]

Prevention of postthrombotic superficial/deep vein incompetence could be a key point of intervention, in view of limited success with valve reconstruction once the valves are damaged in these patients. It has been shown that duration of venous occlusion clearly affects the likelihood of secondary reflux.[107] Multilevel disease and recurrent thrombosis are the two most predictive factors for future CVI.[108] Early spontaneous lysis leads to preserved valve function and fewer symptoms.[109] Therefore, there may be a role for prevention of venous reflux with early thrombus lysis. This is discussed further in Chapter 52. Also, recent data suggest that venous obstruction is more important than valvular incompetence. In a study of 504 patients who underwent iliac vein stenting, stenting was sufficient to control symptoms in the majority of patients with combined outflow obstruction and deep venous reflux, without need to correct underlying reflux.[26]

TREATMENT OF DEEP VEIN OBSTRUCTION

Open surgical reconstructions have been challenging because of multiple factors affecting graft patency,[110] including inadequate graft material, low venous flow, and the thrombophilia that often occurs in these patients. Endovascular stenting is first-line therapy, with excellent midterm and even long-term results in patients with chronic symptomatic venous stenosis and short occlusions,[111] but stenting is not possible or successful in all patients with long femoro-iliocaval venous occlusions.[112]

Femorofemoral Crossover Bypass

Femorofemoral crossover bypass can be performed for unilateral iliofemoral obstruction with suprapubic transposition of the GSV (Palma-Dale procedure; Fig. 55-9). The contralateral GSV is tunneled subcutaneously to the groin incision of the affected limb. An end-to-side anastomosis is performed between the saphenous vein and ipsilateral common femoral vein. This anastomosis can be spatulated onto the ipsilateral GSV if the femoral or deep femoral veins are diseased and the GSV is the predominant outflow in the affected leg. An externally supported 10- to 12-mm diameter polytetrafluoroethylene (PTFE) graft is used if the GSV is inadequate, less than 5 mm in diameter, or of poor quality. An (AVF) is performed between the conduit and SFA in selected cases and marked with a Silastic sheath for easy identification at a later time.

Femoroiliac or Iliocaval Bypass

For femoroiliac or iliocaval bypass, the iliac vein is exposed via a flank incision, and the femoral vein is exposed through a standard groin incision. In cases with CIV occlusion, the infrahepatic cava is used as outflow, exposed through a midline incision. These "short" bypasses have a hemodynamic advantage due to the length and high flow. We prefer an externally supported 10- to 14-mm PTFE graft for these bypasses.

Femorocaval or Complex Bypass

Long bypasses from the femoral vein to the IVC have poor results because of the hemodynamics of flow across the femoral vein. Most of these patients also have extensive postphlebitic changes in the femoral and distal veins, making these procedures technically challenging and prone to failure due to poor inflow. Patients with bilateral disease, or those with obstruction of the suprarenal or suprahepatic IVC who have failed endovascular intervention, are evaluated for a complex reconstruction using either a bifurcated graft or tube graft with contralateral jump graft.

Saphenopopliteal Bypass

Saphenopopliteal bypass is popularly known as the *May-Husni procedure* and is indicated for femoral or proximal popliteal vein obstruction. The GSV, which most commonly is the major outflow from the leg via collaterals in these patients, is exposed above the knee joint, and a direct anastomosis is performed between the GSV and popliteal vein (end to side). Alternatively, a free vein conduit or prosthetic can be used in case the ipsilateral GSV is not suitable.

In a recent report on open surgical reconstruction for chronic iliofemoral occlusion, 50 patients underwent 52 open reconstructive procedures for CVI over a 25-year period.[113] Twenty-nine patients underwent a femorofemoral crossover bypass, and 17 underwent a short bypass (femoroiliac or iliocaval). Early graft occlusion occurred in 17%, requiring reoperation, and discharge patency was 96%. There was no mortality or pulmonary embolism (PE). Five-year primary and secondary patency, respectively, for Palma vein grafts was 70% and 78%; for femoroiliac and ilio-infrahepatic IVC bypasses, 63% and 86%; and for femoro-infrahepatic IVC bypasses, 31% and 57%. May-Thurner's syndrome with associated chronic thrombosis, use of prosthetic grafts, and endoscopic vein harvesting were each

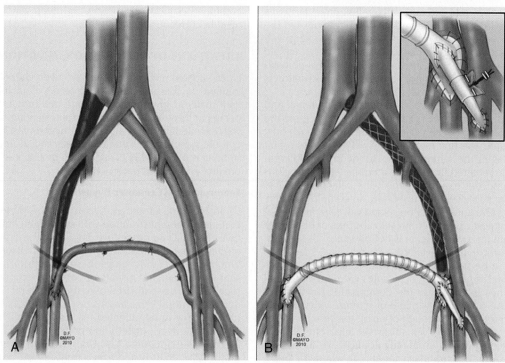

FIGURE 55-9 **Schematic presentation of femorofemoral crossover venous bypass with either the contralateral great saphenous vein (GSV) (A) or prosthetic graft (B).** An arteriovenous fistula (AVF) is shown in inset, with marking Silastic sheath. *(Used with permission of Mayo Foundation for Medical Education and Research.)*

noted to be adversely related to long-term graft patency. More than 60% of patients had no venous claudication and no or minimal swelling. In multiple large series, the Palma procedure has shown good to excellent patency rates of 70% to 85% on mid- to long-term follow-up.[114]

Endovenous Treatment

TREATMENT OF SUPERFICIAL VEIN INCOMPETENCE

Endovenous treatment of superficial vein incompetence using radiofrequency (RFA) or laser (endovenous laser treatment [EVLT]) ablation or foam sclerotherapy has made significant advancement over the last decade and has replaced open surgical treatment in most centers. We again refer readers to Chapter 54 for details on technique and results of endovenous treatment of superficial venous incompetence.

TREATMENT OF PERFORATOR INCOMPETENCE

The emergence of ultrasonographically guided thermal ablation and sclerotherapy in recent years has transformed the techniques of perforator ablation.[96,115-117]

Advantages of *percutaneous ablation of perforators* (PAPS) include the low risk of a minimally invasive procedure that is easily repeatable and can be performed under local anesthesia in an office setting.[118] PAPS is performed under ultrasound guidance, with direct needle puncture of the perforating vein performed under local anesthesia, with the patient in the reverse Trendelenburg position to allow for full venous distention. The tip of the needle should be at or just below the fascia in the vein to minimize deep vessel and nerve injury. After confirmation of probe position, local anesthesia is used to infiltrate surrounding tissues before treatment, and the patient is then placed in the Trendelenburg position.

Radiofrequency ablation of the perforating veins can be accomplished using a new intravascular ablation device (ClosureRFS Stylet, VNUS Medical Technologies, San Jose, Calif.). Intraluminal placement of the RF stylet is confirmed by ultrasonography and also by measuring impedance: values between 150 and 350 ohms indicate the intravascular location of the tip of the probe. Treatment is performed with a target temperature of 85 °C. All four quadrants of the vein wall are treated for 1 minute each. The catheter is then withdrawn 1 to 2 mm, and a second treatment is performed. The treatment is finished with applying compression to the region of the treated perforating vein.

Perforator EVLT is done with a 16-gauge angiocatheter (for 600-μm laser fiber) or a 21-gauge micropuncture needle (for a 400-μm laser fiber).[119] Intraluminal placement of the access catheter is confirmed by ultrasonography and aspiration of blood at or just below the fascial level. Various methods of energy application are used, and perforating veins are treated at three locations, each segment receiving between 60 and 120 joules in 1 or 2 treatments.[117,119] The rest of the procedure is similar to RFA.

Sclerotherapy of perforating veins is done with a 25-, 27-, or 30-gauge needle. A wire may be placed into the deep system for better control of the access. Ultrasonographically guided sclerotherapy can be performed using different agents. Care should be taken to avoid injection of the agent into the accompanying artery; 0.5 to 1 mL of the sclerosant is injected with the leg elevated to avoid flow into the deep system, and compression is applied over the treated perforators.[119]

Outcomes of PAPS are largely unknown. Most publications report small numbers of patients with short follow-up, frequently treated for mild disease (class C2-C3). Most data provided are on safety and surrogate endpoints, such as perforating vein occlusions, but less so on clinical and functional endpoints. A systematic review of five recently published cohort studies and seven unpublished case series found a mean occlusion rate of 80%, with a mean follow-up of less than 2 months.[96] Ultrasonographically guided sclerotherapy is gaining rapid acceptance because perforating veins can be accessed easily with a small needle, without much pain to the patient. Significant improvement in VCSS was noted after ultrasonographically guided sclerotherapy using morrhuate sodium in 80 limbs with predominantly perforator incompetence, and ulcers rapidly healed in 86.5%, with a mean time to heal of 36 days.[116] The ulcer recurrence rate was 32% at a mean of 20 months despite low compliance (15%) with compression hose. New and recurrent perforators were identified in 33% of limbs, and ulcer recurrence was associated with perforator recurrence and the presence of postthrombotic syndrome.

TREATMENT OF DEEP VEIN INCOMPETENCE

Endovascular treatment of deep vein incompetence using stents mounted with native or artificial valves has been fraught with failure. New designs in development are still in infancy, awaiting good clinical data.[120]

TREATMENT OF DEEP VEIN OBSTRUCTION

Deep vein obstruction, either postthrombotic or nonthrombotic, has recently been shown to be significant contributor to CVD. Adequate tests to quantify the exact role of deep vein obstruction are lacking, so experts now recommend routine use of IVUS for detailing venous assessment.[111] In one study, more than one fourth of patients were shown to have more than 50% stenosis based on IVUS, whereas venogram failed to reveal any obstruction.[121]

Endovenous stenting (Fig. 55-10) is performed under local or general anesthesia in an endovascular suite. Access is achieved under ultrasound guidance, either via the femoral or jugular vein. After venography and IVUS (as needed), obstructed segments are crossed using a hydrophilic wire. Predilation is performed with high-pressure balloons, with which the risk of rupture is low to none. Chronic occlusive lesions usually require serial dilation to a final diameter of 12 to 18 mm. Self-expanding stents are used in the entire diseased segment. The Wallstent (Boston Scientific, USA) is used by most interventionalists because of the external compression due to high radial force in the common iliac vein. Large-diameter nitinol stents are used less frequently. Extension of the stent across the inguinal ligament is less of a concern in the venous segment.[122] In cases of IVC obstruction, a large Gianturco (Cook Inc., USA) or Wallstent is used. We prefer to use a large Wallstent, and inside this a Gianturco stent, all the way to the caval bifurcation. Subsequent iliac stenting is performed with a Wallstent or nitinol self-expanding stents.[123] Coverage of the renal veins with Gianturco stents has not been of concern in our experience and that of others.[124]

In patients with common femoral vein obstruction and proximal disease, vascular access could be impossible, so *hybrid reconstruction* may be necessary. Endovenous recanalization and stent placement is combined with femoral vein endophlebectomy and patch angioplasty in these cases. Balloon angioplasty and stenting is performed prior to or at completion of the patch angioplasty. Jugular vein access is obtained for retrograde recanalization as an alternative to or in combination with femoral access. The stent is extended proximally to the healthy vein and across the inguinal ligament distally. With recent experience, we extend the distal end of the stent into the venous patch.[113]

Technical success for endovascular iliac vein recanalization is reported to be 87% to 100% in multiple series.[123] Inferior vena cava occlusion does decrease the ability to cross the occluded segment, and technical success in these cases is reported to be 66% in one series.[124] Mid- to long-term secondary patency is very good in successful cases, ranging from 75% at 48 months to 93% at 36 months.[123] Patients with nonthrombotic obstruction fare much better than those with thrombotic occlusion.[125] Cumulative rate of improvement of pain and swelling at 5 years after treatment of venous outflow obstruction was 78% and 55%, respectively, and reflux parameters did not deteriorate after stenting in one large study.[26] In a study from Mayo Clinic, we also observed marked improvement in hemodynamics, venous function, and symptoms after successful treatment of venous outflow obstruction with stenting[126] (Fig. 55-11). We noted improvement in both venous outflow and calf muscle pump function, and the residual volume fraction had decreased at the expense of venous reflux, which increased (increase of median venous filling index by 24%).

Stenting improved the CEAP class status of the patients. Incapacitating venous claudication, noted in 62.5% of patients before stenting, was eliminated in all after stenting. The Mayo Clinic study concluded that successful treatment of venous outflow obstruction in patients with CVI ameliorates venous claudication, normalizes outflow, and enhances calf muscle pump function,

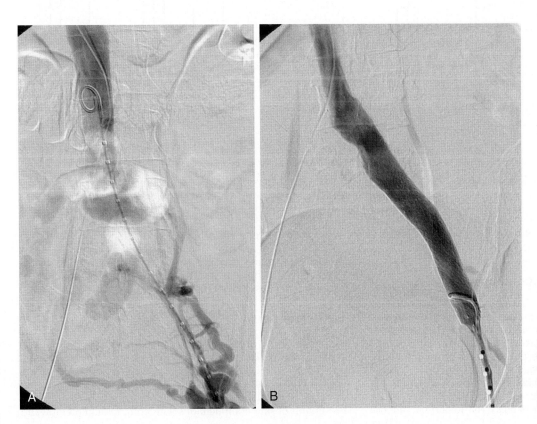

FIGURE 55-10 Successful recanalization and stenting of left iliac vein in a 43-year-old woman, with excellent luminal result and predominant flow through iliac vein (B) rather than pelvic collaterals (A).

CH
55

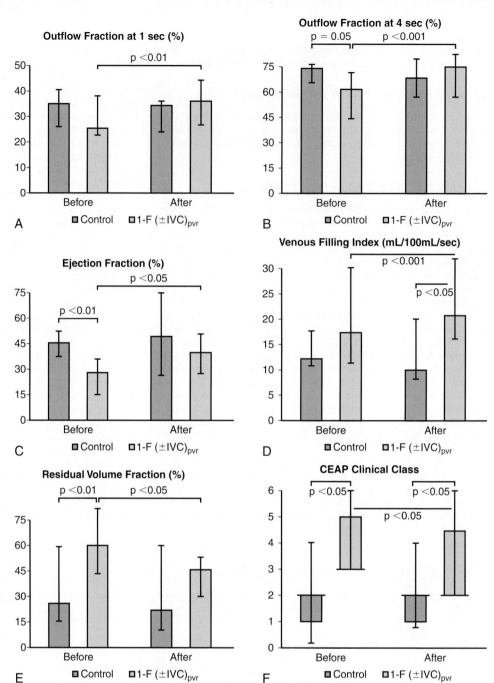

FIGURE 55-11 A-F, Effects of successful treatment of venous outflow obstruction using venous stents. Venous hemodynamics, including venous outflow (outflow fraction at 1 and 4 seconds; **A-B**), calf muscle pump function (ejection fraction; **C**), amount of venous reflux (venous filling index; **D**), and venous hypertension (residual volume fraction; **E**), and the CEAP clinical class (**F**) in 23 limbs with chronic iliofemoral (IF) inferior vena cava (IVC) thrombosis (DVT) and nine control limbs, before (30 days) and after (median, 8.4; interquartile range, 3-11.8 months) successful IF (IVC) venous stenting. Data are median and interquartile range. *(From Delis KT, Bjarnason H, Wennberg PW, et al: Successful iliac vein and inferior vena cava stenting ameliorates venous claudication and improves venous outflow, calf muscle pump function, and clinical status in post-thrombotic syndrome. Ann Surg 245: 130–139, 2007, with permission.)*

resulting in significant clinical improvement of CVD. Increase in the amount of venous reflux of the stented limbs indicated that elastic or inelastic compression support of the successfully stented limbs would be pivotal in preventing disease progression. The study also supports the notion that venous obstruction is likely more important than venous valvular incompetence.[126]

Assessment of Treatment Outcome

Clinical outcome studies evaluate results of procedures on patient-focused outcomes, including symptom improvement, recurrence of varicosities, healing or recurrence of skin ulcers, improvement in the chronic progressive symptoms of CVD, improved QOL, and cosmetic improvement.[127] These can be assessed using multiple questionnaires, including QOL measures for symptom relief and CEAP classification, in combination with revised VCSS for disease severity outcomes (reader is referred to previous section on "Severity of Venous Disease" for details). The Recurrent Varicose

Veins After Surgery (REVAS) classification,[128] a descriptive evaluation of recurrent and residual varicosities based on the physician's assessment, can be used for cosmetic outcome, although it has some limitations.

Surrogate outcome measures are commonly used in reporting outcomes of treatment, although caution should be used. Surrogate outcomes may include patency of the ablated saphenous or perforating vein, patency of a venous bypass or stent, or hemodynamic results after interventions.

Conclusions

Treatment of CVI has progressed markedly over the last decade. This can be attributed to better understanding of the pathophysiology of venous disease, increased awareness of complications among both patients and care providers, and the advent of endovascular techniques and minimally invasive technology. Prevention of skin complications with compression therapy and early treatment of CVI with endovenous thermal ablations are essential. Endovenous ablation therapy has replaced open treatment of superficial reflux and is likely to replace open surgical treatment of perforator incompetence as well. Venous stenting is now the first line of treatment for deep venous outflow obstruction; open surgical reconstruction is indicated only in patients who fail or are not candidates for stenting. Further research is still needed to develop more effective treatment of deep vein valvular incompetence.

REFERENCES

1. Kaplan RM, Criqui MH, Denenberg JO, et al: Quality of life in patients with chronic venous disease: San Diego population study, *J Vasc Surg* 37(5):1047–1053, 2003.
2. Nicolaides AN: Investigation of chronic venous insufficiency: a consensus statement (France, March 5-9, 1997), *Circulation* 102(20):E126–E163, 2000.
3. Gillespie DL, Kistner B, Glass C, et al: Venous ulcer diagnosis, treatment, and prevention of recurrences, *J Vasc Surg* 52(Suppl 5):8S–14S, 2010.
4. Smith JJ, Guest MG, Greenhalgh RM, et al: Measuring the quality of life in patients with venous ulcers, *J Vasc Surg* 31(4):642–649, 2000.
5. Korn P, Patel ST, Heller JA, et al: Why insurers should reimburse for compression stockings in patients with chronic venous stasis, *J Vasc Surg* 35(5):950–957, 2002.
6. Eklof B, Rutherford RB, Bergan JJ, et al: Revision of the CEAP classification for chronic venous disorders: consensus statement, *J Vasc Surg* 40(6):1248–1252, 2004.
7. Kistner R, Eklof B: Classification and etiology of chronic venous disease. In Gloviczki P, editor: *Handbook of venous disorders*, vol 1, ed 3, London, 2009, Hodder Arnold, pp 37–46.
8. Raju S, Neglen P: Clinical practice. Chronic venous insufficiency and varicose veins, *N Engl J Med* 360(22):2319–2327, 2009.
9. Eberhardt RT, Raffetto JD: Chronic venous insufficiency, *Circulation* 111(18):2398–2409, 2005.
10. Labropoulos N, Giannoukas AD, Delis K, et al: Where does venous reflux start? *J Vasc Surg* 26(5):736–742, 1997.
11. Gloviczki P, Bergan JJ, Rhodes JM, et al: Mid-term results of endoscopic perforator vein interruption for chronic venous insufficiency: lessons learned from the North American subfascial endoscopic perforator surgery registry. The North American Study Group, *J Vasc Surg* 29(3):489–502, 1999.
12. Kalra M, Gloviczki P, Noel AA, et al: Subfascial endoscopic perforator vein surgery in patients with post-thrombotic venous insufficiency–is it justified? *Vasc Endovascular Surg* 36(1):41–50, 2002.
13. Caggiati A, Bergan JJ, Gloviczki P, et al: Nomenclature of the veins of the lower limb: extensions, refinements, and clinical application, *J Vasc Surg* 41(4):719–724, 2005.
14. Caggiati A, Bergan JJ, Gloviczki P, et al: Nomenclature of the veins of the lower limbs: an international interdisciplinary consensus statement, *J Vasc Surg* 36(2):416–422, 2002.
15. Delis KT, Knaggs AL, Khodabakhsh P: Prevalence, anatomic patterns, valvular competence, and clinical significance of the Giacomini vein, *J Vasc Surg* 40(6):1174–1183, 2004.
16. Mozes G, Gloviczki P, Menawat SS, et al: Surgical anatomy for endoscopic subfascial division of perforating veins, *J Vasc Surg* 24(5):800–808, 1996.
17. Gloviczki P, Mozes G: Development and anatomy of the venous system. In Gloviczki P, editor: *Handbook of venous disorders*, vol 1, ed 3, London, 2009, Hodder Arnold, pp 12–24.
18. Pang AS: Location of valves and competence of the great saphenous vein above the knee, *Ann Acad Med Singapore* 20(2):248–250, 1991.
19. LePage PA, Villavicencio JL, Gomez ER, et al: The valvular anatomy of the iliac venous system and its clinical implications, *J Vasc Surg* 14(5):678–683, 1991.
20. Labropoulos N, Delis K, Nicolaides AN, et al: The role of the distribution and anatomic extent of reflux in the development of signs and symptoms in chronic venous insufficiency, *J Vasc Surg* 23(3):504–510, 1996.
21. van Rij AM, Solomon C, Christie R: Anatomic and physiologic characteristics of venous ulceration, *J Vasc Surg* 20(5):759–764, 1994.
22. Labropoulos N, Giannoukas AD, Nicolaides AN, et al: The role of venous reflux and calf muscle pump function in nonthrombotic chronic venous insufficiency. Correlation with severity of signs and symptoms, *Arch Surg* 131(4):403–406, 1996.
23. Labropoulos N, Leon M, Geroulakos G, et al: Venous hemodynamic abnormalities in patients with leg ulceration, *Am J Surg* 169(6):572–574, 1995.
24. Hanrahan LM, Araki CT, Rodriguez AA, et al: Distribution of valvular incompetence in patients with venous stasis ulceration, *J Vasc Surg* 13(6):805–811, 1991 discussion 811–802.
25. May R, Thurner J: A vascular spur in the vena iliaca communis sinistra as a cause of predominantly left-sided thrombosis of the pelvic veins, *Z Kreislaufforsch* 45(23–24): 912–922, 1956.
26. Raju S, Darcey R, Neglen P: Unexpected major role for venous stenting in deep reflux disease, *J Vasc Surg* 51(2):401–408, 2010 discussion 408.
27. Gloviczki P, Comerota A, Dalsing M, et al: The care of patients with varicose veins and associated chronic venous diseases: clinical practice guidelines of the Society for Vascular Surgery and the American Venous Forum, *J Vasc Surg* 53(5 Suppl):2S–48S, 2011.
28. Langer RD, Ho E, Denenberg JO, et al: Relationships between symptoms and venous disease: the San Diego population study, *Arch Intern Med* 165(12):1420–1424, 2005.
29. Eklof B, Perrin M, Delis KT, et al: Updated terminology of chronic venous disorders: the VEIN-TERM transatlantic interdisciplinary consensus document, *J Vasc Surg* 49(2):498–501, 2009.
30. Vasquez MA, Rabe E, McLafferty RB, et al: Revision of the venous clinical severity score: venous outcomes consensus statement: special communication of the American Venous Forum Ad Hoc Outcomes Working Group, *J Vasc Surg* 52(5):1387–1396, 2010.
31. Rabe E, Pannier F: Epidemiology of chronic venous disorders. In Gloviczki P, editor: *Handbook of venous disorders*, vol 1, ed 3, London, 2009, Hodder Arnold, pp 105–112.
32. Bradbury A, Ruckley CV: Clinical presentation and assessment of patients with venous disease. In Gloviczki P, editor: *Handbook of venous disorders*, vol 1, ed 3, London, 2009, Hodder Arnold, pp 331–341.
33. Gloviczki P, Driscoll DJ: Klippel-Trenaunay syndrome: current management, *Phlebology* 22(6):291–298, 2007.
34. Cavezzi A, Labropoulos N, Partsch H, et al: Duplex ultrasound investigation of the veins in chronic venous disease of the lower limbs–UIP consensus document. Part II. Anatomy, *Eur J Vasc Endovasc Surg* 31(3):288–299, 2006.
35. Coleridge-Smith P, Labropoulos N, Partsch H, et al: Duplex ultrasound investigation of the veins in chronic venous disease of the lower limbs–UIP consensus document. Part I. Basic principles, *Eur J Vasc Endovasc Surg* 31(1):83–92, 2006.
36. Meissner MH, Moneta G, Burnand K, et al: The hemodynamics and diagnosis of venous disease, *J Vasc Surg* 46(Suppl S):4S–24S, 2007.
37. McMullin GM, Coleridge Smith PD: An evaluation of Doppler ultrasound and photoplethysmography in the investigation of venous insufficiency, *Aust N Z J Surg* 62(4):270–275, 1992.
38. Labropoulos N, Tiongson J, Pryor L, et al: Definition of venous reflux in lower-extremity veins, *J Vasc Surg* 38(4):793–798, 2003.
39. Abai B, Labropoulos N: Duplex scanning for chronic venous obstruction and valvular incompetence. In Gloviczki P, editor: *Handbook of venous disorders*, 1, ed 3 , London, 2009, Hodder Arnold, pp 142–155.
40. Markel A, Meissner MH, Manzo RA, et al: A comparison of the cuff deflation method with Valsalva's maneuver and limb compression in detecting venous valvular reflux, *Arch Surg* 129(7):701–705, 1994.
41. Struckmann J: Venous investigations: the current position, *Angiology* 45(6 Pt 2):505–511, 1994.
42. Struckmann JR: Assessment of the venous muscle pump function by ambulatory strain gauge plethysmography. Methodological and clinical aspects, *Dan Med Bull* 40(4):460–477, 1993.
43. Rooke TW, Heser JL, Osmundson PJ: Exercise strain-gauge venous plethysmography: evaluation of a "new" device for assessing lower limb venous incompetence, *Angiology* 43(3 Pt 1):219–228, 1992.
44. Criado E, Farber MA, Marston WA, et al: The role of air plethysmography in the diagnosis of chronic venous insufficiency, *J Vasc Surg* 27(4):660–670, 1998.
45. Lurie F, Rooke T: Evaluation of venous function by indirect noninvasive tests (plethysmography). In Gloviczki P, editor: *Handbook of venous disorders*, vol 1, ed 3, London, 2009, Hodder Arnold, pp 156–159.
46. Rhodes JM, Gloviczki P, Canton L, et al: Endoscopic perforator vein division with ablation of superficial reflux improves venous hemodynamics, *J Vasc Surg* 28(5):839–847, 1998.
47. Park UJ, Yun WS, Lee KB, et al: Analysis of the postoperative hemodynamic changes in varicose vein surgery using air plethysmography, *J Vasc Surg* 51(3):634–638, 2010.
48. Neglen P, Raju S: Intravascular ultrasound scan evaluation of the obstructed vein, *J Vasc Surg* 35(4):694–700, 2002.
49. Masuda EM, Kistner RL: Long-term results of venous valve reconstruction: a four- to twenty-one-year follow-up, *J Vasc Surg* 19(3):391–403, 1994.
50. Kistner RL, Ferris EB, Randhawa G, et al: A method of performing descending venography, *J Vasc Surg* 4(5):464–468, 1986.
51. Reed NR, Kalra M, Bower TC, et al: Left renal vein transposition for nutcracker syndrome, *J Vasc Surg* 49(2):386–393, 2009 discussion 393–384.
52. Lee BB, Bergan J, Gloviczki P, et al: Diagnosis and treatment of venous malformations. Consensus document of the International Union of Phlebology (IUP)-2009, *Int Angiol* 28(6):434–451, 2009.
53. Labropoulos N, Manalo D, Patel NP, et al: Uncommon leg ulcers in the lower extremity, *J Vasc Surg* 45(3):568–573, 2007.
54. Kahn SR, M'Lan CE, Lamping DL, et al: Relationship between clinical classification of chronic venous disease and patient-reported quality of life: results from an international cohort study, *J Vasc Surg* 39(4):823–828, 2004.
55. Launois R, Reboul-Marty J, Henry B: Construction and validation of a quality of life questionnaire in chronic lower limb venous insufficiency (CIVIQ), *Qual Life Res* 5(6): 539– 554, 1996.
56. Lamping DL, Schroter S, Kurz X, et al: Evaluation of outcomes in chronic venous disorders of the leg: development of a scientifically rigorous, patient-reported measure of symptoms and quality of life, *J Vasc Surg* 37(2):410–419, 2003.
57. Coleridge Smith P: Drug treatment of varicose veins, venous edema and ulcers. In Gloviczki P, editor: *Handbook of venous disorders*, vol 1, ed 3, London, 2009, Hodder Arnold, pp 359–365.
58. Martinez MJ, Bonfill X, Moreno RM, et al: Phlebotonics for venous insufficiency, *Cochrane Database Syst Rev* (3):CD003229, 2005.
59. Pittler MH, Ernst E: Horse chestnut seed extract for chronic venous insufficiency, *Cochrane Database Syst Rev* (1):CD003230, 2006.
60. Nelson EA, Prescott RJ, Harper DR, et al: A factorial, randomized trial of pentoxifylline or placebo, four-layer or single-layer compression, and knitted viscose or hydrocolloid dressings for venous ulcers, *J Vasc Surg* 45(1):134–141, 2007.
61. Dale JJ, Ruckley CV, Harper DR, et al: Randomised, double blind placebo controlled trial of pentoxifylline in the treatment of venous leg ulcers, *BMJ* 319(7214):875–878, 1999.
62. Falanga V, Fujitani RM, Diaz C, et al: Systemic treatment of venous leg ulcers with high doses of pentoxifylline: efficacy in a randomized, placebo-controlled trial, *Wound Repair Regen* 7(4):208–213, 1999.
63. Hirsh J, Guyatt G, Albers GW, et al: Executive summary: American College of Chest Physicians evidence-based clinical practice guidelines (8th edition), *Chest* 133(Suppl 6): 71S–109S, 2008.
64. Coleridge-Smith P, Lok C, Ramelet AA: Venous leg ulcer: a meta-analysis of adjunctive therapy with micronized purified flavonoid fraction, *Eur J Vasc Endovasc Surg* 30(2): 198–208, 2005.
65. Moneta G, Partsch B: Compression therapy for venous ulceration. In Gloviczki P, editor: *Handbook of venous disorders*, vol 1, ed 3, London, 2009, Hodder Arnold, pp 348–358.
66. Partsch B, Partsch H: Calf compression pressure required to achieve venous closure from supine to standing positions, *J Vasc Surg* 42(4):734–738, 2005.
67. Ibegbuna V, Delis KT, Nicolaides AN, et al: Effect of elastic compression stockings on venous hemodynamics during walking, *J Vasc Surg* 37(2):420–425, 2003.

CH
55

68. Zajkowski PJ, Proctor MC, Wakefield TW, et al: Compression stockings and venous function, *Arch Surg* 137(9):1064–1068, 2002.

69. Mayberry JC, Moneta GL, Taylor LM Jr, et al: Fifteen-year results of ambulatory compression therapy for chronic venous ulcers, *Surgery* 109(5):575–581, 1991.

70. Fletcher A, Cullum N, Sheldon TA: A systematic review of compression treatment for venous leg ulcers, *BMJ* 315(7108):576–580, 1997.

71. Partsch H, Flour M, Smith PC: Indications for compression therapy in venous and lymphatic disease consensus based on experimental data and scientific evidence. Under the auspices of the IUP, *Int Angiol* 27(3):193–219, 2008.

72. Amsler F, Willenberg T, Blattler W: In search of optimal compression therapy for venous leg ulcers: a meta-analysis of studies comparing diverse [corrected] bandages with specifically designed stockings, *J Vasc Surg* 50(3):668–674, 2009.

73. Palfreyman S, Nelson EA, Michaels JA: Dressings for venous leg ulcers: systematic review and meta-analysis, *BMJ* 335(7613):244, 2007.

74. Barwell JR, Davies CE, Deacon J, et al: Comparison of surgery and compression with compression alone in chronic venous ulceration (ESCHAR study): randomised controlled trial, *Lancet* 363(9424):1854–1859, 2004.

75. Gohel MS, Barwell JR, Taylor M, et al: Long term results of compression therapy alone versus compression plus surgery in chronic venous ulceration (ESCHAR): randomised controlled trial, *BMJ* 335(7610):83, 2007.

76. Geerts WH, Bergqvist D, Pineo GF, et al: Prevention of venous thromboembolism: American College of Chest Physicians evidence-based clinical practice guidelines (8th edition), *Chest* 133(Suppl 6):381S–453S, 2008.

77. Scriven JM, Hartshorne T, Thrush AJ, et al: Role of saphenous vein surgery in the treatment of venous ulceration, *Br J Surg* 85(6):781–784, 1998.

78. Criado E, Lujan S, Izquierdo L, et al: Conservative hemodynamic surgery for varicose veins, *Semin Vasc Surg* 15(1):27–33, 2002.

79. Pittaluga P, Chastanet S, Rea B, et al: Midterm results of the surgical treatment of varices by phlebectomy with conservation of a refluxing saphenous vein, *J Vasc Surg* 50(1):107–118, 2009.

80. Passman M: Transilluminated powered phlebectomy in the treatment of varicose veins, *Vascular* 15(5):262–268, 2007.

81. Bergan JJ: Varicose veins: hooks, clamps, and suction. Application of new techniques to enhance varicose vein surgery, *Semin Vasc Surg* 15(1):21–26, 2002.

82. Gay J: On varicose disease of the lower extremities and its allied disorders: skin discoloration, induration, and ulcer: being the Lettsomian Lectures delivered before the Medical Society of London in 1867, London, 1868, John Churchill and Sons.

83. Linton RR: The communicating veins of the lower leg and the operative technic for their ligation, *Ann Surg* 107(4):582–593, 1938.

84. Cockett FB: The pathology and treatment of venous ulcers of the leg, *Br J Surg* 43(179):260–278, 1955.

85. Dodd H: The diagnosis and ligation of incompetent ankle perforating veins, *Ann R Coll Surg Engl* 34:186–196, 1964.

86. Homans J: The operative treatment of varicose veins and ulcers, based upon a classification of these lesions, *Surg Gynecol Obstet* 22:143–158, 1916.

87. Mendes RR, Marston WA, Farber MA, et al: Treatment of superficial and perforator venous incompetence without deep venous insufficiency: is routine perforator ligation necessary? *J Vasc Surg* 38(5):891–895, 2003.

88. Stuart WP, Adam DJ, Allan PL, et al: Saphenous surgery does not correct perforator incompetence in the presence of deep venous reflux, *J Vasc Surg* 28(5):834–838, 1998.

89. Wilkinson GE Jr, Maclaren IF: Long term review of procedures for venous perforator insufficiency, *Surg Gynecol Obstet* 163(2):117–120, 1986.

90. Negus D, Friedgood A: The effective management of venous ulceration, *Br J Surg* 70(10):623–627, 1983.

91. Pierik EG, van Urk H, Hop WC, et al: Endoscopic versus open subfascial division of incompetent perforating veins in the treatment of venous leg ulceration: a randomized trial, *J Vasc Surg* 26(6):1049–1054, 1997.

92. Hauer G: Endoscopic subfascial discussion of perforating veins–preliminary report, *Vasa* 14(1):59–61, 1985.

93. O'Donnell TJ Jr: Surgical treatment of incompetent perforating veins. In Bergan JJ, Kistner RL, editors: *Atlas of venous surgery*, Philadelphia, 1992, W. B. Saunders Company, pp 111–124.

94. Gloviczki P, Cambria RA, Rhee RY, et al: Surgical technique and preliminary results of endoscopic subfascial division of perforating veins, *J Vasc Surg* 23(3):517–523, 1996.

95. Conrad P: Endoscopic exploration of the subfascial space of the lower leg with perforator vein interruption using laparoscopic equipment: a preliminary report, *Phlebology* 9(4):154–157, 1994.

96. O'Donnell TF: The role of perforators in chronic venous insufficiency, *Phlebology* 25(1):3–10, 2010.

97. Gloviczki P, Bergan JJ, editors: *Atlas of endoscopic perforator vein surgery*, London, 1998, Springer.

98. Tenbrook JA Jr, Iafrati MD, O'Donnell TF Jr, et al: Systematic review of outcomes after surgical management of venous disease incorporating subfascial endoscopic perforator surgery, *J Vasc Surg* 39(3):583–589, 2004.

99. Luebke T, Brunkwall J: Meta-analysis of subfascial endoscopic perforator vein surgery (SEPS) for chronic venous insufficiency, *Phlebology* 24(1):8–16, 2009.

100. Kistner RL: Surgical repair of a venous valve, *Straub Clin Proc* 34:41–43, 1968.

101. Kistner RL: Surgical repair of the incompetent femoral vein valve, *Arch Surg* 110(11):1336–1342, 1975.

102. Raju S: Surgical repair of deep vein valve incompetence. In Gloviczki P, editor: *Handbook of venous disorders*, vol 1, ed 3, London, 2009, Hodder Arnold, pp 472–482.

103. Gloviczki P, Merrell SW, Bower TC: Femoral vein valve repair under direct vision without venotomy: a modified technique with use of angioscopy, *J Vasc Surg* 14(5):645–648, 1991.

104. Raju S, Fountain T, Neglen P, et al: Axial transformation of the profunda femoris vein, *J Vasc Surg* 27(4):651–659, 1998.

105. Lugli M, Guerzoni S, Garofalo M, et al: Neovalve construction in deep venous incompetence, *J Vasc Surg* 49(1):156–162, 162 e151–152, 2009; discussion 162.

106. Raju S, Fredericks R: Valve reconstruction procedures for nonobstructive venous insufficiency: rationale, techniques, and results in 107 procedures with two- to eight-year follow-up, *J Vasc Surg* 7(2):301–310, 1988.

107. Meissner MH, Manzo RA, Bergelin RO, et al: Deep venous insufficiency: the relationship between lysis and subsequent reflux, *J Vasc Surg* 18(4):596–605, 1993 discussion 606–598.

108. Ziegler S, Schillinger M, Maca TH, et al: Post-thrombotic syndrome after primary event of deep venous thrombosis 10 to 20 years ago, *Thromb Res* 101(2):23–33, 2001.

109. O'Shaughnessy AM, Fitzgerald DE: Natural history of proximal deep vein thrombosis assessed by duplex ultrasound, *Int Angiol* 16(1):45–49, 1997.

110. Gloviczki P, Hollier LH, Dewanjee MK, et al: Experimental replacement of the inferior vena cava: factors affecting patency, *Surgery* 95(6):657–666, 1984.

111. Neglen P: Endovascular reconstruction for chronic iliofemoral vein obstruction. In Gloviczki P, editor: *Handbook of venous disorders*, vol 1, ed 3, London, 2009, Hodder Arnold, pp 491–502.

112. Raju S, Neglen P: Percutaneous recanalization of total occlusions of the iliac vein, *J Vasc Surg* 50(2):360–368, 2009.

113. Garg N, Gloviczki P, Karimi KM, et al: Factors affecting outcome of open and hybrid reconstructions for nonmalignant obstruction of iliofemoral veins and inferior vena cava, *J Vasc Surg* 53(2):383–393, 2011.

114. Jost CJ, Gloviczki P, Cherry KJ Jr, et al: Surgical reconstruction of iliofemoral veins and the inferior vena cava for nonmalignant occlusive disease, *J Vasc Surg* 33(2):320–327, 2001 discussion 327–328.

115. Hingorani AP, Ascher E, Marks N, et al: Predictive factors of success following radio-frequency stylet (RFS) ablation of incompetent perforating veins (IPV), *J Vasc Surg* 50(4):844–848, 2009.

116. Masuda EM, Kessler DM, Lurie F, et al: The effect of ultrasound-guided sclerotherapy of incompetent perforator veins on venous clinical severity and disability scores, *J Vasc Surg* 43(3):551–556, 2006 discussion 556–557.

117. Proebstle TM, Herdemann S: Early results and feasibility of incompetent perforator vein ablation by endovenous laser treatment, *Dermatol Surg* 33(2):162–168, 2007.

118. Marks N, Hingorani A, Ascher E: New office-based vascular interventions, *Perspect Vasc Surg Endovasc Ther* 20(4):340–345, 2008.

119. Elias S: Percutaneous ablation of perforating veins. In Gloviczki P, editor: *Handbook of venous disorders*, vol 1, ed 3, London, 2009, Hodder Arnold, pp 536–544.

120. Dalsing M: Artificial venous valves. In Gloviczki P, editor: *Handbook of venous disorders*, vol 1, ed 3, London, 2009, Hodder Arnold, pp 483–490.

121. Neglen P, Berry MA, Raju S: Endovascular surgery in the treatment of chronic primary and post-thrombotic iliac vein obstruction, *Eur J Vasc Endovasc Surg* 20(6):560–571, 2000.

122. Neglen P, Tackett TP Jr, Raju S: Venous stenting across the inguinal ligament, *J Vasc Surg* 48(5):1255–1261, 2008.

123. Bjarnason H: Endovascular reconstruction of complex iliocaval venous occlusions. In Gloviczki P, editor: *Handbook of venous disorders*, vol 1, ed 3, London, 2009, Hodder Arnold, pp 503–513.

124. Raju S, Hollis K, Neglen P: Obstructive lesions of the inferior vena cava: clinical features and endovenous treatment, *J Vasc Surg* 44(4):820–827, 2006.

125. Neglen P, Hollis KC, Olivier J, et al: Stenting of the venous outflow in chronic venous disease: long-term stent-related outcome, clinical, and hemodynamic result, *J Vasc Surg* 46(5):979–990, 2007.

126. Delis KT, Bjarnason H, Wennberg PW, et al: Successful iliac vein and inferior vena cava stenting ameliorates venous claudication and improves venous outflow, calf muscle pump function, and clinical status in post-thrombotic syndrome, *Ann Surg* 245(1):130–139, 2007.

127. Kundu S, Lurie F, Millward SF, et al: Recommended reporting standards for endovenous ablation for the treatment of venous insufficiency: joint statement of the American Venous Forum and the Society of Interventional Radiology, *J Vasc Surg* 46(3):582–589, 2007.

128. Perrin M, Allaert FA: Intra- and inter-observer reproducibility of the Recurrent Varicose Veins after Surgery (REVAS) classification, *Eur J Vasc Endovasc Surg* 32(3):326–332, 2006.

CHAPTER 56   # Pulmonary Arterial Hypertension

Stephen Y. Chan, Joseph Loscalzo

Definition and Classification of Pulmonary Arterial Hypertension

Pulmonary arterial hypertension (PAH) is formally defined as a mean pulmonary artery pressure (PAP) of 25 mmHg or greater at rest or 30 mmHg or greater during exercise. This is accompanied by a pulmonary vascular resistance (PVR) of greater than 3 Wood units (WU), with a normal pulmonary artery wedge pressure (<15 mmHg) in the absence of any known cause of pulmonary hypertension (PH). Pulmonary arterial hypertension encompasses one of the five categories of PH, based on the most recent classification system.[1] The pathophysiology and clinical characteristics of categories 2 through 5 of PH (i.e., PH associated with left-sided heart disease; lung disease/chronic hypoxia; thromboembolic PH; and other groups) are reviewed in Chapter 57. In this chapter, we will focus on category 1, PAH, which includes idiopathic and familial PAH as well as PAH associated with various other diseases (Box 56-1). Until improved therapeutic options became available during the past 2 decades, PAH was considered a rare but rapidly progressive and devastating condition, leading to death from right heart failure by a median of 2.8 years from the time of diagnosis.[2] In recent years, an improved conceptual framework has been developed to better delineate the pathogenesis and clinical presentation of PAH, accompanied by improved directed therapeutic approaches. Nonetheless, PAH still carries a 15% annual mortality rate, and current therapeutics have been mostly effective at slowing illness progression rather than reversing or curing the disease. This chapter will highlight current molecular understanding of the complex disease, via the still incompletely characterized interplay of genetic and exogenous upstream stimuli with downstream vascular effectors. This framework will then be coupled to current understanding of the clinical presentation and progression of PAH and existing and evolving treatment modalities.

Epidemiology

Early epidemiological data from the 1980s estimated the incidence of PAH at one to two cases per million people in the general U.S. population.[2] More recent estimates in Europe[3] place the incidence and prevalence of PAH, respectively, at 2.4 cases per million annually and 15 cases per million in France and 7.6 cases per million annually and 26 cases per million in Scotland. Globally, the prevalence may be much higher given that many risk factors for PAH, such as human immunodeficiency virus (HIV) and schistosomiasis, are also more prevalent in the developing world. An exact number is difficult to estimate on a global scale, given the difficulty of diagnosing PAH and overall limited access to health care worldwide.[4] The disease affects women more frequently than men (1.7:1). This female predominance is exaggerated in the population of African descent (4.3:1), although the overall racial distribution of patients reflects that in the general population.

Primary PAH presents most commonly in the fourth decade of life; ages range from 1 to 81, with 9% of patients older than 60 years of age.[5] Some sources cite a similar gender ratio among children diagnosed with the disease, whereas others note an equal distribution between male and female children.[6] Primary PAH is typically difficult to diagnose, and the average time from onset of symptoms to diagnosis was 2 years in the National Institutes of Health (NIH) Registry.[2] More recently, however, thanks to improved clinical awareness and more sophisticated invasive and noninvasive techniques for PAP measurements, time to diagnosis has decreased considerably, at least in the developed world.

Molecular Pathogenesis of Pulmonary Arterial Hypertension

In humans, the natural history of PAH lesions is unknown because patients usually present when the disease is advanced. The pathological appearance of severe PAH is similar regardless of cause and reflects the end stage of a common response to pulmonary vascular injury. Common histological features in nearly all types of PAH occur at the level of the small peripheral pulmonary arteries (100-1000 μm) (Fig. 56-1); these include intimal fibrosis, distal localization and proliferation of vascular smooth muscle, and pulmonary arterial occlusion.[7] A hallmark of severe end-stage disease is the formation of a vessel "neointima," characterized by increased deposition of extracellular matrix (ECM) and myofibroblasts. Plexiform lesions can predominate, characterized by over-proliferation of endothelial-like cells encroaching upon the vessel lumen.

Multiple cell types in the pulmonary arterial wall and pulmonary arterial circulation contribute to the specific response to injury and development of vessel remodeling[8] (Fig. 56-2). The endothelium serves as a central sensor of injurious stimuli such as hypoxia, shear stress, inflammation, and toxins. Dysregulation of numerous downstream vascular effectors may be the result of initial endothelial cell (EC) injury or dysfunction. It has been hypothesized that endothelial apoptosis early in PAH initiates selection of apoptosis-resistant ECs that can further proliferate via monoclonal amplification in plexiform populations. This has led to speculation of a model of end-stage PAH similar to that of progression to cancer, with dysregulation of the cell cycle and apoptosis as predominant features. Similarly, dysregulated growth of pulmonary artery smooth muscle cells (SMCs) also plays a key role in PAH progression because apoptosis is suppressed while proliferation increases.

In addition to the endothelium and vascular smooth muscle, dysfunction of alternative vascular components may participate in these processes. Most notably, adventitial fibroblasts display increased proliferative capacity in PAH as well as carry an increased sensitivity to serotonin. Metalloproteinase activation in the ECM can induce cellular migration and leads to production of additional mitogenic factors. As a result, an

Box 56-1   Clinical Classification of Pulmonary Arterial Hypertension

Idiopathic
Familial
Associated with:
  Collagen vascular disease
  Congenital systemic-to-pulmonic shunt
  Portal hypertension
  Human immunodeficiency virus (HIV) infection
  Drugs and toxins
  Other: thyroid disorders, glycogen storage disease, Gaucher's disease,
    hereditary hemorrhagic telangiectasia (HHT), hemoglobinopathies,
    myeloproliferative disorders, splenectomy
Associated with significant venous or capillary involvement:
  Pulmonary veno-occlusive disease
  Pulmonary capillary hemangiomatosis
Persistent pulmonary hypertension of the newborn (PPHN)

Adapted with permission from Simmoneau G, Galiè N, Rubin L, et al: Clinical classification of pulmonary hypertension. J Am Coll Cardiol 43:5 S—12 S, 2004.

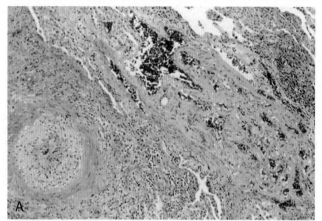

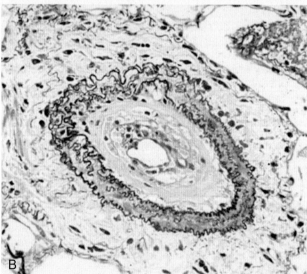

FIGURE 56-1 Histopathology of pulmonary arterial hypertension **(PAH). A,** Hematoxylin and eosin stain of histological section of lungs showing characteristic idiopathic PAH vascular lesions: completely occluded vessel with severe concentric intimal fibrosis and medial thickening *(left)* and plexiform lesion with multiple lumina *(right)*. **B,** Elastin von Gieson stain of internal and external elastic laminae demonstrates medial hypertrophy and neointimal formation in a small muscular pulmonary artery in patient with idiopathic PAH. *(Courtesy JL Faul, MD, Stanford University.)*

imbalance of a multitude of downstream secreted vasoactive factors ensues and directs vascular remodeling via pathological cellular processes. These further exacerbate dysregulated cell proliferation, vasoconstriction, and thrombosis, which are associated with more complex patterns of inflammation and angiogenesis. Transdifferentiation of ECs to vascular smooth muscle cells (VSMCs) may also contribute to the process. Inflammatory cells and activated platelets appear to predominate in later stages of PAH and in PAH associated with connective tissue disease and parasitic infections like schistosomiasis; but our understanding is limited regarding the mechanistic role of these cellular populations in disease progression. Finally, circulating or resident progenitor cells have been proposed to factor significantly in vessel wall injury and repair; dysregulation of these functions may also contribute to PAH.

Genetic Association

An understanding of the mechanism of genetic predisposition to PAH is of paramount importance for identifying the root pathogenesis (Fig. 56-3). The familial variety of idiopathic PAH accounts for at least 6% of all cases of PAH.[7] Pedigree analysis has demonstrated an autosomal dominant inheritance but with variable penetrance; only 10% to 20% of putative genetic carriers develop clinical PAH. Genetic anticipation is present, since each successive generation of affected families is afflicted at a younger age and greater severity compared with the preceding generation.

BONE MORPHOGENETIC RECEPTOR-II

Mutations in the transforming growth factor (TGF)-β receptor superfamily have been genetically linked to PAH and likely play a causative role in disease development. A rare group of patients with hereditary hemorrhagic telangiectasia (HHT) and idiopathic PAH harbor specific mutations in ALK1 or endoglin, genes encoding for two such members of the TGF-β receptor superfamily.[9,10] However, a more prevalent cohort of PAH patients carries mutations in the bone morphogenetic protein receptor type II (BMPR2 gene which encodes for BMPR2).[11,12] Over 140 mutations in BMPR2 have been reported in patients with familial PAH,[13] mainly located in the extracellular ligand-binding domain, cytoplasmic serine/threonine kinase domain, or long carboxyterminal domain. These account for 70% of all familial pedigrees of PAH and 10% to 30% of idiopathic PAH cases.[8] BMPR2 loss-of-function mutations have only been found in the heterozygous state. The absence of BMPR2 mutations in some familial cohorts and in most sporadic cases indicates that additional unidentified genetic mutations can also predispose to development of PAH. Furthermore, the presence of incomplete penetrance (approximately 25% of carriers in affected families develop clinical PAH) and genetic anticipation suggests that BMPR2 mutations are necessary but insufficient alone to result in clinically significant disease.

The mechanism of action of BMPR2 is complex, and its role in PAH progression is still unclear (Fig. 56-4A). It functions as a receptor with serine/threonine kinase activity, and it activates a broad and complex range of intracellular signaling pathways (as reviewed in[14]). Upon binding one of many possible bone morphogenetic protein (BMP) ligands, BMPR2 forms a heterodimer with one of three type-I receptors. BMPR2 phosphorylates the bound type-I receptor, which in turn phosphorylates one of the Smad family of proteins to allow for nuclear translocation, binding to deoxyribonucleic acid (DNA), and regulation of gene transcription. Alternatively, BMPR2 activation can also lead to signaling via the LIM kinase pathway, p38/mitogen-activated protein kinase/extracellular signal regulated kinase/c-jun NH 2-terminal kinase (MAPK/ERK/JNK) pathways, or c-Src pathway, independent of Smad activation.

Cellular effects of BMPR2 activation are multiform. In the adult, BMPR2 is expressed predominantly in pulmonary endothelium, medial SMCs, and macrophages.[15] Under normal conditions, BMP

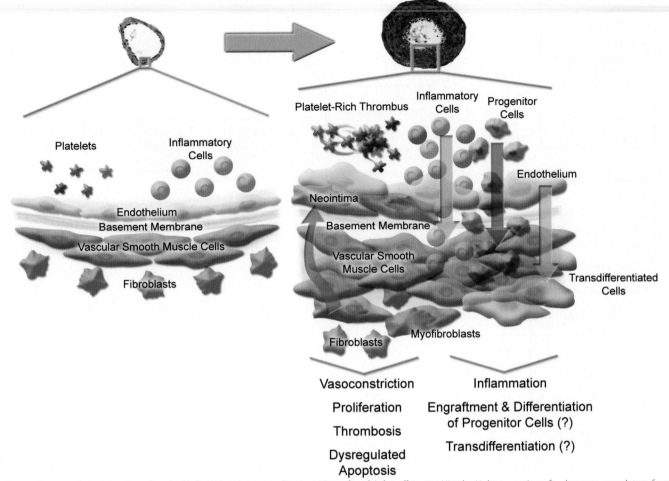

FIGURE 56-2 **Pulmonary arterial pathobiology involves coordinate action of multiple cell types.** Histological progression of pulmonary vasculature from quiescence to pathogenic activation in pulmonary arterial hypertension (PAH) involves numerous vascular cell types and phenotypic responses. Initial injury to endothelium and/or adventitial fibroblasts may initiate pathogenic signaling pathways. These activate an imbalance of secreted vascular mediators that drive vascular responses of vasoconstriction, proliferation, thrombosis, and dysregulation of apoptosis, leading to formation of a layer of "neointima." Bloodborne inflammatory cells and platelets also likely play prominent roles in these processes, but their exact mechanistic actions are unclear. Pathological phenotypes that may influence disease progression include transdifferentiation of endothelial cells (ECs) to vascular smooth muscle cells (VSMCs) and transdifferentiation of fibroblasts and VSMCs to myofibroblasts. Engraftment and differentiation of vascular progenitor cells may contribute as well. *(Adapted with permission from Chan S, Loscalzo J: Pathogenic mechanisms of pulmonary arterial hypertension. J Mol Cell Cardiol 44:14–30, 2008. Micrographs of pulmonary arteries courtesy www.scleroderma.org and Humbert M, et al: Treatment of pulmonary arterial hypertension. N Engl J Med, 2004, 351:1425–1436, 2004. Copyright 2004, Massachusetts Medical Society. All rights reserved.)*

ligands bind BMPR2 to suppress growth of VSMCs. In contrast, binding of BMP2 and BMP7 to BMPR2 in pulmonary endothelium protects against apoptosis. A widely held hypothesis contends that failure of the suppressive effects of BMP ligands on vascular smooth muscle and failure of the protective effects of BMP ligands on endothelium may trigger vascular proliferation and remodeling. Accordingly, in VSMCs derived from patients with familial PAH harboring BMPR2 mutations, exposure of BMP ligands does not suppress proliferation. Unlike the response in wild-type endothelium, exposure of ECs cultured from patients with idiopathic PAH to BMP2 does not protect against apoptosis.[16] These dysfunctional signaling pathways have been corroborated in some rodent models of PAH. In correlation, pulmonary levels of BMPR2 are reduced both in familial cases of PAH without any BMPR2 mutation and in cases of secondary PAH.[15] Thus, dysregulation of the BMP signaling pathway may be a common pathogenic finding in multiple types of PAH due to genetic or exogenous stimuli, but the definitive *in vivo* effects of these mutations have been difficult to decipher. Specifically, mouse models harboring specific BMPR2 heterozygous mutations have failed to exhibit robust PAH under static conditions,[17,18] again suggesting that dysfunctional BMPR2 is likely insufficient alone to cause disease. As a result, a clear mechanistic explanation of the impact of BMPR2 mutations on pathogenesis remains elusive.

ADDITIONAL GENETIC PATHWAYS

In addition to BMPR2 haploinsufficiency, alternative mechanisms involving complementary "modifier" genes may also contribute to a genetic predisposition to PAH. The most promising data identifying such modifier genes have analyzed the association of particular single nucleotide polymorphisms (SNPs) with the development of PAH. Thus far, SNP variants have suggested certain genes such as the serotonin transporter (SERT), Kv1.5, and the trp cation channel, subfamily C, member 6 (TRPC6).[3] Such associations do not always suggest a causal relationship, so additional mechanistic data are necessary for proper interpretation.

In the case of SERT and serotonin signaling, supportive data are more prevalent. Serotonin is both a vasoconstrictor and mitogen that promotes smooth muscle hyperplasia and hypertrophy (see Fig. 56-4B). Primarily stored in platelet granules, secreted serotonin binds G protein–coupled serotonin receptors (GPCRs) present on pulmonary artery SMCs. Activation of these receptors leads to a decrease in adenylyl cyclase and cyclic adenosine monophosphate (cAMP), resulting in increased contraction. Furthermore, the cell-surface SERT allows for transport of extracellular serotonin into the cytoplasm of SMCs, thereby activating cellular proliferation directly through the action of serotonin or indirectly via potential pleiotropic mechanisms.

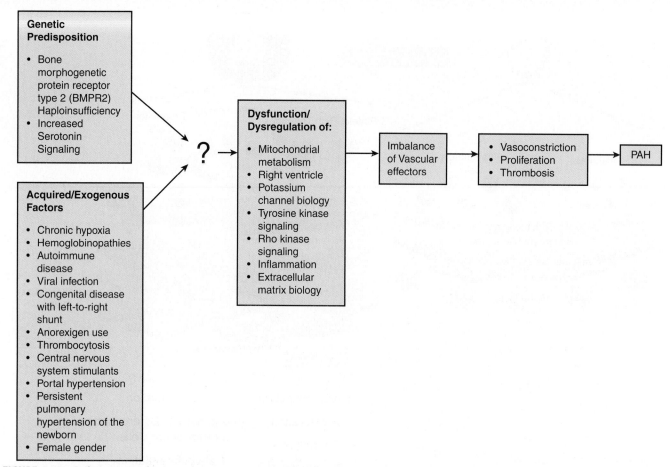

FIGURE 56-3 Pathogenic mechanisms that connect genetic and exogenous triggers of pulmonary arterial hypertension (PAH) to downstream dysregulated phenotypes are beginning to be explored at the molecular level. Although numerous clinical risk factors in PAH exist, mechanisms that lead to imbalance of vascular mediators and a relatively stereotyped phenotype of vascular dysregulation have only recently begun to be elucidated. CNS, central nervous system; ECM, extracellular matrix; PPHN, persistent pulmonary hypertension of the newborn; RV, right ventricle.

A number of observations in idiopathic and familial disease, congenital disease, and environmental exposure have implicated the proliferative effects of serotonin in PAH.[19] In idiopathic PAH, pulmonary expression of serotonin receptors is increased, and plasma levels of serotonin are chronically elevated. A mouse model of hypoxic PH parallels these changes.[20] A positive association has been noted among patients with congenital platelet defects in serotonin uptake (i.e., delta storage pool disease) and development of PAH. Chronic exposure to anorexigens, such dexfenfluramine (an inhibitor of serotonin reuptake and stimulator of serotonin secretion), leads to increased levels of circulating free serotonin. In mice, these changes are accompanied by increased 5HT receptor type 2B response and inhibition of SERT responses. In humans, these changes correlate with an increased risk for development of PAH. In addition, the L-allelic variant of SERT is associated with increased expression of the transporter and enhanced smooth muscle proliferation. In some human studies,[21] this variant has been associated with an increased risk of PAH in the homozygous population.

Animal models of PH have also implicated the activated serotonin pathway in disease progression. Treatment with serotonin and chronic hypoxia in a rat model led to worsened hemodynamics and increased vessel remodeling.[22] Exposure to increased serotonin led to worsened PH in a BMPR2[+/−] heterozygote murine model.[23] Similarly, overexpression of SERT in mice resulted in spontaneous development of PAH in the absence of hypoxia and exaggeration of PH after a hypoxic stimulus.[24] Conversely, vessel remodeling and hypoxic PH are reduced in a 5HT1B receptor–null mouse[25] and are abrogated in a 5HT2B receptor–null mouse.[20] As a result, serotonin signaling modulates pulmonary smooth muscle function in both normal and disease states

and likely contributes to disease progression of PAH. However, attempts at using selective serotonin reuptake inhibitors (SSRIs) as a therapeutic approach have yielded mixed results[3] to date. The exact contribution of this mechanism in PAH requires further clarification.

Acquired/Exogenous Factors

In addition to genetic predisposition, development of PAH likely depends on a variety of physiological, acquired, and/or exogenous stimuli. Some of these factors have been studied to a sufficient degree to hypothesize potential pathogenic mechanisms (see Fig. 56-3).

CHRONIC HYPOXIA

Pulmonary vascular response to hypoxia has been well studied in cell culture and animal models,[26] but its impact on PAH is unclear. In general, pulmonary vascular responses in acute and chronic hypoxia likely allow for the propagation of PAH, and therefore may contribute to later stages of the disease. Acute hypoxia induces vasodilation in systemic vessels but induces vasoconstriction in pulmonary arteries. This acute and reversible effect is mediated in part by up-regulation of endothelin-1 (ET-1) and serotonin, and in part by hypoxia- and redox-sensitive potassium channel activity in pulmonary VSMCs. Coordinately, these events lead to membrane depolarization in SMCs, increase in cytosolic calcium, and vasoconstriction.[27] In contrast, chronic hypoxia induces vascular remodeling and less reversible changes, including migration and proliferation of VSMCs and deposition of ECM. These cellular events in chronic hypoxia correlate with the remodeling events in

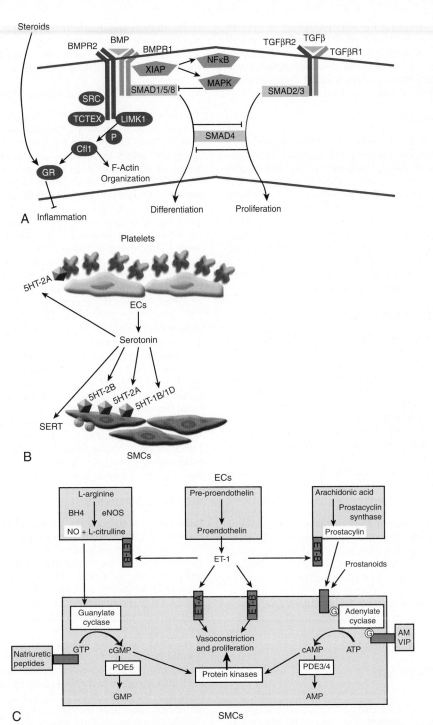

FIGURE 56-4 **Molecular signaling mechanisms of pulmonary arterial hypertension (PAH). A,** Bone morphogenetic protein receptor type II (BMPR2) signaling in pulmonary vasculature. Heterozygous loss-of-function mutations in BMPR2 are found throughout the gene, leading to a complex cascade of dysregulated signaling that predisposes to PAH. When activated by a BMP ligand, BMPR2 heterodimerizes with BMPR1 to activate SMAD transcription factors. SMAD activity can control cellular differentiation, vascular tone, and proliferation, among other functions. BMPR1 can also activate signaling through XIAP (X-linked inhibitor of apoptosis), which controls activation of nuclear factor (NF)-κB and mitogen-activated protein kinase (MAPK), both of which facilitate proinflammatory signaling. BMPR2 also carries a long cytoplasmic tail that binds to numerous signaling molecules including SRC, TCTEX, RACK1 (receptor for activated C-kinase 1), and LIMK1 (LIM domain kinase 1). LIMK1 can phosphorylate cofilin (Cfl1), which influences F-actin organization and glucocorticoid receptor (GR) nuclear translocation, important in inflammation. **B,** Serotonin signaling in pulmonary vasculature. Increased serotonin bioavailability is observed during PAH progression. This stems from increased release by platelets and increased production by endothelial cells (ECs). On vascular smooth muscle cells (VSMCs), serotonin receptors (5HT-2A, 5HT-2B, 5HT-1B/1D) are activated and induce vasoconstriction and remodeling. Overexpression of serotonin transporter (SERT) enhances the mitogenic effect of serotonin. Serotonin receptors on platelets potentiate aggregation. **C,** Nitric oxide (NO), endothelin-1 (ET-1), and prostacyclin are dysregulated vasoactive effectors in PAH. In pulmonary vasculature, NO is predominantly generated in ECs and transported to VSMCs; there, it stimulates production of cyclic guanosine monophosphate (cGMP) to induce vasorelaxation and decrease proliferation. Endothelin-1 is also predominantly synthesized and released from ECs. It activates endothelin receptor subtype A (ET-A) on smooth muscle cells (SMCs) to induce vasoconstriction and proliferation, while it stimulates NO and prostacyclin release via endothelin receptor subtype B (ET-B) on endothelial cells. Prostacyclin is produced from arachidonic acid and released from endothelial cells. In vascular smooth muscle cells, it activates production of cyclic adenosine monophosphate (cAMP) to promote vasorelaxation and inhibit proliferation. In PAH, NO and prostacyclin levels are significantly reduced while ET-1 levels are markedly elevated. This leads to a profound imbalance of these vasoactive effectors and exaggerated vasoconstriction and abnormal vascular smooth muscle proliferation. AM, adrenomedullin; AMP, adenosine monophosphate; ATP, adenosine triphosphate; BH4, tetrahydrobiopterin; eNOS, endothelial nitric oxide synthase; GMP, guanosine triphosphate; PDE, phosphodiesterase; TGFβ, transforming growth factor beta; TGFβR, transforming growth factor beta receptor; VIP, vasoactive intestinal peptide. *(Adapted from Archer SL, Weir EK, Wilkins MR: Basic science of pulmonary arterial hypertension for clinicians: new concepts and experimental therapies. Circulation 121:2045–2066, 2010.)*

end-stage PAH; however, because the histopathology of hypoxic PH does not recapitulate all aspects of PAH, some mechanistic differences in pathogenesis certainly exist but have not yet been fully identified. These are important considerations, especially in the context of interpreting studies of hypoxic PH and extrapolating those findings to the pathogenesis of PAH.

HEMOGLOBIN DISORDERS

Pulmonary arterial hypertension is associated with hemoglobinopathies, especially thalassemias and sickle cell anemia.[28] Hemolysis accompanying these disorders may lead to destruction of bioactive nitric oxide (NO) by free hemoglobin or reactive oxygen species (ROS). Furthermore, ROS may lead to increased levels of oxyhemoglobin, which further impairs delivery of NO to the vessel wall. As a result of the lack of available NO, an inflammatory and proliferative cascade may ensue, with culmination in PAH. Accordingly, decreased NO bioavailability with development of PH has been reported after hemolysis in a murine model of sickle cell disease (SCD),[29] and acutely in a murine model of intravascular hemolysis.[30] In vivo correlation to human disease is pending.

PORTOPULMONARY HYPERTENSION

Portopulmonary hypertension is defined as PAH associated with portal hypertension (portal pressure >10 mmHg), with or without hepatic disease.[31] Approximately 9% of patients with severe PAH are reported to have portal hypertension. Portopulmonary hypertension affects 4% to 6% of patients referred for liver transplantation. Liver transplantation perioperative mortality is significantly increased in patients with a mean PAP above 35 mmHg. Diagnosis of PH is usually made 4 to 7 years after the diagnosis of portal hypertension, but it has occasionally been reported to precede onset of portal hypertension. Risk of PH increases with duration of disease. The correlation between severity of portal hypertension and development of PH is debated. The female predominance of primary PAH is not seen in portopulmonary hypertension.

Survival is much worse than in PAH of other causes, with a median survival of 6 months. Because patients with nonhepatic causes of portal hypertension have been reported with this entity, it appears that portal hypertension, not cirrhosis, triggers development of PAH, yet the mechanism of portopulmonary hypertension is unknown. Hypotheses include inability of the liver to metabolize serotonin and other vasoactive substances. Alternatively, shear stress from increased pulmonary blood flow may result in endothelial injury, triggering a cascade of events that result in the characteristic adverse remodeling described earlier.

COLLAGEN VASCULAR DISEASE

Pulmonary arteriopathy complicates autoimmune diseases, especially in the setting of the CREST (calcinosis, Raynaud phenomenon, esophageal dysfunction, sclerodactyly, telangiectasia) variant of limited systemic sclerosis and, to a lesser degree, in mixed connective tissue disease, systemic lupus erythematosus (SLE), and rheumatoid arthritis.[32] Pulmonary arterial hypertension has been reported in approximately 10% to 30% of patients with mixed connective tissue disease, 5% to 10% of patients with SLE, and more rarely in the settings of rheumatoid arthritis, dermatomyositis, and polymyositis.[33] Sjögren syndrome may rarely be complicated by rapidly progressive PAH. It is particularly important to distinguish between PAH and thromboembolic PH in patients with SLE and antiphospholipid syndrome. Occurrence of PAH in each disease has been associated with Raynaud phenomenon, suggesting at least some similarities in pathogenesis.[34] Presence of interstitial lung disease and pulmonary fibrosis, seen at varying frequency in these autoimmune syndromes, may represent a common pathogenic factor in development of PAH. Accordingly, in the setting of pulmonary fibrosis and hypoxia, significant perivascular inflammation and deposition of ECM have been observed, which may increase vasoconstriction, proliferation, and vessel remodeling. Murine models of interstitial lung disease may prove important in further elucidating pathogenic mechanisms.

HUMAN IMMUNODEFICIENCY VIRUS

An association between HIV infection and PH has been noted in approximately 0.5% of all patients with HIV infection, a rate 6 to 12 times higher than the general population.[35] Notably, HIV does not infect pulmonary arterial endothelium, but mechanisms of disease have been proposed that directly stem from effects of HIV infection.[36] These include infection of SMCs with subsequent dysregulation of proliferation, imbalance of vascular mitogens in response to systemic HIV infection, and endothelial injury precipitated by HIV-infected T cells. The direct actions of HIV-encoded proteins may also factor into PAH development.[8] The HIV gp120 protein may induce pulmonary endothelial dysfunction and apoptosis. In a macaque model of simian immunodeficiency virus infection, a pathogenic interaction of the viral Nef protein with the pulmonary vessel wall has been reported, leading to pulmonary arteriopathy. Cell culture studies have also demonstrated a role for the HIV Tat protein in repression of BMPR2 transcription, potentially provoking a proliferative response in the vessel wall.

It had been proposed that human herpesvirus 8 (HHV-8), the causative agent of Kaposi sarcoma and an opportunistic pathogen highly associated with HIV infection, may play a role in PAH development with progression to plexiform lesions. Although it was initially reported that HHV-8 infection is associated with idiopathic PAH,[37] that link has not been consistently validated after study of additional populations. Nonetheless, PAH in the setting of HIV infection likely results from multifactorial effects, and the underlying pathogenesis may involve both direct results of viral infection and indirect consequences of associated pathogens.

SHUNT PHYSIOLOGY

Increased flow through the pulmonary circulation has long been associated with development of PAH. Certain types of congenital heart disease with functional systemic-to-pulmonary shunts, such as unrestricted ventricular septal defects (VSDs) and large patent ductus arteriosus (PDA), invariably lead to pulmonary vascular remodeling and the clinical syndrome of PAH during childhood (Eisenmenger's syndrome).[38] Approximately a third of patients with uncorrected VSDs and PDAs die from PAH. The timing of surgical repair greatly influences the outcome. If the shunt is repaired within the first 8 months of life, patients tend to have normal pulmonary pressures regardless of pathological findings; by contrast, patients operated on after age 2 tend to have persistent PAH. Importantly, when PVR equals or exceeds systemic vascular resistance, surgical correction of a shunt will increase the load on an already overburdened right ventricle (RV), worsen the patient's clinical condition, and not reverse PAH.

The presence of atrial septal defects (ASD) with systemic-to-pulmonary shunts may also lead to PAH over time.[39] Yet, in contrast to cases of unrestricted VSD and PDA, only 10% to 20% of all persons with ASDs progress to PAH. This observation may reflect differences in the response of the pulmonary vasculature to pressure overload (as seen in shunts with VSD and PDA) as compared to volume overload (as seen in shunts with ASD). Furthermore, patients with ASD may harbor a specific unidentified genetic predisposition to the development of PAH that may exacerbate the increased volume load to the pulmonary circulation.

At the molecular level, the physiological flow patterns of laminar shear stress, turbulent flow, and cyclic strain are all recognized by ECs, leading to transduction of intracellular signals and modulation of a wide variety of phenotypic changes.[40] Significant prior work has focused mainly on the endothelium of the peripheral vasculature, suggesting that laminar flow induces a vasoprotective quiescent vascular state, whereas turbulent flow leads to a proinflammatory and thrombogenic state. It is unclear whether these flow-dependent phenotypes are recapitulated in the pulmonary vasculature. In part, this stems from the difficulty of directly studying directly the *in vivo* flow patterns at the anatomical level of the pulmonary arteriole. Ex vivo modeling of pulsatile flow with high levels of shear stress and chronic vascular endothelial growth factor (VEGF) inhibition has demonstrated apoptosis of pulmonary artery ECs, followed by outgrowth and selection for proliferating apoptosis-resistant cells.[41] Therefore, chronically elevated flow may allow for selection of cells with dysregulated EC growth and resulting clonal or polyclonal expansion to plexiform lesions.

PERSISTENT PULMONARY HYPERTENSION OF THE NEWBORN

Persistent pulmonary hypertension of the newborn (PPHN) is characterized by persistent elevation of PVR, right-to-left shunting, and severe hypoxemia. It can occur with pulmonary parenchymal diseases including sepsis, meconium aspiration, pneumonia, maladaptation of the pulmonary vascular bed, or without an apparent cause.[42] Persistent PH in newborns may lead to death during the neonatal period, or it may be transient, leading to spontaneous and complete recovery. Inadequate production of NO may be an important contributor to persistent PH in infants, and inhaled NO is useful in treating this disorder.

MISCELLANEOUS DISORDERS

Pulmonary arterial hypertension is more rarely reported in patients suffering from other clinical syndromes such as pulmonary veno-occlusive disease, chronic myelodysplastic syndromes with thrombocytosis, and idiopathic thrombocythemia, as well as in persons exposed to stimulants of the central nervous system, such as methamphetamines and cocaine. Dysregulation of serotoninergic signaling may contribute[8] but does not explain these associations entirely. Finally, idiopathic PAH demonstrates a gender predilection of unclear etiology, with a high predominance of affected females.[43]

Vascular Effectors

Downstream of the genetic and acquired triggers of PAH, the histopathological processes that predominate later stages of disease include vasoconstriction, cellular proliferation, and thrombosis. These processes are influenced by a complex and dysregulated balance of vascular effectors controlling vasodilation and vasoconstriction, growth suppressors and growth factors, and pro- vs. antithrombotic mediators. Most of these effectors have been described in previous comprehensive reviews and will be described here specifically in regard to their known roles in PAH pathogenesis (Table 56-1).

NITRIC OXIDE

Gaseous vasoactive molecules regulate pulmonary vascular homeostasis, and alterations in their endogenous production have been linked to progression of PAH. Nitric oxide is the best described of these factors (see Fig. 56-4C).[44] It is a potent pulmonary arterial vasodilator as well as a direct inhibitor of platelet activation and VSMC proliferation. Nitric oxide diffuses into recipient cells (e.g., vascular muscle), where it activates soluble guanylyl cyclase (sGC) to produce cyclic guanosine monophosphate (cGMP). In turn, cGMP interacts with at least three different groups of effectors: cGMP-dependent protein kinases, cGMP-regulated phosphodiesterase (PDE), and cyclic nucleotide-gated ion channels. Synthesis of NO is mediated by a family of NO synthase (NOS) enzymes. In the pulmonary vasculature, the endothelial (eNOS) isoform figures most prominently and is regulated by a multitude of vasoactive factors and physiological stimuli including hypoxia, inflammation, and oxidative stress. Reduced levels and reduced activity of eNOS, reduced NO bioavailability, dysregulated intracellular NO transport via caveolae, and increased degradation of cGMP all aggravate PAH progression in human studies and/or animal models.

Dysregulation of NO may also depend upon still incompletely characterized processes of NO transport in blood.[45] Specific polymorphisms of NOS have also been associated with pulmonary hypertension. Together, these effects indicate a coordinated mechanism of dysregulated vasoconstriction. Correspondingly, murine models that genetically lack eNOS, GTP cyclohydrase-1 (the rate limiting enzyme for synthesis of an essential cofactor of NOS, tetrahydrobiopterin), or dimethylarginine dimethylaminohydrolase (DDAH, an enzyme important in degradation of NOS inhibitors) all display exaggerated susceptibility to developing PH in response to other endogenous stimuli.[3] Finally, the impact of NO has been reflected in its therapeutic role in PAH, such as inhaled NO[46] and the NO-dependent phosphodiesterase type-5 (PDE5) inhibitors (discussed later in detail).

PROSTACYCLIN/THROMBOXANES

The arachidonic acid metabolites prostacyclin and thromboxane A_2 (TxA_2) also play crucial roles in vasoconstriction, thrombosis, and to a certain degree, vessel wall proliferation (see Fig. 56-4C). Prostacyclin (prostaglandin I_2) activates cAMP-dependent pathways and serves as a vasodilator, antiproliferative agent for vascular smooth muscle, and inhibitor of platelet activation and aggregation. In contrast, TxA_2 increases vasoconstriction and activates platelets.[47] Protein levels of prostacyclin synthase are decreased in small and medium-sized pulmonary arteries in patients with PAH, particularly with the idiopathic form.[48] Biochemical analysis of urine in patients with PAH has shown decreased levels of a breakdown product of prostacyclin (6-ketoprostacyclin $F_2\alpha$), accompanied by increased levels of a metabolite of TxA_2 (thromboxane B_2).[49]

TABLE 56-1	Roles of Vascular Effectors in Pathogenesis of Pulmonary Arterial Hypertension			
VASCULAR EFFECTOR	**CHANGE IN ACTIVITY IN PAH**	**EFFECT ON VASOCONSTRICTION**	**EFFECT ON CELL PROLIFERATION**	**EFFECT ON THROMBOSIS**
Serotonin	Increased	Increased	Increased	Increased
Nitric oxide	Decreased (Increased in plexiform lesions)	Increased	(?) Increased in plexiform lesions	Increased
Thromboxane A_2	Increased	Increased	Increased	Increased
Prostacyclin	Decreased	Increased	Increased	Increased
Endothelin-1	Increased	Increased	Increased	(N/A)
Vasoactive intestinal peptide (VIP)	Decreased	Increased	Increased	Increased
Peroxisome proliferator-activated receptor (PPAR)-γ	Decreased	(N/A)	Increased	(N/A)

Therefore, it appears that production of these effectors is coordinately regulated, with the imbalance toward TxA$_2$ favored in the development of PAH. The mode of this regulation remains to be characterized. Nonetheless, recognition of this imbalance has led to the success of prostacyclin therapy and improvement of hemodynamics, clinical status, and survival in patients with severe PAH.[50]

ENDOTHELIN-1

Endothelin-1 is expressed by pulmonary ECs and has been identified as a significant vascular mediator in PAH (see Fig. 56-4C).[51] It acts as both a potent pulmonary arterial vasoconstrictor and mitogen of pulmonary smooth muscle cells. The vasoconstrictor response relies upon binding to the endothelin receptor A (ET-A) on vascular smooth muscle cells. This leads to an increase in intracellular calcium, along with activation of protein kinase C (PKC), mitogen-activated protein kinase (MAPK), and the early growth response genes c-fos and c-jun.[52] The mitogenic action of ET-1 on pulmonary VSMCs can occur through either the ET-A and/or the ET-B receptor subtype, depending on the anatomical location of cells. Endothelin receptor A predominantly mediates mitogenesis in the main pulmonary artery, whereas mitogenesis in resistance arteries relies upon contributions from both subtypes. The resulting vasoconstriction, mitogenesis, and vascular remodeling are thought to lead to significant hemodynamic changes in the pulmonary vasculature and to PAH. Plasma levels of ET-1 are increased in animal and human subjects suffering from PAH due to a variety of etiologies[53] and correlate with disease severity.[54] Again, improvement in hemodynamics, clinical status, and survival of PAH patients treated with chronic ET receptor antagonists highlights the significance of these effects.[55]

VASOACTIVE INTESTINAL PEPTIDE

Down-regulation of vasoactive intestinal peptide (VIP) may also play a pathogenic role. Vasoactive intestinal peptide is a pulmonary vasodilator, an inhibitor of proliferation of VSMCs, an inhibitor of platelet aggregation, and free radical scavenger. Decreased concentrations of VIP and VIP receptors have been reported in serum and lung tissue of patients with PAH.[56] Vasoactive intestinal peptide-null mice suffer from moderate pulmonary hypertension.[57] Both pulmonary arterial pressure (PAP) and PVR in humans decrease after treatment with VIP.[58,59] Key questions regarding the mode(s) of regulation of VIP expression and its putative causative role in PAH remain unanswered.

PEROXISOME PROLIFERATOR-ACTIVATED RECEPTOR γ

Peroxisome proliferator-activated receptor gamma (PPAR-γ) and apolipoprotein E (apoE) may function as integral factors in PAH.[60,61] PPARs are ligand-activated nuclear transcription factors that heterodimerize with the retinoid X receptor for subsequent binding to PPAR response elements in the promoters of target genes. Idiopathic PAH patients carry reduced pulmonary transcript levels of PPAR-γ and apoE. PPAR-γ in particular is a direct target of BMP2 in human PASMCs, leading to stimulation of apoE synthesis and downstream inhibition of vascular smooth muscle proliferation. PPAR-γ also regulates a host of protein kinases implicated in PASMC proliferation and migration. PPAR-γ agonists are antiinflammatory and induce pro-apoptotic phenotypes, both theoretically inhibitory to the pathogenesis of PAH. Mice deficient in smooth muscle–specific PPAR-γ are prone to PAH. Similarly, when fed a high-fat diet, male mice deficient in apoE develop PAH. This condition is reversed by rosiglitazone, a PPAR-γ agonist. Nonetheless, less robust results have been seen when using rosiglitazone hypoxic-PH rats, suggesting that these results offer a partial explanation to the complex molecular pathogenesis of BMPR2 signaling and PAH pathogenesis.

NATRIURETIC PEPTIDES

The atrial and brain natriuretic peptides (ANP and BNP) are produced by myocardium in response to stretch. They bind guanylyl cyclase receptors (NPR-A and NPR-B) that induce production of cGMP. Increased plasma concentrations of these peptides in PAH have been used as markers of the extent of RV dysfunction.[62] Genetic inactivation of NPR-A in mice is associated with PH[63]; in contrast, administration of atrial natriuretic peptide (ANP) ameliorates PAH in rodent models.[64] Additionally, inhibition of the metabolic breakdown of natriuretic peptides via neutral endopeptidase inhibitors has shown promise in animal studies of PAH. Human studies have yet to confirm efficacy.

ADRENOMEDULLIN

Adrenomedullin is an endogenous peptide that activates signaling pathways (i.e., cAMP, NO-cGMP, phosphatidylinositol-3-kinase/Akt) to induce vasodilation and inhibit proliferation. It decreases mean PAP and RV hypertrophy in hypoxic rats.[65] A related peptide, adrenomedullin-2, binds the same cellular receptors as adrenomedullin, and it is elevated in some rodent forms of PAH.

MISCELLANEOUS EFFECTORS

Other potential contributing factors include angiopoietin-1, the vasodilatory gases carbon monoxide and hydrogen sulfide, phosphodiesterase I, survivin, the calcium binding protein S100A4/Mts, the transient receptor potential channels, and Notch 3.[66] These may represent important but as yet incompletely described pathogenic contributors.[8] Other mitogenic and angiogenic growth factors, such as VEGF, platelet-derived growth factor (PDGF), basic fibroblast growth factor (bFGF)-2, insulin-like growth factor (IGF)-1, and epidermal growth factor (EGF) all may play downstream roles in later stages of PAH.

Pathogenic Pathways

Our understanding of specific actions of individual effectors has improved, but how they relate to upstream genetic or exogenous triggers of PAH remains unclear. In fact, none of these factors has yet been definitively linked to the root pathogenesis of disease. Insight into this topic is offered by the fact that known effectors are likely subject to upstream, overarching regulatory pathways that affect the action of multiple vasoactive molecules.[67] Characterization of these regulatory mechanisms may eventually allow for identification of primary molecular triggers of disease and offer novel therapeutic targets for drug development (see Fig. 56-3).

MITOCHONDRIAL METABOLISM

Mitochondrial and metabolic dysfunction may be common in PAH. Endothelial and VSMCs from human PAH tissue display dysmorphic and hyperpolarized mitochondria.[68] Metabolically, these cells preferentially exhibit a down-regulation of mitochondrial metabolism with an induction of glycolysis for energy production.[69] Under hypoxic conditions, this so-called Pasteur effect is a normal adaptive event that improves cellular survival by optimizing adenosine triphosphate (ATP) production while reducing oxygen radicals generated from the mitochondrial electron transport chain. Under normoxic conditions, however, such a shift to glycolysis (the Warburg effect) is thought to confer inappropriate resistance to apoptosis and is prominently seen in various cancer lineages. Such metabolic changes in the mitochondria are dependent upon a master transcription factor of hypoxia, hypoxia inducible factor 1 alpha (HIF-1α), and its critical downstream targets such as pyruvate dehydrogenase kinase (PDK1), among others.[70] In PAH, HIF-1α and PDK1 are dysregulated; conversely, treatment with dichloroacetate, a PDK inhibitor, ameliorates multiple forms of PAH in rodent models (chronic hypoxic PH, monocrotaline PAH, and fawn-hooded rat PAH).[71] It is conceivable that therapies aimed at reversing this metabolic dysregulation may result in improvement and/or regression of the PAH phenotype.

RIGHT VENTRICULAR DYSFUNCTION

After birth, PAPs typically decline, leading to involution of the RV to a thin-walled structure in the adult. During pathological conditions of increased PAPs in PAH, however, RV hypertrophy (RVH) and strain ensue, followed by RV failure if left untreated. Historically, the molecular pathways governing left ventricular (LV) failure, which have been better characterized, had been assumed to play primary roles in RV failure as well. Contemporary evidence suggests there may be distinct molecular and physiological differences between LV and RV failure that are just beginning to be explored.[72] For instance, PDE5, which is expressed in the fetal RV, is selectively up-regulated in the hypertrophied RV. Interestingly, inhibition of PDE5 enhances RV contractility without affecting the LV, where PDE5 expression is absent.

Unique metabolic changes in the RV have also been reported. The normal RV can use either fatty acids or glucose as needed for energy production. In RVH, the RV nearly exclusively relies upon glycolysis. Adenosine monophosphate (AMP)-activated protein kinase is activated in RVH, which preserves ATP levels by increasing glucose transport and glycolysis while inhibiting the tricarboxylic acid (TCA) cycle via repression of acetyl-coenzyme A carboxylase.[73] Furthermore, during RVH, PDK is activated, inducing a metabolic switch away from oxidative phosphorylation to glycolysis. As a result, the hypertrophied RV has been hypothesized to behave as "hibernating myocardium," which may suggest that the RV can be targeted therapeutically in PAH.[3]

POTASSIUM CHANNEL BIOLOGY

Modulation of voltage-gated potassium channels (Kv) may also represent an overarching pathogenic mechanism of PAH.[71] Kv channels are tetrameric membrane-spanning channels that selectively conduct potassium ions; in PASMCs, Kv channels aid in regulation of the resting membrane potential. In response to Kv inhibition or down-regulation, depolarization leads to the opening of voltage-gated calcium channels, increase in intracellular calcium, and initiation of a number of intracellular signaling cascades promoting vasoconstriction and proliferation and inhibiting apoptosis. Expression array analysis has demonstrated a depletion of Kv1.5 channels in pulmonary tissue derived from PAH patients.[74] It is currently unknown whether these Kv channel abnormalities are congenital or acquired, but a number of polymorphisms in the Kv1.5 channel gene (KCNA5) have been described, which may suggest a genetic predisposition to channel depletion.[75] Appetite suppressants (e.g., dexfenfluramine, aminorex) that are risk factors for development of PAH can also directly inhibit Kv1.5 and Kv2.1. A variety of transcription factors (HIF-1α, NFAT, and c-Jun) are increased in PAH, with resulting down-regulation of Kv1.5 expression in PASMCs. Inhibition of these factors consequently increases Kv1.5 expression, with resulting improvements in Kv current and in some cases, improved pulmonary arterial remodeling in hypoxic rodent models of PH. Inhibition of Kv currents in pulmonary SMCs may be regulated by serotonin, TxA_2, and perhaps NO. Furthermore, BMP signaling can regulate Kv receptor expression. Taken together, the Kv pathway may represent a common point of regulation in pathogenesis. Accordingly, augmentation of Kv activation would be predicted to induce vasodilation and perhaps allow for regression of vessel remodeling. In vivo gene transfer of Kv channels in chronically hypoxic rats has led to improvement of PH and suggests its therapeutic potential.[76]

TYROSINE KINASES

End stages of PAH are marked by exaggerated expression or activity of multiple growth factors, including PDGF, fibroblast growth factor 1 (FGF-1), FGF-2, EGF, and VEGF. All appear to contribute substantially to the overall obstructive arterial remodeling characteristic of PAH, via synergistic and combinatorial pathways. Some of the receptors for these growth factors are transmembrane receptor tyrosine kinases that activate a diverse and overlapping set of intracellular signaling pathways. Inhibition of EGF[77] and PDGF[78] receptors demonstrates improved hemodynamics and survival in PAH. Case reports exist of a beneficial effect of adding imatinib (a nonselective tyrosine kinase inhibitor)[79] or sorafenib (a "multikinase inhibitor")[80] to baseline PAH therapy; however, further mechanistic clarity of the specific role of tyrosine kinases in the pathogenesis of PAH is needed.

RHO-KINASE SIGNALING

Multiple vascular cell types rely upon the rho kinase signaling pathway for homeostatic function and response to injury.[81] Rho is a guanosine triphosphate (GTP) binding protein that activates its downstream target, rho-kinase, in response to activation of a variety of GPCRs (including those related to BMP/SMAD signaling and serotonin signaling). In vitro activation of these signaling cascades results in modulation of multiple cellular processes, including enhanced vasoconstriction, proliferation, impaired endothelial response to vasodilators, chronic pulmonary remodeling, and up-regulation of vasoactive cytokines via the nuclear factor kappa beta (NFκB) transcription pathway. Rho-kinase activity has also been linked specifically to a number of known effectors of PAH, including ET-1, serotonin, and eNOS, among others. Elevated rho-kinase activity has been demonstrated in animal models of PAH,[82,83] and intravenous fasudil, a selective rho-kinase inhibitor, has induced pulmonary vasodilation and regression of PAH in various animal models (as reviewed in[8]), as well as in patients with severe PAH who were otherwise refractory to conventional therapies.[84,85] Taken together, these data suggest that rho-kinase may control a master molecular "switch" in the pulmonary artery, initiating an activated state in disease from a quiescent state in health. As a result, rho-kinase represents an attractive and novel upstream therapeutic target for treatment of PAH.

INFLAMMATION

As reflected by a strong association of PAH with various autoimmune and infectious states as well as a significant presence of T cells, B cells, and macrophages in plexiform lesions, a severe inflammatory state predominates end-stage PAH. Athymic nude rats, which lack functioning T cells, display greater sensitivity to PAH.[86] T-cell dysregulation may figure prominently because regulatory T cells (T_{reg}) are increased, whereas CD8+ cytotoxic cells are decreased, in idiopathic PAH.[87] In addition, a number of soluble chemoattractants and proinflammatory cytokines from the pulmonary artery are up-regulated in human and animal models of severe PAH. These include interleukin (IL)-1β, TGF-β_1, bradykinin, monocyte chemotactic protein-1, fractalkine, RANTES, and leukotrienes, among others. 5-Lipoxygenase (5-LO) regulates synthesis of leukotrienes, which in turn can promote cytokine release. 5-Lipoxygenase may represent a possible upstream factor involved in inciting this proinflammatory state, and elevated levels of 5-LO have been detected in macrophages and pulmonary endothelium derived from patients suffering from idiopathic PAH.[88] In various murine models of PAH, overexpression of 5-LO has worsened PH and vascular remodeling,[89] while 5-LO inhibitors have attenuated PH. It is thus tempting to speculate that 5-LO itself may possess an upstream regulatory role in PAH progression.

EXTRACELLULAR MATRIX BIOLOGY

Vascular-specific serine elastase activity has been implicated in PAH pathogenesis via regulation of the remodeling response in the extracellular matrix.[90] In pulmonary arterioles, serine elastases are secreted into the extracellular space to activate matrix metalloproteinases (MMP) and inhibit tissue inhibitors of MMP (TIMP). Both MMP and elastases degrade most components of the ECM leading to an up-regulation of fibronectin (FN) and subsequent enhancement of cellular migration. Matrix degradation also increases integrin signaling, with resulting expression of the glycoprotein tenascin C. Tenascin C acts cooperatively with other factors to enhance smooth muscle proliferation. Increased degradation of elastin[91] has been observed in pulmonary arteries from patients suffering from congenital heart disease and resultant PAH. In pulmonary tissue of PAH patients harboring BMPR2 mutations and rat models of PAH, increased production and activity of vascular elastases[92] and tenascin C[93] have been reported. This up-regulation of elastase function may be induced by a number of vascular effectors implicated in PAH, including NO, serotonin, and theoretically, the BMP pathway. Elastase inhibitors can induce apoptosis of SMCs in cell culture and can improve PAH in animal models.[94,95] Thus, elastase function may also represent a novel therapeutic target.

Clinical Pathophysiology

The pulmonary vascular bed has a remarkable capacity to dilate and recruit unperfused vessels, adapting easily to large increases in blood flow. In PAH, these properties are lost. Right ventricle function is highly afterload dependent and works less efficiently with increases in PVR. With increased afterload, the RV hypertrophies and dilates. In the early stages of PAH, resting PAP remains normal and cardiac output (CO) is maintained, but with exercise, PAP becomes abnormally high and the RV is unable to increase CO. With progressive PH there may eventually be a decrease in measured PAP due to a decrease in CO, while the PVR remains elevated. Cardiac function is characterized by RV systolic and diastolic overload from tricuspid regurgitation. The LV is not directly affected by pulmonary vascular disease, but when PAP rises to the extent that the RV changes from its normal crescent shape to expand into the LV, it can impair LV filling, increase LV end-diastolic pressure, and decrease CO, a phenomenon described as the *reverse Bernheim effect*.

The two most frequent causes of death in PAH are progressive RV failure and sudden death. Right ventricle failure may be exacerbated by pneumonia, and alveolar hypoxia can cause further vasoconstriction and greater impairment of CO. Sudden death may be caused by arrhythmias that arise in the setting of hypoxemia and acidosis, acute pulmonary emboli, massive pulmonary hemorrhage, and subendocardial RV ischemia.[96]

Diagnostic Evaluation

Initial Approach

There is no pathognomonic finding in PAH; thus the diagnosis is one of exclusion. A thorough evaluation must be performed to reveal potentially contributing factors, including causes of secondary forms of PH that require a different treatment approach. It is important to probe for a family history of PH, early unexplained deaths, congenital heart disease, and collagen vascular disease. A thorough history should also include all associated risk factors of PH to uncover a possible explanation for the onset of PAH and exclude secondary causes of PH. A functional assessment should be made on the basis of the New York Heart Association (NYHA) functional classification of heart failure adopted for PAH at the World Health Organization (WHO)-sponsored symposium.[1] In addition to a comprehensive history, diagnostic evaluation should include physical examination, exercise testing (e.g., 6-minute walk), chest radiograph, electrocardiography, pulmonary function tests, arterial blood gas and other blood tests, noninvasive cardiac and pulmonary imaging, and cardiac catheterization with measurement of response to vasodilator administration (Fig. 56-5).

SYMPTOMS

By the time patients develop symptoms, PAH is usually advanced, and CO is often reduced. The nonspecificity of presenting symptoms can cause a long delay in diagnosis in most patients. The most common presenting symptom is dyspnea on exertion, which affects nearly all patients as disease progresses. Other presenting symptoms include fatigue, syncope or near syncope, chest pain, lower-extremity edema, or palpitations. Dyspnea may be due to impaired oxygen delivery during exercise, secondary to inability to increase CO to accommodate increased oxygen demand. Syncope occurs when CO is severely limited and inadequate cerebral blood flow with exertion ensues. Chest pain in PAH may be caused by subendocardial RV ischemia.

PHYSICAL FINDINGS

Clinical findings in PAH are initially subtle. The first signs of disease may be an RV heave, a loud pulmonic second heart sound, and a right-sided fourth heart sound. Eventually a right-sided third heart sound and a left parasternal systolic murmur of tricuspid regurgitation may be audible. Findings of jugular venous distension, ascites, and peripheral edema indicate overt right heart failure. Physical examination must include evaluation for signs associated with specific diseases associated with PAH, including collagen vascular disease, liver disease, HIV, HHT, thyroid disease, and all secondary causes of PH.

LABORATORY STUDIES

Secondary causes of PAH should be sought with serology for HIV and collagen vascular diseases, liver function tests (LFTs), and toxic exposures. Thyroid function should be evaluated. Thrombocytopenia may be present in severe PAH and has multiple contributing causes, including platelet activation and aggregation, pulmonary vascular sequestration, hepatosplenomegaly with splenic sequestration, and an autoimmune-mediated syndrome similar to idiopathic thrombocytopenic purpura.[97] Thrombocytopenia may accompany microangiopathic hemolysis when blood flows through fibrin deposits in plexiform lesions, with subsequent shearing of red blood cells and platelets. Prostacyclin may also induce thrombocytopenia. Thrombocytosis may be present in patients following splenectomy.

In patients with PH, high levels of ANP and BNP parallel decreased RV function. Levels of both peptides decrease with prostacyclin treatment and ensuing hemodynamic improvement. A subsequent increase in plasma BNP has been demonstrated to be an independent predictor of mortality.[98]

RADIOGRAPHIC STUDIES

Chest radiographs in PH usually show an enlarged pulmonary trunk and hilar pulmonary arteries, pruning of peripheral vessels, and obliteration of the retrosternal clear space by the enlarged RV (Fig. 56-6). Occasionally the chest radiograph may appear normal.[5] High-resolution computed tomography (CT) is used to evaluate lung parenchyma for interstitial lung disease. Helical CT is used to evaluate the central pulmonary arteries for presence of thrombi. Ventilation/perfusion scans are used to rule out chronic pulmonary thromboemboli. In patients with PAH, these scans are normal or show only patchy defects. If inconclusive, a pulmonary angiogram, which will show pruning of peripheral vessels in PAH, must be performed to definitively exclude thromboembolic disease. Use of pulmonary magnetic resonance angiography (MRA) has not been widely reported, but has recently been shown to identify patients with PAH with high sensitivity and negative predictive values.[98]

ELECTROCARDIOGRAM

The electrocardiogram (ECG) is not a sensitive or specific screening tool. In advanced disease, the ECG usually shows signs of right heart strain and enlargement, including right axis deviation and evidence of RV hypertrophy. Presence of a conduction abnormality is not typical of PAH. Electrocardiogram evidence of right heart strain has been associated with decreased survival.[2]

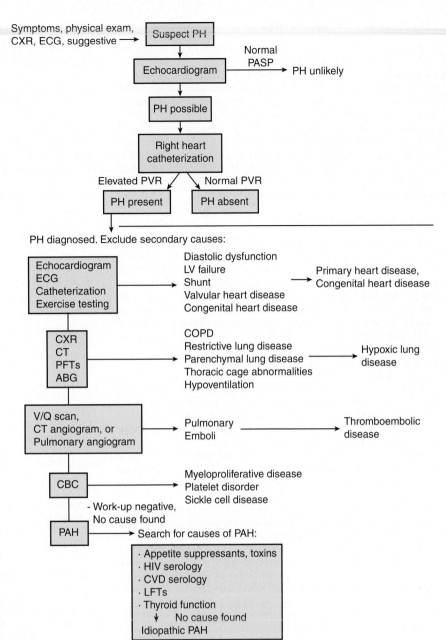

FIGURE 56-5 Diagnostic evaluation for suspected pulmonary arterial hypertension (PAH). (SeeChapter58 for a discussion of secondary pulmonary hypertension.) ABG, arterial blood gas; CBC, complete blood cell count; COPD, chronic obstructive pulmonary disease; CPET, cardiopulmonary exercise test; CT, computed tomography scan; CVD, collagen vascular disease; CXR, chest x-ray; ECG, electrocardiogram; HIV, human immunodeficiency virus; LFTs, liver function tests; LV, left ventricle; PAH, pulmonary arterial hypertension; PASP, pulmonary arterial systolic pressure; PFTs, pulmonary function tests; PH, pulmonary hypertension; PVR, pulmonary vascular resistance; SCD, sickle cell disease; V/Q scan, ventilation/perfusion nucleotide scan.

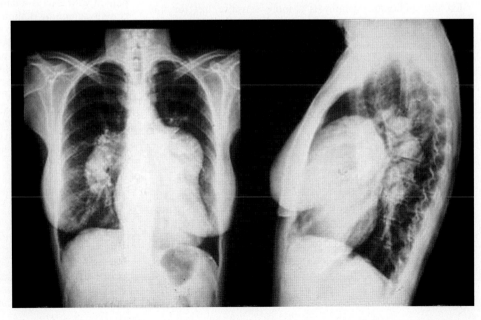

FIGURE 56-6 Chest radiograph in pulmonary arterial hypertension (PAH). Pulmonary arteries are highly prominent bilaterally, with abrupt tapering (or "pruning") of vessels due to increased peripheral vascular resistance (PVR) and diminished flow. There is right atrial and ventricular enlargement. Lung parenchyma is normal.

PULMONARY FUNCTION TESTS

Pulmonary function tests (PFTs) are important in excluding secondary causes of PH, particularly chronic obstructive airways disease. Airway obstruction is not typical of PAH, although cases of bronchial obstruction due to enlarged pulmonary arteries have been reported. Pulmonary arterial hypertension patients typically demonstrate borderline restrictive physiology, a reduced diffusing capacity for carbon monoxide (DLCO), and hypoxemia with hypocapnea.[5] Reduction in DLCO results from reduced blood volume in alveolar capillaries. In a study of pulmonary function in 79 patients presenting with PAH, significantly reduced DLCO (mean 68% of predicted values) was observed in 75% of patients, and mild restrictive physiology was seen in 50%.[99]

ECHOCARDIOGRAPHY

Transthoracic echocardiography is a crucial diagnostic tool in evaluating patients for PH.[96] It can determine the presence of left-sided heart disease, valvular disease, and intracardiac shunts, and it allows noninvasive measurement of PAP. A finding of elevated PAP must be further evaluated with pulmonary artery catheterization. Echocardiography of PAH patients frequently shows RV hypertrophy and dilation, right atrial enlargement, and decreased LV cavity size due to bowing of the interventricular septum in advanced disease. The inferior vena cava is typically distended and does not collapse during inspiration in advanced disease. Systolic PAP can be estimated using Doppler measurement of the tricuspid regurgitant flow velocity. The upper limit of normal systolic PAP is generally considered 40 to 50 mmHg at rest, corresponding to a tricuspid regurgitant velocity of 3 to 3.5 m/s (although this value varies with age, body mass index [BMI], and right atrial pressure).

Limitations to Doppler measurement of PAP do exist, however; false-negative studies are possible in patients with poor-quality views or moderate elevations in PAP. Doppler estimates of pressures are also operator dependent. Studies comparing Doppler-derived PAP values with pressures determined by catheterization yield varying results, with some reporting underestimation of systolic PAP by Doppler.[98] Echocardiography is probably best employed for its negative predictive value, although a number of echocardiographic features of PAH suggest worsened prognosis.[100] These mostly include echocardiographic markers of RV dysfunction (i.e., right atrial or ventricular size, septal shift toward the LV during diastole, tricuspid annular plane excursion to approximate RV ejection fraction, RV myocardial index). Notably, however, echocardiographic estimates of RV systolic pressure do not predict survival.[101]

Exercise echocardiography is a more sensitive test for the presence of early PAH, which is particularly valuable in pediatric cases where it may influence decisions regarding surgery. Exercise echocardiography has been studied as a screening tool to identify asymptomatic carriers of BMPR2 mutations in PAH families.[102] A resting echocardiogram demonstrating normal PA pressure usually excludes a diagnosis of PH. When PAH is strongly suspected or a patient has unexplained dyspnea, however, exercise echocardiography performed during exercise may reveal exercise-induced PAH.

CARDIAC CATHETERIZATION

Cardiac catheterization remains the gold standard for establishing the diagnosis and type of PAH. This procedure can directly measure right heart and PA pressures, as well as pulmonary capillary wedge pressure and CO. It can also be used to assess vasodilation reserve (see explanation later in the section on vasodilator therapy) and is the major determinant in prognosis of PH. Cardiac catheterization can also be performed with exercise to assess the possibility of exercise-induced PH, in which the resting PAP is normal, but PAP during exercise is abnormally high.

EXERCISE TESTING

Exercise testing is not required for a diagnosis of PH, but it may provide valuable information regarding prognosis. The most widely used and reproducible exercise test is the 6-minute walk test. This test is usually done after the diagnosis is confirmed by cardiac catheterization, and at regular intervals to monitor functional status. The distance walked in 6 minutes has been shown to decrease in proportion to the NYHA functional class and is a strong independent predictor of mortality. Patients with PAH who walk 300 or fewer meters and display decreased arterial oxygen saturation by 10% at maximal distance suffer from a significantly increased rate of mortality.[98] Maximal exercise testing must be avoided because syncope and sudden death have been reported. Cardiopulmonary exercise testing with or without echocardiography has been increasingly used in research studies and can be helpful in distinguishing PAH from PH secondary to diastolic heart failure.

SCREENING

Screening asymptomatic patients at high risk for PAH is recommended.[103] The exact population recommended for screening is controversial, since the prevalence of disease is low even in categories of patients at increased risk. Patient groups who likely benefit from screening include those with already known genetic mutations predisposing to PAH, first-degree relatives in a familial PAH cluster, patients with scleroderma, portal hypertension prior to liver transplantation, and patients with congenital systemic-to-pulmonary shunts.[104] Some patients should be evaluated for PAH only if they present with symptoms suggestive of the disease, including those with collagen vascular disease other than scleroderma, HIV, intravenous drug users, patients exposed to appetite-suppressant drugs, and patients with portal hypertension who are not being considered for transplantation. Screening asymptomatic or minimally symptomatic patients should begin with a thorough history and physical examination to elicit symptoms or signs consistent with PH, followed by diagnostic testing if inconclusive. Transthoracic echocardiogram is the best noninvasive test used for screening patients.

GENETIC TESTING

Genetic testing of asymptomatic individuals is not currently advocated as an effective method for diagnosis, considering the low penetrance of disease manifestation even if a predisposing mutation is present. The risk for disease in first-degree relatives of a patient with PAH is relatively low, which has led to uncertainty in genetic screening of their family members. Advocates suggest that screening asymptomatic patients may enhance knowledge of the prevalence of familial PAH and shed light on whether early treatment influences disease pathogenesis. Screening also allows at-risk individuals to be aware of known risks that theoretically may augment penetrance of the disease.[105] However, genetic testing results can be confusing; even if family members have inherited a predisposing mutation, about an 80% chance exists that no discernible disease phenotype will manifest. Notably, such circumstances may result in detrimental psychological, employment, and insurance effects and, if pursued, must be supported by appropriate genetic counseling.

Treatment

There is no known cure for PAH, but current therapeutic options have dramatically improved survival and quality of life for PAH patients. Recently the American Heart Association (AHA) and American College of Cardiology, in collaboration with the American College of Chest Physicians, American Thoracic Society, and Pulmonary Hypertension Association, released consensus recommendations for treatment of PAH[103] (Fig. 56-7).

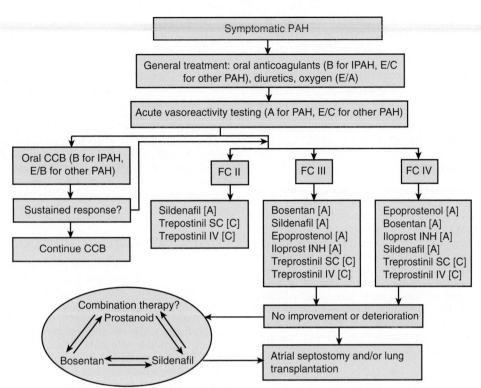

FIGURE 56-7 Algorithm for treatment of pulmonary arterial hypertension (PAH), adapted from 2007 AHA/ACC/ACCP Guidelines. Letters following recommendations are based on a combination of level of evidence and perceived benefit: A, strong recommendation; B, moderate recommendation; C, weak recommendation. Recommendations with an E are based on expert opinion rather than clinical trial evidence. CCB, calcium channel blocker; FC, functional class; INH, inhaled; IPAH, idiopathic pulmonary arterial hypertension; IV, intravenous; SC, subcutaneous. *(Adapted from Badesch DB, Abman SH, Simonneau G, et al: Medical therapy for pulmonary arterial hypertension: updated ACCP evidence-based clinical practice guidelines. Chest 131:1917–1928, 2007.)*

General Measures

Any behavior that increases oxygen demand or CO can worsen PAH symptoms and RV failure. Heavy physical exertion should be avoided. High altitude and nonpressurized airplane cabins can induce hypoxia and hypoxia-induced PH. Supplemental oxygen should be used if it is necessary for the patient to be exposed to high altitude. Pulmonary arterial hypertension is an absolute contraindication to pregnancy because it may precipitate fatal right heart failure. Oral contraceptives theoretically can increase the risk of hypercoagulability, leading to thromboembolic events that could exacerbate PAH. Nonetheless, oral contraceptives are often used in nonsmoking women with PAH without a history of thromboembolic disease.

Anticoagulation

Anticoagulation has been incorporated into PAH treatment on the basis of presence of thrombosis in small PAs, risk of compounding PAH with a thromboembolic component, and increased risk of deep venous thrombosis (DVT) in the setting of a low CO. No controlled trial of anticoagulation in PAH currently exists, but anticoagulation is based on improved survival of patients who received warfarin in historical smaller studies.[106] The usual recommended International Normalized Ratio (INR) is 2 to 2.5.[107] Although prostacyclin inhibits platelet aggregation, additional anticoagulation is typically used in the absence of a contraindication. Since patients with congenital systemic-to-pulmonary shunts are at greater risk for hemoptysis, however, some practitioners do not recommend anticoagulation in those cases.[108]

Oxygen Therapy

Use of supplemental oxygen therapy should be considered in patients with hypoxemia at rest (partial pressure of oxygen in arterial blood [Pao_2] <55 mmHg or arterial blood oxygen saturation

[Sao_2] <88%). Shunt-induced hypoxemia in patients with patent foramen ovale or intracardiac shunt is refractory to supplemental oxygen therapy. A controlled trial has not been performed, but oxygen therapy can improve quality of life by improving dyspnea and exercise capacity, although oxygen equipment can limit mobility.

Treatment of Right Heart Failure

Diuretics are used to reduce intravascular volume and hepatic congestion. Cautious use of loop and thiazide diuretics may be required for adequate management. Overdiuresis must be avoided; it can impair CO by decreasing RV preload. Digoxin is generally not used in PAH except for rate control of arrhythmias. Intravenous inotropes may acutely improve symptoms of right heart failure but are not feasible as chronic agents.

Pulmonary Vascular—Specific Therapies

INITIAL SCREENING FOR VASODILATOR RESERVE

Acute vasoreactivity testing is generally used as an initial screen to assess for vasodilator reserve and potential response to vasodilator therapy.[109] A significant response to vasodilator testing is generally accepted as a decrease in PVR by at least 25%, with a decrease in mean PAP to less than 40 mmHg. Other parameters include a greater than 20% decrease in systolic PAP, a greater than 10 mmHg drop in mean PAP, or an increase in cardiac index by 30% or more. The most widely used drugs for acute vasoreactivity testing include inhaled NO and intravenous prostacyclin (epoprostenol), adenosine, and iloprost, a prostacyclin analog with less effect on the systemic vasculature. Testing more than one drug offers no advantage. Vasodilator challenge must be performed with care because drug-induced systemic hypotension (e.g., with prostacyclin) may reduce RV coronary blood flow and cause RV ischemia.

Most studies on PAH report the proportion of responders to vasodilators as between 12% and 25%.[96] There is no particular clinical or disease characteristic that reliably predicts vasodilator response. Lack of response to acute vasodilators predicts response to oral vasodilator therapy (i.e., nonresponders to inhaled NO do not respond to oral calcium channel blockers). Response to acute vasodilators, however, does not predict a response to prostacyclin. A trial of long-term calcium channel blocker therapy is usually recommended in PAH patients who respond to vasodilator challenge with a decrease in PVR of 50 or more.

CALCIUM CHANNEL BLOCKERS

Calcium channel blockers are the oral drugs of choice for treating patients who have a significant response to acute vasodilators.[109] These agents have been shown to improve hemodynamics, RV function, and survival in the subpopulation of PAH patients responding to acute vasoreactivity testing.[110] Empirical therapy without vasodilator testing is not recommended because of the high rate of treatment failure. Both nifedipine and diltiazem are effective in appropriate patients, and the choice between these two drugs is guided by resting heart rate. Doses of these drugs required to lower PVR are much higher than those used for other indications, which makes systemic side effects a significant problem, particularly hypotension and lower-extremity edema. Verapamil is not used because of its greater negative inotropic effects. Acute administration of amlodipine causes pulmonary vasodilation, but its long-term efficacy has not been studied.

ENDOTHELIN-1 RECEPTOR ANTAGONISTS

Presently, three endothelin receptor antagonists are approved for oral use in PAH: two in the United States (bosentan [Tracleer] and ambrisentan [Letairis]) and one in Europe and Canada (sitaxsentan [Thelin]).[111] Bosentan is a nonspecific antagonist recognizing both endothelin receptor subtypes A (ET-A) and B (ET-B), and ambrisentan and sitaxsentan are specific for ET-A. It is thought that specific inhibition of ET-A may provide more benefit by decreasing the vasoconstrictor effects of ET-A while allowing the vasodilator and ET-1 clearance functions of ET-B receptors. All three agents have been found to improve exercise capacity and hemodynamics in 12- to 16-week clinical trials.[112–114] Bosentan has also improved survival in open-label studies and comparison with historical control data.[96] Long-term survival data for the selective endothelin inhibitors appear favorable as well, with some preliminary data suggesting that time to clinical worsening favors sitaxsentan over bosentan. No clear survival data are yet available from properly designed clinical trials. Because of its efficacy and ease of use, bosentan is currently recommended for stable functional class III PAH patients as first- or second-line agents.

A major complication of bosentan includes a dose-dependent increase in liver transaminases, which necessitates discontinuation in 2% and dose adjustment in 8% to 12% of patients. Hepatic toxicity can occur. Teratogenicity is a class effect of these medications. Delayed hemodynamic benefit, compared to the immediate effect of prostacyclins, should also be expected. Bosentan can alter levels of concurrently dosed oral contraceptives, PDE inhibitors, or HIV antiretroviral drugs. Sitaxsentan use has been complicated by supertherapeutic anticoagulation.

PHOSPHODIESTERASE INHIBITORS

Originally marketed for erectile dysfunction (ED), oral PDE5 inhibitors such as sildenafil (Revatio) selectively inhibit the cGMP-specific enzyme PDE5, enabling endogenous NO to exert a more sustained effect.[115] This PDE is highly abundant in pulmonary vasculature, making such medications relatively selective pulmonary vasodilators. A more recently approved PDE5 inhibitor for use in PAH includes tadalafil. In patients with lung fibrosis and PAH, acute administration of sildenafil surpasses the vasodilating effect of NO. The effect is similar to intravenous epoprostenol, except sildenafil is more selective for better ventilated areas of the lung, resulting in improved gas exchange. Clinical efficacy has been reported with use of sildenafil in patients with primary PAH and PAH associated with congenital shunts, SLE, and HIV. Benefits with treatment include improved symptoms and hemodynamics, and increased 6-minute walk distance. In a multicenter double-blinded, randomized, placebo-controlled study of sildenafil treatment for PAH, significant improvements in exercise ability and quality of life have been observed; in the open-label follow-up study, 95% survival was measured at 1 year.[116]

Major side effects of PDE5 inhibitors include systemic hypotension, especially in the setting of nitroglycerin use. Approved dosing of sildenafil for PAH is three times daily, whereas tadalafil is typically a once-daily medication. Currently, PDE inhibitors are approved for functional class II-III PAH patients as first-line agents, and for class IV patients as second-line agents.

PROSTACYCLIN AND PROSTACYCLIN ANALOGS

Prostacyclin is an endogenous prostaglandin (prostaglandin I$_2$) that causes vasodilation and inhibits platelet aggregation. It also has antiproliferative and weak fibrinolytic activities. Intravenous prostacyclin (epoprostenol [Flolan]) was first used to treat PAH in the early 1980s. Since then, multiple trials of epoprostenol have demonstrated improved survival, exercise capacity, and hemodynamics in patients with PAH compared with conventional treatment.[117] Epoprostenol was approved for use in PAH in 1995; it is now considered the treatment of choice in patients with functional class IV PAH and is an alternative to lung transplantation.[107] A chronic, perhaps remodeling, effect of epoprostenol has additionally been suggested by several findings. Patients who have no acute response may demonstrate a delayed hemodynamic improvement. Hemodynamic improvement increases in patients who show an initial response, and RV dysfunction improves after long-term therapy.

Epoprostenol has an extremely short half-life (approximately 3-6 minutes), must be kept cold, and must be administered through a central venous catheter. It is started in the hospital, employing a PA catheter with continuous monitoring. Some clinicians continue the dose escalation until limited by side effects or until there is a plateau in the hemodynamic response. Notably, initiation of epoprostenol can lead to increased CO with LV strain, or isolated pulmonary edema, with rapid clinical deterioration. Long-term dose requirements are highly variable among patients, and further dose increases are made on an outpatient setting on the basis of clinical symptoms, exercise testing, and hemodynamic measurements. Common side effects include jaw pain, headache, diarrhea, flushing, leg pain, nausea, and vomiting. Patients also tend to develop tachyphylaxis to epoprostenol over time.

Major limitations to use of epoprostenol include the need for permanent central venous access, with the associated small risk of catheter-related infection or air embolism, the capacity to handle the catheter and pump, and the high cost of the drug. Complexities of epoprostenol administration have led investigators to search for alternative agents.[118]

The prostacyclin analogs treprostinil (Remodulin), iloprost (Ventavis), and beraprost have been tested in 12-week placebo-controlled trials.[117] All these agents have demonstrated significant improvements in mean exercise capacity. Treprostinil (Remodulin, UT-15) has a longer half-life (≈4 hours) than epoprostenol and can be delivered intravenously or subcutaneously with a pump system similar to that used with subcutaneous insulin. Treprostinil does not require reconstitution or cold temperature. Pain at the site of subcutaneous infusion is a frequent problem that requires cessation of the drug in 8% to 12% of patients. Iloprost is another chemically stable analog that can be given intravenously and by inhaled routes. Iloprost can be used in a nebulized form that must be inhaled 6 to 9 times daily for a continuous effect. Beraprost is an oral analog taken four times daily. Treprostinil and iloprost are approved for PAH therapy—treprostinil for functional class II-IV and iloprost for functional class II-IV.

Treatment of Pulmonary Arterial Hypertension Associated with Specific Diseases

Current treatment guidelines do not distinguish between PAH sub-groups in initial therapy recommendations, but most of the cited data supporting vasodilator therapies have originated from patient populations suffering from idiopathic PAH. Additionally, vasodilator therapy in PAH patients with collagen vascular diseases has been substantially studied with good evidence for benefit.[119] As in idiopathic PAH, baseline hemodynamic data do not predict a response to epoprostenol in PAH associated with scleroderma. The acute vasodilator response is present in an even smaller proportion of patients with collagen vascular diseases than with idiopathic PAH. Accordingly, calcium channel blockers are not beneficial in this group of patients.[120] Nonetheless, epoprostenol can be effective in improving symptoms, hemodynamics, and survival. Skin lesions in patients with scleroderma may also improve substantially with this treatment.[121] Case reports of successful epoprostenol treatment of PAH in patients with SLE also exist, but treatment in this group has been complicated by severe thrombocytopenia. Patient outcomes with CREST/scleroderma have also been studied, with improved symptoms and hemodynamics after use of oral endothelin receptor antagonists.

Efficacy of such treatment in other PAH subgroups has been studied, but in smaller numbers of patients. Epoprostenol has been shown to improve functional capacity, oxygen saturation, and hemodynamics in a group of adults with Eisenmenger's syndrome who were suffering from NYHA class III and IV heart failure.[122] Small numbers of adults with repaired or unrepaired congenital heart disease have also been included in clinical trials of endothelin receptor blockers and PDE5 inhibitors; improvement in hemodynamics, exercise capacity, and symptoms have been demonstrated.[123–125] Epoprostenol has also been used successfully in patients with PAH secondary to HIV infection. In patients suffering from portopulmonary hypertension, such treatment has facilitated successful liver transplantation.[96] There are additional reports of improvement in PAH secondary to portopulmonary hypertension with the use of β-blockers and nitrates, which may also decrease the incidence of variceal bleeding. Yet, caveats to PAH treatment exist for this special patient population. Anticoagulation in these patients is controversial because of the risk of hemorrhage. Furthermore, the liver toxicity associated with bosentan and sitaxsentan make these unacceptable choices for patients with hepatic disease.

Disease Course, Prognosis, and Monitoring

Prior to the introduction of vasodilator therapies, median survival among patients diagnosed with PAH in the United States between 1981 and 1985 was 2.8 years, with single-year survival rates of 68% at 1 year, 48% at 3 years, and 34% at 5 years.[2] Given such a bleak prognosis, most patients were referred for lung transplantation at the time of diagnosis. With the advent of effective medical therapies to ameliorate disease, survival and quality of life have improved substantially. Currently, at the time of diagnosis, patients begin medical therapy with serial reassessments. Five-year survival among epoprostenol-treated patients is now 47% to 55%, with better than 70% 5-year survival among those improving to functional class I or II.[126,127]

After starting medical therapy, only a small subset of patients benefit from immediate hemodynamic improvement.[96] Most, however, display a slow improvement in hemodynamics over several months, as evidenced by increases in 6-minute walk distance and reduced symptoms. These improvements typically peak around 12 to 16 weeks of treatment and can be maintained for years, although significant variability and deterioration is not unexpected.

Frequent evaluations at 3-month intervals, with detailed evaluation of PAP and RV function annually, are necessary to identify patients failing therapy and consider lung transplantation. Patients who develop signs or symptoms of right heart failure have much lower survival rates than those with only elevations of PAP.

Evidence of poor prognosis after treatment include elevated right atrial pressure, low cardiac index, low mixed venous oxygen saturation, continued functional class III/IV symptoms, poor exercise capacity, pericardial effusion, or elevated B-type natriuretic peptide levels.[100,126,128] In early NIH registry data, lower DLCO and presence of Raynaud phenomenon also portended a worse outcome.[2] Increased PAP itself may also predict worse outcomes when RV function is still relatively normal. Finally, failure to demonstrate improvements after treatment in symptoms, hemodynamics, and exercise capacity correlate with worse outcomes. In these cases, consideration for combination therapy, atrial septostomy, or lung transplantation should be pursued.

Management of Refractory Pulmonary Arterial Hypertension

Combination Therapy

Combination therapy using at least two separate classes of PAH medications has been advocated, based on the potential for additive or synergistic effects. Improvement in hemodynamics, exercise capacity, and symptoms over 12- to 16-week periods have been reported in nonresponders who failed standard drug regimens.[129] Typically, improvement in 6-minute walk distance is modest (20-26 meters) compared to initial response to monotherapy. A single long-term but uncontrolled trial studying protocol-driven combination therapy for patients failing to achieve exercise test goals while on monotherapy reported good survival rates (93%, 83%, and 80% at 1, 2, and 3 years) that are better than historical controls on monotherapy.[130] More rigorous and better controlled long-term studies comparing rates of survival and morbidity indices are ongoing. Currently, combination therapy can be considered for patients with signs of right heart failure, 6-minute walk distance less than 380 meters, and persistent functional class III-IV symptoms despite monotherapy for more than 6 months.

Atrial Septostomy

The rationale for surgical creation of an interatrial orifice to improve survival is based on the observation that survival in PAH depends critically upon RV function, and relieving stress on the RV theoretically improves PAH in general.[131] For example, PAH patients with a patent foramen ovale or Eisenmenger's syndrome tend to carry better cardiac function and survive longer compared with patients without intracardiac defects. A review of 64 cases who underwent atrial septostomy prior to contemporary treatment regimens reported improved clinical status in 47 of 50 patients. Median survival of the 54 patients who survived the procedure was 19.5 months (range, 2-96 months), which represents an improvement compared to treatments available before epoprostenol. However, because of the improved efficacy of currently available vasodilators, atrial septostomy is only considered as a palliative procedure for patients with severe PAH and clinical deterioration despite maximal medical therapy, or as a bridge to transplantation. It should only be attempted in centers with experience in the procedure.

Lung Transplantation

Before the introduction of epoprostenol, transplantation was the treatment of choice for severe PAH. It is still the last option in treating severe PAH and the only available cure.[132] Patients with persistent functional class III or IV symptoms, right atrial pressure above 15 mmHg, or cardiac index below 2 L/min/m² should be considered for lung transplantation. Hemodynamic responses to a 3-month epoprostenol infusion may also aid in identifying a subset of PAH patients who might benefit from being considered earlier for lung transplantation. Poor survival has been noted in patients with NYHA functional classes III and IV who remained in that class or failed to achieve a 30% decrease in PVR after 3 months on continuous IV epoprostenol.

CH
56

Heart-lung and single- and double-lung transplantations have been successfully performed in patients with PAH. Lung transplantation alone has demonstrated that severe RV dysfunction is reversible, indicating that heart transplantation is not necessary unless the patient has cardiac disease unrelated to PH. Availability of single-lung transplantation is greater, considering the scarcity of donor organs, but there are disadvantages in marked ventilation/perfusion mismatching and potential for injury. There may be less functional recovery and higher graft-related complications with single-lung transplant. There may be a slightly higher long-term survival rate with double-lung transplantation.

Survival in the early postoperative period is lower for PAH patients than other patients undergoing lung transplantation. However, long-term outcome in patients with PAH is similar to general transplantation patients.[133] Survival rates at 1, 3, and 5 years after transplantation have been reported as 65%, 55%, and 44%, respectively. Pulmonary arterial hypertension has not been reported to recur after transplantation, although a careful examination of those with genetic predisposition has not been performed.

Previously, patients with collagen vascular disease were excluded from transplantation, but they have recently demonstrated survival rates similar to those of other patient groups. Transplantation can be considered for collagen vascular disease patients in whom extrapulmonary manifestations are not severe. Because of the high intraoperative and perioperative risks, liver transplantation has generally not been offered to patients with portopulmonary hypertension. Pulmonary hemodynamics have been reported to improve with liver transplantation, however, and the risk of mortality at surgery is minimal if the mean PAP is less than 35 mmHg. If the PAP is greater than 35 mmHg, pretransplantation management with epoprostenol may decrease mortality risk, and it has been used as a bridge to transplantation.

Experimental Therapies

In addition to the more established therapies for PAH, additional intriguing yet still developing therapeutic approaches are under investigation (Table 56-2). Unlike current medical therapies that at best ameliorate disease, there is optimism that regression of pulmonary vascular remodeling and cure for PAH is possible with these evolving treatment paradigms.

ALTERNATIVE NITRIC OXIDE–BASED THERAPY

In addition to PDE5 inhibitors, a number of therapeutic approaches designed to improve NO production, release, and activity in the pulmonary vasculature are under investigation. Inhaled NO gas has been successfully used to decrease PAP and improve oxygenation and hemodynamics in diverse forms of PAH. However, long-term

TABLE 56-2 Established and Experimental Therapies in Pulmonary Arterial Hypertension

TARGET	GOAL	DRUG
L-type Ca^{2+} channels	Decrease SMC Ca^{2+}	L-type Ca^{2+} channel blockers
Coagulation cascade	Decrease thrombosis	Warfarin
Prostacyclin receptors	Increase cAMP	Epoprostenol
Endothelin receptors A and B	Inhibit constriction and proliferation	Bosentan
Endothelin receptor A	Inhibit constriction and proliferation	Sitaxsentan
PDE5 inhibitors	Increase cGMP	Sildenafil
Guanylate cyclase activators	Increase cGMP	iNO
Novel Targets		
Rho kinase	Decrease Ca^{2+} sensitivity in SMCs	Rho kinase inhibitors: fasudil
Rho A prenylation	Decrease Ca^{2+} sensitivity in SMCs	Statins
Serine elastases	Decrease MMP activation	Elastase inhibitors
Kinase-associated receptors	Inhibit PDGF or EGF activity	Tyrosine kinase inhibitors
PDF kinase	Normalize mitochondrial function	Dichloroacetate
NFAT	Decrease antiapoptotic bcl-2; slow proliferation	Cyclosporine A
Immune system	Immunosuppression	Mycophenolate mofetil
Survivin	Inhibits antiapoptotic effect of survivin	Transfection of dominant negative
Guanylate cyclase	Increase cGMP	Direct sGC activators (e.g., Riociguat [BAY 63-2521]- DHEA)
COX	Inhibit TxA_2	Aspirin
Ornithine decarboxylase	Inhibit polyamine synthesis	α-Difluoromethylornithine
CDKI γ27	Inhibit SMC proliferation	Heparin
PPAR-γ	Increase PPAR-γ activity	Rosiglitazone
Angiopoietin and TIE2	Inhibit SMC proliferation	Adenoviral gene transfection
Serotonin transporter	Inhibit SMC proliferation	SSRI
VPAC 1 and 2 receptors	Inhibit SMC proliferation	VIP, inhaled
Adrenomedullin receptors	Inhibit SMC proliferation, vasodilation	Adrenomedullin
BMPR2	Enhance BMPR2 signaling	Adenoviral transfection and/or enhancing receptor trafficking to membrane
eNOS	Increase cGMP and NO signaling	eNOS-transfected EPCs
eNOS	Increase cGMP and NO signaling	VEGF-transfected fibroblasts

NO therapy is cumbersome, necessitates continuous inhalation, and must be monitored carefully to avoid toxicity with nitrogen oxides and methemoglobin. Alternative strategies to deliver NO include the use of NONOates, compounds that release predictable levels of NO when exposed to physiological pH. Such compounds have been used by daily nebulization in rodent PAH models, with reduction of PAP without systemic hypotension.[134]

Another avenue of increasing NO levels in PAH relies upon enhancing NOS activity. Tetrahydrobiopterin (BH4) is an important NOS cofactor that enzymatically links oxygenation of L-arginine to create NO and L-citrulline. BH4 levels may be decreased in PAH patients, so administration of BH4 in its synthetic form (sapropterin) may hold promise in PAH to increase NOS activity and NO levels in the pulmonary vasculature.[3]

Finally, NO-independent sGC activators have been developed for PAH patients.[44] Both heme-dependent (BAY 41-2272) and heme-independent (BAY 58-2667 and HMR-1766) sGC activators exist.[135] BAY 41-2272 stimulates sGC directly and sensitizes sGC to NO, resulting in synergism. It improves pulmonary hemodynamics in models of PH. NO-independent sGC activators appear to provide an additive rather than synergistic effect when combined with NO donors. Both BAY 41-2272 and BAY 58-2667 ameliorate PAH in rodent models, yet this benefit is partially dependent on endogenous NOS activity. BAY 63-2521 is an oral agent, has a favorable safety profile, and is currently under phase III clinical study in PAH. Interestingly, dehydroepiandrosterone (DHEA), an endogenous steroid, also increases sGC expression, activates vasodilatory calcium-sensitive potassium channels (BKCa) in vascular smooth muscle, and inhibits hypoxic PH in rats.[136] More data are necessary before testing in human trials.

SEROTONIN AND SEROTONIN TRANSPORTER INHIBITORS

Terguride is a potent antagonist of 5-hydroxytryptamine receptors and is currently in a phase II study for PAH patients.[3] It has already received orphan drug status in Europe. PRX-08066 is a selective 5-hydroxytryptamine 2B receptor antagonist that inhibits hypoxia-mediated increases in PAP in humans and is also under phase II trial study. Given the importance of SERT in the biology of serotonin signaling, synergistic inhibition of both SERT and serotonin receptors may represent a potent future strategy for therapeutic benefit.

BMPR2-TARGETED THERAPIES

Recent advances linking BMPR2 haploinsufficiency to PAH suggests that enhancing BMPR2 expression or activity may benefit or reverse PAH progression. Gene replacement therapy has been proposed but has yet to show success in animal models. It has also been found that some mutant forms of BMPR2 in PAH result in impaired trafficking to the cell surface rather than decreased expression.[137] In that case, medications that improve protein trafficking (e.g., sodium 4-phenybutyrate as used in cystic fibrosis) may be useful; however, it remains uncertain how much mutant BMPR2 must reach the cell membrane to result in a relevant effect in vivo. Finally, dysfunction of BMPR2 can lead to increased signaling via other TGF receptor superfamily members such as the TGF-β/activin receptor-like kinase 5. Notably, SB525334, an inhibitor of TGF-β/activin receptor-like kinase 5, reverses PAH and RVH in a rodent model and may have therapeutic benefit.[138]

TYROSINE KINASE INHIBITORS

Initial experience with the tyrosine kinase inhibitor imatinib and the "multikinase inhibitor" sorafenib in PAH patients have been encouraging but results are still preliminary. In humans, there are case reports of beneficial effects in adding imatinib to conventional therapy.[79] Sorafenib reverses PAH and RV remodeling in monocrotaline-treated rats.[80] Phase I clinical trials studying both medications have been performed recently.

RHO KINASE INHIBITORS

Rho kinase inhibitors (i.e., Y-27632, fasudil) have been developed for study in the PAH population.[139] These medications reduce PAP in multiple rodent models of PAH. In humans, fasudil induces modest but immediate reductions in PVR. However, a common adverse side effect includes systemic vasodilation and hypotension. Alternative delivery options such as inhaled or nebulized formulations may allow circumvention of this side effect.

Interestingly, one of the pleiotropic effects of HMG CoA reductase inhibitors (statins) includes inhibition of rho kinase activity. In some rodent studies, simvastatin reduces PAH and demonstrates a significant improvement in survival[140,141]; however, these beneficial effects have not been replicated in all rodent models.[142] Nonetheless, several statin trails in human PAH are underway.

MISCELLANEOUS PATHWAYS

Therapeutic targets in several additional pathogenic pathways have been studied to varying degrees. Inhaled adrenomedullin modestly reduces PVR and increases peak oxygen consumption during exercise in humans with PAH.[143] Nebulized VIP improves pulmonary hemodynamics in PAH to a larger degree, and if continued for 3 months, reduces PVR and improves 6-minute walk distance[56]; however, VIP is susceptible to rapid degradation. A sustained-release liposomal VIP preparation is currently under development. Heparins and inhibitors of angiopoietin 1, STAT3, polyamines, survivin, and the cell cycle have also been proposed for therapeutic benefit, but with varying degrees of success.[3]

ENDOTHELIAL PROGENITOR CELLS

Progenitor cell infusion represents a potentially powerful, but currently nebulous, therapeutic possibility. Specifically, endothelial progenitor cells (EPCs) arise from mesodermal stem cells or hemangioblasts in the bone marrow. From there, they are released and circulate in blood until they engraft into sites of ischemia or injury, leading to angiogenesis and revascularization. Circulating EPCs (defined by CD34+/KDR+ and CD34+/CD133+/KDR+ cells) are lower in patients with Eisenmenger's syndrome.[144] Some reports have indicated reduced levels of EPCs in idiopathic PAH patients.[145] Furthermore, the functions of EPCs in cell culture (i.e., colony forming activity, adherence, migration, apoptotic potential) differ from those isolated from PAH patients as compared with normal controls.[144–146] Administration of EPCs in rats has resulted in improvement in pulmonary hemodynamics, vascular remodeling, and survival in models of PAH.[147] Additionally, two small studies in which adults[148] and children[149] with idiopathic PAH were given a single infusion of autologous mononuclear cells provides support for the therapeutic potential of such therapy. A therapeutic trial has begun to assess the safety of administering such cells in patients with PAH.

Much still remains unclear regarding regenerative cell-based therapy. Differences in markers used to identify EPCs have complicated interpretation of results. The complex biology of EPCs upon engraftment has not been delineated and may carry detrimental consequences in certain clinical contexts. Previously reported beneficial effects of progenitor cells may very likely result from paracrine effects of secreted factors, rather than true engraftment and transdifferentiation to healthy endothelium. In addition, some investigators argue that EPCs promote development of plexogenic lesions, suggesting that their use may worsen end-stage disease. Caution is certainly warranted before such a therapeutic avenue can be pursued on a large scale.

Conclusions

Pulmonary arterial hypertension is a clinical syndrome of vascular disease with a stereotyped pattern of histopathology and is related to a variety of secondary disease states. It has become increasingly clear that development of PAH entails a complex multifactorial

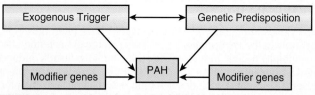

FIGURE 56-8 **Paradigm for the "multiple-hit" hypothesis promoting pulmonary arterial hypertension (PAH).** Susceptible persons with genetic or acquired traits do not progress to PAH without suffering from additional insults that are synergistic in the pathogenesis of disease.

pathophysiology. Although genetic mutations, exogenous exposures, and acquired disease states can predispose to PAH, no one factor identified thus far is sufficient alone to fully drive the pathogenic process. Similar to carcinogenesis, in which a susceptible person with a specific genetic mutation requires additional injuries to manifest disease, a "multiple-hit" hypothesis has emerged to explain progression to clinical PAH (Fig. 56-8). More delineated mechanisms of disease have focused on the end-stage condition and the effects of the imbalance of multiple vascular effectors. Some unifying mechanisms of disease have become more apparent, linking regulation of these effectors into a more cohesive model. As a result, effective therapeutic approaches have been developed to ameliorate disease and improve survival.

Nonetheless, our understanding of these complex cellular processes is incomplete. In part, this fact stems from the great complexity of overlapping pathogenic mechanisms that drive this unique disease. In the postgenomic era, it is conceivable that complex clinical syndromes such as PAH can be redefined based on growing genomic, transcriptional, and proteomic data. A systems-based network analysis may therefore be helpful in identifying common overarching pathways of pathogenesis and aid understanding of the genetic and mechanistic links among primary disease triggers and end-stage disease.

Additionally, a challenge of research in PAH is lack of a small animal model that can be followed and genetically manipulated from initiation through progression to severe disease. There has been some success in physiological study of PAH in larger mammals, but identification of contributors in the molecular process of pulmonary remodeling has been difficult, owing to incomplete genetic data and tools specific for these models.[150,151] Conversely, although genetic and molecular studies in the mouse are more tractable, induction of significant PAH in murine models has been challenging. Nonetheless, recent advances have hinted at the possibility of more tractable animal models of PAH, which would be useful for combining genetic study and pathophysiological exposures.

Finally, with decreasing numbers of PAH patients undergoing transplantation, the ability for the researcher to obtain human PAH tissue for molecular analysis via traditional routes is dwindling. Nonetheless, with advances in fields such as pulmonary artery catheterization, inducible stem cell biology and others, the intricate molecular study of even complex human diseased tissue such as in PAH may be much more feasible in the coming years. The next decade of research will hopefully lead to vast improvements in disease prevention for at-risk individuals, diagnosis of disease at earlier time points, and perhaps identification of therapeutic targets useful for regression of the pathogenic process itself.

REFERENCES

1. Simonneau G, Robbins IM, Beghetti M, et al: Updated clinical classification of pulmonary hypertension, *J Am Coll Cardiol* 54(1 Suppl):S43–S54, 2009.
2. D'Alonzo GE, Barst RJ, Ayres SM, et al: Survival in patients with primary pulmonary hypertension. Results from a national prospective registry, *Ann Intern Med* 115(5):343–349, 1991.
3. Archer SL, Weir EK, Wilkins MR: Basic science of pulmonary arterial hypertension for clinicians: new concepts and experimental therapies, *Circulation* 121(18):2045–2066, 2010.
4. Butrous G, Ghofrani HA, Grimminger F: Pulmonary vascular disease in the developing world, *Circulation* 118(17):1758–1766, 2008.
5. Rich S, Dantzker DR, Ayres SM, et al: Primary pulmonary hypertension. A national prospective study, *Ann Intern Med* 107(2):216–223, 1987.
6. Widlitz A, Barst RJ: Pulmonary arterial hypertension in children, *Eur Respir J* 21(1):155–176, 2003.
7. Farber H, Loscalzo J: Pulmonary arterial hypertension, *N Engl J Med* 351(16):1655–1665, 2004.
8. Chan SY, Loscalzo J: Pathogenic mechanisms of pulmonary arterial hypertension, *J Mol Cell Cardiol* 44(1):14–30, 2008.
9. Trembath R, Thomson JJ, Machado R, et al: Clinical and molecular genetic features of pulmonary hypertension in patients with hereditary hemorrhagic telangiectasia, *N Engl J Med* 345(5):325–334, 2001.
10. Chaouat A, Coulet F, Favre C, et al: Endoglin germline mutation in a patient with hereditary haemorrhagic telangiectasia and dexfenfluramine associated pulmonary arterial hypertension, *Thorax* 59(5):446–448, 2004.
11. Lane K, Machado R, Pauciulo M, et al: Heterozygous germline mutations in BMPR2, encoding a TGF-beta receptor, cause familial primary pulmonary hypertension. The International PPH Consortium, *Nat Genet* 26(1):81–84, 2000.
12. Newman J, Wheeler L, Lane K, et al: Mutation in the gene for bone morphogenetic protein receptor II as a cause of primary pulmonary hypertension in a large kindred, *N Engl J Med* 345(5):319–324, 2001 [Erratum, *N Engl J Med* 2345:1506, 2001, 2346:1258, 2002].
13. Aldred M, Machado R, James V, et al: Characterization of the BMPR2 5′-untranslated region and a novel mutation in pulmonary hypertension, *Am J Respir Crit Care Med* Epublication.
14. Shi Y, Massagueé J: Mechanisms of TGF-beta signaling from cell membrane to nucleus, *Cell* 113(6):685–700, 2003.
15. Atkinson C, Stewart S, Upton P, et al: Primary pulmonary hypertension is associated with reduced pulmonary vascular expression of type II bone morphogenetic protein receptor, *Circulation* 105(14):1672–1678, 2002.
16. Teichert-Kuliszewska K, Kutryk M, Kuliszewski M, et al: Bone morphogenetic protein receptor-2 signaling promotes pulmonary arterial endothelial cell survival: implications for loss-of-function mutations in the pathogenesis of pulmonary hypertension, *Circ Res* 98(2):209–217, 2006.
17. Beppu H, Ichinose F, Kawai N, et al: BMPR-II heterozygous mice have mild pulmonary hypertension and an impaired pulmonary vascular remodeling response to prolonged hypoxia, *Am J Physiol Lung Cell Mol Physiol* 287(6):L1241–L1247, 2004.
18. West J, Fagan K, Steudel W, et al: Pulmonary hypertension in transgenic mice expressing a dominant-negative BMPRII gene in smooth muscle, *Circ Res* 94(8):1109–1114, 2004.
19. Morrell NW, Adnot S, Archer SL, et al: Cellular and molecular basis of pulmonary arterial hypertension, *J Am Coll Cardiol* 54(1 Suppl):S20–S31, 2009.
20. Launay J, Herveé P, Peoc'h KT, et al: Function of the serotonin 5-hydroxytryptamine 2B receptor in pulmonary hypertension, *Nat Med* 8(10):1129–1135, 2002.
21. Eddahibi S, Chaouat A, Morrell N, et al: Polymorphism of the serotonin transporter gene and pulmonary hypertension in chronic obstructive pulmonary disease, *Circulation* 108(15):1839–1844, 2003.
22. Eddahibi S, Raffestin B, Launay J, et al: Effect of dexfenfluramine treatment in rats exposed to acute and chronic hypoxia, *Am J Respir Crit Care Med* 157(4 Pt 1):1111–1119, 1998.
23. Long L, MacLean M, Jeffery T, et al: Serotonin increases susceptibility to pulmonary hypertension in BMPR2-deficient mice, *Circ Res* 98(6):818–827, 2006.
24. MacLean M, Deuchar G, Hicks M, et al: Overexpression of the 5-hydroxytryptamine transporter gene: effect on pulmonary hemodynamics and hypoxia-induced pulmonary hypertension, *Circulation* 109(17):2150–2155, 2004.
25. Keegan A, Morecroft I, Smillie D, et al: Contribution of the 5-HT(1B) receptor to hypoxia-induced pulmonary hypertension: converging evidence using 5-HT(1B)-receptor knockout mice and the 5-HT(1B/1D)-receptor antagonist GR127935, *Circ Res* 89(12):1231–1239, 2001.
26. Moudgil R, Michelakis E, Archer S: Hypoxic pulmonary vasoconstriction, *J Appl Physiol* 98(1):390–403, 2005.
27. Sweeney M, Yuan J: Hypoxic pulmonary vasoconstriction: role of voltage-gated potassium channels, *Respir Res* 1(1):40–48, 2000.
28. Vij R, Machado RF: Pulmonary complications of hemoglobinopathies, *Chest* 138(4):973–983.
29. Hsu L, Champion H, Campbell-Lee S, et al: Hemolysis in sickle cell mice causes pulmonary hypertension due to global impairment in nitric oxide bioavailability, *Blood* 109(7):3088–3098, 2007.
30. Hu W, Jin R, Zhang J, et al: The critical roles of platelet activation and reduced NO bioavailability in fatal pulmonary arterial hypertension in a murine hemolysis model, *Blood* 116(9):1613–1622.
31. Stauber RE, Olschewski H: Portopulmonary hypertension: short review, *Eur J Gastroenterol Hepatol* 22(4):385–390.
32. Le Pavec J, Humbert M, Mouthon L, et al: Systemic sclerosis-associated pulmonary arterial hypertension, *Am J Respir Crit Care Med* 181(12):1285–1293.
33. Hassoun PM: Pulmonary arterial hypertension complicating connective tissue diseases, *Semin Respir Crit Care Med* 30(4):429–439, 2009.
34. Peacock A: Primary pulmonary hypertension, *Thorax* 54(12):1107–1118, 1999 [*Thorax* 1155(1103):1254, 2000].
35. Degano B, Sitbon O, Simonneau G: Pulmonary arterial hypertension and HIV infection, *Semin Respir Crit Care Med* 30(4):440–447, 2009.
36. Galiè N, Manes A, Uguccioni L, et al: Primary pulmonary hypertension: insights into pathogenesis from epidemiology, *Chest* 114(3 Suppl):184S–194S, 1998.
37. Cool C, Rai P, Yeager M, et al: Expression of human herpesvirus 8 in primary pulmonary hypertension, *N Engl J Med* 349(12):1113–1122, 2003.
38. Beghetti M, Tissot C: Pulmonary arterial hypertension in congenital heart diseases, *Semin Respir Crit Care Med* 30(4):421–428, 2009.
39. Webb G, Gatzoulis M: Atrial septal defects in the adult: recent progress and overview, *Circulation* 114(15):1645–1653, 2006.
40. Topper J, Gimbrone MJ: Blood flow and vascular gene expression: fluid shear stress as a modulator of endothelial phenotype, *Mol Med Today* 5(1):40–46, 1999.
41. Sakao S, Taraseviciene-Stewart L, Lee J, et al: Initial apoptosis is followed by increased proliferation of apoptosis-resistant endothelial cells, *FASEB J* 19(9):1178–1180, 2005.

42. Cool CD, Deutsch G: Pulmonary arterial hypertension from a pediatric perspective, *Pediatr Dev Pathol* 11(3):169–177, 2008.

43. Robles A, Shure D: Gender issues in pulmonary vascular disease, *Clin Chest Med* 25(2):373–377, 2004.

44. Coggins MP, Bloch KD: Nitric oxide in the pulmonary vasculature, *Arterioscler Thromb Vasc Biol* 27(9):1877–1885, 2007.

45. Gladwin M, Schechter A: NO contest: nitrite versus S-nitroso-hemoglobin, *Circ Res* 94(7):851–855, 2004.

46. Griffiths M, Evans T: Inhaled nitric oxide therapy in adults, *N Engl J Med* 353(25):2683–2695, 2005.

47. Gerber J, Voelkel N, Nies A, et al: Moderation of hypoxic vasoconstriction by infused arachidonic acid: role of PGI2, *J Appl Physiol Respir Env Exercise Physiol* 49:107–112, 1980.

48. Tuder R, Cool C, Geraci M, et al: Prostacyclin synthase expression is decreased in lungs from patients with severe pulmonary hypertension, *Am J Respir Crit Care Med* 159(6):1925–1932, 1999.

49. Christman B, McPherson C, Newman J, et al: An imbalance between the excretion of thromboxane and prostacyclin metabolites in pulmonary hypertension, *N Engl J Med* 327(2):70–75, 1992.

50. Strauss W, Edelman J: Prostanoid therapy for pulmonary arterial hypertension, *Clin Chest Med* 28(1):127–142, 2007.

51. Davie NJ, Schermuly RT, Weissmann N, et al: The science of endothelin-1 and endothelin receptor antagonists in the management of pulmonary arterial hypertension: current understanding and future studies, *Eur J Clin Invest* 39(Suppl 2):38–49, 2009.

52. Jeffery T, Morrell N: Molecular and cellular basis of pulmonary vascular remodeling in pulmonary hypertension, *Prog Cardiovasc Dis* 45(3):173–202, 2002.

53. Allen S, Chatfield B, Koppenhafer S, et al: Circulating immunoreactive endothelin-1 in children with pulmonary hypertension. Association with acute hypoxic pulmonary vasoreactivity, *Am Rev Respir Dis* 148(2):519–522, 1993.

54. Giaid A, Yanagisawa M, Langleben D, et al: Expression of endothelin-1 in the lungs of patients with pulmonary hypertension, *N Engl J Med* 328(24):1732–1739, 1993.

55. Langleben D: Endothelin receptor antagonists in the treatment of pulmonary arterial hypertension, *Clin Chest Med* 28(1):117–125, 2007.

56. Petkov V, Mosgoeller W, Ziesche R, et al: Vasoactive intestinal peptide as a new drug for treatment of primary pulmonary hypertension, *J Clin Invest* 111(9):1339–1346, 2003.

57. Said S, Hamidi S, Dickman K, et al: Moderate pulmonary arterial hypertension in male mice lacking the vasoactive intestinal peptide gene, *Circulation* 115(10):1260–1268, 2007.

58. Söderman C, Eriksson L, Juhlin-Dannfelt A, et al: Effect of vasoactive intestinal polypeptide (VIP) on pulmonary ventilation-perfusion relationships and central haemodynamics in healthy subjects, *Clin Physiol* 13(6):677–685, 1993.

59. Haydar S, Sarti J, Grisoni E: Intravenous vasoactive intestinal polypeptide lowers pulmonary-to-systemic vascular resistance ratio in a neonatal piglet model of pulmonary arterial hypertension, *J Pediatr Surg* 42(5):758–764, 2007.

60. Hansmann G, Wagner R, Schellong S, et al: Pulmonary arterial hypertension is linked to insulin resistance and reversed by peroxisome proliferator-activated receptor-gamma activation, *Circulation* 115(10):1275–1284, 2007.

61. Hansmann G, de Jesus Perez VA, Alastalo TP, et al: An antiproliferative BMP-2/PPARgamma/apoE axis in human and murine SMCs and its role in pulmonary hypertension, *J Clin Invest* 118(5):1846–1857, 2008.

62. Nagaya N, Nishikimi T, Okano Y, et al: Plasma brain natriuretic peptide levels increase in proportion to the extent of right ventricular dysfunction in pulmonary hypertension, *J Am Coll Cardiol* 31(1):202–208, 1998.

63. Zhao L, Winter RJ, Krausz T, et al: Effects of continuous infusion of atrial natriuretic peptide on the pulmonary hypertension induced by chronic hypoxia in rats, *Clin Sci (Lond)* 81(3):379–385, 1991.

64. Baliga RS, Zhao L, Madhani M, et al: Synergy between natriuretic peptides and phosphodiesterase 5 inhibitors ameliorates pulmonary arterial hypertension, *Am J Respir Crit Care Med* 178(8):861–869, 2008.

65. Qi JG, Ding YG, Tang CS, et al: Chronic administration of adrenomedullin attenuates hypoxic pulmonary vascular structural remodeling and inhibits proadrenomedullin N-terminal 20-peptide production in rats, *Peptides* 28(4):910–919, 2007.

66. Li X, Zhang X, Leathers R, et al: Notch3 signaling promotes the development of pulmonary arterial hypertension, *Nat Med* 15(11):1289–1297, 2009.

67. Loscalzo J, Kohane I, Barabasi A: Human disease classification in the postgenomic era: complex systems approach to human pathobiology, *Mol Syst Biol* 3:124, 2007.

68. Bonnet S, Michelakis ED, Porter CJ, et al: An abnormal mitochondrial-hypoxia inducible factor-1alpha-Kv channel pathway disrupts oxygen sensing and triggers pulmonary arterial hypertension in fawn hooded rats: similarities to human pulmonary arterial hypertension, *Circulation* 113(22):2630–2641, 2006.

69. Xu W, Koeck T, Lara AR, et al: Alterations of cellular bioenergetics in pulmonary artery endothelial cells, *Proc Natl Acad Sci U S A* 104(4):1342–1347, 2007.

70. Semenza GL: Hypoxia-inducible factor 1: regulator of mitochondrial metabolism and mediator of ischemic preconditioning, *Biochim Biophys Acta* 2010; Aug 21 [Epub ahead of print].

71. Archer SL, Gomberg-Maitland M, Maitland ML, et al: Mitochondrial metabolism, redox signaling, and fusion: a mitochondria-ROS-HIF-1alpha-Kv1.5 O2-sensing pathway at the intersection of pulmonary hypertension and cancer, *Am J Physiol Heart Circ Physiol* 294(2):H570–H578, 2008.

72. Sharma S, Taegtmeyer H, Adrogue J, et al: Dynamic changes of gene expression in hypoxia-induced right ventricular hypertrophy, *Am J Physiol Heart Circ Physiol* 286(3):H1185–H1192, 2004.

73. Young LH, Li J, Baron SJ, et al: AMP-activated protein kinase: a key stress signaling pathway in the heart, *Trends Cardiovasc Med* 15(3):110–118, 2005.

74. Yuan X, Wang J, Juhaszova M, et al: Attenuated K+ channel gene transcription in primary pulmonary hypertension, *Lancet* 351(9104):726–727, 1998.

75. Remillard C, Tigno D, Platoshyn O, et al: Function of Kv1.5 channels and genetic variations of KCNA5 in patients with idiopathic pulmonary arterial hypertension, *Am J Physiol Cell Physiol* 292(5):C1837–C1853, 2007.

76. Pozeg Z, Michelakis E, McMurtry M, et al: In vivo gene transfer of the O2-sensitive potassium channel Kv1.5 reduces pulmonary hypertension and restores hypoxic pulmonary vasoconstriction in chronically hypoxic rats, *Circulation* 107(15):2037–2044, 2003.

77. Merklinger SL, Jones PL, Martinez EC, et al: Epidermal growth factor receptor blockade mediates smooth muscle cell apoptosis and improves survival in rats with pulmonary hypertension, *Circulation* 112(3):423–431, 2005.

78. Schermuly RT, Dony E, Ghofrani HA, et al: Reversal of experimental pulmonary hypertension by PDGF inhibition, *J Clin Invest* 115(10):2811–2821, 2005.

79. Ghofrani HA, Seeger W, Grimminger F: Imatinib for the treatment of pulmonary arterial hypertension, *N Engl J Med* 353(13):1412–1413, 2005.

80. Moreno-Vinasco L, Gomberg-Maitland M, Maitland ML, et al: Genomic assessment of a multikinase inhibitor, sorafenib, in a rodent model of pulmonary hypertension, *Physiol Genomics* 33(2):278–291, 2008.

81. Shimokawa H, Takeshita A: Rho-kinase is an important therapeutic target in cardiovascular medicine, *Arterioscler Thromb Vasc Biol* 25(9):1767–1775, 2005.

82. Nagaoka T, Morio Y, Casanova N, et al: Rho/Rho kinase signaling mediates increased basal pulmonary vascular tone in chronically hypoxic rats, *Am J Physiol Lung Cell Mol Physiol* 287(4):L665–L672, 2004.

83. Oka M, Homma N, Taraseviciene-Stewart L, et al: Rho kinase-mediated vasoconstriction is important in severe occlusive pulmonary arterial hypertension in rats, *Circ Res* 100(6):923–929, 2007.

84. Fukumoto Y, Matoba T, Ito A, et al: Acute vasodilator effects of a Rho-kinase inhibitor, fasudil, in patients with severe pulmonary hypertension, *Heart* 91(3):391–392, 2005.

85. Ishikura K, Yamada N, Ito M, et al: Beneficial acute effects of rho-kinase inhibitor in patients with pulmonary arterial hypertension, *Circulation J* 70(2):174–178, 2006.

86. Taraseviciene-Stewart L, Nicolls MR, Kraskauskas D, et al: Absence of T cells confers increased pulmonary arterial hypertension and vascular remodeling, *Am J Respir Crit Care Med* 175(12):1280–1289, 2007.

87. Ulrich S, Nicolls MR, Taraseviciene L, et al: Increased regulatory and decreased CD8+ cytotoxic T cells in the blood of patients with idiopathic pulmonary arterial hypertension, *Respiration* 75(3):272–280, 2008.

88. Wright L, Tuder R, Wang J, et al: 5-Lipoxygenase and 5-lipoxygenase activating protein (FLAP) immunoreactivity in lungs from patients with primary pulmonary hypertension, *Am J Respir Crit Care Med* 157(1):219–229, 1998.

89. Song Y, Coleman L, Shi J, et al: Inflammation, endothelial injury, and persistent pulmonary hypertension in heterozygous BMPR2-mutant mice, *Am J Physiol Heart Circ Physiol* 295(2):H677–H690, 2008.

90. Rabinovitch M: Pathobiology of pulmonary hypertension. Extracellular matrix, *Clin Chest Med* 22(3):433–449, 2001.

91. Rabinovitch M: Elastase and the pathobiology of unexplained pulmonary hypertension, *Chest* 114(3 Suppl):213S–224S, 1998.

92. Zhu L, Wigle D, Hinek A, et al: The endogenous vascular elastase that governs development and progression of monocrotaline-induced pulmonary hypertension in rats is a novel enzyme related to the serine proteinase adipsin, *J Clin Invest* 94(3):1163–1171, 1994.

93. Jones P, Rabinovitch M: Tenascin-C is induced with progressive pulmonary vascular disease in rats and is functionally related to increased smooth muscle cell proliferation, *Circ Res* 79(6):1131–1142, 1996.

94. Cowan K, Jones P, Rabinovitch M: Elastase and matrix metalloproteinase inhibitors induce regression, and tenascin-C antisense prevents progression, of vascular disease, *J Clin Invest* 105(1):21–34, 2000.

95. Zaidi S, You X, Ciura S, et al: Overexpression of the serine elastase inhibitor elafin protects transgenic mice from hypoxic pulmonary hypertension, *Circulation* 105(4):516–521, 2002.

96. Chin KM, Rubin LJ: Pulmonary arterial hypertension, *J Am Coll Cardiol* 51(16):1527–1538, 2008.

97. Nef HM, Mollmann H, Hamm C, et al: Pulmonary hypertension: updated classification and management of pulmonary hypertension, *Heart* 96(7):552–559, 2010.

98. Chemla D, Castelain V, Herve P, et al: Haemodynamic evaluation of pulmonary hypertension, *Eur Respir J* 20(5):1314–1331, 2002.

99. Sun XG, Hansen JE, Oudiz RJ, et al: Pulmonary function in primary pulmonary hypertension, *J Am Coll Cardiol* 41(6):1028–1035, 2003.

100. Raymond RJ, Hinderliter AL, Willis PW, et al: Echocardiographic predictors of adverse outcomes in primary pulmonary hypertension, *J Am Coll Cardiol* 39(7):1214–1219, 2002.

101. McLaughlin VV, Presberg KW, Doyle RL, et al: Prognosis of pulmonary arterial hypertension: ACCP evidence-based clinical practice guidelines, *Chest* 126(1 Suppl):78S–92S, 2004.

102. Grunig E, Janssen B, Mereles D, et al: Abnormal pulmonary artery pressure response in asymptomatic carriers of primary pulmonary hypertension gene, *Circulation* 102(10):1145–1150, 2000.

103. McLaughlin VV, Archer SL, Badesch DB, et al: ACCF/AHA 2009 expert consensus document on pulmonary hypertension: a report of the American College of Cardiology Foundation Task Force on Expert Consensus Documents and the American Heart Association: developed in collaboration with the American College of Chest Physicians, American Thoracic Society, Inc., and the Pulmonary Hypertension Association, *Circulation* 119(16):2250–2294, 2009.

104. McGoon M, Gutterman D, Steen V, et al: Screening, early detection, and diagnosis of pulmonary arterial hypertension: ACCP evidence-based clinical practice guidelines, *Chest* 126(1 Suppl):14S–34S, 2004.

105. Humbert M, Trembath RC: Genetics of pulmonary hypertension: from bench to bedside, *Eur Respir J* 20(3):741–749, 2002.

106. Johnson SR, Mehta S, Granton JT: Anticoagulation in pulmonary arterial hypertension: a qualitative systematic review, *Eur Respir J* 28(5):999–1004, 2006.

107. Badesch DB, Abman SH, Simonneau G, et al: Medical therapy for pulmonary arterial hypertension: updated ACCP evidence-based clinical practice guidelines, *Chest* 131(6):1917–1928, 2007.

108. Herveé P, Humbert M, Sitbon O, et al: Pathobiology of pulmonary hypertension: the role of platelets and thrombosis, *Clin Chest Med* 22(3):451–458, 2001.

109. Tonelli AR, Alnuaimat H, Mubarak K: Pulmonary vasodilator testing and use of calcium channel blockers in pulmonary arterial hypertension, *Respir Med* 104(4):481–496

110. Sitbon O, Humbert M, Jais X, et al: Long-term response to calcium channel blockers in idiopathic pulmonary arterial hypertension, *Circulation* 111(23):3105–3111, 2005.

111. Price LC, Howard LS: Endothelin receptor antagonists for pulmonary arterial hypertension: rationale and place in therapy, *Am J Cardiovasc Drugs* 8(3):171–185, 2008.

112. Channick R, Badesch DB, Tapson VF, et al: Effects of the dual endothelin receptor antagonist bosentan in patients with pulmonary hypertension: a placebo-controlled study, *J Heart Lung Transplant* 20(2):262–263, 2001.

113. Rubin LJ, Badesch DB, Barst RJ, et al: Bosentan therapy for pulmonary arterial hypertension, *N Engl J Med* 346(12):896–903, 2002.

114. Barst RJ, Langleben D, Badesch D, et al: Treatment of pulmonary arterial hypertension with the selective endothelin-A receptor antagonist sitaxsentan, *J Am Coll Cardiol* 47(10):2049–2056, 2006.

115. Archer SL, Michelakis ED: Phosphodiesterase type 5 inhibitors for pulmonary arterial hypertension, *N Engl J Med* 361(19):1864–1871, 2009.

116. Galiè N, Ghofrani H, Torbicki A, et al: Sildenafil citrate therapy for pulmonary arterial hypertension, *N Engl J Med* 353(20):2148–2157, 2005.

117. Mubarak KK: A review of prostaglandin analogs in the management of patients with pulmonary arterial hypertension, *Respir Med* 104(1):9–21, 2010.

118. Boutet K, Montani D, Jais X, et al: Therapeutic advances in pulmonary arterial hypertension, *Ther Adv Respir Dis* 2(4):249–265, 2008.

119. Badesch DB, Tapson VF, McGoon MD, et al: Continuous intravenous epoprostenol for pulmonary hypertension due to the scleroderma spectrum of disease. A randomized, controlled trial, *Ann Intern Med* 132(6):425–434, 2000.

120. Galie N, Manes A, Farahani KV, et al: Pulmonary arterial hypertension associated to connective tissue diseases, *Lupus* 14(9):713–717, 2005.

121. Mathai SC, Hassoun PM: Therapy for pulmonary arterial hypertension associated with systemic sclerosis, *Curr Opin Rheumatol* 21(6):642–648, 2009.

122. Rame JE: Pulmonary hypertension complicating congenital heart disease, *Curr Cardiol Rep* 11(4):314–320, 2009.

123. Galie N, Beghetti M, Gatzoulis MA, et al: Bosentan therapy in patients with Eisenmenger syndrome: a multicenter, double-blind, randomized, placebo-controlled study, *Circulation* 114(1):48–54, 2006.

124. Singh TP, Rohit M, Grover A, et al: A randomized, placebo-controlled, double-blind, crossover study to evaluate the efficacy of oral sildenafil therapy in severe pulmonary artery hypertension, *Am Heart J* 151(4):851, e851–e855, 2006.

125. Apostolopoulou SC, Manginas A, Cokkinos DV, et al: Long-term oral bosentan treatment in patients with pulmonary arterial hypertension related to congenital heart disease: a 2-year study, *Heart* 93(3):350–354, 2007.

126. Sitbon O, Humbert M, Nunes H, et al: Long-term intravenous epoprostenol infusion in primary pulmonary hypertension: prognostic factors and survival, *J Am Coll Cardiol* 40(4):780–788, 2002.

127. McLaughlin VV, Shillington A, Rich S: Survival in primary pulmonary hypertension: the impact of epoprostenol therapy, *Circulation* 106(12):1477–1482, 2002.

128. McLaughlin VV, Sitbon O, Badesch DB, et al: Survival with first-line bosentan in patients with primary pulmonary hypertension, *Eur Respir J* 25(2):244–249, 2005.

129. Abraham T, Wu G, Vastey F, et al: Role of combination therapy in the treatment of pulmonary arterial hypertension, *Pharmacotherapy* 30(4):390–404, 2010.

130. Hoeper MM, Markevych I, Spiekerkoetter E, et al: Goal-oriented treatment and combination therapy for pulmonary arterial hypertension, *Eur Respir J* 26(5):858–863, 2005.

131. Corris PA: Atrial septostomy and transplantation for patients with pulmonary arterial hypertension, *Semin Respir Crit Care Med* 30(4):493–501, 2009.

132. Keogh AM, Mayer E, Benza RL, et al: Interventional and surgical modalities of treatment in pulmonary hypertension, *J Am Coll Cardiol* 54(1 Suppl):S67–S77, 2009.

133. Trulock EP, Christie JD, Edwards LB, et al: Registry of the International Society for Heart and Lung Transplantation: twenty-fourth official adult lung and heart-lung transplantation report-2007, *J Heart Lung Transplant* 26(8):782–795, 2007.

134. Hampl V, Tristani-Firouzi M, Hutsell TC, et al: Nebulized nitric oxide/nucleophile adduct reduces chronic pulmonary hypertension, *Cardiovasc Res* 31(1):55–62, 1996.

135. Evgenov OV, Pacher P, Schmidt PM, et al: NO-independent stimulators and activators of soluble guanylate cyclase: discovery and therapeutic potential, *Nat Rev Drug Discov* 5(9):755–768, 2006.

136. Oka M, Karoor V, Homma N, et al: Dehydroepiandrosterone upregulates soluble guanylate cyclase and inhibits hypoxic pulmonary hypertension, *Cardiovasc Res* 74(3):377–387, 2007.

137. Sobolewski A, Rudarakanchana N, Upton PD, et al: Failure of bone morphogenetic protein receptor trafficking in pulmonary arterial hypertension: potential for rescue, *Hum Mol Genet* 17(20):3180–3190, 2008.

138. Thomas M, Docx C, Holmes AM, et al: Activin-like kinase 5 (ALK5) mediates abnormal proliferation of vascular smooth muscle cells from patients with familial pulmonary arterial hypertension and is involved in the progression of experimental pulmonary arterial hypertension induced by monocrotaline, *Am J Pathol* 174(2):380–389, 2009.

139. McMurtry IF, Abe K, Ota H, et al: Rho kinase-mediated vasoconstriction in pulmonary hypertension, *Adv Exp Med Biol* 661:299–308, 2010.

140. Nishimura T, Faul J, Berry G, et al: Simvastatin attenuates smooth muscle neointimal proliferation and pulmonary hypertension in rats, *Am J Respir Crit Care Med* 166(10):1403–1408, 2002.

141. Hu H, Sung A, Zhao G, et al: Simvastatin enhances bone morphogenetic protein receptor type II expression, *Biochem Biophys Res Commun* 339(1):59–64, 2006.

142. McMurtry MS, Bonnet S, Michelakis ED, et al: Statin therapy, alone or with rapamycin, does not reverse monocrotaline pulmonary arterial hypertension: the rapamycin-atorvastatin-simvastatin study, *Am J Physiol Lung Cell Mol Physiol* 293(4):L933–L940, 2007.

143. Nagaya N, Kyotani S, Uematsu M, et al: Effects of adrenomedullin inhalation on hemodynamics and exercise capacity in patients with idiopathic pulmonary arterial hypertension, *Circulation* 109(3):351–356, 2004.

144. Diller GP, van Eijl S, Okonko DO, et al: Circulating endothelial progenitor cells in patients with Eisenmenger syndrome and idiopathic pulmonary arterial hypertension, *Circulation* 117(23):3020–3030, 2008.

145. Junhui Z, Xingxiang W, Guosheng F, et al: Reduced number and activity of circulating endothelial progenitor cells in patients with idiopathic pulmonary arterial hypertension, *Respir Med* 102(7):1073–1079, 2008.

146. Asosingh K, Aldred MA, Vasanji A, et al: Circulating angiogenic precursors in idiopathic pulmonary arterial hypertension, *Am J Pathol* 172(3):615–627, 2008.

147. Zhao YD, Courtman DW, Ng DS, et al: Microvascular regeneration in established pulmonary hypertension by angiogenic gene transfer, *Am J Respir Cell Mol Biol* 35(2):182–189, 2006.

148. Wang XX, Zhang FR, Shang YP, et al: Transplantation of autologous endothelial progenitor cells may be beneficial in patients with idiopathic pulmonary arterial hypertension: a pilot randomized controlled trial, *J Am Coll Cardiol* 49(14):1566–1571, 2007.

149. Zhu JH, Wang XX, Zhang FR, et al: Safety and efficacy of autologous endothelial progenitor cells transplantation in children with idiopathic pulmonary arterial hypertension: open-label pilot study, *Pediatr Transplant* 12(6):650–655, 2008.

150. Medhora M, Bousamra MN, Zhu D, et al: Upregulation of collagens detected by gene array in a model of flow-induced pulmonary vascular remodeling, *Am J Physiol Heart Circ Physiol* 282(2):H414–H422, 2002.

151. Botney M: Role of hemodynamics in pulmonary vascular remodeling: implications for primary pulmonary hypertension, *Am J Respir Crit Care Med* 159(2):361–364, 1999.

CHAPTER 57

Pulmonary Hypertension in Non-Pulmonary Arterial Hypertension Patients

Bradley A. Maron, Joseph Loscalzo

Overview of Pulmonary Hypertension

Definition and Nomenclature

Pulmonary hypertension (PH) is defined as a sustained mean pulmonary arterial blood pressure above 25 mmHg and pulmonary vascular resistance (PVR) of above 3 Wood units (240 dyne/s/cm^{-5}) at rest in the setting of a pulmonary capillary wedge pressure (PCWP) less than 15 mmHg.[1] Pulmonary hypertension is a clinical syndrome typically characterized by hypoxemia, diminished exercise capacity, and dyspnea. In the vast majority of patients, PH develops as a consequence of hypoxic pulmonary vasoconstriction, vascular congestion, or impedance to pulmonary blood flow in the setting of primary lung, cardiac, or pulmonary vascular thromboembolic disease.

In contrast, mean pulmonary arterial hypertension (mPAH), a rare form of PH, results from an interplay between genetic and molecular factors that promotes pulmonary vascular endothelial dysfunction, vascular smooth muscle cell (VSMC) hypertrophy, and negative remodeling of small- and medium-sized pulmonary arteries in the absence of other cardiopulmonary disease.[2] In PAH, pulmonary artery pressure (PAP) is often over 40 mmHg and may reach suprasystemic levels in severe cases; however, this occurs uncommonly in PH from non-PAH etiologies.[3] Thus, PH and PAH are distinct pathophysiological entities, and although clinical signs and symptoms often overlap between these conditions, the terms are not synonymous.[1]

The contemporary PH classification system was created by an international panel of world experts at the 4th World Symposium on PH in 2008 (Dana Point, California) and broadly divides PH patients into two groups: those with PAH or PAH-associated conditions (i.e., formerly *primary* pulmonary hypertension) and PH that occurs in the setting of another cardiopulmonary disease (i.e., formerly *secondary* pulmonary hypertension).[4]

Chapter 56 is devoted to a discussion of PAH and PAH-associated conditions, whereas the current chapter provides an overview of the pathophysiology and treatment of disorders associated with secondary forms of PH. Specifically, this chapter will review primary diseases that modulate PH by causing (1) pulmonary venous hypertension, (2) chronic hypoxia, (3) pulmonary thromboembolism, and (4) mechanical disruption to the normal pulmonary vasculature (i.e., World Health Organization [WHO] PH classification groups 2-5; Box 57-1).[5] In clinical practice and throughout the published literature, the designation *nonpulmonary arterial hypertension pulmonary hypertension* is often invoked to describe these patients.

Epidemiology, Diagnosis, and Natural History

The prevalence of PH in the general population is not well established, and PH incidence varies substantially according to primary disease subtype. A recent report of 455 patients with an elevated left ventricular (LV) end-diastolic pressure (but without left-sided valvular disease) observed that over half had comorbid PH,[6] whereas PH is present in more than 90% of selected chronic obstructive pulmonary disease (COPD) patients.[7,8] Rates of PH vary significantly within a specific primary disease subpopulation as well. For example, Handa et al. reported a 5% PH prevalence rate

in one cohort of asymptomatic or mildly symptomatic sarcoidosis patients despite abnormal chest radiography, restrictive pattern on pulmonary function testing (PFT), and decreased peripheral oxygen saturation levels. If persistent dyspnea is present in sarcoidosis, however, PH prevalence rates increase to over 50%.[9,10]

The likelihood of developing *clinically evident* PH is often tightly linked to comorbid cardiac or lung disease characteristics. For example, symptomatic PH due to impaired LV diastolic function from chronic systemic hypertension is an indolent process that progresses with respect to decline in myocardial compliance.[11] In contrast, severe PH from acute altitude sickness occurs via sudden hypoxia-mediated pulmonary microvascular vasoconstriction and hyperemia, which may occur independently of pulmonary reserve.[12]

Pulmonary hypertension prognosis, treatment choice, and clinical response to therapy are strongly associated with PH disease subtype. At present, goal-directed medical therapy for restoration of pulmonary microvascular function with calcium channel blockers, endothelin receptor antagonists (ERAs), inhaled nitric oxide (iNO), selective phosphodiesterase type 5 (PDE5) inhibition, or prostanoid replacement therapy is approved by the U.S. Food and Drug Administration (FDA) for use only in PAH patients. As is discussed in greater detail later, conclusions from small clinical trials have demonstrated a favorable effect of various PAH therapies on pulmonary hemodynamics and exercise tolerance in some WHO Class 2 thorough 5 conditions,[13] but *inappropriate* administration of advanced PAH therapies to non-PAH patients with PH is likely to be ineffective and possibly harmful.[1,6] Therefore, the emphasis of contemporary diagnostic algorithms is on discrimination of PAH from non-PAH patients[1] (Fig. 57-1A). Comprehensive clinical, radiographic, serological, echocardiographic, and/or invasive hemodynamic testing is often necessary to confirm the absence of disease states that predispose to PH prior to making the diagnosis of PAH[7] (Fig. 57-1B).

Pulmonary hypertension is underrecognized in clinical practice.[14] Initiation of diagnostic testing for PH therefore requires a low index of clinical suspicion among practitioners who must recognize clues that suggest PH pathophysiology, such as familial or genetic risk factors for PAH, or comorbid conditions known to promote elevations in PAP.

Pulmonary Venous Hypertension

Pathophysiology of Pulmonary Hypertension due to Left-Sided Heart Disease

ACUTE LEFT HEART FAILURE

Among the most common causes of PH is left-sided cardiac disease from LV systolic or diastolic dysfunction, or left-sided valvular disease (Table 57-1). In nonvalvular forms of left-sided heart disease, increased LV end-diastolic filling pressure is transmitted retrograde to the pulmonary venous and arterial circulatory beds. Acute changes to normal LV pressure-volume hemodynamics, such as occurs during an acute myocardial infarction (MI) or as a consequence of mitral valve leaflet rupture, predispose to sudden and dramatic increases in left atrial pressure and PAP[15] (Fig. 57-2). Owing to the noncompacted, thin-walled architecture of the right ventricle (RV), acute pressure loading is poorly tolerated and

Box 57-1 Clinical Classification of Pulmonary Hypertension by Etiology*

1. Pulmonary arterial hypertension (PAH)
   1.1 Idiopathic pulmonary arterial hypertension (IPAH)
   1.2 Familial pulmonary arterial hypertension (FPAH)
   1.3 PAH-associated diseases
       1.3.1 Collagen vascular disease
       1.3.2 Congenital systemic-to-pulmonary shunts
       1.3.3 Portal hypertension
       1.3.4 Human immunodeficiency virus (HIV) infection
       1.3.5 Drug and toxins (e.g., anorexogenins)
       1.3.6 Others (e.g., hereditary hemorrhagic telangiectasia, glycogen storage diseases)
   1.4 Associated with primary pulmonary venous or capillary involvement
       1.4.1 Pulmonary veno-occlusive disease (PVOD)
       1.4.2 Pulmonary capillary hemangiomatosis
   1.5 Persistent pulmonary hypertension of the newborn (PPHN)
2. Pulmonary hypertension (PH) with left heart disease
   2.1 Left-sided atrial or ventricular heart disease
   2.2 Left-sided valvular disease
3. PH associated with lung disease and/or hypoxemia
   3.1 Chronic obstructive pulmonary disease (COPD)
   3.2 Interstitial lung disease (ILD)
   3.3 Sleep-disordered breathing (SDB)
   3.4 Alveolar hypoventilation disorders
   3.5 Chronic exposure to high altitude (HA)
   3.6 Developmental abnormalities
4. PH due to chronic thrombotic and/or embolic disease
   4.1 Thromboembolic obstruction of proximal pulmonary arteries (chronic thromboembolic pulmonary hypertension [CTEPH])
   4.2 Thromboembolic obstruction of distal pulmonary arteries (CTEPH)
   4.3 Nonthrombotic pulmonary embolism (PE) (e.g., parasites, foreign body)
5. Miscellaneous causes of PH (sarcoidosis, malignancy, fibrosing mediastinitis, Takayasu's arteritis, iatrogenic)

* Diseases in groups 2 to 5 are reviewed in the current chapter.
Adapted from Simonneau G, Robbins IM, Beghetti M, et al: Updated clinical classification of pulmonary hypertension. J Am Coll Cardiol 54(1 Suppl):S43–S54, 2009.

results in RV systolic dysfunction, a major determinant of outcome in PH.[16] Acute increases in PAP results in a congestive vasculopathy characterized by decreased pulmonary arteriolar compliance and loss of normal autoregulation of pulmonary vasomotor tone.[17] These pathophysiological changes are generally reversible with pharmacotherapies that promote pulmonary vasodilation, reduce cardiac preload (e.g., nitric oxide [NO] donors), or directly alleviate pulmonary vascular congestion (e.g., loop diuretics).

CHRONIC NONVALVULAR LEFT-SIDED HEART FAILURE

In addition to passive pulmonary vascular congestion, circulating levels of the vasoactive peptide endothelin-1 (ET-1) positively correlate with PH severity in chronic left-sided heart failure.[18] Pathophysiological concentrations of ET-1 disrupt normal vasomotor tone via activation of $ET_{A/B}$ receptors on VSMCs that increases intracellular $[Ca^{+2}]_i$ levels. Endothelin-1 also promotes release of catecholamines (e.g., norepinephrine).[19,20] Together, these processes are linked to VSMC contraction and in PH offset vasodilatory cell signaling pathways, resulting in pulmonary VSMC vasoconstriction.

Chronically elevated pulmonary venous pressure induces a cellular environment in pulmonary arterioles characterized by inflammation and increased levels of reactive oxygen species (ROS) generation. Over time, these maladaptive molecular processes are implicated in the development of irreversible pathological changes to normal pulmonary blood vessel architecture, including intimal fibrosis and VSMC hypertrophy and proliferation. Chronic RV pressure overload is also linked to the propagation of worsening *left-heart* failure by promoting abnormal changes in RV chamber deformation that adversely influences LV geometry.[21]

Diagnosis, Treatment, and Natural History

The diagnosis of PH from left-sided heart failure is often evident on clinical grounds alone. Complaints of decreased exercise tolerance, dyspnea, and lower-extremity edema are common in PH but do not necessarily discriminate right- from left-sided congestive heart failure. Therefore, echocardiography is used to estimate PA systolic pressure and evaluate RV size and function. Invasive hemodynamic monitoring with right heart catheterization confirms the diagnosis of PH and excludes alternate etiologies of PH-like symptoms, such as constrictive pericardial disease, in which PVR is usually normal.

Pulmonary artery pressure, PVR, and RV systolic function are independent predictors of outcome in patients with chronic left-sided heart failure. In one study of 377 patients undergoing right heart catheterization with low LV ejection fraction and a history of congestive heart failure, mean pulmonary artery pressure (mPAP) over 29 mmHg portended about a threefold higher 36-month mortality rate (irrespective of RV function) compared to patients with normal mPAP.[22] Interpretation of pulmonary hemodynamics, however, must occur according to an individual patient's specific clinical scenario. Although typically, PAP positively correlates with PH severity in chronic left-sided heart failure, this is not always the case. Since the generation of PAP is dependent on RV systolic function, abnormally low PAP may be observed in severe PH with RV failure. In this scenario, left-sided heart failure–mediated pulmonary vascular congestion results in an increased PVR even if PAP is normal or low.[18] Pulmonary hemodynamic indices commonly used in clinical practice are provided in Table 57-2.

Conventional heart failure pharmacotherapy is the cornerstone treatment strategy for PH from nonvalvular left-sided cardiac disease. Angiotensin-converting enzyme (ACE) inhibitors, β-adrenergic receptor antagonists, loop diuretics, and vasodilators (e.g., hydralazine) often effectively decrease PVR and PAP, thereby promoting favorable responses in RV systolic function. A subset of chronic left-sided heart failure patients tends to exhibit a degree of PH that seems clinically and hemodynamically out of proportion to the severity of LV dysfunction, raising suspicion that alternative processes beyond passive vascular congestion alone are in play.[1,7] Overall, sufficiently powered randomized clinical trials evaluating the effect of iNO, prostacyclin replacement, and ERAs for PH due to chronic left-sided heart failure have either failed to demonstrate a beneficial effect on pulmonary vascular hemodynamics or did so, but at the cost of significant adverse clinical events, including increased early mortality in one large trial of intravenous epoprostenol.[23] Sildenafil, which promotes vasodilation by inhibiting PDE5 in lung VSMCs that consume cyclic guanosine monophosphate (cGMP), appears to decrease PAP and PVR safely without compromising cardiac output[13] (Fig. 57-3). The effect of sildenafil on long-term outcome and survival in chronic heart failure patients is not yet known.

Pulmonary Hypertension due to Left-Sided Valvular Disease

Pulmonary hypertension due to left-sided valvular disease most often occurs as a consequence of mitral regurgitation (MR) or mitral stenosis and less commonly from severe aortic regurgitation. In aortic stenosis, initial pressure loading–induced LV hypertrophy is protective against PH. However, in decompensated aortic stenosis, LV cavitary dilation due to volume overload is associated with progressive PH.[24] The final common pathway in the pathophysiology of PH, irrespective of valve lesion, is pulmonary venous hypertension. In only MR, however, PH is a key determinate for the timing of surgical valve therapy. The American College of Cardiology/American Heart Association (ACC/AHA) guidelines recommend mitral valve surgery (class IIa, level of evidence C) in *asymptomatic* patients with severe MR, preserved LV function, and PH (systolic PAP >50 mmHg).[25] Magne et al. reported that in a cohort of 78 asymptomatic patients with at least moderate MR from

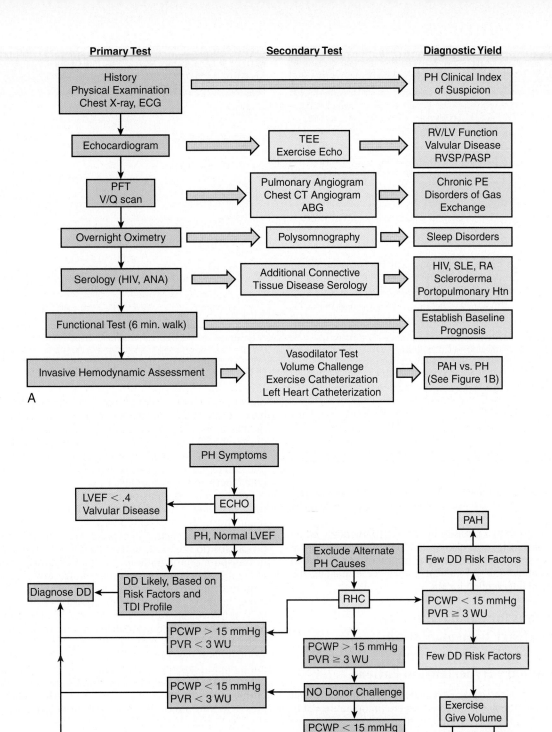

FIGURE 57-1   Pulmonary hypertension (PH) diagnostic algorithm. A, Low clinical index of suspicion initiates clinical evaluation for PH. Primary test results aid the clinician in establishing the diagnosis of PH and determining the most likely PH classification. Secondary tests are based on results from primary tests and provide additional information for determination of PH etiology. **B,** One possible diagnostic algorithm for discriminating pulmonary arterial hypertension (PAH) vs. PH from primary left-heart disease. ABG, arterial blood gas; ANA, antinuclear antibody; CT, computed tomography; CXR, chest x-ray; DD, diastolic dysfunction; ECG, electrocardiogram; ECHO, echocardiogram; HIV, human immunodeficiency virus; LV, left ventricle; LVEF, left ventricular ejection fraction; NO, nitric oxide; PASP, pulmonary artery systolic pressure; PCWP, pulmonary capillary wedge pressure; PE, pulmonary embolism; PFT, pulmonary function test; PVR, pulmonary vascular resistance; RHC, right heart catheterization; RV, right ventricle; RVSP, right ventricular systolic pressure; SLE, systemic lupus erythematosus; TEE, transesophageal echocardiogram; V/Q, ventilation/perfusion; WU, Wood units. (*A adapted from McLaughlin VV, Archer SL, Badesch DB, et al: ACCF/AHA 2009 expert consensus document on pulmonary hypertension: a report of the American College of Cardiology Foundation Task Force on Expert Consensus Documents and the American Heart Association: developed in collaboration with the American College of Chest Physicians, American Thoracic Society, Inc., and the Pulmonary Hypertension Association. J Am Coll Cardiol 53:1573–1619, 2009. B adapted from Hoeper MM, Barbera JA, Channick RN, et al: Diagnosis, assessment, and treatment of non-pulmonary arterial hypertension pulmonary hypertension. J Am Coll Cardiol 54[1 Suppl]:S85–S96, 2009.*)

TABLE 57-1	Cardiovascular Diseases That Predispose to Pulmonary Hypertension	
CLINICAL FEATURE	**MECHANISM**	
Chronic systemic hypertension	↑ Left ventricular (LV) afterload → LV hypertrophy → ↓ LV compliance → ↑ LV end-diastolic filling pressure → pulmonary venous hypertension	
Diabetes mellitus	Intramyocardial microcirculatory and epicardial coronary vascular dysfunction → LV systolic or diastolic dysfunction → pulmonary venous hypertension	
Coronary artery disease (CAD)	Myocardial ischemia → LV systolic or diastolic dysfunction → pulmonary venous hypertension	
Atrial fibrillation	Loss of "atrial kick" → ↑ left atrial and pulmonary venous congestion	
Impaired diastolic function	↑ End-diastolic filling pressure secondary to restrictive, infiltrative, or genetic cardiomyopathy → pulmonary venous hypertension	
Mitral stenosis	↑ Transmitral valve pressure ± atrial fibrillation → ↑ pulmonary venous hypertension	
Mitral regurgitation (MR)	Chronic LV volume overload → LV cavitary dilation → ↑ LV end-diastolic filling pressure → pulmonary venous hypertension With elevated mitral regurgitant fraction, pulmonary artery pressure (PAP) is elevated secondary to pulmonary circulatory volume and pressure overload, particularly during exercise	
Aortic insufficiency	Chronic LV volume overload → LV cavitary dilation → ↑ LV end-diastolic filling pressure → pulmonary venous hypertension	

TABLE 57-2	Pulmonary Hemodynamic Measurements and Normal Ranges	
MEASUREMENT	**EQUATION**	**NORMAL RANGE**
Mean RA BP	Directly measured (PA catheter)	0-8 mmHg
Pulmonary artery (PA) BP	Directly measured (PA catheter)	Systolic (PASP): 15-25 mmHg Diastolic (PADP): 4-12 mmHg mPAP 10-20 mmHg
PA capillary wedge pressure	Directly measured (PA catheter) PASP + (2 × PADP)]/3	6-12 mmHg
Cardiac output	Heart rate × Stroke volume/1000	4-7 L/min
PVR	80 × (mPAP − PCWP)/ cardiac output	20-130 dyne/s/cm^{-5} or 0.25-1.6 Wood units
Transpulmonary gradient	Mean SBP − Mean RABP	5-8 mmHg

BP, blood pressure; mPAP, mean pulmonary artery pressure; PA, pulmonary artery; PADP, pulmonary artery diastolic pressure; PASP, pulmonary artery systolic pressure; PCWP, pulmonary capillary wedge pressure; PVR, pulmonary vascular resistance; RA, right atrial; SBP, systolic blood pressure.

degenerative mitral valve disease, resting PH (systolic PAP >60 mmHg) and exercise-induced PH were associated with a significantly lower 2-year symptom free survival rate (36 ± 14% vs. 59 ± 7% and 35 ± 8% vs. 75 ± 7%, respectively). Exercise-induced PH (particularly when systolic PAP >56 mmHg) was also an independent risk factor for development of symptoms.[26] These data support exercise-induced PH as one potentially useful clinical marker for estimating the timing of surgical intervention for MR.

Considerations for Cardiac Surgery, Orthotopic Heart Transplantation, and Heart-Lung Transplantation in the Pulmonary Hypertension Patient

In contrast to select end-stage PAH patients for whom bilateral lung transplantation may be indicated, severe preoperative PH in non-PAH patients is associated with an increased rate of adverse

outcome in cardiac surgery patients who require cardiopulmonary bypass (CPB).[27] In the case of orthotopic heart transplant candidates, a transpulmonary gradient greater than 15 mmHg or PVR greater than 5 Wood units that is unchanged despite preoperative NO donor or selective PDE5 inhibitor pharmacotherapy is an absolute contraindication to surgery, owing to high rates of premature graft failure and early mortality.[28]

Pulmonary hypertension reversibility in response to pulmonary vasodilator therapy appears to improve 30-day posttransplant mortality rates compared to patients with fixed PH.[29] Although universally accepted pulmonary hemodynamic thresholds do not exist, a target PVR of less than 2.5 Wood units or transpulmonary gradient less than 12 mmHg is often used in clinical practice to define preoperative optimization for CPB-requiring surgery. For patients with fixed PH requiring cardiac transplantation, left ventricular assist device (LVAD) therapy may improve operative candidacy. Zimpfer and colleagues reported that in 35 consecutive cardiac transplant candidates with fixed PH receiving LVAD therapy, PVR decreased from 5.1 Wood units at baseline to 3.2 Wood units 3 days following device implantation, an effect sustained over 6 weeks.[30] Larger clinical trials are necessary to determine the complete risk/benefit profile (including financial costs) of LVAD implantation under these circumstances. The role of right ventricular assist device (RVAD) therapy in improving PH is unknown.

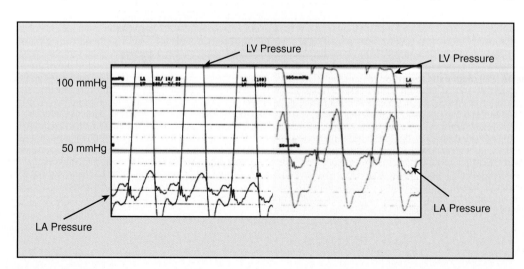

FIGURE 57-2 Effect of acute mitral regurgitation (MR) on left atrial pressure. Intraprocedural hemodynamic tracing obtained during mitral balloon valvotomy captures dramatic increase in mean left atrial (LA) pressure from 20 to 48 mmHg due to acute mitral insufficiency. Sudden changes in LA or pulmonary pressure are poorly tolerated by right ventricle and may induce cor pulmonale. LV, left ventricle. (*Adapted from Ha JW, Chung N, Chang BC, et al: Acute mitral regurgitation due to leaflet tear after balloon valvotomy. Circulation 98:2095–2097, 1998.*)

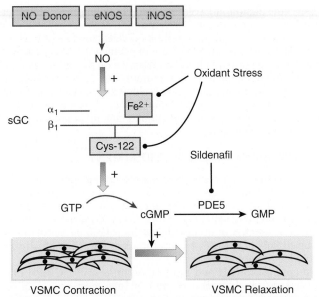

FIGURE 57-3 **Nitric oxide (NO)-soluble guanylyl cyclase signaling in vascular smooth muscle cells (VSMCs).** NO generated from nitric oxide synthase (NOS) or pharmacological sources (e.g., nitroglycerin, inhaled NO [iNO]) activate the heterodimer soluble guanylyl cyclase (sGC) to catalyze conversion of cytosolic guanosine triphosphate (GTP) to cyclic guanosine monophosphate (cGMP), which results in VSMC relaxation. In pulmonary vasculature, phosphodiesterase-5 (PDE5) hydrolyzes cGMP to form guanosine monophosphate (GMP), thereby decreasing bioactive cGMP levels. Sildenafil is a selective PDE5 inhibitor that increases cGMP levels to promote VSMC dilation. Increases in pulmonary vascular reactive oxygen species (ROS) formation, which occurs in various forms of pulmonary hypertension (PH), may also impair sGC activation via oxidation of the prosthetic heme group or cysteine-122 located in the catalytically active β_1-subunit of sGC. eNOS, endothelial nitric oxide synthase; iNOS, inducible nitric oxide synthase.

Pulmonary Hypertension Under Conditions of Hypoxemia

Pulmonary hypertension is a potential component of most chronic lung disease syndromes that cause hypoxemia. It has long been established that PH severity in COPD, interstitial lung disease (ILD), cystic fibrosis, and bronchiectasis is predictive of morbidity and mortality.[1,31] A stronger appreciation developed over the previous decade regarding the central role of PH in the natural history of sleep-disordered breathing (SDB) and alveolar hypoventilation disorders.

Hypoxic pulmonary vasoconstriction is the cornerstone pathophysiological process common to lung disease–associated forms of PH. Small and precapillary blood vessel vasoconstriction in response to hypoxia distinguishes pulmonary from coronary, cerebral, and skeletal circulations; a fall in alveolar partial pressure of oxygen (Po_2) to less than 50 mmHg results in an increase in PVR by 50%.[32,33]

A multitude of cell signaling mechanisms modulated by hypoxia have been implicated in pulmonary vasoconstriction, including increased ET-1 production, intracellular $[Ca^{+2}]_i$-mediated activation of oxygen-sensitive Ca^{+2} channels in VSMC, and local activation of α-adrenergic receptors. In addition, hypoxia inducible factor (HIF)-1α, a "master" transcription factor activated in response to hypoxia, may modulate the pathogenesis of PH in chronic lung disease via nuclear factor (NF)-κB-mediated pulmonary VSMC proliferation, among other pathological cell signaling pathways that promote negative pulmonary vascular remodeling.[34] Alternatively, suppression of HIF-1α requires iron (Fe[II]), raising speculation that iron supplementation is a potential therapeutic target for attenuation of pathogenic HIF-1α-dependent cell signaling in PH. For example, Smith et al. recently reported that iron infusion (Fe[III]-hydroxide sucrose, 200 mg) administered to healthy individuals who developed PH following exposure to hypoxic conditions at elevated altitudes decreased PA systolic from a mean of 37 to 31 mmHg ($P = 0.01$).[35]

Late-stage findings in hypoxia-mediated PH include arteriole VSMC hypertrophy and hyperplasia, which lead to medial thickening and may contribute to PH via a reduction in the pulmonary vessel lumen area.

Chronic Obstructive Pulmonary Disease

Chronic obstructive pulmonary disease is the most common cause of hypoxemia-induced PH and cor pulmonale, accounting for more than 80% of cases.[36] A mPAP "cutoff" of 20 mmHg captured 91% of 120 severe emphysema patients in one widely cited retrospective analysis.[1,8] It is uncommon for PAP to exceed 40 mmHg in patients with COPD, and if this value is used to define PH, disease prevalence drops substantially.[1]

DIAGNOSIS

Jugular venous pressure assessment or detection of a loud pulmonic component of the second heart sound may be obscured in COPD patients with PH due to chest hyperinflation. Echocardiography is generally sufficient for diagnosis of PH in COPD patients, but rotational changes to normal heart anatomy in severely hyperinflated patients may distort acoustic windows and limit detection of the tricuspid regurgitant jet envelope required for PA systolic pressure estimation. In these patients, right heart catheterization is indicated.

NATURAL HISTORY

Progression of PH in COPD patients is indolent, with an average change in mPAP of 0.5 mmHg/year.[37] In one case series of 84 patients undergoing right heart catheterization after initiation of long-term oxygen therapy for severe COPD, the 5-year mortality rate for patients with a PAP above 25 mmHg was 36%, vs. 62% for the remainder of the study population.[38] Identification of COPD patients at risk for RV dysfunction does not, however, necessarily require echocardiography or invasive hemodynamic monitoring. The presence of one or more electrocardiographic signs of cor pulmonale in COPD patients is associated with a significantly decreased lifespan.[39]

Interstitial Lung Disease

Interstitial lung disease is characterized by impaired gas exchange, patchy collagen fibrosis, fibroblastic foci deposition, and in certain instances, noncaseating granulomas on lung histopathological analysis.[40] Owing to pulmonary blood vessel compression from fibrosis, PH is a potential complication in most forms of ILD. In idiopathic pulmonary fibrosis (IPF), the most aggressive ILD subtype, histopathological findings include adverse vascular remodeling of small muscular pulmonary arteries, destruction of capillary beds, peripulmonary vessel adventitial thickening, and VSMC hypertrophy with increased collagen and elastin accumulation.[41] Together, these changes contribute to low diffusion capacity (DLCO) and development of PH that are classic features of this condition.

DIAGNOSIS AND TREATMENT

A mean PA diameter greater than 29 mm on computed tomography (CT) scan is suspicious for PH, but echocardiography or right heart catheterization remain the gold standard diagnostic tests for PH in ILD.[42] Universal guidelines for iNO, PDE5 inhibitors, ERAs, or prostacyclin replacement therapy in ILD do not exist; current management emphasizes alleviation of hypoxemia with supplemental oxygen and improvement in alveolar gas exchange (e.g., corticosteroids if appropriate). A randomized clinical tria l to evaluate iloprost in IPF patients with PH is complete, but results have not yet been published (clinicaltrials.gov; NCT00109681).

Pulmonary Hypertension in Obstructive Sleep Apnea

Obstructive sleep apnea (OSA) is a clinical syndrome resulting from involuntary collapse of pharyngeal muscles during sleep. Decreases in the arterial partial pressure of oxygen (Pao_2) and increased sleep arousal and sympathetic tone adversely affect cardiovascular function by increasing LV afterload, systemic blood pressure, and heart rate. The aggregate effect of these pathological adaptations results in increased rates of OSA-associated ischemic heart disease, congestive heart failure, and arrhythmias. Furthermore, these processes in turn promote PH via left-sided heart failure–induced passive pulmonary vascular congestion. Obesity, which is associated with increases in cardiac output compared to lean individuals, correlates positively with PAP, irrespective of OSA status.[43] This observation suggests that high cardiac output, perhaps by inducing reactive pulmonary vasoconstriction from increased circulating blood volume, may contribute to elevated rates of PH observed in patients with obesity, OSA, or both.

Continuous positive pressure airway pressure (CPAP), which in OSA patients is associated with improvement in LV diastolic function, decreases PAP ($\approx$5 mmHg over 4 months of CPAP use) and is associated with decreased mortality and hospitalization rates in OSA patients.[43–45]

Chronic High-Altitude Exposure

Over 140 million people live at high altitude (HA) (>2500 m above sea level).[46] A parabolic inverse relationship between PAP and peripheral oxygen saturation (Sao_2) exists in populations of native HA dwellers.[46] It is believed that chronic hypoxia-mediated vasoconstriction from low oxygen tension at HA results in several cardiopulmonary adaptations, which include RV hypertrophy, VSMC hypertrophy of small and distal pulmonary arterioles, increased oxygen carrying capacity due to reactive erythrocytosis, and increased heart rate at baseline and on exertion.[46] If these protective responses are disrupted, typically from hypoventilation-mediated worsening of hypoxia, a cascade of maladaptive responses may ensue, resulting in chronic mountain sickness syndrome (CMS). Severe PH, cor pulmonale, and excessive polycythemia are hallmark clinical features of CMS. In contrast to acute altitude sickness, pulmonary edema from severe PH is not typical. Altitude descent is usually required to cure CMS.[47]

Pulmonary Hypertension Secondary to Pulmonary Thromboembolic Disease

Chronic Thromboembolic Pulmonary Hypertension

Chronic thromboembolic pulmonary hypertension (CTEPH) is characterized by luminal obliteration of central and distal pulmonary arteries, which results in PH and RV failure. Epidemiological data describing the frequency of CTEPH in the general population is limited; however, 0.5% to 5% of patients surviving an acute pulmonary embolism (PE) tend to develop this condition.[48] Histopathological analysis demonstrates intraluminal and *in situ* thrombus, and stenosis from associated fibrous deposition in the wall of pulmonary arteries.[49,50] Pulmonary hypertensive arteriopathy is present in vessels that are distinct from the site of thrombus, suggesting thrombus potentiation of diffuse injury to the pulmonary vasculature.

It is parsimonious to speculate that this syndrome is merely a consequence of incompletely recanalized PE but up to 50% of CTEPH patients have not been previously diagnosed with a pulmonary embolism. Furthermore, a surprisingly strong association between CTEPH and asplenism exists. In one case-controlled analysis of 257 patients, splenectomy was present in 8.5% of CTEPH patients, compared with 2.5% of PAH patients and 0.5% of patients with chronic parenchymal lung disease.[51] The precise mechanisms to account for this association remain speculative. Loss of hematopoietic filtering in asplenic patients may generate a prothrombotic environment in vascular tissue, owing to elevated circulating levels of platelets and abnormal erythrocytes. One hypothesis suggests that the platelet-derived vascular effector serotonin, implicated in microthrombus formation and

VSMC constriction in PAH-associated conditions, may contribute to PH in asplenic patients. Alternatively, in asplenic patients, unfiltered structurally abnormal red blood cells may function as procoagulant intermediaries because of expression of the negatively charged phospholipid phosphatidylserine on the outer cell membrane, which interacts with thrombin (see Hemoglobinopathy, later).[52,53] Additional risk factors include a history of venothromboembolism, positive anticardiolipin antibody status, osteomyelitis, surgically placed ventriculoatrial shunt, inflammatory bowel disease, and malignancy.[54]

DIAGNOSIS AND MEDICAL TREATMENT

CTEPH often presents with progressive exertional dyspnea. Late in the disease course, signs and symptoms of decreased right-sided cardiac output, such as exertional chest pain, increased abdominal girth and lower-extremity edema, and syncope or near-syncope may be present. A bruit auscultated over the lung fields, present in up to 30% of patients, reflects turbulent flow through partially occluded pulmonary vessels.[55]

In contrast to PAH and most other forms of PH, CTEPH often involves proximal pulmonary arteries. Thus, the presence of one or more ventilation/perfusion (V/Q) mismatched segmental (or larger) defects detected by V/Q scintigraphy is often a key finding that distinguishes CTEPH from PAH. In up to 45% of patients with CTEPH, lower-extremity venous duplex ultrasound examination suggests venothromboembolism.[55] Although pulmonary angiography has traditionally been the gold standard diagnostic imaging modality in this condition, multidimensional CT or magnetic resonance angiography (MRA) is at least equally effective in determining proximal, segmental, and subsegmental clot burden, and is superior for detecting alternative PH-associated lung disease (e.g., fibrosing mediastinitis, adenopathy, tumors of the pulmonary artery)[56] (Fig. 57-4). Nevertheless, pulmonary angiography is necessary for defining CTEPH type, which predicts operative success, and is therefore recommended for all surgical intervention candidates (see later discussion).

For inoperable CTEPH patients, a systolic PAP over 40 mmHg, elevated PVR (>584 dyne/s/cm^{-5}), and/or elevated right atrial pressure (>12 mmHg) is associated with a poor prognosis. One study conducted prior to the era of modern PAH pharmacotherapy demonstrated that in CTEPH patients with mPAP over 50 mmHg treated only with anticoagulation, the 2-year survival rate was below 20%.[57] In contrast, data from contemporary trials in nonoperative CTEPH patients suggest that therapy with PDE5 inhibitors, ERAs, or prostacyclin replacement therapy improves outcome. For example, one recently published retrospective analysis of 84 inoperable CTEPH patients on maximal medical therapy reported a survival rate of 68% at 5 years.[58] In the BENEFiT trial, 157 patients with inoperable or surgically refractory CTEPH were randomized to receive ERA therapy with the $ET_{A/B}$ receptor antagonist bosentan or placebo. Bosentan was well tolerated and resulted in a statistically significant 24% decrease in PVR from baseline, but did not influence exercise tolerance.[59] Pilot studies evaluating the effects of iNO and/or selective PDE5 inhibition have demonstrated similar beneficial effects on pulmonary vascular hemodynamics.[60] At present, initiation of PAH therapies in CTEPH is generally recommended for poor surgical candidates or those with disease refractory to surgery awaiting lung transplantation.

SURGICAL TREATMENT

Primary treatment for CTEPH is pulmonary thromboendarterectomy for excision of thromboembolic and fibrotic tissue adherent to the lung vessel wall[61,62] (Table 57-3). Deep hypothermic circulatory arrest with CPB is a strategy used to minimize bleeding in the surgical field, and at experienced centers has been met with low neurological morbidity rates and favorable outcomes.[63] Factors favoring operative success include a proximal clot burden and a decrease in mPAP in response to preoperative iNO treatment.[64] When successful, surgery results in a substantial reduction in clot burden and PVR[65] (see Fig. 57-4). In one prospective analysis of

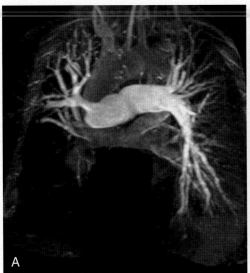
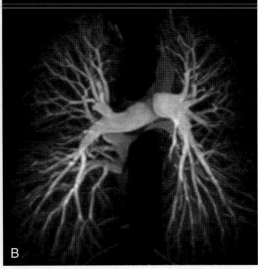

FIGURE 57-4 **A,** Preoperative pulmonary magnetic resonance angiography (MRA) in patient with chronic thromboembolic pulmonary hypertension (CTEPH). **B,** Images acquired from same patient following surgical endarterectomy. *(Adapted from Hamilton-Craig C, Kermeen F, Dunning JJ, et al: Cardiovascular magnetic resonance prior to surgical treatment of chronic thromboembolic pulmonary hypertension. Eur Heart J 31:1040, 2010.)*

TABLE 57-3	**Classification of CTEPH According to Intraoperative Findings***		
CLASSIFICATION	**DISTRIBUTION**	**ANATOMIC INVOLVEMENT**	**PATHOLOGY**
Type I	30% of surgical cases	Main or lobar pulmonary arteries	Fresh thrombus Vessel wall disease Clot propagation into primary and secondary pulmonary blood vessels
Type II	60% of surgical cases	Proximal to segmental pulmonary arteries	Intimal thickening Vessel wall fibrosis ±Organized thrombus
Type III	10% of surgical cases	Distal segmental and subsegmental pulmonary arteries	Vessel fibrosis Intimal webbing Blood vessel thickening ±Organized thrombus
Type IV	<1% of surgical cases	Distal arterioles	Microscopic arteriolar vasculopathy No evidence of visual thrombus

*A higher likelihood of elevated postoperative pulmonary arterial pressure (PAP) and pulmonary vascular resistance (PVR) exists with type III or IV disease.
Data from Jamieson SW: Pulmonary thromboendarterectomy. Heart 79:118–120, 1998; Thistlethwaite PA, Madani M, Jamieson SW: Pulmonary thromboendarterectomy surgery. Cardiol Clin 22:467–478, vii, 2004; and Jamieson SW, Kapelanski DP, Sakakibara N, et al: Pulmonary endarterectomy: experience and lessons learned in 1,500 cases. Ann Thorac Surg 76:1457–1462; discussion 1462–1454, 2003.

181 CTEPH patients, compared with nonsurgical treatment, pulmonary thromboendarterectomy was associated with a significantly lower PVR (586 ± 248 vs. 269 ± 201 dyne/s/cm^{-5}) and mPAP, (45 ± 12 vs. 25 ± 11 mmHg).[66] In this study, surgeries performed within the last decade were associated with a 6% or lower mortality rate. Lung transplantation should be considered for those with inoperable disease or an incomplete response to thromboendarterectomy.[55] Lifelong anticoagulation is recommended for all patients irrespective of operative candidacy.

Pulmonary Hypertension with Hemoglobinopathies

Pulmonary hypertension from primary blood dyscrasias that are characterized by abnormal erythrocyte structure or hemolysis occurs as a consequence of decreased bioavailable NO, increased microthrombi formation, and possibly, increased vascular endothelial ET-1 synthesis (see mechanism details later). Examples include sickle cell disease (SCD), hereditary spherocytosis, β-thalassemia (particularly in patients with splenectomy), and stomatocytosis.

Pulmonary hypertension is a part of the SCD syndrome in about 40% of patients. The 4-year mortality rate is 40% in SCD patients with PH; when RV systolic pressure is above 30 mmHg, there is a 10-fold increase in mortality compared with non-PH SCD patients.[67] Histopathological findings in SCD and hemolysis-associated PH demonstrate a pulmonary arteriopathy similar to that observed in PAH. Specifically, the presence of pulmonary VSMC hypertrophy, neomuscularization of small- and medium-sized pulmonary arteries, luminal microthrombi, and plexiform lesions are described at autopsy in patients with these various primary disorders of erythrocyte structure[68] (Fig. 57-5).

Potential Mechanisms Linking Pulmonary Hypertension and Sickle Cell Disease

DECREASED BIOAVAILABLE NITRIC OXIDE

In the pulmonary vasculature, NO is a critical intermediary that promotes vasodilation, decreases platelet aggregation, and is a potent antagonist of vascular inflammation. In SCD and hemolytic anemias, erythrocyte deformity or rupture results in release of free hemoglobin (Hb) into plasma. In the microcirculation, free Hb interacts with NO to form methemoglobin and nitrate (NO_3^-) [$Hb - Fe^{2+} = O_2 + NO \rightarrow Hb\text{-}Fe^{3+} + NO_3^-$], thereby decreasing bioavailable levels of NO, which increases pulmonary vascular reactivity.

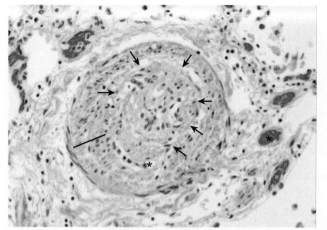

FIGURE 57-5 Histopathological findings in sickle cell disease (SCD)–associated pulmonary hypertension (PH). Hematoxylin and eosin preparation of distal pulmonary blood vessel in patient with sickle cell anemia reveals vascular smooth muscle cell (VSMC) hypertrophy, intimal thickening *(line)*, and subtotal obliteration of vessel lumen due to a plexiform lesion *(outlined by arrows)*. Microvessel thrombus is also noted *(star)*. *(From Machado RF, Gladwin MT: pulmonary hypertension in hemolytic disorders: pulmonary vascular disease: the global perspective. Chest 137[6 Suppl]:30 S–38 S, 2010.)*

Ischemia-reperfusion injury in small pulmonary arterioles and capillaries is a hallmark feature in the pathophysiology of SCD occlusive crises.[69,70] The downstream molecular effect of these events includes scavenging of bioavailable NO by superoxide O_2^- in a reaction that generates peroxynitrite anion (ONOO−).[71] Superoxide is generated during ischemia-reperfusion injury via (1) direct activation of ROS generating enzymes (e.g., xanthin oxidase), (2) increased NADPH oxidase activity modulated by enhanced leukocyte recruitment to the vascular endothelium, (3) uncoupling of endothelial nitric oxide synthase (eNOS) due to enzyme cofactor depletion (e.g., BH_4), and (4) inducible nitric oxide synthase (iNOS)-dependent NO-mediated ROS formation.[70] In addition to scavenging NO, O_2^- is converted to hydrogen peroxide (H_2O_2), which has been shown *in vitro* to disrupt endothelium-independent vasodilatory signaling pathways by oxidatively modifying a key cysteinyl thiol involved in normal NO sensing by sGC[72] (see Fig. 57-3).

Intracellular levels of arginase, which converts L-arginine to ornithine, are elevated in sickled erythrocytes and released into plasma upon hemolysis.[73] It has been postulated, therefore, that since L-arginine is a substrate for NO synthesis, this may represent an additional mechanism by which bioavailable NO is decreased in SCD. Data examining arginine replacement therapy, PDE5 inhibition with sildenafil, or iNO to treat PH in SCD, although encouraging, are at this time limited to case reports or very small patients series.[74]

The role of arginase in modulating PH in other primary blood dyscrasias has been evaluated. In paroxysmal nocturnal hemoglobinuria (PNH), an acquired mutation results in the absence of erythrocyte membrane-bound glycosylphosphatidylinositol-anchored proteins, which predisposes to compliment-mediated hemolysis and free Hb scavenging of NO. Patients with PNH express a low bioactive NO state in several ways, including PH, gastrointestinal smooth muscle cell (SMC) hyperactivity, and erectile dysfunction (ED).[75] Data extracted from patients enrolled in the Transfusion Reduction Efficacy and Safety Clinical Investigation Using Eculizumab in Paroxysmal Nocturnal Hemoglobinuria (TRIUMPH) study demonstrated that plasma arginase activity levels were 10-fold higher compared with the normal range, a finding associated with a roughly 30-fold increase in NO consumption. Interestingly, by blocking compliment C5 and thereby decreasing erythrocyte hemolysis, eculizumab treatment resulted in a significant decrease in hemolysis, N-terminal pro-brain natriuretic peptide levels, and patient-reported dyspnea.[76]

Less well-established mechanisms that may influence NO bioavailability may involve asymmetrical dimethylarginine (ADMA), a NOS inhibitor, which is present at elevated concentrations in plasma of SCD patients.[77]

HYPERCOAGULABLE STATE

In SCD, stroke, veno-occlusive crises, and PH are believed to occur in part from thrombus formation in the cerebral and pulmonary microcirculations. Decreased bioavailable NO (through loss of platelet aggregation antagonism), increased whole blood tissue factor expression and thrombin formation, and decreased levels of the coagulation pathway inhibitors activated protein C (APC) and its cofactor protein S contribute to a hypercoagulable state. In SCD, β-thalassemia, and/or asplenic patients, erythrocyte membrane dyssymmetry results in abundant exposure of phosphatidyl choline, which is linked to increased erythrocyte vascular endothelial cell (ED) adhesion and thrombin activation.[78] Antiplatelet therapy with aspirin is recommended in selected high-risk SCD patients for primary prevention of ischemic stroke; however, the effect of these agents in modulating a decrease in PAP has not been adequately tested.

Despite these observations, the attributable contribution to the pathophysiology of PH by free Hb scavenging of NO remains unresolved. A surprisingly low difference in reticulocyte count and lactate dehydrogenase (LDH) levels between non-PH and PH patients with SCD; lack of a positive association between extent of hemolysis and PH disease severity; and an absence of extrahematological clinical signs or symptoms indicative of decreased bioactive NO, such as esophageal spasm or ED (i.e., impotence but not priapism), has led some to suggest that alternative mechanisms may play an underrecognized role in promoting PH in SCD.[52]

INCREASED ENDOTHELIN-1 SYNTHESIS

A threefold increase in circulating ET-1 levels are observed in patients with SCD compared to age-matched normal controls.[79] This presumably occurs as a consequence of microvascular hypoxia and increased sheer stress in SCD that triggers pulmonary vascular endothelial secretion of ET-1. *In vitro*, exposure of vascular ECs to sickled erythrocytes significantly increases ET-1 gene transcription, suggesting that ET-1 may act as a vasoconstrictor intermediary in SCD.[80] Because of the central role of ET-1 in the pathophysiology of PAH, investigators have tested the hypothesis that $ET_{A/B}$ receptor antagonism may attenuate PH disease severity in SCD. Early data from small clinical trials have demonstrated about a 10% increase in distance performed during a 6-minute walk test in SCD patients with PH treated with bosentan therapy for 6 months. In the same study, a mean fall of 6 mmHg in estimated systolic PAP (by echocardiography) was also observed.[81] Larger randomized double-blinded placebo-controlled clinical trials to investigate further bosentan therapy in a similar patient cohort are ongoing (ASSET-1 and -2 at clinicaltrials.gov).[82]

Other Secondary Causes of Pulmonary Hypertension

Numerous other less common disease states are associated with PH by causing direct compression of the pulmonary vasculature via mass effect or vessel wall infiltration. Fibrosing mediastinitis, which is associated with granulomatous diseases such as histoplasmosis, is an immunologically mediated response to caseous nodes. Fibrotic encroachment of large and small pulmonary arteries and veins has been observed at necroscopy of patients when this condition includes severe PH. A similar PH pathophysiology has been implicated in sarcoidosis, where impedance to pulmonary blood flow occurs secondary to fibrosis of the pulmonary vasculature in the setting of extensive parenchymal lung disease or direct invasion of the intima and media of the pulmonary arteries with noncaseating granulomas, resulting in blood vessel encroachment.

Primary inflammatory vascular diseases including pulmonary capillary hemangiomatosis, characterized by uncontrolled proliferation of capillaries infiltrating vascular, bronchial, and interstitial pulmonary structures, and Takayasu's arteritis (see Chapter 42) are rare causes of PH. An important iatrogenic etiology of PH is secondary to pulmonary vein stenosis as a complication of pulmonary vein isolation radiofrequency ablation for treatment of atrial fibrillation. In the previous decade, pulmonary vein stenosis was reported in up to 20% of patients undergoing this procedure. However, improved technology and enhanced awareness among operators appears to have resulted in a substantial downward trend in the frequency of this potentially devastating procedural complication, with contemporary case series reporting event rates of 1% to 3%.[83]

REFERENCES

1. McLaughlin VV, Archer SL, Badesch DB, et al: ACCF/AHA 2009 expert consensus document on pulmonary hypertension a report of the American College of Cardiology Foundation Task Force on Expert Consensus Documents and the American Heart Association developed in collaboration with the American College of Chest Physicians; American Thoracic Society, Inc.; and the Pulmonary Hypertension Association, J Am Coll Cardiol 53(17):1573–1619, 2009.

2. Farber HW, Loscalzo J: Pulmonary arterial hypertension, N Engl J Med 351(16):1655–1665, 2004.

3. Benza RL, Miller DP, Gomberg-Maitland M, et al: Predicting survival in pulmonary arterial hypertension: insights from the Registry to Evaluate Early and Long-Term Pulmonary Arterial Hypertension Disease Management (REVEAL), Circulation 122(2):164–172, 2010.

4. Proceedings of the 4th World Symposium on Pulmonary Hypertension, February 2008, Dana Point, California, USA, J Am Coll Cardiol 54(1 Suppl):S1–S117, 2009.

5. Simonneau G, Robbins IM, Beghetti M, et al: Updated clinical classification of pulmonary hypertension, J Am Coll Cardiol 54(1 Suppl):S43–S54, 2009.

6. Leung CC, Moondra V, Catherwood E, et al: Prevalence and risk factors of pulmonary hypertension in patients with elevated pulmonary venous pressure and preserved ejection fraction, Am J Cardiol 106(2):284–286, 2010.

7. Hoeper MM, Barbera JA, Channick RN, et al: Diagnosis, assessment, and treatment of non-pulmonary arterial hypertension pulmonary hypertension, J Am Coll Cardiol 54(1 Suppl):S85–S96, 2009.

8. Scharf SM, Iqbal M, Keller C, et al: Hemodynamic characterization of patients with severe emphysema, Am J Respir Crit Care Med 166(3):314–322, 2002.

9. Handa T, Nagai S, Miki S, et al: Incidence of pulmonary hypertension and its clinical relevance in patients with sarcoidosis, Chest 129(5):1246–1252, 2006.

10. Baughman RP, Engel PJ, Taylor L, et al: Survival in sarcoidosis associated pulmonary hypertension: the importance of hemodynamic evaluation, Chest 2010.

11. Damy T, Goode KM, Kallvikbacka-Bennett A, et al: Determinants and prognostic value of pulmonary arterial pressure in patients with chronic heart failure, Eur Heart J 31(18):2280–2290, 2010.

12. Maggiorini M, Melot C, Pierre S, et al: High-altitude pulmonary edema is initially caused by an increase in capillary pressure, Circulation 103(16):2078–2083, 2001.

13. Lewis GD, Shah R, Shahzad K, et al: Sildenafil improves exercise capacity and quality of life in patients with systolic heart failure and secondary pulmonary hypertension, Circulation 116(14):1555–1562, 2007.

14. Pengo V, Lensing AW, Prins MH, et al: Incidence of chronic thromboembolic pulmonary hypertension after pulmonary embolism, N Engl J Med 350(22):2257–2264, 2004.

15. Ha JW, Chung N, Chang BC, et al: Acute mitral regurgitation due to leaflet tear after balloon valvotomy, Circulation 98(19):2095–2097, 1998.

16. Zafrir N, Zingerman B, Solodky A, et al: Use of noninvasive tools in primary pulmonary hypertension to assess the correlation of right ventricular function with functional capacity and to predict outcome, Int J Cardiovasc Imaging 23(2):209–215, 2007.

17. Hirakawa S, Suzuki T, Gotoh K, et al: Human pulmonary vascular and venous compliances are reduced before and during left-sided heart failure, J Appl Physiol 78(1):323–333, 1995.

18. Moraes DL, Colucci WS, Givertz MM: Secondary pulmonary hypertension in chronic heart failure: the role of the endothelium in pathophysiology and management, Circulation 102(14):1718–1723, 2000.

19. Furutani H, Zhang XF, Iwamuro Y, et al: Ca2+ entry channels involved in contractions of rat aorta induced by endothelin-1, noradrenaline, and vasopressin, J Cardiovasc Pharmacol 40(2):265–276, 2002.

20. Kaddoura S, Firth JD, Boheler KR, et al: Endothelin-1 is involved in norepinephrine-induced ventricular hypertrophy in vivo. Acute effects of bosentan, an orally active, mixed endothelin ETA and ETB receptor antagonist, Circulation 93(11):2068–2079, 1996.

21. Puwanant S, Park M, Popovic ZB, et al: Ventricular geometry, strain, and rotational mechanics in pulmonary hypertension, Circulation 121(2):259–266, 2010.

22. Ghio S, Gavazzi A, Campana C, et al: Independent and additive prognostic value of right ventricular systolic function and pulmonary artery pressure in patients with chronic heart failure, J Am Coll Cardiol 37(1):183–188, 2001.

23. Califf RM, Adams KF, McKenna WJ, et al: A randomized controlled trial of epoprostenol therapy for severe congestive heart failure: The Flolan International Randomized Survival Trial (FIRST), Am Heart J 134(1):44–54, 1997.

24. Malouf JF, Enriquez-Sarano M, Pellikka PA, et al: Severe pulmonary hypertension in patients with severe aortic valve stenosis: clinical profile and prognostic implications, J Am Coll Cardiol 40(4):789–795, 2002.

25. Bonow RO, Carabello BA, Chatterjee K, et al: 2008 focused update incorporated into the ACC/AHA 2006 guidelines for the management of patients with valvular heart disease: a report of the American College of Cardiology/American Heart Association Task Force on Practice Guidelines (Writing Committee to revise the 1998 guidelines for the management of patients with valvular heart disease). Endorsed by the Society of Cardiovascular Anesthesiologists, Society for Cardiovascular Angiography and Interventions, and Society of Thoracic Surgeons, J Am Coll Cardiol 52(13):e1–e142, 2008.

26. Magne J, Lancellotti P, Pierard LA: Exercise pulmonary hypertension in asymptomatic degenerative mitral regurgitation, Circulation 122(1):33–41, 2010.

27. Murali S, Kormos RL, Uretsky BF, et al: Preoperative pulmonary hemodynamics and early mortality after orthotopic cardiac transplantation: the Pittsburgh experience, Am Heart J 126(4):896–904, 1993.

28. Gorlitzer M, Ankersmit J, Fiegl N, et al: Is the transpulmonary pressure gradient a predictor for mortality after orthotopic cardiac transplantation? Transpl Int 18(4):390–395, 2005.

29. Chen JM, Levin HR, Michler RE, et al: Reevaluating the significance of pulmonary hypertension before cardiac transplantation: determination of optimal thresholds and quantification of the effect of reversibility on perioperative mortality, J Thorac Cardiovasc Surg 114(4):627–634, 1997.

30. Zimpfer D, Zrunek P, Sandner S, et al: Post-transplant survival after lowering fixed pulmonary hypertension using left ventricular assist devices, Eur J Cardiothorac Surg 31(4):698–702, 2007.

31. Hopkins N, McLoughlin P: The structural basis of pulmonary hypertension in chronic lung disease: remodelling, rarefaction or angiogenesis? J Anat 201(4):335–348, 2002.

32. Harris P, Heath D: Influence of respiratory gases. In Harris P, Heath D, editors: The human pulmonary circulation, ed 2, London, 1986, Churchill Livingston, pp 456–483.

33. Dumas JP, Bardou M, Goirand F, et al: Hypoxic pulmonary vasoconstriction, Gen Pharmacol 33(4):289–297, 1999.

34. Diebold I, Djordjevic T, Hess J, et al: Rac-1 promotes pulmonary artery smooth muscle cell proliferation by upregulation of plasminogen activator inhibitor-1: role of NFkappaB-dependent hypoxia-inducible factor-1alpha transcription, Thromb Haemost 100(6):1021–1028, 2008.

35. Smith TG, Talbot NP, Privat C, et al: Effects of iron supplementation and depletion on hypoxic pulmonary hypertension: two randomized controlled trials, JAMA 302(13):1444–1450, 2009.

36. Hyduk A, Croft JB, Ayala C, et al: Pulmonary hypertension surveillance–United States, 1980–2002, MMWR Surveill Summ 54(5):1–28, 2005.

37. Weitzenblum E: Chronic cor pulmonale, Heart 89(2):225–230, 2003.

38. Oswald-Mammosser M, Weitzenblum E, Quoix E, et al: Prognostic factors in COPD patients receiving long-term oxygen therapy. Importance of pulmonary artery pressure, Chest 107(5):1193–1198, 1995.

39. Incalzi RA, Fuso L, De Rosa M, et al: Electrocardiographic signs of chronic cor pulmonale: a negative prognostic finding in chronic obstructive pulmonary disease, Circulation 99(12):1600–1605, 1999.

40. Ryu JH, Daniels CE, Hartman TE, et al: Diagnosis of interstitial lung diseases, Mayo Clin Proc 82(8):976–986, 2007.

41. Patel NM, Lederer DJ, Borczuk AC, et al: Pulmonary hypertension in idiopathic pulmonary fibrosis, Chest 132(3):998–1006, 2007.

42. Tan RT, Kuzo R, Goodman LR, et al: Utility of CT scan evaluation for predicting pulmonary hypertension in patients with parenchymal lung disease. Medical College of Wisconsin Transplant Group, Chest 113(5):1250–1256, 1998.

43. McQuillan BM, Picard MH, Leavitt M, et al: Clinical correlates and reference intervals for pulmonary artery systolic pressure among echocardiographically normal subjects, Circulation 104(23):2797–2802, 2001.

44. Devaraj A, Wells AU, Meister MG, et al: Detection of pulmonary hypertension with multidetector CT and echocardiography alone and in combination, Radiology 254(2):609–616, 2010.

45. Shahar E, Whitney CW, Redline S, et al: Sleep-disordered breathing and cardiovascular disease: cross-sectional results of the Sleep Heart Health Study, Am J Respir Crit Care Med 163(1):19–25, 2001.

46. Penaloza D, Arias-Stella J: The heart and pulmonary circulation at high altitudes: healthy highlanders and chronic mountain sickness, Circulation 115(9):1132–1146, 2007.

47. Penaloza D, Sime F: Chronic cor pulmonale due to loss of altitude acclimatization (chronic mountain sickness), Am J Med 50(6):728–743, 1971.

48. Ribeiro A, Lindmarker P, Johnsson H, et al: Pulmonary embolism: one-year follow-up with echocardiography Doppler and five-year survival analysis, Circulation 99(10):1325–1330, 1999.

49. Hoeper MM, Mayer E, Simonneau G, et al: Chronic thromboembolic pulmonary hypertension, Circulation 113(16):2011–2020, 2006.

50. Klepetko W, Mayer E, Sandoval J, et al: Interventional and surgical modalities of treatment for pulmonary arterial hypertension, J Am Coll Cardiol 43(12 Suppl S):73S–80S, 2004.

51. Jais X, Ioos V, Jardim C, et al: Splenectomy and chronic thromboembolic pulmonary hypertension, Thorax 60(12):1031–1034, 2005.

52. Bunn HF, Nathan DG, Dover GJ, et al: Pulmonary hypertension and nitric oxide depletion in sickle cell disease, Blood 116(5):687–692, 2010.

53. Eldor A, Rachmilewitz EA: The hypercoagulable state in thalassemia, Blood 99(1):36–43, 2002.

54. Bonderman D, Jakowitsch J, Adlbrecht C, et al: Medical conditions increasing the risk of chronic thromboembolic pulmonary hypertension, Thromb Haemost 93(3):512–516, 2005.

55. Fedullo PF, Auger WR, Kerr KM, et al: Chronic thromboembolic pulmonary hypertension, N Engl J Med 345(20):1465–1472, 2001.

56. Tardivon AA, Musset D, Maitre S, et al: Role of CT in chronic pulmonary embolism: comparison with pulmonary angiography, J Comput Assist Tomogr 17(3):345–351, 1993.

57. Riedel M, Stanek V, Widimsky J, et al: Long-term follow-up of patients with pulmonary thromboembolism. Late prognosis and evolution of hemodynamic and respiratory data, Chest 81(2):151–158, 1982.

58. Saouti N, de Man F, Westerhof N, et al: Predictors of mortality in inoperable chronic thromboembolic pulmonary hypertension, Respir Med 103(7):1013–1019, 2009.

59. Jais X, D'Armini AM, Jansa P, et al: Bosentan for treatment of inoperable chronic thromboembolic pulmonary hypertension: BENEFiT (Bosentan Effects in iNopErable Forms of chronIc Thromboembolic pulmonary hypertension), a randomized, placebo-controlled trial, *J Am Coll Cardiol* 52(25):2127–2134, 2008.

60. Suntharalingam J, Hughes RJ, Goldsmith K, et al: Acute haemodynamic responses to inhaled nitric oxide and intravenous sildenafil in distal chronic thromboembolic pulmonary hypertension (CTEPH), *Vasc Pharmacol* 46(6):449–455, 2007.

61. Jamieson SW: Pulmonary thromboendarterectomy, *Heart* 79(2):118–120, 1998.

62. Thistlethwaite PA, Madani M, Jamieson SW: Pulmonary thromboendarterectomy surgery, *Cardiol Clin* 22(3):467–478, vii, 2004.

63. Jamieson SW, Kapelanski DP, Sakakibara N, et al: Pulmonary endarterectomy: experience and lessons learned in 1,500 cases, *Ann Thorac Surg* 76(5):1457–1462, 2003; discussion 1462–1454.

64. Skoro-Sajer N, Hack N, Sadushi-Kolici R, et al: Pulmonary vascular reactivity and prognosis in patients with chronic thromboembolic pulmonary hypertension: a pilot study, *Circulation* 119(2):298–305, 2009.

65. Hamilton-Craig C, Kermeen F, Dunning JJ, et al: Cardiovascular magnetic resonance prior to surgical treatment of chronic thrombo-embolic pulmonary hypertension, *Eur Heart J* 31(9):1040, 2010.

66. Bonderman D, Skoro-Sajer N, Jakowitsch J, et al: Predictors of outcome in chronic thromboembolic pulmonary hypertension, *Circulation* 115(16):2153–2158, 2007.

67. Gladwin MT, Sachdev V, Jison ML, et al: Pulmonary hypertension as a risk factor for death in patients with sickle cell disease, *N Engl J Med* 350(9):886–895, 2004.

68. Haque AK, Gokhale S, Rampy BA, et al: Pulmonary hypertension in sickle cell hemoglobinopathy: a clinicopathologic study of 20 cases, *Hum Pathol* 33(10):1037–1043, 2002.

69. Gibson WH, Roughton FJ: The kinetics and equilibria of the reactions of nitric oxide with sheep haemoglobin, *J Physiol* 136(3):507–524, 1957.

70. Aslan M, Freeman BA: Redox-dependent impairment of vascular function in sickle cell disease, *Free Radic Biol Med* 43(11):1469–1483, 2007.

71. Hammerman SI, Klings ES, Hendra KP, et al: Endothelial cell nitric oxide production in acute chest syndrome, *Am J Physiol* 277(4 Pt 2):H1579–H1592, 1999.

72. Maron BA, Zhang YY, Handy DE, et al: Aldosterone increases oxidant stress to impair guanylyl cyclase activity by cysteinyl thiol oxidation in vascular smooth muscle cells, *J Biol Chem* 284(12):7665–7672, 2009.

73. Iyamu EW, Cecil R, Parkin L, et al: Modulation of erythrocyte arginase activity in sickle cell disease patients during hydroxyurea therapy, *Br J Haematol* 131(3):389–394, 2005.

74. Morris CR, Morris SM Jr, Hagar W, et al: Arginine therapy: a new treatment for pulmonary hypertension in sickle cell disease? *Am J Respir Crit Care Med* 168(1):63–69, 2003.

75. Brodsky RA: Advances in the diagnosis and therapy of paroxysmal nocturnal hemoglobinuria, *Blood Rev* 22(2):65–74, 2008.

76. Hill A, Rother RP, Wang X, et al: Effect of eculizumab on haemolysis-associated nitric oxide depletion, dyspnoea, and measures of pulmonary hypertension in patients with paroxysmal nocturnal haemoglobinuria, *Br J Haematol* 149(5):414–425, 2010.

77. Kato GJ, Wang Z, Machado RF, et al: Endogenous nitric oxide synthase inhibitors in sickle cell disease: abnormal levels and correlations with pulmonary hypertension, desaturation, haemolysis, organ dysfunction and death, *Br J Haematol* 145(4):506–513, 2009.

78. Manodori AB, Barabino GA, Lubin BH, et al: Adherence of phosphatidylserine-exposing erythrocytes to endothelial matrix thrombospondin, *Blood* 95(4):1293–1300, 2000.

79. Werdehoff SG, Moore RB, Hoff CJ, et al: Elevated plasma endothelin-1 levels in sickle cell anemia: relationships to oxygen saturation and left ventricular hypertrophy, *Am J Hematol* 58(3):195–199, 1998.

80. Phelan M, Perrine SP, Brauer M, et al: Sickle erythrocytes, after sickling, regulate the expression of the endothelin-1 gene and protein in human endothelial cells in culture, *J Clin Invest* 96(2):1145–1151, 1995.

81. Minniti CP, Machado RF, Coles WA, et al: Endothelin receptor antagonists for pulmonary hypertension in adult patients with sickle cell disease, *Br J Haematol* 147(5):737–743, 2009.

82. Barst RJ, Mubarak KK, Machado RF, et al: Exercise capacity and haemodynamics in patients with sickle cell disease with pulmonary hypertension treated with bosentan: results of the ASSET studies, *Br J Haematol* 149(3):426–435, 2010.

83. Holmes DR Jr, Monahan KH, Packer D: Pulmonary vein stenosis complicating ablation for atrial fibrillation: clinical spectrum and interventional considerations, *JACC Cardiovasc Interv* 2(4):267–276, 2009.

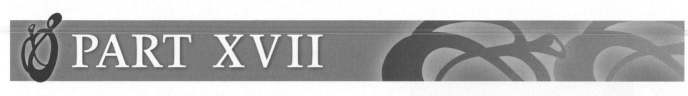

PART XVII

LYMPHATIC DISORDERS

CHAPTER **58** **Diseases of the Lymphatic Circulation**

Stanley G. Rockson

Diseases of the lymphatic circulation may be developmental or acquired. Developmental disorders may be due to impaired or disordered development of the lymphatic vasculature, with accompanying disorders of lymph transit. The acquired lymphatic vascular diseases most often occur following disruption of lymphatic channels, typically in the setting of trauma, infection, neoplasia, or surgical interventions.

Without regard to the prevailing specific cause, interstitial fluid accumulates and swelling ensues when regional lymphatic flow is insufficient to maintain tissue homeostasis. When lymph stasis is chronic, variable degrees of cutaneous and subcutaneous fibrosis typically ensue, often accompanied by substantial deposition of adipose tissue within the subcutis. Collectively, these pathological alterations characterize the lymphatic disorder known clinically as *lymphedema*. Lymphedema may also accompany proliferative disorders of the lymphatic microvasculature that in turn lead to a functionally incompetent vasculature. Lymphatic insufficiency of the viscera can also lead to profound metabolic disturbances. The lymphatic vasculature subserves physiological requirements for both fluid homeostasis and immune traffic. Accordingly, in addition to edema, lymphatic disease is characterized by distinct regional and systemic immune functional compromise.

Historically, the rather limited therapeutic options for lymphatic disease have reflected an incomplete understanding of the pathophysiology of lymphedema; nevertheless, recent advances in imaging and therapeutics, as well as insights gained from vascular biology, hold promise for elaboration of more definitive therapies.

Anatomy of Lymphatic Circulation

Recognition of the lymphatic system and comprehension of its importance came relatively late to the medical and scientific communities. It was not until the 17th century that Gasparo Aselli recognized the lymphatics as a distinct anatomical entity.[1] The gifted professor of anatomy and surgery from Milan was frequently asked by friends and colleagues to perform his elegant vivisections, and on July 23, 1622, he intended to demonstrate to them the action and innervation of the canine diaphragm.

"While I was attempting this, and for that purpose had opened the abdomen and was pulling down with my hand the intestines and stomach…I suddenly beheld a great number of cords, as it were, exceedingly thin and beautifully white, scattered over the whole of the mesentery and the intestine, and starting from almost innumerable beginnings…I noticed that the nerves belonging to the intestine were distinct from these cords, and wholly unlike them, and besides, were distributed quite separately from them. Wherefore struck by the novelty of the thing, I stood for some time silent…When I gathered my wits together for the sake of the experiment, having laid hold of a very sharp

scalpel, I pricked one of these cords and indeed one of the largest of them. I had hardly touched it, when I saw a white liquid like milk or cream forthwith gush out. Seeing this, I could hardly restrain my delight."[1]

The chylous return from the intestine of the recently fed animal allowed Aselli to recognize the lymphatics; when he repeated the demonstration several days later, no vessels were to be seen. Aselli eventually realized the relation between feedings and the visibility of the mesenteric lymphatics and duplicated the work in several species (Fig. 58-1). Over the following half century, Aselli's work was extended by Pecquet, Bartholinus, and Rudbeck, who defined the gross anatomy of the lymphatic system *in toto*.[1] By the 18th century, smaller lymphatic channels were visualized by Anton Nuck using mercury injections. Using those techniques, Sappey observed and recorded the human lymphatic system in exquisite detail (Fig. 58-2). Even greater resolution of the anatomy was provided by von Recklinghausen in 1862 with his discovery that the lymphatic endothelium stained darkly with silver nitrate. Using that technique, he differentiated lymphatic capillaries from blood vessel capillaries. Most recently, substantial advances in the techniques of immunohistochemistry and transmission electron microscopy have enabled the certain identification of the lymphatic microcirculation and discrimination from blood vasculature.[2,3]

It is now well established that lymphatic capillaries are blind-ended tubes formed by a single layer of endothelial cells (ECs). The ECs of lymphatic capillaries closely resemble those of blood vessels and have a common embryonic origin.[4] Like blood vascular endothelium, cultured lymphatic ECS form confluent "cobblestone" monolayers that "sprout" to form tubules. They demonstrate identical histological markers (von Willebrand factor (vWF), F-actin, fibronectin (FN), and Weibel-Palade bodies). Unlike systemic capillaries, the basement membrane of lymphatic capillaries is absent or widely fenestrated, allowing greater entry of interstitial proteins and particles.

The capillaries join to form larger vessels (100-200 μm) that are invested with smooth muscle and capable of vasomotion. Those vessels in turn merge to form larger conduits composed of three distinct layers: intima, media, and adventitia. Those conduits possess intraluminal valves located a few millimeters to centimeters apart that ensure lymph flow is directed centrally.[5,6]

In the lower limbs, the larger conduits form a system of lymphatic return that is divided into superficial and deep components. The superficial component comprises medial and lateral channels. The medial channel originates on the dorsum of the foot and runs along the course of the saphenous vein. The lateral channel begins on the lateral aspect of the foot and ascends to the mid-leg, where the tributaries cross anteriorly to the medial side to follow the course of the medial lymphatics up to the inguinal nodes. Deep lymphatics do not usually communicate with the superficial system except through the popliteal and

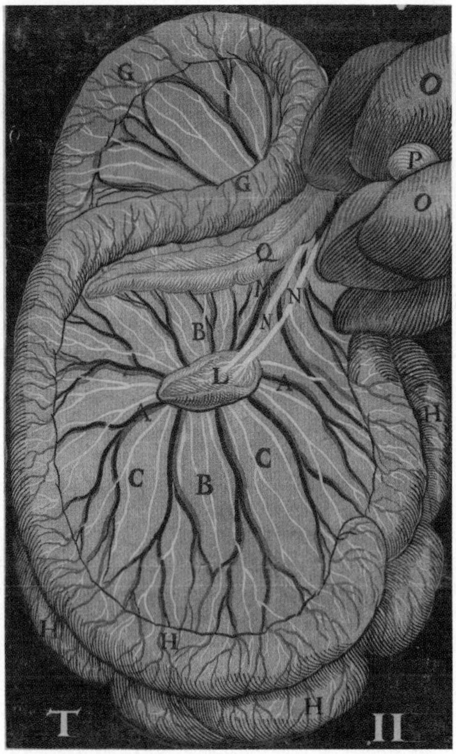

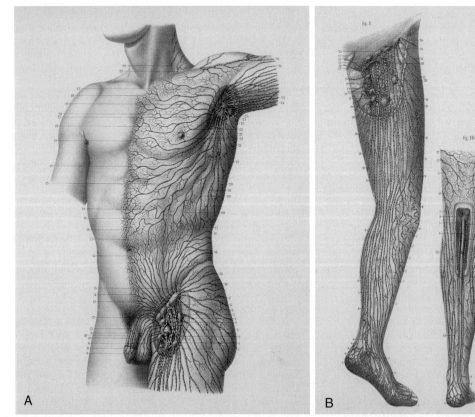

FIGURE 58-1 **Original anatomical illustration of visceral lymphatics by Gasparo Aselli.** *(From the monograph* De Lactibus Sive Lacteis Venis, *courtesy Harvard Medical Library, Francis A. Countway Library of Medicine.)*

inguinal lymph nodes. Those vessels originate subcutaneously, follow the course of the deep blood vessels, and eventually pass through the inguinal nodes.

Small- and medium-sized lymphatic vessels empty into main channels, of which the thoracic duct is the largest. That vessel, roughly 2 mm wide and 45 cm long, ascends from the abdomen through the lower chest just to the right of and anterior to the vertebral column. At approximately the level of the fifth thoracic vertebra, it crosses to the left of the spine, where it continues to ascend through the superior mediastinum to the base of the neck and eventually empties into the left brachiocephalic vein. Other large right- and left-sided lymphatic ducts may exist, although their arrangement, size, and course are highly variable. Those vessels join with the main thoracic duct or empty directly into great veins; they provide important collateral conduits should the thoracic duct become obstructed.

Physiology of Lymphatic Circulation

In 1786, William Hunter and two of his pupils, William Cruikshank and William Hewson, published the results of their work, laying a foundation for the physiology of the lymphatic system.[1] They correctly inferred from clinical observation that the lymphatics were involved in the response to infection, as well as in the absorption of interstitial fluid. A century later, their theories received experimental support from the physiological studies of Karl Ludwig and Ernest Starling. Ludwig cannulated lymph vessels, collected and analyzed the lymph, and proposed that it was a filtrate of plasma. Starling elucidated the forces governing fluid transfer from the blood capillaries to the interstitial space and offered evidence that the same forces apply to the

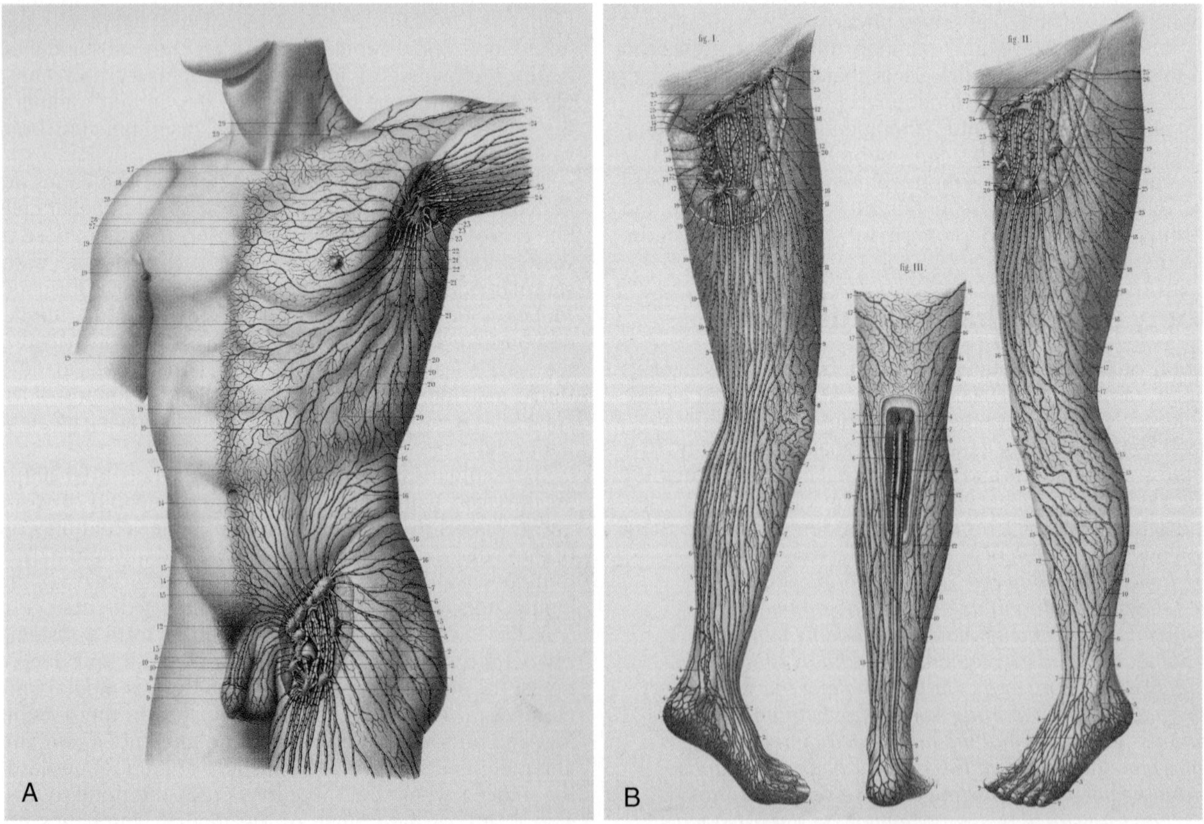

FIGURE 58-2 **Nineteenth-century anatomical delineation of the cutaneous lymphatics of the human trunk (A) and lower extremity (B).** *From the text* Anatomie, Physiologie, Pathologie des Vaisseaux Lymphatiques *by P.C. Sappey [1874], courtesy Harvard Medical Library, Francis A. Countway Library of Medicine.)*

lymphatic capillaries. He proposed that an imbalance in those forces could give rise to edema formation:

> *"In health, therefore, the two processes, lymph production and absorption are exactly proportional. Dropsy depends on a loss of balance between these two processes—on an excess of lymph-production over lymph-absorption. A scientific investigation of the causation of dropsy will therefore involve, in the first place, an examination of the factors which determine the extent of these two processes and, so far as is possible, the manner in which these processes are carried out."[7]*

As first enunciated by Starling, interstitial fluid is largely an ultrafiltrate of blood. Its rate of production reflects the balance between factors that favor filtration out of capillaries (capillary hydrostatic pressure and tissue oncotic pressure) and those that favor reabsorption (interstitial hydrostatic pressure and capillary oncotic pressure).[7] Under normal conditions, filtration exceeds reabsorption at a rate sufficient to create 2 to 4 L of interstitial fluid per day. There is a net filtration of protein (primarily albumin) from the vasculature into the interstitium; approximately 100 g of circulating protein may escape into the interstitial space daily. The interstitial fluid also receives the waste products of cellular metabolism, as well as foreign matter or microbes that enter through breaks in the skin or by hematogenous routes.

The volume and composition of interstitial fluid are kept in balance by the lymphatic system. The functions of that system include (1) transport of excess fluid, protein, and waste products from the interstitial space to the blood stream; (2) distribution of immune cells and substances from the lymphoid tissues to the systemic circulation; (3) filtration and removal of foreign material from the interstitial fluid; and (4) in the viscera, promoting absorption of lipids from the intestinal lumen.

Not surprisingly, the lymphatics require a complex interplay of specific anatomy and function to meet physiological requirements. Several forces drive fluid through the lymphatic system. The lymphatic vessels in skeletal muscle are compressed by extrinsic muscular contractions that propel the fluid centrally through the unidirectional valves. In other tissues, such as the splanchnic and cutaneous systems, it is primarily contractions of lymphatic smooth muscle that generate the driving force.[8,9] These contractions are increased in frequency and amplitude by elevated filling pressure, sympathetic nerve activity, and shock, and they may be modulated by circulating hormones and prostanoids.[10–12] Considerable force can be generated by those contractions; experimentally induced obstruction of the popliteal lymphatic system augments the strength and frequency of contraction, generating pressures of up to 50 mmHg.[13] Other factors that may contribute to lymphatic flow include intermittent compression from arterial pulsations and gastrointestinal peristalsis. In addition, it has most recently been proposed that the initial lymphatics (small lymphatic capillaries that begin blindly in the tissues) most likely possess a two-valve system.[14,15] In addition to the classically described secondary intralymphatic valves, the initial lymphatics are thought to possess a primary valve system at the level of the endothelium to ensure unidirectional flow at this level. Once lymph enters the thorax, negative intrathoracic pressure generated during inspiration aspirates fluid into the thoracic duct (the "respiratory pump").[13] Failure of adequate lymph transport promotes lymphedema and likely contributes to the pathological presentation of a wide variety of lymphatic vascular diseases.

Lymphatic Insufficiency (Lymphedema)

Pathogenesis of Edema

Edema develops when production of interstitial fluid (lymph) exceeds its transport through the lymphatic system. Thus, overproduction of lymph (enhanced lymphatic load) or decreased ability to remove fluid (defective transport) from the interstitium may result in edema. Conditions associated with overproduction of lymph include elevated venous pressures, increased capillary permeability, and hypoproteinemia. Elevated hydrostatic pressure in the veins results in increased filtration of plasma from venules and blood capillaries (as seen in right-sided congestive heart failure (CHF), tricuspid regurgitation, and deep vein thrombosis [DVT]). Conversely, local inflammation increases capillary permeability, accelerating loss of protein and fluid to the interstitium despite a normal capillary hydrostatic pressure. Lymph production may increase by 10- to 20-fold, exceeding lymphatic transport and resulting in marked edema.[16] Hypoproteinemia also may lead to marked edema, in which case hydrostatic pressure and capillary permeability are normal, but capillary oncotic pressure is reduced, favoring osmotic flow to the interstitium. The edema that ensues in these conditions can, strictly speaking, be called *lymphedema* only when there is objective evidence of impaired lymphatic clearance or physical evidence of consequences of impaired lymphatic function in the skin or subcutaneous tissues.

Pathogenesis of Lymphedema

Lymphedema occurs whenever lymphatic vessels are absent, underdeveloped, or obstructed. Impedance to lymphatic flow may be due to an inborn defect (primary lymphedema) or an acquired loss of lymphatic patency (secondary lymphedema).

PRIMARY LYMPHEDEMA

Prevalence estimates for the heritable causes of lymphedema are difficult to ascertain and vary substantially. Primary lymphedema is thought to occur in approximately 1 of every 6 to 10,000 live births. Females are affected 2- to 10-fold more commonly than males.[17,18] Primary lymphedema represents a heterogeneous group of disorders, and therefore its classification schemata are numerous. Affected individuals can be classified by age of onset, functional anatomical attributes, or clinical setting.

Age of Onset

When distinguished by age of clinical onset, primary lymphedema can typically be divided into the following categories[19]:
1. Congenital lymphedema, clinically apparent at or near birth.
2. Lymphedema praecox, with onset after birth and before age 35; *lymphedema praecox*, a term used by Allen in 1934, most typically appears in the peripubertal years.
3. Lymphedema tarda appears after the age of 35.

Anatomical Patterns

An alternative classification scheme relies on an anatomical description of the lymphatic vasculature[20,21]:
1. Aplasia: no collecting vessels identified.
2. Hypoplasia: a diminished number of vessels are seen.
3. Numerical hyperplasia (as defined by Kinmonth): an increased number of vessels are seen.
4. Hyperplasia: in addition to an increase in number, the vessels have valvular incompetence and display tortuosity and dilation (megalymphatics).

Approximately one third of all cases are secondary to agenesis, hypoplasia, or obstruction of the distal lymphatic vessels, with relatively normal proximal vessels.[26,27] In those cases, swelling is usually bilateral and mild and affects females much more frequently than males. The prognosis in such cases is good. Generally after the first year of symptoms, there is little extension in the same limb or to uninvolved extremities. Although the extent of involvement is established early in the disease in about 40% of patients, the girth of the limb continues to increase.

In more than half of all cases, the defect primarily involves obstruction of the proximal lymphatics or nodes, with initial lack of involvement of distal lymphatic vessels. Pathological studies reveal intranodal fibrosis.[15] In those cases, swelling tends to be unilateral and severe; there may be a slight predominance of females in this group. In patients with proximal involvement, the extent and degree of the abnormality is more likely to progress and require surgical intervention. Initially uninvolved distal lymphatic vessels may become obliterated with time.

A minority of patients have a pattern of bilateral hyperplasia of the lymphatic channels or tortuous dilated megalymphatics. In these less common forms of primary lymphedema, there is a slight male predominance. Megalymphatics are associated with a greater extent of involvement and a worse prognosis.

Clinical Characteristics

As a third alternative, the primary lymphedemas can often be characterized by associated clinical anomalies or abnormal phenotype.[21] Although sporadic instances of primary lymphedema are more common, the tendency for congenital lymphedema to cluster in families is significant. The syndrome of a familial predisposition to congenital lymphedema, ultimately determined to ensue from an autosomal dominant form of inheritance with variable penetrance, was first described by Milroy in 1892.[22] He reported "hereditary edema" affecting 22 individuals of one family over six generations. Although Milroy ultimately came to consider not only congenital lymphedema but also praecox and tarda forms as variants of the syndrome that bears his name,[23] the praecox form of primary lymphedema more often carries the eponym of *Meige's disease*.[24]

In fact, a long list of disorders are associated with heritable forms of lymphedema. Increasingly these disorders have yielded to chromosomal mapping techniques. Lymphedema-cholestasis, or *Aagenaes' syndrome*, has been mapped to chromosome 15q.[25] In several family cohorts of *Milroy's disease*, it has been determined that the disorder reflects missense inactivating mutations in the tyrosine kinase domain of vascular endothelial growth factor receptor 3 (VEGFR3),[26,27] thus underscoring the likelihood that the pathogenesis of this condition likely reflects an inherited defect in lymphatic vasculogenesis. Several additional lymphedema syndromes have recently lent themselves to successful genetic mapping.[21] *Lymphedema-distichiasis*, an autosomal dominant dysmorphic syndrome in which lymphedema presents in association with a supplementary row of eyelashes arising from the meibomian glands, has been linked to truncating mutations in the forkhead-related transcription factor FOXC2[28]; mutations in FOXC2 have subsequently been associated with a broad variety of primary lymphedema presentations.[29] Similarly, a more unusual form of congenital lymphedema, *hypotrichosis-lymphedema-telangiectasia*, has been ascribed to both recessive and dominant forms of inheritance of mutations in the transcription factor gene SOX18.[30] Most recently, linkage analysis of three affected family cohorts has associated the occurrence of autosomal recessive congenital lymphatic dysplasia (*Hennekam's syndrome*) to the gene CCBE1,[31,32] also identified as critical to lymphangiogenesis in zebrafish.[31] It is altogether plausible that further elucidation of the molecular pathogenesis of these diseases linked to FOXC2, SOX18, and CCBE1 mutations will lead to enhanced insights into mechanisms of normal and abnormal lymphatic development. Furthermore, mutational analysis of families expressing inherited forms of lymphedema have disclosed specific mutations in hepatocyte growth factor (HGF) (which encodes HGF) and MET (the HGF receptor).[33] GJC2, the gene that encodes connexin-47 has also been implicated in the familial occurrence of lymphedema.[34]

In general, autosomal or sex-linked recessive forms of congenital lymphedema occur less commonly than the dominant forms of inheritance. Nevertheless, the list of heritable lymphedema-associated syndromes is long and growing (Box 58-1). Primary lymphedema has been described in association with various forms of chromosomal aneuploidy (e.g., Turner's and Klinefelter's syndromes), various dysmorphogenic genetic anomalies (e.g., Noonan's syndrome, neurofibromatosis), and with various as yet unrelated disorders such as yellow nail syndrome, intestinal lymphangiectasia, lymphangiomyomatosis, and arteriovenous malformation (AVM).[35] The association of lymphedema with vascular anomalies likely derives from the shared embryological origin of the lymphatic and venous vasculature.

Box 58-1 Hereditary Conditions Associated with Lymphedema

Chromosomal Aneuploidy
Trisomy 13
Trisomy 18
Trisomy 21
Triploidy
Klinefelter's syndrome
Turner's syndrome

Dysmorphogenic-Genetic Disturbances
Noonan's syndrome
Nonne-Milroy hereditary lymphedema
Meige lymphedema (lymphedema praecox)
Lymphedema-distichiasis
Cholestasis-lymphedema syndrome (Aagenaes' syndrome)
Lymphedema-microcephaly-chorioretinopathy
Neurofibromatosis type I (von Recklinghausen)
Lymphedema-hypoparathyroidism syndrome
Klippel-Trénaunay-Weber's dr syndrome

From Rockson SG: Syndromic lymphedema: keys to the kingdom of lymphatic structure and function? Lymph Res Biol 1:181, 2003.[21]

SECONDARY LYMPHEDEMA

Secondary lymphedema is an acquired condition that can arise after loss or obstruction of previously adequate lymphatic channels. A wide variety of pathological processes may lead to such lymphatic obliteration.

Infection

Recurrent bacterial lymphangitis leads to thrombosis and fibrosis of the lymphatic channels and is one of the most common causes of lymphedema.[36] The responsible bacteria are almost always streptococci, which tend to enter through breaks in the skin or fissures induced by trichophytosis. Recurrent bacterial lymphangitis is also a frequent complicating factor of lymphedema from any cause.

Filariasis, a nematode infection endemic to regions of South America, Asia and Africa, is the most common cause of secondary lymphedema in the world. The World Health Organization (WHO) estimates that more than 130 million people may be affected by filarial infections; in India alone there are up to 14 million symptomatic cases. Common tropical filaria include *Wuchereria bancrofti* and *Brugia malayi* or *timori*. Other *Brugia* species are found in North America and occasionally cause lymphatic obstruction.

The microfilaria are transmitted by a mosquito vector and induce recurrent lymphangitis and eventual fibrosis of lymph nodes. It is unclear whether filaria themselves produce the lymphangitis or simply predispose those afflicted to recurrent episodes of bacterial lymphangitis. The filaria also can be identified in blood specimens of tissue obtained by fine-needle biopsy of affected areas, and eosinophilia is a common local and systemic feature. Diethylcarbamazine remains the most popular drug for treating filariasis; although side effects are frequent, it is extremely efficacious.[37] Ivermectin is a newer antifilarial agent that may replace diethylcarbamazine; it is less toxic, and a single oral dose (25 μg/kg) appears to be as efficacious as a 2-week course of diethylcarbamazine.[38]

Lymphatic Trauma

Within this category, by far the most common mechanism of lymphedema relates to surgical excision of lymph nodes.[39] This occurs most commonly in the setting of cancer staging and therapeutics. Breast cancer–associated lymphedema is the most common form of lymphedema in the United States. Both axillary lymph node dissection and adjuvant radiation therapy, particularly to the breast and axilla, predispose to development of secondary lymphedema of the upper extremity.[40] In clinical follow-up after periods of up to 13 years following invasive treatment of breast cancer, a late incidence of lymphedema of 14% can be expected in surgically treated patients with adjuvant postoperative irradiation.[41] Even less radical surgery (e.g., lumpectomy) can occasionally be complicated by lymphedema. Despite improvements in surgical and radiotherapeutic techniques, lymphedema remains a potential complication.[42,43] Similarly, edema of the leg may occur after surgery for pelvic or genital cancer, particularly when there has been inguinal and pelvic lymph node dissection or irradiation.[44] Its reported frequency varies between 1% and 47%.[45,46] Pelvic irradiation increases the frequency of leg lymphedema after cancer surgery[47] for such conditions as malignant melanoma, prostate cancer, and gynecological malignancies.

Lymphedema can also ensue from other mechanisms of lymphatic trauma, among them burns, large or circumferential wounds of the extremity, or other iatrogenic causes.[48]

Malignant Diseases

In addition to cancer therapeutics, various malignancies may induce secondary lymphedema. Tumor cells may obstruct lymphatic vessels, inducing lymphedema directly or predisposing the patient to bacterial lymphangitis. In males, the most common neoplastic etiology is prostate cancer; in females it is lymphoma.

Other Causes

Other conditions leading to or associated with obstruction of lymphatic channels include tuberculosis, contact dermatitis, rheumatoid arthritis, and pregnancy.[49] Autoimmune destruction of the lymphatics remains an interesting but unproven etiology.[50] Factitious lymphedema ("oedema bleu") also occurs. The condition usually affects the hand, arm, or both; is unilateral; and is induced by applications of tourniquets, self-inflicted cellulitis, or maintenance of the limb in an immobile and dependent state. Chronic subcutaneous injections of drugs (most notably, pentazocine hydrochloride) also may lead to lymphatic sclerosis and obstruction.

Pathology of Lymphedema

Early in the natural history of lymphedema, there is variable thickening of the epidermis; the skin becomes rough with hyperkeratosis and accentuation of skin folds. Organization and fibrosis may lead to development of papillomatosis. Early on, substantial edema of the dermis may occur. On cut section of gross specimens, the dermis is firm and gray, as is the deep fascia. Usually later in the course, but sometimes quite early, there may be expansion of the subcutaneous adipose tissue, often septated by prominent fibrous strands. In some specimens, compression causes lymph to exude from the dermis and subcutaneous tissue, although this is not a prominent feature. Microscopic examination reveals hyperkeratosis with prominent dermal fibrosis, as well as variable degrees of dermal edema (Fig. 58-3). Abundant subcutaneous fat with prominent fibrous septa is apparent in all cases. Often, perivascular inflammatory cells (lymphocytes, plasma cells, and occasionally eosinophils) can be seen. The lymphatic vessels often are difficult to visualize and may be obliterated or thrombosed by previous inflammatory episodes or may be congenitally absent or hypoplastic. Dilation of the lymphatics may be seen.

Clinical Presentation

Clinical signs of lymphedema largely depend on duration and severity of the disease. Initially the interstitial space is expanded by an excess accumulation of relatively protein-rich fluid volume. The swelling produced by that fluid collection typically is soft, is easily displaced with pressure ("pitting edema"), and may substantially decrease with elevation of the limb. In the lower extremities, the edema typically extends to the distal aspects of the feet, resulting in the characteristic "square toes" seen in this condition. Over a period of years, the limb may take on a woody texture as the surrounding tissue becomes indurated and fibrotic (Fig. 58-4). In these

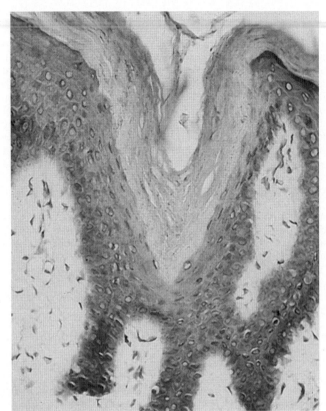

FIGURE 58-3 Skin biopsy in chronic lymphedema discloses characteristic hyperkeratosis and hypercellularity.

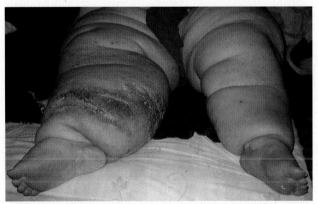

FIGURE 58-4 Profound cutaneous and subdermal changes in chronic lower-extremity lymphedema.

later stages, pitting edema is no longer a major component, and limb elevation or external compression is much less successful at reducing the girth of the extremity.

Proliferation of subcutaneous connective and adipose tissue leads to thickening of the skin and loss of flexibility; the affected limb is grossly enlarged, and a mossy or cobblestone skin texture may develop. Correlates of these changes that can be sought on physical examination include the peau d'orange that reflects cutaneous and subcutaneous fibrosis, and the so-called Stemmer sign (inability to tent the skin at the base of the digits), which is considered to be pathognomonic of lymphedema when present in a swollen limb.[51] In many cases of long-standing lymphedema, deposition of substantial amounts of subcutaneous adipose tissue has been described,[52] hypothetically ascribable to abnormalities of adipogenesis or lipid accumulation that accompany chronic stagnation of lymph.[53] However, the mechanisms of this consequence of chronic lymphatic circulatory insufficiency have not yet been delineated.

Natural History and Differential Diagnosis

The natural history of lymphedema is quite variable and often may encompass a substantial interval of subclinical asymptomatic disease. For example, even 3 years following modified radical mastectomy and axillary lymph node dissection, more than 80% of women remain free of any overt clinical evidence of lymphatic impairment despite extensive iatrogenic destruction of the lymphatic architecture in these patients. Similarly, in many forms of primary lymphedema, there may be a protracted phase of apparently adequate lymphatic function despite the inherited anatomical or functional pathology. Precipitating factors for the appearance of overt lymphedema are unknown. At the onset of clinical lymphedema, swelling of the involved extremity is typically described as puffy, and at times, the edematous changes may even be intermittent. With chronicity, the involved structures develop the characteristic features of induration and fibrosis.[54] In many of these patients, the maximal volume increase of the involved limb is determined within the first year after clinical onset unless there are supervening complications like recurrent cellulitis. The propensity to recurrent soft-tissue infection is one of the most troublesome aspects of long-standing lymphedema. In addition to the proinfectious features of accumulated fluid and proteins, lymphatic dysfunction also impairs local immune responses.[55,56] With recurrent infections, there is progressive damage of lymphatic capillaries.

In rare cases, long-standing chronic lymphedema may be complicated by local development of malignant tumors. Although it is unnecessary to burden patients about the possibility of malignancy, they should be alerted to report any changes in appearance of the limb. Neoplastic transformation of blood or lymph vessels can develop in long-standing lymphedema of any cause, including primary or secondary lymphedema.[57,58] Angiosarcomas or lymphangiosarcomas are potentially devastating but fortunately uncommon complications of long-standing lymphedema, occurring in less than 1% of cases.[59] Lymphangiosarcomas can be either sclerotic plaques or multicentric lesions with blue-tinged nodules or bullous changes. Early detection and amputation can be lifesaving, but recognition of the condition is often delayed by a lack of awareness on the part of the patient and physician. Other malignancies including lymphoma, Kaposi sarcoma, squamous cell cancer, and malignant melanoma have been reported in association with chronic lymphedema.

The hypertrophied limb with thickened skin seen in chronic lymphedema has little similarity to the edematous limb of deep venous insufficiency (see Chapter 55). In the latter case, a soft-pitting edema is prominent and seen in association with stasis dermatitis, hemosiderin deposition, and superficial venous varicosities. The history and examination easily differentiate chronic lymphedema from venous disorders and other causes of limb swelling (see Fig. 58-4). Earlier in the presentation, however, it may be more difficult to distinguish lymphedema from venous disease, reflex sympathetic dystrophy, or other causes of limb swelling.

Myxedema can be characterized by lower-extremity edema that superficially resembles lymphedema. In hypothyroidism, edema arises when abnormal mucinous deposits accumulate in the skin. Hyaluronic acid–rich protein deposition in the dermis produces edema with resulting abnormal structural integrity and reduced skin elasticity. In thyrotoxicosis, this process is localized to the pretibial region. Myxedema is characterized by roughening of the skin of the palms, soles, elbows, and knees; brittle, uneven nails; dull, thinning hair; yellow-orange discoloration of the skin; and reduced sweat production.

Lipedema is a condition that affects women almost exclusively, although it can be seen in men with a feminizing disorder. Edema is caused by accumulation of subcutaneous adipose tissue in the leg, with sparing of the feet. Although the pathophysiology of lipedema is uncertain, it does involve an increase of subcutaneous adipocytes with structural alterations in the small vascular structures within the skin. Indeed, regional abnormalities of the circulation may cause the initial accumulation of fat in affected regions. The characteristic distribution, with sparing of the feet, should suggest the correct diagnosis. Absence of a Stemmer sign is an additional clue. Most often, lipedema arises within 1 to 2 years after the onset of puberty. In addition to the near-lifelong history of heavy thighs and hips, affected patients often complain of painful swelling. In addition, these individuals are commonly predisposed to easy bruising, perhaps a result of increased fragility of capillaries within the adipose tissue.

Diagnostic Modalities

Sometimes it is necessary to obtain more information about the nature and degree of lymphatic involvement when (1) the etiology of a swollen limb remains uncertain, (2) the diagnosis is evident but the etiology is unclear, or (3) a surgical drainage procedure is being considered.

LYMPHANGIOGRAPHY

Human lymphatics were first visualized *in vivo* by Hudack and McMaster at the Rockefeller Institute in 1933.[1] They used one another as subjects to demonstrate superficial lymphatic plexuses along the forearm and inner thigh, using subcutaneous injection of vital dyes. In 1948, Glenn cannulated a lymphatic vessel in the dog hindlimb and injected contrast media to produce a lymphangiogram in the canine leg and groin.[1] Subsequently, Servelle and Deysson visualized the lymphatics in patients with elephantiasis, using retrograde injection.[1] Visualization of the dilated lymph channels, however, depended on partial or complete valvular incompetence. Direct contrast lymphangiography was developed by Kinmonth and coworkers in 1952.[60] The technique involves identification of a distal vessel made visible by an intradermal injection of a vital dye into the metatarsal web spaces. The vessel is isolated and cannulated, and iodinated contrast material is injected. Following the injection, the contrast material is visualized radiographically as it progresses proximally through lymphatic channels.

There are several drawbacks to the procedure, including frequent requirements for surgical exposure in the edematous limb, microsurgical techniques to achieve direct cannulation, and occasionally the need for general anesthesia.[27] Of greater importance is the fact that the irritation caused by the contrast agent results in lymphangitis in one third of the studies and potentially can worsen the lymphedema.[61] For these reasons, the use of lymphangiography as a diagnostic modality for the edematous limb has largely been abandoned and is contraindicated in patients with lymphedema.

LYMPHOSCINTIGRAPHY

Lymphoscintigraphy involves injection of radiolabeled macromolecules, such as sulfur colloid or albumin, into the distal subcutaneous tissue of the affected extremity (e.g., dorsum of foot). The progress of the radionuclide through the lymphatic system is followed by a radioscintigraphic camera. In primary lymphedema, channels are obliterated or absent; in a small percentage of cases, they are ectatic and incompetent. In secondary lymphedema, often with dilation of the vascular channels, the level of obstruction can be determined.[62] In lymphedema of any cause, the proximal progression of the radionuclide is delayed, and its accumulation distally in the dilated channels of the dermis is manifested as a "dermal backflow" pattern (Fig. 58-5).

Lymphoscintigraphy is easier to perform than lymphangiography and is not reported to cause lymphangitis. It lacks the spatial resolution of lymphangiography; resolution is maximized by reducing the swelling of the extremity as much as possible before the study (reducing dilution of the radionuclide in stagnant lymph). Effective use of lymphoscintigraphy to plan therapeutic interventions requires an understanding of the pathophysiology of

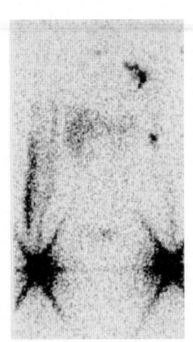

FIGURE 58-5 **Bilateral upper-extremity lymphoscintigraphy is accomplished by subcutaneous interdigital injection of radiolabeled sulfur colloid.** Study illustrates absence of nodal uptake in right axilla, along with prominent "dermal backflow" in right forearm. These findings confirm diagnosis of unilateral lymphedema.

lymphedema and the influence of technical factors, such as selection of the radiopharmaceutical, imaging times after injection, and patient activity after injection on the images.[63]

COMPUTED TOMOGRAPHY

Computed tomography (CT) scans of a lymphedematous limb are characterized by a honeycomb pattern in the affected area.[64] Computed tomography cannot directly localize the level of obstruction.[65] This technique can, however, provide insight into volume changes within various compartments visualized on cross-sectional images of the affected limb.[66] The greatest utility of CT is its ability to distinguish some of the causes of secondary lymphedema (e.g., lymphoma, pelvic tumor). Certainly, the typical honeycomb pattern of lymphedema can be sought. In addition, elements of the differential diagnosis (venous obstruction, obesity, hematoma, ruptured popliteal cyst) can be further delineated through CT images.

MAGNETIC RESONANCE IMAGING

Magnetic resonance imaging (MRI) is an alternative, and most likely superior, technique to image the soft tissues in edema.[67] Among the discernible attributes by MRI are: cutaneous thickening with a honeycomb pattern in the subdermis, dilated lymphatic channels (when present as a consequence of lymphangioma or lymph reflux), and dermal accumulation of free fluid with surrounding fibrosis. This technique has particular virtue in differentiating lymphedema from lipedema. In addition, more recently it has been demonstrated that nonenhanced three-dimensional (3D) heavily T2-weighted images obtained with two-dimensional (2D) prospective acquisition and correction has the capacity to visualize the thoracic duct, cisterna chyli, and lumbar lymphatics, at least in healthy volunteers.[68]

Treatment

MEDICAL THERAPY

Successful treatment of lymphedema requires close collaboration between patient and physician. To that end, the physician should (1) carefully instruct the patient in the details of the

medical program and (2) attend to the psychological impact of the disease. Associated emotional problems are not uncommon and are often neglected by physicians.[24] The need to address the psychological aspects of long-term disfigurement, especially with adolescent patients, cannot be overemphasized. In discussing these issues with the patient, the physician should be realistic about the possibility of progression but should emphasize the patient's ability to modulate the course of the disease by careful attention to the details of the medical program.

The physiotherapeutic approach to lymphedema has been termed *decongestive lymphatic therapy*. Meticulous attention to control of edema may reduce the likelihood of disease progression and limit the incidence of soft-tissue infections.[69] The elements of this therapeutic approach have been designed to accomplish the initial reduction in edematous limb volume, maintain these therapeutic gains, and ensure optimal health and functional integrity of the skin.[70,71] In addition to the acute reduction in limb volume that is attainable, a well-maintained therapeutic program has been demonstrated to accelerate lymph transport and enhance dispersal of accumulated protein. Decongestive lymphatic therapy integrates elements of meticulous skin care, massage, bandaging, exercise, and use of compressive elastic garments.

To hydrate and soothe the skin, water-soluble emollients should be applied in a consistent and diligent manner. For excessive hyperkeratosis, these emollients can be supplemented with application of salicylic acid ointments. Where skin cracking is prominent, meticulous attention to hygiene can be coupled with topical antiseptic agents.

The specialized massage technique for these patients (socalled manual lymphatic drainage or therapy) is an empirically derived technique. Its goal is to enhance lymphatic contractility and to augment and redirect lymph flow through the unobstructed cutaneous lymphatics. Manual lymphatic drainage should not be confused with other forms of therapeutic massage that do not share this ability to augment lymphatic contractility and may in fact be detrimental to lymphatic function (e.g., athletic massages). The mild tissue compression during manual lymphatic drainage results in enhanced filling of the initial lymphatics and improves transport capacity through cutaneous lymphatic dilation and development of accessory lymph collectors.[71] Typically, 8 to 15 consecutive daily sessions of manual lymphatic drainage are required to achieve optimal reduction of limb volume in a previously untreated patient.

During this acute approach to volume reduction, nonelastic compressive bandages should be applied in multiple layers after each session of manual lymphatic drainage (Fig. 58-6). These are worn during muscular exertion (which is encouraged) to prevent reaccumulation of fluid and promote lymph flow during exertion. Multilayer bandaging can also help reverse skin changes, soften subcutaneous tissues, and reduce the degree of lymphorrhea when present. In the maintenance phase of lymphedema care, use of multilayer bandages is most often supplanted by daily use of compressive elastic garments.

Elastic support hose should be fitted to the patient's limb after edema in the extremity has been maximally reduced by compression and elevation.[36] This is an important detail. The stocking or sleeve does not reduce the size of the limb but maintains the circumference to which it is fitted. However, if the limb is fitted for a stocking while in a swollen state, the limb will be maintained by the stocking in a swollen state. The prescription of compressive garments is a necessary adjunct to all other forms of maintenance lymphedema therapy. Relatively inelastic sleeves, stockings, and underwear that transmit high-grade compression (40-80 mmHg) will prevent reaccumulation of fluid after successful decongestive treatments. Garments must be fitted properly and replaced when they lose their elasticity (every 3-6 months). In addition to standard fitted garments for upper and lower extremities, various additional appliances are now available. They provide the capacity to maintain limb volume during sleep, when the sleeve or stocking is removed, and during various forms of activity.

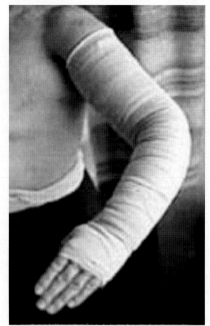

FIGURE 58-6 **Short-stretch multilayer compression bandaging in secondary lymphedema of the upper extremity.**

Without guidance from the physician, some patients become sedentary in response to uncomfortable or heavy sensations in the affected limb. Reduced physical activity at work and home leads to apathy and malaise; that consequence can be averted by encouraging physical activity with proper support hose. Regular exercise appears to reduce lymphedema as long as elastic support (or hydrostatic pressure) is applied. Swimming is a particularly good physical activity for these patients because the hydrostatic pressure of the surrounding water negates the need for compressive support.

Although the elements of decongestive lymphatic therapy were initially derived empirically, the efficacy of these interventions has now been demonstrated in numerous prospective observations.[72–74] Long-term efficacy is particularly enhanced when there is attention to focused patient instruction in maintenance self-care.[73]

Various adjunctive treatment approaches have been investigated. Of these, perhaps the most useful is intermittent pneumatic compression (IPC). Multichamber pneumatic devices are available that intermittently compress the limb; techniques that employ sequential graduated compression (in which the cuffs are inflated sequentially from distal to proximal sites with a pressure gradient from the most distal cuff to the most proximal) are the most efficacious.[75] Pneumatic compression techniques cannot, however, clear edema fluid from adjacent noncompressed sections of the limb. Consequently, as fluid shifts occur during pneumatic compression, the root of the limb must be decompressed with the aforementioned manual techniques.

Incorporation of IPC into a multidisciplinary therapeutic approach has long been advocated empirically by some physiotherapeutic schools.[75] Individual reports of complications and lack of efficacy have reduced enthusiasm for the use of pneumatic compression as stand-alone therapy. More recently, it has been demonstrated that when IPC is used adjunctively with other established elements of decongestive lymphatic therapy, it enhances therapeutic response, both in the initial and maintenance approaches to the patient. Pneumatic compression is well tolerated and remarkably free of complications.[76,77] However, it must be stressed that any form of compressive therapy requires sufficient arterial blood supply to the limb. In cases where severe peripheral artery disease (PAD) coexists, any form of sustained compression can further compromise arterial blood flow.

Other physical forms of therapy are under investigation. Low-level laser therapy may be effective in postmastectomy lymphedema; in one small series, subjective improvement accompanied an objective documentation of improved bioimpedance and reduced extracellular and intracellular fluid accumulation.[78] In other hands, such techniques as local hyperthermia or intraarterial injection of autologous lymphocytes[79] have independently produced favorable results. In the latter approach, it is postulated that regression of edema is linked to the expression of L-selectin, a lymphocyte-specific adhesion molecule.[79] Observations in these pilot studies must be confirmed in larger controlled trials.

Additional standard treatment approaches are directed toward prevention and control of infection. Recurrent cellulitis and local infections pose a constant threat of exacerbation. Skin hygiene is essential. In addition to the application of emollients to the skin, trauma must be avoided (when ambulatory, the feet should be covered by slippers or shoes; a podiatrist should attend to nail care as needed). Fungal infections should be aggressively treated with topical antifungal agents. The patient should be instructed to take antibiotics at the earliest sign of cellulitis and should be given a prescription for a course of an oral semisynthetic penicillin or (for penicillin-sensitive patients) erythromycin. In lymphedema, acute inflammatory episodes may not elicit typical clearly demarcated erythematous skin responses or associated systemic evidence of infection. Nevertheless, these more subtle presentations should be treated aggressively with antibiotics. After a course of therapy, the edema once again responds to compressive therapy, and the tenderness resolves. Various broad-spectrum oral antibiotics can be used to good effect, particularly with attention to the spectrum of activity against streptococcal and staphylococcal species.

Other than antibiotic therapy where needed, pharmacotherapy has little role in the management of lymphedema. Diuretics, although widely prescribed for this chronic edematous condition, are rarely useful and may in fact be deleterious. On the other hand, in edema of mixed origin, diuretics may have a beneficial effect through their ability to reduce circulating blood volume and thereby reduce capillary filtration. An understanding of the mechanisms inducing the proliferation of subcutaneous connective tissue and lymphedema may lead to more definitive treatment. Agents might then be designed to alter the relationship between the deposition and lysis of collagen fibers such that lysis is favored, thereby reducing fibrosis.[5]

Benzopyrones (coumarin, hydroxyethylrutin) represent a class of agents that have been reported to reduce volume in affected limbs, purportedly by stimulating tissue macrophages, which in turn increase interstitial proteolysis. Although initial trials appeared favorable,[80,81] subsequent evaluation suggests that the therapeutic gains are small[82]; furthermore, the utility of coumarin is significantly hampered by the risk of drug-related hepatotoxicity.[83] An important question left unanswered is whether coumarin is additive in its effects to the usual compressive measures. The agent is not yet approved by the U.S. Food and Drug Administration (FDA) for use in the United States.

Another experimental therapy is intralymphatic injections of steroids, which may help by inhibiting proliferation of connective tissue. Development of angiogenic steroids that have some tissue specificity could make this a feasible approach. Alternatively, flavonoids such as hesperidin and diosmin have been employed to beneficial effect. Their use is supported by preclinical experimental investigations that suggest the agents have the capacity to improve microvascular permeability and augment lymphatic contractile activity. Extract of horse chestnut seed containing escin, a bioflavonoid, has been shown to reduce venular capillary permeability and edema of lymphatic or venous etiology.

SURGICAL TREATMENT

Surgery is a last resort and only for selected cases. It should not be considered lightly. When the lymphatic obstruction is of a proximal type and the lymphatic channels distal to the obstruction are of adequate diameter, a drainage procedure is occasionally feasible under certain well-defined circumstances, and only by skilled operators. Even then, successful drainage is gained in only about 50% of cases and is often temporary.

Flaps of tissue rich in lymphatics have been implanted into the edematous region. In theory, if the lymphatic vessels in the flap remain functional, they eventually may anastomose with the surrounding lymphatics and provide an alternative pathway for drainage from the edematous area. The myocutaneous flap (using latissimus dorsi) has been reported to be useful for the upper extremity, and the intestinal flap (enteromesenteric bridge) may improve drainage in the lower extremity.

Direct microsurgical anastomotic procedures also have been used.[84] Lymphovenous anastomoses can be made between lymphatic vessels distal to an obstruction in nearby small veins; these allow lymph from the obstructed region to flow directly into the venous system. Anastomoses also can be made from the lymph nodes to the adjacent vein. One of the latest techniques involves harvesting normal autogenous lymphatic vessels for use as bypass grafts around a lymphatic obstruction. All these microsurgical techniques require the presence of dilated lymphatic vessels distal to the obstruction. These operations obviously are of no value when the lymphatic obstruction is at the level of the smaller distal vessels. The argument has been made, however, that lymphatic bypass operations should be performed as soon as possible after the onset of obstruction to avoid the cutaneous changes of chronic lymphedema, as well as the gradual destruction of the distal lymphatic channels. An appropriate candidate for such surgery would be an individual with a recent onset of lymphedema secondary to trauma and with an otherwise normal lymphatic system proximal and distal to the area of obstruction. In a recently published large series of such appropriately selected patients, microsurgical lymphatic-venous anastomosis accomplished objective reduction of limb volume in 85% of cases.[85]

Reduction procedures have generally been employed for limbs that have become so bulky or unsightly they constitute a significant impairment to daily living. Such procedures are generally considered a patient's last resort and, by themselves, result in a limb that is scarred and disfigured, albeit more mobile. Reduction procedures involve resection of a portion of the skin and subcutaneous tissue and subsequent closure of the wound to reduce the limb diameter. Acute complications include wound infection or necrosis of the skin flaps; late complications include recurrent cellulitis or verrucous hyperplasia of the skin grafts. Swelling of the extremity is more likely to progress if recurrent bouts of cellulitis are not adequately controlled or if adequate compressive support is not provided postoperatively (the procedure does not correct the obstruction to lymph efflux). These limbs require lifelong compressive support and, because of their vulnerability to infection, fastidious attention to hygiene. Some of the most challenging patients cared for by a lymphedema center are those who have had aggressive reduction surgery, producing a painful mutilated limb that is immunocompromised and ravaged by recurrent fungal and bacterial infections.

Currently, medical therapy is directed at preventing complications and retarding progression of the disorder, whereas surgery is palliative. Of interest are recent reports of therapeutic success of liposuction in advanced stable lymphedema. Surgical liposuction of chronic postmastectomy lymphedema has been reported to produce excellent results, with sustained reduction of excess volume. In one series, an average long-term reduction of edema volume of 106% was observed in 28 patients with an average edema volume of 1845 mL.[52] Liposuction combined with long-term decongestive compression therapy reduces edema volume more successfully than compression therapy alone. However, the volume reduction is unsuccessful unless compression therapy is maintained after the surgical intervention.[52]

PROSPECTS FOR MOLECULAR THERAPY

Although many therapeutic strategies for lymphedema effectively reduce excess volume, minimize complications, and optimize function, the disease currently lacks a cure. For these reasons, there has been emphasis on the possible application of effective molecular therapies. Among these, the most exciting to date is therapeutic lymphangiogenesis, which is based on insights into the developmental biology of the lymphatics.

Among the mitogenic substances that initiate and regulate the growth of vascular structures, those in the VEGF family play a central role.[86,87] VEGF-C and VEGF-D direct the development and growth of the lymphatic vasculature in embryonic and postnatal life through binding to VEGFR-3 receptors on lymphatic endothelia.[88–90] Exogenous administration of VEGF-C upregulates the VEGFR-3 receptor, leading to a lymphangiogenic response,[92] and in transgenic mice that overexpress VEGF-C, the lymphatic vessels demonstrate a hyperplastic proliferative response with secondary cutaneous changes.[90]

These molecular observations have shed light on the mechanisms that contribute to disease expression in the most common heritable form of lymphedema, the autosomal dominant condition known as *Milroy's disease*. This disease has been linked to the FLT4 locus encoding vascular VEGFR-3.[26] Disease-associated alleles contain missense mutations that produce an inactive tyrosine kinase, thereby preventing downstream gene activation. It is believed that the mutant form of the receptor is excessively stable as well as inactive, so the normal signaling mechanism is blunted, leading to hypoplastic development of the lymphatic vessels.[93]

The prospects for therapeutic lymphangiogenesis in human lymphedema have been underscored by the recent description of a mouse model of inherited limb edema based on mutations in the VEGFR-3 signaling mechanism and pathology that resembles human disease.[91] In this model, therapeutic overexpression of VEGF-C using a viral vector induces the generation of new functional lymphatics and the amelioration of lymphedema. Similarly, in rodent models of acquired postsurgical lymphatic insufficiency (i.e., resembling postmastectomy lymphedema), exogenous administration of human recombinant VEGF-C restores lymphatic flow (as assessed by lymphoscintigraphy), increases lymphatic vascularity, and reverses the hypercellularity that characterizes the untreated lymphedematous condition[94–97] (Fig. 58-7).

Intensive future investigation is necessary to verify the therapeutic potential of such approaches, as well as to establish dose-response relationships and durability of the therapeutic response. As with other forms of angiogenic therapy, the relative virtues of growth factor (gene product) therapy versus gene therapy must be established.

Diseases of the Lymphatic Vasculature

Complex Vascular Pathology with Lymphatic Anomalies

There is a broad constellation of developmental anomalies of the arteriovenous circulation that concurrently distort lymphatic anatomy, function, or both. These mixed vascular deformities are best characterized by the dominant vascular anomaly, whether angiomatous, venous, or arteriovenous.[20] The reader is referred to Chapter 64 for more on vascular anomalies.

KLIPPEL-TRÉNAUNAY'S SYNDROME

Klippel-Trénaunay's syndrome is the most common congenital venous anomaly to affect the entire limb. It is a congenital disorder in which varicose veins, cutaneous nevi, and limb hypertrophy are observed. Lymphedema is reported in 5% of these patients. It has been suggested that this syndrome reflects a generalized disturbance of mesodermal development, thereby engendering the commonly associated anomalies: bony overgrowth, soft-tissue hypertrophy, syndactyly, hypospadias, and lymphatic hypoplasia. Treatment is generally restricted to meticulous skin care (e.g., hydration, protection from trauma), compressive therapy for the associated lymphedema and venous insufficiency, prevention of superficial bleeding from the varicose veins, and prophylaxis against DVT.

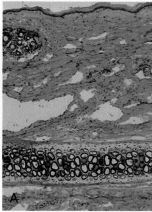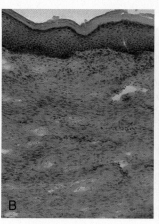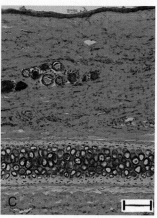

FIGURE 58-7 Postmortem histology (H&E stained frozen sections) of rabbit skin after recombinant human vascular endothelial growth factor (VEGF)-C therapy **(A)** and in untreated lymphedema (saline control) **(B)**. Histology of normal skin specimen **(C)** is provided for comparison. Thickening of dermal and epidermal structures in untreated lymphedema is so profound that, in contrast to both normal and VEGF-C–treated specimens, visualization of subdermal cartilage within the microscopic field is rendered impossible. All three panels were photographed at the same magnification (scale = 100 μm). (From Szuba A, Skobe M, Karkkainen MJ, et al: Therapeutic lymphangiogenesis with human recombinant VEGF-C. FASEB J 16:1985, 2002.)

MAFFUCCI'S SYNDROME

Maffucci's syndrome is described as severe dyschondroplasia in association with multiple lymphangiomata (see later discussion). In this condition, lymphatic vasculature and nodes are typically hypoplastic.[20]

PARKES WEBER'S SYNDROME

Parkes Weber's syndrome is characterized by the presence of multiple arteriovenous fistulae (AVFs) with associated enlargement of the girth of a single limb. The condition can be ascribed at least in part to concomitant dilated tortuous lymphatics and consequent lymphedema. The pathophysiology of this disorder likely reflects the enormous increase in blood flow consequent to multiple arteriovenous fistulae; this increase in capillary filtration would then lead to an increase in lymphatic load, producing first vascular dilatation and, ultimately, insufficiency. Lymph reflux in the limb may lead to the appearance of lymph vesicles in the skin, which should be treated conservatively. We have had some initial success with percutaneous and intravascular catheter-based embolization of associated AVFs (unreported observations).

Proliferative Growth of Lymphatic Vascular Structures and Neoplasm

LYMPHANGIOMA

Lymphangioma is a developmental malformation first detectable in infants. Strictly speaking, these are not, despite their name, tumors. Rather, these lesions are composed of profuse numbers of dilated thin-walled lymphatic vascular structures. They can occur throughout the body, but are seen most commonly on the proximal extremities and at the limb girdle. Small clear vesicles are observed in the skin, sometimes with associated cutaneous bleeding. When these lesions are encountered in the setting of dyschondroplasia, the designation of *Maffucci's syndrome* is applied.

CAVERNOUS LYMPHANGIOMA AND CYSTIC HYGROMA

Cavernous lymphangioma and cystic hygroma are hamartomatous lesions that if not present at birth, appear within the first years of life. Like lymphangiomata, these lesions contain dilated lymphatic vascular structures. The cavernous lesions are typically found in the mouth, mesentery, and on the extremities; cystic hygromas present in the neck, axilla, and groin. These lesions are often surgically resected to prevent complications.

LYMPHANGIOMATOSIS

Lymphangiomatosis is a rare developmental condition in which proliferation of lymphatic vascular structures involves dermis, soft tissue, bone, and parenchyma in a diffuse manner. The organs most typically affected are liver, spleen, lung, and pleura.

Associated lymphangiectasia can be observed in numerous additional organs including liver, kidney, testes, lymph nodes, adrenals, and intestines. Involvement of the viscera typically confers a poor prognosis. When chylothorax is present, repeated thoracentesis and pleurodesis is often required. In one small series, all patients died within 6 to 33 months of clinical presentation.[98]

LYMPHANGIOSARCOMA

Lymphangiosarcomas, malignant angiosarcomas that develop in association with lymphedema, develop as multicentric lesions that have a high propensity for systemic metastasis. The vast majority of such lesions have been observed in lymphedema patients that are breast cancer survivors with chronic significant edema. It is seen only rarely in other forms of lymphedema. Whatever the clinical substrate, the prognosis for survival is poor, even following radical amputation. The reader is referred to Chapter 64 for more on vascular tumors.

Visceral Lymphatic Disorders

CHYLOUS REFLUX, CHYLOTHORAX, CHYLOUS ASCITES

When the lymphatics are incompetent, obstructed, or hypoplastic, fluid has the capacity to reflux. In visceral disease, this fluid can be lymph or chylous lymph. The presence of chylous lymph denotes incompetence of lymphatic flow that extends to the level of the lacteals, at the point where they join the preaortic lymphatics and the cisterna chyli. The anatomical substrate of this problem can be either primary or secondary. In the former case, hypoplastic or dilated incompetent lymphatics reflect the inherited defect of lymphatic development; in secondary forms, thoracic duct obstruction occurs through surgical mishap, trauma, malignancy, or the damage created by filariasis.

Lymph or chyle reflux can occur directly into the lower limbs. The abnormal fluid drains directly from vesicles on the surface of the leg or on the genitalia. Variants of this same presentation can produce chylothorax, chylous ascites, chylous arthritis, and chyluria. In general, if chyle is present in the refluxing body fluid, the therapeutic approach should include a fat-restricted diet with supplementation of medium-chain triglycerides. If the response is not satisfactory, complete elimination of chyle from the fluid can be accomplished at least temporarily with total parenteral nutrition.

The prognosis for such presentations is not favorable. The natural history of reflux reflects the tendency for the condition to worsen with the passage of time. In some patients, there may be an episodic pattern of leakage with sudden exacerbations. Others experience a steady increasing tendency to lymphorrhea and reflux. In patients with the secondary form, an assiduous search for predisposing malignancy or extrinsic lymphatic obstruction should always be undertaken. In patients with the various forms of visceral involvement, complex surgical interventions are sometimes required to mitigate the functional and symptomatic consequences of reflux into the serous cavities.

PROTEIN-LOSING ENTEROPATHY

The presence of visceral lymphatic vascular disease can predispose to a life-threatening form of metabolic insufficiency called *protein-losing enteropathy*. When chyle refluxes back into the villi as a consequence of the effective blockade of its passage into the central lymphatics, this condition engenders weight loss, diarrhea, and steatorrhea as protein, fat, calcium, and fat-soluble vitamins are malabsorbed. In addition to the secondary forms of lymphatic obstruction (usually malignant), the primary hypoplastic and lymphangiectatic disorders can also predispose to enteropathy; in these cases, lymphedema of an extremity often precedes or accompanies the appearance of the enteropathy. As with other forms of reflux, the initial therapeutic strategy should entail medium-chain triglyceride supplementation, with restriction of total dietary fat intake. Where the response to conservative therapy is insufficient, it has been suggested that systemic treatment with octreotide may help alleviate the severity of the disorder, although the mechanism of benefit is not entirely understood.[99–102]

REFERENCES

1. Kanter MA: The lymphatic system: an historical perspective, *Plast Reconstr Surg* 79:131, 1987.
2. Rockson SG: Preclinical models of lymphatic disease: the potential for growth factor and gene therapy, *Ann N Y Acad Sci* 979:64, 2002.
3. Shin WS, Szuba A, Rockson SG: Animal models for the study of lymphatic insufficiency, *Lymphat Res Biol* 1:159, 2003.
4. Oliver G: Lymphatic vasculature development, *Nat Rev Immunol* 4:35, 2004.
5. Baldwin M, Stacker S, Achen M: Molecular control of lymphangiogenesis, *Bioessays* 24:1030, 2002.
6. Gashev A: Physiologic aspects of lymphatic contractile function: current perspectives, *Ann N Y Acad Sci* 979:178, 2002.
7. Sparks HV, Rooke TW: *Essentials of cardiovascular physiology*, Minneapolis, 1987, University of Minnesota Press.
8. Cotton KD, Hollywood MA, McHale NG, et al: Outward currents in smooth muscle cells isolated from sheep mesenteric lymphatics, *J Physiol* 503(pt 1):1, 1997.
9. von der Weid PY, Zawieja DC: Lymphatic smooth muscle: the motor unit of lymph drainage, *Int J Biochem Cell Biol* 36:1147, 2004.
10. Gashev AA, Zawieja DC: Physiology of human lymphatic contractility: a historical perspective, *Lymphology* 34:124, 2001.
11. Muthuchamy M, Gashev A, Boswell N, et al: Molecular and functional analyses of the contractile apparatus in lymphatic muscle, *FASEB J* 17:920, 2003.
12. McHale NG, Thornbury KD, Hollywood MA: 5-HT inhibits spontaneous contractility of isolated sheep mesenteric lymphatics via activation of 5-HT(4) receptors, *Microvasc Res* 60:261, 2000.
13. Hall JL, Morris B, Wooley L: Intrinsic rhythmic propulsion of lymph in anesthetized sheep, *J Physiol* 180:336, 1965.
14. Trzewik J, Mallipattu SK, Artmann GM, et al: Evidence for a second valve system in lymphatics: endothelial microvalves, *FASEB J* 15:1711, 2001.
15. Mendoza E, Schmid-Schonbein GW: A model for mechanics of primary lymphatic valves, *J Biomech Eng* 125:407, 2003.
16. Szuba A, Shin WS, Strauss HW, et al: The third circulation: radionuclide lymphoscintigraphy in the evaluation of lymphedema, *J Nucl Med* 44:43, 2003.
17. Rockson SG: Primary lymphedema. In Ernst CB, Stanley JC, editors: *Current therapy in vascular surgery*, ed 4, Philadelphia, 2000, Mosby.
18. Rockson SG: Lymphedema, *Am J Med* 110:288, 2001.
19. Szuba A, Rockson SG: Lymphedema: classification, diagnosis and therapy, *Vasc Med* 3:145, 1998.
20. Kinmonth JB: *The lymphatics*, ed 2, London, 1982, Arnold.
21. Rockson SG: Syndromic lymphedema: keys to the kingdom of lymphatic structure and function? *Lymphat Res Biol* 1:181, 2003.
22. Milroy WF: An undescribed variety of hereditary edema, *N Y Med J* 56:505, 1892.
23. Milroy WF: Chronic hereditary edema: Milroy's disease, *JAMA* 91:1172, 1928.
24. Smeltzer DM, Stickler GB, Schirger A: Primary lymphedema in children and adolescents: a followup study and review, *Pediatrics* 76:206, 1985.
25. Bull LN, Roche E, Song EJ, et al: Mapping of the locus for cholestasis-lymphedema syndrome (Aagenaes syndrome) to a 6.6-cM interval on chromosome 15q, *Am J Hum Genet* 67:994, 2000.
26. Karkkainen MJ, Ferrell RE, Lawrence EC, et al: Missense mutations interfere with VEGFR-3 signalling in primary lymphoedema, *Nat Genet* 25:153, 2000.
27. Irrthum A, Karkkainen MJ, Devriendt K, et al: Congenital hereditary lymphedema caused by a mutation that inactivates VEGFR3 tyrosine kinase, *Am J Hum Genet* 67:295, 2000.
28. Fang J, Dagenais SL, Erickson RP, et al: Mutations in FOXC2 (MFH-1), a forkhead family transcription factor, are responsible for the hereditary lymphedema distichiasis syndrome, *Am J Hum Genet* 67:1382, 2000.
29. Finegold DN, Kimak MA, Lawrence EC, et al: Truncating mutations in FOXC2 cause multiple lymphedema syndromes, *Hum Mol Genet* 10:1185, 2001.
30. Irrthum A, Devriendt K, Chitayat D, et al: Mutations in the transcription factor gene SOX18 underlie recessive and dominant forms of hypotrichosis-lymphedema-telangiectasia, *Am J Hum Genet* 72:1470, 2003.
31. Alders M, Hogan BM, Gjini E, et al: Mutations in CCBE1 cause generalized lymph vessel dysplasia in humans, *Nat Genet* 41:1272, 2009.
32. Connell F, Kalidas K, Ostergaard P, et al: Linkage and sequence analysis indicate that CCBE1 is mutated in recessively inherited generalised lymphatic dysplasia, *Hum Genet* 127:231, 2010.
33. Finegold DN, Schacht V, Kimak MA, et al: HGF and MET mutations in primary and secondary lymphedema, *Lymphat Res Biol* 6:65, 2008.
34. Ferrell RE, Baty CJ, Kimak MA, et al: GJC2 missense mutations cause human lymphedema, *Am J Hum Genet* 86:943, 2010.
35. Wheeler ES, Chan V, Wassman R, et al: Familial lymphedema praecox: Meige's disease, *Plast Reconstr Surg* 67:362, 1981.
36. Schirger A: Lymphedema, *Cardiovasc Clin* 13:293, 1983.
37. Bockarie M, Tisch D, Kastens W, et al: Mass treatment to eliminate filariasis in Papua, New Guinea, *N Engl J Med* 347:1841, 2002.
38. Kumaraswami V, Ottesen eA, Vijayasekaran V, et al: Ivermectin for the treatment of Wuchereria bancrofti filariasis: efficacy and adverse reactions, *JAMA* 259:3150, 1988.
39. Szuba A, Rockson S: Lymphedema: a review of diagnostic techniques and therapeutic options, *Vasc Med* 3:145, 1998.
40. Rockson SG: Precipitating factors in lymphedema: myths and realities, *Cancer* 83:2814, 1998.
41. Hojris I, Andersen J, Overgaard M, et al: Late treatment-related morbidity in breast cancer patients randomized to postmastectomy radiotherapy and systemic treatment versus systemic treatment alone, *Acta Oncol* 39:355, 2000.
42. Tengrup I, Tennvall-Nittby L, Christiansson I, et al: Arm morbidity after breast-conserving therapy for breast cancer, *Acta Oncol* 39:393, 2000.
43. Petrek JA, Heelan MC: Incidence of breast carcinoma-related lymphedema, *Cancer* 83(Suppl 12):2776, 1998.
44. Fiorica JV, Roberts WS, Greenberg H, et al: Morbidity and survival patterns in patients after radical hysterectomy and postoperative adjuvant pelvic radiotherapy, *Gynecol Oncol* 36:343, 1990.
45. Werngren-Elgstrom M, Lidman D: Lymphoedema of the lower extremities after surgery and radiotherapy for cancer of the cervix, *Scand J Plast Reconstr Surg Hand Surg* 28:289, 1994.
46. Soisson AP, Soper JT, Clarke-Pearson DL, et al: Adjuvant radiotherapy following radical hysterectomy for patients with stage IB and IIA cervical cancer, *Gynecol Oncol* 37:390, 1990.
47. Lynde CW, Mitchell IC: Unusual complication of allergic contact dermatitis of the hands-recurrent lymphangitis and persistent lymphoedema, *Contact Dermatitis* 8:279, 1982.
48. Rockson SG, Rivera KK: Estimating the population burden of lymphedema, *Ann N Y Acad Sci* 1131:147, 2008.
49. Nagai Y, Aoyama K, Endo Y, et al: Lymphedema of the extremities developed as the initial manifestation of rheumatoid arthritis, *Eur J Dermatol* 17:175, 2007.
50. Majeski I: Lymphedema tarda, *Cutis* 38:105, 1985.
51. Stemmer R: Ein klinisches Zeichen zur fruh-und differential-Diagnose des Lymphodems. [A clinical symptom for the early and differential diagnosis of lymphedema], *Vasa* 5:261, 1976.
52. Brorson H, Ohlin K, Olsson G, et al: Breast cancer-related chronic arm lymphedema is associated with excess adipose and muscle tissue, *Lymphat Res Biol* 7:3, 2009.
53. Rosen E: The molecular control of adipogenesis, with special reference to lymphatic pathology, *Ann N Y Acad Sci* 979:143, 2002.
54. Schirger A, Harrison EG, Janes JM: Idiopathic lymphedema: Review of 131 cases, *JAMA* 182:124, 1962.
55. Mallon E, Powell S, Mortimer P, et al: Evidence for altered cell-mediated immunity in postmastectomy lymphoedema, *Br J Dermatol* 137:928, 1997.
56. Beilhack A, Rockson SG: Immune traffic: a functional overview, *Lymphat Res Biol* 1:219, 2003.
57. Muller R, Hajdu SI, Brennan MF: Lymphangiosarcoma associated with chronic filarial lymphedema, *Cancer* 59:179, 1987.
58. Benda JA, Al Jurf AS, Benson AB III: Angiosarcoma of the breast following segmental mastectomy complicated by lymphedema, *Am J Clin Pathol* 87:651, 1987.
59. Servelle M: Surgical treatment of lymphedema: a report on 652 cases, *Surgery* 101:485, 1987.
60. Kinmonth JB, Taylor GW, Harper RK: Lymphangiography: a technique for its clinical use in the lower limb, *Br Med J* 1:940, 1955.
61. O'Brien BM, et al: Effect of lymphangiography on lymphedema, *Plast Reconstr Surg* 68:922, 1981.
62. Vaqueiro M, et al: Lymphoscintigraphy in lymphedema: an aid to microsurgery, *J Nucl Med* 27:1125, 1986.
63. Szuba A, Shin WS, Strauss HW, et al: Lymphoscintigraphy in the evaluation of lymphedema, *J Nucl Med* 44:43, 2003.
64. Hadjis NS, Carr DH, Banks L, et al: The role of CT in the diagnosis of primary lymphedema of the lower limb, *AJR Am J Roentgenol* 144:361, 1985.
65. Gamba JL, Silverman PM, Ling D, et al: Primary lower extremity lymphedema: CT diagnosis, *Radiology* 149:218, 1983.
66. Vaughan BF: CT of swollen legs, *Clin Radiol* 41:24, 1990.
67. Liu NF, Wang CG: The role of magnetic resonance imaging in the diagnosis of peripheral lymphatic disorders, *Lymphology* 31:319, 1998.
68. Matsushima S, Ichiba N, Hayashi D, et al: Nonenhanced magnetic resonance lymphoductography: visualization of lymphatic system of the trunk on 3-dimensional heavily T2-weighted image with 2-dimensional prospective acquisition and correction, *J Comput Assist Tomogr* 31:299, 2007.
69. Gniadecka M: Localization of dermal edema in lipodermatosclerosis, lymphedema, and cardiac insufficiency: high-frequency ultrasound examination of intradermal echogenicity, *J Am Acad Dermatol* 35:37, 1996.
70. Rockson SG, Miller LT, Senie R, et al: American Cancer Society Lymphedema Workshop. Workgroup III: diagnosis and management of lymphedema, *Cancer* 83:2882, 1998.
71. Kubik S: The role of the lateral upper arm bundle and the lymphatic watersheds in the formation of collateral pathways in lymphedema, *Acta Biol Acad Sci Hung* 31:191, 1980.
72. Ko DS, Lerner R, Klose G, et al: Effective treatment of lymphedema of the extremities, *Arch Surg* 133:452, 1998.

DISEASES OF THE LYMPHATIC CIRCULATION

73. Szuba A, Cooke JP, Yousuf S, et al: Decongestive lymphatic therapy for patients with cancer-related or primary lymphedema, *Am J Med* 109:296, 2000.

74. Badger CM, Peacock JL, Mortimer PS: A randomized, controlled, parallel-group clinical trial comparing multilayer bandaging followed by hosiery versus hosiery alone in the treatment of patients with lymphedema of the limb, *Cancer* 88:2832, 2000.

75. Leduc O, Leduc A, Bourgeois P, et al: The physical treatment of upper limb edema, *Cancer* 83:2835, 1998.

76. Szuba A, Achalu R, Rockson SG: Decongestive lymphatic therapy for patients with breast carcinoma-associated lymphedema: a randomized, prospective study of a role for adjunctive intermittent pneumatic compression, *Cancer* 95:2260, 2002.

77. Mayrovitz HN: The standard of care for lymphedema: current concepts and physiological considerations, *Lymphat Res Biol* 7:101, 2009.

78. Piller NB, Thelander A: Treatment of chronic postmastectomy lymphedema with low level laser therapy: a 2.5 year follow-up, *Lymphology* 31:74, 1998.

79. Ogawa Y, Yoshizumi M, Kitagawa T, et al: Investigation of the mechanism of lymphocyte injection therapy in treatment of lymphedema with special emphasis on cell adhesion molecule (L-selectin), *Lymphology* 32:151, 1999.

80. Casley-Smith JR, Morgan RG, Piller NB: Treatment of lymphedema of the arms and legs with 5,6-benzo-(alpha)-pyrone, *N Engl J Med* 329:1158, 1993.

81. Casley-Smith JR, Wang CT, Zi-hai C: Treatment of filarial lymphoedema and elephantiasis with 5,6-benzo-alpha-pyrone (coumarin), *BMJ* 307:1037, 1993.

82. Mortimer PS, Badger C, Clarke I, et al: A double-blind, randomized parallel-group, placebo-controlled trial of o-(b-hydroxyethyl)-rutosides in chronic arm oedema resulting from breast cancer treatment, *Phlebologie* 10:51, 1995.

83. Loprinzi CL, Kugler JW, Sloan JA, et al: Lack of effect of coumarin in women with lymphedema after treatment for breast cancer, *N Engl J Med* 340:346, 1999.

84. Damstra RJ, Voesten HG, van Schelven WD, et al: Lymphatic venous anastomosis (LVA) for treatment of secondary arm lymphedema. A prospective study of 11 LVA procedures in 10 patients with breast cancer related lymphedema and a critical review of the literature, *Breast Cancer Res Treat* 113:199–206, 2009.

85. Campisi C, Boccardo F: Microsurgical techniques for lymphedema treatment: derivative lymphatic-venous microsurgery, *World J Surg* 28:609, 2004.

86. Olofsson B, Jeltsch M, Eriksson U, et al: Current biology of VEGF-B and VEGF-C, *Curr Opin Biotechnol* 10:528, 1999.

87. Veikkola T, Karkkainen M, Claesson-Welsh L, et al: Regulation of angiogenesis via vascular endothelial growth factor receptors, *Cancer Res* 60:203, 2000.

88. Joukov V, Pajusola K, Kaipainen A, et al: A novel vascular endothelial growth factor, VEGF-C, is a ligand for the Flt4 (VEGFR-3) and KDR (VEGFR-2) receptor tyrosine kinases, *EMBO J* 15:1751, 1996.

89. Kaipainen A, Korhonen J, Mustonen T, et al: Expression of the fms-like tyrosine kinase 4 gene becomes restricted to lymphatic endothelium during development, *Proc Natl Acad Sci U S A* 92:3566, 1995.

90. Jeltsch M, Kaipainen A, Joukov V, et al: Hyperplasia of lymphatic vessels in VEGF-C transgenic mice, *Science* 276:1423, 1997.

91. Oh SJ, Jeltsch MM, Birkenhager R, et al: VEGF and VEGF-C: specific induction of angiogenesis and lymphangiogenesis in the differentiated avian chorioallantoic membrane, *Dev Biol* 188:96, 1997.

92. Enholm B, Karpanen T, Jeltsch M, et al: Adenoviral expression of vascular endothelial growth factor-C induces lymphangiogenesis in the skin, *Circ Res* 88:623, 2001.

93. Karkkainen MJ, Petrova TV: Vascular endothelial growth factor receptors in the regulation of angiogenesis and lymphangiogenesis, *Oncogene* 19:5598, 2000.

94. Karkkainen MJ, Saaristo A, Jussila L, et al: A model for gene therapy of human hereditary lymphedema, *Proc Natl Acad Sci U S A* 98:12677, 2001.

95. Szuba A, Skobe M, Karkkainen MJ, et al: Therapeutic lymphangiogenesis with human recombinant VEGF-C, *FASEB J* 16:1985, 2002.

96. Tabibiazar R, Cheung L, Han J, et al: Inflammatory manifestations of experimental lymphatic insufficiency, *PLoS Med* 3:e254, 2006.

97. Jin D, An A, Liu J, et al: Therapeutic responses to exogenous VEGF-C administration in experimental lymphedema: immunohistochemical and molecular characterization, *Lymphat Res Biol* 7:47, 2009.

98. Ramani P, Shah A: Lymphangiomatosis: histologic and immunohistochemical analysis of four cases, *Am J Surg Pathol* 17:329, 1993.

99. Makhija S, von der Weid PY, Meddings J, et al: Octreotide in intestinal lymphangiectasia: lack of a clinical response and failure to alter lymphatic function in a guinea pig model, *Can J Gastroenterol* 18:681, 2004.

100. Lee HL, Han DS, Kim JB, et al: Successful treatment of protein-losing enteropathy induced by intestinal lymphangiectasia in a liver cirrhosis patient with octreotide: a case report, *J Korean Med Sci* 19:466, 2004.

101. Tibballs J, Soto R, Bharucha T: Management of newborn lymphangiectasia and chylothorax after cardiac surgery with octreotide infusion, *Ann Thorac Surg* 77:2213, 2004.

102. Bliss CM, Schroy IP: Primary intestinal lymphangiectasia, *Curr Treat Options Gastroenterol* 7:3, 2004.

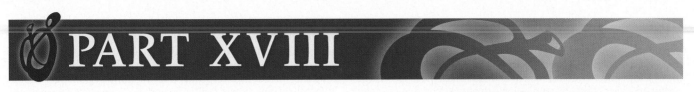

CHAPTER **59**   # Vascular Infection

R. James Valentine, Mitchell M. Plummer

Vascular infection is a rare but serious problem associated with potentially disastrous complications. Considering the numerous episodes of bacteremia humans experience in a lifetime, it is somewhat surprising that vascular infection is so uncommon in the general population. Resistance to infection is attributable to a number of teleological mechanisms, many of which can be conveniently grouped into immune, architectural, and anatomical themes. The reticuloendothelial and immune systems rapidly clear organisms from the circulation, providing excellent first-line protection against bloodborne invasion. The continuous endothelial cell (EC) lining of the arterial tree represents an important barrier to organism invasion. The tough adventitial outer lining and the deep anatomical location of most arteries make external penetration unlikely. There are many other resistance mechanisms related to arterial wall function that are considered elsewhere in this text. Overall, resistance to vascular infection is comprehensive, redundant, and efficient.

The presence of arterial infection implies profound homeostatic failure. Risk factors include arterial injury, underlying arterial pathology, EC dysfunction, immune deficiency, and the presence of a foreign body, such as prosthetic graft material. Prosthetic graft infections are far more common than primary arterial infections, and there are important differences in presentation, treatment, and outcome between the two. This chapter describes current concepts of vascular infection, considering primary arterial infections and secondary graft infections separately. The continuously evolving experience in both areas promises better understanding of prevention and treatment of these difficult problems.

Primary Arterial Infections

The first published experience with primary arterial infection is generally credited to Koch, who reported a patient with a ruptured superior mesenteric artery (SMA) aneurysm in 1851.[1] Arterial infections were not well appreciated before this time because the basic tenets of bacteriology and infection were not yet developed. Breakthroughs in human bacteriological research by Pasteur and others in the mid-19th century set the stage for a basic understanding of the pathophysiology and classification of vascular infections.

Classification and Etiology

Nearly all primary arterial infections result in the formation of aneurysms or pseudoaneurysms. Osler coined the term *mycotic aneurysm* in 1885 to describe infected aortic arch aneurysms containing "fresh fungal vegetation" in a patient who had concomitant aortic valve vegetations.[2] While "mycotic" aneurysms apply only to the subset of individuals with infected aneurysms caused by septic emboli, the term has been loosely applied to include all infected aneurysms, regardless of etiology. This practice is confusing and prevents meaningful comparison of the numerous small series of infected aneurysms reported in the modern literature.

The most widely accepted classification of arterial infections was introduced by Wilson et al. in 1978.[3] In keeping with the traditional definition introduced by Osler, the authors classified a *mycotic aneurysm* as one that occurred in an otherwise normal, nonaneurysmal artery as a result of septic emboli of endocardial origin. A preestablished aneurysm that became infected as a result of bacteremia is classified as an *infected aneurysm. Microbial arteritis* refers to infection of a normal or atherosclerotic (i.e., nonaneurysmal) artery that has become infected as a result of bacteremia. This most often results in rupture with formation of a pseudoaneurysm. *Traumatic infected aneurysms* include infected aneurysms due to trauma or iatrogenic injury (e.g., complications of arteriography). *Contiguous arterial infection* is due to direct extension of an adjacent infection into the wall of the artery, such as infected aortitis associated with vertebral osteomyelitis. The specific classification based on etiology will be acknowledged wherever appropriate in this chapter. However, for purposes of clarity and simplification, the generic term *infected aneurysm* will be applied to include all arterial infections discussed.

The etiology of infected aneurysms has changed in the past 150 years. In the pre-antibiotic era, 86% of patients with arterial infections had evidence of endocarditis.[4] Following widespread use of antibiotics, the incidence of infective endocarditis has relegated the true mycotic aneurysm to a rare entity. In 1984, Brown and associates reported a collective series of infected aneurysms based on a search of the English literature.[5] The etiology could be determined in 75% of the 180 subjects. The authors separated the reported experience into cases occurring before 1965 and those occurring since that time. Accuracy of the results suffers because of important differences in diagnosis and reporting frequency between the two periods. Nevertheless, this collective experience remains the largest comparative analysis of infected aneurysms to date. In the earlier part of the series, endocarditis was still the leading cause of infected aneurysms, but arterial trauma of all types became the leading cause after 1965. The authors attributed this etiological shift to a substantial change in the pattern of antibiotic use for treatment of sepsis and trauma.[5] Other explanations include an increased prevalence of intravenous drug abuse and the widespread application of transarterial interventional procedures. The increase in interventional procedures was particularly notable after the pioneering work of Grunzig and others in the 1970s. The enthusiasm for endovascular technology seen in recent years suggests that arterial trauma may soon become an even more important cause of arterial infection.

Pathogenesis of Infected Aneurysms

The basic mechanisms leading to formation of infected aneurysms have been studied most extensively in the abdominal aorta. Chronic uninfected abdominal aortic aneurysms (AAAs) are thought to form as a result of both destruction of medial elastin and adventitial collagen (see Chapter 37).[6] Elastolytic matrix metalloproteinases (MMPs) play a central role, leading to initial aortic dilation.[6]

Collagenase MMP leads to collagen failure that eventually leads to gross enlargement and eventual rupture of the AAA. The extensive transmural infiltration typically seen in noninfected AAAs suggests that inflammation and immune responses play a significant role in AAA formation.[7] Interestingly, infectious causes have also been postulated: histochemical studies have demonstrated that as many as 55% of AAAs harbor *Chlamydia pneumoniae*.[7] Thus, it appears that infected and noninfected AAAs may represent two ends of the same spectrum, with progression to infection depending on organism virulence and host resistance.

A number of important clinical differences have been noted between infected and uninfected aneurysms of the abdominal aorta. In contrast to chronic AAA, infected AAAs follow a more rapid course, have a predilection for the suprarenal aorta, and may be isolated to a small segment of an otherwise normal aorta. Recent studies have revealed a number of interesting findings related to the etiology of infected AAA. First, Buckmaster et al. have shown that elastolytic activity is derived from host leukocytes, not from the infectious organisms.[8] However, infectious organisms play a central role in collagen degradation. Many bacterial isolates produce collagenases,[9] and bacteria are capable of activating the collagenase promoter in macrophage-like cells.[10] Furthermore, a variety of bacterial proteases activate MMP-1, MMP-8, and MMP-9.[9] Therefore, infected AAAs appear be the consequence of bacterial proteases causing rapid collagen breakdown in a previously normal aorta.[9] The collagenase activity may be relatively localized, leading to formation of a saccular AAA or pseudoaneurysm in an otherwise normal appearing vessel. Collagenase activity may also be intensive, which may explain the rapid course associated with infected AAAs. The reason infected AAAs are predisposed to the suprarenal aorta has not been elucidated.

Pathological findings of infected aortic aneurysms have been described by Hsu and Lin.[11] Typical findings included aortic atherosclerosis, acute suppurative inflammation, neutrophil infiltration, and bacterial clumps. Two thirds of patients in their series showed acute inflammation superimposed on severe chronic atherosclerosis; the remainder showed atherosclerosis with chronic inflammation or pseudoaneurysms.

Anatomical Location

In their classic 1984 study, Brown and associates documented 243 infected aneurysms in 180 patients in the following distribution: 38% femoral artery, 31% abdominal aorta, 8% SMA, 7% brachial artery, 6% iliac artery, 5% carotid artery, 3% ulnar/radial arteries, 1% hepatic artery, less than 1% subclavian artery, and less than 1% popliteal artery.[5] Notably, there were no cases involving the suprarenal or thoracoabdominal aorta in this series. More recent reports have documented a much higher prevalence of infected aortic aneurysms involving the segments proximal to the renal arteries,[12-15] suggesting the aorta is the most frequent site of involvement.

Bacteriology

Approximately 75% of clinically infected aneurysms are associated with positive culture results.[5] There have been significant shifts in the bacteriological patterns of infected aneurysms that have paralleled the changes in etiology. Prior to 1960, gram-positive organisms predominated, particularly *Streptococcus pneumoniae*, *Streptococcus*, and *Staphylococcus aureus*.[3] More recent series have reported a higher prevalence of gram-negative organisms, paralleling the increasing number of arterial infections due to bacteremia, particularly *Salmonella* species.[13,16] Gram-negative sepsis in elderly patients is a frequent clinical scenario in these circumstances.[17] It appears that the bacteriological pattern is continuing to evolve: several reports have identified *S. pneumoniae* as an increasingly frequent cause of infected aortic aneurysms.[14,18,19] The prevalence of organisms associated with opportunistic infections such as fungus and *Mycobacterium* species may also be on the rise owing to the increasing prevalence of chronic diseases associated with impaired immunity.

Salmonella infections deserve special emphasis. For uncertain reasons, *Salmonella* organisms have a tendency to infect the abdominal aorta. Up to 36% of all infected aneurysms of the aorta are due to *Salmonella* species; conversely, 65% of *Salmonella* vascular infections are localized to the aorta.[20] Humans become infected by ingestion of contaminated food or water. Of the patients who develop *Salmonella* gastroenteritis, a small proportion will develop bacteremia that may result in extraintestinal seeding and infection. The interval between the onset of gastrointestinal symptoms and development of aortic infection may be several weeks.[20] Diagnosis can be difficult because the signs and symptoms are nonspecific: more than half of patients have ruptured aneurysms before the diagnosis is made.[20] Common isolates from aortic wall specimens have included *Salmonella choleraesuis*, *Salmonella typhimurium*, and *Salmonella enteritidis*. *Salmonella* aortitis is an extremely morbid condition that has historically been associated with mortality rates of 50% and a high rate of reinfection after revascularization.[20] However, this trend appears to be reversing: in a more recent series, Hsu et al. documented an 11% mortality rate and showed that *Salmonella* was a predictor of survival compared to other microorganisms.[21] Much of this effect may have been due to the fact that the *Salmonella* infected patients in this series were significantly younger than patients who died with other infections.

Syphilitic aneurysms, once a common cause of death due to aortic arch rupture, are now very rare. In a review of the literature on infected aortic aneurysms, Leon and Mills reported that syphilitic aneurysms occur most commonly in the ascending and arch aorta; they are uncommon below the sixth vertebral body.[22] These aneurysms result from the intense inflammatory response associated with the treponemes that lodge in vasa vasorum.

Infected Aortic Aneurysms

The definition of aortic aneurysm infection has been confounded by the fact that 10% to 15% of patients with uninfected chronic AAA will have positive culture results from intraluminal thrombus removed at the time of aneurysm repair. Fortunately, positive culture results are not associated with an increased risk of late graft infection.[23,24] However, this underscores the fact that the definition of infected AAA relies on other criteria such as operative findings (inflammation and purulence), clinical symptoms (fever, pain, leukocytosis), aneurysm architecture (saccular or localized), and positive aneurysm wall culture.[13]

Modern series of infected aortic aneurysms reveal that the majority of affected patients have comorbid conditions associated with immunosuppression such as diabetes, chronic renal failure, chronic steroid use, human immunodeficiency virus (HIV), or cancer.[13,25] Nearly 50% of patients have had a recent documented infection such as pneumonia or urinary tract infection,[13] and several reports have documented direct extension of vertebral osteomyelitis.[14,26,27]

Features

Infected aneurysms of the aorta may involve any segment from the ascending arch to the distal infrarenal area. In a series of 43 patients with infected aortic aneurysms treated at the Mayo Clinic over a 25-year period, Oderich et al. documented a wide distribution of lesions.[13] No segment of the aorta was spared. As can be seen in Figure 59-1, 40% of infected aneurysms were localized to the infrarenal aorta, and the remaining lesions were almost evenly distributed in the juxta/pararenal, paravisceral, thoracoabdominal, and descending thoracic segments. A similar distribution has been observed by others.[14,28,30]

The majority of aortic infections can be classified as bacterial aortitis.[11] Most lesions are saccular and well localized in an otherwise normal-appearing aorta (Fig. 59-2). This appearance is highly suggestive of a ruptured aortic pseudoaneurysm, which is pathognomonic for aortic infection. In a minority of cases, infection of a preexisting aortic aneurysm may make diagnosis difficult. In these circumstances, suspicion of infection is completely reliant on clinical information.

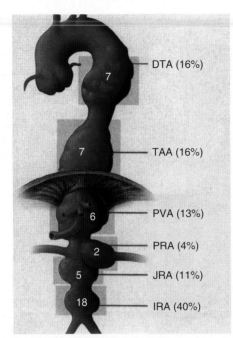

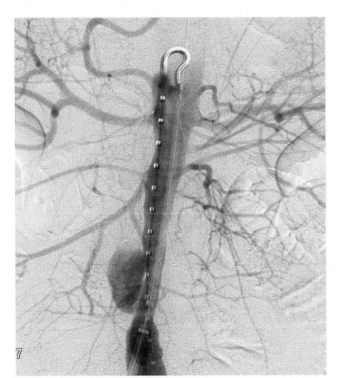

FIGURE 59-1 **Distribution of infected aortic aneurysms in a series of 43 patients treated at the Mayo Clinic.** *(From Oderich GS, Panneton JM, Bower TC, et al: Infected aortic aneurysms: aggressive presentation, complicated early outcome, but durable results. J Vasc Surg 34:900, 2001, with permission from the Society for Vascular Surgery and the American Association for Vascular Surgery.)*[13]

FIGURE 59-2 **Arteriogram of infected aneurysm in infrarenal abdominal aorta.** Note saccular shape of pseudoaneurysm and normal appearance of aorta above and below the lesion.

Diagnosis

The majority of patients with infected aortic aneurysms are symptomatic. In the series by Oderich et al., 93% of patients had symptoms, the most common of which were fever, back pain, and leukocytosis (Table 59-1).[13] Blood cultures are positive in approximately 75% of cases.[13] The degree of symptomatology may be an important indicator of prognosis. Recent data suggest that the

TABLE 59-1	Clinical Presentation and Laboratory Findings in 43 Patients Treated at the Mayo Clinic for Infected Aortic Aneurysms	
		NO. PATIENTS (%)
Symptomatic		40 (93)
Fever		33 (77)
Pain (abdominal or back)		28 (65)
Leukocyte count >12,000/mm³		23 (54)
Chills		22 (51)
Sweats		12 (28)
Enlarging aneurysm		12 (28)
Nausea/vomiting or diarrhea		10 (25)
Pulsatile mass		7 (16)
Hemodynamic instability		3 (7)

Adapted from Oderich GS, Panneton JM, Bower TC, et al: Infected aortic aneurysms: aggressive presentation, complicated early outcome, but durable results. J Vasc Surg 34:900, 2001.[13]

systemic inflammatory response syndrome (SIRS), a marker for sepsis, is associated with increased morbidity and mortality in patients with infected aortic aneurysms.[14,29] Diagnostic criteria for SIRS include the presence of two or more of the following: body temperature above 38°C or below 36°C; heart rate over 90 beats/min; respiratory rate over 20 breaths/min or a partial pressure of carbon dioxide in arterial blood ($Paco_2$) less than 32 torr; and white blood cell (WBC) over 12,000 cells/mm³, less than 4000 cells/ mm³, or 10% immature (band) forms.[29]

Diagnosis of infected aortic aneurysms relies on a number of imaging techniques. The presence of a saccular aneurysm in a patient with typical symptoms is pathognomonic, and the diagnosis is confirmed if blood cultures are positive. Gas bubbles and periaortic fat stranding on magnetic resonance imaging (MRI) or enhanced computed tomography (CT) scans are also diagnostic for infection (Fig. 59-3) but are not universally present. More subtle signs include periaortic stranding, proximity to abnormal fluid collections or nearby infections such as vertebral osteomyelitis, and rapid aneurysm expansion over several days.[15] Indium-111-labeled WBC scans have been used in some patients, but the 80% sensitivity and specificity of this test suggest that it has limited usefulness. Angiography has been recommended to localize the infection and plan appropriate operative treatment in all patients. As an alternative, newer imaging techniques such as CT angiography (CTA) can be used to assess periaortic tissues, localize the

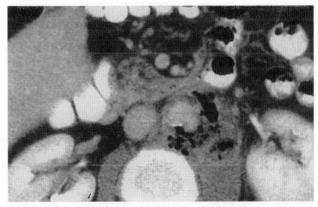

FIGURE 59-3 **Enhanced computed tomography (CT) scan demonstrating gas bubbles and periaortic fat stranding suggestive of an infected aortic aneurysm.** *(From Oderich GS, Panneton JM, Bower TC, et al: Infected aortic aneurysms: aggressive presentation, complicated early outcome, but durable results. J Vasc Surg 34:900, 2001, with permission from the Society for Vascular Surgery and the American Association for Vascular Surgery.)*[13]

infectious process, and evaluate vascular anatomy. This technique has the advantage of being minimally invasive compared to standard angiography, and it essentially combines two tests into one.

Clinical Course

The natural history of infected aortic aneurysms depends on the classification. The more common bacterial aortitis is associated with inexorable expansion of the pseudoaneurysm and eventual rupture. Rapid expansion over 2 to 3 days has been documented; in more than half of cases, the pseudoaneurysm has already ruptured at the time of diagnosis. Contiguous and traumatic infections of the aorta, also associated with pseudoaneurysms, have a similar natural history. Urgent repair of these lesions is always indicated. Infections involving preexisting aortic aneurysms are relatively rare, and the natural history is unknown, but because of the potential for rapid expansion and rupture as well as recurrent bacteremia, urgent repair is indicated for these lesions as well. Patients with true mycotic aneurysms have two problems: the aortic aneurysm and the primary cardiac valvular lesion. Treatment may require extensive preoperative stabilization before the aneurysm is repaired.

Treatment

Treatment of infected aortic aneurysms is surgical. Although treatment with broad-spectrum antibiotics may "sterilize" an infected aneurysm, the aneurysm still requires treatment because of the significant risk of rupture. In a series of 22 high-risk patients treated with antibiotics but without resection, Hsu et al. reported that 50% had in-hospital mortality, and 59% of those who survived to leave the hospital died of aneurysm rupture in late follow-up.[30]

The urgent nature of infected aortic aneurysms cannot be overstated because of the potential for rupture with exsanguination. In a recent series, nearly half of all patients with infected AAAs had already ruptured at the time of surgery, including free ruptures in 20%.[31] Once the diagnosis is confirmed with appropriate imaging, preoperative preparation should be completed as rapidly as possible—preferably within 2 or 3 hours. Patients with hemodynamic instability should be transported immediately to the operating room. Stable patients should be admitted to an intensive care unit for rapid fluid repletion, institution of broad-spectrum intravenous antibiotics, and placement of appropriate monitoring devices. Blood should be typed and crossmatched, and at least four units of packed red blood cells should be available in the operating room.

Surgical treatment of infected aortic aneurysms depends on the location and extent of the infection. The most common operation is ligation and débridement of the infected arterial segment, with revascularization of the lower extremities using grafts brought through uninfected tissues remote from the infected site (extra-anatomical bypass).[28,32] For example, infected aneurysms of the infrarenal aorta can be treated with ligation of the abdominal aorta distal to the renal arteries and revascularization of the lower extremities using axillofemoral bypass grafts. However, proximal aortic aneurysms involving the renal arteries, visceral aorta, or descending thoracic aorta are much more complicated. These aortic segments require direct revascularization to preserve blood flow to the kidneys, intraabdominal organs, and the spinal cord. In these cases, aortic débridement with direct revascularization of the affected segment within the infected bed (*in situ* reconstruction) is appropriate.

In situ reconstruction has been performed with prosthetic grafts, but the reinfection rate of up to 20% makes this option unattractive except in patients who are unstable at the time of operation.[33,34] Prolonged administration of antibiotics is generally recommended in these patients.[35] As an alternative, a rifampin-bonded gelatin-impregnated Dacron has been recommended in patients with arterial infections caused by susceptible organisms such as *S. aureus*[36]; however, these grafts are not effective against methicillin-resistant *S. aureus* or *Escherichia coli* infections.[37] Additional alternatives

include human allografts and autogenous vein grafts. The mid-term results of cryopreserved human allografts are encouraging: Brown et al. reported a series of 52 patients with infected aortas or aortic grafts who underwent replacement with cryopreserved allografts.[38] At 20 months follow-up, three patients had graft thrombosis or stenosis, and one developed a recurrent ilioenteric fistula; the remainder had no evidence of aneurysmal change or reinfection. The experience with autogenous superficial femoral-popliteal vein (SFPV) grafts is also encouraging. Several small series attest to the negligible reinfection rates and excellent durability associated with *in situ* SFPV reconstruction.[14,39] The early enthusiasm for this option is buoyed by excellent experience using the SFPV to replace infected prosthetic grafts of the aorta (see later discussion).

The modern enthusiasm for endovascular therapy has extended to infected aortic aneurysms. Several small series have suggested that placement of endografts in combination with long-term antibiotics represent definitive treatment of infected aortic aneurysms with similar outcomes to open aortic repair.[40,41] However, these data are countered by reports of a high rate of graft infection requiring removal, or extension of the aortic infection to more proximal segments.[42,43] This appears to be a particular risk in patients with *Salmonella* infections. Therefore, we suggest that endovascular repair might be a good option to treat acute complications from infected aortic aneurysms such as aerodigestive fistulas. However, these grafts should not be considered definitive treatment, and additional surgical therapy is indicated after resolution of the acute problem.[42]

Infected Femoral Artery Aneurysms

The superficial location of the femoral artery makes it an excellent choice for access to the central arterial circulation, but it also provides a convenient route of access for drug abusers. Femoral artery infections tend to be extensive and are often associated with virulent organisms or those that are resistant to standard antibiotics. Proper treatment requires radical débridement and careful consideration of the options for revascularization. Errors in surgical decision often result in recurrent femoral artery infections, with disastrous complications.

Femoral Artery Infections Associated with Invasive Procedures

Compared to alternative approaches involving direct puncture of the axillary artery or the abdominal aorta, the transfemoral approach is associated with the lowest risk of complications. Modern results indicate that the overall arterial complication rate of transfemoral catheterizations is less than 1%; the risk of femoral artery infection is exceedingly rare.[44,45] However, the increasing popularity of transcatheter techniques suggests that the absolute number of patients with catheter-related complications is likely to rise.

In an effort to reduce the incidence of pseudoaneurysms, many interventionalists use percutaneous closure devices to mechanically seal the arterial puncture site. Compared to manual compression, these devices have resulted in earlier mobilization and discharge of patients after arterial catheterization. However, these devices have been associated with a slightly higher risk of femoral artery infection. In a recent meta-analysis, Biancari et al. reported that the risk of access site infection is 0.6% after closure devices, compared to 0.2% without closure devices.[46] Risk factors for infection include diabetes, obesity, therapeutic intervention, and groin hematoma.

Primary femoral artery infections present as pseudoaneurysms. Common findings include pain at the puncture site, fever with chills, and a pulsatile groin mass. The onset of symptoms may be delayed up to several weeks after the original puncture. Gram-positive organisms predominate, especially *S. aureus*, but gram-negative bacteria are common isolates. Treatment involves institution of broad-spectrum antibiotics, débridement of the infected arterial segment, removal of all closure device material, and excision of grossly infected adjacent tissues. Direct revascularization with autogenous saphenous vein has been associated with a high risk of reinfection and vein graft blowout.[47] Alternatively, use of SFPV has been associated with excellent durability and resistance to infection in two small series.[48,49] Simple ligation of the common femoral artery (CFA) may be preferable if the femoral bifurcation is uninvolved.[50] If revascularization is necessary, the bypass should be routed through extra-anatomical tissues to avoid infected areas. A transobturator bypass is ideally suited to this situation.[51]

Femoral Artery Infections in Intravenous Drug Abusers

These complex lesions are extremely difficult to treat. In addition to the acute infection-related problems, many affected patients have serious comorbidities such as seropositivity for HIV and hepatitis B. Psychiatric disorders associated with chronic addiction can cause these individuals to be notoriously unreliable, and most do not return for follow-up after hospital discharge. Therefore, most authorities recommend conservative treatment approaches that emphasize avoidance of reinfection and late complications.

Approximately three fourths of all admissions for accidental intravenous drug injections involve the lower extremity, and the femoral artery is the most common site of involvement.[52] Most patients present with a painful, pulsatile groin mass, often associated with overlying cellulitis. The most commonly cultured organism is *S. aureus*. Appropriate treatment involves ligation of the affected arterial segment to reduce the risk of hemorrhage and débridement of all grossly contaminated tissue to remove the septic focus. The advisability of subsequent revascularization remains controversial.

Many authors recommend ligation without revascularization, even if this leads to amputation. Repeated use of superficial veins for drug injection eliminates available autogenous conduits, necessitating the use of prosthetic material in many cases. The incidence of reinfection is extremely high in these circumstances, risking graft disruption and life-threatening hemorrhage.

Avoidance of revascularization rarely leads to amputation. Earlier reports documented an 11% amputation rate when one artery was ligated and a 33% amputation rate after triple-vessel ligation.[53] More recent reports suggest that the incidence of amputation is much lower. Ting and Cheng performed routine ligation in 34 infected femoral pseudoaneurysms, including 24 that involved the femoral bifurcation.[54] The mean postoperative ankle-brachial index was .43 after triple ligation and .52 with single-vessel ligation. Although 88% of patients had some degree of intermittent claudication after discharge, there were no instances of delayed limb loss. Cheng and colleagues reported a similar rate of claudication after single- or triple-vessel ligation, but one patient (5%) required above-knee amputation.[55] Mousavi et al. reported the results of femoral artery ligation for infected pseudoaneurysms in 134 illicit drug users. There were no amputations in this series.[56]

Modern consensus is that infected femoral aneurysms in drug addicts are best treated with ligation alone. Most patients will suffer some degree of claudication, but the risk of early and late amputation is low. Immediate revascularization should be limited to cases in which no Doppler signal is detected at the ankle after femoral artery ligation.[57] In the vast majority, staged revascularization should be considered in patients with limiting claudication after the infection has been completely cleared. The known propensity for prosthetic graft infection from a remote injection site suggests that autogenous tissue is preferable in these circumstances. In the absence of usable saphenous vein, the SFPV represents an excellent alternative.[48]

Infected Aneurysms of the Superior Mesenteric Artery

The SMA is the third most common site of visceral aneurysms from all causes, but it is the most common site for infected aneurysms in the splanchnic circulation.[58,59] Original studies from more than 20 years ago reported that approximately 60% of SMA

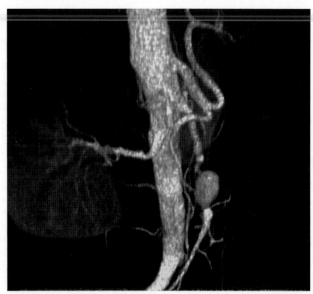

FIGURE 59-4 Computerized tomographic (CT) arteriogram demonstrating an infected superior mesenteric aneurysm in a 32-year-old female with endocarditis.

aneurysms had an infectious etiology,[60] but this proportion appears to be decreasing. More recent series have reported an infectious etiology in 5% to 33% of reported cases.[58,59,61] Infected SMA aneurysms usually occur secondary to subacute bacterial endocarditis, and the most commonly isolated organism is nonhemolytic *Streptococcus*.[58,62]

Most infected SMA aneurysms occur in patients younger than 50 years; men and women are equally affected.[58,60] Only 10% of patients are completely asymptomatic.[58] Some degree of abdominal discomfort is present in two thirds, and up to half have a tender, mobile, pulsatile mass.[60] Fever, nausea, vomiting, gastrointestinal hemorrhage, and jaundice may also be present.

Superior mesenteric artery aneurysms tend to occur within 5 cm of the SMA origin, but any segment may be affected. Aneurysms may be suspected when vascular calcifications are seen on plain radiographs of the abdomen. Diagnosis should be confirmed with appropriate imaging studies that also localize the extent of the aneurysm such as standard mesenteric angiography or CTA (Fig. 59-4). Most infected SMA aneurysms are single, with variable involvement of visceral branches.

The natural history of infected SMA aneurysms is one of progression and eventual rupture; in fact, rupture has occurred at the time of presentation in 38% to 50% of patients.[58] Reported mortality rate after rupture approaches 30%.[61] Treatment includes transabdominal exploration and ligation of the arterial segments proximal and distal to the aneurysm. Complete excision is hazardous due to the proximity of the superior mesenteric vein and pancreas; therefore, débridement should be limited to exposed portions of the aneurysm wall and to the aneurysm sac contents. In the vast majority of cases, extensive mesenteric collateralization preserves bowel viability after SMA ligation. Therefore, ligation with resection of short segments of nonviable intestine is almost always appropriate. Direct revascularization is necessary in approximately 15% of cases. Bypass should be performed with autogenous tissue; we have found the SFPV to be an excellent alternative with superior patency compared to saphenous vein.[63]

Infected Carotid Artery Aneurysms

Infected aneurysms are rare in the extracranial carotid circulation. In a series of 67 carotid artery aneurysms treated over a 35-year period at the Texas Heart Institute, only one was infected.[64] Most patients present with fever and a tender pulsatile neck mass. Medial deviation of the pseudoaneurysm may lead to clinical findings suggestive of a parapharyngeal mass. Before the antibiotic era, most carotid artery infections were the consequence of direct spread from pharyngeal infections. Most lesions are currently due to septicemia from bacterial endocarditis.

Gram-positive organisms, especially *S. aureus* and *S. pyogenes*, are common isolates from infected carotid aneurysms, but *Salmonella* infections have also been reported.[65,66] Treatment involves ligation of all infected segments, even if this requires ligation of the internal and external carotid branches. Owing to the potential for graft disruption and exsanguinating hemorrhage, revascularization is rarely indicated. To prevent propagation of the internal carotid thrombus into the middle cerebral artery circulation, systemic anticoagulation with warfarin is recommended. Anticoagulation should theoretically be continued until the thrombus becomes stable, a period not longer than 6 weeks. Although most patients can be expected to tolerate internal carotid ligation without sequelae, temporary occlusion with a balloon catheter should be performed in the preoperative period. Patients who develop neurological deficits during balloon occlusion should be considered for prophylactic extracranial-intracranial bypass through remote uninfected tissues. As an alternative, some patients may benefit from hypertensive therapy combined with hypervolemia and hemodilution.[66] To decrease the risk of exsanguination during carotid exposure, Wales et al. have advocated staged repair using a covered endovascular stent to temporarily exclude the pseudoaneurysm before proceeding to early definitive surgical management.[67]

Other Infected Aneurysms

Primary arterial infections of the upper extremity are rare and generally the consequence of arterial trauma. Infected aneurysms of the axillary, brachial, radial, and ulnar arteries have been reported most frequently in intravenous drug abusers, but these lesions are also seen after percutaneous catheterization for diagnostic procedures. Infected radial artery aneurysms are frequently associated with indwelling catheters used for arterial monitoring. The most common isolates are gram-positive organisms, usually *S. aureus*. Patients may present with a tender mass and overlying cellulitis, but digital embolization has been the first manifestation in many cases. Treatment involves ligation of the arteries proximal and distal to the aneurysm, followed by excision of infected tissues. Following excision, single involvement of the radial or ulnar artery does not often require revascularization; collateral flow in the hand is usually adequate. However, revascularization may be required in rare cases of incomplete hand circulation. More proximal arteries should be revascularized using autogenous tissue such as saphenous vein.

Aside from femoral artery aneurysms, infected aneurysms of the lower extremity are exceedingly rare. The vast majority of infected popliteal artery aneurysms are a consequence of septic embolization from infective endocarditis.[68] Mycotic aneurysms of the tibioperoneal trunk and tibial vessels have also been reported. Most infections involve gram-positive organisms such as *Streptococcus*, but *Salmonella* species have been recovered in a significant number of recently reported cases. The most common presentation is rupture, although thrombosis with foot ischemia has also been described. Treatment involves excision of the infected arterial segment and revascularization using autogenous bypass grafts.

Prosthetic Graft Infections

Development of a prosthetic graft infection remains a daunting complication. Despite improvements in diagnosis and management, modern morbidity and mortality rates remain prohibitively high. Even after successful treatment, the recovery from operative therapy is often prolonged, and many patients require extensive rehabilitation. Clinical diagnosis remains challenging, because many graft infections follow an insidious course. In fact, most patients will present with complications of latent graft infections such as graft occlusions or pseudoaneurysms months to years after implantation.

Despite the improvements in imaging modalities, radiological diagnosis remains exceedingly difficult. A high index of suspicion is required to diagnose graft infections prior to otherwise inevitable catastrophic complications. Once the diagnosis is made, careful operative planning is required to minimize the risk of loss of life and limb and to assure that recurrent infection does not occur. The advent of new endovascular approaches to the management of arterial disease has not eliminated the problem of graft infections; rather, these devices have created a new set of diagnostic and management challenges for surgeons and internists alike.

Risk Factors and Pathogenesis

The pathogenesis of graft infections is multifactorial and partly related to the site of implantation. Contamination prior to implantation due to failed sterilization techniques or breaks in packaging is thought to occur very infrequently. Likewise, gross breaks in sterile technique are rare. Most graft infections occur as a result of unrecognized bacterial contamination at the time of implantation. Exposure of the graft material to surrounding skin is a likely source; viable bacteria remain in the dermis of the skin despite antiseptic preparation.[69] Graft contamination can also occur from remote infections such as cellulitis or pyelonephritis. Wet gangrene of a toe can increase the risk of infection in a prosthetic femoropopliteal bypass graft. Similarly, concurrent intraabdominal procedures such as cholecystectomy or appendectomy can expose an aortic graft to the patient's enteric flora, thereby increasing the risk of graft infection.

A number of specific risk factors have been associated with aortic graft infections. Colonic ischemia following the repair of ruptured and nonruptured aortic aneurysms is associated with a high risk of graft infection due either to direct contamination or to hematogenous seeding from bacterial translocation.[70] It has long been recognized that graft infections are more common after emergency repair of ruptured aortic aneurysms compared to elective operations.[71] The emergent nature of ruptured AAA repair likely leads to inadvertent breaks in sterile techniques as the surgical team rushes to gain vascular control. In addition, patients presenting with either acute occlusion of the aorta or rupture of an aortic aneurysm are at high risk to develop postoperative SIRS. This SIRS response leads to an initial production of a proinflammatory cytokine response followed by a compensatory antiinflammatory cytokine response. This response renders the patient immunocompromised and at risk for nosocomial infections. Theoretically, this immunocompromised state may contribute to the increased risk of graft infection by hematogenous seeding during episodes of bacteremia.

Aortic grafts are uniquely prone to primary bacterial colonization at the time of aortic aneurysm repair. As already noted, many studies have demonstrated that the mural thrombus found in aneurysms is frequently colonized with bacteria. Macbeth et al. found that up to 43% of arterial walls were culture-positive for bacteria at the time of surgery.[72] In this series, all of the aortic graft infections (.9%) occurred exclusively in patients with positive aortic wall cultures. The most common isolate was *Staphylococcus epidermidis* (71%) followed by *Streptococcus* species (13%) and other isolates (16%).[72] Similarly, Buckels et al. in 1985 found that graft infection occurred more frequently in patients with positive cultures of aortic contents compared to those with negative cultures.[73] More contemporary studies have failed to confirm an absolute association between positive aortic cultures and subsequent graft infections. Farkas et al. reported positive cultures in 37% of 500 aortic aneurysms.[24] However, only one patient with a positive culture developed a graft infection. In contrast, 6 of 296 patients with negative cultures developed aortic graft infections during follow-up.[24] Based on these observations, it is clear that colonization of the mural thrombus by bacteria plays, at most, a minor role in the pathogenesis of aortic graft infection. Results from more contemporary experiences may be due to the consistent use of perioperative antibiotic therapy.

Local and regional factors may also play a role in development of graft infections. Use of groin incisions (e.g., aortobifemoral bypass) can more than double the risk of graft infection compared to aortic grafts that remain completely intraabdominal (e.g., aortobiiliac bypass or aortic tube graft repairs). This may be related to the local environment of the groin, an area associated with one of the highest concentrations of *Staphylococcus* species found on the body.[69] In addition, dissection in the groin disrupts abundant femoral lymphatics, leading to risk of lymph leak, groin wound breakdown, and direct graft contamination. Furthermore, the lymphatic system transports bacteria from distal sites of infection to the groin lymph nodes; opening these channels exposes the graft to potential contamination. Translocated bacteria have been demonstrated in animals and humans. In patients presenting with complex foot infections, positive lymphatic cultures at the time of amputation have been demonstrated in up to 20% of patients.[74] Cultures of groin lymph nodes at the time of vascular reconstruction have revealed bacteria in 11%. However, these cultures do not correlate with subsequent groin wound infections.[75]

Recurrent operations in the same location, particularly the groin, represent a significant risk for graft infection. Repeated catheter access also increases the overall risk. Aortofemoral bypass grafts placed for treatment of occlusive disease, while durable, do thrombose and are frequently revised by either lysis or thrombectomy. Procedures used to reestablish flow through occluded grafts, whether surgical or endovascular, expose the graft to potential contamination. It is common to find that patients with late graft infections have had multiple procedures to reestablish arterial flow through such grafts.

Graft material also plays a role in the pathogenesis of graft infections. The immune system responds to the foreign body by walling off the offending agent. The initial response is an acute inflammation, with influx of neutrophils followed by macrophages. These inflammatory cells produce cytokines and release proteases in an attempt to eliminate the foreign body. This initial response has a negative effect on bacterial survival; however, if the inoculum is large, some bacteria may survive. The graft interstices may offer a safe haven for bacteria and allow them to survive the initial inflammatory phase. After the acute inflammatory response, a reparative phase begins. This stage is characterized by fibroblasts depositing collagen in response to locally secreted cytokines. A resulting connective tissue barrier shields bacterium from detection and obliteration by immune competent cells. This results in a closed space for the bacteria to thrive and grow on exudative proteins existing in an acidic and ischemic environment. In the absence of infection, the reparative phase culminates in tissue ingrowth and incorporation of the graft. However, if bacterial colonization is present, the graft fails to incorporate, and chronic inflammation continues. Failure to incorporate may be due to fibroblast inhibition by the bacterial components found in the perigraft fluid.[76] This results in the failure to obliterate the closed space around the graft and failure of incorporation. Bacteria are left to thrive in this closed space, eventually becoming an abscess. This can manifest as perigraft fluid that may express through incisions with sinus tract formation. In addition, the artery may be degraded at suture lines, resulting in pseudoaneurysm formation.

Clearly, multiple factors play a role in establishment of graft infections following vascular reconstructions. Despite this, the incidence of graft infection remains low, at less than 5% for all reconstructions. Vascular graft infections can be categorized into two general groups: aortic graft infections and graft infections following infrainguinal arterial reconstruction. These two broad groups can be further subdivided into prosthetic and autogenous graft infections. Virtually all graft infections following aortic reconstructions are prosthetic graft infections, but infection following infrainguinal reconstructions can occur in both autogenous and synthetic grafts. The anatomical configuration of the graft and the material that composes the graft alter both the diagnostic and therapeutic modalities. Diagnosis and management of aortic and infrainguinal graft infections will be considered separately in the sections that follow.

Aortic Graft Infection

Over the last 2 decades, refinements in diagnosis and operative management of aortic graft infections have resulted in improved mortality and morbidity. Mortality during the early experience of aortic graft infection approached 50%, and limb loss rates were as high as 75%. With refinement in technique, the respective mortality and limb loss rates have decreased to 20% or less in many series.[77]

Incidence

The exact incidence of graft infection following aortic reconstruction is not precisely known because most series are retrospective and suffer from lack of inclusive follow-up. The best estimates suggested that the incidence of graft infection following aortic reconstructions ranges from 1% to 5%.[77-79] More contemporary data can be abstracted from the U.K. Small Aneurysm Trial, a randomized study of AAA repair in patients with small aneurysms. Although this study did not directly report the incidence of aortic graft infection, a number of graft-related complications were documented. Three patients in the trial had late aortic rupture following AAA repair, and four patients died following development of aortoenteric fistula. Most of these complications can be assumed to represent complications from aortic graft infection and represent 2% of the total patients.[80] The true incidence of aortic graft infection remains inadequately described, but most authorities agree the incidence is quite low and certainly less than 2% in the contemporary experience.

Classification

To better understand the pathogenesis and natural history of graft infections, classification systems have been developed. Wound complications following vascular reconstruction were first classified by Szilagyi et al. in 1972.[81] The authors characterized wound complications following prosthetic graft placement in terms of anatomical involvement. Grade I lesions involved only the dermis. Grade II lesions extended into the subcutaneous tissue without involvement of the graft, while grade III lesions involved the graft by direct extension.[81] Grade III lesions can be considered technical problems associated with wound closure. Certainly, local factors such as ischemic tissue play a significant role in wound infections, but they may be avoidable. This grading scheme is important only for early graft infections, which account for less than 1% of all graft infections.[82] It does not take into account graft infections that present during late follow-up after aortic reconstruction. This grading scheme is more relevant to infections that follow infrainguinal arterial reconstructions, which result most frequently from complications of wound infections.

More relevant to the understanding of aortic graft infection is the scheme developed by Bandyk, who categorized aortic graft infections according to time of presentation after graft implantation.[82] This classification scheme offers better insight into the origin of graft infections and is a better predictor of the type of bacteria that will be found infecting the graft. Bandyk defined an early graft infection as one that occurred less than 4 months after implantation, and late graft infections manifested after 4 months. Graft infections are subcategorized in terms of presentation: perigraft infection, graft-enteric erosion, and graft-enteric fistula. Most early perigraft infections represent the sequela of Szilagyi grade III wound infection; that is, extension of local wound infections to involve the graft. Remote sites of infection (e.g., wet gangrene) or immunosuppression are thought to play a minor role in early graft infections.[82] The diagnosis of an early perigraft infection is usually obvious: most patients present with purulent drainage from the wound, signs of sepsis with bacteremia, acute pseudoaneurysm formation, or anastomotic disruption with hemorrhage. Early infections will be manifest almost exclusively in wounds located at or below the femoral level. These infections can be expected to contain any one of a variety of organisms including gram-positive and gram-negative organisms. In contrast, late perigraft infections tend to occur months to years following implantation. Most will present more than 1 year following implantation, and the majority result from *S. epidermidis* infection with biofilm production.

Bandyk further subdivided graft enteric fistulas into graft enteric erosions and graft enteric fistulas. *Graft enteric erosions* are aorto-enteric communications that do not involve an anastomosis. Many affected patients do not have evidence of gastrointestinal bleeding. These lesions appear late and are thought to be the result of erosion of the graft into a contiguous loop of bowel by mechanical forces. Most graft enteric erosions occur in the body of the graft, and some consider the erosions to be a preliminary step in the process that ultimately extends to involve an anastomosis and leads to aortoenteric fistula. Bacterial cultures from these graft infections will yield predominantly gram-negative pathogens. Yeast is also a commonly isolate. Graft enteric erosions are attributed to inadequate retroperitoneal closure over the prosthetic graft at the time of aortic reconstruction. However, graft enteric erosions may be a manifestation of unrecognized perigraft infection. The infective process involves the overlying retroperitoneum with extension to the bowel and eventual graft enteric erosion. Mechanical forces and inadequate coverage of the graft likely contribute, but in the authors' opinion, most erosions are the result of latent perigraft infections. Regardless of the etiology, the graft associated with enteric erosion should be considered infected.

Graft enteric fistulas communicate with a vascular anastomosis and present with gastrointestinal bleeding. These fistulas rarely occur in the early postoperative period. In contrast to erosions, graft enteric fistulas are the result of a perigraft infection that leads to anastomotic breakdown and pseudoaneurysm formation at a suture line. The pseudoaneurysm then erodes into the overlying bowel, leading to fistula formation and the potential for exsanguinating hemorrhage. Like erosions, cultures of graft enteric fistulas yield predominantly gram-negative enteric pathogens.

These classification systems are not all-encompassing. All aortic graft infections will not fall into a single category, but such systems serve as a useful guide and allow one to anticipate the pathogens likely to be encountered.

Etiology

Most aortic graft infections are thought to occur by direct contamination or extension of adjacent infections. No good evidence exists confirming that bacteremia contributes to aortic graft infection in humans. However, there is ample evidence from animal studies that bacteremia can result in prosthetic graft infections.[83,84] Antibiotic therapy during bacteremia in dog models prevents prosthetic graft infections.[84] All these models consist of bacteremia immediately following graft implantation. In humans, bacteremia frequently occurs after aortic surgery, yet the rate of acute graft infection is very low. Bacteremia likely plays only a minor role in acute aortic graft infections. The role of bacteremia in late-occurring graft infection is not known, but it is thought to be a rare cause of late graft infection.

Should patients with vascular grafts receive prophylactic antibiotics before procedures associated with bacteremia, such as dental or genitourinary instrumentation? Although past case reports have suggested a possible association, there is little evidence to indicate that these procedures lead to graft infection. Late-occurring graft infections are caused only rarely by organisms found in mouth flora.[85] Graft incorporation may act as a barrier to bacteremia and prevent late graft infections. In contrast to patients with prosthetic cardiac valves, current American Heart Association (AHA) guidelines do not recommend antibiotic prophylaxis after vascular graft placement for patients undergoing dental, respiratory, gastrointestinal, or genitourological procedures.[86]

Clinical Presentation

The signs of aortic graft infection are highly variable. As noted previously, early graft infections can be easy to identify because they represent complications of wound infections. Affected patients usually present with induration and cellulitis at the wound, purulent wound drainage, and/or wound dehiscence with exposed graft. In patients with aortic reconstructions confined to the abdomen, presenting symptoms tend to manifest without wound involvement. Typical symptoms include failure to thrive, ileus, fever, elevated WBC count, or frank sepsis. Similarly, malaise, weight loss, and vague constitutional symptoms may be the only manifestations of graft infection. Graft infections can be difficult to diagnose in these patients, and the diagnosis is often made fortuitously during workup of more common sources. Alternatively, the patient may present with pseudoaneurysm formation or catastrophic rupture of the aortic anastomosis.

Any patient with a wound infection overlying a prosthetic graft requires careful wound exploration. The authors examine these wounds in the operating room unless the infection manifests solely as cellulitis. Operative exploration is mandatory because the exterior wound can be deceptive; only direct exploration can reveal that the infective process involves the body of the graft. Cellulitis with drainage requires exploration for an underlying abscess. In the operating room, the wound is explored and opened to the deepest depth of involvement. If the deep tissues are unaffected (Szilagyi grade II), most grafts are not contaminated.

The clinical presentation of late graft infection can be subtle. Latent graft infections can present as chronic femoral pseudoaneurysms. At repair, the graft will be poorly incorporated, with surrounding perigraft fluid. These findings are considered diagnostic for graft infection and have been associated with positive cultures in 71% of cases.[87] Lack of graft incorporation is more sensitive for graft infection; Padberg et al. found that 97% of incorporated grafts were not infected.[87] Infection may be a primary process for the formation of anastomotic femoral pseudoaneurysm. Up to 60% of clinically uninfected femoral pseudoaneurysms will be culture positive at repair.[88] The presence of a latent graft infection should be considered in all cases of femoral pseudoaneurysms. Another subtle sign of latent graft infection is graft thrombosis. This is particularly true if the graft has failed in the past, requiring revision either surgically or by thrombolysis. All patients with graft limb thrombosis or femoral pseudoaneurysms should have CT scan imaging of the graft to rule out infection prior to repair or revision.[89] Hydronephrosis may also herald a latent graft infection.[89] All patients with prior aortic surgery should have a CT to evaluate for latent graft infection when hydronephrosis is encountered.

Less subtle presentations of latent graft infections include draining sinuses from groin wounds (Fig. 59-5) and a history of bleeding from a groin pseudoaneurysm. Bleeding from the groin in the presence of a pseudoaneurysm is a surgical emergency and must be addressed immediately. Such bleeding episodes are herald bleeds and portend life-threatening hemorrhage if not dealt with expeditiously. Graft infection may also present as gastrointestinal bleeding in a patient with prior aortic surgery. All such patients should be considered to have an aortoenteric fistula until proven otherwise. Rupture of a previously repaired aneurysm or pseudoaneurysm at the proximal anastomosis should be considered the sequelae of graft infection. An updated summary of the clinical manifestations of aortic graft infections in 187 patients with aortic graft infections treated at University of Texas Southwestern Medical Center is found in Table 59-2. This experience is similar to other published series.[85,90]

Diagnosis

Numerous modalities have been used to diagnose aortic graft infection, including CT, MRI, tagged WBC scans, ultrasound, sinography, percutaneous aspiration, arteriography, and operative exploration. Each method has inherent strengths and weaknesses, and often several tests are used in concert to assure accurate diagnosis.

COMPUTED TOMOGRAPHY SCAN

The CT scan remains the gold standard for diagnosis of aortic graft infections. Findings on CT that are suggestive of graft infections include loss of continuity of the aortic wrap (i.e., the residual native aortic wall closed over the graft at the time of repair), pseudoaneurysms, perigraft fluid, perigraft inflammation with loss of

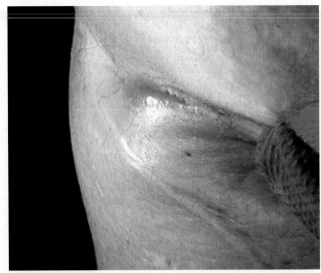

FIGURE 59-5 Draining sinus from the right groin in a patient with a late aortic graft infection.

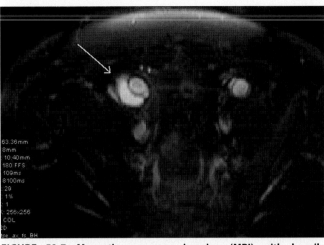

FIGURE 59-7 Magnetic resonance imaging (MRI) with heavily T2-weighted images of patient with infected aortobifemoral bypass. Perigraft fluid is seen as a bright *(white)* signal surrounding graft *(arrow)*. Note bright fluid "halo" surrounding infected graft.

TABLE 59-2	Clinical Manifestations of Aortic Graft Infections* in 187 Patients: University of Texas Southwestern Medical Center Experience
CLINICAL MANIFESTATION	**NO. PATIENTS (%)**
Open groin sinus	81 (43)
Femoral pseudoaneurysm	68 (36)
Constitutional/weight loss	61 (32)
Ischemia	52 (29)
Sepsis	40 (21)
AE erosion/fistula	26 (14)
Bleeding	23 (12)

*Many patients had more than one sign.
AE, aortoenteric.
Adapted from Ali AT, Modrall JG, Hocking J, et al: Long-term results of the treatment of aortic graft infection by *in situ* replacement with femoral popliteal vein grafts. J Vasc Surg 50:30, 2009.[124]

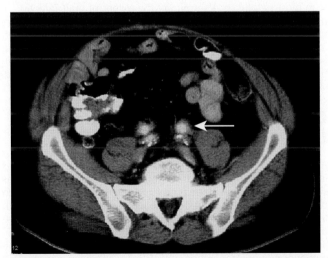

FIGURE 59-6 Computed tomography (CT) scan of patient with infected aortobifemoral bypass demonstrating presence of perigraft fluid. Arrow points to perigraft fluid.

tissue planes, perigraft air, and focal bowel wall thickening. Presence of any of these findings is highly suggestive of aortic graft infection. Figure 59-6 demonstrates the presence of perigraft fluid in a patient with an infected aortic graft. The same patient was found to have bilateral femoral artery pseudoaneurysms (Fig. 59-7).

The reported sensitivity and specificity of CT scans to diagnose all graft infections is 95% and 85%, respectively.[91] Sensitivity and specificity approaches 100% when findings of perigraft fluid, perigraft inflammation, or ectopic gas are present.[89,91] However, CT scanning may not be able to accurately diagnose subtle graft infections manifest solely by the presence of perigraft fluid. While CT imaging of low-grade aortic graft infection has a specificity of 100%, the sensitivity is only 55%.[89] The other disadvantage of CT scanning is the requirement for intravenous contrast. This may be contraindicated in patients with chronic renal insufficiency or dye allergies. However, the CT modality is readily available, safe, inexpensive, and familiar to clinicians; it remains the imaging modality of choice for initial evaluation.

MAGNETIC RESONANCE IMAGING

The major advantage of MRI, in comparison to CT scanning, is the ability to diagnose small fluid collections and differentiate inflammatory changes from chronic hematomas. Perigraft fluid has low to medium signal intensity on T1-weighted images and high intensity on T2-weighted images. Noninfected aortic grafts will have perigraft fibrosis without the characteristic bright fluid "halo" seen surrounding infected grafts on heavily T2-weighted images. Tissue surrounding infected aortic grafts frequently exhibits heterogeneous increased signal intensity that is not seen in association with sterile grafts.[92] Olofsson et al. found the sensitivity and specificity of MRI for diagnosing graft infections to be 85% and 100%, respectively.[93] The ability of MRI to detect small fluid collections on T2-weighted images gives this modality a distinct advantage over CT scanning to diagnose low-grade *S. epidermidis* graft infections. The authors use CT scans as the initial imaging modality, and MRI is used to find latent graft infections not detected by CT.

RADIONUCLIDE SCANNING

Radionuclide scanning relies on labeled WBCs to localize areas of infection and inflammation. A variety of scanning techniques have been developed to aid in diagnosis. The major pitfall of such imaging techniques is false-positive results. Initially, gallium-67 and indium-111 were used without WBC labeling. The sensitivities and specificities of imaging with gallium and indium were quite high, but these tracers have been largely abandoned owing to uptake by the gastrointestinal tract and kidneys that obscures the aorta and makes analysis difficult. More recently, WBC labeling techniques have become the norm. Indium-111-oxine–labeled WBC scans have been found to be very sensitive (82%-100%) but have a lower specificity (80%-83%).[94–96] The low specificity of this technique is due to co-labeling of platelets that can deposit on noninfected graft surfaces, resulting in an unacceptably high false-positive rate.

Other techniques have been employed in an attempt to increase the sensitivity of radionuclide scanning. These include labeling WBC with technetium-99 m hexametazime or technetium-99 m D,L-hexamethylpropylene amine oxide (Tc-99 m-HMPAO). These techniques are less expensive and do not suffer from the co-labeling problems seen with indium. Liberatore et al. reported a sensitivity for Tc-99 m-HMPAO of 100% and a specificity of 92%.[97] Other techniques included indium-111-labeled immunoglobulin (Ig)G and avidin/indium-111-labeled biotin scintigraphy.[92] Both of these techniques appear to have increased specificity compared to indium labeled WBCs, but the published experience has been limited. The role of radionuclide scanning is not entirely clear; some centers use radionuclide scanning as the primary mode of imaging for graft infections. Perera et al. have suggested that these scans are most useful when diagnosis by CT is equivocal or there is a low-grade infection.[77] Like all nuclear medicine imaging techniques, the results can be dependent on the skill and experience of the interpreting radiologist. The most rational approach is to use such scanning techniques as an adjunct to both CT scanning and MRI.

ULTRASOUND

Ultrasonography has a limited role in the diagnosis of aortic graft infection. Although ultrasound can accurately diagnose the presence of perigraft fluid (Fig. 59-8), the intraabdominal portion of grafts is not readily imaged. The primary utility of ultrasound is to diagnose femoral pseudoaneurysms and perigraft fluid around infrainguinal grafts or aortic grafts that extend to the groin.

SINOGRAPHY

Injection of draining sinuses associated with aortic grafts has been reported. A positive study will demonstrate contrast tracking from the sinus to fill a perigraft fluid collection around an unincorporated graft. The utility of such studies is not known, and it is doubtful such studies add any new information from what can be gleaned from CT or MRI. In addition, injection of contrast into an infected perigraft fluid collection could result in bacteremia or bleeding.

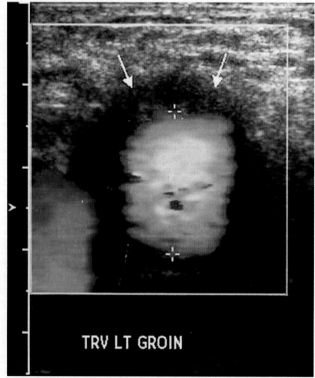

FIGURE 59-8 Duplex ultrasound of femoral anastomosis in patient with infected aortofemoral bypass graft. Note hypoechoic rim surrounding graft, consistent with perigraft fluid ("halo" sign).

Almost all draining sinuses after vascular prosthetic grafting represent external expression of an infection and, thus sinography is unlikely to yield any information not already known to the clinician.

PERCUTANEOUS ASPIRATION

Some authors have advocated percutaneous aspiration to confirm the diagnosis of a suspected graft infection.[98,99] In the routine diagnosis of graft infection, this modality offers little additional information beyond conventional noninvasive imaging techniques, and percutaneous aspiration can lead to introduction of bacteria into an otherwise sterile fluid collection. Percutaneous aspiration may offer some assistance in the high-risk patient to confirm the diagnosis prior to embarking on surgical repair. Concurrent placement of an external drainage catheter can be used as a therapeutic measure. Belair et al. reported a series of 11 patients treated with percutaneous drainage and antibiotic therapy.[98] In this retrospective series, four patients were successfully treated with percutaneous drainage and antibiotic therapy. The remaining patients required adjunctive procedures (two surgical drainage, four graft excision), and one patient died as a complication of hemorrhage following drainage.[98] Percutaneous drainage with lifelong antibiotic therapy may be an option for the very high-risk patient who is not anticipated to survive graft excision.

ARTERIOGRAPHY

Arteriography has little role in the diagnosis of aortic graft infection. Unsuspected pseudoaneurysm may be uncovered on arteriography, but the images obtained will give little insight to potential infectious etiologies. However, arteriography is vital for preoperative planning and should be obtained prior to any planned surgical therapy for infected grafts.

OPERATIVE EXPLORATION

In rare circumstances, there may be a high index of suspicion for graft infection, with no supporting evidence on imaging of graft infection. In such situations, operative exploration may be the only way to determine the presence of a latent graft infection.[78] As noted earlier, the finding of a nonincorporated graft is not necessarily diagnostic for graft infection, but the finding of a well-incorporated graft does rule out the diagnosis of infection. Operative exploration may most helpful in determining the extent of graft infection. If preservation of a portion of a graft is entertained, operative exploration is often the only mechanism to determine whether a graft infection is isolated to a segment of the graft or the entire graft is infected. Careful preoperative planning is required before such operative explorations to ensure that noninvolved graft is not inadvertently contaminated.

Diagnostic Pitfalls with Early Graft Infection

Although most early graft infections are obvious, normal findings in the immediate postoperative period may be misconstrued as signs of graft infection. There is no good diagnostic solution in such cases. Fluid and air surrounding the graft are common findings in the early postoperative period and are not necessarily indicative of infection. The finding of air around the graft is seen routinely until 1 week following implantation; air is not considered to be pathognomonic for infection until 4 to 7 weeks have elapsed.[100,101] Likewise, fluid around the graft is a common finding. Virtually all patients will have some degree of hematoma around the graft in the early postoperative period, but fluid persisting past 3 months is abnormal and highly suspicious for graft infection.[89]

Magnetic resonance imaging evaluation for early graft infection suffers from the same pitfalls as CT scanning. Magnetic resonance imaging cannot distinguish between air and calcium in the wall aortic wall remnant and thus depends on the finding of perigraft fluid. Labeling of WBCs for scintigraphy is also unreliable in the early postoperative period. Ramo et al. found that 29% of Tc-99 m-HMPAO–labeled WBC scans were positive in 24 patients examined 2 weeks following surgery.[102] At 3 months, 4 of 24 studies continued to be positive. Only one patient was ultimately found to have an infected graft. Sedwitz et al. found a similar lack of specificity for the diagnosis of early graft infection (<3 months) using indium-labeled WBC scintigraphy.[103]

Direct aspiration of perigraft fluid is not helpful in diagnosis of early graft infection and is not recommended in the early postoperative period owing to the potential for introducing bacteria into an otherwise sterile fluid collection.[92] Any of these imaging modalities may be helpful in the early postoperative period if they are negative. A negative study will lead the clinician to entertain other diagnoses to explain the clinical findings that have raised the suspicion of an early graft infection. However, a positive study is not useful; the clinician will have to rely on judgment, and operative exploration may be the only solution to this vexing clinical dilemma.

Diagnosis of Aortoenteric Fistula

The diagnosis of aortoenteric fistula can be as challenging as diagnosing an early graft infection. Any patient presenting with gastrointestinal hemorrhage and a history of aortic reconstruction should be considered to have an aortoenteric fistula until proven otherwise. Both MRI and CT can fail to diagnose graft enteric fistulas. Magnetic resonance imaging can fail to clearly demonstrate ectopic air that may be misinterpreted as aortic wall calcifications. Computed tomography scanning may fail to diagnose fistulas because of limited inflammation or fluid around the graft, resulting in misinterpretation.[92] If the patient is stable, either MRI or CT should be obtained. Concerning findings are absence of a soft-tissue plane between adjacent bowel and the graft, as well as ectopic air or perigraft fluid. Extravasation of contrast into the bowel is virtually never seen. All stable patients should undergo upper endoscopy to include the fourth portion of the duodenum. Endoscopy rarely demonstrates visible graft, but endoscopy should be performed to rule out other causes of upper gastrointestinal hemorrhage, such as peptic ulcer disease or gastroesophageal varices. Colonoscopy may be indicated in selected patients suspected of having graft erosions into the colon (Fig. 59-9). In unstable patients

or patients in whom no other source of bleeding is found, operative exploration is needed to rule out graft-enteric fistula. During exploration, the entire duodenum and any other adherent bowel must be entirely dissected free to rule out a fistula.

Bacteriology

A wide variety of bacterial pathogens can be cultured from infected grafts. The type of pathogen that will be isolated can be anticipated from the timing of presentation. The culture results from Yeager and colleagues' experience treating 60 infected grafts[104] are typical and presented in Table 59-3. In late-occurring graft infections, staphylococcal species are predominant, with *S. epidermidis* found most frequently. Bandyk et al. reported that 60% of late-occurring graft infections were culture positive for *S. epidermidis*.[105] Although the most commonly cultured organism responsible for early graft infection is *S. aureus*,[106] early graft infections will have a higher frequency of gram-negative rods and atypical organisms such as anaerobes and yeast. Aortoenteric fistulas and graft erosions are characterized by gram-negative rod and yeast infections. Pseudomonal infections are notorious for their virulent course. Graft and arterial disruption are common. This is related to production of elastase and alkaline proteases by *Pseudomonas*, leading to arterial degradation and eventual disruption.[69] Time of presentation of the graft infection and the pathogens found at the time of therapy will guide antibiotic therapy.

Optimal length of treatment with antibiotics after graft excision is not known. Some authorities have recommended a 6-week course of parenteral antibiotics followed by 6 months of suppressive therapy to treat concurrent arterial wall infection.[72] Macbeth et al. based his treatment decision on cultures from pathological specimens and aortic biopsies at the time of infected graft excision.[72] Patients with positive arterial wall cultures who were treated with only minimal débridement and short-term antibiotics all suffered aortic stump disruption or other arterial wall disruption. Consequent to these findings, the authors advocated 6 weeks of parenteral antibiotics, followed by 6 months of oral suppressive therapy in patients with positive arterial wall cultures.

Our practice has been to administer a brief period of perioperative antibiotics after graft excision and autogenous superficial femoral/popliteal vein (SFPV) reconstruction (see later discussion). We do not routinely treat patients for 6 weeks with parenteral antibiotics.

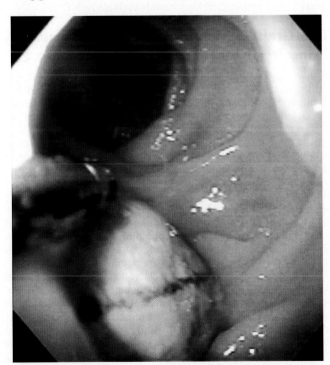

FIGURE 59-9 Colonoscopy in patient with suspected graft enteric erosion, showing visible graft material in sigmoid colon.

TABLE 59-3	Cultures from Infected Aortic Grafts in 32 Patients
ORGANISM	**NO. CASES (%)**
Staphylococcus aureus	14 (44)
Staphylococcus epidermidis	14 (44)
Bacteroides	3 (9)
Escherichia coli	2 (6)
Streptococcus	2 (6)
Klebsiella	1 (3)
Pseudomonas	1 (3)
Enterococcus	1 (3)
Clostridium	1 (3)
Serratia	1 (3)
Candida	1 (3)
Corynebacterium	1 (3)
Propionibacterium	1 (3)
No growth	2 (6)
Multiple organisms	10 (31)

Adapted from Yeager RA, Taylor LM Jr, Moneta GL, et al: Improved results with conventional management of infrarenal aortic infection. J Vasc Surg 30:76–83, 1999.[104]

With autogenous replacement and adequate operative débridement of the infected perigraft tissue, long-term antibiotic therapy does not appear to be necessary. We have experienced one reinfection in a patient culture positive for *Candida*. In our practice, only patients with virulent infections such as *Pseudomonas* or opportunistic infections such as yeast are considered for long-term antibiotic therapy following reconstruction with autogenous SFPV.

Treatment of Aortic Graft Infections

The basic tenet of management of infected arterial grafts is excision of the infected graft and revascularization through uninvolved tissue planes (extra-anatomical bypass). The traditional management of infected aortic grafts has been axillary-to-femoral bypass followed by graft excision and ligation of the aortic stump. This technique is plagued by the poor graft durability, risk of bypass infection, and aortic stump blowout. More recent innovations have included in-line reconstruction with antibiotic-impregnated grafts, arterial homografts, and reconstruction with autogenous SFPVs. Each approach has its advantages and disadvantages, and operative therapy must be tailored to suit the individual patient.

Antibiotic Therapy

Limited treatment using lifelong antibiotic therapy or percutaneous drainage and antibiotic therapy are options for the most high-risk patient with a limited life expectancy. There are little data to support such treatment regimens. Roy and Grove reported a series of high-risk patients treated with antibiotic therapy alone for proven or suspected graft infections.[106] Only two of the patients had proven infections of preexisting grafts. All patients were alive at the median follow-up of 36 months without systemic symptoms of infection. Although this appears to be a reasonable option, it should be stressed that this therapy is appropriate only for latent graft infections due to low-virulence organisms, particularly *S. epidermidis*. This therapy should be condemned in all but the most high-risk patients. Infection by more virulent bacteria has a grave prognosis, and antibiotic therapy alone will have little impact on the natural history of the infection.

Total Graft Excision without Revascularization

In the early experience of management of aortic graft infections, graft excision without arterial reconstruction was commonly done. The infected graft would be excised, and a wait-and-see strategy would be used to determine whether the limbs required revascularization. This approach led to unacceptably high rates of amputation and death. Graft excision alone can be considered in patients with occluded grafts who do not have limb-threatening ischemia. Most patients will tolerate excision of a thrombosed infected graft without worsening of the preexisting ischemia; however, the risk of interrupting important collaterals during graft excision should be borne in mind.

Patients who underwent aortic grafting for claudication may tolerate graft excision without revascularization. Such patients can be expected to return to their preoperative degree of ischemia after graft removal, assuming that important collaterals are not interrupted. This technique should be reserved for patients that have had end-to-side aortic grafting for aortoiliac occlusive disease. Preoperative arteriography must be obtained to determine whether native circulation remains intact. Thrombosis of the native aorta is common following end-to-side aortobifemoral bypass graft and must be ruled out prior to graft excision. In most patients and virtually all patients operated on for aortic aneurysmal disease, graft excision without revascularization can be expected to result in lower-extremity amputation.

Total Graft Excision and Extra-Anatomical Revascularization

Total graft excision with extra-anatomical bypass is the traditional treatment for infected aortic graft. This treatment strategy consists of extra-anatomical bypass by axillary-femoral-femoral bypass or bilateral axillary to femoral bypasses with total graft excision. The sequence of operations is very important to prevent cross-contamination of the new graft. The extra-anatomical bypass should be performed first through noninfected tissues, and the wounds should be closed and dressed prior to exposing the infected graft. In addition to avoiding contamination of the new graft, this sequencing has the advantage of limiting leg ischemia.

Axillary-femoral-femoral bypasses are employed for treatment of infected grafts that do not involve the femoral arteries; bilateral axillary-to-femoral bypasses are used to treat infected aortobifemoral bypass grafts. The approach for infected aortobifemoral bypass requires careful planning and inventive tunneling. To prevent cross-contamination of the new graft, the femoral vessels are approached through uninvolved tissue planes, typically lateral to the sartorius muscle. Bypasses are performed from the axillary artery to the profunda femoris artery or to the superficial femoral artery if it is disease free. Axillary-to-popliteal bypasses have very poor patency and have largely been abandoned.

After completing the extra-anatomical bypass, the infected graft is removed. Timing of the two stages is controversial. The extra-anatomical bypass can be performed just prior to removal of the infected graft during the same operative procedure, or the procedures can be staged with extra-anatomical bypass performed several days prior to removal of the infected graft. Staging procedures give the patient time to recover from the initial bypass and avoid a long procedure. Proponents of the staged procedure purport a lower operative morality and increased limb salvage than the single-stage operative strategy.[107,108]

There are several disadvantages to extra-anatomical bypass with total graft excision. The most worrisome complication is infection of the new bypass graft. Reinfection rates can be as high as 20%, but most series report a low reinfection rate of less than 10%.[67,68,108] The notoriously poor durability of the extra-anatomical bypasses is also a concern. The highest reported primary patency rate for axillary-femoral-femoral bypasses is over 75%, but the reported primary patency rates of unilateral axillary-femoral bypasses average approximately 60% at 3.5 years.[107,109] The most devastating complication of this procedure is disruption of the oversewn aortic stump (aortic stump blowout). Fortunately, this lethal complication is rare. Because of these disadvantages, a number of other options for graft excision and revascularization have been introduced.

Total Graft Excision with *In Situ* Replacement Using Prosthetic Graft

In situ replacement of an infected graft with a new prosthetic graft is technically the simplest method of revascularization and avoids the potential for aortic stump blowout. However, replacing an infected prosthetic graft with a new prosthesis poses the very real potential for recurrent graft infection. *In situ* prosthetic replacement may be best used as a salvage operation for unstable patients with either aortoenteric fistula or ruptured proximal pseudoaneurysms. Fortunately, the reported rates of clinically apparent reinfection following *in situ* replacement for aortoenteric fistula is surprisingly low (<15%).[110,111] Replacement with new graft may be appropriate for localized graft infections such as those found in the setting of aortoenteric fistula. Recurrent infection in the setting of gross graft infection has been disappointing. The authors use *in situ* replacement with prostheses as a bridge to definitive therapy with autogenous replacement at a later operation.

The advent of antibiotic-bonded Dacron grafts appeared to offer improved results for *in situ* prosthetic replacement. This modality seems to be most appropriate for treatment of graft infections with biofilm-producing *S. epidermidis* or *S. aureus*. Young et al. reported a series of nine patients treated with rifampin-soaked grafts and found that the reinfection rate was 11%.[111] Bandyk et al. and Hayes et al. both concluded that rifampin-bonded grafts are acceptable for treatment of low-grade biofilm graft infections by *S. epidermidis* and *S. aureus*.[112,113] Bandyk et al. found that recurrent infection occurred in less than 10% of patients.[112] Hayes et al. only reported reinfection in patients with meticillin-resistant *S. aureus* (MRSA) infections.[113] It appears that antibiotic-bonded grafts may offer improved results, but only in selected patients with low-grade *S. epidermidis* and possibly *S. aureus* infections. They are usually not appropriate in cases involving more virulent organisms. Similar findings have recently been reported using silver-coated polyester grafts for *in situ* replacement. In a series of 24 patients with a variety of polymicrobial graft infections, Batt et al. documented a 40% prevalence of graft reinfections.[114]

Total Graft Excision with *In Situ* Replacement Using Arterial Allograft

An alternative to *in situ* replacement with prosthetic graft is replacement with arterial allograft. Animal studies have demonstrated the allograft is relatively resistant to infection when antibiotic loaded.[115] The experience in humans has confirmed this finding. Leseche et al. reported a series of 28 patients treated with allografts for graft infection or infected aortic aneurysms.[116] They reported no recurrent infection. In a series of 49 patients, Vogt et al. reported two patients with recurrent infections that resulted in death.[117] However, in this series there were four deaths related to allograft technical complications. In three patients, allograft side branch rupture resulted in three aortoenteric fistulas that were uniformly fatal. A fourth patient died intraoperatively from rupture of a friable allograft. In a recent study of 110 consecutive patients with aortic infections, Bisdas et al. reported a 9% overall operative mortality. During a mean follow-up of 36 months, 6% required reoperation for graft deterioration, but no recurrence of infection was noted.[118] Others have noted that reoperation for reinfection or degenerative changes in allografts is common (9%-17%) and that pathological changes are seen in up to 26% of patients.[38,116] *In situ* allograft and prosthetic graft replacement may be best used a temporizing technique until more definitive therapy can be undertaken.

Total Graft Excision with *In Situ* Replacement Using Autogenous Veins

Perhaps the best solution for management of prosthetic graft infection is *in situ* reconstruction with SFPV. This conduit has proven to be the most resistant conduit to infection, has unchallenged patency rates, avoids the risk of aortic stump blowout, and rarely degenerates. Operative mortality following aortic reconstruction with SFPV has been reported as less than 10%.[119–123] Reinfection is very rare. In our experience, only one patient suffered infection of an SFPV graft, and the offending organism was *Candida*. Franke noted two cases of SFPV infection that occurred in the face of overwhelming *Pseudomonas* infection.[123] In our experience, all patients with pseudomonal infections have been treated successfully, but it should be pointed out that none of our patients presented with overwhelming sepsis. Patients with overwhelming sepsis may be better served by extra-anatomical bypass and graft excision. SFPV is very durable, with primary patency rates of greater than 80% and less than 5% of grafts requiring revision.[122,124] Venous morbidity is minimal.[125]

Most patients are suitable for aortic reconstruction with SFPV regardless of the bacterial pathogen. The only downside to this management strategy is the length of the operative procedure. Harvest of the SFPV requires two teams, and mean operative time is 8 hours. Because of the length of time required, SFPV aortic reconstruction is not appropriate for unstable patients, particularly patients with bleeding aortoenteric fistulas. However, such patients can be treated with *in situ* prosthetic replacement with delayed conversion to SFPV after a period of stabilization and recovery. We have had very pleasing results with this strategy. Extra-anatomical bypass with graft excision has been the standard for treatment of aortic graft infection, but we believe that autogenous replacement with SFPV has earned a place as the new gold standard for management of such patients.

Partial Graft Excision

With the improvement in imaging techniques, some authors have advocated partial graft excision if the aortic graft infection can be localized to the femoral portion on preoperative imaging. Reconstruction can be carried out by extra-anatomical bypass or *in situ* grafting. This technique is most appropriate for patients with late *S. epidermidis* infections. It is not appropriate for patients with early graft infections because the entire graft is almost invariably involved.[82] Towne et al. described treating 14 patients with confirmed *S. epidermidis* or *S. aureus* infection using partial graft excision, wide local débridement, and *in situ* replacement with PTFE graft.[126] Only 2 of the 14 patients ultimately developed infection in the remaining graft, but the new PTFE grafts remained uninfected. Calligaro et al. demonstrated that graft patch remnants on infrainguinal vessels can be safely left *in situ* at the time of graft excision in over 92% of patients.[127] Reilly et al. have described good results with partial graft excision and extra-anatomical bypass.[77] In the authors' most recent experience, only 63% of patients require total graft excision. In our experience, subtotal graft excision can be attempted if the body of the graft is found to be incorporated at the time of surgical exploration. In these situations, planned reconstruction with SFPV has a real advantage. The body of the graft can be explored prior to violating the clearly infected portion. If the entire graft is infected, total graft excision and reconstruction with SFPV can be undertaken. If the body of the graft is not infected, the graft can be divided and sewn to the SFPV. The wound is closed, the infected portion of the graft is removed, and the reconstruction completed. Subtotal graft excision should only be considered in high-risk patients with late-occurring graft infections. Such patients should be followed closely, and infection of the residual graft should be anticipated.

Graft Infection Following Endovascular Repair

Graft infection following stent graft repair of aneurysm is becoming more frequently reported. As of 2010, there have been 102 reports of abdominal endograft infections in the literature.[128] In a series of 494 consecutive stent grafts (389 abdominal aorta and 105 thoracic aorta), Heyer et al. reported a prevalence of abdominal endograft and thoracic endograft infection of 0.26% and 4.8%, respectively.[129] All affected patients suffered significant morbidity. While rare, endograft infections are extremely difficult to diagnose. The typical clinical presentation and radiographic finding associated with stent graft infections are not well described and await a more mature experience with these endovascular techniques. Infected grafts have been associated with highly virulent organisms including *Propionobacterium*, *Staphylococcus*, *Streptococcus*, and *Enterobacter*.[129] Treatment for infected abdominal aortic endografts includes complete graft excision and extra-anatomical or *in situ* bypass. We have used the SFPV for *in situ* replacement with gratifying results in these circumstances. On the other hand, treatment of infected thoracic endografts should include graft excision and bypass with antibiotic-soaked prosthetic graft or cryopreserved allograft if more virulent organisms are present.

Treatment of Peripheral Graft Infections

The incidence of graft infection following infrainguinal peripheral arterial reconstruction ranges from 2%-5%.[130] Most peripheral graft infections occur subsequent to extension of local wound infections. Late infections of autogenous grafts are very rare and most frequently occur in thrombosed grafts. Late infections occur more commonly in prosthetic grafts. Since most infections result from extension of a local wound infections (Szilagyi grade III), the microbiology can be varied, with gram-negative rods playing a prominent role. In a series of 68 patients with infected infrainguinal autogenous grafts, Treiman et al. found *S. aureus* and *S. epidermidis*, most commonly followed closely by *Pseudomonas*.[131]

Peripheral graft infections can present as drainage of pus from the wound, graft occlusion, or graft disruption with hemorrhage. A patient presenting with bleeding from the site of an infrainguinal arterial reconstruction should be considered to have a graft infection, and operative exploration is mandatory. In less obvious cases, the diagnosis of such infections is similar to that of aortic graft infections. Computed tomography scanning is most helpful, and will demonstrate perigraft fluid collections and inflammation. Magnetic resonance imaging can successfully diagnose infected prosthetic grafts that have surrounding perigraft fluid. Ultrasound may also be helpful in such cases. The grafts are easily accessible, and ultrasound is particularly good at identifying perigraft fluid.

The mainstay of therapy is arterial reconstruction through uninfected fields and graft removal. In patients with occluded grafts who do not have limb-threatening ischemia, the graft can be excised without arterial reconstruction. However, patients who were operated on for limb-threatening ischemia who undergo graft excision can be anticipated to need revascularization or face inevitable amputation.

In patients who will require concurrent revascularization at the time of infected graft excision, the management options are different for prosthetic grafts versus autogenous graft. In virtually all cases of prosthetic graft infection, the entire graft is involved in the infectious process. This requires total graft excision with revascularization through uninfected tissues. Revascularization is performed first with autogenous conduit if possible. Careful planning and inventive tunneling are required if cross-contamination is to be avoided. If the graft originates from the femoral artery, the profunda femoris artery, approached lateral to the sartorius muscle, can be used as the site of the proximal anastomosis. If the profunda femoris artery is diseased, the iliac vessels can be used, and the graft can be tunneled through the obturator foramen into the thigh. The recipient artery or run off artery must be one level below the infective process. If the popliteal artery above the knee is involved in the infective process, the new runoff vessel will have to be the below-the-knee popliteal artery or the tibial vessels. More distal reconstruction to uninvolved tibial vessels will be required if the infected graft terminates at the popliteal vessel below the knee or more distal. Often the graft will have to be tunneled through the lateral thigh to avoid the previously violated medial thigh. The below-the-knee popliteal artery, peroneal artery, and the anterior tibial artery can all be approached through lateral leg incisions. After reestablishing flow and closing the wounds, the prosthetic graft is excised through a separate incision. If possible, the entire graft should be excised with autogenous patching of the donor and recipient arteries to avoid late complications from infected graft remnants. Well-incorporated remnants of prosthetic grafts can be left in place with successful healing and few late complications, but these patients will require close observation.[127]

Virtually all autogenous graft infections occur at the site of a wound infection. An autogenous graft infection is often localized to segment of the graft located directly beneath the infected wound. In these cases, the uninvolved portion of the graft can be left in place, and a new autogenous graft can originate from these uninvolved portions. As with prosthetic graft infections, the best option is revascularization through uninfected tissue planes. However, new autogenous grafts can be placed in the infected tissue planes, with concurrent coverage by well-vascularized muscle flaps. In patients with infected grafts but without graft disruption, graft preservation may be attempted. The graft may be left *in situ*, covered with muscle flaps, and treated with intravenous antibiotics.

In a series of 16 patients with autogenous graft infections without disruption, Calligaro et al. were able to successfully salvage 11 grafts.[132] Of these patients, six were treated with muscle flap coverage, with only one failure and no graft associated mortality. Patients treated with operative débridement and antibiotic-soaked dressing changes had more complications and higher mortality from graft complications. Limb salvage was obtained in 6 of 10 patients. In this series, the overall operative mortality was 19%, and the amputation rate was 8%.[132] Tukiainen et al. reported improved results with graft preservation, aggressive débridement, and muscle flap coverage in a series of 14 patients with autogenous graft infections.[133] One patient required a late amputation because of ongoing graft infection, and four patients had late graft occlusions. All four patients with late graft occlusions had *in situ* replacement with new graft for graft disruption and hemorrhage. There were no graft-related mortalities and no graft disruptions from recurrent infection.[133] Treiman identified graft disruption with bleeding, elevated WBCs, fever, and renal insufficiency as the only predictors for graft failure and limb loss following selective graft preservation.[131]

In the authors' experience, wound infections that involve autogenous grafts without graft disruption represent graft contamination rather than graft infections. Such grafts can be treated by graft preservation and muscle flap coverage. It is imperative that well-vascularized muscle be used to cover such grafts. If the graft is not covered by muscle, continued wound sepsis with progression to frank graft infection and disruption can be anticipated. True graft infections manifest as graft degradation and hemorrhage. Invariably, pathological examination of such grafts will reveal pathogens in the wall of the graft. Such grafts should be treated by graft ligation with revascularization through uninfected tissue planes; uninfected portions of the graft may be left place. *In situ* reconstruction with new autogenous graft such as contralateral saphenous vein or arm vein[134] has been reported. In the face of graft degradation and hemorrhage, muscle flap coverage is not a good option and should be reserved only for patients with limited autogenous conduit. In these rare circumstances, close observation with prolonged antibiotic therapy is needed. Such patients should be observed in the intensive care unit setting until wound healing and absence of recurrent graft infection is assured. Graft ligation with or without primary amputation may be the safest course in such patients.

Suppurative Thrombophlebitis

Widespread use of intravenous therapy in hospital patients has made primary venous infections more common than their arterial counterparts. The term *suppurative thrombophlebitis* implies a localized infection of the vein wall associated with intraluminal thrombosis, which should be differentiated from catheter-related sepsis. While the two may be temporally related in the same patient, they can usually be distinguished by the following characteristics: (1) catheter sepsis is not usually associated with vein wall suppuration, and (2) in catheter sepsis, the intraluminal thrombus is adherent to the catheter, not the vein wall. The following discussion will focus on diagnosis and management of suppurative thrombophlebitis; more complete information on catheter sepsis is available elsewhere.[135]

Suppurative thrombophlebitis can be classified into five areas: superficial, central/pelvic, portal (pylephlebitis), cavernous sinus, and jugular (Lemierre's syndrome).

Peripheral Vein Suppurative Thrombophlebitis

Thrombophlebitis is the most common complication of peripheral vein infusion, occurring in up to a fourth of hospitalized patients receiving intravenous therapy via veins of the forearm or hand.[136] Pathogenesis has been related to irritation of the vein from the catheter material, infusate, or bacteria. Thrombosis occurs as a result of localized stasis and prostaglandin-mediated activation of the coagulation cascade.[137] Suppurative superficial thrombophlebitis results from infection of the thrombus, which is estimated to occur in 0.2% to 2% of peripheral vein catheter insertions.[138] Onset of infection is a serious development, resulting in significant morbidity and prolonged hospital stay. Development of life-threatening infections such as osteomyelitis or endocarditis may occur after a single episode of superficial suppurative thrombophlebitis. This complication is more common with plastic catheters than with steel ("scalp vein") cannulas and is related to duration of intravenous catheterization.[139] Prolonged catheterization is the most important predictor of peripheral vein infusion thrombophlebitis; this has led to the recommendation by the Centers for Disease Control and Prevention (CDC) that short peripheral intravenous catheters should be changed every 72 hours.

Although there is a higher risk of suppurative superficial thrombophlebitis from catheters inserted in the lower extremity, upper-extremity involvement is the more common presentation. Affected patients have signs of local inflammation, including tenderness, erythema, induration, and warmth over the involved superficial vein. Differentiation between noninfected and suppurative thrombophlebitis may be difficult. Systemic signs of infection such as fever, tachycardia, and leukocytosis are not universally present. Bacteremia occurs in the majority of patients, and gross pus within the vein lumen may be found in up to half the cases.[139] Diagnosis often relies on a positive culture of the indwelling catheter tip. S. aureus is the most common isolate, but gram-negative organisms are becoming more frequent. Antibiotic resistance is common.

Treatment of superficial suppurative thrombophlebitis involves removal of the intravenous catheter, institution of broad-spectrum antibiotics, and excision of the involved vein. The involved vein should be explored proximal to the highest anticipated site of involvement—usually several centimeters above the inflamed area. The infected vein segment and its tributaries should be completely excised using a patent noninflamed vein segment as the endpoint. Incisions should be left open to heal by secondary intention. Postoperatively, antibiotics should be continued for an undetermined period of time. Empirical recommendations suggest continuation of culture-directed antibiotics for at least 2 to 3 weeks.

Central Vein Suppurative Thrombophlebitis

Two classic scenarios have been described for suppurative thrombophlebitis of central veins: (1) residual central thrombosis following central line sepsis and (2) pelvic suppurative thrombophlebitis associated with gynecological complications. Suppurative thrombophlebitis of thoracic veins occurs in the chronic setting, whereas suppurative pelvic thrombophlebitis occurs more acutely.

CENTRAL SUPPURATIVE THROMBOPHLEBITIS FOLLOWING INTRAVENOUS LINE SEPSIS

Suppurative thrombophlebitis often follows prolonged intravenous therapy in immunocompromised patients. The condition is most common in patients receiving total parenteral nutrition, in critically ill patients receiving intravenous therapy through central venous catheters, and in those with long-term cannulation devices such as Hickman or Broviac catheters. Central suppurative thrombophlebitis may also be the consequence of intravenous drug abuse (see earlier discussion). Catheter infections are usually due to microorganisms that migrate from the skin entry site, but hematogenous seeding and contaminated fluids have also been implicated.[135] Suppurative thrombophlebitis occurs subsequent to infection of the thrombus that typically develops around the intravenous device. The thrombus becomes attached to the central vein wall and causes localized inflammation.

Central suppurative thrombophlebitis should be suspected in any patient who fails to improve after removal of an infected central venous catheter. Systemic signs of infection are more common than venous obstructive symptoms such as arm edema. Diagnosis can be made by demonstrating a deep vein thrombosis (DVT) (by duplex ultrasonography, venography, or MRI) in a septic patient with positive blood cultures who does not have other sources of primary infection.[140] Computed tomography scans may be useful to demonstrate a vein thrombosis, especially if gas is detected in the vein lumen.[139]

Treatment of central suppurative thrombophlebitis involves removal of central catheters, use of broad-spectrum antibiotics, and anticoagulation with heparin. In some cases, fibrinolytic therapy[141] or surgical thrombectomy[142] may be required. Long-term anticoagulation with warfarin is recommended to reduce the risk of embolization and recurrent thrombosis. A 2- to 3-week course of culture-directed antibiotics is usually appropriate.

PELVIC SUPPURATIVE THROMBOPHLEBITIS

Infection of the deep pelvic veins usually develops 2 to 3 weeks postpartum or after gynecological complications such as criminal abortions or other severe pelvic infections. Diagnosis of pelvic suppurative thrombophlebitis should be suspected in a postpartum woman with high fevers, chills, and abdominal pain. Large veins may cause ureteral obstruction, resulting in severe flank pain.[139] Nearly 80% of cases are on the right side due to compression of the right ovarian vein at the pelvic brim by the gravid uterus.[139] Although a tender vein can be palpated on pelvic examination in up to 30% of women, physical examination may be normal.[139] Computed tomography scanning and MRI have both been useful to confirm deep pelvic vein thrombosis; a positive test in the clinical setting of sepsis confirms the diagnosis. Pelvic suppurative thrombophlebitis usually responds to broad-spectrum intravenous antibiotics. It remains controversial whether patients benefit from anticoagulation with heparin. Occasionally, patients do not respond to conservative treatment, and drainage of a pelvic abscess or ligation of the affected vein has been required.

Suppurative Thrombophlebitis of the Portal Vein (Pylephlebitis)

Suppurative thrombophlebitis of the portal vein usually follows infection of an organ drained by the portal vein or a contiguous structure. Historically, pylephlebitis was most commonly due to appendicitis.[143] Widespread use of antibiotics and early diagnosis and intervention for abdominal infections have made the condition rare. Most modern cases occur as a complication of diverticulitis, but it has also followed other intraabdominal infections such as appendicitis, acute cholecystitis, and foreign body perforation.[144] However, some are due to secondary infection of portal vein thrombosis associated with a hypercoagulable disorder such as cirrhosis or malignancy.[145]

The clinical presentation of patients with pylephlebitis is nonspecific: most have fevers of unknown origin with variable signs of systemic toxicity. Abdominal pain occurs in about three fourths of affected patients, and up to 20% have severe sepsis.[144] Ultrasound may be helpful to detect thrombus within the lumen of the portal vein, but CT is the more common test to confirm the diagnosis. Magnetic resonance imaging with angiography may be able to discern acute from chronic thrombus.[144,145] Many patients have other intraabdominal processes such as abscesses or common bile duct stones. Small intrahepatic liver abscesses may also be present.

Treatment of pylephlebitis involves use of broad-spectrum intravenous antibiotics and eradication of the underlying infection. Early treatment is critical to reduce the risk of ischemic bowel infarction from mesenteric vein thrombosis. Although systemic administration of broad-spectrum antibiotics is usually adequate, catheter infusion of antibiotics directly into the portal vein may result in more prompt improvement.[146] Intraabdominal infections should be treated promptly by percutaneous drainage or surgical intervention. In rare cases, laparotomy and thrombectomy of the portal system have been used in severely ill patients.[144] In all cases, antibiotics should be continued until complete resolution or cavernous transformation of the thrombus, as confirmed with CT or MRI.[144] This usually requires at least 4 to 6 weeks. Fortunately, development of acute portal hypertension with variceal hemorrhage is uncommon.

Septic Thrombosis of the Cavernous Sinuses

Widespread use of antibiotics has dramatically reduced the incidence of cavernous sinus thrombophlebitis, but it is still occasionally seen in patients with severe head and neck infections. Infection of the ethmoid and sphenoid sinuses is the most common primary source that leads to cavernous sinus thrombophlebitis.[147] S. aureus is isolated in approximately 60% to 70% of cases, followed by

S. pneumoniae, gram-negative bacilli, and anaerobes.[147] Early diagnosis and treatment are extremely important; mortality rates of 20% to 30% are still reported in the modern era.[147]

Patients with cavernous sinus thrombophlebitis typically present with fever, ptosis, proptosis, chemosis, and external ophthalmoplegia.[147] Ocular signs are due to damage of nerves that traverse the cavernous sinus. Headache, papilledema, and periorbital swelling are present in more than half of affected patients. Diagnosis may be established by high-resolution CT scans or by MRI. Management includes treatment of the underlying infection (sinusitis, dental abscess, tonsillitis) and use of broad-spectrum antibiotics. Cavernous sinus drainage is almost never performed.[147] At least one study[148] suggests that anticoagulation with heparin may reduce the mortality rate in survivors. Severe sequelae have been reported in most survivors, including lung, brain, and orbital abscesses and prolonged cranial nerve dysfunction. Early diagnosis and treatment remain the keys to reducing potential disasters in these patients.

Septic Thrombophlebitis of the Internal Jugular Vein

This disorder was first described in 1936 by Lemierre, who reported a 90% mortality rate in his patients.[149] Widespread use of antibiotics has reduced the prevalence and mortality of septic thrombophlebitis of the internal jugular vein (also known as *postanginal septicemia* or *Lemierre's syndrome*), but the rarity of the syndrome also means that it is often overlooked. Several stages have been described.[144] Septic thrombophlebitis of the internal jugular vein usually follows an acute oropharyngeal infection; a sore throat is the most common presentation. In the second stage, local invasion of the parapharyngeal space leads to septic thrombophlebitis of the internal jugular vein. This most commonly presents as swelling and tenderness of the neck, which should be considered a serious development in a patient with pharyngitis. Metastatic infections occur in the third stage, most commonly the lungs and joints.

Diagnosis of Lemierre's syndrome should be considered in any patient with current or recent pharyngitis who presents with tenderness in the anterior cervical triangle. Clinical signs during the course of disease include fever, abdominal pain, and hyperbilirubinemia.[144] Most patients have already developed metastatic infections at the time of diagnosis. A triad of pharyngitis, tender/swollen neck, and noncavitating pulmonary infiltrates has been described.[150] The most common isolate is *Fusobacterium necrophorum*, an anaerobic gram-negative rod that is a normal inhabitant of the oral cavity.[144,150] Diagnostic tests such as ultrasonography, CT, or MRI should be used to confirm the presence of internal jugular vein thrombosis. Computed tomography or MRI may be helpful to delineate the presence of neck abscesses that require drainage; these tests are also useful to follow the local anatomy once treatment has been instituted. Treatment involves a 3- to 6-week course of intravenous antibiotics; surgical excision of the internal jugular vein is only necessary in patients with uncontrolled sepsis or recurrent septic emboli despite appropriate antibiotic therapy (<10% of cases).

Conclusions

Primary arterial infections and graft infections remain a daunting problem for clinicians. A high index of suspicion and modern imaging techniques are required to make the diagnosis of arterial infection, whether primary or following arterial reconstruction. With the advent of inventive management strategies, the mortality and morbidity associated with such infections has steadily improved. SFPV is the conduit of choice for reconstruction of large arteries with primary infections such as the carotid and mesenteric vessels. Aortic reconstruction with SFPV is the optimal management strategy for most patients with primary aortic infections or prosthetic aortic graft infections. Long-term administration of antibiotics represents the mainstay of treatment for primary venous infections; surgical excision is reserved for infections involving superficial veins and for deep veins in patients who do not improve on appropriate antibiotic therapy.

REFERENCES

1. Koch L: *Ueber aneurysma der arterial mesenterichae superioris. Inag Di Erlangen*, 1851.
2. Osler W: The Gulstonian lectures on malignant endocarditis, *Br Med J* 1:467, 1885.
3. Wilson SE, Van Wagenen P, Passaro E Jr: Arterial infection, *Curr Probl Surg* 15:1, 1978.
4. Stengel A, Wolferth CC: Mycotic (bacterial) aneurysms of intravascular origin, *Arch Intern Med* 31:527, 1923.
5. Brown SL, Busuttil RW, Baker JD, et al: Bacteriologic and surgical determinants of survival in patients with mycotic aneurysms, *J Vasc Surg* 1:541, 1984.
6. Thompson RW: Reflections on the pathogenesis of abdominal aortic aneurysms, *Cardiovasc Surg* 10:389, 2002.
7. Ailawadi G, Eliason JL, Upchurch GR: Current concepts in the pathogenesis of abdominal aortic aneurysm, *J Vasc Surg* 38:584, 2003.
8. Buckmaster MJ, Curci JA, Murray PR, et al: Source of elastin-degrading enzymes in mycotic aortic aneurysms: bacteria or host inflammatory response? *Cardiovasc Surg* 7:16, 1999.
9. Tilson MD: Pathogenesis of mycotic aneurysms, *Cardiovasc Surg* 7:1, 1999.
10. Pierce RA, Sandefur S, Doyle GA, et al: Monocytic cell type-specific transcriptional induction of collagenase, *J Clin Invest* 97:1890, 1996.
11. Hsu RB, Lin FY: Surgical pathology of infected aortic aneurysm and its clinical correlation, *Ann Vasc Surg* 21:742, 2007.
12. Gomes MN, Choyke PL, Wallace RB: Infected aortic aneurysms. A changing entity, *Ann Surg* 215:435, 1992.
13. Oderich GS, Panneton JM, Bower TC, et al: Infected aortic aneurysms: aggressive presentation, complicated early outcome, but durable results, *J Vasc Surg* 34:900, 2001.
14. Fillmore AJ, Valentine RJ: Surgical mortality in patients with infected aortic aneurysms, *J Am Coll Surg* 196:435, 2003.
15. Macedo TA, Stanson AW, Oderich GS, et al: Infected aortic aneurysms: imaging findings, *Radiology* 231:250, 2004.
16. Oz MC, Brener BJ, Buda JA, et al: A ten-year experience with bacterial aortitis, *J Vasc Surg* 10:439, 1989.
17. McNamara MF, Roberts AB, Bakshi KR: Gram-negative bacterial infection of aortic aneurysms, *J Cardiovasc Surg (Torino)* 28:453, 1987.
18. Brouwer RE, van Bockel JH, van Dissel JT: *Streptococcus pneumoniae*, an emerging pathogen in mycotic aneurysms? *Neth J Med* 52:16, 1998.
19. Goswami R, Cleveland KO, Gelfand MS: Evolving infectious aortitis caused by *Streptococcus pneumoniae*, *South Med J* 97:1004, 2004.
20. Katz SG, Andros G, Kohl RD: *Salmonella* infections of the abdominal aorta, *Surg Gynecol Obstet* 175:102, 1992.
21. Hsu RB, Chen RJ, Wang SS, et al: Infected aortic aneurysms: clinical outcome and risk factor analysis, *J Vasc Surg* 40:30, 2004.
22. Leon LR Jr, Mills JL Sr: Diagnosis and management of aortic mycotic aneurysms, *Vasc Endovasc Surg* 44:5, 2010.
23. van der Vliet JA, Kouwenberg PP, Muytjens HL, et al: Relevance of bacterial cultures of abdominal aortic aneurysm contents, *Surgery* 119:129, 1996.
24. Farkas JC, Fichelle JM, Laurian C, et al: Long-term follow-up of positive cultures in 500 abdominal aortic aneurysms, *Arch Surg* 128:284, 1993.
25. Gouny P, Valverde A, Vincent D, et al: Human immunodeficiency virus and infected aneurysm of the abdominal aorta: report of three cases, *Ann Vasc Surg* 6:239, 1992.
26. McHenry MC, Rehm SJ, Krajewski LP, et al: Vertebral osteomyelitis and aortic lesions: case report and review, *Rev Infect Dis* 13:1184, 1991.
27. Hagino RT, Clagett GP, Valentine RJ: A case of Pott's disease of the spine eroding into the suprarenal aorta, *J Vasc Surg* 24:482, 1996.
28. Muller BT, Wegener OR, Grabitz K, et al: Mycotic aneurysms of the thoracic and abdominal aorta and iliac arteries: experience with anatomic and extra-anatomic repair in 33 cases, *J Vasc Surg* 33:106, 2001.
29. Ihaya A, Chiba Y, Kimura T, et al: Surgical outcome of infectious aneurysm of the abdominal aorta with or without SIRS, *Cardiovasc Surg* 9:436, 2001.
30. Hsu RB, Chang CI, Wu IH, et al: Selective medical treatment of infected aneurysms of the aorta in high risk patients, *J Vasc Surg* 49:66, 2009.
31. Dubois M, Daenens K, Houthoofd S, et al: Treatment of mycotic aneurysms with involvement of the abdominal aorta: single-centre experience in 44 consecutive cases, *Eur J Vasc Surg* 2010 Aug 16 (Epub ahead of print).
32. Woon CY, Sebastian MG, Tay KH, et al: Extra-anatomic revascularization and aortic exclusion for mycotic aneurysms of the infrarenal aorta and iliac arteries in an Asian population, *Am J Surg* 195:66, 2008.
33. Robinson JA, Johansen K: Aortic sepsis: is there a role for *in situ* graft reconstruction? *J Vasc Surg* 13:677, 1991.
34. Hollier LH, Money SR, Creely B, et al: Direct replacement of mycotic thoracoabdominal aneurysms, *J Vasc Surg* 18:477, 1993.
35. Fichelle JM, Tabet G, Cormier P, et al: Infected infrarenal aortic aneurysms: when is *in situ* reconstruction safe? *J Vasc Surg* 17:635, 1993.
36. Gupta AK, Bandyk DF, Johnson BL: *In situ* repair of mycotic abdominal aortic aneurysms with rifampin-bonded gelatin-impregnated Dacron grafts: a preliminary case report, *J Vasc Surg* 24:472, 1996.
37. Koshiko S, Sasajima T, Muraki S, et al: Limitations in the use of rifampicin-gelatin grafts against virulent organisms, *J Vasc Surg* 35:779, 2002.
38. Brown KE, Heyer K, Rodriguez H, et al: Arterial reconstruction with cryopreserved human allografts in the setting of infection: a single-center experience with midterm follow-up, *J Vasc Surg* 49:660, 2009.
39. Benjamin ME, Cohn EJ Jr, Purtill WA, et al: Arterial reconstruction with deep leg veins for the treatment of mycotic aneurysms, *J Vasc Surg* 30:1004, 1999.
40. Berchtold C, Eibl C, Seelig MH, et al: Endovascular treatment and complete regression of an infected abdominal aortic aneurysm, *J Endovasc Ther* 4:543, 2002.

41. Kan CD, Lee H, Luo CY, et al: The efficacy of aortic stent grafts in the management of mycotic abdominal aortic aneurysm–institute case management with systemic literature comparison, *Ann Vasc Surg* 24:433, 2010.
42. Lew WK, Rowe VL, Cunningham MJ, et al: Endovascular management of mycotic aortic aneurysms and associated aortoaerodigestive fistula, *Ann Vasc Surg* 23:81, 2009.
43. Forbes TL, Harding GJ: Endovascular repair of *Salmonella* infected abdominal aortic aneurysms: a word of caution, *J Vasc Surg* 44:198, 2006.
44. Oweida SW, Roubin GS, Smith RB III, et al: Postcatheterization vascular complications associated with percutaneous transluminal coronary angioplasty, *J Vasc Surg* 12:310, 1990.
45. McCann RL, Schwartz LB, Pieper KS: Vascular complications of cardiac catheterization, *J Vasc Surg* 14:375, 1991.
46. Biancari F, D'Andrea V, Di Marco C, et al: Meta-analysis of randomized trials on the efficacy of vascular closure devices after diagnostic angiography and angioplasty, *Am Heart J* 159:518, 2010.
47. Whitton HH Jr, Rehring TF: Femoral endarteritis associated with percutaneous suture closure: new technology, challenging complications, *J Vasc Surg* 38:83, 2003.
48. Bell CL, Ali AT, Brawley JG, et al: Arterial reconstruction of infected femoral artery pseudoaneurysms using superficial femoropopliteal vein, *J Am Coll Surg* 200:831, 2005.
49. Schneider JR, Oskin SI, Verta MJ Jr: Superficial femoral vein graft interposition *in situ* repair for femoral mycotic aneurysm, *Ann Vasc Surg* 23:147, 2009.
50. Arora S, Weber MA, Fox CJ, et al: Common femoral artery ligation and local débridement: a safe treatment for infected femoral artery pseudoaneurysms, *J Vasc Surg* 33:990, 2001.
51. Patel A, Taylor SM, Langan EM III, et al: Obturator bypass: a classic approach for the treatment of contemporary groin infection, *Am Surg* 68:653, 2002.
52. Buerger R, Benitez P: Surgical emergencies from intravascular injection of drugs. In Bergan JJ, Yao JST, editors: *Vascular surgical emergencies*, Orlando, 1987, Grune & Stratton, pp 309–318.
53. Reddy DJ, Smith RF, Elliott JP Jr, et al: Infected femoral artery false aneurysms in drug addicts: evolution of selective vascular reconstruction, *J Vasc Surg* 3:718, 1986.
54. Ting AC, Cheng SW: Femoral pseudoaneurysms in drug addicts, *World J Surg* 21:783, 1997.
55. Cheng SW, Fok M, Wong J: Infected femoral pseudoaneurysm in intravenous drug abusers, *Br J Surg* 79:510, 1992.
56. Mousavi SR, Saberi A, Tadayon N, et al: Femoral artery ligation as treatment for infected for pseudoaneurysms secondary to drug injection, *Acta Chir Belg* 110:200, 2010.
57. Padberg F Jr, Hobson R, Lee B, et al: Femoral pseudoaneurysm from drugs of abuse: ligation or reconstruction? *J Vasc Surg* 15:642, 1992.
58. Lorelli DR, Cambria RA, Seabrook GR, et al: Diagnosis and management of aneurysms involving the superior mesenteric artery and its branches–a report of four cases, *Vasc Endovascular Surg* 37:59, 2003.
59. Stone WM, Abbas M, Cherry KJ, et al: Superior mesenteric artery aneurysms: is presence an indication for intervention? *J Vasc Surg* 36:234, 2002.
60. Stanley JC, Wakefield TW, Graham LM, et al: Clinical importance and management of splanchnic artery aneurysms, *J Vasc Surg* 3:836, 1986.
61. Messina LM, Shanley CJ: Visceral artery aneurysms, *Surg Clin North Am* 77:425, 1997.
62. Zimmerman-Klima PM, Wixon CL, Bogey WM Jr, et al: Considerations in the management of aneurysms of the superior mesenteric artery, *Ann Vasc Surg* 14:410, 2000.
63. Modrall JG, Sadjadi J, Joiner DR, et al: Comparison of superficial femoral vein and saphenous vein as conduits for mesenteric arterial bypass, *J Vasc Surg* 37:362, 2003.
64. El Sabrout R, Cooley DA: Extracranial carotid artery aneurysms: Texas Heart Institute experience, *J Vasc Surg* 31:702, 2000.
65. Grossi RJ, Onofrey D, Tvetenstrand C, et al: Mycotic carotid aneurysm, *J Vasc Surg* 6:81, 1987.
66. Nader R, Mohr G, Sheiner NM, et al: Mycotic aneurysm of the carotid bifurcation in the neck: case report and review of the literature, *Neurosurgery* 48:1152, 2001.
67. Wales L, Kruger AJ, Jenkins JS, et al: Mycotic carotid pseudoaneurysm: staged endovascular and surgical repair, *Eur J Vasc Endovasc Surg* 39:23, 2010.
68. Safar HA, Cina CS: Ruptured mycotic aneurysm of the popliteal artery. A case report and review of the literature, *J Cardiovasc Surg (Torino)* 42:237, 2001.
69. Seabrook GR: Pathobiology of graft infections, *Semin Vasc Surg* 3:81, 1990.
70. Woodcock NP, el Barghouti N, Perry EP, et al: Is bacterial translocation a cause of aortic graft sepsis? *Eur J Vasc Endovasc Surg* 19:433, 2000.
71. Reilly LM, Altman H, Lusby RJ, et al: Late results following surgical management of vascular graft infection, *J Vasc Surg* 1:36, 1984.
72. Macbeth GA, Rubin JR, McIntyre KE Jr, et al: The relevance of arterial wall microbiology to the treatment of prosthetic graft infections: graft infection vs. arterial infection, *J Vasc Surg* 1:750, 1984.
73. Buckels JA, Fielding JW, Black J, et al: Significance of positive bacterial cultures from aortic aneurysm contents, *Br J Surg* 72:440, 1985.
74. Fisher DF Jr, Clagett GP, Fry RE, et al: One-stage versus two-stage amputation for wet gangrene of the lower extremity: a randomized study, *J Vasc Surg* 8:428, 1988.
75. Josephs LG, Cordts PR, DiEdwardo CL, et al: Do infected inguinal lymph nodes increase the incidence of postoperative groin wound infection? *J Vasc Surg* 17:1077, 1993.
76. Henke PK, Bergamini TM, Watson AL, et al: Bacterial products primarily mediate fibroblast inhibition in biomaterial infection, *J Surg Res* 74:17, 1998.
77. Perera GB, Fujitani RM, Kubaska M: Aortic graft infection: update on management and treatment options, *Vasc Endovasc Surg* 40:1, 2006.
78. Valentine RJ: Diagnosis and management of aortic graft infection, *Semin Vasc Surg* 14:292, 2001.
79. Hallett JW Jr, Marshall DM, Petterson TM, Gray DT, et al: Graft-related complications after abdominal aortic aneurysm repair: reassurance from a 36-year population-based experience, *J Vasc Surg* 25:277, 1997.
80. The United Kingdom Small Aneurysm Trial Participants: Long-term outcomes of immediate repair compared with surveillance of small abdominal aortic aneurysms, *N Engl J Med* 346:1445, 2002.
81. Szilagyi DE, Smith RF, Elliott JP, et al: Infection in arterial reconstruction with synthetic grafts, *Ann Surg* 176:321, 1972.
82. Bandyk DF: Aortic graft infection, *Semin Vasc Surg* 3:122, 1990.
83. White JV, Freda J, Kozar R, et al: Does bacteremia pose a direct threat to synthetic vascular grafts? *Surgery* 102:402, 1987.
84. Goeau-Brissonniere O, Leport C, Lebrault C, et al: Antibiotic prophylaxis of late bacteremic vascular graft infection in a dog model, *Ann Vasc Surg* 4:528, 1990.
85. Jones L, Braithwaite BD, Davies B, et al: Mechanism of late prosthetic vascular graft infection, *Cardiovasc Surg* 5:486, 1997.
86. Baddour LM, Bettman MA, Bolger AF, et al: Nonvalvular cardiovascular device-related infections, *Circulation* 108:2015, 2003.
87. Padberg FT Jr, Smith SM, Eng RH: Accuracy of disincorporation for identification of vascular graft infection, *Arch Surg* 130:183, 1995.
88. Seabrook GR, Schmitt DD, Bandyk DF, et al: Anastomotic femoral pseudoaneurysm: an investigation of occult infection as an etiologic factor, *J Vasc Surg* 11:629, 1990.
89. Orton DF, LeVeen RF, Saigh JA, et al: Aortic prosthetic graft infections: radiologic manifestations and implications for management, *Radiographics* 20:977, 2000.
90. Sharp WJ, Hoballah JJ, Mohan CR, et al: The management of the infected aortic prosthesis: a current decade of experience, *J Vasc Surg* 19:844, 1994.
91. Low RN, Wall SD, Jeffrey RB Jr, et al: Aortoenteric fistula and perigraft infection: evaluation with CT, *Radiology* 175:157, 1990.
92. Modrall JG, Clagett GP: The role of imaging techniques in evaluating possible graft infections, *Semin Vasc Surg* 12:339, 1999.
93. Olofsson PA, Auffermann W, Higgins CB, et al: Diagnosis of prosthetic aortic graft infection by magnetic resonance imaging, *J Vasc Surg* 8:99, 1988.
94. Brunner MC, Mitchell RS, Baldwin JC, et al: Prosthetic graft infection: limitations of indium white blood cell scanning, *J Vasc Surg* 3:42, 1986.
95. Reilly DT, Grigg MJ, Cunningham DA, et al: Vascular graft infection: the role of indium scanning, *Eur J Vasc Surg* 3:393, 1989.
96. Lawrence PF, Dries DJ, Alazraki N, et al: Indium 111-labeled leukocyte scanning for detection of prosthetic vascular graft infection, *J Vasc Surg* 2:165, 1985.
97. Liberatore M, Iurilli AP, Ponzo F, et al: Clinical usefulness of technetium-99m-HMPAO-labeled leukocyte scan in prosthetic vascular graft infection, *J Nucl Med* 39:875, 1998.
98. Belair M, Soulez G, Oliva VL, et al: Aortic graft infection: the value of percutaneous drainage, *AJR Am J Roentgenol* 171:119, 1998.
99. Harris KA, Kozak R, Carroll SE, et al: Confirmation of infection of an aortic graft, *J Cardiovasc Surg (Torino)* 30:230, 1989.
100. Qvarfordt PG, Reilly LM, Mark AS, et al: Computerized tomographic assessment of graft incorporation after aortic reconstruction, *Am J Surg* 150:227, 1985.
101. O'Hara PJ, Borkowski GP, Hertzer NR, et al: Natural history of periprosthetic air on computerized axial tomographic examination of the abdomen following abdominal aortic aneurysm repair, *J Vasc Surg* 1:429, 1984.
102. Ramo OJ, Vorne M, Lantto E, et al: Postoperative graft incorporation after aortic reconstruction–comparison between computerised tomography and Tc-99m-HMPAO labelled leucocyte imaging, *Eur J Vasc Surg* 7:122, 1993.
103. Sedwitz MM, Davies RJ, Pretorius HT, et al: Indium 111-labeled white blood cell scans after vascular prosthetic reconstruction, *J Vasc Surg* 6:476, 1987.
104. Yeager RA, Taylor LM Jr, Moneta GL, et al: Improved results with conventional management of infrarenal aortic infection, *J Vasc Surg* 30:76, 1999.
105. Bandyk DF, Berni GA, Thiele BL, et al: Aortofemoral graft infection due to *Staphylococcus epidermidis*, *Arch Surg* 119:102, 1984.
106. Roy D, Grove DI: Efficacy of long-term antibiotic suppressive therapy in proven or suspected infected abdominal aortic grafts, *J Infect* 40:184, 2000.
107. Seeger JM, Pretus HA, Welborn MB, et al: Long-term outcome after treatment of aortic graft infection with staged extra-anatomic bypass grafting and aortic graft removal, *J Vasc Surg* 32:451, 2000.
108. Reilly LM, Stoney RJ, Goldstone J, et al: Improved management of aortic graft infection: the influence of operation sequence and staging, *J Vasc Surg* 5:421, 1987.
109. Yeager RA, Moneta GL, Taylor LM Jr, et al: Improving survival and limb salvage in patients with aortic graft infection, *Am J Surg* 159:466, 1990.
110. Walker WE, Cooley DA, Duncan JM, et al: The management of aortoduodenal fistula by *in situ* replacement of the infected abdominal aortic graft, *Ann Surg* 205:727, 1987.
111. Young RM, Cherry KJ Jr, Davis PM, et al: The results of *in situ* prosthetic replacement for infected aortic grafts, *Am J Surg* 178:136, 1999.
112. Bandyk DF, Novotney ML, Back MR, et al: Expanded application of *in situ* replacement for prosthetic graft infection, *J Vasc Surg* 34:411, 2001.
113. Hayes PD, Nasim A, London NJ, Sayers RD, Barrie WW, Bell PR, et al: *In situ* replacement of infected aortic grafts with rifampicin-bonded prostheses: the Leicester experience (1992 to 1998), *J Vasc Surg* 30:92, 1999.
114. Batt M, Jean-Baptiste E, O'Connor S, et al: *In situ* revascularization for patients with aortic graft infections: a single centre experience with silver coated polyester grafts, *Eur J Vasc Endovasc Surg* 236:182, 2008.
115. Knosalla C, Goeau-Brissonniere O, Leflon V, et al: Treatment of vascular graft infection by *in situ* replacement with cryopreserved aortic allografts: an experimental study, *J Vasc Surg* 27:689, 1998.
116. Leseche G, Castier Y, Petit MD, et al: Long-term results of cryopreserved arterial allograft reconstruction in infected prosthetic grafts and mycotic aneurysms of the abdominal aorta, *J Vasc Surg* 34:616, 2001.
117. Vogt PR, Brunner-LaRocca HP, Lachat M, et al: Technical details with the use of cryopreserved arterial allografts for aortic infection: influence on early and midterm mortality, *J Vasc Surg* 35:80, 2002.
118. Bisdas T, Bredt M, Pichlmaier M, et al: Eight-year experience with cryopreserved arterial homografts for the *in situ* reconstruction of abdominal aortic infections, *J Vasc Surg* 2010:323, 2010.
119. Valentine RJ, Clagett GP: Aortic graft infections: replacement with autogenous vein, *Cardiovasc Surg* 9:419, 2001.
120. Cardozo MA, Frankini AD, Bonamigo TP: Use of superficial femoral vein in the treatment of infected aortoiliofemoral prosthetic grafts, *Cardiovasc Surg* 10:304, 2002.
121. Daenens K, Fourneau I, Nevelsteen A: Ten-year experience in autogenous reconstruction with the femoral vein in the treatment of aortofemoral prosthetic infection, *Eur J Vasc Endovasc Surg* 25:240, 2003.

122. Ehsan O, Gibbons CP: A 10-year experience of using femoro-popliteal vein for revascularization in graft and arterial infections, *Eur J Vasc Endovasc Surg* 38:172, 2009.

123. Franke S, Voit R: The superficial femoral vein as arterial substitute in infections of the aortoiliac region, *Ann Vasc Surg* 11:406, 1997.

124. Ali AT, Modrall JG, Hocking J, et al: Long-term results of the treatment of aortic graft infection by *in situ* replacement with femoral popliteal vein grafts, *J Vasc Surg* 50:30, 2009.

125. Modrall JG, Hocking JA, Rosero E, et al: Late incidence of chronic venous insufficiency after deep vein harvest, *J Vasc Surg* 46:520, 2007.

126. Towne JB, Seabrook GR, Bandyk D, et al: *In situ* replacement of arterial prosthesis infected by bacterial biofilms: long-term follow-up, *J Vasc Surg* 19:226, 1994.

127. Calligaro KD, Veith FJ, Valladares JA, et al: Prosthetic patch remnants to treat infected arterial grafts, *J Vasc Surg* 31:245, 2000.

128. Setacci C, De Donato G, Setacci F, et al: Management of abdominal endograft infection, *J Cardiovasc Surg* 51:33, 2010.

129. Heyer KS, Modi P, Morasch MD, et al: Secondary infections of thoracic and abdominal aortic endografts, *J Vasc Interv Radiol* 20:173, 2009.

130. Chang JK, Calligaro KD, Ryan S, et al: Risk factors associated with infection of lower extremity revascularization: analysis of 365 procedures performed at a teaching hospital, *Ann Vasc Surg* 17:91, 2003.

131. Treiman GS, Copland S, Yellin AE, et al: Wound infections involving infrainguinal autogenous vein grafts: a current evaluation of factors determining successful graft preservation, *J Vasc Surg* 33:948, 2001.

132. Calligaro KD, Veith FJ, Schwartz ML, et al: Management of infected lower extremity autologous vein grafts by selective graft preservation, *Am J Surg* 164:291, 1992.

133. Tukiainen E, Biancari F, Lepantalo M: Deep infection of infrapopliteal autogenous vein grafts–immediate use of muscle flaps in leg salvage, *J Vasc Surg* 28:611, 1998.

134. Parmar CD, Kumar S, Torella F: Autogenous basilic vein for *in situ* replacement of infected prosthetic vascular grafts: initial experience, *J Vasc Surg* 17:158, 2009.

135. Chitticki P, Sherertz RJ: Recognition and prevention of nosocomial vascular device and related bloodstream infections in the intensive care unit, *Crit Care Med* 38:S363, 2010.

136. Tagalakis V, Kahn SR, Libman M, et al: The epidemiology of peripheral vein infusion thrombophlebitis: a critical review, *Am J Med* 113:146, 2002.

137. Lewis GBH, Hecker JF: Infusion thrombophlebitis, *Br J Anaesth* 57:220, 1985.

138. Stratton CW: Infection related to intravenous infusions, *Heart Lung* 11:123, 1982.

139. Bayer AS, Scheld WM: Endocarditis and intravascular infections. In Mandell GL, Bennett JE, Dolen R, editors: *Principles and practice of Infectious Diseases*, ed 5, New York. 2000, Churchill Livingstone, pp 857–902.

140. Miceli M, Atoui R, Thertulien R, et al: Deep septic thrombophlebitis: an unrecognized cause of relapsing bacteremia in patients with cancer, *J Clin Oncol* 22:1529, 2004.

141. Andes DR, Urban AW, Archer CW, et al: Septic thrombosis of the basilic, axillary, and subclavian veins caused by a peripherally inserted central venous catheter, *Am J Med* 105:446, 1998.

142. Kuiemeyer HW, Grabitz K, Buhl R, et al: Surgical treatment of septic deep venous thrombosis, *Surgery* 118:49, 1995.

143. Plemmons RM, Dooley DP, Longfield RN: Septic thrombophlebitis of the portal vein (pylephlebitis): diagnosis and management in the modern era, *Clin Infect Dis* 2:1114, 1995.

144. Chirinos JA, Garcia J, Alcaide ML, et al: Septic thrombophlebitis, diagnosis and management, *Am J Cardiovasc Drugs* 6:9, 2006.

145. Singh P, Yadav N, Visvalingam V, et al: Pyelophlebitis – diagnosis and management, *Am J Gastroenterol* 96:1312, 2001.

146. Pelsang RE, Johlin F, Dhada R, et al: Management of suppurative pyelophlebitis by percutaneous drainage: placing a drainage catheter into the portal vein, *Am J Gastroenterol* 96:3192, 2001.

147. Ebright JR, Pace MT, Niazi AF: Septic thrombosis of the cavernous sinuses, *Arch Intern Med* 161:2671, 2001.

148. Levine SR, Twyman RE, Gilman S: The role of anticoagulation in cavernous sinus thrombosis, *Neurology* 28:517, 1988.

149. Lemierre A: On certain septicemias due to anaerobic organisms, *Lancet* 1:701, 1936.

150. Chirinos JA, Lichtstein DM, Garcia J, et al: The evolution of Lemierre syndrome: report of two cases and review of the literature, *Medicine* 81:458, 2002.

CHAPTER 60

Lower-Extremity Ulceration

Bauer E. Sumpio, Peter Blume

Ulceration of the lower extremity is a common condition that causes significant discomfort and disability.[1] An *ulcer* is defined as a disruption of the skin with erosion of the underlying subcutaneous tissue. This breach may extend further to the contiguous muscle and bone. The pathophysiological mechanisms underlying ulcer formation are multifactorial and include neuropathy, infection, ischemia, and abnormal foot structure and biomechanics. It is not surprising then that management of the diabetic foot is a complex clinical problem requiring an interdisciplinary approach.[2,3] Minor trauma, often footwear related, is a frequent inciting event. A *chronic ulcer* is defined as a full-thickness skin defect with no significant reepithelialization for more than 4 weeks.

Three etiologies of leg ulcerations are responsible for almost 95% of leg ulcers: about 40% to 80% are due to underlying venous disease, 10% to 20% are due to arterial insufficiency, and 15% to 25% are secondary to diabetes mellitus; in 10% to 15% of patients, a combination of two or more causes exists. Prolonged pressure and local infection are common causes of leg ulcers with minimal vascular compromise. Rare causes are responsible for less than 5% of all leg ulcers[4] (Box 60-1). The disease entities that usually underlie leg ulceration (e.g., venous insufficiency, peripheral artery disease (PAD), diabetes mellitus) are associated with significant patient morbidity and mortality. A detailed knowledge of the clinical picture, pathogenesis, relevant diagnostic tests, treatment modalities, and differential diagnosis of leg ulcerations is essential in planning the optimal treatment strategy (Table 60-1). An incorrect or delayed initial diagnosis may harm the patient and increase the risk of serious complications, including permanent disability and amputations.

The exact prevalence of lower-extremity ulcers in the United States is unknown. The prevalence of leg ulceration in the general population of Western nations is 1% to 3.5%, with the prevalence increasing to 5% in the geriatric population.[5–8] Data from these studies most likely underestimate the true prevalence because they do not include patients with leg ulcers who are not known to the healthcare system.

The cost of treating leg ulceration is staggering. Epidemiological studies from Sweden estimated annual costs of treatment of lower-extremity ulcers at $25 million. In England, the estimated cost of care for patients with leg ulcers in a population of 250,000 is about $130,000 annually per patient.[9] Items factored into the equation include physician visits, hospital admissions, home health care, wound care supplies, rehabilitation, time lost from work, and jobs lost. Adding to the cost is the chronic nature of these wounds, high rate of recurrence, and propensity for infection. A true accounting of the cost is difficult because of the unknown prevalence of disease.

Because the disease affects a patient's lifestyle and attitude, the social cost of leg ulcers accrue. The ability to work may be temporarily or permanently affected by the condition,[8] and the reduction in work capacity adds to the medical cost to society. An estimated 10 million workdays are lost from lower-extremity ulcers in the United States annually, and this figure may be low.[10,11] A report in 1994 focused on the financial, social, and psychological implications of lower-extremity lesions in 73 patients.[12] Among the study patients, 68% reported feelings of fear, social isolation, anger, depression, and negative self-image because of the ulcers. In addition, 81% of the patients felt that their mobility was adversely affected. Within the younger population that was still actively working, there was a correlation between lower-extremity ulceration and adverse effect on finances, time lost from work, and job loss. In addition, there was a strong correlation between time spent on ulcer care and feelings of anger and resentment. These factors combined to have a negative emotional impact on their lives.

Biomechanics of Walking and Ulcer Formation

An appreciation of the biomechanics required for walking is essential to understanding the etiology of foot ulcers. The foot is a complicated biological structure containing 26 bones, numerous joints, and a network of ligaments, muscles, and blood vessels. *Gait* is a complex set of events that requires triplanar foot motion and control of multiple axes for complete bipedal ambulation[13] (Fig. 60-1A). When the heel hits the ground, its outer edge touches first; the foot is in a supinated position, which makes it firm and rigid. The soft-tissue structures (muscles, tendons, and ligaments) then relax, allowing the foot to pronate. The foot becomes less rigid and is able to flatten, absorb the shock of touchdown, and adapt to uneven surfaces. During midstance, the heel lies below the ankle joint complex, the front and back of the foot are aligned, and the foot easily bears weight. Toward the end of midstance, the soft-tissue structures begin to tighten; the foot resupinates and regains its arch. The foot is again firm, acting as a rigid lever for propulsion. The heel lifts off the ground, swings slightly to the inside, and the toes push weight off the ground.

Sensory input from the visual, vestibular, and proprioceptive systems is necessary to modify learned motor patterns and muscular output to execute the desired action. Various external and internal forces affect foot function.[14] The combination of body weight pushing down and ground reactive force pushing up creates friction and compressive forces. *Shear* results from the bones of the foot sliding parallel to their plane of contact during pronation and supination. Foot deformities or ill-fitting footwear enhance pressure points because they focus the forces on a smaller area. When the foot flattens too much or overpronates, the ankle and heel do not align during midstance, and some bones are forced to support more weight. The foot strains under the body's weight, causing the muscles to pull harder on these areas, making it more difficult for tendons and ligaments to hold bones and joints in proper alignment. Over time, swelling and pain on the bottom of the foot or near the heel may occur. Bunions can form at the great toe joint, and hammertoe deformities can form at the lesser toes. Abnormal foot biomechanics resulting from limited joint mobility and foot deformities magnify shearing forces, resulting in increased plantar pressure on the foot during ambulation (see Fig. 60-1B-C). This can represent critical causes for tissue breakdown.

Pathophysiology of Ulcer Formation

Venous Disorders

Venous leg ulcers are the most frequently occurring chronic lower-extremity wounds (Fig. 60-2A) (also see Chapter 56). The prevalence of lower-extremity ulceration resulting from chronic venous disease (CVD) in European and Western populations is estimated to be 0.5% to 1%. In the United States, it is estimated that between 600,000 and 2.5 million patients have venous ulcerations; treatment costs are estimated at $2.5 to $3 billion dollars, with a corresponding loss of 2 million workdays per year.[15] Ten years ago, the estimated annual cost of treatment for venous ulcer patients was almost $40,000 per patient.[16] This cost has risen since then. The pathophysiology of venous ulceration is straightforward. Blood returns from the lower extremities against gravity to the inferior vena cava (IVC) through the deep and superficial venous systems. The deep veins are

Box 60-1 Causes of Lower-Extremity Ulcers

Vascular
Common
Venous disease and insufficiency
Peripheral atherosclerotic disease

Rare
Vasculitis
Autoimmune disease (scleroderma)
Hypertension (Martorell ulcer)
Thromboangiitis obliterans (TAO) (Buerger's disease)
Lymphedema
Hematological disorders (sickle cell anemia)
Clotting disorders (antiphospholipid syndrome)

Neurotrophic
Diabetes mellitus
Uremia
Acquired immunodeficiency syndrome (AIDS)
Nutritional deficiencies

Biomechanical
Charcot foot
Rheumatoid arthritis (Felty's syndrome)
Fracture, dislocations

Others
Infectious diseases
Physical or chemical injury (trauma, pressure ulcers, burns, frostbite)
Metabolic diseases (porphyria, calciphylaxis)
Neoplastic (melanoma, basal cell carcinoma, squamous cell carcinoma, sarcomas)
Drug reactions or side effects (steroids, Coumadin)
Ulcerating skin diseases (pyoderma gangrenosum)

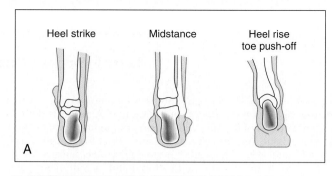

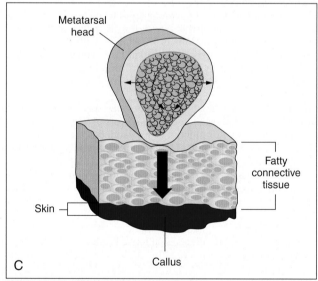

located within the muscles and deep fascia of the legs. The superficial system consists of the great saphenous vein and the small saphenous vein and is located within the subcutaneous fat. Valves are present within all three systems and prevent retrograde flow of blood. A portion of blood from the superficial system is directed to the deep system through the communicating perforators. While standing, about 22% of the total blood volume is localized to the lower extremities, and hydrostatic pressure in the foot veins can reach 80 mmHg. In healthy individuals with competent venous valves, the efficient calf muscle pump can reduce venous pressure by two thirds during exercise. Venous insufficiency occurs when any of these elements do not function adequately. Pressure in the venous system increases, and (most importantly) ambulatory venous pressure rises during leg exercise. The primary cause of venous hypertension is insufficiency of the valves of the deep venous system and perforating veins of the lower leg.

The exact mechanism by which ulcerations develop in patients with venous insufficiency is not clear. One theory is that ulceration is due to increased intraluminal pressure within the capillary system of the leg. The capillaries become dilated and elongated, and blood flow is sluggish, resulting in microthrombi formation

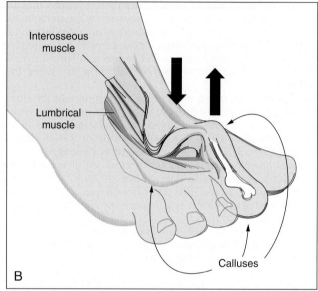

FIGURE 60-1 Biomechanics of ulceration.

TABLE 60-1	Lower-Extremity Ulcers Characterized by Etiology			
	SITE	**SKIN APPEARANCE**	**ULCER CHARACTERISTICS**	**OTHER FINDINGS**
Venous	Lower third of leg; malleolar area	Edema, hemosiderin, dermatitis, eczema	"Weeping," irregular borders, painful	Varicose veins, "bottle leg," ABI normal
Arterial	Most distal areas, toes	Thin, atrophic, dry, "shiny," hair loss	Round, regular borders, no bleeding, dry base, very painful	Weak/absent pulse, poor capillary refill, ABI <0.8
Neurotrophic (diabetes mellitus)	Pressure sites; heel and metatarsal heads	Cellulitis	Round, deep, purulent discharge, painless	Sensory deficit; ABI often >1.3 due to vascular calcification

ABI, ankle-brachial index.

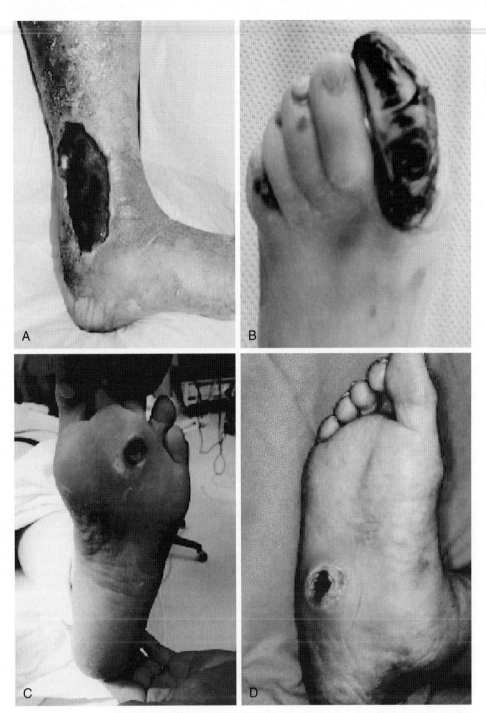

FIGURE 60-2 Various foot ulcers. A, Venous stasis. **B,** Ischemic. **C,** Neurotrophic. **D,** Charcot foot.

and frequently leading to capillary occlusion. Fibrin, albumin, and various macromolecules leak into the dermis, where they bind to and trap growth factors, making them unavailable for the tissue repair process.[17] Leakage of fibrinogen through capillary walls results in deposition of pericapillary fibrin cuffs,[18] which has been suggested as a physical barrier impeding passage of oxygen.[10] Iron deposition, white blood cell (WBC) accumulation, decreased fibrinolytic activity, and a myriad of inflammatory responses to vascular damage are all postulated to be the final pathways leading to venous ulcerations, but it is still not clear whether they represent causative factors.

Tissue hypoxia appears to be the major underlying factor in developing venous ulceration. Unlike ulcers associated with arterial insufficiency, this hypoxic state is not caused by decreased blood flow to the legs. Patients with venous insufficiency usually have

adequate blood flow to their lower extremities. Direct measurements of transcutaneous oxygen levels on the lower leg have demonstrated that exercise produces a marked rise in skin oxygen tension in normal legs, but not in those affected by venous insufficiency. Exercise reduces venous pressure in patients with competent valves, thus removing the stimulus for reflex vasoconstriction. In patients with compromised valves, venous pressure remains high during exercise, and reflex vasoconstriction persists.[19]

On the basis of these findings, it is clear that management of lower-extremity ulcers secondary to venous insufficiency must include measures that improve the abnormal venous blood return from the affected extremity. Leg elevation, compression therapy, local wound care, and surgical correction of selected underlying pathology are all important components of the treatment plan.

Arterial Disease

The incidence of lower-extremity ulcers caused by PAD (see Fig. 60-2B) is increasing in Western nations.[8] The general aging of the population and better diagnostic techniques may provide possible explanations for this observation. Risk factors for development of atherosclerotic lesions causing leg ischemia include diabetes mellitus, smoking, hyperlipidemia, hypertension, obesity, and age.[20] Lack of perfusion decreases tissue resilience, leads to rapid death of tissue, and impedes wound healing (see Chapter 17). Wound healing and tissue regeneration depend on adequate blood supply to the region. Ischemia due to vascular disease impedes healing by reducing the supply of oxygen, nutrients, and soluble mediators involved in the repair process.[21]

The Diabetic Foot

Persons with diabetes mellitus are particularly prone to foot ulcers. The *diabetic foot* is a common and serious clinical condition that has its specific characteristics. The American Diabetes Association Consensus Group found that among persons with diabetes, the risk of foot ulceration was increased among men, patients who had had diabetes for more than 10 years, and patients with poor glucose control or cardiovascular, retinal, or renal complications.[22] It is estimated that 15% of U.S. patients with diabetes will develop manifestations of diabetic foot disease in their lifetime.[23,24] In this population, the prevalence of lower-extremity ulcers ranges from 4% to 10%, with an annual incidence of 2% to 3%.[25] Although representing only 6% of the population, patients with diabetes account for 46%[25] of the 162,000 hospital admissions for foot ulcers annually. Foot ulcers occur in up to 25% of patients with diabetes and precede more than 8 in 10 nontraumatic amputations. In 2005, approximately 1.6 million people were living with limb loss; this number is expected to more than double by 2050.[26] Diabetic foot ulcers and their sequelae, amputations, are the major cause of disability, morbidity, mortality, and costs for these patients.[23] Ulceration and infection of lower extremities are a leading cause of hospitalization in patients with diabetes.[25] Treatment of pedal soft-tissue deficits in the diabetic patient population continues to be a medical and surgical challenge, thereby extending the length of their disability and significantly increasing the cost of medical care. Nearly half of all patients who undergo amputation will develop limb-threatening ischemia in the contralateral limb, and many will ultimately require an amputation of the opposite limb within 5 years. In 2000, the Centers for Disease Control and Prevention (CDC) estimated that 12 million Americans were diagnosed with diabetes, and the estimated annual direct and indirect costs of diabetes treatment in the United States was approximately $174 billion, with 1 in 5 diabetes dollars spent on lower-extremity care. Preventing ulcerations and/or amputations is critical from both medical and economical standpoints.[2]

Development of diabetic foot disease can be attributed to several primary risk factors, including neuropathy, ischemia, infection, and immune impairment. Four foot-related risk factors have been identified in the genesis of pedal ulceration: altered biomechanics, limited joint mobility, bony deformity, and severe nail pathology.[22]

NEUROPATHY

Neuropathy is the most common underlying etiology of foot ulceration and frequently involves the somatic and autonomic fibers. Although there are many causes of peripheral neuropathy, diabetes mellitus is by far the most common (see Box 60-1). Neuropathy is present in 42% of diabetic patients after 20 years[27] and is usually a distal symmetrical sensorimotor polyneuropathy. Peripheral neuropathy is postulated to result from abnormalities in metabolism, one of which is a deficiency in sorbitol metabolism via the polyol pathway.[28,29]

Neurotrophic ulcers typically form on the plantar aspect of the foot at areas of excessive focal pressures. These are most commonly encountered over the bony prominences of the metatarsal heads and forefoot region because of the requirements of midstance and heel-off during the gait cycle (see Fig. 60-2C). Loss of protective sensation in the foot can lead rapidly to ulceration if patient education and preventive measures are not taken. Diabetic patients are especially prone to development of a neuro-osteoarthropathy known as *Charcot foot*.[30] This condition is thought to involve autonomic nerve dysfunction that results in abnormal perfusion to foot bones, which leads to bony fragmentation and collapse (see Fig. 60-2D). The resulting "rocker-bottom foot" is prone to tissue breakdown and ulceration.[23,30]

Several investigators[23,30,31] have demonstrated that there is an increase in both static and dynamic foot pressures.[32] To date, high pressures alone have not been shown to cause foot ulceration. Rheumatoid patients with high plantar foot pressures but no sensitivity deficit have almost no evidence of foot ulceration.[33]

Type A sensory fibers are responsible for light touch sensation, vibratory sensation, pressure, proprioception, and motor innervation to the intrinsic muscles of the foot. Type C sensory fibers detect painful stimuli, noxious stimuli, and temperature. When these fibers are affected, protective sensation is lost. This manifests as a distal symmetrical loss of sensation described in a "stocking" distribution and proves to be the primary factor predisposing patients to ulcers and infection.[34] Patients are unable to detect increased loads, repeated trauma, or pain from shearing forces. Injuries such as fractures, ulceration, and foot deformities therefore go unrecognized. Repeat stress to high-pressure areas or bone prominences, which would be interpreted as pain in the non-neuropathic patient, also go unrecognized. Sensory dysfunction results in increased shearing forces and repeated trauma to the foot.[35,36] Patients have inadequate protective sensation during all phases of gait, so high loads are undetected owing to loss of pain threshold, which results in prolonged and increased forces.[31,35] These problems manifest as abnormal pressure points, increased shearing, and greater friction to the foot. Because this goes unrecognized in the insensate foot, gait patterns remain unchanged, and the stresses eventually cause tissue breakdown and ulceration.

Motor neuropathy is associated with demyelinization and motor end-plate damage, which contribute to conduction defects. The distal motor nerves are the most commonly affected, resulting in atrophy of the small intrinsic muscles of the foot. Wasting of the lumbrical and interosseous muscles of the foot results in collapse of the arch and loss of stability of the metatarsal-phalangeal joints during midstance of the gait. Overpowering by extrinsic muscles can lead to depression of the metatarsal heads, digital contractures, and cocked-up toes; equinus deformities of the ankle; or a varus hindfoot.[37]

Autonomic involvement causes an interruption of normal sweating at the epidermal level and arteriovenous shunting at subcutaneous and dermal levels. Hypohidrosis leads to a noncompliant epidermis that increases the risk of cracking and fissuring. Arteriovenous shunting diminishes delivery of nutrients and oxygen to tissue regions, and skin and subcutaneous tissues become more susceptible to breakdown.[38]

MUSCULOSKELETAL DEFORMITIES

Atrophy of the small muscles within the foot results in nonfunctioning intrinsic foot muscles referred to as an *intrinsic minus foot*[39] (see Fig. 60-1B). Muscles showing early involvement are the flexor digitorum brevis, lumbricales, and interosseous muscles. These muscle groups act to stabilize the proximal phalanx against the metatarsal head, preventing dorsiflexion at the metatarsal phalangeal joint (MTPJ) during midstance in the gait cycle. With progression of the neuropathy, these muscles atrophy and fail to function properly. This causes the MTPJs to become unstable, allowing the long flexors (flexor digitorum longus and flexor hallucis longus) and extensors (extensor digitorum longus and extensor hallucis longus) to act unchecked on the digits. Dorsal contractures develop at the MTPJs, with development of hammer digit syndrome, also known as *intrinsic minus disease*.

The deformity acts to plantarflex the metatarsals, making the heads more prominent and increasing the plantar pressure created beneath them (see Fig. 60-1B). It also acts to decrease the amount of toe weight-bearing during the gait cycle, which also increases pressure on the metatarsal heads. In normal foot anatomy, a metatarsal fat pad located plantar to the MTPJs helps dissipate pressures on the metatarsal heads from the ground. When *hammer digit deformity* occurs, this fat pad migrates distally and becomes nonfunctional, resulting in elevated plantar pressures that increase the risk of skin breakdown and ulceration due to shearing forces.[1]

Overpowering by the extrinsic foot muscles also leads to an equinus deformity at the ankle and a varus hindfoot. A *cavovarus foot type* can develop, leading to decreased range of motion of the pedal joints, inability to adapt to terrain, and low tolerance to shock. In essence, a mobile adapter is converted to a rigid lever. Pressure is equal to body weight divided by surface area, thus decreasing surface area below a metatarsal head with concomitant rigid deformities and leading to increased forces or pressure to the sole of the foot. When neuropathic foot disease is associated with congenital foot deformities such as long or short metatarsals, a plantarflexed metatarsal, abnormalities in the metatarsal parabola, or a Charcot foot[30] (see Fig. 60-2D), there is a higher propensity toward breakdown as a result of increased and abnormal plantar foot pressures.

Increased body weight and decreased surface area of contact of the foot components with the ground increase pressure. A low pressure but constant insult over an extended period can have the same ulcerogenic effect as high pressure over a shorter period. This is typical of the effect of tight-fitting shoes. If the magnitude of these forces in a given area is large enough, either skin loss or hypertrophy of the stratum corneum (callus) occurs (see Fig. 60-1C). Presence of callus in patients with neuropathy should raise a red flag because the risk of ulceration in a callused area is increased by two orders of magnitude.

ARTERIAL DISEASE

One of the major factors affecting diabetic foot disease is development of lower-extremity arterial disease.[26] Peripheral artery disease is estimated to be two to four times more common in persons with diabetes than in others[23,40] (see Chapter 14). Atherosclerosis occurs at a younger age in persons with diabetes than in others, and its hallmark is involvement of the tibioperoneal vessels, with sparing of the pedal vessels. In addition to being more prevalent in diabetes, atherosclerosis is more accelerated and results in a higher rate of amputations.[41–43] Lesions in persons with diabetes tend to localize to the infracrural region. Relative sparing of the pedal vessels often assists pedal bypass. Occlusive lesions affecting the foot and precluding revascularization are not common in diabetic patients.[23]

Purely ischemic diabetic foot ulcers are uncommon, representing only 10% to 15% of ulcers in patients with diabetes. More commonly, ulcers have a mixed ischemic and neuropathic origin, representing 33% of diabetic foot ulcers.[23] Initiation of an ischemic

ulcer usually requires a precipitating factor such as mechanical stress. Ulcers often develop on the dorsum of the foot over the first and fifth metatarsal heads. A heel ulcer can develop from constant pressure applied while the heel is in a dependent position or during prolonged immobilization and bed rest. Once formed, the blood supply necessary to allow healing of an ulcer is greater than that needed to maintain intact skin. This leads to chronic ulcer development unless the blood supply is improved.

INFECTION

Patients with diabetes appear to be more prone to various infections than their nondiabetic counterparts.[44] Several factors increase the risk of developing diabetic foot infections, including diabetic neuropathy, peripheral artery disease, and immunological impairment. Several defects in immunological response relate to increased infection risk in diabetics. Diabetic patients demonstrate a decrease in function of polymorphonuclear leukocytes that can manifest as a decrease in migration, phagocytosis, and decreased intracellular activity. Evidence suggests impaired cellular immune response as well as abnormalities in complement function.[45,46] Some of the defects appear to improve with control of hyperglycemia.[47]

Undiagnosed clean neuropathic foot ulcers often convert to acute infections with abscess and/or cellulitis.[48] Diabetic foot infections can be classified into those that are nonthreatening and those that are life or limb threatening. Non–limb-threatening diabetic foot infections are often mild infections associated with a superficial ulcer. They often have less than 2 cm of surrounding cellulitis and demonstrate no signs of systemic toxicity. These infections have on average 2.1 organisms[48] (Table 60-2). Aerobic gram-positive cocci are the sole pathogens in 42% of these cases, with the most notable organisms being *Staphylococcus aureus*, coagulase-negative *S. aureus*, and streptococci. These less severe infections can often be managed with local wound care, rest, elevation, and oral antibiotics on an outpatient basis. A foot infection in a diabetic patient can present with a more severe, life- or limb-threatening picture. In these patients, there is usually a deeper ulceration or an undrained abscess, gangrene, or necrotizing fasciitis. Methicillin-resistant *S. aureus* (MRSA) is an increasingly common isolate.[44] They tend to have greater than 2 cm of surrounding cellulitis, as well as lymphangitis and edema of the affected limb. These more severe cases generally present with fever, leukocytosis, and hyperglycemia.

In contrast to nondiabetic individuals, complex foot infections in diabetic patients usually involve multiple organisms with complex biofilm environments.[49] Studies report an average of five to eight different species per specimen.[50–53] These include a combination of gram-positive and gram-negative aerobic and anaerobic organisms. The most prevalent organisms identified were *S. aureus*, coagulase-negative *Staphylococcus*, group B *Streptococcus*, *Proteus*, *Escherichia coli*, *Pseudomonas*, and *Bacteroides*. Recently, MRSA infection has become more common in diabetic foot ulcers and is associated with previous antibiotic treatment and prolonged

TABLE 60-2 Percent Frequency of Bacterial Isolates from Diabetic Foot Infection

ORGANISM	LOUIE (20)	SAPICO (32)	GIBBONS (100)	WHEAT (54)	CALHOUN (850)	SCHER (65)	GRAYSON (96)	LEICHTER (55)
Staphylococcus aureus	35	25	54	37	45.9	35.4	56	27.3
Coagulase-negative staphylococci	30	9.3	32	32	22.6	27.7	12.5	40
Enterococcus	45	40.6	32	27	28.7	N/A	29	29
Proteus mirabilis	55	28.1	22	17	26.1	55.8	7.3	12.4
Pseudomonas aeruginosa	20	15.6	14	7	15.9	23.1	7.3	9.1
Bacteroides spp.	85	67	67	33	15.6	84.6	31	9.1

Modified from Caballero E, Frykberg R: Diabetic foot infections. J Foot Ankle Surg 37:248, 1998.

time to healing.[44,54,55] Anaerobic infections with *Clostridium* are also common. These patients require immediate hospitalization, broad-spectrum intravenous (IV) antibiotics, and aggressive surgical débridement. Superficial wound cultures are often unreliable because they may demonstrate organisms responsible for colonization that do not affect the associated infection. Deep wound or bone cultures are the best way to accurately assess the microbiology in a diabetic foot infection and assess for osteomyelitis.

Assessment of the Patient with a Lower-Extremity Ulcer

Accurate diagnosis of the underlying cause of lower-extremity ulceration is essential for successful treatment. The etiology of most leg ulcers can be ascertained quite accurately by careful problem-focused history taking and physical examination.[32] Diagnostic and laboratory studies are occasionally necessary to establish the diagnosis, but are more often performed to guide treatment strategy.[56]

History

Patients with ulcers due to venous insufficiency usually complain of aching and swelling of the legs (see Chapter 55). They may recount a history of recurrent cellulitis, previous deep vein thrombosis (DVT), or previous superficial venous surgery. Symptoms are often worse at the end of the day, exacerbated when the leg is dependent, and relieved by leg elevation.

Arterial insufficiency is suggested by a history of underlying cardiac or cerebrovascular disease, complaints of leg claudication or impotence, or pain in the distal foot when supine (rest pain; see Chapter 18). Symptoms of arterial insufficiency are due to inadequate perfusion to the lower extremity relative to its metabolism. Tissue hypoxia and the subsequent increase in concentration of lactic acid produce pain. Patients may complain of pain in the buttocks or calves brought on with activity and relieved with rest (*intermittent claudication*), or pain in the forefoot aggravated by elevation and relieved by dependency (*rest pain*). Presence of an extremity ulcer is an easily recognized but late sign of peripheral vascular insufficiency. Patients with lower-extremity ulcers resulting from atherosclerotic disease usually have a risk factor profile that includes older age, male sex, smoking, diabetes mellitus, hypertension, hypercholesterolemia, and obesity.[20,23] Patients with leg ulcers and multiple atherosclerotic risk factors often have atherosclerosis in other arterial beds.[57]

Up to one third of patients with diabetes mellitus can have significant atherosclerotic disease without specific symptoms. The common complaints are those of neuropathic disease, which include history of numbness, paresthesias, and burning pain in the lower extremities. Patients often report previous episodes of foot ulcers and chronic skin infections.

Physical Examination

A complete examination can only be performed with the patient supine in an examination gown. The patient's vital signs are recorded and abnormalities noted; temperature, respiratory rate, heart rate, and blood pressure in both upper extremities should be obtained. Fever may indicate the presence of an infected ulcer, and tachycardia and tachypnea may support the diagnosis of a septic foot.

A classic look, listen, and feel examination includes inspection of the skin of the extremities, palpation of all peripheral pulses, measurement of ankle-brachial indices (ABIs), assessment of extremity temperature, auscultation for bruits, and a thorough neurological examination.[32]

Visual inspection coupled with an accurate history can determine the presence of a chronic vascular condition (Fig. 60-3A). Color of the skin is conferred by the blood in the subpapillary layer and varies with position of the extremity, temperature of the skin, and degree of blood oxygenation (reduced hemoglobin (Hb) → blue).

Also in chronic arterial insufficiency, the arterioles are maximally dilated as a compensatory response to the chronic ischemia, intensifying color changes. In acute arterial occlusion, the venules empty, leading to a chalky white appearance regardless of extremity position. Partial but inadequate perfusion from either an incomplete acute or chronic occlusion allows for pooling of blood in the venules, which may be red in the cold or blue at higher temperatures.

When the extremity is at the level of the heart, the pooled blood masks the color imparted by arterial flow. Elevation of the extremity above the level of the central venous pressure (rarely >25 cm) allows the pooled venous blood to drain, enabling an accurate assessment of the degree of arterial flow. A normal extremity remains pink, whereas one with arterial insufficiency becomes pallid. Conversely, allowing the extremity to become dependent causes an intense rubor or cyanosis. Time of return of blood to the dependent extremity is a useful marker of the severity of the deficit (normally <20 seconds). With diminished nutritional supply to the skin, there is thinning and functional loss of dermal appendages, evident as dry, shiny, and hairless skin. Nails may become brittle and ridged. Comparison of color and trophic changes between extremities gives a good indication of the severity of the process unless a bilateral deficit is present, in which case the experience of the examiner is required to make an accurate diagnosis.

Skin temperature is a reliable indicator of blood flow rate in the dermal vessels, although flow is governed primarily by constriction or dilation of the arterioles to maintain a constant core temperature. Nevertheless, the temperature of the skin as a marker of perfusion is useful and can be assessed by lightly palpating the skin with the back of the hand and comparing similar sites from one extremity to the other. An ischemic limb is cool, and demarcation of temperature gives a rough indication of the level of the occlusion. Again, assessment of temperature differences is confounded when both extremities are affected.

In limbs of patients with venous insufficiency, there is evidence of chronic edema. Venous hypertension causes transudation of serous fluid and red blood cells (RBCs) into the subcutaneous tissue. Hemoglobin from the RBCs breaks down to produce the pigment hemosiderin, leading to hyperpigmentation, especially in the medial paramalleolar areas. Patients with venous insufficiency commonly develop stasis dermatitis. This eczematous process may spread from the area of the medial malleolus and involve the leg circumferentially. Recurrent cellulitis can cause contraction of subcutaneous tissue in the lower third of the leg below the knee, and together with the chronic edema can produce a "bottle leg" appearance.

ULCER EVALUATION

A thorough evaluation of ulcers of the lower extremity is critical in ascertaining etiology and instituting an appropriate treatment strategy. Specific characteristics of the ulcer, such as location, size, depth, and appearance, should be recorded during the initial evaluation and with each subsequent follow-up visit to record progress and evaluate the treatment regimen.[58] Ulcers of the foot should be gently examined with a cotton-tipped probe to establish the presence of a sinus tract. The margins of the ulcer should be undermined to evaluate the extent of tissue destruction. Ulcer extension to tendon, bone, or joint should be sought. A positive probe-to-bone finding (see Fig. 60-3B) has a high predictive value for osteomyelitis and is an extremely sensitive and cost-effective screen.[59]

Extremity ulcerations have a characteristic appearance depending on their origin. Ulcerations due to ischemia are typically located on the tips of the toes (see Fig. 60-2B) and between the digits. These lesions often appear punched out and are painful but exhibit little bleeding. Ischemic ulcers are characterized by absence of bleeding, pain, precipitating trauma, or underlying foot deformity. They also often develop on the dorsum of the foot and over the first and fifth metatarsal heads. Ischemic ulcers are uncommon on the plantar surface because pressure is usually less sustained and perfusion better. A heel ulcer can develop

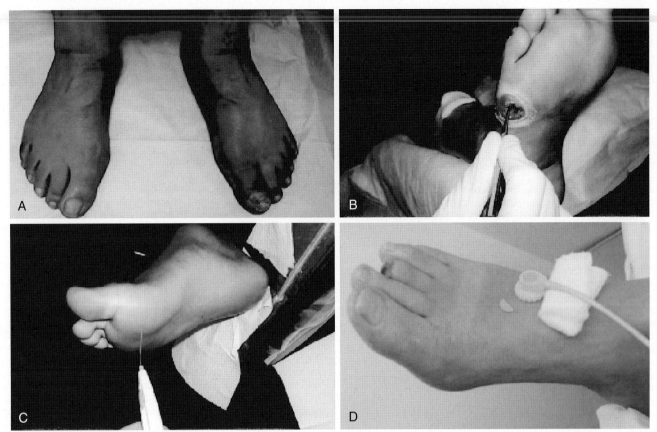

FIGURE 60-3 **Examination of the foot. A,** Visual. **B,** Probing the wound. **C,** Using Semmes-Weinstein monofilament. **D,** Transcutaneous oximetry.

from constant pressure applied while the heel is in a dependent position or during prolonged immobilization and bed rest. It should not be a surprise that a patient with relatively mild symptoms of arterial insufficiency develops limb-threatening extremity ulcers. This is because once an ulcer is present, the blood supply necessary to heal the wound is greater than that needed to maintain intact skin. A chronic ulcer will develop unless blood supply is improved.

Elevated venous pressure due to perforator or deep vein incompetency or venous thrombosis reduces the pressure gradient for perfusion. Inadequate tissue perfusion results because elevated venous pressure and venous stasis hinder clearance of breakdown products. However, venous ulcers rarely present in the foot; they are more commonly located in the "gaiter" distribution of the leg around the medial malleolus, where venous pressures are highest. These are associated with a swollen leg with a distinctive skin appearance (see Fig. 60-2A). Venous ulcerations occur most commonly on the medial aspect of the ankle and are surrounded by areas with induration and brown pigmentation of the surrounding area (brawny induration) and scaling skin. These ulcers are often exquisitely tender and weep copious serous fluid.

The appearance of the extremity in venous insufficiency is distinctive and rarely poses a problem distinguishing between it and arterial insufficiency. It is important to differentiate the rubor associated with vascular insufficiency and cellulitis accompanying an infective process. Cellulitic color changes will persist despite extremity elevation. With isolated venous insufficiency, the extremity is warm and variably swollen, with the characteristic skin changes described earlier. Acute or chronic arterial vascular insufficiency may be superimposed on the changes of chronic venous insufficiency (CVI), impairing healing of the venous ulcer. In these situations, lower-extremity revascularization may be required to assist in healing a venous ulceration that is not responding

appropriately to compression therapy. Furthermore, the presence of significant lower-extremity swelling or skin changes can complicate arterial reconstructions by altering the surgical approach to distal arterial target sites.

Neuropathic ulcerations typically occur at the heel or over the metatarsal heads on the plantar surface at pressure points (mal perforans ulcer; see Fig. 60-2C) but may also occur in less characteristic locations secondary to trauma. They usually are painless. Sensory neuropathy in the diabetic patient may allow the destructive process to go unchecked, with extension into the deep plantar space and minimal appreciation by the patient.

In addition to ulcers, patients may present with varying degrees of tissue loss or frankly gangrenous digits, forefoot, or hindfoot. Presence of dry gangrene is a relatively stable process allowing for a complete vascular evaluation; however, any progression to an infected wet gangrene requires immediate surgical débridement.

VASCULAR EXAMINATION

A careful physical examination should be performed in patients with leg ulcers to elucidate their underlying cause (see Chapter 11). Handheld Doppler ultrasound should be used in case of inability to easily palpate a given vessel. These can be supplemented with noninvasive vascular tests (see Chapter 12) and other diagnostic tests as necessary for each clinical situation. An ABI is an important tool for assessing perfusion to the foot. Patients with an ABI less than 0.6 often experience claudication, and those with an ABI less than 0.3 may complain of rest pain; in patients with tissue loss, the ABI is often less than 0.5.[60] In patients with diabetes and renal failure due to calcification of the vessel, ABI may be falsely elevated and is unreliable for evaluating level of ischemia.

If the physical examination suggests venous insufficiency, a Trendelenburg test should be performed to assess valve function of the deep venous system and perforators. The patient is placed in a supine position and the legs elevated. After decompression of the superficial veins occurs, a tourniquet is placed around the patient's thigh and he or she is asked to stand. If the varicose veins do not fill within 60 seconds below the tourniquet, the valves in the deep system and perforators are not compromised, and proximal saphenous vein incompetence is likely.

NEUROLOGICAL EXAMINATION

The lower-extremity neurological examination is essential and should include testing for motor strength, deep-tendon reflexes, and vibratory, proprioceptive, and protective sensation.[61] Chronic ischemia can cause varying patterns of sensory loss that is usually within the affected arterial distribution. Neuropathy occurs in 42% of patients with diabetes within 20 years after diagnosis of the disease[27] and alters motor, sensory, and autonomic function, which directly affect the dynamic function of the foot during gait. The gait of the patient should be observed to detect any gross asymmetry or unsteadiness.

Motor neuropathy is associated with demyelinization and motor end-plate damage, which contribute to conduction defects. Atrophy of the small intrinsic muscles of the foot occurs secondary to distal motor nerve damage. Wasting of the lumbrical and interosseous muscles of the foot results in collapse of the arch and loss of stability of metatarsal-phalangeal joints during midstance of the gait.[1] Overpowering by extrinsic muscles can lead to depression of the metatarsal heads, digital contractures, and cocked-up toes. These changes result in abnormal pressure points, increased shearing, and ulcer formation.

Diabetic sensory neuropathy is typically a stocking-glove distribution and is associated with a decrement in vibration and two-point discrimination. Loss of protective sensation due to peripheral neuropathy is the most common cause of ulceration in the diabetic population. The use of monofilament gauges (Semmes-Weinstein) is a good objective way of assessing diabetic neuropathy[61] (see Fig. 60-3C). Patients with normal foot sensation usually can feel a 4.17 monofilament (equivalent to 1 g of linear pressure). Patients who cannot detect a 5.07 monofilament when it buckles (equivalent to 10 g of linear pressure) are considered to have lost protective sensation.[62,63] Several cross-sectional studies have indicated that foot ulceration is strongly associated with elevated cutaneous pressure perception thresholds.[61] Magnitudes of association, however, were provided in a case-control study[64] where an unadjusted sevenfold risk of ulceration was observed in those patients (97% male) with insensitivity to the 5.07 monofilament. Screening is vital in identifying diabetic neuropathy early, thus enabling earlier intervention and management to reduce the risk of ulceration and lower-extremity amputation. Although a nerve conduction velocity test (also called *nerve conduction study* [NCS]) is the gold standard, its expense and limited availability prevent its widespread application as a screening tool for diabetic neuropathy. Semmes-Weinstein monofilament is a convenient, inexpensive, painless alternative to NCS that should be used in the initial evaluation of all patients with diabetes mellitus as a screen for peripheral neuropathy. A positive Semmes-Weinstein monofilament result is a significant predictor of future ulceration and likely lower-extremity amputation as well in patients with diabetes mellitus.[65] If diabetic patients have positive monofilament results, their chances of ulceration increase by 10% to 20%, corresponding to a 2.5 to 5 times higher risk than patients with normal sensation as determined by monofilament. Additionally, the risks of leg amputation increase 5% to 15%, which corresponds with a 1.5 to 15 times higher risk for patients with diabetes mellitus with positive monofilament results compared to those with negative monofilament results. The Semmes-Weinstein monofilament is an important evidence-based tool for determining which patients are at increased risk of complications during follow-up, leading to improved patient selection for early intervention and management. Ultimately, screening

with Semmes-Weinstein monofilament may lead to improved clinical outcomes for patients with diabetes.[65]

The presence of neuropathy mandates attention to the biomechanics of the foot. The role of the podiatrist or foot surgeon in evaluating these patients cannot be underscored enough.[2] Use of a computerized gait analysis system to assess abnormally high-pressure areas has led to greater use of orthotic devices to prevent skin breakdown. For example, an F-scan system uses an ultra-thin Tekscan sensor (Tekscan Inc., South Boston, Mass.) consisting of 960 sensor cells (5 mm^2 each). The sensor is used in a floor mat system designed to measure barefoot or stocking-foot dynamic plantar pressures, indicating those individuals with pressures of 6 kg/cm^2 or greater. Abnormal mechanical forces that can result in ulcerations should be addressed with the use of offloading devices or other modalities to assist wound healing.

Particular attention should be paid to documenting a complete neurological examination on patients who have suffered from a previous stroke; much of the rationale for extremity salvage hinges on potential for rehabilitation. The remainder of the physical examination should be undertaken with attention to the presence of comorbidities that may influence the decision-making process.

Tests and Imaging Techniques

Use of nondiagnostic imaging techniques by duplex ultrasound has been covered in depth in Chapter 12. Other noninvasive imaging methods useful in the assessment of patients with leg ulcers include plain radiography, magnetic resonance imaging (MRI), and magnetic resonance angiography (MRA; see Chapter 13).[66] Imaging techniques can be used to diagnose osteomyelitis and confirm the presence of bony deformities. Plain film radiography is used primarily to exclude bony lesions as a cause of a patient's pain complaints, assess the presence of osteomyelitis beneath a ulcerated foot lesion, and assess the degree of vascular wall calcification (usually in concert with standard IV contrast angiography). Plain films of the foot are relatively inexpensive and can show soft-tissue swelling, disruption of bone cortex, and periosteal elevation. Magnetic resonance imaging can provide details of pathological anatomical features and has high sensitivity for assessment of deep space infection and presence of osteomyelitis in the diabetic foot.

Assessment of a patient with foot ulcers stemming from PAD encompasses a thorough history and physical examination with adjunctive use of the noninvasive vascular laboratory to confirm, localize, and grade lesions.[60] Although multiple noninvasive and invasive methods are available to assess the peripheral vasculature, it should be obvious that not every patient requires an exhaustive battery of tests to evaluate his or her vascular status. In general, only those tests likely to provide information that alters the course of action should be performed. Differing clinical syndromes mandate the extent of peripheral vascular testing. It is imperative that flow-limiting arterial lesions be evaluated and reconstructed or bypassed if ischemic foot ulcers are to heal.

Management of Ulcers

General

Aggressive mechanical débridement, systemic antibiotic therapy, and strict non–weight-bearing are the cornerstones for effective wound care.[67] Sharp débridement in the operating room or at the bedside, when applicable, allows for thorough removal of all necrotic material and optimizes the wound environment.[68] All necrotic bone plus a small portion of the uninvolved bone, soft tissue, and devascularized structures should be excised, and the degree of penetration of the infection should be established.[68] Curettage of any exposed or remaining cartilage is important to prevent this avascular structure from becoming a nidus of infection. Foot soaks, whirlpool therapy, or enzymatic débridement provide modest benefit but are rarely effective and may lead to further skin maceration or wound breakdown. No prospective randomized studies have demonstrated the superiority of dressing products compared with standard saline wet-to-dry sterile gauze in establishing a granulation bed. Use of moist dressings in clean granulating wounds is recommended to enhance the wound environment.[21,69] An ideal dressing not only provides protection against further bacterial contamination but also maintains moisture balance, optimizes wound pH, absorbs fibrinous fluids, and reduces local pain. Various dressings are currently available to target specific characteristics of the wound[70]; however, moist normal saline dressings are probably sufficient for most wounds. These inexpensive dressings are highly absorptive of exudative drainage and maintain the moist environment.

In the presence of infection and cellulitis, oral antimicrobial therapy should be instituted on the basis of the suspected pathogen and clinical findings. Severe infections should be treated with broad-spectrum IV antibiotics,[71] with particular emphasis on the role of biofilms.[49] After bacterial contamination has been controlled, small ulcers can usually be excised and closed immediately. Large open wounds, however, are treated with a staged approach with frequent débridement and establishment of a granulation base. The clean wounds can then be closed with healthy tissue, with the use of local or free-flap coverage and soft-tissue repair. Meticulous surgical reconstruction of these wounds can help avert the production of inelastic scar tissue over weight-bearing surfaces. Any remaining extrinsic or intrinsic pressures can be reduced with the postoperative use of orthoses.

Surgical correction of biomechanical defects, plastic and soft-tissue reconstruction, and appropriate measures to minimize foot pressure are all essential to enable the patient to walk effectively again. In cases of gross wound infections and rampant cellulitis, use of a silver-containing medication such as Silvadene may be necessary in the initial setting to reduce bacterial load. Oral antimicrobial therapy should be instituted on the basis of the suspected pathogen and clinical findings. Intravenous antimicrobials should be administered for severe infections. Use of bioactive drugs (e.g., recombinant platelet-derived growth factor [PDGF], Regranex) or skin substitutes (e.g., Apligraf, Dermagraft) show promising results and have proven useful under specific circumstances. Likewise, the use of negative pressure wound therapy has been a big advance in the care of advanced wounds.[72–74] A clinical practice algorithm for foot ulcers[75] is seen in Figure 60-4.

Off-loading strategies such as total contact casting or removable walkers has resulted in significant decreases in healing times.[76,77] Stresses placed on the foot can be intrinsic, as was previously described with respect to digital contractures, or extrinsic in nature. These external forces can result from inappropriate footwear, traumatic injury, or foreign bodies. Shoes that are too tight or too shallow are a frequent yet preventable component to development of neuropathic ulcers. Various shoe modifications such as the rocker-sole design and different types of insoles have made it possible to reduce plantar foot pressures, thus decreasing the risks of ulceration.[78–80]

Venous Ulcers

Elevation of the leg is a simple maneuver that can effectively (but temporarily) eliminate venous hypertension. All patients should be encouraged to elevate the affected leg above the level of the heart for 2 to 3 hours during the day and when lying in bed at night. Compression therapy is also effective in controlling edema and accelerates healing of ulcerations. However, before compression is applied to the limb, significant occlusive arterial disease should be excluded. Compression therapy is generally contraindicated in patients with an ABI less than 0.7 or with other signs and symptoms of compromised blood supply to the leg. Many different types of compression devices are available, including elastic and nonelastic bandages, graduated compression stockings (GCS), and compression pumps. The most effective way of delivering compression must be decided on an individual basis.

Compression should be applied just before arising from bed and removed at bedtime.

Treatment of stasis dermatitis minimizes further trauma to the skin from scratching. Pruritus can be controlled by topically applied corticosteroids, orally administered antihistamines, or both. The goal of local wound care in patients with venous ulcers is to minimize stasis, decrease bacterial contamination of the ulcer, and provide a healthy moist wound environment that promotes healing. Heavily contaminated venous ulcers with surrounding cellulitis may require systemic antibiotic therapy in addition to local wound control. The predominant organisms cultured from chronic ulcers are gram-positive pathogens like *S. aureus* and *Streptococcus pyogenes*. The most common gram-negative bacteria are *Pseudomonas aeruginosa*, especially in the diabetic population. Various moisture retentive dressings can be used in conjunction with compression therapy to relieve pain, débride necrotic tissue, and promote granulation tissue formation.

The goal of surgical treatment in venous insufficiency is to correct underlying pathology. Surgical intervention can result in healing up to 90% of ulcers and modest long-term results if diagnostic studies can adequately characterize and localize the incompetent superficial or perforating system valves.[81] Ulcer recurrence is significantly less after superficial venous surgery and use of compression stockings when compared with compression therapy alone.[82,83] If reflux exists in the deep venous system, ligation and stripping of the superficial veins has a poor result and high ulcer recurrence rate. For patients who are young and understand the importance of long-term compression therapy and adjunctive antiplatelet or anticoagulant therapy, reconstruction of vein valves can be recommended.[84,85]

Ischemic Ulcers

Management of ischemic ulcers follows some basic guiding principles. It is imperative that flow-limiting arterial lesions be evaluated and reconstructed or bypassed.[86] In general, the optimal strategy is to perform revascularization, if indicated, as soon as possible. Closure of the ulcer by primary healing or secondary reconstructive surgery will then be expedited. If revascularization of an ischemic ulcer is not possible for medical or technical reasons, amputation of the foot or limb will most likely result. Contraindications to revascularization include nonambulatory patients and a foot phlegmon with sepsis or excessive foot gangrene, precluding a functional foot despite adjunctive plastic surgical procedures such as skin grafts and free flaps.

Nonoperative management of patients with lower-extremity ischemia consists of general wound care measures. As a rule, however, severe ischemia of the lower limb generally requires an interventional approach. The method of revascularization of the affected limb depends on several factors, among the most important being the indications for surgery, the patient's operative risk, arteriographic findings, and available graft material. Chapter 21 reviews these important issues.

Diabetic Ulcers

The role of a multidisciplinary group of consultants in the management of diabetic ulcers cannot be overemphasized.[87] Successful management of foot ulcers involves recognition and correction of the underlying etiology, as well as appropriate wound care and prevention of recurrence. Assessment of the ulcer consists of determining the size and depth of the wound and inspection of the surrounding area for local signs of infection or gangrene. Several classification systems have been devised for descriptive purposes and act as prognostic indicators.[88]

The absence of systemic manifestations such as fever, chills, or leukocytosis is an unreliable indicator of underlying infection, especially in the diabetic immunocompromised population. The use of plain films to rule out osteomyelitis or deep culture of the wound is frequently necessary.

CH
60

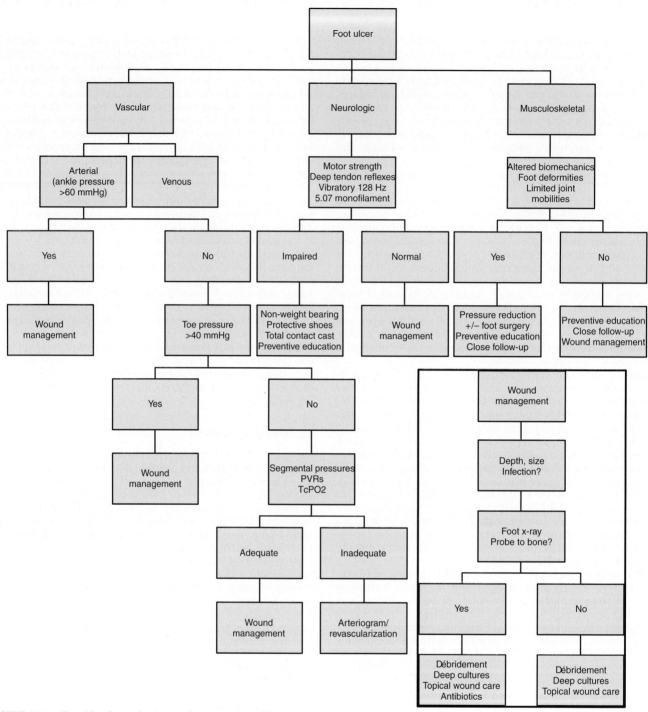

FIGURE 60-4 Algorithm for evaluation and management of foot ulcers.

Neuropathic and Musculoskeletal Management

To avoid major amputations in these chronic neuropathic wounds, reconstructive foot surgery may often become the conservative treatment. The endpoint for chronic diabetic foot wounds should include reduction in the number of major amputations, prevention of infection, decreased probability of ulceration, maintenance of skin integrity, and improvement of function. Successful outcomes for diabetic foot reconstruction should result in less intrinsic pressures via minor amputations, arthroplasties, osteotomies, condylectomies, exostosectomies, tendon procedures, and joint arthrodesis.[87] Open wounds can be treated in one stage and are primarily closed with premorbid tissue using local flap reconstruction and soft-tissue repair.[89] Plastic surgical repair of these wounds can

help avoid production of inelastic scar tissue over weight-bearing surfaces.[90] Extrinsic and intrinsic pressures can be further neutralized with postoperative accommodative shoe gear.[76,77] Prophylactic diabetic foot surgery is an increasingly used option to prevent recurrent ulceration and reduce the risk of major amputations.[91,92] Surgical biomechanics, plastic and soft-tissue reconstruction, and appropriate offloading are all essential to creating a stable platform from which to keep these difficult patients free from tissue breakdown and as functional as possible.

Treatment of pedal soft-tissue deficits in the diabetic patient population continues to be a medical and surgical challenge that extends the length of the patient's disability and significantly increases the cost of medical care. Simple closure of these wounds is often difficult because of preexisting bone deformity, tissue inelasticity, location of the defect, and superimposed osteomyelitis. Clinical pathways related to diabetic foot ulcers frequently involve persistent sharp débridement, expensive wound care products, long-term IV antibiotics, total contact casting, total contact casting with Achilles tendon lengthening, use of skin equivalents, electrical stimulation, multiple offloading orthopedic devices, and even amputation.

Wounds are often allowed to granulate, contract, and heal by secondary intention. Use of negative pressure wound therapy has increased the armamentarium of wound specialists and has significantly improved outcomes.[74,87] When these wounds occur on the plantar aspect of the foot, they frequently recur, since the resulting scar has decreased extensibility and mobility. Attempted primary wound closure of diabetic pedal defects is frequently unsuccessful and may be a sequela of inadequate wound assessment, lack of proper evaluation of comorbidities, and an inadequate treatment plan.[93] Reconstructive surgery has traditionally been performed on selected patients with severe deformities that cannot be accommodated by custom footwear. Some authors have stressed the importance of addressing the underlying bony pathology in treating diabetic foot problems and have dispelled the unfounded fear of performing surgery on diabetic feet.[89,91,92]

Reconstructive surgery can range from simple metatarsal head resections to subtotal calcanectomies. Local flaps that are often difficult to elevate and inset are more easily mobilized and incised when concomitant bone resection is achieved at the time of flap creation. In addition, a local flap results in greater exposure and direct visualization of the underlying osseous structures compared with a single linear or semielliptical incision. Implementation of local random flaps can eliminate the need for additional incisions often deemed necessary to gain access to a forefoot, midfoot, or rearfoot bony defect. Use of negative pressure wound therapy has greatly enabled salvage of these complex limb wounds.[74,87]

Summary

Chronic leg ulcers are frequently encountered in clinical practice. The cost of chronic nonhealing wounds is enormous. Considerable morbidity and mortality are associated with ulcerations of the lower limbs in both diabetic and nondiabetic patients. The role of the primary care physician in evaluation, diagnosis, and management of lower-extremity wounds is critical. Careful assessment of vascular disease, evaluation and management of biomechanical and metabolic abnormalities, and aggressive treatment of any infections are required. A multidisciplinary approach provides a comprehensive treatment protocol and significantly increases the chances of successfully healing the ulcer and preventing recurrence.

ACKNOWLEDGMENT

Bauer E. Sumpio is supported by grants from the National Institutes of Health (R01-HL47345) and the Veterans Administration (Merit Review). This work was supported in part by an unrestricted grant from the North American Foundation for Limb Preservation.

REFERENCES

1. Sumpio BE: Foot ulcers, N Engl J Med 343:787–793, 2000.
2. Sumpio BE, Armstrong DG, Lavery LA, et al: The role of interdisciplinary team approach in the management of the diabetic foot: a joint statement from the Society for Vascular Surgery and the American Podiatric Medical Association, J Vasc Surg 51:1504–1506, 2010.
3. Sumpio BE, Aruny J, Blume PA: The multidisciplinary approach to limb salvage, Acta Chir Belg 104:647–653, 2004.
4. Mekkes JR, Loots MA, Van Der Wal AC, et al: Causes, investigation and treatment of leg ulceration, Br J Dermatol 148:388–401, 2003.
5. Beauregard S, GB: A survey of skin problems and skin care regiments in the elderly, Arch Dermatol 123:1638–1643, 1987.
6. Clement DL: Venous ulcer reappraisal: insights from an international task force. Veines International Task Force, J Vasc Res 36(Suppl 1):42–47, 1999.
7. De Wolfe V: The prevention and management of chronic venous insufficiency, Pract Cardiol 6:187–202, 1980.
8. Phillips TJ: Chronic cutaneous ulcers: etiology and epidemiology, J Invest Dermatol 102:38S–41S, 1994.
9. Ellison DA, Hayes L, Lane C, et al: Evaluating the cost and efficacy of leg ulcer care provided in two large UK health authorities, J Wound Care 11:47–51, 2002.
10. Browse NL: The etiology of venous ulceration, World J Surg 10:938–943, 1986.
11. Goldman M, Fronek A: The Alexander House Group: consensus paper on venous leg ulcers, J Dermatol Surg Oncol 18:592, 1992.
12. Phillips T, Stanton B, Provan A: A study of the impact of leg ulcers on quality of life: financial, social, and psychological implications, J Am Acad Dermatol 31:49–53, 1994.
13. Hutton W, Stokes I: The mechanics of the foot. In Klenerman L, editor: The foot and its disorders, Oxford, 1991, Blackwell Scientific Publications, p 11.
14. Murray H, Boulton A: The pathophysiology of diabetic foot ulceration, Clin Podiatr Med Surg 12:1, 1995.
15. Phillips TJ: Leg ulcer management, Dermatol Nurs 8:333–340, 1996; quiz 41–42.
16. O'Donnell TF Jr, Browse NL, Burnand KG, et al: The socioeconomic effects of an iliofemoral venous thrombosis, J Surg Res 22:483–488, 1977.
17. Falanga V, Eaglstein WH: The "trap" hypothesis of venous ulceration, Lancet 341:1006–1008, 1993.
18. Burnand KG, Clemenson G, Whimpster I, et al: Proceedings: extravascular fibrin deposition in response to venous hypertension-the cause of venous ulcers, Br J Surg 63:660–661, 1976.
19. Dodd HJ, Gaylarde PM, Sarkany I: Skin oxygen tension in venous insufficiency of the lower leg, J R Soc Med 78:373–376, 1985.
20. Sumpio B, Pradhan S: Atherosclerosis: biological and surgical considerations. In Ascher E, Hollier L, Strandness DE Jr, editors: Haimovici's vascular surgery, Malden, Mass, 2004, Blackwell Science, p 137.
21. Singer AJ, Clark RA: Cutaneous wound healing, N Engl J Med 341:738–746, 1999.
22. American Diabetes Association: Preventive foot care in people with diabetes [position statement], Diabetes Care 26(Suppl 1):78, 2003.
23. Knox RC, Dutch W, Blume P, et al: Diabetic foot disease, Int J Angiol 9:1–6, 2000.
24. Reiber GE, Lipsky BA, Gibbons GW: The burden of diabetic foot ulcers, Am J Surg 176(2A Suppl):5S–10S, 1998.
25. Boulton AJ: The diabetic foot: a global view, Diabetes Metab Res Rev 16(Suppl 1):S2–S5, 2000.
26. Weiss JS, Sumpio BE: Review of prevalence and outcome of vascular disease in patients with diabetes mellitus, Eur J Vasc Endovasc Surg 31:143–150, 2006.
27. O'Brien IA, Corrall RJ: Epidemiology of diabetes and its complications, N Engl J Med 318:1619–1620, 1988.
28. Kamal K, Powell RJ, Sumpio BE: The pathobiology of diabetes mellitus: implications for surgeons, J Am Coll Surg 183:271–289, 1996.
29. Laing P: The development and complications of diabetic foot ulcers, Am J Surg 176(2A Suppl):11S–9S, 1998.
30. Lee L, Blume PA, Sumpio B: Charcot joint disease in diabetes mellitus, Ann Vasc Surg 17(5):571–580, 2003.
31. Veves A, Fernando D, Walewski P, et al: A study of plantar pressures in a diabetic clinic population, Foot 2:89, 1991.
32. Boulton AJ, Armstrong DG, Albert SF, et al: Comprehensive foot examination and risk assessment: a report of the task force of the foot care interest group of the American Diabetes Association, with endorsement by the American Association of Clinical Endocrinologists, Diabetes Care 31:1679–1685, 2008.
33. Masson E, Hay E, Stockley I, et al: Abnormal foot pressures alone may not cause ulceration, Diabet Med 6:426–428, 1989.
34. Levin ME: Diabetes and peripheral neuropathy, Diabetes Care 21:1, 1998.
35. Boulton AJ, Hardisty CA, Betts RP, et al: Dynamic foot pressure and other studies as diagnostic and management aids in diabetic neuropathy, Diabetes Care 6:26–33, 1983.
36. Fernando DJ, Masson EA, Veves A, et al: Relationship of limited joint mobility to abnormal foot pressures and diabetic foot ulceration, Diabetes Care 14:8–11, 1991.
37. Morag E, Pammer S, Boulton A, et al: Structural and functional aspects of the diabetic foot, Clin Biomech (Bristol, Avon) 12:S9–S10, 1997.
38. Saltzman C, Pedowitz W: Diabetic foot infection, AAOS Instructional Course Lectures 48: 317–323, 1999.
39. Habershaw G, Chzran J: Management of diabetic foot problems. Biomechanical considerations of the diabetic foot, Philadelphia, 1995, WB Saunders, pp 53–65.
40. Bullock G, Stavosky J: Surgical wound management of the diabetic foot, Surg Technol Int 6:301–310, 1997.
41. Bild DE, Selby JV, Sinnock P, et al: Lower-extremity amputation in people with diabetes. Epidemiology and prevention, Diabetes Care 12:24–31, 1989.
42. Kannel WB, McGee DL: Diabetes and cardiovascular disease. The Framingham study, JAMA 241:2035–2038, 1979.
43. Melton LJ 3rd, Macken KM, Palumbo PJ, et al: Incidence and prevalence of clinical peripheral vascular disease in a population-based cohort of diabetic patients, Diabetes Care 3:650–654, 1980.
44. Dang CN, Prasad YD, Boulton AJ, et al: Methicillin-resistant Staphylococcus aureus in the diabetic foot clinic: a worsening problem, Diabet Med 20:159–161, 2003.
45. Hostetter MK: Handicaps to host defense. Effects of hyperglycemia on C3 and Candida albicans, Diabetes 39(3):271–275, 1990.
46. Hostetter MK, Krueger RA, Schmeling DJ: The biochemistry of opsonization: central role of the reactive thiol ester of the third component of complement, J Infect Dis 150:653–661, 1984.
47. MacRury SM, Gemmell CG, Paterson KR, et al: Changes in phagocytic function with glycaemic control in diabetic patients, J Clin Pathol 42:1143–1147, 1989.
48. Caballero E, Frykberg RG: Diabetic foot infections, J Foot Ankle Surg 37:248–255, 1998.
49. Davis SC, Martinez L, Kirsner R: The diabetic foot: the importance of biofilms and wound bed preparation, Curr Diab Rep 6:439–445, 2006.
50. Louie TJ, Bartlett JG, Tally FP, et al: Aerobic and anaerobic bacteria in diabetic foot ulcers, Ann Intern Med 85:461–463, 1976.
51. Sapico FL, Canawati HN, Witte JL, et al: Quantitative aerobic and anaerobic bacteriology of infected diabetic feet, J Clin Microbiol 12:413–420, 1980.

52. Sapico FL, Witte JL, Canawati HN, et al: The infected foot of the diabetic patient: quantitative microbiology and analysis of clinical features, *Rev Infect Dis* 6(Suppl 1): S171–S176, 1984.

53. Wheat LJ, Allen SD, Henry M, et al: Diabetic foot infections. Bacteriologic analysis, *Arch Intern Med* 146:1935–1940, 1986.

54. Day MR, Armstrong DG: Factors associated with methicillin resistance in diabetic foot infections, *J Foot Ankle Surg* 36:322–325, 1997 discussion 31.

55. Tentolouris N, Jude EB, Smirnof I, et al: Methicillin-resistant *Staphylococcus aureus*: an increasing problem in a diabetic foot clinic, *Diabet Med* 16:767–771, 1999.

56. Adam DJ, Naik J, Hartshorne T, et al: The diagnosis and management of 689 chronic leg ulcers in a single-visit assessment clinic, *Eur J Vasc Endovasc Surg* 25:462–468, 2003.

57. Weitz JI, Byrne J, Clagett GP, et al: Diagnosis and treatment of chronic arterial insufficiency of the lower extremities: a critical review, *Circulation* 94:3026–3049, 1996.

58. Pressley Z, Foster J, Kolm P, et al: Digital image analysis: a reliable tool in the quantitative evaluation of cutaneous lesions and beyond, *Arch Dermatol* 143:1331–1333, 2007.

59. Grayson ML, Gibbons GW, Balogh K, et al: Probing to bone in infected pedal ulcers. A clinical sign of underlying osteomyelitis in diabetic patients, *JAMA* 273:721–723, 1995.

60. Collins KA, Sumpio BE: Vascular assessment, *Clin Podiatr Med Surg* 17:171–191, 2000.

61. Feng Y, Schlosser FJ, Sumpio BE: The Semmes-Weinstein monofilament examination as a screening tool for diabetic peripheral neuropathy, *J Vasc Surg* 50:675–682, 2009 682 e1, 2009.

62. Armstrong DG, Lavery LA: Diabetic foot ulcers: prevention, diagnosis and classification, *Am Fam Physician* 57:1325–1332, 37–38, 1998.

63. Birke J, Sims D: Plantar sensory threshold in the ulcerative foot, *Leprosy Rev* 57:261, 1986.

64. McNeely M, Boyko E, Ahroni J, et al: The independent contributions of diabetic neuropathy and vasculopathy in foot ulceration: how great are the risks? *Diabetes Care* 18:216–219, 1995.

65. Feng Y, Schlosser FJ, Sumpio BE: The Semmes Weinstein monofilament examination is a significant predictor of the risk of foot ulceration and amputation in patients with diabetes mellitus, *J Vasc Surg* 53:220–226 e1–5, 2010.

66. Sumpio BE, Lee T, Blume PA: Vascular evaluation and arterial reconstruction of the diabetic foot, *Clin Podiatr Med Surg* 20:689–708, 2003.

67. Steed DL, Donohoe D, Webster MW, et al: Effect of extensive debridement and treatment on the healing of diabetic foot ulcers. Diabetic Ulcer Study Group, *J Am Coll Surg* 183:61–64, 1996.

68. Granick M, Boykin J, Gamelli R, et al: Toward a common language: surgical wound bed preparation and debridement, *Wound Repair Regen* 14(Suppl 1):S1–S10, 2006.

69. Bergstrom N, Bennett M, Carlson C: *Treatment of pressure ulcers. Clinical practice guidelines*, no. 15. (AHCPR publication no. 95-0652.). Rockville, Md., 1994, Agency for Health Care Policy and Research, pp 1–102.

70. Bello YM, Phillips TJ: Recent advances in wound healing, *JAMA* 283:716–718, 2000.

71. Joshi N, Caputo GM, Weitekamp MR, et al: Infections in patients with diabetes mellitus, *N Engl J Med* 341:1906–1912, 1999.

72. Orgill DP, Manders EK, Sumpio BE, et al: The mechanisms of action of vacuum assisted closure: more to learn, *Surgery* 146:40–51, 2009.

73. Sumpio BE, Allie DE, Horvath KA, et al: Role of negative pressure wound therapy in treating peripheral vascular graft infections, *Vascular* 16:194–200, 2008.

74. Blume PA, Walters J, Payne W, et al: Comparison of negative pressure wound therapy using vacuum-assisted closure with advanced moist wound therapy in the treatment of diabetic foot ulcers: a multicenter randomized controlled trial, *Diabetes Care* 31:631–636, 2008.

75. Frykberg RG, Armstrong DG, Giurini J, et al: Diabetic foot disorders. A clinical practice guideline. For the American College of Foot and Ankle Surgeons and the American College of Foot and Ankle Orthopedics and Medicine, *J Foot Ankle Surg* 39:S1–S60, 2000.

76. Bus SA, Valk GD, van Deursen RW, et al: The effectiveness of footwear and offloading interventions to prevent and heal foot ulcers and reduce plantar pressure in diabetes: a systematic review, *Diabetes Metab Res Rev* 24:S162–S180, 2008.

77. Bus SA, Valk GD, van Deursen RW, et al: Specific guidelines on footwear and offloading, *Diabetes Metab Res Rev* 24:S192–S193, 2008.

78. Barrow J, Hughes J, Clark P: A study of the effect of wear on the pressure-relieving properties of foot orthosis, *Foot* 1:195–199, 1992.

79. Nawoczenski D, Birke J, Coleman W: Effect of rocker sole design on plantar forefoot pressures, *J Am Podiatr Med Assoc* 78:455–460, 1988.

80. Tang PC, Ravji K, Key JJ, et al: Let them walk! Current prosthesis options for leg and foot amputees, *J Am Coll Surg* 206:548–560, 2008.

81. Bello M, Scriven M, Hartshorne T, et al: Role of superficial venous surgery in the treatment of venous ulceration, *Br J Surg* 86:755–759, 1999.

82. Barwell JR, Taylor M, Deacon J, et al: Surgical correction of isolated superficial venous reflux reduces long-term recurrence rate in chronic venous leg ulcers, *Eur J Vasc Endovasc Surg* 20:363–368, 2000.

83. Ghauri AS, Nyamekye I, Grabs AJ, et al: Influence of a specialised leg ulcer service and venous surgery on the outcome of venous leg ulcers, *Eur J Vasc Endovasc Surg* 16:238–244, 1998.

84. Eriksson I: Reconstruction of deep venous valves of the lower extremity, *Surg Annu* 24 (Pt 2):211–229, 1992.

85. Plagnol P, Ciostek P, Grimaud JP, et al: Autogenous valve reconstruction technique for post-thrombotic reflux, *Ann Vasc Surg* 13:339–342, 1999.

86. Sarage A, Yui W, Blume P, et al: Aggressive revascularization options using cryoplasty in patients with lower extremity vascular disease. In Geroulakos G, editor: *Re-do vascular surgery*, London, 2009, Springer Verlag, pp 79–84.

87. Sumpio B, Driver V, Gibbons G, et al: A Multidisciplinary approach to limb preservation- the role of VAC Therapy, *Wounds Oct Suppl* 1–19, 2009.

88. Frangos S, Kilaru S, Blume P, et al: Classification of diabetic foot ulcers: improving communication, *Int J Angiol* 11:158–164, 2002.

89. Blume P, Partagas L, Attinger C, et al: Single stage surgical treatment of noninfected diabetic foot ulcers, *J Plastic Reconstr Surg* 109:601–609, 2002.

90. Blume P, Salonga C, Garbalosa J, et al: Predictors for the healing of transmetatarsal amputations: retrospective study of 91 amputations, *Vascular* 15:126–133, 2007.

91. Armstrong D, Lavery L, Stern S, et al: Is prophylactic diabetic foot surgery dangerous? *J Foot Ankle Surg* 35:585–589, 1996.

92. Catanzariti A, Blitch E, Karlock L: Elective foot and ankle surgery in the diabetic patient, *J Foot Ankle Surg* 34:23–41, 1995.

93. Blume PA, Key JJ, Thakor P, et al: Retrospective evaluation of clinical outcomes in subjects with split-thickness skin graft: comparing V.A.C. therapy and conventional therapy in foot and ankle reconstructive surgeries, *Int Wound J* 7:480–487, 2010.

CHAPTER 61

Vascular Trauma

Chandler A. Long, Christopher J. Kwolek, Michael T. Watkins

Treatment of vascular trauma in the civilian and military venues has had a symbiotic relationship. Although German surgeons accomplished a limited number of arterial repairs in the early part of World War I, ligation of major arterial injuries was not abandoned until the Korean Conflict in the 1950s. Until that time, arterial ligation was used preferentially, and some experts of the day felt there was little place for definitive arterial repair of the combat wound. Review of the arterial injuries during World War II revealed that arterial ligation was followed by gangrene and amputation in half the cases.[1] After World War II, significant advances made in civilian hospitals included atraumatic vascular clamps, monofilament sutures, arteriography, and prosthetic grafting. These advances made it possible to repair arterial injuries in the battlefield, such that during the Korean conflict, the overall amputation rate was reduced to 13%.[2] The latest innovation in vascular surgery, the "endovascular revolution," is rapidly changing our approach to managing some components of vascular trauma in the civilian setting.[3] It is unclear to what extent these techniques will facilitate care in the battlefield.

Trauma remains the leading cause of death in the 15- to 44-year-old age group in the United States. The prevalence of iatrogenic vascular injury has increased in tandem with the number of catheter-based invasive procedures.[4] Overall, arteries in the lower extremities are injured more than other anatomical areas. In this chapter, the basic definitions and treatment strategies for vascular trauma are described.

Basic Concepts and Definitions

Vascular trauma occurs in a finite number of archetypes that are directly dependent on the mechanism of injury. Vascular trauma can be related to two major categories of injury: penetrating and blunt. The resulting injury to the artery and its treatment can vary dramatically based on mechanism of injury. The clinical presentation of arterial injury may include external or internal bleeding, regional ischemia, pulsatile hematoma, and shock. The clinical presentation depends as much on location of the injured vessel(s) as on the mechanism itself.

Penetrating trauma, usually by way of stab or missile wounds, creates varying degrees of laceration to a vessel, with the most severe being transection. Complete transection of a vessel allows the ends of the vessel to retract and spasm, and in some scenarios is associated with arterial thrombosis. In this instance, thrombosis prevents hemorrhage, thus preserving circulatory homeostasis. It should be noted that most often, vessel spasm minimizes bleeding in an underresuscitated patient. However, once the patient has been adequately resuscitated (with intravenous [IV] fluid or blood products) and normal blood pressure and systemic perfusion are restored, bleeding from the transected ends may resume. Vessels with incomplete transection or laceration tend to bleed more profusely because of their inability to retract and spasm.

Blunt injury to an artery disrupts the integrity and structure of the wall. Severity of the injury ranges from small intimal disruption to focal dissection to transmural injury with thrombosis or extravasation. Blunt injuries can be more indolent in their presentation but result in just as devastating outcomes as those seen in penetrating trauma. Arteries that are tethered at a portion or segments in their course through the body are more susceptible to blunt injury because of the shearing force associated with acceleration and deceleration. *Shear forces* associated with injury often cause deformation of the vessel wall that may cause transmural disruption or dissection, frequently in the proximal descending aorta. Smaller arteries subjected to shear forces (e.g., renal arteries) develop focal intimal flaps.

Pseudoaneurysm/Traumatic Arteriovenous Fistula

False aneurysms, or *pseudoaneurysms*, differ from true aneurysms in that they lack all three normal elements of the arterial wall. The most common etiology of false aneurysms is trauma, related to either catheter-based interventions or injury. Vascular trauma to the artery wall that can result in false aneurysms can be either penetrating or blunt in nature. Infection can complicate the clinical course of pseudoaneurysms when there is inadvertent puncture of arteries associated with drug abuse, contamination or secondary seeding after percutaneous intervention, or as a consequence of bacterial seeding in the presence of a prosthetic vascular anastomosis. *Arteriovenous fistulae* (AVFs) are abnormal direct communications between an artery and vein. These communications can be iatrogenic, congenital, or acquired.

Signs of Vascular Trauma

The hard signs of vascular trauma warrant urgent or immediate operative exploration and intervention (Box 61-1). In many instances, these patients present with systemic shock, and resuscitative efforts are best coordinated in the operating room. The soft signs of vascular injury (see Box 61-1) require further diagnostic evaluation to plan intervention if needed. Depending on the hemodynamic status of patients with soft signs of vascular injury, subsequent evaluation may include invasive or noninvasive imaging techniques.

Hemorrhagic Shock

Hemorrhagic shock is a condition of reduced tissue perfusion due to inadequate delivery of oxygenated blood, resulting in anaerobic metabolism, acidosis, and deleterious alterations to cell function. Because bleeding may be a major complication associated with vascular trauma, it is important to provide information on the kinds of shock that may be associated with these injuries. There are four types of hemorrhagic shock, ranging in severity based on the amount of blood lost. Clinical characteristics associated with the degree of hemorrhagic shock are described in Table 61-1.

Ischemia/Reperfusion Injury

Ischemia/reperfusion is a complex pathological process involving intracellular and extracellular processes that result in metabolic, thrombotic, and inflammatory changes in brain, intestine, heart, kidney, and skeletal muscle. A devastating component of ischemia/reperfusion injury is the paradoxical increase in tissue injury associated with restitution of blood flow to ischemic tissues. The *myonephropathic-metabolic syndrome* was described by Haimovici in a few patients who underwent lower-extremity revascularization following acute ischemia in the late 1950s, providing one of the first published clinical observations of limb ischemia and reperfusion.[5,6] These patients experienced ongoing lower-extremity necrosis and myoglobin-induced renal failure in the presence of palpable pulses.

One of the most severe components of ischemia/reperfusion injury, the paradoxical decrease in blood flow following restoration of perfusion, was described initially as a *no-reflow phenomenon* in the brain,[7] and May et al. described the same phenomenon 10 years later in skin flaps.[8] These investigators described cellular swelling, intravascular aggregation of cellular components of blood (platelets, neutrophils), and leakage of intravascular fluid into the interstitial space as basic mechanisms whereby tissue flow

Box 61-1 Hard and Soft Signs of Vascular Injury

Hard Signs
Pulsatile bleeding
Expanding or pulsatile hematoma
Absent distal pulse
Signs of distal ischemia (six Ps*)
Palpable thrill or audible bruit

Soft Signs
Wound in close proximity to known vessel
Stable hematoma
History of hemorrhage
Peripheral nerve deficit

*Pain, pallor, pulselessness, paresthesias, poikilothermia, paralysis.

is decreased during reperfusion, providing the first definitive histological evidence to support the existence of the no-reflow phenomenon. From a biochemical perspective, it is useful to discuss this process in terms of its components: ischemic injury and reperfusion injury.

ISCHEMIC INJURY

There is a differential degree of tissue ischemia tolerance for various organs that is dependent on each tissue's baseline metabolic demand. Critical ischemia of human skeletal muscle under normothermic conditions is more than 2 hours, whereas jejunum develops histological changes after approximately 30 minutes of ischemia. Decreased oxygen delivery to tissue results in decreased mitochondrial energy production (adenosine triphosphate [ATP] synthesis, oxidative phosphorylation) and a marked decrease in cellular energy stores (ATP content). Inadequate energy stores result in disturbances of cellular ion homeostasis, activation of hydrolases, and increases in permeability of cellular membranes. As ischemia progresses, there is a logarithmic increase in adverse ion homeostasis and activation of hydrolases. As ATP is degraded, cellular lysosomes leak hydrogen ions, and cells increase their glycolytic rate, resulting in cellular acidosis. Acidosis impairs the function of Na^+/K^+-ATPase and other enzymes responsible for managing cellular ion homeostasis, resulting in increased cytosolic Na^+ and Ca^{2+} concentrations. Increased levels of Ca^{2+} concentration activate phospholipases (especially phospholipase A_2) and proteases (calpains), which enhance tissue injury. Activated phospholipases and calpains respectively degrade membrane phospholipid moieties and cytoskeletal proteins to exacerbate tissue injury.

Key events occur during ischemia that set the stage for worsening injury during reperfusion. One of these is the conversion of xanthine dehydrogenase (D) to xanthine oxidase (O). Xanthine dehydrogenase uses NAD^+ as an electron acceptor during the oxidation of xanthine and hypoxanthine. Heat, proteolysis, and reducing agents such as sulfhydryl compounds can transform the D to the O form, which is incapable of using $NAD+$ as an electron acceptor. The O form uses oxygen as an electron acceptor, and generates superoxide anion and hydrogen peroxide during the oxidation

of hypoxanthine and xanthine. Some investigators have proposed that calcium mediated activation of proteases converts the dehydrogenase form to the oxidase form.

REPERFUSION INJURY

There are metabolic, thrombotic, and inflammatory components of reperfusion injury. The degree to which reperfusion either restores tissue integrity or exacerbates ischemic injury is dependent primarily on the duration of ischemia. It is indeed paradoxical that moderate ischemia followed by reperfusion may cause a more fulminant postischemic tissue injury than ischemia alone. However, without reperfusion, the loss of function in the brain, gut, heart, or limb may have more catastrophic outcome than seen with reperfusion.

Vascular endothelium plays a major role in modulating the tissue response to reperfusion. The generation of reactive oxygen metabolites by calcium-mediated xanthine oxidase–dependent pathways in vascular endothelium during reperfusion contribute to local injury, vascular permeability, and autocrine and paracrine signaling. The increased generation of reactive oxygen metabolites during reperfusion compromises production of nitric oxide (NO) and prostaglandins (PGs), which contributes to alteration of vascular tone. Decreased endothelial ATP levels results in a loss of the apposition of endothelial monolayers, which triggers both an increase in vascular permeability and a decrease in vascular tone.

It is the induction of inflammatory mediator protein synthesis/deposition, decreased vascular tone, and endothelial cell (EC) apposition that leads to the development of the no-reflow phenomenon. A variety of inflammatory mediators are delivered by bloodborne cells (macrophages, lymphocytes, neutrophils, mast cells, platelets) to reperfused tissues. Noncellular elements, such as the complement system, reactive oxygen species (ROS), nitric oxide, and pro- and antiinflammatory cytokines, are also believed to modulate the complex scenario of reperfusion injury. Ischemia/reperfusion injury is believed to manifest clinically as development of cardiac arrhythmias, the evolution of stroke, translocation of bacteria across the bowel wall following revascularization, early organ dysfunction following transplant, and compartment syndrome.

Compartment Syndrome

Acute compartment syndrome is a surgical emergency. *Compartment syndrome* may be defined as increased tissue pressure in a closed myofascial space, resulting in disturbed microcirculation that leads to irreversible neuromuscular ischemic damage.[9] Acute compartment syndrome most commonly occurs following lower-limb trauma. Emergency decompression through open and extensive fasciotomies is the treatment of choice. The cardinal clinical feature is severe pain, greater than would be expected from the original insult. The pain may be exacerbated by passive extension of the tendons crossing the symptomatic compartment or arising from the muscles within it. Among other clinical features, the first is usually hypoesthesia, followed by compartment distension and muscle weakness in the later stages. The need for prompt intervention

TABLE 61-1	Classification of Hemorrhagic Shock			
	COMPENSATED (I)	**MILD (II)**	**MODERATE (III)**	**SEVERE (IV)**
Blood loss (mL)	<1000	1000-1500	1500-2000	>2000
Heart rate (bpm)	<100	>100	>120	>140
Blood pressure	Normal	Orthostatic change	Marked hypotension	Significant hypotension
Capillary refill	Normal	Sometimes delayed	Usually delayed	Delayed
Respiratory rate	Normal	Mild increase	Moderate tachypnea	Significant tachypnea
Urinary output	>30 mL/h	20-30 mL/h	5-20 mL/h	Anuria
Mental status	Normal or agitated	Agitated	Confused	Lethargic, obtunded

and the benefits of timely surgical decompression require a high index of suspicion and effective clinical assessment to make the diagnosis. Clinical assessment may be supported by compartment pressure measurements, in which a needle is inserted into the compartment and pressure monitored using a pressure transducer. The pressure that indicates a need for fasciotomy has not been universally established, although a pressure greater than 30 mmHg is widely accepted as abnormal. Other authors advocate a threshold that relates to the diastolic blood pressure, with compartment pressures within 30 mmHg of the diastolic pressure indicating a need for fasciotomy.

A recent 10-year review of the incidence of compartment syndrome in a mature level I trauma center indicated that after lower-extremity trauma, 2.8% of patients will require fasciotomy. A stepwise logistic regression identified the presence of vascular injury (arterial, venous, or combined), need for packed red blood cell (RBC) transfusion, male gender, open fracture, elbow or knee dislocation, and age younger than 55 as independent predictors for the need for fasciotomy after extremity trauma. Combined arterial and venous injury resulted in fasciotomy in 42% of patients.[10]

TECHNIQUE OF FASCIOTOMY

A single method of fasciotomy is not universally suitable for all indications. Fasciotomy through limited skin incisions has been both advocated and denounced by many specialists. The rationale for limited skin incisions is based on the concept that the fascia is the limiting constrictive tissue, whereas the skin contributes to the tamponade in certain instances. Limited skin incision fasciotomy is associated with minimal or no morbidity. Infection is less likely, and this technique does not leave large open wounds that can be troublesome in the setting of anticoagulant therapy. In the performance of limited fasciotomy, the skin is not incised along the length of the extremity. By two or three short vertical incisions, the investing fascia can be identified and incised. Long skin incisions are necessary when there is massive swelling and when, on clinical examination, the skin contributes to the constrictive process. The incisions are planned such that vascular or nerve repairs are not exposed. In the posterior medial long incision, it is necessary to release the deep compartment by retracting the gastrocnemius and soleus muscles. In the anterolateral incision, the investing fascia is incised, and the extensor digitorum and peroneal muscles are separated where the deep peroneal nerve can be seen. In the upper extremities, the incisions are made from just proximal to the wrist to the elbow.

Thoracic Vascular Injury

With the heart, great vessels, brachiocephalic vessels, and descending aorta housed within the confines of the thorax, mortality following vascular injury is associated with exsanguinating hemorrhage at the scene. Hemothorax associated with penetrating trauma can be managed with a chest tube, but if a major vascular structure is involved, patient survival is largely dependent on whether there is free hemorrhage or a contained hematoma. It is estimated that over 80% of patients suffering blunt trauma to the aorta will die at the scene of the accident.[11]

Thoracic/Cardiac Box

Penetrating wounds to the thoracic, or cardiac, "box" are concerning for injury to the heart, bronchial tree, esophagus, and great vessels. Injuries to these structures can be devastating, and delay in diagnosis has morbid consequences. The *thoracic box* is anatomically bordered by the level of the thoracic outlet superiorly, the midclavicular lines laterally, and the costal margin inferiorly. These wounds should be explored operatively. All precordial penetrating injuries occurring between the nipple lines laterally, the clavicles superiorly, and the epigastrium inferiorly should be assumed to involve the heart until ruled out.

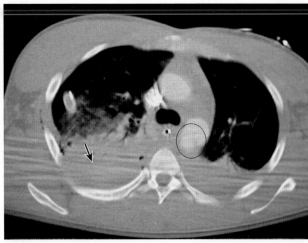

FIGURE 61-1 Thoracic aortic injury and associated nonvascular injuries. Spiral thoracic computed tomography (CT) image demonstrating aortic transection 2 cm distal *(circled)* to subclavian artery origin, with surrounding traumatic thoracic pseudoaneurysm and an intraparenchymal tear of right lung *(arrow)*.

THORACIC AORTA

Traumatic aortic rupture is a devastating clinical problem that is difficult to manage owing to the need to approach aortic repair in concert with management of complex associated injuries to nonvascular organ systems (Fig. 61-1). The natural history of aortic transection is relatively self-selective, with a significant majority of patients exsanguinating at the scene. Of those who make it to the hospital alive, upwards of 38% die largely as a result of associated injuries.[12] Fabian et al. estimate the incidence of traumatic aortic disruptions in the United States to be between 7500 and 8000 patients annually; about 1000 to 1500 of these patients arrive at hospitals alive.[13] It took 50 centers 2.5 years to generate 274 patients for this prospective report. This averages just over two patients per year per center. Despite the low volume, contemporary analysis reveals that of the 9% to 19% who reach the hospital alive,[14] approximately 30% will die within the next 6 hours, and a total of 50% within 24 hours.[15]

Until recently, open operative intervention for these traumatic injuries required thoracotomy, anticoagulation, and application of an aortic cross-clamp. These operative maneuvers conceded the potential of exacerbating associated injuries and spinal cord injury.[13,16,17] Proximal-to-distal aortic bypass using a Gott Shunt, left heart bypass with heparin-bonded circuits, and cardiopulmonary bypass (CPB) may all significantly reduce the likelihood of paraplegia.[18,19] Thus, the current status of traumatic aortic disruption and traditional repair is not ideal. Advances in endovascular repair techniques for traumatic rupture have resulted in a major change in the approach to treatment of this devastating clinical entity.[20-22] This change in approach is based on and supported by improved mortality associated with repair by endovascular vs. open techniques in patients with multiple trauma[23] (Fig. 61-2).

Open Surgical Approach

Open repair may be accomplished either with direct cross-clamping alone or with circulatory assistance (left-sided heart bypass with heparin-coated conduits, cardiopulmonary bypass, or femoral-femoral bypass).[19,24,25] Optimal exposure of the thoracic aorta is gained through a posterolateral thoracotomy with an incision in the fourth intercostal space. The aortic arch may be controlled either with clamping between the left common carotid and left subclavian, or just distal to the left subclavian artery. The descending thoracic aorta is controlled distally immediately after the traumatic injury to avert sacrifice of the intercostal arteries. The aorta can then be repaired with direct suturing or graft interposition.

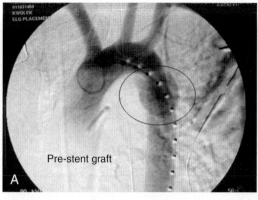

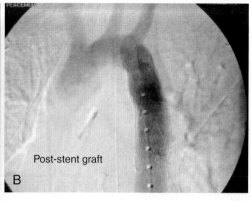

Pre-stent graft

A

Post-stent graft

B

FIGURE 61-2 Thoracic aortic disruption. A, Thoracic aortogram illustrating a 4-cm pseudoaneurysm *(circled)* in descending thoracic aorta, 2 cm from subclavian artery. **B,** Post-deployment aortogram revealing no endoleak or extravasation.

Endovascular Approach

Trauma centers equipped with radiographic fixed or mobile C-arms and angiographic equipment in the operating rooms would be ideal. This affords the opportunity for patients to be treated for their vascular injury(s) via open cutdown or percutaneously in a setting where surgical interventions for associated injuries may also be treated if indicated at that time.[26] Though not specifically designed to treat thoracic aortic transections, the use of endoluminal abdominal aortic extension cuffs has been shown to be technically feasible in several small series.[26-28] This has been particularly evident in young individuals with normal-sized aortas. Broad prepping and draping of the patient should be undertaken so that emergent intervention for associated abdominal or thoracic injuries can be pursued while the patient is under anesthesia. Patients should be placed supine on the appropriate x-ray table, with slight rotation to a decubitus position. This orientation of the patient provides access to the femoral and iliac vessels and the abdominal aorta if needed.

The diameter of stent grafts should be oversized at least 20% based on sizing obtained from computed tomographic angiography (CTA). Unlike treatment of patients with degenerative aneurysms, the aortic diameter proximal to the injured aorta is most often in the 18- to 26-mm range. Generous oversizing can lead to collapse of a stent graft.[29]

At times, the turn radius in the arch of young patients may be too tight for the Lunderquist wire. The smallest thoracic endograft available commercially in the United States is the 26 mm–diameter Gore TAG device. We have used proximal and distal Zenith TX2 thoracic endograft extensions, Gore TAG thoracic endografts, and Medtronic extensions from aortic endografts. Precise placement of the stent graft can be facilitated by adjusting the mean arterial pressure to 70 mmHg during implantation. Depending on the patient's heart rate, the device being implanted, and associated injuries, IV administration of adenosine to induce transient bradycardia/asystole may be used immediately prior to deployment of the graft.

Completion angiography should be performed after the stent graft has been deployed to ensure that the false aneurysm has been properly excluded. After removing the introducer delivery systems, the arteriotomy in the femoral artery is repaired. Computed tomography (CT) scans are performed prior to discharge, at 3 and 6 months, then yearly thereafter. Systemic anticoagulation should be used selectively to avoid thromboembolic complications associated with transient occlusion of the femoral vessels and wire/catheter manipulations in the aortic arch. This is often a major issue in patients with extensive associated injuries, particularly in those with associated head trauma.

THORACIC VENAE CAVAE

The superior vena cava is formed by the confluence of the left and right brachiocephalic veins in the superior mediastinum at the level of the right first costal cartilage. It descends down 5 to 7 cm to where it enters the posterior aspect of the right atrium at the

level of the third costochondral cartilage. The inferior vena cava (IVC) enters the chest at the level of T8 and has a short posterior course to the right atrium. Because of the location and short segments of these structures, the intrathoracic venae cavae rarely suffer traumatic injury. The low-pressure system and distendabilty of the vessels make blunt trauma a rare etiology of injury. Penetrating injury to the chest or iatrogenic injury are more common etiologies. Cardiac tamponade can be a frequent presentation following injury to the thoracic venae cavae, owing to the pericardium's extension and envelopment of the proximal portions of the vessels prior to entering the heart.

Simple isolated injuries to the thoracic venae cavae can be managed with lateral venorrhaphy. Partial-occluding clamps or temporary inflow occlusion can be used in these circumstances to facilitate repair.[30] Complex injuries to the venae cavae or associated injuries to the heart may require CPB and/or interposition grafts for exposure and repair.

PULMONARY VESSELS

Trauma to the main right or left pulmonary arteries is extremely rare and almost exclusively found after penetrating traumatic injury. Some case reports have described blunt traumatic injury to the main pulmonary arteries, but it remains exceedingly rare.[31] As with many of the great vessel injuries, cardiac tamponade or hemopericardium is the common presenting finding. Usually the diagnosis is made in the operating room during an empirical thoracotomy for hemopericardium. Distal pulmonary vascular injuries beyond the mediastinum can be seen following both blunt and penetrating trauma. Extensive vascular injury or significant injury to the hilar region may necessitate a pneumonectomy, which bears a significantly high mortality rate in trauma situations.[32]

Carotid and Vertebral Vascular Trauma

Penetrating Carotid Artery Trauma

Stab and low-velocity missile wounds account for the vast majority of civilian penetrating carotid artery injuries. Demographics of the injured generally include young, healthy males and associated alcohol and/or illegal drug use precipitating the injury. Studies have shown that carotid injuries occur in roughly 17% of all penetrating neck trauma.[33] Common carotid artery (CCA) injury is more frequent than internal carotid injuries. Iatrogenic injury to the carotid artery is most commonly due to attempted central venous catheter insertion.

DIAGNOSTIC EVALUATION

With penetrating injuries to the neck, the depth, location, and presence or absence of hard/soft signs of vascular trauma dictate the progression and trajectory of care. If the platysma muscle has not been violated by the penetrating insult, no immediate operative exploration is warranted. The presence of soft vascular injury signs in this scenario may necessitate further diagnostic imaging to rule out occult injury. If the injury traverses the platysma and/or hard signs of vascular injury are present, operative intervention or diagnostic interrogation (e.g., CTA) should not be delayed.

Imaging

Catheter-based angiography remains the gold standard for evaluation of vascular lesions, regardless of etiology. The benefit to angiography over other diagnostic imaging modalities is the capacity for therapeutic intervention during evaluation. With advances in non-invasive imaging, modalities such as helical CT with multidetector-row scanners and color Doppler ultrasonography have created fast, easily accessible means of diagnosing vascular injury.

ANATOMICAL CONSIDERATIONS

The neck is divided anatomically into three zones of injury (Box 61-2). Zone I comprises the area from the thoracic outlet (the level of jugular notch) to the cricoid cartilage, zone II begins at level of the cricoid cartilage and terminates at the angle of the mandible, and zone III extends from the angle of the mandible to the skull base. The zone divisions were based on the anatomical relationships of the neurovascular and aerodigestive tract structures, as well as the surgical approach for exposure.

Zone II Injuries

In stable patients, the management of zone II injuries of the neck is the source of some debate among trauma centers. Historically, all zone II injuries were operatively explored because of improved mortality rates with immediate operative intervention, as opposed to delayed or expectant intervention.[34] The relative ease of operative exposure in zone II and low morbidity rate with operation, coupled with the many vital structures passing through this region, made it the mainstay of treatment for many years, despite the high negative exploration rate. With advancements in diagnostic imaging, selective exploration has become more popular in stable patients. Thus, the decision whether operative exploration is necessary can be predicated on further diagnostic evaluation and imaging to confirm or rule out vascular injury. Usually this evaluation includes serial physical examinations, esophagoscopy, bronchoscopy, and imaging studies (i.e., catheter-based angiography, CTA, magnetic resonance angiography [MRA], or duplex ultrasound scanning) when vascular injury is suspected.[33,35-37] Centers that have used angiography to evaluate penetrating neck injuries in hemodynamically stable patients have found that only 13% to 17% of these patients have major vascular (carotid and vertebral) injuries requiring repair.[33,37] Because of this, some have begun to advocate angiography only in cases of suspected vascular injury and report very few missed injuries with this approach. More recent studies have also advocated CT scanning as an adjunct to the physical examination in zone II neck injuries, but angiography remains the gold standard.

Zone I and III Injuries

In zone I and III injuries, hemodynamic and neurologically stable patients usually undergo catheter-based angiography or a CTA to diagnose/define the presence and location of injury in these anatomically complex areas. Zone III vascular injuries are frequently amenable to coil embolization or stent grafting. Both zone I and III injuries, similar to zone II, usually require evaluation of the naso-pharynx and upper aerodigestive tract via laryngoscopy, bronchoscopy, and rigid esophagoscopy to diagnose occult injuries. Concomitant injuries to nonvascular structures can carry significant morbidity if not identified early.

OPERATIVE APPROACH/OPEN SURGICAL MANAGEMENT

Surgical exposure of the neck differs markedly depending on the zone of injury. Exposure of a zone II injury is straightforward and typically accomplished through a standard oblique incision along the anterior border of the sternocleidomastoid. This affords appropriate exposure and easy accessibility to the carotid sheath and its neurovascular contents.

The surgical approaches for zone I and III injuries can be significantly more complicated and challenging. To obtain adequate proximal vascular control and exposure, vascular injuries within zone I frequently require a median sternotomy or supraclavicular "trap-door" incision in addition to the standard cervical oblique incision. Zone III injuries may necessitate cephalad extension of the exposure to attain distal vascular control. Maneuvers such as dislocation or partial resection of the mandible are not infrequent, especially in high zone III injuries. Temporary control of bleeding at or near the skull base can be accomplished through insertion and inflation of a Fogarty catheter into the injured vessel.[38]

ENDOVASCULAR MANAGEMENT

Though endovascular management is less prevalent in blunt carotid injury, it has provided some promising results in the management of penetrating carotid trauma, especially in zone I and high zone III (internal carotid artery [ICA]) injuries.[39,40] Traditionally, ICA injuries (pseudoaneurysm and dissections), albeit rare, warrant anatomical reconstruction to prevent devastating ischemic neurological insults. Operating high in the neck is technically demanding and can be associated with cranial nerve injury; thus, endovascular stenting and coiling has the potential to limit iatrogenic damage associated with open exploration. Recent reviews have demonstrated that stent graft placement for traumatic ICA pseudoaneurysms have been successful in neurologically symptomatic patients following trauma.[41,42] Consideration must be given to thromboembolic events associated with stent graft placement, the potential for intimal hyperplasia formation, and restenosis. The anatomical tortuosity of the vessel may prevent safe crossing of the traumatic lesion with a guidewire. A recent retrospective review of 113 patients with blunt or penetrating carotid injury demonstrated a promising short-term patency (up to 2 years) of carotid stent grafts (80%).[43]

Blunt Carotid/Vertebral Artery Injury

Blunt carotid and vertebral artery injury (BCVI) is diagnosed roughly once in every 1000 patients.[44] Though BCVI is considered a rare occurrence, without prompt and appropriate care, cerebral ischemia rates range from 40% to 80%, and mortality rates from 25%

Box 61-2 Anatomical Structures in Each Zone of the Neck

Zone I
Aortic arch
Subclavian vessels
Proximal carotid arteries
Jugular veins
Trachea
Esophagus
Vagus nerve
Vertebral arteries
Thoracic duct
Thyroid gland

Zone II
Common carotid arteries (CCAs)
Internal jugular veins
Vertebral arteries
External jugular vein
Larynx/vocal cords
Esophagus
Vagus nerve

Zone III
Internal and external carotid arteries
Salivary and parotid glands
Cranial nerves IX-XII

to 60%.[44,45] BCVI lesions vary in mechanism and location; skull base fractures, for example, can contuse the intrapetrous/cavernous portion of the internal carotid artery. Blunt trauma to the carotid artery can be induced via a stretching, twisting, or shearing effect to the neck. BCVI after strangulation and choking has been described as well.[45] Several authors have proposed signs, symptoms, or injury patterns that should raise the suspicion for BCVI.[44,46,47] Skull base, midface, mandible, and cervical spine fractures are associated with BCVI and should raise a healthy concern. Significant blunt trauma to the chest and neck in a patient with a Glasgow Coma Scale score of 8 or less represents another clinical scenario that warrants further investigation. Note that these injuries can also be insidious in their presentation, so in a patient with a Glasgow Coma Scale score above 8 but a history of a high-risk mechanism (motor vehicle accident/deceleration injury) and/or trauma to the face and neck, suspicion for BCVI should remain.

DIAGNOSTIC EVALUATION

In most emergency situations, multidetector CTA remains the initial tool for evaluation of carotid injuries because it can often be performed expeditiously near or in the emergency room. Adequacy of the older single-slice helical CTA in diagnosing BCVI was limited by sensitivities and specificities of 68% and 67%, respectively.[48] However, several studies have shown the effectiveness of 16-channel multislice CTA in diagnosis of BCVI,[44,49] with sensitivities and specificities each greater than 94%. The somewhat subtle nature of blunt carotid injury makes digital subtraction angiography (DSA) the gold standard for the diagnosis of blunt carotid injury. Imaging by CTA may be compromised in situations where metallic artifact is present (shrapnel, plates, prosthesis, etc.). Although DSA is an invasive method, it not only depicts the extent and severity of vessel injury, it can also provide information about the integrity of cerebral circulation. Magnetic resonance angiography is another safe, noninvasive technique that can provide data concerning vessel morphology and blood flow. Its accuracy in diagnosing BCVI may rival that of CTA, but time required for the examination, difficulty monitoring the patient during the study, and high cost limit its use.[45] Duplex ultrasonography is used more in penetrating carotid trauma but is not sensitive enough to be the screening modality of choice in BCVI.[44]

CLASSIFICATION OF BLUNT CAROTID INJURY: THE DENVER SCALE

The Denver Scale (Table 61-2) has been widely accepted and used to classify blunt carotid injury.[50] It was employed to standardize and direct care for the different grades of vessel injury based on multiplanar CTA or DSA findings. Grade I to IV injuries typically warrant anticoagulation as the mainstay of treatment, with consideration of surgical intervention if contraindication of anticoagulation or further neurological deterioration exists. Grade V injury, which represents complete transection with extravasation, is most appropriately treated through surgical intervention, whether it be an endovascular or open approach.

TABLE 61-2	Denver Scale for Blunt Carotid Injury
TYPE/ GRADE	RADIOLOGICAL/ANGIOGRAPHIC FINDINGS AND CRITERIA
I	Vessel wall irregularity or dissection/intramural hematoma with <25% luminal stenosis
II	Presence of intraluminal thrombus, raised intimal flap, or dissection/intramural hematoma with ≥25% luminal stenosis
III	Presence of pseudoaneurysm
IV	Vessel occlusion
V	Complete transection with extravasation

From Biffl WL, Moore EE, Offner PJ, et al: Blunt carotid arterial injuries: Implications of a new grading scale. J Trauma 47:845–853, 1999.

CLINICAL MANAGEMENT

Despite increased awareness of blunt carotid injury, there is no agreement on the best therapeutic approach. Accumulated data suggest that conservative therapy using antithrombotic therapy with heparin prevents cerebral infarction. Similarly, antiplatelet therapy and anticoagulation with warfarin (international normalized ratio [INR] 2-3) were equally effective in reducing risk of stroke following BCVI.[45,51] In a recent analysis of the national trauma database, a comparison of functional independence following BCVI in patients treated conservatively (anticoagulation and/or antiplatelet agents) vs. operatively (open and endovascular treatment) was performed.[52] There was no difference in functional outcome in these patients, regardless of conservative or operative intervention. The only demographic difference among the groups was greater injury severity score in patients undergoing endovascular repair. In most studies, BCVI in surgically accessible areas are treated operatively; however, the vast majority of BCVI lesions occur in surgically challenging areas high within the carotid canal or foramen transversarium. Such locations make standard operative approaches for thrombectomy or reconstruction difficult.[53]

Venous Injury in the Neck

Major cervicothoracic venous injury can pose added complexity to a trauma situation, especially when concomitant arterial injury is present. Venous bleeding can be temporized with direct pressure, and in scenarios of troublesome hemorrhage, the brachiocephalic, internal jugular, or subclavian veins can be ligated with relative impunity. If primary repair can be accomplished without compromising more than 50% of the injured vessel, a lateral venorrhaphy is appropriate. Repair/reconstruction should always be done in the presence of obvious venous hypertension or for one of the brachiocephalic or internal jugular veins if bilateral injury is present.

Abdominal Vascular Injuries

Abdominal vascular injury represents 5% to 25% of all abdominal traumatic injuries[54] and carries a mortality rate of 31% to 87%.[55] With penetrating trauma overwhelmingly the most common etiology of traumatic vascular injury (>90% of cases), any penetrating injury to the torso from the upper thigh to the level of the nipples should generate high suspicion for vascular injury.[56] Most patients with major abdominal vascular injury present with a contained or partially contained retroperitoneal hematoma. Patients who suffer major free intraperitoneal hemorrhage frequently die at the scene of injury. Patients with free retroperitoneal or intraabdominal hemorrhage who make it to the hospital usually present with profound hypotension in class IV hemorrhagic shock.[56] The incidence of arterial and venous injury is similar and depends on the location, force, and mechanism of the insult. The association of abdominal vascular trauma with assault and aggressive behavior accounts for a shocking 90% to 95% of cases.[55]

When vascular injury is present in the abdomen, the aorta and IVC are most commonly injured—25% and 33%, respectively.[57] The overall mortality rate from penetrating abdominal vascular injuries is 45%, but associated injuries to the abdominal aorta, hepatic veins, retrohepatic vena cava, and/or the portal vein can elevate it to as high as 90%.[35,54] Despite our advances in technology and surgical/medical techniques, no significant changes have occurred with regard to mortality associated with abdominal vascular trauma over the last 20 to 30 years. This reflects the lethal potential of these injuries and the fact that patients presenting in shock with vascular injury continue to have a high mortality rate.[58]

Clinical Presentation and Evaluation

Of those patients with abdominal vascular injury who make it to the hospital, about 14% will lose vital signs en route; thus, minimizing the time from injury to delivery at a medical care facility can result in a significant improvement in outcomes.[59] In addition to prehospital time, the clinical presentation will depend on the mechanism of injury, vessel injured, severity of the injury, and presence of other associated injuries. Blunt trauma causes vascular injury through rapid deceleration, anterior/posterior crushing, or laceration from sharp bony fractures. These patients often initially present with stable vital signs, but may rapidly decompensate because of the insidious evolution of blunt abdominal trauma. In contrast, penetrating vascular trauma to the abdomen presents in a less subtle manner.

Regardless of the mechanism, operative exploration is paramount and must be done expeditiously, foregoing any diagnostic imaging in a hemodynamically unstable patient with suspected abdominal vascular injury. Cautious resuscitation is prudent in hemodynamically unstable patients. Excessive fluid resuscitation of an actively hemorrhaging patient can potentiate ongoing blood loss and coagulopathy.[60–62] To maintain end-organ perfusion until definitive control of hemorrhaging is obtained, cessation of bleeding and permissive hypotension should be the initial goals of resuscitation.

RETROPERITONEAL HEMATOMAS

Retroperitoneal hematomas occur in more than 90% of abdominal vascular injuries.[59] The retroperitoneum is divided into three main zones of injury: zone I is the central/midline retroperitoneum, zone II encompasses the perinephric space, and zone III comprises the pelvic retroperitoneum. Treatment of retroperitoneal hematomas varies depending on the anatomical location and mechanism of injury.

Zone I injuries mandate exploration for both penetrating and blunt injury because of the major vascular structures residing in this region and the unforgiving consequences if injury diagnosis is delayed. The transverse mesocolon subdivides this zone into the central supra- and infra-mesocolic spaces. Hematomas in the central supramesocolic space develop behind the lesser omentum and push the stomach forward. These hematomas result from injury to the suprarenal aorta, celiac axis, proximal superior mesenteric artery (SMA), or proximal renal arteries. Thus, for surgical exploration, proximal control of the aorta should be obtained at the level of the diaphragm, and exposure carried out with a left-sided medial visceral rotation (Mattox maneuver). Central infra-mesocolic hematomas present behind the root of the small-bowel mesentery are a consequence of either infrarenal aorta or IVC injury. Exposure is obtained through a retroperitoneal opening on the midline, and control of the aorta is gained above the celiac axis.

Zone II retroperitoneal hematomas are commonly due to injury to the renal vasculature or parenchyma. All zone II hematomas secondary to penetrating trauma necessitate operative exploration because of the risk for vascular laceration. Stable zone II hematomas following blunt trauma are best managed conservatively because exploration entails opening the Gerota fascia, which under these conditions bears a high likelihood of causing further injury to an already damaged kidney.

Pelvic retroperitoneal hematomas, or zone III hematomas, are typically managed nonoperatively. Iliac vessel injury or suspicion of it represents the only true indication for surgical exploration. This is more common following penetrating injury to the pelvis, as opposed to those of blunt mechanisms. Hematomas arising from blunt means typically result from pelvic fractures, where external fixation and angiographic coil embolization represent the best treatment modalities.

Diagnostic Imaging

In many instances of penetrating abdominal vascular injury with clinical instability, imaging studies are irrelevant because the diagnosis will be made in the operating room. However, for a patient who is hemodynamically stable and not in need of urgent surgical intervention, it is appropriate to use imaging modalities for further evaluation. Plain radiographs provide information regarding the location of ballistic or shrapnel fragments in the abdomen. This information, in conjunction with the location of the penetrating wounds, can give some idea of the trajectory/path of the missile, and thus the imperiled vascular structures.

Ultrasonography is an easy and readily accessible means of acutely assessing for hemoperitoneum following trauma to the abdomen.[63] The FAST exam, which is an acronym for Focused Assessment with Sonography in Trauma, is performed immediately after the primary survey per the Advanced Trauma Life Support (ATLS) protocol. The confirmation of fluid in the abdomen during the FAST exam, coupled with hemodynamic instability, affirms the plan of immediate laparotomy. Ultrasonography is limited in its ability to delineate the presence of retroperitoneal hematomas and the morphology of visceral vasculature injury. Therefore, it is not the modality of choice to assess the extent of vascular injury in the abdomen. However, its use is significantly valuable in assessing morphology of vascular injury elsewhere in the body.

Multidetector CT scanners remain the mainstay for fast, reliable imaging in the setting of trauma, where sound clinical decisions have to be made in a timely fashion. Contrast CT of the abdomen reveals the integrity of solid organs, confirms presence or absence of free air/fluid, delineates vasculature morphology, and can illustrate traumatic pathology in the retroperitoneum. This means of imaging provides the largest amount of accurate information noninvasively in the shortest amount of time. In abdominal vascular trauma, angiography plays a more substantial role in therapeutic means, such as coil embolization of hemorrhage with pelvic fractures. In hemodynamically stable patients who are found to have vascular injury on contrast CT imaging, subsequent angiography coupled with endovascular techniques may provide therapeutic options.

Operative Management and Damage Control

There should be no delay in getting a patient who meets the criteria for surgery to the operating room. The room should prewarmed and appropriate IV fluid, blood products, and infusion mechanisms should be ready for ongoing resuscitation efforts during surgery. The patient should be placed in the supine position with their entire torso from neck to knees prepped. The abdomen should be opened on the midline. If concern for concomitant vascular injuries in the thorax and abdomen exist, a pad or roll can be placed under the left torso and back to make abdominal and thoracic approaches equally accessible.

Varying degrees of intraperitoneal hemorrhage and/or retroperitoneal hematomas will be found, depending on the mechanism of trauma. Blunt injury is more likely to produce retroperitoneal hematomas, and a distinction must be made as to whether the hematoma is stable or expanding and/or pulsatile. Penetrating injury is more likely to produce intraabdominal hemorrhage or a combination of the two. The operative approach and management are dependent on the location of the injured vessel, location and characteristics of the retroperitoneal hematoma, and overall condition of the patient.

Aortic cross-clamping can be a means of obtaining comprehensive proximal control in the face of massive hemorrhage and as an adjunct to resuscitation. Control should be gained at the supraceliac aorta at the level of the diaphragm. This location is easily accessible and less likely to be a site of iatrogenic injury to neighboring structures. If the injury is proximal in the abdominal aorta, control of the aorta may have to be obtained through the chest via a left lateral thoracotomy. Cross-clamping the aorta will help control hemorrhage and elevate blood pressure, but causes ischemia to the abdominal viscera and lower extremities. Thus, aortic cross-clamping should only be employed in the most extreme circumstances.

Different maneuvers can be undertaken to gain the needed exposure for particular regions and structures in the abdomen. To expose the entire length of the abdominal aorta and most of its branches, a left-sided medial visceral rotation was described by Mattox et al. in 1974.[64] The only artery not accessible via this approach is the right renal artery. The *Mattox maneuver* is implemented by taking down the lateral peritoneal attachments of the sigmoid and left colon. The left colon, left kidney, and spleen are then swept/mobilized medially toward the midline, exposing the retroperitoneum and aorta. A right-sided medial visceral rotation can also be done, providing exposure to the infrarenal vena cava and iliac vessels. This is called an *extended Kocher maneuver*. The right colon along with the third and fourth portion of duodenum may be released from their lateral attachments, then reflected medially and superiorly using the *Cattell-Braasch maneuver*.[65] This maneuver provides additional exposure to the suprarenal IVC and makes the portal venous system accessible. This exposure is extensive and provides access to most of the structures in the retroperitoneum.

Appropriate operative management for the different zones of the retroperitoneum and for specific vascular injuries are covered elsewhere in the chapter. However, once the extent of injury has been identified, the American Association for the Surgery of Trauma Organ Injury Scale (AAST-OIS) for abdominal vascular injury should be used to determine the severity of injury and overall prognosis (Table 61-3). This grading scale has demonstrated excellent correlation between mortality and extent of vascular damage following trauma.[66] Understanding the extent of injury and risk of mortality should be factored into the treatment plan that ensues.

Many patients with abdominal vascular injury who warrant immediate surgery will also face the "trauma triad of death": acidosis, hypothermia, and coagulopathy. Under these conditions, a definitive repair or reconstruction of the injured vessel(s) may place an insurmountable burden on the patient. In these circumstances, a damage-control philosophy is the most appropriate therapeutic management.[67] In a damage-control scenario, major venous injuries are ligated, retroperitoneal bleeding/oozing is packed off tightly, and arterial injuries are temporarily shunted. The abdomen is temporarily closed with a prosthetic material,

and the patient is transferred to the intensive care unit (ICU) for resuscitation. Definitive vascular repair and abdominal closure are deferred until the patient has been adequately resuscitated and his/her condition has stabilized.

Specific Abdominal Vascular Injuries

ABDOMINAL AORTA

The aorta is the largest artery in the body, and its abdominal portion spans from where it traverses the diaphragm at the level of T12 to where it bifurcates into the iliac arteries at the L4/L5 level. It is the most commonly injured artery in the abdomen following trauma; many times, aortic injury presents as a lethal condition. Blunt injury to the abdominal aorta is most often associated with motor vehicle accidents, followed by falls and direct blows to the abdomen. The mortality associated with blunt aortic injury is estimated to be around 30%.[56,68] Penetrating trauma remains the most common method of injury to the abdominal aorta and carries a significantly higher mortality than blunt injury. Mortality following penetrating injury (e.g., fire arm blasts, knife stab wounds, etc.), has been estimated to be between 67% and 85%.[69]

Many patients with significant aortic injury never make it to the hospital. The fortunate few who make it to a medical care facility present with injuries such as intimal disruptions, thrombosis, and/or contained retroperitoneal hematomas.[54,55,59,63,70] The clinical presentation will depend on the mechanism of trauma, type of aortic injury, prehospital time, and associated traumatic vascular and nonvascular injuries. Penetrating injuries typically present in a dramatic fashion with profound hypotension, shock, and hemodynamic collapse. Under certain conditions, an emergency resuscitative thoracotomy can temporize cardiovascular collapse in order to get the patient to the operating room for definitive surgical intention.

Ultrasonography during the FAST exam can immediately inform the trauma team of the presence of free intraperitoneal fluid and, in the setting of hemodynamic instability, the affirmative need for operative intervention. Blunt injuries tend to have a less dramatic presentation with normotensive patients but can still have significant injury leading to visceral, renal, or lower-extremity ischemia. Multidetector CT scans provide a fast, accurate method of evaluating aortic injuries in hemodynamically stable patients. The diagnosis in unstable patients should be made during laparotomy. Depending on the findings from clinical examination and imaging studies, endovascular techniques can be implemented to treat both penetrating and blunt acute traumatic injuries.[3,71-74]

The significantly high incidence of associated injuries following penetrating abdominal trauma (>90%)[75] make open surgical intervention the gold standard for repair, in part because assessing and treating bowel and solid-organ injuries are critical. When the abdomen is explored, all four quadrants should be packed off, then examination of the quadrants should be done meticulously to identify all injuries, vascular and nonvascular alike. For supramesocolic zone I injuries, proximal control is obtained by clamping or compressing the aorta as it traverses the diaphragm. If the injury to the aorta resides high on the abdominal aorta, proximal control can be gained above the diaphragm through a left thoracotomy. The injured portion of the aorta or associated injured vessels can be exposed by means of a left-sided medial visceral rotation (Mattox maneuver). Infra-mesocolic zone I hematomas result from injury to either the infrarenal aorta or IVC. In this scenario, proximal control is gained at the supraceliac aorta, and exposure is provided by opening the posterior peritoneum in the midline.

Endovascular management is becoming far more frequently used with aortic trauma, and is more common following blunt injury than penetrating injury.[3,73,74] Much of the impetus for its use in trauma has been drawn from the success of stent grafting in the treatment of nontraumatic aortic disease (e.g., aneurysms, ruptures, dissections, fistula formations, thrombosis). The extension of endovascular techniques into the setting of trauma is logical and has provided more treatment options for patients presenting with contained retroperitoneal hematomas.[73] If a patient has a perforated

TABLE 61-3	American Association for the Surgery of Trauma Organ Injury Scale for Vascular Injury*
GRADE	**EXTENT OF VASCULAR INJURY**
I	Injury to an unnamed branch of the superior mesenteric artery or vein
	Injury to an unnamed branch of the inferior mesenteric artery or vein
	Phrenic artery or vein injury
	Lumbar artery or vein injury
	Gonadal artery or vein injury
	Ovarian artery or vein injury
	Unnamed small artery or vein requiring ligation
II	Right hepatic, left hepatic or common hepatic artery injury
	Splenic artery or vein injury
	Right or left gastric artery injury
	Gastroduodenal artery injury
	Inferior mesenteric artery, trunk, or vein injury
	Primary named branches of mesenteric artery or vein injury
	Other named vessels requiring ligation of repair
III	Superior mesenteric vein, trunk injury
	Renal artery or vein injury
	Iliac artery or vein injury
	Hypogastric artery or vein injury
	Vena caval, infrarenal injury
IV	Superior mesenteric artery, trunk injury
	Celiac axis proper injury
	Vena caval, suprarenal, and infrahepatic injury
	Aortic, infrarenal injury
V	Portal vein injury
	Extraparenchymal hepatic vein injury
	Vena caval, retrohepatic, or suprahepatic injury
	Aortic, suprarenal, and subdiaphragmatic injury

*Classification system applicable for extraparenchymal vascular injury. Increase one grade for multiple grade III or grade IV injuries involving >50% of the vessel circumference. Downgrade one grade if the laceration is <25% of the vessel circumference for grade IV or V injuries.

viscous, small-bowel anastomosis, partial colectomy, or ostomy, endoluminal treatment of associated arterial injuries avoids opening the retroperitoneum and placing a prosthetic conduit in a contaminated field.

CELIAC AXIS INJURY

Celiac artery injuries are rare and almost always a result of penetrating trauma. In a review of 302 patients with abdominal vascular injuries, the celiac artery was injured in only 3.3% of cases.[59] The celiac axis gives rise to the left gastric, splenic, and common hepatic arteries. Injuries amenable to primary repair should be carried out, but ligation of the artery can be done without ischemic sequelae because of the robust collateral circulation of the proximal gastrointestinal tract. That being said, endovascular coiling and embolization is a frequently used technique for controlling hemorrhage from the hepatic and splenic vasculature following blunt trauma.[76] The mortality rate for celiac axis injuries has been reported to range between 38% and 75%.[56] However, many of these patients have associated vascular injuries that contribute to the high mortality rate; isolated celiac injury likely carries a much lower mortality rate.

SUPERIOR MESENTERIC ARTERY AND VEIN INJURY

Superior mesenteric artery injury presents as either free intraperitoneal hemorrhage, a central (zone I) supramesocolic retroperitoneal hematoma, ischemic proximal small bowel, or any combination of the three. Superior mesenteric artery injuries account for roughly 10% of all abdominal vascular injuries[59] and are diagnosed in less than 0.1% of total trauma admissions.[77] It is the second most commonly injured abdominal vascular structure following blunt trauma, but penetrating trauma accounts for the significant majority of SMA injuries.[77] The mortality rate associated with SMA injury is estimated to be as high as 47% to 67%.[54,56,59,77]

The SMA is divided into four anatomical zones of injury, which were first described by Fullen et al.,[78] who also correlated grade of ischemia with injury location (Table 61-4). The affected zone, ischemic grade, and AAST-OIS for abdominal vascular trauma correlate well with mortality.[77,79] The surgical approach is driven by the location of the injury. Injuries to the first two zones should undergo primary repair whenever possible. Ligation of the artery at these levels would result in significant small-bowel ischemia and a poor prognosis without revascularization. Revascularization with autogenous or prosthetic conduits is another option and sometimes necessitates extra-anatomical routes. Zone III and IV injuries should be primarily repaired as well. Should ligation at these levels or of the segmental branches prove necessary for hemostasis, only local ischemia to the small bowel will follow, which segmental bowel resection can remedy. A second-look laparotomy is mandatory to asses the viability and integrity of the small bowel following any surgical manipulation of the SMA. Endovascular techniques have been implemented in limited cases but have demonstrated promise.[80]

Superior mesenteric vein (SMV) injuries are infrequent but incur high mortality rates due to the difficulty in obtaining prompt exposure and hemorrhage control, combined with the high incidence of concomitant portal vein injury.[81] Lateral venorrhaphy is the preferred surgical means of repair for an isolated SMV injury. Graft conduits can restore flow, but thrombosis can be a devastating complication. Ligation of the vein is a plausible surgical option, especially in hemodynamically unstable patients,[81] but carries a risk of venous mesenteric ischemia secondary to splanchnic sequestration. Aggressive resuscitation is vital following venous ligation, and a second-look laparotomy is again standard, as with SMA injuries.

INFERIOR MESENTERIC ARTERY AND VEIN INJURY

Injury to the inferior mesenteric artery (IMA) is typically managed by ligation.[56] In rare cases, collateral circulation to the descending and sigmoid colons and the upper rectum may be inadequate and result in ischemia to these regions of bowel. Again, this is a very rare occurrence because of the rich collateral flow via the marginal artery and its arcade. Ligation of the inferior mesenteric vein is tolerated much better than that of the SMV and can be done with impunity.

RENOVASCULAR INJURIES

Renovascular injury is relatively uncommon following trauma. The kidney itself is injured in only 1.2% of all trauma cases, and vascular injury only accounts for 2.5% to 4% of those cases.[82] It does, however, represent roughly 16% of all abdominal vascular trauma.[59] Renovascular injury is more common following blunt as opposed to penetrating trauma, with blunt trauma making up almost 80% of cases.

The clinical presentation is most often subtle with regard to the vascular injury itself, but associated injuries can cause a more concerning clinical picture, frequently taking precedence over the renovascular injuries. Unlike many other vascular injuries, exsanguination from the renal vasculature is uncommon and is usually contained in the retroperitoneum. Flank pain, proteinuria, and hematuria (gross and microscopic) are findings that indicate the presence of renal vascular injury, but are neither always present nor specific for vascular injury itself. Computed tomography is the best first-line imaging modality for renovascular injuries.[83] It can illustrate the extent of parenchymal damage and perfusion, along with the morphology of the retroperitoneal hematoma. Angiography coupled with endovascular techniques is frequently needed to confirm and sometimes treat the vascular injuries.

Renal function is diminished significantly following just 3 to 6 hours of ischemic insult. If revascularization is to be done, it should be accomplished within this window, despite a success rate of 28% for renal function preservation.[84] Revascularization can be done via primary repair, vein patch angioplasty, interposition grafting, or segmental resection with reanastomosis. This is usually performed if the injury is found during operative exploration or when there is bilateral vascular injury in an attempt to preserve some renal function. A nephrectomy is an accepted surgical treatment/option for devastating unilateral renovascular injuries. Studies support that nephrectomy in the setting of major unilateral vascular injury has comparable mortality, posttreatment renal function, transfusion requirements, and level of service as that of repair.[82,85] Renal vein injury can be repaired similarly to the artery. If devastating injury occurs to the left renal vein, ligation is acceptable. Ligation of the left renal vein near its confluence with the IVC can be tolerated because

TABLE 61-4	**Fullen's Anatomical Classification of Superior Mesenteric Artery Injury by Zone and Grade**				
ZONE	**SEGMENT OF ARTERY**	**GRADE**	**ISCHEMIC CATEGORY**	**ISCHEMIC BOWEL SEGMENTS**	
I	Trunk proximal to first major branch (inferior pancreaticoduodenal artery)	1	Maximal	Jejunum, ileum, right colon	
II	Trunk between inferior pancreaticoduodenal artery and middle colic artery	2	Moderate	Major segment, right colon, small bowel, or both	
II	Trunk distal to middle colic artery	3	Minimal	Minor segment(s), small bowel or right colon	
IV	Segmental braches; jejunal, ileal, or colic arteries	4	None	No ischemic bowel	

Adapted from Fullen WD, Hunt J, Altemeier WA: The clinical spectrum of penetrating injury to the superior mesenteric arterial circulation. J Trauma 12:656–664, 1972.

of accessory venous drainage through the left gonadal, left adrenal, and lumbar veins. Attempts to repair the right renal vein should be made, since the absence of adequate venous collateral flow on the right side will lead to a right nephrectomy. Endovascular approaches to manage renovascular trauma have been useful in selected instances of pseudoaneurysm formation, intimal tears, or AVFs.[85-87]

Mortality is hard to estimate because of the significant occurrence of major associated injuries that drive the data. Rates of posttraumatic renal failure and hypertension are low and in two studies were estimated to be 6.4% and 4.5%, respectively.[85,88]

ILIAC VESSEL INJURY

Exsanguination from iliac vessel injuries is common and associated with high mortality resulting from refractory hemorrhage and associated injuries.[89-91] Mortality rates range from 25% to 40%, but the incidence of iliac vessel injury represents 10% of all abdominal vascular injuries and less than 2% of all vascular trauma.[91] Gaining surgical control of the bleeding can be challenging, and many of these patients present acidotic, coagulopathic, and hypothermic from extensive blood loss.[90,91] The close proximity and shared course of the iliac veins make combined arteriovenous injuries a frequent occurrence. The small bowel, colon, urinary bladder, and ureters intimately cohabitate the microenvironment of the iliac vessels, and concomitant injury to these structures are the rule rather than the exception. Extent of injury to the surrounding structures and degree of enteric contamination are principal factors that can increase the complexity of management with regard to repair and/or revascularization.

Injury to the iliac artery or suspicion of it is a clear indication for surgery in zone III retroperitoneal injuries. Proximal control is gained at the infra-mesocolic aorta, with distal control gained at the external iliac at the level of the inguinal ligament. The ascending colon is reflected medially via a Kocher or Cattell-Braasch maneuver, exposing the pelvic retroperitoneum. Primary arteriorrhaphy is the preferred method of repair for a simple injury. Reconstruction can also be accomplished with end-to-end anastomosis of autogenous saphenous vein or polytetrafluoroethylene (PTFE) grafts.[90] It is important to be cognizant of the fact that prosthetic grafts may be problematic in an environment contaminated by associated small-bowel or colon injury. Iliac injuries are amenable to bailout or damage-control procedures in the circumstance of a patient critically ill due to other traumatic injuries, where an extensive operation is too high risk. Temporary shunt insertion, arterial ligation with delayed extra-anatomical reconstruction, or balloon

tamponade of venous injury may be employed in this situation. Iliac vein injury can be even more complex with regard to gaining access and control of the vessel. Occasionally, the iliac artery must be divided to allow adequate access to the venous structures, and then reconstructed following venous repair. Concerns of edema and compartment syndrome following prolonged ischemic time or vein ligation merit a low threshold for lower-extremity fasciotomies. Endovascular techniques have shown utility in selected cases of isolated iliac artery injury. Patients with AVFs, pseudoaneurysms, or major intimal tears may benefit from endovascular stenting and/or coiling rather than open exploration[92,93] (Fig. 61-3).

INFERIOR VENA CAVA

The IVC is the most commonly injured vessel in the abdomen, accounting for one fourth of abdominal vascular injuries.[59] About 90% of injuries to the IVC are a result of penetrating trauma, and approximately 18% have associated aortic injury.[94,95] More than half of patients with IVC injuries will die before reaching the hospital. Of those who make it to a medical care facility, more than half are in class III hemorrhagic shock.[95] The most important prognostic factors following IVC injury are the grade of hemorrhagic shock, anatomical level of IVC injury, and associated vascular injuries.[58,94-96] Supra- and retrohepatic lacerations have the worst prognosis, and their management can be challenging.

Some IVC injuries present with a contained zone I retroperitoneal hematoma, and the patient will remain hemodynamically stable. In this circumstance, a decision for expectant management for lesions in the retro- or suprahepatic vena cava would be reasonable, despite the dogma of zone I retroperitoneal hematoma treatment. There is a considerable degree of difficulty and mortality associated with surgical exploration.[95,96] Surgical exploration for lesions behind the liver may involve combined entry into the chest and abdomen and require extensive mobilization of the liver, atriocaval shunting, total vascular occlusion, or hepatic vascular isolation. In extreme circumstances, direct exposure of the IVC can also be accomplished through division of the liver along the Cantlie line, though it is rarely employed and only if there is already significant injury to the liver.

Infrarenal caval ligation can be an acceptable treatment in a hemodynamically unstable patient with significant associated traumatic injuries. Ligation above the level of the renal veins would lead to fulminant renal failure and is not an appropriate option. Reconstruction with autogenous vein or prosthetic conduits are the most appropriate treatments despite the low success rate due

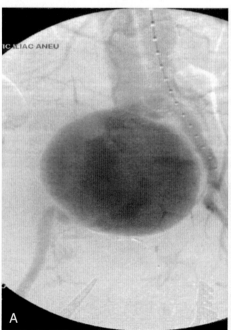

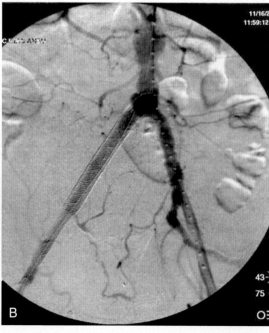

FIGURE 61-3 Penetrating iliac artery injury. A, Arteriogram revealed 10-cm right common iliac artery (CIA) aneurysm with iliocaval fistulae following gunshot wound to abdomen. **B,** Arteriogram following successful deployment and placement of a covered stent.

to the extreme condition of the patient. If ligation of the infrarenal IVC is done, the patient's bilateral lower extremities should be wrapped and elevated to prevent morbid lower-extremity edema. Patients can experience transient edema in the lower extremities following primary repair of the IVC that causes stenosis. Older patients with IVC stenosis following repair are at increased risk for a pulmonary embolus, so some have advocated vena cava filter placement superior to the repair.[95]

PORTAL VEIN INJURY

The portal vein is made up by the confluence of the superior mesenteric and splenic veins behind the neck of the pancreas. It constitutes 80% of the hepatic blood flow and provides 50% of the hepatic oxygen demand. Its injury accounts for 5% of all abdominal vascular injuries.[59] The vast majority are a result of penetrating trauma (90%) and associated with other vascular injuries 70% to 90% of the time.[97] Following penetrating injury, patients usually present with hemorrhagic shock and require an emergent laparotomy. Blunt trauma causing a direct blow to the abdomen or severe deceleration forces can injure the portal vein, usually in combination with the SMV.

The operative exposure for these injuries can be extensive, using an extensive right-sided medial visceral rotation of the ascending colon and duodenum. In some circumstances, especially with combined SMV injuries, this exposure may not be adequate, warranting division of the neck of the pancreas to increase exposure. These patients present in such poor condition that complex reconstructions are rarely feasible or advisable. Primary repair, if acquiescent, is the best surgical treatment. Complex reconstructions should only be done in patients with associated hepatic artery injury not amenable to repair. The combined absence of blood flow through the portal vein and hepatic artery is not compatible with life. These situations merit revascularization with autogenous saphenous vein graft.[97] Ligation is another option that should be considered for devastating retropancreatic injuries. Similar to ligation of the SMV, splanchnic bed sequestration can lead to patchy bowel-wall necrosis. Massive fluid resuscitation should be expected postoperatively. Historical data indicate survival rates between 55% and 85% following ligation.[97-99] The abdomen should be left open and vacuumed packed, with a planned return visit to the operating room in roughly 48 hours. The mortality rate associated with portal vein injuries can be as high as 50% to 72%.[59,98,99]

Extremity Vascular Injury

Males 20 to 40 years of age represent the majority the population affected by peripheral vascular trauma. Trauma to peripheral vascular structures accounts for roughly 80% of all vascular trauma and poses significant disability to a relatively young population. Arterial ligation had been the standard of care from the time of Galen and the gladiatorial games of Rome through World War II. Advances in technique and surgical philosophy during the Korean and Vietnam Wars with regard to arterial revascularization and limb salvage fostered a significant reduction in amputation rates. This revolutionized vascular management of trauma, decreased morbidity, and significantly improved outcomes.

Evaluation of patients with suspected peripheral vascular injury should be performed promptly and thoroughly. Special attention should be paid to the hard and soft signs of vascular injury, as well as the viability of the extremity. Despite the fact that over 80% of patients with vascular injury will present with absent pulses, shock, or neurological deficits, some will have arterial injuries yet also have distal pulses in the affected extremity and be hemodynamically stable.[100]

Mangled Extremity Score

Assessing the viability of an extremity following trauma can be difficult. Some patients require a primary amputation because of the unsalvageable nature of their limb after trauma. The Mangled Extremity Severity Score (Table 61-5) is an objective set of criteria used to predict the need for amputation in the upper and lower extremities following trauma. It takes into account the extent of soft-tissue/skeletal damage, degree of ischemia, level of systemic hypotension, and age. A score of 7 or higher is the threshold for performing an amputation.

Noninvasive Studies

Doppler ultrasonography has been a valuable resource in the acute assessment of extremity vascular injury. Its accuracy in detecting vascular injury is high, but limited in its ability to detect intimal defects and small false aneurysms. B-mode ultrasonography is also an easily accessible and inexpensive study that provides good resolution and the ability to diagnose small vascular defects that would otherwise be missed by Doppler or physical examination.[100]

Measuring the *ankle-brachial index* (ABI) is always helpful. The ABI is a ratio of the systolic blood pressure at the ankle relative to that of the brachial artery. An ABI of less than 0.9 is indicative of vascular disease and, in the setting of trauma, vascular injury.

Computed tomography angiography and MRA are more expensive studies but offer the most accurate noninvasive anatomical assessment of peripheral vascular injury. Computed tomography angiography is used more frequently because of the presence of multiplanar CT scanners within close proximity to most level I trauma/emergency bays.

Angiography

In hemodynamically stable patients, catheter-based contrast angiography is an excellent modality for evaluation and provides the opportunity for therapeutic measures as indicated. In general, angiography is commonly used following blunt extremity injury but may prove useful in many circumstances. For example, it can be extremely useful in cases with extensive global damage to the limb, multiple complex fractures, gunshot wounds, and injuries resulting in extensive soft-tissue defects.[100] Its use intraoperatively and even for postoperative evolution makes it the gold standard of most vascular evaluation and treatment modalities.

TABLE 61-5	Mangled Extremity Severity Score	
	FACTOR	SCORE
Skeletal/Soft-Tissue Injury		
Low energy (stab, simple fracture, low-energy GSW)		1
Medium energy (open or multiple fractures, dislocation)		2
High energy (close-range shotgun or "military" GSW, crush)		3
Very high energy (above conditions plus contamination, avulsion)		4
Limb Ischemia (Score Double For >6 Hours of Ischemia)		
Pulse reduced but perfusion normal		1
Pulseless, paresthesias, decreased capillary refill		2
Cool, paralyzed, insensate, numbness		3
Hypotension		
Systolic BP >90 mmHg		0
Transient hypotension		1
Persistent hypotension		2
Age (Years)		
<30		0
30-50		1
>50		2

BP, blood pressure; GSW, gunshot wound. Adapted from Johansen K, Daines M, Howey T, et al: Objective criteria accurately predict amputation following lower extremity trauma. J Trauma 30: 568–572, 1990.

Specific Peripheral Vascular Injuries

SUBCLAVIAN-AXILLARY INJURY

Much of the course of the subclavian/axillary artery and vein are covered by the clavicle and overlying pectoralis musculature, making injury to these structures uncommon. Penetrating trauma accounts for the overwhelming majority of cases.[101] Concomitant injury of artery and vein occurs in roughly 20% of cases.[102] Blunt injury to these structures are rare, but clavicle and first rib fractures/dislocations have been associated with blunt vascular injury in multiple studies.[102-104]

Minimizing prehospital time is key to successful management of these injuries. Upon presentation, critical ischemia of the upper extremity is uncommon, and a palpable pulse may be present in the extremity owing to the rich collateral circulation around the axillary artery. Uncontained hemorrhage from these injuries can be devastating and result in mortality at the scene. One study demonstrated an overall mortality rate of 39% in a series of 54 consecutive subclavian artery injuries.[101] Another review of 79 patients illustrated that more than 20% of patients with subclavian/axillary injuries arrived at a medical care facility with no vital signs or imminent cardiac arrest due to massive hemorrhage.[102]

If a proximal venous injury from a neck or chest wound is suspected, the patient should be placed in the Trendelenburg position to avoid an embolus (based on the Bernoulli principle of fluid dynamics). In the presence of profound hypotension, major hemorrhage, or an ischemic/threatened limb, surgical intervention should not be delayed. In a hemodynamically stable patient, a careful pulse examination of the upper extremities should be coupled with a low index of suspicion for further evaluation with ABI and/or color-flow Doppler studies.

Similar to other types of vascular injury, multidetector CT scanners are a useful modality, especially with penetrating missile injuries. One study demonstrated that multidetector CT scans were helpful in avoiding unnecessary angiography in 85% of cases involving transmediastinal gunshot wounds.[105] Angiography is less used in the diagnostic setting because of the utility and efficacy of color-flow Doppler and CT, but it continues to have a vital role in the therapeutic arena for managing subclavian and axillary injuries.[3,73,105-107]

The standard incision for a proximal axillary or midsubclavian artery injury extends from the jugular notch along the clavicle and then downward in the deltopectoral groove. This incision can be combined with a median sternotomy to gain exposure for proximal subclavian injuries. A trap-door incision has been described for proximal left subclavian injuries but carries a host of complications that can be avoided with anterolateral thoracotomy.

Endovascular therapy has been used with high success in both blunt and penetrating trauma in selected patients. Those who are hemodynamically stable and found to have traumatic AVFs, false aneurysms, and focal dissections are ideal candidates. It is important to note that lesions in close proximity to the origins of the vertebral and/or right CCAs may preclude safe deployment of an endovascular stent graft without covering the origin. One series reviewed 23 patients who underwent intervention for traumatic subclavian/axillary artery injuries. Patients who met the criteria for and underwent endovascular stenting had shorter operative time, less blood loss, and similar patency rates.[107]

BRACHIAL AND FOREARM VESSEL INJURY

The incidence of upper-extremity vascular trauma historically represents 30% of vascular trauma. The upper-arm arterial supply is made up by the brachial and deep brachial arteries. The forearm blood supply consists of the radial, ulnar, and interosseous arteries. Penetrating trauma is the most common etiology of injury, and the brachial artery is damaged more than half the time in upper-extremity vascular injuries.[108] The vascular component of upper-extremity trauma per se does not play a large role in overall mortality, compared to associated traumatic injuries. Nerve injury is widely accepted as the most important prognostic factor/indicator of function.[108] Concomitant bone, nerve, or venous injury has been observed to be as high as 73% in some studies.[109]

Angiography remains the gold standard for evaluation/diagnosis of upper-extremity injuries, but noninvasive studies provide good utility in the acute setting. Physical examination and duplex ultrasound studies can diagnose most significant injuries but may miss smaller or more subtle injuries. Compared to conventional angiography, small series have shown CTA to approach 95% sensitivity and 98% specificity for upper-extremity vascular lesions.[108] That accuracy, combined with the easy accessibility of CTA, makes it one of the most common modalities used in evaluating these injuries.

Expedient repair of all brachial or forearm arterial injuries is vital. Critical limb ischemia may develop in as short as 4 hours following injury if not repaired.[108] Furthermore, studies of arterial injuries of the upper extremity repaired more than 12 hours after the traumatic insult suggest that only 25% return to normal arm function.[110] Isolated injury to the radial or ulnar artery can usually tolerate ligation without subsequent ischemia because of the rich collateral circulation of the forearm and hand. However, it is important to remember that only 80% to 85% of the population has an intact palmer arch. Under these circumstances, the patient will need repair to the ulnar or radial artery to prevent hand ischemia. Although compartment syndrome is less commonly seen in the upper extremity than the lower extremity, a fasciotomy should be considered following any arterial repair in the arm.

FEMORAL VESSELS

Femoral vessel injury is among the most common vascular injuries, constituting approximately 70% of all peripheral vascular injuries.[111] More than 90% of femoral artery injuries result from penetrating trauma, primarily gunshot wounds.[100] Exsanguination does occur following these injuries, but the superficial course of the vessel allows for prehospital control of hemorrhage through direct pressure.

Obvious injury to the femoral vessels warrants transfer to a surgical suite for repair. Control of the external iliac vessels may be obtained before accessing the contents in the femoral triangle. Exposure of the femoral vessels can be gained through a linear incision along the medial edge of the sartorius muscle below the inguinal ligament. Combined vein and arterial injury can prove challenging, with venous bleeding occasionally proving more challenging than that of the arterial circuit. Historically, the most commonly injured extremity veins include the superficial femoral vein (42%), the popliteal vein (23%), and common femoral vein (14%).[112] The contralateral limb should be prepared in case autogenous vein grafts are needed for repair of the injured artery or vein.

In the case of small intimal flaps and pseudoaneurysms, observation, nonoperative management, or endovascular techniques (stenting, coiling, etc.) may provide effective therapy. Anticoagulation may not be an option in trauma patients, depending on the associated injuries, but if the decision for observation or nonoperative management is made, reevaluation by invasive (angiography) or noninvasive (ultrasound, CTA, MRA) methods should be performed to confirm convalescence.

Early diagnosis and aggressive management of femoral vessel injury has led to an amputation rate of less than 9%.[100] In contrast to the strategy employed for venous injury in other parts of the body, femoral vein repair is preferred to ligation. If the femoral vein is ligated, early fasciotomy and meticulous monitoring of compartment pressures should be performed.

CALF VESSEL INJURIES

The calf vessels include the vascular circuit starting and extending distally from the popliteal fossa. These vessels include the popliteal, anterior and posterior tibial, and peroneal arteries. Popliteal artery injuries represent one of the most challenging of all vascular extremity injuries to manage. The popliteal artery is the second most commonly injured artery in the leg, and more commonly results from penetrating injury. Blunt popliteal injury is most commonly seen following posterior knee dislocations,[113] which can have significant orthopedic and neurological consequences.

The outcome from popliteal injury depends importantly on the mode of injury. Amputation rates may reach as high as 20% to 50% following a high-velocity gun or shotgun blast, which may lead to significant soft-tissue injury and septic sequelae. A recent review of 24 published series demonstrated a much lower amputation rate of 11%, indicating the marked improvement in limb salvage in modern civilian series.[113,114] The rate of associated injury of local neurovascular structures (popliteal vein, tibial nerve, tibial/peroneal arteries, etc.) involved with penetrating popliteal injury ranges from 20% to 38%.[113,115–117]

The operative approach taken depends on the location of associated injuries. Popliteal vein injuries should be taken very seriously, with repair or reconstruction performed whenever possible. Because of the significant risk of reperfusion injury and venous congestion, a low threshold should be maintained for fasciotomy in the setting of severe popliteal vessel injury associated with prolonged ischemia or combined arterial/venous injury.

Injury to one of the three infrapopliteal arteries rarely results in limb ischemia in the absence of preexisting occlusive disease. In the setting of isolated hemorrhage from one of these vessels, ligation or embolization is an option. However, when the tibioperoneal truck or two or more of the infrapopliteal arteries are injured, repair or revascularization is vital for limb salvage. Nerve, bone, and soft-tissue damage in this region of the body plays a major role in limb salvage. Historical data demonstrate an amputation rate of 54% when associated orthopedic, nerve, and soft-tissue injuries are present.[118]

EXTREMITY VENOUS INJURY

The aggressive approach to arterial injury in the extremities has not been matched in the approach to venous repair. Venous ligation may result in thrombosis and venous insufficiency, ultimately leading to significant chronic disability. A balanced approach should include ligation for injury to minor veins, and repair or reconstruction for larger veins when possible.

Iatrogenic Vascular Injury

An increased incidence of iatrogenic vascular injury has been associated with the development of catheter-based cardiac and peripheral interventions to treat cardiovascular disease. Most of these injuries fall within the realm of penetrating vascular injuries. In a recent observational series, the commonest cause of vascular trauma (and with the lowest mortality rate) was catheter-based iatrogenic injury. While noniatrogenic injury occurred with the same incidence as penetrating/blunt trauma, it was associated with a fourfold excess mortality.[119] Many iatrogenic injuries have therapeutic solutions that can depend on catheter-based intervention, but direct surgical repair is occasionally required. The need for surgical intervention is usually dependent on the hemodynamic status of the patient at the time of injury, or the presence of significant ischemia due to the injury.

Pseudoaneurysms and Arteriovenous Fistulae

FALSE ANEURYSM

Suspicion of an iatrogenic pseudoaneurysm should occur in the setting of a swollen groin, excessive pain at the insertion site, or soft-tissue hematoma at the puncture site. Presence of a bruit and ongoing pulsatile bleeding are highly suggestive of a pseudoaneurysm. Arterial duplex examination has nearly 100% diagnostic accuracy, and if suspicion is present, no hesitation should delay obtaining the examination (also see Chapter 12). The test is simple, quick, and has excellent sensitivity and specificity. Duplex

ultrasonography can be performed at any location in the hospital but may be less efficacious in conditions of morbid obesity or when a very large hematoma is present. The location of certain vessels, including the subclavian, profunda femoris, and visceral arteries can make imaging by duplex ultrasound challenging owing to depth of the vessel, overlying bone, or bowel gas. Duplex ultrasound evaluation in the longitudinal and transverse planes is essential to identify the neck, confirm flow outside the artery, and accurately measure the size of the pseudoaneurysm. Typical characteristics seen on duplex ultrasound imaging include swirling of color flow in a mass distinct from the underlying artery, color flow signal through a tract leading to a sac, and to-and-fro Doppler waveform in the pseudoaneurysm neck. The precise definition of the false aneurysm size and neck is one of the most important parameters for determining treatment options. Larger neck and width often correlates directly with larger arterial defects that are generally more refractory to treatment with minimally invasive techniques. In the setting of a significant drop in blood pressure, decreasing hematocrit, or an obese patient, where duplex ultrasound examination is technically difficult, a CT scan with contrast may be useful to confirm the diagnosis of a pseudoaneurysm and exclude the presence of a large retroperitoneal hematoma.

ARTERIOVENOUS FISTULA

Although physical examination alone is not diagnostic for femoral pseudoaneurysm, it can be highly accurate and specific for detecting the presence of an AVF. A to-and-fro holosystolic/diastolic bruit at the puncture site is both diagnostic and pathognomonic for an AVF. In addition, the intensity of the sounds correlates with the size of the fistula. An ultrasound is unlikely to better characterize the extent of arteriovenous flow in the presence of these clinical findings. In the acute setting, femoral AVFs after groin interventions tend to be small in size and have significantly less flow than AVFs constructed for patients requiring hemodialysis. In certain situations, days, months, or years after trauma or a groin intervention, the insidious onset of heart failure, limb swelling, or claudication can be the initial presentation for an AVF.[120] The diagnosis of an AVF can be made by duplex ultrasound when the characteristic physical findings are not clearly present (also see Chapter 12). There are strict duplex ultrasound criteria for establishing a diagnosis of AVF:

1. A colorful speckled mass at the level of the fistula, with turbulent flow in the arteriovenous connection.
2. Increased venous flow in the proximal common femoral vein as compared to the contralateral side of the fistula.
3. No augmentation of venous flow with Valsalva.
4. Decreased arterial flow distal to the suspected fistula.

Computed tomography scans do not provide great efficacy in confirming the diagnosis of a femoral AVF, but in patients who have a more central fistula (aortocaval, iliac artery–iliac vein AVF), CT scanning is essential to delineate the arterial location of the connection and adjacent structures.

Treatment Options

FALSE ANEURYSMS

In the absence of impending cutaneous necrosis, femoral nerve compression symptoms, and continued bleeding despite local compression, most pseudoaneurysms can be managed conservatively with observation. In a study of femoral aneurysms 3 cm or less in diameter, not associated with severe pain, and in the setting of no systemic anticoagulation, there was an 89% spontaneous thrombosis rate with no complications. The mean time for thrombosis was 23 days, with a mean number of 2.6 duplex examinations per patient.[121] Loss or compromise of distal circulation, necrosis of overlying skin, uncontrolled bleeding despite compression, and reversal of anticoagulation mandates emergent surgical intervention to repair the femoral pseudoaneurysm.

Ultrasound-Guided Compression

Usually, direct compression should be performed in an unfed patient (to limit the risk of aspiration due to a vagal response) whose tissue is infiltrated with copious amounts of Xylocaine. A C-clamp or FemoStop can be applied to the apex of the false aneurysm for 30 to 40 minutes and slowly released over time.

Thrombin Injection

Ultrasound-guided thrombin injection (bovine and human thrombin) is currently the preferred treatment method in many centers. Because of the risk of immunoglobulin (Ig)E-mediated anaphylaxis, the bovine form should be used with caution in patients with a history of previous exposure. Some evidence exists to suggest that considerably lower doses of human thrombin are needed to treat pseudoaneurysms, so there is reduced risk for complications. Thrombin injection is accomplished by inserting a 22-gauge needle under direct ultrasound visualization through the superficial aspect of the pseudoaneurysm. Thrombin (usually 50-1000 units) is injected until blood flow ceases on color Doppler ultrasound imaging. Recurrence rates range from 0% to 9%; therefore, a repeat or serial ultrasounds are obtained within 24 hours of the initial injection. Intraarterial occlusion with thrombosis or embolization is estimated to be 2% and can be managed expectantly depending on the clinical situation. Thrombin injection is contraindicated in the presence of an AVF or a pseudoaneurysm with a very short, broad neck because of the risk of embolizing thrombin clot into the artery and down the leg.

Endovascular Repair

Traumatic injury to visceral and pelvic vessels can lead to false aneurysms that are best treated with percutaneous methods including microvascular coils, thrombotic agents, and covered stents. In many circumstances, prostheses developed to treat aneurysms can be modified to treat traumatic rupture and pseudoaneurysms of vessels on an individualized basis. To date, these endovascular repairs have been durable, and in the absence of life-threatening bleeding should be considered in light of many significant associated injuries.[3,122] Endovascular repair of iatrogenic injury to femoral vessels can be achieved quickly, but could inadvertently occlude the common femoral artery (CFA) because of kinking. The groin is an area of repetitive flexion, which can lead to stent fracture and thrombosis.

Surgical Intervention

In patients with impending skin necrosis or compression of the adjacent nerve or vein, urgent open repair of a pseudoaneurysm is indicated. On rare occasion, especially when the presentation is delayed or there is suspicion of an infectious process, access to the retroperitoneum may be necessary to achieve proximal control of lower-extremity inflow at the level of the iliac vessels. Regardless, exposure should be obtained proximal and distal to the puncture site, and digital control of the bleeding can be obtained. In most cases, the defect in the artery can be repaired primarily. It is essential to check the back wall of the artery to be sure there is not another source of bleeding. Rarely, when significant injury is present in a significantly diseased artery, a patch may be required to avoid compromising the lumen. Interrupted rather than continuous suture repair may be preferable because it allows precise placement of individual sutures and avoids excessive tension on the repair of the arterial suture line.

ARTERIOVENOUS FISTULAE

Femoral AVFs tend to persist in patients who are on steroids or suffer from chronic renal insufficiency. Implantation of covered stents in the femoral artery has been reported but appears to be contraindicated. As previously mentioned, there is considerable concern regarding complications of this approach, risks for restenosis, stent fracture due to frequent flexion in the groin region, and possible limitations for future femoral intervention.[123] Ongoing investigations will provide definitive understanding of the utility of this technique for managing femoral AVFs. In contrast to healthy concern about the durability of covered stent repairs in common femoral AVFs, the use of covered stents to manage iliac vein–iliac artery or aortocaval fistulas have been very effective.[124,125] Operative repair of a chronic AVF can be hazardous because of the friable nature of the vessels and the risk for considerable blood loss. Optimal treatment requires obliteration of the fistula and restoration of arterial and venous flow. At times, interposition grafting or patch angioplasty is needed to preserve flow without narrowing vessels. If there is a large defect in the vein, preoperative placement of arterial or venous balloons for intraoperative occlusion may help decrease hemorrhage during repair of the vessels feeding the fistula.

Pediatric Vascular Trauma

Vascular trauma in the pediatric population is uncommon, occurring in only 0.6% of all pediatric trauma patients. Although less frequent than in adults, penetrating trauma is responsible for a slight majority of pediatric vascular injuries.[126,127] Vascular trauma in children presents a unique challenge based on the characteristics of small, thin-walled vessels with poor tissue support and pronounced tendency for vasospasm in the setting of small intravascular volumes.[127,128] Vessels of the upper extremity are the most commonly injured and are associated with low mortality. Injuries of the thoracic aorta and great vessels are rare. Injury to the carotid artery is exceedingly rare but can have devastating morbidity and mortality if not recognized and managed promptly.[129] Decisions regarding operative management in the pediatric population must take into account vessel size and future growth potential, which may require future vascular revision. Amputations are usually reserved for severely mangled extremities; all attempts should be made for limb salvage. Overall, pediatric patients have an improved adjusted mortality when compared to adults.[130]

ACKNOWLEDGEMENTS

Dr. Long is the Visiting Surgical Research Fellow from the Department of Surgery, University of Tennessee–Knoxville. Dr Kwolek is the Program Director in Vascular and Endovascular Surgery at the Massachusetts General Hospital and Chief of Vascular Surgery at the Newton Wellesley Hospital. The authors acknowledge funding from the National Institutes of Health (1R01AR055843), the Foundation for Advanced Vascular Research (Wylie Scholar Award), and the Division of Vascular and Endovascular Surgery, Massachusetts General Hospital (The Geneen Fund). Dr. Watkins is the Isenberg Scholar in Academic Surgery at the Massachusetts General Hospital.

REFERENCES

1. DeBakey ME, Simeone FA: Battle injuries of the arteries in World War II; an analysis of 2,471 cases, *Ann Surg* 123:534–579, 1946.
2. Hughes CW: Arterial repair during the Korean war, *Ann Surg* 147(4):555–561, 1958.
3. Starnes BW, Arthurs ZM: Endovascular management of vascular trauma, *Perspect Vasc Surg Endovasc Ther* 18(2):114–129, 2006.
4. Giswold ME, Landry GJ, Taylor LM, et al: Iatrogenic arterial injury is an increasingly important cause of arterial trauma, *Am J Surg* 187(5):590–592, 2004; discussion 592–593.
5. Haimovici H: Arterial embolism with acute massive ischemic myopathy and myoglobinuria: evaluation of a hitherto unreported syndrome with report of two cases, *Surgery* 47:739–747, 1960.
6. Haimovici H: Myopathic-nephrotic-metabolic syndrome and massive acute arterial occlusions, *Arch Surg* 106(5):628–629, 1973.
7. Ames A 3rd, Wright RL, Kowada M, et al: Cerebral ischemia. II. The no-reflow phenomenon, *Am J Pathol* 52(2):437–453, 1968.
8. May JW Jr, Chait LA, O'Brien BM, et al: The no-reflow phenomenon in experimental free flaps, *Plast Reconstr Surg* 61(2):256–267, 1978.
9. Elliott KG, Johnstone AJ: Diagnosing acute compartment syndrome, *J Bone Joint Surg Br* 85(5):625–632, 2003.
10. Branco BC, Inaba K, Barmparas G, et al: Incidence and predictors for the need for fasciotomy after extremity trauma: a 10-year review in a mature level I trauma centre, *Injury*.
11. Yamane BH, Tefera G, Hoch JR, et al: Blunt thoracic aortic injury: open or stent graft repair? *Surgery* 144(4):575–580, 2008; discussion 580–572.

12. Camp PC, Shackford SR: Outcome after blunt traumatic thoracic aortic laceration: identification of a high-risk cohort. Western Trauma Association Multicenter Study Group, *J Trauma* 43(3):413–422, 1997.

13. Fabian TC, Richardson JD, Croce MA, et al: Prospective study of blunt aortic injury: multicenter Trial of the American Association for the Surgery of Trauma, *J Trauma* 42(3):374–380, 1997; discussion 380–373.

14. Richens D, Kotidis K, Neale M, et al: Rupture of the aorta following road traffic accidents in the United Kingdom 1992–1999. The results of the co-operative crash injury study, *Eur J Cardiothorac Surg* 23(2):143–148, 2003.

15. Jamieson WR, Janusz MT, Gudas VM, et al: Traumatic rupture of the thoracic aorta: third decade of experience, *Am J Surg* 183(5):571–575, 2002.

16. Cowley RA, Turney SZ, Hankins JR, et al: Rupture of thoracic aorta caused by blunt trauma. A fifteen-year experience,, *J Thorac Cardiovasc Surg* 100(5):652–660, 1990 discussion 660–651.

17. von Oppell UO, Dunne TT, De Groot MK, et al: Traumatic aortic rupture: twenty-year metaanalysis of mortality and risk of paraplegia, *Ann Thorac Surg* 58(2):585–593, 1994.

18. Jahromi AS, Kazemi K, Safar HA, et al: Traumatic rupture of the thoracic aorta: cohort study and systematic review, *J Vasc Surg* 34(6):1029–1034, 2001.

19. Weiman DS, Gurbuz AT, Gursky A, et al: Comparison of spinal cord protection utilizing left atrial-femoral with femoral-femoral bypass in patients with traumatic rupture of the aortic isthmus, *World J Surg* 30(9):1638–1641, 2006; discussion 1641–1633.

20. Kato N, Dake MD, Miller DC, et al: Traumatic thoracic aortic aneurysm: treatment with endovascular stent-grafts, *Radiology* 205(3):657–662, 1997.

21. Lebl DR, Dicker RA, Spain DA, et al: Dramatic shift in the primary management of traumatic thoracic aortic rupture, *Arch Surg* 141(2):177–180, 2006.

22. Dake MD, Miller DC, Semba CP, et al: Transluminal placement of endovascular stent-grafts for the treatment of descending thoracic aortic aneurysms, *N Engl J Med* 331(26):1729–1734, 1994.

23. Lettinga-van de Poll T, Schurink GW, De Haan MW, et al: Endovascular treatment of traumatic rupture of the thoracic aorta, *Br J Surg* 94(5):525–533, 2007.

24. Pate JW, Fabian TC, Walker WA: Acute traumatic rupture of the aortic isthmus: repair with cardiopulmonary bypass, *Ann Thorac Surg* 59(1):90–98, 1995; discussion 98–99.

25. Benckart DH, Magovern GJ, Liebler GA, et al: Traumatic aortic transection: repair using left atrial to femoral bypass, *J Card Surg* 4(1):43–49, 1989.

26. Peterson BG, Matsumura JS, Morasch MD, et al: Percutaneous endovascular repair of blunt thoracic aortic transection, *J Trauma* 59(5):1062–1065, 2005.

27. Amabile P, Collart F, Gariboldi V, et al: Surgical versus endovascular treatment of traumatic thoracic aortic rupture, *J Vasc Surg* 40(5):873–879, 2004.

28. McPhee JT, Asham EH, Rohrer MJ, et al: The midterm results of stent graft treatment of thoracic aortic injuries, *J Surg Res* 138(2):181–188, 2007.

29. du MM, Reekers JA, Balm R, et al: Collapse of a stent-graft following treatment of a traumatic thoracic aortic rupture, *J Endovasc Ther* 12(4):503–507, 2005.

30. Bakaeen FG, Wall MJ Jr, Mattox KL: Successful repair of an avulsion of the superior vena cava from the right atrium inflicted by blunt trauma, *J Trauma* 59(6):1486–1488, 2005.

31. Ambrose G, Barrett LO, Angus GL, et al: Main pulmonary artery laceration after blunt trauma: accurate preoperative diagnosis, *Ann Thorac Surg* 70(3):955–957, 2000.

32. Mattox KL, Feliciano DV, Burch J, et al: Five thousand seven hundred sixty cardiovascular injuries in 4459 patients. Epidemiologic evolution 1958 to 1987, *Ann Surg* 209(6):698–705, 1989; discussion 706–697.

33. Mittal VK, Paulson TJ, Colaiuta E, et al: Carotid artery injuries and their management, *J Cardiovasc Surg (Torino)* 41(3):423–431, 2000.

34. Fogelman MJ, Stewart RD: Penetrating wounds of the neck, *Am J Surg* 91(4):581–593, 1956 discussion, 593–586.

35. Davis TP, Feliciano DV, Rozycki GS, et al: Results with abdominal vascular trauma in the modern era, *Am Surg* 67(6):565–570, 2001; discussion 570–561.

36. McIntyre WB, Ballard JL: Cervicothoracic vascular injuries, *Semin Vasc Surg* 11(232):1998.

37. van As AB, van Deurzen DF, Verleisdonk EJ: Gunshots to the neck: selective angiography as part of conservative management, *Injury* 33(5):453–456, 2002.

38. Demetriades D, Asensio JA, Velmahos G, et al: Complex problems in penetrating neck trauma, *Surg Clin North Am* 76(4):661–683, 1996.

39. Duane TM, Parker F, Stokes GK, et al: Endovascular carotid stenting after trauma, *J Trauma* 52(1):149–153, 2002.

40. McNeil JD, Chiou AC, Gunlock MG, et al: Successful endovascular therapy of a penetrating zone III internal carotid injury, *J Vasc Surg* 36(1):187–190, 2002.

41. Tsai YH, Wong HF, Weng HH, et al: Stent-graft treatment of traumatic carotid artery dissecting pseudoaneurysm, *Neuroradiology* 52(11):1011–1016, 2010.

42. Maras D, Lioupis C, Magoufis G, et al: Covered stent-graft treatment of traumatic internal carotid artery pseudoaneurysms: a review, *Cardiovasc Intervent Radiol* 29(6):958–968, 2006.

43. DuBose J, Recinos G, Teixeira PG, et al: Endovascular stenting for the treatment of traumatic internal carotid injuries: expanding experience, *J Trauma* 65(6):1561–1566, 2008.

44. Bromberg WJ, Collier BC, Diebel LN, et al: Blunt cerebrovascular injury practice management guidelines: the Eastern Association for the Surgery of Trauma, *J Trauma* 68(2):471–477, 2010.

45. Moulakakis KG, Mylonas S, Avgerinos E, et al: An update of the role of endovascular repair in blunt carotid artery trauma, *Eur J Vasc Endovasc Surg* 40(3):312–319, 2010.

46. Berne JD, Cook A, Rowe SA, et al: A multivariate logistic regression analysis of risk factors for blunt cerebrovascular injury, *J Vasc Surg* 51(1):57–64, 2010.

47. Ringer AJ, Matern E, Parikh S, et al: Screening for blunt cerebrovascular injury: selection criteria for use of angiography, *J Neurosurg* 112(5):1146–1149, 2010.

48. Biffl WL, Ray CE Jr, Moore EE, et al: Noninvasive diagnosis of blunt cerebrovascular injuries: a preliminary report, *J Trauma* 53(5):850–856, 2002.

49. Biffl WL, Cothren CC, Moore EE, et al: Western Trauma Association critical decisions in trauma: screening for and treatment of blunt cerebrovascular injuries, *J Trauma* 67(6):1150–1153, 2009.

50. Biffl WL, Moore EE, Offner PJ, et al: Blunt carotid arterial injuries: implications of a new grading scale, *J Trauma* 47(5):845–853, 1999.

51. Edwards NM, Fabian TC, Claridge JA, et al: Antithrombotic therapy and endovascular stents are effective treatment for blunt carotid injuries: results from longterm followup, *J Am Coll Surg* 204(5):1007–1013, 2007; discussion 1014–1005.

52. Li W, D'Ayala M, Hirshberg A, et al: Comparison of conservative and operative treatment for blunt carotid injuries: analysis of the National Trauma Data Bank, *J Vasc Surg* 51(3):593–599, e592.

53. Cothren CC, Biffl WL, Moore EE, et al: Treatment for blunt cerebrovascular injuries: equivalence of anticoagulation and antiplatelet agents, *Arch Surg* 144(7):685–690, 2009.

54. Tyburski JG, Wilson RF, Dente C, et al: Factors affecting mortality rates in patients with abdominal vascular injuries, *J Trauma* 50(6):1020–1026, 2001.

55. Asensio JA, Forno W, Roldan G, et al: Abdominal vascular injuries: injuries to the aorta, *Surg Clin North Am* 81(6):1395–1416, xiii–xiv, 2001.

56. Asensio JA, Forno W, Roldan G, et al: Visceral vascular injuries, *Surg Clin North Am* 82(1):1–20, xix, 2002.

57. Bowley DM, Degiannis E, Goosen J, et al: Penetrating vascular trauma in Johannesburg, South Africa, *Surg Clin North Am* 82(1):221–235, 2002.

58. Paul JS, Webb TP, Aprahamian C, et al: Intraabdominal vascular injury: are we getting any better? *J Trauma* 2010.

59. Asensio JA, Chahwan S, Hanpeter D, et al: Operative management and outcome of 302 abdominal vascular injuries, *Am J Surg* 180(6):528–533, 2000; discussion 533–524.

60. Rhee P, Koustova E, Alam HB: Searching for the optimal resuscitation method: recommendations for the initial fluid resuscitation of combat casualties, *J Trauma* 54(5 Suppl):S52–S62, 2003.

61. Santry HP, Alam HB: Fluid resuscitation: past, present, and the future, *Shock* 33(3):229–241, 2010.

62. Stern SA: Low-volume fluid resuscitation for presumed hemorrhagic shock: helpful or harmful? *Curr Opin Crit Care* 7(6):422–430, 2001.

63. Chapellier X, Sockeel P, Baranger B: Management of penetrating abdominal vessel injuries, *J Visc Surg* 147(2):e1–e12, 2010.

64. Mattox KL, McCollum WB, Jordan GL Jr, et al: Management of upper abdominal vascular trauma, *Am J Surg* 128(6):823–828, 1974.

65. Cattell RB, Braasch JW: A technique for the exposure of the third and fourth portions of the duodenum, *Surg Gynecol Obstet* 111:378–379, 1960.

66. Moore EE, Cogbill TH, Jurkovich GJ, et al: Organ injury scaling. III: chest wall, abdominal vascular, ureter, bladder, and urethra, *J Trauma* 33(3):337–339, 1992.

67. Asensio JA, Petrone P, O'Shanahan G, et al: Managing exsanguination: what we know about damage control/bailout is not enough, *Proc (Bayl Univ Med Cent)* 16(3):294–296, 2003.

68. Aladham F, Sundaram B, Williams DM, et al: Traumatic aortic injury: computerized tomographic findings at presentation and after conservative therapy, *J Comput Assist Tomogr* 34(3):388–394, 2009.

69. Degiannis E, Levy RD, Florizoone MG, et al: Gunshot injuries of the abdominal aorta: a continuing challenge, *Injury* 28(3):195–197, 1997.

70. Inaba K, Kirkpatrick AW, Finkelstein J, et al: Blunt abdominal aortic trauma in association with thoracolumbar spine fractures, *Injury* 32(3):201–207, 2001.

71. Ding X, Jiang J, Su Q, et al: Endovascular stent graft repair of a penetrating aortic injury, *Ann Thorac Surg* 90(2):632–634, 2010.

72. Yeh MW, Horn JK, Schecter WP, et al: Endovascular repair of an actively hemorrhaging gunshot injury to the abdominal aorta, *J Vasc Surg* 42(5):1007–1009, 2005.

73. Arthurs ZM, Sohn VY, Starnes BW: Vascular trauma: endovascular management and techniques, *Surg Clin North Am* 87(5):1179–1192, x–xi, 2007.

74. Reuben BC, Whitten MG, Sarfati M, et al: Increasing use of endovascular therapy in acute arterial injuries: analysis of the National Trauma Data Bank, *J Vasc Surg* 46(6):1222–1226, 2007.

75. Demetriades D, Theodorou D, Murray J, et al: Mortality and prognostic factors in penetrating injuries of the aorta, *J Trauma* 40(5):761–763, 1996.

76. Durai R, Ng PC: Role of angio-embolisation in trauma--review, *Acta Chir Belg* 110(2):169–177, 2010.

77. Asensio JA, Berne JD, Chahwan S, et al: Traumatic injury to the superior mesenteric artery, *Am J Surg* 178(3):235–239, 1999.

78. Fullen WD, Hunt J, Altemeier WA: The clinical spectrum of penetrating injury to the superior mesenteric arterial circulation, *J Trauma* 12(8):656–664, 1972.

79. Asensio JA, Britt LD, Borzotta A, et al: Multiinstitutional experience with the management of superior mesenteric artery injuries, *J Am Coll Surg* 193(4):354–365, 2001; discussion 365–356.

80. Patel T, Kuladhipati I, Shah S: Successful percutaneous endovascular management of acute post-traumatic superior mesenteric artery dissection using a transradial approach, *J Invasive Cardiol* 22(4):E61–E64, 2010.

81. Asensio JA, Petrone P, Garcia-Nunez L, et al: Superior mesenteric venous injuries: to ligate or to repair remains the question, *J Trauma* 62(3):668–675, 2007; discussion 675.

82. Elliott SP, Olweny EO, McAninch JW: Renal arterial injuries: a single center analysis of management strategies and outcomes, *J Urol* 178(6):2451–2455, 2007.

83. Smith JK, Kenney PJ: Imaging of renal trauma, *Radiol Clin North Am* 41(5):1019–1035, 2003.

84. Bruce LM, Croce MA, Santaniello JM, et al: Blunt renal artery injury: incidence, diagnosis, and management, *Am Surg* 67(6):550–554, 2001; discussion 555–556.

85. Tillou A, Romero J, Asensio JA, et al: Renal vascular injuries, *Surg Clin North Am* 81(6):1417–1430, 2001.

86. Lee JT, White RA: Endovascular management of blunt traumatic renal artery dissection, *J Endovasc Ther* 9(3):354–358, 2002.

87. Weiss VJ, Chaikof EL: Endovascular treatment of vascular injuries, *Surg Clin North Am* 79(3):653–665, 1999.

88. Knudson MM, Harrison PB, Hoyt DB, et al: Outcome after major renovascular injuries: a Western trauma association multicenter report, *J Trauma* 49(6):1116–1122, 2000.

89. Asensio JA, McDuffie L, Petrone P, et al: Reliable variables in the exsanguinated patient which indicate damage control and predict outcome, *Am J Surg* 182(6):743–751, 2001.

90. Asensio JA, Petrone P, Roldan G, et al: Analysis of 185 iliac vessel injuries: risk factors and predictors of outcome, *Arch Surg* 138(11):1187–1193, 2003; discussion 1193–1184.

91. Lee JT, Bongard FS: Iliac vessel injuries, *Surg Clin North Am* 82(1):21–48, xix, 2002.

92. Kiguchi M, O'Rourke HJ, Dasyam A, et al: Endovascular repair of 2 iliac pseudoaneurysms and arteriovenous fistula following spine surgery, *Vasc Endovascular Surg* 44(2):126–130, 2010.

93. Lyden SP, Srivastava SD, Waldman DL, et al: Common iliac artery dissection after blunt trauma: case report of endovascular repair and literature review, *J Trauma* 50(2):339–342, 2001.

94. Kuehne J, Frankhouse J, Modrall G, et al: Determinants of survival after inferior vena cava trauma, *Am Surg* 65(10):976–981, 1999.

95. Buckman RF, Pathak AS, Badellino MM, et al: Injuries of the inferior vena cava, *Surg Clin North Am* 81(6):1431–1447, 2001.

96. Formisano V, Di Muria A, Muto G, et al: Inferior vena cava gunshot injury: case report and a review of the literature, *Ann Ital Chir* 77(2):173–177, 2006.

97. Buckman RF, Pathak AS, Badellino MM, et al: Portal vein injuries, *Surg Clin North Am* 81(6):1449–1462, 2001.

98. Stone HH, Fabian TC, Turkleson ML: Wounds of the portal venous system, *World J Surg* 6(3):335–341, 1982.

99. Pachter HL, Drager S, Godfrey N, et al: Traumatic injuries of the portal vein. The role of acute ligation, *Ann Surg* 189(4):383–385, 1979.

100. Carrillo EH, Spain DA, Miller FB, et al: Femoral vessel injuries, *Surg Clin North Am* 82(1): 49–65, 2002.

101. Lin PH, Koffron AJ, Guske PJ, et al: Penetrating injuries of the subclavian artery, *Am J Surg* 185(6):580–584, 2003.

102. Demetriades D, Asensio JA: Subclavian and axillary vascular injuries, *Surg Clin North Am* 81(6):1357–1373, xiii, 2001.

103. Phillips EH, Rogers WF, Gaspar MR: First rib fractures: incidence of vascular injury and indications for angiography, *Surgery* 89(1):42–47, 1981.

104. Richardson JD, McElvein RB, Trinkle JK: First rib fracture: a hallmark of severe trauma, *Ann Surg* 181(3):251–254, 1975.

105. du Toit DF, Strauss DC, Blaszczyk M, et al: Endovascular treatment of penetrating thoracic outlet arterial injuries, *Eur J Vasc Endovasc Surg* 19(5):489–495, 2000.

106. Janne d'Othee B, Rousseau H, Otal P, et al: Noncovered stent placement in a blunt traumatic injury of the right subclavian artery, *Cardiovasc Intervent Radiol* 22(5):424–427, 1999.

107. Xenos ES, Freeman M, Stevens S, et al: Covered stents for injuries of subclavian and axillary arteries, *J Vasc Surg* 38(3):451–454, 2003.

108. Fields CE, Latifi R, Ivatury RR: Brachial and forearm vessel injuries, *Surg Clin North Am* 82(1):105–114, 2002.

109. Borman KR, Snyder WH 3rd, Weigelt JA: Civilian arterial trauma of the upper extremity. An 11 year experience in 267 patients, *Am J Surg* 148(6):796–799, 1984.

110. Hunt CA, Kingsley JR: Vascular injuries of the upper extremity, *South Med J* 93(5):466–468, 2000.

111. Asensio JA, Kuncir EJ, Garcia-Nunez LM, et al: Femoral vessel injuries: analysis of factors predictive of outcomes, *J Am Coll Surg* 203(4):512–520, 2006.

112. Meyer J, Walsh J, Schuler J, et al: The early fate of venous repair after civilian vascular trauma. A clinical, hemodynamic, and venographic assessment, *Ann Surg* 206(4):458–464, 1987.

113. Mullenix PS, Steele SR, Andersen CA, et al: Limb salvage and outcomes among patients with traumatic popliteal vascular injury: an analysis of the National Trauma Data Bank, *J Vasc Surg* 44(1):94–100, 2006.

114. Frykberg ER: Popliteal vascular injuries, *Surg Clin North Am* 82(1):67–89, 2002.

115. Rowe VL, Salim A, Lipham J, et al: Shank vessel injuries, *Surg Clin North Am* 82(1):91–104, xx, 2002.

116. Wagner WH, Calkins ER, Weaver FA, et al: Blunt popliteal artery trauma: one hundred consecutive injuries, *J Vasc Surg* 7(5):736–743, 1988.

117. Wagner WH, Yellin AE, Weaver FA, et al: Acute treatment of penetrating popliteal artery trauma: the importance of soft tissue injury, *Ann Vasc Surg* 8(6):557–565, 1994.

118. Shah DM, Corson JD, Karmody AM, et al: Optimal management of tibial arterial trauma, *J Trauma* 28(2):228–234, 1988.

119. Bains SK, Vlachou PA, Rayt HS, et al: An observational cohort study of the management and outcomes of vascular trauma, *Surgeon* 7(6):332–335, 2009.

120. Vagefi PA, Kwolek CJ, Wicky S, et al: Congestive heart failure from traumatic arteriovenous fistula, *J Am Coll Surg* 209(1):150, 2009.

121. Toursarkissian B, Allen BT, Petrinec D, et al: Spontaneous closure of selected iatrogenic pseudoaneurysms and arteriovenous fistulae, *J Vasc Surg* 25(5):803–808, 1997; discussion 808–809.

122. Reed AB, Thompson JK, Crafton CJ, et al: Timing of endovascular repair of blunt traumatic thoracic aortic transections, *J Vasc Surg* 43(4):684–688, 2006.

123. Thalhammer C, Kirchherr AS, Uhlich F, et al: Postcatheterization pseudoaneurysms and arteriovenous fistulas: repair with percutaneous implantation of endovascular covered stents, *Radiology* 214(1):127–131, 2000.

124. Gandini R, Ippoliti A, Pampana E, et al: Emergency endograft placement for recurrent aortocaval fistula after conventional AAA repair, *J Endovasc Ther* 9(2):208–211, 2002.

125. Zhou W, Bush RL, Terramani TT, et al: Treatment options of iatrogenic pelvic vein injuries: conventional operative versus endovascular approach–case reports, *Vasc Endovascular Surg* 38(6):569–573, 2004.

126. Klinkner DB, Arca MJ, Lewis BD, et al: Pediatric vascular injuries: patterns of injury, morbidity, and mortality, *J Pediatr Surg* 42(1):178–182, 2007; discussion 182–173.

127. Shah SR, Wearden PD, Gaines BA: Pediatric peripheral vascular injuries: a review of our experience, *J Surg Res* 153(1):162–166, 2009.

128. Mommsen P, Zeckey C, Hildebrand F, et al: Traumatic extremity arterial injury in children: epidemiology, diagnostics, treatment and prognostic value of Mangled Extremity Severity Score, *J Orthop Surg Res* 5:25, 2010.

129. Chamoun RB, Mawad ME, Whitehead WE, et al: Extracranial traumatic carotid artery dissections in children: a review of current diagnosis and treatment options, *J Neurosurg Pediatr* 2(2):101–108, 2008.

130. Barmparas G, Inaba K, Talving P, et al: Pediatric vs adult vascular trauma: a National Trauma Databank review, *J Pediatr Surg* 45(7):1404–1412, 2010.

CHAPTER 62   Vascular Compression Syndromes

Timothy K. Williams, Nancy Harthun, Herbert I. Machleder,
Julie Ann Freischlag

Neurovascular structures can be compressed by adjacent tissues in several areas in the body. Although not common, there are clinical sequelae to these situations. The anatomical regions most associated with compression syndromes are the thoracic outlet, popliteal fossa, and proximal portion of the celiac artery as it passes the arcuate ligament. The basic pathophysiology behind these lesions is occasionally seen elsewhere in unusual diseases such as the nutcracker syndrome (compression of the left renal vein between the aorta and superior mesenteric artery [SMA]), adductor canal compression syndrome (abnormal bands from the adductor magnus compressing the superficial femoral artery [SFA]), or compression of the distal external iliac artery (EIA) just proximal to the inguinal ligament in bicyclists. This chapter focuses on the more commonly encountered syndromes.

Thoracic Outlet Syndrome

Thoracic outlet syndrome (TOS) describes a broad spectrum of symptoms and signs all related to compression or injury of the key anatomical structures that traverse this narrow aperture on their way to the upper extremity. This syndrome manifests in three main forms on the basis of the tissues involved: neurogenic, venous, and arterial. Neurogenic thoracic outlet is by far the most common, accounting for 98% of cases.[1] At a distant second, venous thoracic outlet occurs in 1.5%, followed by arterial at 0.5%. Considerable controversy surrounds the diagnosis of TOS, especially the neurogenic form. However, decades of research have served to better establish pathophysiology, diagnosis, and treatment of this syndrome.

In 1956, Peet et al. caused a major shift in the modern conception of TOS when they coined the term *thoracic outlet syndrome* and described a therapeutic exercise program, essentially the first physical therapy program for TOS.[2] This coincided with a shift of therapeutic focus to surgical intervention. In 1962, Clagett described high thoracoplasty for first rib resection, an operation requiring division of the trapezius and rhomboid muscles.[3] In 1966, Roos described what has become for many the modern treatment of choice for TOS, the transaxillary first rib resection.[4] This operation was fashioned after the transaxillary sympathectomy. First rib resection by this route offered reasonable exposure and minimal morbidity, especially when compared with previously employed techniques.

Anatomy of the Thoracic Outlet

The limited space and large number of important structures that must traverse the neck and chest areas on their way to the upper arm make the thoracic outlet an area like no other in the body. Although any number of anatomical anomalies predispose or directly cause compression to the neural, venous, or arterial structures within its confines, the normal anatomy itself does not leave much room for stress positioning.

Definitions may vary from author to author, but it is generally accepted that the thoracic outlet is the area from the edge of the first rib extending medially to the upper mediastinum and superiorly to the fifth cervical nerve. The clavicle and subclavius muscles can be pictured as forming a roof, and the superior surface of the first rib forms the floor. Machleder's description of the thoracic outlet as a triangle with its apex pointed toward the manubrium is helpful in visualizing the three-dimensional (3D) orientation of the structures, as well as the dynamic changes that can lead to injury.[5] In this model, the clavicle and its underlying subclavius muscle and tendon form the superior limb, and the base is the first thoracic rib.

The point at which these two structures "overlap" medially can be pictured as the fulcrum of a pair of scissors that opens and closes as the arm moves, potentially causing compression of the thoracic outlet contents (Fig. 62-1).

Although most TOS symptoms are related to nerve compression, almost any structure that travels through the thoracic outlet can be involved. Moving from anterior to posterior, one first encounters the exiting subclavian vein, usually positioned adjacent to the region where the first rib and clavicular head fuse to form a fibrocartilaginous joint with the manubrium. Immediately posterior to the vein is the anterior scalene muscle, which inserts onto a prominence on the first rib. Next encountered is the subclavian artery, with the anterior scalene muscle lying between the artery and vein. The brachial plexus is the next structure encountered, oriented superior, posterior, and lateral to the artery. The C4-C6 roots are superiorly oriented, and the C7-T1 roots inferior. Posterior and lateral to the plexus, there is a generally rather broad attachment of the middle scalene muscle to the first rib (Fig. 62-2).

Other structures encountered in the thoracic outlet include the phrenic and dorsal scapular nerves, stellate ganglion, long thoracic nerve (as it emerges through the middle scalene), thoracic duct, and the cupola of the lung. The thoracic duct may be encountered if a left supraclavicular approach is undertaken, and care must be taken not to injure or ligate it if injury occurs. Finally, one must watch for pleural injury in any approach to TOS and be prepared to evacuate pneumothoraces when indicated.

Some authors further classify the thoracic outlet on the basis of three anatomical apertures within this broader space: the interscalene triangle, costoclavicular space, and subpectoral space.[6] The most medial aperture that can result in neurovascular compression is within the interscalene triangle. The artery and brachial plexus together pass through this space formed by the anterior scalene anteriorly, middle scalene posteriorly, and first rib inferiorly. Abnormalities of the anterior or middle scalene, presence of a scalenus minimus muscle (seen in <50% of patients, originating between the T1 nerve root and the anterior and inserting onto the pleura and first rib), presence of a cervical rib (0.5% incidence), and presence of fibrous bands (scarring or congenital) can lead to neurovascular compression in this space.[6]

Lateral and anterior, one can describe the costoclavicular space, bound by the clavicle with its subclavius muscle and tendon anteromedially, the first rib, anterior and middle scalene muscles posteromedially, and the scapula posterolaterally. Bony abnormalities, either congenital or acquired, can narrow this space and result in neurovascular compression. The subclavian vein is especially susceptible to compression in this region as it passes through the narrow space created by the confluence of the clavicle, subclavius muscle and tendon, and the first rib.[6]

Just deep to the insertion of the pectoralis minor muscle on the coracoid process is the subpectoral aperture. Rarely, neurovascular compression can occur in this space, usually as a result of hyperabduction of the arm, compressing the structures against the chest wall.[6]

Pathophysiology of Thoracic Outlet Syndrome

Fundamentally, the pathophysiology of TOS is based on the presence of one or more anatomical abnormalities that narrow the thoracic outlet and extrinsically compress the neurovascular structures contained within. Anatomical abnormalities associated with TOS can be broadly classified as *soft tissue* or *bony* and may be acquired or congenital. Acquired may be related to bony or soft-tissue injury, as well as physical activity leading to muscle hypertrophy.

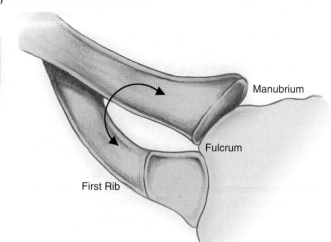

FIGURE 62-1 Useful schematic for visualizing the thoracic outlet, demonstrating "scissoring" effect between clavicle and first rib. Although a simplification, it suggests how removal of either the clavicle or first rib can decompress the region.

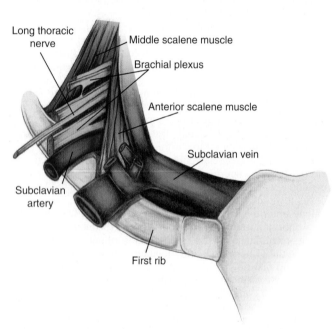

FIGURE 62-2 Diagram showing complex anatomical relationships within thoracic outlet, including broad-based attachment of middle scalene muscle. Clavicle has been removed for exposure.

The congenital soft-tissue anomalies believed to predispose one to TOS have been well described in the literature. Cadaver studies done by Juvonen, Raymond, and others shed light on the incidence of specific anatomical anomalies in the general population.[7] This work is based on the initial observations of Roos, who extensively classified the muscular and fibrous band anomalies seen in patients presenting with TOS.[8]

Many acquired soft-tissue injuries leading to TOS are the direct result of physical trauma. Studies suggest that soft-tissue injury following motor vehicle trauma (e.g., whiplash) may be the most common underlying etiology.[9,10] Other injury patterns include falling onto one's head and shoulder, causing a lateral stretch injury. In a review of operative TOS patients by Sanders and Hammond,[11] 86% had a history of trauma. This prevalence of trauma is considerably higher than in many other reports, but stresses the role trauma can play in the disorder.[11]

Repetitive stress and poor postural habits are also leading causes of TOS.[10] Vocations associated with TOS include typists, violinists, or assembly line workers. Other activities include weight lifting or strenuous sports, which lead to hypertrophied scalene musculature. Anatomical studies have documented compression of the subclavian vein into the costoclavicular notch by this muscle.[12] This has clear implications for axillosubclavian vein thrombosis. Additionally, some surgeons see a link between Paget-Schroetter's syndrome and subclavius tendon hypertrophy, particularly in the presence of an enlarged insertion tubercle. Others have implicated a role for the pectoralis minor muscle.[13] Rarely, connective tissue disorders have been implicated as a direct causative agent, namely localized scleroderma.[14]

A number of bony abnormalities are found in association with TOS, with the presence of a cervical rib being most common. Autopsy studies indicate that approximately 0.5% of the general population has this structure[15] (Fig. 62-3). Further, routine chest radiography demonstrates a cervical rib in roughly 0.7% of individuals.[16] Historically, series from the United States report cervical ribs in 10% to 65% of TOS patients, while the European literature reports 25%.[15,17] The reason for this discrepancy is not known. It may be at least in part due to variable recognition of neurogenic thoracic outlet in the general population, thus adding bias to these figures. Modern data suggest the percentage of TOS patients with cervical ribs is much lower.

Cervical ribs can be completely formed or rudimentary. In the latter case, there is almost always a compressive band of tissue extending to the first thoracic rib. As they project from transverse processes, cervical ribs displace the involved structures forward. The subclavian artery is particularly vulnerable to damage in this configuration, and some surgeons feel that arterial changes secondary to TOS rarely occur in the absence of a cervical rib. Another common bony anomaly is the presence of an elongated C7 transverse process, which can similarly impinge on the neurovascular structures. Fibrous bands may also be present from an elongated C7 transverse process to the first rib, further worsening the problem.[9] Posttraumatic changes following clavicular or first rib fractures are commonly reported, with callous formation at the clavicle and pseudoarthroses of the first rib.[18] These changes can frequently be appreciated radiographically.

Presentation of Thoracic Outlet Syndrome

NEUROGENIC THORACIC OUTLET SYNDROME

Patients can present with the symptoms of neurogenic TOS at any age, although it most commonly occurs in otherwise healthy young to middle-aged individuals. Women are affected three times more frequently than men.[1] Neurogenic symptoms can range in severity from nuisance to severely debilitating pain. The most common symptom is pain in an arm, shoulder, and/or the neck. Paresthesias are also commonly present to varying degrees. Although less common, perceived weakness or loss of dexterity can be seen. This occasionally

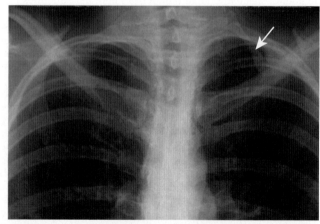

FIGURE 62-3 Chest radiogram demonstrating a left cervical rib (arrow).

manifests as a decrease in grip strength.[1] However, gross motor dysfunction and wasting of the upper extremity is unusual. Gilliat and colleagues description of classic neurogenic TOS with muscle wasting in the hand is seldom seen.[19]

Pain may originate anywhere in the upper extremity, but the most common site is the back of the shoulder. The suprascapular portion of the trapezius may be involved. From the shoulder, pain can spread up the ipsilateral extremity along the back and neck, or even up the face. This situation can lead to hemicranial headaches that can be labeled as migraines.

Pain involving the arm can be focused to a particular nerve distribution or generalized. When localized, ulnar symptoms tend to be the most common, leading to pain and/or paresthesias involving the ring and small fingers. These so-called lower plexus (C8-T1) symptoms are commonly seen. However, upper plexus (C5-C7) manifestations can also be seen, manifesting as pain in the lateral arm and forearm, lateral neck, and deltopectoral region.[1]

Patients may report pain at rest that is not relieved by positioning. However, the typical patient reports that stress positioning exacerbates symptoms. This is particularly the case with work-related situations. People who must perform tasks with elevated arms or hold their arms in other awkward positions note they are no longer able to perform these tasks. Examples include waitresses, mechanics, and truck drivers. With prolonged stress positioning, patients may report finger discoloration, coolness of the extremity, or even swelling. Driving an automobile can be difficult with the concomitant numbness and tingling in the fingers that can occur.

Patients often report that their symptom complex started after a traumatic event. These can be chronic repetitive-type injuries, such as seen with pitchers and other athletes. Direct injury to the chest wall or shoulder can also precipitate symptoms, particularly if associated with a clavicular fracture or acromioclavicular joint dislocation. As mentioned previously, whiplash-type injuries are also associated with TOS. Even a minor injury can unmask the syndrome in a previously completely asymptomatic individual.

VENOUS THORACIC OUTLET SYNDROME (PAGET-SCHROETTER'S SYNDROME)

Paget-Schroetter's syndrome (axillosubclavian vein thrombosis or "effort" thrombosis) usually presents suddenly in a previously healthy patient without antecedent symptoms. Typically the patient is a young athlete or worker with a component to their sport or job that requires prolonged or repetitive stressful positioning of the arm. Examples include baseball players, swimmers, weight lifters, volleyball players, and mechanics. The presentation is usually acute and dramatic, often prompting urgent medical care.

The involved extremity becomes acutely swollen with varying degrees of discoloration ranging from rubor to cyanosis. The redness may be confused with the erythema of an infection, leading to a delay in diagnosis. Physical examination may reveal the presence of dilated collateral veins around the shoulder and upper arm. The remainder of the physical examination is usually normal.

Occasionally, aching pain due to tightness of the skin may also be present, but is absent in the majority of patients.[20] However, the typical spectrum of symptoms seen in patients with neurogenic TOS are not usually associated with Paget-Schroetter's syndrome. Although uncommon, ipsilateral sympathetic hyperactivity can be seen with this condition.

An alternate presentation may occur with an acute traumatic injury. Typically, after an injury to the shoulder area, a few days pass and ipsilateral arm swelling occurs. The natural history of this variant of Paget-Schroetter's syndrome is the same, reflecting the fact that the injury most likely contributed to compression in the thoracic outlet. Thus, the thrombosis associated with injury is really the same insult seen in "spontaneous" thrombosis.

If the condition is left untreated, the swelling typically resolves over the course of days or weeks. The patient typically does not have symptoms at rest but cannot use the arm for any period of time, particularly in a stressed (abducted, externally rotated) position. The collateral channels that develop and allow the swelling to abate are rarely adequate to accommodate the increased venous return that occurs with activity.

ARTERIAL THORACIC OUTLET SYNDROME

Arterial TOS is the most rare and varied form of TOS. Chronic compression of the artery leads to insidiously progressive inflammatory changes and scarring of the vessel. These patients rarely present early in the course of this process. Even after they seek medical care, many will have a history that supports the diagnosis, including symptoms such as episodic pallor, cyanosis, and cold intolerance. Patients may present with an array of complaints and physical findings, ranging from intermittent arm claudication to signs of distal embolization or frank ischemia. Rarely, patients may present with aneurysm rupture from long-standing poststenotic dilatation.[16]

Patients not infrequently are misdiagnosed with collagen vascular disease, various forms of arteritis, or Raynaud's disease. However, when symptoms are unilateral and isolated to circulation distal to the subclavian artery, one should be alerted to the possibility of arterial TOS. Because there is overlap between the clinical presentation of arterial insufficiency and neurogenic disorders, patients may be misdiagnosed with carpal tunnel syndrome, cervical disc disease, or even neurogenic TOS. It is important to maintain a high index of suspicion for this entity because its clinical presentation is not straightforward.[16]

Diagnosis of Thoracic Outlet Syndrome

No generally accepted battery of tests must be performed to confirm the presence of TOS. Most physicians and surgeons familiar with the disorder require, at minimum, a physical examination consistent with the symptoms, cervical radiographs to rule out disc disease, and a chest radiograph to visualize any bony abnormalities. Other tests may be applied as needed when the diagnosis is not clear. The need for invasive or expensive tests is an area of considerable debate.

HISTORY AND PHYSICAL EXAMINATION

Because the overwhelming majority of patients who present with a suspected diagnosis of TOS will be of the neurogenic type, this section mainly focuses on this type of TOS. Venous and arterial forms will be discussed later. As with any initial evaluation, an extensive history should be taken, including any injuries and the patient's occupation. Exacerbating and ameliorating factors should be identified if present. In conjunction with a good history, most cases of TOS can be diagnosed on the basis of physical examination. A thorough examination should focus not only on the site of complaints but also on other areas commonly involved in neurological conditions. This includes the patient's general appearance and other signs of symptom impact. Deep tendon reflexes, grip strength, and pulses should also routinely be assessed. Palmar hyperhidrosis should be noted if present. Machleder points out that even in neurogenic TOS, changes in pulses can occasionally be detected.[21]

Note should be made of symmetry of the muscle groups of the shoulders and upper extremities. Although serratus anterior atrophy is occasionally present with TOS (as demonstrated by a winged scapula), patients generally do not have obvious muscle atrophy. In fact, they often have essentially normal gross baseline sensory and motor examinations. However, useful information can still be obtained if one uses an organized approach. Initial palpation of the structures of the chest wall, cervical region, and shoulder can be useful before undertaking provocative testing. The region overlying the anterior scalene muscle is often exquisitely tender in the face of brachial plexus entrapment or irritation. In addition, percussion of the clavicle can reproduce pains and paresthesias in TOS patients. Point tenderness can sometimes be elicited along the anterior border of the trapezius at the junction of the neck and shoulder (band spot). These simple maneuvers should be performed before more complex maneuvering of the patient, which may cloud later findings.

The physical examination also plays an important role in ruling out other causes of a patient's symptoms. Although cervical symptoms are common with TOS, limited cervical range should not be seen, nor should there be excessive tenderness over the vertebral bodies. The presence of either of these suggests an alternate diagnosis. Specific neurological evaluations such as the Spurling test, eliciting a Tinel sign, and the Phalen maneuver can also be used to rule out other diagnoses.

After this general neurological assessment, tests more specific for the presence of TOS can be undertaken. The most useful test to aid in the diagnosis of TOS is the elevated arm stress test (EAST), which was originally described by Roos in 1966 as a means of eliciting upper-extremity claudication and neurological symptoms.[22] In the test, the patient's arms are placed in 90 degrees of abduction and external rotation, with 90 degrees of flexion at the elbow ("hold-up position"). The patient is then asked to repeatedly clench and unclench the hands. This positioning is designed to constrict the space within the thoracic outlet in an effort to reproduce the patient's symptoms. When positive in patients with TOS, this test should bring on weakness and paresthesias in the ulnar and median nerve distributions within 3 minutes. Inability to complete testing owing to symptoms is also considered a positive result. Attention should also be made to the color of the hands during the EAST because one may become pale and ischemic if arterial compromise is involved. Proponents of EAST argue that it is specific for TOS and that the length of time to onset of symptoms correlates with severity of TOS. However, some question the anatomical basis for the test, particularly how clenching and unclenching the hand can lead to stress on the brachial plexus.[23] This test is not without its detractors. Although anecdotally reported to have excellent specificity, a study from 1985 found a positive test in more than 80% of patients with carpal tunnel syndrome. Other studies conducted using healthy subjects have also reported a high rate of false positives.[24,25]

Closely related to the EAST is the abduction and external rotation (AER) test. The arm is abducted and rotated and held in that position. This test works by a similar mechanism and likewise produces the weakness and numbness seen with EAST in a similar distribution, namely the C8 to T1 fibers supplying the median and ulnar nerves. In addition, one can sometimes detect a bruit below the lateral portion of the clavicle that is attributable to partial compression of the axillary artery. Both of these tests appear particularly suited to work-related and repetitive motion–associated TOS.[26]

Although many clinicians routinely assess for pulse changes with these provocative maneuvers, this adds little useful information to such testing. The original Adson test (chin elevation and head rotation toward affected side) consisted of assessment of the radial pulse; *Adson sign* is subsequent loss of the radial pulse. Although it has historically been used to screen for TOS, Adson sign is also frequently seen in patients without TOS and is unreliably present in those with confirmed TOS. Therefore, it should not be used to establish the diagnosis.[1,27] Additionally, Wright described the hyperabduction position back in 1945, which is also of little clinical utility, given its positive result in most healthy individuals. Furthermore, as many as 60% of healthy subjects who undergo EAST will have diminution of the radial pulse.[25]

None of these aforementioned tests is pathognomonic, but the presence of one or more of them can help support the diagnosis of TOS. Combined with a proper history, the diagnosis of TOS can be established, other disorders can be effectively ruled out, and further tests avoided.

OBJECTIVE TESTING

Although numerous objective modalities have proven useful in the diagnosis of TOS, none are diagnostic and remain adjuncts to a proper history and physical examination. Perhaps the most

useful study is a plain chest radiograph. This inexpensive study can readily identify cervical ribs, evidence of previous rib or clavicular fracture, or other chest wall abnormalities that have been linked to TOS. It is also important to exclude other potential etiologies for the patient's symptoms, namely cervical spine disease, so cervical spine imaging is commonly used. Cervical spine x-rays can be obtained, although this modality has been widely supplanted by computed tomography (CT) and magnetic resonance imaging (MRI) in the diagnosis of cervical spine pathology.

Use of objective neurodiagnostic tests for TOS has met with some success, although it continues to be an area of considerable controversy. This modality came to the forefront in the early 1960s, but the anatomical constraints of attempting to measure changes across the brachial plexus have always made its application in this position difficult. Specific techniques vary, but principally these studies evaluate nerve conduction velocity as well as amplitude. The most common and basic electrophysiological studies involve direct motor and sensory nerve testing at the root, cord, trunk, and/or nerve level. Tests are considered abnormal when the velocities and amplitudes deviate from accepted norms. Perhaps the main criticism of these tests is that they only tend to be positive in patients with advanced disease, in whom history and physical examination should be sufficient. Roos suggests they offer "little definitive diagnostic information" and that one "still must rely on careful history and physical."[24] All of this reflects the fact that most electrophysiological tests evaluate larger myelinated nerve fibers, not the smaller fibers whose injury mediates the pain associated with TOS. A study by Franklin et al. found that of 158 TOS patients, only 7.6% had abnormalities in their electrodiagnostic tests.[28] Furthermore, this diagnostic modality is subject to significant interobserver bias. No standardized easily reproducible technique has been adopted, nor has any been extensively studied and proven useful in suspected TOS patients. Beyond the limited role of establishing the diagnosis of TOS, these studies can result in significant discomfort for the patient who is already suffering from disabling pain. They should therefore be used only in special instances. These techniques can be useful, however, to exclude the diagnosis of TOS in cases where another neurological process is suspected (e.g., carpal tunnel syndrome).

Let us look closer at some specific techniques that have been used in patients with neurological disorders of the upper extremity. First, several authors have described their experience using ulnar conduction velocity from Erb's point (above the clavicle and lateral to the insertion of the sternocleidomastoid muscle) to the elbow to assess for TOS, but this technique has been criticized.[21] However, if there is severe disease with concomitant axonal damage, changes in ulnar action potentials can be demonstrated. A reasonable approach to conduction studies includes sensory testing of the median and ulnar nerves at the wrist to screen for carpel tunnel syndrome and TOS, respectively.

Electromyography is capable of providing objective data supporting the diagnosis of TOS in a setting of advanced disease. This study demonstrates spontaneous firing of acutely denervated muscle fibers (positive sharp waves, fibrillation potentials), but this is not the usual clinical situation for TOS. Rather, after reinnervation, prolonged and irregular potentials are seen. Because this is a reflection of previous denervation injury, many of these patients have atrophy of the involved muscle groups, and the electromyogram (EMG) can confirm that the lower trunk of the brachial plexus was injured. However, in patients without evidence of atrophy, this test is not likely to reveal these findings. This fact is supported by studies showing that standard EMG tests are negative in 62% of TOS patients.[29] However, these tests can be used to examine the paraspinal muscles, which can be important in ruling out radiculopathy as the cause of the patient's symptoms.

F-wave studies are an attractive concept for evaluating TOS because they allow for propagation of the stimulus back to the spinal cord, thus crossing the brachial plexus and obviating the need for proximal nerve access. In this technique, nerve stimulation at the wrist leads to not only an immediate action potential in the affected muscle groups, but also to this proximal propagation with a concomitant reflection from the cord, leading to a secondary action potential. This returning potential is the F-wave. Generally, multiple trials are recorded, and the shortest period between percutaneous stimulus and the secondary response is taken as the latency. This period is delayed if the nerve fibers are damaged, as can be seen with TOS. These tests tend to be poorly tolerated by many patients, and it is prudent to avoid their use unless other tests have proved unrewarding and further diagnostic information is required.

Somatosensory evoked potentials (SSEPs) can play a role in the workup of TOS. Currently, assessment of the ulnar and median nerves can be used for evidence of their compression at the thoracic outlet. When abnormal, these studies tend to show lower plexus injury (ulnar) with normal median function. This is seen primarily as a blunting of Erb's point peak. Machleder et al.[30] showed that 74% of their patients carrying a clinical diagnosis of TOS had abnormal evoked responses. Furthermore, when these patients were studied following operative decompression of their thoracic outlets, more than 90% had correlation between improved symptoms and normalization of their SSEPs.[30] Increases of the sensitivity of these tests can be achieved with provocative maneuvers such as arm positioning, although these maneuvers can also cause SSEP changes in patients with no clinical evidence of TOS. Although neurodiagnostic testing remains useful as exclusionary testing, its role in establishing the diagnosis of neurogenic TOS remains limited.

One diagnostic technique that has proven quite useful in suspected TOS patients is anterior scalene muscle blockade. This is typically accomplished by injecting lidocaine into the anterior scalene muscle to induce muscle relaxation. Essentially this test simulates the decompression achieved with first rib resection and scalenectomy. It is therefore believed that symptomatic improvement with blockade is predictive of a positive response to surgical intervention. Imprecise needle placement can contribute to false-negative results of this test, as well as confound the problem by causing nerve injury or inadvertent somatic or autonomic denervation. Electromyogram with ultrasound or CT guidance can be used to localize the anterior scalene muscle, thus facilitating proper needle placement.

In a study by Jordan and Machleder, 122 patients underwent EMG-guided scalene blockade for a suspected diagnosis of TOS. Reduction in pain was then assessed with provocative maneuvers (generally the EAST); 38 patients went on to have surgical decompression, 32 of whom had a positive result with muscle blockade. The 94% of patients who had a positive response to blockade had a positive long-term result with surgery, as opposed to only 50% of patients with a negative block.[31]

Beyond its utility as a predictor of good outcome following surgery, lidocaine blockade does offer patients some transient relief while awaiting surgery. However, this effect rarely lasts beyond 1 month. Some groups advocate botulinum toxin injection over lidocaine because of its longer duration of action. This is particularly useful in patients who may have a delay between scalene block and surgery. Jordan et al. also demonstrated in a cohort of 22 patients that botulinum injection results in a 50% reduction of symptoms for a least 1 month in 64% of patients (mean duration of 88 days). This is in contrast to only 12% of patients with continued symptomatic relief beyond 1 month when receiving lidocaine alone.[32]

Finally, some centers advocate the use of duplex ultrasonography to assess for the presence of TOS. To perform this test, provocative maneuvers in conjunction with color Doppler are used to assess blood flow velocities in the subclavian artery and vein. In theory, patients without TOS will have minimal velocity changes within the subclavian artery during varying degrees of abduction of the arm. If the patient's symptoms are related to TOS, one would expect to see velocity changes. First, as the artery becomes partially compressed, velocity in the artery increases. Further abduction will worsen compression to the point where flow is diminished, and one should see a resultant decrease in velocities. Finally, with hyperabduction the compression may be so severe that the vessel becomes occluded, with cessation of flow. Recent data have given support to this modality. In a small cohort of patients suspected of having TOS on the basis of symptoms and physical examination, all patients demonstrated the anticipated hemodynamic changes described. With 120 degrees of abduction, mean peak systolic velocities increased greater than 50%. At 180 degrees of abduction, velocities were reduced below baseline values, and hyperabduction revealed absent flow in all patients for whom data were available. As anticipated, venous duplex revealed changes suggestive of venous compression, namely loss of atrial and respiratory dynamics, increased velocities, and increased turbulence.[33] Although this study was underpowered to definitively establish duplex ultrasonography as a proven diagnostic modality in TOS, it does offer promising data. Validating studies should be conducted to further our understanding of the role of ultrasound in TOS.

DIAGNOSIS OF VENOUS THORACIC OUTLET SYNDROME

In the TOS patient who presents with upper-extremity swelling, the diagnosis of axillosubclavian vein thrombosis is suggested by the history and physical examination described earlier. Assessment of the venous system is usually initiated with noninvasive duplex ultrasonography and dynamic phlebography (also see Chapter 12). Provocative positioning, such as external rotation and abduction, can increase the sensitivity of these tests. Other authors describe a two-position technique, with the arms fully adducted and then 90 degrees abducted. It is not clear at this time how useful magnetic resonance venography (MRV) is for axillosubclavian evaluation. It appears to have anatomical limitations similar to duplex ultrasonography, with poor quality of images in the retroclavicular space.

Many patients undergo a diagnostic venogram, which is the gold standard for thrombosis in this situation (Fig. 62-4). Occlusion of the axillosubclavian vein is readily identified with this diagnostic modality. Typically, patients will also have numerous venous collaterals not seen in normal individuals without thrombosis. Although this test confirms the diagnosis of venous thrombosis, the occasional patient needs further clarification as to its cause. Neurogenic symptoms are usually not present, and one must often rely on exclusion of causes of venous thrombosis other than TOS in this situation.

DIAGNOSIS OF ARTERIAL THORACIC OUTLET SYNDROME

As discussed earlier, a number of symptoms and signs are a consequence of arterial involvement in TOS. Thus the diagnostic algorithm is not straightforward. A careful physical examination may be extremely helpful in patients with suspected arterial TOS. Pulse changes with provocative positioning, subclavian bruits, and blood pressure differentials between the extremities may be seen. The stress positions described previously can be used. Depending on the degree of arterial involvement, patients may have absence of a brachial pulse and/or radial pulse. Patients may initially be evaluated with digital plethysmography or upper-extremity arterial duplex ultrasonography. Computed tomographic angiography (CTA) is also useful in detecting thromboembolic events in these patients. As experience has been gained with magnetic resonance angiography (MRA), this technique has also been applied with utility. Arteriography remains the gold standard and is almost always required in this setting. When arterial compression is suspected, attention should first be toward an arch study, which also includes the subclavian and axillary arteries more distally.

Frequently, arterial compression can be better visualized if the arm is abducted 90 degrees, and most studies are obtained with the arms in two positions (Fig. 62-5). When distal embolization is suggested, the angiography should encompass the target sites, often requiring studies of the hand on the affected side. Provocative positioning (abduction) can be used in conjunction with angiography to demonstrate arterial compression.

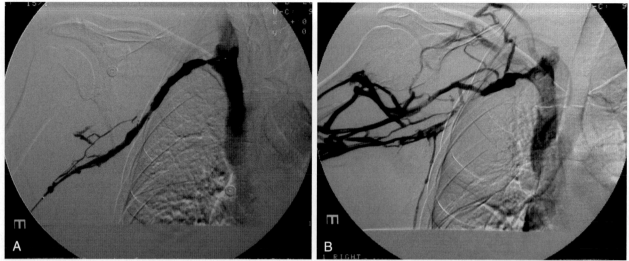

FIGURE 62-4 **These two images clearly display compression of axillosubclavian vein when arm is placed in neutral position (A) and stressed abducted position (B).** Images must be obtained with and without stress positioning to confirm diagnosis of venous thoracic outlet syndrome (TOS).

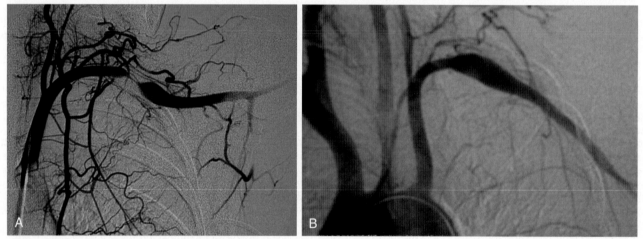

FIGURE 62-5 **Angiogram demonstrating occlusion of subclavian artery when arm is abducted (A) and resumption of flow when arm is returned to neutral position (B).** Note presence of poststenotic dilation when arm is fully adducted.

Treatment of Thoracic Outlet Syndrome

In all likelihood, the vast majority of patients with neurogenic TOS go undiagnosed and thus receive no therapy. This reflects the range of severity inherent in the spectrum of symptoms associated with TOS. For those seeking medical intervention, it is clear that most have substantial improvement without operation. Although the numbers are controversial and dependent on the modalities used to make the diagnosis, more than 95% of patients avoid operation. Currently, considerable debate surrounds neurogenic TOS surgery, with several groups reporting no long-term benefit from operation versus physical therapy. Nonetheless, most surgeons with considerable experience with neurogenic TOS report good surgical results with properly selected patients.

For many TOS surgeons, referral patterns are such that patients have already undertaken unsuccessful conservative therapy before seeking further consultation. It is important for surgeons to be aware of this selection bias. It is also important to have an algorithm for conservative treatment so that the correct patients are selected for operation. A minimum of 6 weeks of physical therapy is required before its effects can be evaluated. It is also important that the correct program be used because it has been recognized that inappropriate physical therapy can worsen TOS symptoms. In general, these programs are designed to relax muscle groups that tighten the thoracic outlet while conditioning those that open it. Aligne and Barral described a program in which the trapezius,

levator scapulae, and sternocleidomastoid muscles are strengthened and the middle scalene, subclavius, and pectoralis muscles relaxed.[34]

Other nonsurgical interventions are available. Following the concept of diagnostic scalene blocks, attempts have been made at therapeutic blockade of the scalene muscles. Although steroid injection has not been successful, temporary symptomatic relief with selective botulinum toxin injection can be employed successfully in those reluctant to pursue surgical intervention. Additionally, this technique may allow the patient to tolerate an extended period of physical therapy or other adjustments such as work-related ergonomic modifications.

SURGICAL TREATMENT

When a symptomatic patient who has sought treatment fails to improve with physical therapy, surgical intervention is warranted. Resection of the first rib and anterior scalenectomy can be performed via either the transaxillary or supraclavicular approach. In our practice, we preferentially use the transaxillary approach owing to its excellent exposure of the first rib, minimal morbidity, and better cosmetic appearance. The patient is placed in the lateral decubitus position, with the head neutral. No paralytic agents are used beyond short-acting agents for induction. Various devices are available for elevation of the arm on the operative side, all of

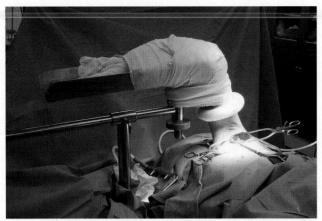

FIGURE 62-6 Proper positioning of patient for transaxillary first rib resection. Although it is possible to perform procedures using an assistant to support ipsilateral upper extremity, customized retractor systems are the preferred method. There should be a mechanism for convenient intermittent lowering of arm to allow perfusion in a less stressed position during course of operation.

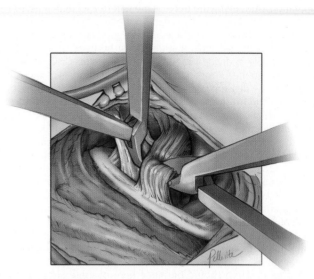

FIGURE 62-8 Division of anterior scalene muscle. Care is taken to develop the tissue plane on either side of anterior scalene muscle to avoid injury to subclavian artery and vein.

which should permit easy lowering of the extremity intermittently throughout the procedure to allow periods of increased arterial inflow and decreased tension on stretched nerves (Fig. 62-6). The incision is placed between the pectoralis major and the latissimus dorsi in the lower aspect of the axilla. Dissection is carried down to the chest wall, with care taken to identify intercostal brachial cutaneous nerves. These structures should be avoided and preserved when possible, but it is preferable to sacrifice them rather than leave them injured, thereby subjecting the patient to possible causalgic pain.

Deep dissection begins by bluntly exposing the external surface of the first rib. Using a periosteal elevator, intercostal muscle and soft-tissue attachments to the first rib are cleared (Fig. 62-7). The parietal pleura is then bluntly dissected away from the internal surface of the first rib. The anterior surface of the first rib is cleared of soft tissue and middle scalene fibers, again using the periosteal elevator. Care is taken to not cut the fibers of the middle scalene. The long thoracic nerve often traverses the muscle in this region, and injury to the long thoracic nerve will result in a winged scapula and is associated with significant long-term disability. Tissue is

then cleared bluntly overlying the nerve, artery, and vein. The anterior scalene muscle is now carefully separated from the subclavian vessels, and its attachment to the first rib is divided (Fig. 62-8). The subclavius tendon is also divided.

A rib shear is next positioned anteriorly over the rib, which is divided almost at the level of the costal cartilage. Care must be taken to avoid the subclavian vein in this location. Following clearing of residual muscle and any fibrous attachments remaining, the rib is divided posteriorly just anterior to the brachial plexus. The rib is now free and is removed from the patient. Considerable care must be taken following removal of the rib to smooth the posterior stump to prevent any subsequent T1 injury. At this point, any further encountered anomalies (fibromuscular bands, scalenus minimus muscles) should be resected. Cervical ribs are resected in a similar fashion to the first rib, requiring division of their attachments to the middle scalene and intercostal muscles.

Before closure, irrigation is placed into the wound, and inspection is made for a pleural leak. In the presence of a leak, a small chest tube can be used for pleural drainage but is rarely needed. It can usually be removed the following day. A postoperative chest radiograph is obtained. Most patients are discharged home on postoperative day 1 or 2. Careful follow-up and physical therapy are also employed in the early postoperative period.

The supraclavicular approach for scalenectomy (with or without first rib resection) is considered in three situations. The first is when the patient's symptoms are particularly suggestive of upper brachial plexus involvement (as opposed to the more common lower plexus). As described by Roos,[35] it is reasonable to use an approach in which these nerves can be more directly decompressed. The second situation is in patients who have undergone transaxillary operation but now have upper plexus symptoms. The third situation is a matter of preference when a surgeon feels the supraclavicular approach is as effective as and safer than the transaxillary operation. The first rib can also be resected as a component of this procedure, although some argue that it cannot be done with the same margins as the transaxillary approach.

As with the transaxillary approach, no paralytics are used so that nerve function can be assessed intraoperatively. The patient is placed in the semi-Fowler position, with the head turned away from the operative side. An incision is placed two fingerbreadths above the clavicle, extending from the external jugular vein to the sternocleidomastoid muscle. This muscle is subsequently mobilized medially, and the omohyoid muscle is usually transected. The scalene fat pad is carefully divided, taking care to avoid the underlying phrenic nerve. This nerve must be protected throughout the course of the

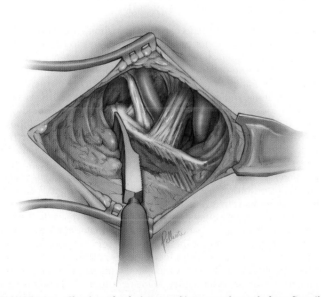

FIGURE 62-7 Clearing of soft tissue and intercostal muscle from first rib. Note anatomical arrangement of neurovascular structures within thoracic outlet, with vein, anterior scalene, artery, and nerve positioned from anterior to posterior.

operation. Underlying the nerve is the anterior scalene muscle. This is divided inferiorly at its insertion on the first rib. There are usually adhesions between the muscle and the subclavian artery and brachial plexus components that also must be freed. The origin end of the muscle is divided medially to expose the C5-C7 roots. The area between the C7 root and the subclavian artery is next cleaned, including the division of a subclavius minimus muscle if present. At this point, the five roots should be completely cleaned and tested using a nerve stimulator, although many surgeons have noted that it is often difficult to assess the T1 nerve root in this manner.

If the operation is to include first rib resection, the middle scalene muscle must be divided. The rib is divided posteriorly and a finger used to dissect it from the pleura while elevating the divided end. The subclavian artery must be freed from the anterior portion of the rib before it is divided. It can then be carefully extracted.

Irrigation is placed in the wound to assess for pleural leak. If present, the soft closed suction drain can be positioned so that the tip drains the pleural space. Otherwise, the drain can be placed to drain the wound. Postoperative chest radiograph is obtained, and the patient is usually discharged home within 1 or 2 days.

A brief mention should be made here of some alternative surgical approaches for patients with TOS. Some advocate for a thoracoscopic approach to rib resection and scalenectomy. Although offered at several centers, this procedure has not gained widespread acceptance. Many question the stated benefits over the transaxillary approach.[36] Also reported in the literature is endoscopic-assisted transaxillary rib resection and scalenectomy. Again, this has not been demonstrated in any large series to be superior to the traditional approaches.

TREATMENT OF VENOUS THROMBOSIS

Venous occlusion at the thoracic outlet should be treated expeditiously. Although this disease was historically treated with a conservative approach of anticoagulation and arm elevation, most therapeutic protocols now emphasize thrombolysis, anticoagulation, and surgical decompression as the key components of treatment. When patients present acutely, as is often the case, they should undergo catheter-directed fibrinolysis of the clot expeditiously. Currently, fibrinolytics such as alteplase and reteplase are used and have largely replaced streptokinase and urokinase, owing to improved safety profiles. Patients tend to respond better to thrombolytic therapy instituted within days of the onset of symptoms, but many may still benefit as far out as 4 to 6 weeks.[37] Following thrombolytic therapy, patients should receive systemic anticoagulation.

Traditionally, clinicians would advocate for a 1- to 3-month period of anticoagulation following thrombolysis, prior to surgical intervention. Previous work by Machleder and Kunkle demonstrated that this protracted time frame allowed for intimal healing of the damaged vein and reduction in the inflammatory response, thus facilitating a successful surgical outcome.[38] In the modern era, most clinicians advocate for earlier surgical intervention in attempts to decrease the period of disability.[39,40] Some authors even promote first rib resection during the initial hospitalization. Moreover, this approach has been demonstrated to be safe. Angle et al.[41] recently reported a series of patients treated in this fashion and noted no increased morbidity compared with patients with delayed operation. In particular, none of the theoretical concerns for bleeding following the use of thrombolytics were realized, nor were there particular technical problems secondary to the thrombosis-mediated inflammatory response seen in these patients. In 2007, Molina et al. reported a series of 97 patients undergoing immediate surgical decompression following thrombolysis, with only one bleeding complication.[42] Conversely, many suggest that early surgical intervention minimizes the incidence of residual symptoms, postthrombotic syndrome, and rethrombosis.[37,43]

Although controversial, recent data published by our group suggest that thrombolysis may not even be necessary. In a series of 110 first rib resection and scalenectomies, the number of patent vessels at 1 year was equal at 91% in patients undergoing preoperative thrombolysis and those who only had anticoagulation.[44] This needs to be validated by additional studies, but may further evolve the management approach to patients presenting with this disease in the future.

Beyond details outlined earlier for surgical treatment of TOS, it is important to emphasize a few points specific to venous TOS. Because venous compression commonly occurs within the costoclavicular aperture, it is imperative to adequately decompress this space. Complete lysis of the subclavius tendon is integral in this process. Furthermore, the first rib should be cut as far anterior as possible, well into the costal cartilage. Many advocate lysis of any fibrotic tissue surrounding the vein, although this may increase the incidence of a vein injury. Some authors even remove a portion of the medial clavicle, although most clinicians do not advocate this aggressive approach.[40] In some cases, the vein is so severely damaged that the only operative repair possible is a jugular-subclavian bypass, although this is rarely undertaken.[45]

Following surgical intervention, most clinicians use routine venography to both diagnose and treat residual disease.[39,46] Angioplasty for residual strictures appears to work quite well after surgical decompression.[41] Although enticing from a theoretical perspective, intravascular stenting for residual stenosis following angioplasty has been shown to be detrimental. Multiple authors report higher rethrombosis rates with stent placement compared to patients undergoing angioplasty alone.[47-49]

Most authors agree that anticoagulation is a key component in the treatment of venous TOS, but no consensus exists on the duration of anticoagulation following surgery. In most cases, patients who present to the vascular specialist after the diagnosis of venous TOS have already been placed on anticoagulation (usually in the form of warfarin). In our practice, patients discontinue warfarin and start low-molecular-weight heparin (LMWH) beginning 5 days prior to planned surgery. Low-molecular-weight heparin is then restarted 3 days post surgery. We routinely continue LMWH until a venogram is obtained 2 weeks after surgery. If the vein is patent and no intervention is required, anticoagulation is then discontinued. If the vein is stenotic, thrombosed, or undergoes intervention in the form of angioplasty, LMWH is restarted as a bridge to warfarin. At the 1-month follow-up visit, patients undergo duplex ultrasonography. In patients with evidence of complete thrombosis or increased velocity with EAST, anticoagulation is continued for an additional month. If the vessel appears widely patent, anticoagulation is discontinued at that time.

TREATMENT OF ARTERIAL COMPLICATIONS OF THORACIC OUTLET SYNDROME

A number of arterial problems can arise from thoracic outlet obstruction, although they are not common. Therapy has to be tailored to the individual patient on the basis of severity and extent of arterial compromise. These patients are rare and varied in presentation, so no standardized algorithm has been established to guide therapy.

Most patients will present in a subacute fashion. Just as with the other forms of TOS, the mainstay of treatment is thoracic outlet decompression. Most patients can safely undergo decompression with either the supraclavicular or transaxillary approach. The need for arterial reconstruction, however, dictates the approach and extent of exposure. Standard approaches are used, with a high anterior thoracotomy for proximal lesions on the left and a median sternotomy for proximal lesions on the right. For more distal lesions, various supra- and infraclavicular incisions may be used. Aneurysms or long-segment occlusions are typically treated with resection and graft reconstruction. Graft material is a matter of surgeon preference, but synthetic material, vein grafts, and arterial grafts all have been used with success in this position. Postoperative anticoagulation usually is not indicated, and patients tend to do well if the thoracic outlet is adequately decompressed and the vessel is no longer subjected to trauma.

Various catheter-based approaches can be used in the management of these patients. Focal areas of stenosis can be managed successfully with angioplasty and stent placement. In patients presenting with peripheral embolization, as commonly occurs, catheter-directed thrombolysis may be of benefit. However, distal emboli are often chronic in nature and may be resistant to lysis. These cases pose unique challenges, and depending on severity, frequently require open mechanical thrombectomy or even distal arterial reconstruction.

An additional consideration in these patients is the presence of reflex sympathetic dystrophy, causalgia, or other autonomic dysfunction. Cervicodorsal or cervicothoracic sympathectomy may be helpful in these patients and can often be performed at the time of the arterial repair by standard approaches.

Outcomes for Thoracic Outlet Syndrome

For the majority of patients diagnosed with TOS, conservative management yields positive results. Following physical therapy and modifications to inciting activities such as work postures and repetitive motions, patients can experience a significant reduction or resolution of symptoms. However, for patients with more debilitating symptoms who have undergone surgical intervention, the long-term prognosis remains poorly defined. There have been a few recent outcome-based studies that do offer promising results.

In a recent series published by our group, quality-of-life (QOL) measures were prospectively assessed in both neurogenic and venous TOS patients using the short form (SF)-12 and DASH (Disabilities of the Arm, Shoulder, and Hand) instruments.[50] Patients completed QOL surveys preoperatively and then at 3, 6, 12, 18, and 24 months. Of an eligible 105 patients, 2-year follow-up data were available for 70 patients, with 44 subjects having neurogenic TOS. These patients were followed out to 2 years postoperatively, with promising results. At baseline, the physical component score of the SF-12 was the most notably decreased score, with a median of 33.8 points. Postoperatively, this value increased on average 0.24 points per month over the 2-year follow-up period, with return to normal QOL for the physical component by 23 months on average. Notably, the return to normal quality for the mental component score was on average 12 months.[50]

For the venous TOS patients in the study, mean recovery period was notably shorter. Recovery to normal QOL occurred at a mean of 11 months for the physical component score and 8 months for the mental component score. Return to full activity or work in both groups occurred earlier than complete functional recovery (50% at 4 months and 77% at 5 months). Notably, fewer patients in the venous subset had return to full activity at 2 years (77%), since only 8% of patients were disabled or unemployed preoperatively. Reasons for this are unclear.[50]

In line with this study, Cordobes-Gual et al. similarly reported prospective results, also using the DASH instrument. A full 78% of neurogenic patients reported significant improvement in functional status and reduction in symptoms over the study period. There was a significant reduction in mean DASH scores from 54 preoperatively to 18 postoperatively at a mean follow-up interval of 40 months.[51]

Scali et al. also recently reported promising retrospective results on a small cohort of neurogenic patients. They noted a 91% reduction in the use of therapeutic adjuncts (e.g., narcotics, physical therapy, scalene blocks) following surgical decompression. Furthermore, patients' self-assessment of functional status was rated as good or excellent in 68% of patients postoperatively, compared to only 14% reporting a status of good or fair preoperatively.[52]

Despite these encouraging results, others have reported poorer outcomes. In a series of 254 procedures performed for neurogenic TOS, only 46% had a successful outcome after the first operation, defined as greater than 50% reduction in symptoms. Furthermore, 80 patients underwent a repeat procedure for "failure," with an overall secondary success rate of 66%. Of the failures, 89% occurred within 12 months of surgery.[53] The reasons for variable success rates are unclear, but likely related to variability in patient selection, operative intervention, and lack of standardized outcome measures.

A study by Sharp et al. focused on patients' ability to return to work following TOS surgery, noting that 80% of the patients in their study were able to do so, and that 85% of the patients subjectively described their outcomes as good to excellent.[54] Employment and disability issues complicate outcomes in TOS. In the Washington State workers' compensation study done by Franklin et al., 40% of postoperative TOS patients were still not working 2 years after their operations; this percentage was actually worse at 5 years (44%).[28] Interestingly, the conservatively treated patients in this study did better in this regard, although this was a retrospective study where the cohorts were not particularly well matched. Numerous other studies have shown worse outcomes when the patients have work-related or legal issues related to their TOS.[55]

Other factors predicting outcome following TOS surgery have been studied. Trauma as the event precipitating TOS is associated with poor outcomes in several series, but not in others.[56,57] Preoperative depression has been linked to worse outcome as well. In a report by Axelrod et al., those patients with preoperative depression were more likely to have continued functional and vocational disability following operation.[58] This study combined preoperative and postoperative interviews, psychological evaluations, and patient examinations; overall, 67% subjectively reported good or average outcome. At an average of 47 months' follow-up, 64% of patients were satisfied with their outcomes, and 69% reported they would undergo operation again if faced with the same symptoms. Eighteen percent of the patients considered themselves disabled.

In one of the largest series of TOS patients, Roos reported that in 1844 transaxillary first rib resections, 90% of patients were able to return to performing tasks they had been unable to perform preoperatively. In addition, 97% said that they would recommend rib resection to other patients with symptoms from TOS. There was a 5% recurrence, which was better than the 19% seen with scalenectomy (although this was without rib resection).[35] Green et al. also reported higher recurrence following anterior approach, although other authors have reported that the two approaches yielded equivalent recurrence rates.[56,59]

The prognosis for untreated axillosubclavian venous thrombosis had been one of progressive disability. Recurrence rates of 58% to 75% have been reported for patients receiving only anticoagulation.[60,61] Following modern treatment protocols, most patients can expect an excellent functional recovery and can resume normal activities in a relatively short period of time. Urschel and Patel reported 96% of 506 patients experiencing a good to excellent response to the current treatment paradigm of early thrombolysis with prompt rib resection and scalenectomy.[61] These promising results are of particular importance to this group of predominantly young and otherwise healthy patients. The most important factor is the time to treatment following thrombosis, with most treatment failures occurring if treatment is delayed. Feugier et al. reported that all treated patients were asymptomatic after an average follow-up of 45 months.[62] Long-term sequelae are not common if patients are treated expeditiously and if complete recanalization of the vein is achieved and the compressive rib is removed. If this cannot be accomplished, repeated venous problems occur, and these can lead to debilitating outcomes.

The prognosis for patients with arterial involvement in TOS is highly variable and depends on the pattern of disease. If the compressive element of the process is removed, the principal issue affecting prognosis is the result of the arterial repair. The outcomes of subclavian artery repairs generally mirror those of repairs done for other disease processes and are generally good.

May-Thurner's Syndrome

Presentation

May-Thurner's syndrome is the clinical condition caused by extrinsic compression of the left common iliac vein (CIV) by the right common iliac artery (CIA). Typically the presentation of this syndrome involves left lower-extremity swelling, pain, or other signs of venous hypertension as a manifestation of deep venous thrombosis (DVT).[63,64] This condition usually manifests in early adulthood, and there is a female predominance. Children can develop May-Thurner's syndrome, although this is infrequent.[65,66] Interestingly, patients with a patent foramen ovale have experienced stroke as the first symptom of the syndrome, with occult pelvic deep venous thrombus crossing the foramen and traveling to the brain.[67,68] Pregnancy can also precipitate DVT in patients with this mechanical finding, likely due to the added compression on the pelvic veins caused by a gravid uterus. Rupture of the left iliac vein has also been reported as an initial presentation.[69]

Pathophysiology

The right CIA crosses anterior to the left CIV at the confluence with the aorta and vena cava. Mechanical compression of the left CIV can occur, with resultant left lower-extremity venous hypertension and thrombosis. However, mechanical compression of the left CIV is frequently identified in patients who are asymptomatic, thus calling into question the contribution of mechanical compression in the syndrome.[70,71] Prothrombotic states have been implicated in the occurrence of this syndrome,[72–74] and it is not known whether mechanical compression is the sole instigator of symptoms or if other factors are involved for most patients.

Diagnosis

Diagnosis can be delayed until symptoms persist or multiple thrombotic events occur, because computed tomography (CT) venography,[75] MR venography,[76] or conventional venography of the pelvis are needed to confirm the presence of May-Thurner's syndrome. Lower-extremity ultrasound frequently fails to confirm the diagnosis, especially in the setting of extensive iliofemoral DVT.[77] Although quite rare, right-sided and vena cava compression have also been reported.[67,78–80]

Treatment

Symptomatic extensive iliofemoral DVT in a young low-risk patient is treated with thrombolytic therapy with increasing frequency. If the lytic therapy is successful, completion venography would confirm the diagnosis of May-Thurner syndrome. Two options exist for relief of the mechanical compression. The traditional method is to perform an open surgical procedure where the right CIA is divided and transposed beneath the left common iliac artery. The two ends of the artery are reanastomosed in an end-to-end fashion. Fibrous bands frequently cross the left CIV and attach to the underlying lumbar vertebra. These have to be divided sharply before the artery is reattached.

Endovenous stents for May-Thurner's syndrome have gained increasing popularity to avoid the laparotomy and arterial transection required for the open procedure.[81–85] Stents appear to have the radial force necessary to overcome the compression, and stent fractures from repeated trauma have not been reported. Stents are subject to migration and restenosis that may require reintervention.[86] Stents are frequently deployed in the left CIV and extended into the vena cava. This placement can lead to thrombosis of the right iliac venous system. Endovascular treatment may be preferable when patients presenting with acute complications due to May-Thurner's syndrome are also pregnant.[87,88] No randomized trials have been performed to compare endovascular stenting to open surgery, and treatment options are typically individualized for each patient.

Outcomes

Endovascular outcomes have been excellent, with reported initial technical success greater than 90% and an equally high rate of symptom resolution.[82,83,89,90] Complications included mainly bleeding, usually related to administration of thrombolytic agents.

Over an average of 2 years of follow-up, stent thrombosis occurs in approximately 10% of patients. Most of these stents are reopened using endovascular techniques.

Reports of open surgical procedures for May-Thurner's syndrome are scarce. Frequently the results are reported for a mix of clinical presentations including May-Thurner's syndrome. The Mayo Clinic has published two reports in the past 10 years.[91,92] These show secondary patency rates of 70% at 5-year follow-up. Most of these patients received surgical bypass or a hybrid procedure and had received other interventions before the surgical bypass was performed.

Nutcracker Syndrome
Presentation

Nutcracker syndrome is a clinical condition that results from venous hypertension of the left renal vein and its branches. When found radiographically in its asymptomatic form, it is referred to as *nutcracker phenomenon*. Both males and females are affected, with a slight female preponderance. Age of presentation is quite variable, but most commonly is young adulthood.[93–95] There are many reports documenting childhood presentation.[96,97] Symptoms can include hematuria (micro- and macroscopic), orthostatic proteinuria, left flank pain, abdominal pain, left lower-extremity varicose veins, left varicocele (males), and pelvic congestion syndrome (females). Pelvic congestion syndrome symptoms include dyspareunia, dysuria, dysmenorrhea, vulvar varicosities, and vaginal tenderness. Children and adolescents with nutcracker syndrome frequently have associated medical problems that include urolithiasis,[98] Henoch-Schönlein purpura,[99] immunoglobulin (Ig)A nephropathy,[100] hypercalciuria,[101] and familial Mediterranean fever.[102]

Pathophysiology

The course of the left renal vein passes between the SMA and the aorta before emptying into the inferior vena cava (IVC). The gap between the SMA and the aorta is variable, and mechanical compression of the left renal vein can develop when the angle between the two arteries is too sharp. Acute weight loss, which diminishes the amount of mesenteric and retroperitoneal soft tissue, can lead to shrinking of the angle between the aorta and SMA. However, acute weight loss is a variable of unpredictable importance; many patients with this problem do not experience antecedent weight loss. Hypertension of the renal vein can cause hematuria and hypertension of the veins that empty into the left renal vein, which include the left gonadal vein. Retroaortic location of the left renal vein is also associated with nutcracker syndrome, with the left renal vein being entrapped between the aorta and the adjacent vertebral body. This is known as *posterior nutcracker syndrome*.[103] A left-sided vena cava can also lead to nutcracker syndrome.[104]

Diagnosis

Cross-sectional imaging that demonstrates left abdominal and pelvic venous hypertension can confirm the diagnosis of nutcracker syndrome. Ultrasound, CT, MRI, and traditional venography with pressure measurements have all been used for this purpose. Typically, demonstration of increased pressures distal to the area of compression is sought before invasive treatment is recommended. Ultrasound findings suggestive of nutcracker syndrome include elevated peak systolic velocities in the aortomesenteric portions of the left renal vein as compared to the hilar portion, typically with a ratio of >5.[105]

Left renal vein acute angle (beak sign) and a diameter ratio of greater than 4.9 between the hilum and the aortomesenteric segment are CT findings that demonstrate the highest correlation with venographic pressure gradients.[106] Computed tomography findings correlate with proteinuria in children.[107] Computed tomography has also demonstrated usefulness when patients have a presentation consistent with nutcracker syndrome where compression of the left renal vein is caused by unusual structures such as the splenic vein, pancreas, duodenum, and the right diaphragmatic cruz.[108] Magnetic resonance fast-spin echo (FSE) T2-weighted imaging can demonstrate stagnant venous flow in the left renal vein and associated varicosities, potentially obviating the need for venography.[109]

Treatment

Conservative management has proven effective in selected cases.[110,111] In particular, pediatric patients with minimal hematuria may improve with further growth. Weight gain may also enlarge the aorto-SMA angle. For patients with concomitant medical problems that may induce acute weight loss, supportive treatment and attainment of weight gain may trigger spontaneous recovery. Use of angiotensin-converting enzyme (ACE) inhibitors has demonstrated efficacy in pediatric patients for relief of proteinuria.[112,113]

For patients whose symptoms are too severe for conservative management, or for those who do not improve with conservative measures, a wide variety of percutaneous minimally invasive and open surgical techniques are available to address symptoms of nutcracker syndrome. A large number of surgical procedures have been employed for relief of left renal vein compression. These include left renal vein transposition (to an area lower on the vena cava),[111,114] autotransplantation of the kidney,[115,116] laparoscopic placement of external left renal vein stent,[117] laparoscopic splenorenal vein bypass,[118] laparoscopic left renal vein transposition,[119] and laparoscopic transposition[120] and ligation[121] of the left ovarian vein. Synthetic bypass of the left renal vein has also been performed.[122] Rarely is nephrectomy indicated for this condition.

Endovascular stenting has also been performed and may be gaining in popularity.[123–126] This treatment is controversial because many treated patients are very young, and the implanted stent must last for many years.

Interventions performed should be chosen to address the patient's specific symptoms. Varicocele and pelvic congestion symptoms can be addressed by gonadal vein embolization or open surgical and laparoscopic resection of the affected engorged venous structures. Treatment of the left renal vein in isolation frequently does not improve pelvic symptoms and secondary procedures are needed to address these symptoms directly.[111]

Outcomes

The rarity of nutcracker syndrome, fairly recent recognition of this entity, and the success of conservative management for some patients means that outcomes data from large series are lacking. A few small reports regarding long-term outcomes following interventions for nutcracker syndrome do exist.[94] Two series and two reviews for open surgical techniques document that the most frequently performed procedure is left renal vein transposition.[93,111,127,128] Outcomes reported are excellent, with no mortality and minimal morbidity. Symptom resolution was seen in more than 80% of treated patients. Follow-up has been inconsistent but ranges over the course of many years. In certain instances, secondary procedures were needed for additional treatment of pelvic symptoms or recanalization of left renal veins that occluded after initial treatment. This rethrombosis occurred exclusively in patients with left renal vein occlusion at the time of initial presentation.[111]

Outcomes for stenting also show a very high rate of symptom resolution and similarly low rates of complications.[127,129,130] No procedure-related deaths have been reported. However, two stents have embolized and required retrieval.[127,130] Stent thrombosis and stenosis have also been reported.[93] As with other endovascular modalities, left renal vein stenting offers a significantly shorter recovery time. However, more data are needed to determine the optimal treatment for nutcracker syndrome.

Popliteal Entrapment Syndrome

Presentation

Popliteal entrapment is a rare syndrome caused by congenital anomalous pathology of the popliteal artery and presents with claudication-like symptoms. Patients most commonly present in early adulthood, although the syndrome has been diagnosed in children.[131,132] The most frequent symptom is unilateral lower-extremity pain with exertion. This pain resolves within minutes of activity cessation. The physical examination is typically normal at rest. Provocative maneuvers, which include forced plantar and passive dorsiflexion, will cause diminution or loss of pedal pulses. The presentation may also be bilateral.[133] If the syndrome has been long-standing, patients may present with total occlusion or aneurysmal degeneration of the popliteal artery. Occlusion of the popliteal artery aneurysm may cause significant ischemia.[134,135] The popliteal vein is involved rarely in the entrapment, so below-knee DVT may be a presenting symptom as well.[136,137] Functional entrapment of the popliteal artery has also been reported and is seen in asymptomatic patients as well.[138–140]

Pathophysiology

The congenital anomalies seen in popliteal entrapment syndrome disturb the normal relationship between the popliteal artery and the muscular structures within the popliteal fossa.[141] There are six distinct anatomical presentations of this syndrome (Box 62-1). The most common type (type I) causes the popliteal artery to traverse the popliteal fossa medial to the medial head of the normally configured gastrocnemius muscle. This configuration results in compression of the artery against the head of the tibia when the muscle contracts (typically during ambulation). One variant also causes entrapment of the popliteal vein either in combination with the artery or in isolation.

Diagnosis

MRI/MRA is the study of choice for popliteal entrapment syndrome owing to its excellent visualization of both the soft tissue and arterial anatomy in this region. It is not only diagnostic but also provides enough anatomical information to facilitate operative planning.[142–144] Catheter-based angiography may also be performed, but forced plantar or dorsiflexion may be required to demonstrate the abnormality, since flow may be normal in a neutral position[145] (Fig 62-9). A medial course of the popliteal artery during angiography also suggests the diagnosis. In cases of suspected popliteal artery occlusion, angiography may be necessary for operative planning of a distal bypass. Computed tomography angiography has also been used and studied for its utility in diagnosing popliteal entrapment syndrome.[146,147] Like MRA, Computed tomography angiography demonstrates both the vascular structures and soft-tissue relationships, ideal for confirming the diagnosis and planning treatment.[148]

Box 62-1 Types of Popliteal Entrapment	
Type I	Popliteal artery deviates medial to medial head of normally configured gastrocnemius
Type II	Abnormally lateral insertion of medial head of gastrocnemius displacing popliteal artery medially
Type III	Normal popliteal artery is compressed by accessory "slips" of gastrocnemius muscle
Type IV	Compression of popliteal artery by popliteus muscle, nerve tissue, or fibrous bands
Type V	Any of the above also involving compression of the popliteal vein
Type VI	Functional entrapment

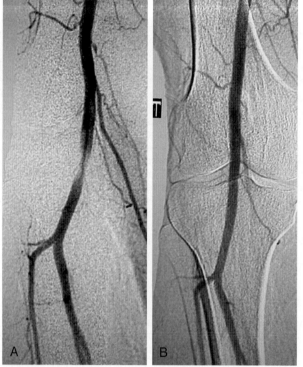

FIGURE 62-9 These two angiograms clearly show compression of popliteal artery with forced dorsiflexion of foot (A) and subsequent filling when leg is relaxed (B). Note presence of underlying disease in both affected segment of artery and runoff vessels.

Treatment

Open surgical repair is typically required to relieve the mechanical compression. Prone positioning is commonly used, and an S-shaped incision is made over the popliteal fossa. Ligation of the offending muscular segments is usually tolerated with no subsequent loss of function. In instances where the entire medial head of the gastrocnemius muscle must be divided, it should be relocated and reattached to the tibial condyle. If indicated, arterial reconstruction can easily be performed through this approach as well. For patients with short-segment disease, repair can be performed with resection of the affected segment, mobilization of the vessels distally and proximally, and construction of an end-to-end anastomosis. If the affected segment is too long, thus precluding primary repair, reconstruction using an interposition saphenous vein graft should be performed.[149]

Endovascular treatment can include thrombolysis when thrombus is present and the clinical presentation is not advanced irreversible ischemia.[150] Decompression of the mechanical compression should be performed during the same hospitalization. Stenting the arterial abnormality is contraindicated, especially if decompression of the compression has not been performed.[151,152] In this circumstance, the stent is subjected to the same mechanical trauma that produced the arterial injury, thus leading to stent fracture and the potential for further arterial injury. This approach may lead to a more substantial open repair (e.g., distal bypass) when decompression alone, with or without primary repair, may have sufficed.

Outcomes

Outcomes following intervention for popliteal artery entrapment syndrome depend significantly on the amount of vascular damage that has been incurred prior to diagnosis. The rarity of the syndrome and the low index of suspicion for arterial insufficiency in this atypical patient population frequently delay diagnosis until significant arterial damage has occurred and signs of advanced ischemia are present. In these situations, complex repair may be required,[153] and eventual limb loss may be unavoidable. When the syndrome is diagnosed in early stages, with symptoms of claudication and no arterial occlusion, simple decompression of the offending musculotendinous structures should be curative.[149]

Cystic Adventitial Disease

Presentation

Cystic adventitial disease is a rare entity characterized by accumulation of mucin within the adventitia, resulting in vascular compression. In its most common form, the cyst compresses the popliteal artery. However, many case reports demonstrate the occurrence of these cysts in other locations,[154,155] sometimes resulting in compression of veins[156-159] instead of arteries. Presenting symptoms are typically those of unilateral claudication. Cases with bilateral cysts have been reported, which can result in bilateral symptoms.[160,161] Occasionally, acute occlusion of the popliteal artery may be the event causing someone to initially seek medical care.[162] The age of presentation is younger than patients with lower-extremity atherosclerosis, but more varied than patients with popliteal entrapment.[163,164] There appears to be a male predominance in patients with this disorder.[165] The cyst is benign but has a tendency to recur. The quality of substance within the cyst is gelatinous.

Pathophysiology

The cause of the cyst remains unknown, but there are suggestions that they occur as mucin-producing cells relocate from an adjacent joint.[164,166] There is also the possibility that the cyst communicates directly with the synovium of the joint.[167]

Diagnosis

Cross-sectional imaging including ultrasound,[168] CT,[169] and MRI[170,171] are all useful in establishing the diagnosis of cystic adventitial disease by demonstrating the cyst in close proximity to the vascular structures being compressed. Catheter angiography can confirm arterial compression. Signs typical of cystic adventitial disease include a scalloped appearance of the artery wall.

Treatment

Treatment is directed at full resection or enucleation of the cyst, which also involves the artery wall. Revascularization is typically performed with a saphenous vein interposition graft where appropriate. Despite the goal of treatment being full resection of the cyst, they are known to recur. Alternatives to surgical resection and revascularization include aspiration of the cyst[172] and aspiration combined with introduction of a sclerosing agent into the cyst.[173] Endovascular stenting in isolation has not been successful in treating cystic adventitial disease,[174,175] although treatment of recurrence with angioplasty alone has been reported.[176]

Outcomes

Determining outcomes of treatment for cystic adventitial disease is difficult owing to the rarity of this disease process. Most available literature consists of case reports. Long-term resolution has been reported with image-guided cyst aspiration.[172] Small series (three patients) document good outcomes with surgical resection and revascularization.[163,164]

Median Arcuate Ligament Syndrome

Presentation

Median arcuate ligament syndrome (MALS) is a rare syndrome characterized by celiac artery compression by the diaphragmatic crura and median arcuate ligament. This syndrome is essentially a diagnosis of exclusion, so many patients have experienced symptoms for many years before a diagnosis of MALS is established. It presents at variable ages (adolescence to late adulthood), with a female preponderance.[177-179] The most common symptoms are abdominal pain and weight loss. Vomiting is frequent, and an epigastric bruit is frequently present on physical examination. The pain can be episodic, postprandial, or constant. Exercise-related abdominal pain has also been reported.[180] Recently the suggestion that MALS may be a familial syndrome has been made.[177,181]

Pathophysiology

The celiac artery is the first branch originating from the aorta in the abdomen. The celiac take-off forms a 90-degree angle with the aorta. In this location, it is susceptible to compression by the diaphragmatic crura during thoracic motion throughout respiration. The median arcuate ligament connects the two crura. This compression can result in stenosis or occlusion of the celiac artery. In most patients, this is asymptomatic and can frequently be found incidentally.[182,183] Symptoms may manifest in those patients who do not have adequate collateral flow from the SMA to carry the demand of the foregut structures. Some patients experience chronic pain, likely due to compression of neural structures surrounding the celiac artery, and their symptoms are unrelated to visceral perfusion. Increased flow through the SMA can rarely lead to aneurysm formation or rupture in branches of the SMA.[184-186]

Diagnosis

Presenting symptoms for MALS are very nonspecific. As mentioned, celiac stenosis can be seen in asymptomatic patients. These two factors make it mandatory that these patients go through a thorough evaluation to eliminate other possible explanations for their symptoms.[187-189] There is no standard battery of examinations, but any structural or functional abnormality of the upper abdomen should be evaluated and treated first. Following exclusion of other pathologies, it is important to document the celiac artery stenosis or occlusion. If the artery is not occluded, demonstrating that the stenosis varies with respiration is important to rule out other more typical causes of celiac artery stenosis such as atherosclerosis.[189] Some clinicians recommend injection of vasodilators[190] during angiography or measurement of gastric exercise tonometry[191] as adjunctive diagnostic tools. The anatomy can be imaged using catheter angiography, MRI,[192] CT,[193-197] and ultrasound.[198] Ultrasound has the advantage of also providing information about flow through the celiac artery. When angiography is performed, images should be captured during both inspiration and expiration because the degree of celiac compression is worse during full expiration (Fig. 62-10). However, compression of the celiac axis during expiration can be demonstrated in asymptomatic individuals and further underscores the challenge of establishing this diagnosis.

Treatment

Two primary goals must be addressed for treatment of MALS. The first is to divide the median arcuate ligament and all the dense fibrotic tissue that surrounds the celiac artery. This relieves mechanical compression on the artery. The second goal is to perform revascularization for patients who require this as well. Traditionally, both these steps are performed in one open surgical procedure. Less invasive interventional methods proliferated recently and have probably increased the number of patients with this disease who undergo treatment. Many publications have advocated laparoscopic surgery to treat the mechanical compression by skeletonizing the celiac artery (removing all crural components and other investing tissue).[189,199-204] If revascularization is needed, it is performed in a second endovascular or surgical procedure. Robotic surgery[205] and retroperitoneal endoscopic release[206] have also been utilized to treat MALS.

It is unclear when clinicians should perform revascularizations of the celiac artery. The most straightforward scenario would be an occluded celiac artery with minimal collateral flow and symptoms of postprandial pain and weight loss. However, many patients present with varying degrees of celiac stenosis that may not be flow-limiting, a widely patent SMA, and symptoms that are not typical of intestinal malperfusion. With the increasing use of laparoscopic techniques to treat MALS, there is a corresponding increase in experience in patients where celiac revascularization is not performed.

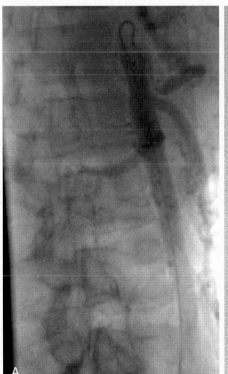
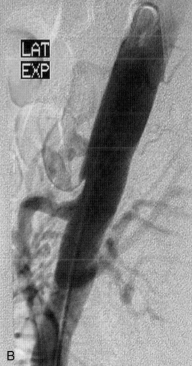

FIGURE 62-10 Lateral angiograms of celiac axis in both inspiration (A) and expiration (B) demonstrate characteristic compression of artery.

CH
62

Some authors advocate decompression alone with minimally invasive techniques, whereas others decompress and revascularize all or most patients immediately via an open approach.[207,208]

Rupture or aneurysm of an SMA branch associated with celiac stenosis or occlusion is extremely rare, and treatment of this is difficult. Patients may present with sudden and severe abdominal pain in hypovolemic shock. Endovascular embolization of this entity is preferable to open surgery[184,185] because these aneurysms are very difficult to locate and expose surgically. Gastroduodenal branches are frequently involved, and definitive open surgery may include a pancreatic resection because of the rich collateral network of arteries in this location.

Outcomes

Patient selection is a key component of obtaining good outcomes for invasive treatment of MALS. Improvement in symptoms is unlikely if the original diagnosis is incorrect. Symptoms can recur even after initial improvement.[206] Minimally invasive approaches to MALS are technically difficult and prone to bleeding complications, requiring conversion to an open procedure.[189,203] However, when successful, laparoscopic approach to MALS reduces length of stay and significantly decreases recovery time. It also prevents future complications from a laparotomy.

Regardless of approach and procedures performed, most series show favorable outcomes. The majority of patients experience valuable symptom relief. There is generally limited morbidity and mortality. One report documented that in a series of six patients with long-term follow-up, all patients would have the surgery again.[209] Contemporary management for this disease is still evolving, as is the ability to accurately recognize it. Future outcomes research will hopefully shed light on the ideal intervention for patients with this challenging and elusive disorder.

REFERENCES

1. Brantigan CO, Roos DB: Diagnosing thoracic outlet syndrome, Hand Clin 20:27–36, 2004.
2. Peet RM, Henriksen JD, Anderson TP, et al: Thoracic-outlet syndrome: evaluation of a therapeutic exercise program, Proc Staff Meet Mayo Clin 31:281–287, 1956.
3. Clagett O: Research and prosearch, J Thorac Cardiovasc Surg 44:153–166, 1962.
4. Roos DB: Transaxillary approach for first rib resection to relieve thoracic outlet syndrome, Ann Surg 163:354–358, 1966.
5. Machleder H, editor: Vascular disorders of the upper extremity, ed 2, Mt Kisco, NY: 1989, Futura Press.
6. Atasoy E: Thoracic outlet syndrome: anatomy, Hand Clin 20:7–14, v, 2004.
7. Juvonen T, Satta J, Laitala P, et al: Anomalies at the thoracic outlet are frequent in the general population, Am J Surg 170:33–37, 1995.
8. Roos D: Congenital anomalies associated with thoracic outlet syndrome: anatomy, symptoms, diagnosis, and treatment, Am J Surg 132:771–778, 1976.
9. Brantigan CO, Roos DB: Etiology of neurogenic thoracic outlet syndrome, Hand Clin 20:17–22, 2004.
10. Sanders RJ, Hammond SL: Etiology and pathology, Hand Clin 20:23–26, 2004.
11. Sanders RJ, Hammond SL: Management of cervical ribs and anomalous first ribs causing neurogenic thoracic outlet syndrome, J Vasc Surg 36:51–56, 2002.
12. Daskalakis E, Bouhoutsos J: Subclavian and axillary vein compression of musculoskeletal origin, Br J Surg 67:573–576, 1980.
13. Dijkstra P, Westra D: Angiographic features of compression of the axillary artery by the musculus pectoralis minor and the head of the humerus in the thoracic outlet compression syndrome. Case report, Radiol Clin 47:423–427, 1978.
14. Le EN, Freischlag JA, Christo PJ, et al: Thoracic outlet syndrome secondary to localized scleroderma treated with botulinum toxin injection, Arthritis Care Res (Hoboken) 62:430–433, 2010.
15. Roos D: Historical perspectives and anatomic considerations. Thoracic outlet syndrome, 1996.
16. Patton GM: Arterial thoracic outlet syndrome, Hand Clin 20:107–111, viii, 2004.
17. Firsov G: Cervical ribs and their distinction from under-developed first ribs, Arkh Anat Gistol Embriol 67:101, 1974.
18. Terabayashi N, Ohno T, Nishimoto Y, et al: Nonunion of a first rib fracture causing thoracic outlet syndrome in a basketball player: a case report, J Shoulder Elbow Surg 19:e20–e23, 2010.
19. Gilliatt R, Le Quesne P, Logue V, et al: Wasting of the hand associated with a cervical rib or band, J Neurol Neurosurg Psych 33:615–624, 1970.
20. Sanders RJ, Hammond SL: Venous thoracic outlet syndrome, Hand Clin 20:113–118, viii, 2004.
21. Machleder HI: Thoracic outlet syndromes: new concepts from a century of discovery, Cardiovasc Surg 2:137–145, 1994.
22. Roos D, Owens J: Thoracic outlet syndrome, Arch Surg 93:71–74, 1966.
23. Wilbourn A: The thoracic outlet syndrome is overdiagnosed, Arch Neurol 47:328–330, 1990.
24. Costigan D, Wilbourn A: The elevated arm stress test: specificity in the diagnosis of thoracic outlet syndrome, Neurology 35:74, 1985.
25. Plewa M, Delinger M: The false-positive rate of thoracic outlet syndrome shoulder maneuvers in healthy subjects, Acad Emerg Med 5:337–342, 1998.
26. Toomingas A, Nilsson T, Hagberg M, et al: Predictive aspects of the abduction external rotation test among male industrial and office workers, Am J Ind Med 35:32–42, 1999.
27. Roos D: The place for scalenectomy and first-rib resection in thoracic outlet syndrome, Surgery 92:1077–1085, 1982.
28. Franklin G, Fulton-Kehoe D, Bradley C, et al: Outcome of surgery for thoracic outlet syndrome in Washington state workers' compensation, Neurology 54:1252–1258, 2000.
29. Abe M, Ichinohe K, Nishida J: Diagnosis, treatment, and complications of thoracic outlet syndrome, J Orthop Sci 4:66–69, 1999.
30. Machleder H, Moll F, Nuwer M, et al: Somatosensory evoked potentials in the assessment of thoracic outlet compression syndrome, J Vasc Surg 6:177–184, 1987.
31. Jordan SE, Machleder HI: Diagnosis of thoracic outlet syndrome using electrophysiologically guided anterior scalene blocks, Ann Vasc Surg 12:260–264, 1998.
32. Jordan SE, Ahn SS, Freischlag JA, et al: Selective botulinum chemodenervation of the scalene muscles for treatment of neurogenic thoracic outlet syndrome, Ann Vasc Surg 14:365–369, 2000.
33. Wadhwani R, Chaubal N, Sukthankar R, et al: Color Doppler and duplex sonography in 5 patients with thoracic outlet syndrome, J Ultrasound Med 20:795–801, 2001.
34. Aligne C, Barral X: Rehabilitation of patients with thoracic outlet syndrome, Ann Vasc Surg 6:381–389, 1992.
35. Cronenwett, editor: Rutherford's vascular surgery, ed 3, Philadelphia, 1989, WB Saunders. Roos DB, ed.
36. Ohtsuka T, Wolf RK, Dunsker SB: Port-access first-rib resection, Surg Endosc 13:940–942, 1999.
37. Alla V, Natarajan N, Kaushik M, et al: Paget-Schroetter syndrome: review of pathogenesis and treatment of effort thrombosis, West J Emerg Med 11:358–362, 2010.
38. Kunkel JM, Machleder HI: Treatment of Paget-Schroetter syndrome. A staged, multidisciplinary approach, Arch Surg 124:1153–1157, 1989; discussion 1157–1158.
39. Brooke B, Freischlag J: Contemporary management of thoracic outlet syndrome, Curr Opin Cardiol 25:535–540, 2010.
40. Illig KA, Doyle AJ: A comprehensive review of Paget-Schroetter syndrome, J Vasc Surg 51:1538–1547, 2010.
41. Angle N, Gelabert HA, Farooq MM, et al: Safety and efficacy of early surgical decompression of the thoracic outlet for Paget-Schroetter syndrome, Ann Vasc Surg 15:37–42, 2001.
42. Molina J, Hunter D, Dietz C: Paget-Schroetter syndrome treated with thrombolytics and immediate surgery, J Vasc Surg 45:328–334, 2007.
43. Molina J, Hunter D, Dietz C: Protocols for Paget-Schroetter syndrome and late treatment of chronic subclavian vein obstruction, Ann Thorac Surg 87:416–422, 2009.
44. Guzzo JL, Chang K, Demos J, et al: Preoperative thrombolysis and venoplasty affords no benefit in patency following first rib resection and scalenectomy for subacute and chronic subclavian vein thrombosis, J Vasc Surg 52:658–662, 2010.
45. Thompson R: Venous thoracic outlet syndrome: paraclavicular approach, Op Tech Gen Surg 10:113–121, 2008.
46. de Leon RA, Chang DC, Hassoun HT, et al: Multiple treatment algorithms for successful outcomes in venous thoracic outlet syndrome, Surgery 145:500–507, 2009.
47. Lee J, Karwowski J, Harris E, et al: Long-term thrombotic recurrence after nonoperative management of Paget-Schroetter syndrome, J Vasc Surg 43:1236–1243, 2006.
48. Meier GH, Pollak JS, Rosenblatt M, et al: Initial experience with venous stents in exertional axillary-subclavian vein thrombosis, J Vasc Surg 24:974–981, 1996; discussion 981–973.
49. Kreienberg P, Chang B, Darling R: Long-term results in patients treated with thrombolysis, thoracic inlet decompression, and subclavian vein stenting for Paget-Schroetter syndrome, J Vasc Surg 33:100–105, 2001.
50. Chang DC, Rotellini-Coltvet LA, Mukherjee D, et al: Surgical intervention for thoracic outlet syndrome improves patient's quality of life, J Vasc Surg 49:630–635, 2009.
51. Cordobes-Gual J, Lozano-Vilardell P, Torreguitart-Mirada N, et al: Prospective study of the functional recovery after surgery for thoracic outlet syndrome, Eur J Vasc Endovasc Surg 35:79–83, 2008.
52. Scali S, Stone D, Bjerke A, et al: Long-term functional results for the surgical management of neurogenic thoracic outlet syndrome, Vasc Endovasc Surg 44:550–555, 2010.
53. Altobelli GG, Kudo T, Haas BT, et al: Thoracic outlet syndrome: pattern of clinical success after operative decompression, J Vasc Surg 42:122–128, 2005.
54. Sharp WJ, Nowak LR, Zamani T, et al: Long-term follow-up and patient satisfaction after surgery for thoracic outlet syndrome, Ann Vasc Surg 15:32–36, 2001.
55. Lepäntalo M, Lindgren K: Long-term outcome after resection of the first rib for thoracic outlet syndrome, Br J Surg 76:1255–1256, 1989.
56. Green R, McNamara J, Ouriel K: Long-term follow-up after thoracic outlet decompression: an analysis of factors determining outcome, J Vasc Surg 14:739–745, 1991.
57. Sanders R, Pearce W: The treatment of thoracic outlet syndrome: a comparison of different operations, J Vasc Surg 10:626–634, 1989.
58. Axelrod DA, Proctor MC, Geisser ME, et al: Outcomes after surgery for thoracic outlet syndrome, J Vasc Surg 33:1220–1225, 2001.
59. Sessions R: Recurrent thoracic outlet syndrome: causes and treatment, South Med J 75:1453–1466, 1982.
60. Tilney N, Griffiths H, Edwards E: Natural history of major venous thrombosis of the upper extremity, Arch Surg 101:792–796, 1970.
61. Urschel H, Patel A: Surgery remains the most effective treatment for Paget-Schroetter syndrome: 50 years' experience, Ann Thorac Surg 86:254–260, 2008.
62. Feugier P, Aleksic I, Salari R, et al: Long-term results of venous revascularization for Paget-Schroetter syndrome in athletes, Ann Vasc Surg 15:212–218, 2001.
63. Dhillon RK, Stead LG: Acute deep vein thrombus due to May-Thurner syndrome, Am J Emerg Med 28(254):e253–e254, 2010.
64. Dogan O, Boke E: Three cases with May-Thurner syndrome: a possibly under-reported disorder, Vasa 34:147–151, 2005.

65. Oguzkurt L, Tercan F, Sener M: Successful endovascular treatment of iliac vein compression (May-Thurner) syndrome in a pediatric patient, *Cardiovasc Interv Radiol* 29:446–449, 2006.

66. Vyas S, Roberti I, McCarthy C: May–Thurner syndrome in a pediatric renal transplant recipient—case report and literature review, *Pediatr Transplant* 12:708–710, 2008.

67. Im S, Lim SH, Chun HJ, et al: Leg edema with deep venous thrombosis-like symptoms as an unusual complication of occult bladder distension and right May-Thurner syndrome in a stroke patient: a case report, *Arch Phys Med Rehabil* 90:886–890, 2009.

68. Kiernan TJ, Yan BP, Cubeddu RJ, et al: May-Thurner syndrome in patients with cryptogenic stroke and patent foramen ovale: an important clinical association, *Stroke* 40:1502–1504, 2009.

69. Kim Y, Ko S, Kim H: Spontaneous rupture of the left common iliac vein associated with May Thurner syndrome: successful management with surgery and placement of an endovascular stent, *Br J Radiol* 80:e176–e179, 2007.

70. Kibbe MR, Ujiki M, Goodwin AL, et al: Iliac vein compression in an asymptomatic patient population, *J Vasc Surg* 39:937–943, 2004.

71. Raju S, Neglen P: High prevalence of nonthrombotic iliac vein lesions in chronic venous disease: a permissive role in pathogenicity, *J Vasc Surg* 44:136–144, 2006.

72. De Bast Y, Dahin L: May-Thurner syndrome will be completed? *Thromb Res* 123:498–502, 2009.

73. Sharma R, Joshi W: A case of May-Thurner syndrome with antiphospholipid antibody syndrome, *Conn Med* 72:527–530, 2008.

74. Murphy EH, Davis CM, Journeycake JM, et al: Symptomatic iliofemoral DVT after onset of oral contraceptive use in women with previously undiagnosed May-Thurner syndrome, *J Vasc Surg* 49:697–703, 2009.

75. Jeon UB, Chung JW, Jae HJ, et al: May-Thurner syndrome complicated by acute iliofemoral vein thrombosis: helical CT venography for evaluation of long-term stent patency and changes in the iliac vein, *Am J Roentgenol* 195:751–757, 2010.

76. Gurel K, Gurel S, Karavas E, et al: Direct contrast-enhanced MR venography in the diagnosis of May-Thurner syndrome, *Eur J Radiol* 80:533–536, 2011.

77. Oguzkurt L, Ozkan U, Tercan F, et al: Ultrasonographic diagnosis of iliac vein compression (May-Thurner) syndrome, *Diagn Interv Radiol* 13:152–155, 2007.

78. Fretz V, Binkert C: Compression of the inferior vena cava by the right iliac artery: a rare variant of May-Thurner syndrome, *Cardiovasc Interv Radiol* 33:1060–1063, 2010.

79. Abboud G, Midulla M, Lions C, et al: Right-sided May-Thurner syndrome, *Cardiovasc Interv Radiol* 33:1056–1059, 2010.

80. Burke RM, Rayan SS, Kasirajan K, et al: Unusual case of right-sided May-Thurner syndrome and review of its management, *Vascular* 14:47–50, 2006.

81. Grunwald M, Goldberg M, Hofmann L: Endovascular management of May-Thurner syndrome, *AJR Am J Roentgenol* 183:1523–1524, 2004.

82. Kwak HS, Han YM, Lee YS, et al: Stents in common iliac vein obstruction with acute ipsilateral deep venous thrombosis: early and late results, *J Vasc Interv Radiol* 16:815–822, 2005.

83. Kim JY, Choi D, Guk Ko Y, et al: Percutaneous treatment of deep vein thrombosis in May-Thurner syndrome, *Cardiovasc Interv Radiol* 29:571–575, 2006.

84. Moudgill N, Hager E, Gonsalves C, et al: May-Thurner syndrome: case report and review of the literature involving modern endovascular therapy, *Vascular* 17:330–335, 2009.

85. Canales JF, Krajcer Z: Intravascular ultrasound guidance in treating May-Thurner syndrome, *Tex Heart Inst J* 37:496–497, 2010.

86. Mullens W, De Keyser J, Van Dorpe A, et al: Migration of two venous stents into the right ventricle in a patient with May-Thurner syndrome, *Int J Cardiol* 110:114–115, 2006.

87. Hartung O, Barthelemy P, Arnoux D, et al: Management of pregnancy in women with previous left ilio-caval stenting, *J Vasc Surg* 50:355–359, 2009.

88. Zander KD, Staat B, Galan H: May-Thurner syndrome resulting in acute iliofemoral deep vein thrombosis in the postpartum period, *Obstet Gynecol* 111:565–569, 2008.

89. O'Sullivan GJ, Semba CP, Bittner CA, et al: Endovascular management of iliac vein compression (May-Thurner) syndrome, *J Vasc Interv Radiol* 11:823–836, 2000.

90. Titus J, Moise MA, Bena J, et al: Iliofemoral stenting for venous occlusive disease, *J Vasc Surg* 53:706–712, 2011.

91. Jost CJ, Gloviczki P, Cherry KJ: Surgical reconstruction of iliofemoral veins and the inferior vena cava for nonmalignant occlusive disease, *J Vasc Surg* 33:320–328, 2001.

92. Garg N, Gloviczki P, Karimi KM, et al: Factors affecting outcome of open and hybrid reconstructions for nonmalignant obstruction of iliofemoral veins and inferior vena cava, *J Vasc Surg* 53:383–393, 2011.

93. Ahmed K, Sampath R, Khan M: Current trends in the diagnosis and management of renal nutcracker syndrome: a review, *Eur J Vasc Endovasc Surg* 31:410–416, 2006.

94. Kurklinsky AK, Rooke TW: Nutcracker phenomenon and nutcracker syndrome, *Mayo Clinic Proc* 85:552–559, 2010.

95. Menard M: Nutcracker syndrome: when should it be treated and how? *Perspect Vasc Surg Endovasc Ther* 21:117–124, 2009.

96. Park YH, Choi JY, Chung HS, et al: Hematuria and proteinuria in a mass school urine screening test, *Pediatr Nephrol* 20:1126–1130, 2005.

97. Shin JI, Lee JS: Unexpected superimposition of nutcracker effect in various conditions: is it an unrecognized confounding factor? *Eur J Pediatr* 166:1089–1090, 2007.

98. Altugan FS, Ekim M, Fitöz S, et al: Nutcracker syndrome with urolithiasis, *J Pediatr Urol* 6:519–521, 2010.

99. Shin J, Park J, Shin Y, et al: Superimposition of nutcracker syndrome in a haematuric child with Henoch Schönlein purpura, *Int J Clin Pract* 59:1472–1475, 2005.

100. Shin JI, Park JM, Shin YH, et al: Nutcracker syndrome combined with IgA nephropathy in a child with recurrent hematuria, *Pediatr Int* 48:324–326, 2006.

101. Shin JI, Park JM, Lee JS, et al: Superimposition of nutcracker syndrome in a hematuric child with idiopathic hypercalciuria and urolithiasis, *Int J Urol* 13:814–816, 2006.

102. Ozcan A, Gonul II, Sakallioglu O, et al: Nutcracker syndrome in a child with familial Mediterranean fever (FMF) disease: renal ultrastructural features, *Int Urol Nephrol* 41:1047–1053, 2009.

103. Ali-El-Dein B, Osman Y, El-Din ABS, et al: Anterior and posterior nutcracker syndrome: a report on 11 cases, *Transplant Proc* 35:851–853, 2003.

104. Fitoz S, Yalcinkaya F: Compression of left inferior vena cava: a form of nutcracker syndrome, *J Clin Ultrasound* 36:101–104, 2008.

105. Mohamadi A, Ghasemi-Rad M, Mladkova N, et al: Varicocele and nutcracker syndrome: sonographic findings, *J Ultrasound Med* 29:1153–1160, 2010.

106. Kim KW, Cho JY, Kim SH, et al: Diagnostic value of computed tomographic findings of nutcracker syndrome: correlation with renal venography and renocaval pressure gradients, *Eur J Radiol* 80:648–654, 2011.

107. Cho BS, Suh JS, Hahn WH, et al: Multidetector computed tomography findings and correlations with proteinuria in nutcracker syndrome, *Pediatric Nephrol* 25:469–475, 2010.

108. Karaosmanoglu D, Karcaaltincaba M, Akata D, et al: Unusual causes of left renal vein compression along its course: MDCT findings in patients with nutcracker and pelvic congestion syndrome, *Surg Radiol Anat* 32:323–327, 2010.

109. Wong HL, Chen MCY, Wu CS, et al: The usefulness of fast-spin-echo T2-weighted MR imaging in nutcracker syndrome: a case report, *Korean J Radiol* 11:373–377, 2010.

110. Shin JI, Park JM, Lee SM, et al: Factors affecting spontaneous resolution of hematuria in childhood nutcracker syndrome, *Pediatr Nephrol* 20:609–613, 2005.

111. Reed NR, Kalra M, Bower TC, et al: Left renal vein transposition for nutcracker syndrome, *J Vasc Surg* 49:386–394, 2009.

112. Ha TS, Lee EJ: ACE inhibition can improve orthostatic proteinuria associated with nutcracker syndrome, *Pediatr Nephrol* 21:1765–1768, 2006.

113. Shin JI, Lee JS: ACE inhibition in nutcracker syndrome with orthostatic proteinuria: how about a hemodynamic effect? *Pediatr Nephrol* 22:758, 2007.

114. Kim J, Joh J, Choi H, et al: Transposition of the left renal vein in nutcracker syndrome, *Eur J Vasc Endovasc Surg* 31:80–82, 2006.

115. Salehipour M, Rasekhi A, Shirazi M, et al: The role of renal autotransplantation in treatment of nutcracker syndrome, *Saudi J Kidney Dis Transpl* 21:237–241, 2010.

116. Xu D, Liu Y, Gao Y, et al: Management of renal nutcracker syndrome by retroperitoneal laparoscopic nephrectomy with *ex vivo* autograft repair and autotransplantation: a case report and review of the literature, *J Med Case Reports* 3:82, 2009.

117. Zhang Q, Zhang Y, Lou S, et al: Laparoscopic extravascular renal vein stent placement for nutcracker syndrome, *J Endourol* 354–357, 2010.

118. Chung BI, Gill IS: Laparoscopic splenorenal venous bypass for nutcracker syndrome, *J Vasc Surg* 49:1319–1323, 2009.

119. Hartung O, Azghari A, Barthelemy P, et al: Laparoscopic transposition of the left renal vein into the inferior vena cava for nutcracker syndrome, *J Vasc Surg* 52:738–741, 2010.

120. Hartung O, Barthelemy P, Berdah SV, et al: Laparoscopy-assisted left ovarian vein transposition to treat one case of posterior nutcracker syndrome, *Ann Vasc Surg* 23:413, 2009.

121. Rogers A, Beech A, Braithwaite B: Transperitoneal laparoscopic left gonadal vein ligation can be the right treatment option for pelvic congestion symptoms secondary to nutcracker syndrome, *Vascular* 15:238–240, 2007.

122. Shaper K, Jackson J, Williams G: The nutcracker syndrome: an uncommon cause of haematuria, *Br J Urol* 74:144–146, 1994.

123. Basile A, Tsetis D, Calcara G, et al: Percutaneous nitinol stent implantation in the treatment of nutcracker syndrome in young adults, *J Vasc Interv Radiol* 18:1042–1046, 2007.

124. Chen W, Chu J, Yang J, et al: Endovascular stent placement for the treatment of nutcracker phenomenon in three pediatric patients, *J Vasc Interv Radiol* 16:1529–1533, 2005.

125. Cohen F, Amabile P, Varoquaux A, et al: Endovascular treatment of circumaortic nutcracker syndrome, *J Vasc Interv Radiol* 20:1255–1257, 2009.

126. Gagnon LO, Ponsot Y, Benko A, et al: Nutcracker syndrome in a 20-year-old patient treated with intravascular stent placement: a case report, *Can J Urol* 16:4765–4769, 2009.

127. Hartung O, Grisoli D, Boufi M, et al: Endovascular stenting in the treatment of pelvic vein congestion caused by nutcracker syndrome: lessons learned from the first five cases, *J Vasc Surg* 42:275–280, 2005.

128. Wang L, Yi L, Yang L, et al: Diagnosis and surgical treatment of nutcracker syndrome: a single-center experience, *Urology* 73:871–876, 2009.

129. Kim S, Kim CW, Kim S, et al: Long-term follow-up after endovascular stent placement for treatment of nutcracker syndrome, *J Vasc Interv Radiol* 16:428–431, 2005.

130. Zhang H, Li M, Jin W, et al: The left renal entrapment syndrome: diagnosis and treatment, *Ann Vasc Surg* 21:198–203, 2007.

131. Bernheim JW, Hansen J, Faries P, et al: Acute lower extremity ischemia in a 7-year-old boy: an unusual case of popliteal entrapment syndrome, *J Vasc Surg* 39:1340–1343, 2004.

132. Haidar S, Thomas K, Miller S: Popliteal artery entrapment syndrome in a young girl, *Pediatr Radiol* 35:440–443, 2005.

133. Ferreira J, Canedo A, Graça S, et al: Thrombosed popliteal aneurysm-first manifestation of bilateral popliteal entrapment syndrome, *Int Angiol* 29:83–86, 2010.

134. Tercan F, Oguzkurt L, Kizilkilic O, et al: Popliteal artery entrapment syndrome, *Diagn Interv Radiol* 11:222–224, 2005.

135. Beuthien W, De Potzolli O, Mellinghoff HU, et al: Popliteal artery entrapment with peripheral thromboembolism, *J Clin Rheumatol* 10:147–149, 2004.

136. Misselbeck T, Dangleben D, Celani V: Isolated popliteal vein entrapment by the popliteus muscle: a case report, *Vasc Med* 13:37–39, 2008.

137. Nottingham JM, Haynes JL: Isolated popliteal vein entrapment by a fibrous band, *Vasc Endovasc Surg* 35:487–490, 2001.

138. Pillai J, Levien LJ, Haagensen M, et al: Assessment of the medial head of the gastrocnemius muscle in functional compression of the popliteal artery, *J Vasc Surg* 48:1189–1196, 2008.

139. Turnipseed WD: Functional popliteal artery entrapment syndrome: a poorly understood and often missed diagnosis that is frequently mistreated, *J Vasc Surg* 49:1189–1195, 2009.

140. Pillai J: A current interpretation of popliteal vascular entrapment, *J Vasc Surg* 48: 61s–65s, 2008.

141. Aktan Ikiz ZA, Ucerler H, Ozgur Z: Anatomic variations of popliteal artery that may be a reason for entrapment, *Surg Radiol Anat* 31:695–700, 2009.

142. Holden A, Merrilees S, Mitchell N, et al: Magnetic resonance imaging of popliteal artery pathologies, *Eur J Radiol* 67:159–168, 2008.

143. Kim HK, Shin MJ, Kim SM, et al: Popliteal artery entrapment syndrome: morphological classification utilizing MR imaging, *Skeletal Radiol* 35:648–658, 2006.

144. Özkan U, Oguzkurt L, Tercan F, et al: MRI and DSA findings in popliteal artery entrapment syndrome, *Diagn Interv Radiol* 14:106–110, 2008.

145. Kukreja K, Scagnelli T, Narayanan G, et al: Role of angiography in popliteal artery entrapment syndrome, *Diagn Interv Radiol* 15:57–60, 2009.

146. Anil G, Tay K, Howe T, et al: Dynamic computed tomography angiography: role in the evaluation of popliteal artery entrapment syndrome, *Cardiovasc Interv Radiol* 34:259–270, 2011.

147. Zhong H, Liu C, Shao G: Computed tomographic angiography and digital subtraction angiography findings in popliteal artery entrapment syndrome, *J Comput Assist Tomogr* 34:254–259, 2010.

148. Hai Z, Guangrui S, Yuan Z, et al: CT angiography and MRI in patients with popliteal artery entrapment syndrome, *AJR Am J Roentgenol* 191:1760–1766, 2008.

149. Goh BKP, Tay KH, Tan SG: Diagnosis and surgical management of popliteal artery entrapment syndrome, *Aust N Z J Surg* 75:869–873, 2005.

150. Shen J, Abu-Hamad G, Makaroun MS, et al: Bilateral asymmetric popliteal entrapment syndrome treated with successful surgical decompression and adjunctive thrombolysis, *Vasc Endovasc Surg* 43:395–398, 2009.

151. di Marzo L, Cavallaro A, O'Donnell SD, et al: Endovascular stenting for popliteal vascular entrapment is not recommended, *Ann Vasc Surg* 24:1135, 2010.

152. Meier T, Schneider E, Amann-Vesti B: Long-term follow-up of patients with popliteal artery entrapment syndrome treated by endoluminal revascularization, *Vasa* 39: 189–195, 2010.

153. Paraskevas N, Castier Y, Fukui S, et al: Superficial femoral artery autograft reconstruction for complicated popliteal artery entrapment syndrome, *Vasc Endovasc Surg* 43:165–169, 2009.

154. Gagnon J, Doyle D: Adventitial cystic disease of common femoral artery, *Ann Vasc Surg* 21:84–86, 2007.

155. Jindal R, Majed A, Hamady M, et al: Cystic adventitial disease of the iliofemoral artery: case reports and a short review, *Vascular* 14:169–172, 2006.

156. Dix FP, McDonald M, Obomighie J, Chalmers, et al: Cystic adventitial disease of the femoral vein presenting as deep vein thrombosis: a case report and review of the literature, *J Vasc Surg* 44:871–874, 2006.

157. Gasparis AP, Wall P, Ricotta JJ: Adventitial cystic disease of the external iliac vein presenting with deep venous thrombosis, *Vasc Endovasc Surg* 38:273–276, 2004.

158. Morizumi S, Suematsu Y, Gon S, et al: Adventitial cystic disease of the femoral vein, *Ann Vasc Surg* 24:1135e5–1135e7, 2010.

159. Seo JY, Chung DJ, Kim JH: Adventitial cystic disease of the femoral vein: a case report with the CT venography, *Korean J Radiol* 10:89–92, 2009.

160. França M, Pinto J, Machado R, et al: Case 157: Bilateral adventitial cystic disease of the popliteal artery, *Radiology* 255:655–660, 2010.

161. Ortiz MWR, Lopera JE, Giménez CR, et al: Bilateral adventitial cystic disease of the popliteal artery: a case report, *Cardiovasc Interv Radiol* 29:306–310, 2006.

162. Ortmann J, Widmer M, Gretener S, et al: Cystic adventitial degeneration: ectopic ganglia from adjacent joint capsules, *Vasa* 38:374–377, 2009.

163. Asciutto G, Mumme A, Marpe B, et al: Different approaches in the treatment of cystic adventitial disease of the popliteal artery, *Chir Ital* 59:467–473, 2007.

164. Setacci F, Sirignano P, de Donato G, et al: Adventitial cystic disease of the popliteal artery: experience of a single vascular and endovascular center, *J Cardiovasc Surg* 49:235–239, 2008.

165. Chappel P, Gielen J, Salgado R, et al: Cystic adventitial disease with secondary occlusion of the popliteal artery, *JBR–BTR* 90:180–181, 2007.

166. Tsilimparis N, Hanack U, Yousefi S, et al: Cystic adventitial disease of the popliteal artery: an argument for the developmental theory, *J Vasc Surg* 45:1249–1252, 2007.

167. Buijsrogge MP, van der Meij S, Korte JH, et al: "Intermittent claudication intermittence" as a manifestation of adventitial cystic disease communicating with the knee joint, *Ann Vasc Surg* 20:687–689, 2006.

168. Taurino M, Rizzo L, Stella N, et al: Doppler ultrasonography and exercise testing in diagnosing a popliteal artery adventitial cyst, *Cardiovasc Ultrasound* 7:23, 2009.

169. Nano G, Dalainas I, Casana R, et al: Case report of adventitial cystic disease of the popliteal artery presented with the "dog-leg" sign, *Int Angiol* 26:75–78, 2007.

170. Maged IM, Turba UC, Housseini AM, et al: High spatial resolution magnetic resonance imaging of cystic adventitial disease of the popliteal artery, *J Vasc Surg* 51:471–474, 2010.

171. Tomasian A, Lai C, Finn JP, et al: Cystic adventitial disease of the popliteal artery: features on 3T cardiovascular magnetic resonance, *J Cardiovasc Magn Reson* 10:38, 2008.

172. Keo HH, Baumgartner I, Schmidli J, et al: Sustained remission 11 years after percutaneous ultrasound-guided aspiration for cystic adventitial degeneration in the popliteal artery, *J Endovasc Ther* 14:264–265, 2007.

173. Johnson JM, Kiankhooy A, Bertges DJ, et al: Percutaneous image-guided aspiration and sclerosis of adventitial cystic disease of the femoral vein, *Cardiovasc Interv Radiol* 32: 812–816, 2009.

174. Khoury M: Failed angioplasty of a popliteal artery stenosis secondary to cystic adventitial disease, *Vasc Endovasc Surg* 38:277–280, 2004.

175. Rai S, Davies RSM, Vohra RK: Failure of endovascular stenting for popliteal cystic disease, *Ann Vasc Surg* 23:410, 2009.

176. Maged IM, Kron IL, Hagspiel KD: Recurrent cystic adventitial disease of the popliteal artery: successful treatment with percutaneous transluminal angioplasty, *Vasc Endovasc Surg* 43:399–402, 2009.

177. Foertsch T, Koch A, Singer H, et al: Celiac trunk compression syndrome requiring surgery in 3 adolescent patients, *J Pediatr Surg* 42:709–713, 2007.

178. Gander S, Mulder DJ, Jones S, et al: Recurrent abdominal pain and weight loss in an adolescent: celiac artery compression syndrome, *Can J Gastroenterol* 24:91–93, 2010.

179. Okten RIS, Kucukay F, Tola M, et al: Is celiac artery compression syndrome genetically inherited?: a case series from a family and review of the literature, *Eur J Radiol* 2011; epub ahead of print.

180. Desmond C, Roberts S: Exercise-related abdominal pain as a manifestation of the median arcuate ligament syndrome, *Scand J Gastroenterol* 39:1310–1313, 2004.

181. Said SM, Zarroug AE, Gloviczki P, et al: Pediatric median arcuate ligament syndrome: first report of familial pattern and transperitoneal laparoscopic release, *J Pediatr Surg* 45: e17–e20, 2010.

182. Loukas M, Pinyard J, Vaid S, et al: Clinical anatomy of celiac artery compression syndrome: a review, *Clin Anat* 20:612–617, 2007.

183. Soman S, Sudhakar SV, Keshava SN: Celiac axis compression by median arcuate ligament on computed tomography among asymptomatic persons, *Ind J Gastroenterol* 29:121–123, 2010.

184. Akatsu T, Hayashi S, Yamane T, et al: Emergency embolization of a ruptured pancreaticoduodenal artery aneurysm associated with the median arcuate ligament syndrome, *J Gastroenterol Hepatol* 19:482–483, 2004.

185. Ogino H, Sato Y, Banno T, et al: Embolization in a patient with ruptured anterior inferior pancreaticoduodenal arterial aneurysm with median arcuate ligament syndrome, *Cardiovasc Interv Radiol* 25:318–319, 2002.

186. Tsai YS, Lee CH, Pang KK: Electronic clinical challenges and images in GI, *Amb Pediatr* 136:e3–e4, 2009.

187. Duncan AA: Median arcuate ligament syndrome, *Curr Treat Options Cardiovasc Med* 10:112–116, 2008.

188. Gloviczki P, Duncan AA: Treatment of celiac artery compression syndrome: does it really exist? *Perspect Vasc Surg Endovasc Ther* 19:259–263, 2007.

189. Roseborough GS: Laparoscopic management of celiac artery compression syndrome, *J Vasc Surg* 50:124–133, 2009.

190. Kalapatapu VR, Murray BW, Palm-Cruz K, et al: Definitive test to diagnose median arcuate ligament syndrome: injection of vasodilator during angiography, *Vasc Endovasc Surg* 43:46–50, 2009.

191. Mensink PBF, van Petersen AS, Kolkman JJ, et al: Gastric exercise tonometry: the key investigation in patients with suspected celiac artery compression syndrome, *J Vasc Surg* 44:277–281, 2006.

192. Aschenbach R, Basche S, Vogl TJ: Compression of the celiac trunk caused by median arcuate ligament in children and adolescent subjects: evaluation with contrast-enhanced MR angiography and comparison with Doppler US evaluation, *J Vasc Interv Radiol* 2011; epub ahead of print.

193. Horton K, Talamini M, Fishman E: Median arcuate ligament syndrome: evaluation with CT angiography, *Radiographics* 25:1177–1182, 2005.

194. Ilica AT, Kocaoglu M, Bilici A, et al: Median arcuate ligament syndrome: multidetector computed tomography findings, *J Comput Assist Tomogr* 31:728–731, 2007.

195. Karahan Ö, Kahr man G, Y k Imaz A, et al: Celiac artery compression syndrome: diagnosis with multislice CT, *Diagn Interv Radiol* 13:90–93, 2007.

196. Manghat N, Mitchell G, Hay C, et al: The median arcuate ligament syndrome revisited by CT angiography and the use of ECG gating–a single centre case series and literature review, *Br J Radiol* 81:735–742, 2008.

197. Özbülbül NI: CT angiography of the celiac trunk: anatomy, variants and pathologic findings, *Diagn Interv Radiol* 2010; epub ahead of print.

198. Wolfman D, Bluth EI, Sossaman J: Median arcuate ligament syndrome, *J Ultrasound Med* 22:1377–1380, 2003.

199. Baccari P, Civilini E, Dordoni L, et al: Celiac artery compression syndrome managed by laparoscopy, *J Vasc Surg* 50:134–139, 2009.

200. Baldassarre E, Torino G, Siani A, et al: The laparoscopic approach in the median arcuate ligament syndrome: report of a case, *Swiss Med Wkly* 137:353–354, 2007.

201. Mirkia K, Subin B: Minimally invasive approach to median arcuate ligament syndrome in a patient with HIV/AIDS, *Int J STD AIDS* 20:209–210, 2009.

202. Riess KP, Serck L, Gundersen SB, et al: Seconds from disaster: lessons learned from laparoscopic release of the median arcuate ligament, *Surg Endosc* 23:1121–1124, 2009.

203. Tulloch AW, Jimenez JC, Lawrence PF, et al: Laparoscopic vs. open celiac ganglionectomy in patients with median arcuate ligament syndrome, *J Vasc Surg* 52:1283–1289, 2010.

204. Vaziri K, Hungness ES, Pearson EG, et al: Laparoscopic treatment of celiac artery compression syndrome: case series and review of current treatment modalities, *J Gastrointest Surg* 13:293–298, 2009.

205. Jaik N, Stawicki S, Weger N, et al: Celiac artery compression syndrome: successful utilization of robotic-assisted laparoscopic approach, *J Gastrointest Liver Dis* 16:93–96, 2007.

206. van Petersen AS, Vriens BH, Huisman AB, et al: Retroperitoneal endoscopic release in the management of celiac artery compression syndrome, *J Vasc Surg* 50:140–147, 2009.

207. Grotemeyer D, Duran M, Iskandar F, et al: Median arcuate ligament syndrome: vascular surgical therapy and follow-up of 18 patients, *Langenbecks Arch Surg* 394:1085–1092, 2009.

208. Wang X, Impeduglia T, Dubin Z, et al: Celiac revascularization as a requisite for treating the median arcuate ligament syndrome, *Ann Vasc Surg* 22:571–574, 2008.

209. Kohn GP, Bitar RS, Farber MA, et al: Treatment options and outcomes for celiac artery compression syndrome, *Surg Innov* 18:338–343, 2011.

CHAPTER 63

Congenital Anomalies and Malformations of the Vasculature

Renu Virmani, Naima Carter-Monroe, Allen J. Taylor

Anomalous Venous Connections

An anomalous venous connection abnormally connects a systemic or pulmonary vein to another venous structure or directly to the left or right atrium. The connections arise from failed development of normal embryological venous communications or persistence, lack of regression of normal embryological venous communications, or both.

Anomalous Pulmonary Venous Connections

Anomalous pulmonary venous connection refers to the absence of one or more pulmonary venous connections to the left atrium, without reference to the subsequent drainage of the anomalously disconnected pulmonary vein(s). *Total anomalous pulmonary venous connection* (TAPVC) refers to the bilateral absence of a connection of both pulmonary veins of each lung to the left atrium. The pulmonary veins connect directly into the right atrium or into one of its tributaries. TAPVC is almost always associated with some type of atrial septal defect (ASD) for life to be sustained beyond the newborn period.[1] *Partial anomalous pulmonary venous connection* (PAPVC) is the presence of connection of one or more—but not all—pulmonary veins to the right atrium or one of its tributaries. TAPVC is found in about 2% of autopsied cases with congenital heart disease and has a male predominance. PAPVCs constitute about 0.6% of autopsied cases of congenital heart disease.[1] TAPVC is an isolated anomaly in two thirds of patients, and is associated with complex congenital heart disease in the remaining third, especially the heterotaxy syndromes (so-called isomeric TAPVC).

EMBRYOLOGY

In the human embryo, the lung buds and their pulmonary veins connect to the veins of the foregut, the splanchnic plexus. With growth, a new pulmonary venous channel, the primary pulmonary vein, grows as a bulging of the left atrium. At the same time, the intrapulmonary veins lose their connections with the splanchnic plexus and fuse with the primary pulmonary vein. The intrapulmonary veins eventually form the four pulmonary veins and are absorbed into the left atrium (Fig. 63-1). Failure of severance of the connection between the intrapulmonary and splanchnic veins results in anomalous pulmonary venous connections that may be total, partial, bilateral, or unilateral.

The drainage site of pulmonary veins may be supradiaphragmatic or infradiaphragmatic (Fig. 63-2). When drainage is supradiaphragmatic, both lungs may drain into a confluence, which may then drain into the left innominate vein and the superior vena cava (SVC), or the supradiaphragmatic drainage may be directly into the left SVC, or indirectly to the SVC via azygos or hemiazygos veins[1] (see Fig. 63-2).

Maternal exposure to environmental teratogens such as lead paint or pesticides has been described to cause a familial susceptibility for TAPVC, largely in the presence of a positive family history of cardiac and noncardiac anomalies.[2,3] Familial total anomalous pulmonary venous return is most likely an X-linked inheritance and autosomal dominant with variable expression and incomplete penetrance. Until now, two candidate genes have been proposed. The TAPVR1 gene, playing a role in vasculogenesis, maps to 4q12, in which the centromeric regions contain receptor tyrosine kinase genes as a kinase domain receptor (KDR). Recently it has been shown that dysregulation of the PDGFRA (platelet-derived growth factor receptor-α) gene causes PV inflow tract anomalies, including TAPVR.[4]

TOTAL ANOMALOUS PULMONARY VENOUS CONNECTION

The level of the anomaly relative to the heart or diaphragm classifies TAPVC. Type I denotes anomalous connection at the supracardiac level; type II, anomalous connection at the cardiac level; type III, anomalous connection at the infracardiac level; and type IV, anomalous connection at two or more of those levels.[5] The common forms of TAPVC are illustrated in Figure 63-3. In a recent multicenter study[6] from the United Kingdom, Ireland, and Sweden with a cohort of 422 liveborn cases, the frequency of supracardiac TAPVC (type I) was 48.6%, infracardiac 26.1%, cardiac level 15.9%, and mixed connections 8.8%. Two cases (0.5%) had common pulmonary vein atresia, and 60 (14.2%) had associated cardiac anomalies. Of the supracardiac TAPVC cases, 73.2% showed connection to the innominate vein, 21% connected to various portions of the SVC, 2.9% connected to the azygos vein, and in 2.9% the connection was unknown (undocumented or unable to determine). The majority of cardiac-type TAPVC cases demonstrated connection to the coronary sinus (86.6%), followed by connections to the right atrium at 11.9%, and no identified connection site in 1.5% of cases. In the case of infracardiac TAPVC, the majority of cases demonstrated pulmonary venous connection to the portal system.[6]

Size of the ASD has been shown to relate to longevity in TAPVC; the larger the ASD, the longer the survival. Individual pulmonary vein size at diagnosis also is a strong independent predictor of survival in patients with TAPVC.[7]

Associated cardiac anomalies include transposition of the great arteries, small ventricular septal defects (VSDs),[6] pulmonary atresia, coarctation of the aorta (COA), and anomalies of systemic veins. There is a high frequency of TAPVC in patients with congenital heart disease and asplenia (heterotaxy syndromes). In a recent autopsy series of TAPVC associated with asplenia, anomalous pulmonary venous connection to a systemic vein was total in 42 (58%) of 72 and partial in 2 (3%) of 72, with obstruction in 24 (55%) of 44.[8]

In patients with a widely patent foramen ovale or ASD, which allows free communication between the two atria and mixing of the venous blood, the flow of blood depends on the resistance in the pulmonary and systemic arterial circuits. In cases without pulmonary venous obstruction, the resistance at birth is equal; therefore, the distribution of blood is equal between the pulmonary and systemic circuits. However, within a few weeks of birth, the pulmonary resistance decreases, and a larger proportion of the mixed venous blood returns to the pulmonary circuit, resulting in a nearly three to five times greater pulmonary-to-systemic flow ratio of 3:1 to 5:1, and an equalization of oxygen saturation between the right and left heart. In the presence of pulmonary venous obstruction, there is elevated pulmonary venous pressure that results in pulmonary edema, a decrease in pulmonary flow, pulmonary hypertension (PH), right ventricular (RV) hypertrophy, and ultimately right heart failure.

The signs and symptoms, therefore, depend on the underlying hemodynamics—that is, presence or absence of pulmonary venous obstruction and the extent of mixing of blood between the right and left atrium. If interatrial mixing is inadequate, symptoms occur at birth or shortly thereafter. In TAPVC without pulmonary venous obstruction, patients are usually asymptomatic at birth, but at least 50% become symptomatic within 1 month of life (usually not in the first 12 hours of life). Once symptoms appear, however, they are rapidly progressive. Diagnosis may be established by angiography, echocardiography, or T1-weighted spin-echo magnetic resonance imaging (MRI).[9]

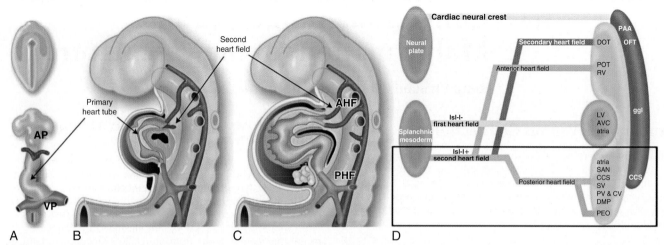

FIGURE 63-1 Schematic representation of sequential stages of cardiac development and the contribution from first and second heart field. The primary heart tube is depicted in brown and the myocardium derived from the second heart field (and incorporated later in the heart) in yellow. **A,** Primary heart tube is formed after fusion of bilateral plates of splanchnic mesoderm in the primitive plate. This tube already has a venous pole *(VP)*, and an arterial pole *(AP)*. **B,** Lateral view of embryo (≈23 days in human), showing primary heart tube surrounded by cardiac jelly *(blue)*, and second heart field situated dorsally to heart. **C,** Human embryo at 25 days. Primary heart tube has expanded at both VP and AP, with myocardium derived from second heart field *(yellow)*. **D,** Scheme of nomenclature primary and second heart field. At VP of heart, myocardium is derived from posterior heart field, which contributes to posterior wall of atria, sinoatrial node *(SAN)*, myocardium of sinus venosus *(SV)*, pulmonary veins *(PV)*, and cardinal veins *(CV)* including the coronary sinus, part of the central conduction system *(CCS)* and the dorsal mesenchymal protrusion *(DMP)*. The second heart field contribution to VP is discussed in more detail later on in this review. *(Reproduced with permission from Crawford MH, DiMarco JP, Paulus WJ: Cardiology: expert consult, ed 3, St. Louis, 2009, Mosby.)*

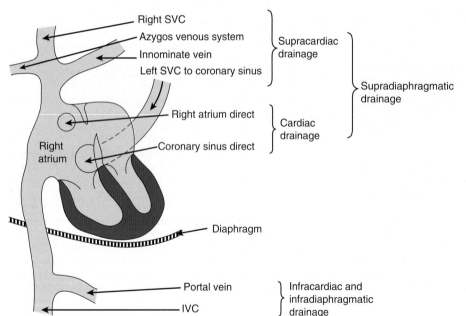

FIGURE 63-2 Possible sites of drainage for anomalous pulmonary venous connections into the venous system. IVC, inferior vena cava; SVC, superior vena cava. *(Reproduced with permission from Becker AE, Anderson RH: Pathology of congenital heart disease, London, 1981, Butterworths, pp 47–66, 333.)*

PARTIAL ANOMALOUS PULMONARY VENOUS CONNECTION

PAPVC is defined when one or more, but not all, pulmonary veins are connected to the right atrium or to a systemic vein. Usually only one lung or part of a lung is involved. The right pulmonary veins are six times more commonly involved than the left pulmonary veins, and the upper lobes of the lung are more commonly involved than the lower. The left-sided pulmonary veins usually connect to the derivatives of the left cardinal system (i.e., coronary sinus and left innominate vein). The right pulmonary veins connect to the derivatives of the right cardinal system (i.e., SVC and inferior vena cava [IVC]) or right atrium. The most common connections are right pulmonary veins to SVC, right pulmonary veins to right atrium, veins of the right lung to the IVC, and left pulmonary veins to the left innominate vein.

The heart usually exhibits mild dilation and hypertrophy of the right atrium and ventricle, with dilation of the pulmonary artery. The left-sided chambers are normal. Usually, ASD accompanies PAPVC; conversely, 9% of cases of ASD have PAPVC. In the case of the right pulmonary vein connecting to the SVC, the right upper and middle lobe veins connect to the SVC. The vein of the right lower lobe usually enters the left atrium but may connect to the right atrium. The lower part of the SVC, below the azygos vein and above the right atrium, is dilated approximately twice the normal size. Most cases have associated ASD of the sinus venosus type, but occasionally a secundum or, rarely, a primum ASD may occur (Fig. 63-4).

Associated cardiovascular defects are common, occurring in up to 80% of patients.[10] Major cardiac anomalies are found in about 20% of cases and include tetralogy of Fallot, VSD, single ventricle, COA, transposition of the great arteries, and hypoplastic left heart

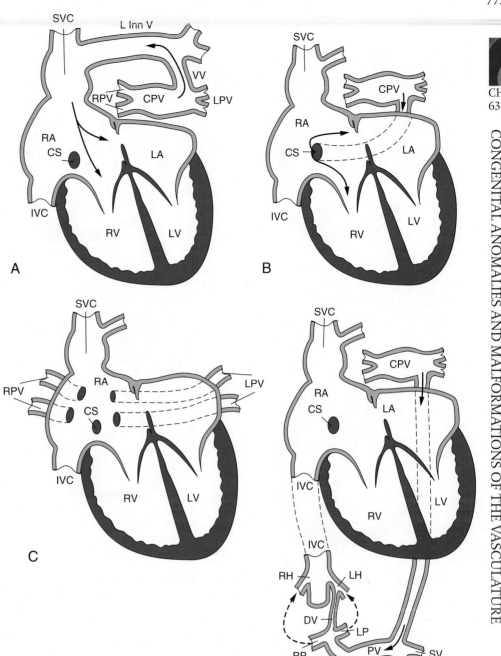

FIGURE 63-3 The most common patterns of circulation in total anomalous pulmonary connection (TAPVC). A, TAPVC to left innominate vein by way of a vertical vein. **B,** TAPVC to coronary sinus. **C,** TAPVC to right atrium. Right and left pulmonary veins usually enter right atrium separately. **D,** TAPVC to portal vein. CPV, common pulmonary vein; CS, coronary sinus; DV, ductus venosus; IVC, inferior vena cava; LA, left atrium; LH, left hepatic vein; L Inn V, left innominate vein; LP, left portal vein; LPV, left pulmonary vein; LV, left ventricle; PV, portal vein; RA, right atrium; RH, right hepatic vein; RP, right portal vein; RPV, right pulmonary vein; RV, right ventricle; SMV, superior mesenteric vein; SV, splenic veins; SVC, superior vena cava; VV, vertical vein. *(Reproduced with permission from Lucas RV, Krabill RA: Anomalous venous connections, pulmonary and systemic. In Adams FH, Emmanouilides GC, editors: Moss' heart disease in infants, children and adolescents, ed 4, Baltimore, 1989, Williams & Wilkins, p 580.)*

syndrome. Indications for surgery for isolated PAPVC include pulmonary-to-systemic flow ratio of over 2.0.[10]

When all right pulmonary veins drain the right middle and lower lobes and enter the IVC, either above or below the diaphragm, the pattern of the pulmonary veins is altered, giving a "fir tree" appearance (see Fig. 63-4). This malformation is called *scimitar syndrome*, as initially described by Chassinat in 1836,[11,12] and derives its name from the shape of the anomalous vein on chest radiographs.[13] Classically, this syndrome is associated with right lung anomalies, dextrocardia of the heart, hypoplasia of the right pulmonary artery, and anomalous connection between aorta and right lung. In the European Congenital Heart Surgeons Association (ECHSA) multi-center study, 65% of patients also presented with secundum-type ASDs, and 16% had a concomitant VSD.[14]

In connection of left pulmonary veins to the left innominate vein, the veins of the left upper lobe or the whole left lung connect to the left innominate vein via the vertical vein. Atrial septal defect of the

secundum type usually is present, and the septum is rarely intact (see Fig. 63-4). Other sites of PAPVC are the left pulmonary veins draining into the coronary sinus, IVC, right SVC, right atrium, or left subclavian vein. In rare cases, veins of both lungs drain anomalously, but a small segment of the pulmonary venous system drains normally. That condition has been termed by Edwards *subtotal anomalous pulmonary venous connection.*

Cor Triatriatum

Cor triatriatum is a relatively rare cardiac anomaly (0.4% of autopsied cases with congenital heart disease, ratio of males to females 1.5:1).[15] In this condition, the pulmonary veins enter an accessory chamber lying posterior to the left atrium and joining the left atrium through a narrow opening. The following broad classification has been suggested by a number of authors[16,17]:

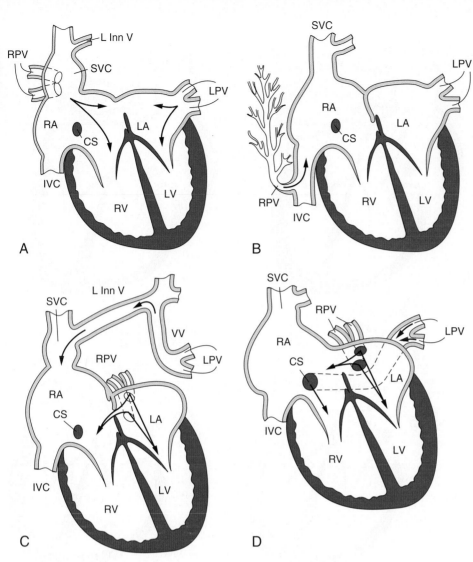

FIGURE 63-4 The most common patterns of circulation in partial anomalous pulmonary connection (PAPVC). A, Anomalous connection of right pulmonary veins to superior vena cava. **B,** Anomalous connections of right pulmonary veins to inferior vena cava in the presence of an intact atrial septum. **C,** Anomalous connection of left pulmonary veins to left innominate by way of a vertical vein. **D,** Anomalous connection of left pulmonary veins to coronary sinus. CS, coronary sinus; IVC, inferior vena cava; LA, left atrium; L Inn V, left innominate vein; LPV, left pulmonary vein; LV, left ventricle; RA, right atrium; RPV, right pulmonary vein; RV, right ventricle; SVC, superior vena cava; VV, vertical vein. *(Reproduced with permission from Lucas RV, Krabill RA: Anomalous venous connections, pulmonary and systemic. In Adams FH, Emmanouilides GC, editors: Moss' heart disease in infants, children and adolescents, ed 4, Baltimore, 1989, Williams & Wilkins, p 580.)*

1. Accessory atrial chamber that receives all pulmonary veins and communicates with the left atrium; no other connections (classic cor triatriatum).
2. Accessory atrial chamber that receives part of pulmonary veins and does not communicate with left atrium.
3. Subtotal cor triatriatum:
   a. Accessory atrial chamber that receives part of the pulmonary veins and connects to the left atrium.
   b. Accessory atrial chamber that receives part of the pulmonary veins and connects to the right atrium.

Physiologically, when blood from the accessory atrial chamber drains into the right atrium, the hemodynamic features are those of TAPVC. A stenotic opening between the accessory atrium and the left atrium, however, results in features of severe pulmonary obstruction. In subtotal cor triatriatum when obstruction affects only one lung, the result is reflex pulmonary arterial obstruction with decreased flow through that portion of the lung. The rest of the unobstructed lung receives increased flow, but there is no elevation in pulmonary arterial pressure (PAP).[17]

The classic cor triatriatum patients have onset of symptoms in the first few years of life. Patients usually have history of breathlessness and frequent respiratory infections. Right heart failure is usually present along with signs of pulmonary hypertension. Surgery has been advocated as early as the neonatal period,[18] and balloon dilation may be successful in older children.[19]

Some patients remain asymptomatic until adulthood[20] or may present with sick sinus syndrome in advanced years.[21] In adults, clinical features on presentation can mimic those of mitral stenosis

because of the obstructive properties of the membrane[22]; they include dyspnea with increased pulmonary capillary wedge pressure (PCWP) on exertion.[23] As with other anomalies of the pulmonary venous system, associated anomalies may occur, including atrioventricular septal defect.[24]

Pulmonary vascular changes in cor triatriatum are progressive medial thickening and intimal fibrosis in pulmonary arteries and veins, accompanied by lymphangiectasia. In contrast to persistent left-to-right shunts, no plexiform lesions or more advanced stages of pulmonary vascular disease occur, which may explain the reversibility of PH due to congenital pulmonary venous obstruction.[25]

Congenital Stenosis of Pulmonary Veins

Congenital pulmonary vein stenosis is often associated with other anomalies, such as anomalous connections, cor triatriatum, and VSDs.[26] The isolated form generally comes to clinical attention because of symptoms related to pulmonary hypertension.[27] In its most severe form, congenital pulmonary vein stenosis is a progressive disease with rapid PH and rare survival beyond the first year of life.[28]

There are two types of stenosis of pulmonary veins. One is localized stenosis of the pulmonary veins at the junction of the left atrium, which may involve one or more pulmonary veins; the other is characterized by narrowing of the lumen of the pulmonary vein, either intra- or extrapulmonary in location, and is called *hypoplasia of the pulmonary veins.* The latter type is occasionally present in patients with pulmonary artery atresia or hypoplastic left heart syndrome. Clinically, patients have a history of respiratory symptoms, which may progress to right heart failure. Because of poor surgical results, balloon angioplasty and stenting currently are being evaluated as noninvasive treatments for pulmonary artery stenosis. In the most severe forms, lung transplantation appears to be an important option.[28]

Anomalous Systemic Venous Connections

Anomalous systemic venous connections, especially persistent left SVC, are usually asymptomatic and of little functional significance because systemic venous flow to the right atrium is not impaired. However, if they are not recognized, systemic venous anomalies may be accidentally severed during cardiac surgery. A classification based on embryological principles includes anomalies of the cardinal venous system, anomalies of the IVC, and anomalies of the valves of the sinus venosus.[16]

Anomalies of the cardinal venous system include persistent left SVC; persistent left SVC connecting to the right or left atrium, with and without failure of development of coronary sinus; right SVC connected to the left atrium; and anomalies of the coronary sinus. Anomalies of the IVC include double IVC, left IVC, and many lesser anomalies that are usually of no clinical significance, except that they may present problems to the surgeon.[29,30] Infrahepatic interruption of the IVC with drainage via the enlarged azygous vein to the SVC has been found to occur in 2.9% of congenital heart defects.[16] Anomalies of the valves of the sinus venosus involve the eustachian and thebesian valves and crista terminalis. Minor abnormal persistence results in larger valves and a Chiari network. Large outgrowth of the valve of the sinus venosus may result in complete or partial subdivision of the right atrium.

As with anomalous pulmonary veins, anomalous systemic venous return is a hallmark of the heterotaxy syndromes, especially asplenia. In a recent autopsy review of 72 cases of asplenia, the SVC was bilateral in 51 cases (71%) and unilateral in 21 (29%). In nine cases of bilateral SVC, one of the SVCs was partly or totally atretic. Although the IVC was never interrupted, a prominent azygos vein was found in six cases (8%). An intact coronary sinus was rare.[8]

Cor Triatriatum Dexter

Cor triatriatum dexter is an unusual cardiac abnormality with division between the sinus and primitive atrial portions of the right atrium. Symptoms in adults with isolated cor triatriatum dexter include lifelong exertional cyanosis and dyspnea.[31]

Congenital Coronary Artery Anomalies

The incidence of coronary artery anomalies is between 0.46% and 1.55% in angiographic series and 0.3% in autopsy series. The major anomalies will be discussed briefly.

Anomalous Left Main Coronary Artery

The most common coronary anomaly resulting in clinical symptoms is an aberrant left main coronary artery arising in the right coronary sinus of Valsalva. There is a male/female ratio of 4:1 to 9:1. Sudden death occurs in up to two thirds of individuals with this anomaly, 75% of which occur during exercise.[32] Most patients are adolescents or young adults, although death may occur as young as 1 month of age. There are often premonitory symptoms of syncope or chest pain, but stress electrocardiograms (ECGs) and stress echocardiograms are often negative.

Pathologically, there are several variants to this anomaly. The common feature is the presence of the left main ostium within the right sinus. This ostium is typically near the commissure, and in some cases actually lies above the commissure between the right and left sinuses. Often the ostium is somewhat malformed and slit-like, and an ostial ridge is present. The proximal artery lies within the aortic media and traverses between the aorta and pulmonary trunk.

The pathophysiology of sudden death in patients with aberrant left main coronary artery may be related to compression of the left main by the pulmonary trunk and aorta, diastolic compression of the vessel lying within the aortic media, and poor filling during diastole because of ostial ridges or slitlike ostia.

Anomalous Right Coronary Artery

In contrast to anomalous left main coronary artery, anomalous right coronary artery from the left sinus is usually an incidental finding, although up to one third of patients may die suddenly. In the majority of cases (67%), the anomalous vessel courses between the aorta and pulmonary trunk, with the remainder usually coursing posterior to the aorta.[32] Almost 50% of sudden deaths are exercise related, and most deaths occur in young and middle-aged adults (<35 years).

Grossly, there are two ostia located in the left sinus of Valsalva. The ostium supplying the right coronary artery may have features similar to anomalous left ostia located in the right sinus. Namely, there may be upward displacement, location near the commissure, and slitlike ostia with ostial ridges. The proximal anomalous right coronary generally also courses between the aorta and pulmonary trunk. The pathophysiology of sudden death is similar to that of anomalous left coronary artery, and like that anomaly, evidence of acute or remote ischemia in the ventricular myocardium is not often found.

Anomalous Left Circumflex Artery

Anomalous left circumflex artery is the most common anomaly of the origin of a coronary artery, accounting for 28% of anomalies identified by cardiac catheterization and with an incidence of 1 in 300.[33] This anomaly is considered benign. Awareness of this anomaly is important during cardiac surgery to avoid problems with myocardial protection or during prosthetic valve replacement.

Origin from Pulmonary Trunk

The left main coronary artery arises from the pulmonary trunk in 1/50,000 to 1/300,000 autopsies. Most cases are identified in the first year of life, and sudden death occurs in approximately 40% of cases. In a minority of cases (≈20%), sufficient myocardial collaterals develop from the normally structured right coronary artery, enabling potential survival into adulthood. In these cases, a continuous murmur may be present with other symptoms including angina pectoris, myocardial infarction (MI), dyspnea (MI), and syncope. Sudden death usually occurs at rest, but may occur after strenuous activity in older children. Pathologically, the aberrant artery arises in the left pulmonary sinus in 95% of cases. Typically, the artery appears thin-walled and veinlike, and the right coronary artery, although normal in location, is tortuous.

Angiographic and Other Imaging in Diagnosis of Anomalous Coronary Arteries

Angiographically identifying an anomalous right or left main coronary artery from the contralateral coronary sinus depends on the vessel's course between the aorta and pulmonary trunk. This particular course is angiographically distinct in the right anterior oblique projection when the left main forms a cranial-posterior loop (Fig. 63-5). An alternative method is to perform simultaneous pulmonary and coronary arteriography, or more practically, insert a pulmonary artery catheter as an angiographic marker for the location of the pulmonary vessels, and then perform an angiogram of the aberrant coronary artery in the steep anteroposterior caudal projection.

Standard two-dimensional (2D) echocardiography has been used as a screening procedure for coronary anomalies in athletes. An echocardiographic screening study of 3650 athletes found 3 cases of anomalous right (*n* = 2) and left (*n* = 1) coronary artery from

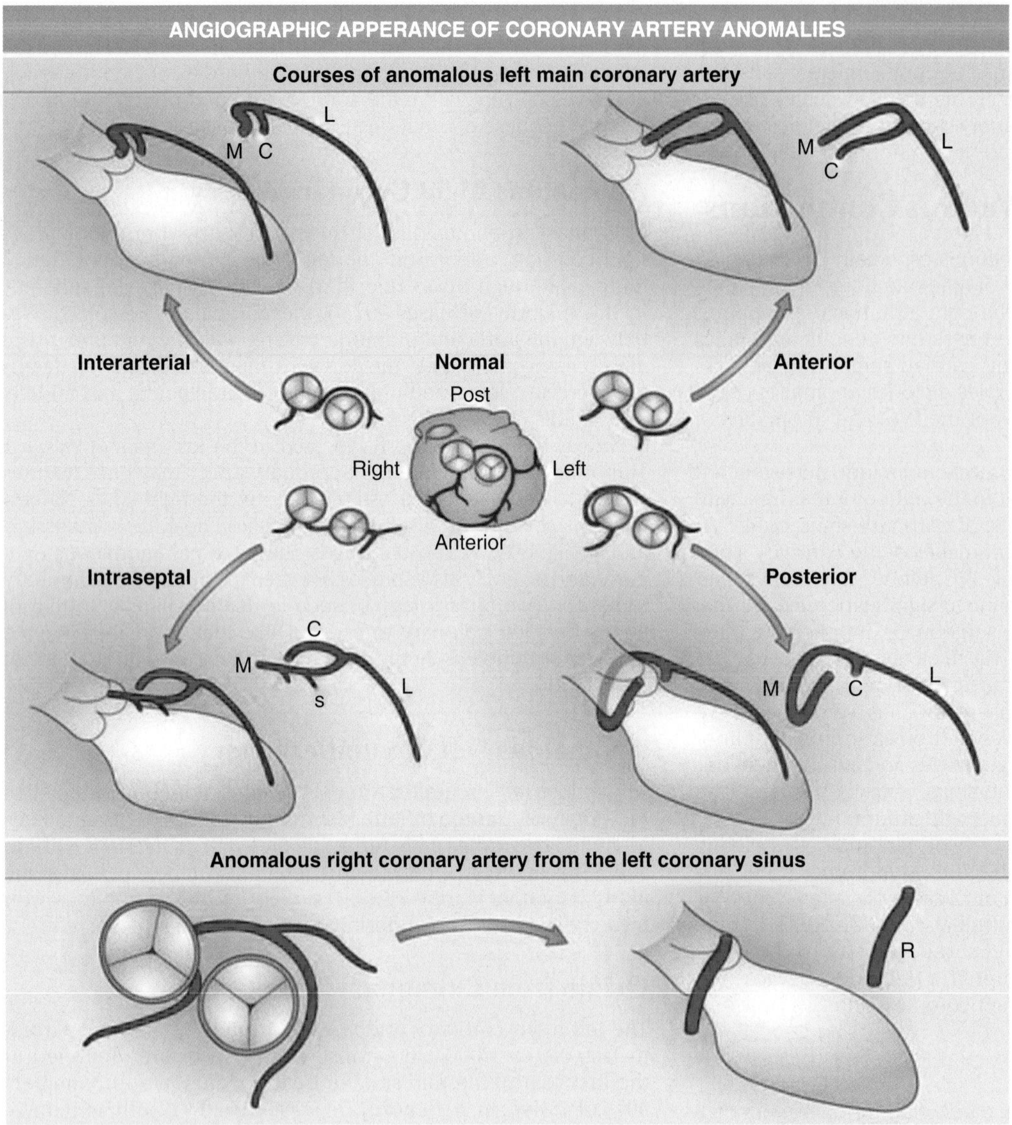

FIGURE 63-5 Development of coronary arteries. *Top,* Movement of the proepicardial organ (PEO) to and over the heart. *Bottom,* Mesenchymal migration and differentiation. The PEO *(blue)* is seen as an outgrowth from the dorsal body wall that moves to the looping heart *(red)*. Next, migrating epithelium is seen spreading over the heart. In cross-section, the epithelium is seen as a single cell layer. Epithelial/mesenchymal transition provides cells that migrate into the myocardium. Vasculogenic cell differentiate and link to form plexi that induce other mesenchymal cells to become smooth muscle. These plexi are remodeled into definitive arteries, and the most proximal points of the major coronaries finally link up with the aorta. *(Reproduced with permission from Reese DE, Mikawa T, Bader DM: Development of the coronary vessel system. Circ Res 91:761–768, 2002.)*

the contralateral aortic sinus.[34] However, the specificity of transthoracic echocardiography (TTE) is insufficient for this test to serve as an accurate screening tool.[35] Alternative noninvasive procedures in the case of inadequate screening echocardiograms include transesophageal echocardiography (TEE) and the recent use of three-dimensional coronary magnetic resonance angiography (3D-CRMA). In one study, 3D-CRMA confirmed the anomalous origin of coronary arteries in 8 out of 15 (53%) pediatric cases, without the use of contrast medium or β-blockers, which could prove advantageous in the evaluation of younger patients.[36]

Malformations Affecting the Great Vessels

Coarctation of the Aorta

Coarctation of the aorta occurs as a congenital narrowing of the aortic arch, either as a discrete narrowing or one of some length that is usually located adjacent to the junction of the ductus arteriosus.[37] The obstruction may be in the form of uniform tubular narrowing of some part of the aortic arch system, usually the isthmus (which lies between the left subclavian artery and the ductus arteriosus) or as a shelflike coarctation within the arch (Box 63-1). The latter is the more common of the two lesions. The narrowing may vary in severity but becomes significant only when there is a pressure gradient across the area of narrowing. That usually occurs when there is greater than 50% cross-sectional area reduction, but there may be lesser narrowing for tubular coarctation.

INCIDENCE

Isolated COA is the fifth or sixth most common anomaly of all the congenital heart diseases, with estimates of 1 in 3000 to 4000 live births.[38-41] In the New England regional study of congenital heart defects, COA accounted for 7.5% of anomalies in infants younger than 1 year of age.[42] That may be an underestimation, since COA in newborn infants may not be detected because of similar blood pressure in the upper and lower extremities.[43] The male-to-female ratio is 1.74:1.[44] In older patients with isolated COA, the incidence is also higher in males. Most cases of COA appear to be sporadic, with no evidence of a mendelian pattern of inheritance.[38] However, congenital heart disease has been reported in approximately 4% of the offspring of female COA patients.[40] In addition, a recent nonparametric linkage analysis suggests a genetic basis for a subset of COA cases. McBride et al. demonstrated possible susceptibility loci on chromosomes 2p23, 10q21, and 16p12 in a cohort of 289 individuals from 43 separate families.[40,45] Coarctation of the aorta is the most common cardiovascular defect found in Turner's syndrome. Noncardiac abnormalities that have been reported with COA are hypospadias, clubfoot, and ocular defects.[44]

PATHOLOGY

The severity of luminal narrowing in the region of the coarctation at autopsy reveals 42% severe (pinhole) stenosis, 25% atresia, and 33% moderate narrowing in individuals 2 years of age and older.[46] In cases of COA containing a contraductal shelf, there is an infolding

Box 63-1 Classification of Coarctation of Aorta

Discrete Coarctation of Aorta (COA)

Coarctation distal to ductus arteriosus:
  With closed ductus
  With patent ductus
Coarctation proximal to ductus arteriosus:
  With closed ductus
  With patent ductus
Coarctation with anomalies of subclavian arteries or aortic arches:
  Atresia or stenosis of left subclavian artery
  Stenosis of right subclavian artery
  Anomalous origin of right subclavian artery:
    Distal to coarctation
    Proximal to coarctation
  Double aortic arch with stenosis of right and coarctation of the left
Coarctation of unusual locations
  Proximal to left subclavian artery:
    With normal branches
    With anomalous origin of right subclavian artery
  At multiple sites
  Of lower thoracic

Tubular Hypoplasia (Isolated or Coexistent with Discrete COA)

Involving aorta beyond the origin of innominate to the origin of ductus arteriosus
Involving only part of the segment of the aorta

Modified from JE Edwards: Congenital malformations of the heart and great vessels. In Gould SE, editor: Pathology of the heart and blood vessels, ed 3, Springfield, Ill., 1968, Thomas, pp 391–454.

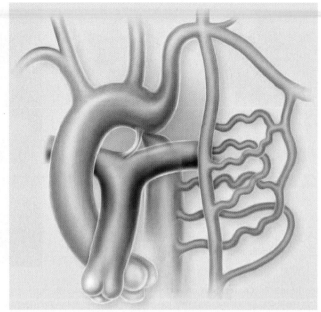

FIGURE 63-6   Coarctation of the aorta (COA). Coarctation causes severe obstruction of blood flow in descending thoracic aorta. Descending aorta and its branches are perfused by collateral channels from axillary and internal thoracic arteries through intercostal arteries. *(Reproduced with permission from Brickner ME: Congenital heart disease in adults. N Engl J Med 342:256–263, 2000.)*

of the aortic media into the lumen located opposite the ductus arteriosus, marked on the adventitial side by a localized indentation like a waist in the aortic wall.[47] The aorta distal to the coarctation shows poststenotic dilation, and the wall of the aorta is thinner, whereas proximally where the pressure is higher, the wall is thicker. The shelf of the coarctation may be pre- or postductal, but most often is juxtaductal.[48] Flow patterns in the fetus with various congenital defects determine the development of the aortic isthmus. In a normal fetus, the level of blood flow across the aortic isthmus is lower (25% of the combined total ventricular output) than after birth; therefore, the aortic isthmus at birth is narrower than the descending thoracic aorta.[48] In congenital heart disease with reduced pulmonary arterial flow (pulmonary stenosis), the diameter of the isthmus is wider than normal because it carries greater flow in the fetus, and coarctation is virtually unknown. In lesions interfering with left ventricular (LV) outflow (mitral and aortic stenosis), the aortic isthmus is underdeveloped. When localized juxtaductal coarctation is present, aortic obstruction is not present during fetal life, but when the ductus arteriosus begins to close at birth, obstruction will appear after birth.[49] The ductus closes from the pulmonary end; obstruction of the aortic end and a gradient across the coarctation may be delayed.

The ductal tissue itself plays an important role in the mechanism of coarctation formation. Normally, ductal tissue, composed mostly of smooth muscle cells (SMCs), extends only partially around the circumference of the aorta. In a patient with left-sided obstruction, there is right-to-left flow through the ductus *in utero*. This results in the migration of ductal tissue into the adjacent aortic wall, resulting in a circumferential distribution.[48] Ho and Anderson, using a serial section technique, have confirmed that ductal tissue completely surrounds the juxtaductal aorta such that "the ductal and descending aorta form a common channel of structural continuity, and the isthmus enters this channel" rather than the ductus entering the isthmus descending aortic region.[50,51]

COLLATERAL CIRCULATION

Olney and Stephens and Bahn et al. have reported that collateral circulation in infants who die with coarctation is poorly developed[52,53] (Fig. 63-6). Bahn et al. noted that this depends on the

location of the coarctation in relation to the ductus arteriosus; if the blood from the ductus enters the aorta proximal to the coarctation (preductal), then collateral circulation will develop[53] (Fig. 63-7). If the ductal blood flow enters below the coarctation (postductal), however, there is little stimulation during fetal life for development of collateral circulation. In that situation, postnatal closure of the ductus results in obstructive hypertension and hypovolemia, which together result in LV failure.

The collateral circulation in COA between the proximal aorta and the distal aorta usually is present to some extent at birth but develops further as the patient ages. Collateral circulation primarily involves branches of both subclavian arteries, especially the internal mammary, vertebral, costocervical, and thyrocervical trunks, which carry blood to the lower limbs, usually through the third and fourth intercostal arteries and subscapular arteries. The subclavian arterial branches become greatly enlarged and are responsible for the classic signs of coarctation, such as rib notching, which extends from the third to the eighth rib, and parascapular pulsations.[37,54,55] Collateral circulation also reaches the lower limbs through the internal mammary to the superior epigastric, which in turn connects with the inferior epigastric and joins the iliac arteries. The anterior spinal artery may provide additional collateral channels through its communication with the vertebral arteries above the coarctation and with intercostals and vertebral arteries below the coarctation.[37,54]

Development of good collateral circulation and clinical manifestations vary depending on the presence of stenosis of the left subclavian artery, which is an important source of collateral circulation; rib notching is seen only on the right side. If the right subclavian artery arises as a fourth branch and is distal to the coarctation, it is not a source of collateral flow, and rib notching occurs only on the left side.[38]

ASSOCIATED CONDITIONS

Coarctation of the aorta is commonly associated with bicuspid aortic valve (BAV), but the exact incidence remains speculative (27%-46%).[51,56] Among 250 patients with COA studied by Tawes et al.,[56] bicuspid valve disease was present in 32 (13%). The most common lesion is stenosis and, unusually, incompetence, which occurs on the basis of bicuspid valve with persistent hypertension.[57]

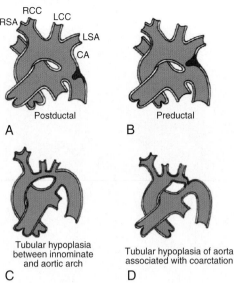

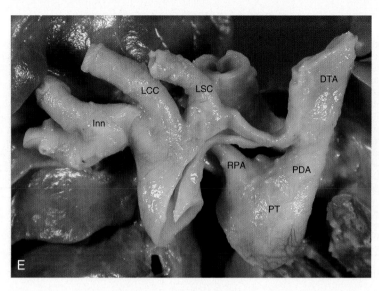

FIGURE 63-7 Coarctation of aorta (COA). A, Postductal. **B,** Preductal with patent ductus arteriosus (PDA). **C,** Tubular hypoplasia of aortic arch between innominate and subclavian artery with patent ductus arteriosus. **D,** Tubular hypoplasia (between common carotid and left subclavian) associated with COA *(arrow)*. **E,** Gross photography of heart and aorta with preductal COA. DTA, descending thoracic aorta; Inn, innominate artery; LCC, left common carotid artery; LSC, left subclavian artery; PT, pulmonary trunk; RPA, right pulmonary artery. *(A-D modified from Moller JH, Amplatz K, Edwards JE: Congenital heart disease, Kalamazoo, Mich., 1974, Upjohn, pp 46–51.)*

There is a high incidence (85%) of major cardiac defects associated with COA in neonates[48]; and infants aged 1 to 11 months, however, the incidence drops to 52%. After 1 year of age, the incidence drops further to 40% (excluding bicuspid valve), as reported by Kirklin and Barratt-Boyes.[57] Infants undergoing operation in the first 3 months of life have a 60% incidence of other congenital cardiac anomalies, compared to 25% of those between 6 and 12 months.[57]

Patent ductus arteriosus (PDA) is present in virtually all neonates and is considered part of the coarctation complex.[57] Ventricular septal defect occurs in 30% to 36% of cases of COA.[38,54] Coarctation of the aorta in transposition of the great arteries occurs in 10%, and ASD in 6% to 7%.[58] Mitral valve disease, which causes mitral stenosis and regurgitation, is present in fewer than 10%.[58]

COMPLICATIONS

Aortic rupture usually occurs in the second or third decade and normally involves the ascending aorta, with resultant tamponade. Aortic rupture also may occur distal to the coarctation where the aorta is thin and dilated (poststenotic dilation).[57] Some ruptures may be accompanied by aortic dissection.[57] Women with coarctation are at high risk of aortic dissections during pregnancy. Stroke, as reported by Liberthson et al., usually occurs in older patients: older than age 40, 21%; age 11 to 39, 8%; and younger than age 11, less than 1%.[58] The main cause is usually rupture of a congenital berry aneurysm in the circle of Willis and is secondary to the presence of hypertension.[59]

Aortic Arch Anomalies

Malformations of the aortic arch are a complex group of lesions first described in the 18th century. Classification of the aortic arch malformations is presented in Box 63-2. *Vascular ring* is the broad term used to describe an aortic arch malformation in which the trachea and esophagus are compressed. The first clinical description of tracheal and esophageal compression by a double aortic arch is credited to Wolman in 1939.[60]

INCIDENCE

The true incidence of aortic arch malformations and vascular rings is difficult to determine because so many lesions are asymptomatic. Congenital heart defects involving the outflow tract, aortic

---

Box 63-2 Aortic Arch Malformations

Vascular Rings
Double aortic arch
Right aortic arch:
  Without retroesophageal component
  With retroesophageal component
Left aortic arch:
  Aberrant right subclavian artery
Ductus arteriosus sling

Cervical Aorta
Complete Interruption of Aortic Arch

---

arch, ductus arteriosus, and pulmonary arteries account for 20% to 30% of all congenital heart defects.[61] The incidence of vascular rings is thought to be approximately 1% of congenital heart disease. Conotruncal malformations, including interrupted aortic arch and isolated anomalies of the aortic arch, are included in the constellation of findings in patients with the 22q11.2 deletion syndrome (del 22q11.2).[62]

In 1948, Edwards proposed the hypothetical double aortic arch model to conceptualize all the known and possible aortic arch malformations.[63] Today there is a better understanding of the embryology, and it has been shown that the final arrangement and morphology of the great arteries requires reciprocal signaling between endothelial cells (ECs) lining the pharyngeal aortic arteries and their surrounding SMCs and mesenchyme, derived from neural crest cells (NCC)[64] (Fig. 63-8). Septation of the truncus into the aorta and pulmonary artery is accompanied by migration of the cardiac NCC into the pharyngeal arches and the heart, and this occurs in the mouse embryo at 9 (E9.0) days onwards. The NCC also contribute to the bilateral symmetrical aortic arches that arise from the aortic sac and undergo extensive remodeling, resulting in formation of the aorta, ductus arteriosus, and proximal subclavian, carotid, and pulmonary arteries. The NCC are remodeled to give rise to segments of the mature aortic arch, which is present from E12.5 days onwards.[61] The left and right third arch arteries form the common carotid arteries (CCAs), the right fourth arch artery forms the proximal portion of the right subclavian artery, the left sixth arch artery forms the ductus arteriosus, and the right sixth arch artery regresses.[65] Recent work with transgenic mice has shown which factors may be important for normal development of the

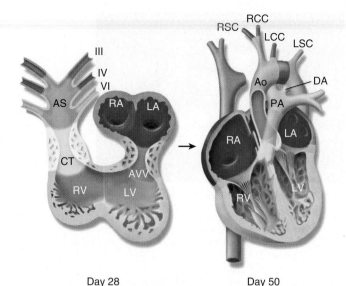

Day 28   Day 50

FIGURE 63-8   Schematic of development of arch vessels and outflow tract of the heart. Neural crest cells populate the bilaterally symmetrical aortic arch arteries *(III, IV, and V)* and aortic sac *(AS)* that together contribute to specific segments of the mature aortic arch, also color coded. Mesenchymal cells form the cardiac valve from the conotruncal *(CT)* and atrioventricular valve *(AVV)* segments. Corresponding days of human embryonic development are indicated. Ao, aorta; DA, ductus arteriosus; LA, left atrium; LCC, left common carotid; LSC, left subclavian artery; LV, left ventricle; PA, pulmonary artery; RCC, right common carotid artery; RSC, right subclavian artery; RV, right ventricle. *(Reproduced with permission from Srivastava D, Olson EN: A genetic blueprint for cardiac development. Nature 407:221–226, 2000.)*

arch vessels. For example, disruption of the forkhead transcription factor Mfh1 causes hypoplasia of the fourth aortic arch artery in mice, resulting in absence of the transverse aortic arch, resembling the interruption of the aortic arch in man.[66]

As already noted, aortic arch vascular ring malformations can encircle and compress the trachea, esophagus, or both.[67]

DOUBLE AORTIC ARCH

The double aortic arch is the most frequent type of aortic arch malformation to result in a vascular ring. The ascending aorta arises normally, and as it leaves the pericardium it divides into two branches, a left and a right aortic arch that join posteriorly to form the descending aorta. The left arch passes anteriorly and to the left of the trachea in the usual position and then becomes the descending aorta by the ligamentum arteriosum or the ductus arteriosus. The right aortic arch passes to the right and then posterior to the esophagus to join the left-sided descending aorta, thereby completing the vascular ring.[67] From each arch arise a carotid and a subclavian artery (Fig. 63-9). The arches are usually not equal in size, the right arch commonly the larger of the two. One arch may be represented by a single atretic segment; in that case, the right arch usually persists.

It is theoretically possible, using the double aortic arch model, that the ductus arteriosus could be bilateral or on the right or left side only. No case of functional double arch with bilateral ductus arteriosus has been reported. The descending aorta may be on the right, on the left, or occasionally in the midline.[63,67–69] Associated cardiac anomalies in most series are low but were reported to be as high as 45% in the series by Kocis et al. in 1997,[70] and these include tetralogy of Fallot and transposition of the great arteries.[68]

Most patients present at the time of diagnosis with many symptoms, the most common being those arising from the respiratory system. Wheezing is the most common, followed by stridor, pneumonia, upper respiratory tract infection, respiratory distress, cough, and respiratory cyanosis. If such symptoms occur in the newborn or young infant and occur recurrently, it should alert the

physician to the possibility of the presence of arch anomalies.[71] Surgical repair is the ideal and is usually performed approximately 18 months after the initial diagnosis.

RIGHT AORTIC ARCH

A right aortic arch is present when the ascending aorta and arch pass anterior to the right mainstem bronchus. There are two main types of right aortic arch: without a retroesophageal component (mirror-image branching) and with a retroesophageal component. Right aortic arch exists in 0.1% of the population.[72]

Right Aortic Arch without Retroesophageal Component

In the usual right aortic arch, there is mirror-image branching of the arch vessels compared to the normal left arch. The first vessel is a left innominate artery, the second and third are the right common carotid and right subclavian arteries (Fig. 63-10). The majority of patients have a left ductus arteriosus arising from the left pulmonary artery and inserting into the left subclavian artery. Bilateral patent ductus is associated with congenital cardiac anomalies, usually tetralogy of Fallot or truncus arteriosus.[69] This abnormality does not produce symptoms but may be picked up radiographically.

Right Aortic Arch with Retroesophageal Component

A vascular ring is usually present in the right aortic arch with retroesophageal component. The right aortic arch extends to the left, behind the esophagus, in the form of a diverticulum. The vascular ring is formed from the right arch and a left-sided ductus arteriosus arising from the left pulmonary artery, with extension into the upper descending thoracic aorta. This group of abnormalities also includes anomalous retroesophageal left subclavian artery. Right aortic arch with mirror-image pattern is associated with congenital heart anomalies, and the most common are tetralogy of Fallot and truncus arteriosus.[73]

LEFT AORTIC ARCH

A vascular ring is frequently associated with left aortic arch.

Aberrant Right Subclavian Artery

The most common left arch abnormality is aberrant right subclavian artery. The right subclavian artery arises as the fourth branch of the aortic arch, distal to the left subclavian artery. Aberrant right subclavian artery does not result in a vascular ring unless there is a right ductus arteriosus extending from the right pulmonary artery to the right subclavian artery (Fig. 63-11). This anomaly is of importance because of its frequent association with tetralogy of Fallot and the difficulty of using this vessel for the Blalock-Taussig anastomosis.[74] Aberrant right subclavian artery is also associated with COA.[68]

DUCTUS ARTERIOSUS SLING

An aberrant ductus arteriosus extending from the right pulmonary artery between the trachea and esophagus to the aorta near the origin of an aberrant right subclavian artery has been reported.[75] The patient may have dyspnea and wheezing, which are relieved by surgical division of the vessel.

CERVICAL AORTIC ARCH/INTERRUPTED AORTIC ARCH

Complete interruption of the aortic arch is different from coarctation of the aortic arch in that there is no continuity of the aorta. *Interrupted aortic arch* is a rare congenital malformation occurring in 3 per million live births. It is defined as a loss of continuity between the ascending and descending thoracic aorta and has poor prognosis without surgical treatment. Almost all cases have a PDA and associated intracardiac anomalies such as VSD, subaortic stenosis, and truncus arteriosus. The symptoms of complete interruption of the aortic arch are

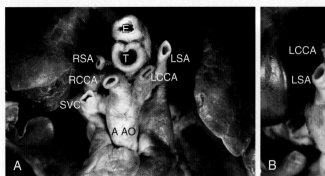

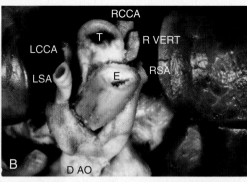

FIGURE 63-9 A, Double aortic arch, anterior/cranial view. Ascending aorta bifurcates into an anterior left branch, supplying left common carotid artery and left subclavian artery, and a posterior right branch, supplying right common carotid and right subclavian arteries. **B,** Double aortic arch, posterior/cranial view. Continuation of aorta viewed from behind demonstrates anterior left branch wrapping around trachea and esophagus, as well as right posterior branch emerging from under esophagus. Distal aorta continues as a centrally located structure. Aao, ascending aorta; DAo, descending aorta; E, esophagus; LCCA, left common carotid artery; LSA, left subclavian artery; RCCA, right common carotid artery; RSA, right subclavian artery; Rvert, right vertebral artery; SVC, superior vena cava; T, trachea.

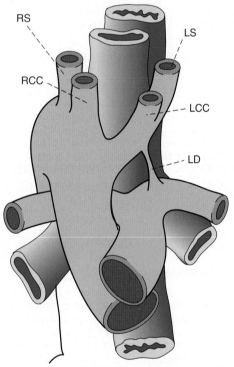

FIGURE 63-10   Right aortic arch with mirror-image branching and left ductus arteriosus. LCC, left common carotid artery; LD, left ductus arteriosus; LS, left subclavian artery; RCC, right common carotid artery; RS, right subclavian artery. *(Reproduced with permission from Bankl H: Congenital malformations of the heart and great vessels. Synopsis of pathology, embryology, and natural history, Baltimore, 1977, Urban & Schwarzenberg, pp 159–166.)*

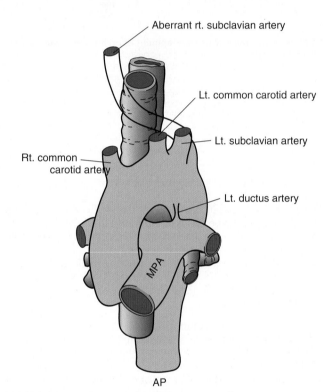

FIGURE 63-11   Aberrant right subclavian artery from an anteroposterior *(AP)* view. *(Reproduced with permission from Stewart JR, Kincaid OW, Edwards JE: An atlas of vascular rings and related malformations of the aortic arch system, Springfield, Ill., 1964, Thomas.)*

severe right-to-left shunting. In infants, the clinical presentation is severe congestive heart failure (CHF). If untreated, 90% of infants will die at a median age of 4 days. Only rare cases in adults have been reported.[76]

CLINICAL PRESENTATION AND DIAGNOSIS

Patients with vascular rings present within the first 6 months of life, and close to 50% have symptoms at birth. Those with associated cardiac defects may present earlier. The signs and symptoms of tracheal and esophageal compression vary with the severity of compression. Infants may present with stridor, wheeze, and recurrent respiratory infections. They often demonstrate poor feeding and dysphagia for solid foods.[56] Surgery is indicated when esophageal and tracheal compression symptoms are severe.

Anomalies of the Pulmonary Trunk and Arteries

Isolated pulmonary artery abnormalities are rare and can be divided into (1) those with anomalous arterial supply to one lung in the presence of separate aortic and pulmonary valves (and without inherent interposition of ductal tissue) and (2) those with lungs receiving normally connected pulmonary arteries.

Origin of Right or Left Pulmonary Artery from Ascending Aorta

When the right pulmonary artery arises from the aorta, it usually arises from the right or posterior aspect of the ascending aorta.[77] The origin is usually within 1 to 3 cm of the aortic valve, and the right pulmonary artery is larger than the left.[77] The pulmonary vascular bed of both lungs may be similar, especially in patients dying within the first 6 months of life.[78] In older patients, however, hypertensive vascular disease is usually present and similar in extent in both lungs.[77] This lesion is seen as an isolated defect in 20% of cases, but most often it is associated with PDA (50%).[79,80] Occasionally, the lesion coexists with left pulmonary vein stenosis.[77] The pulmonary stenosis may be tubular or membraneous.[77]

The origin of the left pulmonary artery from the ascending aorta is more rare than the right pulmonary artery from the aorta, and is usually seen in association with right aortic arch.[77] This anomaly is isolated in 40% of cases, and the most commonly associated lesion is tetralogy of Fallot. Part of one lung may receive anomalous vascular supply, called *sequestration* of the lung. A distinct form of sequestration, *scimitar syndrome* (see earlier under "Partial Anomalous Pulmonary Venous Connection"), involves abnormal arterial supply as well as venous drainage into the IVC.[81] The more severe type of sequestration occurs when one lung is supplied completely from a systemic source.

Pulmonary arteries may arise from the pulmonary trunk, but the left artery connects to the right lung and vice versa.[81] This anomaly has been described in truncus arteriosus, as well as when the pulmonary trunk is normally connected to the right ventricle.[81]

Aortopulmonary Communication

Aortopulmonary communication or window is a distinct anatomical lesion with communication between the ascending aorta and the pulmonary trunk, and the presence of separate aortic and pulmonary valves.[82] The defect is a true window, with no length to the communication between the aorta and pulmonary trunk. Usually the defect is single, large, and oval; infrequently (<10% of cases) the defect is small.[83] The communication is usually situated in the left lateral wall of the ascending aorta (close to the origin of the left coronary artery) in communication with the right wall of the pulmonary trunk (inferior to the origin of the right pulmonary artery).[83,84] It is not surprising, therefore, that the right or, more rarely, the left coronary arteries may be seen arising from the pulmonary trunk. Rarely, the communication may be more downstream.[83–85] Because the defect is often large, it is not surprising that pulmonary vascular disease may develop early, similar to that seen in VSDs and patent ductus arteriosus.[82,83] Aortopulmonary window is associated with other cardiovascular malformations, such as VSDs, tetralogy of Fallot, subaortic stenosis, and infrequently, right aortic arch, ASD, or patent ductus arteriosus.[83–86]

Vascular Anomalies

Before the advent of the system proposed by Mulliken and Glowacki in 1982, proper classification of vascular anomalies was replete with inaccurate and misleading terminology. In 1996, building on the Mulliken and Glowacki system, the International Society for the Study of Vascular Anomalies (ISSVA) established a more appropriate classification system, dividing benign vascular anomalies into two major categories: (1) vascular tumors and (2) vascular malformations (VM)[87] (also see Chapter 64). Although there are several types of vascular tumors, hemangiomas represent the overwhelming number of vascular tumors encountered in pediatrics, are considered benign vascular neoplasms characterized by endothelial proliferation (initially rapidly progressing), and are not considered to cause significant arteriovenous shunting. Vascular malformations, on the other hand, are considered slow-growing congenital anomalies associated with arteriovenous shunting, and histologically are characterized by a proliferation of heterogeneous and often dysplastic vascular elements, including arteries, dysplastic arteries, veins, and arterialized veins. Vascular malformations are further subdivided according to the Modified Hamburg Classification, including a (1) primary classification based on the predominant vascular defect, and (2) an embryological subclassification based on anatomy and the stage of developmental

arrest.[88–91] Vascular malformations can be further divided into groups based on vessel type and flow characteristics. Capillary, venous, and lymphatic malformations are slow-flow lesions, and arteriovenous malformations (AVMs) and fistulas (AVFs) are fast-flow lesions; further combined lesions may also occur. Either proliferation (i.e., VMs, hemangiomas) may be associated with syndromes, especially when multiple.

Vascular Malformations

SLOW-FLOW MALFORMATIONS

Capillary Malformations

Clinically, the most well known of the capillary malformations are known as *fading capillary stains, port-wine stains,* or *venocapillary malformations,* which represent some of the most common vascular malformations of the skin.[87] As a group, *capillary malformations* are a generic term to describe a heterogenous group of vascular stains of the skin, also including lymphaticovenous malformations and the malformations observed in Klippel-Trénaunay's and Parkes-Weber's syndromes. In the case of the facial port-wine stain or the facial nevus flammeus, histological sections may show only rare dilated capillary-like vessels in young children, or collections of haphazardly arranged dilated vessels in the papillary and reticular dermis in older patients[92] (Fig. 63-12).

TELANGIECTASIAS
According to the updated ISSVA classification, telangiectasias are considered a slow-flow type of capillary malformation manifesting as localized dilations of capillaries and venules that are presumed congenital and may form part of an inherited syndrome. Unlike hemangiomas, there is no proliferation of vessels, but rather an idiopathic dilation of preexisting capillaries and venules. However, the term *hemangioma* has often been used, especially clinically, for these lesions. Most forms of telangiectasias are present in the skin, but internal organs including the brain can be affected. There are generally few or no symptoms attributable to the telangiectasia itself, other than cosmetic problems when it involves the skin, or hemorrhagic complications of gastrointestinal hemangiomas. Incidental telangiectasias of the brain are found predominantly in the pons, and have only rarely been reported to cause symptoms by bleeding.

CUTANEOUS TELANGIECTASIAS. The most common congenital cutaneous telangiectasia is the *nevus flammeus,* or ordinary birthmark. Nevus flammeus appears as mottled macular lesion on the head and neck, and usually regresses. The *nevus vinosus,* or *port-wine stain,* is a specialized form of nevus flammeus that demonstrates no tendency to fade and often becomes elevated, reminiscent of a true hemangioma. Unlike true hemangiomas, telangiectasias appear histologically as congested normal vessels that are separated by intervening tissue. Indeed, in most cases there is no detectable histopathological abnormality after processing the tissue for examination.

TELANGIECTASIA SYNDROMES. *Ataxia telangiectasia* is an autosomal dominant inherited disease that is characterized by cerebellar degeneration, immunodeficiency, oculocutaneous telangiectasia, cancer risk, and radiosensitivity. The vascular manifestations are heralded by appearance in childhood of telangiectasias of the bulbar conjunctivae and skin of the face and extremities.[93] Ocular telangiectasias often do not appear until several years after the ataxia. The patients generally succumb to an underlying immunological abnormality that results in recurrent infections and the development of lymphoproliferative disorders. The most common type of malignancy is lymphoma, usually of the B-cell type. Leukemias also occur.[94] Histological examination of the telangiectasias demonstrates the presence of dilated subpapillary venous channels.

Currently, the genetic basis is believed related to mutations in the ataxia-telangiectasia gene (ATM). Since the cloning of ATM in 1995,[95] more that 100 ATM mutations occurring in ataxia-telangiectasia patients have been documented. The mutations are broadly distributed throughout the ATM gene.[96] The

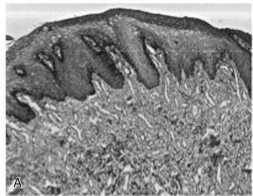 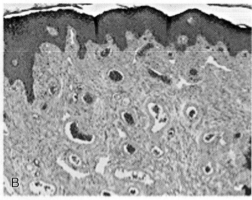

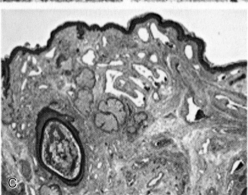

FIGURE 63-12 Capillary malformations (CM). A, Facial CM with lip hypertrophy in a 4-year-old boy, showing an excessive number of thin-walled venule-like channels with narrow lumens (hematoxylin-eosin [H&E] stain × 100). **B,** Facial CM with lip hypertrophy in a 17-year-old boy has an increased number of enlarged vein-like channels with both thin and thick, mostly fibrous walls. Intervascular fibrous tissue is increased (H&E stain × 100). **C,** Facial CM with thickening and nodules in a 35-year-old man with Sturge-Weber's syndrome. Nasal skin shows a nodular cluster of large, abnormal veinlike channels. Fibrosis and follicular dilation and keratin plugging are present (H&E stain × 40). *(Reproduced with permission from Gupta A, Kozakewich H: Histopathology of vascular anomalies. Clin Plast Surg 38:31–44, 2011.)*

product of the ATM gene is a 350-kD protein. ATM is involved in DNA damage recognition and cell cycle control in response to ionizing radiation damage. There is evidence that ATM may also have a more general signaling role.[97] Affected homozygotes are at increased risk for a wide range of malignancies; however, the elevated risk of malignancy is not observed among A-T heterozygotes, with the possible exception of breast carcinoma.[98]

Generalized essential telangiectasia is another localized form of telangiectasia associated with recurrent cutaneous telangiectasis.[99] Another form of telangiectasia that can result in gastrointestinal bleeding is *watermelon stomach*, or *gastric antral vascular ectasia*. Watermelon stomach has been increasingly recognized as an important cause of occult gastrointestinal blood loss and anemia. The histological hallmark of this entity is superficial capillary ectasia of gastric antral mucosa and microvascular thrombosis in the lamina propria. Endoscopic findings of the longitudinal antral folds containing visible columns of tortuous red ectatic vessels (watermelon stripes) are pathognomonic.[100] Watermelon stomach is usually isolated, but has been reported in patients with autoimmune diseases, especially scleroderma.[101–103] The precise nature of the vascular defects is unclear, but underlying fibromuscular dysplasia (FMD) of the gastric arteries has been suggested as a cause for the superficial lesions.[100]

Venous Malformations

Unlike AVMs, vascular malformations are slow-flow lesions composed entirely of veins, which do not show significant enhancement by radiographic procedures.[104] The imaging characteristics, especially those of magnetic resonance (MR), are otherwise similar to those of hemangiomas; hence the past use of the terms *cavernous hemangioma, venous hemangioma*, and *cavernous angioma* still present in textbooks.[105] Typically, there is a focus of attachment to muscle in those occurring in deep sites. Venous hemangiomas have been reported in a variety of sites, including the mediastinum, mesentery, skeletal muscle, and retroperitoneum.[106–111]

Venous malformations histologically are composed of nodules of irregular venous-type vascular channels that may vary in size. This lobular or grouped arrangement of vessels is helpful for distinguishing these benign from malignant vascular proliferations. Mast cells and factor XIII–positive interstitial cells are a consistent feature. The spaces are lined by a mitotically inactive flat endothelium highlighted by CD31, surrounded by smooth muscle that appears attenuated or absent relative to the size of the vessel.[105]

The *blue rubber bleb nevus syndrome* (BRBNS) is a developmental disorder originally identified by the presence of distinctive cutaneous blue nevi, especially of the tongue, lips, neck, and gastrointestinal system, with a predilection for the small bowel.[112] The cutaneous blue nevi are in fact nodular venous malformations involving the dermis and subcutaneous tissue.[105] More recently, central nervous system (CNS) vascular malformations, including venous anomalies, have been associated with BRBNS.[113,114] Colonoscopy with laser photocoagulation is a nonoperative method of controlling bleeding from colonic hemangiomas, although surgical resection may be necessary to control chronic gastrointestinal blood loss.[115] Virtually all internal organs, including the orbit,[116] have been reported as involved in BRBNS, as well as multiple cutaneous sites. There is often a diffuse, mild, consumptive coagulopathy.[117]

BRBNS can be considered a particular manifestation of venous malformation that has been shown to be either sporadic or familial. In the latter, it is inherited in an autosomal dominant fashion. A genetic basis for BRBNS remains inconclusive. Analyses from differing groups have identified a locus chromosome, 9p, responsible for venous malformation in a single large kindred,[118] an activating mutation in the gene that encodes for the kinase domain of the EC receptor TIE2 in another familial genetic analysis,[119,120] and sporadic somatic mutations in TIE2.[121]

FAST-FLOW VASCULAR MALFORMATIONS

Arteriovenous Malformations

Arteriovenous malformations are rare fast-flow lesions consisting of abnormal vascular communications between arteries and veins that occur without an intervening capillary bed and that result in the formation of a mass. These malformations are also referred to as *arteriovenous fistulas, arteriovenous hemangiomas, arteriovenous aneurysms*, and *racemose* or *cirsoid aneurysms*.

ARTERIOVENOUS MALFORMATIONS OF THE CENTRAL NERVOUS SYSTEM, HEAD, AND NECK

Although AVMs are described in almost every organ of the body, approximately 50% are located in the head and neck region, including the CNS.[122–129] Congenital AVMs are often multiple and have a female predominance. Occasionally, there may be familial AVMs in the absence of a defined syndrome.[130] Arteriovenous malformations of the CNS may result in seizures or subarachnoid hemorrhage (SAH) and are treated with a combination of surgery, radiosurgery, embolization, and radiation.[130,131] When the malformation results in vein of Galen steal, treatment consists of coil embolization.[132] There can be an associated venous malformation within the brain.[133] Presenting symptoms of oral and maxillary AVMs vary, including soft-tissue swelling, pain, changes in skin and mucosal color, erythematous and bleeding gingiva, bruit, and paresthesias. The radiological appearance is not pathognomonic. Arteriovenous malformations of the cranial bones can cause bleeding after dental surgery and are also treated with embolization.[134] Some are thought to be hamartomas[134] and can be associated with other vascular anomalies, such as persistent trigeminal artery.[135] Treatment of osseous AVMs of the head and neck include direct transosseous injection of cyanoacrylate.

ARTERIOVENOUS MALFORMATIONS OF THE LUNG

Pulmonary AVMs were first described at autopsy in the 19th century, but the first clinical diagnosis based on the triad of cyanosis, clubbing, and polycythemia was made in 1939.[136] Pulmonary AVM causes a shunt of venous blood from the pulmonary arteries to the pulmonary veins, thus decreasing arterial oxygen saturation. Although most patients are asymptomatic, pulmonary AVMs can cause dyspnea from right-to-left shunts. Because of paradoxical emboli, various CNS complications have been described, including stroke and brain abscesses. There is a strong association between pulmonary AVMs and hereditary hemorrhagic telangiectasia (HHT). Up to 36% of patients with solitary pulmonary AVM and 60% of patients with multiple pulmonary AVMs have associated HHT.[137,138]

Chest radiography and contrast-enhanced computed tomography (CT) are essential initial diagnostic tools, but pulmonary angiography is the gold standard to establish the presence of shunting. Contrast echocardiography is useful for diagnosis and monitoring after treatment. Most patients should be treated. Therapeutic options include angiographic embolization with metal coil or balloon occlusion and surgical excision.[139]

Occasionally a pulmonary AVM receives blood from a systemic artery in addition to a pulmonary artery.[140] Pulmonary AVMs may be single or multiple, small or large enough to involve an entire lung. These can be associated with cerebral AVMs in patients with HHT.[141] They may present during pregnancy with hemoptysis, often heralding HHT, and treatment with embolization is indicated if the patient is symptomatic.[133]

Cyanosis is present since childhood and occasionally since birth. Neurological symptoms may be due to brain abscesses resulting from a loss of the filtering function of the lung.[142] A decrease in arterial oxygen saturation occurs with pulmonary AVM, and pulmonary angiography demonstrates the malformation with early filling of the left atrium.

The frequency of fatal complications is significant in pulmonary AVM.[137] These include rupture, hemorrhage, endocarditis, and brain abscess. Surgery is indicated with segmental resection whenever possible to preserve the maximum amount of lung tissue, but lobectomy may be necessary.[142]

ARTERIOVENOUS MALFORMATIONS OF OTHER SITES

Other locations for AVM include the gastrointestinal tract, heart, liver, and kidney. Those of the gastrointestinal tract typically present with bleeding or mucosal ulceration.[143] They may occur anywhere in the gastrointestinal tract, and endoscopically are raised lesions that may show nonspecific histological alterations.[144] Those of the kidney and pelvis may present with a variety of symptoms and are initially treated with embolization.[145]

Multiplicity and early age at onset are signs that the lesion may be part of a syndrome, especially Klippel-Trénaunay's syndrome or HHT.

The physical findings in AVM are closely related to the location and size of the lesion. Patients may present with swelling, pain, or hemorrhage. If located near the skin, the lesion is often a pulsatile mass with a thrill or bruit. There may be erythema or cyanosis distal to the lesion. Cutaneous or mucosal AVMs may ulcerate and bleed, or there may be thrombosis or cellulitis or both superficially. Hypertrophy of an extremity can occur if a large shunt is present. Cardiomegaly in infancy is occasionally due to an unsuspected AVM, and large aneurysms, particularly in the brain or liver, may cause neonatal heart failure. Central nervous system AVMs may present as repeated episodes of intracranial hemorrhage or as seizure disorders secondary to gliosis or atrophy of the adjacent cortex.

Angiographically, the lesions have multiple anomalous arterial branches and anastomoses with early filling of the venous system. Vessels are dilated, elongated, and tortuous. Magnetic resonance imaging is capable of differentiating AVMs from other types of hemangiomas, both in the CNS and the skin and subcutaneous tissue.[122] Arteriovenous malformations may be present at birth, become apparent soon after birth, or remain asymptomatic until adulthood.[125] Unlike capillary hemangiomas in infants, AVMs do not regress but grow with the growth of the child.

A specialized form of AVM that occurs in the gastric mucosa is termed *Dieulafoy's disease* and is prone to massive upper gastrointestinal hemorrhage. Indications for the treatment of AVMs include congestive heart failure, cosmetic deformity, hemorrhage, or ulceration. Coil embolization of hepatic AVMs may improve heart failure, although there is risk of hepatic damage.[104] Other complications of embolization therapy include stroke,[128] skin slough, and blindness.[123] Treatment of AVMs is tailored to the particular location and size of the lesion. A variety of therapeutic modalities have been used to treat AVMs, including radiation, surgery, and embolization techniques. Surgical treatment of AVMs involves resection. Isolated ligation of the vessel is not curative; collateral circulation can reestablish flow to the lesion.[123,128]

Arteriovenous malformations can recur if not completely excised.[127] The morbidity of surgery relates to hemorrhage, disseminated intravascular coagulation (DIC), and cosmetic deformity.[127] A variety of materials have been used for embolization, including autologous materials such as fat or muscle, hemostatic agents such as gelatin sponges or polyvinyl alcohol, and methyl methacrylate or silicon spheres. More recently, coils and balloons have been used. The amount of shunting and the diameter of shunts determine the size of the embolization particles.

PATHOLOGY

The pathological diagnosis of AVM rests on the presence of communicating arteries and veins in a vascular lesion. In the larger AVM, the gross appearance of the specimen is one of multiple blood-filled spaces, often aneurysmally dilated (Fig. 63-13). A smaller AVM removed for pathological examination may require extensive sectioning to demonstrate the lesion, and ultimately the diagnosis may rest on radiological correlation. Microscopically, AVM is marked by the presence of arteries and veins with little intervening tissue. The direct communication between an artery and a vein may be difficult to locate. Vessels are often elongated and dilated, and the structure of the vessel walls in AVM is usually abnormal. Artery walls are thinned or may be hypertrophied, with disruption and loss of elastic lamina and medial smooth muscle (Fig. 63-14). The medial smooth muscle may also form nodules projecting into the vessel lumen. Vein walls become thickened or arterialized, with the acquisition of internal elastic lamina. Rarely, the malformation may be composed entirely of veins, representing the so-called venous hemangioma. Elastic stains can be helpful, but it is not always possible in AVM to classify a vessel as an artery or a vein.

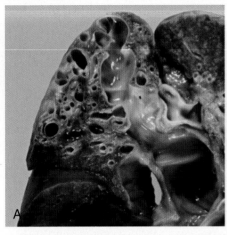
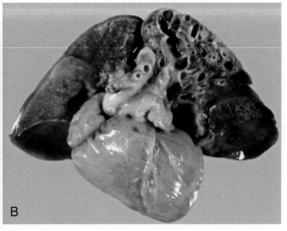

FIGURE 63-13 Pulmonary arteriovenous malformations (AVM). A, Gross image of a large pulmonary AVM demonstrating aneurysmally dilated spaces. **B,** Pulmonary AVM in left upper lobe of lung from a 4-day-old male infant born with low Apgar scores and cyanosis. The infant died in congestive heart failure (CHF).

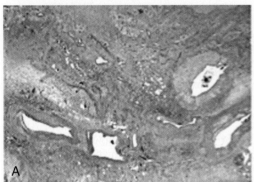
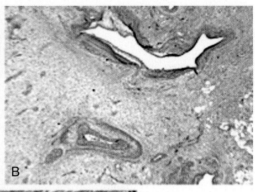

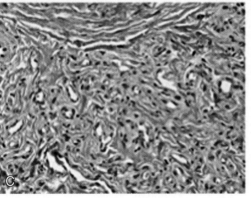

FIGURE 63-14 Arteriovenous malformations (AVM). A, AVM shows malformed arteries and veins (hematoxylin-eosin [H&E] stain × 20). **B,** AVM with Verhoeff-van Gieson (VVG) stain highlights the disrupted internal elastic lamina in arteries, with transition to indeterminate type elastic pattern (top vessel, VVG special stain ×4). **C,** Small vessel (proliferative component) in AVM has foci of small channels with plump endothelium and pericytes (H&E stain × 400). *(Reproduced with permission from Gupta A, Kozakewich H: Histopathology of vascular anomalies. Clin Plast Surg 38:31–44, 2011.)*

Combined Vascular Malformations: Capillary-Venous-Lymphatic Malformations

This category encompasses lesions with a complex combination of vessel types, thus the designation of capillary-lymphatic-venous malformations (CLVMs).[87] CLVMs are the most common vascular malformation associated with Klippel-Trénaunay's syndrome (also see Chapter 64).

CARDIAC HEMANGIOMAS/ARTERIOVENOUS MALFORMATIONS

Vascular malformations within the heart include coronary-cameral fistula and cardiac hemangiomas. Hemangiomas involving the myocardium are a diverse group of lesions that represent either hamartomatous malformations or, less likely, benign neoplasms, despite the designation of a "hemangioma." The histological classification includes those composed of multiple dilated thin-walled vessels (cavernous type), smaller vessels resembling capillaries (capillary type), and dysplastic malformed arteries and veins (arteriovenous

hemangioma, cirsoid aneurysm). Cardiac hemangiomas often have combined features of cavernous, capillary, and arteriovenous hemangiomas, and many contain fibrous tissue and fat. These features are reminiscent of intramuscular hemangiomas of skeletal muscle.

An *intramuscular cardiac hemangioma* has a superficial resemblance to an AVM, with the presence of heterogeneous vessel types, including muscularized arteries, veins, and capillaries. In contrast to capillary hemangiomas, they are infiltrative lesions and occur within the myocardium. They are histologically identical to intramuscular hemangiomas within skeletal muscle and may possess, in addition to the vessels, fat and fibrous tissue. Because of the latter features, some intramuscular cardiac hemangiomas are misclassified as lipomas or fibrolipomas.

Most cardiac hemangiomas are discovered incidentally, but patients may present with dyspnea on exertion, arrhythmias, right-sided heart failure, pericarditis, pericardial effusion, and failure to thrive.[146] Patients may have associated vascular syndromes (e.g., Kasabach-Merritt; see Chapter 64).

Whereas chest roentgenograms are abnormal in the majority of cases, the diagnosis of a cardiac tumor is rarely made on the basis of plain radiographs alone. A characteristic tumor blush on coronary arteriography suggests the diagnosis of a cardiac hemangioma.[147] Echocardiography usually directs the diagnosis toward a cardiac mass. An enhanced-contrast CT scan or MRI can establish the diagnosis of hypervascularized cardiac tumor.

The most frequent locations are the lateral wall of the left ventricle (21%), the anterior wall of the right ventricle (21%), the interventricular septum (17%), and occasionally the RV outflow tract.[148]

Cardiac hemangiomas are often large, and gross appearance depends on the size of the vascular spaces in the tumor. The capillary type is frequently slightly raised from the endocardial surface and appears red to purple. Intramuscular types will appear infiltrative. Cavernous hemangiomas are usually large and are also poorly circumscribed.

Vascular Tumors

According to the modified ISSVA classification, vascular tumors include infantile hemangiomas, congenital hemangiomas, tufted angiomas, pyogenic granulomas, kaposiform hemangioendotheliomas, and the capillary hemangioblastoma/hemangioma associated with von Hippel-Lindau's syndrome (see Chapter 64). Readers are also referred to a recent histological review.[92]

Fibromuscular Dysplasia

Fibromuscular dysplasia is a generic term for a group of structural abnormalities of one or more layers of medium-sized and large arteries that result in luminal narrowing by fibrous, smooth muscle, or fibromuscular tissue, with or without associated aneurysms and dissections of the media. Fibromuscular Dysplasia is an uncommon noninflammatory and nonatherosclerotic angiopathy with a predilection for the renal and carotid arteries. Young to middle-aged predominantly Caucasian females are most commonly affected. Renal involvement is the most common (60%-75%), followed by cervicocranial arteries (25%-30%), visceral arteries (9%), and the arteries of the extremities (5%). The disease consists of a heterogeneous group of histological changes that ultimately lead to arterial narrowing. Clinical manifestations reflect the arterial bed involved, most commonly hypertension (renal), stroke (carotid), and abdominal pain. Classification is based on the histopathological localization and pattern of structural abnormalities. The latter determines the angiographic appearance.

Fibromuscular dysplasia is a pathological diagnosis and has been classified into intimal, medial, and periarterial subtypes. The characteristic angiographic changes described as "string of beads," focal, and tubular can be used to make the diagnosis in the appropriate clinical setting. The most common lesions become symptomatic as high-grade stenosis producing renovascular hypertension, or as an embolic source in the cerebral circulation. Treatment is reserved for symptomatic lesions. Most simple lesions are effectively treated by catheter-based intervention. Surgical therapy is warranted for more complex lesions. Both produce durable long-term results.[149]

The cause(s) of FMD remains obscure and may include estrogen exposure, mechanical factors, ischemic factors, environmental toxins such as cigarette smoke, and autoantibodies. There is an underlying genetic predisposition to the development of FMD. Caucasians are much more likely to develop FMD than blacks, and many cases are familial, with an autosomal dominant transmission and variable penetrance. However, no specific genetic abnormalities have been reported up to now.

Histological Subtypes

The traditional histological classification of FMD has been established based on the layer of vessel involved[150] (Fig. 63-15). Classically, FMD has been divided into medial (Fig. 63-16), intimal (Fig. 63-17), and adventitial types (Fig. 63-18). Medial FMD accounts for up to 95% of cases and has been further subdivided into medial fibroplasia,

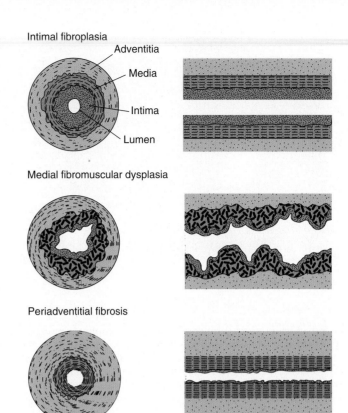

FIGURE 63-15 Schematic showing transverse and longitudinal patterns of involvement of the arteries by the major types of fibromuscular dysplasia (FMD). *(Modified from Harrison EG Jr, McCormack LJ: Pathologic classification of renal arterial disease in renovascular hypertension. Mayo Clin Proc 46:161–167, 1971; and Luschner TF, Lie JT, Stanson AW, et al: Arterial fibromuscular dysplasia. Mayo Clin Proc 69:931–952, 1987.)*

perimedial fibroplasia, and medial hyperplasia.[151] Medial fibroplasia is shown to correlate with either a string-of-beads appearance or multiple stenoses on angiography in 62% of cases. The tubular type with long, concentric stenosis is seen in 14%, and the focal type with solitary stenosis less than 1 cm in length occurs in 7%.

Medial fibroplasia is characterized by fibromuscular ridges of hyperplastic SMCs and fibrous tissue, which project into the lumen

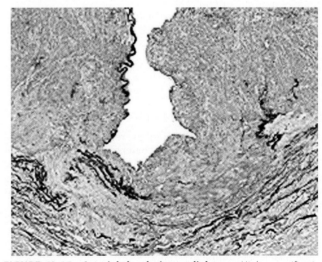

FIGURE 63-16 Arterial dysplasia, medial type. High magnification demonstrates a gap in the arterial media. A succession of such defects results in the string-of-beads appearance on angiogram. *(Reproduced with permission from Virmani R, Burke AP, Farb A: Arterial dysplasia, aneurysms, and dissections. In Virmani R, Burke AP, Farb A, editors: Atlas of cardiovascular pathology, Philadelphia, 1996, Saunders, pp 184–193.)*

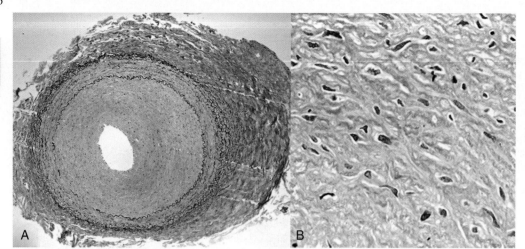

FIGURE 63-17 Fibromuscular dysplasia (FMD), primarily intimal. A 55-year-old woman underwent coronary artery bypass graft (CABG) surgery. Her internal mammary artery (demonstrated histologically) was grossly cordlike, as were other arteries in the mediastinum. **A,** Low magnification shows marked concentric thickening of the intima, with a relatively normal media. There is also a degree of adventitial scarring. **B,** Higher magnification of the intima shows smooth muscle cells (SMCs) within a proteoglycan matrix.

of the affected artery. Perimedial hyperplasia implies a predominance of fibrous tissue, and the proliferation is primarily in the outer layer of the media. Pure medial hypertrophy is quite rare, and represents a concentric hypertrophy of the medial wall. The wall is relatively smooth, lacks fibrosis, and causes severe stenosis. Angiographically and grossly, the stenosis is usually subtotal, tubular, and smooth.

Intimal hyperplasia, which represents less than 5% of lesions, is characterized by proliferation of fibrous tissue, including smooth muscle cells, within the intima. There is no lipid deposition or inflammatory cell infiltrate, and the internal elastic lamina is preserved. Endarteritis secondary to inflammatory conditions or trauma may be associated with intimal fibroplasia in muscular arteries that may mimic the histological picture of intimal fibroplasias. The morphological appearance may be virtually indistinguishable from that of secondary or reactive intimal fibroplasia seen after endarterectomy or in the initial proliferative stage of atherosclerosis. Intimal fibroplasia may also occur concomitantly with medial FMD. In adventitial or periarterial fibroplasia, the primary lesion is a dense collagenous replacement of the loose fibrous tissue of the arterial adventitia. This fibrosis may extend into the surrounding adipose and connective tissues. In periarterial fibroplasia, the media and intima are normal.

The histological classification of FMD is generally based on the layer of vessel involved. Although this classification is well established in the literature, we, as well as others,[152] have not always found this classification useful and reproducible. A simplified classification based on the presence of smooth muscle hyperplasia has recently been proposed.[152]

Fibromuscular Dysplasia of Renal Arteries

In children and young adults, FMD of the renal arteries is the most common cause of renovascular hypertension.[153] The renal arteries are the most common site of symptomatic FMD, accounting for about 75% of cases. Multivessel FMD, which involves renal as well as other arteries, occurs in approximately 25% of patients with renal FMD.

The potential of FMD involving transplant kidneys and affecting the remaining donor kidney has led to the routine use of digital subtraction (DSA) and magnetic resonance angiography (MRA) in potential kidney donors.[154-158]

Although the cause of FMD of the renal arteries is unknown, there is an association with the HLA-DRw6 antigen. In one series of patients, this HLA antigen was more common in the 33 FMD patients than in the 61 renal transplant donor control subjects (odds ratio (OR), 2.5; $P = 0.03$).[159]

Patients with renal FMD are often young women. The diagnosis of FMD is usually made upon investigation for unexplained hypertension. The right renal artery is more often involved than the left, and cases of bilateral involvement are often associated with extrarenal FMD. In a large recent series of 104 unrelated hypertensive patients (94 women) with renal artery FMD, 81 patients had multifocal, 16 had unifocal, and 7 patients both types of stenosis. Fifty-four patients had bilateral FMD. The documented prevalence of familial cases was 11% in this series; familial cases all exhibited the multifocal type and were more commonly bilateral.[160] The distal two thirds of the artery is typically involved, with frequent extension into the branch arteries. Helical CT angiography (CTA), especially the combination of transverse sections and maximum-intensity projection (MIP) reconstructions, can reliably reveal renal artery FMD.[161] Complications of arterial occlusion and renal infarction may result from arterial dissection, embolization originating in the aneurysm, and aneurysmal thrombosis.

Fibromuscular Dysplasia of Aortic Arch Vessels

Fibromuscular dysplasia has been described involving the carotid, subclavian, and vertebral arteries.[162-164] The internal carotid artery (ICA) is typically involved at the level of C1-C2 and is usually "typical" medial FMD, resulting in a classic string-of-beads angiographic appearance. Heterozygous α_1-antitrypsin deficiency may be a genetic risk factor for the development of FMD of the internal carotid artery.[165] Fibromuscular dysplasia is a rare cause of cerebral ischemia; however, FMD of the ICA is typically diagnosed after symptoms such as transient ischemic attacks (TIAs), amaurosis fugax, minor stroke, or nonfocalized ischemic cerebral symptoms. Fibromuscular dysplasia of the arch vessels is increasingly being found incidentally. Surgical intervention in symptomatic cases includes thromboendarterectomy of the bifurcation, venous interposition graft, and venous patching.[166] Recently, endovascular therapy has been applied with increasing frequency. Stent placement has been used for FMD-related aneurysms, and balloon angioplasty for patients with TIA or stroke.[167]

Patients with cerebrovascular FMD have a high incidence of berry aneurysms of the circle of Willis, especially the intracranial ICA and the middle cerebral artery (MCA). Aneurysms in these locations are likely to be found in females with other vascular lesions caused by FMD or other aneurysms. In contrast, aneurysms of the anterior cerebral artery (ACA) are more likely sporadic and found in men. The prevalence of intracranial aneurysms in patients with cervical ICA and/or vertebral artery FMD is approximately 7%, which is not as high as the 21% to 51% prevalence previously reported.[168]

Subclavian and vertebral FMD is less likely to have a characteristic angiographic appearance and has been termed *atypical*

there is significant stenosis of major cephalic or subclavian arteries or embolization from thrombosed areas of FMD. Symptoms include transient ischemic attacks, strokes, and SAH from associated berry aneurysms of the circle of Willis, subclavian steal syndrome, and weakness or claudication of the arms. Complications of cerebrovascular FMD include arterial dissections and carotid cavernous fistulas. Fibromuscular dysplasia of the cerebrovascular circulation and subclavian arteries is more often multifocal and bilateral than isolated renal artery FMD. Patients with subclavian FMD often have systemic FMD, including FMD of the renal arteries.[170]

Fibrous Dysplasia of Miscellaneous Sites

Fibromuscular dysplasia has been described in the visceral arteries,[171-173] iliac,[174] axillary, brachial and coronary arteries, and aorta.[175] Typical arteries involved in FMD of the visceral arteries are the celiac artery, mesenteric arteries, hepatic artery,[176] and splenic artery. These are often found in association with renal artery FMD.[173,177]

Segmental arterial mediolysis, a rare form of mesenteric arteriopathy that typically results in spontaneous dissections and hemoperitoneum in hypertensive patients, may be a form of mesenteric arterial dysplasia. Symptoms related to stenotic lesions of the visceral arteries are rare owing to well-developed collateral vessels. Fibromuscular dysplasia of miscellaneous arteries are prone to similar complications of renal FMD and FMD of the aortic arch, including dissection and embolization.

REFERENCES

1. Burroughs JT, Edwards JE: Total anomalous pulmonary venous connection, *Am Heart J* 59:913–931, 1960.
2. Jackson LW, Correa-Villasenor A, Lees PS, et al: Parental lead exposure and total anomalous pulmonary venous return, *Birth Defects Res A Clin Mol Teratol* 70:185–193, 2004.
3. Ruggieri M, Abbate M, Parano E, et al: Scimitar vein anomaly with multiple cardiac malformations, craniofacial, and central nervous system abnormalities in a brother and sister: familial scimitar anomaly or new syndrome? *Am J Med Genet* 116A:170–175, 2003.
4. Bleyl SB, Saijoh Y, Bax NA, et al: Dysregulation of the PDGFRA gene causes inflow tract anomalies including TAPVR: integrating evidence from human genetics and model organisms, *Hum Mol Genet* 19:1286–1301.
5. Darling RC, Rothney WB, Criaig JM: Total pulmonary venous drainage into the right side of the heart. Report of 17 autopsied cases not associated with other major cardiovascular anomalies, *Lab Invest* 6:44–64, 1957.
6. Seale AN, Uemura H, Webber SA, et al: Total anomalous pulmonary venous connection: morphology and outcome from an international population-based study, *Circulation* 122:2718–2726, 2010.
7. Jenkins KJ, Sanders SP, Orav EJ, et al: Individual pulmonary vein size and survival in infants with totally anomalous pulmonary venous connection, *J Am Coll Cardiol* 22:201–206, 1993.
8. Rubino M, Van Praagh S, Kadoba K, et al: Systemic and pulmonary venous connections in visceral heterotaxy with asplenia. Diagnostic and surgical considerations based on seventy-two autopsied cases, *J Thorac Cardiovasc Surg* 110:641–650, 1995.
9. Masui T, Seelos KC, Kersting-Sommerhoff BA, et al: Abnormalities of the pulmonary veins: evaluation with MR imaging and comparison with cardiac angiography and echocardiography, *Radiology* 181:645–649, 1991.
10. Hijii T, Fukushige J, Hara T: Diagnosis and management of partial anomalous pulmonary venous connection. A review of 28 pediatric cases, *Cardiology* 89:148–151, 1998.
11. Chassinat R: Observations d'anomalies anatomiques remarquables de l'appareil circulatoire, avec hépatocéle congéniale, symptom particulier, *Arch Gen Med* 11:80–91, 1836.
12. Sehgal A, Loughran-Fowlds A: Scimitar syndrome, *Indian J Pediatr* 72:249–251, 2005.
13. Midyat L, Demir E, Askin M, et al: Eponym. Scimitar syndrome, *Eur J Pediatr* 169:1171–1177, 2010.
14. Vida VL, Padalino MA, Boccuzzo G, et al: Scimitar syndrome: a European Congenital Heart Surgeons Association (ECHSA) multicentric study, *Circulation* 122:1159–1166, 2010.
15. Perry LW, Scott LP 3rd: Cor triatriatum: clinical and pathophysiological features, *Clin Proc Child Hosp Dist Columbia* 23:294–304, 1967.
16. Herlong JR, Jaggers JJ, Ungerleider RM: Congenital Heart Surgery Nomenclature and Database Project: pulmonary venous anomalies, *Ann Thorac Surg* 69:S56–S69, 2000.
17. Buchholz S, Jenni R: Doppler echocardiographic findings in 2 identical variants of a rare cardiac anomaly, "subtotal" cor triatriatum: a critical review of the literature, *J Am Soc Echocardiogr* 14:846–849, 2001.
18. Tueche S: Cor triatriatum dextrum. Surgical treatment in a neonate, *Acta Cardiol* 58:39–40, 2003.
19. Huang TC, Lee CL, Lin CC, et al: Use of Inoue balloon dilatation method for treatment of cor triatriatum stenosis in a child, *Catheter Cardiovasc Interv* 57:252–256, 2002.
20. Chen Q, Guhathakurta S, Vadalapali G, et al: Cor triatriatum in adults: three new cases and a brief review, *Tex Heart Inst J* 26:206–210, 1999.
21. Jeong JW, Tei C, Chang KS, et al: A case of cor triatriatum in an eighty-year-old man: transesophageal echocardiographic observation of multiple defects, *J Am Soc Echocardiogr* 10:185–188, 1997.

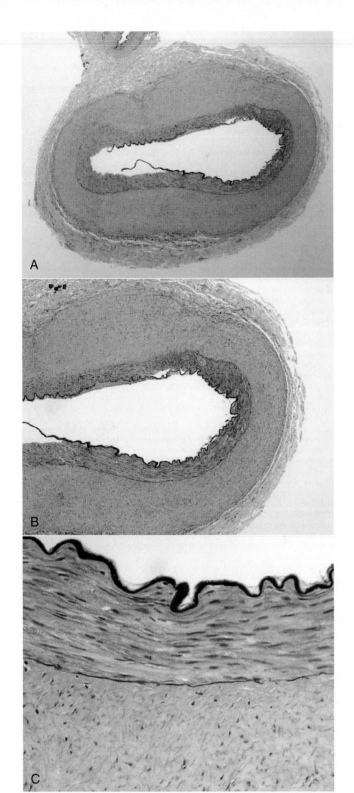

FIGURE 63-18 Fibromuscular dysplasia (FMD), primarily adventitial. A, Low magnification of an artery with normal media and intima but markedly thickened adventitia. **B,** Adventitial scarring is seen at intermediate magnification. **C,** Normal internal elastic lamina, relatively normal media and cellular adventitia.

FMD on the basis of radiological findings. Fibromuscular dysplasia involving more distal branches of the aortic arch, such as the brachial artery, is unusual.[169]

Cerebrovascular FMD and FMD of the subclavian arteries are often asymptomatic and may be an incidental angiographic finding. The overall incidence of this disease, and therefore the proportion of cases that are asymptomatic, are unknown. Symptoms occur if

788

CH
63

22. Slight RD, Nzewi OC, Sivaprakasam R, et al: Cor triatriatum sinister presenting in the adult as mitral stenosis, *Heart* 89:e26, 2003.
23. Rorie M, Xie GY, Miles H, et al: Diagnosis and surgical correction of cor triatriatum in an adult: combined use of transesophageal echocardiography and catheterization, *Catheter Cardiovasc Interv* 51:83–86, 2000.
24. Goel AK, Saxena A, Kothari SS: Atrioventricular septal defect with cor triatriatum: case report and review of the literature, *Pediatr Cardiol* 19:243–245, 1998.
25. Endo M, Yamaki S, Ohmi M, et al: Pulmonary vascular changes induced by congenital obstruction of pulmonary venous return, *Ann Thorac Surg* 69:193–197, 2000.
26. Victor S, Nayak VM: Deringing procedure for congenital pulmonary vein stenosis, *Tex Heart Inst J* 22:166–169, 1995.
27. Omasa M, Hasegawa S, Bando T, et al: A case of congenital pulmonary vein stenosis in an adult, *Respiration* 71:92–94, 2004.
28. Spray TL, Bridges ND: Surgical management of congenital and acquired pulmonary vein stenosis, *Semin Thorac Cardiovasc Surg Pediatr Card Surg Annu* 2:177–188, 1999.
29. Yee ES, Turley K, Hsieh WR, et al: Infant total anomalous pulmonary venous connection: factors influencing timing of presentation and operative outcome, *Circulation* 76:III83–87, 1987.
30. Lincoln CR, Rigby ML, Mercanti C, et al: Surgical risk factors in total anomalous pulmonary venous connection, *Am J Cardiol* 61:608–611, 1988.
31. Dobbertin A, Warnes CA, Seward JB: Cor triatriatum dexter in an adult diagnosed by transesophageal echocardiography: a case report, *J Am Soc Echocardiogr* 8:952–957, 1995.
32. Taylor AJ, Rogan KM, Virmani R: Sudden cardiac death associated with isolated congenital coronary artery anomalies, *J Am Coll Cardiol* 20:640–647, 1992.
33. Yamanaka O, Hobbs RE: Coronary artery anomalies in 126,595 patients undergoing coronary arteriography, *Cathet Cardiovasc Diagn* 21:28–40, 1990.
34. Zeppilli P, dello Russo A, Santini C, et al: In vivo detection of coronary artery anomalies in asymptomatic athletes by echocardiographic screening, *Chest* 114:89–93, 1998.
35. Frescura C, Basso C, Thiene G, et al: Anomalous origin of coronary arteries and risk of sudden death: a study based on an autopsy population of congenital heart disease, *Hum Pathol* 29:689–695, 1998.
36. Clemente A, Del Borrello M, Greco P, et al: Anomalous origin of the coronary arteries in children: diagnostic role of three-dimensional coronary MR angiography, *Clin Imaging* 34:337–343, 2010.
37. Edwards JE: Anomalous pulmonary venous connections. In Gould SE, editor: *Pathology of the heart and blood vessels*, 1968.
38. Gersony WM: Coarctation of the aorta. In Adams FH, Emmanouilides GC, editors: *Heart disease in infants, children and adolescents*, Baltimore, 1989, William & Wilkins, p 243.
39. Fixler DE, Pastor P, Chamberlin M, et al: Trends in congenital heart disease in Dallas County births. 1971–1984, *Circulation* 81:137–142, 1990.
40. Tanous D, Benson LN, Horlick EM: Coarctation of the aorta: evaluation and management, *Curr Opin Cardiol* 24:509–515, 2009.
41. Grech V: Diagnostic and surgical trends, and epidemiology of coarctation of the aorta in a population-based study, *Int J Cardiol* 68:197–202, 1999.
42. Fyler DC, Rothman KJ, Buckley LP, et al: The determinants of five year survival of infants with critical congenital heart disease, *Cardiovasc Clin* 11:393–405, 1981.
43. Edwards JE: Anomalous pulmonary venous connection. In Gould SE, editor: *Pathology of the heart and blood vessels*, ed 3 Springfield, 1968, Thomas, pp 455–478.
44. Campbell M, Polani PE: The aetiology of coarctation of the aorta, *Lancet* 1:463–468, 1961.
45. McBride KL, Zender GA, Fitzgerald-Butt SM, et al: Linkage analysis of left ventricular outflow tract malformations (aortic valve stenosis, coarctation of the aorta, and hypoplastic left heart syndrome), *Eur J Hum Genet* 17:811–819, 2009.
46. Reifenstein GH, Levine SA, Gross RE: Coarctation of the aorta: a review of 104 autopsied cases of the "adult type", 2 years of age or older, *Am Heart J* 33:146, 1947.
47. Pellegrino A, Deverall PB, Anderson RH, et al: Aortic coarctation in the first three months of life. An anatomopathological study with respect to treatment, *J Thorac Cardiovasc Surg* 89:121–127, 1985.
48. Shinebourne EA, Elseed AM: Relation between fetal flow patterns, coarctation of the aorta, and pulmonary blood flow, *Br Heart J* 36:492–498, 1974.
49. Rudolph AM, Heymann MA, Spitznas U: Hemodynamic considerations in the development of narrowing of the aorta, *Am J Cardiol* 30:514–525, 1972.
50. Ho SY, Anderson RH: Coarctation, tubular hypoplasia, and the ductus arteriosus. Histological study of 35 specimens, *Br Heart J* 41:268–274, 1979.
51. Becker AE, Becker MJ, Edwards JE: Anomalies associated with coarctation of aorta: particular reference to infancy, *Circulation* 41:1067–1075, 1970.
52. Olney MB, Stephens HB: Coarctation of the aorta in children: observations in fourteen cases, *J Pediatr* 37:192–203, 1950.
53. Bahn RC, Edwards JE, DuShane JW: Coarctation of the aorta in children: observations in fourteen cases, *Pediatrics* 8:192–203, 1951.
54. Moller JH, Amplatz K, Edwards JE: *Congenital heart disease*, Kalamazoo, 1974, Upjohn.
55. Edwards JE: Pathologic considerations in coarctation of the aorta, *Proc Staff Meet Mayo Clin* 23, 1948.
56. Tawes RL Jr, Berry CL, Aberdeen E: Congenital bicuspid aortic valves associated with coarctation of the aorta in children, *Br Heart J* 31:127–128, 1969.
57. Kirklin JW, Barratt-Boyes BG: Coarctation of the aorta and interrupted aortic arch. In: *Cardiac surgery*, ed 2, New York, 1993, Wiley.
58. Liberthson RR, Pennington DG, Jacobs ML, et al: Coarctation of the aorta: review of 234 patients and clarification of management problems, *Am J Cardiol* 43:835–840, 1979.
59. Lucas RV, Krabill RA: Anomalous venous connections, pulmonary and systemic. In Adams FH, Emmanouilides GC, editors: *Heart disease in infants, children, and adolescents*, Baltimore, 1989, Williams & Wilkins, p 580.
60. Wolman LJ: Syndrome of constricting double aortic arch in infancy report of a case, *J Pediatr* 14:527, 1939.
61. Creazzo TL, Godt RE, Leatherbury L, et al: Role of cardiac neural crest cells in cardiovascular development, *Annu Rev Physiol* 60:267–286, 1998.
62. McDonald-McGinn D, Emanuel BS, Zackai EH: *22q11.2 Deletion syndrome. GeneReviews*, Seattle, 2005, University of Washington.
63. Edwards JE: Anomalies of the derivatives of the aortic arch system, *Med Clin North Am* 6:925, 1948.
64. High FA, Jain R, Stoller JZ, et al: Murine jagged1/notch signaling in the second heart field orchestrates Fgf8 expression and tissue-tissue interactions during outflow tract development, *J Clin Invest* 119:1986–1996, 2009.
65. Conway SJ, Kruzynska-Frejtag A, Kneer PL, et al: What cardiovascular defect does my prenatal mouse mutant have, and why? *Genesis* 35:1–21, 2003.
66. Iida K, Koseki H, Kakinuma H, et al: Essential roles of the winged helix transcription factor MFH-1 in aortic arch patterning and skeletogenesis, *Development* 124:4627–4638, 1997.
67. Kirklin JW, Baratt-Boyes BG: *Vascular rings and slings, cardiac surgery*, New York, 1986, Wiley.
68. Stewart JR, Kincaid OW, Edwards JE: *An atlas of vascular rings and related malformations of the aortic arch system*, Springfield, 1964, Thomas.
69. Sissman NJ: Anomalies of the aortic arch complex. In Adams FH, Emmanouilides GC, editors: *Heart disease in infants, children, and adolescents*, Baltimore, 1983, Williams & Wilkins, pp 199–215.
70. Kocis KC, Midgley FM, Ruckman RN: Aortic arch complex anomalies: 20-year experience with symptoms, diagnosis, associated cardiac defects, and surgical repair, *Pediatr Cardiol* 18:127–132, 1997.
71. Woods RK, Sharp RJ, Holcomb GW 3rd, et al: Vascular anomalies and tracheoesophageal compression: a single institution's 25-year experience, *Ann Thorac Surg* 72:434–438, 2001; discussion 438–439.
72. Moes CA, Freedom RM: Rare types of aortic arch anomalies, *Pediatr Cardiol* 14:93–101, 1993.
73. Gil-Jaurena JM, Murtra M, Goncalves A, et al: Aortic coarctation, vascular ring, and right aortic arch with aberrant subclavian artery, *Ann Thorac Surg* 73:1640–1642, 2002.
74. Taussig HB: *Congenital malformations of the heart*, ed 2, vol 2, Cambridge, Mass, 1960, Harvard University Press.
75. Binet JP, Conso JF, Losay J, et al: Ductus arteriosus sling: report of a newly recognised anomaly and its surgical correction, *Thorax* 33:72–75, 1978.
76. Messner G, Reul GJ, Flamm SD, et al: Interrupted aortic arch in an adult single-stage extra-anatomic repair, *Tex Heart Inst J* 29:118–121, 2002.
77. Kirklin JW, Baratt-Boyes BG: *Origin of the right or left pulmonary artery from the ascending aorta, cardiac surgery*, New York, 1993, Wiley.
78. Keane JF, Maltz D, Bernhard WF, et al: Anomalous origin of one pulmonary artery from the ascending aorta. Diagnostic, physiological and surgical considerations, *Circulation* 50:588–594, 1974.
79. Calder AL, Brandt PW, Barratt-Boyes BG, et al: Variant of tetralogy of Fallot with absent pulmonary valve leaflets and origin of one pulmonary artery from the ascending aorta, *Am J Cardiol* 46:106–116, 1980.
80. Penkoske PA, Castaneda AR, Fyler DC, et al: Origin of pulmonary artery branch from ascending aorta. Primary surgical repair in infancy, *J Thorac Cardiovasc Surg* 85:537–545, 1983.
81. Becker AE, Anderson RH: *Malformations of the pulmonary trunk and arteries, pathology of congenital heart disease*, London, 1981, Butterworths.
82. Becker AE, Anderson RH: Aortopulmonary communications, Pathology of Congenital Heart Disease, London, 1981, Butterworths.
83. Kirklin JW, Baratt-Boyes BG: Aortopulmonary window. In: *Cardiac surgery*, ed 2, New York, 1993, Wiley.
84. Neufeld HN, Lester RG, Adams P Jr, et al: Aorticopulmonary septal defect, *Am J Cardiol* 9:12–25, 1962.
85. Luisi SV, Ashraf MH, Gula G, et al: Anomalous origin of the right coronary artery with aortopulmonary window: functional and surgical considerations, *Thorax* 35:446–448, 1980.
86. Blieden LC, Moller JH: Aorticopulmonary septal defect. An experience with 17 patients, *Br Heart J* 36:630–635, 1974.
87. Huang JT, Liang NG: Vascular malformations, *Pediatr Clin North Am* 57:1091–1110, 2010.
88. Gloviczki P, Duncan A, Kalra M, et al: Vascular malformations: an update, *Perspect Vasc Surg Endovasc Ther* 21:133–148, 2009.
89. Belov S: Anatomopathological classification of congenital vascular defects, *Semin Vasc Surg* 6:219–224, 1993.
90. Lee BB, Laredo J, Lee TS, et al: Terminology and classification of congenital vascular malformations, *Phlebologie* 22:249–252, 2007.
91. Rutherford RB: Classification of peripheral congenital vascular malformations. In Ernst C, Stanley J, editors: *Current therapy in vascular surgery*, vol 22, St. Louis, 1995, Mosby.
92. Gupta A, Kozakewich H: Histopathology of vascular anomalies, *Clin Plast Surg* 38:31–44, 2011.
93. Woods CG, Taylor AM: Ataxia telangiectasia in the British Isles: the clinical and laboratory features of 70 affected individuals, *Q J Med* 82:169–179, 1992.
94. Gatti RA: Ataxia-telangiectasia, *Dermatol Clin* 13:1–6, 1995.
95. Uhrhammer N, Bay JO, Bignon YJ: Seventh International Workshop on Ataxia-Telangiectasia, *Cancer Res* 58:3480–3485, 1998.
96. Concannon P, Gatti RA: Diversity of ATM gene mutations detected in patients with ataxia-telangiectasia, *Hum Mutat* 10:100–107, 1997.
97. Lavin MF, Khanna KK: ATM: the protein encoded by the gene mutated in the radiosensitive syndrome ataxia-telangiectasia, *Int J Radiat Biol* 75:1201–1214, 1999.
98. Yuille MA, Coignet LJ: The ataxia telangiectasia gene in familial and sporadic cancer, *Recent Results Cancer Res* 154:156–173, 1998.
99. Checketts SR, Burton PS, Bjorkman DJ, et al: Generalized essential telangiectasia in the presence of gastrointestinal bleeding, *J Am Acad Dermatol* 37:321–325, 1997.
100. Novitsky YW, Kercher KW, Czerniach DR, et al: Watermelon stomach: pathophysiology, diagnosis, and management, *J Gastrointest Surg* 7:652–661, 2003.
101. Elkayam O, Oumanski M, Yaron M, et al: Watermelon stomach following and preceding systemic sclerosis, *Semin Arthritis Rheum* 30:127–131, 2000.
102. Watson M, Hally RJ, McCue PA, et al: Gastric antral vascular ectasia (watermelon stomach) in patients with systemic sclerosis, *Arthritis Rheum* 39:341–346, 1996.
103. Goel A, Christian CL: Gastric antral vascular ectasia (watermelon stomach) in a patient with Sjogren's syndrome, *J Rheumatol* 30:1090–1092, 2003.

104. Hisamatsu K, Ueeda M, Ando M, et al: Peripheral arterial coil embolization for hepatic arteriovenous malformation in Osler-Weber-Rendu disease; useful for controlling high output heart failure, but harmful to the liver, *Intern Med* 38:962–968, 1999.

105. Abbot ME: Coarctation of the aorta of the adult type II. A statistical study and historical retrospect of 200 recorded cases with autopsy of stenosis or obliteration of the descending aorta in subjects over the age of two years, *Am Heart J* 3:574–618, 1928.

106. Abe K, Akata S, Ohkubo Y, et al: Venous hemangioma of the mediastinum, *Eur Radiol* 11:73–75, 2001.

107. Igarashi J, Hanazaki K: Retroperitoneal venous hemangioma, *Am J Gastroenterol* 93:2292–2293, 1998.

108. Ichikawa MM, Ishida-Yamamoto A, Hashimoto Y, et al: Venous hemangioma. An immunohistochemical and ultrastructural study, *Acta Derm Venereol* 77:382–384, 1997.

109. Itosaka H, Tada M, Sawamura Y, et al: Vanishing tumor of the temporalis muscle: repeated hemorrhage in an intramuscular venous hemangioma, *AJNR Am J Neuroradiol* 18:983–985, 1997.

110. Tada M, Sawamura Y, Abe H, et al: Venous hemangioma of the temporalis muscle, *Neurol Med Chir (Tokyo)* 36:23–25, 1996.

111. Hanatate F, Mizuno Y, Murakami T: Venous hemangioma of the mesoappendix: report of a case and a brief review of the Japanese literature, *Surg Today* 25:962–964, 1995.

112. Bedocs PM, Gould JW: Blue rubber-bleb nevus syndrome: a case report, *Cutis* 71:315–318, 2003.

113. Gabikian P, Clatterbuck RE, Gailloud P, et al: Developmental venous anomalies and sinus pericranii in the blue rubber-bleb nevus syndrome, case report, *J Neurosurg* 99:409–411, 2003.

114. Eiris-Punal J, Picon-Cotos M, Viso-Lorenzo A, et al: Epileptic disorder as the first neurologic manifestation of blue rubber bleb nevus syndrome, *J Child Neurol* 17:219–222, 2002.

115. Morris L, Lynch PM, Gleason WA Jr, et al: Blue rubber bleb nevus syndrome: laser photocoagulation of colonic hemangiomas in a child with microcytic anemia, *Pediatr Dermatol* 9:91–94, 1992.

116. McCannel CA, Hoenig J, Umlas J, et al: Orbital lesions in the blue rubber bleb nevus syndrome, *Ophthalmology* 103:933–936, 1996.

117. Rodrigues D, Bourroul ML, Ferrer AP, et al: Blue rubber bleb nevus syndrome, *Rev Hosp Clin Fac Med Sao Paulo* 55:29–34, 2000.

118. Gallione CJ, Pasyk KA, Boon LM, et al: A gene for familial venous malformations maps to chromosome 9p in a second large kindred, *J Med Genet* 32:197–199, 1995.

119. Calvert JT, Riney TJ, Kontos CD, et al: Allelic and locus heterogeneity in inherited venous malformations, *Hum Mol Genet* 8:1279–1289, 1999.

120. Vikkula M, Boon LM, Carraway KL 3rd, et al: Vascular dysmorphogenesis caused by an activating mutation in the receptor tyrosine kinase TIE2, *Cell* 87:1181–1190, 1996.

121. Limaye N, Wouters V, Uebelhoer M, et al: Somatic mutations in angiopoietin receptor gene TEK cause solitary and multiple sporadic venous malformations, *Nat Genet* 41:118–124, 2009.

122. Awad IA, Robinson JR, Mohanty S, et al: Mixed vascular malformations of the brain: clinical and pathogenetic considerations, *Neurosurgery* 33:179–188, 1993.

123. Coleman CC: Diagnosis and treatment of congenital arteriovenous fistulas of the head and neck, *Am J Surg* 126:424–428, 1973.

124. Finn MC, Celowack J, Mulliken JB: Congenital vascular lesions: clinical application of a new classification, *J Pediatr Surg* 18:894–900, 1983.

125. Garcia-Gonzalez R, Gonzalez-Palacios J, Maganto-Pavon E: Congenital renal arteriovenous fistula (cirsoid aneurysm), *Urology* 24:495–498, 1984.

126. Jellinger K: Vascular malformations of the central nervous system: a morphologic overview, *Neurosurg Rev* 9:177–216, 1986.

127. Trout HH 3rd, McAllister HA Jr, Giordano JM, et al: Vascular malformations, *Surgery* 97:36–41, 1985.

128. Trout HH: Management of patients with hemangiomas and arteriovenous malformations, *Surg Clin North Am* 66:333–345, 1986.

129. Watson WL, McCarthy WD: Blood and lymph vessel tumors–a report of 1,056 cases, *Surg Gynecol Obstet* 71:569–583, 1940.

130. Herzig R, Burval S, Vladyka V, et al: Familial occurrence of cerebral arteriovenous malformation in sisters: case report and review of the literature, *Eur J Neurol* 7:95–100, 2000.

131. Irie K, Nagao S, Honma Y, et al: Treatment of arteriovenous malformation of the brain–preliminary experience, *J Clin Neurosci* 7:24–29, 2000.

132. Brunelle F: Arteriovenous malformation of the vein of Galen in children, *Pediatr Radiol* 27:501–513, 1997.

133. Yanaka K, Hyodo A, Nose T: Venous malformation serving as the draining vein of an adjoining arteriovenous malformation. Case report and review of the literature, *Surg Neurol* 56:170–174, 2001.

134. Kacker A, Heier L, Jones J: Large intraosseous arteriovenous malformation of the maxilla - a case report with review of literature, *Int J Pediatr Otorhinolaryngol* 52:89–92, 2000.

135. Nakai Y, Yasuda S, Hyodo A, et al: Infratentorial arteriovenous malformation associated with persistent primitive trigeminal artery–case report, *Neurol Med Chir (Tokyo)* 40:572–574, 2000.

136. Smith HL, Horton BT: Arteriovenous fistula of the lung associated with polycythemia vera; report of a case in which the diagnosis was made clinically, *Am Heart J* 18:589–594, 1939.

137. Burke CM, Safai C, Nelson DP, et al: Pulmonary arteriovenous malformations: a critical update, *Am Rev Respir Dis* 134:334–339, 1986.

138. Hodgson CEA: Hereditary hemorrhagic telangiectasia and pulmonary arteriovenous fistula: survey of a large family, *N Engl J Med* 26:625–638, 1959.

139. Khurshid I, Downie GH: Pulmonary arteriovenous malformation, *Postgrad Med J* 78:191–197, 2002.

140. Bosher LH, Blake A, Byrd BR: An analysis of the pathologic anatomy of pulmonary arteriovenous aneurysms with particular reference to the applicability of local excision, *Surgery* 45:91–104, 1959.

141. Tripathy U, Kaul S, Bhosle K, et al: Pulmonary arteriovenous fistula with cerebral arteriovenous malformation without hereditary hemorrhagic telangiectasia. Unusual case report and literature review, *J Cardiovasc Surg (Torino)* 38:677–680, 1997.

142. Chow LT, Chow WH, Ma KF: Pulmonary arteriovenous malformation. Progressive enlargement with replacement of the entire right middle lobe in a patient with concomitant mitral stenosis, *Med J Aust* 158:632–634, 1993.

143. Aida K, Nakamura H, Kihara Y, et al: Duodenal ulcer and pancreatitis associated with pancreatic arteriovenous malformation, *Eur J Gastroenterol Hepatol* 14:551–554, 2002.

144. Hayakawa H, Kusagawa M, Takahashi H, et al: Arteriovenous malformation of the rectum: report of a case, *Surg Today* 28:1182–1187, 1998.

145. Game X, Berlizot P, Hassan T, et al: Congenital pelvic arteriovenous malformation in male patients: a rare cause of urological symptoms and role of embolization, *Eur Urol* 42:407–412, 2002.

146. Kojima S, Sumiyoshi M, Suwa S, et al: Cardiac hemangioma: a report of two cases and review of the literature, *Heart Vessels* 18:153–156, 2003.

147. Grebenc ML, Rosado de Christenson ML, Burke AP, et al: Primary cardiac and pericardial neoplasms: radiologic-pathologic correlation, *Radiographics* 20:1073–1103, 2000; quiz 1110–1071, 1112.

148. Burke A, Johns JP, Virmani R: Hemangiomas of the heart. A clinicopathologic study of ten cases, *Am J Cardiovasc Pathol* 3:283–290, 1990.

149. Curry TK, Messina LM: Fibromuscular dysplasia: when is intervention warranted? *Semin Vasc Surg* 16:190–199, 2003.

150. Slovut DP, Olin JW: Fibromuscular dysplasia, *N Engl J Med* 350:1862–1871, 2004.

151. Hata J, Hosoda Y: Perimedial fibroplasia of the renal artery, *Arch Pathol Lab Med* 103:220–223, 1979.

152. Alimi Y, Mercier C, Pellissier JF, et al: Fibromuscular disease of the renal artery: a new histopathologic classification, *Ann Vasc Surg* 6:220–224, 1992.

153. Fenves AZ, Ram CV: Fibromuscular dysplasia of the renal arteries, *Curr Hypertens Rep* 1:546–549, 1999.

154. Andreoni KA, Weeks SM, Gerber DA, et al: Incidence of donor renal fibromuscular dysplasia: does it justify routine angiography? *Transplantation* 73:1112–1116, 2002.

155. Indudhara R, Kenney, Bueschen AJ, et al: Live donor nephrectomy in patients with fibromuscular dysplasia of the renal arteries, *J Urol* 162:678–681, 1999.

156. Williams ME, Shaffer D: ACE inhibitor-induced transplant acute renal failure due to donor fibromuscular dysplasia, *Nephrol Dial Transplant* 14:760–764, 1999.

157. Wolters HH, Vowinkel T, Schult M, et al: Fibromuscular dysplasia in a living donor: early post-operative allograft artery stenosis with successful venous interposition, *Nephrol Dial Transplant* 17:153–155, 2002.

158. Blondin D, Lanzman R, Schellhammer F, et al: Fibromuscular dysplasia in living renal donors: still a challenge to computed tomographic angiography, *Eur J Radiol* 75:67–71.

159. Sang CN, Whelton PK, Hamper UM, et al: Etiologic factors in renovascular fibromuscular dysplasia. A case-control study, *Hypertension* 14:472–479, 1989.

160. Pannier-Moreau I, Grimbert P, Fiquet-Kempf B: v Possible familial origin of multifocal renal artery fibromuscular dysplasia, *J Hypertens* 15:1797–1801, 1997.

161. Beregi JP, Louvegny S, Gautier C, et al: Fibromuscular dysplasia of the renal arteries: comparison of helical CT angiography and arteriography, *AJR Am J Roentgenol* 172:27–34, 1999.

162. Luschner TF, Lie JT, Stanson AW, et al: Arterial fibromuscular dysplasia, *Mayo Clin Proc* 62:931–952, 1987.

163. Perry MO: Fibromuscular dysplasia, *Surg Gynecol Obstet* 97:104, 1974.

164. Sato S, Hata J: Fibromuscular dysplasia. Its occurrence with a dissecting aneurysm of the internal carotid artery, *Arch Pathol Lab Med* 106:332–335, 1982.

165. Schievink WI, Meyer FB, Parisi JE, et al: Fibromuscular dysplasia of the internal carotid artery associated with alpha1-antitrypsin deficiency, *Neurosurgery* 43:229–233, 1998; discussion 233-224.

166. Van Damme H, Sakalihasan N, Limet R: Fibromuscular dysplasia of the internal carotid artery. Personal experience with 13 cases and literature review, *Acta Chir Belg* 99:163–168, 1999.

167. Olin JW, Sealove BA: Diagnosis, management, and future developments of fibromuscular dysplasia, *J Vasc Surg* 53:826–836, e821, 2011.

168. Cloft HJ, Kallmes DF, Kallmes MH, et al: Prevalence of cerebral aneurysms in patients with fibromuscular dysplasia: a reassessment, *J Neurosurg* 88:436–440, 1998.

169. Suzuki H, Daida H, Sakurai H, et al: Familial fibromuscular dysplasia of bilateral brachial arteries, *Heart* 82:251–252, 1999.

170. Leventer RJ, Kornberg AJ, Coleman LT, et al: Stroke and fibromuscular dysplasia: confirmation by renal magnetic resonance angiography, *Pediatr Neurol* 18:172–175, 1998.

171. Kojima A, Shindo S, Kubota K, et al: Successful surgical treatment of a patient with multiple visceral artery aneurysms due to fibromuscular dysplasia, *Cardiovasc Surg* 10:157–160, 2002.

172. Safioleas M, Kakisis J, Manti C: Coexistence of hypertrophic cardiomyopathy and fibromuscular dysplasia of the superior mesenteric artery, *N Engl J Med* 344:1333–1334, 2001.

173. Sandmann W, Schulte KM: Multivisceral fibromuscular dysplasia in childhood: case report and review of the literature, *Ann Vasc Surg* 14:496–502, 2000.

174. Verhelst H, Lauwers G, Schroe H: Fibromuscular dysplasia of the external iliac artery, *Acta Chir Belg* 99:171–173, 1999.

175. Suarez WA, Kurczynski TW, Bove EL: An unusual type of combined aortic coarctation due to fibromuscular dysplasia, *Cardiol Young* 9:323–326, 1999.

176. Jones HJ, Staud R, Williams RC Jr: Rupture of a hepatic artery aneurysm and renal infarction: 2 complications of fibromuscular dysplasia that mimic vasculitis, *J Rheumatol* 25:2015–2018, 1998.

177. Ebaugh JL, Chiou AC, Morasch MD, et al: Staged embolization and operative treatment of multiple visceral aneurysms in a patient with fibromuscular dysplasia–a case report, *Vasc Surg* 35:145–148, 2001.

CHAPTER 64 Peripheral Vascular Anomalies, Malformations, and Vascular Tumors

Francine Blei

Nonmalignant vascular anomalies can be functionally divided into two groups: proliferative vascular lesions and static vascular malformations. Unfortunately, this distinction is not universally appreciated, and diagnoses are often incorrect in the literature and clinical practice because of knowledge gaps and lack of clarity. Box 64-1A delineates a classification initially proposed by Mulliken and Glowaki,[1] and Box 64-1B is an updated version published by the International Society for the Study of Vascular Anomalies (access at www.issva.org/). Functional classification helps guide management and prognosis. This chapter discusses peripheral (i.e., not central nervous system [CNS] or cardiac) vascular anomalies, including vascular tumors and syndromic vascular disorders, and offers new genetic information and insights into putative signaling pathways implicated in their development.

Proliferative Vascular Anomalies and Tumors

Hemangiomas are considered the most common tumors of childhood. They are benign growths of endothelial cells (ECs), with a unique natural history characterized by a rapid growth phase usually beginning in the first weeks of life and continuing until 9 to 12 months of age (Fig. 64-1). The majority of hemangiomas subsequently undergo spontaneous gradual (but extensive) involution. Histological correlation with the growth phase demonstrates involution and is characterized by increased connective tissue in the dermis and fat in the subcutaneous tissues.[2] An important exception to this growth/regression pattern is the group of *rapidly involuting congenital hemangiomas* (RICH), which are generally present in full at birth (or even detected prenatally), and *noninvoluting congenital hemangiomas* (NICH), which do not change size postnatally.[3] Growth curves for these hemangiomas are illustrated in Figure 64-2. A subset of patients with RICH may have high-flow lesions with prenatal or postnatal high-flow characteristics and/or transient coagulopathy[4,5] (Fig. 64-3). Congenital nonprogressive hemangiomas have been shown by North et al. to be histologically and immunophenotypically distinct from classical hemangiomas of infancy and are speculated to have a differing pathogenesis.[6] NICH-type lesions were found to have high flow clinically (as assessed by Doppler), and inferred histologically, in that small arteries were seen shunting into lobular vessels or abnormal veins.[7] Another subtype of hemangiomas are those with minimal or arrested growth, presenting as areas of telangiectasia with peripheral bulkiness. In one series, the majority of this type of hemangioma was present on the lower extremities.[8]

Typical hemangiomas are known to be most common in females, premature infants, and in the facial region. Results of the multicenter Hemangioma of Infancy Study of over 1000 children with hemangiomas showed an increased incidence in white non-Hispanic infants, multiple gestations, infants born to older mothers, and in association with placenta previa and/or preeclampsia.[9] Other studies have shown (1) a threefold increased risk of hemangiomas in infants born to mothers who had transcervical chorionic villous sampling compared to amniocentesis (the incidence of hemangiomas in the amniocentesis group was equivalent to the incidence of hemangiomas in the general population)[10,11] and (2) a correlation with placental anomalies with abnormal uteroplacental circulation.[12,13] Waner et al. noted a nonrandom distribution of facial hemangiomas and found two patterns of growth: focal lesions (in 76.3% of the 205 patients assessed) and diffuse lesions (in 23.7%). The focal hemangiomas

correlated to 22 sites of occurrence, all near lines of mesenchymal or mesenchymal-ectodermal embryonic fusion. The diffuse hemangiomas were in a segmental distribution and were specified as frontonasal (27%), maxillary (35%), or mandibular (38%). There was a threefold increased incidence of ulceration in patients with diffuse hemangiomas compared to that in patients with focal hemangiomas.[14] Haggstrom et al. expanded the observation of nonrandom distribution, designating four primary segments (Seg1-Seg4) to correspond with cutaneous location[15] (Fig. 64-4). Large hemangioma size, facial location, and/or segmental hemangiomas were more likely to require medical intervention.[16] Segmental hemangiomas can be associated with a higher incidence of PHACE(S) syndrome, visceral hemangiomas, and underlying lumbosacral anomalies (e.g., occult spinal dysraphism, including lipomyelomeningocele with tethered cord).[17–20] *PHACE(S) Association* is an acronym for posterior fossa structural malformations, hemangiomas (segmental), arterial anomalies, cardiac defects, eye abnormalities, (and sternal and other midline deformities)[21] (Fig. 64-5). A patient with a segmental hemangioma and one or more of these criteria has PHACES. In one series, approximately one third of patients with facial segmental hemangiomas were found to have PHACES, those at higher risk having large hemangiomas involving more than one anatomical segment, and in the frontonasal or frontotemporal distribution. Of those with PHACES, most (90%) had more than one extracutaneous finding (most commonly CNS arteriopathy or cardiac anomaly).[22] Similarly, Oza et al. observed that patients with large facial segmental cutaneous (Seg1-Seg4) hemangiomas were especially at risk of CNS structural and cerebrovascular anomalies, those with Seg1 distribution hemangiomas had a higher incidence of ocular anomalies, and those with Seg3 distribution had airway, ventral, and cardiac anomalies. In this series, all patients with CNS structural anomalies had concomitant CNS arteriopathies. Also identified were supratentorial CNS anomalies (cortical dysgenesis and migration abnormalities). Arteriopathies are most commonly dysplastic vessels with an aberrant course involving the internal cerebral artery and its embryonic branches ipsilateral to the side of the cutaneous hemangioma.[23] Hypoplasia, agenesis, or absence of normal arteries can also occur. In one review, some 20% of patients had arterial occlusions and stenoses.[24] Progressive changes can lead to aneurysm formation.[23]

Most hemangiomas are asymptomatic and require no therapy. Despite this clinical course, hemangiomas nonetheless may be the source of significant psychosocial morbidity (although this has not been well studied). Early intervention may be considered to prevent morbidity and/or preclude the need for future surgery. Hemangiomas may cause complications requiring medical therapy to catalyze the involution phase. These complications may include obstruction of the upper airway, ophthalmological disturbances, ulceration or bleeding, persistent soft-tissue deformity, cerebral vasculopathy, and/or high-output congestive heart failure (CHF); all are discussed below.

Kasabach-Merritt Phenomenon, Kaposiform Hemangioendothelioma, and Tufted Angioma

Trapping of platelets and other blood elements (*Kasabach-Merritt phenomenon*) has been known to occur in association with a subset of vascular anomalies since it was first described in 1940.[25] This is an extremely important diagnosis because early detection and rapid evaluation and treatment (if clinically symptomatic) are essential. Kasabach-Merritt phenomenon is not associated with

Box 64-1A Functional Classification of Vascular Anomalies

Proliferative Nonmalignant* Vascular Lesions and Tumors

Hemangiomas of infancy:
  Rapidly involuting congenital hemangiomas of infancy (RICH)
  Noninvoluting congenital hemangiomas of infancy (NICH)
Kaposiform hemangioendothelioma
Tufted angioma
Pyogenic granuloma
Kaposi sarcoma

Static Vascular Lesions (Vascular Malformations)

Simple or combined
Arteriovenous
Capillary
Venous
Lymphatic

*Mitotic figures absent or rare.

Box 64-1B Updated ISSVA Classification of Vascular Anomalies

Vascular Tumors

Infantile hemangiomas:
  Congenital hemangiomas
  RICH
  NICH
Tufted angioma (± Kasabach-Merritt's syndrome)
Kaposiform hemangioendothelioma (± Kasabach-Merritt's syndrome)
Spindle cell hemangioendothelioma
Other rare hemangioendotheliomas (epithelioid, composite, retiform, polymorphous, Dabska tumor, lymphangioendotheliomatosis, etc.)
Acquired vascular tumors (pyogenic granuloma, targetoid hemangioma, glomeruloid hemangioma, microvenular hemangioma, etc.)

Vascular Malformations

CM
Port-wine stain
Telangiectasia
Angiokeratoma
VM
Common sporadic VM
Familial cutaneous and mucosal venous malformation (VMCM)
GVM (glomangioma)
Blue rubber bleb syndrome
Maffucci's syndrome
LM
Fast-flow vascular malformations:
AM
AVF
AVM
Complex-combined vascular malformations: CVM, CLM, LVM, CLVM, AVM-LM, CM-AVM

A, arterial; AVF, arteriovenous fistula; AV, arteriovenous; C, capillary; G, glomovenous; ISSVA, International Society for the Study of Vascular Anomalies; L, lymphatic; M, malformation; NICH, noninvoluting congenital hemangioma; RICH, rapidly involuting congenital hemangioma; V, venous.
From Enjolras O, Wassef M, Chapot R: Color atlas of vascular tumors and vascular malformations, Cambridge, 2007, Cambridge University Press.

common hemangiomas of infancy, but with kaposiform hemangioendothelioma (KHE) or tufted angiomas.[26,27] On examination, the lesion is often edematous, boggy, and ecchymotic (Fig. 64-6). Anatomical predilection is for the chest wall and shoulder, groin extending down the leg, retroperitoneum, or face. Gender distribution tends to be equal. Hematological features of Kasabach-Merritt phenomenon include thrombocytopenia, hypofibrinogenemia, elevated fibrin degradation products, and D-dimers. Radiological hallmarks of KHE are cutaneous thickening, diffuse enhancement with ill-defined margins, small feeding/draining vessels, stranding, and hemosiderin deposits. The histological features of KHE are spindled ECs resembling Kaposi sarcoma (but not associated with human immunodeficiency virus [HIV] infection), abnormal lymphatic-like vessels, microthrombi, hemosiderin, and decreased mast cells and pericytes (which are often seen in hemangiomas). There may be residual tumor after resolution of hematological abnormalities, and radiological studies often demonstrate persistent vascular tumors. Residua of KHE-associated tumors may be dormant vascular tumors rather than scars. Clinically as well as histologically, they differ considerably from involuted hemangiomas. A subset of patients with KHE do not have an associated coagulopathy.[28] Treatment of KHE is not standardized but depends on the morbidity, location, and radiological features. Multimodal therapy may include steroids, chemotherapy (most commonly vincristine),

interferon (IFN), antifibrinolytic agents, antiplatelet agents, and/or embolization. Diffuse intramuscular involvement often makes surgery not an option. Treatment with Rapamune (sirolimus) has been reported in one case[2,29] and is currently being studied in a clinical trial (http://clinicaltrials.gov/ct2/show/NCT00975819?term=sirolimus&rank=82; see Table 64-4).

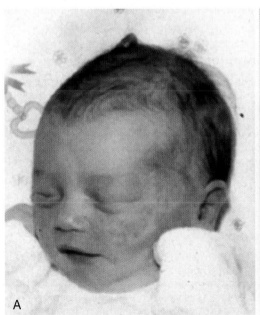

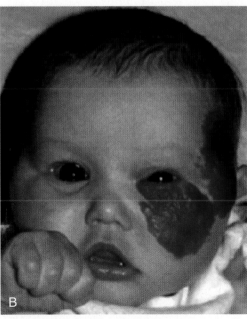

FIGURE 64-1 Hemangioma of infancy. A-B, Sequential photos of infant who developed aggressive proliferative hemangioma with ophthalmological as well as cosmetic issues. In early phases **(A),** this lesion is not easily differentiated from a capillary malformation.

CH
64

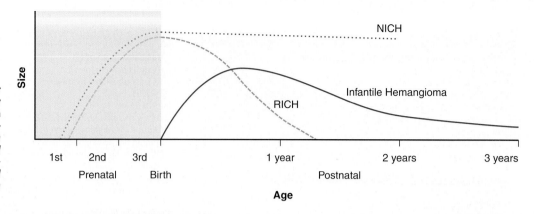

FIGURE 64-2 Growth curves for infantile hemangioma, rapidly involuting congenital hemangioma (RICH), and noninvoluting congenital hemangioma (NICH). *(From Mulliken J, Enjolras O: Congenital hemangiomas and infantile hemangioma: missing links. J Am Acad Dermatol 50:875–882, 2004; used with permission.)[3]*

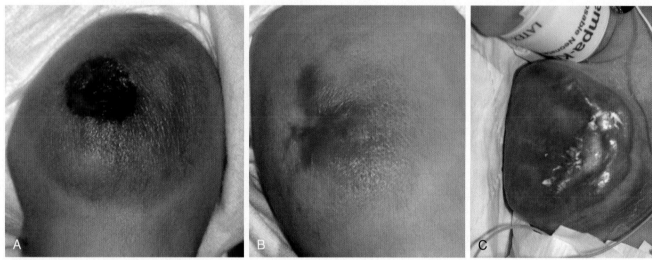

FIGURE 64-3 Rapidly involuting congenital hemangioma (RICH). RICH of thigh with ulceration **(A)** and during natural involution **(B)**. C. RICH of chest wall will high-flow component necessitating inotropic agents, intubation, and embolization. Infant had transient coagulopathy. Notice circumferential halo in both cases.

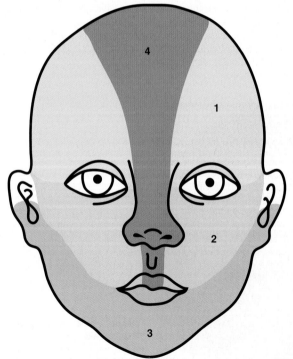

FIGURE 64-4 Distribution patterns of facial segmental hemangiomas. *(From Haggstrom AN, Lammer EJ, Schneider RA, et al: Patterns of infantile hemangiomas: new clues to hemangioma pathogenesis and embryonic facial development. Pediatrics 117:698–703, 2006.) Reproduced with permission, copyright by the AAP.*

Tufted angioma, first described in the late 1980s, is a benign vascular tumor typified by tufts of capillaries in the dermis. The clinical appearance ranges from erythematous indurated annular nodules to plaques, with or without hypertrichosis (Fig. 64-7). They commonly occur on the trunk and extremities, and they may be associated with Kasabach-Merritt phenomenon. Chu et al. suggest that KHE and tufted angioma may represent a continuum; they report a case of transformation between both tumors within a single patient.[30]

Pyogenic Granuloma

Pyogenic granuloma (also termed *lobular capillary hemangioma*) is an acquired vascular lesion of the skin and mucous membranes seen in pediatric patients (Fig. 64-8). The lesions have a cervicofacial propensity but can also be located on the trunk or extremities. The majority occur on the skin, and less frequently the mucous membranes (oral cavity and conjunctivae). These lesions are small and papular and tend to bleed. Treatment includes: (1) excision and linear closure, (2) shave excision, (3) cauterization, (4) cryotherapy, (5) carbon dioxide (CO_2) or pulsed dye laser, or (6) sclerotherapy.[31]

Kaposi Sarcoma

Kaposi sarcoma is a neoplasm commonly but not exclusively seen in patients with acquired immunodeficiency syndrome (AIDS).[32,33] It is an unusual vascular neoplasm originally described in 1872. The clinical appearance begins as violaceous macules that progress to plaques and papules and then nodules. Kaposi sarcoma is thought

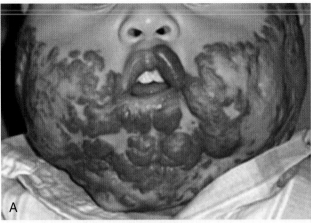

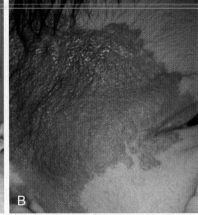

FIGURE 64-5 Segmental hemangiomas. Note beard distribution and Seg3 distribution **(A)**. Patient also had subglottic hemangioma. **B,** Partial Seg1&2 hemangioma that extended to neck and back. Patient was also found to have PHACE (posterior fossa structural malformations, hemangiomas [segmental], arterial anomalies, cardiac defects, eye abnormalities) arteriopathy.

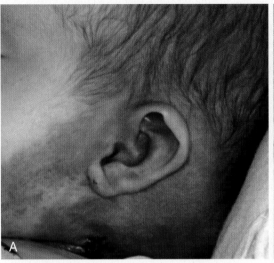

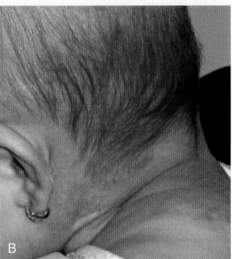

FIGURE 64-6 A, Kaposiform hemangioendothelioma presenting with boggy diffuse mass, thrombocytopenia, and coagulopathy. **B,** After several courses of vincristine therapy.

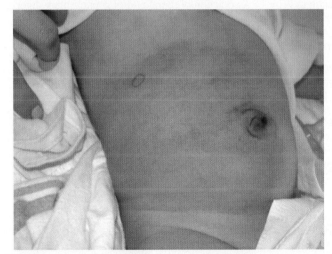

FIGURE 64-7 Tufted angioma on abdominal surface. Patient had Kasabach-Merritt phenomenon. Note site that was biopsied.

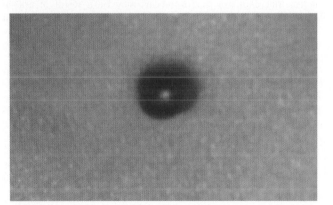

FIGURE 64-8 Pyogenic granuloma, an acquired vascular lesion often seen in children. Lesions are prone to bleeding.

to be multifocal rather than metastatic, with multiple lesions occurring simultaneously at different anatomical locations. Histological features include spindle cells and ECs with rare mitotic figures. Evidence indicates that Kaposi sarcoma is monoclonal, although these data are conflicting. A novel human herpesvirus known as *Kaposi sarcoma–associated herpesvirus* (KSHV), or *human herpesvirus type 8* (HHV8), has been identified in Kaposi sarcoma tissue, supporting a viral etiology. Growth factors and cytokines

are also believed to be involved in Kaposi sarcoma development. Therapies directed against Kaposi sarcoma include antiviral agents, antiangiogenic drugs, and immunosuppressive agents. Recent studies show the effectiveness of antiretroviral therapy suppressing HIV/AIDS-associated Kaposi sarcoma growth.[34]

Vascular Malformations

Vascular malformations are present at birth and grow in parallel with the rate of growth of the child, with no propensity to spontaneous involution. They are due to developmental anomalies of the

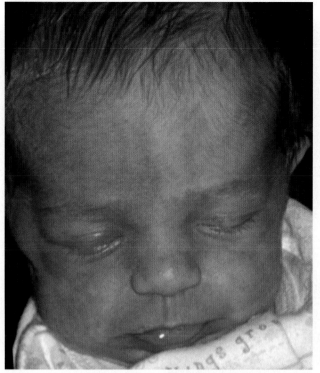

FIGURE 64-9 Capillary malformations. Patient has facial capillary malformation and Sturge-Weber's syndrome.

vasculature and may involve one or several types of vessels (arteries, veins, capillaries, or lymphatics). Vascular malformations are properly described according to the affected anomalous vascular channel. They can range from capillary malformations (commonly referred to as *port-wine stains*; Fig. 64-9) to large bulky growths that can distort the normal structures of the body and potentially lead to a high-output cardiac state (arterial malformations). Studies suggest that capillary malformations may be a result of abnormal innervation of discrete capillary beds causing chronic focal vascular ectasia.[35,36] In one study, nerve density was significantly decreased in biopsies of capillary malformations, as compared to uninvolved skin.[37]

Lymphatic malformations may cause focal or generalized lymphedema, depending on the magnitude of aberrant lymphatics (Fig. 64-10). Abnormal growth of lymphatic circulation encompasses overdevelopment (in lymphangiodysplasias, lymphangiomas, and lymphangiomatosis), underdevelopment of lymphatic vasculature, or both. Disorders of the lymphatic circulation are common, diverse, and often devastating in their functional consequences. Clinical issues common to lymphatic anomalies reflect the tendency of these malformations to develop: (1) local

and systemic infections/cellulitis (infectious and aseptic); (2) leakage (e.g., superficial blebs, chylous ascites, chylothorax, peritonitis, pleural effusions); (3) malabsorption syndromes with significant metabolic consequences; (4) craniofacial distortion interfering with swallowing, airway, or causing significant visceral dysfunction; (5) recurrences or complications after surgery; and (6) swelling of the affected anatomy, with functional limitation.[38]

Syndromic Vascular Anomalies

There is a spectrum of vascular malformations with dysregulated skeletal/adipose/soft-tissue growth (Table 64-1). Klippel-Trénaunay's syndrome (capillary-lymphatic-venous malformation with ipsilateral limb enlargement or hypoplasia, venous varicosities or developmental anomalies, or both) is one of the most common peripheral vascular malformation syndromes (Fig. 64-11). Males and females are affected in equal proportion, and the lower limb is the most frequent site of the anomaly. In severe cases, there may be an accompanying bleeding diathesis characterized by a normal to slightly decreased platelet count, decrease in fibrinogen, and increased D-dimers and fibrin degradation products[39] (Fig. 64-12).

Sturge-Weber's syndrome includes a capillary malformation in the trigeminal distribution, intracranial angiomatosis and dysplasia, seizures, and glaucoma (see Fig. 64-9). Other examples of dysmorphic syndromes associated with vascular malformation are Turner's and Noonan's syndromes, Parkes Weber's syndrome, hereditary hemorrhagic telangiectasia (HHT), blue rubber bleb nevus syndrome (Fig. 64-13), Maffucci's syndrome, CLOVES syndrome (congenital lipomatous overgrowth, vascular malformations, epidermal nevi, spinal/skeletal anomalies or scoliosis), Proteus's syndrome, Bannayan-Riley-Ruvalcaba's syndrome, and Cowden's syndrome (see Table 64-1). Syndromes noted for CNS vascular anomalies include von Hippel-Lindau, ataxia-telangiectasia, Sturge-Weber, and tuberous sclerosis; however, CNS and spinal arterial or venous anomalies are now known to occur in association with a number of vascular anomalies.[23,40–45]

Dysmorphic syndromes associated with hemangiomas are predominantly associated with superficial segmental hemangiomas such as PHACES Association or sacral and/or genitourinary defects, associated with hemangiomas in the lumbar area.[19,46]

PTEN-Associated Hamartoma Syndromes

PTEN (phosphatase and tensin homolog protein) is a tumor suppressor gene. Patients with a PTEN mutation are susceptible to cancers and warrant early and regular screening. Some patients with vascular anomalies (arteriovenous, lymphatic, venous) have the PTEN mutation, such as those with Cowden's and Bannayan-Riley-Ruvalcaba's syndromes.[47] A family history or presence of lipomas, thyroid disorders, tricholemmas, macrocephaly, and penile lentigines may point to a PTEN mutation. Consultation with a geneticist and family screening for mutations is indicated, and early

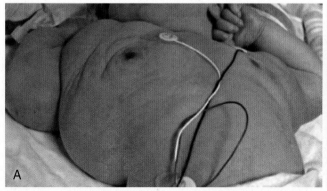
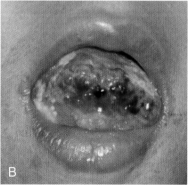
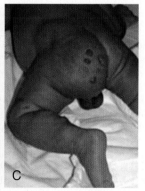

FIGURE 64-10 Lymphatic malformations of chest wall (A), tongue (B), and buttocks/leg (C).

TABLE 64-1   Syndromic Vascular Anomalies and Genetic Information

NAME	FEATURES	OMIM
Blue rubber bleb nevus syndrome Bean syndrome	Multiple small soft venous malformations on skin, gastrointestinal tract, elsewhere	112200
CLOVES syndrome	Congenital lipomatous overgrowth, vascular malformations, and epidermal nevi, skeletal/spinal anomalies	612918
Gorham's syndrome Gorham-Stout's syndrome Cystic angiomatosis of bone, diffuse disappearing bone disease	Lymphangiomatosis, bony destruction	123880
Klippel-Trénaunay's syndrome	Capillary, venous, ± lymphatic malformation, hypertrophy of the related bones and soft tissues ± atretic deep venous system of affected extremity	149000
Maffucci's syndrome (osteochondromatosis/dyschondroplasia with vascular lesions)	Enchondromatosis and subcutaneous spindle cell hemangioendotheliomas, risk of chondrosarcoma, other malignancies including CNS	166000
Proteus' syndrome	Gigantism (partial) of hands and feet, nevi, asymmetrical and disproportionate overgrowth, hemihypertrophy, macrocephaly, dysregulated adipose tissue, vascular malformations	176920
CM-AVM; CMC1 5q13-22 RASA-1 (RAS p21 protein activator 1) loss of function	Multifocal small macular CMs + AVM	608354
Venous malformations, multiple cutaneous and mucosal; VMCM 9p21 TIE2/TEK gain of function AD (most are sporadic)	Focal venous dilation with sparse vascular smooth muscle cells, cutaneous, mucosal, ± underlying areas	600195
Hennekam syndrome 18q21.32 CCBE1 Collagen and calcium-binding EGF domain–containing protein 1	Intestinal lymphangiectasia, severe lymphedema, mental retardation	235510
Hypotrichosis-lymphedema-telangiectasia syndrome HLTS 20q13.33 SOX18	Alopecia and/or areas of sparse hair, transparent skin, lymphedema, telangiectasia	607823
Lymphedema-distichiasis syndrome 16q24.3 AD or *de novo* FOXC2 loss of function	Limb edema and double rows of eyelashes (distichiasis) ± other associated anomalies including cardiac, renal, vascular, CNS gene mutation	153400
Milroy's disease 5q35.3 AD, AR, or *de novo* FLT4 vascular endothelial growth factor receptor 3; VEGFR3 loss of function	Primary congenital hereditary lymphedema type Ia	153100
Lymphedema praecox Meige's disease Late-onset lymphedema	Hereditary lymphedema type II Peripubertal onset	153200
Lymphangioleiomyomatosis LAM 16p13.3, 9q34	Pulmonary (and extrapulmonary) lymphangiomyomatosis; female predominance, adult onset	606690
HHT Osler-Weber-Rendu AD Loss of function HHT type I 9q34.1 Endoglin (131195) Part of TGF-β receptor complex HHT type 2 12q11-q14 ALK1 Activin A receptor, type II-like kinase-1; ACVRLK1 cell surface receptor for TGF-β superfamily HHT type 3 5q31.3-q32 HHT type 4 7p14 Juvenile polyposis/HHT syndrome; JPHT 18q21.1 SMAD4 tumor suppressor; mutations affect TGF-β signaling	Cutaneous, mucosal and visceral telangiectasias and AVMs, epistaxis, and gastrointestinal bleeding, ± pulmonary AV fistulas, hepatic, CNS, spinal AVM HHT1: cerebral AVMs > pulmonary AVMs HHT2: hepatic AVMs more common	187300 600376 601101 610655 175050

Continued

TABLE 64-1   Syndromic Vascular Anomalies and Genetic Information—Cont'd

NAME	FEATURES	OMIM
Cutis marmorata telangiectatica congenita CMTC Macrocephaly-cutis marmorata telangiectatica congenita	Cutaneous reticulated mottling, telangiectasia, and phlebectasia, undergrowth or overgrowth of an involved extremity ± other anomalies	219250
Glomovenous malformation GVM AD 1p22-p21 Glomulin (601749) FKBP (FK506 binding proteins)-associated protein, 48-KD; FAP48	Glomovenous malformations Cutaneous venous malformations with glomus cells surrounding distended vein-like channels	138000
PHACES Association	Posterior fossa brain malformations Segmental facial hemangiomas Arterial anomalies Cardiac anomalies Eye abnormalities Sternal or midline anomalies	606519
Bannayan-Riley-Ruvalcaba 10q23.31 PTEN Phosphatase and tensin homolog; tumor suppressor	Macrocephaly, multiple lipomas, vascular anomalies, pigmented macules of the penis	153480
Cowden's syndrome 10q23.31 AD PTEN Phosphatase and tensin homolog; tumor suppressor PHTS	Macrocephaly, multiple hamartomas, cutaneous verrucous lesions, gingival/buccal papules, facial trichilemmomas, risk of breast/thyroid/renal/endometrial malignancies, cerebelloparenchymal disorder VI (Lhermitte-Duclos' disease)	158350

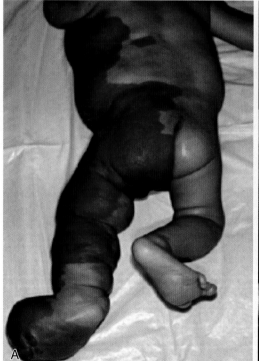 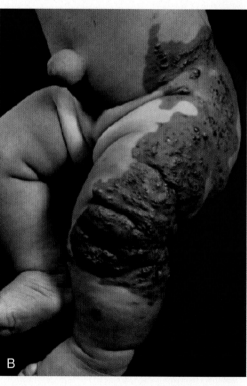

FIGURE 64-11 A, Patient with Klippel-Trénaunay's vascular malformation syndrome complicated by leg-length discrepancy, asymmetrical foot size requiring custom orthotics, lymphopenia, and frequent septic episodes due to abnormal lymphatic communications. **B,** Patient with Klippel-Trénaunay's vascular malformation syndrome, leg length discrepancy with cutaneous capillary malformation, and blebs prone to bleeding.

screening for thyroid, breast, brain, gynecological, and other cancers should be initiated for all individuals with the PTEN mutation.[47,48] Tan et al. recommend screening for PTEN mutations in patients with vascular malformations and the described findings and/or multiple vascular anomalies with a characteristic angiographic appearance, adipose-containing intramuscular lesions, and multiple intracranial developmental venous anomalies.[40]

Patients with Cowden's syndrome have typical skin growths that may resemble small, uniform, cutaneous and mucosal warts or skin tags, as well as macrocephaly and cognitive delay. Malignancies seen in patients with Cowden's syndrome are usually breast, thyroid, or endometrium. Additional findings are benign tumors, thyroid nodules, breast masses, and Lhermitte-Duclos' disease, a benign noncancerous brain tumor, which is pathognomonic. Often the suspicion of Cowden's syndrome begins with a family history of thyroid nodules, lipomas (benign fatty lumps), and/or cancers. If the family history and clinical spectrum (macrocephaly, hamartomas, skin tag–appearing lesions) are present, the patient and family should be referred to a genetics specialist for further discussion and blood testing for the presence of the PTEN mutation. Since not

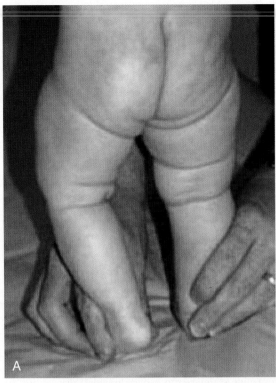

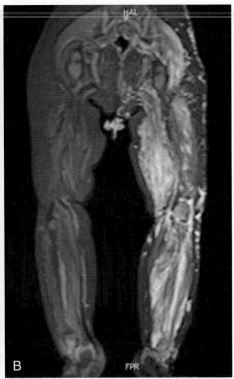

FIGURE 64-12 Patient with venous vascular malformation of left leg (A), with leg length discrepancy and extensive involvement, as noted on magnetic resonance imaging (MR) (B). Patient later developed knee contractures, pain, and coagulopathy.

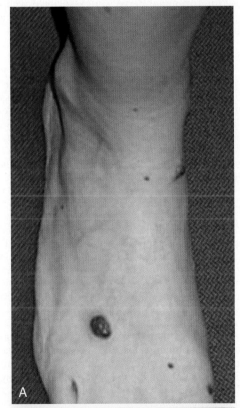

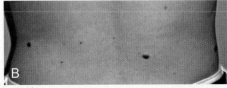

FIGURE 64-13 Patient with blue rubber bleb nevus syndrome. Patient has large vascular malformation of neck and history of severe gastrointestinal bleeding due to similar vascular malformations in gastrointestinal tract.

all the mutations are available for testing, more sophisticated tests may be required if the initial test is negative and the patient/family fulfills the criteria for the disorder. Upon the suspicion or diagnosis of Cowden's syndrome, individuals should be placed in a cancer surveillance program to facilitate early detection and prompt referral for further evaluation and treatment.

Bannayan-Riley-Ruvalcaba's syndrome is characterized by macrocephaly, noncancerous fatty masses (lipomas), vascular malformations, intestinal polyps, thyroid disorders, pectus excavatum, hyperextensible joints, proximal muscle abnormalities, and predisposition to breast and thyroid cancers. Male patients have penile lentigines. Bannayan-Riley-Ruvalcaba's syndrome, which is often diagnosed in childhood, is also associated with mutations of the PTEN gene, thus the same guidelines hold true for patients suspected of having this disorder, as well as their family members.

Prenatal Diagnosis of Vascular Anomalies

With the availability of improved techniques in fetal ultrasound and magnetic resonance imaging (MRI), prenatally diagnosed vascular anomalies are becoming increasingly recognized. Most prenatally diagnosed vascular lesions are vascular malformations. Vascular lesions detected prenatally are generally identified by asymmetrical limbs and/or high-flow lesions (e.g., arteriovenous malformations [AVMs] or high-flow RICH-type lesions).[49] If symptomatic *in utero*, such as high-flow vascular lesions compromising fetal hemodynamic status, prenatal therapy with maternal steroids or digoxin can be instituted. Maternal steroid therapy may be helpful in the management of fetal hemangiomas.[50,51]

Etiology of Hemangiomas and Vascular Malformations

Why do vascular anomalies occur? The simple answer is that they are due to many causes—mechanical, environmental, hormonal, and genetic—although no single etiology is thematic. Within the last several years, major research breakthroughs are unraveling potential etiological factors leading to formation of vascular anomalies, as detailed in excellent reviews.[52–55]

As subtypes of hemangiomas with segmental cutaneous distribution and associated visceral anomalies became evident, researchers speculated involvement of neural crest–derived cells, further supported by identification of neural crest cell markers (neurotrophin receptor p75) in proliferating hemangioma tissue.[56] Several studies demonstrated markers for progenitor mesodermal stem cells (brachyury, GATA) or endothelial and hematopoietic cells (platelet endothelial adhesion molecule [PECAM]-1 [CD31]), intracellular adhesion molecule (ICAM)-3, bcl-2 gene expression, KDR+, CD133+, CD34+, endothelial precursor cells, lymphatic endothelial hyaluronan receptor-1, von Willebrand factor (vWF), and Snrk-1 in hemangioma tissue.[57-60] Constitutive activation of the endothelial tie-2 receptor and vascular endothelial growth factor receptor (VEGFR)-2-related signaling pathways have been identified in human hemangiomas of infancy.[52,54,61]

Clonality of ECs was demonstrated,[62,63] and the potential role of ECs in hemangioma development elucidated.[64-66] Bischoff et al. isolated hemangioma-derived stem cells, which unlike other precursor cells, grew in vitro and differentiated in vivo into cells with properties of hemangiomas, including the eventual presence of adipocytes, as seen in involuting hemangiomas.[2] Hemangiomas and placental vessels express common proteins including glucose transporter (GLUT)-1.[67] This discovery is of diagnostic utility and spearheaded insights into placenta-based hypotheses. For example, Mihm and Nelson proposes a metastatic niche theory for hemangioma development, suggesting the placenta prepares hemangioma precursor cells that "home" to sites of hemangioma growth[68] (Fig. 64-14). Proliferating hemangiomas have been shown to express VEGF-A as well as genes involved with nuclear factor (NF)-κB-related pathways.[69,70]

In addition, proapoptotic factors and appearance of adipocytes during the involution phase support a role for inflammation and immunoregulation in this process[71] (Fig. 64-15). The vast majority of hemangiomas appear to be sporadic; however, familial cases harboring germline mutations of angiogenesis-related genes (VEGF2 and tumor endothelial matrix marker [TEM8]) have been identified.[72] A secondary somatic event appears to be necessary for hemangioma development. Box 64-2 summarizes features of hemangioma endothelial cells.

Genetics and Vascular Malformations

Newly identified genetic mutations are present in many hereditary vascular anomalies, as are well-defined genetic mutations and inheritance patterns (see Table 64-1). Although modes of inheritance are not consistently straightforward, genetic counselors have an increasing role consulting with patients and family members. Furthermore, identification of genes associated with vascular anomalies has greatly contributed to the windfall of basic research studying the signaling mechanisms involved with these disorders.

The gene for hereditary lymphedema has been linked to distal chromosome 5q, an area where a VEGF-C receptor (FLT4) has been mapped. The FLT4 gene is a marker for lymphatic endothelium during development, and VEGF-C receptor has been detected in lymphatic vasculature. Distichiasis is the presence of a second row of eyelashes arising from the meibomian glands of the eyelids. This can be inherited alone or as a component of lymphedema-distichiasis syndrome. Mutations in the FOXC2 gene (a forkhead, or Fox-box gene, coding for winged helix transcription factors) have been identified in the lymphedema-distichiasis syndrome.[65] Additionally, Brooks et al.[73] identified the same mutation in patients with isolated distichiasis, suggesting that hereditary distichiasis and lymphedema-distichiasis may represent the same disorder with different phenotypic expression. Levinson et al. reported genotype-phenotype correlations, with FLT4 mutations associated with congenital lymphedema and FOXC2 mutations in pubertal-onset lymphedema. Both groups had similar male and female penetrance.[74]

Mutations that are passed through the germline and predispose family members to hemangioma development may also be involved in sporadic hemangiomas. Consistent with this speculation,

two recent studies indicate clonality, demonstrating nonrandom X-inactivation and loss of heterozygosity.[62,63] Furthermore, Walter et al. identified two unique somatic mutations of the VEGFR genes, VEGFR2 (FLK1/KDR) and VEGFR3 (FLT4) in hemangioma specimens.[63]

Capillary malformations–arteriovenous malformations (CM-AVM) have been correlated with RASA-1 mutations, characterized by AVMs in the brain, limbs, or spine and evolving cutaneous capillary malformations[44,75,76] (Fig. 64-16). Mutations in the angiopoietin receptor TIE2/TEK, causing up-regulation of Tie-2, are associated with multifocal cutaneomucosal venous malformation (VMCM) with phenotypic heterogeneity.[77-79]

Clinical Issues

Clinical issues warranting evaluation and treatment of hemangiomas and vascular malformations can be found in Tables 64-2 and 64-3, and clinical trials are listed in Table 64-4.

Facial Port-Wine Stains

When an infant has a macular vascular stain covering the trigeminal distribution, the diagnosis may not initially be apparent. If the lesion remains static, the diagnosis is capillary malformation, and the child is at risk for Sturge-Weber's syndrome (dysmorphogenesis of cephalic neuroectoderm) and must be followed for development of glaucoma, seizures, and developmental delay. The risk of ophthalmological sequelae is highest in patients with lesions located in the ophthalmic (or V1 trigeminal) cutaneous area. In one study, port-wine stains of the eyelids, bilateral distribution of the birthmark, and unilateral port-wine stains involving all three branches of the trigeminal nerve were associated with a significantly higher likelihood of having eye or CNS complications, or both.[80] Open studies assessing imaging, laser, epilepsy, and other assessments are listed at http://www.sturge-weber.org/research/current-studies-seeking-participants.html.

Patients with segmental facial and upper trunk hemangiomas, especially of plaque-like quality, should be evaluated for PHACES Association, with (1) cervicofacial MRI evaluation for assessment of structural and vascular abnormalities, (2) magnetic resonance angiography (MRA) of brain, neck, and upper chest for identification of arteriopathies, (3) cardiac evaluation, (4) ophthalmological evaluation, (5) thyroid function studies, and (6) thorough examination to assess for clefting or other anomalies (e.g., sternum, palate, midline supraumbilical raphe).

Airway Symptoms

Recurrent stridor with progressive worsening of symptoms (in an infant with or without cutaneous hemangiomas) should alert the physician to the possibility of a subglottic hemangioma. Definitive diagnosis is made by bronchoscopy with direct visualization of the airway. Orlow et al. reported increased risk of symptomatic airway hemangiomas in association with a distinctive cutaneous beard hemangioma distribution.[81] However, even in the absence of cutaneous signs, one should also entertain this diagnosis. Controversies in management of subglottic hemangiomas include surgery (submucous resection); laser (CO_2 vs. potassium titanyl phosphate [KTP]); oral propranolol; steroids (intralesional vs. systemic); and interferon alpha (IFN-a) or tracheotomy, or both. Carbon dioxide or KTP laser may be helpful for noncircumferential subglottic hemangiomas.[82]

Periocular Vascular Anomalies

Periocular lesions present unique management problems. What is visible externally is the tip of the iceberg. Thus early radiological evaluation by MRI, ophthalmological evaluation, and follow-up are essential, since vascular lesions put patients at risk for blepharoptosis, amblyopia, strabismus, proptosis, optic nerve compression, and anisotropia. Early intervention is essential to minimize ocular

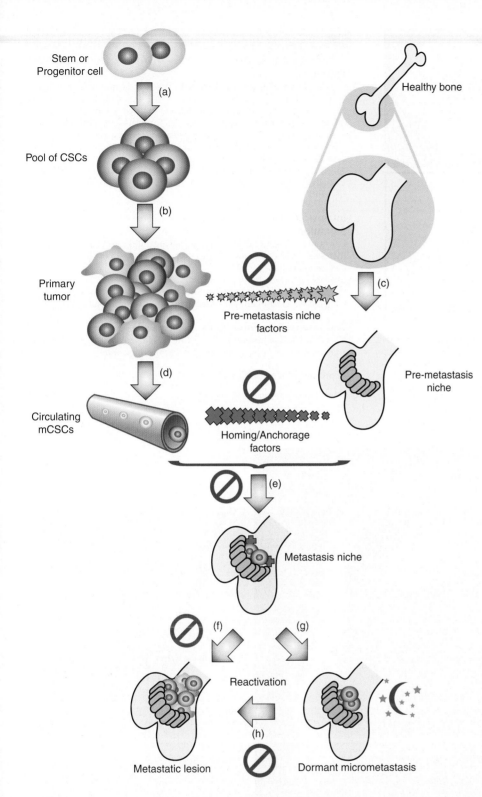

FIGURE 64-14 Metastatic niche theory of hemangioma development. *(From Mihm MC, Nelson JS: Hypothesis: the metastatic niche theory can elucidate infantile hemangioma development. J Cutan Pathol 37:83–87, 2010; used with permission.)*

sequelae. Patients with PHACES or Sturge-Weber's syndrome must be monitored for glaucoma. PHACES patients may also have retinopathies and other anomalies. Periocular hemangiomas belong to the class of hemangiomas that warrant close evaluation and early, active treatment because some have the potential to threaten or permanently compromise vision. Failure to do so can lead to severe and permanent visual disturbances by occluding the visual axis, compressing the globe, or expanding into the retrobulbar space.

Complications such as amblyopia, significant refractive errors, and strabismus are seen in up to 80% of patients with untreated periocular hemangiomas. Hemangioma size (>1 cm in largest diameter) and diffuse segmental hemangiomas were associated with amblyopia in one study,[83] and prompt treatment resulted in reversal of ophthalmological sequelae.[84] Thus, all children with periocular hemangiomas warrant early evaluation and serial follow-up by regular serial cycloplegic refractions performed by a physician skilled in retinoscopy of preverbal children. Therapies include patching of the contralateral eye, topical or systemic pharmacotherapy, and/or surgery. Unique risks of intralesional steroids for periocular hemangiomas include central retinal artery occlusion or iris depigmentation.[85,86]

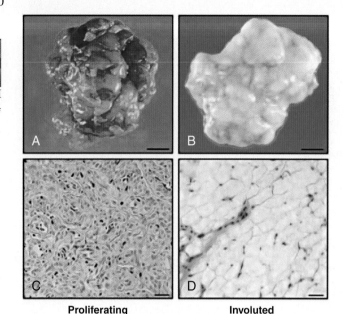

FIGURE 64-15 Adipocytes in hemangioma involution. Photographs and hematoxylin & eosin–stained frozen sections of resected proliferating hemangioma from 3-month-old child **(A, C)** and involuted hemangioma of 7-year-old child **(B, D)**. Note presence of adipocytes in involuted hemangioma. *(From Yu Y, Fuhr, J, Boye, E, Gyorffy, S, Soker, S, Atalia, A, Mulliken, J, Bischoff. Mesenchymal Stem Cells and Adipogenesis in Hemangioma Involution. Stem Cells 2006;24:1605–1612.[2] used with permission.)*

Box 64-2 Summary of Properties of Hemangioma Endothelial Cells*

Express

Glut-1, vascular endothelial growth factor (VEGF) receptors, CD 31, CD34, VEGF-A, β-FGF, IGF-2, HIF-1α, Snrk-1, Tie-2, angiopoietin-2
Markers for progenitor mesodermal stem cell (brachyury, GATA)
Endothelial and hematopoietic cell markers (platelet endothelial adhesion molecule [PECAM]-1; CD31), intracellular adhesion molecule-2 (ICAM-3), bcl-2 gene expression, KDR+, CD133+, CD34+
Lymphatic endothelial hyaluronan receptor-1 (LYVE-1)
Angiotensin-converting enzyme (ACE) and angiotensin receptor 2 (ATR2)
Partially differentiated, resembling fetal endothelial cells in culture
Clonality

Intrinsic Vascular Endothelial Growth Factor Signaling

Calcitonin gene-related peptide (CGRP)—containing nerve fibers
Increased TIE-2 expression/enhanced response to angiopoietin-1
Mesenchymal cells
Increased pericytes during involution
Increased mast cells (produce tissue inhibitors of metalloproteinases [TIMPs], interferon, transforming growth factor [TGF]-β during involution)

Endothelial Progenitor Cells or Stem Cells

Monocyte chemoattractant protein-1 (MCP-1) in perivascular cells and monocytes; may recruit macrophages during proliferation

?Embolic Placental Cells?

* Summary of several reviews and manuscripts.

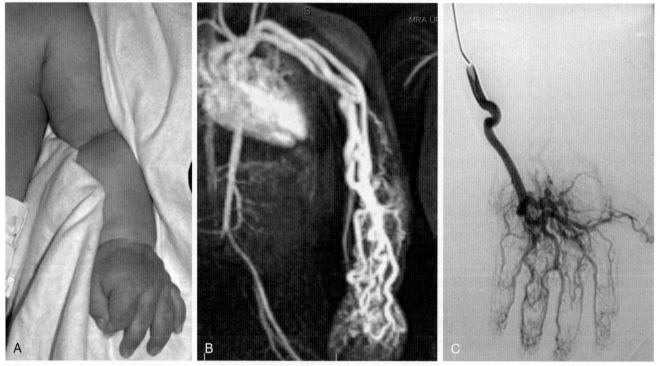

FIGURE 64-16 Arteriovenous malformation (AVM) with RASA1 mutation. A, AVM of arm noted at birth. Patient had thrill and bruit of right arm and high-output cardiac failure. **B,** Magnetic resonance image (MRI) of patient. **C,** Angiogram. Patient was later found to have scattered multiple, small, macular, cutaneous red lesions, and RASA1 mutation was identified.

Hepatic Hemangiomas

Hepatic hemangiomas represent a special category. Although many hepatic hemangiomas are asymptomatic, a subset carries a high morbidity and mortality rate. They may be solitary or multiple and may be seen in association with cutaneous hemangiomatosis or be an isolated finding. Even if radiologically extensive, the clinical spectrum ranges from asymptomatic to life threatening, with high-output CHF or profound consumptive hypothyroidism due to elaboration of type 3 iodothyronine deiodinase by the mass.[87] Therapies include steroids, propranolol, interferon, embolization, antifibrinolytic therapies, surgical resection, and liver transplantation, with inconsistent results.[88]

TABLE 64-2   Significant Clinical Issues Warranting Evaluation of Hemangiomas

CLINICAL FINDING	RECOMMENDED EVALUATION
Hemangiomatosis—multiple small cutaneous hemangiomas	Evaluate for parenchymal hemangiomas, especially hepatic/CNS/gastrointestinal
Cutaneous hemangiomas in beard distribution	Evaluate for airway hemangioma, especially if presenting with stridor
Facial hemangioma involving significant area of face	Evaluate for PHACES MRI ± contrast for orbital hemangioma ± posterior fossa malformation MRA brain, neck to thoracic aorta Cardiac, ophthalmological evaluation Evaluate for midline abnormality—supraumbilical raphe, sternal atresia, cleft palate, thyroid abnormality Evaluate thyroid function MRA evaluation of craniocervical vessels for anomaly
Periocular hemangioma	MRI ± contrast of orbit Ophthalmological evaluation
Paraspinal midline vascular lesion	Ultrasound (if <6 months of age) or MRI to evaluate for occult spinal dysraphism ± underlying vascular lesion
Thrill or bruit, or both, associated with hemangioma	Cardiac evaluation and echo to rule out diastolic reversal of flow of aorta MRI/Doppler of vascular lesion to evaluate flow characteristics
Large hemangioma, especially hepatic	Ultrasound with Doppler flow MRI ± contrast Thyroid function studies
Preferential position (e.g., torticollis, flexure contracture)	Consider physical therapy evaluation
Delayed milestones	Consider side effect of corticosteroids (myopathy, weight related) or interferon (especially spastic diplegia), CNS issue, hearing assessment

CNS, central nervous system; MRA, magnetic resonance angiography; MRI, magnetic resonance imaging.

TABLE 64-3   Clinical Findings and Treatment of Hemangiomas and Vascular Malformations

CLINICAL FINDING	RECOMMENDED TREATMENT
Hemangiomas	
Segmental Distribution	
Severe ulceration/maceration	Encourage cleansing regimen twice daily Sterile saline soaks/air drying/nonstick gauze ± Flashlamp-pulsed dye laser ± Oral propranolol ± Metronidazole gel Analgesics
Bleeding (not Kasabach-Merritt's phenomenon)	Gelfoam (Pharmacia Pfizer, New York)/Surgifoam (Johnson & Johnson, Somerset, NJ) Compression therapy Kids QR Powder (Biolife Inc., Sarasota, FL) ± Embolization
Hemangioma with ophthalmological sequelae	Patching therapy as directed by ophthalmologist Topical timolol maleate gel-forming solution (Merck & Co., Whitehouse Station, NJ) vs. oral propranolol vs. surgery
Subglottic hemangioma	Propranolol ± KTP laser ± surgery Tracheotomy if required
Kasabach-Merritt's phenomenon	Corticosteroids, aminocaproic acid, vincristine, ± chemotherapy, interferon alfa ± Embolization
High-flow hepatic hemangioma	Propranolol or corticosteroids ± embolization ± chemotherapy, ± surgery, ± Synthroid Transplantation
Vascular Malformations	
Swelling	If airway, consider tracheotomy vs. surgery Massage, compression therapy Look for source of infection and treat
Phlebolith	Antiinflammatory agent
Limb-length discrepancy	Shoe insert vs. epiphysiodesis vs. serial observation
Shoe-size discrepancy	Wear two different shoe sizes Epiphysiodesis vs. ray resection
Pain	Evaluate for phlebolith or deep venous thrombosis Analgesics Anticoagulation if thrombosis ± Nerve block, ± sclerotherapy (if not thrombosis)
Recurrent infections/swelling	Local hygienic care Rotating oral antibiotic prophylaxis
Chylous ascites	Drainage/low-fat diet/parenteral nutrition/albumin ± Immunoglobulin replacement

TABLE 64-4 Clinical Trials

TITLE OF STUDY	SITE	CLINICAL TRIALS.GOV IDENTIFIER	DETAILS
Phase 2 Study - Clinical Trial Assessing Efficacy and Safety of the mTOR Inhibitor Sirolimus in the Treatment of Complicated Vascular Anomalies	Children's Hospital Medical Center, Cincinnati	NCT00975819	Age up to 31 years Kaposiform (hemangioendotheliomas, tufted angioma, capillary venous lymphatic malformation, venous lymphatic malformation, microcystic lymphatic malformation, mucocutaneous lymphangiomatosis and thrombocytopenia, capillary lymphatic arterial venous malformations, PTEN overgrowth syndrome with vascular anomaly, lymphangiectasia syndromes)
Vascular Malformations and Abnormalities of Growth	Medical College of Wisconsin	NCT01105676	Skin biopsy of vascular malformation and of normal skin Identification of genes
Registry for Multifocal Lymphangioendotheliomatosis with Thrombocytopenia (MLT)	Medical College of Wisconsin	NCT00576888	Buccal swab, tissue biopsy if available Questionnaire, clinical information
A Pilot Study of Sirolimus (Rapamycin, Rapamune) in Subjects with Cowden Syndrome or Other Syndromes Characterized by Germline Mutations in PTEN		NCT00971789	Persons 18 years of age and older with Cowden's syndrome or other PHTS

REGISTRIES	SPONSOR	LINK	DETAILS
PHACES Patient Registry	Texas Children's Hospital	http://www.texaschildrens.org/carecenters/dermatology/phace.aspx	
National Lymphatic Disease and Lymphedema Registry	Lymphatic Research Foundation	http://lymphaticresearch.org/main.php?menu=research&content=patient-reg-new	
Registry for Vascular Anomalies Associated with Coagulopathy (VAC)	Medical College of Wisconsin	NCT00576888	Multifocal lymphangioendotheliomatosis with thrombocytopenia (MLT) or with a vascular anomaly with coagulopathy
Vascular Malformations and Abnormalities of Growth	Medical College of Wisconsin	NCT01105676	Two skin biopsies taken one time
Genetic Basis of Hemangiomas	Medical College of Wisconsin	NCT00466375	Buccal smear or blood sample
Efficacy and Safety of Bevacizumab for the Treatment of Hemorrhagic Hereditary Telangiectasia (HHT) Associated with Severe Hepatic Vascular Malformations. Phase II Study (METAFORE)	Hospices Civils de Lyon	NCT00843440	Age 18 to 70 years 5 mg/kg every 14 days, with a total of 6 injections A two-phase Gehan method will be used, with a first phase designed to eliminate a noneffective treatment quickly and a second phase allowing assessment of efficacy
The Effects of Aldara (Imiquimod) as an Adjunct to Laser Treatment	University of Kentucky	NCT00979550	Age 2 to 60 years Randomized controlled double-blinded study Unlabeled product (drug or placebo) applied to half of treated lesion beginning the night after laser surgery for 4 weeks
Combined Photodynamic and Pulsed Dye Laser Treatment of Port Wine Stains (PDT/PDL)	University of California, Irvine	NCT00556946	Age 18 years and older Combine photodynamic therapy (verteporfin IV) and pulsed dye laser treatment
Combined Alexandrite and Pulsed Dye Laser Treatment of Port Wine Stain Birthmarks	University of California, Irvine	NCT00580944	Age 12 years and older
Propranolol in Capillary Hemangiomas (HEMANGIOMA)	University Hospital, Bordeaux	NCT00744185	<4 months old Randomized double-blinded control study Placebo vs. propranolol × 30 days (3 mg/kg/day × 15 days and 4 mg/kg/day × 15 days) in nonendangering hemangiomas
Propranolol versus Prednisolone for Treatment of Symptomatic Hemangiomas	Children's Research Institute	NCT00967226	Randomized single blind Drug: propranolol 0.5 mg/kg orally QID × 4-6 months vs. Drug: prednisolone 1 mg/kg orally BID × 4-6 months

Continued

TABLE 64-4 Clinical Trials—Cont'd

REGISTRIES	SPONSOR	LINK	DETAILS
Nadolol for Proliferating Infantile Hemangiomas	The Hospital for Sick Children	NCT01010308	1 month to 1 year of age, with head and neck hemangiomas (not PHACES) with impending or documented morbidity, comparing to historical controls treated with propranolol
Topical Timolol 0.5% Solution for Proliferating Infantile Hemangiomas: a Prospective Double-Blinded Placebo-Controlled Study	Oregon Health and Science University	NCT01147601	Randomized placebo controlled Small uncomplicated infantile hemangiomas
Hemangioma Growth During the First 6 Months of Life	Mayo Clinic Medical College of Wisconsin University of California, San Francisco	NCT00911781	Age 3 months to 5 years Retrospective review of serial photographs of hemangioma
Corticosteroids with Placebo versus Corticosteroids with Propranolol Treatment of Infantile Hemangiomas (IH)	Seattle Children's Hospital	NCT01074437	Age up to 9 months Prospective randomized double-blind study to compare the clinical efficacy of infantile hemangioma treatment using propranolol with corticosteroids vs. corticosteroids and placebo
Study to Demonstrate the Efficacy and Safety of Propranolol Oral Solution in Infants with Proliferating Infantile Hemangiomas Requiring Systemic Therapy (HEMANGIOL)	Pierre Fabre Dermatology	NCT01056341	Age 35-150 days Randomized placebo-controlled double-blind Facial proliferating IH (target hemangioma) with a diameter of at least 1.5 cm, requiring systemic therapy
A Study of CCCTC-binding Factor (CTCF) in Infantile Hemangiomas	Yale University	NCT00974129	Up to 1 year of age One blood draw for genetic analysis of the genotype of CTCF, a transcription factor, in patients with infantile hemangiomas, to determine if the CTCF genotype is an early and reliable predictor of tumor growth
Genetic Analysis of PHACE Syndrome (Hemangioma with Other Congenital Anomalies)	Oregon Health and Science University	NCT01016756	Blood (4 mL) for lymphocyte cell lines and DNA and tissue collection from tissue that would otherwise be discarded after surgery
A Prospective Study Comparing the Incidence of Infantile Hemangiomas Following Normal Pregnancies versus Pregnancies Complicated by Placental Abnormalities	Rady Children's Hospital, San Diego	NCT00490607	Maternal serum and placental and cord blood samples will be obtained for each subject Postnatally, if a hemangioma is diagnosed in the offspring, a blood sample form the infant will be obtained
Longitudinal Study of Neurologic, Cognitive, and Radiologic Outcomes of PHACE Syndrome	Medical College of Wisconsin	NCT01018082	Age 4-6 years Cohort of 30 patients 4-6 years of age, define the functional and neurodevelopmental outcome of PHACE syndrome, and identify potential biomarkers that predict progressive vasculopathy, ischemic stroke, and neurodevelopmental impairment
Thalidomide Reduces Arteriovenous Malformation–Related Gastrointestinal Bleeding	Northport Veterans Affairs Medical Center Medical College of Georgia University of Massachusetts, Worcester	NCT00389935	Age 18 years and older

Hemangiomatosis

The child with multiple hemangiomas may have diffuse neonatal hemangiomatosis (DNH), a dermatosis with a graver prognosis, or benign neonatal hemangiomatosis. A subset of babies with numerous (small) cutaneous hemangiomas is predisposed to parenchymal hemangiomas, especially of the liver (also CNS, eye, pancreas, gastrointestinal tract, lungs, or other organs).

Ulcerating Lesions

Hemangiomas in mucosal (perineum, lip) or intertriginous areas or at pressure points (e.g., back) are prone to ulceration, generally during the proliferative phase.[89] Local wound care may be adequate (e.g., metronidazole or other antibiotic cream, Vaseline gauze, hydrocolloid gels). If infected, topical or systemic antibiotics, or both, are indicated. Other required therapies may be intralesional or systemic steroids or flashlamp pulsed dye laser. Topical Imiquimod[90,91] and platelet-derived growth factor (PDGF)[92,93] have been reported as successful therapies for ulcerated hemangiomas, but the latter carries a black box warning. Topical eosin was reported to be efficacious for ulcerated hemangiomas.[94] Pain management can be achieved with topical and oral analgesics. Simple but helpful measures to comfort the infant with a painful ulcerating hemangioma include twice-daily sitz baths, air drying, and construction of foam rubber cushions with custom-designed cutout areas to relieve direct pressure on the painful area.

Bleeding Associated with Coagulation and Other Abnormalities in Patients with Vascular Anomalies

As noted earlier, bleeding due to Kasabach-Merritt phenomenon (thrombocytopenia, hypofibrinogenemia, and increased fibrinolysis) is often associated with KHE or tufted angioma. In addition to therapy directed toward the primary tumor, antifibrinolytic agents, antiplatelet agents, and heparin are helpful. A transient coagulopathy may be seen in a subgroup of RICH-type lesions.[5] Bleeding may occur with ulcerated hemangiomas. Topical hemostasis may be achieved with QR Powder, Surgifoam, or Gelfoam. Consensus guidelines have been established for management of hereditary hemorrhagic telangiectasia, including bleeding problems.[95]

Hemodynamic Sequelae

Rarely, hemangiomas may demonstrate transient high-flow functionally (until they have undergone significant involution), mimicking AVMs. Hemangiomas with high flow are most frequently located in the liver. These lesions can lead to significant morbidity with high-output cardiac failure. Nonhepatic hemangiomas, prone to develop a high-flow component, include those involving the parotid gland, upper arm, chest wall, scalp, and (rarely) upper lip. These lesions appear to behave as transiently arterialized hemangiomas. During this time, patients may have a failure to thrive–type picture, hyperdynamic precordium, tachycardia, bounding pulses with a widened pulse pressure, and a thrill/bruit over the hemangioma. These findings should alert the treating physician to monitor the hemodynamic status of these patients by careful physical examination and frequent follow-up evaluation. RICH-type hemangiomas may have arterial flow diagnosed pre- or postnatally. Overall, a minority of patients develop high cardiac output states requiring intervention, including diuretics, inotropic agents, or an embolization procedure.

Orthopedic Concerns

Orthopedic issues associated with vascular anomalies involve those relating to limb-dimension discrepancies (e.g., limb length, hypertrophy, atrophy, macrodactyly, polydactyly, gigantism), scoliosis, and other less common orthopedic problems (e.g., foot and hand deformities, joint abnormalities). Limb-length discrepancies may be associated with quadriceps fatigue, hip and lower back pain, or secondary scoliosis. Serial assessment of limb-length data and bone ages at regular intervals is recommended. Interventions include shoe lifts or epiphyseodesis (surgical growth plate closure) for more modest discrepancies; however, for discrepancies predicted to be greater than 5 cm, or in patients who have already reached skeletal maturity, limb shortening and lengthening are the only options to equalize limb lengths.[96] Macrodactyly and gigantism may cause functional problems and difficulty with shoe fit. Therapeutic options include custom shoes, ray or digital resection for macrodactyly of the fingers or toes, debulking procedures, and amputation for severe and otherwise unmanageable cases of hypertrophy.[96] These procedures include removal of subcutaneous fat and ray resection, removal of one or more metatarsals and the associated phalanges. Patients with vascular anomalies can also develop joint contractures due to a mass effect from the lesion. Physical therapy with stretching exercises may be adequate to relieve symptoms; however, direct sclerotherapy plus or minus surgical excision may be required.

Gynecological Issues in Patients with Vascular Malformations

Some women with vascular anomalies have such severe menorrhagia that they undergo hysterectomy. Furthermore, pregnancy is not often seen as an option for women with severe vascular anomalies of the lower extremities, owing to exacerbation of leg swelling, pain, and bleeding from the increased pressure of a gravid uterus. The normal physiological changes of pregnancy include increased plasma volume and cardiac output, increased venous pressure, leg edema, and venous stasis. Additionally, during pregnancy there is a 5.5 times increased risk of thromboembolism; this risk is augmented in patients with vascular anomalies, who already have an increased prothrombotic risk. Increased risk of thrombosis with oral contraceptives limits these patients' choices of contraception. This is also an issue when oral contraceptives are considered to treat dysmenorrhea or other gynecological problems.[97]

Pregnancy for women with vascular anomalies, especially those in the lower extremities, may cause unique problems related to hormonal changes and compression of venous structures by the enlarging uterus. Preliminary data suggest that the risk of obstetric complications, especially preeclampsia and thrombotic events, is higher in women with vascular anomalies of the lower extremities.[83] It is recommended that management of pregnancy be under the direction of an obstetrician who is aware of these risks. Therapy with daily injections of low-molecular-weight heparin (LMWH) during pregnancy may prevent some prothrombotic complications.[97] In addition to pregnancy, other hormonal changes, such as those associated with puberty (in males or females) or the menstrual cycle, may present an increased risk of thrombosis within vascular lesions, necessitating medical intervention with anticoagulants.

Psychosocial Issues

Despite the benign clinical course of infantile hemangiomas in the majority of patients, and the tendency of these lesions to naturally involute, families of patients frequently undergo stress related to social interactions and medical care.[98,99] Tanner et al. conducted interviews of parents of 25 children (5 months to 8 years of age) with facial hemangiomas.[100] They found great variability in parental emotion regarding the lesion. However, support from extended family appeared to be an important factor in coping. Interactions with strangers were a major stress in the majority of cases. Oster studied mother-infant interactions, comparing facial expressions in infants with facial anomalies (including vascular anomalies) and controls, showing that affected infants were capable of effective emotional communication by showing a wide range of facial expressions.[101] Earlier studies by this researcher recognized the role of maternal emotion on affective communication.

Contact with stable familiars (e.g., family members, friends, preschool) appeared to be the least stressful. Many families were dissatisfied with medical care for two reasons: (1) imprecise treatment plans, which are inherent with the nature of many hemangiomas, and (2) what the parents perceived as insensitivity on the part of physicians. Williams et al. assessed the psychological profile of children with hemangiomas and their families in a survey distributed to parents of children with hemangiomas. The results suggested that the families, rather than the infants, experienced emotional and psychological distress.[102]

Contact with other families who are going through or have gone through the same experience enables families to see the light at the end of the tunnel of this curable disorder. In this sense, local family support groups organized at some medical centers, as well as national support networks and meetings, are increasingly providing the necessary stability for families and patients.

Psychosocial stress related to lymphedema is reviewed by Ridner.[103] Although the focus of this review is primarily patients with cancer-related secondary lymphedema, the issues apply to patients with vascular anomalies and lymphedema as well. The Internet has played an enormous role in assisting the exchange of information, as well as enabling families and physicians to connect with one another (Table 64-5). As the field becomes more familiar, older patients who had hemangiomas as infants and children are becoming role models, publishing their experiences and speaking at meetings—further enforcing the optimistic outcome. Furthermore, adult patients with vascular malformations are networking with younger patients.

TABLE 64-5	Web Resources for Patients and Physicians
PROGRAM	**WEBSITE**
Medline Plus	www.medlineplus.gov
Genetics Home Reference	http://ghr.nlm.nih.gov/
About Face	http://www.aboutfaceinternational.org
Arkansas Children's Hospital Vascular Anomalies Program	http://www.birthmarks.org
Boston Children's Hospital Vascular Anomalies Program	http://web1.tch.harvard.edu
Children's Hospital of Wisconsin	http://www.chw.org
Cincinnati Children's Hospital Vascular Anomalies Program	http://www.cincinnatichildrens.org/svc/prog/vascular http://ghr.nlm.nih.gov
Hereditary Hemorrhagic Telangiectasia (HHT) Foundation International	www.hht.org (includes link to: International Guidelines for the Diagnosis and Management of HHT J Med Genet 2009))
Klippel-Trénaunay Foundation	http://www.ktfoundation.com/
Klippel-Trénaunay Support Group	http://www.k-t.org/
Lymphatic Research Foundation	http://www.lymphaticresearch.org/
Lymphatic Disorders	http://www.littleleakers.com/
National Foundation for Facial Reconstruction	http://www.nffr.org/
National Lymphedema Network	http://www.lymphnet.org/
National Organization for Rare Diseases	http://www. rarediseases.org
National Organization of Vascular Anomalies	http://www.novanews.org
Proteus Syndrome	http://www.proteus-syndrome.org
Sturge-Weber Foundation	http://www.sturge-weber.com
UCSF Vascular Anomalies Program	http://dermatology.medschool.ucsf.edu/
Vascular Birthmarks Foundation	http://www.birthmark.org

Malignancies

Treatment-related secondary malignancies due to radiation or chemotherapy may arise in patients with vascular anomalies. Thyroid adenoma, thyroid carcinoma, angiosarcoma, or breast cancer may arise in patients who received radiation therapy (an outdated treatment) for cutaneous hemangiomas of infancy.[104-106] Acute myeloid leukemia occurred in one case of severe hemangiomatosis treated with multiple medications including chemotherapy.[107]

Malignancies such as infantile fibrosarcoma, hemangiopericytoma, rhabdomyosarcoma, glioma, neurofibroma, neuroblastoma, leukemia, and lymphoma in infants may mimic benign hemangiomas of infancy.[108-117] An atypical history and/or physical examination and/or a fixed nonmotile firm mass should alert the practitioner to obtain histological confirmation of the diagnosis.

Concomitant cutaneous hemangiomatosis with hepatic type 2 infantile hepatic hemangioendothelioma (angiosarcoma) has been reported.[118] Additional reports include cases of angiosarcoma in adulthood arising at sites of hemangiomas or vascular malformations,[119] as well as a case of metastatic hepatic lymphangiosarcoma in a child with multiple benign cutaneous and visceral capillary-lymphatic-venous malformations.[108] A higher rate of malignancies can also be seen in young adulthood in patients with PTEN hamartoma syndromes and Maffucci's syndrome.

Treatment of Hemangiomas

Cautious observation is recommended for the majority of hemangiomas, providing there is no impending danger associated with the lesion. Various reviews and guidelines for treatment are available in the medical literature.[86,120] Flashlamp pulsed dye laser is a therapeutic option for some cutaneous hemangiomas, especially in the early phase. Via selective photothermolysis, flashlamp pulsed dye laser selectively destroys superficial dermal vessels while sparing surrounding tissue.[121-125] Pulsed dye laser therapy may also be an effective means of treating ulcerated hemangiomas, although this remains controversial. Further information regarding laser therapy of subglottic hemangiomas is discussed later.

Previously, corticosteroids were the most common medication for proliferating hemangiomas necessitating medical intervention. Along with reports supporting their use[126,127] are concerns of undue side effects such as hypertension, pseudotumor cerebri, and *Pneumocystis carinii* pneumonia,[128-130] as well as iris depigmentation, failure to thrive, adrenal suppression, cellulitis, and retinal artery occlusion with intralesional use.[85,131-135]

Steroid therapy has been supplanted by oral propranolol, a nonselective β-blocker. In 2008, Leaute-Labreze et al. serendipitously noted a dramatic effect of propranolol as a treatment for proliferating infantile hemangioma.[136] Two patients who were treated with oral corticosteroids developed cardiac issues necessitating treatment with propranolol. An immediate improvement in the hemangiomas led to a pilot study that confirmed this perceptive observation. This has revolutionized therapy for infantile hemangioma warranting treatment, and since then several papers have been published, the majority documenting its efficacy.[137-141] Topical β-blockers have also been shown to catalyze involution of superficial hemangiomas.[142,143]

Side effects are cool extremities, gastrointestinal symptoms, hypotension, and bradycardia, with rare but significant reports of hypoglycemia.[144-146] The medication should be held during intercurrent illnesses associated with diminished oral intake and/or respiratory symptoms, as well as prior to any procedures where the child will be fasting.[147]

The mechanism of propranolol-induced involution is under investigation. Inhibition of (1) proliferation (via G0/G1 cell cycle arrest) and chemotactic mobility and differentiation of cultured endothelial cells, and (2) VEGF-induced phosphorylation of VEGFR-2 and other angiogenesis-related pathways were demonstrated by Lamy et al.[148] Itinteang et al. identified angiotensin-converting enzyme (ACE) and angiotensin receptor 2 (ATII) in proliferating hemangioma cells, and suggest a propranolol-induced effect on the renin-angiotensin system of proliferating infantile hemangiomas,[149] as shown in Figure 64-17. Other putative mechanisms involve vasoconstriction resulting from decreased nitric oxide (NO) release, cyclic adenosine monophosphate (cAMP)-induced inhibition of VEGF- and fibroblast growth factor (FGF)-β-induced EC proliferation, or inducing apoptosis.[150,151]

Ulcerated hemangiomas may respond to oral propranolol[152]; however, local management with various medications has been used. Recombinant PDGF has been effective for ulcerated hemangiomas, but a black box warning asserting a higher incidence of cancer fatality in adult patients who used three or more tubes of this medication limits its use (http://www.ncbi.nlm.nih.gov/pubmedhealth/PMH0001057).[92,93] Various combinations of local and systemic therapies for ulcerated hemangiomas are included in the reviews noted earlier. Topical or systemic antibiotics may be warranted for superinfected ulcerated hemangiomas. Topical and/or systemic analgesics, as well as hemostatic agents (e.g., Kids QR Powder, Biolife Inc., Sarasota, Fla.) for bleeding, may also be needed. A study by Lapidoth et al. demonstrated topical application of eosin, a triphenylmethane dye traditionally used as a topical antibiotic and for treatment of diaper dermatitis, hastened healing of ulcerated hemangioma. *In vitro* studies demonstrated angiotensin (Ang-2) messenger ribonucleic acid

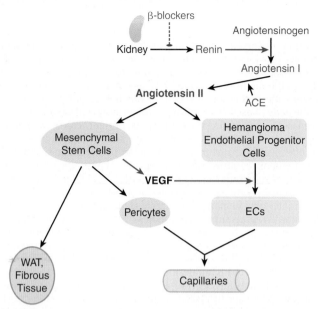

FIGURE 64-17 Proposed model for mechanism of action of propranolol via effect on renin-angiotensin system on hemangioma endothelial cell (EC) proliferation and differentiation. Proliferating hemangiomas were shown to express angiotensin-converting enzyme (ACE) and angiotensin receptor 2 (ATR2). Premature infants, Caucasians, and females (groups with predilection to hemangiomas) have high renin levels, contributing to ATII production. Propranolol, by inhibiting renal renin production, blocks this process. EC, endothelial cell; VEGF, vascular endothelial growth factor. *(From Itinteang T, Brasch HD, Tan ST, Day DJ: Expression of components of the renin-angiotensin system in proliferating infantile haemangioma may account for the propranolol-induced accelerated involution. J Plast Reconstr Aesthet Surg 64:759–765, 2011; used with permission.)*

(mRNA) suppression in cultured ECs.[94] Other agents include topical Imiquimod,[90,91] IFN, and vincristine. Interferon alpha was used in the 1990s, with improvement of endangering hemangiomas, but use of this agent has fallen out of favor, primarily because of concerns about potential neurotoxicity.[153–155] Vincristine has been used for problematic hemangiomas, but the necessity for indwelling intravenous (IV) access and potential toxicities limit its use for straightforward hemangiomas.[156]

Recently, Lazaridou et al. reported treatment of six patients with superficial vascular lesions with topical tacrolimus or pimecrolimus, calcineurin inhibitors.[157] Although the cases are listed as hemangiomas based on the age of the patients, results, and photographs, some of these patients may have had vascular malformations. Calcineurin activates NFATCA (nuclear factor of activated T cell, cytoplasmic), leading to interleukin (IL)-2 expression and T-cell activation. Calcineurin inhibitors block this activation pathway. The Down syndrome critical region 1 (DSCR1) gene provides endogenous feedback inhibition of the calcineurin/VEGF-mediated NFAT signaling pathway in ECs.[158,159]

Surgery

Indications for and timing of surgery for hemangiomas remain controversial. Some surgeons prefer to defer surgery until the hemangioma has undergone substantial involution, with the rationale that the surgery will be less complex and esthetically more favorable. Other surgeons advocate early intervention to possibly prevent medical complications or avert psychological stresses on the patient and/or family. In any case, a well-planned strategy with medical, laser, and surgical management decisions discussed amongst multidisciplinary physicians can provide excellent results.[160–171] Surgical techniques are not discussed in this chapter.

Treatment of Vascular Malformations

Because vascular malformations represent a more chronic condition and fewer specific therapies are available for it, a more supportive approach is often taken (see Tables 64-2 and 64-3). The general rule is, "If it's not broken, don't fix it." If there are no clinical symptoms, alert observation is often adequate. Patients with venous vascular malformations (see Fig. 64-12) often experience painful episodes—this is often in conjunction with a *phlebolith*, or local clot. Therapy with ibuprofen usually suffices. Bleeding from cutaneous blebs may respond to laser cauterization. More severe bleeding from the genitourinary tract may require a combined approach with angiography-guided embolization, laser, or sclerotherapy. Large symptomatic thromboses may require anticoagulation, as might the coagulopathy associated with severe cases. Marimastat, a matrix metalloproteinase (MMP) inhibitor, provided symptomatic relief and reversed bony destruction in a child with intraosseous AVM.[172] The clinical trial Safety and Efficacy Study of Sirolimus in Complicated Vascular Anomalies is assessing the effectiveness and safety of the mammalian target of rapamycin (mTOR) inhibitor, rapamycin, in the treatment of children and young adults diagnosed with complicated vascular anomalies (http://clinicaltrials.gov/ct2/show/NCT00975819).

Patients with arterial and venous abnormalities must be cautioned about triggers. Quiescent vascular anomalies may become more problematic secondary to local trauma, infections, or hormonal fluctuations such as puberty, menstruation, and pregnancy. These changes usually manifest as increased fullness of the malformation as well as pain. The etiology of these difficulties is not clearly understood, but in the hormonally mediated settings it is likely related to hormonal stimulation of EC surface receptors. Use of hormonal birth control can elicit undesirable thromboses and/or pain, thus alternative means of contraception are advised.

Lymphatic malformations are among the most frustrating cases encountered. Evaluation of patients with lymphedema involves physical examination and radiological studies including lymphoscintigraphy for extremity involvement. Lymphatic abnormalities involving the mouth and gastrointestinal tract are prone to infection, so patients with lymphatic malformation in these sites benefit from diligent oral hygiene and, occasionally, rotating prophylactic antibiotic regimens. Microcystic lymphatic malformations of the head and neck may respond well to sclerotherapy (doxycycline, bleomycin, picibanil) or surgery, or a combined approach.[173] Picibanil (OK-432) is a sclerosing agent derived from a low-virulence strain of *Streptococcus pyogenes*. A multicenter prospective nonrandomized trial demonstrated the efficacy of picibanil in the treatment of macrocystic cervicofacial lymphatic malformations, and the results were corroborated by further reports.[174–176] Breakthroughs in the embryology and biology of lymphatic vasculature provide insights into the therapeutic potential for lymphangiogenesis with lymphangiogenic growth factors (e.g., VEGF-C).[177,178]

Therapy is generally supportive, with hygienic skin care, sclerotherapy when possible, complete decompressive physiotherapy with compression bandaging, and intermittent pneumatic compression (IPC) therapy.[179,180] Rockson and Mayrovitz provide detailed reviews of these therapies.[181,182] To date, pharmacological intervention (other than antibiotics when indicated) has not been fruitful. Liposuction for lymphedema has been successful in selected patients with recalcitrant disease.[183] Future molecular-based therapies may evolve from laboratory studies, such as those that demonstrated VEGF-C, a lymphatic growth factor, improved lymphedema in a mouse model.[184]

ACKNOWLEDGMENTS

The author extends gratitude to the patients with vascular anomalies and their families, as well as the staff of the Vascular Birthmark Institute of New York, the Institute for Reconstructive Surgery, and the Stephen D. Hassenfeld Children's Center.

REFERENCES

1. Mulliken JB, Glowacki J: Classification of pediatric vascular lesions, *Plast Reconstr Surg* 70(1):120–121, 1982.
2. Yu Y, Fuhr J, Boye E, et al: Mesenchymal stem cells and adipogenesis in hemangioma involution, *Stem Cells* 24(6):1605–1612, 2006.
3. Mulliken JB, Enjolras O: Congenital hemangiomas and infantile hemangioma: missing links, *J Am Acad Dermatol* 50(6):875–882, 2004.
4. Konez O, Burrows PE, Mulliken JB, et al: Angiographic features of rapidly involuting congenital hemangioma (RICH), *Pediatr Radiol* 33(1):15–19, 2003.
5. Baselga E, Cordisco MR, Garzon M, et al: Rapidly involuting congenital haemangioma associated with transient thrombocytopenia and coagulopathy: a case series, *Br J Dermatol* 158(6):1363–1370, 2008.
6. North PE, Waner M, James CA, et al: Congenital nonprogressive hemangioma: a distinct clinicopathologic entity unlike infantile hemangioma, *Arch Dermatol* 137(12):1607–1620, 2001.
7. Enjolras O, Mulliken JB, Boon LM, et al: Noninvoluting congenital hemangioma: a rare cutaneous vascular anomaly, *Plast Reconstr Surg* 107(7):1647–1654, 2001.
8. Suh KY, Frieden IJ: Infantile hemangiomas with minimal or arrested growth: a retrospective case series, *Arch Dermatol* 146(9):971–976, 2010.
9. Haggstrom AN, Drolet BA, Baselga E, et al: Prospective study of infantile hemangiomas: demographic, prenatal, and perinatal characteristics, *J Pediatr* 150(3):291–294, 2007.
10. Burton BK, Schulz CJ, Angle B, et al: An increased incidence of haemangiomas in infants born following chorionic villus sampling (CVS), *Prenat Diagn* 15(3):209–214, 1995.
11. Bauland CG, Smit JM, Bartelink LR, et al: Hemangioma in the newborn: increased incidence after chorionic villus sampling, *Prenat Diagn* 30(10):913–917, 2010.
12. Lopez Gutierrez JC, Avila LF, Sosa G, et al: Placental anomalies in children with infantile hemangioma, *Pediatr Dermatol* 24(4):353–355, 2007.
13. Colonna V, Resta L, Napoli A, et al: Placental hypoxia and neonatal haemangioma: clinical and histological observations, *Br J Dermatol* 162(1):208–209, 2010.
14. Waner M, North PE, Scherer KA, et al: The nonrandom distribution of facial hemangiomas, *Arch Dermatol* 139(7):869–875, 2003.
15. Haggstrom AN, Lammer EJ, Schneider RA, et al: Patterns of infantile hemangiomas: new clues to hemangioma pathogenesis and embryonic facial development, *Pediatrics* 117(3):698–703, 2006.
16. Haggstrom AN, Drolet BA, Baselga E, et al: Prospective study of infantile hemangiomas: clinical characteristics predicting complications and treatment, *Pediatrics* 118(3):882–887, 2006.
17. Metry DW, Hawrot A, Altman C, et al: Association of solitary, segmental hemangiomas of the skin with visceral hemangiomatosis, *Arch Dermatol* 140(5):591–596, 2004.
18. Metry DW: Potential complications of segmental hemangiomas of infancy, *Semin Cutan Med Surg* 23(2):107–115, 2004.
19. Stockman A, Boralevi F, Taieb A, et al: SACRAL syndrome: spinal dysraphism, anogenital, cutaneous, renal and urologic anomalies, associated with an angioma of lumbosacral localization, *Dermatology* 214(1):40–45, 2007.
20. Drolet B, Garzon M: SACRAL syndrome, *Dermatology* 215(4):360, 2007 author reply -1.
21. Metry DW, Haggstrom AN, Drolet BA, et al: A prospective study of PHACE syndrome in infantile hemangiomas: demographic features, clinical findings, and complications, *Am J Med Genet A* 140(9):975–986, 2006.
22. Haggstrom AN, Garzon MC, Baselga E, et al: Risk for PHACE syndrome in infants with large facial hemangiomas, *Pediatrics* 126(2):e418–e426, 2010.
23. Oza VS, Wang E, Berenstein A, et al: PHACES association: a neuroradiologic review of 17 patients, *AJNR Am J Neuroradiol* 29(4):807–813, 2008.
24. Heyer GL, Dowling MM, Licht DJ, et al: The cerebral vasculopathy of PHACES syndrome, *Stroke* 39(2):308–316, 2008.
25. Kasabach H, Merritt K: Capillary hemangioma with extensive purpura, *Am J Dis Child* 59:1063, 1940.
26. Sarkar M, Mulliken JB, Kozakewich HP, et al: Thrombocytopenic coagulopathy (Kasabach-Merritt phenomenon) is associated with kaposiform hemangioendothelioma and not with common infantile hemangioma, *Plast Reconstr Surg* 100(6):1377–1386, 1997.
27. Enjolras O, Wassef M, Mazoyer E, et al: Infants with Kasabach-Merritt syndrome do not have "true" hemangiomas, *J Pediatr* 130(4):631–640, 1997.
28. Gruman A, Liang MG, Mulliken JB, et al: Kaposiform hemangioendothelioma without Kasabach-Merritt phenomenon, *J Am Acad Dermatol* 52(4):616–622, 2005.
29. Blatt J, Stavas J, Moats-Staats B, et al: Treatment of childhood kaposiform hemangio-endothelioma with sirolimus, *Pediatr Blood Cancer* 55(7):1396–1398, 2010.
30. Chu CY, Hsiao CH, Chiu HC: Transformation between kaposiform hemangioendothelioma and tufted angioma, *Dermatology* 206(4):334–337, 2003.
31. Gilmore A, Kelsberg G, Safranek S: Clinical inquiries. What's the best treatment for pyogenic granuloma, *J Fam Pract* 59(1):40–42, 2010.
32. Greene W, Kuhne K, Ye F, et al: Molecular biology of KSHV in relation to AIDS-associated oncogenesis, *Cancer Treat Res* 133:69–127, 2007 PMCID: 2798888.
33. Patrikidou A, Vahtsevanos K, Charalambidou M, et al: Non-AIDS Kaposi's sarcoma in the head and neck area, *Head Neck* 31(2):260–268, 2009.
34. Barbaro G, Barbarini G: HIV infection and cancer in the era of highly active antiretroviral therapy (Review), *Oncol Rep* 17(5):1121–1126, 2007.
35. Rosen S, Smoller BR: Port-wine stains: a new hypothesis, *J Am Acad Dermatol* 17(1):164–166, 1987.
36. Smoller BR, Rosen S: Port-wine stains. A disease of altered neural modulation of blood vessels? *Arch Dermatol* 122(2):177–179, 1986.
37. Chang CJ, Yu JS, Nelson JS: Confocal microscopy study of neurovascular distribution in facial port wine stains (capillary malformation), *J Formos Med Assoc* 107(7):559–566, 2008.
38. Blei F: Congenital lymphatic malformations, *Ann N Y Acad Sci* 1131:185–194, 2008.
39. Mazoyer E, Enjolras O, Bisdorff A, et al: Coagulation disorders in patients with venous malformation of the limbs and trunk: a case series of 118 patients, *Arch Dermatol* 144(7):861–867, 2008.
40. Tan WH, Baris HN, Burrows PE, et al: The spectrum of vascular anomalies in patients with PTEN mutations: implications for diagnosis and management, *J Med Genet* 44(9):594–602, 2007 PMCID: 2597949.
41. Bisdorff A, Mulliken JB, Carrico J, et al: Intracranial vascular anomalies in patients with periorbital lymphatic and lymphaticovenous malformations, *AJNR Am J Neuroradiol* 28(2):335–341, 2007.
42. Viswanathan V, Smith ER, Mulliken JB, et al: Infantile hemangiomas involving the neuraxis: clinical and imaging findings, *AJNR Am J Neuroradiol* 30(5):1005–1013, 2009.
43. Hess CP, Fullerton HJ, Metry DW, et al: Cervical and intracranial arterial anomalies in 70 patients with PHACE syndrome, *AJNR Am J Neuroradiol* 31(10):1980–1986, 2010.
44. Thiex R, Mulliken JB, Revencu N, et al: A novel association between RASA1 mutations and spinal arteriovenous anomalies, *AJNR Am J Neuroradiol* 31(4):775–779, 2010.
45. Pascual-Castroviejo I, Alvarez-Linera J, Coya J, et al: Pascual-Castroviejo type II syndrome (P-CIIS). Importance of the presence of persistent embryonic arteries, *Childs Nerv Syst* 27(4):617–625, 2011.
46. Metry DW, Garzon MC, Drolet BA, et al: PHACE syndrome: current knowledge, future directions, *Pediatr Dermatol* 26(4):381–398, 2009.
47. Hobert JA, Eng C: PTEN hamartoma tumor syndrome: an overview, *Genet Med* 11(10):687–694, 2009.
48. Blumenthal GM, Dennis PA: PTEN hamartoma tumor syndromes, *Eur J Hum Genet* 16(11):1289–1300, 2008.
49. Elia D, Garel C, Enjolras O, et al: Prenatal imaging findings in rapidly involuting congenital hemangioma of the skull, *Ultrasound Obstet Gynecol* 31(5):572–575, 2008.
50. Morris J, Abbott J, Burrows P, et al: Antenatal diagnosis of fetal hepatic hemangioma treated with maternal corticosteroids, *Obstet Gynecol* 94(5 Pt 2):813–815, 1999.
51. Schmitz R, Heinig J, Klockenbusch W, et al: Antenatal diagnosis of a giant fetal hepatic hemangioma and treatment with maternal corticosteroid, *Ultraschall Med* 30(3):223–226, 2009.
52. Arbiser JL, Bonner MY, Berrios RL: Hemangiomas, angiosarcomas, and vascular malformations represent the signaling abnormalities of pathogenic angiogenesis, *Curr Mol Med* 9(8):929–934, 2009.
53. Bischoff J: Progenitor cells in infantile hemangioma, *J Craniofac Surg* 20(Suppl 1):695–697, 2009 PMCID: 2810465.
54. Boye E, Olsen BR: Signaling mechanisms in infantile hemangioma, *Curr Opin Hematol* 16(3):202–208, 2009 PMCID: 2895461.
55. Jinnin M, Ishihara T, Boye E, et al: Recent progress in studies of infantile hemangioma, *J Dermatol* 37(4):283–298, 2010.
56. Itinteang T, Tan ST, Brasch H, et al: Primitive mesodermal cells with a neural crest stem cell phenotype predominate proliferating infantile haemangioma, *J Clin Pathol* 63(9):771–776, 2010.
57. Dadras SS, North PE, Bertoncini J, et al: Infantile hemangiomas are arrested in an early developmental vascular differentiation state, *Mod Pathol* 17(9):1068–1079, 2004.
58. Nguyen VA, Kutzner H, Furhapter C, et al: Infantile hemangioma is a proliferation of LYVE-1-negative blood endothelial cells without lymphatic competence, *Mod Pathol* 19(2):291–298, 2006.
59. Khan ZA, Boscolo E, Picard A, et al: Multipotential stem cells recapitulate human infantile hemangioma in immunodeficient mice, *J Clin Invest* 118(7):2592–2599, 2008 PMCID: 2413184.
60. Itinteang T, Tan ST, Brasch H, et al: Haemogenic endothelium in infantile haemangioma, *J Clin Pathol* 63(11):982–986, 2010.
61. Perry BN, Govindarajan B, Bhandarkar SS, et al: Pharmacologic blockade of angiopoietin-2 is efficacious against model hemangiomas in mice, *J Invest Dermatol* 126(10):2316–2322, 2006.
62. Boye E, Yu Y, Paranya G, et al: Clonality and altered behavior of endothelial cells from hemangiomas, *J Clin Invest* 107(6):745–752, 2001 PMCID: 208946.
63. Walter JW, North PE, Waner M, et al: Somatic mutation of vascular endothelial growth factor receptors in juvenile hemangioma, *Genes Chromosomes Cancer* 33(3):295–303, 2002.
64. Yu Y, Flint AF, Mulliken JB, et al: Endothelial progenitor cells in infantile hemangioma, *Blood* 103(4):1373–1375, 2004.
65. Khan ZA, Melero-Martin JM, Wu X, et al: Endothelial progenitor cells from infantile hemangioma and umbilical cord blood display unique cellular responses to endostatin, *Blood* 108(3):915–921, 2006 PMCID: 1895853.
66. Kleinman ME, Blei F, Gurtner GC: Circulating endothelial progenitor cells and vascular anomalies, *Lymphat Res Biol* 3(4):234–239, 2005.
67. North PE, Waner M, Mizeracki A, et al: A unique microvascular phenotype shared by juvenile hemangiomas and human placenta, *Arch Dermatol* 137(5):559–570, 2001.
68. Mihm MC, Nelson JS: Hypothesis: the metastatic niche theory can elucidate infantile hemangioma development, *J Cutan Pathol* 37:83–87, 2010.
69. Greenberger S, Adini I, Boscolo E, et al: Targeting NF-kappaB in infantile hemangioma-derived stem cells reduces VEGF-A expression, *Angiogenesis* 13(4):327–335, 2010.
70. Greenberger S, Boscolo E, Adini I, et al: Corticosteroid suppression of VEGF-A in infantile hemangioma-derived stem cells, *N Engl J Med* 362(11):1005–1013, 2010 PMCID: 2845924.
71. Sun ZJ, Zhao YF, Zhang WF: Immune response: a possible role in the pathophysiology of hemangioma, *Med Hypotheses* 68(2):353–355, 2007.
72. Jinnin M, Medici D, Park L, et al: Suppressed NFAT-dependent VEGFR1 expression and constitutive VEGFR2 signaling in infantile hemangioma, *Nat Med* 14(11):1236–1246, 2008 PMCID: 2593632.
73. Brooks BP, Dagenais SL, Nelson CC, et al: Mutation of the FOXC2 gene in familial distichiasis, *J AAPOS* 7(5):354–357, 2003.
74. Levinson KL, Feingold E, Ferrell RE, et al: Age of onset in hereditary lymphedema, *J Pediatr* 142(6):704–708, 2003.
75. Eerola I, Boon LM, Mulliken JB, et al: Capillary malformation-arteriovenous malformation, a new clinical and genetic disorder caused by RASA1 mutations, *Am J Hum Genet* 73(6):1240–1249, 2003 PMCID: 1180390.
76. Boon LM, Mulliken JB, Vikkula M: RASA1: variable phenotype with capillary and arteriovenous malformations, *Curr Opin Genet Dev* 15(3):265–269, 2005.

77. Wouters V, Limaye N, Uebelhoer M, et al: Hereditary cutaneomucosal venous malformations are caused by TIE2 mutations with widely variable hyper-phosphorylating effects, *Eur J Hum Genet* 18(4):414–420, 2010 PMCID: 2841708.
78. Hershkovitz D, Bercovich D, Sprecher E, et al: RASA1 mutations may cause hereditary capillary malformations without arteriovenous malformations, *Br J Dermatol* 158(5): 1035–1040, 2008.
79. Hershkovitz D, Bergman R, Sprecher E: A novel mutation in RASA1 causes capillary malformation and limb enlargement, *Arch Dermatol Res* 300(7):385–388, 2008.
80. Comi AM: Update on Sturge-Weber syndrome: diagnosis, treatment, quantitative measures, and controversies, *Lymphat Res Biol* 5(4):257–264, 2007.
81. Orlow SJ, Isakoff MS, Blei F: Increased risk of symptomatic hemangiomas of the airway in association with cutaneous hemangiomas in a "beard" distribution, *J Pediatr* 131(4): 643–646, 1997.
82. Balakrishnan K, Perkins JA: Management of airway hemangiomas, *Expert Rev Respir Med* 4(4):455–462, 2010.
83. Schwartz SR, Blei F, Ceisler E, et al: Risk factors for amblyopia in children with capillary hemangiomas of the eyelids and orbit, *J AAPOS* 10(3):262–268, 2006.
84. Schwartz SR, Kodsi SR, Blei F, et al: Treatment of capillary hemangiomas causing refractive and occlusional amblyopia, *J AAPOS* 11(6):577–583, 2007.
85. Al-Mahdi H: Iris depigmentation: an unusual complication of intralesional corticosteroid injection for capillary hemangioma, *Middle East Afr J Ophthalmol* 17(1):100–102, 2010 PMCID: 2880367.
86. Maguiness SM, Frieden IJ: Current management of infantile hemangiomas, *Semin Cutan Med Surg* 29(2):106–114, 2010.
87. Huang SA, Tu HM, Harney JW, et al: Severe hypothyroidism caused by type 3 iodothyronine deiodinase in infantile hemangiomas, *N Engl J Med* 343(3):185–189, 2000.
88. Christison-Lagay ER, Burrows PE, Alomari A, et al: Hepatic hemangiomas: subtype classification and development of a clinical practice algorithm and registry, *J Pediatr Surg* 42(1):62–67, 2007 discussion 7–8.
89. Chamlin SL, Haggstrom AN, Drolet BA, et al: Multicenter prospective study of ulcerated hemangiomas, *J Pediatr* 151(6):684–689, 9 e1, 2007.
90. Ho NT, Lansang P, Pope E: Topical imiquimod in the treatment of infantile hemangiomas: a retrospective study, *J Am Acad Dermatol* 56(1):63–68, 2007.
91. McCuaig CC, Dubois J, Powell J, et al: A phase II, open-label study of the efficacy and safety of imiquimod in the treatment of superficial and mixed infantile hemangioma, *Pediatr Dermatol* 26(2):203–212, 2009.
92. Sugarman JL, Mauro TM, Frieden IJ: Treatment of an ulcerated hemangioma with recombinant platelet-derived growth factor, *Arch Dermatol* 138(3):314–316, 2002.
93. Metz BJ, Rubenstein MC, Levy ML, et al: Response of ulcerated perineal hemangiomas of infancy to becaplermin gel, a recombinant human platelet-derived growth factor, *Arch Dermatol* 140(7):867–870, 2004.
94. Lapidoth M, Ben-Amitai D, Bhandarkar S, et al: Efficacy of topical application of eosin for ulcerated hemangiomas, *J Am Acad Dermatol* 60(2):350–351, 2009.
95. Faughnan ME, Palda VA, Garcia-Tsao G, et al: International guidelines for the diagnosis and management of hereditary hemorrhagic telangiectasia, *J Med Genet* 48(2):73–87, 2011.
96. Scher DM: Orthopedic issues in patients with vascular anomalies, *Lymphat Res Biol* 2(1):51–55, 2004.
97. Rebarber A, Roman AS, Roshan D, et al: Obstetric management of Klippel-Trenaunay syndrome, *Obstet Gynecol* 104(5 Pt 2):1205–1208, 2004.
98. Cohen SG: Hemangiomas in infancy and childhood: psychosocial issues require close attention, *Adv Nurse Pract* 13(11):41–44, 2005.
99. Lande RG, Crawford PM, Ramsey BJ: Psychosocial impact of vascular birthmarks, *Facial Plast Surg Clin North Am* 9(4):561–567, 2001.
100. Tanner JL, Dechert MP, Frieden IJ: Growing up with a facial hemangioma: parent and child coping and adaptation, *Pediatrics* 101(3 Pt 1):446–452, 1998.
101. Oster H: Emotion in the infant's face: insights from the study of infants with facial anomalies, *Ann N Y Acad Sci* 1000:197–204, 2003.
102. Williams EF 3rd, Hochman M, Rodgers BJ, et al: A psychological profile of children with hemangiomas and their families, *Arch Facial Plast Surg* 5(3):229–234, 2003.
103. Ridner SH: The psycho-social impact of lymphedema, *Lymphat Res Biol* 7(2):109–112, 2009 PMCID: 2904185.
104. Cabo H, Cohen ES, Casas GJ, et al: Cutaneous angiosarcoma arising on the radiation site of a congenital facial hemangioma, *Int J Dermatol* 37(8):638–639, 1998.
105. Haddy N, Andriamboavonjy T, Paoletti C, et al: Thyroid adenomas and carcinomas following radiotherapy for a hemangioma during infancy, *Radiother Oncol* 93(2):377–382, 2009.
106. Haddy N, Dondon MG, Paoletti C, et al: Breast cancer following radiotherapy for a hemangioma during childhood, *Cancer Causes Control* 21(11):1807–1816, 2010.
107. Sovinz P, Urban C, Hausegger K: Life-threatening hemangiomatosis of the liver in an infant: multimodal therapy including cyclophosphamide and secondary acute myeloid leukemia, *Pediatr Blood Cancer* 47(7):972–973, 2006.
108. Al Dhaybi R, Agoumi M, Powell J, et al: Lymphangiosarcoma complicating extensive congenital mixed vascular malformations, *Lymphat Res Biol* 8(3):175–179, 2010.
109. Al-Mubarak L, Al-Khenaizan S: A wolf in sheep's disguise: rhabdomyosarcoma misdiagnosed as infantile hemangioma, *J Cutan Med Surg* 13(5):276–279, 2009.
110. Assen YJ, Madern GC, de Laat PC, et al: Rhabdoid tumor mimicking hemangioma, *Pediatr Dermatol* 28(3):295–298, 2011.
111. Boon LM, Fishman SJ, Lund DP, et al: Congenital fibrosarcoma masquerading as congenital hemangioma: report of two cases, *J Pediatr Surg* 30(9):1378–1381, 1995.
112. Hassanein A, Fishman S, Mulliken J, et al: Metastatic neuroblastoma mimicking infantile hemangioma, *J Pediatr Surg* 45(10):2045–2049, 2010.
113. Hayward PG, Orgill DP, Mulliken JB, et al: Congenital fibrosarcoma masquerading as lymphatic malformation: report of two cases, *J Pediatr Surg* 30(1):84–88, 1995.
114. Martinez-Perez D, Fein NA, Boon LM, et al: Not all hemangiomas look like strawberries: uncommon presentations of the most common tumor of infancy, *Pediatr Dermatol* 12(1):1–6, 1995.
115. Megarbane H, Doz F, Manach Y, et al: Neonatal rhabdomyosarcoma misdiagnosed as a congenital hemangioma, *Pediatr Dermatol* 28(3):299–301, 2011.
116. Requena C, Miranda L, Canete A, et al: Congenital fibrosarcoma simulating congenital hemangioma, *Pediatr Dermatol* 25(1):141–144, 2008.
117. Yan AC, Chamlin SL, Liang MG, et al: Congenital infantile fibrosarcoma: a masquerader of ulcerated hemangioma, *Pediatr Dermatol* 23(4):330–334, 2006.
118. Nord KM, Kandel J, Lefkowitch JH, et al: Multiple cutaneous infantile hemangiomas associated with hepatic angiosarcoma: case report and review of the literature, *Pediatrics* 118(3):e907–e913, 2006.
119. Rossi S, Fletcher CD: Angiosarcoma arising in hemangioma/vascular malformation: report of four cases and review of the literature, *Am J Surg Pathol* 26(10):1319–1329, 2002.
120. Buckmiller L, Richter G, Suen J: Diagnosis and management of hemangiomas and vascular malformations of the head and neck, *Oral Dis* 16(5):405–418, 2010.
121. Stier MF, Glick SA, Hirsch RJ: Laser treatment of pediatric vascular lesions: port wine stains and hemangiomas, *J Am Acad Dermatol* 58(2):261–285, 2008.
122. Rizzo C, Brightman L, Chapas AM, et al: Outcomes of childhood hemangiomas treated with the pulsed-dye laser with dynamic cooling: a retrospective chart analysis, *Dermatol Surg* 35(12):1947–1954, 2009.
123. Hunzeker CM, Geronemus RG: Treatment of superficial infantile hemangiomas of the eyelid using the 595-nm pulsed dye laser, *Dermatol Surg* 36(5):590–597, 2010.
124. Li DN, Gold MH, Sun ZS, et al: Treatment of infantile hemangioma with optimal pulse technology, *J Cosmet Laser Ther* 12(3):145–150, 2010.
125. Frieden IJ: Commentary: early laser treatment of periorbital infantile hemangiomas may work, but is it really the best treatment option? *Dermatol Surg* 36(5):598–601, 2010.
126. Greene AK: Corticosteroid treatment for problematic infantile hemangioma: evidence does not support an increased risk for cerebral palsy, *Pediatrics* 121(6):1251–1252, 2008.
127. Greene AK: Systemic corticosteroid is effective and safe treatment for problematic infantile hemangioma, *Pediatr Dermatol* 27(3):322–323, 2010.
128. Ray WZ, Lee A, Blackburn SL, et al: Pseudotumor cerebri following tapered corticosteroid treatment in an 8-month-old infant, *J Neurosurg Pediatr* 1(1):88–90, 2008.
129. Maronn ML, Corden T, Drolet BA: *Pneumocystis carinii* pneumonia in infant treated with oral steroids for hemangioma, *Arch Dermatol* 143(9):1224–1225, 2007.
130. Aviles R, Boyce TG, Thompson DM: *Pneumocystis carinii* pneumonia in a 3-month-old infant receiving high-dose corticosteroid therapy for airway hemangiomas, *Mayo Clin Proc* 79(2):243–245, 2004.
131. Deboer MD, Boston BA: Failure-to-thrive in an infant following injection of capillary hemangioma with triamcinolone acetonide, *Clin Pediatr (Phila)* 47(3):296–299, 2008.
132. Goyal R, Watts P, Lane CM, et al: Adrenal suppression and failure to thrive after steroid injections for periocular hemangioma, *Ophthalmology* 111(2):389–395, 2004.
133. Kushner BJ, Lemke BN: Bilateral retinal embolization associated with intralesional corticosteroid injection for capillary hemangioma of infancy, *J Pediatr Ophthalmol Strabismus* 30(6):397–399, 1993.
134. Ang LP, Lee MW, Seah LL, et al: Orbital cellulitis following intralesional corticosteroid injection for periocular capillary haemangioma, *Eye* 21(7):999–1001, 2007.
135. Buckmiller LM, Francis CL, Glade RS: Intralesional steroid injection for proliferative parotid hemangiomas, *Int J Pediatr Otorhinolaryngol* 72(1):81–87, 2008.
136. Leaute-Labreze C, Dumas de la Roque E, Hubiche T, et al: Propranolol for severe hemangiomas of infancy, *N Engl J Med* 358(24):2649–2651, 2008.
137. Leboulanger N, Fayoux P, Teissier N, et al: Propranolol in the therapeutic strategy of infantile laryngotracheal hemangioma: a preliminary retrospective study of French experience, *Int J Pediatr Otorhinolaryngol* 74(11):1254–1257, 2010.
138. Haider KM, Plager DA, Neely DE, et al: Outpatient treatment of periocular infantile hemangiomas with oral propranolol, *J AAPOS* 14(3):251–256, 2010.
139. Rosbe KW, Suh KY, Meyer AK, et al: Propranolol in the management of airway infantile hemangiomas, *Arch Otolaryngol Head Neck Surg* 136(7):658–665, 2010.
140. Tan ST, Itinteang T, Leadbitter P: Low-dose propranolol for infantile haemangioma, *J Plast Reconstr Aesthet Surg* 64:2929, 2011.
141. Mazereeuw-Hautier J, Hoeger PH, Benlahrech S, et al: Efficacy of propranolol in hepatic infantile hemangiomas with diffuse neonatal hemangiomatosis, *J Pediatr* 157(2):340–342, 2010.
142. Pope E, Chakkittakandiyil A: Topical timolol gel for infantile hemangiomas: a pilot study, *Arch Dermatol* 146(5):564–565, 2010.
143. Guo S, Ni N: Topical treatment for capillary hemangioma of the eyelid using beta-blocker solution, *Arch Ophthalmol* 128(2):255–256, 2010.
144. Bonifazi E, Acquafredda A, Milano A, et al: Severe hypoglycemia during successful treatment of diffuse hemangiomatosis with propranolol, *Pediatr Dermatol* 27(2):195–196, 2010.
145. Breur JM, de Graaf M, Breugem CC, et al: Hypoglycemia as a result of propranolol during treatment of infantile hemangioma: a case report, *Pediatr Dermatol* 28(2):169–171, 2011.
146. Holland KE, Frieden IJ, Frommelt PC, et al: Hypoglycemia in children taking propranolol for the treatment of infantile hemangioma, *Arch Dermatol* 146(7):775–778, 2010.
147. Allford MA, Brown JL: Case report: intraoperative hypoglycaemia in a child treated with propranolol following a short preoperative fast, *Eur J Anaesthesiol* 28(1):71–72, 2011.
148. Lamy S, Lachambre MP, Lord-Dufour S, et al: Propranolol suppresses angiogenesis *in vitro*: inhibition of proliferation, migration, and differentiation of endothelial cells, *Vascul Pharmacol* 53(5–6):200–208, 2010.
149. Itinteang T, Brasch HD, Tan ST, et al: Expression of components of the renin-angiotensin system in proliferating infantile haemangioma may account for the propranolol-induced accelerated involution, *J Plast Reconstr Aesthet Surg* 64(6):759–765, 2011.
150. Sans V, de la Roque ED, Berge J, et al: Propranolol for severe infantile hemangiomas: follow-up report, *Pediatrics* 124(3):e423–e431, 2009.
151. Storch CH, Hoeger PH: Propranolol for infantile haemangiomas—insights into the molecular mechanisms of action, *Br J Dermatol* 163(2):269–274, 2010.
152. Naouri M, Schill T, Maruani A, et al: Successful treatment of ulcerated haemangioma with propranolol, *J Eur Acad Dermatol Venereol* 24(9):1109–1112, 2010.
153. Barlow CF, Priebe CJ, Mulliken JB, et al: Spastic diplegia as a complication of interferon alfa-2a treatment of hemangiomas of infancy, *J Pediatr* 132(3 Pt 1):527–530, 1998.

154. Michaud AP, Bauman NM, Burke DK, et al: Spastic diplegia and other motor disturbances in infants receiving interferon-alpha, *Laryngoscope* 114(7):1231–1236, 2004.

155. Chao YH, Liang DC, Chen SH, et al: Interferon-alpha for alarming hemangiomas in infants: experience of a single institution, *Pediatr Int* 51(4):469–473, 2009.

156. Perez-Valle S, Peinador M, Herraiz P, et al: Vincristine, an efficacious alternative for diffuse neonatal haemangiomatosis, *Acta Paediatr* 99(2):311–315, 2010.

157. Lazaridou E, Giannopoulou C, Apalla Z, et al: Calcineurin inhibitors in the treatment of cutaneous infantile haemangiomas, *J Eur Acad Dermatol Venereol* 24(5):614–615, 2010.

158. Yao YG, Duh EJ: VEGF selectively induces Down syndrome critical region 1 gene expression in endothelial cells: a mechanism for feedback regulation of angiogenesis? *Biochem Biophys Res Commun* 321(3):648–656, 2004.

159. Gollogly LK, Ryeom SW, Yoon SS: Down syndrome candidate region 1-like 1 (DSCR1-L1) mimics the inhibitory effects of DSCR1 on calcineurin signaling in endothelial cells and inhibits angiogenesis, *J Surg Res* 142(1):129–136, 2007 PMCID: 1995402.

160. Serena T: Wound closure and gradual involution of an infantile hemangioma using a noncontact, low-frequency ultrasound therapy, *Ostomy Wound Manage* 54(2):68–71, 2008.

161. Spector JA, Blei F, Zide BM: Early surgical intervention for proliferating hemangiomas of the scalp: indications and outcomes, *Plast Reconstr Surg* 122(2):457–462, 2008.

162. Waner M, Kastenbaum J, Scherer K: Hemangiomas of the nose: surgical management using a modified subunit approach, *Arch Facial Plast Surg* 10(5):329–334, 2008.

163. Warren SM, Longaker MT, Zide BM: The subunit approach to nasal tip hemangiomas, *Plast Reconstr Surg* 109(1):25–30, 2002.

164. Watanabe S, Takagi S, Sato Y, et al: Early surgical intervention for Japanese children with infantile hemangioma of the craniofacial region, *J Craniofac Surg* 20(Suppl 1):707–709, 2009.

165. Wu JK, Rohde CH: Purse-string closure of hemangiomas: early results of a follow-up study, *Ann Plast Surg* 62(5):581–585, 2009.

166. Zide BM, Glat PM, Stile FL, et al: Vascular lip enlargement: part I. Hemangiomas--tenets of therapy, *Plast Reconstr Surg* 100(7):1664–1673, 1997.

167. Canavese F, Soo BC, Chia SK, et al: Surgical outcome in patients treated for hemangioma during infancy, childhood, and adolescence: a retrospective review of 44 consecutive patients, *J Pediatr Orthop* 28(3):381–386, 2008.

168. Levi M, Schwartz S, Blei F, et al: Surgical treatment of capillary hemangiomas causing amblyopia, *J AAPOS* 11(3):230–234, 2007.

169. Mandrekas AD, Zambacos GJ, Hapsas DA: Pediatric nasal reconstruction for nasal tip hemangioma, *Plast Reconstr Surg* 125(5):1571–1572, 2010 author reply 3.

170. Mehta M, Waner M, Fay A: Amniotic membrane grafting in the management of conjunctival vascular malformations, *Ophthal Plast Reconstr Surg* 25(5):371–375, 2009.

171. Mulliken JB, Rogers GF, Marler JJ: Circular excision of hemangioma and purse-string closure: the smallest possible scar, *Plast Reconstr Surg* 109(5):1544–1554, 2002 discussion 55.

172. Burrows PE, Mulliken JB, Fishman SJ, et al: Pharmacological treatment of a diffuse arteriovenous malformation of the upper extremity in a child, *J Craniofac Surg* 20(Suppl 1):597–602, 2009.

173. Niramis R, Watanatittan S, Rattanasuwan T: Treatment of cystic hygroma by intralesional bleomycin injection: experience in 70 patients, *Eur J Pediatr Surg* 20(3):178–182, 2010.

174. Smith MC, Zimmerman MB, Burke DK, et al: Efficacy and safety of OK-432 immunotherapy of lymphatic malformations, *Laryngoscope* 119(1):107–115, 2009.

175. Narkio-Makela M, Makela T, Saarinen P, et al: Treatment of lymphatic malformations of head and neck with OK-432 sclerotherapy induce systemic inflammatory response, *Eur Arch Otorhinolaryngol* 268:123-1219, 2011.

176. Greene AK, Burrows PE, Smith L, et al: Periorbital lymphatic malformation: clinical course and management in 42 patients, *Plast Reconstr Surg* 115(1):22–30, 2005.

177. Oliver G, Srinivasan RS: Lymphatic vasculature development: current concepts, *Ann N Y Acad Sci* 1131:75–81, 2008.

178. Oliver G, Srinivasan RS: Endothelial cell plasticity: how to become and remain a lymphatic endothelial cell, *Development* 137(3):363–372, 2010 PMCID: 2858906.

179. Perkins JA, Manning SC, Tempero RM, et al: Lymphatic malformations: review of current treatment, *Otolaryngol Head Neck Surg* 142(6):795–803, e1, 2010.

180. Perkins JA, Manning SC, Tempero RM, et al: Lymphatic malformations: current cellular and clinical investigations, *Otolaryngol Head Neck Surg* 142(6):789–794, 2010.

181. Rockson SG: Current concepts and future directions in the diagnosis and management of lymphatic vascular disease, *Vasc Med* 15(3):223–231, 2010.

182. Mayrovitz HN: The standard of care for lymphedema: current concepts and physiological considerations, *Lymphat Res Biol* 7(2):101–108, 2009.

183. Brorson H: From lymph to fat: complete reduction of lymphoedema, *Phlebology* 25(Suppl 1):52–63, 2010.

184. Rockson SG: Diagnosis and management of lymphatic vascular disease, *J Am Coll Cardiol* 52(10):799–806, 2008.

INDEX

Note: Page numbers followed by *f* indicate figures, *t* indicate tables, and *b* indicate boxes.

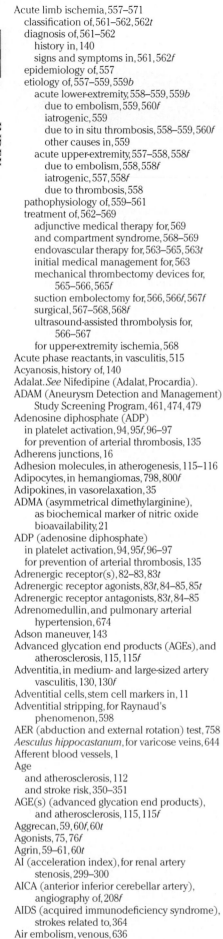

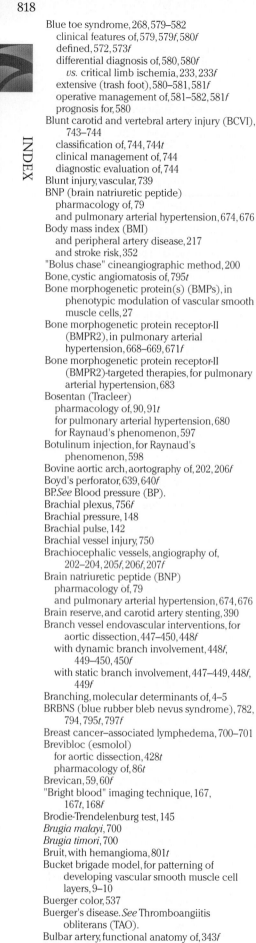

G

844

INDEX